EMERGENCY AND TRAUMA CARE 2e

FOR NURSES AND PARAMEDICS

Australian and New Zealand Edition

D1597174

EMERGENCY AND TRAUMA CARE 2e

FOR NURSES AND PARAMEDICS

Australian and New Zealand Edition

Kate Curtis

RN, BN, Grad Dip (Crit Care), MNurs (Hons), PhD

Trauma Clinical Nurse Consultant, St George Hospital, Sydney, NSW, Australia

Associate Professor, Sydney Nursing School, The University of Sydney, NSW, Australia

Registered Nurse (Casual), Emergency Department, Wollongong Hospital, NSW, Australia

Honorary Professorial Fellow, The George Institute for Global Health, Sydney, NSW, Australia

Conjoint Associate Professor, St George Clinical School, Faculty of Medicine, UNSW, Sydney, Australia

Visiting Associate Professor, Faculty of Health Sciences and the Organisation and Delivery of Care Research Group, University of Southampton, UK

Fellow, College of Emergency Nurses Australasia

Clair Ramsden

RN, MA Healthcare Ethics, MA Health Service Management

Executive Director of Nursing and Midwifery, Nepean Blue Mountains Local Health District, NSW Health, Sydney, NSW, Australia

Associate Professor, Faculty of Health, University of Technology Sydney, NSW, Australia

ELSEVIER

ELSEVIER

Elsevier Australia, ACN 001 002 357
(a division of Reed International Books Australia Pty Ltd)
Tower 1, 475 Victoria Avenue, Chatswood, NSW 2067

Sheehy's Emergency Nursing: Principles and Practice
Copyright Elsevier Inc, 2010, 2003, 1998, 1992, 1985, 1981.
ISBN: 978-0-323-05585-7

This adaptation of Sheehy's Emergency Nursing: Principles and Practice, Sixth Edition, edited by Patricia Kunz Howard and Rebecca A. Steinmann was undertaken by Elsevier Australia and is published by arrangement with Elsevier Inc.

Emergency and Trauma Care for Nurses and Paramedics, 2nd edition
Copyright © 2016 Elsevier Australia; 1st edition © 2011 Elsevier Australia.
ISBN: 978-0-7295-4205-0

Notice

This publication has been carefully reviewed and checked to ensure that the content is as accurate and current as possible at time of publication. We would recommend, however, that the reader verify any procedures, treatments, drug dosages or legal content described in this book. Neither the author, the contributors, nor the publisher assume any liability for injury and/or damage to persons or property arising from any error in or omission from this publication.

National Library of Australia Cataloguing-in-Publication Data

Curtis, Kate, author.

Emergency and trauma care : for nurses and paramedics / Kate Curtis, Clair Ramsden. Second edition.

9780729542050 (paperback)

Emergency nursing—Handbooks, manuals, etc.
Emergency medical technicians—Handbooks, manuals, etc.
Traumatology—Handbooks, manuals, etc.
Hospitals—Emergency services—Handbooks, manuals, etc.

Ramsden, Clair, author.

616.025

Senior Content Strategist: Melinda McEvoy
Content Development Specialist: Tamsin Curtis
Senior Project Manager: Karthikeyan Murthy
Edited by Margaret Trudgeon
Permissions editing and photo research by Sarah Thomas
Proofread by Tim Learner
Design by Natalie Bowra
Index by Robert Swanson
Typeset by Midland Typesetters, Australia
Printed by CTPS, China

Cover page—Main image:
Courtesy of the University of Sydney
Helicopter & patient transfer image:
Courtesy of Ambulance NSW

CENA DISCLAIMER

This book is not written or published by the College for Emergency Nursing Australasia ("CENA"). While CENA endorses this book as a complete work it is not responsible for its content.

CONTENTS

SECTION 4

EMERGENCIES

SECTION 5
MAJOR TRAUMA

SECTION 6
END OF LIFE

FOREWORD

As a specialty area of practice, emergency care focuses on the care of patients presenting with multitudes of conditions ranging from acute to chronic disease, minor to major trauma and those with critical, life-threatening illnesses. *Emergency and Trauma Care for Nurses and Paramedics 2e* provides information that underpins what makes emergency nursing and pre-hospital care a specialty in its own right.

Written by emergency nurses, specialist clinicians, educators, academics and researchers from across the spectrum of emergency care, this textbook provides an Australasian context to care delivery and provides readers with contemporary information on clinical assessment, physiology, management and rationale for a wide variety of emergency presentations. It is written in a logical, easy-to-read style and provides relevant, structured information on emergency concepts using an evidence-based approach. The book has become the preferred text for many tertiary emergency nursing courses across Australia, as well as the College of Emergency Nursing Australasia's (CENA) Trauma Nursing Program.

CENA is the peak professional college representing emergency nurses, and our mission is to foster excellence in emergency nursing. CENA has endorsed this text in recognition of the relevance it has to emergency nursing across Australasia. Many of its contributors are members or Fellows of the College and contribute to our specialty every day. It is my pleasure to congratulate the editors—Kate Curtis and Clair Ramsden—in addition to all the contributors, for providing high quality contributions to this text. The new edition of *Emergency and Trauma Care for Nurses and Paramedics 2e* will become a valuable resource for those working in pre-hospital and emergency department environments, irrespective of the setting.

Lee Trenning
RN, Cert (Emerg Nurs), Grad Dip (Crit Care), Grad Dip (Clin Ed),
FCENA, MACN, MACCCN
National Executive Director
College of Emergency Nursing Australasia
The leaders for emergency nursing: A leader of emergency care.

PREFACE

This book is intended to provide a practical and evidence-based resource for pre-hospital care providers, rural and urban emergency and trauma nurses, students or those with an interest in these specialisations. It offers information specific to clinicians practising in their local environment, while maintaining the clinical elements experienced by our colleagues worldwide. Each of the 80 contributors have been clinicians in Australia or New Zealand and were chosen for their expertise in their chapter area, to ensure relevant, practical information.

The book is organised into six sections. Section 1 discusses the foundation and development of paramedic, emergency and trauma nursing practice as well as the implications on professional practice, such as ethics, law, management and leadership and culture. Section 2 focuses on the fundamentals of emergency care, including professional development, patient education and research. Section 3 addresses the clinical and health service system concepts of scene assessment, patient assessment, triage, resuscitation, pain management and the physiology of emergency care; there is also a chapter featuring essential clinical skills, which are cross-referenced throughout this edition.

Section 4 then progresses to the emergency management of specific body systems emergencies, such as cardiology, respiratory, neurological and endocrine. Other groups of emergency presentations are also covered in depth; these include toxicology, envenomation and ocular and environmental emergencies. Unique population groups, including the elderly, disabled, obstetric and paediatric patients, are also presented in Section 4. Major Trauma assessment and management is covered in detail in Section 5, with an overview of trauma systems, trauma assessment, blast injury and trauma to specific body regions. The final section, Section 6, provides the pre-hospital and emergency clinician with relevant information on end-of-life care and considerations, such as organ donation.

Throughout the 54 chapters, cross references are made to other areas of the book that contain further information pertaining to that subject. The 581 figures and 294 tables support the 'hands-on' clinical approach of the book. Clinical assessment, physiology, management and rationale for intervention of common and not-so-common emergency presentations are provided.

The information contained in this book reflects the knowledge, published research and literature at the time of production. It is important that readers continue to search for the most recent sources of appropriate information to guide their practice. The editors welcome feedback from readers to help ensure that the content remains relevant and is disseminated in a way that suits paramedics, emergency and trauma nurses.

This book is a resource to support clinicians in their provision of care to emergency and trauma patients, and promote the paramedical profession and specialties of emergency and trauma nursing.

Kate Curtis
Clair Ramsden
July 2015

ACKNOWLEDGMENTS

A textbook of this size requires the professional dedication and personal support of many people. An incredible amount of work is necessary to ensure the content is comprehensive and correct, and that the book is completed within specified timeframes. The level of commitment and effort for this second edition has been phenomenal. The editors would like to thank:

- the chapter contributors, some of whom have written for the first time. Their patience, persistence, expertise and knowledge are greatly valued. This book has been written by an extremely skilled group of clinicians and academics

- the team at Elsevier; in particular Tamsin Curtis, Melinda McEvoy, Karthikeyan Murthy, Sarah Thomas and Margaret Trudgeon

- the reviewers who spent time and effort ensuring the content is accurate, relevant and up-to-date and that the editors had not overlooked any pertinent subject matter.

On a more personal note, we would particularly like to thank our husbands (George and Gary), children (Sarah, Beatrix, Edward, Grace and Lewis), family and friends who have endured the many months of hard work and been tremendously patient and encouraging. You have our sincere appreciation and gratitude.

CONTRIBUTORS

Trish Allen RN BN, PostGradDip(Emerg Nurs), MN

Assistant Director of Nursing—Clinical Systems Improvement, Acute Health Services Planning and Design, Department of Health and Human Services, Tasmania, Australia

Carrie Alvaro DipAppSc(Nursing)

Nurse Educator, Western Sydney Local Health District, NSW, Australia

Stephen Edward Asha BSc, MBBS, MMed(Clin Epi), FACEM

Conjoint Associate Professor, Faculty of Medicine, UNSW, Sydney, NSW, Australia

Emergency Physician, Emergency Department, St George Hospital, Sydney, NSW, Australia

Ann Bonner BAppSc(Nursing), MA, PhD

Professor, School of Nursing, Queensland University of Technology, Brisbane, Queensland, Australia

James Brinton RN, BN, GradCertCritCare(Emergency)

Clinical Nurse Specialist, Orthopaedic Trauma and Emergency Surgery, Division of Surgery, Wollongong Hospital, NSW, Australia

Thomas Buckley RN, BSc(Hons), GradCertICU, MN, PhD

Coordinator MA Nursing (Clinical Nursing and Nurse Practitioner); Senior Lecturer, Sydney Nursing School, University of Sydney, NSW, Australia

Erica Caldwell RN, BA, RM, PsychCert

Trauma Clinical Nurse Consultant, Trauma, Liverpool Hospital, NSW, Australia

Julie Considine RN, RM, BN, CertAcuteCareNurs, GradDipNurs, GradCertHigherEd, MN, PhD, FACN, FFCENA

Professor of Nursing, Deakin University—Eastern Health, School of Nursing and Midwifery, Deakin University, Victoria, Australia

Dianne Crellin BN, CertEmerg, PostGradAdvNurs(Paed), MN

Nurse Practitioner, Emergency Department, Royal Children's Hospital, Melbourne, Victoria

Research Associate, Murdoch Childrens Research Institute, Victoria

Lecturer, Nursing, The University of Melbourne, Australia

Allison Cummins RM, MA(Adult Education)

Course Coordinator, Graduate Diploma of Midwifery, University of Technology Sydney, Australia

Lynette Cusack RN, BN, GradDipNurs, PhD, MHA

School of Nursing, University of Adelaide, South Australia, Australia

Suzanne Robyn Davies BAppSc(Med Biotech), MPH

Senior Lecturer, School of Medicine, University of Tasmania, Sydney, Australia

Charlotte F C de Crespigny BN, GradDipPHC(Addictions), PhD

Professor of Drug and Alcohol Nursing, School of Nursing, The University of Adelaide, South Australia, Australia

Ruth Dunleavey BSc(Hons) Nursing, Oncology Diploma

St Vincents Hospital, Sydney, NSW, Australia

Janice Elliott RN, GradDip(Emergency Nursing), MA(Nursing Science)

Registered Nurse, Emergency Department, Royal Adelaide Hospital and Clinical Title Holder, School of Nursing, University of Adelaide, SA, Australia

Julie Evans RN, RM, Grad Dip, Grad Cert(Emergency)

Trauma Clinical Nurse Consultant, John Hunter/John Hunter Children's Hospital, Newcastle, NSW, Australia

Wendy Fenton RN, MA Nursing(Nurse Practitioner)

Emergency Nurse Practitioner, Emergency Department, Wollongong Hospital, Australia

Monika Ferguson BPsych(Hons), PhD

Research Associate, School of Nursing and Midwifery, University of South Australia, Adelaide, South Australia, Australia

David Foley RN, BSc, A&E Cert, MNS, PhD

Director of Nursing Simulations, School of Nursing, University of Adelaide, South Australia, Australia

Margaret Fry NP BSc, MEd(Adult Education), PhD

Northern Sydney Local Health District

Professor Research and Practice Development, Faculty of Health, University of Technology, Sydney, NSW, Australia

Marie Frances Gerdtz BN, A&E Cert, GradDipAdultEd, PhD

Associate Professor, Nursing, The University of Melbourne, Victoria, Australia

Associate Professor, Nursing, Melbourne Health, Victoria, Australia

Honorary Professor, Health Sciences, University Central Lancashire, UK

Kellie Gumm DipNursing, GradCertNursing(Intensive Therapy), GradDipHlthProm, MA(Adult Ed)

Trauma Program Manager, Trauma Service, The Royal Melbourne Hospital, Melbourne, Victoria, Australia

Senior EMST Coordinator, Skill Training, Royal Australasian College of Surgeons, Melbourne, Victoria, Australia

Trauma Education Project Officer, Adult Retrieval Victoria, Ambulance Victoria, Melbourne, Australia

Kane Guthrie BNurs

Clinical Nurse, Sir Charles Gairdner Hospital, Perth, WA, Australia

Karel Habig BSc(Med), MBBS, DipRTM, FACEM

Lead Clinician, Greater Sydney Area HEMS, NSW Ambulance Service, Sydney, NSW, Australia

Andrea Herring RN, GradCertBioethics

Manager, Nursing and Midwifery Education, Western Sydney Local Health District, Westmead, NSW

National Executive, Australasian Trauma Society, Australia

Celine Hill RN, DipAppSc(Nursing), GradCert(Orthopaedcis), MN(Trauma)

Clinical Nurse Consultant Orthopaedics and Trauma, Orthopaedics, Westmead Hospital, PACE/CERS Clinical Nurse Consultant, Shoalhaven District Memorial Hospital, NSW, Australia

Alister Hodge BN, MA Nursing(Nurse Practitioner), MA Nursing(Emergency), GradCertCriticalCare

Nurse Practitioner, Emergency Department, The Sutherland Hospital, Australia

Clinical Lecturer, School of Nursing, University of Sydney, Australia

Andrew JA Holland BSc, MB/BS, GradCertEdStudies, PhD, FACS, FRCS, FRACS

Professor of Paediatric Surgery, Discipline of Paediatrics and Child Health, The University of Sydney, NSW, Australia

Senior Clinical Academic, Douglas Cohen Department of Paediatric Surgery, The Children's Hospital, Westmead, NSW, Australia

Caroline SE Homer RM, MN, MScMed(ClinEpi), PhD

Professor of Midwifery, Centre for Midwifery, Child and Family Health, Faculty of Health, University of Technology Sydney, NSW, Australia

Keryn Jones BNurs, MEd

Nurse Practitioner—Emergency, South Eastern Sydney Local Health District

Lecturer and Subject Assessor, Post Graduate Nurse Practitioner Program, Faculty of Health University of Technology, Sydney, NSW, Australia

Jeff Kenneally BA Bus, DipHealthSc(Paramedic), Mobile Intensive Care Paramedic Cert

Intensive Care Senior Team Manager, Victoria Ambulance Services, Australia

Kirsten Kennedy DipHealthSc(Nursing), GradCert Spinal Nursing, MA(Adult Ed)

Nurse Educator, Spinal Unit, Prince of Wales Hospital, Sydney, NSW, Australia

Kate King BN, MN

Clinical Nurse Consultant—Trauma, John Hunter Trauma Service, Newcastle, NSW, Australia

Conjoint Lecturer Faculty of Health, University of Newcastle, NSW, Australia

Leigh Kinsman RN, BHSc, MHSc, PhD

Professor of Healthcare Improvement (joint appt), University of Tasmania and the Tasmanian Health Organisation (North), Tasmania, Australia

David Koop DipFireTech, AdvCert Safety&OHM, CertHumanRes

AusMat Team Member and AusMat Logistics trained

State Manager, Health Emergency Response Capability and Countermeasures, NSW Health Emergency Management Unit, NSW Ambulance, NSW, Australia

Mary Langcake BMBS, BSC(Hons), FRACS

Director of Trauma, St George Hospital, Kogarah, NSW, Australia

Jennifer Ann Leslie BAppSc(Nursing), PostGradDip Clin Nurs

Trauma Research Nurse, Trauma Services, Royal Perth Hospital, WA, Australia

Bill Lord BHlthSc(PreHospCare), GradDipCBL, MEd, PhD

Associate Professor, Paramedic Science, School of Health and Sport Sciences, University of the Sunshine Coast, Sippy Downs, Queensland, Australia

Jonathan Magill RN, BSc(Hons), MSc

Manager, Nursing and Midwifery Professional Development and Education, Nursing and Midwifery Directorate, Northern NSW Local Health District, NSW, Australia

Coordinator, NNSW LHD CEC Clinical Leadership Program, NSW, Australia

Bronte Martin BNurs, CritCareCert, GradDipNursSc(Emerg), MNurs(Clin)

Nursing Director (Trauma & Disaster), National Critical Care and Trauma Response Centre, Darwin, NT, Australia

Daniel Martin BN, BNursingPrac(Emerg), Grad Cert(Emerg), GradCertNursingSc(Retrieval), PostGradCert(Aeromed Retrieval)

Senior Lecturer (Professional), School of Public Health, Tropical Medicine and Rehabilitation Sciences, James Cook University, Townsville, Queensland, Australia

Jane Mateer BA, GradDipNursePrac, GradDipDefence, GradCertEmergNurs, GradCertClinTeach, MPublicHlth, MAIntSecurStud

Lecturer, Nursing and Midwifery, RMIT University, Victoria, Australia

Nursing Officer, Army, Australian Defence Force

Joanna McCulloch RN, BA(Psych), BA(Hlth Sc), MA Nursing(Nurse Practitioner),

Nurse Educator, Ophthalmology/Programs, Sydney/Sydney Eye Hospital, NSW, Australia

Course Co-ordinator, Post Graduate Certificate in Ophthalmic Nursing, Notre Dame University, Sydney, NSW, Australia

Leigh McKay BAppSc(Nursing), MPubHlth

Education Coordinator, NSW Organ and Tissue Donation Service, Sydney, NSW

James McManus DipParaSci, DipProfDev, HCPC Registered Paramedic, MPA, MANZCP, ASA

Critical Care Paramedic and Senior Clinical Educator, Queensland Ambulance Service, Queensland Health, Queensland, Australia

Eleanor Milligan BA(Hons1), BSc, GradDipEd, PhD

Associate Professor, School of Medicine, Griffith University, Gold Coast, Queensland, Australia

Jacqui Morarty BAppScOT, MAOT

Manager ABI Community and Transitional Living Services, Alfred Health, Melbourne, Victoria, Australia

Judy Rozana Mullan BA, BPharm, PhD, FSHPA

Academic Leader, Research and Critical Analysis Theme; Senior Lecturer, Graduate School of Medicine, University of Wollongong, NSW, Australia

Belinda Munroe RN, BN, MNurs(AdvPrac)

PhD(cand), Sydney Nursing School, University of Sydney, Camperdown, NSW, Australia

Clinical Nurse Specialist—Emergency Department, Wollongong Hospital, Wollongong, NSW, Australia

Margaret Murphy RN, GradDip(CritCarePsych), GradDipChangeMgtGovt, MHsEd

Clinical Nurse Consultant, Emergency, Westmead Hospital, NSW

Clinical Lecturer, Sydney Nursing School, The University of Sydney, NSW

Stuart Andrew Newman RN, ICCert, DipTeach(Nursing), BEd(Nursing), MHA

Lecture in Health Services Management, Sydney Nursing School, The University of Sydney, NSW, Australia

Peter O'Meara BHA, MPP, PhD
Professor, La Trobe Rural Health School, La Trobe University, Bendigo, Victoria, Australia

Linda Ora BN, MPallC, MACN
Clinical Nurse Consultant Palliative Care, Primary Care and Community Health, Nepean Blue Mountains Local Health District, Australia

Lucy Patel RN
Nurse Triage—Director of Nursing, Medibank Health Solutions, Osborne Park, WA, Australia

Andrew Pearce BSc(Hons), BM/BS, PostGradCert(Aeromed Ret) DRTM(RCSEd) MAICD, FACEM
Clinical Director, Education and Training, MedSTAR Emergency Medical Retrieval Service
Senior Consultant and Emergency Physician, Royal Adelaide Hospital, South Australia, Australia
Associate Professor, School of Public Health and Tropical Medicine, James Cook University, Darwin, NT, Australia

Nicholas G Procter RN, BA, GradDipAdultEd, MBA, PhD
Professor and Chair, Mental Health Nursing, School of Nursing and Midwifery, University of South Australia, Adelaide, Australia

Linda Ann Quinn RN, Paediatric Cert, GradDipNursing (Burns)
Burns Advanced Clinical Practice Consultant, Surgical Services, Women's and Children's Hospital, South Australia, Australia

Jamie Ranse BNurs, GradCert(ClinEpi), GradCertClinEd, MCritCareNurs, PhD(cand)
Assistant Professor, Faculty of Health, University of Canberra, Australia

Terri Rebmann RN, PhD, CIC
Director, Institute for Biosecurity; Associate Professor, Environmental and Occupational Health, College for Public Health and Social Justice, Saint Louis University, St. Louis, MO, USA

Dwight Andrew Robinson B Nurs, Grad Cert Emergency Nursing
Registered Nurse, Intensive Care Unit, Nepean Hospital, NSW

Tessa Rogers RN
Emergency Nurse Practitioner, St George Hospital, Sydney, NSW, Australia

Adam Rolley BA(CCJ), DipHlthSci(PreHospCare), GDIntCareParamedicPrac
Senior Educator (Critical Care Paramedics), Queensland Ambulance Service, Brisbane, Queensland, Australia
School of Medicine, The University of Queensland, Queensland, Australia

Manoj Saxena BSc(Hons), MBBChir, MRCP (UK), FRACP, FCICM
Intensive Care Physician, St George Hospital Clinical School, UNSW, Sydney, Australia
Research Fellow, The George Institute for Global Health, Camperdown, NSW, Australia

Lesley Seaton BN, MN, PhD
Senior Lecturer/Coordinator International Relations, Sydney Nursing School, UNSW, Australia

Myra Sgorbini MN(Hons)
Clinical Nurse Consultant, Organ and Tissue Donation Program, Royal Prince Alfred Hospital, Sydney, NSW, Australia

Ramon Z Shaban RN, CICP, BSc(Med), BN, AssDipAppSc(Amb), GradCertInfCon, PostGradDipPHTM, MEd, MCHealthPrac(Hons), PhD, FCENA, FACN
Professor, Centre for Health Practice Innovation, Menzies Health Institute Queensland, School of Nursing and Midwifery, Griffith University, Queensland, Australia

Editor-in-Chief, Australasian Emergency Nursing Journal, Australia

Tony Skapetis BDS, MEd(Adult Ed), PhD
Clinical Director Education—Oral Health, Education Unit, Westmead Centre for Oral Health, Westmead
Clinical Senior Lecturer, Faculty of Dentistry, University of Sydney, Sydney

Jacinta Stewart BA(Nursing), MA(Trauma and Emergency Nursing)
Emergency Clinical Coordinator, Emergency, Royal Hobart Hospital, Tasmania, Australia

Ruth Townsend BN, LLB, LLM, GradDipLegalPrac, GradCertVET, DipParaSc

Jane Treloggen RN, MHSc(Nurs), BHSc(Nurs), DipManagement, ICUCert
Manager, Lions NSW Eye Bank and NSW Bone Bank, NSW, Australia

Alex Tzannes BSc(Med), MBBS, FACEM
Retrieval Consultant, Greater Sydney Area HEMS, NSW Ambulance, Sydney, Australia
Emergency Physician, Emergency Department, St George Hospital, Sydney, Australia

Amber Van Dreven BN, DipAppSc (Nursing), GradDipMid, GradCert(Crit Care), GradCert(Tert Ed), MN (Research)
Clinical Skills and Simulation Instructor, Clinical School, Deakin University, Ballarat, Victoria, Australia

Wayne Varndell BSc(Hons) Nursing, PostGradDip(AP), PostGradCertEd, MN(Research)
Clinical Nurse Consultant, Emergency Department, Prince of Wales Hospital, Randwick, NSW, Australia
Clinical Lecturer, Faculty of Health, University of Technology, Sydney, NSW, Australia

Adrian Verrinder BSc(Hons), PhD(UCL)
Lecturer, La Trobe University (retired)

Ioana Vlad MD, FACEM, DCH, VGDWH
Emergency Consultant and Clinical Toxicologist, Sir Charles Gairdner Hospital, Perth, WA, Australia

Elizabeth Walter BN, GradCert(Emergency Nursing), MEmergNurs
Clinical Nurse Coordinator, South Eastern Sydney Local Health District, Sydney, NSW, Australia

Martin Ward RN, RMN GradDipPubSectMgmnt (Health), MA(Management)
Associate Fellow, University of Technology, Sydney, Australia
Fellow, College of Nursing, NSW
Clinical Nurse Consultant, Emergency Department, Royal North Shore Hospital, St Leonard's, Sydney, NSW, Australia

Anthony Weber AssDipAppSci(Ambulance), AdvDipHlthSci(Advanced Prehospital Care), BHlth (Nursing), MHlthSci (Research)
Deputy Dean (Learning and Teaching) and Paramedic Discipline Lead, School of Medical and Applied Science, Central Queensland University, Rockhampton, Queensland, Australia

Diana Williamson RN, DipHealth Sc(Nursing), GradCert(Emergency), MA ClinNurs(Emergency)
Clinical Nurse Consultant—Metropolitan Emergency Services, District Facilitator CEC Clinical Leadership Program, Hunter New England Local Health District, NSW, Australia
Conjoint Lecturer, School of Nursing and Midwifery, University of Newcastle, NSW, Australia

Sarah Winch RN, BA(Hons), PhD
Senior Lecturer Health Care Ethics, Integrity Officer MBBS/MD, The University of Queensland, School of Medicine, Australia
CEO, Health Ethics Australia

REVIEWERS

Stéphane Bouchoucha BSc(Hons), ENB 100, GradCertTeachingLearning, MSc, PhD

Lecturer, School of Nursing and Midwifery, Deakin University, Melbourne, Victoria, Australia

Lisa Bowerman BHlthSC (Pre-hospital Care), MHlthSC (Ed), PhD(cand)

Senior Lecturer, Paramedic Practice; Course Coordinator, BA Paramedic Practice, School of Medicine, University of Tasmania, Tasmania, Australia

Naomi Bunker RN, BN, MPhil(cand)

Clinical Coordinator (Academic); Lecturer Nursing, School of Health, University of New England, Australia

Michael Crossan RN, MSc Nursing (Hons), GradCertEmergNurs

Professional Teaching Fellow, Nursing, School of Nursing, University of Auckland, Australia

Jenny D'Antonio RN/Midwife, BAppSc (Nursing), GradCert Emerg Nurs, GradDipMid, MPET, MACN, CENA

University Course Coordinator, B Nursing, B Nursing/B Paramedicine, Australian Catholic University, Ballarat, Victoria, Australia

Terri Downer RN, PostGradCertNurseEducation(Clinical Teaching), MAdvPrac, PhD(cand), RM, ACM, CAPEA

Lecturer in Nursing and Midwifery, University of the Sunshine Coast, Australia

Bev Ewens RN, BSc(Hons), PostGradCertEd, PostGradDip(Critical Care), PostGradCert(Management), PhD(cand)

Postgraduate Courses Coordinator, Lecturer, Post Graduate Nursing, Edith Cowan University, Australia

Lyn Francis BN, CM, MHM, LLB, LLM, GradCertTT, PhD(cand), ACM, NTEU

Lecturer, Nursing, University of Newcastle, Australia

Merridy Gina RN, CertIVTAE, GradCertHSc Ed, BHSc(Nursing), A&ECert(NSWCN), DipAppSc(Nursing), ACN, CENA, RAAF

Nurse Educator, Australian College of Nursing, Cairns, Queensland, Australia

Melanie Greenwood RN, MN, GradCertUnivLearnTeach, Cert Intensive Care, Cert Neuroscience

Course Coordinator Postgraduate Studies, University of Tasmania, Hobart, Tasmania, Australia

Peter Hartley PhD

Associate Professor, Director Teaching and Learning/Clinical Learning, Victoria University, Melbourne, Victoria, Australia

Paramedics Australasia (President), Council of Ambulance Authorities, American Education Research Association

David Kelly BPod, BHlthSc(Paramedic), GradDipHlthSc (Pre-hospital Care)

MICA Paramedic, Ambulance Victoria

Clinical Tutor, School of Medicine, University of Queensland, Brisbane, Queensland, Australia

Shane Lenson BNurs, MNursSci(Nurse Practitioner), MA Public Hlth (Major Biosecurity and Disaster Preparedness), FCENA

School of Nursing, Midwifery and Paramedicine, Australian Catholic University, Canberra, ACT, Australia

Martha Mansah RN, BN(Hons), PhD

Course Coordinator and Lecturer, Emergency Nursing; Contemporary Nursing Practice, Gerontology Nursing, Griffith University, NSW, Australia

Thomas Mathew RN, BScNursing, MSc Nursing, Cert Tertiary Teaching, MACN

Lecturer in Nursing (Acute and Critical Care), University of Melbourne, Victoria, Australia

Alexander (Sandy) MacQuarrie BSc, MBA, CCP(F), PhD(cand)

Lecturer Paramedicine, Charles Sturt University, NSW, Australia

Kiri Matiatos RN (Comprehensive), BHSc(Nursing), PGDip (Distinction) (Advanced Nursing)

Professional Teaching Fellow, School of Nursing, University of Auckland, New Zealand

ED Nurse, Adult Emergency Department, Auckland City Hospital, Auckland, New Zealand

Alison McDonald BN, PGCert, MA(Emerg Nurs)

Clinical Nurse Specialist, Emergency Department, Armidale Hospital, NSW, Australia

University of New England, Armidale, NSW, Australia

Hunter New England Health, NSW, Australia

Paula McMullen RN, BSN, MHPEd, PhD, MANZCP

Associate Head of School, Faculty of Health, School of Medicine, Division of Paramedicine, University of Tasmania, Australia

Jonathan Mould PhD, RGN, RMN, RSCN

Lecturer in Nursing, Curtin University, Bentley Campus, WA, Australia

Australian College of Children and Young People's Nurses (ACCYPN)

Leigh Parker DipNursing, PGCertICParamedic, PGCertEdLeadership

Lecturer, Paramedic Practice, University of Tasmania, Hobart, Tasmania, Australia

Virginia Plummer BN, MidwiferyCert, CriticalCareCert, GradCertEmergHth (Disaster Preparedness & Mgmt), GradCert (Health Professional Education), GradDip (Health Admin), MSc (Health Policy & Management), PhD

Associate Professor, Disaster and Emergency Nursing Management, Monash University and Peninsula Health, Victoria, Australia

Sandra Richardson BA, RGON, DipSocSci, PostGradDipHealthSci, DipTertTeach, PhD

Senior Lecturer, University of Otago; Nurse Researcher, Emergency Department, CDHB, Christchurch, New Zealand

Liz Ryan RN, BN, GradCertACN, GradDipACN (Trauma and Crit Care), MN (Clin Educ), MACN, MACEN

Lecturer, University of New England, NSW, Australia

Natashia Scully BA, BN, GradCertTertiaryEd, PGDipNSc, MPH

School of Health, University of New England, NSW, Australia

SECTION I

OVERVIEW OF EMERGENCY CARE

CHAPTER 1
EMERGENCY NURSING IN AUSTRALIA AND NEW ZEALAND

MARGARET FRY

Essentials

- Emergency departments (EDs) are a key entry point for patients entering the acute hospital system.
- Clinical care demands mean that EDs share similar characteristics.
- To meet service demand and optimise workforce supply and retention staff roles and new models of care need further consideration and evaluative research.
- Clinical performance indicators provide an opportunity to compare services, quality and strive for consistency.
- The cultural context of care has embedded beliefs and values which drive behaviour, activities and interactions.
- Emergency nurses are responsible for direct patient care and management, policy, education and research within the specialty of emergency nursing.
- Emergency nurses need to champion the translation of research and thereby anchoring practice in best evidence.

INTRODUCTION

This introductory chapter provides an overview of emergency departments (EDs) and the development of Australasian emergency nursing. The key challenges, research and professional and management issues confronting emergency-care providers today are explored. A brief overview of Australasian ED role delineation is provided. Given that emergency nursing occurs within a specific context of care, embedded cultural beliefs which drive and motivate behaviour and interaction are discussed. The development of the different nursing clinical roles and specialist education and industrial awards is described.

The challenge for those in (re)designing the Australasian healthcare system is to consider how service delivery can better accommodate an ageing population, population growth, increased chronic disease rates and workforce shortages. The challenge to reform the landscape of healthcare provision requires new ways of thinking that will reshape and define roles, activities and the clinician expertise necessary to reduce the fragmentation of care that exists within and between sectors, while leading to greater consistency of practice and healthcare accessibilities and equity for patients.

Emergency nursing: Historical background

Australasian designated EDs were first set up in the early 1970s and functioned mainly as an after-hours patient entry point where a ward nurse came to monitor the patient's condition until the arrival of a doctor.[1] However, the increasing number of patients presenting to EDs, demand for more emergency care, advances in technology and improvements in resuscitation procedures led to the need to expand services and create a specialty area for the delivery of emergency care. By 1985 these changes raised the expectation that both nursing and medical staff needed to become highly trained, specialised and permanently based in EDs.

Emergency nursing as a specialty practice has evolved over the past 40 years. Emergency nurses deliver care to a diverse population experiencing episodic, abrupt, potentially life-threatening health or psychosocial conditions. Emergency care may require minimal intervention or advanced life-support practices. Emergency nurses require in-depth knowledge, skills and clinical expertise to provide care and to manage situations such as patient overcrowding and the use of complex technology.

Emergency nurses can collectively be described as individuals who function well when working in stressful environments, possessing the ability to make sound decisions, even when they are under considerable amounts of stress. They are proactive individuals who enjoy challenges and actively strive to professionally develop themselves. Emergency nurses are friendly, easy-going individuals who possess the ability to engage and develop a rapport with individuals from a diverse range of cultural and socioeconomic backgrounds.[2]

Emergency practice requires nurses to blend theoretical knowledge systems, past experiences, collated patterns of knowing and ways of doing with a patient's physiological, interpersonal and communicative signs.[3,4] Convergences of these knowledge systems with cognitive domains that include assessment, diagnosis, treatment and evaluation skills enable greater accuracy and speed in the decision-making, troubleshooting, prioritisation and delivery of emergency care.[5]

The practice environment of emergency nursing is as diverse as the nursing profession itself. Box 1.1 identifies some of the practice environments of Australasian emergency nurses.

BOX 1.1 Emergency nursing practice environments

Emergency departments
Emergency treatment areas
Minor injury units
Military services
Community health clinics
Remote and very remote health clinics
Industrial areas
Multipurpose centres
Māori health providers
Medical centres
Pre-hospital/retrieval services
Disaster response teams

In keeping with the nursing profession as a whole, emergency nursing roles include assessment, diagnosis, patient care and management, referral, education, consultation, advocacy and research.

In Australasia, emergency nursing practice is guided by various professional and government bodies which include the Nursing Council of New Zealand (NCNZ), New Zealand Nurses Organisation, Australian Nurses Boards, the Nursing and Midwifery Board of Australia, Australian Health Practitioner Regulation Agency (APHRA), the Australian Nursing and Midwifery Council (ANMC), the Australian Nursing and Midwifery Federation, the College of Emergency Nursing Australasia (CENA), the Council of Remote Area Nurses of Australia (CRANA), state and territory emergency nurse associations and local, state, territory and federal governments. However, the demands of the clinical environment also determine the scope of practice roles in emergency nursing. Consequently, role function may vary between and within service providers. For example, emergency nurse roles in a teaching tertiary hospital may vary from those in remote, rural or regional areas.

Emergency department environment

The geographical landmass of Australasia (Australia and New Zealand) is vast—7,955,530 square kilometres—with a combined population in 2009 of over 27 million.[6,7] Throughout Australia the roles of EDs differ depending on the type of hospital, geographical location and position within the healthcare system network (Table 1.1). Within each designated level, physical design, function, staffing and resources are similar. New Zealand's ED role delineation structure is similar to Australia's (Box 1.2).

In the urban setting, most metropolitan and regional areas have a designated ED. However, rural, remote and very remote health centres have designated treatment areas/rooms, which provide limited resuscitation practices. To be designated as an emergency department or service relates to the availability of specialist medical officer and nurse cover and on-site diagnostic services, intensive care and surgical operating services.[10] While rural, remote and very remote centres have access to medical officers, nurses often assess and manage patients.

The New Zealand healthcare system is currently structured as 20 district health boards across 16 regions. These boards, inclusive of emergency services, were established to ensure the delivery, monitoring and evaluation of health services.[11] Similarly, Australian state and territory governments are responsible for health services, although service models vary. Australia has 129 and New Zealand 42 designated public EDs.[12,13] Australia and New Zealand have a national healthcare system that provides universal free access to emergency services, free public hospital care, subsidised pharmaceuticals and out-of-hospital care. A reciprocal healthcare agreement exists between Australia and New Zealand.

Emergency care throughout Australasia is considered a right of citizens, and care should be of an appropriate standard and quality. The challenge for clinicians is the increasing complexity of the emergency environments and of the care being delivered against rising patient presentation rates, an ageing population and comorbidities.

TABLE I.I Australian emergency department distribution[8]

TYPE OF HOSPITAL	NUMBER
Major referral and specialist women's and children's*	30
Metropolitan (urban districts)†	54
Major rural and regional	45
Total*†	129

Australian Health Workforce Advisory Committee: Health workforce planning and models of care in emergency departments. Canberra: National Health Workforce Secretariat, 2006.

Does not include 23 private hospital EDs, although 86% (19) are located in capital cities.

†*Does not include multipurpose rural centres (n = 66); excluded as they are not designated EDs.*

BOX I.2 New Zealand emergency department distribution[9]

T1 Higher-level tertiary
T2 Lower-level tertiary
S1 Secondary
S2 Subacute
Health centre/Rural and remote

The ED is one of the key entry points for patients entering the hospital system and provides an interface between the primary health and acute care sectors. Throughout Australasia, the increased patient attendance rate is largely due to an ageing population, decreased availability of general practitioner (GP) services, increased chronic disease rates and the availability of new technologies and procedures.[14] The need to deliver care for all age groups and respond to patients with minor injuries and illness through to critical or life-threatening conditions requires EDs to be responsive by having specifically designated clinical areas. Hence, EDs are largely configured in the same way, although size may differ between individual departments.

Clinical environment

The clinical environment needs to meet the demands of a range of patient conditions and injuries across the life span, and so all EDs share similar architectural commonalities between sites that make them recognisable and consistent with each other. The organisation of ED work, purpose and function is shaped and ordered by patient case-mix and architecture. Emergency department patient care is usually provided in a range of specifically designated geographical areas which are configured into areas such as waiting and ambulance arrival areas, triage, resuscitation, acute, sub-acute and/or fast-track/consultation areas. For mixed adult and paediatric EDs, best practice requires children to be allocated to a separate waiting, clinical and resuscitation area away from adult patients. Increasingly, assessment or 24-hour short-stay units are being co-located

within or near EDs, for example short-stay mental health or medical aged assessment units.

Patients with critical and/or life-threatening conditions are best managed in resuscitation areas with appropriate lifesaving and continuous-monitoring equipment and enough room in which a range of skilled staff can provide care. Designated resuscitation areas are often resourced to provide care for both paediatric and adult patients. Urgent patient conditions, with the potential for deterioration, need close monitoring for a period of time and are often located in an acute area where there is provision for continuous vital signs, and invasive and cardiac monitoring. In contrast, patients who self-present with minor injuries and illnesses can be managed in a fast-track and/or consultation-type area with equipment targeting minor procedure and/or illness management. However, some patient groups that might require isolation, privacy and/or reduced stimulation may be more appropriately managed in a single room, with or without continuous-monitoring capabilities. The diverse clinical environment of the ED is challenging, given the requirement for clinicians to provide care for patients across the life span and with diverse clinical presentations and comorbidities.

The primary distinguishing feature of emergency nursing is the prominence of patients with undifferentiated diagnoses in a time-pressured environment, so the process of patient assessment is vital in these circumstances. Nurses require in-depth knowledge and clinical expertise to provide care and manage situational events, such as patient overcrowding and complex technology.

Emergency department workforce

The ED workforce is largely driven by patient case-mix, local demand and presentation rates. Therefore, workforce planning and staff ratios, development and work practice (re-)design should be focused on the challenge of making the patient's journey through the ED as efficient, safe and satisfying as possible.

The most appropriate staff ratio profile for an ED is unclear, and development of staffing models remains an urgent priority.[15] Greater clarity is required to understand and define the appropriate workforce model for EDs, which would also give shape to possible advanced practice emergency nursing roles.[10,16] Nevertheless, roles within EDs are diverse and staff include nursing, medical, allied health, transport, and administrative support and communication staff members.[8,9] The workforce profile of an ED is usually individually responsive to local demands and need, and to patient presentation rates and acuity. The emergency department workforce analysis tool may assist in reviewing workforce profiles and future requirements.[17]

A diverse range of staff is needed to sustain ED services' delivery. The emergency doctor's primary role is to assess, stabilise, manage and refer patients. They also oversee/supervise other junior medical staff providing care, including emergency medicine and other specialty trainees, career medical officers, locum practitioners, GPs and junior medical officers.[18] Emergency nurses undertake patient assessment, prioritise nursing care, initiate interventions and provide ongoing nursing management for the range of patients. EDs now offer a range of nursing roles that require varying levels of advanced knowledge, expertise and skills.[15] For example, the nurse practitioner[19] and clinical initiative nurse (CIN).[20]

The ED workforce is a major resource of and for the department. Hence, work practices may be one of the chief areas of attention for redesign in the future. Government and service strategies and policies need to focus on: increasing interdisciplinary teamwork and promotion of collaboration between disciplines; staff development to enable the acquisition of advanced skills and experience required for alternative models of care; building staff capacity and expertise of staff in allocating innovative tasks and roles while recognising experience, knowledge, skills, competencies and qualifications; and using technologies, if proven to enhance efficiency and ensure there is adequate support for implementation.

Workforce is clearly a crucial aspect of ED infrastructure. Across Australasia various EDs are developing innovative approaches to the deployment of clinicians, examples including extended practice for experienced nurses, nurse practitioners and allied health professionals being employed to provide autonomous assessment and treatment. The delivery of effective ED care, in a collaborative system, may require fresh thinking and research about the range and roles of staff working in the area.

Support officers

The complexity of the ED environment requires dedicated support staff who can assist directly or indirectly with patient management, admission, disposition and/or discharge processes. The range of dedicated support staff essential to improve ED services and efficiency include clerical staff, clinical and communication support staff, orderlies, transport/transfer staff and cleaners. Support staff require appropriate education and development and are essential for the efficient provision of ED services. Support staff are necessary to release healthcare workers from non-clinical tasks, enabling their focus to remain on patient care and management.

Optimising work practices

Optimising patient service, flow and management has led to diverse extended practice roles being undertaken by nursing and allied health staff; roles and/or activities that were traditionally undertaken by medical staff. The ability of emergency nurses to undertake a range of extended patient-management activities has been through the establishment of reference tools such as clinical practice guidelines, clinical pathways and standing orders.[19,20] The medically endorsed patient-management guidelines have enabled emergency nurses to undertake an extended range of activities, including assessment, pharmacological and investigative interventions, and targeted management activities such as the commencement of intravenous fluids.[21] By initiating these care activities and interventions for a range of patients, the experienced emergency nurse optimises work practices.[20] Significant improvements in ED services' flow and costs have been demonstrated in many EDs that have established such reference tools.[21,22] Reference tools such as clinical guidelines go some way to securing consistency within practice, and offer clinicians and managers the opportunity to make comparisons with other like services.

Communication support

Communication, both non-clinical and clinical, consumes a significant proportion of ED staff time.[23,24] The need to better coordinate and centralise non-medical communication is growing. Within many EDs the coordination of patient and staff communications requires a dedicated communications support role.

In addition, communication processes concerning patient care and management are also growing in complexity as increasing numbers of healthcare clinicians and hospital managers become involved.[25] Shared decision-making about high-quality patient treatment, care and disposition has led to complex and multilayered communication processes. The communication support role provides a pivotal conduit to better facilitate the patient's journey and provide a consistent link between local, hospital and community engagement. Greater integration of communication processes between primary care and the acute care sector is needed.

A secondary advantage to having a centralised ED communication role is the ability for patients and relatives/family to have access to a consistent communication portal. Providing high-quality patient care is challenged by the pressures of communication in the stressful ED work environment. Communication processes need to be considered within all stages of the patient's journey (pre-hospital to hospital) to alleviate patient, family and/or carer stress and anxiety. Clear information about emergency processing and care while in the ED should be provided systematically and consistently to patients, families and/or carers.

Performance improvement

With the increasing demand and expectation on service delivery, EDs are challenged to provide consistent, safe and timely high-quality care. EDs have been proactively examining ways to provide a more satisfying and appropriate service. Hence much has been done through examination of various practice models, at federal, state and local levels, to improve service delivery. However, consistency in ED practice remains elusive, as organisational comparisons are often difficult given the (often significant) variation in local demand, population mix, geographical location, workforce characteristics and resource availability between sites.

Across Australasia, national accreditation organisations have sought to champion high-quality improvement programs for healthcare. These national accreditation bodies have provided various quality frameworks for healthcare evaluation, which are focused on demonstrating appropriate and consistent patient care practices, staff development and education practices, and patient safety review processes. For example, The Australian Council on Healthcare Standards (ACHS) has introduced quality frameworks (such as the Evaluation and Quality Improvement Program National–EQuIPNational) which aim to facilitate evaluation and review of organisational practices to achieve greater consistency, safety and standardisation of care.[26]

Traditionally, throughout Australasia ED comparisons relating to service delivery have largely focused on triage code allocation and the associated 'seen by doctor' times, patient case-mix and mortality and presentation rates. However, ED staff have been concerned that service comparisons have often failed to accommodate the different levels of service providers. For example, rural EDs may not have a doctor on-site and so triage code benchmarks can be an unreliable indicator for service comparison between metropolitan/urban and rural EDs.

Clinical performance indicators are important, and enable services to make comparisons between themselves throughout Australasia. However, it is timely that consideration be given to the development of other system indicators. Examples may include time to analgesia and time to first antibiotic.[27] Additional performance indicators need to be identified that will maximise equitable comparisons while focusing on the patient's journey and drivers of quality and satisfaction for staff and patients. In addition, many external services (for example, radiology, surgery and pathology) contribute directly or indirectly towards the ED patient flow. These external services are often outside the control of ED staff, but may limit, impede or reduce the capacity for ED patient flow. Many external services are critical to ED patient management and decision-making, and so future external service benchmarking is needed to enhance patient flow broadly.

Emergency service redesign models of care

Workload demands and workforce issues have dominated the recent healthcare debate. For example, governments have sought to drive service change through policies such as the Australian National Emergency Access Targets (NEAT).[28] The NEAT policy was introduced to improve service consistency, delivery and reduce overcrowding in the ED. The impact of governmental policies on emergency workforce, models of care and ED function remain unclear.

While there has been significant increase in ED demand, there has been little debate about the use and appropriateness of current and future emergency staff roles, including the contribution of allied health and paramedical staff within the ED. Optimising ED workforce models to better meet service need is important given workforce projections concerning supply, distribution and skill mix needed to meet future demands for services.

In Australasia, 10–60% of ED presentations have been estimated as primary healthcare patients.[29–31] A proportion of this group could be redirected to new models of care or other healthcare agencies.[32–34] Between 1970 and 2008, extensive research was undertaken of new models of care in many countries, particularly in the UK, the USA, Ireland, Canada, Denmark and Sweden, and to a lesser degree in Australasia. A literature review[35] identified six practice-based new models of care:

- minor injuries units
- walk-in centres
- telephone triage and advice services
- GP cooperatives services
- primary care health centres
- ambulance services ('see and treat' and 'treat and refer').

Models were not mutually exclusive from each other, EDs or GP clinics. The outcomes of these models of care demonstrated a positive impact on acute service use patterns.

While there was a wide range of care models beyond traditional GPs and EDs, telephone triage advice centres, minor injury units and walk-in centres were the most effective models due to ease of access, convenience and prompt service

delivery. The evidence of impact was stronger for services co-located or streamed with EDs. In 2010, Australia opened the first walk-in centre in Canberra, ACT.[36]

A collaborative and integrative relationship between emergency staff, paramedics, GPs, nurse practitioners and other primary healthcare clinicians would enhance the timely delivery of services. Studies in the UK by Ward,[37] Dale et al[38] and Murphy et al[39] demonstrated that GPs based within an ED significantly reduced investigations, referrals, radiology and costs, and managed 16.8% of non-urgent ED presentations. Further exploration of the GP role within ED is needed, as there was UK evidence of reduced hospital costs and emergency doctor workload. While the research is difficult to quantify, ED redesign models globally have had a significant impact on GP workload, hospital admissions and costs.

For those in geographically isolated areas throughout Australasia, concerns remain about healthcare equity and access, and limited healthcare options.[40] The application or impact that redesign models may have in rural, remote and regional areas is unclear. While the different models of care may benefit those living in more-isolated regions, it is difficult to extrapolate the findings of research to these areas. While a portion of these new models could be considered, others would be difficult and/or impractical to implement in geographically isolated areas. Implementation barriers and enablers have been identified within the literature.[35]

Paramedical service redesign models of care

In the UK, preliminary evidence has identified that extended paramedical 'see and treat' and 'treat and refer' protocols may reduce ED activity. In 2007, paramedical 'see and treat' protocols for assessing and treating minor injury or illness in the community were evaluated.[41] This cluster-randomised controlled trial involved 56 UK urban ambulance stations and 3018 patients. The patients treated by a paramedic were less likely to be transported to an ED or need hospital admission within 28 days. The 'see and treat' paramedical model had a positive impact on healthcare agencies, and paramedics reported high levels of satisfaction. Extended paramedical roles were shown to redirect activity away from acute care services.

Similarly, Snooks et al[42] evaluated a 'treat and refer' paramedical protocol. Patients could be assessed, managed and left at the scene with either a referral plan or self-care advice. The evaluation identified that there was no difference in the proportion of patients left at the scene in the intervention or control groups, although job time was longer for the 'treat and refer' group. Paramedical 'treat and refer' protocols were found to be used appropriately. Further testing and validation of protocols, decision support systems and training was required.

Another paramedical redesign model included a minor injuries unit (MIU) referral protocol.[43] This 12-month UK study introduced a protocol aimed at reducing ED activity by enabling paramedic crews to directly refer patients to an MIU. In the randomised-cluster control group, 37 people attended an MIU, 327 attended an ED and 61 were not transported. For the intervention group, 41 people attended an MIU, 303 attended an ED and 65 patients were not transported. Ambulance service job times were shorter for those attending an MIU compared with an ED. The MIU patients were

7.2 times as likely to rate care as excellent. The results suggest that paramedics make appropriate referrals to alternative healthcare agencies and thereby reduce ED activity. Extending the role of paramedics could build service capacity and job satisfaction while redirecting activity away from acute care services.[44] The shift of paramedic education into the tertiary sector will potentially facilitate the extended-care practitioner (ECP) role. Postgraduate courses are now becoming available as well as industry-based ECP training. However, it is unclear exactly how the role of the ECP will develop in Australasia. This is discussed further in Chapter 11.

Australasian nurse competency standards

Emergency nurses require skills, knowledge and expertise to meet the challenge of delivering emergency care. Assisting to define these care dimensions has been the various iterations of Australasian competency standards which detail the combination of skills, knowledge, attitudes, values and abilities that underpin effective performance within a profession/ occupational area. Competency standards have therefore been defined as a set of core standards that describe the current practice of nurses. Such standards can be developed to the professional levels expected of both the beginning nurse and the advanced nurse practitioner (see also Ch 7).[45]

CENA (the College of Emergency Nursing Australasia) has released competency standards in order to provide broad practice and performance guidelines.[46] The emergency nursing specialist standards cover nine domains: clinical expertise, communication, teamwork, resources and environment, professional development, leadership, legal, professional ethics and research and quality improvement.[46] The standards represent the unique character- istics that give shape to the specialty of emergency practice. National competences have been developed within Australasia for registered nurses, enrolled nurses and nurse practitioners by the ANMC and the NCNZ.[47–51] Many peak nursing and midwifery bodies have given support for these competencies.

Within Australasia, nursing and midwifery regulating authorities have established standards of competency that apply to the registration of nurses and midwives, with a focus on safety of practice. These competency standards accommodate the diverse roles that nurses and midwives undertake, provide a framework for undergraduate and postgraduate curriculums, define behaviour and are a means of ensuring high-quality care through safe and effective work practices. In Australia and New Zealand, the developed and endorsed enrolled nurse, registered nurse, nurse practitioner and midwife competency standards provide a framework for ongoing professional development.

In July 2010 the Australian states and territories transferred responsibility for nursing and midwifery registration to the Australian Health Practitioner Regulation Agency (AHPRA). However, ANMC competency standards will continue to provide the national framework for professional registration, conduct and performance.

Development of emergency nurse associations

To support nurses in this new specialty area, professional organisations such as the Emergency Nurses Association (ENA) were formally established in the USA (1970), UK (1972), Australia (1983) and New Zealand (1990).[52] These associations promote clinical, educational and professional development of emergency nurses by producing policy statements on levels of role performance and by fostering specialty recognition. The associations publish newsletters and provide financial sponsorship for ED nurses to attend conferences and conduct research. Many also provide introductory specialty education courses to update knowledge and skills. The Australasian Emergency Nursing Journal, first published in 1996 by the New South Wales ENA, became Australasia's first international, peer-reviewed emergency nursing journal. State and territory ENAs have merged to form the College of Emergency Nursing Australasia (CENA), the peak professional body for emergency nurses throughout Australia with professional links to New Zealand and Singapore emergency nursing groups.[53]

Emergency nurse specialisation

Nursing specialisation was necessary because of the recognition that nurses could no longer master the volume of knowledge and skills required to work in all clinical areas.[54] To assist emergency nurses in gaining in-depth knowledge and clinical expertise, specialty postgraduate courses were developed. By 1979, professional bodies such as the New South Wales College of Nursing had extended their nursing education profile to include advanced emergency nursing programs. By 1995, the Emergency Nursing Graduate Certificate course had been established in Australia.[54]

In 1985, Australian hospital-based pre-registration nurse education began to transfer to the tertiary sector, with com- pletion for all states and territories by 1994. With the shift to tertiary education there was a corresponding demand for postgraduate tertiary qualifications.[55,56] To meet this demand, tertiary programs were developed to articulate with specialist certificate courses and extend nursing knowledge, attributes and clinical skills beyond mere technical competence. Today, Australasian universities provide postgraduate courses in specialty areas such as emergency nursing. Registered nurses can now pursue graduate diploma, master and/or doctoral degrees in their area of specialisation.[55]

Cultural context of care

Today nurses are recognised and defined by their area of specialty practice, such as emergency. While all types of nursing have similar characteristics, in each specialty there is a unique collection of individuals who share knowledge systems including values, beliefs and ways of being that make them and their work distinct from other communities of practice.[57–59] Nurses who work in EDs share common knowledge sets that provide understanding and bring meaning to activities, shape the boundary of emergency work and make them recognisable to each other.[60,61] This creates systems of meaning which allow people to build conceptual maps and orientate activity and behaviour during interaction.[60] Thus, shared information contributes towards a level of stability and coherence.[62] Within an ED, notions of efficiency, timeliness and equity shape meaning through which expectations of patient behaviour are conveyed and a culture of ED care sustained.[60] Through these knowledge sets of meaning, emergency staff come to learn, communicate and understand how practice is viewed and conducted, and how the notion of care is perceived.[22,60]

A cultural context of ED care is reflected in a standard geography of care that is orientated towards the notions of efficiency and timeliness that are shared and understood through patient movement. Patient movement is normalised by architecture, embedded expectations, urgency codes and bed allocations, and creates a spatial web recognisable to all emergency staff. These embedded cultural mores make explicit a particular cadence of care from which a culture of ED care emanates and within which emergency nursing is enacted.[3]

Clinical roles

To keep pace with nursing specialisation across Australasia local, state, territory and regional governments and nurse associations introduced industrial nursing awards which recognised, supported and financially rewarded advanced clinical nurses. For example, the industrial award classification of Clinical Nurse Specialist (CNS) was introduced in New South Wales in 1986. Inherent in this classification is the recognition that advanced-level practitioners deliver and coordinate care appropriate to the needs of the patient, act as clinical resource people, provide leadership and support less-experienced staff. However, CNS award classifications did not mandate an academic qualification for the position, preferring instead to maintain the focus on clinical experience.[63] By the 1990s, other award classifications such as Clinical Nurse Consultant (CNC) and Nurse Practitioner (NP) had been introduced and have added to the clinical career pathways open for registered nurses.[56]

These industrial award classifications meant that experienced nurses no longer had to move away from direct patient care to gain career advancement and financial incentives.[5,64] However, specialty definition, qualifications, levels of competency, accreditation processes and extended practice roles have developed without consistency or national unification throughout Australasia.[5,64] For example, emergency nurses in Australasia can expand their area of chosen professional development and can develop extended clinical nurse roles, such as a Clinical Initiatives Nurse (CIN)[21] or an Advanced Practice Nurse (APN), which are often referred to under several role titles—such as Clinical Nurse Specialist (CNS), Clinical Nurse Educator (CNE), Clinical Nurse Consultant (CNC) and Nursing Unit Manager (NUM).[5,25] However, the extended practice role is not an autonomous advanced role, as extended practice can only be undertaken through the implementation of advanced standing orders.[19]

Across Australia and New Zealand emergency nurses have implemented innovative extended clinical practice roles to meet service demands. Hence, a wider range of patient diagnoses are being managed by nurses with specialist education to ensure safe care.[64] Australian emergency nurses have implemented extended practice roles with a focus on the provision of episodic care; for example, in New South Wales, the 'clinical initiatives nurse' (CIN) or 'advanced practice nurse' (APN). Emergency nurses rely on delegated responsibility to enable the commencement of episodic care for extended practice roles.[21] A significant example of episodic care includes pain management interventions.[65,66] Given the range of extended practice roles within Australasian EDs, there is little doubt regarding the positive impact on patient and system services.[35]

Emergency nurse practitioners

Nationally and internationally, NPs are recognised as undertaking advanced practice roles. Nurse practitioners provide leadership, expertise, support and direction within clinical settings; they undertake assessments, make diagnoses and initiate treatment within their scope of practice, and provide monitoring and care coordination for particular patient groups. Emergency NPs are expert clinicians with advanced skills and theoretical knowledge that enable them to autonomously treat, manage, refer and discharge a range of patient conditions in partnership with medical and other allied health workers.[67,68] Nurse practitioner authorisation requires the nurse or midwife to hold general registration, demonstrate extensive advanced clinical expertise and recency of practice, hold a Master's degree and have competency in the competency standards.[69]

The NP role is well established in the USA (1960s), UK (1980s), Canada (2000) and to a lesser extent Australia (1995) and New Zealand (2000). In a USA Census survey, there were 141,209 (5.8%) authorised NPs with 6000 being educated annually.[70] Within the role, 39% hold hospital privileges and 13% have long-term care privileges, 96.5% usually prescribe medications and write a mean of 19 prescriptions per day.[70] Within Australia (2013) there were 248,578 registered nurses[71] and approximately 966 (0.4%) authorised NPs.[71] In New Zealand (2011) there were 48,563 registered nurses and 89 authorised NPs.[72]

There is national and international evidence of NP impact in relation to: contribution to workload;[19,73–75] appropriate care;[76–78] patient satisfaction;[79–81] documentation and guideline adherence;[83] and efficiency and timeliness.[82,83] No clinical difference was found between NPs and doctors in patient health outcomes.[84–86] Nurse practitioners were found to be more reliable in following practice guidelines and completing medical record documentation. Of note has been the positive economic impact of NP models compared with 'routine medical care'.[86–88] Cost reductions related specifically to resource use, shorter hospital length of stay, and reduced patient complication and (re-)admission rates.

In Australia, regulation of NP authorisation is promoted and maintained by the Australian Health Practitioner Regulating Agency. The Australian statutory authority (the National Registration and Accreditation Scheme) and the NCNZ in New Zealand have established competency standards that apply to the authorisation of NPs.[49,51] Practice areas include metropolitan, district, regional and rural and remote centres with minimal or no doctor coverage. In 2010, Australasian NPs gained prescribing and investigation privileges which should be co-endorsed by their scope of practice and organisation. Within Australasian universities, NP curricula cover care practices for acute and non-acute patient conditions and situations, physical assessment, pharmacology, procedures and ethics and the law (see Chs 3 and 4).

A lack of clarity, internationally, surrounds the NP name. The term 'nurse practitioner' was often used interchangeably with 'clinical nurse specialist' (USA), 'clinical nurse consultant' (UK) and 'advanced practice nurse'.[89–91] Consequently, for consistency greater clarity is needed to define, understand and measure advanced practitioners. Nonetheless, emergency

NPs are caring for patients, from preterm to aged care, and managing acute and chronic conditions in a variety of different models of care and services. The volume, breadth, depth and consistency of research findings provide strong support for expansion of NP roles and numbers.

Management practices

Those in leadership and management positions face increasing challenges in meeting service provision demand and consumer expectation. Current challenges include: sustainable access planning; overcrowding; staff recruitment and retention; and the redesign of models of care to include emergency roles, referrals and redirecting care options. While there are innovative strategies being explored to meet the challenge of service provision, success is often dependent on the ability of clinical leaders and managers to motivate, enthuse and engage with staff to drive new visions of practice.[92,93] Refer to Chapter 6 for more information on leadership.

In Australasia, sustainable access planning remains a major ED management issue.[94,95] Part of sustainable access planning is resolving access block issues. An 'access block' is defined as a patient who is ready to go to a ward bed but remains in the ED for longer than 8 hours because of the lack of an inpatient bed.[84,96] This leads to overcrowding. There is an association between overcrowding, increased hospital length of stay and mortality in Australian hospitals.[94,97,98] Known effects of overcrowding include delays in patient management, poor hospital processes, poor infection control, patients not being placed on the appropriate ward, and so forth.[99]

Hospital strategies which aim to improve inpatient bed access include medical admission units, reforming bed management practices, discharge planning and patient processing. Other complementary strategies include the development of rapid assessment teams, emergency medical units and the use of CINs, APNs, NPs, aged-care assessment teams, and community and chronic disease initiative programs.[20,100,101]

The delivery of emergency care is dependent on sustaining a sufficient nursing workforce. It is essential that the complexities of patient safety, staff recruitment, retention and the development of emergency nursing roles be made explicit to enable strategic planning to sustain and/or enhance nursing workforce density. To this end, transactional leadership provides the basis for responding creatively to workforce issues and the reshaping of emergency nursing roles. Transactional leadership is discussed in Chapter 6.

Contemporary management issues are focused on reshaping models of care that better accommodate and adjust to the ED context, patient safety and processing, fostering clinical expertise and a changing case-mix.[102] One popular UK model being explored throughout Australasia is 'see and treat'. The model aims to reduce waiting times and improve the ED experience by grouping complex and simple patient conditions into separate areas.[67] These patient groups are then treated at the 'right time', in the 'correct area' and by appropriately 'qualified staff' on the initial consultation.[103] Emergency managers and clinical leaders everywhere are continually finding new and innovative ways to provide timely and equitable emergency care, and meet the challenging demands of contemporary service provision.

Integrating research

Research findings can provide insight into and understanding of the complexity of emergency practice and the challenges experienced by emergency care staff. By researching everyday nursing practice, insight is gained into the experience of emergency nurses and how they make sense of reality. From this insight, new ways to educate and support nurses can be developed. From a broad research perspective, six main issues are driving workforce changes and healthcare services:[104]

- patient safety
- declining healthcare infrastructure and funding
- ageing population
- increasing rate of chronic and complex disease
- emerging and re-emerging communicable diseases
- increasing threat of bioterrorism.

Much of the Australasian research healthcare debate and responsive innovative strategies arises out of a response to these issues.

Prevailing nursing research can be categorised into three broad areas: clinical, professional and organisational management. Within clinical research there is a need for greater awareness of the different roles nurses undertake and how these roles differ, improve and impact on patient outcomes.[104] Through clinical research, the factors that determine behaviour and interaction can be made transparent and provide further insight into the consistency of practice. There is also a need for greater clarity regarding advanced and extended practice and how it may be best defined and measured.[5,106] Increasingly, clinicians need to inform their practice through the use of evidence if clinical work is to be defined and shaped by the best available evidence.

Professional research needs to foster greater interdisciplinary collaboration with colleagues and consumers. Greater inter-disciplinary collaboration could improve continuity of care, patient safety and enhance service delivery. Also, by learning what it is that consumers consider important, nurses can learn new ways of being in step with patient need and expectation. Such a research approach will bring about a deeper and more engaging care partnership with consumers.

Organisational management research needs to deconstruct the context of care and, in particular, the dimensions of policy adherence. Shifting contexts of care, such as patient over-crowding, can compromise policy adherence and lead to aggression and violence in the workplace.[107,108] Organisational management research can strategically assist to inform policy development so that policies generate greater relevance, are evidence-based, are workable within practice and accommodate changing contexts of care.

Responsible nursing practice needs to be anchored in best evidence, as this adds to the knowledge of the discipline and contributes towards greater consistency within practice and improved patient outcomes. Refer to Chapter 8 for further information on the importance of evidence-based practice, the research process, practice development and quantitative and qualitative methodologies.

Further research into the ED environment and structures and the drivers of growth in presentation rates would be particularly valuable for service and staff workforce planning.

Implementing new models of care which integrate services between the acute and primary care sectors would add value to the patient experience. Further examination of seamless management plans (acute-primary sectors), specifically for our ageing population and those patients with chronic and complex diseases, may assist to enhance the ED patient journey and better manage this complex and often vulnerable patient group. The impact of overcrowding and long patient stays on satisfaction, mortality and hospital efficiency should also be studied in the Australasian context.

SUMMARY

Emergency care and nursing practice have been shaped by many factors. These factors include advances in resuscitation and technology, recognition of emergency as a specialty practice, increased patient presentation rates, technology, population demands, increased rates of chronic conditions and changing case-mix. These factors and the growing demand on the healthcare system have increased the complexity and demands experienced in emergency nursing. The increasing focus on emergency care provides an opportunity for clinicians to collectively drive the healthcare agenda, management focus, policy direction and research agenda. In this way emergency care services can be strategically directed and reformed. There remains great capacity to reshape and redesign emergency care service delivery within Australasia. Better use of the skills, expertise and qualifications of all healthcare clinicians would go some way towards meeting the challenge for more timely and appropriate healthcare delivery throughout Australasia.

USEFUL WEBSITES

Australian Health Practitioner Regulation Agency (APHRA), www.ahpra.gov.au

Australian Institute for Health and Welfare. Australia's national agency for health and welfare statistics and information, www.aihw.gov.au/index.cfm

Nursing and Midwifery Board of Australia, http://www.nursingmidwiferyboard.gov.au/

Australian Nursing and Midwifery Council, www.anmc.org.au

Australian Nursing and Midwifery Federation. www.anmf.org.au/splash/

College of Emergency Nursing Australasia, www.cena.org.au

Council of Remote Area Nurses of Australia, www.crana.org.au

Emergency Care Institute NSW, www.ecinsw.com.au

National Institute of Clinical Studies (NICS), www.nswnma.asn.au/industrial-issues/awards-and-conditions/public-health-system/

NSW Agency for Clinical Innovation (ARCI), www.aci.health.nsw.gov.au/

New South Wales Health Public Health System Nurses and Midwives (State) Award, www.nswnma.asn.au/industrial-issues/awards-and-conditions/public-health-system/

New Zealand Guidelines Group and Evidence Based Healthcare Bulletin, www.health.govt.nz/about-ministry/ministry-health-websites/new-zealand-guidelines-group

New Zealand Ministry of Health, http://www.health.govt.nz/

New Zealand Nurses Organisation, www.nzno.org.nz

Nursing Council of New Zealand, www.nursingcouncil.org.nz

REFERENCES

1. McKay-Ingalls J, Thayre McCray K. A global perspective on emergency nursing and the new millennium. Journal of Emergency Nursing 1999;25:489–91.
2. Kennedy B, Curtis K, Waters D. The personality of emergency nurses: Is it unique? Australasian Emergency Nursing Journal 2014;17(4):139–45.
3. Fry M. Triage nursing practice in Australian Emergency Departments 2002–2004: An ethnography [PhD]. University of Sydney; 2005.
4. Sbaih L. Shaping the future: reforming routine emergency nursing work. Accident & Emergency Nursing 2001;9:266–73.
5. Gardner G, Chang A, Duffield C. Making nursing work: breaking through the role confusion of advanced practice nursing. Journal of Advanced Nursing 2007;57:382–91.
6. Australian Bureau of Statistics. Population clock. Canberra: Commonwealth of Australia, 2014.
7. Statistics New Zealand. National population estimates. Auckland: New Zealand Ministry Government, 2013.

8. AHWAC. Health workforce planning and models of care in emergency departments. Sydney: Australian Health Workforce Advisory Committee, 2006.

9. Hewitt A, Roos R, Baldwin K. Emergency department use 2011/12. Wellington: New Zealand Ministry of Health, 2012.

10. ACEM. Role delineation for emergency departments. Emergency Medicine 1998;10:65–9.

11. New Zealand Ministry of Health. Annual report for the year ended 30th of June 2013 including the Director-General of Health's Annual Report on the state of public health. Wellington: New Zealand Government, 2013.

12. Australian Health Workforce Advisory Committee. Health workforce planning and models of care in emergency departments. Canberra: National Health Workforce Secretariat, 2006.

13. New Zealand Ministry of Health. Roadside to bedside. Wellington: NZ Ministry of Health, 1999.

14. Australian Commonwealth Government. A national health and hospitals network for Australia's future. Canberra: Commonwealth of Australia, 2010.

15. Williams G, Souter J, Smith C. The Queensland Emergency Nursing Workforce Tool: A prototype for informing and standardising nursing workforce projections. Australasian Emergency Nursing Journal 2010;13.

16. New Zealand Ministry of Health. Recommendations to improve quality and the management of quality in emergency departments. Wellington: New Zealand Ministry of Health, 2008.

17. NSW Health. Emergency Department Workforce Analysis Tool. Sydney: NSW Health, 2010.

18. Cameron P, Jelinek G, Kelly A, Murray L, Brown AF. Textbook of adult emergency medicine, 3rd edn, Sydney: Churchill Livingstone Elsevier, 2009.

19. Fry M, Rogers T. The transitional emergency nurse practitioner role: Implementation study and preliminary evaluation. Australasian Emergency Nursing Journal 2009;12:32–7.

20. Fry M, Jones K. The clinical initiative nurse: extending the role of the emergency nurse, who benefits? Australian Emergency Nursing Journal 2005;8:9–12.

21. Fry M, Ruperto K, Jarrett K, Wheeler J, Fong J, Fetchet W. Managing the wait: clinical initiative nurses' perceptions of an extended practice role. Australasian Emergency Nursing Journal 2013;15:202–10.

22. Fry M, McGregor C, Ruperto K et al. Nursing Praxis, Compassionate caring and Interpersonal Relations: an observational study. Australasian Emergency Nursing Journal 2013;16:37–44.

23. Nugus P, Holdgate A, Fry M, Ferero R et al. Work pressure and patient flow management in the emergency department: Findings from an ethnographic study. Academic Emergency Medicine 2011;18:1045–52.

24. Nugus P, Braithwaite J. The dynamic interaction of quality and efficiency in the emergency department: Squaring the circle? Social Science & Medicine 2010;70:511–17.

25. Nugus P, Greenfield D, Travaglia J et al. How and where clinicians exercise power: Interprofessional relations in health care. Social Science & Medicine 2010;71:898–909.

26. The Australian Council on Healthcare Standards (ACHS). Risk management and quality improvement handbook. Sydney: ACHS, 2013.

27. Fry M, Horvat L, Roche M et al. A four month prospective descriptive exploratory pilot study of patients receiving antibiotics in one emergency department. International Emergency Nursing 2013;21:163–7.

28. COAG Reform Council. National Partnership Agreement on Hospital and Health Workforce Reform. Canberra: Council of Australian Governments (COAG), 2012.

29. Douglas K. New Models of Primary Care—The evidence. In: APHCRI, ed. Canberra: Australian National University 2008.

30. Kelaher M, Dunt D, Feldman P. Effects of financial disadvantage on use and non-use of afterhours care in Australia. Health Policy 2006;79:16–23.

31. Gafforini S, Carson N. Primary-care type presentations to public hospitals. In: Health Do, ed. Victoria: Victoria Government, 2013.

32. Dale J, Williams S, Crouch R, Patel A. A study of out-of-hours telephone advice from an A&E department. British Journal of Nursing 1997;6:171–4.

33. Darnell JC, Hiner SL, Neill PJ et al. After-hours telephone access to physicians with access to computerized medical records. Experience in an inner-city general medicine clinic. Medical Care 1985;23:20–6.

34. Fatovich D, Jacobs I. Emergency department telephone advice: a survey of Australian emergency departments. Emergency Medicine 1998;10:117–21.

35. Fry M. Barriers and facilitators for successful after hours care model implementation: Reducing Emergency Department utilisation. Australasian Emergency Nursing Journal 2009;12:137–44.

36. Parker RLF, Desborough J, McRae I, Boyland T. Independent evaluation of the nurse-led ACT Health Walk in Centre. Canberra: Australian National University, 2011.

37. Ward P, Huddy J, Hargreaves S et al. Primary care in London: an evaluation of general practitioners working in an inner city accident and emergency department. Journal of Accident & Emergency Medicine 1996;13:11–15.

38. Dale J, Green J, Reid F et al. Primary care in the accident and emergency department: II. Comparison of general practitioners and hospital doctors. British Medical Journal 1995;311:427–30.

39. Murphy AW, Bury G, Plunkett PK et al. Randomised controlled trial of general practitioner versus usual medical care in an urban accident and emergency department: process, outcome, and comparative cost. British Medical Journal 1996;312:1135–42.

40. Hargreaves J, Grayson N, Titulaer I. Trends in hospital service provision. Australian Health Review 2002;25:2–18.

41. Mason S, Knowles E, Colwell B et al. Effectiveness of paramedic practitioners in attending 999 calls from elderly people in the community: cluster randomised controlled trial. British Medical Journal 2007;335:919.

42. Snooks H, Kearsley N, Dale J et al. Towards primary care for non-serious 999 callers: results of a controlled study of 'Treat and Refer' protocols for ambulance crews. Quality & Safety in Health Care 2004;13:435–43.

43. Snooks H, Foster T, Nicholl J. Results of an evaluation of the effectiveness of triage and direct transportation to minor injuries units by ambulance crews. Emergency Medicine Journal 2004;21:105–11.

44. Fry M. A systematic review of the impact of afterhours care models on emergency departments, ambulance and general practice services. Australasian Emergency Nursing Journal 2011;14:217–25.

45. Bryant M, Tan G. Seeing primary care patients in emergency departments. Emergency Medicine 1998;10:111–16.

46. CENA. Practice Standards for the Emergency Nursing Specialist. Sydney, 2013;1–20.

47. ANMC. National Competency Standards for the Enrolled Nurse. Canberra: Australian Nursing Midwifery Council, 2002.

48. ANMC. ANMC National Competency Standards for the Registered Nurse. 4th ed. Canberra: ANMC 2006:1–6.

49. ANMC. National Competency Standards for the Nurse Practitioner. Canberra: Australian Nursing Midwifery Council, 2006:1–6.

50. Nursing Council of New Zealand. Competencies for Registered Nurses. New Zealand: Nursing Council of New Zealand, 2007.

51. Nursing Council of New Zealand. Competencies for the Nurse Practitioner Scope of Practice. New Zealand; 2009.

52. Royal College of Nursing. History of the Royal College of Nursing and Emergency Nursing Association. Online. www.icn.ch/echistoryRCN.htm. United Kingdom: RCN, 2004;1–6.

53. CENA. Position Statement Definition of an Emergency Service. Sydney: College of Emergency Nursing Australasia Ltd, 2009.

54. Russell L, Gething L, Convery P. National review of specialist nurse education. Sydney: University of Sydney, 1997.

55. Whyte S. The specialist nurse: a classification system. Contemporary Nurse 2000;9:6–15.

56. Whyte S. Specialist nurses in Australia: the ICN and international regulation. Journal of Professional Nursing 2000;16:210–18.

57. Fry M, Stainton C. An educational framework for triage nursing based on gatekeeping, timekeeping and decision-making processes. Accident and Emergency Nursing 2005;13:214–19.

58. Benkert R, Tanner C, Guthrie B et al. Cultural competence of nurse practitioner students: A consortium's experience. Journal of Nursing Education 2005;44.

59. Taveras EM, Flores G. Why culture and language matter: the clinical consequences of providing culturally and linguistically appropriate services to children in the emergency department. Clinical Pediatric Emergency Medicine 2004;5:76–84.

60. Fry M. An ethnography: Understanding emergency nursing practice belief systems. International Emergency Nursing 2012;20:120–5.

61. Sbaih L. Meanings of immediate: the practical use of the Patients Charter in the accident and emergency department. Social Science & Medicine 2002;54:1345–55.

62. van der Geest S, Finkler K. Hospital ethnography: introduction. Social Science & Medicine 2004;59:1995–2001.

63. Pratt R. The challenge of specialisation: the Australian experience. Collegian: Journal of the Royal College of Nursing 1994;1:6–13.

64. Duffield C, Gardner G, Chang A, Catling-Paull C. Advanced practice nursing: a global perspective. Collegian 2009;16:55–62.

65. Fry M, Ryan J, Alexander N. A prospective study of nurse initiated Panadeine Forte: expanding pain management in the ED. Accident & Emergency Nursing 2004;12:136–40.

66. Fry M, Holdgate A. Nurse initiated intravenous morphine in the emergency department: efficacy, rate of adverse events and impact on time to analgesia. Emergency Medicine 2002;14:249–54.

67. Wilson A, Zwart E, Everett I, Kernick J. The clinical effectiveness of nurse practitioners' management of minor injuries in an adult emergency department: a systematic review. International Journal of Evidence-Based Healthcare 2009;7:3–14.

68. Watts SA, Gee J, O'Day ME et al. Nurse practitioner-led multidisciplinary teams to improve chronic illness care: the unique strengths of nurse practitioners applied to shared medical appointments/group visits. Journal of the American Academy of Nurse Practitioners 2009;21:167–72.

69. Nursing and Midwifery Board of Australia. Nursing and Midwifery Board of Australia Registration Standard for Endorsement of Nurse Practitioners. Sydney: Nursing and Midwifery Board of Australia, 2010.

70. The US Census Bureau. Facts for Features. April 29, 2005 Washington: USA Government, 2005.

71. Nursing and Midwifery Board of Australia. Nurse and Midwifery Registration Data: October 2013. Sydney: Nursing and Midwifery Board of Australia, 2013.

72. Nursing Council of New Zealand. The New Zealand nursing workforce. Wellington: The Nursing Council of New Zealand, 2011.

73. Fry M. Literature review of the impact of nurse practitioners in critical care services. Nursing in Critical Care 2011;16:58–66.

74. Fry M, Fong J, Asha S, Arendts G. A 12-month evaluation of the impact of transitional emergency nurse practitioners in one metropolitan emergency department. Australasian Emergency Nursing Journal 2011;14:4–8.

75. Luttze M, Ratchford A, Fry M. A review of the transitional emergency nurse practitioner. Australasian Emergency Nursing Journal 2011;14:226–31.

76. Sakr M, Kendall R, Angus J et al. Emergency nurse practitioners: a three part study in clinical and cost effectiveness. Emergency Medicine Journal 2003;20:158–63.

77. Chang EM, Daly J, Hancock KM et al. The relationships among workplace stressors, coping methods, demographic characteristics, and health in Australian nurses. Journal of Professional Nursing 2006;22:30–8.

78. Ball S, Walton K, Hawes S. Do emergency department physiotherapy practitioner's [sic], emergency nurse practitioners and doctors investigate, treat and refer patients with closed musculoskeletal injuries differently? Emergency Medicine Journal 2007;24:185–8.

79. Thrasher C, Purc-Stephenson R. Patient satisfaction with nurse practitioner care in emergency departments in Canada. Journal of the American Academy of Nurse Practitioners 2008;20:231–7.

80. Thrasher C, Purc-Stephenson R. Integrating nurse practitioners into Canadian emergency departments: a qualitative study of barriers and recommendations. CJEM: Journal of the Canadian Association of Emergency Physicians 2007;9:275.

81. Drummond AM. Nurse practitioners in Canadian emergency departments: An idea worthy of attention or diverting our attention? CJEM: Journal of the Canadian Association of Emergency Physicians 2007;9:297.

82. Considine J, Martin R, Smit D et al. Emergency nurse practitioner care and emergency department patient flow: case-control study. Emergency Medicine Australasia 2006;18:385–90.

83. Rogers T, Ross N, Spooner D. Evaluation of a 'see and treat' pilot study introduced to an emergency department. Accident and Emergency Nursing 2004;12:24–7.

84. Bunn F, Byrne G, Kendall S. Telephone consultation and triage: effects on health care use and patient satisfaction. Cochrane Effective Practice and Organisation of Care Group, The Cochrane Collaboration: John Wiley & Sons, Ltd, 2009.

85. Laurant M, Reeves D, Hermens R et al. Substitution of doctors by nurses in primary care: A systematic review Cochrane Database of Systematic Reviews 2008.

86. Martin-Misener R, Downe-Wamboldt B, Cain E, Girouard M. Cost effectiveness and outcomes of a nurse practitioner-paramedic-family physician model of care: the Long and Brier Islands study. Primary Health Care Research & Development 2009;10:14.

87. Sylvia ML, Griswold M, Dunbar L et al. Guided care: cost and utilization outcomes in a pilot study. Disease Management 2008;11:29–36.

88. Chenoweth D, Martin N, Pankowski J, Raymond LW. Nurse practitioner services: three-year impact on health care costs. Journal of Occupational & Environmental Medicine 2008;50:1293–8.

89. Duffield C, O'Brien-Pallas L. The nursing workforce in Canada and Australia: two sides of the same coin. Australian Health Review 2002;25:136–44.

90. Duffield C, Pelletier D, Donoghue J. A profile of the clinical nurse specialist in one Australian state. Clinical Nurse Specialist 1995;9:149–54.

91. Glover D, Newkirk L, Cole L et al. Perioperative clinical nurse specialist role delineation: a systematic review. AORN Journal 2006;84:1017–30.

92. Kane-Urrabazo C. Management's role in shaping organizational culture. Journal of Nursing Management 2006;14:188–94.

93. Sellengren S, Ekvall G, Tomson G: Leadership styles in nursing management: preferred and perceived. Journal of Nursing Management 2006;14:348–55.

94. Richardson D, Mountain D. Myths versus facts in emergency department overcrowding and hospital access block. Medical Journal of Australia 2009;190:369–74.

95. Fatovich D, Hughes G, McCarthy S. Access block: it's all about available beds. Medical Journal of Australia 2009;190:362–3.

96. ACEM. Access block and overcrowding in emergency departments. Melbourne: Australasian College for Emergency Medicine, 2004; 1–17.

97. Sprivulis P, Da Silva J, Jacobs I et al. The association between hospital overcrowding and mortality among patients admitted via Western Australian emergency departments. MJA 2006;184:208–12.

98. Richardson D. The access block effect. Medical Journal of Australia 2002;177:492–95.

99. Cameron P. Hospital overcrowding a threat to patient safety? Medical Journal of Australia 2006;184:203–4.

100. NSW Health. Sustainable Access Plan 2004. Sydney: NSW Health Department, 2004.

101. Australian Institute of Health and Welfare. Australian Hospital Statistics 2009–2010. Canberra: AIHW, 2010.

102. Burritt J, Steckle C. Supporting the learning for contemporary nursing practice. Journal Nursing Administration 2009;39:479–84.

103. NHS Modernisation Agency. See and treat. London, 2002.

104. Australian Institute of Health and Welfare. Australia's welfare in 2013 brief. Canberra: Australian Government, 2013.

105. Fairweather C, Gardner G. Specialist nurse: an investigation of common and distinct aspects of practice. Collegian: Journal of the Royal College of Nursing 2000;7:26–33.

106. Gallagher R, Fry M, Duffield C. Nursing: The future in Australia. Contemporary Nurse Journal 2010;36:118–20.

107. Duffield C, Conlon L, Kelly M et al. The emergency department nursing workforce: local solutions for local issues. International Emergency Nursing 2010;18:181–7.

108. Duffield C, Roche M, O'Brien-Pallas L et al. Nursing workload and staffing: Impact on patients and staff. University of Technology, Sydney, 2009.

CHAPTER 2

PRE-HOSPITAL CARE OVERVIEW IN AUSTRALIA AND NEW ZEALAND—PAST, PRESENT AND FUTURE

ANTHONY WEBER AND JAMES McMANUS

Essentials

- The history of organised ambulance services in Australia and New Zealand can be traced back to the late 1800s and the early 1900s. Often these services were of a basic nature, much within the acceptable community standards of the times.
- There were a number of influences that were common in the development of the ambulance services. First-aiders trained by St John Ambulance were often the providers of ambulance services, but—depending upon their location—ambulance services were also provided by hospitals, police, industry groups, government instrumentalities and in some cases commercial operators.
- Initial ambulance services often focused on the means of transport from the scene, rather than treatment at the scene. Over time the mode of transport changed from human-powered Ashford litters to horse-drawn wagons, then progressed to mechanical means of transport on the land and through the air.
- In the late 1960s and early 1970s, a change in the focus of ambulance services occurred as a result of parallel developments in the way the sick and injured were treated before they arrived at hospitals.
- Advances in the care of cardiac and road trauma patients led to the development of the emergency medical services that seem so commonplace today, but were viewed as revolutionary at their inception.

INTRODUCTION

Past

Should you have had the misfortune to be seriously injured around the year 1900, your chances of survival would have been problematic. This was especially true if the type of incident you were involved in required transport to a medical facility for definitive care. You were at the mercy of ambulance services which were part of a fledgling industry. Most of the ambulances services that exist today have long and varied histories. Many have their foundations in the late 1800s and were set up by enthusiastic groups of community-minded people who had an interest in first aid. St John Ambulance was an influential factor in their formation, as they were the providers of the first-aid training for many of the members of these newly created ambulance services.

The increasing number of people with first-aid qualifications who were looking for an opportunity to maintain and utilise their newly acquired skills led to the formation of many St John Ambulance brigades that catered for the treatment and sometimes transport of the sick and injured. However, not all ambulance services in Australia owe their origin to St John Ambulance; there were also a number of community-based groups, government bodies, hospitals and private individuals who initially provided this important function.

In their earliest days, the main role of ambulance services was to facilitate the transport of the sick and injured to hospital. The standard of care for the treatment of these patients was, realistically, at the level of basic first aid when compared with the treatment that is routinely given today. Medical care was within the province of doctors, who, ably assisted by nurses, provided much of the care for the sick or injured when they were admitted to hospital.

Many of the advances that occurred during the early history of ambulance services related to the modes of transport that were available to facilitate the safe arrival of a patient to a hospital. The earliest mode of transport used in Australia and New Zealand was the 'Ashford litter', which could be best described as a stretcher on detachable cart wheels with retractable supporting legs (Fig 2.1). This litter owes its origin to Sir John Furley, one of the founders of the St John Ambulance organisation. His design was patented in 1875 and was known as the 'St John ambulance'. However, the concept of having a system that involved the quick retrieval and transport of the injured can be traced back to Dr Dominique Jean Larrey, a military surgeon in Napoleon's army. In 1792, he developed a system that ensured the treatment and retrieval of injured soldiers from the battle area who were then quickly conveyed to field hospitals where they were treated by military surgeons. The system required the use of lightweight horse-drawn sprung carriages that entered the battlefield and swiftly removed the wounded, taking them to a designated location set up to treat the injured, often situated behind the battle front. These carts were

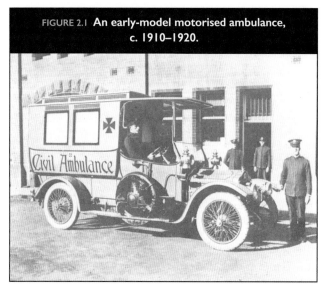

FIGURE 2.1 **An early-model motorised ambulance, c. 1910–1920.**

Courtesy of NSW Ambulance.

called 'flying volantes' and later became known as 'flying ambulances'.[1] Larrey's approach is, in essence, the principle upon which modern-day trauma systems are founded.

Much of the available early history of ambulance services concentrates on the details of advances made in the modes of transport provided by these organisations, as opposed to the care that was provided by them. Over time the Ashford litter was replaced by horse-drawn vans, wagons or carts, but not before the litter was adapted to enable it to become bicycle-powered. The Ashford litter was certainly an improvement on a stretcher carried by two stretcher-bearers, although ultimately its successful utilisation was determined by the patient's proximity to the hospital and by the state of the roads and pathways upon which it was to be deployed.

As motor vehicles became increasingly popular and more affordable, their potential for use in ambulance services was obvious. They were able to transport patients to hospital more quickly and from greater distances and, on occasions, in greater numbers. Initially, trucks, upon whose flat tray the sick and injured were placed, were used by some services, while other services utilised 'fitted out' motorised vans equipped with stretchers. Eventually special vehicles were commissioned by ambulance services and built by coach and body builders on a truck chassis. Much later, passenger vehicles and station wagons were modified to satisfy the unique requirements of ambulance vehicles, thus significantly reducing the cost of new purchases (only modifications were required instead of complete new designs being developed) as demands for service increased and old-model ambulances in fleets that had exceeded their 'use-by' date were replaced.

Over time, ambulances became more specialised, and at times unique vehicles were developed by some ambulance services to meet the specific needs and diverse circumstances of the communities that they served. Converted over-snow vehicles, along with skidoos, have been used in the Australian Alps.[2] During the 1918–19 Spanish flu epidemic and during wartime, tram carriages[3] were transformed into multi-patient modes of transport to move patients to either infectious disease centres or military hospitals. In the Australian outback, motorised rail trikes have been used to transport patients between outlying towns and regional centres.[4] Boats have been adapted to be used in aquatic environments.[5] Planes and helicopters have made a significant contribution to the ability to quickly transport critically ill or seriously injured patients, and this is covered in slightly more detail later on in this chapter.

It is easy to see why the modern-day paramedic was often referred to as an 'ambulance driver' in much earlier days. Staff, either employed or volunteers, who had mechanical ability were highly regarded by ambulance managers. A first-aid certificate was often the only medically related qualification that was needed to become an ambulance driver, the precursor of the modern day paramedic.[6] In some ambulance jurisdictions it was not even necessary for staff to hold a first-aid certificate; conversely, other ambulance service providers required their staff to hold a first-aid medallion.

Historical overview of ambulance service development, by jurisdiction

New South Wales[7]

New South Wales has the earliest recorded/documented ambulance service in Australia dating back to 1881 when the Board of Health, in response to a smallpox epidemic, organised a transport service to a hospital for infectious diseases for patients located on the outskirts of the Sydney urban area. While a number of hospitals developed their own ambulance services, there were also localised, community-based and industrially orientated groups that provided ambulance transport services.[8] One of the largest and best organised of these groups was the Civil Ambulance and Transport Brigade (CATB). It commenced in 1895 and is generally regarded as the original ambulance group from which the present day Ambulance Service of New South Wales developed.

The St John Ambulance Organisation also played a part in the original development of ambulance services in the state. While its main role at this time was to provide first-aid instruction, it did fund the provision of an Ashford litter that could be used to transport the sick and injured. By 1900 St John's had provided 14 such litters, which were strategically positioned around the city of Sydney.

In the early part of the 20th century, the CATB became the Civil Ambulance and Transport Corps (CATC) under the auspices of the St John Ambulance organisation. A number of other ambulance services also existed during these times, and rivalry between the CATC and other suburban services led to the government of the day enacting legislation to create the Ambulance Transport Service Board via the *Ambulance Services Act 1919*. In 1925 the Central District Ambulance Service (CDAS), based in the Sydney region, was formed. In the years that followed, ambulance services in regional areas paralleled the manner of service delivery initiated by CDAS. In 1972 all these services were united together when the Ambulance Service Act came into being. This Act created a statewide ambulance service with a common administrative framework, known as the New South Wales Ambulance Service. Later its name was changed to the Ambulance Service of New South Wales. To this day, it remains under the control of the state's Department of Health.

Victoria[7]

The first ambulance service in Victoria commenced in 1896 when the St John Ambulance Centre placed an Ashford litter at the Eastern Hill Fire Station, Melbourne's main fire station, where it was staffed by trained assistants. It is from this single event that Victoria's state ambulance service grew. Initially the fire brigade provided the service for free, but as demand increased their board sought recompense for the service. Government grants initially assisted the financing of this vital service, but in 1902 the Chief Secretary refused requests for further grants, declaring that police would provide the service using hansom cabs (horse-drawn taxis) and Ashford litters.[9]

Ambulance services continued to be provided, and became increasingly expensive as the method of transport changed from human- and horse-powered transportation to that provided by automobiles. In 1916, the Victorian Civil Ambulance Service (VCAS) was formed. Although legally separate from the St John Ambulance Organisation, there was a high degree of cross-membership between these two organisations. Over time the VCAS became the main provider of ambulance services in Melbourne and its surrounds. In 1922 a 'country division' was formed to service and support the development of ambulance services in rural and regional areas. This 'country division' was a loose alliance/amalgamation of rural and regional ambulance services and continued until the Victorian Hospital and Charities Commission established regional ambulance boards in 1955, making the 'country division' redundant. The VCAS continued until 1973 when the state government restructured ambulance services and created an entity called Ambulance Service Victoria. In 1986, the *Ambulance Service Act* established the Metropolitan Ambulance Service (MAS) and Rural Ambulance Victoria (RAV); RAV was further divided into further administrative and operational regions. In July 2008, MAS, RAV and the Alexandra and District Ambulance Service were amalgamated to form Ambulance Victoria, thus creating a single ambulance service for the entire state.[10]

Queensland[7]

The Queensland Ambulance Transport Brigade (QATB) came into existence in 1902. This organisation has its origins in the City Ambulance Transport Brigade, which was established in 1892. Many of the members of this Brisbane-based group had a strong affiliation with the St John Ambulance Organisation, having gained their first-aid qualification from them. Over time the QATB prospered and enjoyed a great deal of community support, allowing them to extend their operations to other metropolitan locations and regional centres.

In 1916 the QATB took over the St John Ambulance Queensland Centre and became the agent for the Order of St John in Queensland. This resulted in a virtual monopoly right to provide transport services to the sick and injured being given to the QATB. Ambulance services continued to develop as a result of community endeavour and these brigades were very parochial in nature, with the fund-raising activities that supported their services forming part of the social fabric of many communities.[11]

From the time QATB was established until 1967, ambulance services came under the *Hospitals Acts* of 1923 and 1944. The *Ambulance Services Act 1967* provided a separate legislative framework for ambulance services, and specified that local area committees were to be formed and a State Council established as the regulatory body of QATB.

At the time of the creation of the Queensland Ambulance Brigade in 1991 there were 96 brigades. The level of training and equipment available to each brigade differed according to each local committee's fund-raising acumen and the economic conditions of the time. It was once stated that 'when there were 96 brigades the only thing in common was the colour of the shirts'.[12] These brigades amalgamated into a single organisation under the name of the Queensland Ambulance Service.

Western Australia[7]

In 1903 the Perth metropolitan fire brigade began an ambulance service using a horse-drawn van. In the same year the police acquired an Ashford litter. In the following years, ambulance services spread to industrial workplaces as Ashford litters were located at wharves, railway workshops and railway stations. By 1910 all the major railway stations in Perth had an Ashford litter located in their near vicinity. Four Perth municipalities also had their own horse-drawn ambulance services.

As a result of the increasing workload associated with providing ambulance services, the fire brigade decided to concentrate on activities associated with fire-fighting and reduce their involvement in the provision of non-core business. In 1922 St John Ambulance took over formal control of the Perth metropolitan ambulance service, later expanding its activities throughout the state. A second metropolitan ambulance centre was established at Fremantle in 1929. During the 1930s approximately 50 ambulance centres were established throughout the state; by 1970 the number of ambulance locations had risen to 96 and by the late 1980s there were 17 metropolitan ambulance depots and 105 locations outside the metropolitan area. Some ambulance services in remote locations chose to remain outside the St John umbrella, but these were few in number.[13]

South Australia[7]

The early history of ambulance services in South Australia does not appear to be well documented. Up until the early 1950s there was no unified system, as had developed in the other Australian states; rather, there was a 'haphazard series of small, independent and uncoordinated services in the capital city, Adelaide, as well as in the State's other cities and regional centres'.[13]

In 1951, the state government outsourced ambulance services to the St John Council for South Australia Inc. Prior to this government initiative, metropolitan Adelaide was serviced by a collection of organisations. They were South Australia Ambulance Transport Inc (previously Hindmarsh Volunteer Ambulance), Northern Suburbs Ambulance Association, the Civil Ambulance run by the police department and Joe Myren's Private Ambulance. St John Ambulance amalgamated these services, and over the next few decades developed regional and rural services to such a degree that by the 1970s South Australia had a state-wide service similar to those existing in most other states of Australia.[14]

The *Ambulance Service Act 1992* legislated responsibility for ambulance services to a joint venture between the Minister of Health and the Priory in Australia of the Grand Priory of the Most Venerable Order of the Hospital of St John of Jerusalem. In 2005 it became known as the South Australian Ambulance Service (SAAS), and in 2008 SAAS officially became part of South Australia Health.[15]

Tasmania[7]

Tasmania's first ambulance service commenced in Launceston in 1915 when the proprietor of the local livery stable had a horse-drawn ambulance van built. In 1922 the responsibility for this service was transferred to the local municipal authority, which engaged the fire brigade to operate the service. During this time, Hobart City Council had also established an ambulance service to serve that city.

By the 1950s there were 13 regional and local boards operating a total of 33 ambulance vehicles. Each board acted independently of the others with little or no coordination between any of the providers. This lack of coordination,

along with differing standards of training and equipment and widespread community dissatisfaction, finally led to the state government establishing an Ambulance Commission whose role was to oversee all these services.

The state's Minister for Health persuaded the St John Council for Tasmania, based in Hobart, to take control of ambulance services. Within two years, St John provided ambulance coverage to about two-thirds of the state's area, along with services to most cities and main towns. A number of issues affected St John's ability to provide their planned service, and in 1965 they announced that St John would withdraw from the provision of ambulance services. An external consultation reviewed the state's ambulance service and it was recommended that the government should take direct control of ambulance services. Thus the Tasmanian Ambulance Service came into being.

Australian Capital Territory (ACT)[7]

Canberra has had an ambulance service since about 1915 when construction on the nation's capital began. In 1925 the Federal Capital Commission (FCC), whose role was to manage the development of the capital territory, was established. One of its functions was the provision of an ambulance service.

By 1930 the FCC had been abolished and the local fire brigade organised the service that was to be known as the Canberra Fire and Ambulance Service. In 1955 the Canberra Ambulance Service came into existence under the control of the Commonwealth's Department of Interior. It soon changed its name to the ACT Ambulance Service. In the next year, control of the service was handed to the board of the Canberra Community Hospital. In 1989 the ACT became self-governing and the service was brought under the control of the ACT Emergency Services Authority.[16]

Northern Territory[7]

Ambulance services in the Northern Territory were initially provided and run by the local hospitals in its two main towns, Darwin and Alice Springs. The first motorised ambulance commenced in 1929, and continued for some time. In the early 1950s, 'after hours' St John Ambulance provided ambulance services.

The outstanding assistance that St John's Ambulance service was able to provide during Cyclone Tracy (in 1974) and its aftermath became a catalyst to draw together the various Public Health Department ambulances service in an effort to provide a unified service throughout the territory. In 1977 the territory government passed control of the ambulance services to the St John Ambulance Council of the Northern Territory, who proceeded to develop a territory-wide service that today encompasses all the main cities and towns of the territory.[17]

New Zealand[18–20]

There are predominantly four providers of ambulance services in New Zealand: St John Ambulance, Wellington Free Ambulance, and the Taranaki and Wairarapa District Health Boards. St John Ambulance is responsible for ambulance services that cover just over 85% of the nation's land mass. The establishment of St John in New Zealand was first mooted during a public meeting in Christchurch in 1885. By 1889 Christchurch had four Ashford litters based at police and fire stations. This was considerably better than what the people of Auckland had—in 1892 St John reported that the equipment there consisted of a stretcher and a set of bandages, but fortunately by 1903 their fleet had expanded to nine litters. In the same year, the city of Dunedin formed the first division of the St John Ambulance Brigade and begam to provide first-aid services.

St John rapidly established itself throughout New Zealand, proving especially popular in localities where medical services were few and far between and where the local industry was labour-intensive. In 1975 the government of the day revamped the Ambulance Transport Advisory Board, causing St John to review their ambulance service activities. Staff were encouraged to obtain and eventually required to hold formal qualifications. The days of patients being tended to by ambulance personnel who held a basic first-aid certificate were over.[21]

Since 1927, the people of Wellington and its surrounds have been the beneficiaries of free ambulance transport from the Wellington Free Ambulance, an organisation that claims to be the only free ambulance service operating in the southern hemisphere. What started as a single ambulance has grown into a fleet of 24 emergency and 12 patient transport vehicles, operating out of nine ambulance stations covering just over 10% of the population of New Zealand.

The latter-day pioneers of modern pre-hospital care

Peter J Safar MD (1924–2003)[22] made a significant contribution to the development of pre-hospital emergency care throughout the world. He is known as the 'father of CPR' (cardiopulmonary resuscitation) and is credited with identifying the Airway and Breathing elements of the ABC of resuscitation. Some of his notable achievements were: the establishment of the first intensive-care unit in a hospital in the USA; assisting in the development of the first advanced life support (ALS) ambulances; and assisting in the development of the 'Resusci Anne' manikin. Most important, however, was his role in the modern history of emergency medical services—he organised one of the first, if not the first, pre-hospital emergency medical services in the USA.

In 1967, Freedom House Enterprises commenced a paramedics service in Pittsburg, Pennsylvania. It was a welfare project with a two-fold purpose: it was to provide an ambulance service to an impoverished area, and also provide employment and training to unemployed members of a minority group. This project led to a partnership between Dr Safar and Freedom House Enterprises, an outreach of the United Negro Protest Committee. The 'Freedom House Ambulance Service' trainee paramedics were African-American men and women drawn from the ranks of Pittsburg's unemployed.[23,24] The resultant ambulance service provided the most sophisticated emergency care to one of the most disadvantaged groups of people in the USA.

In 1974 Dr Safar appointed Nancy Caroline (1944–2002)[25] as medical director of Freedom House Ambulance Service. She was to become a major author of textbooks for paramedics. Her initial textbook was to be the first, and for many years the only, textbook specifically written for paramedics. It is now in its sixth edition. The 1975 report she prepared for the federal government played a significant role in the development of

the first national paramedic training course. To many she is affectionately known as the 'mother of paramedics'.[26]

In early 1966, in Belfast, Northern Ireland, Frank Pantridge MD (1916–2004), who has sometimes been called the 'grandfather of pre-hospital ALS', set up a mobile intensive-care unit to assist in the management of patients with myocardial infarction. He recognised that in cases of cardiac arrest due to ventricular fibrillation, the defibrillator needed to be brought to the patient rather than the patient brought to the defibrillator (located at the hospital).[27] No portable defibrillators existed at this time, but Pantridge utilised some technology developed by the NASA space program to develop a lightweight, portable defibrillator capable of being carried to the scene of a cardiac arrest by paramedics and thus sufficiently small to be able to be transported in an ambulance.[28] His groundbreaking program confirmed that it was possible to correct cardiac arrest that occurred outside hospitals. As a result of this work, similar programs in many centres were set up throughout the developed world over the next decade.

In 1971, Victoria commenced Mobile Intensive Care Ambulance (MICA). This was the first MICA system in Australia and the third in the world after Belfast, Northern Ireland and Seattle, Washington. Initially a paramedic and a medical registrar staffed the MICA vehicle, but by 1973 the medical officer was replaced by another suitably trained paramedic, making it a 'paramedic only' response.[29]

By the very late 1960s and early 1970s, paramedic programs either had begun planning for their implementation or had commenced in a number of locations. Most notably were the centres of Miami, Florida under the guidance of Eugene Nagel MD; Seattle, Washington overseen by Leonard Cobb MD; Los Angeles, California with medical director Ron Stewart MD; Portland, Oregon; and Nassau County, New York. There were two major influences on the development of such paramedic programs. The work of Pantridge in Northern Ireland inspired a number of cardiologists to become advocates for the advanced treatment of myocardial infarction and cardiac arrest outside the hospital setting. This was to occur in multiple locations throughout the world in the decade following Pantridge's initial research and successful implementation of a coronary care program. Similarly, another quiet revolution occurring in pre-hospital treatment related to the care of the trauma patient. At about the same time Pantridge was implementing pre-hospital coronary care in Belfast, US legislators were enacting laws to improve patient outcomes from automobile trauma. The *National Highway and Safety and Traffic Act 1966* funded the development of a national curriculum for pre-hospital personnel as well as distributing funds to improve emergency medical services in the USA.[30] Importantly, the national curriculum that was developed included CPR instruction. This, considered with the fact that US servicemen injured in Vietnam could be evacuated, on average, in 35 minutes from time of injury and be in surgery within 1–2 hours with an overall mortality rate of just 2.3%[31] added impetus to the call for improvements in pre-hospital trauma care. The stage was now set. The treatment of both trauma and coronary care patients was to become the domain of the modern-day paramedic.

The ALS program that had commenced in Los Angeles became the basis for the TV series *Emergency!* that ran from

1972 to 1977 in the USA and was subsequently syndicated throughout the world. It was inspired by a TV producer who, while scouting a location for a new TV show, heard firefighters who spoke like doctors on a visit to a hospital's emergency department (ED). These firefighters were in fact paramedics in the new ALS program. A seed was planted for a new TV show centred around the exploits of two fictitious fire-fighters, Roy de Soto and John Gage, who worked out of 'Squad 51' in the Los Angeles County Fire Department. The interactions with their patients and the ED staff of the fictional Rampart General Hospital provided the dramatic setting for the new weekly show.[32] The show increased the general public's awareness of the role of a paramedic and by 1975, 46 of the US's 50 states had paramedic programs operating.[30] The technical advisor to the series was, in real life, a fire chief named James O Page (1936–2004).[33] He ensured that artistic licence did not take precedence over authenticity when technical aspects of the paramedic role were part of the storyline. Page was later to become the founder of the widely read *Journal of Emergency Medical Services*.

Air ambulance services

In nations that are either as sparsely populated as Australia or as challenged by its unique topography and weather as New Zealand, it is easy to see why the provision of an aerial ambulance would have become part of the wider provision of ambulance services.

Australia

Australia owes its rich tradition of air ambulance services to the Reverend John Flynn, a member of the clergy. In 1928, he organised an air ambulance service as a year-long trial, based at Cloncurry in Central Queensland. The service proved so successful that it was adopted throughout rural and remote Australia. Within the next decade, operations had extended to Victoria, New South Wales, South Australia, the Northern Territory and Western Australia. Currently the Royal Flying Doctor Service (RFDS) provides aircraft, pilots and engineering resources to the ambulance services of New South Wales, Victoria and Tasmania.[34]

Originally called the Aerial Medical Service, Flynn's concept was to provide a 'mantle of safety' to the residents of the outback where your next-door neighbour might be 100 kilometres away. True to its original charter, the RFDS remains a 'not-for-profit' organisation that provides both emergency assistance and primary healthcare for patients unable to readily gain access either to hospitals or to a general practice.

Australia has embraced the use of helicopters as an adjunct for providing quick transport for the trauma patient to the most appropriate hospital as well as for providing an efficient retrieval service for patients already in hospital but requiring more specialised care at a major referral hospital. A number of public and private enterprises conduct these services throughout Australia and New Zealand. In Australia, some are heavily sponsored by business enterprises, such as large banks and insurance companies, as a community service; others are 'for profit' enterprises contracted by state governments or state ambulance authorities to provide commercial helicopter operations.

New Zealand

New Zealand's air ambulance services began later than those in Australia; it is only over the last three decades that there has been a significant increase in the use of aircraft to complement the largely road-based ambulance sector. The clinical crews manning many of these services are provided primarily by the road-based ambulance services. The driving factor in forming many of these services often occurred as a response to a significant local incident. This led to a high degree of community 'ownership' of the services, with local community donors and corporate and grant funders being key stakeholders.

In 2008 there were at least 41 helicopters and 13 fixed-wing aircraft providing ambulance services throughout New Zealand. Eighteen of the 41 helicopters are 'dedicated' emergency helicopters. The term 'dedicated' in this context means that the aircraft is solely available for ambulance and other emergency response work.[35] These services are operated by a combination of charitable trusts and private companies located throughout the country. Almost 60% of the revenue for emergency helicopters comes from sponsorships, grants and donations. The Crown, along with District Health Boards and the Accident Compensation Commission, provide another 34% of revenue. The government recently commissioned a review[35] of emergency helicopter and other air ambulance services. While finding that the system was functional, the review indicated that there was room for improvement and an opportunity for greater efficiencies was evident. It suggested that a degree of rationalisation of services was possible.

Role of the volunteer in ambulance services

Australia is a large country in terms of land mass, yet has a population density of just under three people per square kilometre—one of the lowest concentrations of people to land mass. Its topography is among the lowest, flattest and driest of the continents with its population highly concentrated on the south-eastern sea border. New Zealand, a nation consisting of two main islands, has a much smaller land mass and a population density of approximately 16 people per square kilometre. Its topography is different from Australia's in that mountainous regions predominate, along with some large coastal plains.[36] Due to the large proportion of sparsely populated areas of Australia and New Zealand, both countries have had a rich tradition of volunteerism from their earliest days to the present time, and this has extended to the provision of ambulance services. The Convention of Ambulance Authorities (CAA; collectively Papua New Guinea, New Zealand St John Ambulance service and Australian St John Ambulance services) estimates that volunteers donate 8.4 million hours per year collectively to their member ambulance services.[37]

The story of volunteers within ambulance services in Australia and New Zealand is a story in two parts: the metropolitan and regional areas, and the rural and remote areas. In urban and metropolitan areas up until the last few decades, volunteers have served their communities alongside their salaried counterparts by assisting in the staffing of after-hours services and making themselves available at times of peak demand. In rural and remote areas, the only cost-effective ambulance service that was available was one staffed either predominantly or entirely by volunteers. In these communities, the role of the volunteer paramedic varied. In some locations, it was a community responder role (Fig 2.2), providing care to the patient prior to the arrival of an ambulance from a location further away, while in other communities there were volunteers who had both treatment and transport capability.

In the metropolitan and regional areas today, volunteers have largely been phased out. When volunteers and salaried staff worked together in the same service, there was often tension between the two groups. In the early years, the salaried staff viewed themselves as 'professionals' and looked down on the volunteers as 'amateurs'.[38] During the working week the salaried staff would attend many more cases than the volunteers and the amount of experience gained by doing so amplified their views of their professional standing. They accepted the volunteers as well-meaning 'interlopers'.[38] The volunteers, on the other hand, thought their motivation superior because it was more altruistic than that of the salaried staff. They were working for the good of their fellow man, whereas the paid staff were primarily working for pecuniary considerations. In times of industrial unrest, the permanent staff viewed the volunteers as potential strikebreakers, should there be a dispute with management. The use of the volunteers meant, in the view of the permanent staff, that working conditions, training and the professional status of the permanent staff would be held to a minimum. In a number of ambulance jurisdictions, the continued use of volunteers in large centres led to union activism, which eventually saw the demise of the position of volunteer at these locations.[39]

In regional and rural areas the story differs. Volunteer paramedics provide a vital first link in the provision of emergency care for many of the residents of Australian and New Zealand rural communities. In 2003 there were over 7000 volunteer paramedics who initially responded to a medical emergency in many of these localities.[40] Given that these areas are sparsely populated and have a low workload, it is easy to understand why a full-time service with paid staff is not justified. The goal for ambulance services will always be to recruit, retain and train volunteers that will serve these communities.

Australian researchers[40] have found that the volunteer paramedic is similar to other Australian volunteers in age and sex, although more volunteer paramedics are employed. What made volunteering enjoyable for them was that they liked both the training and the opportunity to maintain their skills. This, plus the fact that they enjoyed helping people and had made friendships within the group, sustained them. The difficulties facing ambulance volunteers were lack of time and the inadequate provision of resources. To satisfy a duty of care to both the volunteer and the community that they serve, there needs to be a commitment to training by the over-riding ambulance services. For the volunteer, the purpose of training is to gain new skills, have these skills assessed and then to maintain these skills. Most volunteer services now use part of the Australian Qualification Training Framework, associated with the National Training Framework, in a structured approach to ensure that consistent standards and assessments occur in vocational education.

Training done well can be a powerful motivator. Conversely, if done poorly it can be a great deterrent to the process of recruiting, engaging and retaining the volunteer. The challenge for ambulance service managers is to provide the resources that allow just the right amount of training in just the right amount of time to keep the volunteer committed to the role of providing ambulance services in their local community. A balance needs to be maintained to ensure that new volunteers are not kept on as 'observers' for prolonged periods (a powerful demotivator); yet, if required to be deployed, still have the requisite skills to be of assistance to the patient. These issues are similar to those that exist in New Zealand, where some 2600 volunteers assist 900 paid paramedics. The New Zealand Ambulance Service Strategy[41] highlights the need for an improvement in the clinical expertise and sustainability of both the paid and the volunteer workforces. This national strategy acknowledges that an important first step to achieving its goals is support for rural volunteer paramedics to ensure that they receive basic emergency medical training. Interestingly, one of its strategies is to investigate alternative service models and also trial the use of volunteers as just ambulance drivers with minimal medical training to complement paramedics.

Present

The task of any discipline in health and medicine, whether it is emergency medicine, general practice, nursing, allied health or paramedicine, is to reduce pain and suffering and restore health. This goal is supported by most ambulance services' mission statements, which identify that the health and wellbeing of the community is achieved through the efficient delivery of high-quality pre-hospital patient care and specialised patient transport services. Today most ambulance services represent a long history and culmination of modernisation and upgrading of services provided to the community.

An emergency medical system (EMS) is identified as a comprehensive network that delivers prompt health services to victims of sudden illness or injury with their aim being to deliver the patient to the appropriate facility in the appropriate time.

All around the world healthcare providers are trying to create the best emergency medical systems. Some systems focus on how to deliver the best pre-hospital care. While each country has its own systems and protocols, they all can be placed into

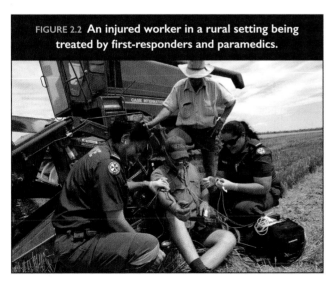

FIGURE 2.2 **An injured worker in a rural setting being treated by first-responders and paramedics.**

Courtesy of NSW Ambulance.

particular categories. With some models of pre-hospital care being the Basic Life Support (BLS) model, Advanced Life Support (ALS) model, and more recently, the emergency care practitioner scheme.[42] However, the most recognised models are the Anglo-American model and the Franco-German models. Many of the models used all over the world today are offshoots of either of these models.[43]

Anglo-American model

The Anglo-American model is widely used by many countries, including the United States, Canada, New Zealand, sultanate of Oman,[42] United Kingdom, Costa Rica, Hong Kong, Iceland, Ireland, Israel, Malaysia, the Netherlands, Nicaragua, the Philippines, Poland, Singapore, South Korea, Taiwan, and Turkey, and according to the Asian Disaster Preparedness Centre it is reportedly growing.[44]

The Anglo-American model is one of a 'Scoop and run' nature.[42] It is based on the simple idea of arriving at the patient and transporting them to hospital for all treatments. As most of the diagnostic treatment is at the hospital's ED, the medical doctors remain there,[44] while the emergency medical tech—nicians or paramedics leave to collect the patient.[44] Because the expectation is for the paramedic to bring the patient back to the ED for treatment, the majority of times the main form of transport used is land ambulance.[42]

As paramedics do not have the qualifications of a doctor they are not classed under a hospital profession, but rather one that delivers fast emergency care and assists public safety. This means they are thought of as being more like police and firefighters.[43] As non-doctors, paramedics are required to make an ED their first port of call due to their apparent inability to diagnose issues. This job is allocated to a hospital ED instead. This model may corporate the BLS method as it also works on the principle of 'load and go'[42]—keeping the patient alive with their basic training until a doctor in an ED can diagnose and offer more specialised and specific care. The interventions usually used in transit include CPR, fracture splinting, full immobilisation and administration of oxygen.[42]

Franco-German model

The Franco-German model does not appear to be as widely used as the Anglo-American model. Some of the countries that use the Franco-German model are Germany, France, Austria, Greece, Malta,[42] Finland, Latvia, Norway, Portugal, Russia, Slovenia, Sweden, and Switzerland.[44]

The Franco-German model works on the principle of 'stay and stabilise',[42] or 'delay and treat'.[42] This model implies its ability to stay on scene longer. This is because essentially it brings the hospital to the patient.[44] As such instead of a basic trained paramedic assisting the patient, the patient would have an ED equivalent doctor come directly to them.[42] Sometimes the doctor would be an anaesthesiologist.[44]

The doctor's attempts to treat on scene can help to cut out the hospital altogether. This removes the need for a hospital ED,[42] as essentially they have a mobile ED in place of an emergency transport system. This also removes the need for a fleet of road ambulances. However, when a patient does need hospitalisation they are directly admitted to the appropriate ward by the attending field doctor.[44] If this happens, the lack of a road ambulance means they need to utilise other modes of transport such as helicopters and the coastal ambulance.[42] This model may be seen to incorporate the advanced life support (ALS) model. It is seen as modelling the 'stay and stabilise' theory.[42] It has ALS-qualified personnel who can perform the same level of care as the BLS personnel and more.[42] On top of Basic Life Support, the ALS team can perform more invasive procedures such as endotracheal intubation, intravenous lines (cannulation), begin fluid replacements and perform chest decompression, as well as have the ability to use many medications.[42]

An example of an EMS mixed model in Australia

In Queensland, paramedics use a mix of the two international models, although the Anglo-American model, 'Scoop and run', is more strongly represented, as the doctor delegates medical care to paramedics.[45]

Paramedics all over Australia, including Queensland, have an extensive fleet of on-road ambulances, which directly transport the patient to an ED for more extensive diagnosis and specialist care, to be delivered by doctors. This is due to the large variety of diagnostic treatments available at the ED.

However, most ambulance services have developed an extended role to deal with medical trauma emergencies. This means that ambulance services, such as the Queensland Ambulance Service, are using some of the features of the Franco-German model. Paramedics have been able to perform more life-saving procedures, such as chest decompression, defibrillation, traction splinting, endotracheal intubation and cannulation (see Tables 2.1 and 2.2). These are all big differences from the traditional Anglo-American model.

Australia's vast rural community, and factors such as severity of injuries and patient location (i.e. rural Queensland), means that more modes of transport must be sought. While road ambulances remain a vital and major form of transport, many instances require fixed-wing aero-medical services such as the Royal Flying Doctor service, state air ambulance, or contracted facilities such as Careflight, or even rotary wing services provided by state- or community-based organisations. These services usually provide a combination of paramedics, nurses and doctors, depending on what is required. This is also reminiscent of the Franco-German system, as doctors are sometimes transported to the patient in severe cases, especially in rural settings.

As the range of clinical interventions utilised by paramedics has expanded in scope, so paramedic education has shifted largely from in-service and vocational education and training (VET) to the university sector, where undergraduate and postgraduate degrees now cater for virtually all Australian and New Zealand ambulance qualifications. Initially the Associate Diploma (AD) was the minimum ambulance qualification. This was then re-accredited as a Diploma of Health Science (Pre-Hospital Care). Advanced Life Support (Intensive Care Paramedic or MICA) programs were also introduced as a VET sector qualification. The minimum qualification expected for all ambulance services is an undergraduate degree, while those wanting to work in higher clinical levels, such as intensive care paramedics, are now required to complete a postgraduate level of education. This approach to educating paramedics in the

TABLE 2.1 Skills, procedures and medication administered by paramedics and intensive-care paramedics in Australia and New Zealand (data from the statutory ambulance services in those countries)[43]

SKILL, PROCEDURE OR MEDICATION	PARAMEDIC		INTENSIVE-CARE PARAMEDIC	
	FEW (3 OR LESS AMBULANCE SERVICES UTILISING)	MOST (4 OR MORE AMBULANCE SERVICES UTILISING)	FEW (3 OR LESS AMBULANCE SERVICES UTILISING)	MOST (4 OR MORE AMBULANCE SERVICES UTILISING)
Intubation	✓			✓
Bougie	Nil			✓
Cricothyroidotomy	✓			✓
CPAP			✓	
Laryngeal mask		✓		✓
Oropharyngeal mask		✓		✓
Nasopharyngeal mask		✓		✓
Defibrillation				
Manual		✓		✓
Semi-auto		✓		✓
Cardioversion	Nil			✓
Fluid administration				
IV cannulation		✓		✓
IO infusion	Nil			✓
IO device	Nil			✓
Mucosal atomiser	✓			✓
Look after IV line		✓		✓
IV fluid management		✓		✓
Interventions				
Decompress tension pneumothorax	✓			✓
Rapid/Delayed Sequence Intubation				✓
Thoracostomy			✓	
Pacing	✓			✓
Radial Arterial Line			✓	
Equipment				
Cervical collars		✓		✓
Extrication device, e.g Extrication board, NEIJ, KED, RED		✓		✓
Pelvic splint	✓			✓
Arterial tourniquet	✓		✓	✓
Traction splint		✓		✓
Pulse oximetry		✓		✓
End-expiratory pressure device	Nil		✓	
PEEP valves	✓		✓	
Colorimetric CO_2 detection	✓			✓
Continuous waveform capnography	✓			✓
Thrombolysis	✓			✓

BG: blood glucose; CO_2: carbon dioxide; GTN: glyceryl trinitrate; KED/RED: Kendrick Extraction device/Russell extraction device; IO: intraosseous; IV: intravenous; MI: myocardial infarction; PEEP: positive end-expiratory pressure

TABLE 2.2 Drugs used by state[47]*									
DRUG/STATE	QLD	NSW	ACT	VIC	TAS	SA	WA	NT	NZ
Activated Charcoal					X				
Adenosine			X	X	X	X	X	X	X
Adrenaline	X	X	X	X	X	X	X	X	X
Amiodarone	X	X	X	X	X	X	X	X	X
Aspirin	X	X	X	X	X	X	X	X	X
Atropine Sulphate	X	X	X	X	X	X	X	X	X
Benztropine	X						X	X	X
Benzyl Penicillin		X				X	X	X	X
Calcium	X	X	X			X			
Ceftriaxone	X		X	X	X		X	X	X
Clopidogrel	X	X	X			X			X
Co-phenylcaine					X	X	X		
Dexamethasone				X	X	X	X	X	
Dextrose 5%	X			X			X	X	X
Dextrose 10%	X	X	X	X	X	X	X	X	X
Dextrose 50%						X	X	X	X
Diazepam						X	X	X	
Dopamine						X			
Enoxaparin	X	X							
Ergometrine					X				
Fentanyl	X	X	X	X	X	X	X	X	X
Fexofenadine		X				X	X	X	
Frusemide		X	X	X	X	X	X	X	
Glucagon	X	X	X	X	X	X	X	X	X
Glucose Gel	X	X	X	X	X	X	X	X	X
Glyceryl Trinitrate	X	X	X	X	X	X	X	X	X
Haloperidol	X				X		X	X	
Heparin	X		X	X			X		X
Hydrocortisone	X		X				X	X	X
Hydroxocobalamin	X								
Hypertonic Saline	X								
Ibuprofen		X					X	X	
Ipratropium Bromide	X	X	X	X	X	X	X	X	X
Isoprenaline						X			
Ketamine	X	X	X	X	X	X	X	X	X
Lignocaine 1%		X		X	X		X	X	X

TABLE 2.2 Drugs used by state[47]*—cont'd

DRUG/STATE	QLD	NSW	ACT	VIC	TAS	SA	WA	NT	NZ
Lignocaine 2%	X	X	X			X	X	X	X
Loratadine							X	X	X
Magnesium Sulphate	X		X	X	X	X			X
Metaraminol				X		X	X	X	
Methoxyflurane	X	X	X	X	X	X	X	X	X
Metoclopramide		X		X	X	X	X		
Metoprolol							X	X	
Midazolam	X	X	X	X	X	X	X	X	X
Morphine Sulphate	X	X	X	X	X	X	X	X	X
Naloxone	X	X	X	X	X	X	X	X	X
Nitrous Oxide								X	X
Noradrenaline				X		X			
Ondansetron	X	X	X	X	X	X	X	X	X
Oxime	X	X	X	X	X	X	X	X	
Oxygen	X	X	X	X	X	X	X	X	X
Pancuronium				X		X	X	X	
Paracetamol	X	X	X	X	X	X	X	X	X
Prasugrel			X						
Prochlorperazine				X	X		X	X	
Promethazine	X					X	X	X	
Propofol							X	X	
Rocuronium	X			X		X	X		
Salbutamol	X	X	X	X	X	X	X	X	X
Sodium Bicarbonate	X	X	X	X	X	X	X	X	X
Sodium Chloride 0.9%	X	X	X	X	X	X	X	X	X
Suxamethonium			X	X		X	X	X	X
Tenecteplase	X	X				X			X
Thiamine							X	X	
Tirofiban	X								
Tramadol							X	X	
Vecuronium							X	X	X
Verapamil				X			X	X	

* *State variations apply to individual drugs being administered by particular levels of clinician. This list is by no means exhaustive as variations to current authorised pharmacology changes monthly, not only state by state but also at each clinical level.*

Other drugs that are authorised to be used by various ambulance services for use by individually accredited intensive care/critical care paramedics, or flight paramedics that are undertaking inter-facillity retrievals include: Acetylcysteine, Insulin, Tranexamic Acid, Packed Red Blood Cells, Phenytoin, and any running infusions under authorisation of their medical co-ordination centres.[46,47]

university environment posits a model where the theoretical and practical learning environments, although separated, allow the candidate to attain a mastery of knowledge that enables them to provide excellent, practical pre-hospital care. In recent times there has been a rapid progression across most ambulance services with change management focusing on patient care, based on current evidence-based medicine (Tables 2.1–2.2).

Level of care offered within ambulance services

The title given to a member of an ambulance service varies across Australia compared with what occurs in New Zealand. Prior to the late 1980s, paramedics were commonly referred to as 'ambulance officers' in most states and territories of Australia. The term 'paramedic' is not enshrined in legislation, so virtually anyone can call him- or herself a paramedic. Their role is to treat trauma and medical emergencies outside the hospital setting and during transport to the most appropriate medical facility. They also transfer patients between various healthcare facilities. A number of services have programs in place that allow paramedics to provide primary health as well as emergency care. Each ambulance authority has titles for their staff based upon the level of care that they can provide, but there is no common nomenclature used across Australia or New Zealand. Many terms are used but there is, in most cases, a degree of similarity between terms for ambulance operatives with similar skill sets. These are outlined below.

First-responder

Either a volunteer or a healthcare professional who provides advanced first aid until a dedicated ambulance crew arrive at the scene.

Patient transport officer

Within Australian ambulance services, the minimum qualification for this role is the nationally recognised Certificate III in Non-Emergency Patient Transport. Operatives in these positions may be employed by the statutory ambulance authorities or by private companies who provide pre-booked non-emergency transports of low-risk patients. It would be rare for them to either attend or respond to an emergency situation.

Ambulance transport officer

Usually an ambulance operative who has been trained to a Certificate IV level that allows them to provide BLS in emergency situations.

Paramedic

Ambulance operatives at this level are well versed in Basic Life Support, with enhanced skills that include advanced airway management, intravenous cannulation, analgesia, antiemetics, hypoglycaemic agents, cardiac and respiratory emergency drug therapies, as well as fluid resuscitation. They are capable of maintaining an infusion, utilising pulse oximetry, taking vital signs, cardiac monitoring (ECG) and defibrillation. Patient assessment is the cornerstone of their practice. Increasingly, a trend in Australia is for most statutory ambulance services to employ only university graduates with a bachelor's degree in a pre-hospital-related course or healthcare professionals with a postgraduate conversion. A small number of ambulance

services still offer the nationally recognised diploma within the Australian vocational education training (VET) framework.

SCOPE OF PRACTICE[48]

- Australian Resuscitation Council—intermediate life support, including use of supraglottic airway devices, e.g. LMA
- New Zealand intermediate life support as defined by Ambulance Service Sector Standard 8156 and New Zealand National Clinical Guidelines
- Use of infection control practices relevant to clinical environment
- Emergency management of the unconscious patient, cardiac arrest, asthma, anaphylaxis, burns, narcotic overdose, chest pain, acute cardiogenic pulmonary oedema (ACPO), hypoglycaemia, pain control (using narcotics), seizures, traumatic brain injury, spinal injury, abnormalities of ventilation, neurovascular incidents and hypovolaemia
- Use of a range of medications (S4 and S8)
- Electrocardiogram (ECG) monitoring and interpretation
- Mental health crisis intervention
- Management of patients across the lifespan, including obstetric emergencies and childbirth
- Use of a stretcher and other patient movement devices
- Emergency driving
- Emergency management and triage
- Extrication and basic rescue
- Access to a range of patient referral pathways (depending upon local circumstance)
- AHPRA Division 2 Registration

Intensive-care paramedic

Ambulance operatives with this level of training have additional training above the level of the paramedic (Fig 2.3). The training for this level of activity will most often be in the form of a university postgraduate diploma or an advanced diploma attained from within the VET framework. They have more advanced airway skills than paramedics and are able to access a wider pharmacology to provide treatment to their patients. They practise under either clinical practice guidelines or approved protocols, depending on their jurisdiction.

SCOPE OF PRACTICE[48]

- Includes paramedic scope of practice
- Australian Resuscitation Council—Advanced Life Support
- New Zealand Advanced Life Support as defined by Ambulance Service Sector Standard 8156 and New Zealand National Clinical Guidelines
- Advanced airway management (including medication facilitated intubation in some jurisdictions)
- Intra-osseous access
- External cardiac pacing and synchronised cardioversion
- Advanced clinical management of pain, ACS and cardiac dysrhythmias, including cardiac arrest, trauma and abnormalities of ventilation
- Use of an expanded range of medications relevant to the role

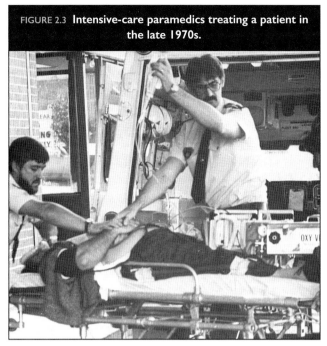

FIGURE 2.3 **Intensive-care paramedics treating a patient in the late 1970s.**

Courtesy of NSW Ambulance.

Rescue paramedic

A few ambulance services have employed paramedics as rescue operatives. In addition to their normal skill set, these paramedics are trained in areas such as road crash rescue, vertical and cliff rescue, confined space and trench rescue, navigation and urban search and rescue. This is being phased out or significantly reduced in ambulance services currently, with the fire service mostly providing the rescue function.

Flight paramedic/Retrieval Paramedic/Critical Care Paramedic[48]

SCOPE OF PRACTICE[48]

- Includes intensive care paramedic scope of practice
- Advanced clinical assessment, including interpretation of blood tests and X-rays
- Specialist clinical management to support the safe transfer of critically injured or ill patients to definitive care
- Rapid sequence intubation
- Use of mechanical ventilators and medication administration devices
- Use of an expanded range of medications relevant to the role

These ambulance operatives work on either fixed-wing or rotary-powered aircraft. They perform emergency, retrieval and routine transports. Most are trained to the level of an intensive-care paramedic but have additional training in rescue techniques and aviation medicine. Registered nurses with postgraduate qualifications staff some fixed-wing air ambulances completing mostly retrieval operations. In some states the rotary-powered aircraft are staffed by a combination of a doctor and a flight paramedic. These doctors are usually emergency or intensive-care doctors. Ambulance services in Australia and New Zealand follow the Anglo-American

model of emergency care, except in the above example, where the healthcare delivery model is more like the Franco-German model.[42]

Extended care paramedic/General care paramedic

The extended care paramedic (ECP) is a relatively new type of paramedic who is able to attend emergency cases and provide advanced care and can also attend patients with subacute and non-acute healthcare needs. The ECP has additional training at a postgraduate level in the application of a range of clinical pathways assessment and management that may not result in the patient being transported to an ED. Health Workforce Australia released a report in June 2014, following an 18-month trial in five key locations across Australia as to national implementation of this low acuity model.[48]

SCOPE OF PRACTICE[48]

- Includes paramedic scope of practice
- Specialist patient assessment, including point-of-care blood testing, ordering plain film X-rays and various specimen testing
- Immunisations, e.g. tetanus, influenza, hepatitis
- Specialist management of wounds (cleaning, closure and dressing), infections (including a broad range of oral and IV antibiotics), dehydration, soft tissue injury, chronic pain and palliative care
- Reduction of common dislocations, e.g. patella, anterior shoulder, finger
- Urinary catheter (male and female) and percutaneous endoscopic gastrostomy (PEG) tube reinsertion
- Use of a wide range of generalist and specialist referral pathways: general medical practitioner, district nurses, palliative care services and community social services

Clinical skills, procedures and pharmacological agents used by paramedics

Tables 2.1 and 2.2 give an overview of skills, medications and treatments used in ambulance services in Australia and New Zealand. They are grouped into paramedic and intensive-care paramedic scopes of practices. The column heading 'Few' indicates that three or fewer ambulance services use the skill, medication or procedure, whereas 'Most' indicates that four or more use it; a 'Nil' response indicates that no ambulance service utilises the practice, procedure or medication within this particular skill grouping. With so much change currently occurring in the pre-hospital environment, this table can at best only be viewed as a collective snapshot of current practice. What it lacks in specific detail is compensated for by its global nature.

Future

As stated previously in this chapter the range of clinical interventions utilised by paramedics has expanded in scope and paramedic education has shifted largely from in-service and

VET training to the university sector with undergraduate and postgraduate degrees with an increased focus on paramedic-driven research leading to evidence-based practice. While there may be advantages and disadvantages to expanding the role of paramedics into the future, the primary overall goal would be to maintain the integrity of services but co-jointly providing effective and efficient care to the public while in the long term reducing the burden on hospital systems. Some expansions in practice are already making positive outcomes (e.g. introduction of FAST into pre-hospital trauma models and pre-hospital thrombolysis). There is certainly room for continuing increases in paramedic scopes associated with community needs. Some projects currently being reviewed around the world include:

- Direct referral of first-time seizure patients to neurology departments
- Mobile stroke units
- Stroke and neuroprotective drug pilot programs.

CASE STUDY

The year was 1917. Australia had a population of approximately five million inhabitants, mostly located in scattered rural areas. A stockman working on a large cattle property was found injured by his co-workers after having fallen from his horse while mustering cattle. Recognising the seriousness of his injuries, his friends took him to the nearest settlement 30 kilometres away, a journey taking over 12 hours by horse and buggy. There was no doctor or hospital in this settlement, and the only person with first-aid qualifications was the postmaster. Aware of how serious the stockman's injuries were, he attempted to make contact with at least one doctor from some of the other local communities via the telegraphic network. This proved unsuccessful, but he persevered in his quest for medical assistance and was eventually successful in contacting a doctor to instruct him in first aid. Unfortunately, the doctor was located almost 3000 kilometres away.

Morse code messages were exchanged, and a diagnosis of a ruptured bladder was made. The only option to save the stockman's life was for the postmaster to operate. The patient was plied with alcohol until he was insensible, and then, with him strapped to the post office counter, the operation commenced using a penknife and a razor. A day later, complications set in and the stockman's expected recovery failed to progress. Upon hearing this, the doctor who had provided the medical advice via Morse code travelled to the patient's location. It took 13 days for this journey, and he arrived only to find that the young stockman had died the day before.

Questions

1. What form of communication would be utilised in a similar situation today?
2. What changes have occurred regarding ambulance transportation from rural and remote areas within Australia and New Zealand?

 Answers to Case Study Questions can be found on evolve
http://evolve.emergencytrauma.curtis

REFERENCES

1. St John Ambulance Australia. 113th Annual report. The Commandery in Western Australia; 30.

2. Rural Ambulance Victoria. (2007) What we do: the RAV fleet. Online. www.rav.vic.gov.au/What-we-do/The-RAV-Fleet.html; accessed 3 Mar 2015.

3. State Records NSW photographic collection. (2007) Ambulance tram, c.1915. Online. www.flickr.com/photos/state-records-nsw/3293684627/; accessed 3 Mar 2015.

4. Queensland Ambulance Service. (2010) Queensland Ambulance Service history and heritage. Online. www.ambulance.qld.gov.au/about/history_and_heritage.asp; accessed 3 Mar 2015.

5. Greenland R, personal communication, January 2008.

6. O'Meara P, Grbich C, eds. Paramedics in Australia—contemporary challenges of practice. Pearson Education Australia; 2009:10.

7. O'Meara P, Grbich C, eds. Paramedics in Australia—contemporary challenges of practice. Pearson Education Australia; 2009:3–27.

8. O'Meara P, Grbich C, eds. Paramedics in Australia—contemporary challenges of practice. Pearson Education Australia; 2009:12–13.

9. O'Meara P, Grbich C, eds. Paramedics in Australia—contemporary challenges of practice. Pearson Education Australia; 2009:4.

10. The Council of Ambulance Authorities. 2007–08 Annual report. Online. http://convention.ambulance.net.au/intranet/docs/doc4805.pdf; 2008:7.

11. Woods S, Clark M, Fitzgerald G. Queensland ambulance service: a case study in organizational reform. Australian Centre for Prehospital Research; 2002:8.

12. Woods S, Clark M, Fitzgerald G. Queensland ambulance service: a case study in organizational reform. Australian Centre for Prehospital Research; 2002:7.

13. O'Meara P, Grbich C, eds. Paramedics in Australia—contemporary challenges of practice. Pearson Education Australia; 2009:16.

14. O'Meara P, Grbich C, eds. Paramedics in Australia—contemporary challenges of practice. Pearson Education Australia; 2009:17.

15. South Australia Ambulance Service. Annual Report 2007–08. Online. www.saambulance.com.au/publicweb/media_pub_june.html; 6.

16. O'Meara P, Grbich C, eds. Paramedics in Australia—contemporary challenges of practice. Pearson Education Australia; 2009:21.

17. O'Meara P, Grbich C, eds. Paramedics in Australia—contemporary challenges of practice. Pearson Education Australia; 2009:20.

18. St John Ambulance Australia. (2010) History of the order. Online. www.stjohn.org.nz/about/history; accessed 17 Mar 2010.

19. Millar D 2001. The history of the ambulance in New Zealand. Online. www.111emergency.co.nz/F-I/history.htm; accessed 14 Dec 2010.

20. Wellington Free Ambulance 2009. A history of Wellington Free Ambulance. Online. www.wellingtonfreeambulance.org.nz/history.htm; accessed 14 Dec 2010.

21. St John. (2010) History of St John in New Zealand. Online. www.stjohn.org.nz/about/history/newzealand_p2.aspx; accessed 14 Apr 2010.

22. Mitka M. Peter J. Safar, MD: 'father of CPR,' innovator, teacher, humanist. JAMA 2003;289(19):2485–6.

23. Freedom House n.d. Street saviours: the documentary. Online. www.freedomhousedoc.com; accessed 14 Dec 2010.

24. Corbett-Bell R 2009. The next page—Freedom House ambulances: 'We were the best'. Online. www.post-gazette.com/pg/09298/1008180-109.stm; accessed 14 Dec 2010.

25. Baskett P, Safar P. The Resuscitation Greats. Nancy Caroline—from mobile intensive care to hospice. Resuscitation 2003;57(2):119–22.

26. Pollak AN. Nancy Caroline's emergency care in the streets. Sudbury MA: Jones and Bartlett; 2008.

27. Pantridge JF, Geddes JS. A mobile intensive care unit in the management of myocardial infarction. Lancet 1967;2(7510):271–3.

28. National EMS Museum Foundation 2010. The virtual EMS Museum. Online. www.emsmuseum.org/virtual-museum/history; accessed 14 Dec 2010.

29. COLAC Ambulance. MICA paramedic. Online. www.colacambulance.com/colac_mica.htm; accessed 14 Dec 2010.

30. Déziel J. Past medical history—paramedics in the United States. Online. http://knol.google.com/k/paramedic-history-in-the-united-states#; accessed 9 Apr 2010.

31. National Association of Emergency Medical Technicians 2008. Scott B Frame Memorial Lecture 'Controversies in Trauma Care'. Online. Via www.naemt.org/about_us/about_home.aspx; accessed 14 Dec 2010.

32. Emergencyfans.com n.d. Biography of Robert A. Cinander. Online. www.emergencyfans.com/people/robert_cinader.htm; accessed 15 Dec 2010.

33. County of Los Angeles Fire Museum 2010. Biography of James O Page, pioneer of paramedicine. Online. www.clafma.org/BioJamesOPage.html; accessed 14 Dec 2010.

34. Royal Flying Doctors Service 2010. Our history. Online. www.flyingdoctor.org.au/About-Us/Our-History; accessed 14 Dec 2010.

35. Report of the air Ambulance Reference Group to the ACC and Health Ministers. (2008) Online. www.moh.govt.nz/moh.nsf/indexmh/report-air-ambulance-reference-group; accessed 14 Apr 2010.

36. Convention of Ambulance Authorities. Australia and New Zealand Ambulance Services—a strategic direction for the future 2009. Annual report. Online. www.caa.net.au/images/stories/2009_Annual_Report.pdf; accessed 14 Dec 2010.

37. Convention of Ambulance Authorities. Australia and New Zealand Ambulance Services—a strategic direction for the future 2009. Annual report. Online. www.caa.net.au/images/stories/2009_Annual_Report.pdf; accessed 14 Dec 2010:7.

38. O'Meara P, Grbich C, eds. Paramedics in Australia—contemporary challenges of practice. Pearson Education Australia; 2009:13.

39. O'Meara P, Grbich C, eds. Paramedics in Australia—contemporary challenges of practice. Pearson Education Australia; 2009:18.

40. Fahey C, Walker J, Lennox G. Flexible, focused training: keeps volunteer ambulance officers. JEPHC 2003;1(1–2).

41. International Roundtable on Community Paramedicine, National Ambulance Sector Office, 2009. The New Zealand Ambulance Service Strategy—the first line of mobile emergency intervention in the continuum of health care. Online. www.ircp.info/LinkClick.aspx?fileticket=RQkuA0dRnRc%3D&tabid=267&mid=761; accessed 14 Dec 2010.

42. Al-Shaqsi S. Models of International Emergency Medical Service (EMS) Systems. Oman Medical Journal, 2010;25:4:320–3.

43. Paramedicine Role Discriptions, Paramedic Australasia. Online. www.paramedics.org/content/2009/07/PRD_211212_WEBONLY.pdf; accessed 20 July 2015.

44. Asian Disaster Preparedness Center, 2003. Online. www.adpc.net/igo/?#; accessed 20 July 2015.

45. FitzGerald GJ, Tippet V, Schuetz M et al. The Queensland Emergency Medical System: A structural and organisational model for the Emergency Medical System in Australia. Emergency Medicine Australasia, 2009;21:6:510–14.

46. Dick WF. Anglo-American vs Franco-German emergency medical services system. Prehosp Disaster Med 2003;18(1):29–35.

47. Caffey, M. Paramedic and Emergency Pharmacology Guidelines, Pearson Education Australia, 2013.

48. Queensland Ambulance Service, Field Reference Guide 2011.

CHAPTER 3
CLINICAL ETHICS FOR EMERGENCY HEALTHCARE

SARAH WINCH, ELEANOR MILLIGAN AND ADAM ROLLEY

Essentials

- Remember that values inform your practice. Why are you in healthcare?
- Slow down … where possible.
- Ethically sensitive care happens in *every* interaction you have with your patients and colleagues, and is not limited to resolving the big dilemmas.
- There are many ways to harm a patient—patients may remember the 'moral harms' (of feeling excluded, ignored, uncared for or misunderstood) long after their physical illnesses subside. Act to minimise *all* harms.
- Every action in an organisation either contributes to or undermines its ethical culture; choose your actions carefully.
- Treat yourself, your colleagues and your patients with kindness.
- Seek help if you are struggling with the ethical aspects of your professional role.

INTRODUCTION

'We are discussing no small matter, but how we ought to live.'
Socrates, Plato's Republic

'Medicine being simultaneously the scientific and humanistic study of man cannot escape being based in an explicit or implicit philosophy of human nature.'
Ed Pellegrino, 'From medical ethics to a moral philosophy of the professions'[1]

Most societies recognise healthcare as a fundamental 'good'—something of great value that is collectively nurtured, protected and preserved. Human communities, even ancient ones, developed traditions of healthcare ranging from the diagnoses and treatments offered by medicine men and shamans within indigenous communities to the healing traditions provided within Chinese medicine, Islamic traditions and the early Western tradition of medicine, derived from the ancient Greeks. These formalised systems of healthcare delivery, and the collective desire to improve and progress medical knowledge, flow from the recognition that the preservation of life and good health is integral to each person's ability to flourish.

While life is valued and we collectively (through the provision of organisational care) and individually (through personal choices) seek to maintain health, the human body is fragile, subject to illness, disease and trauma. In the context of medical emergency, healthcare professionals are called on to respond to the needs of patients at times of unexpected trauma, in addition to expected and unexpected illness. Often patients are in distress, possibly confronting their own (or loved ones') mortality. They enter the healthcare system seeking skilled and competent treatment and, importantly, reassurance, understanding and compassion. The families and loved ones of patients similarly look to emergency healthcare professionals for reassurance that the trust placed in them to provide care is deserved and will not be misused.

At such times when the fragility of life is a stark reality for patients and their families, the ethical response of emergency healthcare professionals is triggered by the personal vulnerability that comes hand-in-hand with illness and trauma. Illness is not simply a matter of physical threat to the body; it is also a threat to a person's sense of identity and wellbeing—who they are, how and as who others regard them, their future possibilities and present capabilities. It is this vulnerability of the ill person that invites a caring response from healthcare professionals. Barry Hoffmaster[2] writes that 'vulnerability is an even more basic feature of our human constitution than rationality, because while all human beings are vulnerable, not all are rational or even possess the potential to become rational … it is our very vulnerability that creates the need for morality'. Thus, healthcare, including the provision of emergency healthcare, occurs in a partnership between the carer and the cared for. It is 'ethically laden practice'[3] because it requires healthcare professionals to respond to the needs of others at times of personal fragility and disempowerment, and to care for patients and families, both in the physical and in the human sense.

While emergency healthcare shares this ethical foundation of providing care and relieving suffering with other healthcare disciplines, it also raises particular and unique ethical challenges. The physical landscape of emergency and trauma care is one in which a pre-existing relationship with the patient often does not exist, potentially impeding critical understandings on both sides. Frequently, organisational resources are limited, creating ethically confronting situations such as 'ramping' (where patients are unable to be handed over from ambulance staff to be triaged in hospital emergency departments (ED)) or poor response times where the best care possible is unable to be given. The inherent unpredictability of emergency, the need to make time-pressured treatment decisions and the professional isolation of emergencies in rural practice can create ethical tension. Similarly, community expectations that emergency healthcare staff will respond to the needs of others and even compromise their own safety in times of pandemic or natural disaster can breed fear and resentment in practitioners. Confusion over what to do when a patient lacks capacity, or does not appear to have given appropriate informed consent, can generate anxiety and unease in healthcare professionals. Decisions concerning the instigation of futile treatment can also generate moral distress. Added to this mix are the hierarchical structures within healthcare organisations that can negatively shape inter-professional communication, sometimes to the detriment of patient care. All of these considerations define the unique and complex environment of emergency and trauma care; all can lead to moral anguish in the individual practitioner; and all can contribute to stress, burnout and even poor retention in the workforce.[4] However, when clinical staff develop the skills and tools to work through, understand and engage with the ethical and human dimensions of their practice, they can become more effective both personally and professionally.

Ethics: An ancient and evolving field

A working knowledge of the approaches available to understand ethical issues is important because it clarifies the emergency healthcare professional's role in ethical situations and the associated decision-making. There are many different ethical perspectives, and considering a clinical scenario through these different lenses can lead to different outcomes.

Ethical concepts drawn from the classical, modern and postmodern centuries of thought are useful tools for understanding, explaining and deciding how to resolve contemporary ethical issues. In this brief review, we consider four of the better-known approaches to understanding ethics: virtue ethics, deontology, utilitarianism and narrative ethics. For a more detailed discussion on ethical theory, a number of good texts are available, such as *Ethics in Nursing: the Caring Relationship*[5] and *Ethics and Law for the Health Professions*.[6] This chapter begins with a brief review of the ethical theory from which the principles for ethical practice and decision-making are drawn, then considers the role of professional codes of ethics and codes of conduct in guiding practice. It concludes with an example of one model of ethical decision-making that may assist health carers in developing their skills of ethical analysis.

Virtue ethics

Ideas from the ancient Greek philosopher Aristotle (384–322 BC) underpin *virtue ethics*, an approach that has seen a resurgence in popularity since the publication of *Modern Moral Philosophy* in 1958.[7] Virtue ethics, in common with Aristotle's thinking, focuses on inner character and/or motives rather than rules or consequences of actions. Virtues are qualities that make their possessor good: a virtuous person is a morally excellent or admirable person who acts and feels well. Virtues are not innate in a person, but can be cultivated. Thus, moral education and the development of a virtuous character are central to virtue ethics.[8] The ethical or moral character of an individual develops over a long period of time and can be encouraged by family, teachers and the peer group. Professional education plays an important role in developing moral character. For example, it is a requirement of a variety of undergraduate health degree programs to teach ethics as part of the core curriculum. The inclusion of ethics tutoring creates an educational space in which healthcare providers can extend and consolidate understanding of how their existing values and beliefs can be actualised in the professional context. Such education can also be an opportunity for personal transformation and growth. Moral training can also be provided by role models, such as senior staff in healthcare organisations who are expected to model ethical behaviour.

Duty-based ethics and utilitarianism

The age of modernity, commonly understood to have begun with the Enlightenment in the 18th century, promoted *rationalism* (the capacity for human reason), *universalism* (truths that can be applied to all) and *individualism* (valuing the individual). These ideas have influenced contemporary approaches to ethical decision-making. Deontology, drawn from the work of Immanuel Kant (1724–1804), takes its name from *deon*, the Greek word for 'duty'. Deontological or duty-based ethics examines the nature of actions and the will of agents, rather than goals achieved. That is, a person has a duty to perform particular actions and to do the right action for its own sake. We see this in the well-accepted notion that healthcarers have a duty to care for patients, no matter what the outcome.

Utilitarianism, conceptualised initially by Jeremy Bentham (1748–1832) and developed further by John Stuart Mill (1806–73), refers broadly to the greatest happiness (or good) for the greatest number. It is known as a consequentialist theory in that it judges an act as morally right or wrong depending on the consequences of that act. This argument is frequently applied to modern resource allocation in the notion of getting the best value out of scarce resources.[9] The ethics of triage can be understood as a form of utilitarianism. If our ultimate goal is to give the best care possible for all patients in the ED, then the sickest patients need to be seen first. If we used an alternative method to prioritise patient care, such as when the patient actually arrived in the ED as opposed to their clinical need, then some patients would suffer significantly poorer outcomes. Resources in the ED are finite and the system of seeing patients according to their clinical urgency actually provides the greatest good for the greatest number in terms of patient outcomes.

Narrative ethics

Narrative ethics acknowledges the *subjective* nature of ethical and moral aspects of any situation. It differs from other philosophical approaches that seek to uncover universal truths through the systematic and objective application of rational thought to ethically challenging circumstances. The narrative approach seeks to uncover each individual stakeholder's personal story as a rich way of understanding their individual perspective and life. Taking a narrative approach, moral rules and principles can be best understood in the context of each person's circumstances, and the subjective meaning each individual places on particular aspects of their situation.[10,11] Narrative ethics draws its concepts and methodologies from literary criticism and phenomenology and is a postmodern approach to understanding ethics.

An example of a clinical situation in which a narrative approach may be useful is in considering the ethical issues surrounding domestic violence that emergency care workers face in their practice.[12] In such cases the emergency care worker needs to hear the patient's story to make sense of the situation and the moral rules that may influence the patient's life, which may be significantly different from the care worker's values, beliefs and expectations. For example, the emergency care worker might be concerned about a young adult patient who frequently calls an ambulance, or presents regularly to the department with injuries that indicate they may be experiencing domestic violence. The care worker feels that it is their moral duty to counsel the patient to leave this situation and seek a safer place to live. Using a narrative approach, the care worker listens to the patient's story and is told that the patient is staying in the situation in order to protect younger siblings. The care worker may use a series of open ended questions such as 'tell me about your stressful situation'. Through such open questioning, an appreciation of the complexity involved can be gleaned, and this is more likely to encourage disclosure than the use of common screening tools.[13] The patient feels they have a moral duty to stay and protect their siblings; the care worker is concerned for the patient. In this case the care worker may decide to support the patient to stay in their situation and put into place actions that help protect them and their siblings.

The ethical framework of emergency healthcare: Our moral commitments and obligations

> Our practices … are the visible manifestations of invisible values.
>
> G HOFSTEDE, IN CULTURE'S CONSEQUENCES: INTERNATIONAL DIFFERENCES IN WORK-RELATED VALUES[14]

A useful starting point for all healthcare workers when confronting ethical decision-making is to examine the values that they hold as individuals. Values are embedded deeply in our psyche, developing from our family, schooling and cultural background. Further education and experience will shape and sharpen these values considerably. These are then expressed consciously or unconsciously in the work environment. Values have three components: emotional, cognitive and behavioural. This means that when our values clash with what we see or hear, we are likely to feel upset or worried about what we see happening. This feeling can be made worse if we feel we have little control over the situation, which may be the case in many emergency presentations. A simple example that may challenge us is the case of the 30-year-old alcoholic single mother who is admitted with liver failure following a wild drinking binge the night before. Her two children are with her and look malnourished and dishevelled. This case challenges values that we hold regarding self-care and monitoring, as well as care of children.

In cases such as these, it is timely to remind ourselves of the professional values we hold. These are often articulated in professional codes of ethics, and are a good reference point to guide our attitudes and subsequent clinical practice. The International Council of Nurses first developed a Code of Ethics in 1953.[15] The Australian Nursing and Midwifery Council initiated their Code of Ethics in 1993, which was revised in 2008; it is applicable to all settings, including the ED. Box 3.1 outlines the broad values that the nursing profession consider essential. These encompass respect for the person, for

---

BOX 3.1 Nursing and Midwifery Board of Australia. Code of Ethics[16]

- Nurses value quality nursing care for all people.
- Nurses value respect and kindness for self and others.
- Nurses value the diversity of people.
- Nurses value access to quality nursing and healthcare for all people.
- Nurses value informed decision-making.
- Nurses value a culture of safety.
- Nurses value ethical management of information.
- Nurses value a socially, economically and ecologically sustainable environment promoting health and wellbeing.

the environment and for the quality of care that is provided. Paramedics Australasia has also developed a Code of Conduct to guide practitioners (see Box 3.2).

These codes encompass the ethical aspects of everyday care. Importantly, they also communicate a shared professional standard to the community. They can provide a framework for determining whether certain behaviours have breached the expected professional standard of care. Codes are often criticised for their broad aspirational statements, for being self-generated and self-monitored within professions and for lacking independent critique. Professional codes of ethics and conduct are not legally binding. They do not provide a means of sanctioning individual professionals who do not abide by them. Legislative pathways to deal with negligent actions or poor professional standards are discussed in Chapter 4. Despite their limitations, however, codes of ethics play a critical role in expressing the underlying values of healthcare practice, while assisting clinicians to develop a shared understanding of their collective moral obligations and to develop a strong professional culture.

In addition to considering aspects of clinical ethical decision-making, healthcare professionals also need to be aware of the research ethics codes that govern the conduct of research involving patients, colleagues and others. In Australia, the Statement on Ethical Conduct in Research Involving Humans, issued by the National Health and Medical Research Council (NHMRC),[18] provides ethical guidance for conducting research. The NHMRC outlines four fundamental principles that must be considered in determining whether any research proposal meets the ethical standards expected by the community. The four principles are that the research must have *merit and integrity*; it must be done *justly* (without unfairly burdening or including/excluding particular groups); it should be carried out with *beneficence* (designed to minimise the risks, harms or discomfort to participants); and should *respect* participants as having intrinsic value, not as a means to a research agenda. A separate document provides guidance for Aboriginal and Torres Strait Islander peoples. For clinicians

in New Zealand, the Health Research Council has published Guidelines on Ethics in Health Research.[19]

Ethical decision-making

While codes provide general guidance for healthcare professionals, specific guides to moral decision-making and problem-solving also exist. The 'four principles' approach developed by Tom Beauchamp and James Childress[20] (see Box 3.3)—also known also as 'principlism'—is popular in the healthcare field because of its accessibility and ease of application.

Based on a combination of common moral theory, virtue ethics and utilitarianism, the four principles seek to guide reflection and decision-making within the context of the specific duties that healthcare professionals owe to patients. These duties are seen to be *prima facie*. This means they are always considered to be in effect, in all situations. While Beauchamp and Childress[20] made it clear that all of the principles should be considered equally, in practice many clinicians tend to place the principle of patient autonomy above the others.

A simple example of how these principles may be applied is to consider a patient who needs a blood transfusion but refuses because this violates her religious beliefs. Using the principlist approach, two ethical principles are in conflict—the right of the patient to decide her own treatment (autonomy) and the duty of the healthcare professional to provide the best assistance possible (beneficence). If the patient is deemed competent to make the decision (that is, she is an adult with capacity), the patient's right to refuse the treatment because of her religious beliefs would be absolute, and to treat without consent, in the name of beneficence, could result in a charge of assault or battery. If the patient in this scenario is a child, the situation would be considered differently. Children are not automatically considered to have the legal capacity to make autonomous decisions. If a parent requests the withholding of a life-sustaining treatment from their child, this poses a very serious situation that emergency staff need to report immediately to senior staff; it may require legal intervention, particularly if the child's life is at risk.

While this approach to ethical decision-making appears straightforward, it has been widely criticised for oversimplifying what are inevitably complex and multifaceted deliberations and viewing the 'problem' primarily from the clinician's perspective.[21,22] The attributes that make this model so accessible, such as the temptation to simplify and reduce the complexity, and to decontextualise difficult ethical decisions, are also its greatest weakness. Pullman[23] suggests that principlism may be better thought of as a sort of 'first aid' response, which

---

BOX 3.2 Paramedics Australasia Code of Conduct[17]

Members of Paramedics Australasia ascribe to the following principles:

- integrity
- respect
- responsibility/accountability
- competence
- consent for patient care
- confidentiality
- research
- ethical review

See Australian and New Zealand College of Paramedicine, www.anzcp.org.au/ for expanded comments on each principle.

Paramedics Australasia Code of Conduct from https://www.paramedics. org/our-organisation/who-we-are/code-of-conduct/

BOX 3.3 The four principles to guide ethical decision-making[20]

Respect for autonomy—respect people's decisions and values.
Beneficence—help people.
Non-maleficence—don't harm people.
Justice—treat like cases alike; distribute benefits and burdens fairly.

may be helpful in the immediate term but cannot fulfil the role of thorough exploration.

Autonomy and informed consent

Seeking informed consent from a patient demonstrates respect for the patient as a person and for their ability to act autonomously when participating in healthcare. For informed consent to occur, the patient (or the patient's representatives if they are a minor or lack capacity) needs to understand:

- the health intervention that is being proposed
- what alternatives are available, and
- the risks attached to any course of action.

In addition, a patient should be able to act freely in choosing or rejecting proposed health interventions without undue influence or control by others.[24,25] Consent may be implied, such as a patient rolling up their sleeve to receive an injection, or assumed in a true emergency situation where delaying care may cause serious or permanent harm.[26,27] The legal aspects of the Doctrine of Necessity (Emergency) are discussed more fully in Chapter 4.

Australian law recognises that individuals aged 18 years and over have full legal capacity, such that they are capable of making decisions relating to their own healthcare. Prior to that age, parents (or legal guardians) are entitled to consent to their child's medical and dental treatment. A parent's authority in this respect is not, however, absolute, as the law in Australia recognises that children become increasingly competent as they move towards adulthood. In New Zealand the age for consent regarding healthcare issues is 16 years. Parents and healthcare professionals should consider the parents' and guardians' response carefully. Childress[28] provides the following guidance for clinicians to evaluate this response. Do they have adequate knowledge and information to make the decision? Are they emotionally stable and able to make reasoned judgements? Is the decision in the best interests of the child? In this complex area of ethical decision-making, junior staff need to alert senior clinicians and managers who can assist them. In turn, senior staff may have to seek legal opinion for the correct course of action. Competent minors may be able to give consent if they demonstrate understanding of the decision and its consequences; however, this must be decided on a case-by-case basis, as there is no prescribed age below 18 at which a child may be considered a 'mature minor' in Australia; similarly, those below the age of 16 in New Zealand can give or refuse consent if considered competent to do so.

Model for ethical decision-making

When healthcare professionals experience competing ethical principles, or a choice between two competing good outcomes, and are not able to resolve them, they are often left feeling burdened.[29] In Box 3.4 we outline an ethical decision-making model that emerges from and is grounded in practice. Initially developed by Kerridge, Lowe and Stewart,[6] it has been modified significantly by Dr Sarah Winch after many clinical ethics consultations in different settings. This revised model includes two new steps which assist the decision-maker to gather and access crucial information.[30] Thus this revised model directs the user to inquire not only into what facts are available, but also into what you as the clinician do not know. Are there crucial

---

BOX 3.4 Ethical decision making model[6] modified by Winch (2015)[30]

1. Identify the ethical problem/s.
2. What facts are available?
3. What facts are still required?
4. Review the ethics literature.
5. Consider the ethical principles.
6. Identify ethical conflicts.
7. Consider the law.
8. Make the decision.

In this model, points '3' and '4' have been added, while the requirement by Kerridge et al 2009 to view the problem using another ethical theory has been deleted. This is because clinicians' knowledge of ethical theories is not always well developed, and in Australia access to a clinical ethicist may be limited. The requirement to review evidence is a skill most clinicians now possess, and can be applied to the ethics literature, which is replete with cases and case discussions. This 'evidence' is likely to be case based, or using qualitative studies. Nevertheless, this process can make a valuable contribution to the decision on how to proceed.

---

elements of this case, of which you are not aware, but that may make a significant difference to the ethical decision-making? A requirement to review the ethics literature replaces Kerridge et al's[6] recommendation to examine the problem using another ethical theory. Knowledge of ethical theory in our experience is reasonably limited among clinicians and few have access to a clinical ethicist. The requirement to review evidence is a skill most clinicians now possess, and can be applied to the ethics literature, which is replete with cases and case discussions. While this 'evidence' is likely to be case-based, or using qualitative studies, it can make a valuable contribution to the decision on how to proceed. Using this model enables a more sophisticated analysis, that builds upon our 'first aid' immediate response of the four ethical principles approach.

In emergency and trauma care, clinical ethics questions arise urgently and often without any prior established relationship with the patient or family. It is sometimes difficult to ascertain the patient's preferences for treatment when they are unaccompanied and unable to speak for themselves. This may hinder the application of ethical decision-making frameworks that are of use in other healthcare settings. One key aspect is to try to slow the decision-making process to allow all the options to be considered for the patient and, if necessary, to secure additional information about the patient's preferences and wishes. In end-of-life situations where the patient may or may not be able to consent or refuse treatment, the emergency care worker needs to be aware of the laws guiding end-of-life intervention in the geographical area where they practise. Chapter 4 considers these issues in more detail.

Ethical decision-making in practice

We will now apply the ethical decision making model to the following case.

CASE STUDY

Paramedics are dispatched code 1 to a 48-year-old male with shortness of breath. On arrival the paramedic crew is met by the patient's wife, Suzanne. She advises that her husband Mark is 48 years of age and has widely disseminated kidney cancer, including multiple abdominal and cerebral secondary tumours. He is experiencing widespread malignant abdominal ascites and pleural effusion, making breathing and communication difficult.

It is apparent to the paramedics that the patient is approaching the end of his life, but has no advanced planning documentation. He is also in pain. The paramedics obtain a history and complete a physical examination. Suzanne advises that she holds his enduring power of attorney and this is confirmed by the patient. Suzanne is adamant that Mark wants to end his life, and requests paramedics administer the patient morphine. Suzanne is anxious, and when paramedics do not immediately administer morphine, she becomes angry.

Meanwhile, Mark's pain is increasing. Despite his brain tumours he appears to have the capacity to make decisions regarding his healthcare and he is also requesting the morphine for his pain. Following a discussion, paramedics decide to administer small aliquots of morphine to assist in the management of the patient's pain, continue to provide oxygen therapy and transport the patient to the local hospital.

On arrival at hospital, ED medical staff are clear that the ascites and pleural effusion should be drained to enable respiration and reduce the pain Mark is feeling. He can then be admitted to the palliative care unit for appropriate end-of-life care. Mark clearly states that he does not want any more tubes stuck in him. Suzanne is adamant that Mark wants to end his life, and again requests increased morphine to make her husband comfortable. Suzanne's anxiety and anger are increasing, leading to her becoming sarcastic with the ED medical staff.

Mark does not consent to the drainage procedures, however doctors argue this is an emergency case and consent is not required. You are aware that patients with capacity can refuse treatment, and feel that the patient and his wife's wishes should be upheld and a morphine infusion started as requested. You communicate these views to the others, who counter that Mark cannot really have capacity because of his cerebral metastasis and that if he was fully competent he would consent to treatment. Meanwhile Mark's lung capacity is now so compromised that his oxygen saturation levels are dropping. He is becoming drowsy and soon will lose capacity to make decisions for himself. Suzanne is getting more and more angry and threatening to call a friend who is a health lawyer to 'sort things out' and 'witness and document' this lack of care and compassion towards her husband. The relationship between Mark and Suzanne and the treating team is becoming fraught. What should happen next?

Identify the ethical problem

Ethical problems may be considered as those arising from an imbalance or misuse of power, or from a clash of underlying values and opinions. In this case we might consider the following points:

- This is an ethically serious matter.
- The patient has refused consent to the proposed medical treatment and this may hasten his death. The aim of the treating team is to preserve life.
- The patient's wishes not to receive any more active treatment are in conflict with the preferred action of the treating team, which is to relieve physical symptoms by draining fluid.
- Can staff override his autonomy, and use their power in this situation to impose the drainage procedure?
- The patient's cognitive capacity, and thus his ability to make healthcare decisions, has been questioned due to the unconfirmed possibility of brain metastasis and low oxygenation.
- Ask yourself whose interests are served by questioning the patient's capacity: the patient or the treating team?
- The patient and his wife are in a very vulnerable position: Mark is dying. They sense there may be an imposition of an unwanted treatment and may be feeling increasingly helpless due to the power imbalance in this context.

A question of central importance that must be answered in this case is, 'does Mark have capacity?' While this is largely a clinical determination, the answer to this question influences all subsequent deliberations. If he has capacity, his refusal to consent to treatment must be respected. If he doesn't, he has a clearly appointed substitute decision-maker in Suzanne, who is affirming his stated position of refusal of the procedure and request for pain relief only.

What facts are available?

- Mark is the patient.
- Mark is in the end stage of a terminal illness.
- He is dying; he appears to know and accept this.
- He has not consented to the drainage procedure.
- He appears to have capacity, but this is being questioned.
- His wife is his substitute decision-maker.
- He is in pain.
- He has requested sedation.
- There is some disagreement among the treating team.

What facts are missing

- Do his cerebral metastases influence his capacity to make a decision to refuse treatment that will prolong but not save his life?
- Do his oxygen saturation levels affect his capacity to make the decision described above?
- Does Suzanne have the legal right to make decisions on Mark's behalf?
- Are there any other family who can speak for Mark?
- Who is his regular treating doctor and team?

Consider the ethical principles

If a patient's autonomy is being respected, they will participate in shared decision-making with clinical staff at all times. This means that all efforts should be made to determine whether the patient is capable of engaging in decisions about their care. ***The law makes the fundamental presumption that all adults have capacity until proven otherwise***. If Mark has capacity, his wishes and refusal to consent must be respected. If he doesn't, we must look for ways to ascertain what his wishes are likely to be. It would appear that he has appointed a substitute decision-maker in his wife, Suzanne, to act in the way he would want. It could be argued that Suzanne's decision-making appears not to be in Mark's best interests, as it will shorten his life. It does appear though from conversations that all the emergency workers have had with Mark before he lost consciousness that he agreed with the decision not to proceed with treatment and that Suzanne was his substitute decision-maker. Both Suzanne and Mark are making the same request for pain relief, even if this shortens his life, and in refusing the drainage procedure.

Acting with beneficence means seeking to do good for the patient. What 'good' means to the patient can only be ascertained by communicating with the patient and his wife, in seeking to understand what aspects of the proposed intervention they perceive as harmful. Occasionally, what the patient perceives as 'good' and what the clinical staff regard as 'good' conflict. Disagreement over what is the best course of action should not be a trigger to question a patient's capacity.

Non-maleficence, or not causing harm, can also only be determined by taking into account what the patient perceives as harmful. Would the drainage procedure inflict additional pain and suffering on a person who has already endured enough? To what end is this procedure being performed? Are we really acting in his best interests by imposing an unwanted procedure, even if this procedure may relieve some of his physical symptoms? Does lengthening the patient's life, perhaps by only a few days, warrant the imposition of this procedure when the extreme discomfort the patient is feeling can be managed another way?

Consideration of justice usually refers to issues of resource allocation and the costs associated with patient care.[6] In a case like this, where the patient is at the end of life, the difference in life span as a consequence of this intervention may not represent a significant cost of care. In our healthcare system, considerations of cost are not usually the primary driving factor in determining what treatments are made available to patients.

Immediate impressions

- The key stakeholders in this case are the patient, his wife and members of the treating team.

- The patient has stated he is tired of being treated, saying he *does not want any more tubes stuck in him*.
- His wife is *anxious, sarcastic and angry*, possibly already in a phase of anticipatory grief.
- Members of the team may feel that their professional relevance and credibility are being undermined by a non-compliant patient.
- Healthcare staff may feel that the patient is under-equipped to make a good decision in such circumstances, and their desire to achieve the best health outcome for the patient may encourage them to act in a paternalistic way—to look for ways to override his stated wishes.
- Paramedical staff may feel guilty that the patient is now in a situation where his options are becoming more limited, and question their role in bringing a palliative care patient to the ED.
- Consider what outcome delivers the best outcome for most people. Answering this question depends upon subjective interpretations of what 'best' means in this circumstance. It also depends on whose perspective is privileged when deciding who among the 'most' count. As Verkerk et al[31] note, 'Man has almost limitless ability to convince him/herself that what s/he wants to do is morally justifiable'. The skill of ethical decision-making is the ability to see the problem from perspectives other than your own, to understand, then respectfully accept and negotiate difference.

Ethical conflicts

- There are a number of ethical conflicts—between the patient, his wife and the treating team. There are also interprofessional conflicts within the treating team, who disagree over the best course of action.
- The powerful voices within the team have a desire to intervene and relieve pain and suffering.
- The patient and his wife are rejecting the intervention.
- The different type of psychological pain and suffering being experienced by the patient and his wife demand equal consideration, but appear not to have been heard by all members of the clinical team.
- In this case, the conflict could be represented as existing between preservation of the autonomy of the patient and the desire of the treating team to do good for the patient.
- Interprofessional disagreement within the clinical team has not yet been resolved constructively.

Consider the law

- The first question that must be clarified is whether the patient has capacity. If he does, his wishes should be respected.
- If he doesn't, his wife, who is his nominated substitute decision-maker, can make healthcare decisions on his behalf, within the law, and in accordance with his values and beliefs. Mark doesn't have an advance healthcare plan, but this would only come into effect if he lacked capacity.
- Suzanne has the legal authority to make decisions for him, as though he were making them.

- Although Mark has arrived in hospital through the ED, this situation may not be a medical emergency negating the need for consent. Treatment in an emergency can *only* be undertaken to the point that averts the emergency; additional treatment without consent should not be initiated.
- Suzanne has requested sedation for her husband. This is not illegal in Australasia: sedation can be given for the purpose of relieving pain. If an unintended consequence of such pain relief is that an imminent death occurs more quickly, this is legally acceptable provided that the primary purpose of administering the drug was for pain relief only.

Consider the ethics literature

There is a very large literature (too long to review here) considering patient autonomy and refusal of treatment at end of life. The consensus of this literature would indicate that patients do have the right to refuse treatment at the end of life, even if it shortens their life. Further, their ongoing care needs still need to be met.

Make the decision

- Mark appears to have capacity and you cannot impose the procedure on him. To do so would constitute an assault or battery. If this is unclear, you may request an independent assessment. In some situations, due to time pressures or lack of appropriate personnel, this might not be possible.
- In general terms, if the patient has made a decision, appears to understand it, was not coerced and can communicate the decision, they are regarded as having capacity.
- You cannot override Mark's request, even in the ED, as he is in a position to make his wishes known. In an emergency, you can only act to the extent that the emergency is averted. You cannot intervene beyond this without patient, or substitute decision-maker, consent.
- A clinician cannot administer morphine for the sole purpose of hastening death. However, pain relief that has the unintended consequence of hastening an imminent death may be administered, but only with the primary intent of relieving pain.
- You should reassure Mark that even though he has rejected the treatment advice of the treating team, he will not be abandoned; he will receive appropriate and ongoing care, including pain relief in the last days of his life.
- Document your decision and conversations with the patient and his wife.
- Reflect on this decision and consider what you can learn for future care of patients in similar situations. You may reflect upon constructive ways to resolve disagreement within the treating team when the immediate pressure has subsided, to equip yourselves as a professional community to better cope in the future.

Initially, this process may seem onerous and overly complex; however, as you become more experienced you will learn to undertake this level of analysis as second nature in your clinical practice. It is also a good idea to de-brief with colleagues when there is a particularly challenging case, as you will learn from each other, and build a supportive and collegial community.

SEQUELAE—Another key value: Taking care of yourself

Clashing professional and personal values, differences in cultural background and expectations and the ongoing pressures of working in frequently under-resourced EDs can increase the personal burden on clinical staff.[32] Frequently when we talk about ethics and morals we have the patient in mind as the focus of our attention. This absolute focus on the patient is important, but sometimes the caregiver can get lost in this process. As we conclude this chapter, we invite you to add another very important value and ethical obligation to the many we have discussed thus far. This is the value of taking care of *you*, of treating yourself well and kindly. Having friends and interests outside of work is important. Making time for exercise and family will not only keep you physically robust, but also mentally able to face the many moral challenges that come your way. This is not entirely selfish, as work stress and overload for healthcarers has been associated with poor patient outcomes in the clinic.[33–35]

Moral distress is described as painful feelings and associated emotional and mental anguish as a result of being conscious of a morally appropriate action that despite all effort cannot be performed due to organisational or other obstacles.[36] Examples of such obstacles may include onerous policies, hierarchical power structures that inhibit action, inadequate numbers of staff, time limitations or legal constraints; all of which can undermine the provision of the best patient care.

Getting support

Empathy and support from colleagues can be most beneficial in times of moral distress and conflict. Ethical dilemmas can be difficult to resolve, and often emerge not from determining what is good or bad but from having to choose between competing 'goods' or competing 'bads'.[37] In Australia and New Zealand there are only a few facilities which have access to a hospital-based ethicist or a facility-based clinical ethics committee. If you work in an area without specialist ethics services, you may wish to discuss any ethical concerns with a team leader, director, nursing manager or trusted senior colleague. Often organisations have pastoral care or staff counselling services, the staff of which often have some ethics training. However, all healthcare staff should strengthen their competence in the area of ethical decision-making by regularly attending education sessions and seminars, or by seeking professional development through organisations such as the Australasian Association of Bioethics and Health Law (see http://aabhl.org for more information).

SUMMARY

In most cases, shared moral values, such as mutual respect, honesty, trustworthiness, compassion and a commitment to pursue shared goals, make the provision of healthcare in emergencies ethically straightforward between the carer and the patient. However, as the healthcare system grows more complex, ethical decision-making will also become more complex. In the context of emergency, anchoring practice to the underlying purpose of healthcare—which is to preserve life and relieve suffering—and considering this goal within the guiding ethical principles and processes for resolving ethical dilemmas are an essential part of practice knowledge. As with any clinical skill, regular training and updates ensure that, when required, emergency healthcare practitioners can act competently in what is likely to be a complex and urgent situation, in a way that does not add a moral burden to the patient or to themselves.

REFERENCES

1. Pellegrino ED. From medical ethics to a moral philosophy of the professions. In: Walter JK, Klein EP, eds. The story of bioethics. Washington DC: Georgetown University Press; 2003:3–15.

2. Hoffmaster B. What does vulnerability mean? Hastings Cent Rep 2006;36(2):38–45.

3. Gastmans C. A fundamental ethical approach to nursing: some proposals for ethics education. Nurs Ethics 2002;9(5):494–507.

4. Schluter J, Winch S, Holzhauser K et al. Nurses' moral sensitivity and hospital ethical climate: a literature review. Nurs Ethics 2008;15(3):304–21.

5. Tschudin V. Ethics in nursing: the caring relationship. 3rd edn. London: Elsevier; 2003.

6. Kerridge I, Lowe M, Stewart C. Ethics and law for the health professions. 3rd edn. Sydney: Federation Press; 2013.

7. Anscombe G. Modern moral philosophy. Philosophy 1958;33:1–19.

8. Aristotle. Nicomachean ethics (Apostle HG, Trans). Grinnell IO: The Peripatetic Press; 1984.

9. Fry ST, Johnstone MJ. Ethics in nursing practice. 2nd edn. Oxford: Blackwell; 2002.

10. Charon R, Montello M. Stories matter: the role of narrative in medical ethics. London: Routledge; 2002.

11. Charon R. Narrative medicine: honoring the stories of illness. New York: Oxford University Press; 2006.

12. Mayer B. Dilemmas in mandatory reporting of domestic violence: carative ethics in emergency rooms. Nursingconnections 1998;11(4): 5–21.

13. Taft A, O'Doherty L, Hegarty K et al. Screening women for intimate partner violence in healthcare settings. Cochrane Database of Systematic Reviews 2013, Issue 4.

14. Hofstede G. Culture's consequences: international differences in work-related values. London: Sage Publications; 1984.

15. International Council of Nurses. The ICN code of ethics for nurses. Geneva: International Council of Nurses; 2000.

16. Nursing and Midwifery Board of Australia. Code of ethics for nurses in Australia. Online. www.nursingmidwiferyboard.gov.au/Codes-Guidelines-Statements/Codes-Guidelines.aspx#codesofethics; accessed 17 Feb 2015.

17. Australian and New Zealand College of Paramedicine. www.anzcp.org.au/code-of-conduct/; accessed 20 July 2015.

18. National Health and Medical Research Council. Statement on ethical conduct in research involving humans. 2007. Online. www.nhmrc.gov.au/health-ethics/history-national-statement-ethical-conduct-human-research-2007; accessed 20 July 2015.

19. Health Research Council of New Zealand. HRC guidance notes on research ethics. 2014. Online. http://www.hrc.govt.nz/sites/default/files/HRC%20Guidance%20Notes%20on%20Research%20Ethics%20-%20November%202014_0.pdf; accessed 20 July 2015.

20. Beauchamp T, Childress J. Principles of biomedical ethics. 5th edn. New York: Oxford University Press; 2001.

21. Dodds S. Choice and control in feminist bioethics. In: Mackenzie C, Stoljar, N, editors. Relational autonomy in context: feminist perspective on autonomy, agency and the social self. New York: Oxford University Press; 2000:213–35.

22. Donchin A. Understanding autonomy relationally: toward a reconfiguration of bioethical principles. J Med Philos 2001;26(4):365–86.

23. Pullman D. Ethics first aid: reframing the role of 'principlism' in clinical ethics education and practice. J Clin Ethics 2005;16(3):223–9.

24. Zawistowski CA, Frader JE. Ethical problems in pediatric critical care: consent. Crit Care Med 2003;31(5):S407–10.

25. Manson NC, O'Neill O. Rethinking informed consent in bioethics. Cambridge: Cambridge University Press; 2007.

26. Luce JM. Ethical principles in critical care. JAMA 1990;263(5):696–700.

27. Townsend R, Luck M. Applied paramedic law and ethics. Elsevier Australia; 2013.

28. Childress JF. Protecting handicapped newborns. In: Milunsky A, Annas G, eds. Genetics and the law III. New York: Plenum Press; 1985.

29. Lützén K, Dahlqvist V, Eriksson S et al. Developing the concept of moral sensitivity in health care practice. Nurs Ethics 2006;13(2): 187–96.

30. Milligan E, Winch S. Practical ethics in clinical care. In Fitzgerald J, Byrne G (eds), Psychosocial dimensions in medicine. Melbourne: IP Communications, 2015.

31. Verkerk M, Lindemann H, Maeckelberghe E et al. Enhancing reflection: an interpersonal exercise in ethics education. Hastings Cent Rep 2004;34(6):31–8.

32. Corley MC, Minick P, Elswick RK et al. Nurse moral distress and ethical work environment. Nurs Ethics 2005;12(4):381–90.

33. Aiken LH, Clarke SP, Sloane DM et al. Hospital nurse staffing and patient mortality, nurse burnout, and job dissatisfaction. JAMA 2002;288(16):1987–93.

34. Cameron ME. Ethical distress in nursing. J Prof Nurs 1997;13(5):280.

35. Sundin-Huard D, Fahy K. Moral distress, advocacy and burnout: theorizing the relationships. Int J Nurs Pract 1999;5(1):8–13.

36. Jameton A. Nursing practice: the ethical issues: New Jersey: Prentice-Hall; 1984.

37. Taylor C. Sources of the self. Cambridge: Harvard University Press; 1989.

CHAPTER 4

EMERGENCY CARE AND THE LAW

RUTH TOWNSEND

Essentials

- It is important to understand the relationship between law, ethics and professionalism to ensure optimum patient care is able to be provided.
- Nurse practitioners and paramedics need to understand the legal framework in relation to privacy, consent, the doctrine of necessity, restraint, negligence, vicarious liability and complaint-making.
- There is a range of processes and procedures that health practitioners need to know in relation to the Coroner's Court.
- Consent is required prior to intervention unless the patient is lacking competence and life saving care is required.
- Health practitioners must work to a standard of competence that is determined by the practitioner peer group and that is 'reasonable' for a practitioner with specific skills.
- There is a hierarchy of people who can be responsible for patients that lack competence. The 'person responsible' must be consulted as the surrogate decision-maker for those who are unable, due to incapacity, to make decisions regarding healthcare for themselves.
- Competent patients have the right to refuse treatment, even if it results in their death.
- If it is necessary to restrict the liberty of a mentally ill patient, it should be carried out in the least restrictive way possible.

Disclaimer: The law recited in this chapter is predominantly NSW and Commonwealth law but reference has been made to general principles. Where possible, reference has been made to corresponding law in other states and it is advisable that practitioners in those states refer directly to that law.

INTRODUCTION

Emergency nurses and paramedics frequently find themselves faced with legal issues within the workplace. These include issues of privacy, consent, negligence and the restriction of personal liberties. It is important that health practitioners understand the law that governs their practice. Our society is structured around a legal system that was adopted from an English system of rules that were essentially designed to govern a community's behaviour and, more specifically, an individual's behaviour within that community. Laws are shaped by societal values and are designed to reflect those. The law is both prescriptive and punitive in the sense that there are laws that establish boundaries of behaviour and there are laws which punish those who do not comply. The system developed into what is now known as common law and statutory or parliamentary-made law.

This chapter will explore the responsibilities of health professionals to comply with the law and the particular pieces of law that most commonly apply to them, and why it is important to do so. We will start with a brief explanation of what the law is.

What is the law?

The law is a system of rules and regulations that are designed to ensure that individual human rights, such as our rights to liberty, justice and equality, are able to be upheld. A law is a rule that comes from a legitimate authority, for example, a democratically elected parliament, and applies to everyone equally. Laws are created to make sure that everyone in a society understands what is expected of them as a member of that society (obligations and duties) and what they can expect from others, including the government (their rights). An example of a law made by the parliament that sets out the rules of behaviour is the Crimes Act.

In addition to setting out the rules by which we live, another function of the legal system is to resolve disputes. The resolution of disputes commonly occurs in civil law matters. For example, contract law is an example of civil law. A contract is an agreement made between two or more parties. Sometimes disputes arise as to the terms of the contract. This dispute can be resolved by the court.

Different types of laws

Common law

Common law is based on principles that have arisen in previous decisions made in cases relating to certain facts and reapplying those principles to new cases. This form of law allows for expansion and development of the law, as each case contributes to the body of law in that area. This is also known as case law or precedent.

Parliamentary law

Parliamentary (or statute) law is also known as legislation and referred to as an Act. This law is made by the people we elect to parliament as our representatives. This law is often written to accommodate the social and technological changes that occur within our society. There are various pieces of statutory law that apply to nurses, midwives and paramedics. There is also subordinate legislation that is referred to as Regulations. Regulations have the force of the law and usually contain a lot of details that are not present in the Act, thus allowing the law to be updated and amended to change with time. This allows the law to be more flexible.

Branches of law

The law is divided into many branches but for the purposes of this chapter we will briefly outline the difference between criminal law and civil law. A criminal case deals with a crime which is an offence against the Crown and punishable by fine or imprisonment, whereas a civil case generally involves disputes between citizens involving liability for damages (such as in a motor vehicle accident) or breach of contract.

Legal jurisdictions

Both criminal and civil cases are dealt with in the general courts (in NSW, the Local Court, the District Court and the Supreme Court), but there are other courts and tribunals which deal with legal issues outside the general courts. There is, for example, a Land and Environment Court, a Workers Compensation Commission, an Administrative Appeals Tribunal. Matters relating to the healthcare decisions of a minor or incompetent patient may be heard by an Administrative Tribunal; matters related to unexpected or unexplained deaths are heard by the Coroner in the Coroner's Court; other criminal or civil matters, like assault or negligence, will be heard by the Supreme Court. There are many others. One legal jurisdiction that is particularly relevant to healthcare staff is the professional regulatory jurisdiction that hears matters pertaining to professional competency and patient safety. We will examine that area first.

Professional competency and patient safety

In July 2010 the National Health Practitioner Regulation Agency (AHPRA) became the national registering body for many health practitioners in Australia, including medical and nursing professionals. The legislation regulating health practitioners is the Health Practitioner Regulation National Law of each state and territory. For example, in the ACT it is called the *Health Practitioner Regulation National Law Act 2010*; in the Northern Territory it is the *Health Practitioner Regulation (National Uniform Legislation) Act 2010*.

Paramedics are not currently included in the scheme. There is a national process considering whether paramedics will be included on the register but, at the time of printing, paramedics are still not included. There have been a number of pieces written that make comment on paramedic registration.[1-3]

The purpose of AHPRA is to offer protection and minimise risks to the public from harm by the actions of registered health professionals by ensuring that health practitioners maintain levels of professional competency, meet core educational standards and are subject to a disciplinary mechanism for those who are underperforming and potentially putting patients at risk. There is a mechanism for practitioners who have an impairment to be offered support to manage their condition while also protecting them from any potential risks to patients. There is also an easily accessible mechanism that allows the public or employers to check whether a paramedic has significant health, conduct or performance issues that may threaten patient safety.

This makes the lack of registration of paramedics, who perform intimate procedures on patients in an unmonitored environment, even more difficult to understand. There are, however, alternative laws that regulate non-registered health practitioners like paramedics in some states. These laws were developed to manage the unscrupulous behaviour of some 'alternative' health practitioners who are commonly not regulated by an employer the way that the bulk of paramedics are. Unregistered providers of health services are regulated by an enforceable statutory code of conduct in NSW and South Australia.[4] Queensland was due to introduce a similar system in 2014. The Victorian government announced in late 2014 that it will consider establishing a state-based registration system for paramedics based on the national AHPRA model.[5]

What is a 'health professional'?

The ACT *Health Professionals Act* defines 'health professional' as anyone who provides a health service, but in explicitly defining a health professional makes no reference to paramedics. The Northern Territory's *Health Practitioners Act* defines health practitioners as those who are registered or enrolled. Paramedics are not registered health practitioners and may therefore not be deemed to be 'professional' for the purposes of some legislation. In NSW the legislation applying to paramedics refers to them as 'ambulance officers', yet the NSW Ambulance Service uses the term 'paramedic'. The lack of consistency in terms used to describe paramedics is a reason for them to become registered with AHPRA, have the title paramedic protected and practitioners recognised as healthcare professionals. For further information see the reference below.[2]

What is in a name? Who is a 'paramedic' at law?

The title 'paramedic' is not protected by law in the way 'registered nurse' or 'medical practitioner' is protected. In essence, this means that any person can lawfully call themselves a paramedic. Not only does the title have no legal meaning, there are no prescribed qualifications that are required to be met in order to call oneself a paramedic. Someone with a first aid certificate is just as legitimately able to call themselves a paramedic as someone with a degree in paramedicine who is employed by a paramedic service. There is a risk that while the title remains unprotected it is open to being abused and causing damage to the reputation of the whole 'paramedic' community. It also risks harm to patients who may have an expectation that someone calling themselves a 'paramedic' will deliver a certain level of care. For the purposes of this text, the term 'paramedics' will refer to those out-of-hospital care workers employed by a private or public ambulance service to provide medical care and transportation.[2]

Complaints handling

Complaints against health professionals and paramedics are referred to the relevant state or territory complaint authority (for example in NSW it is the Health Care Complaints Commission). If the matter is investigated and it is deemed serious enough, it may be referred on to a disciplinary hearing by the respective authority. For example, in Victoria the Victorian Civil and Administrative Tribunal will hear cases regarding the professional actions of medical practitioners and nurses practising in Victoria. In NSW, matters against nurses will be heard by the NSW Nurses and Midwives Tribunal. In South Australia it may be heard by the District or Supreme Court.

Section 140 of the *National Law Act* requires healthcare practitioners to make a mandatory notification to AHPRA if the practitioner forms a reasonably belief that the practitioner has engaged in any of the following. Again the emphasis is placed on protecting patients from harm. Notification is required if you or another practitioner you know has:

a) practised the practitioner's profession while intoxicated by alcohol or drugs; or
b) engaged in sexual misconduct in connection with the practice of the practitioner's profession; or
c) placed the public at risk of substantial harm in the practitioner's practice of the profession because the practitioner has an impairment; or
d) placed the public at risk of harm because the practitioner has practised the profession in a way that constitutes a significant departure from accepted professional standards.

An impairment is defined as 'a physical or mental impairment, disability, condition or disorder (including substance abuse or dependence) that detrimentally affects or is likely to detrimentally affect the person's capacity to practise the profession'. The notification applies to healthcare students who are registered with AHPRA and who suffer an impairment during their clinical training for the program of study they are undertaking and as arranged by their education provider. A voluntary notification can be made by anyone at any time if they believe they are impaired and unable to practise safely.

In March 2014, AHPRA published revised guidelines on mandatory reporting obligations.[6]

Level of professional misconduct

Under the *National Law Act* a registered practitioner may be sanctioned in a number of ways. The Act provides for a determination that a professional has engaged in unsatisfactory professional performance, unprofessional conduct or professional misconduct.[7]

'Unsatisfactory professional performance' is when the practitioner is found to have 'knowledge, skill or judgement possessed, or care exercised by, the practitioner in the practice of the health profession in which the practitioner is registered is below the standard reasonably expected of a health practitioner of an equivalent level of training or experience'.[8] 'Unprofessional conduct' means conduct of a lesser standard than that which might reasonably be expected and includes contravening a condition of registration, conviction of an offence under another Act that may affect the practitioner's suitability to practise, over-servicing, accepting, offering or giving benefit as inducement or reward for a referral to another health service provider or making such a referral when the practitioner has a pecuniary interest in giving it.[8] The most serious disciplinary charge is that of 'professional misconduct' which includes unprofessional conduct that is substantially below the standard reasonably expected of a health professional with equivalent training and experience; or more than one instance of unprofessional conduct; or that the professional's conduct within or outside their professional practice is inconsistent with the professional being a 'fit and proper[9] person' to hold registration in the profession. 'Fit and proper person' has been difficult for the court to define, but in essence it refers to a person's character as having three elements, 'honesty, knowledge and ability',[10] and 'in whom the public … may therefore have confidence'.[11] The Tribunal's decisions are publicly available, which is in part designed to allow the public to maintain their faith in the integrity of the system and to offer reassurance that those practitioners who do pose a risk to the public are made publicly known.[12]

This type of transparency is not currently available when it comes to paramedics. Because paramedics do not fall under the aegis of AHPRA the disciplinary procedures are not undertaken in a public forum. Most paramedic disciplinary matters are dealt with in-house by the employer of the paramedic. If the matter complained of is criminal in nature, it may be subject to a criminal investigation and hearing in a criminal court. This might also apply if the matter is civil in nature, for example, a case of negligence, in which case the matter can be tested in a civil court. The outcome of both those types of matters is quite separate from the employer's authority to retain or dismiss the paramedic. That is, regardless of the outcome of a civil matter for negligence, the paramedic may still be able to be employed by an ambulance service, public or private, somewhere in Australia. Those registered health practitioners who have an adverse finding made against them under the AHPRA scheme will have that finding available for any current or future employer.

The Coroner's Court

The role of the Coroner's Court is an ancient one. The role of the Coroner is to determine the manner and cause of a person's death or to determine the identity of a deceased person where the identity is not known. In general, the Coroner investigates deaths that are violent or unnatural; sudden and of unknown cause; deaths in suspicious or unusual circumstances; deaths during or following surgery or other invasive procedures, or deaths that occur in custody. The role of the Coroner is not to make a finding of guilt or innocence in a case, but to instead establish the way in which a death has occurred and recommend actions that may prevent such a death from occurring in the future. For example, in the past the Coroner has recommended the introduction of the compulsory fencing of swimming pools to prevent toddler drownings.[13] More applicable in the hospital environment are recommendations made by the Coroner that have led to the development of protocols and procedures which may help to reduce the risk of a reoccurrence of an incident that has previously come before the Coroner.

Preparation of body for Coroner

After a patient's death, provided this death falls under the jurisdiction of the coroner, it is necessary for hospital staff to contact the police. The police may wish to take statements from staff and gather evidence. The body should be left exactly as it was at the time death was declared. All interventions should remain in situ, including IV lines, drainage bags, catheters, endotracheal tubes, defibrillation pads, dressings and the like. These should obviously be capped or sealed as necessary. The body can then be transported to the morgue as per hospital procedure and, if necessary, arrangements can be made for a post-mortem. For paramedics working in regional areas, the body may be placed in a body bag and transported to the morgue, but only after the paramedic has contacted the patient's doctor and/or the police. The requirements and circumstances in which this must occur should be set out in procedure manuals.

Appearance at Coroner's Court

If a health practitioner is called to appear before the coroner they can expect that the following processes will occur. Note the points about record-keeping and the stages at which the practitioner is advised to seek advice.

1. They will be approached by police to give a statement pertaining to an event in which they have been a witness or directly involved. The role of the police in Coroner's Court proceedings is to work to assist the coroner by gathering information that will assist the court to identify the circumstances surrounding an event. A practitioner has the right to refuse to give evidence until they have received legal advice. Each person has a right to refuse to give

evidence if they feel they might incriminate themselves. However, this protection was altered by a change in the law in 2000 (s 61 of the NSW Act) which enables the Coroner to require a person objecting to giving evidence on the grounds of self-incrimination to give evidence, but they are given a certificate which prevents that evidence being given against the witness in other court proceedings. If a practitioner does not cooperate with the police, a subpoena may be issued by the court that will compel this witness to attend. If that person does not attend they may be arrested. Note that it is advisable to give evidence or make statements as close to the time of the incident as possible. Contemporaneous evidence is most reliable and is most highly sought. It is advisable to keep a copy of the statement made. If a request for a statement comes some time after the event it may be necessary to access a copy of the patient's notes from records storage and review them. This is where good documentation serves an important purpose.

2. Prior to making a statement it may be necessary to seek legal advice from your employer's legal representatives or, if there is a conflict, contact your own solicitor or union solicitor.

3. A subpoena will be issued stating date, time and location to appear.

4. When the practitioner arrives at court they should check that the case has been listed and in which court it will be heard.

5. The practitioner should notify the court officer they have arrived.

6. The practitioner waits outside the court until called.

7. They are called to the stand to give evidence, at which time they will be asked to take an oath or an affirmation.

8. The practitioner will be asked to give their account of events, which may involve revisiting the contents of their statement.

9. The rules of evidence do not apply in the Coroner's Court as they do in other courts, so the way in which evidence is presented is different. For example, the practitioner may be called upon to give hearsay evidence—evidence of what they have heard someone else say. This is not normally permitted in court, but there are provisions within the Coroner's Act that authorise a Coroner holding an inquest or inquiry to not be bound to observe the rules of procedure and evidence applicable to proceedings before a court of law. This is because the purpose of the Coroner is not to make a determination as to a person's guilt, but rather to establish the truth of a matter.

10. The practitioner may be cross-examined but the purpose of the coroner's inquest is not to put the healthcare practitioner on trial. Instead, its purpose is to ascertain the circumstances surrounding an incident in the hope that such information will lead to a satisfactory explanation of the events that have led to the inquest.

11. Only if the Coroner determines there is enough evidence to suggest that a witness is guilty of a criminal offence will the matter be referred to the Director of Public Prosecutions (DPP) for further examination. There are

very few instances of practitioners being pursued by the DPP in this regard.[14] It is more likely that if the coroner finds the healthcare staff negligent they will refer the matter to the relevant disciplinary body for investigation and possible disciplinary action.[15] In NSW, paramedics may also be referred to the HCCC and in other states referred to their employer's professional standards unit.

Autopsy

A young man dies and the cause of his death is unclear. Ordinarily a matter like this would be referred to the coroner and an autopsy would be conducted to establish the cause of death. The magistrate may exercise his/her discretion in determining whether an autopsy should be performed. If the autopsy would cause the family distress then it may be that no autopsy will be undertaken. However, if the manner of death is unexpected and unexplained, then it is likely that the magistrate would order the autopsy to go ahead because it is in the public's interest that the cause of death be established so that a similar death may be able to be prevented in the future.

Investigations and court

Making a statement

The healthcare system is complex. Mistakes are made and oversights and omissions occur. From time to time this may result in an internal or external investigation being undertaken. The most common way in which an investigator will engage those staff who might be able to help them with their investigation is via an interview. This interview may form part of or remain separate from a formal oral statement that you may also give. You may be asked to provide a written statement of your experience, knowledge and understanding of a certain event or series of events. An affidavit is a written statement sworn as to the truth of its contents before a legal representative or justice of the peace. This statement can be used in court. It is always advisable to seek legal advice before providing a statement, even to your employer, so as to avoid self-incrimination.[16] You may prepare a statement yourself or have your lawyer or other person draft it for you. It is an offence to give a false or misleading statement.[17]

However, although each individual has the right to refuse to give a statement, there may be occasions where remaining silent is not in the healthcare practitioner's best interest. For example, if there is an innocent explanation for a sequence of events that occurred or if the practitioner has a sound alibi, then offering the explanation or alibi may relieve the practitioner of having to engage in any further discussion regarding the events and they should be forthcoming with this information.

If a practitioner is required to give a statement of events, the statement should be precise and factual. It should be written in numbered paragraphs and should commence with the practitioner's name and, if relevant to the inquiry, place of work and role. A chronological recitation of events leading up to and including the event being examined is almost always what is required. Statements may include conversations that the writer has engaged in directly. For instance, 'The patient said "I have some pain in my chest". You [the practitioner] asked, "How long have you had it for?"' Avoid attempting to interpret or explain this direct evidence. Simply recite exactly what happened without embellishment. Where possible, avoid the use of hearsay in statements as hearsay is only admissible as evidence in certain circumstances or in certain jurisdictions, for instance, the Coroner's Court in NSW. An example of hearsay is, 'When I went to the nurses' station, Jill B said that the patient's wife had told her yesterday that the patient was complaining of chest pain.' This is hearsay because the patient's complaint was not heard directly by the nurse making the statement. Just as with any evidence it is advisable to recite only what you heard, saw, did, when and where.

Legal privilege

In some circumstances the issue of privilege arises between professionals and their clients. For healthcare professionals in all states, with the exception of Tasmania,[18] this is not the case. Nurses in these states are compellable and thus required, if asked, to disclose patient information in court. The sharing of confidential patient information with the court is an authorised disclosure of personal information. If the witness has any doubt as to whether it is lawful to share private patient information in court, the witness can ask the judge hearing the matter, or their lawyer, for clarification as to whether the information can or should be disclosed. The exception to this rule is in sexual assault communications. In these cases any counselling communication that is made by, to or about a victim or alleged victim of sexual assault may not be compellable as evidence in court.[19]

Victim impact statements

If the practitioner is the victim of a crime (for instance, is assaulted in the workplace) and the crime is prosecuted, the practitioner will be required to make a statement to police regarding the matter. Once the case has been heard and the offence found proved, the victim (practitioner) may have the opportunity to write a victim impact statement, which can be taken into account by the judge when considering the appropriate sentence.[20] This statement is presented to the court and explains how the crime has harmed the victim. A practitioner may not have been directly injured as a result of the crime but instead have been a witness to it and suffered some loss as a result of witnessing the event. A victim impact statement may also be written in this instance.[21] If someone is physically unable to write the statement themselves then they may have someone else do it for them.

The preservation and collection of evidence

Often patients will present to an emergency department (ED) as a result of being involved in a criminal offence, such as an assault. In this instance it is a healthcare practitioner's first priority and duty to provide care to the patient. However, there may be moments during the care and treatment of the patient when it is possible for healthcare staff to gather and preserve evidence for the police to use at a future time for the purposes of investigating the incident.

Police are generally interested in any object or item left either with a victim, offender or witness at a scene of inquiry, no matter how insignificant it may appear to be. Advances in forensic science, specifically in the area of DNA testing, mean that a wide range of evidence is now suitable for analysis by police, to assist them in determining the events surrounding an offence.

The general rule with the gathering of evidence is simply, 'Don't touch'. However, it is unlikely that in all circumstances this will be possible. The rule then is that if a piece of evidence is handled, the handling is minimised. Staff should wear fresh gloves when handling evidence so as not to contaminate it with DNA from themselves or elsewhere. It should be noted, however, that even gloves can smear fingerprints.

It is important that staff note the placement of certain objects and note who has touched what, where and why. This documentation is important so that the *chain of evidence* remains intact. The chain of evidence is necessary for police to demonstrate that evidence has not been tainted or tampered with. This maintains the integrity of the exhibit so that it may be used in court proceedings. These rules apply equally to all medical professionals, including doctors, nurses and paramedics. It is also important for staff to be aware of the evidence they may inadvertently discard. For instance, the gloves worn by healthcare workers handling materials may come into contact with items of interest, so the gloves themselves can also be gathered as evidence. Other materials used by or taken from a patient suspected of being involved in an event that may be of interest to the police should be placed in a contaminated waste bag assigned to that patient only and passed on to the police at a later time. Almost any item has the potential to hold incriminating evidence so, as a general rule, everything that is used on the patient should be preserved. To wilfully destroy evidence is an offence.[22]

If emergency staff, including paramedics, have reason to believe that their patient has been involved in an event that might be of interest to the police, then they should do all they can to assist the police. For example, a patient presents to emergency with a knife impaled in their body. It is important that someone notes the position of the knife prior to its removal. This position should be documented with the names of all persons who come into contact with the knife and the reasons why it was removed. This procedure should be followed for any piece of evidence removed from a person.

Paper bags are the preferred vessel for storage. Paper preserves evidence for a longer period of time than plastic. Plastic sweats and therefore is more likely to destroy or affect the quality of the evidence. Once clothing, weaponry, drugs, personal items, or the like are gathered by the emergency staff, the items should be placed in a paper bag or box and stored in a secure area. This area could be a safe; alternatively, security staff could be required to supervise the items until police arrive. Refer to local hospital policy in these cases.

It should be noted that police do have the power to seize exhibits if they suspect that an indictable (serious) offence has been committed.[23] Relatives may ask to hold on to a patient's possessions but police do have the authority to seize such items for the purpose of ascertaining information regarding the offence. The only item police are not authorised to seize is the Sexual Assault Investigation Kit. Police are only entitled to seize this item if the patient has signed the relevant documentation permitting them to do so. Police can seize any clothing or other items belonging to the patient. See Chapter 40 for clinical discussion of sexual assault victims.

Paramedics: pre-hospital trauma teams and evidence

Health and emergency service workers in the pre-hospital environment should also be aware that their actions can directly affect the ability of police to gather and preserve evidence. While it is understood that the priority for health workers in this setting is the health and wellbeing of the patient, workers should be mindful of the way in which they enter and work in the environment. If, for instance, paramedics are called to a 'concern for welfare' case or are called to attend a scene by the police, they should be aware of the way their presence at the scene may disturb it. For example, if an intruder has accessed premises unlawfully and is known to have walked across the middle of the room, leaving behind evidence of their presence, and a paramedic, called to that scene, also proceeds across the middle of the room, evidence of this movement will be left as well. It is recommended that rescue parties approaching a scene like this walk around the edge of the room rather than down its centre, thus leaving the evidence of the intruder's pathway undisturbed. Where practicable, pre-hospital care teams should try to preserve as much evidence as possible. This includes items such as the gloves they wear. DNA evidence from the patient may also become embedded in the officer's uniforms. They should be mindful of evidence such as blood splatter and make all attempts to ensure that it remains untouched. Pre-hospital care teams may also take note of anything touched, moved, noticed or smelt at the scene. This may be called upon at a later date as evidence in court.

In the case of *Jackson v Lithgow City Council* [2010] NSW CA 136, the court considered the question of whether the records made by ambulance officers attending the scene of a man who had allegedly fallen 1.5 metres were admissible as evidence of that fact which the man was attempting to prove in his case of negligence against the council. The records showed that the recording officer had written next to Patient History: *"? Fall from 1.5 metres on to concrete."* The question mark appearing in the record suggested that the height and indeed the fall was not confirmed. Neither of the officers were called to give evidence and so the court was asked to consider if the documentation provided any admissible evidence that could contribute to the case. The court accepted that the document added a legitimate opinion (an inference) that from all that he or they could see there was a question whether the plaintiff had fallen off the wall. The inference (and thus the opinion) was based upon what the ambulance officers perceived. This case demonstrates the importance of taking and recording accurate notes of events and findings at the scene as they can later be used and relied upon in court for a variety of reasons.

Blood alcohol testing

If a person over the age of 15 years presents to the ED for examination or treatment as a result of a motor vehicle accident, has been a pedestrian, cyclist, horse rider, motorboat or train driver, then it is the duty of the medical officer to take a sample of the patient's blood for analysis, whether or not the patient consents, and within 12 hours of the patient presenting.[24] If no medical officer is present, the blood or urine sample is to be taken by the Registered Nurse attending the patient. It is an offence to fail to take a sample. The penalty for failing to take a sample is $2200. The defences to the offence include believing that the patient was younger than 15 years, that they had not been involved in a motor vehicle accident or that to take the sample would in some way impair the patient's care and treatment.[25] It is an offence for a person to prevent a health professional from obtaining a sample for the purposes of the Act.[26]

Child victims

In dealing with a child suspected of being the victim of an offence, medical personnel should first treat the child's injuries. However, at no time should medical personnel attempt to elicit evidence from the child about the circumstances surrounding the child's injuries. For example, medical staff should not ask, 'Who did this to you?' To do so could compromise future court proceedings against any offender. It is the responsibility of teams such as the Joint Investigative Response Team (NSW) to gather evidence from the child. This team, made up of Child Protection Unit police officers and Department of Family and Community Services (FACS) staff, are specially trained for this purpose. The medical staff should notify police that they believe such an investigation is required.[27] See Chapter 40 for clinical aspects. All staff have a mandatory duty to report any cases where they believe a child is the victim of abuse.[28]

Child Protection Act[29] and mandatory reporting

Law

Child protection laws fall under the 'protective' jurisdiction of the court. This jurisdiction also covers mental health patients and those under guardianship. Every parent or guardian has responsibility to ensure the care and protection of their child until that child turns 18 years of age. The definition of maltreatment of a child varies in each state and territory, but broadly the term encompasses neglect and sexual, physical or emotional abuse. That is, omitting to provide care is considered maltreatment just as assaulting a child is considered maltreatment. The scope of the area is too large to be effectively covered in this chapter, but each healthcare provider should have a policy in place to assist staff to take action if they suspect that a child is a victim of neglect or abuse.

Mandatory reporting

It is an offence in every state and territory for nominated health professionals to fail to report suspected child abuse or neglect to the authorities. Paramedics are not covered by the legislative requirement to make a mandatory report, but there is the provision for paramedics to make a voluntary report and some ambulance services may have a policy in place that requires staff to make a mandatory report as part of the terms of their employment.[30] The Australian Institute of Family Studies provides a summary of the various legislative provisions around mandatory reporting in its publication titled 'Mandatory reporting of child abuse'.[31]

A person who reports a suspected case of abuse, in good faith, cannot be considered to have breached privacy laws and cannot be sued for defamation. On the contrary, it is more likely there could be ramifications for a healthcare professional if they fail to report.

Prenatal reporting

In some states and territories, a person who reasonably believes that a child, once born, may be at risk of harm and in need of care and protection, may make a report to the Director-General of child-care and protection. It is important to note that a report cannot be made to protect the baby while in utero. This provision only allows for care and protection to be given once the child has been born alive.[32]

Documentation

In nursing and paramedicine there exists a culture of verbal hand-over of information regarding a patient and their condition.[33,34] While the verbal exchange of this information has its place in the healthcare setting, this information should also be recorded in the patient's healthcare record. Records can be used in a variety of ways. For example, they can allow for the exchange of information between different parties, they can be used as evidence that something has or has not been done and they can be used to record incidents that occurred, for the purposes of implementing effective risk management measures. The guide to effective record keeping is:

1. Records should be accurate. Pre-printed fourth-hourly observation charts can cause problems with accuracy. For example, it is not accurate to say the patient's temperature was 38°C at 1800 hrs when the temperature was taken at 1825 hrs.
2. They should be written contemporaneously, that is, at the time of the event.
3. They should be brief and objective. They should not be embellished with interpretation.
4. They should be legible.
5. They should avoid the use of abbreviations and jargon unless this is widely used and accepted in the healthcare community. This avoidance limits misunderstanding among the allied health workforce who all contribute to the patient's integrated record.
6. Errors should be left in the report with a simple line drawn through them.
7. The report should be written for the correct patient. Just as with medication, the notes should be checked to ensure that the notes refer to the patient being written about.
8. Patients should be referred to by name, not number alone.
9. Do not write notes on behalf of someone else. Write only what *you* saw, heard or did.
10. Read the patient's notes. Do not just rely on a verbal hand-over.

The more information recorded in the patient's health record, the better able the healthcare practitioner is to accurately recall issues surrounding the event. Courts will rely on not only oral evidence, but also written evidence. A case may not get to court until some time after the incident that led to the proceedings, and a witness's recollection of events over time can become clouded and unreliable. This can lead the court to question the witness's credibility and the evidence they give may not be able to be relied upon. This highlights the importance of keeping good written records.

In *Micallef & Anor v Minister for Health of the State of Western Australia*,[35] a couple with five children commenced action against the state's Minister for Health for negligence because the wife had undergone a tubal ligation and fallen pregnant two years later. The action was based on failure to inform. The couple argued that they had not been told of the risks of falling pregnant again following a tubal ligation carried out by caesarean section, as opposed to the lower risks of the procedure failing if it were carried out laparascopically. The court dismissed the matter, preferring the doctor's evidence to the applicants'. The doctor was able to show that he had a standard procedure for informing patients of risks associated with procedures, that he personally believed the procedure should be performed laparascopically and that he had made contemporaneous notes regarding the event, unlike the applicants who relied on their memory.

> **PRACTICE TIP**
>
> Complete documentation during and immediately after treating your patient to ensure that it is contemporaneous. This will also help with accuracy and completeness.

Personally Controlled Electronic Health Care Record (PCEHR)

A Personally Controlled Electronic Health Care Record (PCEHR) is an electronic form of medical records that, as the name suggests, is able to be controlled by the patient to some extent. Where previously medical records were only able to be owned, at law, by the creator of that record, under the laws governing the PCEHR, patients are able to legally own and make notes in their own healthcare record. With regard to patient control over the record, there will be a section of the record for personal information that the patient can control and change as they wish. There will also be a clinical component of the record. Within the clinical component of the record, blood test results may be listed on the record. These results cannot be altered by the patient but the patient can control who sees that part of the record. The record will include the patient's prescribed medication, test results, care plans, immunisations and health alerts, such as allergies. The electronic nature of the record means that, with the patient's permission, the record is able to be accessed by the patient or their doctor anywhere in Australia at any time and would be likely to prove invaluable in an emergency.

There are a number of reasons for implementing the e-health system, including to assist in the reduction of high rate of medical errors that occur from inadequate patient information, reduce unnecessary hospital admissions and save doctors from collecting a full medical history each time they see a new patient.

There have been some difficulties in implementing the national opt-in program that has meant the e-health record is not able to be utilised in all health facilities, including paramedic services where a localised form of electronic record-taking is used.

Confidentiality

In order to ascertain the information needed to safely and effectively treat patients, healthcare workers rely on their patients to disclose personal details to them which they would not necessarily disclose to others. Healthcare practitioners encourage their patients to disclose this information on the basis that the information disclosed will remain confidential and will not be discussed with others without the patient's permission. A breach of confidentiality is *any* disclosure of a person's healthcare record without permission. This disclosure may include verbal, written or electronic communication of any sort with respect to the patient and/or the institution's records.[36]

Healthcare workers and public or private health organisations owe a common law duty of confidentiality to their patients. Confidentiality extends to all patients within that facility, whether the healthcare practitioner directly cares for them or not. If confidentiality is breached the healthcare worker can be prosecuted by the patient and/or institution and may be required to pay the injured party damages. They may also face a disciplinary charge by their respective health board.

There are several exceptions to the rule with respect to the disclosure of confidential personal information. Along with the patient agreeing to the disclosure they also include the mandatory reporting of child abuse, the mandatory reporting of infectious diseases (although this may be de-identified information), there is a duty to the public to disclose, by the order of a court for the assistance of police in the investigation of an offence, by subpoena for a civil action or by a government Minister.

Privacy

All public or private sector health service providers are subject to the provisions of the Privacy Act in each state and territory,[37] which aims to regulate the way in which private institutions collect and use personal information. In NSW, the *Health Records and Information Privacy Act 2002 and Regulation 2012* is intended to promote the fair and responsible handling of health information by health service providers and to protect the privacy of an individual's health information, whether it is held by the public or private sector. There is equivalent legislation in South Australia and Victoria. The Act was designed to enhance and promote the individual's ability to be informed about their healthcare and to assist individuals to access their healthcare information. It is designed to allow individuals access to a dispute resolution process regarding the handling of their health information should such a process be required.

In the case of *M v Health Service Provider (2006) PrivCmrA 12* the complainant had undergone a number of tests for a sexually transmitted disease. The patient complained to the health service provider that a staff member had disclosed these tests to the complainant's partner. The matter was investigated and it was discovered that the disclosures had been made by a new employee who knew not to disclose the results but did not understand that the types of tests undertaken should also not be disclosed. An apology was made. This did not satisfy the patient who complained to the Privacy Commissioner stating that they had suffered hurt and embarrassment as a result of the disclosure. The complainant was awarded compensation.

Incident reports

Most health services have an incident management system that is used to improve patient safety and support improvements and maintenance of quality clinical practice. Incident reports allow for the identification of work practices, equipment or environments that can lead to a lower quality of service being provided to a consumer, or that may pose a risk to staff or visitors of a facility. Any accident or near-miss is able to be reported anonymously and able to be investigated by the administration to allow it to put in place policy, procedures and resources to limit the possibility of an accident re-occurring. Once a service becomes aware of an incident or accident they have an obligation to take 'reasonable' measures to address the matter.

Incident reports should contain information on the date, time and place of the incident, the names and details of the parties concerned, a brief but factual and accurate account of the incident with no hearsay or personal interpretation of the events, the harm that the incident caused, any action taken and by whom, including, for example, that faulty equipment has been decommissioned and labelled in compliance with Workplace Safety requirements. They can be relied on as a legal document.

Incident Management Systems are designed to encourage staff to feel that they will not be punished if they admit they have made an error. It stipulates that the obligation of reporting such incidents rests with the individual healthcare worker. It is an attempt when an error is made to move the focus of blame from the individual to the system.

Open disclosure

If an adverse event occurs and the practitioner believes that they have contributed to it, there is provision at law for health practitioners to make an honest expression of regret to a patient.

Assault and consent

Assault

There is a legal requirement that healthcare practitioners obtain the consent of their patient prior to performing any form of intervention upon them. Without this consent any attempt to treat the patient could be considered unlawful and amount to a tort of assault or battery upon that person. Today there are typically few instances where a distinction is made between assault and battery. Assault is the threat of harm one may feel from another. This may not involve any actual physical contact. It is sufficient that a patient simply feels that they will be subjected to a form of treatment to which they have not consented for it to constitute an assault. Battery is the actual physical action of touching someone without consent. The patient does not have to have sustained any injury for it to be a battery. It is the physical contact without consent that constitutes the battery. An assault may fall within the criminal or the civil jurisdiction. Even if a healthcare practitioner states that they contacted the patient with all good intentions, it may not amount to a defence for assault or battery.[38] For the purposes of this chapter assault includes battery.

There are exceptions to the law of assault. Accidentally making contact with someone in public is an example. Another is 'reasonable force' used by police officers in performing their duty.[39] In EDs healthcare staff often deal with patients in a 'time critical' environment where the patient is unable to give consent to contact and in these instances staff must be able to explain their interference with the patient in a legally justifiable

way or risk being charged with assault. This legal justification exists in the form of the 'doctrine of necessity'.

> **PRACTICE TIP**
>
> To avoid issues of assault and as a matter of professional courtesy, it is best, wherever possible, to ask your patient's permission to do something to them before doing it.

Doctrine of necessity

Time-critical life-and-death decisions are made on an almost daily basis in any ED and by paramedics. Often patients who present to emergency are unconscious or incompetent and therefore unable to give or refuse consent to treatment. In these circumstances, under the doctrine of necessity, staff are able to treat patients who are unable to give consent to or refuse treatment, without the risk of litigation for assault.[40] That is, where it is not possible to communicate with the patient and treatment is needed to preserve life or reduce the risk of further harm and where treatment is given in the best interests of the patient, it can be given without the patient's consent (see also below, 'When consent is not required').

Consent

In the medical context, consent is the permission given by one person to another to lawfully touch them. Consent is arguably the strongest representation of patient autonomy and the principle of self-determination is necessary to avoid a claim of battery or charge of assault. Failure to obtain informed consent may also lead to claims of negligence but informed consent is different from consent per se (see below). Consent from a patient is required for direct or indirect touching and both major **and** minor treatment. Consent can be given in writing, verbally or implied. When a patient sees you approaching with a sphygmomanometer and holds out their arm, this constitutes implied consent to perform the blood pressure reading. As a matter of good practice you should tell your patient what you are doing and explain that they may feel a tightness in their upper arm for a minute while you take the pressure reading.

Three elements of valid consent

There are three components that need to be met in order for a consent (or refusal of consent) to be considered valid. The first is that the consent must be given freely by the patient with no coercion,[41] the patient must be informed of the broad nature and effect of the treatment and the risks and benefits associated with it;[42] and the patient must be competent to consent to the treatment.[43]

Competence (capacity)

Any person over the age of 18 years is presumed to be competent to give or refuse consent for medical treatment. If a health professional believes that a patient is not competent to give or refuse consent for treatment, the onus rests on the health professional to show that the patient is not competent. The test for competence has three steps. The patient should be able to take in, retain and understand the treatment information. The patient should believe the information they have been given (for example, some patients with anorexia may not believe that they are unwell at all and therefore not be able to demonstrate competence). Finally, the patient should be able to weigh up the risks and benefits of the treatment and communicate a decision.[44]

Refusal of treatment

The right to consent to or refuse treatment is conferred on all patients by common law.[45] The law acknowledges an individual's right to determine whether they wish to undergo medical treatment or not even if the refusal of treatment results in the patient's death. Professional issues may arise when a health practitioner is confronted by a patient's decision that conflicts with their own. It is a requirement of all health practitioners that they reflect upon and consider carefully their professional position when confronted by such dilemmas. The issue goes beyond just the legal considerations and becomes an ethical and professional concern.

Providing information to patients—informed consent

Prior to commencing a procedure or treatment a clinician is required, as part of their duty of care, to inform the patient about the broad nature and effects of the treatment and has a duty to inform the patient about material risks involved in the treatment so that the patient can give or refuse consent for that proposed treatment/procedure. A material risk is a risk that a reasonable person in the patient's position would, if placed in the patient's position, be likely to attach significance to or that the medical practitioner is or ought reasonably to be aware that the patient would, if warned of the risk, attach significance to. This is distinct from informing the patient of ALL risks. The principle of 'material risk' obviously values the patient's view of what is material over those of the doctor who may think the risk is immaterial and therefore encourages patient autonomy over medical paternalism. These duties developed from the case of *Rogers v Whitaker*.[46]

This case turned largely on the fact that Dr Rogers failed to inform Mrs Whitaker of the material risks involved in a surgical procedure he recommended to her. The causative relationship between the duty of care between the doctor and his patient and the damage that was ultimately done was also examined. This will be discussed later with respect to negligence. Mrs Whitaker had lost sight in her right eye when she was young. She retained normal vision in her good eye and led a normal life. In her mid-40s she consulted Dr Rogers, an ophthalmic surgeon, to see if he could do anything to help her right eye, even if the improvement was just cosmetic. Dr Rogers told Mrs Whitaker that he could operate on her right eye and remove scar tissue from it, thus improving its appearance and possibly restoring some sight. Mrs Whitaker asked Dr Rogers about the risks associated with the operation. None were mentioned despite Mrs Whitaker repeatedly asking and making comments of concern that she had regarding the risk of loss of sight (this was later recognised as a material risk). Mrs Whitaker agreed to the operation. Just after the operation Mrs Whitaker developed complications, not only with her right eye but also with her left in a rare condition called 'sympathetic ophthalmia'. This condition can result in sympathetic inflammation of the untreated eye which can result in loss of sight and this occurred with Mrs Whitaker. Mrs Whitaker brought an action against

Dr Rogers for not warning her of the risk of this complication developing. Mrs Whitaker stated that if she had known that the risk existed she would not have consented to the operation. The causative link between Dr Rogers' negligence and the blindness was provided by Mrs Whitaker relying upon Dr Rogers' advice that there would be no risk. 'But for' this negligent advice Mrs Whitaker would not have had the surgery and would not have suffered the damage.[46]

Children and consent

Unlike with adults, there is a presumption that a person under the age of 18 DOES NOT have capacity to consent or refuse consent for treatment. A parent or guardian can also consent for medical or dental treatment for a child, but they must justify their decisions as being in the child's best interest. If there is some doubt from healthcare staff as to whether healthcare decisions are being made in the child's best interest and that decision is not immediately life threatening, then the matter can be referred to the Supreme Court or Guardianship Division of the Administrative Tribunal for determination. If a parent or guardian of a child under the age of 14 refuses treatment for a child where that treatment is necessary to prevent death or serious injury, treatment may be instituted under Section 174 of the *Children and Young Persons (Care and Protection) Act 1998* (NSW) and in similar provisions in other states, or the common law doctrine of necessity.

There is also a limit to the type of treatment that a parent or guardian can consent to. For example, a parent or guardian does not have the authority to refuse life sustaining treatment to a patient under 18. That is a matter that would have to be determined by a court. A parent or guardian is also not able to consent to gender reassignment surgery. Again, that is a matter for the court operating under its *parens patriae* (protective) jurisdiction. A minor (a person under 18) can consent to minor medical treatment provided they can demonstrate competency. There is a presumption against competency in children and rather than healthcare professionals having the onus to challenge competency, as they do with adults, in the case of children, the onus is on the child to demonstrate that they are competent to make a healthcare decision. This type of competence is referred to as Gillick competency after the case where the issue of competency in children was first established. Gillick competency is most commonly assumed in a minor who is over the age of 14 and is consenting to minor medical treatment. There is no reason why Gillick competency couldn't be established in children under 14, but no child under the age of 18 is able to refuse consent for life-sustaining treatment, even if they demonstrate competence.

When consent is not required

Treatment may be carried out without consent if the treatment is considered necessary, as a matter or urgency, to save a patient's life or to prevent serious damage to the patient's health.[43] The purpose of this part of the Act is to ensure that patients are treated even when they lack the capacity to consent to treatment and that the treatment that is undertaken without their consent is done so for the purposes of promoting and maintaining their health and wellbeing.[47]

Minor treatment, that is, treatment which is not major or special, may be carried out without any consent if there is no person responsible for the patient or that person cannot be contacted or they do not wish to make a decision regarding treatment. However, the clinician carrying out the treatment must certify in writing in the patient's clinical record that the treatment was required to promote the patient's health and wellbeing and that the patient has not made known their objection to the carrying out of the treatment.[48] In short, this means that the clinician must be clear that the patient does not object to the treatment prior to it being initiated.

Who may give consent when the patient cannot

For patients aged 16 years and above where substitute consent is required because the patient is incapable of giving consent to the carrying out of medical or dental treatment, the person responsible is able to consent on the patient's behalf. If a young person is under 16 and without parents, in NSW the Director-General of the Department of Family and Community Services (FACS) is the guardian. In this instance, the child is effectively a ward of the state. If a person responsible is unable to be contacted then the Guardianship Division of the Administrative Tribunal is able to act as the substitute decision-maker. If a patient presents who falls within the jurisdiction of the Mental Health Act, then the provisions of that Act will prevail.

Any person may request a person responsible for a patient to give consent for the carrying out of medical or dental treatment on the patient.[49] This request should specify the following:[49]

1. The condition of the patient and why they require treatment
2. The alternative courses of treatment available in relation to the condition
3. The nature and effect of those courses of treatment
4. The nature and degree of risk associated with those courses of treatment
5. The reason why a course of treatment should be carried out.

The incompetent patient, guardianship and the 'Best Interests' test

Guardianship laws in all states and territories were written for the purposes of providing protection to those within our community who would otherwise be vulnerable to neglect, abuse and exploitation from others. The law essentially applies to patients over the age of 18 who are incapable of consenting to medical treatment and who meet the criteria set out in the law. This law aims to protect and make provisions for a patient 'who is intellectually, physically, psychologically or sensorily disabled, or is of advanced age or who is mentally ill within the meaning of the Mental Health Act or who is otherwise disabled' by ensuring that a surrogate decision-maker is appointed to make those decisions in the person's best interest.

The laws broadly aim to apply a set of principles which essentially serve to ensure that the welfare and interests of people with a disability are observed. Those principles include that the decision making freedom of those with a disability is restricted as little as possible, that they are encouraged to share in decisions that affect their lives and be as independent in this process as possible, that their cultural and family ties

are recognised and preserved, and that the community is encouraged to apply and promote these principles. Similar legislation exists in other states and under the Act[50] that law is recognised as corresponding law in NSW.[51]

Guardians have much of the authority of the individual they advocate for, including consent to medical and dental treatment, provided those treatments do not fall into the category of 'special treatments'. An example of a 'special treatment' includes the sterilisation of a person with a disability. This is to limit the infringement on the human right of those with a disability to have a family.

Guardians can be appointed via an enduring power of attorney document or via the Guardianship Board. The process of appointment varies in each state, but the obligations and powers of the guardian are broadly the same.

The fundamental principle to be applied by guardians making healthcare decisions on behalf of their charge is to act in the best interests of that person. If healthcare staff form a reasonable belief that the guardian is not acting in the best interests of the patient, staff can take the matter to the Supreme Court or Guardianship Tribunal for review.

Offences under the Guardianship Act

It is an offence under the Guardianship Act to perform a medical or dental treatment on a patient without consent. A penalty of imprisonment may be imposed for a special treatment (experimental, including clinical trials) or, with respect to minor or major treatment, imprisonment or a fine or both.

Person responsible/Statutory Health Attorney

In NSW, Queensland, Victoria, Tasmania and Western Australia, there is a hierarchical system whereby a person responsible is authorised to consent to treatment. Under section 33A (4) of the *Guardianship Act* (NSW), a list of the hierarchy of persons who may be considered 'persons responsible' is listed. In descending order of authority the list is:

1. the person's guardian. 'Guardian' means a person who is, whether under this Act or any other Act or law, a guardian of the person of some other person (other than a child who is under the age of 16 years), and includes an enduring guardian. However, this only applies if there is an order or instrument that appoints a guardian for the purpose of giving consent to the carrying out of medical or dental treatment on the person or, if not applicable then
2. the spouse of the person if the relationship is close and continuing. 'Spouse' means a husband or wife, or de facto or, if not applicable, then
3. a person who has the care of the person. A person is deemed to fit this description for the purposes of the Act if on a regular basis they provide domestic services and support to that person or arrange for that person to be provided with that support. This does not apply to those carers who are paid for their services. It also does not include those who care for a person at an institution. The person who has care of the person is that person who cared for the patient prior to them being admitted to that institution, then

4. a close friend or relative of the person. Under the Act a close friend or relative is defined as a person who maintains both a close personal relationship with the other person through frequent personal contact and a personal interest in the other person's welfare. However, a person is not to be regarded as a close friend or relative if that person has any financial interest in any service that is related to the care of that person.[52]

The person responsible should always have regard to the views of the patient (if they are known) when considering any medical or dental treatment of a patient. The information supplied to them from the medical or dental practitioner with respect to the details of the treatment, any alternatives, the nature of the treatment and any risks associated with the treatment must also be considered.

In South Australia powers of consent are able to be given to the closest relative in the absence of a guardian. A relative is a spouse, a parent, a person who acts *in loco parentis* in relation to the person, a brother or sister over 18, a son or daughter over 18.[53] The Northern Territory and the ACT do not have person responsible legislation. This means that family, friends and carers have no immediate legal right to consent to the treatment of incompetent patients and a guardian is required to be appointed if there is no formal instrument doing so. Decisions concerning patients are made by medical practitioners for emergencies, but otherwise require the consent of an administrative tribunal or the Supreme Court. There is a useful guide outlining who can do what at the ACT Public Advocate website.[54]

Enduring guardian

In NSW there exists in the legislation a provision for the enduring guardian to act as the person responsible for a patient who is incapable of consenting to medical or dental treatment. In Schedule 1 of the *Guardianship Regulation 2005* there is a proforma for an enduring guardian appointment form.[55]

Advance care directive

An advance care directive (ACD), or living will, is a document drafted by a patient which contains instructions from the patient outlining their wishes with respect to any medical intervention they may consent to or refuse to consent to, in the event that they are incapable of giving consent directly. ACDs act as the patient's consent. (See Ch 53 for ACDs in relation to death and dying.) The Victorian, Western Australian and ACT laws[56] allow refusal of any treatment, but in the Northern Territory, Queensland and South Australia the laws can only apply to a patient who is terminally ill or permanently unconscious.[57] A failure to comply with an ACD acts in the same way as ignoring a patient's refusal of consent in any other instance. It leaves the healthcare practitioner open to an action of civil or criminal liability. It should be noted that these documents can serve as protection to medical and nursing staff when dealing with issues surrounding withholding and withdrawing of treatment and end-of-life decision-making. They can act as evidence that staff were, for instance, complying with the patient's decision by upholding the patient's refusal of treatment. In NSW this is supported by the Guardianship Act, which states that 'a person shall be taken to object to the carrying out of medical or dental treatment if the person indicates that

they do not want the treatment to be carried out, or if the person has previously indicated, in similar circumstances, that he or she did not then want the treatment to be carried out, and has not subsequently indicated to the contrary'.[58] It should be noted that a lack of formal documentation does not in any way negate the validity of the patient's right to refuse treatment and if they have made their decision known in any form, provided the patient is competent, staff have an obligation to comply. The states, with the exception of Queensland and Tasmania, have legislation which makes specific reference to the patient's right to refuse treatment and offers protection for healthcare staff when complying with this right.

In some instances there may be doubt surrounding the validity of an ACD; for example, whether it applies in the circumstances that exist at the time or if the patient was competent at the time the ACD was made. If there is doubt about the validity or existence of an ACD, the situation is time critical; that is, a life-or-death decision must be made immediately, then healthcare staff should actively treat the patient. In this instance they will be protected by the doctrine of necessity. Once the patient has been stabilised there will be an opportunity for staff to meet with the patient or their person responsible in order to determine the patient's wishes. If healthcare practitioners suspect that the patient has been subjected to undue influence with respect to this decision making process they should seek legal advice and continue to treat the patient according to the patient's best interests. The healthcare practitioner must bear in mind that their primary focus of responsibility is in caring for their patient not their family. Family involvement in treatment discussions is permissible only when the patient gives permission for such involvement or, if they are incapable, with their person responsible or equivalent. All decisions should be documented.

> **PRACTICE TIP**
>
> If there is doubt about whether to treat a patient because of a consent issue, but treatment is required urgently to save a life or prevent further injury, then treat.

Withholding and withdrawing treatment

When a patient refuses treatment, it can be withheld. Health practitioners are lawfully able to withhold treatment at the patient's request provided the patient is competent to refuse consent, and that the healthcare staff do so in good faith and without negligence.

Healthcare staff are also able to withdraw life-sustaining treatment like artificial ventilation, Protections for health practitioners who withdraw treatment that results in the patient's death are provided under a variety of laws.[59]

There are other instances where treatment of the patient is futile and in this instance treatment may also be withheld.[60] There is no obligation on staff to provide treatment that is futile because this treatment would not be in the patient's best interest. There are two situations in which the futility of treatment can be easily determined. The first is when the patient is obviously dead. In NSW the definition of death is contained within s 33 of the *Human Tissue Act 1983*: 'A person has died when there has occurred irreversible cessation of function of the person's brain or irreversible cessation of circulation of blood in the person's body'.[61] The second is when the patient is known to be at the end-stage of a terminal illness, all available avenues for treatment have been exhausted and there is no prospect of a better outcome for the patient. This circumstance may arise when a patient with a known terminal illness suffers a cardiac arrest and for whom resuscitation may be futile. If it is not known that the patient is suffering from a terminal illness and it is not known to the healthcare staff that the patient wishes to refuse treatment, then treatment should be given. If a dispute arises between the parties the matter can be referred to a guardianship authority in an administrative tribunal or application can be made to the Supreme Court.

Palliative care

The legal and ethical basis for treatment of palliative care patients is that the treatment should neither intentionally hasten nor hinder the patient's death.

Medicines

There are strict laws that govern the manufacture, importing, testing, registration, dispensing, storage, supply, possession and prescription of drugs in every jurisdiction in Australia. It is essential that healthcare providers are familiar with these laws and at least be familiar with their employer's policy and procedures about handling medicines.

There are criminal sanctions for the unauthorised possession, supply, administration and self administration of restricted drugs. In addition to criminal sanction, the most common cause for redress by disciplinary tribunals is the wrongful use of drugs by healthcare staff.

Mental health and involuntary detention

Paramedics and ED staff will encounter patients with mental health issues on a regular basis. Every state and territory in Australia has its own legislation with respect to the care and treatment of the mentally ill.[62] The overall purpose of the Acts is to ensure that mentally ill persons will receive the best possible care and treatment in the least restrictive environment. This includes limiting any restriction or interference with their civil liberties, rights, dignity and self-respect to the minimum necessary to effectively provide care and treatment.

Definition of mental illness

Each state and territory has a different definition of mental illness, but they all have similarities and the principles underpinning the legislation are essentially the same. The definition of what constitutes a mental illness in the ACT, NSW, Tasmania and the NT is essentially:

A condition which seriously impairs, either temporarily or permanently, the mental functioning of a person and is charac-terised by the presence in the person of any one or more of the following symptoms:

(a) delusions,

(b) hallucinations,

(c) serious disorder of thought form,

(d) a severe disturbance of mood,

(e) sustained or repeated irrational behaviour indicating the presence of any one or more of the symptoms referred to in paragraphs (a)–(d).

A mentally ill person is defined as:

A person who is suffering from mental illness and, owing to that illness, there are reasonable grounds for believing that care, treatment or control of the person is necessary:

(a) for the person's own protection from serious harm, or

(b) for the protection of others from serious harm.

… In considering whether a person is a mentally ill person, the continuing condition of the person, including any likely deterioration in the person's condition and the likely effects of any such deterioration, are to be taken into account.

In Victoria and Queensland a person is considered mentally ill if he or she has a condition that is characterised by a significant disturbance of thought, mood, perception or memory.[63] In South Australia[64] it is any illness or disorder of the mind and in WA it is a person suffering from a disturbance of thought, mood, volition, perception, orientation or memory that impairs judgement or behaviour to a significant extent.[65]

Mentally disordered

The various Acts also provide a definition for a person who is not mentally ill but may be mentally disordered or disturbed. That is, this section of the Act may apply to a person who is experiencing a crisis which results in behaviour that may be dangerous to themselves or others but which exists only temporarily. That Act defines them as:

A person (whether or not the person is suffering from mental illness) is a mentally disordered person if the person's behaviour for the time being is so irrational as to justify a conclusion on reasonable grounds that temporary care, treatment or control of the person is necessary:

(a) for the person's own protection from serious physical harm, or

(b) for the protection of others from serious physical harm.[66]

The principles of care and treatment of the mentally ill or disordered

In NSW, as in other states, the principles underpinning the care and treatment of people with a mental illness or mental disorder include the following:

(a) people with a mental illness or mental disorder should receive the best possible care and treatment in the least restrictive environment enabling the care and treatment to be effectively given,

(b) people with a mental illness or mental disorder should be provided with timely and high quality treatment and care in accordance with professionally accepted standards,

(c) the provision of care and treatment should be designed to assist people with a mental illness or mental disorder, wherever possible, to live, work and participate in the community,

(d) the prescription of medicine to a person with a mental illness or mental disorder should meet the health needs of the person and should be given only for therapeutic or diagnostic needs and not as a punishment or for the convenience of others,

(e) people with a mental illness or mental disorder should be provided with appropriate information about treatment, treatment alternatives and the effects of treatment,

(f) any restriction on the liberty of patients and other people with a mental illness or mental disorder and any interference with their rights, dignity and self-respect is to be kept to the minimum necessary in the circumstances,

(g) the age-related, gender-related, religious, cultural, language and other special needs of people with a mental illness or mental disorder should be recognised,

(h) every effort that is reasonably practicable should be made to involve persons with a mental illness or mental disorder in the development of treatment plans and plans for ongoing care,

(i) people with a mental illness or mental disorder should be informed of their legal rights and other entitlements under this Act and all reasonable efforts should be made to ensure the information is given in the language, mode of communication or terms that they are most likely to understand,

(j) the role of carers for people with a mental illness or mental disorder and their rights to be kept informed should be given effect.[67]

Detention

There are strict provisions made under the Act for the involuntary detention of a person in a mental health facility. A person may only be detained or continued to be detained involuntarily in a hospital or other place if they meet the criteria of a mentally ill person or mentally disordered person as it is defined under the Act. They may only be detained for the purposes of care and treatment or determining whether the person should be the subject of a community treatment order. This course of action can only be undertaken if there is no other less restrictive course available.[68]

Admission of an involuntary patient to hospital

A doctor or accredited person is able to schedule a mentally ill or mentally disordered patient to a hospital provided that the patient is admitted within a short statutorily defined time from when the admission certificate is issued. The certificate must be in the statutory form. The doctor must have personally examined or observed the patient shortly before completing the certificate and be satisfied that there is no more appropriate way of dealing with the patient. The doctor must not be a near relative of the patient.[69]

Paramedics and involuntary patients

If a paramedic has reasonable grounds to believe that a person appears to be mentally ill or mentally disordered and that it would be beneficial to the person's welfare for them to be treated in accordance with the Mental Health Act, then the paramedic may transport the person to a declared mental health facility. Police may be requested if there are serious concerns about safety of the person or other persons.[70]

Who else can request a patient get help

A relative or friend may submit a written request to the medical superintendent of a hospital to detain a person because it would not be feasible to expect that a medical practitioner should travel a great distance to examine the patient and the matter is urgent.[71]

The police may apprehend a person if they believe that person may harm themselves or others or is committing an offence or has recently committed an offence and police believe it would benefit the welfare of the person to be dealt with under the Mental Health Act. They may take the person to a hospital.[72]

A magistrate, who is of the opinion that a person who appears before them is mentally ill, may order that police take that person to hospital for assessment.[73]

What happens at the hospital?

Once the involuntary patient arrives at the ED, an examination must be undertaken as soon as practicable, but no later than 12 hours after admission to determine if the patient is suffering from a mental illness or mental disorder. Medication prescribed must be the minimum that is able to be given and still preserve the patient's ability to communicate adequately. Before a person is certified they must be informed of their rights both orally and in a written statement. A psychiatrist must perform a second examination. If there is a dispute between the first and second examiners, a third examination must take place. The medical practitioner who wrote the schedule must not perform any of these examinations. If the person is not found to be mentally ill they must be released.[74]

Duration of detention

A mentally disordered person should not be detained for a continuous period in excess of 3 days (this excludes long weekends). A medical officer must examine the person once every 24 hours and the person must not be detained on more than three occasions in 1 month.[75] A mentally ill person must present before a magistrate as soon as practicable after detention so that the court may determine if the person is in fact mentally ill and to confirm, inquire into or overrule the decision made with respect to the period of detention and the care to be given to the patient.[76] Voluntary or involuntary patients retain their right to give or withhold consent for treatment unless they fall under a specific section of the Act that presumes they would be incapable of giving informed consent. In addition, a person is presumed to be incapable of giving informed consent if at the time consent was sought the patient received medication that would impair the patient's ability to give consent. However, it must be remembered that all patients have the right to be informed, the right to the least restrictive environment that is reasonable and the right to an independent review of any decision made regarding their treatment and detention.[77] Under no circumstances is it permissible for health staff to wilfully abuse, neglect or assault a patient. Penalties for this behaviour include imprisonment.[78]

Use of medications

The appropriate use of medications is laid out in the Act.[78] A patient with a mental illness must not be prevented from communicating with any person that may be engaged to represent the person or an authority making enquiries with respect to that person, for example, the Mental Health Review Tribunal. The patient is also able to request details of their medications.

Restraint

There are often times in the healthcare setting when a patient becomes dangerous to themselves or to others. In these instances it may be appropriate for staff to restrain the patient in order to protect them from harming themselves or harming others, including staff. Every workplace should have a policy related to these issues. It is suggested that restraints be used as a last resort and only when the benefits of their use outweigh the potential harm they can cause. There have been cases where the restraint of a patient has contributed to their death. If a person is wrongfully and intentionally restrained it may constitute false imprisonment and this is relevant particularly to paramedics who may transport a patient to hospital against that patient's wishes. Being confined in the back of the ambulance may constitute a form of imprisonment. In order to find for a case of false imprisonment two elements must be met: that the restraint was intentional and that it was a total restraint of the liberty of another person against their will.

In the case of *Sayers v Harlow Urban District Council*[79] Mrs Sayers was inadvertently trapped in a toilet operated by the council when the inside door handle fell off. In an attempt to get out of the toilet cubicle, Mrs Sayers stood on the toilet roll dispenser. Under her weight, the toilet roll dispenser broke from the wall and Mrs Sayers was injured. Mrs Sayers sued the council for false imprisonment and negligence. In hearing her case the court determined that Mrs Sayers had not been falsely imprisoned because there was no intention on the part of the council to restrain her. However, if a person is threatened and consequently believes that their movement is restricted, that may be sufficient to constitute false imprisonment.

If restraint must be used with a patient it should be the minimum restraint required to prevent the patient from harming themselves or others. For instance, if a patient with dementia or confusion was pulling out tubes and intravenous lines then the least restrictive option for a means of restraint would be gloves or bandages of slippery material like 'boxing gloves' to prevent the patient being able to grip and pull at the tubes and lines. This method is preferable to using arm restraints, which tie the patient's arms to the bed, or chemical restraints.

Negligence

Negligence is difficult to define succinctly but in essence it occurs when person/party A (the defendant) has a duty of care to person/party B (the plaintiff) and person/party B suffers damage as a result of a breach of duty by person/party A.[80] Four elements contribute to an act of negligence. The plaintiff must establish on the balance of probabilities that all four elements exist to be successful in their claim. The four elements are:

(a) duty of care—the plaintiff must demonstrate a duty was owed to them by the health practitioner

(b) breach—the health practitioner breached their duty of care by providing treatment that was below the standard expected

(c) damage—that damage was suffered as a result of the breach and the damage suffered by the plaintiff was reasonably foreseeable.[81] That is, any reasonable healthcare professional would have been able to foresee that the breach of duty would result in an injury being suffered

(d) causation—a clear relationship exists between the act or omission that caused the action or omission to act. That is, 'but for' the breach of duty the injury would not have been suffered.

Duty of care

Wherever there is a health practitioner–patient relationship there will exist a duty of care.[82] In *Donoghue v Stevenson*,[82] Lord Atkin stated that it is necessary to give thought to those who 'are so closely and directly affected by my acts that I ought reasonably to have them in contemplation as being so affected when I am directing my mind to the acts or omissions which are called in question'. The duty can also apply to people who are not your patients. The law imposes a duty on a health practitioner to take all reasonable care and skill in the provision of advice and treatment. This extends 'to the examination, diagnosis and treatment of the patient and the provision of information in an appropriate case'.[83]

Duty to rescue

There is no common law duty to attend an emergency when a health practitioner is off-duty. If a health practitioner attends a person in need in good faith and without expectation of a reward—as a 'good Samaritan'—then they are unable to be sued in negligence unless they are under the influence of alcohol, drugs or where they caused the emergency. Tasmania is the only state where this varies, but there are no known cases of rescuers being sued for voluntarily attending an emergency.[84]

Paramedics in NSW and Queensland are offered specific protections under section 67I of the Health Services Act (NSW) and ss 38 and 39 of the *Ambulance Services Act 1991* (Qld) where they are carrying out duties in relation to ambulance service or protecting people from injury or death.

Breach of duty

Once a duty of care is established, the person bringing the action to court (the plaintiff) must provide evidence that the defendant breached their duty of care by failing to provide the requisite standard of care. The standard of care is determined by the *Civil Liability Act* which was introduced into most states in or around 2002. This piece of legislation sets out the 'reasonable man' test, which is the standard used to determine if there has been a breach of duty.[85] The 'reasonable man' test asks what a 'reasonable' person, with equivalent knowledge and resources, would have done if faced with a similar situation. For example, the standard of reasonableness for a paramedic would be to act in accordance with the standard of their peers in the same area. This would apply equally to nurses. In determining what a reasonable standard of care might be for a nurse, the court would have regard to what the 'reasonable' or 'average' nurse might do in a particular situation.

Healthcare workers will also be held to peer group standards of practice, departmental guidelines, policy and procedure directives and responsibilities and obligations as they are set out in other relevant laws like the *Poisons and Therapeutic Goods Act*. If a nurse, for example, were to practise below the reasonable standard of practice for a nurse with an equivalent level of training in an equivalent area and it was reasonably foreseeable that a person would be harmed as a result, and the patient was harmed as a direct result, of that breach of the standard of care, then the nurse would be at high risk of being found negligent in the performance of their duty.

Damage and causation

In any action for negligence there must be not only a breach of the duty of care but also damage sustained as a result of that breach. For example, a nurse may put a prescribed medication in the wrong ear of the patient and this could be considered a breach of her duty because a reasonable nurse would not make such a mistake. However, if no damage has been suffered by the patient because of this breach then there can be no action taken for negligence. Additionally, in order to make a finding of negligence, there must be a link between the breach of the duty owed to the patient and the harm caused to the patient. For example, if an elderly patient presents to emergency with a heavily bleeding leg, is triaged as a low priority and while waiting for medical attention has a stroke, then clearly the triage nurse is in breach of their duty to the patient for prioritising the patient incorrectly with respect to the bleeding leg. However, it is unlikely that the delay in treatment of the leg resulted in the stroke. If it could be established, on the balance of probabilities, that a causal relationship did in fact exist between the two events, then the patient would be entitled to rely on the delay in treatment as a basis for a claim.[86]

Reasonable foreseeability

To be successful in a negligence claim the plaintiff also must establish that a duty of care existed between the parties, that there was a breach in the duty of care, damage occurred as a result of that breach and that the damage should be compensated only to the extent that it was reasonably foreseeable. In the High Court case of *Annetts v Australian Stations Pty Ltd*[87] the court heard that James Annetts, the 16-year-old son of the applicants, left home in August 1986 and went to work as a jackaroo on a Western Australian sheep station. Mrs Annetts (James' mother) was assured by the station manager that James would be constantly supervised. After 7 weeks of work James was assigned to work as a caretaker on a station under the same management about 100 kilometres from the main station. About 8 weeks after that Mr and Mrs Annetts learned that James had gone missing. An intensive search was begun but it was not until April 1987 that Mrs Annetts was telephoned and told that a car had been found with two sets of human remains nearby. Mr and Mrs Annetts were told that James had most likely died not long after moving to the second station as a result of dehydration, exhaustion and hypothermia. James' parents claimed that he had died as a result of the station manager's negligence. The Annetts argued that the station manager owed not only James a duty of care, but that he also owed them a duty of care because he had said that he would constantly supervise James. The Annetts claimed that they had been psychologically damaged as a result of the station manager's breach of his duty of care and that they should be compensated. The issue was not only whether the defendant owed the parents a duty of care (proximity), but also whether the psychological damage sustained by the Annetts was reasonably foreseeable. Could they say, 'but for' the breach of duty of the station manager, the Annetts would not have suffered the harm? The High Court found that the defendant did owe the Annetts a duty of care and it was reasonably foreseeable that a breach of the station manager's duty would lead to a psychological harm to the Annetts.

Vicarious liability

Vicarious liability exists when one person is held legally responsible for the acts or omissions of another. In the healthcare setting, an example of vicarious liability is the employer, for example, the state health department, being responsible for the negligence of its employee—a nurse or paramedic. Although the health department may be completely blameless with respect to its direct involvement with the act or omission to act that has led to the cause of the action, it is vicariously liable for the acts or omissions of those who work for it.

However, where an employee engages in serious or wilful misconduct, or where the act does not arise out of the course of the individual's employment, then an employer does have the right to take action to recover any compensation it has paid out to a claimant from the employee.[88] Essentially this means that if employees fail to comply with guidelines and protocols set down by their employer with respect to the way in which they should conduct their work and as a consequence the employee is found to have been negligent and is required to pay compensation to the injured party, the employer may have a cause of action against them. Paramedics are exempt from personal liability in NSW under section 67I of the Health Services Act. Similar protection for paramedics is found in other jurisdictions.

Triage and negligence

Triage is the system used to sort the order in which patients should be treated. The order in which a patient is treated is determined by need. That is, the patient most in need of treatment will be treated first. As per the Australasian Triage Scale, those most in need will be labelled category 1 patients and should be seen immediately for treatment. These people have life-threatening conditions. Those with a less urgent condition may be classified as category 5 patients and should be seen within 2 hours of presenting. In rural and remote areas where a doctor is not available to see the patient within the time-frame recommended by the guidelines, staff should refer to the health department policy or guidelines on triaging at a location with no on-site doctors. A legal risk associated with triage includes failing to appropriately assess a patient's treatment priority. This could raise the issue of negligence.

Nurse practitioner responsibilities

Nurse practitioners were first recognised in Australia in 2000. Since then many nurses have undertaken further education to become eligible to apply for positions as nurse practitioners throughout Australia. In all states legislation provides for authority for the registration of nurse practitioners.[89] Registered nurses applying to practise as nurse practitioners must meet a certain level of educational and clinical experience requirements. Nurse practitioners are now legally authorised to prescribe some medications and order some diagnostic tests—activities that were previously permitted to be done only by medical practitioners. Nurse practitioners are unable to autonomously define their scope of practice. This is established via state health department guidelines and employer policies and procedures. There are no statutory restrictions on the scope of nurse practitioner practice except in those pieces of legislation that specifically make mention of the responsibilities and obligations of medical practitioners. For example, the ACT Health Act makes provision for abortion to be performed, but it must be undertaken by a suitably qualified medical practitioner.

The scope of practice of nurse practitioners is limited by the qualifications and experience that each individual nurse practitioner holds. For example, if a nurse practitioner has a qualification in mental healthcare, then their scope of practice in the role of the nurse practitioner extends only to mental health. If an emergency situation arises which falls outside the nurse practitioner's usual scope of practice the standard that the practitioner is likely to be held to by a court is that of the registered nurse—not of the nurse practitioner. That is, the nurse practitioner in this example will only be expected to perform the same interventions and provide the same level of care as a registered nurse.[90] A contravention of the approved guidelines may not necessarily constitute a breach of standards, but may result in a finding of professional misconduct or unsatisfactory professional conduct by a professional disciplinary body.[91]

Prescribing medication

In prescribing drugs for a patient the nurse practitioner is expected to inform the patient of everything that is associated with the administration of the medication. This includes the drug's action, its side effects, its interaction with other substances, the importance of compliance, how long the patient can expect to have to take the medication and any specific precautions. The practitioner is also expected to undertake regular monitoring of the drug and its effectiveness.[92]

It should be noted that although over-the-counter drugs do not require a prescription, if the nurse practitioner prescribes an over-the-counter drug to a patient the same responsibilities and accountability applies as if the drug were a prescription-only medication. This also applies to complementary therapies. Nurse practitioner prescribing is governed by the same laws as those that govern the prescribing of drugs by medical practitioners.

SUMMARY

Whole texts have been written on the subject of health law because of its complexities. This chapter has set out to provide only an introduction to the fundamentals of health law. A basic understanding of the law is critical for all professionals including nurses and paramedics because it establishes boundaries on behaviours. The emergency setting provides some exceptions to rules that would apply in other environments and it is critical that practitioners have an understanding of when and to whom those exceptions apply so as not to breach the rights of another person and thus do no harm. The law serves to protect both patients and practitioners and thus a working understanding of it and how it applies to healthcare practice is required of all practitioners.

CASE STUDY

You are called to assess and assist 54-year-old Karen who has kidney disease and is a renal dialysis patient. She has to travel to hospital from her home in the country to undertake dialysis in a regional centre three times a week. The trip takes 3 hours each way. Karen has been making this trip for the past 5 years and is now telling her family that she has had enough and doesn't want to continue this treatment. She says she just wants to stay at home with her family and let nature take its course. Knowing that you are the only health practitioner in town, the family have asked you to come and speak with Karen about her decision.

Questions

Identify the legal issues that arise from this case. Consider the following:

1. What are the issues with respect to consent?
2. a. What are the legal obligations of the care team when it comes to upholding Karen's decision or not?
   b. Is there the potential for assault to be committed? If so, how?
3. What is the final outcome? Does Karen go home or not? Why or why not?

Answers to Case Study Questions can be found on evolve
http://evolve.emergencytrauma.curtis

REFERENCES

1. Australian Health Ministers' Advisory Council. Consultation paper: options for regulation of paramedics, Australian Health Ministers' Advisory Council. 2012. Online. www.paramedics.org.au/content/2012/07/Consultation-Paper-Paramedic-Registration.pdf; accessed 20 July 2015.

2. Eburn M, Bendall J (2010) The provision of ambulance services in Australia: a legal argument for the national registration of paramedics. Journal of Emergency Primary Health Care 8(4).

3. Townsend R, Eburn M. Submission to the AHMAC on Paramedic Registration. 2012. Online. law.anu.edu.au/sites/all/files/users/u4810180/2012_submission_to_the_australian_health_ministers_advisory_council.pdf; accessed 20 July 2015.

4. Health Legislation Amendment (Unregistered Health Practitioners) Act 2006 (NSW); Unregistered Health Practitioners: Code of Conduct 2013 (SA).

5. Department of Health Victoria Paramedic Registration Bill Exposure Draft (2014) www.health.vic.gov.au/paramedicsbill/; Health Ministers' Advisory Council (2011) Options for the regulation of unregistered health practitioners. AMAC. www.coaghealthcouncil.gov.au/

6. AHPRA (2014) Mandatory notifications. www.ahpra.gov.au/Notifications/Who-can-make-a-notification/Mandatory-notifications.aspx

7. Health Practitioner Regulation National Law Act 2009 (Qld).

8. Health Practitioner Regulation National Law Act 2009 (Qld) Sch 1 s 5.

9. Freckelton I. (2008) 'Good Character' and the regulation of medical practitioners. Journal of Law and Medicine 16:1.

10. Hughes and Vale Pty Ltd v New South Wales (No 2) (1955) 93 CLR 127 Dixon CJ, McTiernan and Webb JJ decided [at 156].

11. Edelsten v Medical Practitioners Board (Vic) [2000] VSC 565 [at 36].

12. Nurses and Midwifery Board of Australia v Mundy [2012] SAHPT 5 (25 August 2012) www.austlii.edu.au/cgi-bin/sinodisp/au/cases/sa/SAHPT/2012/5.html?stem=0&synonyms=0&query=title(nursing%20and%20midwifery%20board%20and%20mundy%20)

13. McIlwraith J, Madden B. Health care and the law. 6th edn. Thomson Reuters. 2013:46.

14. Coroners Act 2009 (NSW) s 78; Coroners Act 2003 (Qld) s 48; Coroners Act 1997 (ACT) s 58.

15. For example Coroners Act 2003 (Qld) s 48 (4).

16. Blunt v Park Hotel Lane Ltd (1942) 2 KB 253 at 257.

17. NSW Crimes Act 1900 s 335 www.austlii.edu.au/au/legis/nsw/consol_act/ca190082/s335.html. There are comparable laws in all states and territories.

18. Evidence Act 1910 (Tas).

19. Criminal Procedure Amendment (Sexual Assault Communications Privilege) Act 1999 No 48.

20. Crimes (Sentencing Procedure) Act 1999 s 21.

21. Crimes (Sentencing Procedure) Act 1999 s 26.

22. Crimes Act 1900 s 317.

23. Law Enforcement (Powers and Responsibilities) Act 2002 Part 4 s 21.

24. Road transport (safety and traffic management) Act 1999 (NSW) s 20.

25. Road transport (safety and traffic management) Act 1999 (NSW) s 21.

26. Road transport (safety and traffic management) Act 1999 (NSW) s 22.

27. Children and Young Persons (Care and Protection) Act 1998 (NSW).

28. Mandatory reporting guidelines. www.community.nsw.gov.au/kts/guidelines/reporting/mrg2.htm; accessed 24 June 2015.

29. Children and Young Persons (Care and Protection) Act 1998(NSW); Children and Young People Act 2008 (ACT); Community Welfare Act (NT); Child Protection Act 1999 (Qld); Children's Protection Act 1993 (SA); Children, Young Persons and their Families Act 1997 (Tas); Children Youth and Families Act 2005 (Vic); Children and Community Services act 2004 (WA).

30. Townsend R, Luck M. Applied paramedic law and ethics. Elsevier, Sydney; 2013.

31. Higgins D, Bromfield L, Richardson N et al. (2014) https://www3.aifs.gov.au/cfca/publications/mandatory-reporting-child-abuse-and-neglect

32. Children and Young People Act 2008 (ACT); Children and Young Persons (Care and Protection) Act 1998 (NSW); Children, Youth and Families Act 2005 (Vic); Children, Young Persons and their Families Act 1997 (Tas).

33. The National Nursing Research Unit (2012) What are the benefits and challenges of 'bedside' nursing handovers? Policy+. Issue 36, November 2012. King's College London. https://www.kcl.ac.uk/nursing/research/nnru/policy/By-Issue-Number/Policy--Issue-36.pdf

34. Iedema R, Ball C. (2010) NSW Ambulance/ Emergency Department Handover Project Report. Sydney: NSW Health & UTS Centre for Health Communication. http://www.archi.net.au/documents/resources/qs/clinical/clinical-handover/amb-ed/amb-ed-report.pdf

35. (2006) WASCA 98 (31 May 2006).

36. Breen v Williams (1996) 186 CLR 71.

37. Privacy Act 1988 (Cth); Privacy and Personal Information Protection Act 1998 (NSW); Information Privacy Act 2000 (Vic); Information Privacy Act 2009 (Qld); Freedom of Information Act 1992 (WA); Freedom of Information Act 1991 (SA); Personal Information Protection Act 2004 (Tas); Information Act (NT).

38. Malette v Shulman (1990) 67 DLR (4th) 321.

39. R v Turner (1962) VR 30.

40. In re F (1990) 2 AC 1.

41. Mohr v Williams (1905) 104 NW 12.

42. In re T (1992) 4 All ER 649.

43. In re C (Adult: Refusal of Treatment) [1994] 1 WLR 290.

44. In re C (Adult: Refusal of medical treatment) [1994] 1 All ER 819.

45. Department of Health and Community Services (NT) v JWB and SMB (Marion's Case) (1992) 175 CLR 218.

46. Rogers v Whitaker (1992) 109 ALR 625.

47. Guardianship Act 1987 (NSW) s 32.

48. Guardianship Act 1987 (NSW) s 37(3).

49. Guardianship Act 1987 (NSW) s 40.

50. Section 48A.

51. Guardianship and Management of Property Act 1991 (ACT), Guardianship and Administration Act 2000 (Qld), Guardianship and Administration Act 1993 (SA), Guardianship and Administration Act 1995 (Tas), Guardianship and Administration Act 1986 (Vic), Guardianship and Administration Act 1990 (WA).

52. Guardianship Act 1987 (NSW) s 3.

53. Guardianship and Administration Act 1993 (SA).

54. http://www.publicadvocate.act.gov.au/guardianship

55. Guardianship Regulation 2005 (NSW) s 7.

56. Guardianship and Administration Act 1990 (WA) s 110B; Medical Treatment Act 1994 (Vic) s 5; Medical Treatment Act 1994 (ACT) s 7.

57. Powers of Attorney Act 1998 (Qld) s 36; Consent to Medical Treatment and Palliative Care Act 1995 (SA) s 7; Natural Death Act 1988 (NT) s 4(1).

58. Guardianship Act 1987 (NSW) s 33B.

59. Medical Treatment (Health Directions) Act 2006 (ACT); Natural Death Act 1988 (NT); Powers of Attorney Act 1998 (Qld); Consent to Medical Treatment and Palliative Care Act 1995 (SA); Medical Treatment Act 1988 (Vic).

60. Airedale NHS Trust v Bland (1993) AC 789.

61. Human Tissue Act 1982 (Vic); Transplantation and Anatomy Act 1979 (Qld); Transplantation and Anatomy Act 1983 (SA); Human Tissue Act 1985 (Tas); Human Tissue Transplant Act (NT); Transplantation and Anatomy Act 1978 (ACT).

62. Mental Health Act 1986 (Vic); Mental Health Act 2009 (SA); Mental Health Act 2000 (Qld); Mental Health Act 1996 (WA); Mental Health Act 1996 (Tas); Mental Health (Treatment and Care) Act 1994 (ACT); Mental Health and Related Services Act 1998 (NT); Mental Health Act 2007 (NSW).

63. Mental Health Act 1986 (Vic) s 8.

64. Mental Health Act 2009 (SA) s 3.

65. Mental Health Act 1996 (WA) s 4.

66. Mental Health Act 2007 (NSW) s 15.

67. Mental Health Act 2007 (NSW) s 68.

68. Mental Health Act 2007 (NSW) s 18.

69. Mental Health Act 2007 (NSW) s 19, s 20.

70. Mental Health Act 2007 (NSW) s 20.

71. Mental Health Act 2007 (NSW) s 19, s 26.

72. Mental Health Act 2007 (NSW) s 22.

73. Mental Health (Criminal Procedure) Act 1990 s 33.

74. Mental Health Act 2007 (NSW) s 27.

75. Mental Health Act 2007 (NSW) s 31.

76. Mental Health Act 2007 (NSW) s 34.

77. Mental Health Act 2007 (NSW) s 68.

78. Mental Health Act 1990 (NSW) s 69.

79. [1958] I WLR 623.

80. Donoghue v Stevenson (1932) AC 562 at 580.

81. Jaensch v Coffey (1984) 155 CLR 549 at 579.

82. Donoghue v Stevenson (1932) AC 562.

83. (1992) 109 ALR 625.

84. Civil Liability Act 2002 (WA) Pt ID; Civil Liability Act 1936 (SA) s 74; Civil Liability Act 2003 (Qld) s 26, Law Reform Act 1995 (Qld) s 16; Civil Liability Act 2002 (NSW) ss 56, 57; Civil Law (Wrongs) Act 2002 (ACT) s 5; Wrongs Act 1958 (Vic) s 31B; Personal Injuries (Liabilities and Damages) Act 2005 (NT) s 8.

85. Civil Liability Act 2002 (NSW), Civil Liability Amendment (Personal Responsibility) Act 2002 (NSW).

86. Civil Liability Act 2002 (WA) s 5C; Civil Liability Act 1936 (SA) s 34; Civil Liability Act 2003 (Qld) s 11; Civil Liability Act 2002 (NSW) s 5D; Civil Law (Wrongs) Act 2002 (ACT) s 45; Wrongs Act 1958 (Vic) s 51; Civil Liability Act 2002 (TAS) s 13.

87. [2002] HCA 35.

88. Employees Liability Act 1991 (NSW).

89. Health Practitioner Regulation National Law Act.

90. Rogers v Whitaker (1992) 175 CLR 149.

91. Health Practitioner Regulation National Law Act s 5.

92. Nursing and Midwifery Board of Australia (2014) Nurse practitioner standards for practice. http://www.nursingmidwiferyboard.gov.au/Codes-Guidelines-Statements/Codes-Guidelines/nurse-practitioner-standards-of-practice.aspx

CHAPTER 5

CULTURAL CONSIDERATIONS IN EMERGENCY CARE

LESLEY SEATON

Essentials

- In order to meet the needs of the diverse patient populations that will be encountered in today's multicultural world, a deeper understanding of what is meant by cultural diversity means must be gained by healthcare workers.
- Cultural or personal beliefs, worldviews and traditions espoused by the patient, their family and their community will affect the course and outcome of the health–illness encounter and shape the personal experience of a patient.
- Any social or lifestyle-related issue that might have an impact on a patient's capacity to attain safe, high-quality, effective and equitable personal health care should be considered as being cultural.
- Cultural or social differences can present barriers to the provision and receipt of appropriate treatment and care. All healthcare workers must appreciate that cultural and social difference will have an impact upon their communication and interaction with patients, patients' families and associated other groups.
- Any lack of cross-cultural understanding exhibited by a healthcare worker has the potential to lead to misunderstanding and cause stress, discomfort or distress which in turn may lead to less-than-optimal or even negative health outcomes.
- Healthcare workers in Australasia need to reflect upon the way that they, as a group of professionals, interact with those people who become their patients. Care must be individualised to each patient, and each patient and their family or community's personal or particular worldview and circumstances must be taken into account in a meaningful way during encounters with both healthcare workers and healthcare organisations and systems.

INTRODUCTION

This chapter has been written to assist all healthcare personnel; including pre-hospital healthcare workers, paramedical and ambulance personnel, assistive caregivers and nurses who work with and care for patients and their families in the community, in the hospital emergency and in the acute care setting. It is intended to support them in acquiring insight into and better appreciation of some of the issues, concerns and needs of those patients belonging to the cultural and social (often) minority groups that characterise contemporary society across Australia and New Zealand–Aotearoa. Today the patients, their families and the wider communities of people with whom healthcare workers will meet and work will often belong to cultural and social groups that are perhaps quite different from the healthcare worker's own. This presents a new set of challenges for all healthcare workers, and one which requires that they develop and continue to build on their own knowledge base and skill set to increase their capacity to provide safe, effective and appropriate cross-cultural care.

Healthcare workers need to better appreciate the way in which cultural and social diversity and difference will increasingly have an impact on their interactions and communications with patients, patients' families and associated other groups and communities. This is because culturally determined beliefs affect attitudes and comprehension and will therefore influence the tone and quality of all pre-hospital care and acute care encounters. The potential exists for misunderstanding, distress and even conflict, especially during times of stress such as those that are related to illness, trauma and personal crisis and of the type that will be encountered in the community by pre-hospital healthcare workers and seen in any emergency department (ED) or acute care presentation.

Any lack of understanding exhibited by a healthcare worker has the potential to lead to less than optimal or even negative outcomes. It will contribute to the possibility of non-compliance with care and treatment as well as increase the likelihood and incidence of adverse events. If there is a mismatch between the values, intentions and goals of the healthcare worker and the beliefs, understandings and practices of the patient, unhelpful consequences are more than likely to occur. The intent of this chapter is to assist and enable emergency and healthcare workers to offer high-quality, patient-centred and appropriate care to patients, care that is also culturally safe, therapeutic and effectively individualised.

Culture and what it means for healthcare workers

Meeting and interacting with healthcare workers in a crisis situation or in the ED and acute care areas of a hospital will always be associated with stress and distress. Unfortunately this may also be an individual's first encounter with the healthcare system of Australia or New Zealand–Aotearoa. This initial experience has the potential to affect not only that interaction and its outcomes, but also influence future experiences related to healthcare and may have a long term impact on an individual's health status and health-seeking behaviours.

Most commonly the 'notion' of culture is considered only when healthcare workers encounter an individual from an ethnic group other than their own. However, this is only the most easily recognisable in the spectrum of human social diversity that will be encountered in contemporary Australia and New Zealand–Aotearoa. Healthcare workers will meet individuals from a variety of ethnic and social subgroups and must learn to interact meaningfully and appropriately across a wide range of values–belief systems, behavioural norms and moral codes if positive health outcomes are to be achieved.

Illness or misadventure, as all healthcare workers, para-medical personnel and nurses know, is not only a physical event—it is a total human experience and it will be understood and appreciated in any number of different ways by different individuals. It is important for healthcare workers to have a fundamental understanding of the impact of the cultural or social world of individuals and their interpretations of what takes place in a healthcare encounter and understand the impact of their own interactions with patients and their families. The significance of culturally based beliefs, life-ways and lifestyles

and social traditions should not be underestimated. Such beliefs and traditions are very strong, and affect both the course and the outcome of the health–illness encounter and significantly shape the personal experience of a patient. In a cross-cultural situation, both the patient and the healthcare worker will hold or may encounter points of view, beliefs and self-care practices that might be unfamiliar and very different from their own. While this is an opportunity for growth and enrichment, it also has the potential to cause discomfort, isolation and distress, especially for the patient. Common responses to the unknown or unfamiliar can include anxiety, wariness, fear and even anger, and such potential is on all occasions to be minimised and optimally avoided altogether.

It is also useful to bear in mind that many migrants will arrive or live in Australia or New Zealand–Aotearoa with minimal knowledge of the way that the healthcare system here is fashioned or functions. Many patients and their families will have had a range of different experiences of healthcare in their home country and they may have previously encountered healthcare workers who behave very differently from those in Australia and New Zealand–Aotearoa. Particularly in the case of refugees or asylum seekers, these previous encounters may possibly have even been negative or unpleasant. For other patients, some previous experiences can be 'reawakened' by the hospital environment. For example, those patients or their families who are survivors of torture and trauma might be reminded of previously upsetting or disturbing experiences.

What does the word 'culture' describe?

In Australia and New Zealand–Aotearoa the most common interpretation of 'culture' is that in which social 'difference' is manifested through the concept of ethnic identity. Therefore the perception of culture is invariably associated only with those patients who are different from the healthcare worker in an obvious way. Typically, difference is correlated or linked to the patient's physical appearance or the determination of a different country of origin from the healthcare worker. While defining culture primarily by ethnicity might seem the easiest way to understand culture, it also risks the healthcare worker oversimplifying the real meaning of cultural difference and diversity.[1,2]

If healthcare workers become too focused on what they believe to be the culturally specific beliefs, activities or nuances of a particular ethnic group, there is a tendency to hold ideas that promote a stereotypical view of that group, which then makes it more challenging to respond to individual diversity. For healthcare workers it is important not to treat people according to stereotypes based on physical appearance or ethnic identity—always remember to treat each person as an individual. For example, a patient may have the physical appearance or 'ethnicity' of a Chinese person, but identify with the cultural norms, beliefs, way of life and biases of the general Australian population. In New Zealand–Aotearoa, it is important that patients and their families self-identify, for example as Māori, rather than the healthcare worker making assumptions about an individual's cultural identity or worldview.[3]

In order to meet the needs of the diverse patient populations that are encountered today, a deeper understanding of what cultural diversity might actually mean needs to be gained by healthcare workers. Cultural diversity can and should include, any individuals or groups/communities, that might differ from the healthcare worker in any way, in terms of lifestyle, worldview or beliefs, and includes such differences as, for example, sexuality, age, ability, religion, background or lifestyle. This will also necessarily include any minority social group or sub-culture that can be found represented in contemporary society. In other words any patient should be considered as an *individual* and any categorisation avoided.[1-3]

Quality cross-cultural care is best understood as that care which is individualised to each patient through the healthcare worker seeing them each as unique and different. This approach is suggested, rather than the easy option, which is the previously customary practice of guessing a patient's need using a 'dominant culture mainstream' approach. In this traditional approach, ethnicity was used as the single distinguishing characteristic of an individual or group. The issue here is that patients who belong to similar ethnic groups will probably have different life-ways and values to each other, as well as to the healthcare worker, which are far deeper than is suggested by determining their ethnic origin alone. The term *cross-cultural difference* should be applied to 'any people who might differ from the healthcare provider because of socioeconomic status, age, gender, sexual orientation, ethnic origin, migrant/refugee status, religious belief or disability'.[4] Any social, worldview or lifestyle-related issue that might have an impact on a patient's capacity to receive safe, high-quality, effective and equitable nursing care should be considered as having a cultural source. If this understanding is applied when providing cross-cultural care, then any aspect of diversity or difference must be taken into account by the healthcare worker. All of these elements, which include but are not limited to ethnicity alone, have the potential to significantly influence a healthcare worker's response to a patient.[1-5]

Cultural or social differences can present barriers to the provision and receipt of appropriate treatment and care. Healthcare workers must develop and possess strong skills in communication and remain empathetic, respectful and

---

PRACTICE TIP

Make sure you become familiar with the information available about profession standards in cross-cultural healthcare provision. All professional healthcare providers should become familiar with the relevant standards and conduct code agreements that apply to their professional group. For nurses these can be accessed on the websites of the Australian Nursing and Midwifery Board (available via the APHRA website), the Nursing Council of New Zealand (NCNZ) and the College of Emergency Nursing Australasia (CENA). Ambulance officers, paramedics and emergency personnel should ensure that they consult their own regulatory standards. All such standards are updated regularly and each professional healthcare worker group should have a knowledge of and clear understanding about relevant professional mandates. As well as this, it is important to understand your professional responsibility in terms of equity and diversity legislation, which also changes from time to time.[4,6,7]

---

show understanding towards their patients, as their approach can make a significant difference to the experiences of their patients. The rights of the healthcare consumer have been protected in terms of equity, diversity and anti-discrimination legislation. These rights are also enshrined in the professional practice standards that must be manifested in the practice of all professional healthcare workers in both Australia and New Zealand–Aotearoa. One of the fundamental rights accorded to patients is access to healthcare services which takes into account freedom(s) related to cultural, religious, spiritual and social needs, and accords protection of the associated values and beliefs of the individual. Material outlining these rights and responsibilities should be freely available and easily accessible in all healthcare facilities.[4,6,7]

Understanding the health–illness experience from the patient's perspective

There is clearly a difference in the occurrence patterns of different diseases and responses to illness among the diverse social and cultural groups of Australia and New Zealand–Aotearoa. It is important that healthcare workers understand the way in which individuals, including themselves, are shaped by their social world, and also the way in which healthcare workers shape the environment and context of health and illness care through their actions and interactions with others.

The particular form of Western-based scientific knowledge and the allopathic medical model currently used in healthcare in Australasia is very influential and authoritative. Healthcare knowledge and its associated practices are usually considered by healthcare workers in Australasia to be based on unquestionable 'truths' and supported by sound reasoning and seemingly logical beliefs. When providing care to patients from other cultural groups, especially those who may be unfamiliar with Western ideology, it is important to realise that there can be any number of ways to view the world and that there are many forms of legitimately held but different ideas about health and healthcare. All understanding is appropriate in its context and environment, but some ideas might possibly be unfamiliar to healthcare workers in Australasia and perhaps very different to the views held by individual healthcare workers.

Holding particular ideas about health and illness which are considered socially legitimate in our own country can dominate healthcare workers' thinking about what is right or correct for patients. Gaining an understanding that the 'facts' relied upon in Western healthcare institutions might be sometimes seen very differently by patients belonging to other cultural groups is important if healthcare workers are to work usefully with those who hold alternative ways of thinking and understanding. Commonly, healthcare providers in Western society will consider their own beliefs to be 'common sense' or 'straightforward and unbiased'. Understanding that there are many and different ways to view health and healthcare will assist healthcare professionals to see the world from the point of view of the patient, and may make healthcare workers more understanding of the perspectives of others. What are often presented as facts, for example ideas about 'germ' theory and the associated hand-washing behaviours that arise from it, are ideas not always shared by everyone, especially those from other cultures.

Overseas-qualified healthcare professionals have increasingly become an important part of the Australasian workforce. Those healthcare workers who have not grown up in Australia or New Zealand–Aotearoa but have journeyed or migrated from other countries and contexts might find some significant differences from their home land and its more familiar healthcare setting. Working in a new environment often means that you will encounter new situations and those around you might behave and react differently to how you expect, which may lead to your experiencing a wide variety of different feelings and reactions. When you move somewhere else, naturally you still take your own personality and cultural background with you. It helps in these circumstances to examine your own expectations, keep an open mind and listen to and observe those around you.

Matters specific to Australia

Australia as a modern nation has been historically characterised by successive waves of immigration. The original population is the Indigenous or Aboriginal and Torres Strait Island peoples, but progressively since World War II immigrants from the United Kingdom, Europe and more recently from South-East Asia and the Pacific nations have been arriving here in growing numbers. Australia is now one of the most multicultural countries in the world with people from approximately 200 countries calling the country their home.

On 12 January 2014 the Australian Bureau of Statistics (ABS) recorded the total population at 23,348,424 persons.[8,9] Immigration has for some years exceeded natural population increase, and under current immigration policy this will continue to be the main contributor to Australia's population growth. Some 27.7% of the Australian population, or 6.4 million people currently in Australia, were born overseas; this number has risen from 4.7 million in 2003 and will predictably continue to rise. Within this group the skilled migrant stream accounts for around 43% of all arrivals and family stream migrants for some 26%, with humanitarian program migrants remaining steady at around 9%. Non-program migration (consisting mostly of New Zealand–Aotearoa citizens) comprises about 21% of all settler arrivals. For this reason close to half of the Australian population has now been either born overseas or has at least one parent born overseas. Over 200 languages are spoken in Australia, with the most common languages being English, Italian, Greek, Cantonese, Arabic, Vietnamese and Mandarin. The main religions are Christianity, Buddhism, Islam, Hinduism and Judaism.[8,9]

Australia has built a social infrastructure based in institutions, traditions and processes arising out of a democratic foundation. The cultural diversity of this country is considered to be one of its great social and economic resources. Australian unity in diversity is based on moral values such as respect for difference, tolerance, a common commitment to freedom and an overriding commitment to Australia's national interests. These values are based on the following principles:[10]

- *Civic duty*—obliges all Australians to support those basic structures and principles of Australian society, which guarantee freedom and equality and enable diversity in the society to flourish.

- *Cultural respect*—subject to the law, this gives all Australians the right to express their own culture and beliefs and obliges them to accept the right of others to do the same.
- *Social equity*—entitles all Australians to equality of treatment and opportunity so that they are able to contribute to the social, political and economic life of Australia, free from discrimination on the grounds of race, culture, religion, language, location, gender or place of birth.
- *Productive diversity*—maximises for all Australians the significant cultural, social and economic dividends arising from the diversity of the population.

Aboriginal and Torres Strait Islander health

The poor health of the Indigenous peoples of Australia is one of the more pressing issues facing this country. The Australian National Health and Medical Research Council (2005) asks that Australian healthcare providers begin to recognise the unique position in this country of Aboriginal and Torres Strait Islanders, principally because the Indigenous population is disadvantaged by Australia's current healthcare system.[11] The Australian Productivity Commission's Biennial Review (2009) found that the gap between Indigenous and other Australians, in terms of disadvantage, was actually growing, not diminishing.[5,12] Indigenous Australians do not enjoy the same level of health and wellbeing as other Australians; at all ages and stages, their quality of life is not as good as that of non-Indigenous Australians. This disadvantage has been well documented and is widely recognised as the worst experienced by any population cohort in the country.[13] The life expectancy of an Indigenous Australian is approximately 15 to 20 years lower than the rest of the population, and levels of chronic disease, mental illness, neonatal and child morbidity, mortality and harmful poly-substance abuse and addiction are significantly higher than in the general population.

Much of the negative epidemiology associated with indigeneity is related to economic and social disadvantage. The Indigenous population had a different life experience as a result of Australia's colonial history, with a values system, a language, a religion, a lifestyle, as well as educational, legal, health and social institutions being imposed on their communities that was, and still is, vastly different from that originally in place at the time of British settlement.[14,15] Colonisation has left an enduring legacy into the 21st century, which has been recognised in recent public policy. The long-term effects of colonisation have been characterised as a continued lack of access to health, education, economic power and the resources needed for the Indigenous nation to have the same quality of life as the rest of Australian society.

Despite an increased level of expenditure and a commitment to improving Indigenous health, data regarding health outcomes over the last 15 years demonstrates that progress is slow. Outcomes have not been encouraging and there is only a minimal improvement in the health status of this specific demographic group. This lack of improvement is directly related to the domination of the Western worldview in healthcare research, policy and praxis, the pre-eminence of the biomedical model and personal and institutional racism, which although 'unwitting and systemic' occurs when cultural assumptions become embodied in a society's established institutions and processes. Racism or negative discrimination occurs when a practice or policy appears to be fair because it treats everyone the same, but it actually disadvantages people from one racial or ethnic group.[16] Today, in Australia, Indigenous people appear to have access to the same healthcare services as the rest of the community; however, the impact of the history and issues outlined above must be considered carefully when caring for Indigenous peoples. Healthcare workers need to make this a priority and support the Indigenous effort, recognise the need to develop a deeper understanding of indigenous life-ways and experience, and build trust to genuinely address these healthcare inequalities effectively. Collaborative ventures and increased concern for and consideration of how to work with the Indigenous population can assist pre-hospital carers and healthcare professionals in this process.

Various initiatives have been introduced by state and federal governments in recent years to address concerns and improve Indigenous healthcare. One scheme has been the strengthening of the number of Indigenous healthcare workers, principally in primary healthcare roles and in the community, predominantly in rural and remote communities, but increasingly in high-need areas in urban locations. This strategy has gone some way to improving healthcare access, but further action and reform is required into the future.[17] If there is an Indigenous healthcare worker or a specific support service for Indigenous people associated with or available in your health service, you are encouraged to work closely with and be guided by them.

There is significant evidence confirming that Indigenous health will continue to be a major challenge to healthcare professionals, and in the face of this is an urgent need for healthcare professionals to be better prepared to work with Indigenous patients and communities and to be better educated about the factors related to their health status. In the main, Australian healthcare workers still come from the Eurocentric middle classes and are likely to have had little contact with Indigenous people. Until there is a change on the part of healthcare workers this inequity will remain a reality. This comment is not intended to engender feelings of guilt or anger in non-Indigenous healthcare workers, although it will sound challenging to some; rather it is about healthcare workers developing a concern for and a commitment to social justice—it is really about 'a healing process and acceptance of each other'.[18]

Matters specific to New Zealand–Aotearoa

New Zealand–Aotearoa has a smaller population than Australia, some 4,242,048, people who resided in that country in the 2013 census.[19] It remains legislatively a bicultural rather than a multicultural nation, and is distinguished principally by its indigenous Māori peoples (comprising 14.9% of the population) and the descendants of British settlers—identified as Pakeha. New Zealand–Aotearoa is not considered a multicultural country in the same way as its near neighbour Australia, but it too is beginning to realise that there is a need to develop a means of coping with a changing population demographic.

Nearly three-quarters of the New Zealand–Aotearoa population in the 2013 census identified as European (74%).

Pacific immigration has over time changed the national demographic and will continue to do so, with many former Pacific Island settlers having now become New Zealand–Aotearoa born citizens for several generations. The various immigrant groups seeking to settle in the country has changed and grown in number over the last decade and in 2013 comprised 7.4% of the total population.

Today Pacific Island peoples are well established and South-East Asian immigration increased almost 50%; in 2013 those identifying as 'Asian' accounted for 11.8% of the population, a doubling since 2006.[11] Source countries too are changing for this former British colony; there is a fall in migration from the more traditional sources such as the UK and Europe along with growth in other sectors; for example, immigration from India rose by 48% between 2006 and 2013. Between the 2006 and 2013 census Filipino immigrant numbers doubled[11] and migration from South Korea, South Africa and Fiji has significantly increased.

Māori health

New Zealand–Aotearoa, like Australia, is a former British colony and was recognised as a legally constituted territory during British settlement with the full rights of citizenship being accorded to the indigenous Māori inhabitants. But, like the experience of the Indigenous population of Australia, it became clear that Māori had disproportionately high levels of mortality and morbidity in their population when compared with the non-Māori people of that country. Over the last several decades a more inclusive concept of health has been encouraged, and healthcare professionals have been urged to rethink their attitudes to culture as it pertains to health and healthcare.

The Treaty of Waitangi (1848) is now commonly considered to be the founding document of New Zealand–Aotearoa, and today, after much negotiation, guides all governmental and governing policy and standards in that country relating to healthcare. From this original document, principles were developed by the 1987 Royal Commission on Social Policy, which were and continue to be applied across the healthcare sector and are believed to be integral to future development.[20,21]

They are those of:

- partnership—working together with iwi, hāpu, whānau and Māori communities to develop strategies for Māori health gain and appropriate health and disability services.
- participation—involving Māori at all levels of the sector, in decision-making, planning, development and delivery of health and disability services.
- protection—working to ensure Māori have at least the same level of health as non-Māori, and safeguarding Māori cultural concepts, values and practices.

These concepts have been mandated across the healthcare sector in New Zealand–Aotearoa, and in the last few years have become foundational and integral to the delivery of high-quality and appropriate healthcare services in that country. These concepts are the drivers behind Māori health development and underpin healthcare-based initiatives with a positive correlation to some improvements in mortality and morbidity within this population. Healthcare workers in New Zealand–Aotearoa have specific and collective responsibilities to respond to and address Māori health issues, and considerable value is attached to achieving the goal of offering culturally safe healthcare services.

Nurses in New Zealand–Aotearoa were the forerunners in developing cultural care guidelines in the form of *cultural safety*, a construct unique to that country, which constitutes a mandatory framework for ensuring quality in nursing and healthcare service.[1,2,4,6,22] The formal definition of cultural safety is: 'the effective nursing practice of a person or a family from another culture as determined by that person or family', while unsafe nursing practice is 'any action which diminishes, demeans or disempowers the cultural identity and well being of an individual'.[4] The philosophy of cultural safety, while developed within a nursing framework, nonetheless has much to offer all professional healthcare workers.[1–3,6,22]

Much remains to be done into the future, as Māori remain over-represented in most types of diseases. Higher levels of mental ill health, asthma, diabetes mellitus, drug and alcohol dependency, rheumatic fever, involvement in motor vehicle accidents and rates of sudden infant death syndrome in this population will ensure that this group will be seen commonly in presentations to EDs.

Immigrant health in Australasia

Those from cultural and ethnic backgrounds outside Australasia share with nationals in their new country the same range of biological and physiological responses to disease, illness and dysfunction. Hence the assumption might arise in relation to health that 'we are all the same'. Compared with those who are locally born, on arrival there is an apparent 'healthy' migrant effect that can be seen in those arriving in the Skilled Migrant stream. This is achieved by a government requirement that entry is usually only permitted for those migrants who are determined to be healthy prior to arrival. Epidemiological measures such as mortality, hospitalisation rates and the prevalence of lifestyle-related health risks support this finding of health on arrival for the majority of immigrants.

For humanitarian refugees however, it can be anticipated, they will have pre-arrival experiences that may have a detrimental impact on both their short and their longer-term healthcare needs. Many refugees are likely to have multiple and complex health problems on arrival. Particular concerns are in relation to their probable lack of knowledge about Australasian healthcare availability that leads to the underutilisation of available and appropriate services and a particular need for interpreters. Key issues are generally in relation to mental health, family and social support, sexual health guidance, the enduring impact of long periods of deprivation and of food and nutrition uncertainty; however, the specific needs of individuals and families should be ascertained on a case-by-case basis.

Over time, this relative advantage tends to diminish as length of stay increases and former migrants become integrated into their local community. Evidence is beginning to collect which suggests that morbidity and mortality from certain diseases are increased in certain ethnic minority groups for a number of reasons, one major factor being identified as an avoidance of healthcare services that are perceived as culturally incongruent.[23,24] There is also a range of social, economic and environmental determinants that will have an impact on the experience of ethnic minority groups. Language barriers, financial difficulties, housing problems, unemployment and a range of other social barriers can pose problems. These make it very difficult for migrants, in both the short and the long term, to settle into their new country, and over time this increases their risk in terms of health burden across a range of categories. In spite of the settlement services available to most new migrants and refugees, they often remain at a disadvantage with a very negative correlation to good health.

Issues and concerns

The concerns most commonly articulated by patients about cross-cultural nursing care relate to issues around communication style, variation in beliefs and attitudes and the impact of variability in social custom and differences regarding healthcare knowledge and self-care practices.[2,3,25]

Patients from other cultures will have differing levels of skill in English comprehension and communication that become apparent when presenting to the hospital ED. This can affect the interview process and the provision of care and treatment to these patients. People from some cultures will often answer 'yes' to healthcare workers' questions to avoid further discussion because they are unsure what is being asked or they are trying to disguise poor spoken language skills. Interpreters are available in every major hospital in Australia and New Zealand–Aotearoa and patients should be encouraged to ask for one if they feel that would help. If an interpreter cannot come to the hospital, phone interpreters are available at all times and most languages catered for. Interpreters are well trained in medical terminology.

When it is necessary to use an interpreter, healthcare workers should use a professional interpreter if at all possible. The use of family members to interpret should be discouraged. There are a number of reasons for this: family members might not relay information correctly to the patient, often resulting in a misleading response from the patient; family members might not know the words to use for medical terminology; and when discussing intimate or controversial matters this might cause confusion and distress with a flow-on effect to the patient.

In an Australian study of healthcare workers and culturally and linguistically diverse (CALD) patient groups, Johnstone and Kanitsaki found that while most healthcare workers were informally acquiring the cultural knowledge they needed to care for patients, stereotypical views of patients' culture were often used rather than the perspective of the individual patient.[6,24,25] They describe how the comprehensive assessment of an individual patient's cultural needs was often poorly addressed.[6,24,25]

In another Australasian study,[24,26] it was found that nurses attested to feeling greater uncertainty when caring for patients from other cultures, as a result of being more aware of cultural difference. The participants in this study expressed feelings of inadequacy in establishing relationships with patients who were culturally different from themselves. As a result of this, the participants' perception of their ability to provide individualised and appropriate care was compromised. The inability of the participants to form effective relationships meant that patients failed to divulge crucial information to the nurse. Because of this, the patients' needs were often not clearly understood or utilised in the planning and delivery of care, which inevitably affected adversely the patients' healthcare experience. This demonstrates that apprehension and uncertainty about interacting with minority-group patients affects the ability of nurses to gain a deeper understanding of needs in cross-cultural care. It is likely that this same cause and effect dynamic could be relevant to other healthcare provider groups.

Practical tips

While most healthcare workers acknowledge the importance of issues around culture and appreciate the need for competent and culturally safe nursing care, quite how to achieve this is less certain. In the fast-moving environment of a busy emergency and trauma service, it is easy to become focused on 'what to do' and rather less on 'how to do it'. The 'how' can become eclipsed into the background in the face of multiple presentations, busy triage stations and many demands for attention. Good cross-cultural care is fundamentally good care which is patient-centred and involves using well-developed communication skills.

Working effectively in cross-cultural care encounters will become easier if some time is taken to consider the following points.

Come to understand 'yourself'

Know what your own thoughts and ideas are; these are always apparent to patients as you work alongside and with them. If time is taken in coming to recognise and appreciate your own expectations, by 'seeing yourself' as others might, this means that you will have a fuller understanding of what you bring to each patient encounter. Explore your beliefs and attitudes because you will draw on these to form and shape your reactions and responses to patients. Ramsden[1] identifies the crucial importance of the healthcare worker exploring and understanding that their own attitudes and beliefs and this work (available online) makes worthwhile reading if you want to further develop your skills in this area.[4,7,25,26]

Treat everyone as an individual

It is important to treat each patient as an individual and not make assumptions about their beliefs and customs based on the patient's outward appearance. All healthcare workers should regard each patient and their family as unique and develop the skills to better understand the impact of their individual or personal culture on any situation. The patient and their family might appreciate being asked about their particular cultural or religious beliefs, or they might not. The majority of patients and families are cooperative and helpful when they can see that an effort is being made to understand their culture or belief systems as a means to better understand and meet their needs. Some individuals may adhere closely to the traditional beliefs and practices of a birthplace, while others, born in the same location or country, may be fully acculturated into the way of life of their adopted country.

Communication skills

Develop your communication skills, both spoken and non-verbal. Patients have a sense of healthcare workers as people with personality and presence; in a crisis they are actively seeking out someone in whom they can place trust, find reassurance, depend on for security and gain help and support from to enable them to cope in what might be for them quite an unfamiliar, anxiety-provoking and confronting or frightening emergency presentation and experience. You, as the healthcare professional, will unwittingly be constantly in communication with your patients in terms of your body language and facial expressions, which convey your attitude and expectations every time you meet people. Increasingly, you will work with patients who do not share your spoken language; the best way to be is to have an awareness of and use the full range of communication skills available to you.[1,2,27]

Different cultural groups will communicate with you in different ways; there are many variations in the way that requests can be put to others, the physical or personal space that is comfortable for different people or the extent to which personal information is shared with strangers, however well-intentioned the healthcare provider might be. Patients will remain cautious and apprehensive if they feel they are in an environment that might potentially be unsafe or 'hostile' towards them.

Signage in all health services should, where possible, be written in a number of different and relevant languages to make things as easy as possible for those who are not native English speakers. While it would be impossible to accommodate all the languages used in Australia or New Zealand–Aotearoa, if you know your local population needs well, then a careful and helpful selection used in pamphlets and available resources will assist patients.

How helpful are cultural profiles and checklists?

Using a specific profile or a 'checklist' of how other cultures might be expected to behave, what beliefs they hold or how they are likely to 'think' is not really very efficient, as it is 'best guess' only and is in a real sense just a series of generalisations. Such aids are secondary to making yourself open to the 'real' messages that are being conveyed by patients about what 'works' for them as individuals. There is as much variation within cultural groups as there is between them.

Caution is also advised about assuming what is 'normal' for those with different self-care habits to you. Everyone has their own idiosyncrasies and considers that they know the way to go about things; for example, food choices, bathing preferences and what constitutes an uncomfortable topic of conversation will vary within and across different groups of people. Providing intimate care and touching patients during caregiving is always an activity that must be approached with sensitivity and respect. Take the time to observe what makes your patient comfortable or uncomfortable, and always ask for their preference as a way of showing respect in how you provide care.

Information sharing and patient teaching

Be prepared to negotiate knowledge; much of the information healthcare workers provide to patients is often complex and can be confusing to those unfamiliar with the terminology and concepts you are talking about. Try to establish what information needs your patient or their family has. Understanding and information will be culturally 'filtered' in any attempt by the patient to gain comprehension, and at times of stress language difficulties are magnified and any inability to understand the healthcare professional only leads to greater stress and will cause a deterioration in compliance with your suggestions. Try to give your patients 'think' time—to translate, ascertain meaning, evaluate what words mean and determine what response they need to provide to the healthcare worker. If you cannot establish clear meaning, you can attempt the sentence again and vary your word choice—this provides the patient with a second opportunity to decide what you mean, rather than struggling with the same words they cannot understand already. Be patient and provide positive feedback to the patient—try to avoid displays of impatience or irritation and remember that raising your voice will not assist in a positive way.

Working in a real partnership

Value the importance of working in a real partnership with your patient; try not to make assumptions about what they might need or what they might want. Developing a workable relationship starts with openness, involves remaining receptive to others and relies upon the exchange of trust.

Undertake your work as a professional healthcare provider in the full knowledge that to patients, you have a great deal of 'role power'—use that power wisely. It is unreasonable to assume that patients will have the knowledge and understanding of healthcare in the same way as you, as a healthcare worker.

Cross-cultural care into the future

Goold, an Indigenous Australian nurse, and Ramsden, from New Zealand–Aotearoa, have both voiced concern that nurses and indeed all healthcare workers have to an extent currently failed to ensure that they have a significant impact on healthcare encounters or have been part of effecting any significant improvement on the quality of healthcare service delivery and its related outcomes.[1,15,25,28]

To move forward, professional healthcare workers in Australasia need to reflect upon the way that they, as a body of professionals, interact with people who are marginalised and disempowered and who are accessing the healthcare system of which healthcare workers form an integral part. A people-centred, rather than a task-centred, approach has been advocated as being pivotal for good care to occur. Healthcare workers must begin to individualise care for each patient and consider their personal and particular circumstances more deeply when responding to and caring for patients. Healthcare workers themselves have traditionally articulated this as an important part of their role and must continue to prioritise a patient-centred approach; one which values the individualising of each person's illness experience as a patient.

While tolerance and sensitivity towards cultural difference may be formally espoused, articulated in principle and reflected in policy and standards, there are indications that this is not always easy to accomplish. Despite changes in the population demographic, Australasia has remained largely monocultural in the broader terms of social institutions, norms and attitudes. The same is true for healthcare; it is still rooted in the white Anglo-Celtic origin of the majority culture. There is evidence to suggest that there are valid concerns about what appears to be a 'mainstream' intolerance to diversity on the part of health service providers. The historical tendency for the healthcare system in Australasia to present itself as a place of neutrality has resulted in a 'culture-blind and ethnocentric approach, effectively creating an exclusionary system'.[25,28] There is a lack of acknowledgement of this and a resistance to change in the power structures of healthcare that inhibits adjustment and the changes that are needed to positively advance cross-cultural care in Australia. Although some small gains have been made regarding heightened awareness of the legitimacy of cultural difference, by and large these have only been marginally effective in changing the attitudes of healthcare workers, improving and changing service delivery or in improving health experiences and outcomes for minority group populations.

Healthcare workers need to prioritise cross-cultural care and learn to work within our contemporary multicultural society in an effective, appropriate and ethical way, and this constitutes one of the greatest challenges faced by professional caregivers today. Good health outcomes are 'a product of reciprocal interactions between individuals and the environments that shape their lives'.[4,5,7,15] The need for considerations of 'culture' to become a specific focus in the delivery of emergency healthcare and a priority for the healthcare worker is now undeniable. While this might seem to be just another demand, it is imperative that healthcare workers accommodate such a requirement and it is appropriate that services are responsive to the needs of the patient as those priorities will necessarily change from time to time and over time.

Healthcare workers in Australasia have traditionally been accustomed to working within a predominantly monocultural, historically European workforce; this will change into the future as the demographic of the healthcare workforce begins to mirror that of the wider community. Cross-cultural interaction must be one of the issues considered as important into the future because of this growing heterogeneity in the patient population and in the healthcare provider workforce. Service providers must assume responsibility for becoming more engaged with ideas around culture and culture's place in contemporary society.

SUMMARY

In terms of health, it is well established that cultural beliefs will shape human understanding of and responses to health and illness; that is, the 'culture' of an individual will affect their perceptions and experience of healthcare. Ideas and beliefs about health and illness generally will have a significant impact on individuals, their families and communities, in fashioning their understanding of illness, the treatment of disease and the prevention of ill-health. When individuals seek assistance in times of sickness, their conceptualisation and understanding of social roles and their own personal beliefs and expectations will have an impact on healthcare encounters. Indigenous and minority ethnic group patients have very specific needs across a range of important requirements, for example, levels of linguistic competence, variability in their capacity for comprehension and conceptualisation, different styles of communication, and other specific personal, spiritual or religious needs.

Any healthcare encounter will be influenced by the attitudes and understandings of both the patient and the healthcare worker.

For many minority group patients, there is a risk that there will be a mismatch between their belief systems and understandings and those of the health system or individual service providers they will encounter. All of these might constitute barriers to service appropriateness and quality, and if patient needs are not met this might lead to negative outcomes and adverse events; curative and supportive therapy could potentially be more effective if cultural matters are taken into consideration.

Healthcare workers have an obligation to ensure that all patients are cared for in the best manner possible. This is especially important in relation to illness, death and dying. It is imperative that professional healthcare workers remain open to the idea that there are many different ways of 'thinking, doing and being' in the world. If the healthcare worker is unsure of a patient's customs and practices, the best place to start with is to seek advice from the patient, their family or their social support system. It is also wise to avoid guessing, seeking advice from other healthcare professionals or consulting a text, 'expert' or pamphlet. The best way forward is to ensure that as a professional caregiver and despite the pressures of your workplace, you try to provide the most respectful care possible for individual patients and their families.[4,7,26]

CASE STUDY

It is a busy night and a young female pregnant patient arrives at the ED accompanied by two ambulance (paramedic) officers; the male officer states that this patient's family made a telephone call for help saying the patient was in pain, bleeding and distressed, but her baby is not due yet.

The history is very vague, as are the details of this patient's situation; the accompanying ambulance officers state that they could not really quite understand what was or is actually happening as neither the patient nor her family can speak English very well. Everyone at the home was quite upset, and when the officers tried to examine the patient she became even more distressed and resisted their intervention.

You and the officers take the patient inside the ED—you need to establish what is happening here and determine what to do next.

Questions

1. What issues do you need to consider, in order of priority, about what cultural issues might be having a significant impact on this situation?
2. How can you develop an open and supportive relationship with this patient and her family group?
3. Describe how you might modify the way in which you undertake your physical assessment and history taking.
4. What information will you decide to relay to other staff that will ensure that appropriate care is provided to this patient into the future?

 Answers to Case Study Questions can be found on evolve
http://evolve.emergencytrauma.curtis

USEFUL WEBSITES

Australian Indigenous Health *Info*Net www.healthinfonet.ecu.edu.au

Australian Institute of Aboriginal and Torres Strait Islander Studies www.aiatsis.gov.au

Australian Institute of Health & Welfare www.aihw.gov.au

Central Australian Aboriginal Congress www.caac.org.au/alukura.html

Congress of Aboriginal and Torres Strait Islander Nurses www.indiginet.com.au/catsin

Cultural Safety/Kawa Whakaruruhau culturalsafety.massey.ac.nz

College of Emergency Nursing Australasia, cena.org.au

Hauora.Com—a Māori lead organisation for Māori development at hauora.com

New Zealand Ministry of Health/Manatū Hauora for the health of Pacific peoples, Asian peoples and Māori, disability strategy and the health of New Zealanders www.health.govt.nz

Nganampa Health Council www.nganampahealth.com.au

Nursing and Midwifery Board of Australia (Australian Health Practitioners Regulatory Authority) www.nursingmidwiferyboard.gov.au/

Nursing Council of New Zealand/Te Kaunihera Tapuhi o Aotearoa www.nursingcouncil.org.nz

Public Health Association of New Zealand Inc./Kāhui Hauora Tūmatanui www.pha.org.nz

Statistics New Zealand/Tatauranga Aotearoa www.stats.govt.nz

Te Ora; the Māori Medical Practitioners Association of New Zealand teora.Maori.nz

SECTION I OVERVIEW OF EMERGENCY CARE

REFERENCES

1. Ramsden IM. Cultural safety and nursing education in Aotearoa and Te Waipounamu. Unpublished PhD thesis. New Zealand: Victoria University of Wellington; 2002.

2. DeSouza R. Wellness for all: the possibilities of cultural safety and cultural competence in New Zealand. Journal of Research in New Zealand 2008;13(2):125–35.

3. Durie M. Cultural Competence and Medical Practice in New Zealand. Presented at the Australian and New Zealand Boards and Council Conference. Wellington, New Zealand on 22 November 2001.

4. Nursing Council of New Zealand. Guidelines for cultural safety, the Treaty of Waitangi and Māori health in nursing education and practice. Wellington, New Zealand: NCNZ Whanau Kawa Whakaruruhau; (2005) Updated July 2011.

5. Phiri J, Dietsch E, Bonner A. Cultural safety and its importance to midwifery in Australia. Collegian 2010;17(3):105–11.

6. Richardson S, Williams T, Finlay A, Farrall M. Senior nurses perceptions of cultural safety in an acute clinical practice area. Nursing Praxis in New Zealand. 2009:25(3):27–36.

7. Nursing and Midwifery Board of Australia (Australian Health Practitioner's Regulatory Authority—AHPRA). Regulatory framework, national competency standards and codes of ethics and conduct 2005–2013. Online. www.nursingmidwiferyboard.gov.au/; accessed 17 Feb 2015.

8. Australian Bureau of Statistics. Census Australia 2013. Canberra: Australian Government; 2013.

9. Australian Bureau of Statistics. 2013. Population Estimates: concepts, sources and methods: Census undercount. Online. Available: www.abs.gov.au/ausstats/abs; accessed 17 Feb 2015.

10. Australian Government. The Australian Institute of Health & Welfare (AIHW) and the Institute of Family Studies. Closing the gap: what works to overcome indigenous disadvantage—key learnings and gaps in the evidence. 2011–2012. Published 2013. Online. Available: www.aihw.gov.au/closingthegap/; accessed 17 Feb 2015.

11. National Health and Medical Research Council. Strategic Plan 2013–2015. Road Map II: a strategic framework for improving the health of Aboriginal and Torres Strait Islanders through the support of health research and its translation. Launched June 2010. IBN: 1864963891.

12. Councils of Australian Governments National Reform Agreement. Ratified 25th July 2012. (Agreed August 2011). Online. www.coag.gov.au/; accessed 17 Feb 2015.

13. Australian Medical Association. (AMA) Indigenous Health Report Card 2012–2013. The healthy early years – getting the right start in life. 10th series. Online. https://ama.com.au/policy/indigenous-health; accessed 20 July 2015.

14. Goold S. Transcultural nursing: can we meet the challenge of caring for the Australian Indigenous person? Journal of Transcultural Nursing 2001;12(2):94–9.

15. McMurray A, Clendon, J. Community health and wellness: primary health care in practice. 4th edn. Sydney: Churchill Livingston Elsevier: 2011.

16. Levey GB. The political theories of Australian multiculturalism. University of New South Wales Law Journal 869, 2001. Online. www.austlii.edu.au/au/journals/UNSWLJ/2001/72.html; accessed 17 Feb 2015.

17. Archer F, Spencer C. Paramedics education and teaching on cultural diversity; conventions underpinning practice. Australasian Journal of Paramedicine 2012;4(3). Article 4. http://ro.ecu.edu.au/jephc/vol4/iss4/4; accessed 17 Feb 2015.

18. Hawthorne L. Health Workforce Migration to Australia; policy trends and outcomes 2004–2010. The University of Melbourne. A scoping paper commissioned by Health Workforce Australia. 2012.

19. Statistics New Zealand. Online. www.stats.govt.nz/census.aspx; 2013.

20. Earp R. The Treaty of Waitangi and Māori health: keynote address given to National Forum on Indigenous Health and the Treaty Debate. Sydney: University of New South Wales; 11 Sep 2004. Online. www.gtcentre.unsw.edu.au/sites/gtcentre.unsw.edu.au/files/mdocs/6_RiaEarp.pdf; accessed 17 Feb 2015.

21. Mortenson A. Cultural safety: does the theory work in practice for culturally and linguistically diverse groups. Nursing Praxis in New Zealand 2010;26(3):6–16.

22. MacKay B, Harding T, Jurlina L et al. Utilising the hand model to promote a culturally safe environment for international nursing students. Nursing Praxis in New Zealand 2011;27(1):13–24.

23. Australian Institute of Health and Welfare. Australia's Health 2012. Australian Health series No 13. Catalogue Number Aus. 156. Canberra, Australia. Online. www.aihw.gov.au/publication-detail/?id=10737422172; accessed 17 Feb 2015.

24. Johnstone MJ, Kanitsaki O. Culture, language, and patient safety: making the link. International Journal of Quality in Health Care 2006; 18(5):383–8.

25. Spence D. Nursing people from cultures other than one's own: a perspective from New Zealand. Contemporary Nurse 2003; 15(3):222–31.

26. Stewart S. Ringing in the changes for a culturally competent workforce. 3rd edn. Synergy: Multicultural Mental Health Australia; 2006.

27. Hera J. Cultural competence and patient-centered care. Coles Medical Practice in New Zealand. 2013. Online. www.mcnz.org.nz/assets/News-and-Publications/Coles/Chapter-4.pdf; accessed 17 Feb 2015.

CHAPTER 6
MANAGEMENT AND LEADERSHIP
PETER O'MEARA AND STUART NEWMAN

Essentials

- In the current health system environment, emergency health services face many leadership and management challenges.
- Good management skills are important, but the emergency health environment needs 'leaders' who can anticipate and lead change, build and motivate teams, and implement systems to support evidence-based, patient-centred care.
- Emergency health service leaders are strategic and critical thinkers; they understand organisational challenges, develop and communicate a vision for the future of the services, engage and motivate key stakeholders, build high-performance teams, encourage innovation, share power, engender trust and lead by example.
- Paramedics and nurses at all levels in emergency health services have the potential to be clinical leaders in terms of developing and improving practice to be more evidence-based and to meet the needs of consumers, government agencies, regulatory bodies and the team members with whom they work.
- Leadership development, coaching and support are required to assist clinicians to develop their leadership capacity and emotional, social, cultural intelligence and to actualise their clinical leadership potential.

INTRODUCTION

Emergency health systems (services) are busy microcosms of any healthcare system and they are often the first point of public interface with, or the 'front door' to, many healthcare organisations. The emergency health system is comprised of community first responders and many healthcare professionals, including doctors and allied health providers. However, the emphasis here is on emergency nurses and paramedics who collectively comprise the first point of contact with emergency patients and the people who care about them (consumers).

Healthcare systems in developed countries have experienced significant structural, clinical and socio-political transformations over the last three decades and collectively, these transformations are known as health reform.[1] In the current healthcare environment managers are expected to manage services in an efficient and cost-effective way, build high-performing teams from what are often disparate groups of professionals, refocus care on patient needs and develop innovative ways of improving service provision and patient outcomes. Paramedics and emergency nurses have been directly affected by these transformations and their practice environment is now characterised by increased demand for services from well-informed consumers, continuous change in care delivery systems and demands for safe, high-quality care from consumers, government agencies and regulatory bodies.[2]

The notion of being a 'good manager' in the emergency health system has progressively become insufficient, and organisations have begun to demand and seek out 'manager–leaders'; people who have a vision for the future of clinical practice, can lead change, build and motivate teams and implement systems to support evidence-based, patient-centred care. More than ever, nurses and paramedics need to question the long-held belief that the people traditionally thought to be the leaders (director of nursing, senior operational managers or unit managers) can make a difference at the level of patient care. These 'positions' provide infrastructure and resources and set the standards of care, but the people who are most influential in terms of implementing innovative models of care and improving quality, safety and standards of care are those who interact with consumers to deliver expert emergency healthcare.

Leadership is not something a few anointed people do because they are in certain management positions. On the contrary, leadership can come from any level within an organisation and it is not solely the domain of high-level organisational positions. Nursing and paramedicine needs leaders at the clinical or service delivery interface who can meet the current challenges and lead practice change and development.

In this chapter what it means to be a nurse or paramedic manager and leader in the current healthcare environment is examined. A summary of some of the leadership theories is provided in order to understand the difference between a manager and a leader, and to identify the characteristics that make an effective leader. A number of important contemporary leadership issues are discussed, including the leader–follower relationship and the importance of emotional, social and cultural intelligence. The need for nursing and paramedicine leadership in health politics and policy development and in the implementation of clinical or shared governance and evidence-based practice is explored.

Management challenges

The role of the emergency health manager in paramedic services and emergency departments (ED) is pivotal to the delivery of safe and effective care to patients who present in times of health crisis. As the 'front door' of many health services, the emergency health system is open to scrutiny from the community, consumers who present for services, bureaucrats and politicians who have responsibility for the provision of public health services and the regulators who maintain a watchful eye on the quality and safety of care provided by registered healthcare professionals. While the provision of emergency health services has always been challenging, the level of scrutiny has intensified, underpinned by the health reform agenda and the growing politicisation of the healthcare system.[3] There are two main influences driving the increased level of politicisation and political involvement in healthcare. The first influence represents the flow-on affect of the growing politicisation of the wider public sector in developed countries where the impact of globalisation and New Public Management (viz deregulation and privatisation) is being faced. Healthcare has taken a prominent place within this political agenda.[3–5] The second influence is more specific to healthcare and can

be attributed to the increasing public controversies and overt public and political debate about the quality of the system witnessed predominantly through the media.[3] The management challenges for paramedic and ED services in the contemporary socio-political economic environment in which healthcare is situated are well documented and include:

- increased demand for emergency health services that manifests in overcrowding, difficulties in meeting benchmark waiting times and ambulance response times, ambulance diversions, long-stay or 'boarding' patients and increased levels of inter-personal violence[6]
- culturally diverse, well-informed and vocal consumers who demand that health services become more relationship-centred and service-oriented,[7] and who are now more willing to make complaints to health authorities, the regulators and the media if their needs are not met or if they suffer adverse events during care
- continuous restructure, reform and redesign of the health system in an effort to make care delivery more efficient while meeting the need to address problems of quality and safety and 'dissatisfaction among patients, the public and health professionals' alike[8] (the recent implementation of National Emergency Access Target [NEAT] is a case in point);[9,10]
- workforce shortages and difficulties in recruiting and retaining highly skilled and experienced paramedics and nurses within paramedic services and specialty areas such as EDs to work within new models of care and undertake expanded roles.

Management: concepts and contexts

The development of 'formal management theory' emerged in the early 1900s and is essentially a product of early 20th-century post-industrial society, although management practice is not new and has been traced back to early Egypt, Rome, Greece and China.[11] The existing level of knowledge about organisations and management cannot be attributed to a particular person, but to the work of a number of key theorists. Principal among them are Frederick Taylor's scientific management theory, Max Weber's bureaucratic theory, Frank and Lillian Gilbreth, who studied efficiency and motion, and Mary Parker Follett's human relations theory. Also among these key theorists was French industrialist Henri Fayol, who in 1917 introduced five management functions: planning, organising, commanding (directing), coordinating and controlling. He also developed 14 principles of management (Table 6.1), which were taken at the time to be fundamental or universal truths that could (or should) be taught.[12,13] Fayol was the first management theorist to write about how important it was for employees to understand organisational goals. In 1937, drawing on Fayol's earlier work, Gulick extended Fayol's original five management functions to seven: planning, organising, staffing, directing, coordinating, reporting and budgeting.[14]

Theoretical perspectives developed in the latter half of the 20th century by theorists such as Herzberg, Mintzberg, Carnegie, Silverman and Herbert among others, who articulated the need to have a greater understanding of the person, the centrality of work to our existence and how workplace experiences impact on us. Silverman and Herbert[15–17] led the

TABLE 6.1 Fayol's 14 management principles[12]

PRINCIPLE	UNDERLYING ASSUMPTIONS
1. Division of labour	• Workers who are more specialised can perform their jobs more efficiently. • Greater efficiency increases productivity. • People should be in the job for which they are best suited.
2. Authority	• Management has delegated power and the right to issue commands and compel obedience.
3. Discipline	• Employees must obey rules and regulations. • Managers apply penalties for non-compliance.
4. Unity of command	• Workers should receive instructions from one manager.
5. Unit of direction	• The whole organisation should be moving towards common goals (common direction).
6. Subordination of individual interests to the common good	• The interests of the organisation should take precedence over individual or group interests.
7. Remuneration	• Workers must be paid a fair wage.
8. Centralisation	• Decision-making should be concentrated at a single point or, at the most, employees should only be given enough authority to perform their jobs appropriately.
9. Hierarchy	• Scalar chain – meaning authority must run from top management to the lowest level. • Communication should also follow this chain.
10. Order	• People and materials should be in the right place at the right time. • Order increases efficiency and coordination = increased productivity.
11. Equity	• Managers should practise fairness to all employees.
12. Stability of tenure	• Retention of staff is valued because turnover is both disruptive and costly.
13. Initiative	• Managers should encourage worker initiative (within reason) because this leads to greater work effort.
14. Esprit de corps	• Managers should encourage team spirit (harmony). • Harmony provides a sense of unity.

way in the examination of how work and organisations relate to broader social structures. The ideas expressed by Silverman and Herbert challenged the traditional views of people in organisations because they identified organisations as the product of human action and that organisational order was a negotiated system.

Silverman's social action analysis focused on what people do as they organise their relations with others. That is, how people go about constructing their reality and what the impact of this constructed reality is on the individual, management and the organisation. In Silverman's view, these issues move beyond simple quantifiable data and they require broader consideration because how individuals construct their reality is unique to each person; few, if any, generalisations can be made about individuals within organisations. This view was contrary to the instrumental or functional accounts that identified organisations as collective action in pursuit of organisational goals. As a result, uncertainty, ambiguity, competition and conflict became enduring conditions within the organisational literature.[15,16]

Herbert further addressed the issue of people in organisations and focused on moving away from the rational-economic model. To understand individual behaviour, Herbert argued we should first know something about the influences that make a person behave in a particular way in a particular situation. Herbert called for the suspension of the rational-economic model of human behaviour because it assumed away those factors other than the ones we can calculate the benefits and costs of various alternative choices on how to behave.[17]

Within the more recent theoretical perspectives there is also a strong emphasis on institutional theory, population ecology and strategic management.[18] In many of these theories the common themes are how managers use delegated authority and positional power (authority), rules, regulations and structures.

Various definitions of management have been offered over time and continuing redefinition shows the complexity and dynamism of the concept. In 1973, Henry Mintzberg studied top managers and found that contrary to the popular notion that managers carefully considered all options prior to making a decision, managers spent their time engaged in a large number of 'varied, unpatterned and short-duration activities' or management functions.[19] In his book, *Mintzberg on Management: Inside our Strange World of Organizations*, he divided these ten management functions into three highly integrated and interrelated management categories: the interpersonal role, the informational role and the decisional role (Table 6.2).[20]

Lewis[21] considers that, despite the variations and imprecision of the many definitions of management and the various roles ascribed to managers, it is possible to identify a number of common themes related to management. According to Lewis, management is:

- a formally appointed position that is a separate function in the work process and carries with it delegated decision-making authority and responsibility for meeting performance indicators
- goal-oriented and requires the ability to set and achieve organisational goals and objectives
- a process of getting things done in an organisation through specific functions, activities and groups of people who are employed to perform specialised functions
- achieved through the use of human, material and financial resources
- influenced by the type of organisation and by the knowledge, skills and attributes of the individual who holds the management position

It is clear from these themes that health service managers have a separate role and function from that of providing clinical care. Robbins et al[13] differentiate *managers* from *operatives* (in the case of healthcare, staff who work directly at the frontline delivering care), but they are also quick to point out that there is some blurring of the roles. This blurring can be seen particularly in emergency health services where 24-hour care is provided, for example, when managers sometimes undertake clinical care and when clinicians need to undertake management activities in their roles as team leaders or shift managers.

One of the issues for any organisation is the individuality of particular managers, their interpretation of particular situations and actions that they take in different circumstance given their personal characteristics and previous experience.[22] While organisations can specify requirements related to how resources are used, how policies and procedures are implemented and future directions for service development, the manner in which particular managers go about the business of managing may vary considerably, particularly if they are stronger in some aspects of their role than others.

Management development education has been criticised over the years because of its focus on theory, corporate and political skills, and the 'hard' technical aspects of management such as human resource and financial management.[23,24] According to Kitson,[25] development programs often completely ignore the managers' needs: for the development of critical skills related to leading clinical teams and improving care such as self-management and personal reflection; the ability to critically appraise the many forms of information and evidence available; clinical decision-making; and an understanding of how the context of care and workplace culture can impact on patient outcomes. While in the past strong management skills have been valued, the current healthcare environment is a 'complex adaptive system' and, as Baker states, 'attempting to manage complex adaptive systems using traditional management techniques (more appropriate to simple problems) can be frustrating and counterproductive'.[26] The current healthcare environment requires manager-leaders who can anticipate and lead change, build and motivate teams and implement systems to support evidence-based, patient-centred care.

TABLE 6.2 Mintzberg's ten management roles[20]		
INTERPERSONAL	Figurehead	The person with authority and who has social, ceremonial and legal responsibilities.
	Leader	Responsible for providing leadership (organisational vision, goals, direction, guidance) and for the group's performance.
	Liaison	Responsible for communication between internal and external stakeholders and effective networking on behalf of the organisation.
INFORMATIONAL	Monitor	The organisational 'thermostat'—seeking and monitoring information relevant to the internal and external environments in which the organisation is positioned, as well as monitoring the group's productivity and wellbeing.
	Disseminator	Effective communication of relevant information throughout the organisation.
	Spokesperson	One who speaks on behalf of the organisation (see also Figurehead) in order to communicate with the organisation's external environment and external stakeholders.
DECISIONAL	Entrepreneur	Generating new ideas, implementing change and problem-solving.
	Disturbance Handler	Managing conflict or disruptions to productivity.
	Resource Allocator	Managing both human and financial resources efficiently and effectively.
	Negotiator	Between departments and teams within the organisation and organisations or groups external to the organisation (see also Disturbance Handler).

Leadership

Leadership is a term that is neither well understood nor absolutely defined. Contemporary writers on leadership continue to grapple with a number of questions about what constitutes leadership and the requirements for strong leadership particularly given the more recent research on generations and generational issues in the workforce.[27–29] Equally, they continue to grapple with the question of if and how leadership can be 'taught' or 'learned'. There are no definitive answers to these questions in the literature, which indicates the complexity of the concepts.

Defining leadership

Like definitions of management, many definitions of leadership have been proposed. We have seen these definitions change over time since Dwight Eisenhower's well-known notion of 'getting someone else to do something you want done because he [*sic*] wants to do it'. In the 1980s definitions of leadership focused more on achieving organisational goals and in the 1990s on establishing direction, aligning vision and motivating and inspiring.[30] Peter Drucker proposed one definition that has become particularly influential in the last 10 years, saying 'the only definition of a leader is someone who has followers. Some people are thinkers. Some are prophets. Both roles are important and badly needed. But without followers, there can be no leaders.'[31] In 2007, John Maxwell further emphasised the importance of the leader–follower relationship when he said 'the true measure of leadership is influence—nothing more, nothing less'.[32]

The terms 'leadership' and 'management' are often used interchangeably. Some authors contend that leaders and managers have different roles, while others view leadership and management as two sides of the one coin and that people in management positions also require well-developed leadership skills to be effective in their positions. According to Beech,[33] there is a consensus that 'management implies leadership, but that leaders need not necessarily be managers, which reflects the increasing calls for 'manager–leaders' rather than simply 'managers'. There is however, a stronger distinction to consider in the management/leadership debate—the difference between being in a position of providing leadership and being a leader. As John Maxwell points out,

> when people hear someone has an impressive title or an assigned leadership position, they assume that person is a leader. Sometimes that's true. But titles do not have much value when it comes to leading. True leadership cannot be awarded, appointed or assigned. It comes only from influence, and that cannot be mandated. It must be earned. The only thing a title can buy is a little time—either to increase your level of influence with others or undermine it.[32]

Leadership and management are distinctive, yet complementary, and Kotter argues that the major problem in many organisations is that they are 'overmanaged and underled'.[34] He also points out that strong leadership and poor management is no better. While much has been written about the manager/leader distinction, there is also the school of thought that leaders need to possess good management skills. Strong leaders have good management skills because while they are being visionary, motivating and building high performance teams, among other things, they are also able to get the job done. In addition, the more recent management research is showing that when strong leadership is present, managers also have strong emotional, social and cultural intelligence, which is more important and influential than the cognitive intelligence or technical skill managers may possess.[35–37]

This means that in paramedic services and EDs, where there are appointed managers, other paramedics and nurses at all levels have the potential to be leaders in the clinical setting in terms of developing and communicating a vision, building high-performance teams and improving practice by encouraging innovation and sharing power. In sum, by engendering trust in their teams and leading by example, they have the capacity to influence others and amass followers. This is what leadership is about.

Leadership theories

Like management, leadership has a strong theoretical background. Leadership, and, by association, satisfaction and motivation, are complex concepts, reflected by the number of theoretical positions and critiques developed over the years. In order to understand what it means to be a leader and what constitutes leadership, it is helpful to review the theoretical platform on which leadership is based and how leadership theory and discourse have evolved. Understanding these concepts and what constitutes leadership effectiveness is important to provide support for current clinical leaders and the development of the clinical leaders of the future.

Early theorists attempted to explain leadership on the basis of inherited characteristics, or personality types that resulted in particular leadership behaviours. It was thought that leaders were 'born to lead' and early theorists developed psychological tests, inventories of personality traits and lists of behaviours and compared their findings in relation to people who were said to be leaders.[38] The research identified a large number of traits associated with successful leaders, but there was no consensus on what the essential leadership traits were.[39] There was also a lack of evidence to support the notion that someone who has a particular set of traits would make a good leader.

Later, the behavioural theorists examined leadership behaviours and leadership styles.[39] The theoretical framework moved from describing the personality traits of a leader to one that examined the leader's behaviours and their leadership style (autocratic, democratic, laissez-faire). Theorists soon found that leadership styles and behaviours were not predictive of leadership actions in different contexts and situations.[39]

In the late 1960s, contingency and situational leadership theory (SLT) began to examine the complexity of the workplace and the relationship between it and the leader, rather than just concentrating on the leader's traits and behaviours.[40,41] According to these theorists, no one leadership style is suitable for every work situation or group; an effective leader has the ability to adopt a different leadership style depending upon the type of work, their relationship with the worker and the worker's skill or level of professional maturity. For example, low-skilled or inexperienced workers need direction and close supervision, whereas an experienced group, such as registered nurses and paramedics, need support, not direction. Their professional maturity level means they can take on delegated tasks and work with low supervision.[42] The emergence of SLT saw a shift in emphasis from the characteristics or traits of the leader to recognition of the role that leader/follower relationships played and the importance of the level of development of the followers in this relationship. In the late 1970s attention turned to the interactional theories of leadership when Burns,[43] well known for his work in the area of leader/follower interactions, introduced the notion of transactional and transformational leadership.

Transactional and transformational leadership

Burns[43] maintained that there were two types of leaders: the transactional (TA) leader and the transformational (TF) leader. Since Burns published his groundbreaking work, leadership theory has continued to evolve and a great deal has been published on the differences between these two types of leaders.

The transactional leader is seen as one who is appointed to a position of authority (read a manager), who is most concerned with the structures and systems that support the day-to-day operations and uses the skills of planning and controlling the use of available resources to achieve the vision and strategy of the organisation. Transactional leaders are seen to have a tactical focus, concentrating on managing complexity, allocating resources and focusing on achieving the vision and goals set by the organisation.[44]

In the early transformational leadership literature a number of authors felt strongly that the most essential function of leadership was to bring about adaptive and useful change.[38] In today's fast-paced environment, change has become the one thing that is a constant. The reason many people become 'change weary' and dissatisfied with their working environment is that they are seldom involved in the decisions about the change required or the change process, and as a result cannot see how it will benefit them or their clients. In addition, at a personal level, the more change that confronts an individual combined with their stage of life or career can lead to resistance based on their inability to accommodate yet another transition.[45] Transformational leaders are seen to be more strategic in their style, with the ability to know the organisation and the problems it faces, develop and communicate a vision for the future, engage and motivate key stakeholders, build high-performance teams, encourage innovation, share power, engender trust and lead by example.[41] The transformational theorists agree that leaders do more than 'manage' a situation; they have a special responsibility for understanding complex and changing environments, facilitate dramatic change and energise followers to work towards a shared vision.[38]

So the question is: what sort of person is a transformational leader? The literature[46–48] contains a number of common themes that collectively describe a transformational leader as someone who is:

- able to think critically and strategically
- future oriented and able to articulate a strong and clear vision
- self-aware, reflective and able to manage their emotions
- able to develop people's strengths, build strong teams, motivate and inspire people to achieve shared goals
- able to manage relationships through collaborating, communicating well, developing trust, negotiating,

managing conflict, role modelling and celebrating successes
- politically and culturally aware and able to build strong networks both inside and outside the organisation in order to influence policy and service delivery.

The transformational leadership model is considered to be the current gold standard, but there are some caveats. Although transformational leadership characteristics are highly advantageous there is the potential to subjugate or temper the day-to-day aspects of leadership and the requirements of leaders in organisations. For this reason, some authors propose the need for a combination of transformational approach with the more traditional and day-to-day characteristics of the transactional and situational approaches.[49,50] This idea is premised on the concept that it is highly desirable and valuable to be a visionary and creative, but if the day-to-day needs cannot be met then visions are very hard to achieve. Those who have experienced strong leadership will say that leaders who are visionary and creative are wonderful. However, experience informs us that if leaders are unable to provide leadership on a day-to-day basis to get followers through the immediate issues, uncertainties and crises, then vision and creativity will not motivate people to follow. There needs to be a balance.

The leader–follower relationship

We have established that leadership cannot exist without followers and this leader–follower relationship is based on power. The concept of power has traditionally been a delicate subject and one approached cautiously because of the tendency to associate power with negative or undesirable behaviour. Power is generally described as the capacity to influence others. French and Raven (1959) provided one of the best known and most enduring explanations when they identified five bases of power: coercive, reward, legitimate, expert and referent. While this model is 50 years old, and there has been the addition of information power and opportunity power, the model by French and Raven remains one of the most commonly used models in the management and leadership literature (Table 6.3).[13]

The concept of knowledge-intensive organisations or knowledge-intensive work has gained prominence in the healthcare literature because of increasing acknowledgment of the relationship between leadership and power, in particular expert power and opportunity power. There is now recognition that leadership does not necessarily remain vested in one particular person. It is clear that no single person can necessarily lead a knowledge-intensive group all the time; one may be a leader in one situation but a follower in another.

While strong leaders influence their followers, this influence cannot be achieved without follower willingness or compliance. While the traditional leadership literature considers followers in the conventional way (obedient and relatively uncomplicated),[51] the more recent literature considers leadership to be a participatory activity in which there is mutual benefit because each adds to the other. Subsequently, there is renewed emphasis on the need for leaders to understand the values, beliefs and identity aspects of their followers.[52,53] Therefore, to be a successful leader requires an understanding of what followers need and want. One primary influence affecting the leader–follower relationship is diversity, which refers

TABLE 6.3 Bases of power[13]	
LEGITIMATE	Legitimate or position power is perhaps the most common access to power because it comes with the formal position (authority) a person holds in an organisation.
REWARD	Reward power refers to the ability a person has to reward the effort of others in a meaningful way, either financially or non-financially.
COERCIVE	Coercive power is the opposite of reward power and usually undesirable because it is where compliance (followership) is based on fear (of punishment, retribution, isolation etc.). Coercive power contributes greatly to high levels of dissatisfaction and demotivation and can lead to oppressed group behaviour and horizontal violence.
EXPERT	Expert power refers to power that is gained through knowledge and skills because a leader's expertise gains them respect and compliance. This is a particularly relevant power base in practice disciplines like paramedicine and nursing where skills and knowledge are highly valued.
REFERENT	Referent power is based on the extent to which followers identify with leaders and what they stand for or symbolise. The success of the referent power base depends on the leader's characteristics matching or connecting with the group's fundamental principles. Referent power is also sometimes considered in terms of the ways in which leaders influence others to be like them, that is they role model strong positive behaviours that others replicate.
INFORMATION	Information power refers to the ability of the leader to control the flow of information needed by others to either perform their jobs or make decisions. Leaders gain power by either sharing information openly and transparently or withholding information, which is less desirable. In either case, information power is transient because of the extent to which information needs change in an organisation.
OPPORTUNITY	Opportunity power refers to being in the right place at the right time and recognising the opportunity to gain power. For example, in an emergency or other clinical situation a leader can seize an opportunity to enhance their power base because of their legitimate or expert power coupled with their referent power.

to the nature of the individuals, groups and organisations.[54] In the case of emergency health services this diversity relates to a knowledge intensive and varied workforce and the unique nature of healthcare organisations.

Why then do people follow a certain leader? Rath and Conchie suggest that followers have a clear picture of what they want from and need in a leader. The four most important needs they identify are trust, compassion, stability and hope.[55] They argue, 'whether you are a manager, CEO, or head of state, trust might be the "do or die" foundation for leading'.[55] While skill or competence and vision do not figure in these most important needs, other authors have identified more comprehensive summaries of followers' needs. In relation to nursing leaders, Sherman argues that the key qualities followers look for in leaders are: commitment to excellence, passion about their work, clear vision and strategic focus, trustworthiness, respectfulness, accessibility, empathy and caring, commitment to coaching and developing their staff.[56] What has become increasingly obvious from the leader–follower relationship is the connection between what followers want and the motivation/satisfaction research.[57–59]

Emotional, social and cultural intelligence

One of the strong themes in the current leadership literature is that to be an effective leader requires not only cognitive intelligence and great technical skill, but also emotional, social and cultural intelligence—a triad drawn from aspects of multiple intelligence theory.[37] Cognitive intelligence, often aligned with intelligence quotient (IQ) is broadly defined as the ability to think critically and reason logically without feelings or emotions and it is not concerned with social skills.[60] Emotional intelligence (known as EQ or EI) is different in that it is about self-awareness, self-management, social awareness and relationship management—the ability to understand and manage our emotions to guide decision-making.[61] It is the capacity of a leader to recognise their own emotions and the impact they have on others, to manage those emotions and motivate themselves and to assess, understand and manage the emotions within teams and relationships. If a leader is to inspire and work with people to achieve goals, then they need to have empathy with and a good understanding of the values and emotions of the team members and what motivates and inspires them. Too often in relationships with patients/carers and other professionals, we see negative emotions like anger, fear, frustration and uncertainty, and these emotions can have a powerful effect on working relationships and patient outcomes and contribute to a stressful environment. According to Goleman,[35] 'We are being judged by a new yardstick: not just by how smart we are, or by our training and expertise, but also by how well we handle ourselves and each other.' There is now substantial evidence that supports the view that people with a high emotional intelligence will be better leaders, more successful in business, less stressed and more resilient; they will have more-satisfied staff and customers and higher business profits or, in the case of the healthcare industry, it could be said better teamwork and more efficient workplaces.[62]

The second intelligence in this triad is social intelligence (SI), which is concerned with the ability to think and act wisely in social situations. In the leadership context, the notion of social situations refers to both interaction with followers and the leaders situating practices within the organisational and wider contexts. According to Riggio and Reichard,[36] the components of intelligence include 'the ability to express oneself in social interactions, the ability to "read" and understand different social situations, knowledge of social roles, norms, and scripts, interpersonal problem-solving skills, and social role-playing skills'. The three social skills they identify are: (1) social expressiveness, which is the is ability to communicate and engage others in social interactions; (2) social sensitivity, which is based on knowledge of social rules and norms and the subsequent ability to interpret social situations; and (3) social control, which refers to sophisticated social role-playing skills and tact in social situations.

The concept of cultural intelligence (CQ) is more recent than EI and SI. Cultural intelligence is essentially concerned with the skills leaders have in recognising cultural cues, obtaining cultural knowledge and their understanding of the cultural implications of their actions (interactions) or inactions.[37] The concept of cultural intelligence has become increasingly important in healthcare because, as Groves and Feyerherm[63] point out, the cultural composition of work teams and the values of individual team members in today's organisations has changed dramatically and, given the migratory nature of the healthcare workforce, this trend is likely to continue.

From the discussion above you can see that the leadership literature is replete with long lists of knowledge, skills and attributes required to be an effective leader. This leads to the question: is this type of leadership attainable for paramedicine and nursing today? The good news is that within the contemporary leadership literature there is agreement that present-day leadership is really more about the development of relationships between leaders and followers than about the personality traits or charisma of the leader. Many authors also argue that while leadership cannot be taught per se, it can be learnt through focused development processes that include formal education, guided experience, challenging assignments, coaching, mentoring and reflection.[37] There is also good news about EI, SI and CQ. They are not fixed entities or innate qualities an individual possesses—they can be learned and improved and for effective leadership in contemporary organisations they must be learned!

Integrating service management and leadership of people

While the literature debates the similarities and differences between leadership and management and transactional versus transformational leadership, these two concepts are synergistic.[22] Healthcare, more specifically emergency health services, need transformational leaders who have not only mastered the transactional skills but who can capitalise on the transformational skills of leadership as well.[25] Leadership and management need to be integrated so that people are motivated and empowered to achieve the shared goals, and services are managed to meet the needs of clients in a changing world. As Marquis and Huston[22] point out, integrated leaders/managers think longer term and

are visionary in their decision-making; they look outwards and are aware of how their sphere of practice fits within the 'bigger picture'; they have influence that allows them to have an impact inside and outside the organisation; they are self-aware as well as socially aware; they are politically astute and able to manage conflicting expectations; and they are masterful change agents and reinvent their organisations to meet changing needs. For paramedic and nurse managers, and senior clinicians, to reach their full potential as leaders, they need to work on developing and integrating their management expertise and their leadership capacity. Leadership development programs in the health sector are often aimed at senior management and executive levels, and they fail to offer opportunities for frontline paramedicine and nursing managers and senior clinicians to build the leadership capacity that is required to develop a comprehensive vision for the future of emergency health services.[64]

Contemporary leadership issues for paramedics and emergency nurses

In order for paramedics and clinical nurse leaders, be they clinicians or managers, to be effective in their leadership roles, they need to be politically active in both the internal and the external politics of the healthcare system and keep abreast of new and emerging trends and policy frameworks that will have an impact on their professional roles and responsibilities, service delivery and clinical practice.

Politics, political awareness and policy development

Internal politics is evident in every organisation where key stakeholders, such as paramedic and nurse leaders, use political behaviour and networking to influence decision-making, resource allocation and the management of various systems and processes.[65] However, to be effective, paramedic and nurse leaders need to be directly involved in political activity related to broader health policy agendas so that they can proactively influence policy direction and implementation. They must understand the policy-making process, learn to read the policy agendas and move beyond parochial interests to engage in political action.[65,66] This political activism might be enacted through local, state and national committees, professional organisations and consumer groups. In general, neither the paramedicine nor the nursing voice is consistently heard in the debate regarding the development of health and social policy and its impact on patient care and clinical practice. As Boswell et al[67] suggest in the case of nursing: 'as patient advocates—nurses cannot continue to be spectators in the political arena'. To be politically aware and influential, paramedic and nurse leaders need to understand:

- the bigger political picture about healthcare
- the key political agendas within their own organisations and how they integrate with local, state and national politics and policies
- who has power and authority and how they use it to influence the political agendas, and
- how to influence, being more strategic and proactive rather than reactive to policy change.

Leadership and clinical governance

With the recent focus on patient safety and quality of care, many healthcare systems have implemented clinical governance models to provide a framework for overseeing and monitoring standards of professional practice within organisations and to address the quality and safety issues. Clinical governance (also known as shared governance) is a framework used by healthcare organisations for decentralising accountability for standards of clinical performance, for oversight and monitoring of patient outcomes, for continuous improvement of systems and processes and the effective use of resources.[68]

As pointed out by O'Rourke and Davidson,[68] health professionals are already subject to a number of levels of governance including registration at government level, the development of practice standards by professional bodies and through employment within a particular governing organisation. Clinical governance, however, is a more visible and explicit framework used by organisations for the delegation of accountability for patient care at all levels. According to the Australian Council on Health Care Standards, clinical governance is defined as 'the system by which the governing body, managers and clinicians share responsibility and are held accountable for patient care, minimising risks to consumers and for continuously monitoring and improving the quality of clinical care'.[69]

One of the most important factors in engendering a culture of clinical quality and safety within a clinical governance framework is the establishment of partnerships between senior management and the clinical leaders within an organisation.[70] According to Balding,[69] line managers (such as the nursing unit manager, paramedic operations manager or clinical coordinator in the ED) need to be able to translate the vision of top leaders into an achievable reality for those who deliver patient care and to establish that reality as a part of everyday work. While paramedics may have greater autonomy over their day-to-day clinical practice than nurses, they still have concerns about their limited participation in the decision-making processes of paramedic services and in the development of their clinical practice guidelines.[71] Paramedics are reported to experience structural and cultural challenges when attempting to implement evidence-based practice changes in policy and practice that depart from established clinical protocols or management approaches to service delivery.[71,72]

Clinical leaders in paramedicine and nursing are expert practitioners who have the potential to influence and direct clinical practice using the best available evidence, creativity and innovation. Managers need to establish structures and mechanisms that support the delegation of decision-making authority and accountability, systems for monitoring and reporting outcomes, processes for information sharing and participation and opportunities for staff to enhance their abilities to embrace a more autonomous and accountable style of practice. Clearly this will not happen unless the leader is able to motivate and empower staff in such a way that they readily accept this new level of autonomy and accountability for their practice.

SUMMARY

This chapter has provided an overview of what it means for a paramedic or a nurse to be a manager and leader in the emergency health system today, and how these roles are crucial to the provision of high-quality, safe and efficient care in paramedic and ED services. The challenge for paramedic and nurse managers is to develop their leadership potential, to integrate it with their management expertise and to look beyond day-to-day operations to the future of the emergency health system. It is also essential for managers and organisations to develop the potential of all paramedics and nurses and to empower them to take leadership roles within the clinical environment. Paramedicine and emergency nursing needs politically aware leaders with a clear vision for the future of paramedicine and nursing and how to make that vision reality. As the late Professor Donna Diers[65] said, 'what is exciting about leadership is the way it forces one to have a vision quite beyond the exigencies of the daily grind. Without a vision the work is meaningless'. In her words, 'a vision serves as an energy source, a star to guide us, a hook on which to hang our dreams of glory … a good vision will outlive any leader; it gives one a legacy'.

REFERENCES

1. Bennett CC. Are we there yet? A journey of health reform in Australia. Medical Journal of Australia 2013;199(4):251–5.

2. Lowthian JA, Curtis AJ, Cameron PA et al. Systematic review of trends in emergency department attendances: an Australian perspective. Emergency Medicine Journal 2010;28(5):374–7.

3. Newman S, Lawler J. Managing health care under new public management: a Sisyphean challenge for nursing. Journal of Sociology 2009;45(4):419–32.

4. Deppe H-U. The nature of health care: commodification verses solidarity. Socialist Register 2010;46:29–38.

5. Meadowcroft J. Patients, politics, and power: government failure and the politicization of UK health care. J Med Philos 2008;33(5):427–44.

6. Robinson KS, Jagim MM, Ray CE. Nursing workforce issues and trends affecting emergency departments. Top Emerg Med 2004;26(4):276–86.

7. Vitello-Cicciu JM. Exploring emotional intelligence implications for nurse leaders. J Nurs Adm 2002;32(4):203–10.

8. Locock L. Healthcare redesign: meaning, origins and application. Qual Saf Health Care 2003;12(1):53–7. Online. www.qhc. bmjjournals.com; accessed 19 Apr 2005.

9. Crawford K, Morphet J, Jones T et al. Initiatives to reduce overcrowding and access block in Australian emergency departments: a literature review. Collegian 2013. Online. www.collegianjournal.com/article/S1322-7696(13)00093-0/abstract; accessed 7 November 2013.

10. Emergency Care Institute New South Wales. NEAT—the basics. 2014. Online. www.ecinsw.com.au/NEAT-the-basics; accessed 4 September 2014.

11. Pindur W, Rogers SE, Kim PS. The history of management: a global perspective. Journal of Management History 1995;1(1):59–77.

12. Wren DA, Bedeian AG, Breeze JD. The foundations of Henry Fayol's administrative theory. Management Decision 2002;40(9):906–18.

13. Robbins SP, Bergman R, Stagg I et al. Management. Prentice Hall Sydney; 2000.

14. Gulick LH. Notes on the theory of organization. In: Gulick I, Urwick L, eds. Papers on the science of administration. New York: Institute of Public Administration, 1937:3–35.

15. Silverman D. Formal organisations or industrial sociology: Towards a social action analysis of organisation. Sociology 1968;2:221–38.

16. Silverman D. The theory of organisations. London: Heinemann; 1979.

17. Herbert TT. Dimensions of organizational behaviour. New York: Macmillan; 1976.

18. Courtney M, Nash R, Thornton R. Leading and managing in nursing practice: concepts, processes and challenges. In: Daly J, Speedy S, Jackson D, eds. Nursing leadership. Sydney: Churchill Livingstone; 2004.

19. Mintzberg H. 1973. Cited in Robbins SP, Bergman R, Stagg I et al. Management. Sydney: Prentice Hall; 2000.

20. Mintzberg H. Mintzberg on management: Inside our strange world of organizations. New York: Freedom Press; 1989.

21. Lewis J. Health services management: theory and practice in management. In: Clinton M, ed. Management in the Australian Health Care Industry. 3rd edn. Sydney: Pearson Prentice Hall; 2003.

22. Marquis BL, Huston CJ. Leadership roles and management functions in nursing, theory and application. Philadelphia: Lippincott; 2000.

23. Antrobus S, Kitson A. Nursing leadership: influencing and shaping health policy and nursing practice. J Adv Nurs 1999;29(3):746–53.

24. Darmer P. The subject(ivity) of management. Journal of Organizational Change Management 2000;13(4):334–51.

25. Kitson A. Recognising relationships: reflections on evidence-based practice. Nurs Inq 2002;9(3):179–86.

26. Baker GR. Identifying and assessing competencies: a strategy to improve healthcare leadership. Healthc Pap 2003;4(1):49–58.

27. Kupperschmidt B. Understanding generation X employees. J of Nurs Adm 1998;28(12):36–43.

28. Kupperschmidt, B. Understanding net generation employees, J of Nurs Adm 2000;31(12):570–4.

29. Kupperschmidt B. Addressing multigenerational conflict: mutual respect and carefronting as strategy, The Online Journal of Issues in Nursing 2006;11(2). www.nursingworld.org/MainMenuCategories/ANAMarketplace/ANAPeriodicals/OJIN/TableofContents/Volume112006/No2May06/tpc30_316075.aspx

30. DuBrin AJ. Principles of leadership. 6th edn. Sydney: Cengage Learning International; 2010.

31. Drucker P. The leader of the future: New visions, strategies and practices for the next era. New York: John Wiley; 1996.

32. Maxwell JC. 21 Irrefutable laws of leadership. Tennessee: Thomas Nelson; 2007.

33. Beech M. Leaders or managers: the drive for effective leadership. Nurs Stand 2002;16(30):35–6. Online. http://gateway1.ovid.com/ovidweb.cgi; accessed 4 Mar 2004.

34. Kotter JP. What leaders really do. USA: Harvard Business Review Book; 1999.

35. Goleman D, Boyatzis R. Social intelligence and the biology of leadership. Harvard Business Review 2008;86(9):74–81.

36. Riggio RE, Reichard RJ. The emotional and social intelligences of effective leadership: an emotional and social skill approach. Journal of Management Psychology 2008;23(2):169–85.

37. Crowne KA. The relationships among social intelligence, emotional intelligence and culture intelligence. Organization Management Journal 2009;6:148–63.

38. Van Wart M. Public-sector leadership theory: an assessment. Public Administration Review 2003;63(2):214–28.

39. King K, Cunningham G. Leadership in nursing: more than one way (continuing education credit). Nurs Stand 1995;10(12–14):3–15.

40. Graeff CL. Evolution of situational leadership theory: a critical review. Leadership Quarterly 1997;8(2):153–70.

41. Leatt P, Porter J. Where are the healthcare leaders? The need for investment in leadership development. Healthc Pap 2003;4(1):14–31.

42. Performance and Innovation Unit Strengthening Leadership in the Public Sector. A Research Study by the PIU. Cabinet Office; 2001. Online. www.number-10.gov.uk/su/leadership/00/header.htm; 20 Jan 2004.

43. Burns JM. Leadership. New York: Harper and Row; 1978.

44. De Groot HA. Evidence-based leadership: nursing's new mandate. Nurse Leader 2005;3(2):37–41.

45. Adams JD, Spence SA. People in transition. Training and Development Journal 1988;October:61–3.

46. Govier I, Nash S. Examining transformational approaches to effective leadership in healthcare settings. Nursing Times 2009;105(8):24–7.

47. Murphy L. Transformational leadership: a cascading chain reaction. Journal of Nursing Management 2005;13:128–36.

48. Pieterse AN, van Knippenberg D, Schippers M, Stam D. Transformational and transactional leadership and innovative behaviour: the moderating role of psychological empowerment. Journal of Organizational Behaviour 2010;31:609–23.

49. Firth-Cozens J, Mowbray D. Leadership and the quality of care. Quality in Health Care 2001;10(Suppl II):3–7.

50. Alimo-Metcalf B, Alban-Metcalf J, Bradley M et al. The impact of leadership on performance attitudes to work and wellbeing at work. Journal of Health Organisation and Management 2008;22(6):586–98.

51. Burak O, Bashshur MR. Followership, leadership and social influence. The Leadership Quarterly 2013;24:919–34.

52. Carsten MK, Uhl-Bien M, West BJ et al. Exploring social constructions of followership: a qualitative study. The Leadership Quarterly 2010;21(3):543–62.

53. Uhl-Bein M, Riggio RE, Lowe KB, Carsten MK. Followership theory: a review and research agenda. The Leadership Quarterly 2014; 25:83–104.

54. Lipman-Blumen J. Connective leadership: Managing in a changing world. New York: Oxford University Press; 1996.

55. Rath T, Conchie B. Strengths based leadership: great leaders, teams, and why people follow. New York: Gallup Press; 2009.

56. Sherman RO. What followers want in their nurse leaders. American Nurse Today 2012;7(9):62–4.

57. Fletcher CE. Hospital RNs job satisfactions and dissatisfactions. J of Nurs Adm 2001;31(6):324–31.

58. Densten IL. Clarifying inspirational motivation and its relationship to extra effort. Leadership and Organization Development Journal 2002;23(1):40–4.

59. Sellgren S, Ekvall G, Tomson G. Leadership styles in nursing management: preferred and perceived. Journal of Nursing Management 2006;14:348–55.

60. Côté S, Miners CTH. Emotional intelligence, cognitive intelligence, and job performance, Administrative Science Quarterly 2006;51:1–28.

61. Goleman D. Working with emotional intelligence. New York: Bantam; 1998.

62. O'Rourke M, Davidson P. Governance of practice and leadership. In: Daly J, Speedy S, Jackson D. Nursing leadership. Sydney: Churchill Livingstone; 2004.

63. Groves KS, Feyerherm AE. Leader cultural intelligence in context: testing the moderating effects of team cultural diversity on leader and team performance. Group & Organization Management 2011;36(5):535–66.

64. EMS Chiefs of Canada. The Future of EMS in Canada: Defining the New Road Ahead. Alberta: Canada; 2006. Online. books.google.com.au/books/about/The_Future_of_EMS_in_Canada.html?id=dfqEkgEACAAJ&redir_esc=y; accessed 15th September 2014.

65. Diers D. Speaking of Nursing. Narratives of practice, research, policy and the profession. Boston: Jones and Bartlett; 2004.

66. Parker Ellen B, Ferris GR, Buckley MR. Leader political support: reconsidering leader political behavior. The Leadership Quarterly 2013;24:842–57.

67. Boswell C, Cannon C, Miller J. Nurses' political involvement: responsibility versus privilege. J Prof Nurs 2005;21(1):5–8.

68. O'Rourke MW, Davidson PM. Governance of practice and leadership: implications for nursing leadership. In: Daly J, Speedy S, Jackson D, editors. Nursing Leadership. Sydney: Churchill Livingstone; 2004:327–43.

69. Balding C. Strengthening clinical governance through cultivating the line management role. Aust Health Rev 2005;29(3):353–9.

70. Malcolm L. Achieving best practice leadership and clinical governance: the key role of organisational accountability. ACHSE Health Manager. Summer 2004;15–21.

71. Bigham BL, Kennedy SM, Drennan I, Morrison LJ. Expanding paramedic scope of practice in the community: a systematic review of the literature. Prehospital Emergency Care 2013;17(3):361–72.

72. Dainty KN, Jensen JL, Bigham BL et al. Developing a Canadian emergency medical services research agenda: a baseline study of stakeholder opinions. Canadian J Emerg Med 2013;15(2):83–9.

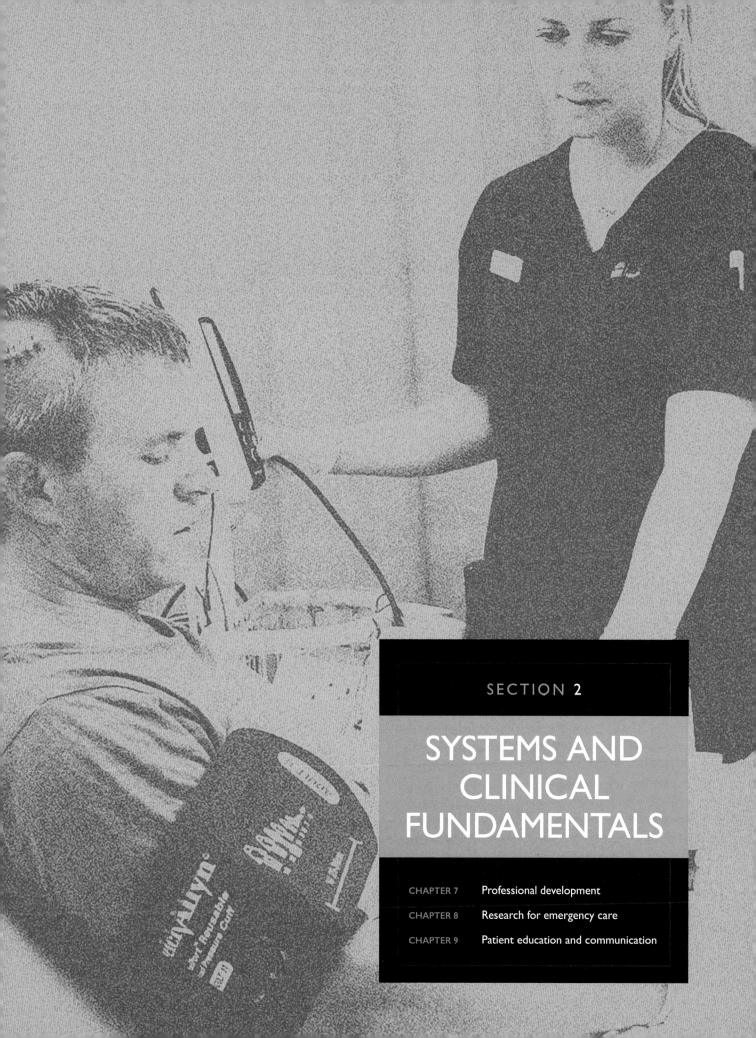

SECTION 2

SYSTEMS AND CLINICAL FUNDAMENTALS

CHAPTER 7

PROFESSIONAL DEVELOPMENT

AMBER VAN DREVEN AND JEFF KENNEALLY

Essentials

- Professional development is the ongoing process by which a practitioner identifies learning needs and addresses them to maintain the competence to practise. It offers advantages to individual healthcare practitioners, healthcare agencies and patients.
- Self-direction and reflection on practice and learning needs are essential to accessing relevant professional development activities.
- Competence is a difficult term to define, and even more difficult to evaluate in individual practitioners. It is up to individual practitioners to reflect on their professional development needs congruent with their attitudes, values and level of skill acquisition.
- Competencies remain useful in providing a framework for tertiary courses and registering bodies to evaluate a practitioner's performance in meeting a defined standard.
- Relevant professional development that has a positive impact on healthcare outcomes relies upon a strong partnership and a shared responsibility between individual practitioners and their employers.
- Professional development can take many forms, not all of which are recognised formally. There are many informal activities that can be effective in their own right or as adjuncts to support formal activities. Mentorship, teaching, instructing, supervising and preceptorship are examples of enabling roles that provide informal professional development support for novice practitioners.
- Changes that have taken place in the tertiary sector have affected formalised postgraduate professional development.

INTRODUCTION

Professional development is a nebulous and somewhat misunderstood concept that pertains to the professional growth of individual healthcare clinicians. While there is some overlap with what determines competence, competencies, attributes and capabilities, professional development encompasses more than that which is mandated by institutions and regulating bodies. In this chapter the responsibilities of individuals and organisations in promoting professional development is outlined. The impact such development can have on individual practitioners, healthcare organisations and, most importantly, the patient healthcare outcomes, are explored. The formal and the informal avenues nursing and paramedic practitioners can pursue to continue professional growth is also examined. A guide outlining the essential elements required to conduct a successful educational session is not included; rather, a brief overview of useful educational theories and strategies is given. A short exploration into the barriers that prevent access to professional development programs and the challenges facing the nursing and paramedic disciplines is also included.

What is professional development?

The term 'professional development' seems synonymous with a variety of other terms such as competencies, evaluation, 'in-service' education, continuing education, self-directed learning, and so on. To many practitioners in the field it may mean little more than the arduous, mandatory slog of annual competency assessments, re-accreditation and performance appraisal. It is helpful, therefore, to define what we actually mean by the term 'professional development'. The Nursing and Midwifery Board of Australia's (2014) interpretation comes in the form of a position statement that is both clear and operational. It states:

> Continuing professional development (CPD) is the means by which members of the professions maintain, improve and broaden their knowledge, expertise and competence, and develop the personal and professional qualities required throughout their professional lives.[1]

Similarly, Martin (2006) describes CPD as 'any activity which follows an outcome based approach to learning, where the individual has reflected on practice and set about identifying an appropriate activity to develop their practice'.[2]

More recently, Martin has added that the aim of CPD should be to promote more competent practitioners able to provide demonstrable improved patient care.[3] Martin further divides continuous professional development into five activities and includes:

- work-based learning activities based on analysis of real work experiences
- professional learning based on mentoring and teaching
- formal activities including structured courses and involvement in research activities
- self-directed learning such as journal reading
- any other diverse activity outside of the other four which may include voluntary or ancillary efforts.[3]

This definition greatly broadens what might constitute professional development activities and reflects the value of 'real life' learning where opportunities for CPD can be spontaneous and varied. It further acknowledges that continuous learning will not be uniform for every person and cannot be achieved by adopting any one strategy. Rather, the ongoing learning must be tailored to meet individual learning needs.

A survey of 1025 nurses in the USA found that nurses rated work experience as the largest contributor to their professional development, followed by their basic professional education, and mentors and preceptors.[4] Interestingly, this study found continuing education, self-study and other factors less helpful in their professional development.[4] Similarly, a small study ($n = 25$) of nurses in the UK highlighted informal learning sources such as working and listening to other professionals or those more experienced, critical incident analysis, professional journals and accessing the internet as the most effective form of continued learning.[5] In an observational case study, Wyatt (2003) considered the role of informal paramedic learning in the context of 'sixth sense' judgement and the value of flexible experience development. Formal education is challenged in the study with informal learning in the workplace considered a legitimate form of 'knowledge acquisition', able to 'develop and refine' sound decision-making.[6] Recognising the value of this type of informal learning is often problematic due to the lack of formal certification or credentialling of such opportunities, but they nonetheless have an important role to play in making professional development accessible to greater numbers of healthcare practitioners.[7]

Interestingly, a preference for pursuing informal avenues of professional development is not limited to healthcare. Similar trends have been noted in academia,[8] and in the digital content industry.[9]

In short, the value of informal professional development should not be underestimated. Informal learning opportunities allow practitioners to meet individual learning needs, are by nature highly flexible and likely to be more clinically relevant in meeting practitioners' immediate learning requirements. This informal learning can be alongside more formal CPD offerings, providing either differing material or a different perspective on similar material. As Deacon[10] points out, it is illogical to argue that CPD only takes place in formal education and training, and if that were the case, then professional experience would not lead to greater professional and organisational expertise. That said, it would be also be illogical to argue that work experience equates to CPD, but rather clinical practice has the potential to enhance CPD in the same way as more formal approaches to education and learning.

Informal methods of CPD have become vital in meeting the learning needs of paramedics as modern paramedic systems are increasingly mobile and away from bases of operation. To maintain maximum coverage availability, paramedics spend increasing time either in moving vehicles or at temporary short-term locations. Similarly, the trend towards increased hospital waiting delays in some jurisdictions can interfere with more traditional informal and formal learning opportunities, such as practical skills practising, coaching opportunities and online learning.

PRACTICE TIP

Informal learning opportunities should be sought and utilised by clinicians to complement more formal learning. Informal avenues are more likely to meet individual clinicians' learning needs due to the diversity, flexibility and reinforcing nature of these learning opportunities.

Competencies

There has been much written and little consensus in the literature as to what constitutes a competency. Part of this confusion relates to the fact that clinical competence is often not clear, obvious, indisputable and visible in the clinical context.[11]

So how does a competency relate to an individual nurse's competence? The Nursing and Midwifery Board of Australia (NMBA)[12] draws a distinction between the terms 'competence' and 'competent'. Competence is defined as the:

> combination of skills, knowledge, attitudes, values and abilities that underpin effective and/or superior performance in a professional/ occupational arena[12]

and a competent nurse is defined as a person who:

> has competence across all the domains of competencies applicable to the nurse, at a standard that is judged to be appropriate for the level of nurse being assessed[12]

—thus encapsulating the very dimensions inherent in a competency. It should be noted that implicit in this definition of a competent practitioner is the provision for various 'levels' of nursing practice, and that a novice's competence, for example, is not compared with that of an expert.

To construct and measure the competence of an emergency nurse, standards must exist against which practice can be measured.[13] Professional organisations, accrediting and regulatory bodies and institutions construct and disseminate standards that may be directed at practice, care outcomes and structure.[14–16] The Australian Nursing and Midwifery Accreditation Council (formerly the Australian Nursing and Midwifery Council) is an independent accrediting authority for the nursing and midwifery professions under a relatively newly formed National Registration and Accreditation Scheme. The NMBA is responsible for the regulation of nurses and midwives and as such takes responsibility for the national competency standards for registered nurses in Australia, providing a framework for assessment both for licensure and for universities developing curricula.[17] The College of Emergency Nursing Australasia (CENA) has developed these standards and from them, competencies and competency assessments may be derived.[18]

Much of the education undertaken by nurses in Australia, both in the tertiary sector and in the employment setting, is shaped by references to stated competencies derived from standards. The reason for the integration of competencies into the educational system arises, in part, from an attraction to outcome-based education, and the perceived need to 'benchmark' areas of expertise in defining nursing practice.[19] Brazen[16] argues that the gap between education and practice is always challenging because it is created by a difference in competence as an outcome-based activity. The graduate student who passes their competency-based course is deemed safe to practise; whereas in the clinical setting, the focus is more directed on how the patient benefits from those actions.[16,20]

How competency and competency standards are viewed in the paramedic discipline is less clear, due in part to the lack of literature surrounding competency and competency standards, but also due to the rapid transition from the vocational education and training (VET) sector to university-based education.

The Council of Ambulance Authorities[21] define professional competency as:

> skills, attitudes or other characteristics (including values and beliefs) attained by an individual based on knowledge (vocational study) and experience (gained through concurrent or subsequent practice). Competence is the consistent application of knowledge and skill to the standard as required by the industry in the workplace; it embodies the ability to adapt to new situations and environments.

Even with the desired stipulation that initial knowledge should be gained at bachelor's degree level, the role of experience and post graduate learning remains an essential component of professional competence. This shifts some of the onus of professionalism from the individual to many workplace factors including formal and informal means of learning.

Competency and competency-based training (CBT) have been central to paramedic education and training since the 1970s. The Kangan Report (1974) and later the Dawkins era (1987) were critical points in time for re-directing paramedic education and training to technical and further education institutions (TAFEs), and later into university-based education. The Kangan Report supported the movement of CBT, ensuring that the VET sector better met the nation's industry and skills requirements, while the Dawkins era saw the abolition of the binary system.[22] Both of these periods ultimately led to the implementation of further educational reforms, overseen by the National Training Board (NTB; now known as the Australian National Training Authority) that fostered and developed competency standards for all workforce occupations while classifying qualifications within a national framework.[23]

These competency standards were also seen as an important facilitator for professional recognition portability and subsequent employability in the paramedic discipline, as well as other healthcare professions.[22] The nature of these health-related training packages and competency standards was (and still is) undoubtedly important in the evolution of paramedic education and training. National accreditation of paramedic programs is currently provided by the Council of Ambulance Authorities making use of these competency standards, and curricula benchmarks, as well as acknowledging the portability of skills and qualifications, the recognition of prior learning and credit transfer.

The relatively recent decision to move paramedic training programs into the university sector has meant that uncertainties surrounding benchmarking of undergraduate paramedic education programs by means of competency standards have yet to be formally addressed. Without national standardised curriculum guidelines, this continues to cause educational duplication, uncertainty, financial inefficiencies and questions surrounding employability and job-readiness. In 2004, a set of 'national ambulance competencies' was created that were benchmarked to an undergraduate diploma level.[24] Fitzgerald and Bange[24] sought to extend this through the preparation of a discussion paper for the Australian College of Ambulance Professionals outlining the case for paramedic national registration. Despite the combination of clear and significant change in paramedic clinical practice and the push for national standard development consistent with other health professionals, national registration and recognition remains elusive.[25] As there are no formal accreditation endorsements of paramedic programs, it is uncertain if, when or how these national competencies will be integrated and assessed in the paramedic curriculum. Currently, the decisions surrounding which competencies are measured are undertaken locally by each individual university and ambulance service, and not on a national basis through a regulatory or registered body such as the Australian College of Ambulance Professionals (ACAP), now known as Paramedics Australasia.

Since the 'national diploma' competencies are not applicable to the bachelor level, learning expectations and requirements of paramedic students have emphasised an urgent need for competency standards reform, particularly as more-complex healthcare models, such as interdisciplinary health management and extended-scope practitioner roles, are currently being considered within the Australian healthcare context. For the most part, however, the goal of competency-based assessment is to evaluate performance and the effective application of knowledge and skill to the practice setting.[15,26]

Measuring competencies

Tertiary institutions in Australia offering nursing education programs incorporate evaluations and assessments based on NMBA competencies. Licensure after successful completion of a course proves minimum competency in that the nurse has learned the theories and standards of nursing practice and is therefore certified as 'competent'.[16] Indeed, such certification of competence appears to be well supported by recent studies, whereby a positive relationship has been noted between nurses who have completed higher tertiary degrees or specialty certification, and better patient outcomes.[27–29] This implies a greater degree of competence among nurses who have pursued further tertiary studies and who have rightfully been certified as competent.

However, there has been some dissent regarding the way in which the tertiary sector has embraced competency-based education. Even if a national competency framework and course accreditation system is in place, educational preparation and work readiness may vary, as the whole concept of 'competence' suffers from a lack of definition and in addition, is difficult to measure.[19,30] Furthermore, after conducting a literature search of 212 articles, Watson et al found that the methods claiming to measure competence have rarely been tested for reliability and validity.[31] Indeed, many factors can detract from a valid and reliable assessment of a nurse's competence, not least of all the influence of situational factors.[32]

An example of how the reliability of a testing tool can affect the perceived 'competence' of nurses can be found in a study conducted with 160 participants undertaking triage assessments. It was found that participants were more accurate in allocating triage categories using triage scenarios containing still photographs on a computer than were those using paper-based scenarios without photographic cues.[33] The choice of assessment tool can certainly colour the perception of an individual's performance; they may well be 'competent' despite poor performance in the assessment. It is difficult enough to validate tests of basic skills and it is not surprising, therefore, that there is little literature validating assessment practices of aspects of competence such as professionalism, teamwork, learning and systems-based care.[34] While testing a practitioner's clinical and technical skills is relatively straightforward, assessing critical thinking and interpersonal skills is certainly more challenging.

At an organisational level, competency-based programs may include tools which require subjective and objective evaluations such as direct observation, chart review, demonstration, return demonstration, written testing, skill validation check lists, professional portfolios and certification.[30] However, there is little consensus on how best to test or assess certain competencies. For example, a paramedic may be deemed competent if a skill or procedure is learnt and demonstrated in a skills laboratory, without the metacognitive aspects of context and clinical judgement being tested. The push for contextual assessment and learning has seen a call from some quarters for nursing to embrace the use of Objective Structured Clinical Evaluations (OSCEs) to evaluate areas of clinical competence that are less readily examined by more traditional methods.[35] Some have argued that clinical competence is an ongoing process, rather than a state, and manifests itself in both an ontological and contextual dimension.[11] Ontologically, competence can be reached through education with measurable categories expressed in learning outcomes. Contextual competence, however, can only be reached after clinical experience, and some would argue, best assessed through contextual assessments such as OSCEs.[35]

PRACTICE TIP

Competency assessment should consider a variety of evaluation methods to best match the mix of skill and knowledge that is to be examined. Subjective methods of assessment should ideally be supported with other more objective measures of competency.

Delivery of knowledge content has rarely embraced measuring the results of learning, such as patient outcomes.[24] Typically, the success of nursing CPD is measured in light of participant satisfaction, but doesn't measure the true effectiveness of the professional development.[36,37] Attending CPD does not alone guarantee sustaining competency,[59] and there is no evidence that nurse attendance at lectures, conferences or presentations improves practice or patient outcomes.[37–39] Yet even evaluating the competence of a registered nurse by monitoring their clinical bedside skills does not guarantee that they possess the actual knowledge, skill and ability to care for patients in changing situations.[16,29,40]

Within the paramedic context, assessing the competence of a practitioner is perhaps even more complex, given the nature of clinical exposure, and uncertainty surrounding:

1. which competencies have been taught
2. whether educators are competent to assess those competencies
3. by what means those competencies should be assessed.

The net result of these issues continues to plague clinical placement learning and increases the theory–practice gap surrounding paramedic education, amplifying the misunderstanding of novice practitioner work-readiness versus adept and able job-readiness,[41] and confusion over whether indeed graduates are actually competent.

Some argue that competencies such as adaptability can only be assessed by subjective means,[42] and while there is some support in the literature for the use of clinical portfolios and self-assessment,[16,43] one solution may be to entrust summative judgements of competence to multi-source feedback, 360-degree feedback, evidence of workplace performance and critical incident review rather than self-assessment.[44]

Nursing and paramedical educators often collaborate in formulating competency assessment tasks conducted in healthcare and educational organisations, and construct the grading requirements and the frequency by which competencies are to be assessed.[20] These decisions are often arbitrary and have little evidence to back them. For example, if someone is judged 90% competent by various assessments tasks or observations, does that mean that they are competent to practise?[31] At what point do we judge the practitioner as incompetent? Based on what?

These complexities also raise further questions surrounding competence and the determination of experience. Should competencies be measured according to call volume, the amount of skills undertaken, or simply time, such as 6 months probation? If a graduate student is not exposed to any significant blunt or penetrating trauma, how can they be assessed as being competent or otherwise in managing such cases? Moreover, can instructors confidently rely on simulation, role-play or oral vivas to achieve these competencies in simulated settings? Are graduate paramedics really competent after the arbitrary 20 intubations, for example? Or should their probation be extended until these 20 intubations are completed?

Similarly, it is not uncommon for emergency departments to conduct annual nursing competency testing, such as Advanced Life Support (ALS). Is annual testing enough to guarantee competent staff? Should testing and refresher training be run every 6 months instead?

There remains a paucity of research to address these questions, and in the absence of hard evidence, individual institutions continue to create their own benchmarking for competence assessment which may or may not reflect accurately the competence of the practitioners, and are unlikely to be transferrable from institution to institution. A small study examining knowledge retention in 14 nurses undertaking a

---

PRACTICE TIP

Competency assessment in nursing and paramedicine must often evaluate infrequently performed skills. This will require the use of simulation or other methods to represent clinical reality. Careful consideration of assessment tool to be used is required to ensure applicability and reliability of assessment outcome.

The variability in assessing educational outcomes has also been reflected in a systematic review of simulation-based learning where Cant and Cooper[46] found some papers tested learning immediately after teaching, some after 1 week, and some after 1 month to determine knowledge retention. It is noteworthy, however, that the main difference between the trauma course and ward restructure studies was that the first one taught trauma knowledge and skills that had little reinforcement in the clinical setting, while the ward restructure group were practising the knowledge and skills learnt in their new ward. A small study of Finnish critical care nurses ($n = 129$) similarly discovered that competence profiles are context-specific and that the frequency of use of competencies correlates significantly with the level of competence.[47] It is clear that to maintain the changes in practice, clinicians require the opportunity to use or practise the newly acquired skill in the clinical setting.[37]

---

trauma course utilised questionnaires conducted immediately post the course and again 3 months later, and concluded that there was very poor knowledge retention at the 3-month mark.[32] However, another study of 36 nurses undertaking an education program to update their skills as a result of a ward restructure found similar improved competency levels immediately after and 3 months post education.[45] It is apparent that even anecdotal evidence may be contradictory in deciding how often to run competency education and assessment programs, let alone how soon after an education program the competencies should be assessed.

In short, the tools used to assess competencies are multifarious, can vary from one institution and organisation to another, and may or may not be reliable or valid. Coupled with this, the practitioners conducting the assessment may risk the validity of an assessment tool and introduce bias. Interpersonal factors such as familiarity, the assessor favouring or disfavouring the person being assessed and nervousness of the person being assessed can also bias assessment observations.[16] These points illustrate the difficulties and complexities surrounding competency measurement and evaluation, which, in the authors' experience, are at odds with curriculum and course development, where evaluation and assessment is generally a secondary consideration in course and objective planning.

It seems somewhat ironic that educators and institutions have embraced the use of competencies as a means by which we could standardise and prove competence of individual practitioners. By linking competencies to job profiles, many employers view competencies as a means of establishing occupational and quality indicators.[48] Competence is also a poorly defined concept, and when examined closely, competencies consist of many facets, most of which are almost untestable individually or objectively. Some claim that the very skills that are at the core of nursing are the most resistant to measurement.[49] And yet we persist, perhaps because we have no better way to determine a practitioner's ability to perform their job in a safe manner and positively influence a patient's outcome. It must be remembered, however, that competency education and assessment is but one of many facets of professional development. Nevertheless, with limited time, money and resources, institutions that have mandated annual competency testing and updates for all staff may find that there are few resources or little time to support professional development of any other kind.

Generally, qualified and graduate paramedic staff undertake between one and as much as five professional development days annually in their respective ambulance service. There is no industry standard, with each state defining their own agreed requirements, typically based on industry agreements with employee representative bodies. Further, the intent of such professional development time is not specifically defined, with frequent competing pressures within any organisation seeking access to the available time. Time dedicated to clinical material will vary and will often be limited by other operational or administrative learning activities. The same issues surrounding measurement apply themselves to university departments, where the focus should be outcome-based, not necessarily scores or attempts before proficiency.

Why bother with professional development?

The literature outlines many reasons why professional development is essential for individual practitioners' professional growth, for organisational integrity and, most importantly, for optimal patient care. The Australian College of Nursing (ACN) recognises that nurses work in a constantly changing and evolving environment that necessitates an 'ongoing engagement with technologies, ideas and advances in professional practice',[50] and so in our fast-paced, ever-changing field of emergency care, it is imperative that our CPD focuses on the latest evidence-based practice.

While CPD is not mandatory for paramedics in Australia, professional development is compulsory in other countries, such as in the UK. Registered paramedics in the UK under the auspices of the Health Professions Council must undertake and provide evidence of professional development activities, such as involvement in journal clubs or short courses.[51,52] Undertaking and maintaining professional development is also important for the paramedic discipline in its quest to become a fully fledged profession.[2,52] The discipline in Australia is still considered a semi-profession because of national curricula inconsistencies caused by the lack of national accreditation, leading to an inability to develop a unique body of knowledge and self-govern on a national basis. The push towards national registration and professional recognition remains slow, although it is widely believed to be inevitable.[25] A crucial component of developing a unique body of knowledge is ongoing or lifelong learning, both of which are central to CPD, and indeed are considered important professional traits.[53–55] Implementing compulsory CPD for paramedics in Australia unquestionably will assist in the professionalisation process. Sibson reinforces the importance of CPD by saying: 'Undertaken by other health professionals over the years, a mandatory CPD system can be considered an indicator of the profession's response to the increasing sense of accountability demanded by today's society' (p. 74).[51]

Clinicians' perspective

From an individual nurse's perspective, engaging in professional development activities is a requirement and an expectation of regulating authorities. Indeed, the Nursing and Midwifery Board of Australia[1] states:

> CPD is the means by which members of the professions maintain, improve and broaden their knowledge, expertise and competence, and develop the personal and professional qualities required throughout their professional lives.

The Australian College of Nursing (ACN, formerly the Royal College of Nursing Australia), while not a regulating authority per se, is a professional nursing organisation that, among other things, supports nurses in their continuing professional development and education. To this end, the ACN has developed an online 'life long learning program' (3LP) which integrates e-learning activities with current research and tools for recording professional development activities undertaken.[50]

It is clear that the onus of maintaining competence and pursuing professional development falls, in large part, to the individual nurse. Nurses' self-recognition of their own levels of competence is essential for maintaining high levels of care,

and in an environment of ever-changing demands, nurses must be diligent to ensure that the quality of care remains excellent.[14,18,39] Indeed, evidence of CPD undertaken is now mandatory to maintain nursing registration. As of 1 July 2010, nursing registration matters will be dealt with through the Australian Health Practitioner Regulation Agency (AHPRA), which represents, among other professions, the Nursing and Midwifery Board of Australia. This unified national registration system does not include the paramedic discipline, despite recent calls for a national register.[56] While proposals for national registration are in process, it is anticipated that progress will be slow, particularly with recent reports.[57,58] Without this national registration, mandated formal CPD requirements for paramedics is unlikely to occur for some time.

All nurses on the new national register will be required to participate in, and keep written documentation of, at least 20 hours of CPD per year,[1] although there are no quality requirements for CPD offerings, nor stipulation regarding the frequency of engagement.[59] In contrast to this, the major CPD certification available within the paramedic profession requires 50 hours per year of professional development. Paramedic members from Paramedics Australasia (PA, previously ACAP) have developed the Certified Ambulance Professional program (CAP) in an attempt to address the CPD requirements of its members. The CAP program is a non-mandatory CPD program whereby paramedics are able to accumulate continuing education points.[60] Points are allocated based on educational activity, which are at the discretion of individual paramedics, but might include, for example, participation in a workshop, seminar or conference. Crediting education opportunities exist outside of the PA, however the PA also offers educational opportunities such as short courses. While the project team and the PA should be commended, without CPD being made mandatory it is unlikely this mode of formal CPD will be sustainable. The discrepancy in the number of hours required to maintain competency within a profession is not surprising as, to date, the exact number of hours required to maintain competency is unknown.

Similarly, the whole notion of mandatory CPD as a way of safeguarding practitioner competency may also be questionable. More than half of the 61 boards of nursing in the USA and its territories have directed that to maintain professional registration, nurses are mandated to accumulate a certain number of hours of professional development per year.[4] However, a study of 1025 nurses found that those who were mandated to attend professional development were more likely to attend education unrelated to their work or interest for the sole purpose of fulfilling that mandate. At the same time, there were no statistical differences between the amount of professional growth and ability of those nurses mandated to attend professional development and those nurses who were not.[4] There are a number of things that might be concluded from such a study: first, that professional development has little impact on professional growth. As unlikely as this seems, there has been no link established between mandatory professional development and the development of competence.[4,39] Second, we could conclude that mandated professional development translates into nurses scrambling to pursue any educational offering simply to get the required number of hours of CPD.[59]

Finally, the results of this study suggests that nurses who are not mandated to attend professional development sessions are more likely to attend education that is relevant to their professional growth, is of high quality and is of interest to them. Indeed, a small study of 289 Australian nurses found that 92% agreed that CPD was important to their nursing practice and over 80% believed it was an important part of reflection and career progression. Conversely, only 17% stated they only participated in CPD to keep their hours up for registration.[61] In light of this, some have argued that mandatory CPD is an invasion of practitioner autonomy, as it removes the practitioners' right to access relevant CPD.[20]

Professional development activities include such things as undertaking policy work, involvement in quality improvement activities, attending conferences and subscription to refereed journals, to name but a few (others can be found in Box 7.1). While these activities may improve standards of care, or enhance professionalism, skills or knowledge, there is no requirement to prove that this is the case. Simply subscribing to a journal does not guarantee that it will be read, or that the topics covered in a conference will be translated into a change of practice, for example.

Mandated professional development, like any other form of professional development, may not guarantee professional growth, nor help to identify ongoing professional development needs. In addressing this, the NMBA requires hard evidence that some form of learning has occurred, mandating written reflections of the learning encounter such as a discussion of the experience, what new knowledge was gained and how this impacts on the clinician's professional role.[1] Interestingly, in the UK, undergraduate and postgraduate medical education is moving away from a credit-point earning system to a CPD system that explicitly links education to change in practice, and is managed and monitored through mandatory peer appraisal.[62]

It is also the responsibility of expert clinicians to guide, mentor and facilitate the professional development of less-skilled clinicians. In any healthcare field, one can find clinicians exemplifying Benner's continuum of skill acquisition, from novice to advanced beginner, to competent, proficient and ultimately to the level of an expert.[48] In most instances graduate paramedics and nurses represent the novice, but Benner also notes that any clinicians entering a clinical setting where she or he has no experience may be limited to the novice level of performance if the goals and tools of patient care are unfamiliar.[63] The continuum of skill acquisition ranges from a novice who is typically taught context-free rules to guide actions and as such display behaviours that are inflexible and limited, to that of an expert clinician who no longer relies on analytical principles (such as rules or guidelines) to connect an understanding of a situation to an appropriate action.[63] Experts have a wealth of experience and have an 'intuitive grasp' of each situation, accurately focusing on problems without wasting time considering other inaccurate, alternative diagnoses and solutions.[63] Expertise, while accompanied by a sound theoretical underpinning, is derived from ongoing education that is grounded in everyday practice, through the process of reflection and clinical supervision.[63] In terms of professional development provision, it is clear that expertise can be derived from ongoing education[64] and that it is up to individual practitioners to reflect on their professional development needs congruent with their level of skill acquisition.

Both nursing and paramedical practitioners should consider the personal rewards that accessing professional development can afford. For example, nurses who continue their education and belong to professional organisations are more likely to be critical thinkers, innovative and to be able to participate in creative problem solving.[64,65] For paramedics, CPD fosters the critical thinking skills crucial to developing a unique body of knowledge and enhancing the discipline. Nurses employed in organisations that have robust professional development programs report an increased level of accountability, and a pride in their profession.[66] In terms of benefits to individual practitioners, it appears that reflecting on professional development needs and then accessing them translates to greater personal satisfaction, clinical competence and enjoyment of work. It is noteworthy that Bradley et al,[67] in a survey of Canadian psychologists, found that practitioner engagement with a variety of CPD activities led to practitioners' similar feelings of competence, value and support. In addition, Pool et al[64] found that CPD-inclined nurses tended to share their knowledge freely and invite others into their development process. This is congruent with CENA's practice standards that emergency nurses should provide support for formal and informal learning opportunities for their colleagues.[18]

Finally, from a medicolegal viewpoint, it can also be noted that accessing professional development and maintaining competency standards may help individual nurses and paramedics to protect themselves from potential litigation and compensation.[68]

Organisational and managerial perspective

There has been much written about the impact a robust professional development program has on recruitment and retention of nursing staff. The term 'magnet hospital' was originally coined by a group of US hospitals that were able to successfully recruit and retain nurses during a nursing shortage in the early 1980s.[42] One of the fundamental requirements of magnet facilities is a strong educational presence, where professional and personal development experiences are valued and opportunities exist for competency-based clinical advancement.[69,70] However, merely providing opportunities for professional development to willing staff may not be enough.

BOX 7.1 Examples of professional development

- Teaching/mentorship/role modelling
- Journal club
- Undertaking clinical auditing/quality improvement activities
- Reflection portfolio
- Clinical review discussion groups
- Seminar, workshop and conference attendance
- Presentation at seminar or conference
- Pursuing formalised education qualifications/accreditation
- Research

Educational outcomes will be strongly influenced by conditions in the workplace.[71] As mentioned earlier in the chapter, education that is not reinforced in the workplace appears to be poorly retained by practitioners, and workplace culture may significantly impede the implementation of new knowledge or skills.[72] Magnet hospitals, by contrast, demonstrate organisational attributes that provide nurses with the support needed to fully use their knowledge and expertise to provide high-quality patient care.[73] As a result, nurses' satisfaction and retention rates are higher and recruitment of new staff is optimised.[37,42,55,69,73]

Organisational structure can also limit opportunities for professional development. For example, opportunities for peer discussions motivate nurses to reflect on their own performance—even the shift hand-over can be seen as an opportunity to gain feedback.[45] In support of this assertion, feedback from 26 South Australian nurses revealed that the use of taped hand-overs and staggered shift times reduced the opportunity for facilitated reflection, self-assessment and professional interaction.[45] In contrast to this, a Canadian study introduced a model of nursing where 80% of the nurses' salaried time was spent in direct patient care and the other 20% of their time was spent on professional development. Outcomes of this study included reduced overtime hours, an increase in workload hours per patient day, sick leave staying low, increased patient and staff satisfaction and non-existent turnover. Interestingly, despite this dramatic change in managerial model, there was noted to be no significant difference in variable direct labour costs.[74] Changes to organisational structure, be they small, apparently insignificant changes or large-scale remodelling, can greatly affect professional development opportunities for nursing staff.

Martin[2] suggests the challenges for paramedic managers largely involve providing and facilitating professional development opportunities. However, providing and facilitating these opportunities may not be enough to ensure a robust CPD program, as he also argues that paramedic staff require personal motivation to undertake defined learning activities. For example, a clinical feedback study in the UK where paramedic staff were involved in tracking patient outcomes following hand-over illustrated the degree of clinical curiosity required to better inform practice.[75] Staff interested in patient progress and their outcomes completed a patient feedback form, which was later mailed back to their ambulance station. This form provided paramedics with a summary of patient progress including pathology investigations and final outcome, offering paramedic staff important learning opportunities not normally available. While preliminary results are anecdotal, this study emphasises the importance of organisational support and an innovative way that management can facilitate the provision of relevant CPD.

The Australian experience is somewhat different to that of the UK in that the clinical curiosity of paramedic staff is often stymied by laws pertaining to patient confidentiality and rights to privacy. Increasing workloads on paramedics also reduce the time available for following up patient outcomes and present further barriers to this form of CPD. Occasionally managers and a very small number of individuals are included in formal hospital case reviews and periodic data analysis, and this may offer an avenue for feedback but the formality precludes many from being able to benefit.

Importantly, learning outcomes should feed back into day-to-day clinical practice, thereby improving clinical practice and individual enthusiasm to undertake similar professional development opportunities. It has been noted that an organisational culture that supports CPD and displays a willingness to change can positively influence clinicians' attitudes towards the value of CPD.[54,61] Similarly it has been found that as the employer payment for CPD increases, the greater the value staff place on ongoing education and professional growth.[61] Given that attending 'face-to-face' CPD offerings can include added costs such as travel, accommodation, time off work and child-minding, all of which can add hundreds of dollars to the total outlay,[59] financial support and partnership with employers in meeting CPD needs is crucial.

Margolis et al[76] identified twelve key factors for the success of paramedic education programs. Recognised high performing educational institutions provided representatives to form a focus group to determine key reasons for success in educational programs. Some of these pertained to continued education and not just initial pre-employment education, and include:

- establishing a philosophy that fosters a culture which values continuous review and improvement
- creating your own examinations
- lesson plans, presentations and course materials using multiple current references
- emphasising basic concepts of paramedic practice
- use of frequent case-based classroom scenarios
- providing staff with frequent detailed feedback regarding their performance.[76]

Patient outcome and continuing care data is vital to paramedic performance review and may offer a rich source of information to further enhance individual practice. However, until privacy laws are reviewed to allow this degree of information sharing, this form of relevant self-reflection remains limited.

More formally, an avenue for organisations to further enhance and augment the professional development of their staff is through performance appraisals. The common denominator for formal and informal performance feedback is the measurement of performance against expectations.[45] Performance might also, as mentioned earlier in this chapter, be guided by a set of standards, either professionally based (such as the ANMC competencies, CENA standards, National Ambulance Competencies, or Clinical Practice Guidelines) or organisationally-specific (such as a position description).[45] Management of poor performance requires specific weaknesses to be identified at an early stage, as competence is often assumed by the practitioner until he or she receives feedback to the contrary.[45] Mechanisms addressing professional development needs should then be agreed upon and instituted to address these weaknesses.[45] It is vitally important, therefore, that the practitioner assessed as not performing to a level of competence expected receives timely feedback, and this is not delayed or omitted lest the potentially unsafe practice is perpetuated.[45] However, instead of a 'name, shame, blame' type of culture, good assessments are a form of learning and should provide guidance and support to address learning needs.[34]

In Australia there is an almost nationwide use of electronic patient care records by paramedics that are capable of producing not only a record for supply to hospitals on hand-over, but also an extensive case database. Known as VACIS (Victorian Ambulance Clinical Information System), this system is being increasingly used for retrospective research and for audit and clinical case review purposes. It is capable of providing reasonable quality data to form part of the future foundation for evidence-based change and the provision of almost real-time case feedback. The challenges posed by reviewing this database is to ensure that managers and educators reviewing the records are mindful that the documentation may not be a perfect reflection of the clinical reality. Issues of poor documentation rather than errors of practice need to be taken into consideration, and feedback should be balanced in this regard. In a period where recruitment of large numbers of paramedic graduates is the norm, clinical and operational managers and educators are often stretched for availability and time. The appeal to be able to manage from afar using electronic records is tempting and, though it will have strengths, remains only one form of professional development that complements other varied approaches.

Accessing professional development should be one of the reliable strategies suggested to improve performance and clinical governance and safeguard patient wellbeing.[52] For further information regarding leadership and management goals, see Chapter 6.

In contrast to performance feedback that identifies individual professional development requirements are annual performance appraisals that contribute little to the professional growth of the individual. Indeed, some practitioners view performance appraisals as an imposition: a management-driven, organisational requirement which merely 'goes through the motions' of improving performance.[45] Workplace managers should recognise and support our future nurse and paramedic leaders by implementing strategies such as mentoring and coaching, where experienced staff help younger or less-experienced staff to develop and progress.[14,44,77] Again operational imperatives can adversely impact on this ambition. For example, in attempting to increase ambulance availability and decrease response time, paramedic response teams are increasingly located in isolation from other teams and from their own base locations. Roaming educators such as clinical support officers find themselves performing in field roles to meet such operational imperatives, as well as juggling competing demands of response coverage, auditing and investigative roles.

PRACTICE TIP

Innovative managerial strategies are often required to ensure learning needs are met of practitioners working in fluid clinical environments. Similarly, educators, instructors and mentors are required to be creative and flexible in educational facilitation.

Professional development opportunities may improve confidence and motivation, but as studies have shown, recognition, encouragement and the relationship with immediate supervisors are the main predictor of job satisfaction and increased morale.[78–80] Given that in the paramedic sector,

annual performance appraisals are limited to middle and upper management levels, mechanisms by which feedback is given to clinical paramedics is somewhat limited and may have a negative impact on relationships with immediate supervisors.

It is apparent, then, that it takes more than salary and fringe benefits to recruit and retain staff; a culture of caring and flexibility with the provision for continuing education and promotion of professionalism should be a priority.[73,74,78] While CPD is important to practising clinicians, it should be viewed as equally important by employers, in that it is crucial in developing a workforce that is required to meet future healthcare needs.[81]

The enabling role

One of the fundamental requirements of magnet facilities is that nurses are expected to be teachers in all aspects of their practice.[69] This may take the form of enabling roles such as mentorship, preceptorship or clinical supervision—indeed, these terms seem interchangeable and difficult to define due to the fluid nature of the roles and overlapping responsibilities. Preceptors have been described as offering clinical supervision, providing opportunities to practise and offering a resource of clinical expertise.[82] Mentors have been described as counsellors, teachers, advocates, confidantes and advisors, a role model and guide who encourages and inspires,[66] yet similar attributes could also just as easily be applied to preceptors. Mentors have been found to be uncommon in paramedic practice and typically only occur between the novice and the expert.[83] Co-locating intensive-care paramedic responders with other paramedic teams has the potential to provide informal professional development opportunities and has anecdotal support from paramedic teams where it occurs.

The role of preceptor has been found to be in increasing demand in paramedicine with fewer people available and necessarily suitable for the role.[84] The lack of role clarity is also reflected in the paramedic profession where the terms 'educators' and 'instructors' are used to embrace many of the aspects implicit in the enabling role.[85] For example, paramedic educators/instructors are characterised by: educating, training, building confidence and friendship, development of socialisation skills, structuring one-on-one partnerships and setting challenging learning tasks. Such a multifarious role may indeed meet individual learning needs, but the lack of role delineation and definition may be a source of inconsistent clinical education, especially in light of the fact that there are now 11 universities offering formative paramedic programs throughout Australia.[86] Willis et al[87] argue that university education of nurses and paramedics produces novices and that with increasing graduate numbers, clearly defined enabling roles are vital for the constancy of educational preparation of paramedic novices and ongoing refresher training for paramedic staff, particularly as exposure to certain clinical cases and skills is often unpredictable. In any case, the enabling roles of mentors, preceptors, educators, instructors and clinical supervisors are indispensable in providing 'novice' clinicians with the support they require to meet professional development goals.

Informal enabling relationships occur in multiple ways at all levels of our professions, and recognise that clinicians across all levels of experience and education have something positive to offer to their colleagues.[65] Andrew[88] suggests that the initial mentoring experience for the novice may be a predictor of progression to competence by the novice. A positive mentoring experience at an early stage may well influence positive behaviour throughout the undergraduate years and beyond, and as such mentoring excellence should be recognised as the 'cornerstone of student development'.[88]

The rewards for performing the enabling role can take many forms, from institutional levels such as financial support[44,89] to personal rewards such as increased levels of intellectual stimulation, personal satisfaction, improved skills and increased motivation.[90] However, being a preceptor can also prove to be an additional workload in an environment where the workload may already be uncontrollable, resulting in a conflict of roles and high stress levels.[43,90] Preceptors may also feel underprepared for the role, lacking educational skills and support in how to manage the 'unsafe' learner, the 'disinterested' learner or the 'challenging' learner.[89] It is therefore imperative that clinicians undertaking formalised preceptor roles receive education and support pertinent to their role, and that only those clinicians with significant clinical experience be chosen to perform formalised enabling roles.[44,89] The additional resources required to support staff in formalising their enabling roles appears to be worth the fiscal investment for health care institutions. Magnet hospitals have reported that mentorship programs can improve recruitment, job satisfaction and retention, thereby reducing organisationsal financial and quality costs linked with staff turnover and disruption of teams.[55]

The patient's perspective

Continuing professional development and lifelong learning skills are essential to providing good quality of care to patients and communities.[2,55,91] However, there has been little research conducted to support this statement. The problematic lack of research may stem in part from the fact that, for simplicity's sake, most continuing education evaluations focus only on participants' perceptions of their meeting the workshop/ conference objectives and not on how the education session has affected daily work practices.[16,92] The latter appears much harder to research than the former.

The link between nursing professional development and patient outcomes has been difficult to establish. A large, multicentred study examining the proportion of hospital registered nurses educated to a baccalaureate level (as opposed to a diploma level) or higher, and risk-adjusted mortality and deaths in surgical patients with serious complications found that there were significantly lower levels of patient mortality and death in hospitals that employed nurses with higher degrees.[93] Despite examining 232,342 patient records across 168 hospitals, the study never stated that the data *proved* that education leads to better patient outcomes or provides a link between educational levels of nurses and the causally related outcomes of patients.[94] Better patient care might be related to the practitioners' ability to advocate for patients with other highly educated professions, for example.[94] Conversely, nurses with better educational backgrounds could be differently attracted to hospitals with better patient outcomes.[94] However, the trend needs to be acknowledged that better-educated nurses are associated with better patient outcomes, with many authors espousing that CPD is crucial to patient safety and quality standards of patient care.[37,54,55,81]

Studies acknowledging the impact that advanced education within the paramedic profession has had on patient outcomes are similarly limited. However, one area that has been extensively researched is the relationship between the practice of endotracheal intubation and adverse patient outcomes.[95–98] The need for this research has been brought about because of questions relating to clinical exposure, inconsistent training programs and inadequate professional development opportunities. Deakin, King and Thompson[99] undertook a retrospective study examining paramedic endotracheal intubation training, maintenance of intubation skills and provision of continuing professional development. They found skill acquisition and skill maintenance was problematic given the limited exposure to intubation, but perhaps more pertinent to this chapter were their findings suggesting that paramedic organisations did not provide adequate CPD programs to compensate for the lack of clinical exposure.[99]

As discussed earlier, there is strong suggestive evidence that inadequacy of professional education can be associated with adverse patient outcomes. In contrast though, where that education can be delivered correctly and effectively, it can be linked to improved patient outcomes.[100,101] It is clearly advantageous to be able to target CPD in areas of clinical need, with learning outcomes that are desired and measurable to be able to demonstrate benefit.

PRACTICE TIP

Improved patient care is the objective of any educational strategy undertaken as a clinician. It is often difficult to measure the impact this education has on patient health outcomes, but evaluation of educational strategies should demonstrate patient benefit.

In addition to nurses' professional development affecting patient morbidity and mortality, nurses' professional development may also affect other important measures such as length of stay and cost of care. Small anecdotal studies have found that short courses and specialist nursing care do indeed have a positive impact on discharge rates and morbidity and mortality.[27,29] However, there exists a paucity of recent, large-scale research studies to prove or disprove the impact professional development may have on healthcare outcomes, within both the nursing and the paramedic spheres of practice. The limited studies that have been conducted imply that there is a positive relationship between the care that patients receive and continued lifelong learning by clinicians. It seems intuitive that this is indeed the case, but further research examining the impact professional development has on healthcare outcomes is greatly needed. In terms of paramedicine, to counter ongoing exposure issues, sufficient education, training and CPD are vital not only for the discipline itself, but to protect public members from incompetent practitioners.[52]

Education access

It is apparent that fiscal imperatives drive much of the professional development available to clinicians, both in the workplace and in the tertiary sector. In relation to the tertiary sector, costs associated with postgraduate courses are a formidable barrier to clinicians wishing to access further education.[102] In Australia in 2002, a government-sponsored National Review of Nursing Education recognised this and recommended that undergraduate courses be taxed at the lowest level of the Higher Education Contribution Scheme (HECS); it was also recommended that scholarships be made available for nurses undertaking postgraduate studies.[103] Having said this, publicly funded healthcare agencies in Australia have state-based forms of qualification allowances as an incentive to undertake further study and in recognition of the value to the workplace that they afford.[103] While government scholarships are not presently available for paramedics, financial support is often provided in part by the employing ambulance service, potentially by the PA and a very limited number of private schemes to undertake postgraduate studies.

In terms of professional development within the workplace, factors such as shift work, high patient acuity and unpredictable patient flow create barriers to the traditional methods for delivering quality education.[104] A literature review of 10 studies examining barriers to CPD identified getting time off work, childcare and home responsibilities as the most frequent deterrents.[105] Additional deterrents included lack of quality or interesting topics, lack of benefit to attending CPD, lack of support from administration and peer opinions and attitudes.[61,105]

Many studies have examined the use of computer-based education packages as a way to deliver education at a time and place convenient to the learner, and have done so with some success.[50,104–106] Such education packages can include webinars ('live' online presentations), e-courses that utilise management systems such as 'Moodle' and 'Blackboard', PowerPoint presentations, lectures, notes and podcasts,[59] as well as interactive CD-ROMs[107] and accessing internet and intranet resources such as e-journals.[108] However, the levels of computer literacy among nurses and paramedics has yet to be thoroughly examined. Skills such as internet browsing, uploading documents and online communication, if lacking, can present a significant barrier to this form of CPD delivery.[59] Similarly, reliability and a lack of standardised web browsers, platforms and computers expose potential problems with technology-mediated teaching.[107] Stoner[109] has coined the term 'technological hardiness' to describe the affective, cognitive and psychomotor skills required to utilise technology in all its forms effectively, and without this hardiness, physical, mental and cognitive stress may be experienced.[109,110] As teachers, we need to be mindful of this diversity in learners' technology skills and enthusiasm for technology.[111] It should also be noted that self-direction, particularly for the inexperienced learner, can appear challenging, especially if the learner has novice technical skills.[112] Difficulties can therefore arise if solely relying on self-directed computer packages to deliver aspects of professional development. It should also be noted that web-based tools raise issues of privacy and dissemination that are not present in more traditional forms of education.[110]

Ideally, uninterrupted professional development time should be allocated and held in an environment removed from the clinical workplace. A secure, trusting and stimulating environment tends to keep learners interested and engaged in learning. Conversely, environmental effects can negatively impact on learners' concentration and readiness to learn.[113] However, recent trends toward busier and continually mobile workforces increase the difficulty in delivering meaningful, high-quality CPD away from the clinical coal face. The operational staff educational email provided by Ambulance Victoria allowed an opportunity to target operational staff with CPD relevant to those individuals, thereby addressing identified knowledge deficits in a timely manner. These briefer communications were readily available on computer or telephone technology with frequent access during delays in hospitals or other brief downtime. They principally complemented formal education to pick up on both repetition for learning, as well as allowing further explanation and clarification where gaps were identified in feedback. Further, those practitioners could in fact tailor future information provision through email and telephone reply avenues ensuring the relevancy and pitch remained accurate. In this way informal education remained clinically focused, relevant and self-directed while still retaining direct link to the original education source.

Other barriers to professional development include time pressures, costs of courses, distance and access issues to courses, difficulty in finding an appropriate course, non-clinician input into senior health decisions, shift work, a lack of CPD funding and research skills.[20,82,121] Similarly, a shortage of relieving staff and workload demands present further significant barriers to professional development[28,61,106] and have implications for both developing and releasing staff for specific courses.

Conducting professional development

The first step in constructing a relevant, accessible, and valued professional development program is to conduct a 'needs assessment' and seek input from clinical practitioners as to the content and processes that are required.[5,13,91] Insisting on involvement in learning will not be successful without understanding what clinicians need.[61] The CPD must be relevant to practise and facilitative of practitioners' ability to provide high standards of care.[114] There may be instances where such apathy exists that practitioners are no longer self-reflective or self-aware of the professional development that would be beneficial to them and their patients. In these cases, a useful starting point might be to stimulate self-awareness through providing opportunities for feedback and professional reflection at work.[34,45] Case study reviews with guided reflection and critical analysis of disease processes, care outcomes, initiatives that worked, and those that didn't, and identifying elements that hindered the provision of optimal care can be very effective and offer multiple learning opportunities to a diverse audience of practitioners.

PRACTICE POINT

CPD should address clearly identified learning needs and educational goals that are directly relevant to quality patient care. Practitioner input is required to establish these goals to ensure relevancy and learner participation.

The learning objectives and teaching techniques must be pitched correctly for the paramedic audience, which, though widely tertiary educated, will within itself have significant variation from novice graduate through to experienced intensive care paramedic. Even correctly pitched, the message within must clearly articulate the clinical relevance of the CPD, such as new item introduction, errors in practice or an important update.

In conducting and facilitating professional development programs, the incorporation of andragogy (adult learning principles) is crucial. Adult learning principles are approaches to adults as learners based on recognition of each individual's autonomy and self-direction, life experiences and readiness to learn, and are useful in the promotion of problem orientation to learning as individuals generally want to apply information applicable to the clinical setting.[30,111,113] Examples of teaching and learning approaches grounded in adult learning principles include problem-based learning, case-based learning, patient-centred learning and simulation. Such andragogical approaches are now common among nursing and paramedic programs, and are seen as effective ways to develop learning empowerment and discovery,[30,113] as well as representing key elements of a successful professional development program.

Education sessions must be designed with the diversity of learners in mind so as to avoid disadvantaging individuals or groups.[112,115] Indeed, nurses are often frustrated with available CPD offerings because they do not match their ability and experience level.[54] Each adult learner brings to the table a variety of skills and experiences, personalities and learning preferences. To begin with, there are clinicians on various stages of Benner's novice to expert continuum. Then there is the diversity in learning preferences more broadly—such as those who prefer visual, auditory or kinesthetic learning styles, or a mixture of all three.[81]

To address these differences, educators need to be mindful of this diversity and be flexible enough to tailor their learning sessions to meet the audience's needs. This can be achieved in large part by making the session as interactive as possible. Learning is described as a collaborative process in which individual understanding is rooted in social interaction,[116,117] and research shows that students learn best when the class is highly interactive.[109] For example, many of us have experienced 'death by PowerPoint'. PowerPoint presentation slides that are overloaded with too much text are often indicative of a 'spray and pray' approach to teaching, inundating learners with copious amounts of information in the hope that some of it sticks.[36] In contrast, PowerPoint presentations that contain only bulleted lists of topical information that is coupled with active learning activities thereby engaging the audience have a better chance of the bulleted information lists being retained.[111]

Diversity can also be found in the differences in ages of clinicians undertaking CPD. The proportion of nurses and midwives aged 50 or older increased from 33% to 38.6% between 2007 and 2011,[118] and the learning preferences of older clinicians will no doubt be different to the oft-written-about Gen-Y or Millennial learner. This diversity in generations of learners brings unique ways of being in the world to the classroom.[111] Gen-Y learners (born 1980–2001) are digital natives, having never experienced the world without the internet. Physiological changes have occurred in response to the intensity and duration of technological bombardment and

have rewired Gen-Y's brains to prefer certain learning styles.[36,119] These neuroplastic changes see Gen-Y learners preferring visual/visual–kinaesthetic processing rather than text processing. They also have a preference for multitasking, are highly social and enjoy group work.[36,119,120] Due to their multitasking preferences, their attention span is often shorter, and as such information should be reduced to small useful chunks[36,120] that is heavily weighted towards visual and kinaesthetic modalities.

Shift workers may also have specific educational needs. Night-shift workers who are required to attend CPD after a long night shift will have less acquisition and retention of material than those on day shifts.[121] Similarly, during the hours of 0200 and 0400 (when the internal circadian rhythm dictates the period of strongest sleep drive) educational initiatives should be avoided.[121]

All emergency nurses and paramedics must have advanced assessment skills, be creative and effective in their problem-solving, have well-developed communication and teaching skills, as well as caring and management expertise. In short, emergency nurses and paramedics need to be constantly critiquing the care being provided and the outcome of that care. Problem based learning (PBL) is an approach to learning that incorporates real-life problems to provide stimulus for critical thinking and self-taught content.[122] PBL encourages clinicians to identify their own gaps in knowledge, which incorporates an active, learner-centred and learner-driven, collaborative, inquiry based learning activity.[107] It is a useful technique to address the learning needs of a diverse range of practitioners with the potential for clinicians to learn from one another. PBL moves the educator away from expert lecturer to being a facilitator of small groups and individual, self-directed learners.[107] Similarly, PBL can foster self-reflection, both in terms of learning needs as well as reflecting on individual clinical performance, which in turn can lead to greater self direction in meeting CPD requirements.

> ## PRACTICE TIP
>
> Problem based learning encourages reflection on practice and critical thinking abilities inherent in real-life clinical scenarios. Content as well as thinking processes can be taught using this method, and variance in the clinical background of the audience can be well catered for.

Part of a professional development charter should include the provision for dissemination of changes in evidence-based practice (EBP). It is imperative that clinicians are up-to-date and implement the latest research findings to provide optimal care for their patients and facilitate cost-effective healthcare.[107] Misconceptions about EBP constitute a barrier to its implementation, and by clarifying those preconceptions and teaching the basics of EBP, we may advance evidence-based care.[123] The skills to retrieve and critically appraise information are not easy to develop and it is desirable that practitioners have the ability to appraise the level of evidence presented in a particular resource, and to understand the worth of the information once interpreted correctly.[111,107] Continued interdisciplinary research projects and the implementation of an interdisciplinary journal club may go some way in addressing these learning needs. By building clinicians' skills in information accessing and processing, they become independent in their ability to identify and answer their own evidence-related practice questions.[107] However, in light of the exponential number of internet resources and other sources of research evidence, it should also be noted that while individual practitioners need to be encouraged to be familiar with current research and clinical trends, they need to be actively involved in bringing that research to the clinical coal face through the official channels of their organisation. Clinicians cannot practise outside of organisation-sanctioned practice guidelines.

There is much support in the literature for an inter-disciplinary approach to professional development and learning.[43,103,124] This is partly in response to awareness that patient outcomes are increasingly determined by how well teams function under pressure,[75] as well as a recognition of the differences in knowledge and expertise other disciplines have to offer. Some have advocated that shared knowledge and supervision help cultivate a learning community in which clinicians share a common interest in gaining knowledge, comprehension or mastery through experience and study, and where staff are encouraged to question practice.[82]

In considering interdisciplinary CPD, we not only support practitioners learning together, but also their being prepared for their future work as diverse clinicians working together in diverse clinical settings.[111] Hurdles such as rostering time for staff of differing disciplines to attend professional development are well worth overcoming, as this also helps promote an appreciation of differing work demands and practices and can result in better team function and bonding. Indeed, a small study of 99 healthcare workers found that work-based interprofessional education was markedly more likely to improve the quality of service and/or bring direct benefit to patients than was college-based education.[125]

Simulation techniques provide great opportunity for inter-disciplinary professional development. Simulations offer such advantages as:

- no patient risk
- errors are allowed to occur
- participants encounter traumatic situations in a safe and controlled environment
- an unlimited choice of scenarios which can be replicated for future groups
- the learning takes place in a team environment which mirrors 'real-life' team function
- participants learn from, and solve problems in, realistic, complex situations, in real time.[109,111,122,126–128]

However, due to the huge spectrum of application, the facilitator of the simulation must make some clear decisions about the purpose of the simulation. Learning objectives need to be made explicit to the participants prior to the commencement of the simulation in order to maximise learning potentials. These learning objectives may be constructed around:

- knowledge (such as conceptual understanding)
- skills (such as psychomotor or technical skill sets)
- behaviours (such as decision-making, leadership, team orientation, communication).[129]

Similarly, technologies and techniques employed to best fit with these learning objectives can range from simple part-task trainers, to role-play, to simulations using high-fidelity mannequins. Debriefing post-simulation facilitates or guides reflection to assist the participants (and the group as a whole) to analyse and assimilate the learning experience.[130] It is worth noting that there is little evidence to indicate whether the learning outcomes for those observing the simulation and participating in the debriefing are the same as those learners who actually played a role in the scenario and participated in the debriefing.[111]

Similarly, what effect, if any, the size of the team taking part in the simulation has on learning outcomes is yet to be determined.[46] The skill of the debriefer is paramount to ensuring the best learning outcome, and therefore training in facilitation and debriefing is vital.[130] Likewise, the skill of the facilitator in debriefing and recognising the vulnerability of the participant is paramount in providing a safe and rich learning environment. In simulations where emotions have run high, ventilation of feelings should be part of the debriefing.[122] Due to the immersive nature of high fidelity simulations, students can become quite distraught if, for example, the simulated patient dies.[111] Immersive simulation is not without risk to the participants and the authors cannot overexaggerate the importance of skilled debriefing. While simulation is indeed a valuable learning modality, it must also be recognised that it can be expensive, both fiscally in the case of high-fidelity, fully immersive simulations, and in the time required to set up (and participate in) a well-constructed, objective-driven simulation.[131]

Much has been written extolling the virtues and superiority of simulation methods of teaching in paramedicine over more traditional methods. Mobile simulation units can take the training units to where the paramedics are.[132] Technical, high risk and infrequently performed procedures such as advanced airway management,[133] including the paediatric patient,[134] can be practised. This is particularly important given the adverse studies demonstrating failures of the ability for paramedics to be able to provide suitable advanced airway care in some circumstances. Bernard et al[101] used simulations to form a major part of the training and the assessment process for endorsement, while Lammers et al (2009) demonstrated the effectiveness of mannequin based simulation in the assessment of paramedic resuscitation skills to allow for future training program development. Byers et al[135] showed not only the effectiveness of simulation training in advanced airway care provision but also in skill retention after one year,[136] while Williams et al[137] demonstrated that undergraduate students found DVD simulation relevant and beneficial highlighting the variety of approaches that can be utilised in simulation training.

Focusing on developing a skill when placed into the context of performing a broader care regimen has been shown to be effective in improving patient outcomes. The integration of teamwork can also be effectively incorporated into simulated scenarios. Siriwardena et al (2009) demonstrated in a non-randomised control group study that an education program delivered through clinical leaders in teams could positively impact on appropriateness and safety in performance of intravenous cannulation practice.[138] Other focused educational programs intending to produce demonstrable outcomes by using a combination of technical skills, theoretical education and practice within a clinical context have been studied, including French et al,[139] who showed an improvement in pre-hospital non-pharmacological pain therapy. Cantwell et al[100] similarly improved appropriateness of paramedic tension pneumothorax decompression where there was considerable emphasis on 'when and why' education to improve skill performance in the context of patient presentation.

The use of simulation as a complementary adjunct to other methods of teaching has also been well documented. Bernard et al[101] demonstrated improved patient outcomes following rapid sequence intubation of patients with traumatic brain injury using a variety of formal educational components, including simulation practice, classroom learning and written and practical assessments. Clearly defined and assessable competencies were included in the training and endorsement for eligibility to perform this procedure and incorporated assessment in simulation, practical skill demonstration, supervised hospital theatre exposure and written questionnaire examination. Considerable use was made of ongoing informal methods including peer review and discussion, bulletin updates and case presentations for discussion. The substantial change in clinical practice was demonstrated a decade after the educational intervention. In contrast there is evidence that failure to provide sufficient initial and ongoing professional education to maintain a clinical skill within a practical context will see inferior outcomes over time.[97–99]

Professional development strategies need to incorporate provision for practitioners to acquire personal strategies that help them to survive emotionally in practice situations. Issues of emotional literacy need to be addressed, as clinician 'burnout' occurs partly because issues that elicit a negative personal response are not identified or are inadequately analysed and evaluated.[7] Peer support programs, case reviews and facilitated, interdisciplinary debriefing can help support practitioners to analyse and evaluate issues, as well as promote personal and aesthetic learning and team bonding.

Professional development and the tertiary sector

Formalised professional development can be undertaken in the tertiary sector in the form of postgraduate awards in chosen specialties. In Australia, the trend of postgraduate courses available and supported by various funding agencies has oscillated from graduate certificate to graduate diploma and back again. Variations in course structures and content have led to a blurred distinction between the different awards, and consequently have led to employer confusion as to the abilities of graduates based not only on award, but also on what year it might have been undertaken.

In the paramedic education and training context, the same uncertainty over course structure and levels of practice also exist, largely due to the issues surrounding registration and accreditation of undergraduate and postgraduate courses. Indeed, a graduate diploma should translate to greater ability, higher thinking processes or metacognition than a graduate certificate; but the passage of time, funding structures, employability and organisational needs has seen the availability and standard of courses vary, and concomitant confusion surrounding the employability of graduates.

With the abolition of the binary system delineating higher research-focused university education from advanced workplace-focused colleges during the Dawkins' era in the late 1980s, the nursing and paramedical education sectors transferred and upgraded their courses to the university sector in 1984 and the late 1990s, respectively.[140,141] This transition undoubtedly has seen both disciplines develop and integrate their own discrete bodies of knowledge and EBP. However, it could also be argued that the current confusion, disparity and lack of uniformity between tertiary courses, tertiary awards, within and between states, and over time has translated to a variation in the preparation of both nurses and paramedics, and has done little for perceived professionalism.

Due to the diversity of set competencies and standards on which courses have been based, there has not been a guaranteed uniformity or standard in tertiary awards, let alone abilities of students. The inconsistency of educational preparation in Australia has not gone unnoticed by government bodies. The Australian Health Ministers Advisory Council has sponsored the formation of a National Nursing and Nursing Education Taskforce (N3ET). In a commentary paper released in 2005, the taskforce noted:

> Whilst there is legislated mandate for regulatory authorities to form standards for courses/education/training programs leading to registration and endorsement, this is problematic at a national level as there are different categories of registration, differences in the recognition of specialist titles and a lack of uniformity in requirements of education (both undergraduate and postgraduate) across the States and Territories.[77]

In response to this, the Council of Australian Governments signed an intergovernmental agreement on the health workforce in 2008 which paved the way for a single national registration and accreditation system for 10 boards of healthcare professionals.[142] It is noteworthy that paramedicine is not included in this system, and struggles to gain recognition as an independent profession requiring registration and accreditation.

In establishing the Australian Health Practitioner Regulation Agency (AHPRA), a nationally-agreed minimum standard for accredited courses is being established, leading to mutual recognition of accredited courses and greater mobility of graduates due in part to a greater acceptance of interstate qualifications by employers.[143] Insofar as nursing is concerned, the AHPRA has adopted the then ANMC (now NMBA) competency standards by which performance is to be assessed to obtain and retain a licence to practise.[12]

Politics aside, undertaking professional development that leads to a tertiary qualification in a specialist area of practice is valuable, and needs to be encouraged as it expands knowledge and skill bases required for nurses and paramedics to better care for patients of increased complexity and acuity.[144] From personal perspectives, advanced or higher-level education also tends to be associated with added self-confidence and real or imagined mobility.[96]

SUMMARY

The nursing and paramedical disciplines have struggled and continue to struggle to prove the worth of professional development programs. While it seems intuitive that ongoing education and professional development translates to more competent practitioners who provide optimum care resulting in better patient outcomes, the link has never been formally established in large-scale studies. There is however evidence that clinically relevant and high-quality formal professional education can be aligned with specific organisational objectives and improved patient outcomes. Outcomes of professional development programs are rarely examined in light of improved clinical outcomes, however, primarily because of methodological constraints. Nevertheless, there is evidence to suggest that undertaking professional development is rewarding for individual clinicians and that the institutions which provide access and facilitate ongoing professional development have higher rates of recruitment and retention of staff.

CPD can take many forms, not all of which are encapsulated by formal educational programs. Informal learning is a rich source of CPD and occurs commonly when clinicians are reflective of their practice and learning needs. Despite the informality of this type of learning, and the difficulty in capturing it in terms of formalised objectives and outcomes, it is a vital component of CPD and perhaps the most clinically relevant in promoting excellence in patient care.

Both nursing and paramedical disciplines in Australia place great emphasis on proving and measuring the competence of their members, ensuring regulatory and registration responsibilities. Assessments of competence that take on a 'tick the box' approach in order to fulfil managerial requirements are at odds with behaviourist teaching methods. Such approaches may be counter-productive in furthering individual professional development, as they may promote 'strategic learning' where the nurse or paramedic only learns what he or she thinks will be examined, rather than learning for comprehension, retention and application.[113] It seems that while competency frameworks are useful in describing what we do, the standards we must maintain and the infrastructure for course development, problems still exist in competency assessment.

Integral to effective professional development is the individual clinician's ability to reflect on his or her own practice and performance, identify learning needs, access education that will meet these needs and ultimately accept responsibility for their own learning.[18,39,81] Current evidence suggests that nurses are adept at self-monitoring and that this process becomes automated over time,[45] and that paramedics are showing similar positive signs. Facilitating the opportunities for self-reflection, through performance feedback, case reviews, PBL, simulation and performance of enabling roles is essential for an ongoing, robust professional development program.

As educators, there is a need to understand the new learner, the evolving technological landscape and the implications for all learners.[36] We must employ contemporary instructional design principles to meet the 21st-century consumer,[36] while not leaving the older, more experienced clinicians behind. Recognition of the diversity of learners can help shape teaching methods to meet learning objectives more effectively. Educators must no longer be seen as the experts imparting pearls of wisdom, but instead are charged with the responsibility of being facilitators of learning, guiding clinicians on an inner journey to realise their own potential to learn.[113]

CASE STUDY

You have been given the portfolio responsibility of professional development at your workplace. This requires you to facilitate the professional development of yourself and your colleagues. Management has also mandated that several key clinical areas require annual competency assessment and need to be incorporated into the program.

Questions

1. What should be your first step in constructing a relevant, accessible and valued professional development program?
2. How would you apply adult learning principles to the professional development program you are conducting?
3. How would you incorporate the latest evidence-based research into the professional development program?
4. What barriers do you expect to encounter in running a successful professional development program?
5. Discuss ways in which knowledge and skills learnt in professional development programs may be more likely to be retained.
6. Competency assessment is multi-dimensional and therefore complex. How could you address the various dimensions that constitute a competency within an assessment framework?

Answers to Case Study Questions can be found on evolve
http://evolve.emergencytrauma.curtis

Acknowledgement

The contributors would like to acknowledge and thank Diane Inglis for her assistance on this chapter.

REFERENCES

1. Nursing and Midwifery Board of Australia. Online. http://www.nursingmidwiferyboard.gov.au/Codes-Guidelines-Statements/Codes-Guidelines.aspx; accessed 20 July 2015.
2. Martin J. The challenges of introducing continuous professional development for paramedics. J Emerg Prim Health Care 2006;4(2).
3. Martin J. The challenge of introducing continuous professional development for paramedics. Australasian Journal of Paramedicine 2012;4(2).
4. Smith JE. Exploring the efficacy of continuing education mandates. JONA's Healthcare Law, Ethics and Regulation 2004;6(1):22–31.
5. Bahn D. Reasons for post registration learning: impact of the learning experience. Nurse Educ Today 2007;27(7):715–22.
6. Wyatt A. Paramedic Practice—Knowledge Invested in Action. Australasian Journal of Paramedicine 2003;1(3).
7. Morton-Cooper A, Palmer A. Mentoring, preceptorship and clinical supervision: a guide to professional roles in clinical practice. 2nd edn. Oxford: Blackwell Science; 2000.
8. Mansvelt J, Suddaby G, O'Hara D. Learning how to e-teach? Staff perspectives on formal and informal professional development activity. In Hello! Where are you in the landscape of educational technology? Proceedings ascilite Melbourne 2008.
9. Capana J. Professional development using informal learning networks: An empirical study in Australia's digital content industry. Queensland University of Technology (QUT) 2012.
10. Deacon M. Being creative about continuing professional development. Mental Health Nursing 2011 Dec; 31(6):14–17.
11. Lejonqvist G, Eriksson K, Meretoja R. Evidence of clinical competence. Scandinavian Journal of Caring Sciences 2012 Jun; 26(2):340–8.
12. Nursing and Midwifery Board of Australia. Online. www.nursingmidwiferyboard.gov.au/Codes-Guidelines-Statements/Codes-Guidelines.aspx#competencystandards; accessed 11 January 2014.
13. Proehl J. Assessing emergency nursing competence. Emergency Nursing 2002;37(1):97–110.
14. Winslow S, Dunn P, Rowlands A. Establishment of a hospital-based simulation skills laboratory. J Nurses Staff Dev 2005;21(2):62–5.
15. McGaughey J. Standardizing the assessment of clinical competence: an overview of intensive care course design. Nurs Crit Care 2004;9(5):238–46.
16. Brazen L. Competence, nursing practice, and safe patient care. Perioperative Nursing Clinics 2008;3(4):297–303.
17. Office of the Queensland Parliamentary Council. Health Practitioner Regulation National Law Act 2009. Online. www.legislation.qld.gov.au/LEGISLTN/CURRENT/H/HealthPracRNA09.pdf; accessed 11 January 2014.
18. College of Emergency Nursing Australasia. Practice Standards for the Emergency Nurse. Online. http://cena.org.au/CENA/Documents/Practice_Standards_for_the_Emergency_Nurse_Specialist_FINALJan%2014[1].pdf; accessed 22 January 2014.
19. Cowin L, Hegstberger-Sims C, Eagar S, Gregeory L, Andrew S, Rolley J. Competency Measurements: Testing convergent validity for two measures. J Adv Nurs 2008; 64(3):272–7.
20. French HP, Dowds J. An overview of continuing professional development in physiotherapy. Physiotherapy 2008;94(3):190–7.
21. Council of Ambulance Authorities. Professional Competency Standards Version 2.2. Online. www.caa.net.au; 12 January 2014, p. 5.
22. Gonczi A, Hager P, Oliver L. Establishing competency-based standards in the professions. Canberra: Australian Government Publishing Service; 1990.
23. Burns R. The adult learner at work. Sydney: Business & Professional Publishing; 1995.
24. FitzGerald G, Bange RF. The road to professional regulation. Brisbane: Queensland University of Technology; 2007.
25. O'Meara P. Paramedics marching towards professionalism. Australian Journal of Paramedicine 2009;7(1).
26. Redman R, Lenburg CB, Walker P. Competency assessment: methods for development and implementation in nursing education and practice. Online J Issues Nurs. Washington DC: American Nurse Association; 1999. Online. www.nursingworld.org/ojin; accessed 9 Sep 2005.
27. Kendall-Gallagher D, Blegen MA. Competence and certification of registered nurses and safety of patients in intensive care units. Am J Crit Care 2009;18(2):106–14.
28. Aiken L, Clarke S, Cheung R et al. Education levels of hospital nurses and surgical patient mortality. JAMA 2003;290:1617–23.
29. Kurtzman ET, Corrigan JM. Measuring the contribution of nursing to quality, patient safety, and health care outcomes. Policy Polit Nurs Pract 2007;8(1):20–36.
30. Harding A, Walker-Cillo G, Duke A, Campos G, Stapleton S. A Framework for Creating and Evaluating Competencies for Emergency Nurses. Journal of Emergency Nursing 2013 May;39(3):252–64.
31. Watson R, Stimpson A, Topping A et al. Clinical competence assessment in nursing: a systematic review of the literature. J Adv Nurs 2002;39(5):421–31.

32. Yanhua C, Watson R. A review of clinical competence assessment in nursing. Nurse Education Today 2011 Nov;31(8):832–6.

33. Considine J, LeVasseur S, Villanueva E. The Australasian triage scale: examining emergency department nurses' performance using computer and paper scenarios. Ann Emerg Med 2004;44(5):516–23.

34. Epstein R, Hundert E. Defining and assessing professional competence. JAMA 2002;287(2):226–35.

35. Walsh M, Bailey P, Koren I. Objective structured clinical evaluation of clinical competence: an integrative review. J Adv Nurs 2009 Aug;65(8):1584–95.

36. Yoder S, Terhorst R. 'Beam Me Up, Scotty': Designing the Future of Nursing Professional Development. J of Continuing Education in Nursing 2012 Oct;43(10):456–62.

37. Covell C. Outcomes achieved from organizational investment in nursing continuing professional development. J of Nursing Administration 2009 Oct;39(10):438–43.

38. Thomas S. The implications of mandatory professional development in Australia. British Journal of Midwifery 2012 Jan;20(1):57–61.

39. Australian Nursing and Midwifery Federations (Victorian Branch): Continuing Professional Development. Online. www.anmfvic.asn.au/multiversions/3455/FileName/Continuing_Professional_Development.pdf; accessed 22 January 2014.

40. Donley R, Flaherty MJ. Promoting professional development: three phases of articulation in nursing education and practice. Online J Issues Nurs 2008;13(3).

41. Willis E, Williams B, Brightwell R et al. Road-ready paramedics and the supporting sciences curriculum. Focus on Health Professional Education: A Multi Discipline Journal 2010;11(2):1–13.

42. Weinstein SM. Certification and credentialing to define competency-based practice. J Infus Nurs 2000;23(1):21–8.

43. Fordham A. Using a competency based approach in nurse education. Nurs Stand 2005;19(31):41–8.

44. Bratt MM. Retaining our next generation of nurses: the Wisconsin nurse residency program provides a continuum of support. J Contin Educ Nurs 2009;40(9):416–25.

45. Fereday J, Muir-Cochrane E. The role of performance feedback in the self-assessment of competence: a research study with nursing clinicians. Collegian 2006;13(1):10–15.

46. Cant R, Cooper S. Simulation-based learning in nurse education: systematic review. J Adv Nurs 2009 Jan;66(1):3–15.

47. Salonen AH, Kaunonen M, Meretoja R et al. Competence profiles of recently registered nurses working in intensive and emergency settings. J Nurs Manag 2007;15(8):792–800.

48. Barton D. How to assess teaching and learning. In Hinchliff S (ed.) The practitioner as teacher. 4th edn. Edinburgh: Elsevier; 2009.

49. Cowan DT, Norman IJ, Coopamah VP. A project to establish a skills competency matrix for EU Nurses. Br J Nurs 2005;14(11):613–17.

50. Australian College of Nursing. Online. www.3lp.rcna.org.au/network/home.php; accessed 2 January 2014.

51. Sibson L. An introduction to CPD for paramedic practice. J Paramed Pract 2008;1(2):73–5.

52. Woollard M. Professionalism in UK paramedic practice. J Emerg Prim Health Care 2009;7(4).

53. Sheather R. Challenges in paramedic practice: professionalisation. In: O'Meara P, Grbich C, eds. Paramedics in Australia: contemporary challenges of practice. Sydney: Pearson Education Australia; 2009.

54. Cooper E. Creating a culture of professional development: a milestone pathway tool for registered nurses. Journal of Continuing Education in Nursing 2009 Nov;40(11): 501–8.

55. Halfer D. Supporting nursing professional development: a magnet hospital's story. Journal for Nurses in Staff Development 2009 May–Jun;25(3):135–40.

56. Government of Western Australia. St John Ambulance inquiry: report to the Ministry for Health Perth. Government of Western Australia: Department of Health; 2009.

57. Burgess S, Boyle M, Chilton M et al. Monash University Centre for Ambulance and Paramedic Studies (MUCAPS) submission to the Department of Human Services (DHS), in response to the DHS discussion paper examining the regulation of the health professions in Victoria. J Emerg Prim Health Care 2003;1(3–4).

58. New South Wales Government. Performance review—ambulance service of NSW. Sydney: Department of Premier and Cabinet; 2008.

59. Ross K, Barr J, Stevens J. Mandatory continuing professional development requirements: what does this mean for Australian nurses? BMC Nursing 2013;12(1):9–15.

60. Australian College of Ambulance Professionals. Certified Ambulance Professional program; 2007.

61. Katsikitis M, McAllister M, Sharman R et al. Continuing professional development in nursing in Australia: Current awareness, practice and future directions. Contemporary Nurse: A Journal for the Australian Nursing Profession 2013;45(1):33–45.

62. Dornan T. Self-assessment in CPD: lessons from the UK undergraduate and postgraduate education domains. J Contin Educ Health Prof 2008;28(1):32–7.

63. Benner P. (1984). From novice to expert: excellence and power in clinical nursing practice. Menlo Park CA: Addison-Wesley; 1984: 13–34.

64. Pool I, Poell R, Cate O. Nurses' and managers' perceptions of continuing professional development for older and younger nurses: A focus group study. International Journal of Nursing Studies 2013;50(1):34–43.

65. Cleaver K. Developing expertise—the contribution of paediatric accident and emergency nurses to the care of children, and the implications for their continuing professional development. Accid Emerg Nurs 2003;11(2):96–102.

66. Hale-Andrews S. Mentoring, membership in professional organizations, and the pursuit of excellence in nursing. J Soc Pediatr Nurs 2001;6(3):147–51.

67. Bradley S, Drapeau M, DeStafano J. The relationship between continuing education and perceived competence, professional support, and professional value among clinical psychologists. Journal of Continuing Education in the Health Professions 2012:32(1):31–8.

68. Way R. Assessing clinical competence. Emerg Nurse 2002;9(9):30–4.

69. Guanci G. Destination magnet: charting a course to excellence. J Nurses Staff Dev 2005;21(5):227–35.

70. Middleton S, Griffiths R, Fernandez R et al. Nursing practice environment: how does one Australian hospital compare with magnet hospitals? Int J Nurs Pract 2008;14(5):366–72.

71. Shanley C. Extending the role of nurses in staff development by combining an organizational change perspective with an individual learner perspective. J Nurses Staff Dev 2004;20(2):83–9.

72. Waxman A, Williams B. Paramedic pre-employment education and the concerns of our future: what are our expectations? J Emerg Prim Health Care 2006;4(3).

73. Heinz D. Hospital nurse staffing and patient outcomes: a review of current literature. Dimens Crit Care Nurs 2004;23(1):44–50.

74. Bournes DA, Ferguson-Paré M. Human becoming and 80/20: an innovative professional development model for nurses. Nurs Sci Q 2007;20(3):237–53.

75. Jenkinson E, Hayman T, Bleetman A. Clinical feedback to ambulance crews: supporting professional development. Emerg Med J 2009;26(4):309.

76. Margolis GS, Romero GA, Fernandez AR, Studnek JR. Strategies of High-Performing Paramedic Educational Programs. Pre-hospital emergency care 2009;13(4):505–11.

77. Australian Health Ministers' Advisory Council. National Nursing & Nursing Education Taskforce (N3ET)—scopes of practice commentary paper. (2005) Online. www.nnnet.gov.au/downloads/n3et_sop_commentary_paper_final.pdf; accessed 23 Jan 2006.

78. Bailey K, Swinyer M, Bard M et al. The effectiveness of a specialized trauma course in the knowledge base and level of job satisfaction in emergency nurses. J Trauma Nurs 2005;12(1):10–15.

79. Ellenbecker CH, Samia L, Cushman MJ et al. Employer retention strategies and their effect on nurses' job satisfaction and intent to stay. Home Health Care Serv Q 2007;26(1):43–58.

80. Melnyk BM. The latest evidence on the outcomes of mentoring. Worldviews Evid Based Nurs 2007;4(3):170–3.

81. Howard S. How to make your teaching effective. In Hinchliff S (ed.) The practitioner as teacher. 4th edn. Edinburgh: Elsevier; 2009.

82. Bassi S, Polifroni E. Learning communities: the link to recruitment and retention. J Nurses Staff Dev 2005;21(3):103–9.

83. Furness S, Pascal J. Focus on health professional education 2013;15(2):30–40.

84. Edwards D. Paramedic preceptor: work readiness in graduate paramedics. The Clinical Teacher 2011;8(2):79–82.

85. Pointer JE. Experience and mentoring requirements for competence in new/inexperienced paramedics. Prehosp Emerg Care 2001;5(4):379–83.

86. Williams B, Onsman A, Brown T. From stretcher-bearer to paramedic: the Australian paramedics' move towards professionalisation. J Emerg Prim Health Care 2009;7(4).

87. Willis E, Williams B, Brightwell R, O'Meara P, Pointon T. Road ready paramedics and the supporting sciences curriculum (online). Focus in health professional education: A multi-disciplinary Journal 2010;11(2):1–13.

88. Andrew N. Clinical imprinting: The impact of early clinical learning on career long professional development in nursing. Nurse Education in Practice 2013;13(3):161–4.

89. Speers A, Strzyzewski N, Ziolkowski L. Preceptor preparation: an investment in the future. J Nurses Staff Dev 2004;20(3):127–33.

90. Dilbert C, Goldenberg D. In: Bassi S, Polifroni EC, eds. Learning communities: the link to recruitment and retention. J Nurses Staff Dev 2005;21(3):103–9.

91. Campbell S. Continuing professional development: what do we need? Nurs Manag 2004;10(10):27–31.

92. Underwood P, Dahlen-Hartfield R, Mogle B. Continuing professional education: does it make a difference in perceived nursing practice? J Nurses Staff Dev 2004;20(2):90–8.

93. Aiken L, Clarke S, Cheung R et al. Education levels of hospital nurses and surgical patient mortality. JAMA 2003;290(12):1617–23.

94. Clarke SP, Connolly C. Nurse education and patient outcomes: a commentary. Policy Polit Nurs Pract 2004;5(1):12–20.

95. von Goedecke A, Herff H, Paal P et al. Field airway management disasters. Anesth Analg 2007;104:481–3.

96. Wang H, Yealy D. Out-of-hospital endotracheal intubation—it's time to stop pretending that problems don't exist. Acad Emerg Med 2005;12(5):417–22.

97. Deakin CD, Clarke T, Nolan J et al. A critical reassessment of ambulance service airway management in prehospital care: Joint Royal Colleges Ambulance Liaison Committee Airway Working group. Emerg Med J 2010;27:226–33.

98. Lossius HM, Roislien J, Lockey DJ. Patient safety in pre-hospital emergency intubation: a comprehensive meta-analysis of the intubation success rates of EMS providers. Critical Care 2012;16:R24.

99. Deakin C, King P, Thompson F. Prehospital advanced airway management by ambulance technicians and paramedics: is clinical practice sufficient to maintain skills? Emerg Med J 2009;26(12):888–91.

100. Cantwell K, Burgess S, Patrick I et al. Improvement in the pre-hospital recognition of tension pneumothorax: the effect of a change to paramedic guidelines and education. Injury 2014;45(1):71–6.

101. Bernard S, Nguyen V, Cameron P et al. Pre-hospital rapid sequence intubation improves functional outcomes for patients with severe traumatic brain injury: a randomized controlled trial. Annals of Surgery 2010:252(6);959–65.

102. Considine J, Hood K. Career development year in emergency nursing: using specific educational preparation and clinical support to facilitate the transition to specialist practice. Nurse Educ Pract 2004;4(3):168–76.

103. The Australian Government's Department of Education, Science and Training. (2006) National review of nursing education—our duty of care. Online. www.nnnet.gov.au/downloads/n3et_final_report.pdf; accessed 18 Feb 2015.

104. Curran-Smith J, Best S. An experience with an online learning environment to support a change in practice in an emergency department. Comput Inform Nurs 2004;22(2):107–10.

105. Schweitzer D, Krassa T. Deterrents to nurses' participation in continuing professional development: an integrative literature review. Journal of Continuing Education in Nursing 2010 Oct;41(10):441–7.

106. Courtney M, Yacopetti J, James C et al. Queensland public sector nurse executives: professional development needs. Online. http://eprints.qut.edu.au/archive/00000258/; accessed 16 Feb 2015.

107. Messecar D. Nursing as a career. In Moyer, B and Wittmann-Price, R. eds. Nursing education: foundations for practice excellence, F.A. Davis Company, Philadelphia; 2008.

108. Pawlyn J. The use of e-learning in continuing professional development. Learning Disability Practice 2012 Feb;15(1):33–7.

109. Stoner M. The nursing resource center. In Moyer, B and Wittmann-Price, R. eds. Nursing education: foundations for practice excellence, F.A. Davis Company, Philadelphia; 2008.

110. Green B, Hope A. Promoting clinical competence using social media. Nurse Educator 2010 May–Jun;35(3):127–9.

111. Bonnell WE, Vogel Smith K. Teaching technologies in nursing and the health professions: beyond dimulation and online courses. Springer Publishing company, New York; 2010.

112. Howatson-Jones L. Designing web-based education courses for nurses. Nurs Stand 2004;19(11):41–4.

113. Bancato V. Management strategies in the educational setting. In Moyer, B and Wittmann-Price, R. eds. Nursing education: foundations for practice excellence, F.A. Davis Company, Philadelphia; 2008.

114. Deacon M. Being creative about continuing professional development. Mental Health Nursing 2011 Dec;31(6):14–17.

115. Zummo K, Kearney G. Staff development story—an innovative approach to 'mandatory nursing education'. J Nurses Staff Dev 2009;25(2):95–7.

116. Williams B, Day R. Context based learning. In Young L, and Paterson, B. eds. Teaching nursing: developing a student-centred learning environment, Lippincott Williams & Wilkins, Philadelphia; 2007.

117. Pratt D, Paterson B. Perspectives on teaching: Discovering BIASes. In Young L, and Paterson B. eds. Teaching nursing: developing a student-centred learning environment, Lippincott Williams & Wilkins, Philadelphia; 2007.

118. Australian Institute on Health and Welfare. Nursing and Midwifery Workforce 2011. Online. www.aihw.gov.au/publication-detail/?id=10737422167; accessed 20 Jan 2014.

119. Jukes I, McCain T, Crockett L. Understanding the digital generation: teaching and learning in the new digital landscape, Kelowna BC: 21st Century Fluency Project Inc; 2010.

120. Mastrian K, McGonigle D, Mahan W, Bixler B. Integrating technology in nursing education: tools for the knowledge era, Jones and Bartlett Publishers, Massachusetts; 2011.

121. Mayes P, Schott-Baer D. Professional development for night shift nurses. Journal of Continuing Education in Nursing 2010 Jan; 41(1):17–24, 49.

122. De Young, S. Teaching strategies for nurse educators 2nd edn, New Jersey: Prentice Hall; 2009.

123. Melnyk B, Fineout-Overholt E. Evidence-based practice in nursing and healthcare: a guide to best practice. Philadelphia: Lippincott Williams & Wilkins; 2005.

124. McClelland HM. Guest editorial: Learning environments. Accid Emerg Nurs 2004;12(4):195.

125. Watcher R. The end of the beginning: patient safety five years after 'To err is human'. Health affairs—Web exclusive. (20 Nov 2004) Online. http://content.healthaffairs.org/cgi/reprint/hlthaff.w4.534v1.pdf; accessed 13 Jan 2014.

126. Lloyd G, Kendall J, Meek S et al. High-level simulators in emergency department education: thoughts from the trainer's perspective. Emerg Med J 2007;24:288–91.

127. Walsh M. Using a simulated learning environment. Emerg Nurse 2010;18(2):12–16.

128. Joel L. Assessment and evaluation strategies. In Moyer B, Wittmann-Price R (eds), Nursing education: foundations for practice excellence. Philadelphia: F.A. Davis Company: 2008.

129. Gaba D. Formal organization for simulation applications in health care: possibilities and actualities. SimTecT—Health and medical symposium. Melbourne, 24–26 May 2004.

130. Fanning R, Gaba D. The role of debriefing in simulation-based learning. Simul Healthcare 2007;2(2):115–25.

131. Thomas S. The implications of mandatory professional development in Australia. British Journal of Midwifery 2012 Jan;20(1):7–61.

132. Alinier G, Newton A. A model to embed simulation training during ambulance shift work. International Paramedic Practice 2013;3(2):35–40.

133. Kennedy CC, Cannon EK, Warner DO, Cook DA. Advanced airway management simulation training in medical education: a systematic review and meta-analysis. Critical Care Medicine 2014;42(1):169–78.

134. Nishisaki A, Nguyen J, Colborn S et al. Evaluation of multidisciplinary simulation training on clinical performance and team behavior during tracheal intubation procedures in a pediatric intensive care unit. Pediatric Critical Care Medicine 2011;12(4):406–14.

135. Lammers RL, Byrwa MJ, Fales WD, Hale RA. Simulation based assessment of paramedic pediatric resuscitation skills. Education and Practice 2009;13(3):345–56.

136. Byers D, Lo B, Yates J. Effect of paramedic utilization of the intubating laryngeal mask airway in high fidelity simulated critical care scenarios. Pre-hospital and disaster medicine 2013;28(6):630–1.

137. Williams B, Brown T, Archer F. Can DVD simulations provide an effective alternative for paramedic clinical placement education? Emerg Med J 2009;26:377–81.

138. Siriwardena AN, Iqbal M, Banerjee S et al. An evaluation of an educational intervention to reduce inappropriate cannulation and improve cannulation technique by paramedics. Emerg Med J 2009;26:831–6.

139. French SR, Salama NP, Baqai S et al. Effects of an educational intervention on pre-hospital pain management. Prehosp Emerg Care 2006:10(1):71–6.

140. Reid J. Nursing education in Australian universities: report of the national review of nurse education in the higher education sector—1994 and beyond. Canberra: Department of Education, Training and Science; 1994.

141. Lord B. The development of a degree qualification for paramedics at Charles Sturt University. J Emerg Prim Health Care 2003;1(1–2):5.

142. Australia's Health Workforce Online. National registration and accreditation scheme. Online. www.nhwt.gov.au; accessed 27 Nov 2009.

143. Australian Health Practitioner Regulation Agency. Online. www.ahpra.gov.au; accessed 25 Nov 2009.

144. American Association of Critical Care Nurses. Safeguarding the patient and the profession: the value of critical care nurse certification. Am J Crit Care 2003;12(2):154–64.

CHAPTER 8

RESEARCH FOR EMERGENCY CARE

JULIE CONSIDINE, RAMON Z SHABAN, MARGARET FRY AND KATE CURTIS

Essentials

- Healthcare practitioners require knowledge, skills and motivation to evaluate research studies and determine that they have sufficient rigour to provide findings that are reliable, useful and safe for practice.
- When formulating a research question, always ask yourself about the significance of the research for knowledge, practice, education, workforce or policy. Your research should answer the following questions: What do we know? What don't we know? What should we know? Why should we know it? In answering these questions, you will be able to discern a research question from the problem statement.
- Some research questions should always be clear and concise. Research may not be viable if:
  - it is expensive to undertake and there is little or no funding
  - it is poorly or incorrectly designed
  - there are barriers to accessing data or sufficient data relative to the methodology
  - data collection procedures are overly complex or onerous.
- Make sure before you attempt even a pilot project that you have sufficient funding or resources to undertake the project.
- Engage a mentor or a supervisor to guide you with your research, especially if you are an inexperienced researcher. Seek out opportunities to join and contribute actively to an established research team or group and begin to establish your own research track record.
- All researchers must act ethically, with honesty and integrity, throughout the research process including publication of the findings.
- When planning your research, make sure you consider how you will disseminate the findings through publications, presentations and professional events.

INTRODUCTION

Research, the systematic search for new knowledge, is essential for the continuing evolution of professional nursing and paramedical practice. Research provides the foundation upon which the actions of nurses and paramedics are evidence-based, and it goes beyond intuition, traditional behavioural norms, opinion or word-of-mouth. Evidence gained from scholarly research informs practice decisions and enables change for its improvement. Evidence-based care, that is practice based on research findings, is essential to safe, effective and efficient healthcare provision and meeting the expectations of patients, families and colleagues. Where the evidence for practice is strong, protocols based on the research findings should guide clinical practice. This chapter overviews the basics of the research process and assists you to read and understand research literature. The chapter encourages paramedics and emergency nurses to support and engage in collaborative research as part of research teams to identify new knowledge and/or evaluate the outcomes of practice change.

The research process

The research process is the acquisition of knowledge through a systematic and logical series of steps that a researcher moves through to understand reality.[1] Research findings in nursing are frequently classified as taking one of two approaches. One way of classifying research is by the type of data generated. Research is regarded as *quantitative* (numerical)—moving from more general concepts to specific observations or hypothesis testing—or *qualitative* (narrative), in which specific subjective observations move to general concepts or theories.[2] Many studies in nursing and midwifery use a combination of both approaches, referred to as 'mixed method'. Field and Morse[3] wrote that while the steps in qualitative research are less encapsulated than those in quantitative research, they are seen to flow in the same directions and together offer a richer understanding of the phenomena under interest.

Within these two classifications there is a variety of methods available to researchers to answer research questions or problems. Clinicians reading journal articles to inform their practice require a basic knowledge of research elements or steps, because these elements are reflected in the way journal articles are traditionally structured and presented. New researchers obviously require a more comprehensive understanding of research processes. It is advisable for new researchers to seek support in selecting an appropriate approach and method from more experienced colleagues or from supervisors, prior to proposal submission to a human research ethics committee and prior to the collection of any data even for a pilot study. Larger research projects are usually undertaken by a research team involving a group of clinicians from one discipline, or members from various disciplinary groups. The term 'collaborative' is used to refer to research groups formed through a varied membership. For example a research team may include doctors, pharmacists, nurses and paramedics as well as a psychologist, a communication expert and a statistician. The following section provides an overview of the elements of the research process as a beginning point. There are many excellent research texts written by experienced researchers which you are encouraged to read for detailed explanations of research concepts, including a small, practical A&E research text.[4] An excellent glossary of research terms is available in the Cochrane Resources Glossary.[5]

Identification of a research problem or phenomenon

Clinical research starts with a question, a problem or a phenomenon of interest. An identified problem may concern patient care or a clinical problem, nurses, systems of administration or any issue of nursing or paramedical interest. Patient care or nursing practice problems generally address practice differences or discrepancies and what clinicians consider is ideal or desirable for the patient. At this stage the question needs to be asked if the problem or difference is something that really matters, is able to be researched and whether it relates to more-general conceptual issues. However, deciding on and formulating a specific research question is often difficult for the beginning researcher. One starting point is for nurses and paramedics to reflect on their personal and clinical experiences as an initial source of potentially researchable problems. An observation and reflection can be turned into a question which can start a research plan. For example:

- I wonder if continuous positive airway pressure (CPAP) applied by face mask would benefit patients with pulmonary oedema during transportation by ambulance from home to the ED?
- I wonder if ED nurses could administer pain medicine on a standing order. Would this decrease the severity of patients' pain prior to seeing a doctor and increase patients' satisfaction with care?

At this early stage of the research process it is usually necessary to 'refine' the problem area or phenomenon to form a question that enables a search of the literature by the use of key terms. It is usually possible to discuss ideas with a colleague who has some research experience, or if you have a mentor from your own or other disciplinary areas, seek their advice.

Using the first example given above, 'patients with pulmonary oedema' could be focused upon using the PICO format—**P**atient (or disease), **I**ntervention (drug, diagnostic test), **C**omparison (other drug, test or intervention) and **O**utcome. This would then read 'In patients with acute cardiogenic pulmonary oedema, does paramedic-initiated CPAP prior to and during transport to hospital reduce mortality (or reduce need for intubation, or reduce length of hospital admission or whatever the outcome of interest may be)?' In addition, logistical and staffing issues may limit the availability of CPAP in rural areas. Therefore, the study might initially need to focus on care in major urban settings. This would be a refinement in the question, which could now read as:

- Does continuous positive airway pressure (CPAP) applied by face mask benefit patients with acute cardiogenic pulmonary oedema during transportation by urban ambulance to the ED?

The refinement process continues until each term (variable) within the research question is defined. Even at this early point it is important to be very clear about each term or variable, and it can be useful to define your use of a term to ensure you are clear about the meaning you are trying to communicate to others.

Other sources of potential research questions are the recommendations for further research in many published research reports. When reviewing research articles, a nurse may identify research questions based on the state of the science about a given area or clinical problem. The same research question answered in a publication can be asked again in a different country to verify the findings of the primary study (replication) or for a different sample of patients or clients. When an aspect of practice is changed, based on the available evidence, it is useful to evaluate the impact of that change by measuring the outcomes of the change in a specific location, institution or service. The evaluation of outcomes could be a measure of cost changes or staff time, as well as the impact on patients or clients.

Searching and reviewing the literature

The purpose of the literature search is to identify published research work conducted previously in the particular area of interest to assist the researcher to clarify and specify the research problem and to identify whether similar studies have already been published. The statement of the problem or research question is used to guide the literature search. Underline keywords in the statement or question and use them as search terms; e.g. family presence, resuscitation, invasive procedures, emergency. A review that uses these keywords provides a good example of how this is done.[6] Electronic searches of databases such as the Cumulative Index for Nursing and Allied Health Literature (CINAHL), Medline, PubMed or EMBASE, normally start with broad terms and then the search is narrowed. It is often worthwhile to ask a librarian to check that you have identified all the appropriate databases, if you are unsure. Once you start the search with specific terms, keywords can be combined to narrow the search output; for example, resuscitation and family presence as a combined search term will provide references containing both terms. You can also limit your search by checking specifications such as the language the article is written in and the year of publication. Once you have a listing of the articles, you move to the next stage of the review process.

It takes practice to read each section of a research article and understand exactly what is meant. If this process is new to you, you might need to do a lot of re-reading to fully comprehend the meaning of the text. Many ways to achieve an informed read have been suggested. For example, some people skim over the article first before focusing on any particular sections. Others read the abstract several times. You will choose your preferred method, which might include making notes in the margins or using a bibliographic software package. When you understand each section, you then need to judge if the sections are consistent in answering the research question. For example, you would consider whether the research design can answer the question asked, whether the sample was selected appropriately and is of a sufficient size, whether data were analysed according to the design and whether the results answered the question/s asked.

After reading and critiquing previous research in a specific area, the reviewer summarises what has been previously studied. This summary of previous research findings is helpful in making decisions about the usefulness or significance of the evidence to inform practice decisions. If the reviewer is interested in undertaking new research, how this new study will contribute to the state of the science can be delineated. A thorough review reinforces the need for the study in light of previous research findings, and what is accepted as truth from other studies is the groundwork on which new studies or replication studies are based. A written literature review will include summaries of articles in which the conclusions may differ from or agree with the proposed point of view. A useful summary of the steps and strategies of this process is provided by Schneider et al.[7] Sources of information for literature reviews can include both primary and secondary sources. A *primary source* of information is the description of an investigation written by the person who conducted it. A *secondary source* is a description of a study written by someone other than the original researcher. Both

sources can be helpful, but written literature reviews should be based on primary sources whenever it is possible to locate those primary sources. A secondary source is useful when the primary source is unavailable, or when the secondary source is providing a different perspective or emphasis to the primary source. At times grey literature is useful and includes sources such as government reports, professional associations and blogs summarising evidence can be useful; however, the cited references and authority of the sources should always be considered.[8–10] If the topic is a general-practice issue, such as the emergency management of patients with abdominal pain, it is important to check whether a systematic review (scientific summary) has been undertaken. Librarians at your local hospital are generally more than willing to assist with the sourcing of literature. If you are enrolled in tertiary education, your college or university faculty librarians can be consulted for assistance.

PRACTICE TIP

Check the literature for a systematic review on the chosen topic before looking for single articles. The review will identify the 'strongest' articles and provide a summary of the evidence for you to read.

In summary, the literature search and review is a comprehensive, systematic and critical review of scholarly papers, government reports, unpublished works and even personal communications. Clinicians require the skill to critically review literature as either a researcher or a reader of research (consumer) to enable the development of evidence-based clinical practice. The critical review process can be assisted by using a series of appraisal questions that are based on the elements of the research process.[11,12] When the literature review process is complete, the reviewer summarises and synthesises all information on the topic into a written summary. If a research study is subsequently conducted, ongoing updates of the literature need to be undertaken to ensure the literature review remains current.

Theoretical and conceptual frameworks

Theoretical and conceptual frameworks provide a structure to guide the study of clinical problems. A *theoretical framework* defines the concepts and proposes relationships among those concepts. It enables the findings of the researcher's study to be linked to existing knowledge. A framework consists of definitions of concepts and propositions about the relationships of those concepts to each other. It helps to interpet beliefs about what is observed, and provide a systematic way to organise information about a particular aspect of interest in a research study.[13]

Two components of a theory are concepts and a statement of propositions. *Concepts*, the building blocks of a theory, are abstract characteristics, categories or labels of things, persons or events. Examples of concepts employed by nurses and paramedics are health, stress, adaptation, caring and pain. *Propositions* are statements that define the relationships among concepts. A set of propositions may state that one concept is associated with another or is contingent upon another. Examples of theories are critical social theory, systems and adaptation theory. The power of theories lies in the ability to explain the relationship of variables and the nature of this relationship. Theories also help stimulate research by giving direction.[13]

Conceptual frameworks represent a less-well-developed system for organising phenomena. Frameworks contain concepts that represent a common theme but lack the deductive system of propositions which gives the relationship among concepts. Research in nursing practice often uses conceptual frameworks rather than theories. These conceptual frameworks can lay the groundwork for more-formal theories.[14]

Each methodology in qualitative research has a basic belief system that is manifest in the particular conventions of sampling, data collection, data management and auditing, analyses and conceptualisation that the researcher is required to follow. If no existing theory or conceptual framework has been applied to the phenomenon of interest, the researcher chooses a methodological approach that will enable the research question to be explored. Examples are Lyneham et al's study that used a hermeneutic phenomenological approach to explicate the experience of intuition in emergency nursing by 14 expert nurses,[15] and Fry's use of ethnography to investigate triage nursing practice in Australian emergency departments (see Research Highlight 8.1).[16] A different qualitative method, the Delphi technique, was used by Rodger and Kristjanson[17] to survey emergency nurses in Western Australia. Using this method, the researchers sent the results of the research question back to the respondents for further refinement. The number of times this process occurs varies for each situation, but the process usually continues until a predetermined consensus rate is reached by all respondents. In this project, 25 research questions were developed by emergency nurses and then ranked according to priority.

Exploratory or explanatory studies may use 'mixed methods'. That is, qualitative data are collected as well as quantitative data, with the intent of achieving a richer understanding of a situation or the phenomena under study. In mixed methods studies the numerical results are further explored and understood through the collection of qualitative data obtained from what participants say or write. For example, in an initial study of the practice of 'ambulance ramping' in 10 EDs in Southern Queensland, the researchers used in-depth interviews, focus groups and chart audits to collect data that provided information not only on the extent of the practice but also on the antecedents to this practice (see Research Highlight 8.2).[18] Interviews and focus groups provided narrative data while chart audits provided numerical data such as response and transportation times, waiting periods at the hospital and patient demographics.

RESEARCH HIGHLIGHT 8.1

Study using an ethnographic design[16]

Title—Triage nursing practice in Australian emergency departments 2002–2004: an ethnography.

Aim—To provide insight and understanding into the triage nurse (TN) role in Australian emergency departments (EDs) to enable appropriate education and support.

Method—A survey of 900 nurses who worked in the triage role in 50 New South Wales EDs was initially undertaken.

Subsequently, purposive sampling of four metropolitan EDs (levels 4 and 6) was undertaken and 10 TNs were observed and interviewed about their role.

Results—Observation and interviews showed that the triage nurse culture incorporated a series of beliefs, for example 'patients should respect the triage space'. The study found that TNs determine patient movement, the timing of care and the initiation of extended activities. To accomplish these tasks, TNs use three major processes: gate-keeping, time-keeping and decision-making. The study went on to examine other contextual ED pressures such as overcrowding and aggressive behaviour towards nurses from people using the ED service.

RESEARCH HIGHLIGHT 8.2

Study using mixed methods[18]

Title—An exploratory study to examine the phenomenon and practice of 'ambulance ramping' at hospitals within Southern Health Districts of Queensland and Queensland Ambulance Service (QAS).

Aim—To understand the antecedents to 'ambulance ramping' in health service delivery.

Method—An exploratory, descriptive study involving QAS and 10 hospital emergency departments was undertaken. Data were collected through in-depth interviews, focus groups and chart audits.

Results—'Ambulance ramping' is a practice primarily of triage nurses. Patients brought to ED by ambulance are not admitted to the ED because of overcrowding or insufficient staffing levels. Patients are left explicitly in the clinical care of ambulance personnel on either a physical or a virtual ambulance ramp out of necessity because of the acuity of their condition. Significant inconsistencies in the practice and reporting of ambulance ramping across all EDs were reported.

Research questions or hypotheses

As previously stated, before a problem can be researched it must be focused and refined, so that it is possible to develop a research design (plan) that can potentially answer the problem or question of interest. The research interest can be stated as a research question or as a hypothesis. The term 'research question' is used in qualitative approaches where findings are presented as narrative themes or theories. A research question also directs the processes of numerical descriptive studies. Quantitative research questions that are used in descriptive studies should be specific and not attempt to describe too much, because data analysis may be complex and confusing to interpret. A research project can (and frequently does) answer more than one question or hypothesis in the same study. As previously mentioned, research questions and hypotheses should define key variables or terms.

Questions formulated about what will occur in specific situations in quantitative approaches are called *hypotheses*. Hypotheses are tested to identify significant associations between variables or significant differences between groups and to determine how results fit existing theory. A hypothesis expands upon a research question because it is a tentative prediction or explanation of the relationship between two or more variables,[12] which the researcher postulates before the initiation of the research study. For example, one hypothesis might be that adults (20–50 years of age) with severe abdominal pain who are managed with a nurse-led pain protocol soon after arrival in the ED will report a perception of better management (satisfaction) than will adults with similar presentations who wait longer to see a doctor and have delayed analgesia. In this example, the researcher is postulating not only a relationship between the time of treating pain and adults' perception of better management (satisfaction), but is also predicting an outcome from this relationship. The null (or 'no effect') hypothesis indicates that the two populations (the sample of adults treated quickly for pain and the sample of adults with delayed pain treatment) have the same perceptions of hospital management (satisfaction) score. Therefore the *null* hypothesis, stated as 'there is no relationship between the length of time waiting for analgesia and satisfaction' or 'there will be no difference in the satisfaction scores between the two groups', is generated as a position of non-bias towards finding the result the researcher seeks, as well as guiding the statistical analyses and discussion.

The terms or variables of a hypothesis have identifying names. An independent variable is what is assumed to cause or thought to be associated with the dependent or outcome variable. Changes in the dependent variable are presumed to depend on the independent variable's effects. The dependent variable is explained through its relationship with the independent variable, and it is what the researcher wants to explain or understand.[13] The dependent variable in the example above is 'adults' perceptions of better management (satisfaction score)'. The independent variable is 'the time taken to provide the adult in pain with analgesia'. It is known that while many factors affect an adult's perception of good hospital management (satisfaction), only one independent variable (time to analgesia) is intended to be measured in the proposed research question to keep the variables under consideration specific and clear.

Often the dependent (outcome) variable can be the result of a number of influences (factors), such as (in our example) age of the participant, gender or pain level. A study might be designed to examine several factors and their impact on a phenomenon or dependent variable. For example, you may want to know whether experience with triage or an educational program concerning triage influences the ability to perform triage adequately. Both independent variables (education and experience) can influence triage performance ability (dependent variable). Another research design could have several dependent or outcome variables designated as measures of treatment effectiveness. An example of multiple dependent variables identified in a research question is, 'Does a comprehensive triage system influence length of stay in the ED, patient satisfaction and patient outcome?' In this question it is proposed that the length of stay in ED, patient satisfaction and patient outcome are all dependent on the system of triage.[1]

Method

The method section of a research study identifies how the researcher plans to implement the research study in order to answer the research questions or hypotheses. The components of the method section include: the research design; participants or subjects in the study, commonly labelled the sample; the study procedure which describes how data will be collected; and the measures used to collect data, including any instruments (tools) such as a questionnaire or an apparatus such as thermometer. It is essential that the validity of an instrument (basically, testing what it purports to be testing) and its reliability (consistency of results over repeated use) is established prior to data collection. In some cases a questionnaire will require testing in a pilot study to establish validity and reliability prior to the main study being conducted. Then these results are reported in the section discussing the instrument. A description of how data will be analysed is also required. Box 8.1 identifies some commonly used quantitative approaches.

Design

The research design tells a reader how the research is planned. A formal design statement may not be provided in qualitative studies, but the research approach and method will be clearly outlined in, for example, the constructivist–interpretive, feminist or critical approaches.[19] Each different approach/method incorporates a way of structuring the study, selecting participants and collecting and analysing data.

In quantitative research the design statement includes information on the variables: whether the variable (also called a factor) has different levels or classes, such as high and low, the number of groups participating in the research, and the occasions on which data will be collected. For example, in a design that is called a pre-test/post-test design, an experimental or treatment group and a control group (two randomly selected or matched groups) will be tested for the variable (e.g. physical fitness) before the experimental group is given a treatment or intervention that the control group will not receive. Following the treatment or intervention, both groups are re-tested within a similar time-frame for physical fitness. The pre-test/post-test design seeks to determine if a treatment or intervention had any effect on physical fitness while controlling for extraneous or outside events the researcher has no control over. The pre-test results from both groups should be similar, or at least not statistically different, indicating that both groups started with a similar level of fitness. Following the intervention, if fitness is statistically different in the two groups (called significantly different), then the researcher can conclude that the treatment or intervention had some effect that changed the level of fitness of the group receiving it. A comparative design has been used in Research Highlight 8.3, where Rickard et al[20] are comparing the use of intranasal fentanyl with the use of intravenous morphine pre-hospital by how patients given the respective drugs verbally rate their pain relief.

RESEARCH HIGHLIGHT 8.3

Study using a randomised controlled trial design[20]

Title—A randomised controlled trial of intranasal fentanyl vs intravenous morphine for analgesia in the prehospital setting.

Aim—To compare intranasal fentanyl (INF) with intravenous morphine (IVM) for pre-hospital analgesia.

Method—Randomised, controlled, open-label trial in which 258 consecutive adult patients requiring analgesia (Verbal Rating Score VRS >2/10 non-cardiac or >5/10 cardiac) were recruited. Patients received INF 180 µg ± 2 doses of 60 µg at ≥ 5-minute intervals, or IVM 2.5–5 mg ± 2 doses of 2.5–5 mg at ≥ 5-minute intervals. The endpoint was the difference in baseline destination VRS.

Results—Groups were equivalent (*p* = not significant) for baseline VRS, mean (SD) was INF 8.3 (1.7); IVM 8.1 (1.6), and minutes to destination mean (SD) was INF 27.2' (15.5'); IVM 30.6' (19.1'). Patients had a mean (95% confidence interval) VRS reduction as follows: INF 4.22 (3.74–4.71), IVM 3.57 (3.10–4.03); *p* = 0.08. Higher baseline VRS (*p* < 0.001), no methoxyflurane use (*p* < 0.01) and back pain (*p* = 0.02) predicted VRS reduction. Safety and acceptability were comparable.

Conclusion—There was no significant difference in the effectiveness of INF and IVM for prehospital analgesia.

Samples—participants and subjects

The sampling of participants or subjects for a quantitative research study depends on the population to be studied and the estimated number of subjects needed to demonstrate a significant difference between experimental and control groups.[20] The definition of a population is not restricted to human subjects. A population can consist of records, animals, blood samples, actions, words, organisations and numbers. Whatever the unit to be studied or sampled, a population is always made up of specific elements of interest. Generally, in a research study it is impossible to include large populations because of expense and the time involved for data collection. Therefore, a quantitative study will usually limit the members of the population to a 'representative' sample. Samples attempt to include subjects that represent a portion of the entire population to be studied to ensure that the sample is 'representative' of that population. If the sample is not representative, then it is not possible to accurately generalise the research outcomes to the whole population.

Researchers use probability and non-probability sampling techniques when designing studies. *Probability sampling* is the use of some method of random selection (e.g. a table of random numbers) to choose the subjects or units to be sampled; any member of the defined population has an equal chance to be selected. A number of inclusion criteria will be identified by the researcher. These might be the participants' (subjects') age, gender, illness diagnosis or language spoken. Potential participants who do not meet the inclusion criteria are excluded from the study. A statistical technique, known as

---

BOX 8.1   Research using quantitative research approaches[21–23]

- *Descriptive research* is a means of discovering new meanings by describing what exists, or the frequency at which something occurs, or the categorising of information. Descriptive studies provide the knowledge base and potential hypotheses to direct correlational or experimental studies subsequently. Descriptive data can be obtained by auditing records, observations of events or by questionnaires. Descriptive studies undertaken over a long time period (months and years) are called *longitudinal*.
- *Correlational research* involves the investigation of relationships between two or more variables. The strength or degree of a relationship between variables can be measured and a numerical coefficient provided that identifies the strength of the relationship. Where two variables are strongly related, by knowing the value of one variable, it is possible to predict the likely value of the other. It is important to note that a significant relationship between two variables does not imply one variable caused the other.
- *Experimental research* is defined as an objective, systematic, controlled investigation for the purpose of examining causality. That is, the intervention and nothing else is responsible for the result. Experimental or comparative studies have three main characteristics: controlled manipulation of the treatment or independent variable (one group gets the treatment and the other group doesn't), treatment and control groups, and each subject has an equal chance of random selection for either the treatment or control group (randomisation). This design is considered to provide the highest level of research evidence for an individual study, when the researcher does not know

what intervention the subject received. That is, the researcher is 'blind' to knowing what group the subject is in or whether the subject received the treatment or not. It is often difficult in nursing for an investigator to be 'blind' to an intervention, because the treatment or intervention can be identified even when the researcher is not informed. An example is a study to compare patient outcomes from the use of peripherally inserted central lines and midline lines for low irritant antibiotic administration. Even when patients are randomly assigned to type, the investigator monitoring the outcomes will know what has been inserted from expert knowledge of the different vascular access devices.

- *Quasi-experimental research* is used to explain relationships and/or clarify why certain events occur. This design is not considered to be as 'controlled' as experimental studies, because there is a lack of control over the setting or the intervention or the subjects have not been assigned randomly. This design is useful in some clinical situations where the population receiving the intervention is very small, or where random assignment of subjects to a control group is not possible because of ethical considerations (see **Research Highlight 8.2**).
- *Mixed methods*: some studies combine both qualitative and quantitative methods. An investigator may choose to do this because of small populations or difficulty sampling from a large population because of access restrictions. In a research study, the method of data collection may include narrative data about a phenomenon provided by a sufferer of an illness combined with physiological measures of the illness. Mixed methods are often used in case study research.

'power analysis', is used by researchers to estimate the sample size required to get an accurate result when data are analysed. In general, as a 'rough' guide, it is recommended that a sample size of 30 be selected for each subset of data or 'cell' of the design.[9]

Non-probability sampling is used in both qualitative and quantitative methods. There are different types of non-probability sampling including accidental or convenience, quota, purposive and snowballing. Accidental samples are based on convenience of gathering subjects, such as surveying the first 100 patients in the ED on a particular day. Quota samples are used when a researcher knows an element of the population and bases sampling on the known representativeness within the population. For example, if a researcher knows that 25% of the ED nurses are males, the researcher attempts to ensure that 25% of the sample of ED nurses selected for a study of ED nurses is male. This technique improves the representativeness of the population within the sample.

Purposive sampling occurs when a researcher 'hand-picks' cases to be included in the sample that represent the typical subjects within a given population. A study may use purposive sampling to ensure a variety of responses or because the choices are judged to be typical of a specific population or matching samples (see Research Highlight 8.4). Purposive sampling is said to provide information-rich cases for in-depth study in qualitative research.[24] *Snowball sampling* is used in qualitative or quantitative research to locate participants who might be difficult for the researcher to identify. When participants who have all the inclusion criteria are identified, they use their networks to locate other participants. Qualitative methods require a direct relationship between the researcher and the research participants because data are collected through in-depth interviews or direct encounters in focus groups. This level of direct relationship may not be required in quantitative research; for example, the use of questionnaires or surveys where the respondent may be anonymous. Participants may not benefit directly from participating in a research study, but give informed consent to be involved because they want to progress the development of knowledge for the benefit of others. Some researchers do provide an incentive, such as a small amount of money or a movie ticket as a token of appreciation for the participant's time.

RESEARCH HIGHLIGHT 8.4

Study using a retrospective cohort design[25]

Title—Trauma case management: improving patient outcomes.

Background—The purpose of the study was to measure the effect of trauma case management (TCM) on patient outcomes, using practice-specific outcome variables such as in-hospital complication rates, length of hospital stay, resource use and allied health service intervention rates.

Method—A retrospective, cohort design was used with purposive sampling.

Procedure—TCM was provided 7 days a week to all trauma patient admissions. Data from 754 patients were collected over 14 months. These data were compared with 777 matched patients from the previous 14 months.

Results—TCM greatly improved time to allied health intervention ($p < 0.0001$). Results demonstrated a decrease in the occurrence of deep vein thrombosis ($p < 0.038$) and a trend towards decreased patient morbidity, unplanned admissions to the intensive care unit and operating suite. A reduced length of hospital stay, particularly in the paediatric and 45–64-year age groups, was noted. A total of 6621 fewer pathology tests were performed and the total number of bed-days was 483 days less than predicted from the control group.

Conclusion—The introduction of TCM improved the efficiency and effectiveness of trauma patient care in the study institution. This initiative demonstrated that TCM resulted in improvements to quality of care, trauma patient morbidity, financial performance and resource use.

Data collection and data measurement

Data collection refers to a description of the processes used or proposed to be used to implement the study and gather data. Different research designs require different methods of data collection. An example of the types and characteristics of data are summarised in Table 8.1.

TABLE 8.1 Types of data, features of data and examples of each type

TYPE OF DATA	FEATURE	EXAMPLE
Biophysical measures	Sensitive and precise	Electronic thermometer to measure temperature
Direct observation	Entities difficult to measure by instruments or interview	Interactions between patients, nurses and doctors are observable
Interview—unstructured or structured; think-aloud technique	Participants can report data about themselves or what they are thinking	People with illicit drug use and pain management following injury. Nurses' decision-making
Questionnaire/scales	Participants can report the degree to which they possess an attitude or trait	Questionnaire about state and trait anxiety. Visual analogue scale for pain
Records or existing databases	Convenient and can provide insight	Information on a patient's chart to identify variance in the clinical pathway

Instruments: data measurement, validity and reliability

When instruments are used for measuring data about subjects, the validity and reliability of instrument needs to be determined by the researcher. *Instruments*, or *tools* as they are more commonly called, used for research measurement refer not only to physiological and psychometric measures, but also to questionnaires and surveys used in studies. *Validity* is the degree to which an instrument measures what it is intended to measure.[1] There are three main types: content, construct or criterion-related. Although an instrument may appear to measure some aspect of a concept or construct, it must be evaluated to determine whether it really does provide such measurement. *Content* validity is the degree to which an instrument measures the total content of the construct that it is said to represent or measure. Content validity is often determined by a panel of experts in the field in which the research is being conducted. If a researcher wanted to measure bereavement behaviours in the ED, for example, a variety of knowledgeable opinions from social workers, members of the clergy and emergency nurses could be sought out to review the instrument that will be used to measure bereavement behaviour. *Construct* validity is the degree to which an instrument measures the construct that is being researched. A construct is an abstraction such as hopefulness, anxiety or coping, developed for a scientific purpose. That is, it can be beneficial to be able to measure a patient's level of anxiety so that it can be managed if it is too high, before adverse physiological symptoms occur. The construct validity of an instrument is usually determined over time after results from several studies demonstrate support for the construct to a greater degree, or question it further. An example might be if a research study was implemented to determine the sense of hope in trauma patients' families. The researcher's instrument must discriminate between families who are hopeful and families who are not hopeful to ensure construct validity. *Criterion-related* validity consists of predictive validity and concurrent validity. The participant's (subject's) performance on one measure is used to infer the likely response on another measure. *Predictive* validity is a measure used to predict future performance. For example, a nurse's score on a content knowledge test in emergency nursing predicts how well he or she might perform in practice. *Concurrent* validity is the degree to which an instrument can distinguish between participants/subjects who differ on a certain criterion measured at the same time.

A reliable instrument consistently produces the same results when it is used to measure a specific criterion or behaviour. A test of reliability is whether the instrument produces the same measurement when a measurement is repeated several times. The less an instrument varies in repeated measurements, the greater the reliability of the instrument.[26] An example for a physiological measurement might be a thermometer that records two different oral temperatures, 37.2°C one moment and 39°C shortly after, in a person with no obvious pyrexia. You would suspect that the instrument (the thermometer) is not giving reliable readings. Problems with reliability can also arise when more than one data collector is used for the same study. When more than one data collector is required to administer the same instrument to measure participants' responses, it is essential that they administer the instrument in the same way. The process, called inter-rater reliability, is the degree of agreement (consistency) between the scores of two or more data collectors for the same observation. Inter-rater reliability should be tested by the researcher prior to formal data collection and throughout data collection for members of the research team collecting data.

PRACTICE TIP

Always check the literature to find if there is an existing instrument with established validity and reliability that measures the construct of your research *before* you try to develop a new instrument.

The accuracy of data is just as important in qualitative research as it is in quantitative research. In qualitative approaches, such as grounded theory, information spoken to the researcher by a participant is summarised by the researcher and provided as narrative for the participant to check that it was an accurate reflection of what was said.[27] Similarly, a researcher can write an account of the observed behaviours of participants in an ethnographic study and ask participants at a later stage, or another observer of the event, to comment on the accuracy of the account of the observations. Criteria used in narrative methods to ensure the 'truthfulness' of data, credibility, auditability and fittingness, are discussed in the section below on data analysis.

Data analysis

After completing data collection the researcher summarises, with the support of a statistician if necessary, quantitative data through statistical procedures to answer the study questions or hypotheses. Researchers who use quantitative methods for data collection should plan the analysis before the research data are collected to ensure there are sufficient participants in the sample to provide an accurate result. Statistical tests give meaning to quantitative data because they reduce, summarise, organise, evaluate, interpret and communicate numerical data. One does not need to know all the statistical tests to understand the common principle that the statistical test will reveal whether the findings are statistically significant. This means the findings are probably valid and replicable with a new sample of subjects. The level of statistical significance is an index of the probability of reliability of the findings. If findings are reported as significant at the 0.05 level, this means that five times out of 100 there is a risk that the result would be different from the reported finding; in other words, 95 out of 100 times the findings would be the same.[27] A researcher can set a higher level of significance: 0.01 means that only one time out of 100 is there a risk that the result has occurred by chance.

Statistical tests are referred to as either descriptive or inferential. *Descriptive statistics* describe and summarise data. Examples are the mode, median, mean, average, percentage and frequency. *Inferential statistics* are used to draw conclusions, to make judgements and to generalise information about a large population based on a sample from a study. Inferential statistics are used to test hypotheses to determine if they are correct. Two categories of inferential statistics are non-parametric and parametric. Most statistical tests undertaken by researchers are parametric tests, which focus on populations, require measurements on at least one interval or ratio scale and make assumptions about the distribution of the variables. The distribution of the scores of a variable should be close to the shape of a bell curve, called a 'normal' distribution, before they are statistically tested. Alternatively, non-parametric tests are used when measured variables are nominal or ordinal (ranked). These tests do not require the assumption that the variables in the research are distributed normally. An example of a study finding a statistical significance is provided in Research Highlight 8.5, in which the length of time in hours or minutes it took for patients to receive pain relief if they were in the nurse-initiated analgesia group (study group) was significantly different to that of the non-nurse-initiated analgesia group (control).

RESEARCH HIGHLIGHT 8.5

Study using a descriptive design[28]

Title—Nurse-initiated intravenous morphine in the emergency department: efficacy, rate of adverse events and impact on time to analgesia.

Aim—(i) To determine whether nurses could autonomously initiate intravenous narcotics in patients presenting with acute pain, without compromising patient safety while awaiting medical assessment; and (ii) To determine whether such a procedure would improve the time to analgesia.

Method—A prospective, convenience sample of patients presenting in acute pain received titrated intravenous morphine by experienced emergency nurses. Pain scores on a 10 cm visual analogue scale and physiological parameters were measured at regular intervals over the following 60 minutes. Demographic, diagnostic and waiting time data were also recorded.

Results—349 patients were enrolled over a 12-month period. The mean initial pain score was 8.46 cm, with a reduction to 3.95 cm at 1 hour. Physiological parameters showed a small but statistically significant reduction over 60 minutes, which reflected a physiological response to pain control. There were no clinically significant episodes of hypotension, respiratory depression or reduced level of consciousness. The mean time to analgesia was 25.56 minutes and the mean time to be seen by a doctor was 58.62 minutes.

Conclusion—The study identified a significant reduction in pain scores and improved delivery of analgesia. Experienced triage nurses initiated analgesia safely, effectively and efficiently.

Qualitative research provides narrative data that are often referred to as 'rich' data. The challenge for researchers collecting qualitative data is to subject what is usually a large amount of observation or narrative to a rigorous and systematic analysis that is not distorted from the initial representation when it is summarised as overarching themes. The process of analysing narrative data usually starts with a transcription of the verbal or observational encounters into a textual account. Then the researcher undertakes an interpretative analysis that is an iterative process whereby data is clustered and re-conceptualised

into a higher level of abstraction (interpretation) that will be presented as overarching themes. The focus of the analysis and the formulation of themes is guided by the theoretical basis of the study—for example, grounded theory, that is trying to distil participants' meanings accurately and without researcher bias. The scientific rigour of qualitative analysis is evaluated by four criteria. The findings should reflect participants' experience of the phenomenon when their feedback is sought.[29] This process is called *credibility*. A second criterion, *auditability*, is the adequacy of information leading from the question and raw data through the analysis and interpretation of findings that is logical and consistent. *Fittingness* is the match between the research findings and other published research, and can indicate the accuracy of interpretation; while *confirmability* is the process of scrutinising the accuracy of data using various ways of checking. Confirmability demonstrates the rigour of the analytical process used.[30]

Ethical considerations in research

Healthcare research raises questions about what is acceptable and 'right' or unacceptable and 'bad'. Before research on humans can be undertaken, it must be evaluated and approved by members of an institutional human research ethics committee (HREC) that manages research proposals in that area or institution. In 2005 there were more than 220 such functional committees.[31] The constitution of an HREC is determined in Australia by the National Health and Medical Research Council (NHMRC). Members of an HREC make decisions about each research project and give approval for specified periods for the research to be conducted. Any person undertaking health-related research on humans is required to submit an ethics application to an HREC. An interactive web-based tool for researchers of all disciplines has been developed to assist researchers to submit well-formulated ethics proposals to HRECs. The use of this National Ethics Application Form (NEAF) aims to increase the efficiency and quality of the ethical review process by providing HRECs with ethics proposals containing consistent information that can be assessed more readily and effectively. The NEAF version 2.0 is available for public use at the NHMRC website (www.nhmrc. gov.au/health_ethics/ahec/neaf/index.htm).

The practices of all those involved in human research is guided by the National Statement on Ethical Conduct in Human Research, a document that has been compiled by the NHMRC, the Australian Research Council and the Australian Vice-Chancellors' Committee. The statement is intended for use by any researcher conducting research with human participants, members of an ethical review body, those involved in research governance and potential research participants. The five sections of the review document are presented in Box 8.2. Further reading on critiquing ethical issues in published research is available in textbooks[12] or on the NHMRC website.

Over the last decade, a much greater appreciation of the ethical and moral dilemmas in conducting clinically based research with colleagues has been discussed. While some researchers indicate that they have little difficulty in complying with the legal requirements of getting informed consent, according to Puchner and Smith[32] they struggle with issues of loyalty, confidentiality and trust in conducting action research

---

BOX 8.2 Sections of the Australian National Statement on Ethical Conduct in Human Research document[31]

- *Section 1* sets out the values and principles of ethical conduct that apply to all human research, and stipulates that researchers and review bodies consider these values and principles and be satisfied that the research proposal addresses and reflects them. E.g. research confidentiality means that any data provided by a participant will not be reported in a way that could identify that person, nor accessible to anyone outside the research team.
- *Section 2* identifies the themes in research ethics: risk, benefit and consent. Research users need to identify the level of risk involved in the planned research, and how to minimise, justify and manage that risk. Researchers must identify the information that needs to be disclosed to participants. The statement will help researchers to draft information for participants and plan the consent process (or develop a proposal for waiver of consent). It will help reviewers to assess the suitability of the proposed consent process and help participants understand what information they are entitled to receive, and what their participation in research will characteristically involve.
- *Section 3* provides ethical considerations specific to research methods or fields to assist researchers and reviewers to identify ethical matters specific to the research methods proposed.
- *Section 4* identifies ethical considerations specific to participants to help researchers and reviewers identify ethical matters relating to specific categories of research participants.
- *Section 5* identifies the processes of research governance and ethical review to help those involved in research governance to understand their responsibilities for research ethics, ethical review and monitoring of human research, as well as criteria for accountability.

---

studies. Additional ethical considerations such as loyalty and trust are now recognised by researchers as important to consider prior to the implementation of research projects.

Results, conclusions and recommendations

Results of quantitative studies are usually organised using the research hypotheses or questions of the study. The research question may be re-stated and the results reported in tables and/or graphs because they can be more easily interpreted. Based on the findings of the study, the research draws conclusions and then uses these conclusions as the foundation for the discussion section of the research report or manuscript. The researcher should attempt to give meaning to 'why' the findings occurred by interweaving the findings of previous related studies.

Recommendations can stem from changes the researcher plans in sample, design or analysis if the study is repeated. Other explanations for results should be discussed so that progress can be made with the research problem in future

studies. The implications of research, such as how findings can be used to improve clinical practice and patients' outcomes or how to advance knowledge through additional research, should be provided.[1,7]

The findings from qualitative research are written up in a carefully categorised and organised way. Data presented as themes can be interpreted at different levels of abstraction.[33] The 'writing up' of results is considered a crucial part of the research process because the act of writing explicates patterns, linkages and themes as the writer reflects within the process. In the grounded theory method, the categorisation continues until a core category emerges from data that provide the basis for a new theory.[34] The objective and dispassionate tone of quantitative research reporting is often replaced by a more personable account that frequently uses the first person in reporting the meaning and interpretation of data.[29] Examples of participants' active speech may be used to demonstrate authenticity and confirmability. While the findings of qualitative research are not considered to be generalisable, they can provide healthcare practitioners with new insight into phenomena that are important to clinical practice.[30]

Publication and presentation of the findings

A researcher's job is not completed until the findings of a study have been written up and attempts made to present the results at a conference or publish them in a peer-reviewed journal. Disseminating the results of a research project often seems to be the hardest part of the research process for many researchers. However, it is no longer acceptable for research to be undertaken with no attempt made to publish the findings. Research is a costly process that involves the thinking and time commitment of a lot of people, including that of the participants. Consequently, researchers have a moral obligation to share the findings of their project with others. Fortunately, there are many opportunities for sharing new knowledge, not only by writing for journals or books, but also by speaking at conferences and other events about the research outcomes. Within any clinical area there will be opportunities for you to assist in maintaining published protocols and practice guidelines with the most recent evidence. Involvement in guideline development or revision is an excellent way to become familiar with new knowledge and publication requirements. Many organisations managing population healthcare have established organisational structures and processes, such as clinical governance committees that support the revision of protocols by clinicians working in specific clinical areas across an institution.

There is support available for clinicians to get assistance in writing for publication if they lack confidence initially. It is very likely there will be at least one colleague in the clinical area or nearby who has published successfully in a journal. If not, then try contacting an academic supervisor or member of staff from a local university to critique a draft of the article. It is important to carefully select several journals that are more likely to be interested in the topic or the research approach prior to writing up the findings, because different journals have specific publication requirements that you need to follow when writing the draft.

When a local review and critique of the draft article from colleagues has been completed (it may take a number of drafts when you are new to this process), then you are ready to submit your article to a journal. When submitting an article for publication to a peer-reviewed journal the article will be reviewed anonymously (the researcher's name won't be used) by professionals who are familiar with writing for publication and possibly expert in the area or topic. The journal editor will send the reviewers' feedback on your article back to you, and you will have an opportunity to make corrections to the manuscript if the editor decides to accept the article for publication. If not successful initially, then persevere. Writing for publication is a skill that needs to be developed and it is important not to be discouraged if one journal sends a rejection letter. Select a journal with a lower impact rating and try again.

Evidence-based practice

Evidence-based practice started with Professor Archie Cochrane who, in the late 1970s made the statement:

> It is a great criticism of our profession that we have not organised a critical summary, by speciality or subspeciality, adapted periodically, of all relevant randomised controlled trials[35]

More contemporary definitions of evidence-based practice include the 'conscientious, explicit and judicious use of current best evidence in making decisions about the care of individual patients'[36] and the 'integration of best research evidence with clinical expertise and patient values'.[37]

Evidence-based practice has changed the way nurses and paramedics make clinical decisions and how they behave in practice. Rather than make decisions about practice actions based on routine or how one was taught, there are professional and consumer expectations that nurses and paramedics will translate the best available evidence as a basis for all clinical decisions and behaviours. Other considerations in the application, evaluation and translation of research evidence include the clinical expertise of the healthcare professional, the acceptability of evidence to specific patients, the context of practice and the availability of resources. Consequently, evidence-based healthcare requires a whole of organisation approach to the translation of evidence, whereby clinicians are engaged across all disciplines and includes support staff, managers and policy makers.

Levels of evidence

Evidence generated from research is classified according to the research design. These classifications are called 'levels of evidence' and organise evidence in a hierarchical structure according to quality.

The levels of evidence reflect the degree of confidence in the research findings. The levels of evidence used by the NHMRC are shown in Box 8.3. In this grading, Level I evidence is regarded as the highest level of evidence and evidence provided from systematic reviews of all the randomised controlled trials undertaken to evaluate an intervention. Recommendations to administer or not administer an intervention are based on the trade-off between benefits on the one hand and risk, burden and potential costs on the other. If benefits outweigh risks and burden, experts will recommend that clinicians offer a

---

BOX 8.3 Research designs and the assigned levels of evidence[38]

- Evidence obtained from a systematic review of all relevant randomised controlled trials is regarded as **Level I** evidence, and data from at least one properly designed randomised control trial is **Level II** evidence.
- **Level III** evidence has three sub-levels:
  - **III-1** is obtained from well-designed pseudorandomised controlled trials
  - **III-2** from comparative studies with concurrent controls and allocation not randomised, cohort studies, case control studies or interrupted time series with a control group
  - **III-3** from comparative studies with historical control, two or more single-arm studies or interrupted time series without a parallel control group.
- Studies obtained from case series, either post-test or pre-test/post-test design, without a control group are regarded as providing **Level IV** evidence.

---

treatment to typical patients. The NHMRC provides evidence-based recommendations for practice as an alphabetical grading (Table 8.2).

Another system of grading evidence that is gaining international momentum is GRADE: Grading of Recommendations, Assessment, Development & Evaluation.[39] The GRADE system classifies the quality of evidence as high, moderate, low or very low. A high recommendation means that further research is unlikely to change our confidence in the estimate of effect, while very low means that any estimate of effect is very uncertain.[39]

TABLE 8.2 Example of NHMRC grades of recommendation and description in a published guideline

GRADE	DESCRIPTION
A	Body of evidence can be trusted to guide practice
B	Body of evidence can be trusted to guide practice in most situations
C	Body of evidence provides some support for recommendation(s) but care should be taken in its application
D	Body of evidence is weak and recommendation must be applied with caution
NA	Not applicable—unable to grade body of evidence
GPP	Good practice point—consensus-based recommendations

To source evidence and enhance your research knowledge and skills:

- enrol in a postgraduate degree that includes coursework in research
- Subscribe to nursing journals such as the *Australasian Journal of Emergency Nursing*
- attend seminars and conferences relevant to emergency practice.

Knowledge translation

While sourcing sufficient evidence to base practice on is an ongoing challenge, so too is identifying established evidence and translating it into practice.[40] The time lapse between the publication of evidence and its implementation into practice is referred to as an *evidence–practice gap*. Addressing this gap required *knowledge translation*. Synonymous terms are used by researchers around the world. For example, similar processes are called *research utilisation* in the UK and Europe, *research dissemination, diffusion* or *knowledge uptake* in the USA and *knowledge translation* and knowledge-to-action in Australia and Canada.[31] Multiple factors influence the uptake of research into practice. The increasing volume of research evidence being produced, access to new evidence, the skills to appraise the quality of the evidence, time to locate and read evidence and the capacity to apply evidence[41] are some of the major factors identified. Strategies to promote the use of research in practice by healthcare workers continue to be devised as the complexity of the application of evidence into practice has been recognised. One strategy now commonly used is *knowledge distillation*. These processes synthesise the findings from the most rigorously conducted research available on a specific topic. These research summaries, called systematic reviews, provide a published summary of the results from reviews of the best research papers available for a specific topic or research question. The synthesis can then be presented to clinicians as practice guidelines or fact sheets (see, for instance, www.nhmrc.gov.au/guidelines/titles_guidelines.htm and www.clinicalguidelines.gov.au for two Australian organisations providing practice guidelines).

The leading global organisation is The Cochrane Collaboration. The Australasian Cochrane Centre (http://acc.cochrane.org) in Melbourne is one of many global Cochrane centres. The Cochrane Collaboration coordinates the Cochrane Library, the production and dissemination of systematic reviews, randomised controlled trials and other information for an international audience. Guidelines provided by the NHMRC produce guidelines to grade the strength of the evidence, as outlined earlier. The Joanna Briggs Institute for Evidence Based Nursing and Midwifery (JBIEBNM) (www.joannabriggs.org) coordinates the conduct and dissemination of systematic reviews of clinical nursing and midwifery research in Australia, New Zealand and Hong Kong. This institute publishes Best Practice Information Sheets based on the findings from systematic reviews, and evaluates the impact these have on nursing and midwifery practice. Emergency nurses are increasingly publishing systematic reviews[42] and reviews of current guidelines.[43]

Translating knowledge and the implementation of the findings of systematic reviews and other research requires strong organisational support and patronage.[44] In Australia, the National Health and Medical Research Council National Institute of Clinical Studies (NICS) undertakes strategic work in partnership with researchers and clinicians to close the theory–practice gap. One key initiative was the NICS Emergency Care Collaborative Initiative which conducted and reported on multicentre emergency department (ED) research.[45]

Research utilisation implies not only the implementation of new knowledge into practice, but also the evaluation of consequent changes in practice.[26] It is no longer acceptable to implement a change in practice and not evaluate the impact of that change. That is, if the research evidence is applied in a given context, the resulting change should be evaluated in terms of the outcomes, for example for patients, consumers, clinicians and the organisation. Outcome research assesses the effectiveness of healthcare services and workforce.[1] Professional standards review organisations such as the Australian Council on Healthcare Standards (ACHS) monitor the delivery of healthcare through their evaluation and quality improvement program (EQuIP), and report on the performance of public hospitals to ensure the maintenance of the highest standards. This process, called accreditation, enables the general public and medical insurers to have confidence in institutional standards, and holds organisations accountable to the recommended standards of patient safety.[46] There are ten Australian National Safety and Quality Health Service Standards that seek to improve the quality of health service provision and minimise risk to patients. In North America, research utilisation was the predecessor to evidence-based practice as a movement from task-oriented to science-based practice.[8] Many proposed theories and frameworks exist currently to support knowledge-to-action or knowledge translation.[47] In Australia and New Zealand, evidence-based nursing has followed on from evidence-based medicine, and the British evidence-based nursing movement has influenced developments in Australia and New Zealand.[48]

Barriers to translation of research into practice

Any attempt to improve the quality of care for patients must incorporate a clear understanding of the associated barriers and facilitators. It is challenging to apply evidence and evidence-based protocols in the context of competing priorities in the challenging pre-hospital and ED environments. Despite high-level recommendations to improve implementation of evidence-based practice, implementation remains variable, with numerous organisational and individual factors influencing healthcare workers' behaviour. These factors include a lack of time, difficulties in developing evidence-based guidelines, a lack of continuing education and an unsupportive organisational culture,[49] the availability of evidence, its relevance to practice, the dissemination of evidence and guidelines, individual motivation, the ability to keep up with current changes, clarity of roles and practice and the culture of specific healthcare practices.[50,51]

Research-focused courses to develop nurses' research skills have become available in Australia and New Zealand since the 1990s, and paramedic education also lacked a research focus until the transition to the higher education sector in the late

1990s. Consequently, there are nurses and paramedics practising who are unfamiliar with research processes or, if they know of the processes, are insufficiently confident to evaluate research findings and apply this evidence in their practice settings. The workloads for some nurses and paramedics are another limiting factor, because there is little time available to read or conduct research during working hours. It is important to build structures within the workplace to provide opportunities for all staff to examine, evaluate and use new knowledge.

Ways to improve clinicians' research use—implementation science

Australian and New Zealand government health departments are making concerted efforts to close the gap between high-standard health-research evidence and everyday clinical practice by setting up and funding programs in the field of implementation science. *Implementation science is the study of methods to promote the integration of research findings and evidence into healthcare policy and practice.* It seeks to understand the behaviour of healthcare professionals and other stakeholders as a key variable in the sustainable uptake, adoption and implementation of evidence-based interventions. Implementation science addresses the major barriers (e.g. social, behavioral, economic, management) that impede effective implementations.[52]

Behaviour change is key to improving healthcare and health outcomes, particularly the implementation of evidence-based practice. Improving implementation of evidence-based practice by healthcare workers depends on changing multiple behaviours of multiple types of people (e.g. health professionals, managers, administrators).[53] Changing behaviour is not easy, but is more effective if interventions are based on evidence-based principles of behaviour change. The validated theoretical domains framework[54] is a well-accepted tool on which to structure implementation strategies to introduce new policies and practice. It provides comprehensive coverage of possible influences on behaviour in 14 domains: 'Knowledge', 'Skills', 'Social/Professional Role and Identity', 'Beliefs about Capabilities', 'Optimism', 'Beliefs about Consequences', 'Reinforcement', 'Intentions', 'Goals', 'Memory, Attention and Decision Processes', 'Environmental Context and Resources', 'Social Influences', 'Emotions' and 'Behavioural Regulation'. The intent of implementation science and related research is to investigate and address major bottlenecks (e.g. social, behavioural, economic, management) that impede effective implementation, test new approaches to improve health programming, as well as determine a causal relationship between the intervention and its impact.[52]

There is a growing expectation in Australian and New Zealand nursing and midwifery that practice evidence will be filtered, disseminated and introduced into the clinical arena by specialists such as clinical nurse/midwifery consultants, nurse practitioners, clinical nurse specialists and nursing/midwifery educators. Some hospitals provide clinical nurses with research support by funding research units that assist nurses to conduct new or replication projects or evaluate the application of evidence in their local context.[55]

Evidence-based practice

Evidence-based nursing is an emergent and significant change to the way nurses make clinical decisions.[56] The Canadian

Institutes of Health Research promote knowledge translation by the use of the model of knowledge-to-action cycle[47] as the preferred approach (Figure 8.1). This seven-action-phase model adds to the well-established clinical improvement PDSA (plan, do, study, act) cycle model promoted by the NSW Health Department[57] with the inclusion of a knowledge-creation cycle.[47]

Practice development

Practice development (PD) is a movement that supports the application of evidence into clinical areas to optimise patient care and has gained recognition in Australia and New Zealand. PD is perceived by a growing number of healthcare professionals as a way to reposition the patient at the centre of care that is evidence-based and contextually flexible. Emanating from the UK, the PD movement advocates the development of nursing work that is patient-centred and evidence-based.[58] Although care decisions are undeniably centred on patients/consumers, PD philosophy also acknowledges the importance of the healthcare professional in the caring relationship. The definition of PD given by McCormack, Manley and Garbett[58] is: 'a continuous process of improvement towards increased effectiveness in patient-centred care. This is brought about by helping healthcare teams to develop their knowledge and skills and to transform the culture and context of care'. These authors go on to explain that the emancipatory and cultural change that can occur for clinicians reflecting the perspectives of service users (that is, the patients) is enabled by facilitator and staff commitment to systematic, rigorous and ongoing process and service evaluation. PD takes commitment by the clinical area and staff to enact technical changes in practice and cultural changes in how clinicians feel about themselves and their work.

Two types of PD have been identified—technical and emancipatory.[59] PD based on technical knowledge focuses on implementing evidence that may benefit patients' care, but largely ignores nurses' ownership of the change or the social context in which change occurs. The approach that focuses on increasing emancipatory knowledge concerns power and seeks to ensure that all staff have a voice in the change process and freedom from constraint and retribution which stifle participation and engagement within service delivery.[60] This approach may use an action research method (see Box 8.4) to reveal discrepancies in beliefs, values and 'rules' that may be driving the problems, issues or concerns experienced in everyday practice.

Transformational research is defined as qualitative research that promotes personal transformation by using creative strategies to foster self-reflection and reflection in others.[61] The transformational capacity of emancipatory PD, facilitating the growth of the whole person, 'human flourishing', as well as the development of new knowledge about effective processes and outcomes[61] has been experienced by many Australasian nurses working in public hospitals. Some PD projects incorporate aspects of both approaches; that is, they start out as emancipatory PD and conclude with not only an emancipatory impact on the participants but also effect a technical, practice change.[62] The importance of PD is that by exploring their values, beliefs and concerns, staff can challenge assumptions and contradictions evident within practice and creating barriers to person-centred

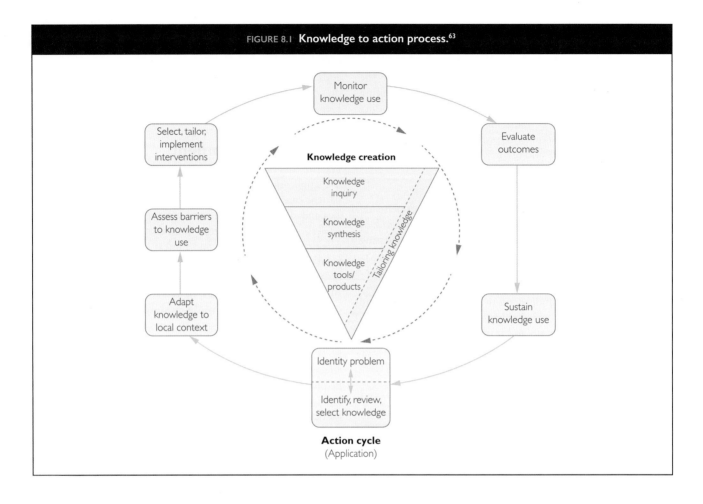

FIGURE 8.1 **Knowledge to action process.**[63]

- *Qualitative research* approaches provide data (information) in a non-numerical form, most commonly as writing (stories) or spoken language obtained during an interview. These methods are used to investigate phenomena that are difficult to categorise or where there has been little previous research conducted. Specific observations and/or interviews are analysed to develop themes and, in some instances, theories to explain a phenomenon.
- *Phenomenological interpretative research* is an inductive, descriptive approach developed from phenomenological philosophy. The aim of the research is to describe experience as it is lived by the person. The focus of the research is an attempt to understand the whole human being rather than specific behaviours or parts, and the numerous ways human beings experience the complexity of their world.
- *Grounded theory research* seeks to identify social problems and the processes people use to manage these problems. Through observations and interviews, the researcher develops an understanding of the relations between variables and formulates propositions that are tested with participants and redeveloped until 'saturation' (no new information arises). The

grounded new theory that emerges from data has its basis in data and it evolves from these propositions.
- *Ethnographic research* seeks to understand the behaviours of people within the context of their culture. It is considered naturalistic research, in that the social milieu is observed without control or manipulation to gain insights into the subjective experiences and actions of people. Analysis of the observations enables the researcher to develop a theory about the culture. An example of ethnographic research is presented in Research Highlight 8.1.
- *Critical social research* seeks to understand how people communicate and how they develop symbolic meanings in a social group. Symbolic meanings may take on factual status and they are not disputed or challenged but taken for granted. In the method of critical social research, the researcher seeks to identify the constraints that impede autonomous and uncoerced participation in the society. Action research, in which the researcher works with a group to effect technical or emancipatory change, is a major method of critical social research. An action research method can be used in practice development projects.

care. In this way PD can positively change the cultural context of practice and the patient experience within clinical areas.

Nurses participating in PD will find that an elementary understanding of research processes is useful for evaluating and exploring practice, and documenting and analysing the processes occurring within the clinical context in a critical way. An experienced, knowledgeable PD facilitator or a person who has worked on quality improvement projects can provide useful guidance for groups new to using PD. The facilitator/s can assist to ensure movement through PD cycles and project development is achieved and outcomes recorded and evaluated.

SUMMARY

Research is critical for paramedic and emergency nursing practice. This chapter has provided a basic overview of the steps of the research process and the language that is used to describe this process for clinicians in the earlier stages of this continuum. The steps in research, guided by either a research question or a hypothesis, collecting narrative or numerical data, have been represented as 'flowing in the same direction'. Both narrative and numerical approaches have value in informing practice to enhance patient care. Well-defined systems, such as evidence-based practice and practice development, exist to support clinicians engaging in the research continuum. While the provision of evidence and methods that support the application of evidence into practice are gaining increased acceptance by managers as well as clinicians, the outcome that most clinicians want from research activity is knowledge to improve the care of patients and clients. It is imperative for all healthcare professionals to understand their professional responsibility to engage in research to ensure that new, useful knowledge is continuously generated, implemented and evaluated for the benefit of the people for whom they care.

CASE STUDY

You are a registered nurse (year 4) employed in the emergency department (ED) of a 500-bed metropolitan tertiary hospital. Within the year you have enrolled in a graduate course at the local university. While undertaking a literature review for an assignment you identify that there are new guidelines for the management of adults presenting to the ED. When you read the new guideline and the practice recommendations by the National Heart Foundation of Australia/Cardiac Society of Australia and New Zealand Guidelines for the Management of Acute Coronary Syndromes (ACS), you realise that the existing practice protocol at your hospital is out of date. Some change in practice needs to occur in the ED where you work.

After careful consideration of the issues, you decide that a technical practice development (PD) project could be undertaken, with support from the Clinical Nurse Consultant (CNC) who is an experienced researcher, as part of your Masters degree. After gaining some knowledge of the action research method and implementation science at university, you agree to facilitate the process in the ED with the help of the CNC. You develop a proposal and attach a copy of the new guideline from the National Heart Foundation website.

Once you have gained the necessary permissions, including approval from the HREC for the project to be conducted, you start to talk to your colleagues about the new guidelines because their engagement in the process is central to effective change. Also, you are fully aware that EDs are busy places most of the time and some colleagues are concerned about the amount of time required to undertake the project. The first meetings are held, and the majority of your colleagues are prepared to discuss the new guideline and decide how practice needs to change to accommodate the new evidence.

Questions

1. Using the steps of the research process, make a list of the information you would include in the proposal.

2. Identify the stakeholders you need to speak with about your proposal to implement a new guideline with a knowledge to action research design.

3. Identify some ways to schedule the first meetings to involve as many of your colleagues as possible in the implementation. How will staff on evening and night duty shifts be involved if the meetings are conducted during the day?

4. What suggestions would you give your colleagues about maintaining records of the processes and outcomes of meetings, particularly as you may not be able to attend every meeting?

5. You are required to write an assignment for your course, evaluating the project. How will you determine the 'success' of your project? How will you know whether clinicians are implementing the new guideline correctly and completely?

Answers to Case Study Questions can be found on evolve
http://evolve.emergencytrauma.curtis

REFERENCES

1. Polit DF, Beck CT, Hungler BP. Essentials of nursing research. Philadelphia: JB Lippincott; 2001.

2. Roberts CA, Burke SO. Nursing research: a quantitative and qualitative approach. Boston: Jones and Bartlett; 1989.

3. Field PA, Morse JM. Nursing research: the application of qualitative approaches. Rockville: Aspen Systems; 1985.

4. Dolan B. The nurse practitioner: real-world research in A&E. London: Whurr Publishers; 2000.

5. The Cochrane Collaboration. Glossary of Cochrane Collaboration and research terms. 2009; Online. http://community.cochrane.org/glossary. Accessed 18 Feb 2015.

6. Hodge AN, Marshall AP. Family presence during resuscitation and invasive procedures. Collegian 2009;16(3):101–18.

7. Schneider Z, Elliott D, LoBiondo-Wood G, Haber J. Nursing research: methods, critical appraisal and utilisation. 2nd edn. Sydney: Mosby; 2004.

8. Estabrooks CA. The conceptual structure of research utilization. Research in Nursing & Health 1999;22(3):203–16.

9. Goode CJ, Piedalue F. Evidenced-based clinical practice. Journal of Nursing Administration 1999;29(6):15–21.

10. Hinshaw AS. Nursing knowledge for the 21st century: Opportunities and challenges. Journal of Nursing Scholarship Second Quarter 2000;32(2):117–23.

11. Brown SJ. Knowledge for health care practice: a guide to using research evidence. Philadelphia: WB Saunders; 1999.

12. Crookes P, Davies S. Research into practice: essential skills for reading and applying research in nursing and health care. 2nd edn. Edinburgh: Baillière Tindall; 2004.

13. Barnason S. Research. In: Newberry L, ed. Sheehy's emergency nursing. 5th edn. Philadelphia: Mosby; 2003.

14. Mateo MA, Kirchhoff KT. Using and conducting nursing research in the clinical setting. 2nd edn. Philadelphia: WB Saunders; 1999.

15. Lyneham J, Parkinson C, Denholm C. Explicating Benner's concept of expert practice: intuition in emergency nursing. Journal of Advanced Nursing 2008;64(4):380–7.

16. Fry MM. Triage nursing practice in Australian emergency departments 2002–2004: an ethnography. Sydney: The University of Sydney; 2004.

17. Rodger M, Hills J, Kristjanson L. A Delphi. Study on Research Priorities for Emergency Nurses in Western Australia. Journal of Emergency Nursing 2004;30(2):117–25.

18. Hammond E, Holzhauser K, Shaban R, Melton N. An exploratory study to examine the phenomenon and practice of 'Ambulance Ramping' at hospitals within the Southern Health Service Districts of Queensland and Queensland Ambulance Service. Australasian Emergency Nursing Journal 2009;12(4):170.

19. Denzin NK, Lincoln YS. The handbook of qualitative research. 2nd edn. Thousand Oaks, CA: Sage Publications; 2002.

20. Rickard C, O'Meara P, McGrail M et al. A randomized controlled trial of intranasal fentanyl vs intravenous morphine for analgesia in the prehospital setting. The American Journal of Emergency Medicine 2007;25(8):911–17.

21. Burns N, Grove S. The practice of nursing research, conduct, critique and utilization. 4th edn. London: Saunders; 2001.

22. Kerlinger FN. Foundations of behavioral research. New York: Holt, Reinhart and Winston; 1986.

23. Yin RK. Case study research: design and methods. 3rd edn. Thousand Oaks, CA: Sage Publications; 2002.

24. Coyne IT. Sampling in qualitative research. Purposeful and theoretical sampling; merging or clear boundaries? Journal of Advanced Nursing 1997;26(3):623–30.

25. Curtis K, Zou Y, Morris R, Black D. Trauma case management: Improving patient outcomes. Injury 2006;37(7):626–32.

26. Jones J. Performance improvement through clinical research utilization: the linkage model. Journal of Nursing Care Quality 2000;15(1):49–54.

27. Glaser B, Strauss A. The discovery of grounded theory: strategies for qualitative research. New York: Aldine; 1967.

28. Fry M, Holdgate A. Nurse-initiated intravenous morphine in the emergency department: Efficacy, rate of adverse events and impact on time to analgesia. Emergency Medicine 2002;14(3):249.

29. Webb C. The use of the first person in academic writing: objectivity, language and gatekeeping. Journal of Advanced Nursing 1992;17(6):747–52.

30. Jackson D, Daly J, Chang E. Approaches in qualitative research. In: Schneider Z, Elliott D, eds. Nursing research: methods, critical appraisal and utilisation. 2nd edn. Sydney: Mosby; 2003.

31. National Health and Medical Research Council, Australian Research Council, Committee AVCs. National statement on ethical conduct in human research 2007. Canberra: Commonwealth of Australia; 2014.

32. Puchner LD, Smith LM. The ethics of researching those who are close to you: the case of the abandoned ADD project. Educational Action Research 2008;16(3):421–8.

33. Van Manen M. Researching lived experience: human science for an action sensitive pedagogy. London: State University of New York Press; 1990.

34. Strauss A, Glaser B, Schatzman L, Morse JM. Developing grounded theory: the second generation. Proceedings of the Advances in Qualitative Methods. Paper presented at: Banff conference 2007; 2009, 2007; Walnut Creek, CA.

35. Cochrane AL. 1931–1971: A critical review, with particular reference to the medical profession. In: Teeling-Smith G, Wells N, eds. Medicines for the year 2000. London: Office of Health Economics; 1979:1–11.

36. Sackett DL, Rosenberg WMC, Gray JAM et al. Evidence based medicine: what it is and what it isn't. BMJ 1996;312(7023):71–2.

37. Sackett DL. Evidence-based medicine: how to practice and teach EBM. 2nd edn. Edinburgh: Churchill Livingstone; 2000.

38. National Health and Medical Research Council. A guide to the development, implementation and evaluation of clinical practice guidelines. In: NHMRC, ed. Canberra: NHMRC: Commonwealth of Australia; 1999.

39. GRADE Working Group. GRADE Working Group. Online. www.gradeworkinggroup.org/index.htm; accessed 16 Feb 2015.

40. Pearson A, Royal College of Nursing Australia. Evidence based nursing: an examination of the role of nursing within the international evidence-based health care practice movement. Deakin, ACT: Royal College of Nursing; 1997.

41. Gravel K, Legare F, Graham I. Barriers and facilitators to implementing shared decision-making in clinical practice: a systematic review of health professionals' perceptions. Implementation Science 2006;1(1):16.

42. Fry MM. Barriers and facilitators for successful after hours care model implementation: Reducing ED utilisation. Australasian Emergency Nursing Journal 2009;12(4):137–44.

43. McGillivray B, Considine J. Implementation of evidence into practice: Development of a tool to improve emergency nursing care of acute stroke. Australasian Emergency Nursing Journal 2009;12(3):110–19.

44. Bate P, Mendel P, Glenn R. Organizing for quality: the improvement journeys of leading hospitals in Europe and the United States. Radcliffe: Abingdon; 2008.

45. National Institute of Clinical Studies. National emergency department report: 2004.

46. Banks G. Australian Council on Healthcare Standards. ACHS 30 years. Ultimo: ACHS; 2004.

47. Straus SE, Tetroe J, Graham I. Defining knowledge translation. Canadian Medical Association Journal 2009;181:3–4.

48. Rosswurm MA, Larrabee JH. A model for change to evidence-based practice. Image: The Journal of Nursing Scholarship Fourth Quarter 1999;31(4):317.

49. Wallis L. Barriers to implementing evidence-based practice remain high for US nurses. The American Journal of Nursing 2012;112(12):15.

50. Newman M, Papadopoulos I, Sigsworth J. Barriers to evidence-based practice. Clinical Effectiveness in Nursing 1998;2(1):11–18.

51. McKenna H, Ashton S, Keeney S. Barriers to evidence based practice in primary care: a review of the literature. International Journal of Nursing Studies 2004;41(4):369–78.

52. Fogarty International Center. What is implementation science? 2013; Online. www.fic.nih.gov/News/Events/implementation-science/Pages/faqs.aspx; accessed 16 Feb 2015.

53. Grol R, Grimshaw J. From best evidence to best practice: effective implementation of change in patients' care. The Lancet 2003;362(9391):1225–30.

54. Cane J, O'Connor D, Michie S. Validation of the theoretical domains framework for use in behaviour change and implementation research. Implementation Science 2012;7:37.

55. Gerrish K, Clayton J. Promoting evidence-based practice: an organizational approach. Journal of Nursing Management 2004;12(2):114–23.

56. New Zealand Guidelines Group. Evidence based health care bulletin. 2009. Online. www.nzgg.org.nz/index.cfm?screensize=1024&ScreenResSet=yes; accessed 16 Feb 2015.

57. NSW Health Department. Easy guide to clinical practice improvement: a guide for healthcare professionals. In: NSW Health Department, ed. North Sydney: NSW Health Department; 2002.

58. Manley K. Practice development: a growing and significant movement. Nursing in Critical Care 1997;2(1):5.

59. McCormack B, Manley K, Garbett R. Practice development in nursing. Oxford: Blackwell; 2004.

60. Manley K, McCormack B. Practice development: purpose, methodology, facilitation and evaluation. Nursing in Critical Care 2003;8(1):22–9.

61. Titchen A, Armstrong H. Re-directing the vision: dancing with light and shadows. In: Higgs J, Titchen A, Horsfall D et al, eds. Being critical and creative in qualitative research. Sydney: Hampden Press; 2007:151–63.

62. Hart E, Bond M. Action research for health and social care: a guide to practice. Philadelphia: Open University Press; 1995.

63. Graham ID, Logan J, Harrison MB et al. Lost in knowledge translation. Time for a Map? J Contin Educ Health Prof 2006; Winter;26(1):13–24.

64. Munhall PL. Philosophical ponderings on qualitative research methods in nursing. Nursing Science Quarterly 1989;2(1):20.

CHAPTER 9

PATIENT EDUCATION AND COMMUNICATION

JUDY MULLAN

Essentials

- Key interventions should be targeted to achieve effective patient education.
- Simple strategies can be used to help improve healthcare professional–patient communication and partnerships.
- It is important to target patient education interventions for patients with poor health literacy skills.
- There is a range of instruments and tools that can be used to assess the readability, presentation, quality and suitability of written patient information.
- Medication compliance and health promotion needs to be encouraged to further improve patient health outcomes.

INTRODUCTION

Since around 2005 the notion of patient-centred care, with patient education as a central focus, has been increasingly incorporated in healthcare models worldwide.[1–6] The Hippocratic Oath, written in Ionic Greek in the 5th century BC, required physicians, among other undertakings to swear that 'I will prescribe regimens for the good of my patients according to my ability and my judgement and never do harm to anyone'. With due respect to history, it is therefore fair to acknowledge that patient-centred care is not a new concept. It is understandable and professionally responsible that today healthcare professionals and many healthcare organisations have been seeking to improve the quality of their patient education by supporting the use of patient-centred communication standards.[1,3–6] These patient-centred communication standards recommend multiple strategies which encourage patients and, where appropriate, their family member(s) to become active participants in the decision-making process about their care.[3,5,7–9] The standards are born of evidence showing that active patient/family participation and partnerships with healthcare professionals can result in reductions in mortality, reductions in healthcare utilisation, improved patient outcomes, improved patient satisfaction and improved patient self-management skills.[10–15]

Since the move towards patient-centred care from a patient's perspective represents high-quality care based on their individual needs and expectations,[12,16] nurses and paramedics are in a good position to foster and practise patient education from a patient-centred viewpoint. This is an important consideration because patient education is one of the crucial roles played by both nurses and paramedics in a wide range of healthcare environments, both within and outside of hospital settings. It is also worth noting that hospital emergency departments (EDs) are becoming more regular healthcare access points for patients suffering from both acute and chronic conditions.[17] As such, there is an increasing need to consider providing effective patient education in these busy settings,[17,18] and during patient transfers by paramedics to these settings.[19–22]

The process of effective patient education begins with the imparting of information, but also includes interpretation and integration of information to bring about attitudinal or behavioural change(s) that benefit the patient's health status.[23] Since effective patient education helps patients to participate in their care and to make informed choices, nurses, paramedics and, for that matter, all members of the healthcare team[23,24] should focus upon providing education based on the needs of the patient and, where appropriate, their family members.[25] These patient and/or family members' needs which should be focused upon include, but are not limited to: their reading and literacy skills; their learning preferences; their religious and cultural beliefs.[1,25] It is also important to consider the needs of 'at-risk' patient populations, such as those who are older (> 65 years of age);[26,27] those with poor health literacy skills;[28–31] and those from culturally and linguistically diverse (CALD) backgrounds.[32–34] These patient populations are considered 'at-risk' because they are often overwhelmed and seldom voluntarily admit that they have not understood the information they received during patient education sessions, making them more susceptible to poor therapeutic outcomes and adverse events.[28,30,34,35]

Effective patient education requires effective communication, which in turn requires a rapport between the healthcare professional and the patient, in order to develop a mutual understanding.[36] Having a mutual understanding is reliant upon establishing respectful and trusting relationships.[36] This in turn will promote collaborative partnerships and effective communications, which are key factors to consider when providing patient education. Other key factors required for effective patient education include the provision of clear verbal communication and simple, easy-to-read written patient information (where appropriate), the promotion of good therapeutic and/or medication compliance and the provision of patient follow-up.

Effective healthcare professional–patient communication

Interventions to help improve healthcare professional–patient communications during patient education sessions

Interventions which target improving healthcare professional–patient communication and partnerships are recognised as important ways to improve patient knowledge and understanding, allowing them to make confident, educated decisions about their healthcare. Ineffective communication places patients at increased risk of poor health outcomes and preventable adverse events.[37] All healthcare professionals, especially nurses and paramedics who are charged with the responsibility of forming relationships often in acute critical situations, should therefore focus on promoting their roles as competent educators by developing good communication skills and collaborating more effectively with patients.[23,38]

Effective communication during healthcare professional–patient interactions can be fostered by using the following guiding principles:[39] (i) making the sessions interactive; (ii) minimising any uncertainties within sessions; (iii) planning and thinking about desired outcomes for each session; and (iv) engaging the patient and/or their family members during each session. All healthcare professionals should encourage patients to become part of the decision-making process by providing important healthcare education and information in a timely manner, as well as by offering encouragement, reinforcement, reassurance and feedback.[40–42] Encouragement can be given to patients by developing a rapport, establishing trust, asking lots of questions, inviting patients to make comments[40] and by respecting their opinions, assumptions and attitudes.[43] Reinforcement can be provided by giving clear, simple and concise verbal and written instructions (where applicable), as well as underlining key points within available written patient information.[44] Reinforcement can also be offered by reiteration and repetition of important patient information.[39] Reassurance can be promoted by addressing patients in a positive, caring and motivating manner, while ensuring that they are as comfortable as possible and confident enough to ask questions.[43] Providing feedback, which is yet another valuable communication tool, can be elicited by asking open-ended questions, which do not require 'yes' or 'no' answers,[45] thereby ensuring that patients have comprehended and understood the information provided. In the event that patients have completely misunderstood or misinterpreted the information provided, they should have the correct information politely and positively reinforced.

Active listening is one of the core components of effective communication which can positively impact upon the patient's health outcomes.[36,39] Healthcare professionals who listen to their patients make them feel more valued and confident,[36] thereby fostering a collaborative and supportive therapeutic relationship. When appropriate, non-verbal cues, such as maintaining appropriate eye contact, direction of gaze, proximity, sitting slightly forward facing the patient, facial expression and nodding, can be used by the healthcare professional to demonstrate active listening.[39,45] Similarly, verbal cues, such as asking questions associated with or subsequent to the patient's last comment, as well as using the appropriate tone, rate and volume of speech can also be used to demonstrate active listening.[39,45] The use of non-verbal and verbal cues will promote a good rapport between the patient and the healthcare professional, which in turn will contribute to effective patient education and communication.

Patient follow-up is another key component of patient education and communication because it has been shown to improve therapeutic outcomes.[46] Patient follow-up interventions, which include individual, group, telephone, letters and/or electronic communication sessions, are useful strategies to support the provision of reassurance and reinforcement of important health information, confirmation of referrals, appointments and appropriate health behaviours, as well as clarification of issues regarding their therapeutic regimens and ongoing healthcare, when appropriate.[47–49] The literature identifies that follow-up, especially after hospital discharge, significantly reduces the incidence of hospital readmission.[46,50] Nurses and paramedics working in both hospital and community healthcare settings are ideally placed to encourage patients to attend the necessary consultations, health checks, screenings, immunisations and all other relevant follow-up appointments to help optimise their health outcomes.

Perhaps one of the more valuable interventions to help improve healthcare professional–patient communication and partnerships is to urge family members and/or significant others to attend patient education sessions.[51–54] The active participation of patients and/or their family members in the learning process helps to ensure the patient understands and comprehends the information imparted to them, which should build on what they already know to improve their health outcomes.[55,56]

Verbal patient information and communication

Guidelines for effective verbal patient education and communication sessions

Verbal communication is the most frequently used education strategy and a key component of effective patient education. Healthcare professionals use verbal communications during both formal and informal patient education sessions with the added bonus of being able to readily tailor their education session(s) based on the patient's needs and their current understanding of their health status. Simple and useful tips to assist in achieving effective patient education during verbal communication sessions are:[30,36,37,39,45,55,57,58]

- use simple language
- avoid medical jargon
- speak slowly in a clear, active voice
- confirm the patient's understanding of information provided by asking them to repeat what they have heard and what it means to them (e.g. teach-back method)
- avoid giving too many directives which may overwhelm the patient
- repeat and reinforce key points
- provide suitable simple and easy-to-read written information (when available)
- encourage patients to ask questions; use an open-ended approach.

When verbally communicating with older patients, as well as those with low literacy skills, it may also be necessary to:[30,51]

- ensure enough time is spent with the patient
- allow for frequent short appointments rather than one long appointment (when possible)
- provide pictures and visual images (when available)
- encourage them to bring along a family member
- demonstrate respect and empathy.

Pitfalls that should be avoided during verbal communication sessions include:[39,45]

- unnecessary disruptions
- not giving patients and/or families enough time to have their say
- asking too many questions
- failing to recognise both verbal and non-verbal cues
- using slang or vague terms which may be misinterpreted.

BOX 9.1 Practice guidelines for effective patient communication[39,41]

- Assess patient's knowledge prior to providing information.
- Address underlying concerns that the patient and/or family member expresses.
- Ensure that the information and explanations relate to the patient's perspectives and/or concerns.
- Provide information and explanations in an organised, logical sequence.
- Engage the patient in an interactive conversation through the use of open-ended questions, simple language and analogies to teach important concepts.
- Encourage patients to be involved in the learning process by contributing their ideas and suggestions.
- Elicit patient's responses, reactions and attitudes regarding information provided and/or therapeutic management plans suggested.
- When tailoring a therapeutic management plan, elicit and address the patient's perspectives, offering suggestions, options and choices.
- When tailoring a therapeutic management plan, negotiate a mutually acceptable plan which takes into consideration the patient's lifestyle, beliefs, cultural background and abilities.
- Encourage patients to be involved in implementing their therapeutic management plans and taking responsibility in the self-management of their health conditions.
- Use appropriate non-verbal encouragement (e.g. when appropriate a pat on the shoulder, nodding, smiling) and verbal encouragement when appropriate.

In addition to the simple and useful tips provided above, Box 9.1 provides some practical guidelines, based on communication principles, which can be used by healthcare professionals during their patient educations sessions.[39,41] The generic nature of these practical guidelines make them suitable for both formal and informal patient education in any healthcare setting.

Written patient information

Health literacy and written patient information

Health literacy is a concept which has emerged because of the well-recognised relationship between poor literacy skills and health status.[59,60] According to the World Health Organisation (WHO) definition:

> Health literacy is linked to literacy and entails people's knowledge, motivation and competence to access, understand, appraise and apply health information in order to make judgements and take decisions in everyday life concerning healthcare, disease prevention and health promotion to maintain or improve quality of life during the life course.[61]

A patient who is health literate is able to read, understand and act on health information provided to them.[30,62] In contrast, however, people with poor health literacy skills cannot read or understand written patient information or prescription guidelines; they cannot fill out consent forms and find it difficult to comply with health information and treatment recommendations.[30,51,63] Moreover, people with poor health literacy skills don't know when to seek appropriate healthcare.[62,64]

Poor health literacy is a pervasive and under-recognised problem in healthcare, both in Australia and overseas.[30,59,61] Data from the Australian Bureau of Statistics indicates that a significant proportion of the Australian population has poor health literacy skills.[65] In 2006, the Adult Literacy and Life Skills Survey (ALLS) identified that 19% of adults had level 1 health literacy skills, with a further 40% having level 2 skills.[66] Given that a skill level of 3 is regarded as the minimum required to allow individuals to meet everyday life demands, 59% of the adults aged 15–74 years who took part in the survey had difficulty with simple tasks, such as locating information on a bottle of medicine and identifying the maximum number of days to take the medicine.[66] Importantly, these people would not be able to read or comprehend commonly available patient information,[63,64,67] which is often written at or above grade 9 readability levels,[68] typically containing lots of medical jargon and terminology.[69,70] This inability may then result in errors in judgement, failure to recognise important signs and symptoms, or even the possibility of completely misunderstanding their healthcare information and treatment recommendations. Consequently, they would be more likely to experience poorer therapeutic outcomes and/or adverse events, while at the same time incurring increased healthcare costs.[55,64,71–74] In view of the extent of poor health literacy skills among Australians,[66] it is important for all healthcare professionals to avail their patients of written information that is simple and easy-to-read. Interestingly, it has also been identified that patients at all literacy levels prefer and better understand simple and easy-to-read written resources, as opposed to more complex resources containing lots of medical jargon and terminology.[75]

Providing simple, easy-to-read written patient information

Evidence suggests that the addition of good quality, simple and easy-to-read written information to verbal information and communication increases the patients' knowledge, understanding, compliance and satisfaction with therapeutic regimens.[58,74,76–78] Written educational materials are also convenient, economical and very useful for providing information and enhancing patient participation in therapeutic regimens.[67,79] Healthcare professionals should therefore always endeavour to provide patients and/or their family members with written information as a supplement to verbal information, especially since patients remember approximately 25% of what they hear, but approximately 65% of what they hear and see.[80]

To ensure that the written information is simple and easy-to-read for all patients, including those with poor health literacy skills, it should be written at or below a grade 8 reading grade level,[81] or where possible at or below a grade 6 reading level.[28] Unfortunately, the latter is not always possible to achieve because of the need to often include specific medical terminology and/or medication names within written patient information materials. Additionally, for patients from CALD, it is also important, whenever possible, to provide written materials that are culturally appropriate.[28,37,49,82–84]

The readability of written patient information

The goal of written patient information is to increase patient knowledge and understanding by providing a cheap, reusable, portable, self-paced learning resource which supplements and reinforces verbal information and communication.[42,85] It is therefore the responsibility of all healthcare professionals, including nurses and paramedics, to ensure that the written information can be read and understood by the patients and/or their family member(s). There are two methods that can be used to assess readability and understandability: (a) assessing the patients' literacy and/or health literacy level to ensure that they can understand the information, and (b) assessing the reading grade level required to read and understand the written patient information.

A number of tests are available to assess patients' literacy and/or health literacy levels. These include simple word recognition tests such as: the Wide Range Achievement Test-Revised (WRAT-R);[86] the Rapid Estimate of Adult Literacy in Medicine (REALM);[87] and the Slosson Oral Reading Test-Revised (SORT-R).[88] For research purposes, another health literacy comprehension test, the Test of Functional Health Literacy in Adults (TOFHLA),[89] is considered the most useful because it has been found to have good content validity and uses text from real healthcare settings,[90] measuring both patients' comprehension and patients' numeracy skills.[91] In December 2005, a tool known as the Newest Vital Sign (NVS),[92] accessible in English and Spanish, was made available as a quick screening test for limited literacy in primary healthcare settings. The NVS consists of a nutrition label with six questions which investigate the participant's ability to read and apply the information from the label. Unlike the other health literacy assessment tests that tend to be time-consuming to administer, the NVS is quick (1–3 minutes) and convenient, which makes it more appealing for busy healthcare professionals. However, despite the availability of these valid and reliable literacy/health literacy assessment tools, most healthcare professionals working in busy clinical settings do not screen for limited literacy.[93] It was for this reason that researchers such as Chew et al[94] identified three questions which are predictive of limited health literacy ('How often do you have someone help you read hospital materials?' 'How confident are you filling out medical forms by yourself?' and 'How often do you have problems learning about your medical condition because of difficulty understanding written information?'),[94] as well as a single screening question which can be used to detect inadequate health literacy ('How confident are you filling out medical forms by yourself?').[95]

Rather than assess the literacy and/or health literacy levels of patients themselves, busy healthcare professionals may prefer to assess the reading grade level required to read and understand specific written patient information. Healthcare professionals should therefore be aware of the different available readability formulae that are designed to make quick and easy readability assessments of written information. Some of the more well-known readability formulae include: the Simple Measure of Gobbledygook (SMOG) index;[96] the Fry Readability Formula (FRY);[97] the Gunning FOG formula;[98] and the Flesch Reading Ease (FRE) formula.[99] Each of these readability formulae has a high correlation with each other, which means that they can all be readily used and interchanged to assess the readability of written information. Thankfully, during recent times, most of these formulae are available as convenient and easy to use online resources (available on http://www.readabilityformulas.com/free-readability-formula-tests.php) and the Flesch-Kincaid program has also been included as a component of the readability statistics available in Microsoft Office Word programs. Perhaps the major limitation for each of these formulae, as far as written patient information is concerned, is that they are not healthcare-specific.

Reliable and reputable sources of written patient information

Suitable written patient information for patients and/or their family members can often be accessed from reliable and reputable electronic sources. Some hospitals and institutions have free access to reliable web based resources, such as the 'Clinical Information Access Program' (CIAP), to support evidence-based practice at the point of care. In the state of New South Wales, for example, Australian healthcare professionals working in the public health system can access CIAP on http://www.ciap.health.nsw.gov.au/. Alternatively, written health information, which could be used to assist with patient education, is available through the internet. It is important, however, to consider the quality and the accuracy of this information, as well as the needs of the patients and/or their family members. Reliable databases and scholarly sites that are particularly useful for healthcare professionals include: CINAHL, Cochrane, Medline, PsychInfo, Proquest, PubMed, Science Direct, Scopus and Web of Science. These are generally accessible from most libraries, including some hospital libraries, and are sometimes available on individual hospital intranets. Other useful sites for patient information resources include: department of health websites, national prescribing websites, university websites and other suitable, reliable and reputable Australian websites found in Box 9.2.

Guides for developing written patient information

In addition to accessing and providing patients with good-quality, simple and easy-to-read patient information, many healthcare professionals are routinely involved in developing and writing patient information resources such as medication instructions, discharge instructions and/or written health information sheets relating to a wide variety of issues.[18,58,77] Unfortunately, the majority of available print materials are written at a reading level well above the average reading level of many patients (i.e. year 6/7).[3,100,101] Consequently, it is important for healthcare professionals to develop new written materials that patients and/or their families can read, understand and relate to.[58,77,102] While developing these written materials, healthcare professionals need to target the information at or below a grade 8 reading grade level,[81] or, better still, where possible, a grade 6 reading level.[28] They also need to take into consideration other factors, such as format, text, print size and the use of pictures/pictograms/illustrations which can impact upon the patient's knowledge, understanding, satisfaction and engagement with the written information.[42,79,103–106] There are a number of functional, practical and easy-to-use tools and guidelines which can be applied to ensure that written

> **BOX 9.2 Examples of suitable, reliable and reputable Australian websites**
>
> - Advisory Committee on the Safety of Medicines (ACSOM) www.tga.gov.au/about/committees-acsom.htm
> - Alzheimer's Australia https://fightdementia.org.au/
> - Arthritis Australia www.arthritisaustralia.com.au/
> - Asthma Foundations Australia www.asthmaaustralia.org.au/
> - Australian Commission on Safety and Quality in Healthcare www.safetyandquality.gov.au/
> - Australian Government Department of Health and Ageing www.health.gov.au/
> - Australian Sports Commission www.ausport.gov.au
> - Beyond Blue www.beyondblue.org.au
> - Clinical Excellence Commission www.cec.health.nsw.gov.au/
> - Diabetes Australia www.diabetesaustralia.com.au/
> - Health Direct Australia www.healthdirect.gov.au/
> - Heart Foundation Australia www.heartfoundation.org.au/
> - National Institutes of Health—National Centre for Complementary and Alternative Medicine https://nccam.nih.gov/health/
> - National Prescribing Service (NPS) www.nps.org.au
> - Pregnancy and Birth Information www.birth.com.au/
> - QUIT—The National Tobacco Campaign www.quit.org.au/
> - The Australian Government National Drugs Campaign www.drugs.health.gov.au
> - The Australian Immunisation Handbook www.immunise.health.gov.au/internet/immunise/publishing.nsf/Content/Handbook10-home
> - The Australian Institute of Health and Welfare www.aihw.gov.au/
> - The Cancer Council of Australia www.cancer.org.au/

information complies with these other factors (i.e. format, colour, text, print size and illustrations). Online resources that can do this include:

- Guidelines for Creating Materials (available on www.hsph.harvard.edu/healthliteracy/practice/innovative-actions/)
- Simply Put: A Guide for Creating Easy-to-Understand Materials (available on www.cdc.gov/healthliteracy/pdf/whatsyourpoint.pdf)
- Plain language: Improving Communication from the Federal Government to the Public (available on www.plainlanguage.gov/)
- Toolkit for making written material clear and effective (available on www.nih.gov/clearcommunication/plainlanguage/resources.htm)
- How to present the evidence for consumers: preparation of consumer publications (available on www.nhmrc.gov.au/_files_nhmrc/publications/attachments/cp66.pdf)

- Health Literacy and Patient Safety: Help patients understand (available on www.ama-assn.org/ama/pub/about-ama/ama-foundation/our-programs/public-health/health-literacy-program/health-literacy-kit.page)

Other useful resources also include: The United Kingdom Department of Health 'Toolkit for Producing Patient Information';[107] 'Guidelines for Writing Patient Information';[28] 'Health literacy and patient safety: Help patients understand: Manual for clinicians';[58] and the 'Clinical Excellence Commission Guide to Health Literacy'.[101]

In addition to the resources suggested above, Box 9.3 contains tips to assist healthcare professionals when developing easy-to-read written materials.

Suitability and presentation of written patient information

In the current information-rich environment, not only is it imperative to offer patients and/or their family members simple easy-to-read information, but it is also important to offer them written information that is both presented clearly and is suitable for their needs. Traditionally, instruments such as the validated 'Suitability Assessment of Materials instrument' (SAM)[28] have been used to evaluate the content, literacy demands, graphics, layout and typography of written materials. Moreover, the SAM[28] instrument has been used to evaluate

---

BOX 9.3 Tips to assist with developing easy-to-read written materials[58,78,107]

Plain language

Organisation
- Information needs to be presented in a logical order
- Include necessary background information or context
- Provide small blocks of text with clear headings
- Emphasise and summarise main points
- Help patients make decisions by giving them facts about risks, side effects and benefits—link information to other reputable and reliable sources

Style
- Use everyday plain conversational language—avoid jargon and acronyms
- Write at or below grade 6–8 reading levels
- Use short sentences—approximately 15 to 20 words long
- Use lower-case letters where possible
- Use present and active tenses
- Use a question and answer format to help engage readers

Layout and design
- Use serif type with a minimum font size of 12
- Ensure a good amount of white space on the page
- Bullets are preferable to blocks of text
- Use appropriate space between lines (e.g. 1.2 to 1.5 spacing between lines)
- Use large bold font to emphasise text. Avoid upper case letters, italics and underlining
- If appropriate provide clearly labelled, simple and instructive visual aids/illustrations.

---

learning stimulation, motivation and cultural appropriateness of the written information for patient populations, inclusive of the low literacy skilled populations. The 'Bernier Instructional Design Scale' (BIDS)[108] was another instrument designed to identify and measure the presence (or absence) of instructional design and learning principles within the written patient information, while the quick and easy-to-use 'Checklist for print materials'[109] was developed to assesses the appropriateness of the written materials for patients. Another instrument, the 'Baker Able Leaflet Design' (BALD)[110] was developed to assess the standardised Australian consumer medicine information leaflets[111] and contributed to the development of the 'Medicine Information Design Assessment Scale' (MIDAS),[112] which assesses the layout, design and quality of written medication information. Tools such as these can be used by healthcare professionals to evaluate the suitability and presentation of written information they are distributing to or developing for their patients and/or family members.

Quality of written patient information

The quality of the written information being presented and/or developed for patients and their family members is another important element to consider. Instruments such as the DISCERN instrument[113,114] can be used to assess the quality of written information. The main advantages of the DISCERN instrument is that the patients themselves can use the instrument. The 'Ensuring Quality Information for Patients' EQIP scale[115] and the EQIP36[116] are two additional instruments which can be used to assess the quality of written information in terms of language, tone and text organisation, as well as the quality of information regarding risk and consequences for medical procedures, procedural steps and other background information for the EQIP36 tool.[116]

Patient comprehension and satisfaction with written information

Ultimately patients and/or their family members need to be satisfied with the written information they receive and they also need to be able to comprehend the written information they are given. Apart from asking the patients themselves about whether or not they are satisfied with and can understand the written information they have been presented with, there are tools such as the 'Satisfaction with Information about Medicines Scale' (SIMS)[117] and the 'Consumer Information Rating Form' (CIRF)[118] which specifically targets written information about medication. Furthermore, the Cloze test[28,119] can be used to assess the patients' understanding, as well as the reading difficulty of the written information.

Additional patient education materials

In addition to verbal and written patient education and communication, it is important for healthcare professionals to consider additional materials that may be very beneficial to assist with patient education. These additional materials can include graphic illustrations, such as pictures, pictographs (using simple line drawings), models, audio compact discs, DVDs and various forms of computer-assisted learning.[58] Studies in the literature have shown that the use of pictures (including cartoons and pictographs) and models in combination with verbal communication and/or written information have helped to improve patient understanding, recall and retention of medical information.[104-106,120] Similarly, the addition of educational materials, available on CDs and/or DVDs, can be used to reinforce important information and improve patient knowledge and understanding about what was communicated during patient education sessions.[121-124] The ready access to modern technology also makes computer-assisted education a viable option for patient education. Research indicates that computer-assisted multimedia modalities are effective in helping patients to understand, retain, comply with and act upon important medical information.[125-132] Notably, many of the computer-assisted multimedia modalities are interactive and can be successfully used by patients with limited experience using computers, including those with low literacy skills.[58] Perhaps one of the most appealing features regarding many computer-assisted multi-media modalities is that they can be tailored to match the patients' needs.[58] Several of the websites identified in Box 9.2 include various multi-media modalities that can be used to effectively assist with patient education.

Patient education and communication with CALD patients

Cultural competence is often used to describe the knowledge, skills and attitudes that healthcare professionals require, when providing effective patient education to patients from various cultural backgrounds.[4,39] This involves sensitivity towards several issues, such as gender, family relationships, religion, spiritual and cultural beliefs,[4,8,30,37] as well as support and a mutual respect for these patients.[37,45] These CALD patients may have certain expectations and beliefs about their healthcare needs, which is why it is important for healthcare professionals to cater for these needs, thereby helping to optimise these patients' health outcomes.[45,133] Moreover, since it is important for healthcare professionals to identify which cultural differences might affect the patient's therapeutic management, it is important to involve the patient by encouraging them to contribute to the session, as well as by asking questions. The healthcare professionals should endeavour to ask open-ended questions during the education sessions to better accommodate for these cultural differences without compromising their quality of care.[36,39,45] They also need to be aware of possible cultural differences in non-verbal behaviours, such as touching, proximity and eye contact which may inadvertently but negatively impact on the education session by making the patient feel uncomfortable.

Healthcare professionals should also be aware that they may need to address additional cultural competency issues when communicating with vulnerable groups, such as Indigenous peoples and/or refugees. For example, when communicating with Indigenous peoples healthcare professionals need to recognise the importance of using appropriate terms and they need to be cognisant of the many factors which may impact upon cultural safety for Indigenous peoples such as communication styles, the notion of family and the imbalance of power.[36] Furthermore, healthcare professionals need to understand that Indigenous peoples may have different approaches to managing illness, that they may react differently to the healthcare environment and that they may have different traditional approaches to managing illness.[36] With regard to refugees, healthcare professionals need to appreciate that in

addition to the language and cultural barriers experienced by many CALD groups,[134] refugees often experience higher rates of psychological and physical health problems, resulting from a lack of access to appropriate healthcare services and possible exposure to trauma prior to their arrival in the country.[134,135] It is important that healthcare professionals recognise that cultural influences may impact on the attitudes and health-seeking behaviours of this vulnerable patient population and that good listening skills are essential when communicating with and caring for this vulnerable patient population.[134]

Verbal communication with CALD patients

Language and communication barriers can be a major contributor to adverse events for many CALD patients.[136,137] For example, CALD patients with limited English proficiency skills experience greater risk of infections, falls, hospital re-admissions, poor medication compliance and surgical delays, as compared to their English speaking counterparts.[137-143] Healthcare professionals should therefore be aware of their legal and ethical requirements to ensure effective patient education and communication with their CALD patients, which may necessitate the use of professional qualified interpreters.[30,49,133,144,145] This is important because the use of family members and friends who may not understand medical terminology, can contribute to these adverse events[83] and longer lengths of hospital stays.[146] Furthermore, the use of qualified interpreters for CALD patients with limited English proficiency has been found to improve information recall, satisfaction and support for the patients.[28,85,147] Certainly access to and use of qualified interpreters could be problematic and logistically difficult in busy healthcare environments, such as emergency departments or during health emergencies in the community setting, but at the same time they are essential to achieve optimal health outcomes for CALD patients. In situations where qualified interpreters are not available on-site, healthcare professionals need to be aware that telephone interpreter services are also available, and are a suitable alternative.[102]

The following include tips which should be considered when communicating with CALD patients via an interpreter:[36]

- If possible, liaise with the interpreter prior to the patient education session to introduce yourselves to each other and to clarify any areas of uncertainty.
- At the beginning of the patient education session introduce everyone and describe their role.
- Speak to the patient and/or their family members rather than the interpreter.
- Use plain language and short sentences and avoid medical jargon.
- Observe non-verbal cues.
- Encourage patient engagement by asking open-ended questions.
- Summarise, highlight and reinforce key issues.

Written information and CALD patients

When selecting and/or developing written information for CALD patients and/or their family members it is important to include information and illustrations that are culturally sensitive.[30] Seeking the advice of cultural group members and, where possible, healthcare professionals who are from similar cultural groups would be beneficial in such circumstances. Similarly, if the patient and/or their family members were literate in their own native language, information which has been translated into their own language would be the preferred option when it comes to choosing suitable written patient information.[102] However, healthcare professionals should recognise that limited health literacy and English-speaking proficiency often co-exist,[148] suggesting that these patients may require additional education sessions with fewer health literacy demands, as well as additional information resources, if available, such as visual aids and multi-media tools.[58,105,149,150]

Learning environments

Learning environments play an important role in patient education. To be effective, learning environments should encourage patients to listen, feel confident enough to ask questions, access information and seek reassurance about their knowledge and understanding.[151] In busy environments, such as EDs and other emergency settings it is not always possible to find a quiet area in which to offer education to patients and/or their family members. It is important, however, to try to ensure that the surroundings are as private and comfortable as possible, thereby facilitating communication between all parties.[18,36] It is not always busy environments that make communication difficult. For example, a patient in a hospital bed, in a shared room, may not wish to discuss personal health-related matters or may be distracted by whatever else is happening within the hospital setting.[152] Education/information sessions should, where possible, take place in an alternative quiet setting with appropriate lighting, seating and temperature arrangements.[36,45] Furthermore, for healthcare professionals working in the community setting the opportunity to provide education in the patient's home would be an excellent opportunity to educate patients in a comfortable and familiar environment that has fewer distractions.

Despite the challenges of providing patient education in busy healthcare settings (e.g. EDs),[17] these settings often present opportunities described as 'teachable moments' where patients and/or their family members can be engaged in education sessions regarding health behaviours to help improve their health status.[153–158] In the main, for healthcare professionals to effectively use these 'teachable moments' they need to engage in using verbal instruction, problem solving, provide up-to-date written information and potentially participate in role playing and/or simulations.[18,159] Additionally, with the rapidly advancing technology available today, these 'teachable moments' may also involve the use of multimedia education programs, interactive computer-assisted patient education programs and access to good quality health information websites.[160–162] Such opportunities would be particularly important to help promote and reinforce positive health behaviours and therapeutic management strategies which can be used to help optimise health outcomes for the patient.[42,56,158] Furthermore, emerging evidence in the literature has identified that patient educational interventions in the ED, using a variety of teaching methods, has been effective and achievable.[17,18]

In addition to the learning environment, the physical proximity of the healthcare professional to the patient and/or their family member can have an impact upon the effectiveness of patient education. A close but comfortable position is important[163] because sitting too close may make them feel threatened, while sitting too far away may suggest disinterest.[45] When communicating with patients in both hospital and community settings, it is also important to be sitting at the same level as the patient, rather than speaking to them from a standing position which could make them feel vulnerable.[45]

Targeting patient education about medication compliance

Medication compliance is a key indicator of the success of many patient education programs, involving medication use as part of the patients' therapeutic regimens and recommendations. Estimates of poor medication compliance range from 20% to 70% for all medications[164,165] and 50% to 65% for long-term medications in chronic disease.[166,167] This indicates there is room for improvement in promoting medication compliance through effective patient education.[168] Consequently, for patients who are taking medications as part of their therapeutic regimens, all healthcare professionals should target the following medication compliance issues when delivering their patient education:[167,169,170]

- inform the patients and/or their family members about the importance of regular medication compliance
- suggest appropriate dosing schedules
- inform the patient about potential medication-related side effects
- identify possible drug-to-drug interactions and/or contraindications
- explain the implications of poor medication compliance
- when appropriate, recommend medication compliance aids and dosage reminders, such as blister packs, dosette boxes, medications alarms or medication cards, for patients with physical (e.g. poor eye sight) and/or cognitive impairments (e.g. dementia).

Health promotion activities

In addition to the provision of patient education, all healthcare professionals working within and outside of the hospital environment should recognise the importance of encouraging health promotion and risk factor reduction activities to promote better health outcomes.[23] Health promotion activities incorporate broad issues relating to health, which enable people to increase their control and management of their own health behaviours, with a view to improving their health.[171] Health promotion interventions can be individual, social and environmental interventions, some of which include disease prevention strategies. Disease prevention strategies can occur on three levels: primary disease prevention strategies which are designed to eradicate health risks (e.g. vaccination); secondary disease prevention strategies which can lead to early diagnosis of disease (e.g. screening); and tertiary disease prevention strategies which refer to rehabilitation activities assisting with the recovery process following ill health (e.g. referral to cardiac rehabilitation clinic).[172] The choice of health promotion interventions, and uptake of disease prevention strategies, can be influenced by many factors which include health priorities, available programs, policies and societal influences.[173] On an individual level, they can also be impacted upon by social factors such as age, sex, gender, socio-economic status, education levels and cultural issues.[173] It is important for healthcare professionals to be aware of these influences when promoting and encouraging the uptake of these health promotion interventions and strategies.

When educating patients and/or their family members, healthcare professionals should take every opportunity to encourage patients to pursue healthy lifestyle behaviours, which are examples of health promotion interventions. These behaviours should include: undertaking regular exercise; eating nutritious foods, minimising alcohol intake, smoking cessation (when and if appropriate), stress management and the development and maintenance of social support systems. When necessary, healthcare professionals should also recommend secondary disease prevention activities such as: immunisation programs for adults and children;

identification of age-appropriate screening examinations (e.g. breast screening, cervical screening, prostate screening); and the clarification of safety issues which include seatbelts, child safety, occupational health and safety issues and safe sex behaviour. Although nurses and paramedics working in ED do not necessarily view their role as supporting secondary disease prevention strategies, they need to recognise that many of the patients that they see regularly would greatly benefit from education about disease-preventive issues.[18] Moreover, despite the challenges of providing patient education in the busy ED environments,[174] it is also important to acknowledge that ED may be the most regular contact for many patients suffering from chronic diseases, such as asthma, diabetes and cardiovascular disease.[17,18] Healthcare professionals should therefore take advantage of these situations to reinforce important information about appropriate health lifestyle behaviours, for example, which could benefit their health outcomes.

SUMMARY

In this chapter, it has been established that through providing effective patient education, healthcare professionals can play a pivotal role in helping patients to achieve optimal therapeutic outcomes, while also reducing a patient's potential to experience adverse events. Effective patient education can be achieved by targeting the following interventions and strategies: the promotion of good healthcare professional–patient communication and partnerships; the provision of good quality simple, easy-to-understand verbal, written and additional patient information; and when applicable, the promotion of good medication compliance and/or relevant health promotion activities. Healthcare professionals should also be mindful of the need to provide CALD patients, with limited English proficiency skills, with a qualified health interpreter and if possible good quality simple, easy-to-understand information that is culturally appropriate during the patient education sessions.

Nurses and paramedics are well placed to make a significant improvement to health outcomes for patients and they need to be particularly aware of problems associated with educating patients in 'high risk' groups. These patients include older patients, patients with low literacy skills and patients from culturally and linguistically diverse speaking backgrounds. In this chapter, it is recommended that a number of simple tests and instruments can be used to assess and ensure that written patient information, given in conjunction with verbal instruction, can be read and understood by a wider patient population, inclusive of the 'high risk' groups. Recommendations are also made about a number of simple instruments, which can be used to ensure the suitability and the quality of the written patient information.

CASE STUDY

Paramedics are called out to the home of Miss PG, a 5-year-old child, who is distressed and experiencing breathing problems, i.e. rapid and shallow breathing. Her mother is extremely agitated and informs the paramedics that her child used to suffer bronchiolitis as a baby, but has never had an experience as bad as this one before. Clinical examination of the child by the paramedics confirms evidence of hypoxaemia associated with impaired ventilation and expiratory wheeze. Following the administration of oxygen, and nebulised salbutamol, Miss PG's condition only improves slightly and she is transported by the paramedics via ambulance to the local hospital emergency department (ED). On route to the hospital, the paramedics gently but firmly reassure

the mother about the child's safety to allay her fears and they also ensure that the child is comfortable, relaxed and continues to receive appropriate care.

On arrival at the hospital, the paramedics inform the triage nurse about the child's condition and as a result she is immediately seen by a paediatric registrar, who diagnoses her with experiencing an acute exacerbation of asthma. The paediatric registrar prescribes a salbutamol (reliever) inhaler and a steroid (preventer) inhaler for the child to use and writes a discharge letter for the mother and child to take to their local doctor. The nurse is then asked to take on the responsibility of educating the mother and the child about the asthma medications, correct inhaler technique, the importance of medication compliance and the importance of follow-up consultations with their local doctor. The nurse is also asked to provide the mother with useful resources for asthma and asthma medication information.

Questions

1. In this scenario, how would both the paramedic and the ED nurse best communicate with the child and her mother?

2. Describe the most appropriate location for the nurse to educate both the mother and the child about the new asthma medications and correct inhaler technique?

3. Where would the nurse search to find the most reliable, valid and appropriate information about asthma, asthma medications and correct inhaler technique?

4. What advice should the nurse provide to the mother for the ongoing monitoring, management and continuity of care for her daughter's asthma following her discharge from the hospital emergency department?

 Answers to Case Study Questions can be found on evolve http://evolve.emergencytrauma.curtis

REFERENCES

1. JCI. Joint Commission International Accreditation Standards for Hospitals: Standards Lists Version; 2011.

2. Euromed Info. Patient/Family Education Standards. www.euromedinfo.eu/patient-family-education-standards.html/; accessed 16 Feb 2015.

3. Clinical Excellence Commission. Partnering with patients. www.cec.health.nsw.gov.au/programs/partnering-with-patients; accessed 16 Feb 2015.

4. Australian Council for Safety and Quality in Healthcare. National Patient Safety Education Framework. Sydney; 2005.

5. Australian Commission on Safety and Quality in Healthcare. National Safety and Quality Service Standards. Sydney; 2011.

6. Institute of Medicine. Crossing the quality chasm: A new health system for the 21st century. Online. www.nap.edu/html/quality_chasm/reportbrief.pdf; accessed 16 Feb 2015.

7. The Joint Commission. Patient-centred communication standards for hospitals. Online. www.jointcommission.org/; accessed 16 Feb 2015.

8. The Joint Commission. Advancing effective communication, cultural competence, and patient- and family-centred care: A roadmap for hospitals. Oakbrook Terrace, IL; 2010.

9. Australian Government Department of Health and Ageing. Consumer Engagement in Healthcare. Online. www.health.gov.au/internet/vcms; accessed 6 June 2005.

10. Meterko M, Wright S, Lin H et al. Mortality among patients with acute myocardial infarction: the influences of patient-centered care and evidence-based medicine. Health services research 2010;45(5):1188–204.

11. Bertakis K, Azari R. Patient-centered care is associated with decreased healthcare utilization. Journal of the American Board of Family Medicine 2011;24(3):229–39.

12. Sidani S. Effects of patient-centered care on patient outcomes: an evaluation. Research and theory for nursing practice 2008;22(1):24–37.

13. Maizes V, Rakel D, Niemiec C. Integrative medicine and patient-centered care. Explore (New York, N.Y.) 2009;5(5):277–89.

14. Robinson JH, Callister LC, Berry JA, Dearing KA. Patient-centered care and adherence: Definitions and applications to improve outcomes. Journal of the American Academy of Nurse Practitioners 2008;20(12):600–7.

15. Saha S, Beach MC. The impact of patient-centered communication on patients' decision making and evaluations of physicians: A randomized study using video vignettes. Patient Education and Counseling 2011;84:386–92.

16. Bergeson SC, Dean JD. A Systems Approach to Patient-Centered Care. JAMA: The Journal of the American Medical Association 2006;296(23):2848–51.

17. Wei H, Camargo CJ. Patient education in the emergency department. Academic Emergency Medicine 2000;7(6):710–17.

18. Szpiro KA, Harrison MB, Van Den Kerkhof EG. Patient education in the emergency department: A systematic review of interventions and outcomes. Advanced Emergency Nursing Journal 2008;30(1):34–49.

19. Macnab AJ, Richards J, Green G. Family-oriented care during pediatric inter-hospital transport. Patient Education and Counseling 1999;36(3):247–57.

20. Lowthian JA, Jolley DJ, Curtis AJ et al. The challenges of population ageing: Accelerating demand for emergency ambulance services by older patients, 1995–2015. Medical Journal of Australia 2011;194(11):574–78.

21. Peacock PJ, Peacock JL, Victor CR, Chazot C. Changes in the emergency workload of the London ambulance service between 1989 and 1999. Emergency Medicine Journal 2005;22(1):56–9.

22. Cummins NM, Dixon M, Garavan C et al. Can advanced paramedics in the field diagnose patients and predict hospital admission? Emergency Medicine Journal 2013;30(12):1043–7.

23. Rankin SH, Duffy Stallings K. Patient education: principles and practice. 4th edn. Philadelphia: Lippincott, Williams & Wilkins; 2001.

24. Redman Klug B. The practice of patient education. 9th edn. Detroit, Michigan: Mosby Inc.; 2001.

25. Euromed Info. JCAHO Patient and Family Education (PF) Standards. www.euromedinfo.eu/patient-family-education-standards.html/; accessed 16 Feb 2015.

26. Gurwitz JH, Field TS, Harrold LR et al. Incidence and preventability of adverse drug events among older persons in the ambulatory setting. The Journal of the American Medical Association 2003;289(9):1107–16.

27. Forster AJ, Murff HJ, Peterson JF et al. The incidence and severity of adverse events affecting patients after discharge from the hospital. Annals of Internal Medicine 2003;138(3):161–8.

28. Doak CC, Doak LG, Root JH. Teaching patients with low literacy skills. 2nd edn. Philadelphia: Lippincott 1996.

29. Feifer R. How a few simple words improve patients' health. Managed Care Quarterly 2003;11(2):29–31.

30. Scudder L. Words and well-being: how literacy affects patient health. The Journal for Nurse Practitioners 2006;2(1):28–35.

31. Sudore RL, Landefeld CS, Pérez-Stable EJ et al. Unraveling the relationship between literacy, language proficiency, and patient–physician communication. Patient Education and Counseling 2009;75(3):398–402.

32. Nadar S, Begum M, Kaur B. Patient's understanding of anticoagulation therapy in a multiethnic population. Journal of the Royal Society of Medicine 2003;96(4):175–9.

33. Shaw J, Hemming MP, Hobson JD et al. Comprehension of therapy by non-English speaking hospital patients. Medical Journal of Australia 1977;2:423–7.

34. Williams A, Manias E, Liew D et al. Working with CALD groups: testing the feasibility of an intervention to improve medication self-management in people with kidney disease, diabetes, and cardiovascular disease. Renal Society of Australasia Journal 2012;8(2):62.

35. Ryan AA. Medication compliance and older people: a review of the literature. International Journal of Nursing Studies 1999;36:153–62.

36. O'Toole G. Communication core interpersonal skills for health professionals: Elsevier; 2008.

37. The Joint Commission. 'What did the doctor say?' Improving health literacy to protect patient safety; 2007.

38. Aslani P, Du Pasquier S. Compliance, adherence or concordance? Australian Pharmacist 2002;21(3):170–4.

39. Silverman J, Kurtz S, Draper J. Skills for communicating with patients. 3rd edn. London: Radcliffe Publishing 2013.

40. Kok G, van den Borne B, Mullen PD. Effectiveness of health education and health promotion: Meta-analyses of effect studies and determinants of effectiveness. Patient Education & Counseling 1997;30:19–27.

41. Clark NM, Gong M, Schork A et al. Impact of education for physicians on patient outcomes. Paediatrics 1998;101:831–6.

42. Hoffmann T, McKenna K. Analysis of stroke patients' and carers' reading ability and the content and design of written materials: Recommendations for improving written stroke information. Patient Education and Counseling 2006;60(3):286–93.

43. The Royal Pharmaceutical Society of Great Britain. From compliance to concordance: Achieving shared goals in medicine taking. London; March 1997.

44. Doak CC, Doak LG, Lorig K. Selecting, preparing, and using materials. In: Patient education: a practical approach. 2nd edn. Thousand Oaks: SAGE Publications; 1996.

45. Lloyd M, Bor R. Communication skills for medicine. 3rd edn. London: Churchill Livingstone Elsevier; 2009.

46. Dudas V, Bookwalter T, Kerr K, Pantilat S. The impact of follow-up telephone calls to patients after hospitalization. The American Journal of Medicine 2001;111(9B):26S–30S.

47. Hendricks LE, Hendricks RT. The effect of diabetes self-management education with frequent follow-up on the health outcomes of African American men. Diabetes Educator 2000;26(6):995–1002.

48. Waterman AD, Milligan PE, Banet GA et al. Establishing and running an effective telephone-based anticoagulation service. Journal of Vascular Nursing 2001;XIX(4):126–34.

49. AHRQ. Health literacy universal precautions toolkit. Rockville: Agency for Healthcare Research and Quality; 2010.

50. Jackson SL, Peterson GM, Vial JH, Jupe DM. Improving the outcomes of anticoagulation: an evaluation of follow-up of warfarin initiation. Journal of Internal Medicine 2004;256(2):137–44.

51. Rajda C, George NM. The effect of education and literacy levels on health outcomes of the elderly. The Journal for Nurse Practitioners 2009(February):115–19.

52. Smith SK, Dixon A, Trevena I et al. Exploring patient involvement in healthcare decision making across different education and functional health literacy groups. Social Science & Medicine 2009;69:1805–12.

53. Australian Commission on Safety and Quality in Healthcare. Safety and Quality Improvement Guide Standard 2: Partnering with consumers. Sydney; 2012.

54. Joint Commission International. Joint Commission International Accreditation Standards for Hospitals. 4th edn. Oakbrook Terrace, Illinois; 2011.

55. Ross J. Health Literacy and its influence on patient safety. Journal of PeriAnesthesia Nursing 2007;22(3):220–2.

56. Gruman J, Rovner MH, French ME et al. From patient education to patient engagement: implications for the field of patient education. Patient Education and Counseling 2010;78(3):350–6.

57. Kripalani S, Weiss BD. Teaching about health literacy and clear communication. Journal of General Internal Medicine 2006;21(8):888–90.

58. Weiss BD. Health literacy and patient safety: Help patients understand: Manual for clinicians. Chicago; 2007.

59. Nutbeam D. The evolving concept of health literacy. Social Science & Medicine 2008;67:2072–8.

60. CHCS. What is Health Literacy? Fact Sheet. Online. www.chcs.org; accessed 25 Jan 2010.

61. WHO. Health literacy: The solid facts. In: Kickbusch I, Pelikan JM, Apfel F, Tsouros AD, eds. World Health Organization: Regional Office for Europe; 2013, p. 4.

62. Jordan JE, Buchbinder R, Osborne RH. Conceptualising health literacy from the patient perspective. Patient Education and Counseling 2010;79(1):36–42.

63. Cameron KA, Ross EL, Clayman ML et al. Measuring patients' self-efficacy in understanding and using prescription medication. Patient Education and Counseling 2010;80(3):372–6.

64. Baker DW, Wolf MS, Feinglass J, Thompson JA. Health literacy, cognitive abilities, and mortality among elderly persons. Journal of General Internal Medicine 2008;23(6):723–6.

65. ABS. Australian Social Trends 4102.0. Online. www.ausstats.abs.gov.au/ausstats/subscriber.nsf/LookupAttach/4102.0Publication30.06.093/$File/41020_Healthliteracy.pdf; accessed 16 Feb 2015.

66. ABS. Adult Literacy and Life Skills Survey 2006 (Cat 4228.0): Australian Bureau of Statistics; 2009.

67. Karnieli-Miller O, Adler A, Merdler L et al. Written notification of test results: meanings, comprehension and implication on patients' health behavior. Patient Education and Counseling 2009;76(3):341–7.

68. Rolland PD. Reading levels of drug information printouts: A barrier to effective communication of patient medication information. Drug Information Journal 2000;34(4):1329–38.

69. Murphy PW, Davis TC. When low literacy blocks compliance. RN 1997;60(10):58–63.

70. Fields AM, Freiberg CS, Fickenscher A, Shelley KH. Patients and jargon: are we speaking the same language? Journal of Clinical Anesthesia 2008;20(5):343–6.

71. Adams RJ, Stocks NP, Hill CL et al. Health Literacy—A new concept for general practice? Australian Family Physician 2009;38(3):144–7.

72. Baker DW, Wolf MS, Feinglass J et al. Health literacy and mortality among elderly persons. Archives of Internal Medicine 2007;167(14):1503–9.

73. Bhasale AL, Miller GC, Reid SE, Britt HC. Analysing potential harm in Australian general practice: an incident-monitoring study. Medical Journal of Australia 1998;169:73–6.

74. Baker DW. The meaning and the measure of health literacy. Gen Intern Med 2006;21(8):878–83.

75. Doak LG, Doak CC, Meade CD. Strategies to improve cancer education materials. Oncology Nursing Forum 1996;23(8):1305–12.

76. Roter DL, Hall JA, Merisca R et al. Effectiveness of interventions to improve patient compliance. A meta-analysis. Medical Care 1998;36(8):1138–61.

77. Rudd RE. How to create and assess print materials. www.hsph.harvard.edu/healthliteracy/materials.html; accessed 25 January 2010.

78. Rudd RE. Guidelines for creating materials. www.hsph.harvard.edu/healthliteracy/creating-materials/; accessed 16 Feb 2015.

79. Clark RB, AbuSabha R, von Eye A, Achterberg C. Text and graphics: manipulating nutrition brochures to maximize recall. Health Education Research 1999;14(4):555–64.

80. Bateman WB, Glassman KS, Kramer EJ. Patient and family education in managed care and beyond: Seizing the teachable moment. New York: Springer Publishing Company; 1999.

81. Buchbinder R, Hall S, Grant G et al. Readability and content of supplementary written drug information for patients used by Australian rheumatologists. Medical Journal of Australia 2001;174(11):575–8.

82. Chang Weir R. Evaluation of culturally appropriate community health education on diabetes outcomes. Oakland: AAPCHO; 2008.

83. AHRQ. Improving patient safety systems for patients with limited English proficiency: A guide for hospitals. Rockville: Agency for Healthcare Research and Quality; 2012.

84. GPCog Tool. www.alz.org/health-care-professionals/cognitive-tests-patient-assessment.asp#cognitive_screening. Accessed 16 Feb 2015.

85. Washington KT, Meadows SE, Elliott SG, Koopman RJ. Information needs of informal caregivers of older adults with chronic health conditions. Patient Education and Counseling 2011;83(1):37–44.

86. Jastak S, Wilkinson G. The Wide Range Achievement test revised: Administration manual (WRAT-3): Jastak Associates; 1993.

87. Murphy PW, Davis TC, Long SW et al. Rapid estimate of adult literacy in medicine (REALM): a quick testing for patients. Journal of Reading 1993;37:124–30.

88. Slosson RL. Slosson oral reading test (SORT) revised. East Aurora, NY: Slosson Educational Publications; 1990.

89. Nurrs JR, Parker RM, Williams MV, Baker DW. Test of Functional Health Literacy in Adults. Atlanta: Centre for the Study of Adult Literacy; 1995.

90. Davis TC, Michielutte R, Askov EN, Williams MV, Weiss BD. Practical assessment of adult literacy in healthcare. Health Education and Behavior 1998;25(5):613–24.

91. Speros C. Health Literacy: Concept Analysis. Journal of Advanced Nursing 2004;50:633–40.

92. Weiss BD, Mays MZ, Martz W et al. The newest vital sign. Annals of Family Medicine 2005;3(6):514–22.

93. Wallace LS, Rogers ES, Roskos SE et al. Brief Report: screening items to identify patients with limited health literacy skills. Journal of General Internal Medicine 2006;21(8):874–7.

94. Chew LD, Bradley KA, Boyko EJ. Brief questions to identify patients with inadequate health literacy. Fam Med 2004;36(8):588–94.

95. Chew LD, Griffin JM, Partin MR et al. Validation of screening questions for limited health literacy in a large VA outpatient population. J Gen Intern Med 2008;23(5):561–6.

96. McLauglin GH. SMOG grading—a new readability formula. Journal of Reading 1969;12:639–46.

97. Fry EB. A readability formula that saves time. Journal of Reading 1968;11:513–16, 578.

98. Gunning R. The technique for clear writing. New York: McGraw-Hill; 1952.

99. Flesch RF. A new readability yardstick. Journal of Applied Psychology 1948;32:221–33.

100. Smith S, McCaffery K. Health Literacy: a brief literature review. Sydney: NSW Clinical Excellence Commission, Australia; 2010.

101. Clinical Excellence Commission. Guide to health literacy. Online. www.cec.health.nsw.gov.au/hlg; accessed 3 March 2014.

102. Dewalt DA, Callahan LF, Hawk VH et al. Health Literacy Universal Precautions Toolkit. In Chapel Hill: North Carolina Network Consortium, Agency for Healthcare Research and Quality; 2010.

103. Koo MM, Krass I, Aslani P. Factors influencing consumer use of written drug information. The Annals of Pharmacotherapy 2003;37(February):259–67.

104. Ngoh LN, Shepherd MD. Design, development, and evaluation of visual aids for communicating prescription drug instructions to nonliterate patients in rural Cameroon. Patient Education and Counseling 1997;31(3):245–61.

105. Houts PS, Doak CC, Doak LG, Loscalzo MJ. The role of pictures in improving health communication: A review of research on attention, comprehension, recall, and adherence. Patient Education and Counseling 2006;64(1–3):393–4.

106. Choi J. Pictograph-based discharge instructions for low-literate older adults after hip replacement surgery: development and validation. Journal of Gerontological Nursing 2011;37(11):47–56.

107. The United Kingdom Department of Health. Toolkit for producing patient information. http://ppitoolkit.org.uk/PDF/toolkit/patient_info_toolkit.pdf; accessed 18 Feb 2015.

108. Bernier MJ. Establishing the psychometric properties of a scale for evaluating quality in printed education materials. Patient Education and Counseling 1996;29:283–99.

109. Bidford Maine Area Health Education Center. Checklist for print materials. In: Doak CC, Doak LG, Root JH, eds. Teaching patients with low literacy skills. 2nd edn. Philadelphia: J.B. Lippincott Co; 1996;43.

110. Baker SJ. Who can read consumer product information? The Australian Journal of Hospital Pharmacy 1997;27(2):126–31.

111. Luk A, Aslani P. Tools used to evaluate written medicine and health information: Document and user perspectives. Health Education and Behavior 2011;38(August):389–403.

112. Krass I, Svarstad BL, Bultman D. Using alternative methodologies for evaluating patient medication leaflets. Patient Education and Counseling 2002;47(1):29–35.

113. Charnock D, Shepperd S et al. DISCERN: an instrument for judging the quality of written consumer health information on treatment choices. Journal of Epidemiology and Community Health 1999;53:105–11.

114. Khazaal Y, Chatton A, Cochand S et al. Brief DISCERN, six questions for the evaluation of evidence-based content of health-related websites. Patient Education and Counseling 2009;77(1):33–7.

115. Moult B, Franck LS, Brady H. Ensuring quality information for patients: development and preliminary validation of a new instrument to improve the quality of written healthcare information. Health expectations: an international journal of public participation in healthcare and health policy 2004;7(2):165–75.

116. Charvet-Berard AI, Chopard P, Perneger TV. Measuring quality of patient information documents with an expanded EQIP scale. Patient Education and Counseling 2008;70(3):407–11.

117. Horne RA, Hankins M, Jenkins R. The Satisfaction with Information about Medicines Scale (SIMS): a new measurement tool for audit and research. Quality in Healthcare 2001;10(3):135–40.

118. Koo MM, Krass I, Aslani P. Evaluation of written medicine information: Validation of the consumer information rating form. Annals of Pharmacotherapy 2007;41(6):951–6.

119. Taylor WL. Cloze procedure: A new tool for measuring readability. Journalism Quarterly 1953;30:415–33.

120. Roberts NJ, Partridge MR. Evaluation of a paper and electronic pictorial COPD action plan. Chronic respiratory disease 2011;8(1): 31–40.

121. Gossey JT. Increasing awareness of colorectal cancer screening through targeted exam room based video messages: UMI Dissertations Publishing; 2011.

122. Katz ML, Slater M, Paskett ED et al. Development of an educational video to improve patient knowledge and communication with their healthcare providers about colorectal cancer screening. American Journal of Health Education 2009;40(4):220.

123. Matsuyama RK, Lyckholm LJ, Molisani A, Moghanaki D. The value of an educational video before consultation with a radiation oncologist. Journal of Cancer Education 2013;28(2):306–13.

124. Anonymous. DVD designed to support the management of incontinence. Irish Medical Times 2007;Sect. 34.

125. Tait AR, Voepel-Lewis T, Moscucci M et al. Patient comprehension of an interactive, computer-based information program for cardiac catheterization: A comparison with standard information. Archives of internal medicine 2009;169(20):1907–14.

126. Cornoiu A, Beischer AD, Donnan L et al. Multimedia patient education to assist the informed consent process for knee arthroscopy. ANZ Journal of Surgery 2011;81(3):176–80.

127. Jerant A, Kravitz RL, Rooney M et al. Effects of a tailored interactive multimedia computer program on determinants of colorectal cancer screening: a randomized controlled pilot study in physician offices. Patient Education and Counseling 2007;66(1):67–74.

128. Huber J, Moll P, Schneider M et al. Multimedia support for improving preoperative patient education: a randomized controlled trial using the example of radical prostatectomy. Annals of Surgical Oncology 2013;20(1):15–23.

129. Shaw MJ, Beebe TJ, Tomshine PA et al. A randomized, controlled trial of interactive, multimedia software for patient colonoscopy education. Journal of clinical gastroenterology 2001;32(2):142–7.

130. Wilson EAH, Park DC, Curtis LM et al. Media and memory: The efficacy of video and print materials for promoting patient education about asthma. Patient Education and Counseling 2010;80(3):393–8.

131. Gysels M, Higginson IJ. Interactive technologies and videotapes for patient education in cancer care: systematic review and meta-analysis of randomised trials. Supportive care in cancer: official journal of the Multinational Association of Supportive Care in Cancer 2007;15(1):7–20.

132. Miller DP Jr, Kimberly JR Jr, Case LD, Wofford JL. Using a computer to teach patients about fecal occult blood screening: A randomized trial. Journal of General Internal Medicine 2005;20(11):984–8.

133. Diamond LC, Jacobs EA. Let's not contribute to disparities: the best methods for teaching clinicians how to overcome language barriers to healthcare. Journal of General Internal Medicine 2010;25(S2):S189–93.

134. Rowe J, Patterson J. Culturally competent communication with refugees. Home Healthcare Management and Practice 2010;22(5): 334–8.

135. Farley R, Askew D, Kay M. Caring for refugees in general practice: perspectives from the coalface. Australian Journal of Primary Health 2014;20:85–91.

136. Divi C, Koss RG, Schmaltz SP, Loeb JM. Language proficiency and adverse events in US hospitals: a pilot study. International Journal for Quality in Healthcare 2007;19(2):60–7.

137. Wilson E, Chen AH, Grumbach K et al. Effects of limited English proficiency and physician language on healthcare comprehension. Journal of General Internal Medicine 2005;20(9):800–6.

138. John-Baptiste A, Naglie G, Tomlinson G et al. The effect of English language proficiency on length of stay and in-hospital mortality. Journal of General Internal Medicine 2004;19(3):221–8.

139. Graham CL, Ivey SL, Neuhauser L. From hospital to home: assessing the transitional care needs of vulnerable seniors. The Gerontologist 2009;49(1):23–33.

140. Jiang HJ, Andrews R, Stryer D, Friedman B. Racial/ethnic disparities in potentially preventable readmissions: the case of diabetes. American Journal of Public Health 2005;95(9):1561–7.

141. Ash M, Brandt S. Disparities in asthma hospitalization in Massachusetts. American Journal of Public Health 2006;96(2):358–62.

142. Alexander M, Grumbach K, Remy L et al. Congestive heart failure hospitalizations and survival in California: patterns according to race/ethnicity. American Heart Journal 1999;137(5):919–27.

143. Traylor AH, Schmittdiel JA, Uratsu CS et al. Adherence to cardiovascular disease medications: does patient-provider race/ethnicity and language concordance matter? Journal of General Internal Medicine 2010;25(11):1172–7.

144. Jacobs EA, Diamond LC, Stevak L. The importance of teaching clinicians when and how to work with interpreters. Patient Education and Counseling 2010;78(2):149–53.

145. Kale E, Syed HR. Language barriers and the use of interpreters in the public health services. A questionnaire-based survey. Patient Education and Counseling 2010;81(2):187–91.

146. Lindholm M, Hargraves JL, Ferguson WJ, Reed G. Professional language interpretation and inpatient length of stay and readmission rates. Journal of General Internal Medicine 2012;27(10):1294–9.

147. Baker D, Hayes R, Fortier JP. Interpreter use and satisfaction with interpersonal aspects of care for Spanish-speaking patients. Medical Care 1998;36(10):1461–70.

148. Sudore RL, Landefeld CS, Perez-Stable EJ et al. Unravelling the relationship between literacy, language proficiency, and patient-physician communication. Patient Education and Counseling 2009;75:398–402.

149. Sobel R, Paasche-Orlow M, Waite K et al. Asthma 1-2-3: A low literacy multimedia tool to educate African American adults about asthma. Journal of Community Health 2009;34(4):321–7.

150. Ngo-Metzger Q, Hayes GR, Yunan C et al. Improving communication between patients and providers using health information technology and other quality improvement strategies: focus on low-income children. Medical Care Research and Review 2010;67(5):246S–67S.

151. Australian Council for Safety and Quality in Healthcare. Second national report on patient safety-improving medication safety; 2002 July.

152. Anderson WG, Winters K, Arnold RM et al. Studying physician-patient communication in the acute care setting: the hospitalist rapport study. Patient Education and Counseling 2011;82(2):275–9.

153. Bischof G, Freyer-Adam J, Meyer C et al. Changes in drinking behavior among control group participants in early intervention studies targeting unhealthy alcohol use recruited in general hospitals and general practices. Drug and Alcohol Dependence 2012;125(1–2):81–8.

154. Holdsworth G, Criddle J, Mohiddin A et al. Maximizing the role of emergency departments in the prevention of violence: developing an approach in South London. Public Health 2012;126(5):394–6.

155. Sommers MS, Lyons MS, Bohn CM et al. Health-compromising behaviors among young adults in the urban emergency department: opportunity for a teachable moment. Clinical Nursing Research 2013;22(3):275–9.

156. Lawson PJ, Flocke SA. Teachable moments for health behaviour change: A concept analysis. Patient Education and Counseling 2009;76:25–30.

157. Lassman J. Teachable moments: A paradigm shift. Journal of Emergency Nursing 2001;27(2):171–5.

158. Johnson SB, Bradshaw CP, Wright JL et al. Characterizing the teachable moment: is an emergency department visit a teachable moment for intervention among assault-injured youth and their parents? Pediatric Emergency Care 2007;23(8):553–9.

159. Szpiro KA. Providing asthma self-management education in the emergency department: A systematic review and feasibility study: ProQuest, UMI Dissertations Publishing; 2007.

160. Fox MP. A systematic review of the literature reporting on studies that examined the impact of interactive, computer-based patient education programs. Patient Education and Counseling 2009;77(1):6–13.

161. Kandula NR, Nsiah-Kumi PA, Makoul G et al. The relationship between health literacy and knowledge improvement after a multimedia type 2 diabetes education program. Patient Education and Counseling 2009;75(3):321–7.

162. White JV, Pitman S, Denny SC. Tool kits for teachable moments. Journal of the American Dietetic Association 2003;103(11):1454–5.

163. Tamparo CT, Lindh WQ. Therapeutic Communications for Health Professionals. 2nd edn. Delmar Thomson Learning; 2000.

164. Barat I, Andreasen F, Damsgaard EMS. Drug therapy in the elderly: what doctors believe and patients actually do. British Journal of Clinical Pharmacology 2001;51:615–22.

165. Heneghan C, Glasziou P, Perera R. Reminder packaging for improving adherence to self-administered long-term medications (Review). The Cochrane Collaboration 2007.

166. Haynes RB, McKibbon KA, Kanani R. Systematic review of randomised trials of interventions to assist patients to follow prescriptions for medications. The Lancet 1996;348:383–6.

167. Haynes RB, Ackloo E, Sahota N et al. Interventions for enhancing medication adherence. The Cochrane database of systematic reviews 2008(2):CD000011.

168. Haynes RB, McDonald H, Garg AX, Montague P. Interventions for helping patients to follow prescriptions for medications. www.ncbi.nlm.nih.gov/pubmed/12076376; accessed 18 Feb 2015.

169. Gibbar-Clements T, Shirrell D, Dooley R, Smiley B. The challenge of warfarin therapy. AJN 2000;100(3):38–40.

170. Hirsh J, Dalen JE, Deykin D et al. Oral anticoagulants: Mechanism of action, clinical effectiveness, and optimal therapeutic range. Chest 1995;108(Suppl 4):231–46.

171. WHO. Health Promotion. Online http://www.who.int/topics/health_promotion/en/; accessed 7 March 2014.

172. Gordis L. Epidemiology. 4th edn. Elsevier Mosby Saunders; 2008.

173. Corcoran N. Communicating health: strategies for health promotion: Sage Publications; 2007.

174. Jenkins J, Calabria E, Edelheim J et al. Service quality and communication in emergency department waiting rooms: Case studies at four New South Wales hospitals: Southern Cross University; 2011.

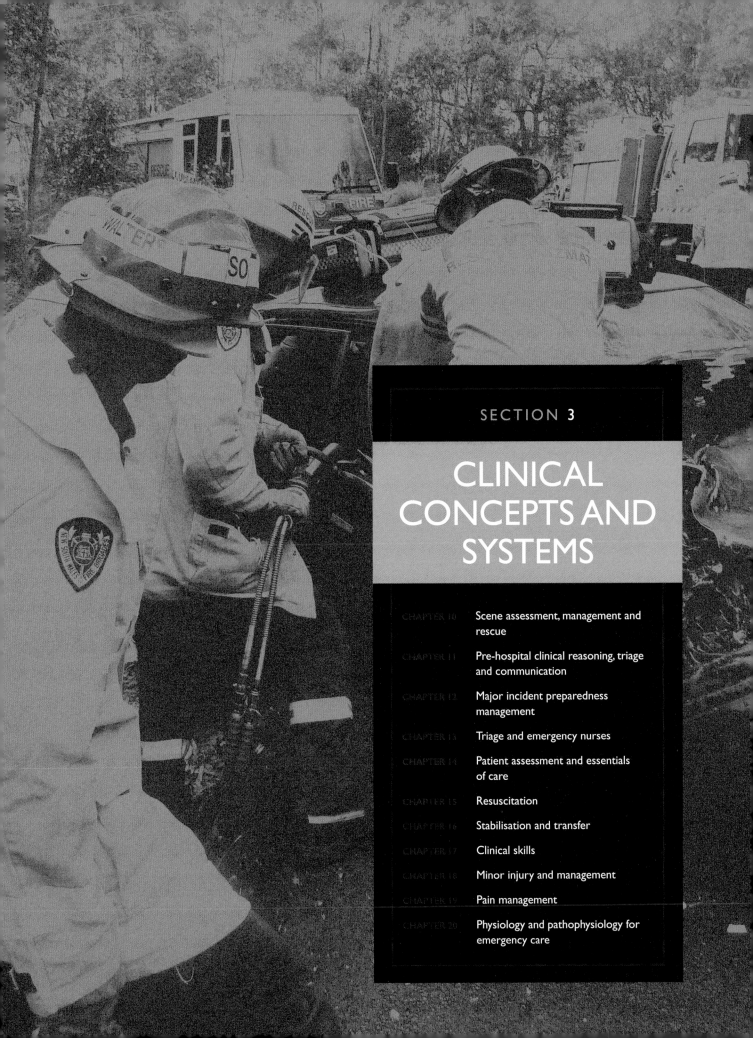

CHAPTER 10
SCENE ASSESSMENT, MANAGEMENT AND RESCUE

KAREL HABIG

Essentials

- Safety comes first in all emergency responses, and is fundamental from the time of the emergency call to the conclusion of scene management.

- Accurate and comprehensive information gathered from the emergency caller is essential, as it determines not only the urgency but also the composition, skill set and degree of the response.

- Personal protective equipment (PPE) should be used routinely as it protects against common hazards such as water, body fluids, chemicals and some variation in temperature, but also has high-visibility characteristics to enable the wearer to be easily seen in traumatic or confused scenes. It should always be worn, and donned prior to approaching or entering a scene.

- Good planning, leadership, command and teamwork, both within the organisation and by the scene responders, should be a priority to ensure the safety and health of personnel and patients.

- Adapting the environment is essential in ensuring safety. Response vehicles should be used, where possible, to enhance safety to rescuers, such as parking in the 'fend-off' position.

- An essential prerequisite to moving in to treat patients is to take control of the scene, then assess, communicate and triage, treat and transport.

- Emergency healthcare providers must maintain a high level of situational awareness of the overall scene, and consider all potential hazards as they approach the patient and while on-scene.

- Crowds present unique challenges to emergency service providers and a cautious approach using 'lights' but not sirens to move slowly through mass gatherings is recommended.

- The principles of vehicle extrication include: protection of the scene, stabilisation of the vehicle, patient assessment, triage and treatment, creation of space and physical extrication of the patient.

- During an extrication the aim is to focus on limiting clinical procedures to 'meaningful interventions' to minimise unnecessary delays on-scene.

Safety first—keeping you and the patient safe

Safety in emergency responses, whether by an ambulance service or by the police or fire services, starts as soon as the emergency call is received and includes appropriate dispatch prioritisation, well-planned procedures and equipment for scene care and clear protocols for high-risk situations.

Dispatch and pre-arrival information

In Australia, a call to 000 (111 in New Zealand) elicits the help of a call-taker who directs the caller to the appropriate service to deal with the call.[1] At this stage of the operation of an emergency paramedic response, the caller is asked a structured set of important questions that are intended to identify and prioritise life-threatening emergencies, elicit essential information to allow dispatch of appropriate resources and give a clear picture of the speed of response necessary by clinicians. In a typical computer-aided dispatch systems like Medical Priority Dispatch System,[2] software prompts call-takers to ask 'case-entry' questions, a process which has been likened to the primary survey: the location and a call-back number for the incident are verified, and the patient's age, status of consciousness, status of breathing and 'chief complaint' are determined. If information is given that the patient is unconscious and not breathing (for any reason), a maximal response is dispatched before any further interrogation or instructions continue. In this way, ambulance services can implement a degree of triage, ensuring that most rapid responses are made to only the most urgent cases that need this, rather than sending an urgent response to all cases, a common occurrence before the implementation of these sorts of triage and decision-support systems.

After these case-entry questions, 'key questions' are asked from the appropriate protocol, which is determined from the chief complaint. These key questions have been described as being equivalent to the secondary survey, and provide an ordered view of the patient complaint, to ensure that the pre-hospital care provided is appropriate and in keeping with the severity of the injury or illness. Finally, the structured elicitation of key facts from a 000 (or 111) caller also allows the delivery of pre-arrival instructions to the caller, including coaching on cardiopulmonary resuscitation, even allowing coaching in non-standard resuscitation.[3] Early research has shown that the proportion of inappropriate advance life support (ALS) responses was able to be reduced significantly by the use of emergency medical dispatch software.[4]

Dispatch information is also essential in ensuring that the paramedic is able to appropriately prepare to manage the scene. Data, such as the type of vehicle and number of patients, can prompt rescuers to consider situations very differently; very different procedures may be needed in a school bus incident compared with a single motorcyclist trauma. The following items of data are extremely useful in ensuring safety en route to an incident:

- traffic congestion, preferred routes and potential delays
- other delays such as raised bridges or blocked railway crossings
- pertinent weather information

- fastest, safest route to follow
- identified alternative routes
- pre-arrival instructions regarding care for the patient.

Essential dispatch information also includes as complete a description of the scene as possible, and enables the paramedic to determine whether the call:

- is a call to a trauma or to a potential medical case
- includes any life-threatening conditions
- involves multiple vehicles if trauma or multiple victims, which may indicate the need for more personnel
- involves fire or unstable building hazards
- involves other hazards such as downed power lines, broken gas lines, chemical spills or dangerous animals
- requires special rescue equipment, personnel or equipment, or the possibility of helicopter evacuation
- involves very hot or cold conditions that may aggravate the patient's condition
- involves any type of reported violence—paramedics are taught never to enter a scene in these circumstances until it is secured by law enforcement officers
- includes pre-arrival instructions, such as CPR coaching, that have been given to the caller to provide care to the patient until paramedics arrive.

The location and type of call help to determine if a need for more than one response unit is required, such as in a cardiac arrest situation where two crews may potentially be needed to transport the patient while continuing effective CPR. They may also help to determine if an immediate need for specialised resources exists, such as Hazmat teams.[5] In Australia, fire services assume the responsibility for managing hazardous materials and have specially trained personnel to handle these types of calls.[5]

Notification of an incident can also come through other sources, such as police or fire services, and it is essential that data can be shared between systems to ensure rapid dispatch of ambulance resource. A shared Computer Aided Dispatch platform, as exists in most states of Australia, is the ideal model.

Travelling to the scene

Collisions involving emergency vehicles are rare, but have resulted in serious injury or death.[6] Most data on this phenomenon comes from the USA when incidents occur when primary responders[7] are using 'lights and sirens'.[8] One study showed that there were 67 ground-transportation-related fatalities in the USA during the six years from 1992 to 1997;[7] another study revealed that the collision rate for emergency medical service (EMS) road transportation was 5 in 10,000 responses.[8]

It has been identified that situations when emergency vehicles are responding to emergencies under lights and sirens are particularly dangerous because they may be performing manoeuvres, such as entering intersections against red lights and using lanes not commonly employed. Most drivers, however, if obeying the road rules stop at red lights and keep to the appropriate lanes. A contradiction is apparent where emergency vehicle drivers believe that they are following the road rules that apply to them in an emergency, believing that other drivers will always yield, whereas a 'civilian' driver is conditioned to believe that other vehicles will give way when he has the right of way.[9] One report into an incident involving a fire engine and a train in the USA described the phenomenon of 'sirencide', 'used to describe the emotional reaction of emergency vehicle drivers when they begin to feel a sense of power and urgency that blocks out reason and prudence, leading to the reckless operation of the emergency vehicle'.[10]

It has been suggested that there should be a set of strict criteria defined for the response to any emergency situation, as paraphrased in Box 10.1.[11]

It has been pointed out that driver training for emergency vehicles is now widely available and should be part of every paramedic's training.[12] The purpose and intent of any well-regarded program is to minimise injury, death and damage to expensive equipment, with a parallel decrease in risk of liability likely to occur as well for agencies that provide driver training. It is recommended that instruction should include all aspects of both non-emergency and emergency vehicle operation, including use of the emergency warning systems, communications system, vehicle locating system, on-board computer system, location of area emergency facilities, proper parking and backing procedures and safe driving practices. It was also proposed that a new driver should have the assistance of a trained driving instructor for a certain number of initial miles (kilometres) of driving, in both emergency and non-emergency modes.

Personal protective equipment

Personal protective equipment (PPE) refers to protective clothing, helmets, goggles and other garments designed to protect the body from injury by blunt impacts, infection, electrical hazards, traffic, caustic substances, extremes of temperature and assault by patients, relatives or bystanders, for job-related occupational safety and health purposes. PPE therefore comprises garments with specific protective properties, and equipment, which may contribute to maximising personal protection for paramedics working in uncontrolled pre-hospital

scenes. Although unpredictability is part of pre-hospital care, the potential harmful effects of factors, such as those described above, need to be minimised to ensure the safety of clinicians. The ability of these articles of protective clothing and equipment to perform their function appropriately is usually mandated through national quality agencies, which are often members of the International Organization for Standardization (www.iso.org) or organisations such as Standards Australia (www.standards.org.au) or the American National Standards Institute (www.ansi.org).

Routinely worn PPE protects against common hazards such as water, body fluids and some variation in temperature, but also has high-visibility characteristics to enable the wearer to be easily seen in traumatic or confused scenes. There are often strips or patches of reflective material that form distinctive patterns seen easily in car headlights etc (Figs 10.1 to 10.3). Added PPE for the purposes of physical safety are safety glasses and helmets. In traumatic incidents these items of protective equipment should always be worn, and donned prior to approaching or entering the scene.

Protection against infection is an essential prerequisite to arrival at any incident, and standard PPE of this nature includes gloves and the safety glasses mentioned earlier, which provide a barrier to protect the healthcare worker from contamination. Medical examination gloves, which may be latex or a latex substitute, are worn in situations where there is direct contact anticipated with blood, body fluids, mucous membranes or non-intact skin. Facial protection such as the glasses and/or fluid-resistant face masks with transparent eye shields should be worn if there is a likelihood of splashing or splattering of body substances or blood.

The performance of hand hygiene has been seen to be essential in the prevention of cross-infection,[13] and has also been shown to be achievable and effective with simple measures.[14]

BOX 10.1 Emergency vehicle response and travel guidelines

1. The first arriving ambulance should be responsible for determining the response status for any additional ambulance vehicles going to the scene of the call.
2. Ambulance service vehicles should not exceed posted speed limits by more than 10 mph (~15 kph).
3. Ambulance service vehicles should not exceed posted speed limits when proceeding through intersections with a green light.
4. Ambulance service vehicles approaching a red light, stop sign or railway crossing must come to a complete stop before proceeding with caution.
5. When traffic conditions require ambulance service vehicles to travel in the oncoming traffic lanes, the maximum speed should be 20 mph (~30 kph).
6. When ambulance service vehicles use the turning lane or oncoming traffic lane to approach intersections, they must come to a complete stop before proceeding through the intersection with caution.

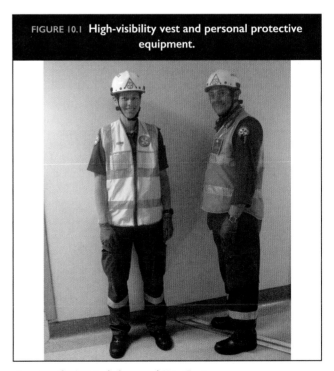

FIGURE 10.1 **High-visibility vest and personal protective equipment.**

Courtesy of NSW Ambulance and Kate Curtis.

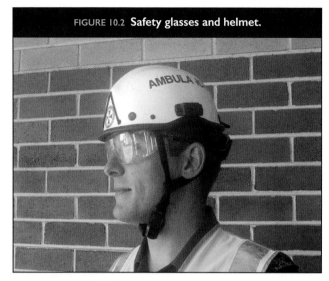

FIGURE 10.2 **Safety glasses and helmet.**

Courtesy NSW Ambulance.

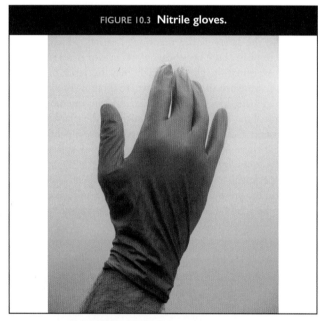

FIGURE 10.3 **Nitrile gloves.**

Courtesy NSW Ambulance.

PRACTICE TIP

Alcohol-based hand rubs are the best way to clean hands and should be available in all vehicles as well as on scene before and after all patient contacts.

Specific PPE may also be used in higher-risk situations where there are defined hazards; these may often be termed Hazmat suits (for hazardous materials), and are discussed in relation to mass-casualty incidents in Chapter 12. The US Department of Homeland Security defines a Hazmat suit as 'an overall garment worn to protect people from hazardous materials or substances, including chemicals, biological agents, or radioactive materials'.[15] These may provide protection from:

- chemical agents—through the use of appropriate barrier materials like Teflon, heavy PVC or rubber

BOX 10.2 **Classifications of Hazmat protective clothing[16]**

Level A
The highest level of protection against vapours, gases, mists and particles is Level A, which consists of a fully encapsulating chemical-entry suit with a full-facepiece self-contained breathing apparatus (SCBA) or a supplied air respirator (SAR) with an SCBA escape cylinder.

Level B
Level B protection requires a garment (including SCBA) that provides protection against splashes from a hazardous chemical. Since the breathing apparatus is worn on the outside of the garment, Level B protection is not vapour-protective.

Level C
The same type of garment used for Level B protection is worn for Level C, but there are differences in the equipment needed for respiratory protection, allowing any of the various types of air-purifying respirators. Level C equipment does not offer the protection needed in an oxygen-deficient atmosphere.

Level D
Level D protection does not protect from chemical exposure and, therefore, this level of protection can only be used in situations where a crew member has no possibility of contact with chemicals. Most fire-fighter gear is considered to be Level D.

- nuclear agents—possibly through radiation shielding in the lining, but more importantly by preventing direct contact with or inhalation of radioactive particles or gas
- biological agents—through fully sealed systems (often at overpressure to prevent contamination even if the suit is damaged)
- fire/high temperatures—usually by a combination of insulating and reflective materials which reduce or retard the effects.[15]

The commonest classification of Hazmat protective clothing uses the US system[16] which classifies as Level A, B, C or D based on the degree of protection the clothing provides; these are outlined in Box 10.2 and discussed in detail in Chapter 12.

Working with other agencies at a scene

Teamwork, whether on a scale involving inter-agency inter-actions with colleagues on-scene or most commonly between individual paramedics forming the two-person treating team, is a fundamental component of pre-hospital care. Although it might be obvious that partners within an ambulance need to work together, good teamwork is also an essential component of successful organisations at every administrative and corporate level. On a small scale, and particularly in longer-term partnerships, teamwork contributes to safety on multiple levels, including improved vigilance for environmental hazards, coordination of patient care and manual handling, dealing with and defusing intense emotional scenes, negotiating traffic safety and recognising stress and burnout. On a multi-agency level, teamwork becomes particularly important as the specialised activities and talents of individual organisations directly affect, and need to be closely coordinated with, each other.

Although ambulance personnel may be an early arrival at the scene of an incident, there are defined responsibilities attributable to and expected of other emergency service personnel. These may be summarised as police being in control of an incident scene, fire services being in control of hazardous materials and situations and ambulances/paramedics being in control of patient management. The discrete responsibilities of each service mean that as the scene evolves different priorities will emerge requiring a high level of communication between agencies. One team may continue a high level of control, such as in a dangerous situation involving weapons, where the police will assume extended control even in the presence of wounded patients (discussed in the section below on scene safety), or one agency may temporarily default to another, such as in the management of violent patients where paramedics may need police assistance to manage them. Some agency interactions may have local variations, such as rescue operations, which may be managed primarily by a range of services including ambulance, fire/rescue services or volunteer agencies such as the State Emergency Service (SES) in rural Australia.[17]

In disaster situations, either a natural calamity or a man-made catastrophe, and defined in health terms as when affected patient load overwhelms the available resources, similar but more formalised arrangements apply: police maintain a defined perimeter around the incident, the fire service takes responsibility for direct rescue operations and healthcare services, including ambulance services, manage immediate trauma scenes, of which there may be several, and the triage, stabilisation and orderly evacuation of casualties. The Major Incident Medical Management and Support (MIMMS)[18] course manual describes this in terms of a major incident, defined as causing so many live casualties that special arrangements are necessary to deal with them, an incident that disrupts the health service or an incident that presents a serious threat to the health of the community.

Scene management priorities—why an organised scene is priceless

A summary of the priorities at an incident scene can be remembered as CONTROL and ACT. An essential prerequisite to moving in to treat patients is to take control of the scene, and then to assess, communicate and triage, treat and transport (Box 10.3). The following sections elaborate on this theme.

Team function

Leadership, command and control are important. In emergency incident terms, a scene without adequate leadership may

> **BOX 10.3 Scene management priorities—the ACT mnemonic[19]**
>
> **A** Assess
> **C** Communicate
> **T** Triage, treat and transport

deteriorate quickly. One approach, which is being adapted to the paramedical environment, is the Incident Management System (IMS), an outgrowth of the US Incident Command System (ICS).[12] The US National Fire Protection Association states that 'the purpose of an incident management system is to provide structure and coordination to the management of emergency incident operations in order to provide for the safety and health of … persons involved in those activities'.[20] It is described[12] as a process for creating order from disorder through a comprehensive approach to leadership and task delegation. Versions of IMS have been used for handling wildland fires, urban fire scenes, Hazmat situations and everyday emergency medical service (EMS) scenes.

Effective, consistent scene leadership is a vital issue in pre-hospital safety, and no matter how a system is organised or functions on a day-to-day basis, this leadership may be routinely achieved through use of the primary principle of defining one leader who makes all scene management decisions. There is no doubt that the presence of this one leader at a pre-hospital scene, no matter how large or small, ensures that the scene is both more orderly and more organised. This has parallels with other team decision-making, such as in the trauma team setting where decisions are based on the big picture rather than piecemeal as new information becomes known, or subsumed in a mass of hands-on detail that prevents perception of the greater picture.

Even when a two-person crew is handling a routine emergency call, this may improve incident coordination. The clinician assuming the leadership role should prepare to take on certain functions, delegating them as needed depending on circumstances; for example, an available first-responder might be asked to scout out the best path from the scene to the ambulance vehicle. The incident commander, even in a single-paramedic response, should be the individual with the best ability to assemble the resources necessary and the experience to take an overview of the scene while allowing the other clinician to attend directly to the patient. Roles should be clearly delineated in standard operating procedures, although allowing for training, mentoring and guidance of more junior staff.

Scene management begins prior to the actual arrival of the paramedical crew at the patient. The NSW Ambulance Service (NSWAS) scene management skill training manual[21] states: 'Scene assessment is commenced as soon as visual contact is made with the scene and is as equally important at medical situations as at trauma scenes.' Communications are also of great value at this point—the NSWAS protocol also directs paramedics arriving at the scene of a motor vehicle accident to provide a brief preliminary report once visual contact is made with the scene. It suggests a script such as 'Car approaching scene. I observe a single motor vehicle crash. Car into a tree.'

Vehicle placement

Pre-hospital scenes, particularly roadside trauma, can be extremely hazardous; many paramedics' lives have been lost in this environment. In an ideal world, police maintain scene control in this sort of incident, but to rely on this would be naïve, as they are not always in a position to provide traffic control. This is particularly true when pre-hospital clinicians are first on the scene, and in many areas assistance is patchy, slow to arrive or unavailable. Paramedics and other pre-hospital clinicians need to know how to provide the safest environment to assure their own protection.

Vehicles should be positioned in a lane that is already blocked or on the same side of the carriageway as the incident, unless there are some specific reasons not to do so; there are several advantages to this apart from being efficient for patient care. First, it prevents clinicians from crossing busy roads to gain access to the patients and possibly being injured themselves; second, as the lane is already blocked, the ambulances and other emergency vehicles occupy little further space. Third, leaving other lanes open ensures that other traffic can move past, albeit at a slower pace, which may in itself prevent further accidents. Passers-by in other vehicles are often a source of further accidents as they drive with their attention on what is happening in the more interesting accident scene. Finally, and related to the last point, if ambulances and other rescue vehicles such as fire engines and police rescue are parked across other lanes, bringing equipment and hydraulic lines across the carriageways would not only block these lanes to other traffic but would effectively stop the egress of emergency vehicles themselves.

Vehicles should be parked in such a way as to create a barrier to oncoming traffic that might cause injury to rescuers,

in the 'fend-off' position (Fig 10.4). The steering wheel should be turned so that any vehicle which is struck by another would move away from the scene, entrapped patients and rescuers. Even this is not that simple, however; there is a belief that it is safest if the ambulance is placed between oncoming traffic and the involved vehicles, providing emergency warning beacons at that end of the crash site, illuminating the scene with the ambulance headlights, and providing a physical barrier from approaching traffic. However, once the patient(s) and paramedics are actually in the ambulance, they are endangered by being closest to oncoming traffic during preparations for leaving the scene. Therefore, although it makes sense to position an emergency vehicle at the end of the crash site, using the ambulance for this is probably not the best choice if another emergency vehicle is available. It is probably better for the ambulance to be moved ahead of the crash site when another vehicle arrives to create a barrier against traffic.

It has been suggested that when parking on the side of a road, one front and one rear wheel should be left on the solid surface of the road, to ensure that there is sufficient traction to move the vehicle when it attempts to leave the scene. It is often safer, even when there are urgent interventions that need to be performed, to briefly move the vehicle and patient to a location away from passing traffic. Considerations when parking the ambulance may include:

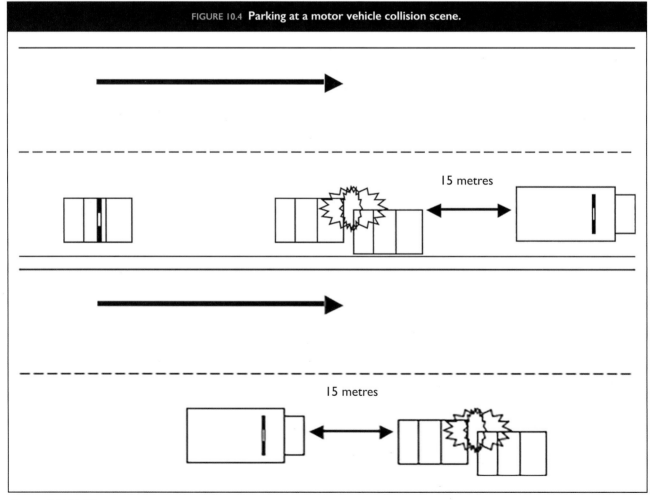

FIGURE 10.4 **Parking at a motor vehicle collision scene.**

Courtesy PM Middleton.

- which spot is safest
- which is most convenient for patient care
- which will best facilitate traffic flow around the scene
- which allows the best outlet for departure
- whether other emergency personnel are already on the scene or will arrive later.

Headlights should be kept on low beam, and if needed to illuminate the scene should be pointed specifically in that direction to avoid blinding other drivers. Exhaust fumes should be considered, and vehicles parked in such a way as to minimise the possibility of these affecting both patients and rescuers.

The following aide memoire for securing safety at the scene is a version of that in the publication *EMS safety: Techniques and Applications*,[20] a guide for fire-fighters that is also very appropriate for all EMS and ambulance personnel. It describes the mnemonic PROTECTION, which is outlined in Box 10.4.

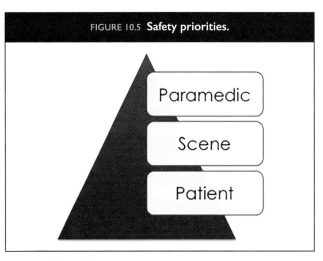

FIGURE 10.5 **Safety priorities.**

Courtesy PM Middleton.

BOX 10.4 The PROTECTION mnemonic[20]

P Proceed slowly, using your vehicle as a safety shield for personnel.

R Remember: passing motorists are watching you, not where they are going.

O Observe types of vehicles, placards, condition of containers and fire hazards.

T Take the time to stabilise all vehicles before beginning operations.

E Evacuate as necessary to ensure the safety of public and EMS personnel.

C Call for additional assistance early. Overtaxed personnel become a safety liability.

T Treat the incident scene with great caution. Wear full protective clothing and use all warning devices.

I In the interests of safety, appoint a safety officer and dedicate adequate resources.

O Once assessment is complete, close the road when necessary to protect personnel.

N Never let your guard down.

Scene assessment

Risk and hazard assessment

One of the first decisions that needs to be made by paramedics arriving at the scene of any sort of incident, whether trauma scene or medical case, is actually whether it is safe to get out of the vehicle or not. There are many factors that make a scene unsafe or potentially hazardous, and in a substantial proportion of these not actually approaching or entering the area without further information or back-up may be recommended. Although it can be seen by some to be contrary to the priorities of routine clinical intervention and behaviour, the priorities for safety are paramedic, scene and patient, in that order (Fig 10.5).

Scene assessment (otherwise known as 'scene size-up'[20] or 'reading the scene'[22]) is a quick analysis of the scene on arrival, and is vital for safe and efficient operations in order to enforce a rapid and accurate evaluation, particularly of obvious hazards. This initial reading of the scene comprises a scan for immediate hazards—fire, power lines and potential assailants with weapons—which need to be mitigated prior to operating at the scene. EMS personnel in the USA are taught that the driver of the rescue vehicle should stay behind the wheel to facilitate rapidly leaving the scene if attacked, and treating clinicians are taught to approach a vehicle from behind, close any opened car boot to prevent attack by a hidden assailant, not to move forward of the B pillar of a car (the rear frame of the front door) and always to keep the hands of the driver or passenger in sight. These precautions are less often required in Australia and other similar regions, although may still be valid and life-saving in particular areas. The 1994 US Department of Transport EMT-Basic National Standard Curriculum[23] lists five key components of the scene size-up process:

1. Number of patients.
2. Mechanism of injury/nature of illness.
3. Resource determination (heavy rescue, Hazmat, etc).
4. Standard precautions before leaving the ambulance.
5. Scene safety.

Environmental factors

Another important aspect of reading the scene is evaluation of environmental hazards, such as rain, snow, ice, bright sunlight, extreme temperatures and humidity. The environment may provide significant physical and mental stress, which can decrease resistance to disease, and decrease emotional tolerance and responsiveness to others. The environment obviously may have a profound impact on the patient's physical condition and ability to maintain core body functions, and heat stress or cold exposure may have increasingly significant effects on both patient and clinician during prolonged incidents.

Hazardous materials have been discussed above in relation to PPE, but their potential or actual presence at a scene may have great importance as they are indiscriminate in causing harm to patients and rescuers alike. Paramedics and other pre-hospital staff need to have a substantial index of suspicion, particularly in motor vehicle accidents involving large vehicles or industrial transport, and also in industrial or rural areas. Hazardous materials are subject to clear labelling, which may be common between countries. In the USA the Department of

Transport and the Environmental Protection Agency regulate transport of hazardous goods[24] as well as their labelling, whereas Australia and the UK follow the Hazchem labelling system which uses standard United Nations codes.[25] Plates that use the Hazchem system are displayed on vehicles and storage facilities, and give coded information describing the hazard, the level of protection needed and the actions required (Figs 10.6 and 10.7).

Correct and adequate illumination of a night-time trauma scene is vital to operations that are safe and efficient for paramedic and patient. Vehicle-mounted or portable lights powered by a generator or 12-volt vehicle supply are in common use, and portable fluorescent or LED lights provide ample light with minimal heat output. Special care should be taken to avoid the use of lights or other appliances that produce heat near either patients or flammable materials.

Using your senses

Less speed, more haste

Pre-hospital work is often intense and stimulates the release of endogenous catecholamines, which often clouds the judgement of inexperienced practitioners. The sense of urgency when another's life is potentially at stake and the perception that resolution of the situation is in the hands of the clinician is often a trigger for rushing, which diminishes the chance of carrying out a well-thought-out and coordinated plan.[20] Although there exists a degree of urgency to any emergency, running to the patient does not allow time to 'absorb' the scene.

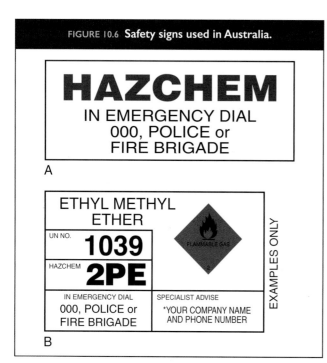

FIGURE 10.6 **Safety signs used in Australia.**

A Simple Hazchem sign. **B** Dangerous goods signage, with UN and Hazchem substance identification numbers in the middle left panels, emergency number in the bottom left panel, warning symbol indicating the danger represented by the hazard in the top right panel, and telephone number for specialist advice in the bottom right panel. *Courtesy Signs of Safety www.signsofsafety. net.au.*

Looking

While walking briskly to the patient, time can be spent not only scanning for hazards, as already described, but also assessing the incident scene for clues to causation, including mechanism of injury pointers such as skid marks, airbag deployment, 'bullseye' fractures of windscreens, deformation of vehicles and distance of patients from vehicles. A rapid global overview of the patients, both in numbers and in appearance, potentially prompts the call for increased resources and back-up, and contributes to the clinician's expectation of the likelihood of significant illness or injury.

Other key visual cues, particularly when responding to a potential crime scene or calls to an assault, may be vital for the safety of clinicians and others. Importantly, when approaching on-scene civilians and bystanders, attempt to 'read' their body language on three levels:[20] their overall body language, their facial expressions and their eyes. Although the most dominant emotion is usually demonstrated, there may be conflict between facial expression, body language and eyes. A typical example might be in the responsibility felt by the parent of an injured child, where potential guilt at contributing or causing an event may conflict with anger, often displaced onto paramedics, and fear for the potential outcome. Weapons of any kind, as well as signs of intoxication with alcohol or drugs, should be actively looked for by paramedics, as should the presence of other emergency service vehicles, particularly police and fire service; and signs of fire, smoke and downed power lines are other essential visual cues to the potential harm in any situation.

Listening

Listening on approach to a scene may give important insights into the potential number of victims, the type of incident and the immediate situation that may be encountered at the scene. Typical auditory cues may be human, animal or environmental, and may obviously include calls for help and cries of pain, crowd noise and voices associated with attempts to help, rescue or organise the scene. Sounds of conflict—loud, argumentative voices or screams—are especially important. Animal noises are less common, but may include dogs barking; this may represent a potentially severe injury risk to clinicians, particularly when attempting to access private or industrial premises where dogs will have a real or perceived guard function. The family dog, however harmless-looking, always has the potential to attack; always summon trained assistance where there is a perceived risk of this. Environmental noise is potentially very significant, and includes traffic noise—or the lack of it, as an unusual silence may have important connotations.

Feeling

Feeling has less of a role in the assessment of a scene, but a great role in the assessment of a patient, as palpation and appropriate movement are two of the key methods to identify injury and some illnesses. Even on approach to an accident scene or into a dwelling, there is a need to use all the senses. Feeling for heat, or cold, is particularly important if there is a possibility of burn injury or hypothermia. The presence of a cold draught has been seen to signify everything from an open window to a gas jet from a leaking propane cylinder.

FIGURE 10.7 **Standard symbols used in hazard warning signs.**

CLASS	LABEL	DESCRIPTION
1	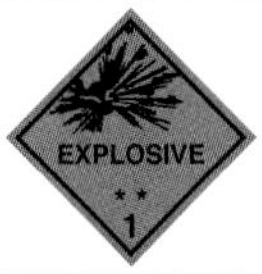	EXPLOSIVE Orange Background Black Text & Symbol
2.1	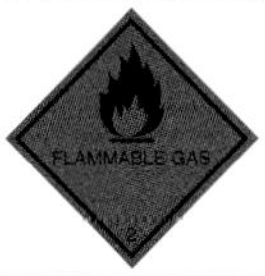	FLAMMABLE GAS Red Background Black Text & Symbol
2.2	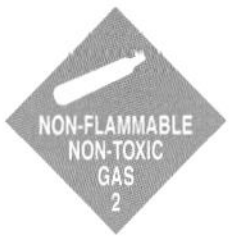	NON-FLAMMABLE NON-TOXIC GAS Green Background White Text & Symbol
2.2	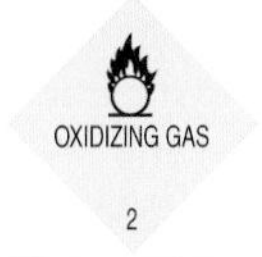	OXIDIZING GAS Yellow Background Black Text & Symbol Subsidiary Risk 5.1
2.3	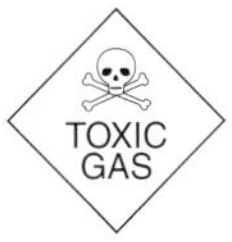	TOXIC GAS White Background Black Text & Symbol
3	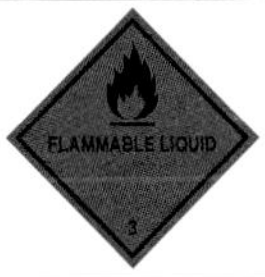	FLAMMABLE LIQUID Red Background Black Text & Symbol
4.1	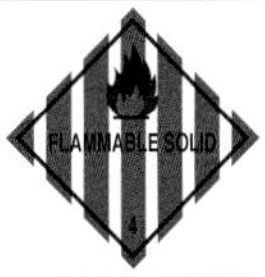	FLAMMABLE SOLID Red/White Vertical Striped Background Black Text & Symbol
4.2	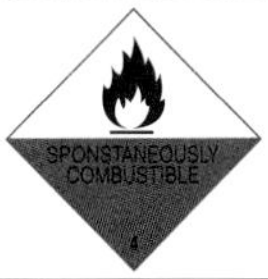	SPONTANEOUSLY COMBUSTIBLE White Upper Background Red Lower Background Black Text & Symbol
4.3	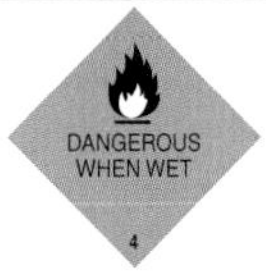	DANGEROUS WHEN WET Blue Background Black Text & Symbol

CLASS	LABEL	DESCRIPTION
5.1	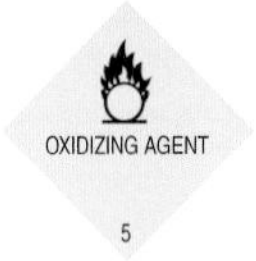	OXIDIZING AGENT Yellow Background Black Text & Symbol
5.2	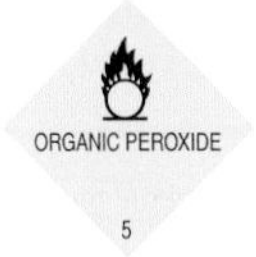	ORGANIC PEROXIDE Yellow Background Black Text & Symbol
6.1(A)	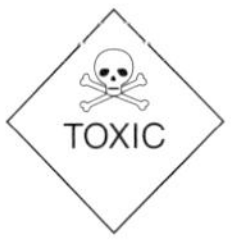	TOXIC White Background Black Text & Symbol
6.1(B)	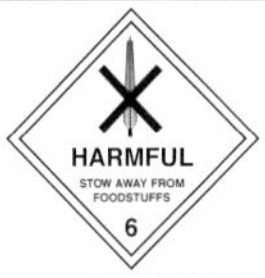	HARMFUL White Background Black Text & Symbol
6.2	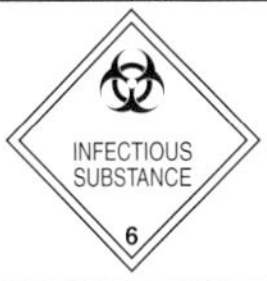	INFECTIOUS SUBSTANCE White Background Black Text & Symbol
7	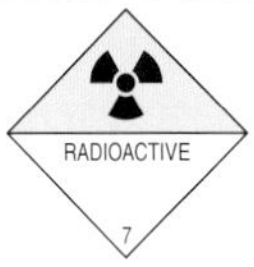	RADIOACTIVE Yellow Upper Background White Lower Background Black Text & Symbol
8	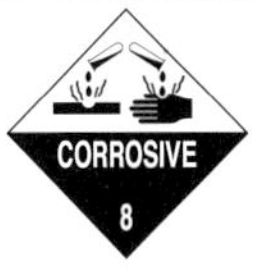	CORROSIVE White Upper Background Black Lower Background White Text & Symbol
9	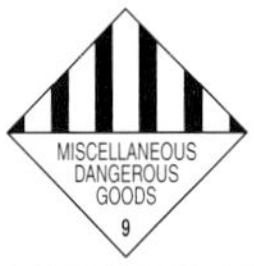	MISCELLANEOUS White & Black Vertical Striped Upper Background Black Text
10	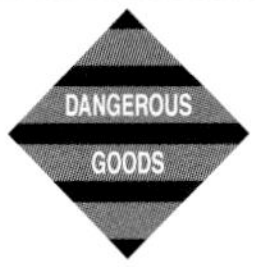	DANGEROUS GOODS Orange & Black Horizontal Striped Background White Text

Courtesy Signs of Safety www.signsofsafety.net.au.

Smelling

Smelling has a vital role in the scene size-up, as there are many things that could give a clue to mechanism of injury, potential harm to rescuers or need for intervention. Some of these are the smell of gas in a house and the smell of caustic chemicals in road traffic incidents and particularly in tanker accidents; remember to look for the Hazchem sign. Smells of smoke and sulfur from discharged firearms, and even the smell of body fluids such as blood, urine or sweat, all may be a pointer to possible hazards, patients or pathologies about to be encountered. The smell of a cigarette or a match being struck where there is a potential fuel spill or gas leak may certainly prove to be a warning of the possibility of harm for all concerned, and prompts urgent action to ensure protection.

BOX 10.5 Preservation of evidence promotion

- Avoid moving furniture or other articles apart from to provide vital medical care.
- Take a picture of the scene prior to moving a body if this is possible in the context of the ambulance system. Many paramedics carry mobile phones that are able to take high-quality digital images, although patient privacy and confidentiality hampers the use of these in many jurisdictions.
- Do not cut through bullet holes or stab holes in clothing when attempting to expose the patient in trauma. Investigators often use minute evidence from these areas in forensic examination relevant to the pursuit of a criminal prosecution.
- Be careful with clothing, and place in a paper bag if possible.
- Try to avoid tracking through blood and other items of evidence; this is a damaging mistake to make at a crime scene.
- Clean up and carry away any debris that is generated from treating the patient, such as wrappings from cannulae, dressings, etc.

BOX 10.6 The ETHANE mnemonic[29]

- E Exact location—the precise location of the incident.
- T Type—the nature of the incident, including how many vehicles, buildings and so on are involved.
- H Hazards—both actual and potential.
- A Access—best route for emergency services to access the site, or obstructions and bottlenecks to avoid.
- N Numbers—numbers of casualties, dead and uninjured on scene.
- E Emergency services—which services are already on scene, and which others are required.

Protecting the scene

Protection of the integrity of a scene of an incident or accident is exceptionally important for several reasons. First, in the short term the environment and the way it displays the habitat or habits of an individual may give valuable information, which can assist in the diagnosis and risk stratification of a newly encountered patient. Ensuring that this is undisturbed until the clinician has had a chance to work through a process of clinical reasoning, structured examination and emergency intervention may prevent vital pieces of diagnostic evidence being found or used. All the senses of a seasoned pre-hospital clinician should be routinely alert to notice factors relevant to safety, medical intervention priorities and interpersonal communication (the 1-2-3 of pre-hospital care). In a similar way, when there is a suspicion of a crime being committed, it is essential to avoid inadvertent disruption or destruction of potential evidence. Preservation of evidence can be promoted by observing some simple rules and principles as outlined in Box 10.5.

Communication from the scene

Communication is important in many aspects of scene and patient management: between clinician and patients, relatives and bystanders; between clinical colleagues; and between emergency services—but absolutely vital is clear and structured communication from ambulance to control or operations centre. It has been shown that lack of structure in information transfer leads to information loss,[26,27] and conversely that applying a structure to the hand-over process results in a decrease in information loss and an improvement in hand-over quality.[28]

There are three situations where a structured set of information has great value. It has already been mentioned that

a situation report ('sitrep') is extremely useful when arriving at the scene of an incident or accident, in order to give a brief overview of the appearance as a crew arrives. This sitrep enables the control centre to gain some sense of the potential scale of the problems encountered by the first clinician crew, and to put other resources on standby. Following an accurate, complete but rapid scene size-up as described above, it is often essential to transmit another set of structured information back to the control centre; this is the result of the systematic patient assessment. Worldwide this is most commonly given in the MIST format:

- M Mechanism of injury
- I Injuries identified
- S Signs. Vital signs including PR, BP, RR, SaO_2, GCS.
- T Treatment. Interventions and medications administered.

Early notification of the severity of illness or injury of the patients assessed by paramedics enables actions to be carried out, including pre-warning of emergency departments and activation of medical teams or retrieval services, not only to increase the level of care available at the scene if necessary but also to shorten the time to definitive care. Finally, in the situation of a major incident or disaster scenario, an accurate picture of the scale of the incident, the actions taken and the need for extra resources, may be summarised by the mnemonic ETHANE (Box 10.6).[29]

Scene access

Following assessment of the scene, it is then time to access the patient; specific considerations and hazards will vary depending on the type of scene and incident. Planning scene access is a critical element of the overall successful management of pre-hospital incidents.[30]

Planning

Emergency healthcare providers must have a high level of situational awareness of the overall scene and consider all potential hazards as they approach the patient.[31] Special circumstances will be dealt with later in the chapter; for most incidents, patient access is straightforward and readily achievable.

Where possible, following the call for an ambulance, the operations centre dispatchers should advise callers to assist EMS staff finding the scene. This may be done by sending a bystander, friend or family member to wait by the road or entrance to escort the team. At night, switching on external lights can be of great assistance; however, patients on their own or incapacitated by their illness or injury may not be able to help in this way.

Houses

Most patients are easily accessed via the front door or main entrance. As the team approaches it is imperative to remain vigilant to hazards, and assess and plan an egress route should this be required urgently. When approaching at night look for lights and listen for voices, which may indicate the number of people inside; knock firmly or ring the door bell, announcing yourself as an emergency healthcare provider. Standing to the side of the door and leaving screen or security doors closed, if present, is a sensible safety measure if there is any concern about personal security. Establish rapport as soon as possible and identify the whereabouts of the patient; it is best to follow the person who met you rather than have them follow you.[31] At night, turn illumination on as you proceed through the house; this will assist with planning the egress of the patients and identification of hazards. Always be aware of your closest egress point as well as an alternative.

Units

Identification of, and gaining access to, units or apartment blocks is often much more challenging for EMS providers than are single dwellings. Locating the correct block of units can be difficult in high-density residential areas, as numbering is often inadequate or absent or insufficient information has been provided by the caller. Security buildings have intercom systems which require the resident to activate to enable access, and if this is not possible due to injury, illness or incapacity then neighbouring residences will need to be tried. As always it is imperative to clearly identify yourself and your organisation. If a lift is available, this is usually the quickest way to access the patient, but take careful note of the internal dimensions in relation to your stretcher as many lifts will not accommodate a stretcher in a standard configuration, necessitating alternative route of egress where patients must be moved using a stretcher. Some units do not have lifts and the team will be required to ascend stairs while carrying their equipment. It is vital that packs and equipment for all likely eventualities are carried by the team to the first contact, as it is rarely easy to rapidly undo an error of omission upon assessing the patient. As one moves through the building it is essential to consider how egress might be accomplished once the patient is loaded as it is always easier to get equipment to a patient than to extricate the patient once loaded on a stretcher or extrication board. On arrival outside the unit, it is important not to block egress with equipment should you need to retreat quickly. Once on-scene seeking local knowledge of alternative routes for egress can be invaluable.

Outdoors

A large proportion of situations requiring emergency medical care occur outdoors. These include simple falls, vehicle collisions, environmental emergencies (such as heat-related illness or envenomation) and sporting injuries or medical illnesses occurring outside. The general principles of access for such scenes include getting the ambulance as close as possible to the patient, and then using the vehicle to protect you and the patient, both in physical terms ('fending off' at motor vehicle accidents on roadways) and as a privacy screen (where crowds of onlookers are present).[31] Experienced EMS providers always consider how they will load the ambulance and egress the scene when choosing a place to park. Where practical and safe to do so, parking with the ambulance facing downhill generally makes loading the patient easier.

Crowds

Crowds present unique challenges, and vary from the quiet and courteous to the angry and anti-social. Individuals within a crowd commonly have reduced awareness of the approach of emergency medical services, even when these arrive in a vehicle the size of an ambulance. Use of sirens is typically unhelpful and can increase the unpredictability of the crowd, and therefore their use is discouraged in close proximity.[2] Judicious use of 'lights' is generally a satisfactory way to move slowly through a crowd. Emergency healthcare providers need to be particularly mindful of children, patrons affected by drugs or alcohol and individuals who seem unaware of your presence and intent. Windows should be closed and doors locked to avoid interference and delay. If proceeding on foot, the notification of your response to your control centre is imperative; move purposefully through the crowd, announcing your approach to indicate the urgent medical nature of your response. A key barrier to moving within crowds is your equipment, which generally significantly increases your width and can cause harm or injury to others; backpacks are helpful, if available, to assist in moving through densely packed people. It may be very challenging to locate a patient requiring assistance among large crowds, and it requires careful observation on the part of the responders and accurate directions by dispatchers. Always have access to a radio and stay together with a partner, keeping a close eye on each other. Inadvertently coming across another person ill or injured is not uncommon, and needs to be managed in accordance with the urgency of your task; priorities should be reconciled with the assistance of the control centre.

Equipment

Choice and carriage of equipment is very important when accessing scenes and will vary greatly depending on the skills of the provider. Typically, a minimum of oxygen, suction, medication kit with approved medications and a monitor/defibrillator would be carried to all scenes. Emergency healthcare professionals will need to consider whether other specialised equipment which is not routinely carried may be required (such as maternity packs, pelvic sheeting, burns dressings, etc). Emergency healthcare responders need to keep a close eye on their equipment, as it is not uncommon for equipment to be left behind or even taken by bystanders. Equipment taken to the side of the patient and opened also requires time to repack, and in certain circumstances it may be prudent to expeditiously load the patient and commence treatment in the ambulance rather than take all equipment to the patient.

BOX 10.7 **Extrication process/steps**[32]

1. Protection of the scene—avoid further collisions by marking the scene and fending off with vehicles, and mitigate obvious risks such as downed power lines, fire or leaking fuel.
2. Stabilisation of the vehicle by blocks or cribbing to prevent unintended movement.
3. Patient assessment, triage and first aid.
4. Creation of space by cutting or opening the structure with tools.
5. Removal of the patient(s) (physical extrication) from the vehicle with the least amount of movement consistent with urgency of their clinical needs. Where patients are physically compressed, this is called disentanglement.

Patient extrication

Theory of extrication

Vehicle extrication is the process of removing or deforming parts of a vehicle from around a person following a motor vehicle accident, where conventional means of exit are impossible or hazardous. There are several steps to all extrications, as outlined in Box 10.7.

A practical approach to extrication is to seek to perform the least effort for the greatest gain. Typically, effort is associated with increased time on scene and often unnecessary delay. For example, if a patient could be safely extricated from a crashed vehicle by simply removing a single door, then this is likely to be more appropriate than removing the roof and the entire side of the vehicle. Extrication must be tailored to meet the specific needs of the patient, the severity of illness or injury, the environment and the available resources (Figs 10.8 to 10.12).

Indications for rapid extrication[32]

Rapid extrication is indicated when the clinical condition of the patient mandates urgent clinical interventions which

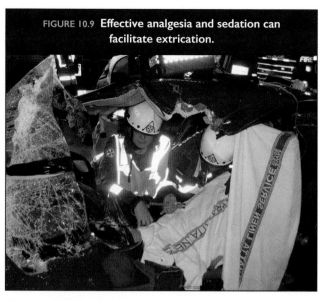

FIGURE 10.9 **Effective analgesia and sedation can facilitate extrication.**

Courtesy of NSW Ambulance.

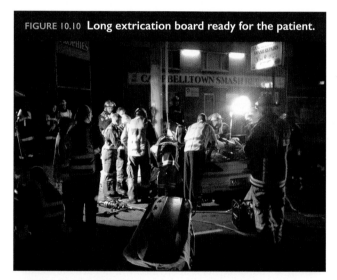

FIGURE 10.10 **Long extrication board ready for the patient.**

Courtesy of NSW Ambulance.

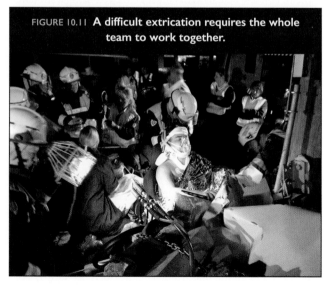

FIGURE 10.11 **A difficult extrication requires the whole team to work together.**

Courtesy of NSW Ambulance.

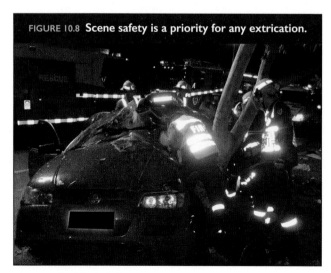

FIGURE 10.8 **Scene safety is a priority for any extrication.**

Courtesy of NSW Ambulance.

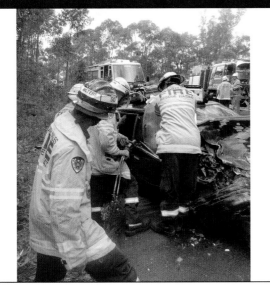

FIGURE 10.12 **Hydraulic cutting tools being used by rescuers.**

Courtesy of NSW Ambulance.

cannot be delivered in situ. Rapid extrication is indicated for the following situations:

1. deteriorating level of consciousness or haemodynamic parameters
2. penetrating trauma to the torso
3. threatened airway unable to be managed on the scene
4. uncontrolled haemorrhage
5. potentially reversible life-threatening medical conditions such as myocardial infarction or cardiac arrhythmia.

Following extrication, the patient should be reassessed and immediately life-threatening conditions treated, followed by rapid transport to a centre able to provide definitive care.

PRACTICE TIP

Decisions about the speed of extrication are inevitably a compromise between reducing patient movement (especially of the spinal column) and enabling life-threatening injuries to be managed effectively. Discussion with the designated rescue agency should ALWAYS include an estimate of time required for standard extrication but with a Plan B briefed in case of patient deterioration.

Techniques of extrication

There are many techniques and types of specialised rescue equipment used for extrication of patients, and it is beyond the scope of this book to describe the more technical aspects. An excellent online resource on vehicle extrication techniques is available at http://www.neann.com/pdf/vet.pdf.

The key role of emergency healthcare providers is to access the patients (where safe to do so) and control and coordinate their clinical management. It is vital to liaise closely with rescue services regarding the extrication plan and have a plan B to expedite in case of sudden clinical deterioration. Emergency medical care providers must have a good understanding of commonly used

extrication equipment such as stretchers and spinal boards, and extrication aids such as the Kendrick Extrication Device (KED) or Neann Immobilisation and Extrication Jacket (NEIJ).

Scene egress

Planning egress from the scene is a key component in the overall management of ill or injured patients, and this planning should begin at the initial scene assessment. The route taken to access the patient may not be the best way of leaving the scene, particularly if the patient is immobile or stretcher-bound.[31] Emergency healthcare providers must carefully plan the egress route considering terrain (surface, gradient, stairs), patient condition, ongoing treatment (oxygen, intravenous fluids etc) and the need for, and manipulation of, a stretcher or carry-chair. Ambulance vehicle egress becomes another important factor, especially in urban environments, and nowhere is this more important than when multiple units respond to an incident, where subsequently arriving vehicles can interfere with egress routes.

Management of specific hazards

Remote clinical access

Remote areas are defined as inaccessible or difficult-to-access places due to their terrain (dense bush, mountains, coastlines, water, etc) or extreme distances from transport infrastructure (Fig 10.13). Remote clinical access refers to the ability to attend, triage, treat and evacuate[33] patients who are ill or injured in areas inaccessible to usual EMS resources such as road ambulances.

The skills and procedures required for remote access overlap significantly with other aspects of 'difficult' access missions such as confined space, safety at heights and helicopter operations; details of these will be considered within their respective sections. The defining nature of remote clinical access missions is that they all require a team approach and thoughtful systematic planning.

The basic principles[33] of such missions are:

1. plan
2. brief
3. execute
4. review.

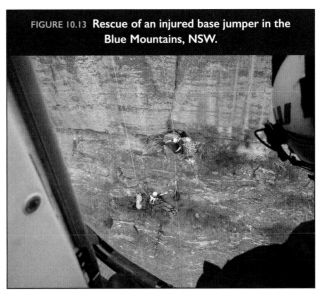

FIGURE 10.13 **Rescue of an injured base jumper in the Blue Mountains, NSW.**

Courtesy of NSW Ambulance.

Mission planning

Planning may be considered on a strategic or operational level, but both levels involve the process of gathering relevant information, determining the key priorities, assessing alternatives and coming to a final decision about the plan which must be executed. Relevant considerations include:

- logistics—requirements for food, water, equipment and additional personnel
- communication methods—direct, radio, cellular phone, satellite phone
- back-up—are there any other resources coming and do they know the 'plan'?
- helicopter resources—are these available?
- alternative/contingency plan—is there another way to do this mission?

Team briefing

The mnemonic SMEACS is a useful one; it has been adapted from the Australian armed forces guide[34] to assist in organising the briefing of a mission:

S   Situation—brief statement of the current situation

M Mission—clear explanation of the goal of the operation

E   Execution—step-by-step list of how the mission will be performed

A   Administration and logistics—description of the stores, job delegations and contingency plans

C   Communications and signals—chain of command, communications and timings

S   Safety—all identified hazards and abatements

Execution

Carry out the plan as briefed.

Review

Constant evaluation and review should take place. A time-frame for completion of the mission and an interim set of goals to work towards can assist in this process.

Safety at heights

Falls from heights are the most common cause of fatal injury to employees in Australia[35] and worldwide,[36] and a growing cause of injury and death in domestic settings as well.[37] Emergency medical service staff must understand the risks of accessing patients at height and ensure that these risks are minimised.

Settings in which to consider safety at heights

There are a broad range of relevant settings, including:

- roof structures
- building sites
- industrial sites
- ladders
- trees
- cliff edges/mountains
- truck or other large vehicle extrications.

The keys to working safely at heights are constant vigilance on the part of each individual team member in regard to their movements and actions, and the use of anchors to secure all personnel and equipment at risk of falling.[33,38]

Casualties who require consideration of safety at heights during their rescue have most commonly fallen from above, and

consequently there is always the risk that an unstable structure (or debris that is about to fall) is directly above the casualty; this must be considered and anticipated on approaching the scene. Wherever possible, the patient should be removed from a dangerous position as early as possible during their treatment. This 'rule' applies to all pre-hospital situations and settings, but vigilance is even more vital where risk of falling from height exists.

As well as individual awareness of the dangers, it is important to appoint a 'safety officer' who is not involved in any other activities to supervise the safety of the team. All staff should remain 2 metres or more from hazardous edges at all times unless secured to an anchor. If there is a need to look over an edge before an anchor is set up, then the safest way is to lie prone and inch slowly up to the edge. Remember that edges that are unstable or undermined may give way when weight is applied from above.

In any situation where there will be prolonged exposure to the risk of falling from a height, it is essential that anchors are

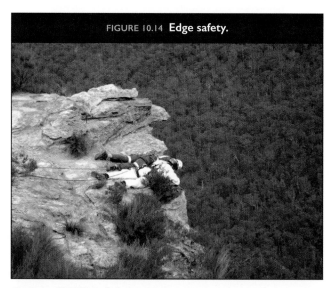

FIGURE 10.14 **Edge safety.**

Courtesy of NSW Ambulance.

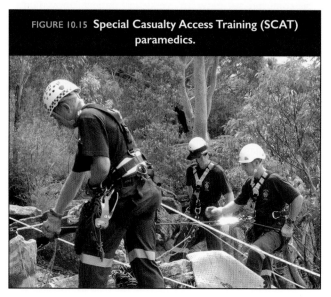

FIGURE 10.15 **Special Casualty Access Training (SCAT) paramedics.**

Courtesy of NSW Ambulance.

secured and all staff and equipment are tied to an anchor in such a way as to avoid or minimise injury should they fall. Anchors should be set up by appropriately trained rescue staff and must be capable of sustaining the intended load of personnel or equipment, including 'shock-loading' due to sudden falls where there is slack in attachment lines. Attachment lines must be kept as short as possible and always shorter than the distance to the edge.

In some cases it is necessary for rescue teams to descend to the casualty by way of roping equipment such as belay systems. This must only be undertaken by appropriately credentialled rescue operators who undertake regular training in the use of ropes, anchors and climbing equipment.[1] Such technical aspects are beyond the scope of this book to describe.

Caves and confined spaces

Caves and other confined spaces pose significant dangers to those who must work within them and those who choose to recreate within them. Access and rescue of patients suffering illness or injury from confined spaces presents many hazards to rescuers and clinical teams, and should only be undertaken by staff with appropriate training and a thorough understanding of the risks.

A confined space is any space of an enclosed nature where there is risk to human health from dangerous conditions or hazardous substances. Some examples of enclosed spaces include:

- mine shafts
- caves
- collapsed buildings
- machinery rooms
- silos
- storage tanks
- drains or sewers
- small, poorly ventilated rooms or compartments.

Possible hazards of enclosed spaces

A range of dangers may exist within enclosed spaces, as listed below,[38,39] and the mnemonic 3TVIPS should be followed (Box 10.8).

- irrespirable atmospheres
- toxic substances or residues
- fires/explosions
- physical injury due to falls, moving equipment, unstable structures, etc
- environmental exposure—hypothermia, hyperthermia

BOX 10.8 Confined space operations mnemonic—3TVIPS[33]

T Test (oxygen)
T Test (flammable)
T Test (toxic)
V Ventilate (prior and after)
I Isolate (lock out/tag out)
P Personal protective equipment
S Safety and standby teams

- electrical hazards
- concentrations of dust
- psychological responses
- confined space operations.

Confined space entry

Prior to entering confined spaces, it is essential to assess the risks involved and be prepared for potential hazards. The following vital elements should be considered.

- *Risk assessment*—the safety of the entry teams must be the prime consideration.
- *Safety officer*—a single individual should be appointed to this role, and they must remain outside the dangerous environment to oversee the operation.
- *Communications*—confirm communication systems and back-up communication plan. Such a plan must also include a specific determination of when to send a back-up team if contact is lost.
- *Team assembly*—ensure that all staff entering the hazardous area have had the relevant training to be competent in confined space access. Such training usually includes hazard identification and mitigation, escape and rescue procedures and confidence with PPE, lighting, communications and environmental monitoring equipment. Record all staff in and out (tag in/out).
- *PPE*—check all staff have appropriate PPE. This must include adequate means of illumination, with back-up in case of failure.
- *Safe atmosphere*—set up atmospheric monitoring and maximise ventilation. Atmospheric monitoring using multi-gas detection systems must be undertaken prior to rescuer access.

Specific hazards of enclosed spaces/caves
Hazardous/irrespirable atmospheres

High concentrations of gases can displace oxygen from the atmosphere in enclosed spaces. This is particularly common in underground settings, where gas may naturally vent from surrounding rocks and where heavier-than-air gases such as carbon dioxide collect in particular areas. Where concentrations

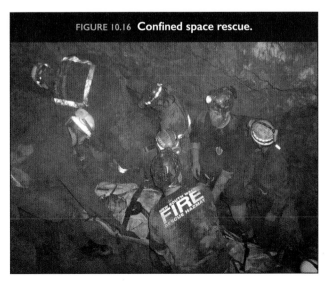

FIGURE 10.16 **Confined space rescue.**

Courtesy K Harbig, NSW Ambulance.

of such gases rise sufficiently to displace a significant proportion of the atmospheric oxygen, there is a risk of hypoxic asphyxia. In addition, any inhaled gases may have their own toxic effects. The most common three such gases are carbon dioxide, carbon monoxide and 'sewer gas'.[39]

- 'Foul air' refers to an atmosphere with a high level of carbon dioxide. Carbon dioxide is a colourless and odourless gas that causes physiological effects in proportion to its concentration. Symptoms begin at concentrations as low as 1%,[39] with initial headache, increased respiratory rate and 'panting' respirations. Death is possible at concentrations as low as 10%. Treatment is removal from the toxic atmosphere and administration of 100% oxygen.

- Carbon monoxide is produced by the incomplete combustion of carbon fuels, and is also odourless and colourless. It may build up due to emissions from internal-combustion engines or from poorly ventilated gas or charcoal fires. Once inhaled, it binds preferentially to circulating haemoglobin and displaces oxygen from red blood cells. Early symptoms include headache, nausea and confusion, followed by coma. Treatment is removal from the source and administration of 100% oxygen.

- Sewer gas[38] comprises a variable combination of hydrogen sulfide, methane, sulfur dioxide and trichloroethylene. These gases are poisonous and highly explosive, making them a particular risk when naked flames or cutting tools are used. Treatment is removal from the source and administration of 100% oxygen.

Fires/explosions

Flammable gases (such as methane) or vapours (such as petroleum vapour) and dusts (such as coal dust or grain dust) are a threat to rescuers in many environments, but particularly in mines and industry. Naked flames pose a high risk in such environments and should never be used unless continuous atmospheric monitoring can be undertaken.

Physical injury

Enclosed spaces present a multitude of ways in which the rescuer can become a victim. These range from rock falls, trip hazards and slippery surfaces in caves to unstable structures and falling debris in damaged buildings. Enclosed spaces with tight passages present a real risk of entrapment due to rescuers becoming physically jammed within tight passages or spaces and unable to extricate themselves. The entrapped person then may succumb to physical restriction on chest excursion, hypothermia or dehydration.

Psychological responses

It is easy for inexperienced staff to become disoriented and lost in enclosed spaces, and particularly in cave systems. Fear and panic can threaten the safety of rescuers unused to these environments.

Helicopter EMS operations

Helicopters are a vital part of EMS responses around the world. There is a large variety of aircraft types, capabilities and crew mix, but in general the utility of helicopters in pre-hospital responses relates to their ability to gain access to difficult scenes, extricate the patient and rapidly transport them 'as the crow flies' to definitive treatment, usually with an enhanced

level of clinical care over typical ground EMS responses. The ability to call for helicopter EMS (HEMS) support can provide a vital link in the chain of survival for patients suffering major trauma[40] or medical illness remote from major hospital resources. An understanding by each EMS provider of the capabilities of their local HEMS response is vital in decision-making about utilising these resources.

PRACTICE TIPS

The indications for calling for a HEMS response comprise:

- Patient access issues (need for winchings, etc)
- Rapid transport requirements (critically ill remote from suitable hospital, etc)
- Provision of enhanced clinical resources (medical teams, etc)

Access problems requiring helicopters

Helicopters are able to take off and land vertically, and can land in unprepared sites distant from road infrastructure. Helicopters equipped with a winch or 'long-line' provide even more flexibility, and allow clinical and/or rescue teams to directly access ill or injured parties where no suitable helicopter landing zone exists near the scene, such as with wilderness areas, mountains, coastal zones, oceans, boats or waterways (Figs 10.17 and 10.18). Access issues requiring helicopter response most commonly involve a patient who is ill or injured in a location remote from roads and therefore remote from a standard road EMS response. Other scenarios where access by helicopter may be preferable include extreme road conditions that inhibit usual road responses, such as following an earthquake, flood, rock fall or extreme road traffic congestion.

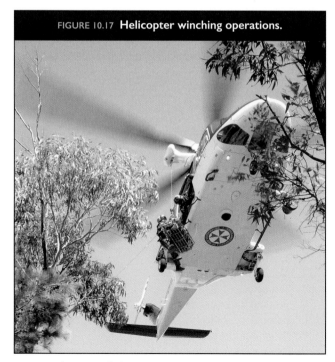

FIGURE 10.17 **Helicopter winching operations.**

Courtesy of NSW Ambulance.

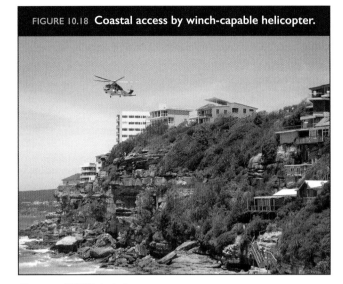

FIGURE 10.18 **Coastal access by winch-capable helicopter.**

Courtesy of NSW Ambulance.

Rapid transport capability

Critically unwell patients likely to have prolonged transport times to definitive care may benefit from aeromedical helicopter transport.[41] In general, helicopters are able to provide faster transfer times (from emergency call to arrival in hospital) where anticipated road transport times exceed 20 minutes or approximately 16 km when tasked simultaneously, and approximately 60 km where helicopter dispatch occurs after road ambulance arrival and report.[42] Transport times must always factor-in the time for engine start-up and spool-down at each end of the transfer. Helicopters have the advantage of travelling 'as the crow flies' at speeds between 220 and 300 kph[42] and are not subject to issues of road traffic congestion or limited by terrain. They can also take the patient from the scene directly to the most appropriate hospital, bypassing smaller hospitals if needed.

Enhanced clinical resources

Worldwide, HEMS typically provides enhanced clinical resources and crewing over standard road-based paramedical systems. In Australia, Europe and the UK, HEMS crew mix is most commonly a doctor and a paramedic or flight nurse team. In the USA, most HEMSs utilise a paramedic or flight nurse team only, though usually these teams have significantly higher levels of training and skills than the road-based EMS systems where they operate. Critical interventions available to HEMSs include emergency pre-hospital anaesthesia, procedural sedation and more-advanced pharmacological interventions, and advanced surgical interventions such as thoracostomy or amputation.

Helicopter landing zones

Once the decision has been made to call for HEMS support the next important step, where possible, is to identify and prepare a suitable helicopter landing zone (LZ). The largest flat, open and unobstructed area close to the accident scene should be chosen for the LZ. Consider carefully hazards to helicopter flight or landing such as buildings, towers, wires, animals, loose objects or debris. Helicopters will always try to land 'into wind' (towards the wind direction), and so wind direction is a crucial

factor in the approach path. The LZ must be a minimum of 25 m × 25 m and preferably 40 m × 40 m in size.

By day, a ground-marshalling officer wearing appropriate PPE (including ear, eye and head protection and safety vest) standing at the upwind end of the area with their back to the wind should indicate the area. If a smoke flare is available, it should be activated when the aircraft approaches overhead to show position, wind direction and wind speed (Fig 10.19). If the area is large enough (40 m × 40 m) and there are sufficient responsible ground personnel, then four people standing one at each corner should indicate the area. At night, the four corners of the area should be indicated using vehicles, lights or 'Cyalume' (glow) sticks. Information helpful to the HEMS team is outlined in Box 10.9 and a landing plan is given in Figure 10.20.

Helicopter safety

Working around helicopters poses risks to EMS providers. Apart from the obvious risk of injury or death due to contact with moving main or tail rotors, hazards also include injury due to 'downwash' (which is proportional to the size of the helicopter), and dust or debris being blown around, particularly into the eyes causing temporary blindness. The same rules of safety around helicopters should apply whether the helicopter's engines and rotors are running or shut down, and are outlined in Box 10.10 and shown in Figures 10.21 to 10.26.

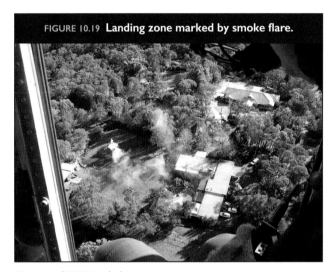

FIGURE 10.19 **Landing zone marked by smoke flare.**

Courtesy of NSW Ambulance.

BOX 10.9 **Information helpful to the HEMS team**

- Location—GPS coordinates (latitude and longitude) if possible or street-grid map reference.
- Weather—wind speed and direction, fog, rain, clouds, temperature.
- Obstacles on approach—wires, towers, buildings, trees, bystanders, animals.
- Supporting resources on scene—ambulance service commander, police, rescue, etc.
- Patient details—e.g. MIST-formatted report (Mechanism, Injuries, Signs and Treatment).
- Landing site—terrain, slope, surface, dust conditions.

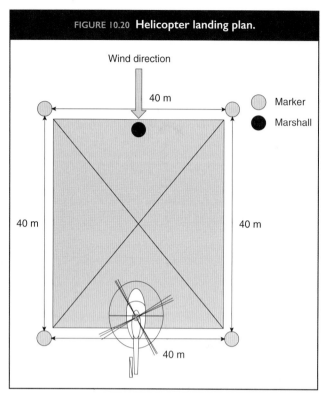

FIGURE 10.20 Helicopter landing plan.

Courtesy Dr Jason Bendall.

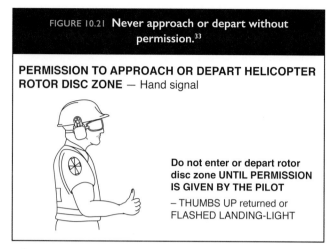

FIGURE 10.21 Never approach or depart without permission.[33]

PERMISSION TO APPROACH OR DEPART HELICOPTER ROTOR DISC ZONE — Hand signal

Do not enter or depart rotor disc zone UNTIL PERMISSION IS GIVEN BY THE PILOT
– THUMBS UP returned or FLASHED LANDING-LIGHT

Edgar C. SCAT (Special Casualty Access Training) reference text. NSW Ambulance, 2006.

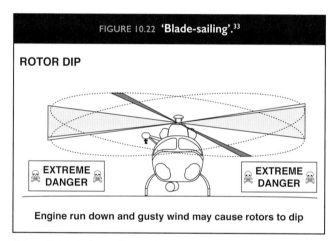

FIGURE 10.22 'Blade-sailing'.[33]

ROTOR DIP

☠ EXTREME DANGER ☠   ☠ EXTREME DANGER ☠

Engine run down and gusty wind may cause rotors to dip

Edgar C. SCAT (Special Casualty Access Training) reference text. NSW Ambulance, 2006.

BOX 10.10 Helicopter safety[33]

- Remain clear of the helicopter at all times unless accompanied by a helicopter crewperson.
- Follow all instructions (verbal or hand signal) given by the helicopter pilot and flight crew.
- During engine shut-down in gusty winds, the helicopter blades may dip below head height ('blade-sailing'). Do not approach the helicopter until the rotor blades have ceased rotating.
- If blinded by helicopter downwash or dust, sit down and await assistance.
- When approaching the helicopter always approach from the front—in the 'ten-to-two-o'clock' safe area of the helicopter—and depart in the same direction.
- Never walk around or approach a helicopter from the tail-rotor area.
- When approaching a helicopter on a slope, always approach from the downhill side.
- Never reach for, especially above head height, or chase after articles which have blown away.
- Intravenous drips or other objects must be carried below shoulder level at all times, and long objects carried parallel to the ground between two officers.

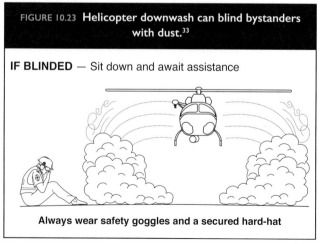

FIGURE 10.23 Helicopter downwash can blind bystanders with dust.[33]

IF BLINDED — Sit down and await assistance

Always wear safety goggles and a secured hard-hat

Edgar C. SCAT (Special Casualty Access Training) reference text. NSW Ambulance, 2006.

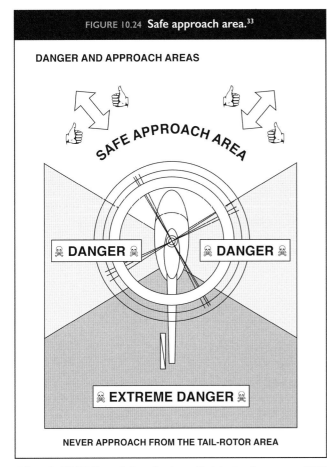

FIGURE 10.24 **Safe approach area.**[33]

Edgar C. SCAT (Special Casualty Access Training) reference text. NSW Ambulance, 2006.

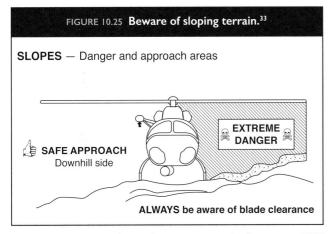

FIGURE 10.25 **Beware of sloping terrain.**[33]

Edgar C. SCAT (Special Casualty Access Training) reference text. NSW Ambulance, 2006.

Railway incidents

Railway incidents present a multitude of dangers to rescuers, and working close to railway lines requires a great deal of common sense, understanding of the components of railway systems and careful coordination of operations. The most common reason for EMSs to need to access railway lines is a person falling or jumping onto tracks. Patients injured or trapped beneath trains

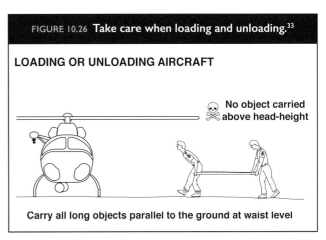

FIGURE 10.26 **Take care when loading and unloading.**[33]

Edgar C. SCAT (Special Casualty Access Training) reference text. NSW Ambulance, 2006.

represent a great challenge to rescuers and require a coordinated multidisciplinary approach.

Possible hazards at railway incidents
Such hazards include:
- contact with moving trains/rolling stock
- electrical injury from overhead systems, the 'third rail', pylons and signalling systems
- mechanical track-switching equipment
- trip/slip hazards
- falling from platforms.

In Australia the majority of railway lines operate with overhead power systems that supply electricity to the engine units through lines at up to 25,000 volts. While the supporting pylons are not electrified, all lines or wires suspended from them should be considered so. Electrical injury can result from contact or even close proximity to overhead power transmission lines due to arcing, and so all personnel, clothing and equipment must be kept back at least 3 m from overhead lines. If there are powered rails—the 'third rail'—then it must be confirmed that power has been cut to all lines prior to anyone accessing the track area.

Never go on or near railway lines or cross rails (except at marked level crossings) unless there is no alternative. Before entering the vicinity of railway tracks, it must be confirmed that the track is safe and that trains have been stopped on those lines. Be aware that electric trains can coast for a significant distance even when the power is cut. If trains cannot be stopped on all lines in the vicinity, then ensure that everyone has a clear understanding of the direction trains will move in, and have a lookout stationed for protection. It is worth assuming that trains can come from either direction at any time. High-visibility vests with reflective markings should be worn whenever accessing the track area.

Besides the obvious dangers of electricity and fast-moving vehicles, working close to or on railway tracks poses serious risks from falls or trips. Rail lines are a tripping hazard and become slippery, particularly in wet weather, as can timber sleepers. It is much safer to walk on the ballast (stone chippings) or use over-bridges or other safer routes where possible. Training and coordination are no substitute for constant vigilance at all times in this challenging environment.

Water rescue

The aquatic environment refers to open ocean/sea, coastal zones, beaches, dams (natural or man-made), lakes, creeks/rivers, swimming pools or flooded urban environments (stormwater drains, flooded streets or buildings). These environments pose a wide variety of hazards to rescuers.

Possible hazards of water rescue include:

- drowning/immersion
- hypothermia
- ocean waves, tides, rips
- hidden sand-bars or rocks
- slip hazards on rocks/rock pools
- whitewater/rapids
- boats—collision, propellers
- debris in running water
- underwater snags
- disease due to contaminated water
- sea creatures—sharks, venomous stingers, etc.

Access to patients in open water or on boats requires very specialised rescue skills and equipment, but rescuers and EMS staff may be called to a casualty requiring rescue in an inland or inshore waterway without immediate access to additional resources.

Inshore/inland waterway rescue

The principle of inshore and inland waterway water rescue is to Reach, Throw, Wade, Row and only finally consider Swim and Tow.[38]

This means that where possible it is much better to reach out to a person using a pole or branch than to enter the water to effect a rescue. If this is not possible, the next best option is to throw a rope, life-preserver or other buoyant object to the person. If you can wade out to the person safely then this is the next option, but rescuers must beware of fast-flowing water in rivers or streams and unseen underwater hazards. If a boat is available, then this may be utilised in the rescue. There is always the risk of capsize, particularly in a small dinghy if a panicked casualty tries to clamber aboard unsafely. In inshore rescues such as at a beach, a boat such as a powered inflatable or water bike may be the only safe way of accessing the patient. Only if all other options are exhausted should one ever consider swimming to the victim and attempting to tow them back to shore. This should only be contemplated with appropriate equipment such as personal inflatable life-preservers and safety lines with enough assistants to pull both the victim and the rescuer out of the water. Finally, a winch-equipped helicopter may be able to access the patient most safely; however, such specialised resources require time to reach the scene (Fig 10.27).

Violent presentations

Apart from dangers posed by the pre-hospital environment, patients themselves can pose a risk to emergency medical crews. There is evidence that violent attacks on paramedics are common and increasing in frequency.[43] Patients or bystanders may be violent for a variety of reasons, including alcohol intoxication, use of drugs such as methamphetamines and cocaine, psychiatric conditions such as schizophrenia,

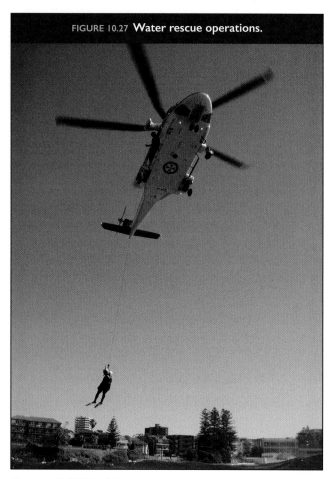

FIGURE 10.27 **Water rescue operations.**

Courtesy of NSW Ambulance.

psychosis or personality disorder, dementia, head injury or medical illness such as hypoglycaemia or epilepsy. The risk of violence to EMS staff increases in cases of domestic dispute, where the patient has been the subject of a violent act such as stabbing or shooting, in large crowds or in episodes of civil disturbance.[43]

Violent behaviour may come after clear warning signs with a period of escalation, but may occasionally come without warning. When approaching a scene it is essential to learn to look beyond the usual physical and environmental threats to safety, and consider risks from patients, family or bystanders. Where a risk of violence is perceived or anticipated, police should be called as early as possible. This should be a routine policy for any incident where a person has been injured by someone else (especially where firearms or knives are suspected), or where there is a previous history of violent or criminal behaviour. Most ambulance service dispatch systems enable flagging of such individuals and incidents so that police are dispatched simultaneously. Never enter such an incident until police are present and have confirmed that the scene is safe. Ask whether the alleged assailant has been secured.

On occasion, EMS providers find themselves arriving at a scene where a domestic or other dispute is occurring or recurs on their arrival. In such cases it is important to have training and knowledge of how to de-escalate an aggressive situation (Ch 37).

De-escalation

Where possible, always position yourself close to an exit and keep yourself and your partner between the aggressor and the exit.[38,44] Lower the tone and volume of speech, to convey calmness. Be polite, and address the person by name if possible. Maintain eye contact in a non-threatening manner. Stand at least 1 m from the person and ask permission before any action which may be seen as an invasion of personal space. People involved in a heated argument are usually highly emotional and not thinking logically. Asking questions relevant to the patient's condition can help the person revert to logical behaviour. Remove distractions from the scene, such as bystanders, and do not allow others to interact with the person.

Mental health considerations

The legislative framework for management of patients with a mental illness or mental disorder differs between states of Australia and throughout the world.[45-47] EMS providers must ensure that they understand the particular rights and obligations of themselves and their patients in the jurisdiction where they work. In all states of Australia and many places in the world, EMS providers have the power under legislation to detain a person against their will for the purposes of transportation to a mental health facility for further evaluation and treatment, where that person refuses voluntary transport and where that patient's behaviour is such that it presents a risk of serious harm to themselves or others. Police will often be involved in assisting with this process. Police generally have similar powers to enact involuntary transport of patients to a mental health service or facility for the purposes of further assessment or treatment. Physical restraint by EMS providers may be allowed under local standard operating procedures, and police have further powers of restraint. Chemical restraint, or administration of psychoactive medications for behavioural control, is generally only permitted under the direction of a medical practitioner (Ch 37).

SUMMARY

Assessment and management begins long before any arrival at the scene of an injury or an illness. The key principles of safety, including dispatch and pre-arrival information, planned and cautious travel to scene, personal protective equipment, planning an approach to the scene and careful and meticulous scene assessment, pave the way for the next stage of systematic patient assessment and structured intervention. Much of this may be summarised in the first stage of Caroline's Six Rs of Paramedic Practice—read the scene (Box 10.11).

BOX 10.11 Caroline's Six Rs of Paramedic Practice[22]

1. **READ THE SCENE**—scan the environment, review the surroundings, gather information regarding mechanisms of injury, identify and resolve dangers or threats to safety.
2. **READ THE PATIENT**—observe the patient, talk with the patient and others, take vital signs, identify life-threatening conditions, obtain complete vital signs through primary and secondary survey.
3. **REACT**—discern the patient's problems, determine provisional diagnosis, provide treatment, develop and implement plan for outcome.
4. **RE-EVALUATE**—obtain revised patient data, examine response to treatment, discern secondary problems and their significance, provide treatment, suitability of outcome.
5. **REVISE THE PLAN**—reconsider the plan and goal for achieving the outcome in light of emerging changes identified during ongoing data collection and analysis.
6. **REVIEW YOUR PERFORMANCE**—reflect on the case using continuous quality improvement. Integrate review outcomes into future practice.

Adapted from Caroline N. Nancy Caroline's Emergency care in the streets. 6th edn. Sudbury, MA: Jones and Bartlett; 2008.

CASE STUDY

You have responded to a three-car motor vehicle collision on the highway approximately 30 minutes south of the regional town where you work. There have been multiple calls and regular updates arriving via the mobile data terminal indicating the severity of the incident. There is a report of one car on fire, multiple patients and one vehicle over a 5-m steep embankment with both the driver and a passenger trapped. As you approach the scene, you find traffic not moving in either direction with a significant amount of smoke in the area. You are the first emergency service to arrive at the scene; however, the police, fire rescue and other emergency service resources are on the way. You find many bystanders already on the scene. The Control Centre has launched the Helicopter Emergency Medical Service (HEMS) from the closest facility, which will be overhead in approximately 45 minutes.

Questions

1. Describe the key principles of your initial scene assessment.
2. Describe key considerations regarding scene access and egress.
3. Describe the principles of patient extrication following vehicular collisions.
4. Describe key considerations when dealing with bystanders and other emergency services.
5. Describe the principles for establishing a landing site for the helicopter.

 Answers to Case Study Questions can be found on evolve
http://evolve.emergencytrauma.curtis

USEFUL WEBSITES

http://ambofoam.wordpress.com—an interesting and insightful blog by a Victorian ICP

http://prehospitalpro.com—another great blog from a Victorian ICP

www.prehospitalblog.com—humourous but enlightening blog by a US-based paramedic

http://prehospitalmed.com—Prehospital and Retrieval Medicine blog by a Queensland-based retrieval doctor

REFERENCES

1. NSW Health. Calling an ambulance. Online. www0.health.nsw.gov.au/hospitals/going_to_hospital/ambulance.asp; accessed 18 Feb 2015.

2. National Academies of Emergency Dispatch. What is MPDS? Online. www.emergencydispatch.org/articles/whatis.html; accessed 18 Feb 2015.

3. Roppolo LP, Pepe PE, Cimon N et al. Modified cardiopulmonary resuscitation (CPR) instruction protocols for emergency medical dispatchers: rationale and recommendations. Resuscitation 2005;65(2):203–10.

4. Bailey ED, O'Connor RE, Ross RW. The use of emergency medical dispatch protocols to reduce the number of inappropriate scene responses made by advanced life support personnel. Prehosp Emerg Care 2000;4(2):186–9.

5. Fire Brigades Act 192 of 1989, Part 3. Fighting and preventing fires and dealing with hazardous material incidents. As at 29 October 2010. Online. www.austlii.edu.au/au/legis/nsw/consol_act/fba1989112/; accessed 18 Feb 2015.

6. Lutman D, Montgomery M, Ramnarayan P et al. Ambulance and aeromedical accident rates during emergency retrieval in Great Britain. Emerg Med J 2008;25(5):301–2.

7. Maguire BJ, Hunting KL, Smith GS et al. Occupational fatalities in emergency medical services: a hidden crisis. Ann Emerg Med 2002;40(6):625–32.

8. Biggers WA Jr, Zachariah BS, Pepe PE. Emergency medical vehicle collisions in an urban system. Prehosp Disaster Med 1996;11(3): 195–201.

9. Solomon SS. Emergency response and vehicle operation. In: Solomon SS, Hill PF, eds. Emergency vehicle accidents: prevention, reconstruction and survey of state law. Tucson, AZ: Lawyers and Judges Publishing Company Ltd; 2002:89–93.

10. National Transportation Safety Board report by Chairman James L. Kolstad dated January 4, 1991 regarding the incident in Catlett, Virginia on September 28, 1989. Further citation in Firefighter's News 1990;Aug–Sep;36–7.

11. Elling R. Dispelling myths on ambulance accidents. J Emerg Med Serv 1989;14(7):60–4.

12. EMS Safety: techniques and applications. US fire administration. Online. www.usfa.dhs.gov/downloads/pdf/publications/fa-144.pdf; accessed 18 Feb 2015.

13. Pittet D, Allegranzi B, Boyce J. World Health Organization, World Alliance for Patient Safety First: Global Patient Safety Challenge core group of experts. The World Health Organization guidelines on hand hygiene in health care and their consensus recommendations. Infect Control Hosp Epidemiol 2009;30(7):611–22.

14. McLaws ML, Pantle AC, Fitzpatrick KR et al. Improvements in hand hygiene across New South Wales public hospitals: clean hands save lives, part III. Med J Aust 2009;191(8 Suppl):S18–24.

15. O'Leary MR, ed. Dictionary of homeland security and defense. iUniverse, Inc; 2006:215. Online. http://en.wikipedia.org/wiki/Splash_suit#cite_note-0.

16. Naval Sea Systems Command. Protective Clothing—Hazmat Gear Online. www.dcfpnavymil.org/Personnel%20Protection/HMUG/OPNAVINST_5100.28_(Previous_HMUG).pdf; accessed 18 Feb 2015.

17. Australasian Fire and Emergency Service Authorities Council (AFAC). How we operate. Online. www.afac.com.au/about/operate; accessed 18 Feb 2015.

18. Advanced Life Support Group. MIMMS: the practical approach at the scene. Online. http://onlinelibrary.wiley.com/book/10.1002/9781444398236; accessed 4 Dec 2010.

19. Greaves I, Hodgetts T, Porter K. Emergency care. A textbook for paramedics. London: WB Saunders; 1997;2.

20. EMS Safety: Techniques and Applications. Federal emergency management agency. United States Fire Administration. Online. Available: www.usfa.dhs.gov/downloads/pdf/publications/fa-144.pdf; 23 Aug 2010.

21. Ambulance Service of New South Wales 2003. Skills Manual Index Section 4, Patient Assessment.104.12 Scene management procedure.

22. Caroline N. Nancy Caroline's Emergency care in the streets. 6th edn. Sudbury, MA: Jones and Bartlett; 2008.

23. National Highway Traffic Safety Administration. Emergency medical technician: basic refresher curriculum instructor course guide. US Department of Transport EMT—Basic National Standard Curriculum, 1994.

24. Dangerous goods. Online. http://en.wikipedia.org/wiki/Dangerous_goods#Classification_and_labeling_summary_tables; 23 Aug 2010.

25. National Chemical Emergency Centre. Dangerous goods emergency actions codes list 2009. AEA Group, Norwich. Online. http://the-ncec.com/hazchem; accessed 19 Dec 2010.

26. Wong K, Levy RD. Interhospital transfers of patients with surgical emergencies: areas for improvement. Aust J Rural Health 2005;13(5):290–4.

27. Mikos K. Monitoring handoffs for standardization. Nurs Manag 2007;38(12):16–20.

28. Alem L, Joseph M, Kethers S et al. Information environments for supporting consistent registrar medical handover. Health Inf Manag J 2008;37(1):9–25.

29. Hodgetts TJ, Abraham K, Homer T, eds. Major incident medical management and support. The practical approach (Australian supplement). Sydney: SWSAHS Staff Development Unit; 1995.

30. Eaton CJ. Essentials of immediate medical care, 2nd edn. Edinburgh: Churchill Livingstone; 2006.

31. Calland V. Safety at scene. A manual. rev. edn 2005 aLL2easyIT Ltd.

32. Moore R. Vehicle rescue life cycle. In: Moore R, ed. Vehicle rescue and extrication. 2nd edn. Mosby: JEMS; 2003.

33. Edgar C. SCAT (Special Casualty Access Training) reference text. Ambulance Service of NSW; 2006.

34. Australian Armed Forces. Procedures guide. Online. www.australianarmedforces.org/AFPG/; accessed 5 Nov 2010.

35. Australian Bureau of Statistics. Australian social trends 2007—work-related injuries. Online. www.abs.gov.au/ausstats/abs@.nsf/0/63ED457234C2F22DCA25732C002080A7?opendocument; accessed 18 Feb 2015.

36. Health and Safety Commission, UK. Statistics of workplace fatalities and injuries—falls from a height. National statistics. Online. www.hse.gov.uk/statistics/pdf/rhsfall.pdf; accessed 18 Feb 2015.

37. Australian Bureau of Statistics. 3303.0 Causes of death, Australia, 2007.

38. Calland V. Safety at scene: safety at scene manual for pre-hospital emergency care providers and police officers. Revised 1st edn. aLL2easyIT August 2008.

39. Queensland Government. A guide to working in confined spaces. 2003.

40. Thomas SH, Harrison TH, Buras WR et al. Helicopter transport and blunt trauma mortality: a multicentre trial. J Trauma 2002;52(1):136–45.

41. Frankema SP, Ringburg AN, Steyerberg EW et al. Beneficial effect of helicopter emergency medical services on survival of severely injured patients. Br J Surg 2004;91(11):1520–6.

42. Diaz MA, Hendey GW, Bivins HG. When is the helicopter faster? A comparison of helicopter and ground ambulance transport times. J Trauma 2005;58(1):148–53.

43. Pozzi C. Exposure of prehospital providers to violence and abuse. J Emerg Nurs 1998;24(4):320–3.

44. Ambulance Service of NSW. Standard operating procedure SOP2007-075. ASNSW safety and security information for ambulance officers 28 Sept 2007.

45. Mental Health Act 2000. Queensland. Online. www.health.wa.gov.au/mhareview/resources/legislation/Qld_Mental_Health_Act_2000.pdf; accessed 19 Jul 2000.

46. NSW Mental Health Act 2007. Online. www.austlii.edu.au/au/legis/nsw/consol_act/mha2007128/.

47. Victorian Mental Health Act 1986. Online. www.mentalhealthvic.org.au/fileadmin/site_files/news_item/Mental_Health_Act_2014_Final.pdf; accessed 18 Feb 2015.

CHAPTER 11

PRE-HOSPITAL CLINICAL REASONING, TRIAGE AND COMMUNICATION

RAMON Z SHABAN AND JULIE CONSIDINE

Essentials

Clinical reasoning and critical thinking

- There is a dichotomous philosophical paradigm of classic and naturalistic decision-making.
- Theoretically, judgement and decision-making may be descriptive, normative and prescriptive.
- When it comes to judgement and decision-making, there is always the risk of irreducible uncertainty, inevitable error and unavoidable injustice.[1]
- In emergency care, clinical reasoning and critical thinking are focused on problem-solving.
- Essential to clinical reasoning is the gathering and organising of information, discerning of relevant from irrelevant data and concept formation of the patient's problem, making comparisons with similar situations and experiences, and maintaining analytical distance.
- Clinical reasoning in the emergency-care setting requires the recognition and management of uncertainty and ambiguity.
- Clinical reasoning and critical thinking must be based on information and evidence.

Protocols and triage for problem-solving

- Protocols and guidelines are designed to assist paramedics and emergency nurses with clinical thinking and clinical reasoning.
- Though important, protocols and guidelines may not always account for the finer details of the context.
- Facilitate and secure safety of the scene to reduce harm, minimise morbidity and prevent mortality.
- Triage and tag all casualties regardless of their injury or status.

Communication

- Effective communication is essential to the delivery of high-quality, pre-hospital emergency care.
- Ambulance clinical records are an essential element of pre-hospital emergency-care practice for patient assessment, care and transportation. They are factual and legal documents, and the healthcare professional's best protection from liability action.
- Ensure records are legible, timely, accurate, complete, original, factual and objective.
- If information is omitted from formal clinical records, then it is largely treated as not having occurred.

Contemporary challenges in pre-hospital emergency care: quality and safety

Within Australia, New Zealand and around the world there is an unprecedented demand for quality and safety in healthcare.[2] The provision of high-quality healthcare ultimately depends on the services provided by individual healthcare professionals. In recent times, individuals and the organisations they work within have been called to account for the quality of their clinical judgements and decisions more than ever before.[3–5] The clinical judgement and decision-making of healthcare professionals and their ability to understand, diagnose and respond to clinical problems are fundamental to the delivery of high-quality healthcare and medical care.[5,6]

The relationship between professional knowledge and research has never been more important for healthcare workers. Evidence-based practice (EBP) is central to establishing, maintaining or increasing the professional status of healthcare workers, and for exercising professional accountability. The demand for professionalism is particularly onerous for clinicians delivering frontline or primary healthcare, such as nurses, paramedics and doctors in emergency departments (EDs), whom Higgs and Jones refer to as *first-contact practitioners*.[4] For many, such as those in medicine and dentistry, achieving profession-hood has been realised through efforts spearheaded by the birth of EBP. There is a well-developed and growing international body of knowledge and research on clinical judgement and decision-making in medicine, nursing, psychology and other healthcare professions, motivated in part by the need for healthcare reform and unprecedented demands for accountability in healthcare. This literature is dominated by analyses of medical decision-making, due largely to rapid technological and biomedical advances.[7,8]

However, for some first-contact practitioners in healthcare professions, such as paramedics, the value of research in driving the demand for professionalism and quality and safety in healthcare is yet to be fully realised. Paramedic clinical judgement and decision-making, like much of ambulance practice, has not been the subject of sustained and systematic research.[9–12] Little is known about how paramedics make and account for their everyday clinical judgements and decisions in the field, or the challenges they face when they do so.[10,11] Compared with other healthcare professions, paramedic clinical judgement and decision-making has attracted little research attention;[12,13] there is an enormous body of research on clinical judgement and decision-making in medicine, psychology, psychiatry and nursing, but published research examining this for paramedics is scant. The scope of practice required of paramedics, described in earlier chapters, continues to expand with new roles, skills and procedures,[14] and this expansion has occurred in the absence of a rigorous body of knowledge grounded in sustained and systematic research. Given the infancy of paramedic practice and pre-hospital care as a recognised discipline in healthcare, this absence is not unexpected.[8,15]

Essential to the delivery of high-quality and safe pre-hospital emergency care are, among other things: (i) the sciences of critical thinking and clinical reasoning; (ii) the application of these sciences to emergency healthcare practice by way of protocols for problem-solving and triage; and (iii) the communication of these within the broader healthcare setting. All of these will be discussed in this chapter.

Clinical reasoning and critical thinking for quality and safety

Critical thinking and clinical reasoning are vital antecedents to high-quality and safe pre-hospital healthcare and professionalism.[13,16,17] Making high-quality clinical judgements is an 'intrinsic and inescapable imperative'[7] for all healthcare professionals if they are to render high-quality and safe healthcare. The ability of healthcare workers to solve clinical problems with clinical judgements and make decisions are skills that are critical features of professionalism.[4] Professionalism requires the possession of a body of knowledge that is the peculiar domain of the group, where its growth is driven by the conduct of appropriate scientific research.[17] Higgs and Jones in citing Heath[18] suggest that professions must build and maintain a formidable store of knowledge and skills. They must learn to absorb information through the various senses and to assess its validity, reliability and relevance, and must acquire the art and culture of their calling. Most importantly, they must learn to use these qualities to solve practical problems.[4]

General definitions and theoretical foundations

The terms 'clinical thinking and clinical reasoning' and 'clinical judgement and decision-making' are used interchangeably within the literature. Generally speaking, the *clinical* care that healthcare professionals provide is concerned with the treatment of patients.[19] Their *judgement* is a critical faculty of discernment, good sense or an opinion or estimate;[19] and a *decision* is the act or process of deciding a conclusion or other future action after consideration.[19] Broadly speaking, *clinical judgement and decision-making* may be viewed as 'an assessment of the alternatives in treatment from which decisions or choices between alternatives for optimal treatment are made'.[20] A healthcare professional's clinical reasoning is a 'series of cognitive processes involving inclusion of evidence to facilitate optimum patients' outcomes'.[21] For brevity, we will refer to these terms collectively as *clinical reasoning*, although we acknowledge that therein exists different philosophical and theoretical perspectives.[7,8]

The ability of healthcare professionals to form clinical judgements, to make clinical decisions and to exercise clinical reasoning is fundamental to the delivery of high-quality healthcare.[5,6] Researchers have focused on the study of clinical reasoning for more than half a century.[22] It is a rapidly evolving field, which makes attempts to understand its full scope a controversial and daunting task.[23] The origins of this work are largely connected to the desire to deal with uncertainty and the unknown,[23,24] and are interconnected with the highly contested and controversial study of emotion, cognition and perception. Moreover, there is no single or universal way to arrange or organise the literature on judgement and decision-making.[7,23] All that is known and recorded cannot be considered as 'singularly paradigmatic, but rather as immersed in a number of competing schools of thought that identify issues as interesting and deem different methods as appropriate'.[23] Each of the theoretical positions is contextually bound, bearing rich, complex and contested philosophical origins emanating from specific professions or disciplines. Many of their meanings and understandings are not sharply demarcated—they overlap, often because of shared theoretical and philosophical positions. One understanding or position does not supersede or silence another.[25] Rather, the sum total of the theoretical positions of judgement and decision-making co-exist as competing accounts.[7,8]

Attempts to arrange the extensive and competing array of theories and positions of clinical judgement and decision-making into a single or definitive theoretical framework are highly problematic, if not impossible. Much of the debate in the literature is about that very issue—how researchers and theorists view, define and categorise the theoretical literature on judgement and decision-making. The problematic and controversial attempts to do so, which many view as inappropriate, is well-documented.[22,23,26–28]

Broadly speaking, theories of human judgement and decision-making are derived from different philosophical positions. The science of decision-making dates back to the early 1950s.[26] The original dominant paradigm of judgement and decision-making was *classical decision-making*. This views the decision-maker as an element in a context of complete certainty.[4] The problems decision-makers face are clearly defined, and they know all the possible alternatives for action, and their consequences. The action they choose provides for an optimum outcome. They are characteristic of laboratory settings, and articulate the correct way to make an optimum decision in an ideal situation, environment or world. Theories derived from this paradigm have been applied to decision-making in many contexts, although Chapman[27] and others note that it does not fit well in chaotic contexts, uncontrolled environments or critical situations. They are most relevant in controlled settings and environments, typically those that are purely theoretical and non-applied.[8,29]

Growing criticism of classical decision-making and its limitations in the 1980s spurred a re-think of judgement and decision-making theory. An alternative position that attracted great attention, namely *naturalistic (or behavioural) decision-making*, was promulgated.[28] Unlike classic decision-making, naturalistic decision-making acknowledges that individuals exist and function within cognitive limitations in a bounded rationality. According to Orasanu and Connolly,[30] within this paradigm individuals are presented with ill-structured problems in uncertain, dynamic environments with shifting, ill-defined and competing goals. Of particular importance here is the significance of time as a constraint, especially when individuals are required to assess, interpret and assimilate multiple data from multiple sources, often in settings where the stakes are high. The problem faced by the naturalistic decision-maker lacks clarity, and he or she has limited knowledge of possible action alternatives and their consequences. The action they undertake is more geared towards achieving a satisfactory outcome rather than the optimal outcome, out of sheer necessity.[28] Naturalistic decision-making holds particular relevance in chaotic environments where conditions are uncertain and individuals have limited information. In these situations, such as in pre-hospital emergency care, individuals most often rely on their experience to resolve patient problems.[29]

Within this dichotomy, classical and naturalistic decision-making, lie three models or theoretical positions of clinical judgement and decision-making: descriptive, normative and prescriptive. The relationship between these and a description of them is illustrated in Box 11.1 and Figure 11.1.

When it comes to pre-hospital emergency care, the clinical reasoning of paramedics and emergency nurses is focused on problem-solving.[8,31]

> **PRACTICE TIP**
>
> A definitive diagnosis is no substitute for comprehensive description of the patients' presenting problems that require intervention.

Foundations for pre-hospital emergency care: problem-solving

Fundamentally, paramedics' and emergency nurses' critical thinking and clinical reasoning is focused on *problem-solving*.[8] In the contemporary context, the problems paramedics are called on to solve are diverse. Some research suggests that the majority of paramedical practice is focused on solving social problems, rather than medical or health problems.[8,13] The emphasis is on early identification of the most serious problems, which enables the paramedic to achieve their core goal of providing the best outcome for the patient. The obligations placed upon paramedics and emergency nurses to provide the best possible care for the patient are explicit.[8] To do so, they are expected to adhere to the relevant evidence-based guidelines to achieve what is in the best interests of the patient.[8] This requires paramedics and emergency nurses to, among other things, draw on information from the patient and the field, from which they then develop a plan of action.

Modern standards for paramedic clinical thinking and reasoning draw on the US Department of Transportation's Emergency Medical Technician Paramedic National Standards Curriculum.[32] These underpin practice standards for paramedic clinical thinking and reasoning globally. Most standards adopt a fundamental schema, consisting of the elements illustrated in Figure 11.2.

When it comes to clinical practice and solving problems in pre-hospital emergency care, paramedics' and emergency nurses' clinical reasoning and critical thinking are exercised in two key ways: (i) protocols for problem-solving, and (ii) triage.

Paramedic applications: patterns and protocols and triage for problem-solving

Paramedic pattern recognition and protocols for problem-solving

Much of the related ambulance literature conceptualises clinical judgement and decision-making for paramedics and nurses as *problem-solving*. In the contemporary context, paramedics solve a diverse range of problems, for which they are expected to arrive at a single, correct solution. The emphasis is on the early identification of the most serious problems, which in turn enables the paramedic to achieve their core goal of providing

---

BOX 11.1 Descriptive, normative and prescriptive models[8,29]

Descriptive theories

Naturalistic and behavioural in nature, these theories originate from the philosophies and professions of psychology and behavioural science.[22,26] Specifically, descriptive theories are concerned with understanding how individuals actually make judgements and decisions. Descriptive theories place no restriction on whether the individual is rational and logical or irrational and illogical, and seek to understand how individuals make judgements and decisions in the real world, focusing on the actual conditions, contexts, ecologies and environments in which they are made.[26] Irrationality in this context refers to instances where individuals have not given any thought to the process of judgement or decision-making (JDM), and, even if they have, are unable to implement the desired process.[22] These theories seek to understand the learning and cognitive capabilities of 'ordinary people' and aim to determine if their behaviour is consistent or 'rational'.[26] Context, interactions and ecology are central to the interpretation.

Normative theories

These are classical and positivist in nature, and are born from the statistical, mathematical and economic philosophies.[26] In this domain, researchers (often referred to as decision theorists) seek to propose rational procedures for decision-making that are logical and may be theorised. The focus of normative theory is to discover how rational people make decisions with the aim of determining how decisions *should be made* in an ideal or optimal world, where decisions are based on logical and known conclusions supported by clear or probable evidence. Normative theories, often based on statistics and probabilities within the positivist domain, propose to evaluate how good judgements should be made and how good outcomes should be

achieved.[22,26] Normative theories give little or no consideration to how judgements are made by 'ordinary people' in reality and everyday practice, and place little or no emphasis on the context or ecology of the judgement.[22] They are concerned only with optimal conditions and environments, and assume that decision-makers are 'super-rational',[30] with little or no emphasis on how JDM occurs in the 'real' world.[26]

Prescriptive theories

These theories set out to 'improve' the clinical reasoning of individuals by investigating how people make decisions.[22,26] The focus of prescriptive theories is to *help* or *improve* individuals' judgements. In evaluating the application of prescriptive models and theories that attempt to aid in the JDM process, the central question asked is pragmatic—did it make the judgement any better? Prescriptive theories have been applied in multiple settings and contexts. Decision analysis and decision trees (described later in the chapter) are used commonly in prescriptive modelling in medicine to improve clinician reasoning.[22] A recently introduced but now common prescriptive model for assisting JDM in clinical settings is the use of clinical guidelines and clinical policies. Clinical guidelines are prescriptive tools used to assist practitioner and patient decisions about appropriate healthcare for specific circumstances.[22] They are largely guidelines that outline operational information, procedures and guidelines with options, and are often referred to as 'protocols'. Primarily aimed at improving the quality of care or standardising care, guidelines are mechanisms for reducing variations in clinical practice and discouraging practices that are not based on sufficient evidence.[22] While they have been found to provide improvements in the quality of care,[22] the effects of their application are significantly variable and the extent to which they are routinely applied is not clear.[26]

---

the best outcome for the patient.[33] The obligations placed on paramedics to provide the best possible care for the patient are explicit. Contemporary models of paramedic problem-solving, clinical thinking and reasoning and clinical judgement and decision-making draw on the Emergency Medical Technician Paramedic National Standards Curriculum.[34] Most recently, in 2013, the Convention of Ambulance Authorities and Paramedics Australasia[35] established professional competency standards for paramedics. These underpin practice standards for paramedic curriculum and practice. Bendall and Morrison[33] describe clinical judgement and decision-making as 'fundamental to the role of a professional paramedic' and 'core business'.[33] In their view, the acquisition of good quality information and its synthesis is essential to clinical judgement and decision-making, where the 'best information → best judgement'.[33] Bendall and Morrison describe how expertise is developed in paramedic decision-making, citing Billett's[36] work which characterises key attributes of an expert's performance. In addition, they suggest that there are five cognitive decision-making strategies that are common to emergency medical services, these being algorithmic, pattern recognition, worst-case scenario (rule out), event-driven and hypothetico-deductive. They suggest that algorithms are common in ambulance services, and that use

of pattern recognition is 'rife'.[33] Bendall and Morrison offer a description of paramedic critical thinking consistent with the model for paramedic problem-solving described by Sanders.[37] Bendall and Morrison argue that when problem-solving, paramedics make use of the model and its five elements and 'pull it all together',[33] which is consistent with guidelines in popular paramedic textbooks from the United States.[37–39]

A cognitive assessment of paramedics' problem-solving and judgement practice has been reported in a recent study by Alexander,[40] who examined the cognitive processes by which paramedics in the United States undertook clinical reasoning to solve clinical problems. Verbal protocol analysis and thinking aloud were used to analyse the current and retrospective clinical reasoning of 10 paramedics when solving two vignettes. The theoretical framework for the study was based on information-processing theory, and drew on information in the United States Paramedic National Standard Curriculum,[34] and literature on emergency medicine doctors' problem-solving processes. Alexander argues that paramedic clinical decision-making is derived from the practice of emergency medicine, which renders the cognition literature on medicine and emergency medicine a suitable comparison for research purposes in the absence of paramedic-specific literature. Moreover, Alexander argues that

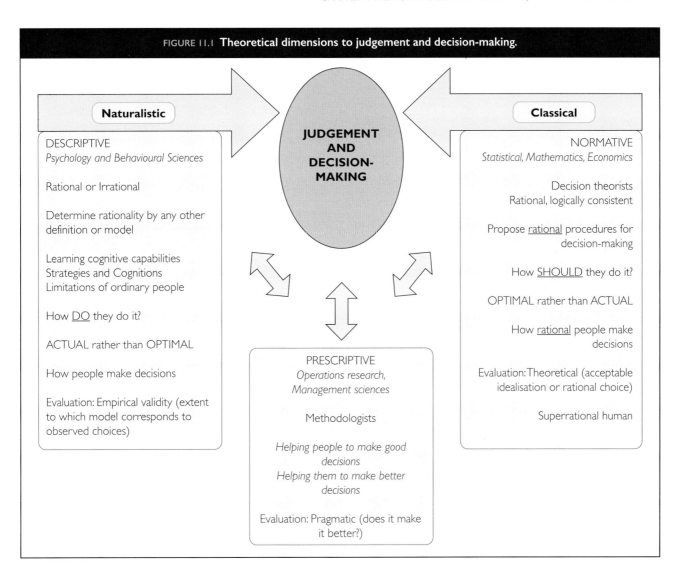

FIGURE 11.1 **Theoretical dimensions to judgement and decision-making.**

Naturalistic

DESCRIPTIVE
Psychology and Behavioural Sciences

Rational or Irrational

Determine rationality by any other definition or model

Learning cognitive capabilities
Strategies and Cognitions
Limitations of ordinary people

How <u>DO</u> they do it?

ACTUAL rather than OPTIMAL

How people make decisions

Evaluation: Empirical validity (extent to which model corresponds to observed choices)

JUDGEMENT AND DECISION-MAKING

Classical

NORMATIVE
Statistical, Mathematics, Economics

Decision theorists
Rational, logically consistent

Propose <u>rational</u> procedures for decision-making

How <u>SHOULD</u> they do it?

OPTIMAL rather than ACTUAL

How <u>rational</u> people make decisions

Evaluation: Theoretical (acceptable idealisation or rational choice)

Superrational human

PRESCRIPTIVE
Operations research, Management sciences

Methodologists

Helping people to make good decisions
Helping them to make better decisions

Evaluation: Pragmatic (does it make it better?)

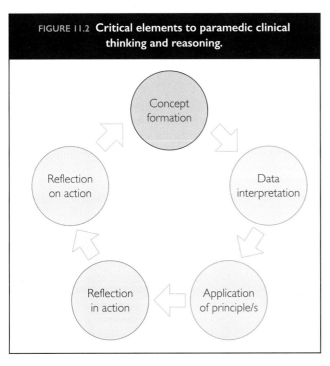

FIGURE 11.2 **Critical elements to paramedic clinical thinking and reasoning.**

Concept formation

Data interpretation

Application of principle/s

Reflection in action

Reflection on action

emergency doctors are intimately involved with all aspects of paramedic practice, are the primary authors and content editors of paramedic training textbooks and are required to approve all accredited paramedic training programs and all paramedic provider services. Paramedics in Alexander's[40] study were found to solve problems primarily by pattern recognition without adequate hypothesis testing. According to Alexander, paramedics' patient assessment and illness scripts for both sets of vignettes were 'inadequately developed, disorganised, and, in some ways, faulty'.[40] Moreover, in the absence of adequate illness scripts for pattern recognition and adequate hypothesis testing, paramedics in the study generated pseudo-information and used cognitive biases in their problem-solving. For the vignettes presented, the paramedics had a low threshold for initiating treatment, and provided inappropriate treatment. Alexander has called for additional research and argues that 'changes [in] paramedic education practice should focus on providing meaningful learning experiences, promoting learner reflection on problem-solving and giving feedback on clinical reasoning processes in order to improve the quality of paramedics' illness scripts and clinical reasoning processes'.[40]

The use of pattern recognition by paramedics is underpinned by clinical guidelines and protocols. Individuals and organisations use clinical guidelines and protocols to limit the occurrence and impact of error. Ambulance services provide paramedics with case-management guidelines and protocols to assist them in achieving the desired outcome in the best interests of the patient.

PRACTICE TIP

Review guidelines and protocols systematically based on evidence and the extent to which they enable timely, effective problem-solving.

Clinical guidelines and protocols and other forms of decision support are fundamental to paramedic clinical judgement and decision-making and practice. Research supporting the use of this kind of decision support exists for many of the classic areas of pre-hospital emergency care, including telephone triage,[41] ambulance service telemedicine,[42] ambulance dispatch,[43] triage,[44] management of trauma,[45] recognition of cardiac injury and death,[46–49] cardiac arrest and resuscitation,[50,51] disasters and mass gatherings[52,53] and determining the need for further treatment and transport.[54,55] The findings of the majority of this research recommend the use of decision-support processes, such as protocols and guidelines, for paramedic judgement practice.

Much of this existing research advocates the use of computer-assisted decision support systems. The use of computer-assisted decision-making software for accurate ambulance call taking and the management of emergency health services is common internationally.[56,57] Farrand et al[58] examined the introduction of a computerised dispatch system into an emergency medical system call centre traditionally staffed by nurses. The study found that in attempting to formalise nurse decision processes using artificial intelligence, the complexities of the decision processes therein were revealed. An assessment of the accuracy of the decision process—using an expert panel review of 1006 calls—found almost perfect sensitivity with telephone triage and decision as to whether to send an EMS resource or not. In this instance, the study demonstrated that nurses' clinical judgement and decision-making processes in this setting were sophisticated.[59] Other studies have reported similar findings.[60,61] Researchers[46,62,63] have suggested that paramedics' clinical judgement and decision-making regarding the futility of resuscitation is best supported by the use of an algorithm and doctor-guided clinical guidelines. Dunne et al[64] conducted a study to estimate the proportion of patients transported by paramedics who do not need emergency medical care. They found that paramedics could not reliably identify those patients in need of emergency medical treatment when unaided by protocols or specific training. Although the use of computer-aided decision-support is common for call-taking and ambulance dispatch, recent research reveals a poor uptake of electronic decision-support and information systems for evidence-based practice by Australian paramedics.[65]

Clinical guidelines and other decision support is often presented as decision trees. Decision trees are a direct application of normative theories of judgement and decision-making. They outline how decisions *should* be made. Decision trees, such as the one illustrated in Figure 11.3, work by breaking down problems into smaller decisions and choices.[8] Traditionally,

determining how judgements and decisions should be made requires comprehensive risk analyses so as to identify all possible risks, which are then weighted.[22] The decisions alluded to within the tree are based on the predictability of events using probability and statistical occurrence. Once each choice has been assigned a probability—assuming this is possible—the option with the highest utility for the decision-maker can be calculated.[22] Such models attempt to quantify the probability of the most likely and most desirable event in an attempt to assist the individual or group in making that judgement or decision by making this probability known.

PRACTICE TIP

When developing and reviewing a clinical decision tree, both qualify and quantify the clinical problem that it seeks to solve.

Decision trees also assist paramedics and emergency nurses to make decisions about the transportation and transfer of patients. Relevant factors include:

- location—remote, rural or urban, and is there any choice of hospital?
- access to additional facilities—whether other modes of transportation, such as by air, sea or land, are available
- the stability of the patient's condition—whether the patient is transport or time/treatment critical
- the demands or requests of the patient
- resources available at the receiving facility. Is the proposed receiving facility currently available? Is there access block or ambulance ramping?
- local ambulance/hospital policy.

There is considerable evidence in the literature that supports, in principle, the notion that demonstrates the improvement clinical guidelines can have on practice and standard of care.[8,22,66] Though intended to guide judgement and decision-making to obtain high-quality outcomes, protocols and procedures, and their implementation, are far from infallible. An often under-recognised feature of clinical guidelines and protocols is that they are socially constructed. They are forms of social policy—that is, they 'propose regulatory principles of action for adoption by individuals, groups and organisations'.[1] Protocols, policies and procedures are a form of social policy, and the 'uncertainty in the creation of social policy makes error inevitable, and error makes the injustice unavoidable'.[1] Being socially constructed, they provide accounts and representations of people, events and contexts at one point in time in a given set of circumstances. They are crafted communicative objects. Culturally and ideologically, they stand somewhere; the crafting process serves to position the users in certain ways.[67] Many factors influence the ways in which individuals interpret and enact these texts. Their universal use and enactment will inevitably precipitate problems in practice.[8]

Although clinical guidelines are at the heart of quality-improvement strategies, Rycroft-Malone argues that they are not the panacea (or a replacement) for professional clinical decision-making or judgement, nor should ever be viewed as such.[66] They are often used to flag high-quality practice, particularly

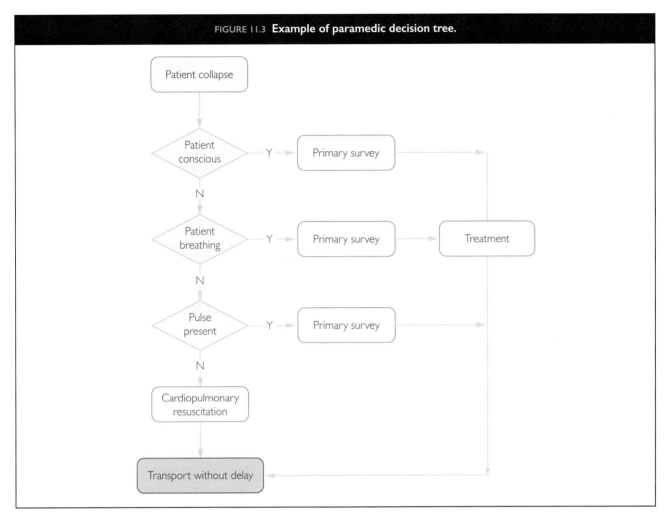

FIGURE 11.3 **Example of paramedic decision tree.**

when promulgated by professional bodies, associations and governments. They are official texts designed to assist individuals in making quality judgements and decisions about patient care. In principle, they are 'systematically developed statements to assist practitioner and patient decisions about appropriate health care for specific circumstances'.[68] Clinical guidelines that are not evidence-based, uncomprehensive, without context or applied incorrectly or inconsistently, can have detrimental effects on the quality and safety of care. Their use is intentionally universal, with all practitioners required to practise within the scope outlined within all clinical guidelines. With that mandate, their use is intended to reduce variability in individual decision-making, to deal with notions of uncertainty and therefore to minimise risk and the generation of error. Recent research illustrates that protocols only provide part of the answer for clinical judgement and decision-making for emergency health professionals. A study of how Australian paramedics accomplish clinical judgement and decision-making of mental illness in the field and the factors that influence this aspect of their work revealed that paramedic clinical judgement and decision-making of mental illness is not a simple, technicist activity. The research, an in-depth case study of paramedics' accounts of actual clinical judgement and decision-making of mental illness in the field, revealed that their practice is not wholly governed by protocols, legislation, policies, guidelines and other normative and prescriptive instruments. Rather, their practice has been shown

to be highly individualised and influenced by the contextual and mediating elements, as illustrated in Figure 11.4.[8]

Conceptually, paramedic clinical judgement and decision-making of mental illness was found to be comprised of three different interconnected elements—contextual, practice and mediating. Fundamental to judgement practice was the *contextual element*, an amalgam of organisational and occupational factors associated with various historical, cultural, educational, political and regulatory dimensions of the Queensland pre-hospital emergency care setting. The Contextual Element established the framework for the formal roles of paramedics within a hierarchy of medical treatment. The *practice element* consisted of field actions for problem-solving and a range of individual-specific factors. The paramedics' field actions consisted of an individualised, enacted systematic approach that articulated their expectations of protection and transport of the patient. Actions included gathering and assessing data, describing the problem in objective detail, assessing the nature and severity of the problem, making a provisional diagnosis, and implementing actions to achieve the best possible outcome. Coupled with field actions were individual factors, namely knowledge, experience, interpersonal skills and personal traits. These individual factors augmented the paramedics' field actions for problem-solving in differing measure according to the individual jobs and patients they encountered. The *mediating element* was comprised of paramedics' interactions

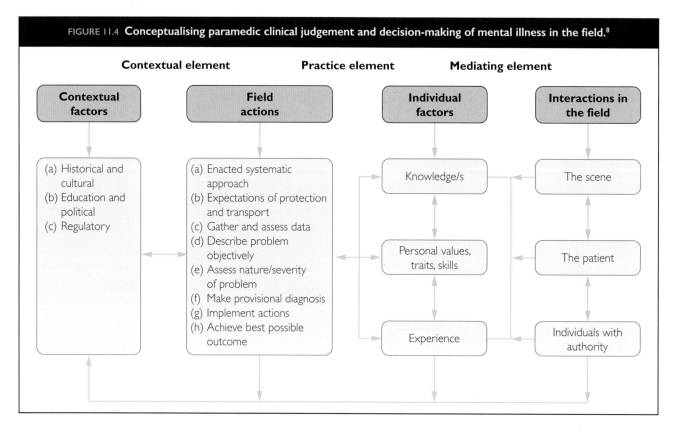

FIGURE 11.4 **Conceptualising paramedic clinical judgement and decision-making of mental illness in the field.**[8]

within the scene, with the patient and with individuals in authority. These interactions influenced the success of their clinical judgement and decision-making, in particular their interactions with the patient, doctors, relatives, bystanders and other individuals in authority. The roles paramedics ascribed to those individuals were integral to their actual judgement practice.[8] Critically, interactions in the field, which were also fundamental to actual judgement practice, did not feature strongly in the formal regulatory expectations of practice such as protocols. The use of an interpretive, naturalistic case study that adopted a descriptive theoretical framework unearthed the complex mix of elements and the interplay among them that characterises the paramedics' accounts of their own judgement practice. More specifically, the study provided the opportunity for the paramedics themselves to reflect on, and talk about, their in-the-field judgement practice, and generating insights into what had previously been private and unpublished. That is, their judgement and decision-making had not been subject to formal critical inquiry, nor has this aspect of paramedic work been the subject of sustained research. At issue in this study was the preparedness of paramedics to recognise, assess and manage mental illness in everyday practice and the sufficiency of education and training programs, clinical standards, policy and legislation for ensuring quality practice and accountability in the field.[8]

> ### PRACTICE TIP
>
> Clinical reasoning should always feature more than the individual nurse or paramedic, and includes the patient and others.

(In)sufficiency and errors

Sometimes the clinical judgements and decisions made by healthcare professionals are insufficient or inaccurate, and sometimes they get it wrong.[7] Problems with the quality of clinicians' judgement and decision-making and subsequent mistakes have been the focus of attention for both clinicians and researchers for decades. The fallibility of clinical judgement and decision-making has always presented problems for individuals, professions, communities and societies.[1] Broadly speaking, when it comes to judgement and decision-making, there is always the risk of 'irreducible uncertainty, inevitable error and unavoidable injustice'.[1] Because of this, research into judgement and decision-making has for decades focused heavily on reducing uncertainty and risk of error, particularly in professional practice settings.[7]

The focus on reducing uncertainty and risk of error in the Australian medical and healthcare context is, however, comparatively recent. In recent times the media, particularly in Western societies, has focused on highlighting failures and mistakes in healthcare. There has been little impetus in Australia within the medical or healthcare professions to study or question the ways in which clinical decisions are made.[6,69] In 1995, the Medical Journal of Australia published a groundbreaking study—The Quality of Australian Health Care Study. The study presented disturbing findings that 'seared patient safety into the public's psyche'[70] and subsequently crystallised quality and safety within the healthcare agenda in Australia. More than 10 years later, Wilson and van der Weyden[70] suggested that most patients in Australia's healthcare system receive good care and do not suffer preventable harm. Such commentary is contradictory to recent events in Australia's healthcare system, particularly in Queensland. The

Bundaberg Hospital Commission of Inquiry and subsequent Queensland Public Hospitals Commission of Inquiry[71] and the Queensland Health Systems Review[72] made serious findings of gross substandard and unsafe care in Queensland. Similar events have been documented in other jurisdictions.[73] The impetus for these investigations was complaints from patients and healthcare professionals about individual instances of care. The investigations uncovered a chronic and systematic failure of organisational health service delivery systems, which was attributed mainly to individual error.[71,72]

There have been investigations and reviews[74–78] into ambulance and emergency services and paramedic practices, although these are relatively few in number when compared with the medical and nursing practice context. In recent times, independent commissions for quality and safety in healthcare across Australia and New Zealand have had their terms of reference and jurisdiction extended to include unregulated healthcare professions such as paramedics.[79] As these commissions of inquiry and investigations unfold, greater insight into the sufficiency of protocols and guidelines for paramedics and their scope of practice will emerge. Recent research[8,10,13,80] has called into question the sufficiency of protocols in ambulance practice.

When there is little evidence: best guess

Although an 'intrinsic and inescapable imperative',[7] accomplishing clinical judgement and decision-making is far from simple.[8] Formulating clinical judgements and making decisions for high-quality and safe healthcare are complex processes. Making judgements and decisions about 'which diagnosis, whose version or account of the troubles they find most convincing, or morally robust'[7] is challenging. There are multiple competing priorities for healthcare professionals in formulating clinical judgement and decision-making. One notable priority for healthcare professionals for ensuring quality healthcare is the mandate for EBP. Production and use of the best available evidence are central to all efforts to improve the quality of healthcare around the world.[81]

PRACTICE TIP

The absence of evidence is not always evidence of absence.

Providing evidence-based healthcare may be a contemporary imperative, but there are many challenges to achieving this goal. In some healthcare disciplines, such as paramedics, there is little evidence on which to base practice and the evidence–practice gap is substantial.[81] Some kinds of evidence—namely randomised controlled trials, systematic reviews and meta-analyses—carry greater weight in the hierarchy of evidence. Knowledge generated in this way often limits or undervalues the influence of context in generating the best available evidence. The context in which some healthcare professionals work can make providing evidence-based care particularly challenging. Emergency healthcare is one such area. The context in which emergency healthcare professionals practise is one in which they are required to attend to 'a serious, unexpected, and potentially dangerous situation requiring immediate action'.[19] The demands that the context of emergency healthcare places on doctors, nurses and paramedics to render life-saving care

to the sick and injured are complex, time-pressured and high-stakes.[82–86] These kinds of healthcare professionals, or first-contact practitioners,[4] often have scant evidence to support their clinical practice. Nevertheless, they 'go about their ordinary but complicated business of making sense of the symptoms and troubles of their patients and clients'.[7]

Contemporary practices

In the contemporary pre-hospital emergency-care setting, the application of the theoretical principles of critical thinking and clinical reasoning are translated into key skills and processes for action. The key skills and abilities of paramedics include:[16]

- ability to deal with uncertainty with respect to aetiology
- sound knowledge of anatomy, physiology, pathophysiology and pathology
- data and information-gathering
- discerning information-gathering and assessment skills
- differentiating relevant and irrelevant data
- analysing similar and contrary situations
- articulate reasoning and constructing of arguments for practice.

In the international setting, a popular permeation of this is that proposed by the late Nancy Caroline, outlined in Box 10.11 on page 161.

In Australian and New Zealand jurisdictions, variations of this exist.[79] For example, in Queensland the paramedic's approach to clinical judgement and decision-making and problem-solving is referred as the 'systematic approach'.[8] This approach is:

a systematic means of analysing the patient's problems, determining how to solve them, carrying out a plan of action, and then evaluating the effectiveness of that plan and responding to it accordingly. Paramedics' clinical judgement is expected to consist of a combination of knowledge, skill, experience, attitudes and intuition. In most circumstances, paramedics should attempt to identify the physiological linkages to presenting injury or illness and manage the presenting primary and potential secondary patient problems accordingly. The paramedic must endeavour to correctly analyse each situation and select actions that produce the best long-term patient outcomes.[8]

Box 11.2 provides practical tips for minimising error in clinical judgement and decision-making, particularly in emergency healthcare.

Pre-hospital triage

Key principles

Triage is central to quality and safety in emergency care and paramedic practice. Healthcare workers in emergency care routinely use triage to prioritise patients according to their level of clinical urgency. The philosophical underpinnings of triage are *utilitarian*—arguing for the rational use of limited resources to ensure the greatest good for the greatest number; and *egalitarian*—intended to achieve fair treatment of patients. As a clinical tool, triage is enacted when the resources on hand are inadequate for the number or nature of those injured, such as during a multi-casualty event. In instances where demand exceeds supply, the allocation of resources for care is aimed at achieving the best possible clinical outcome for the greatest number of patients.

BOX 11.2 Tips for minimising error in judgement practice

- Maintain a systematic assessment and judgement practice.
- Gather and organise data, and form concepts and patterns of injury and illness.
- Focus on specific and multiple elements of data concurrently.
- Identify and deal with uncertainty as much as is possible.
- Differentiate between relevant and irrelevant data.
- Analyse events and situations in light of past experience.
- Recall cases in which judgements and decisions were incorrect or inaccurate.
- Construct and articulate arguments in support of your judgement practice and clinical reasoning.
- Seek the advice and opinion of others, particularly those with different skills and expertise.
- Communicate your assessments and plans to others in a clear and concise manner.
- Test and critically evaluate your assessment and assumptions with your peers and colleagues.

Under normal circumstances where the number of patients is manageable in terms of the resources available, triage is egalitarian and patients with a high degree of clinical urgency are treated first and are allocated the most resources. In circumstances where resources are overwhelmed by the numbers of patients (for example, in a disaster or mass casualty situation—see Ch 12), triage serves a different purpose and a utilitarian approach is taken to ensure optimal use of limited resources to ensure the greatest good for the greatest number. Under disaster triage, patients with a high degree of clinical urgency may be the lowest priority. The aim in both settings, the emergency department (ED) and the pre-hospital emergency-care setting, is to satisfy the utilitarian principle of providing the best possible care to the greatest number of patients.

In hospital settings, the outcomes of triage are used during clinical audit to assess the suitability, or otherwise, of the patient's outcome.[87] The quality of triage influences patient length of stay, rates of admission to intensive care units and rates of morbidity and mortality. The majority of research literature related to triage has come from ED triage by expert emergency nurses where triage decision-making has been studied from a number of perspectives. Studies to date have focused on inter-rater and intra-rater reliability of triage decisions;[88–95] influences on triage decision-making, including triage nurse characteristics;[89–91,94,96,97] ED workload;[98,99] financial incentives;[100] and patient populations.[101,102] Knowledge and experience of triage personnel are two factors that have dominated research related to triage decision-making. Although numerous studies have examined the role of experience as an independent influence on triage decisions, none have found a significant relationship between experience and triage decision-making.[90,91,94,96,97,103] Factual knowledge appears to be more important than years of triage experience in improving the accuracy of triage decisions.[90,92,103,104]

PRACTICE TIP

Review triage decisions systematically, particularly in light of the deteriorating patient.

In the pre-hospital emergency-care setting, one sentinel performance measure for ambulance services is response times.[105] For example, the response time to Code 1 incidents (requiring at least one immediate response under lights and sirens) is measured from the time of the commencement of recording details of the incident at the ambulance communications centre (call-taker's first keystroke) to the time the first ambulance service response arrives at the incident scene. First-responder and community volunteer responses are not included.[105] Ambulance services measure response times aggregately to triage code, and assess performance against agreed yet arbitrary standards adopted by the Council of Ambulance Authorities.[105] Such systems are fundamental characteristics of the corporate governance in contemporary ambulance services in Australia and New Zealand.

Contemporary practices

In pre-hospital care, triage is a continuous process but one which is emphasised at key points in the continuum of care. These points include extrication from the scene, on arrival at the ED, upon admission to hospital and on presentation to operating theatres. Assessment of the patient and judgement of the urgency of their condition will determine the treatment and the ongoing care of the patient. Triage is a necessary element of the system-wide organisation. Assignment of urgency is necessary to determine the priority of dispatch of ambulances, to determine the priority of treatment in the field, to determine the priority of extrication and transport and to determine the optimal location for ongoing care.

In EDs, nurses and doctors assess the patients and determine their clinical urgency for treatment, which is reflected in a triage score.[106–109] In the pre-hospital care setting, ambulance response is based on a scale of clinical urgency, and paramedics use triage to assign clinical urgency to patients during multi-casualty situations where there are insufficient resources to manage all patients immediately.[8,109] Although in most circumstances paramedics in the field are faced with a one-to-one therapeutic relationship, triage remains a critical element of pre-hospital care.

Triage in the field is usually performed by the most clinically and operationally experienced paramedics. Important principles that guide triage in the pre-hospital emergency care setting are listed in the Essentials section at the start of the chapter. Triage scales designed for pre-hospital care seek to determine the rapidity of extrication from the scene and the priority for further treatment.[87] Many factors influence this priority, including not only the clinical urgency of the patients but also the capacity of care and the practical ability to maximise the extrication of patients. Thus, the walking wounded may be extricated quickly and encouraged to 'keep walking'. Second priority may be given to those requiring rapid interventions and who can be extricated quickly, while those who are difficult to extricate (trapped) or those for whom survival is not expected may be assigned the lowest priority for extrication and may require resuscitation on scene.

The nature of the patient's complaint and potential severity of their condition is related to the priority of ambulance dispatch. Most ambulance services utilise a medical protocol to determine the priority of dispatch within an electronic dispatch system. The need to do so is determined by the mismatch of demand and resources available. These, now computerised, protocolised systems guide the call-taker through a series of questions which ultimately determine a priority for dispatch. In Australia and New Zealand,[105] systems adopted nationally determine priority into one of four categories as described in Table 11.1.

Similarly, the nature of the patient's clinical problem, as determined and expressed by the paramedic via provisional diagnosis, is material to their response procedures in the field. Paramedics communicate the nature and severity of the patient's condition to hospital staff, both on arrival at hospital and en route, using scales. Values on the scale do not relate to initial on-scene triage, as for mass-casualty situations, but rather to the officer's assessment of patient severity while in transit.

Triage is also critical to the management of multiple patients. In these circumstances, paramedics at the scene have the reasonability to determine the priority of extrication from the scene. In mass-casualty situations, and all situations where the number of patients exceeds the capability of the initial ambulance response, the field triage process is necessary. In such situations, the standard (initial triage) codes are Red, Yellow, Green and Black, corresponding to Emergency (immediate treatment), Urgent (delayed treatment), Non-urgent (walking wounded) and Dying or Deceased.[110] This is discussed in detail in Chapter 12.

The ultimate aim of triage is to determine the priority and extent of ongoing care. Part of the priority for pre-hospital triage is to determine the most appropriate source of ongoing care. Most patients will be taken to the nearest appropriate hospital. However, with the development of super-specialisation of health services, paramedics are confronted with the need to triage patients from the scene directly to super-specialised services, where practicable. Thus appropriate cardiac patients may need to be taken to catheter laboratories and stroke patients to stroke units. The most common example is the specialisation of trauma services and the development of major trauma units. Major gaps in this approach are acknowledgement of the need for pain relief, mental health issues[13] and acute behavioural disturbance. These issues have been addressed in EDs by revision of the National Triage Scale to the Australasian Triage Scale, but are still absent in the descriptors used in paramedical practice.

Communicating for quality and safety in the emergency setting

The particular geography and demography of Australia and New Zealand is characterised by urban concentration and sparse rural dispersal of the population. As a result, servicing of people's healthcare needs is heavily dependent on retrieval of patients to an appropriate source of medical care and the transfer of patients between the various levels of care, including primary, secondary and tertiary care. Nurses and paramedics are extensively involved in this system, both in terms of utilisation of the system in the interests of their patients and in terms of patient care during transport and retrieval. Timely, efficient and effective communication is essential to the high-quality functioning of a contemporary emergency medical system.

Key principles

Important elements of communication in healthcare include information about the patient's current state and future events or goals.[111] A possible strategy for improving information transfer is the use of standardised systems for communication.[18] Advantages of such standardised systems and use of a predetermined structure are a decrease in omission of important information and clear expectations about the order in which information will be conveyed.[111] Studies of interprofessional communication comparing standard information transfer with communication using the ISBAR mnemonic (see Table 11.4 later in the chapter) showed that the content and clarity of communication was higher when ISBAR was used, and that use of a structured method improved communication during telephone referral in a simulated clinical setting.[112] The Australian Commission on Safety and Quality in Health Care has established standards and implementation tool kits for quality clinical hand-over via the National Safety and Quality Health Service Standard for Clinical Handover, which adopts the ISBAR framework.[113]

TABLE 11.1	Council of Ambulance Authorities 2011–2012 dispatch data definitions[105]	
CODE	DEFINITION	DESCRIPTOR
1	Immediate response under lights and sirens	Incident is potentially life-threatening
2	Urgent dispatch un-delayed response without lights and sirens	Arrival desirable within 30 minutes
3	Time-based non-urgent	Non-emergency
4	Non-urgent	Non-urgent response by required ambulance or patient transport service
–	Casualty room attendance	

(a) An incident is an event that results in one or more responses by an ambulance service. Incidents are prioritised using the codes listed above.

(b) A response is the dispatch of an ambulance service vehicle. There may be multiple responses to a single incident. Responses are prioritised as per incidents, but in some instances responses to the same incident may be dispatched with different priorities (e.g. a Code 1 response to a Code 1 incident may be supported by an additional Code 2 response as a back-up).

(c) A patient is an individual who is attended by the ambulance service and transported or treated; there may be multiple patients at an incident. Treatment includes clinical assessment of the patient (recording of observations), even when it is determined that no further clinical intervention is required.[105]

To provide quality pre-hospital emergency care, paramedics and emergency nurses rely on communication centre staff, comprising experienced and highly trained telephonists, call-takers, dispatchers and clinicians.[114] The dynamic nature of the pre-hospital emergency-care setting makes communications challenging. Communicating in the emergency medical system is typically event or incident centred, and occurs in five stages, as illustrated in Figure 11.5.

Methods of communicating

The ability to receive, understand and forward information within the pre-hospital emergency-care setting is critical to patient welfare and the quality and safety of the care that paramedics and emergency nurses provide. Communicating information in the emergency medical system requires the use of a variety of methods and equipment, all of which have advantages and limitations, as described in Table 11.2. This is also discussed in Chapter 14.

Importance of communication

The importance of communication to providing high-quality and safe pre-hospital emergency care is most evident when providing clinical hand-over and patient- and family-centred pre-hospital emergency care.

Ensuring high-quality clinical hand-over

One of the most important forums for information transfer in pre-hospital emergency care is clinical hand-over. Clinical hand-over is defined as 'the transfer of professional responsibility and accountability for some or all aspects of care for a patient, or group of patients, to another person or professional group on a temporary or permanent basis'.[115] Clinical hand-over processes are also referred to as hand-off, shift report and patient

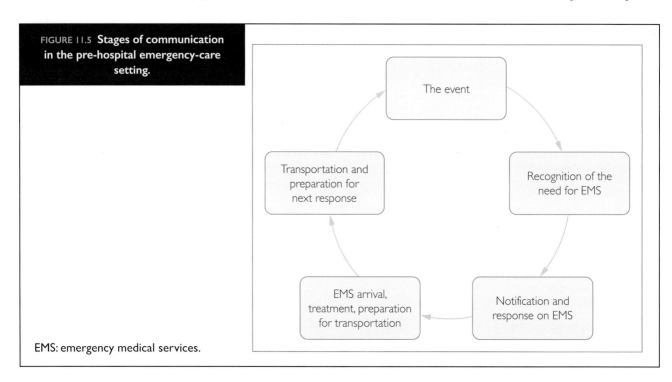

FIGURE 11.5 **Stages of communication in the pre-hospital emergency-care setting.**

EMS: emergency medical services.

TABLE 11.2 Methods of communicating in the field		
TYPE	ADVANTAGES	LIMITATIONS
Short-wave radio	Inexpensive	Limited to voice
	Timely	
	Portable	
Biotelemetry	Transmit high volumes of complex data	Expensive
	Rapid	Requires integrated infrastructure
		Network-access dependent
Telephone	Inexpensive	Network-access dependent
	Portable	Limited to voice or text data
Mobile internet	Access to servers for data transmission	Network-access dependent

transfer.[116] The aim of clinical hand-over is efficient transfer of high-quality clinical information and transfer of responsibility for patient care.[115]

> **PRACTICE TIP**
>
> Role clarification and delineation is critical to timely and effective clinical hand-over.

A rigorous approach to clinical hand-over protects both patients and clinicians.[115] Benefits of competent hand-over practices for patients include increased safety, decreased error, decreased morbidity and mortality, increased continuity of care, decreased repetition and increased satisfaction. For clinicians, high quality affords professional protection, makes accountability and responsibility transparent, decreases stress associated with feeling ill-informed, provides opportunity for education and improves job satisfaction by enabling provision of a high standard of care.[115]

Numerous studies clearly show that clinical hand-over is a high-risk event with potential for fragmentation of care and for adverse events.[116] A review of the literature[116] identified a number of major themes related to high-risk scenarios in clinical hand-over, summarised in Table 11.3. The elements of hand-over in the pre-hospital emergency-care setting include a verbal report, the handing-over of documented accounts and the physical hand-over of the patient from ambulance to the hospital, which one study claims is symbolic.[117] Clinical hand-over, as a form of formal communication, is most successful when a structured approach is adopted.[117]

Providing patient- and family-centred care

It is well documented that effective communication with patients and families and between healthcare professionals is a significant factor in the quality and safety of care.[118] Communication failures (either between staff and patients or between staff and other staff) are a well-documented factor in adverse events, and as many as 70% of serious incidents in healthcare are related to communication failure.[119–122] Despite clear evidence of gaps in communication between patients and healthcare professionals, the majority of safety and quality initiatives focus on improving communication between doctors and nurses, and tend to exclude patients.[123]

A recent systematic review of the literature related to nurse–patient communication showed that the terms 'interaction' and 'communication' are often used interchangeably without consideration of the true theoretical definition.[123] In the nurse–patient context, the main intent of communication and interaction is to promote a positive patient health outcome or state of wellbeing.[123] Though not a subject of systematic research, similar phenomena apply in the pre-hospital care setting.

Involving patients and families in their care and using understandable language free from medical jargon are both important aspects of effective communication between patients, families and healthcare professionals.[123,124] There are many challenges to effective communication between healthcare professionals and patients/families. Time constraints, patient stress and poor health literacy may mean that patients often do not understand their care.[125] One study found that 78% of ED patients did not understand one or more critical element of their treatment,[125] and a study of surgical patients showed that 40–80% of information covered in a consultation is immediately forgotten.[126] Poor or inappropriate communication between patients and healthcare professionals has significant clinical consequences: patients who do not fully understand their care have longer lengths of hospital stay and higher mortality rates.[127,128] Further, patients from diverse and particularly minority cultural and language backgrounds, or those who have physical communication problems, are at increased risk of preventable adverse events.[129,130]

Documenting and communicating for quality outcomes

In a democratic society, such as those in Australia and New Zealand, patients have the right to receive timely and appropriate pre-hospital emergency care. Moreover, a variety of common law and statute law places obligations and a duty of care on paramedics and emergency nurses to provide appropriate pre-hospital emergency care, as outlined in Chapter 4. The consequences of poor documentation of the care provided and the events surrounding the care are significant for the patient, paramedics and emergency nurses. Not only does poor documentation present a significant risk to patient safety and the quality of their health experience and outcomes, but it also exposes the paramedic and emergency nurse to actions for negligence and breaches in tort. There is perhaps no greater professional risk to paramedics and emergency nurses than failure to adequately document patient refusal of treatment and/or transportation.

There are a variety of systems used by paramedics for gathering and documenting information for high-quality and safe pre-hospital emergency care within Australia and New Zealand. The more common of these are described in Table 11.4. Recent research into the practices of Australian paramedics shows that paramedics' gathering and reporting of information follows the requirements of the formal document, particularly with the move to electronic ambulance records. Such systems prompt paramedics for the information required.[8]

Regardless of the individual system or method used, there are critical features of the gathering, documenting and communicating of information for providing high-quality and safe pre-hospital emergency care. These include:

- accuracy
- timeliness
- completeness
- legibility
- originality
- objectivity.

Attention to such measures will ensure that paramedics and emergency nurses augment efforts to provide high-quality and safety in pre-hospital emergency care.

> **PRACTICE TIP**
>
> Ensure records are legible, timely, accurate, complete, original, factual and objective.

TABLE 11.3 Risks during clinical hand-over[116]

ASPECT OF HAND-OVER	RISKS IDENTIFIED IN THE LITERATURE
Hand-over risks generally	Risks related to: • seniority/experience of medical staff • nature/type of communication behaviours • quality/content of information recorded and/or exchanged • discontinuity in patient care • lack of standardised protocols • healthcare professional fatigue
Interprofession hand-over	Risks related to hand-over between: • ambulance and emergency department • paramedics and first-responders
Interdepartment hand-over	Risks related to hand-over: • between emergency department and intensive care • between emergency department and inpatient team • in which interdepartmental boundaries/responsibilities are unclear
Shift-to-shift hand-over	Risks related to: • lack of structure/policy/procedures • role of medical discretion, particularly during weekend hand-over • poor quality of information in emergency department hand-over • uncertainty over responsibility in an intensive care unit • importance of the maintenance of core values/relationships in nursing hand-over • lack of guidelines for hand-over of anaesthetised patients • impact of fragmentation of hand-over among mental health nurses • information overload • dangers of long hand-overs
Hospital-to-community hand-over	Risks related to: • poor hospital-to-community discharge processes due to shift-to-shift hand-over • poor communication and differences in information quantity/quality depending on a patient's community destination • increased incidence of medical errors and re-hospitalisations
Provision of verbal hand-over only	Risks related to: • limitations of human memory • loss of information across each hand-over
Use of abbreviations in hand-over	Risks related to: • use of non-standard abbreviations by specific groups of clinicians (paediatrics) that were not understood by other healthcare professionals
Patient characteristics affecting hand-over	Risks related to: • varying responses by emergency staff to hand-over information from paramedics depending on patient condition • complex patient problems receiving poorer quality hand-over than more-defined patient conditions • failures in communicating patients' mental health status during transfer between hospital and residential aged care
Characteristics of hand-over	Risks related to: • lack of clarity over the effectiveness of verbal versus tape-recorded versus face-to-face hand-over • communication failures • hand-over being complex and cognitively taxing • interruptions

Wong MC, Yee KC, Turner P. (2008) Clinical Handover Literature Review. eHealth Services Research Group, University of Tasmania, Australia.

TABLE 11.4 Popular mnemonics for gathering and documenting information				
ISBAR[111]	SOAP[131]	SAMPLE[131]	CHART[131]	IMIST-AMBO[132]
Identify	**S**ubjective data	**S**igns and symptoms	**C**hief complaint	**I**dentification of the patient
Situation	**O**bjective data	**A**llergies	**H**istory	**M**echanism/Medical complaint
Background	**A**ssessment data	**M**edications	**A**ssessment	**I**njuries/Information relative to the complaint
Assessment/Agreed plan	**P**lan for patient management	**P**ast medical history	**T**reatment	**S**igns vitals and GCS
Recommendations/**R**ead back		**L**ast meal or intake	**T**ransport	**T**reatment and trends/ response to treatment—
		Events pre-emergency		**A**llergies
				Medications
				Background history
				Other (social) information

SUMMARY

Pre-hospital clinical reasoning, triage and communication are fundamental elements of the practice of paramedics and emergency nurses. At the core of contemporary paramedic and emergency nursing clinical reasoning and triage practice is the mandate to provide high-quality, safe and evidence-based care to patients, their families and communities. An understanding of the theoretical basis of clinical reasoning and the emerging research and evidence-base therein, coupled with timely and appropriate communication for practical problem-solving of patients, informs quality care and practice. Moreover, quality care is reliant on effective communication, especially during periods in the care continuum which traditionally are high risk, such as clinical hand-over. Continuing to extend the research and evidence-base will contribute to the increasing scope and complexity of paramedic clinical reasoning and triage practice.

CASE STUDY

You are an emergency nursing member of a mobile emergency medical team attending a large annual music festival of approximately 35,000 party goers. You and your colleague, an intensive care paramedic from the local ambulance services, respond to a report of a patient in cardiac arrest following a drug overdose. On arrival, the patient has a Glasgow Coma Scale score of 3 and is in respiratory arrest. There is a party going on at the house, with multiple bystanders, and you elicit from a bystander that the patient has used heroin. You successfully resuscitate the patient, who becomes conscious and combative following your administration of naloxone. He refuses to receive any further treatment and transportation. Your assessment of the patient indicates that he has consumed a large quantity of alcohol and other unknown illicit substances. He appears intoxicated, is unsteady of gait and his speech is slurred.

Questions

1. What are some of the environmental challenges this incident presents with respect to your clinical reasoning and judgement practice?

2. How would you go about performing a clinical assessment of the patient?

3. What process would you follow with respect to clinical judgement and decision-making about this patient, the condition and your actions in managing the case?

4. What are the foreseeable risks to this patient should he not receive further treatment and transport?

5. What are the risks to the emergency nursing and paramedic when patients refuse treatment?

6. What communication strategies should you employ when managing a patient and bystanders on scene?

Answers to Case Study Questions can be found on evolve
http://evolve.emergencytrauma.curtis

REFERENCES

1. Hammond KR. Human judgment and social policy: irreducible uncertainty, inevitable error, unavoidable justice. London: Oxford University Press; 1996.

2. Australian Commission on Safety and Quality in Health Care. Windows into Safety and Quality in Health Care 2008. Sydney: ACSQHC; 2008.

3. Higgs J. Physiotherapy, professionalism and self-directed learning. Journal of the Singapore Physiotherapy Association 1993;14:8–11.

4. Higgs J, Jones M. Clinical reasoning in the health professions. 2nd edn. Melbourne: Butterworth–Heinemann; 2000.

5. Groves MA. The clinical reasoning process: a study of its development in medical students [Doctoral Thesis], University of Queensland; 2002.

6. de Dombal T. Medical decision-making, clinical judgment and decision analysis. In: Llewelyn H, Hopkins A, eds. Analysing how we reach clinical decisions. London: Royal College of Physicians; 1993.

7. White S, Stancombe J. Clinical judgment in the health and welfare professions: extending the evidence base. Philadelphia, USA: Open University Press; 2003.

8. Shaban RZ. Paramedic clinical judgment of mental illness: a case study of accounts of practice [PhD]. Brisbane: Arts, Education and Law Group, Griffith University; 2011.

9. Shaban RZ. Mental health assessments in paramedic practice: a warrant for research and inquiry into accounts of paramedic clinical judgment and decision-making. Journal of Emergency Primary Health Care 2004;2:3–4.

10. Snooks HA, Kearsley N, Dale J et al. Gaps between policy, protocols and practice: a qualitative study of the views and practice of emergency ambulance staff concerning the care of patients with non-urgent needs. Quality and Safety in Health Care 2005;14(4): 251–7.

11. Shaban RZ. Paramedics and the mentally ill. In: Grbich C, O'Meara P, eds. Paramedics in Australia: contemporary challenges. Melbourne: Pearson Education; 2009.

12. Alexander M. Reasoning processes used by paramedics to solve clinical problems [Dissertation], George Washington University; 2010.

13. Shaban RZ. Paramedics and the mentally ill. In: Grbich C, O'Meara P, eds. Paramedics in Australia: contemporary challenges of practice. Melbourne: Pearson Education; 2009.

14. Raven S, Tippett V, Ferguson JG, Smith S. An exploration of expanded paramedic health roles for Queensland. Brisbane: Queensland Department of Emergency Services; 2006.

15. Lord B. Book review: clinical reasoning in the health professions. Journal of Emergency Primary Health Care 2003;1:3–4.

16. Caroline N. Nancy Caroline's emergency care in the streets. 6th ed. Sudbury, MA: Jones and Bartlett; 2009.

17. Fitzgerald GJ. Research in pre-hospital care. Journal of Emergency Primary Health Care 2003;1:2.

18. Heath T. Education for the professions: Contemplations and reflections. In: Moses I, ed. Higher education in the late twentieth century: reflections on a changing system—a Festschrift for Ernest Rose. Sydney: Higher Education Research and Development Society of Australia; 1990.

19. Oxford University Press Australia. The Australian Oxford Dictionary. 3rd edn. Melbourne: Oxford University Press Australia; 2006.

20. Dowie J. Clinical decision analysis: background and introduction. In: Llewelyn H, Hopkins A, eds. Analysing how we reach clinical decisions. London: Royal College of Physicians; 1993.

21. Ritter B. Why evidence-based practice? CCNP Connection 1998;1(5):1–8.

22. Thompson C, Dowding D. Clinical decision making and judgment in nursing. London: Churchill Livingstone; 2002.

23. Goldstein WM, Hogarth RM. Judgment and decision research: some historical context. In: Goldstein WM, Hogarth RM, eds. Research on judgment and decision making: currents, connections and controversies. Cambridge: Cambridge University Press; 1997.

24. Bell DE, Raiffa H, Tversky A. Descriptive, normative and prescriptive interactions in decision-making. In: Bell DE, Raiffa H, Tversky A, eds. Decision making: descriptive, normative and prescriptive interactions. Cambridge: Cambridge University Press; 1988.

25. Berg M. Problems and promises of the protocol. Social Science & Medicine 1997;44(8):1081–8.

26. Bell DE, Raiffa H, Tversky A. Decision making: descriptive, normative and prescriptive interactions. Cambridge: Cambridge University Press; 1988.

27. Chapman GB, Sonnenberg FA. Decision making in health care: theory, psychology and applications. Cambridge: Cambridge University Press; 2000.

28. Clemen RT. Naturalistic decision making and decision analysis. Journal of Behavioral Decision Making 2001;14(5):359.

29. Shaban RZ. Theories of judgment and decision-making: a review of the theoretical literature. Journal of Emergency Primary Health Care 2005;3:1–2.

30. Pruitt JS, Cannon-Bowers JA, Salas E. In search of naturalistic decisions. In: Flin R, Salas E, Strub M, Martin L, eds. Decision making under stress: emerging themes and applications. Aldershot, England: Ashgate Publishing Ltd; 1997.

31. Bendall J, Morrison A. Clinical judgment. In: O'Meara P, Grbich C, eds. Paramedics in Australia: contemporary challenges of practice. Melbourne: Pearson Education; 2009.

32. US Department of Transportation. National Highway Traffic Safety Administration: Emergency Medical Technician Paramedic; national standards curriculum. 1998.

33. Bendall J, Morrison A. Clinical judgement. In: O'Meara P, Grbich C, eds. Paramedics in Australia: Contemporary challenges of practice. Frenchs Forest, NSW: Pearson Education Australia; 2009:96–111.

34. United States Department of Transportation. Emergency Medical Technician Paramedic (EMT-P) national standards curriculum. In: National Highway Traffic Safety Administation, ed. 1998. www.nhtsa.gov/people/injury/ems/emt-p/disk_1%5B1%5D/intro.pdf; accessed 3 March 2009.

35. Convention of Ambulance Authorities and Paramedics Australasia. Professional Competency Standards—Paramedics. St Kilda, Victoria, Australia: Convention of Ambulance Authorities and Paramedics Australasia; 2013.

36. Billett S. Learning in the workplace: Strategies for effective practice. Crows Nest, Australia: Allen & Unwin; 2001.

37. Sanders MJ, ed. Mosby's paramedic textbook. 3rd edn. St Louis, Missouri: Mosby JEMS Elsevier; 2006.

38. Elling B, Smith MG, Pollack AN, eds. Nancy Caroline's emergency care in the streets. 6th edn. Sudbury, Massachusetts: Jones and Bartlett; 2009.

39. Bledsoe BE, Porter RA, Cherry RA. Paramedic care: Principles and practice. 2nd edn. Upper Saddle River, New Jersey: Prentice Hall; 2006.

40. Alexander M. Reasoning processes used by paramedics to solve clinical problems. Columbia, United States, The George Washington University; 2010.

41. Marks PJ, Daniel TD, Afolabi O et al. Emergency (999) calls to the ambulance service that do not result in the patient being transported to hospital: An epidemiological study. Emergency Medicine Journal 2002;19:449–52.

42. Karlsten R, Sjoqvist BA. Telemedicine and decision support in emergency ambulances in Uppsala. J Telemed Telecare 2000;6(1):1–7.

43. Dale J, Higgins J, Williams S et al. Computer assisted assessment and advice for 'non-serious' 999 ambulance service callers: The potential impact on ambulance despatch. Emergency Medicine Journal Mar 2003;20(2):178–83.

44. Marks P, Daniel T. Emergency ambulance triage. J R Soc Med 2002;95(5):270.

45. Grzybowski M, Zalenski RJ, Ross MA, Bock B. A prediction model for prehospital triage of patients with suspected cardiac ischemia. J Electrocardiol 2000;33 Suppl:253–8.

46. Donnelly PD, Weston CF. Editorial—Ambulance staff exercise discretion over resuscitation decision. British Medical Journal Sep 1995;311(7009):877–8.

47. Figgis K, Slevin O, Cunningham JB. Investigation of paramedics' compliance with clinical practice guidelines for the management of chest pain. Emergency Medicine Journal Feb 2010;27(2):151–5.

48. Jones T, Woollard M. Paramedic accuracy in using a decision support algorithm when recognising adult death: A prospective cohort study. Emergency Medicine Journal Sept 2003;20(5):473–6.

49. Rittenberger JC, Beck PW, Paris PM. Errors of omission in the treatment of prehospital chest pain patients. Prehosp Emerg Care Jan–Mar 2005;9(1):2–7.

50. Hein C, Owen H, Plummer J. A proposed framework for deciding suitable extraglottic airway devices (EAD) for paramedics to use. Resuscitation Jul 2010;81(7):914.

51. Nurmi J, Pettila V, Biber B et al. Effect of protocol compliance to cardiac arrest identification by emergency medical dispatchers. Resuscitation 2006;70(3):463–9.

52. Neal D. Prehospital patient triage in mass casualty incidents: An engineering management analysis and prototype strategy recommendation. USA, The George Washington University; 2009.

53. Feldman MJ, Lukins JL, Verbeek PR et al. Use of treat-and-release medical directives for paramedics at a mass gathering. Prehosp Emerg Care Apr–Jun 2005;9(2):213–17.

54. Schmidt T, Atcheson R, Federiuk C et al. Evaluation of protocols allowing emergency medical technicians to determine need for treatment and transport. Acad Emerg Med Jun 2000;7(6):663–9.

55. Yeh EL, Cone DC. Cancellation of responding ALS units by BLS providers: A national survey. Prehosp Emerg Care Jul–Sep 2000;4(3):227–33.

56. Clawson J, Olola C, Heward A et al. Ability of the medical priority dispatch system protocol to predict the acuity of 'unknown problem' dispatch response levels. Prehosp Emerg Care Jul–Sep 2008;12(3):290–6.

57. Clawson J, Olola CH, Heward A et al. Accuracy of emergency medical dispatchers' subjective ability to identify when higher dispatch levels are warranted over a medical priority dispatch system automated protocol's recommended coding based on paramedic outcome data. Emergency Medicine Journal Aug 2007;24(8):560–3.

58. Farrand L, Leprohon J, Kalina M et al. The role of protocols and professional judgement in emergency medical dispatching. Eur J Emerg Med 1995;2(3):136–48.

59. Thompson C, Dowding D. Clinical decision making and judgement in nursing. London: Churchill Livingstone; 2002.

60. Watcher DA, Brillman JC, Lewis J, Sapien RE. Pediatric telephone triage protocols: Standardized decision making or a false sense of security. Ann Emerg Med 1999;33(4):388–94.

61. Poole SR, Schmitt BD, Caruth T et al. After-hours telephone coverage: An application of area-wide telephone triage and advice system for paediatric illness. Paediatrics 1993;92(5):670–9.

62. Hick JL, Mahoney BD, Lappe M. Factors influencing hospital transport of patients in continuing cardiac arrest. Ann Emerg Med Jul 1998;32(1):19–25.

63. Marsden AK, Ng GA, Dalziel K, Cobbe SM. When is it futile for ambulance personnel to initiate cardiopulmonary resuscitation? British Medical Journal 1995;311:49–51.

64. Dunne RB, Compton S, Welch RD et al. Prehospital on-site triaging. Prehosp Emerg Care 2003;7(1):85–8.

65. Westbrook JI, Westbrook MT, Gosling AS. Ambulance officers' use of online clinical evidence. BMC Med Inf Decis Mak 2006;6:31.

66. Rycroft-Malone J. Clinical guidelines. In: Thompson C, Dowding D, eds. Clinical decision making and judgement in nursing. London: Churchill Livingstone: 2002.

67. Freebody P. Qualitative research in education: interaction and practice. 1st ed. London: SAGE Publications; 2004.

68. Grimshaw JM, Russell T. Effect of clinical guidelines on medical practice: a systematic review of rigorous evaluations. Lancet 1993;342:1317–22.

69. Wilson RM, Runciman WB, Gibberd RW et al. The quality in Australian health care study. Medical Journal of Australia 1995;163(9): 458–71.

70. Wilson RM, Van Der Weyden MB. The safety of Australian healthcare: 10 years after QAHCS. Medical Journal of Australia 2005;182(6):260–1.

71. Davies G. Queensland Public Hospital Commission of Inquiry. Brisbane: Queensland Government; 2005.

72. Forster P. Queensland health systems review. Vol 430: The Consultancy Bureau; 2005.

73. Australian Institute of Health and Welfare (AIHW), Australian Commission on Safety and Quality in Health Care (ACSQHC). Sentinel events in Australian public hospitals 2004–2005. Canberra: AIHW; 2007.

74. Staib L. Staib Report: Queensland Ambulance Service. Brisbane: Queensland Ambulance Service; 1996.

75. Department of Health. WA Ambulance Service Inc Inquiry. Perth: Government of Western Australia; 2009.

76. Minister for Health. Investigation into Rural Ambulance Victoria. Melbourne: State Government of Victoria; 2006.

77. Kelty M. Sustaining the unsustainable: Police and Community Safety Review Final Report. Brisbane: Queensland Government; 2013.

78. Audit Office of New South Wales. New South Wales Auditor-General's Report Performance Audit—Reducing ambulance turnaround time at hospitals. Ambulance Service of NSW, NSW Ministry of Health. Sydney: New South Wales Government; 2013.

79. Australian Health Ministers' Advisory Council Health Workforce Principal Committee. Consultation paper—Options for regulation of paramedics. Canberra: Australian Health Ministers' Advisory Council 2012.

80. Shaban RZ. Invited submission—Review of Western Australia mental health policy and mental health services. Perth: Minister for Mental Health: Government of Western Australia; 2009.

81. National Institute of Clinical Studies. Implementation of a state-wide emergency department mental health triage tool in Victoria. Melbourne: National Institute of Clinical Studies; 2006.

82. Kovacs G, Croskerry P. Clinical decision making: an emergency medicine perspective. Academic Emergency Medicine 1999;6(9):947–52.

83. Croskerry P, Sinclair D. Emergency medicine: A practice prone to error? Journal of the Canadian Association of Emergency Physicians 2001;3(4):271–6.

84. Campbell SG, Croskerry P, Bond WF. Profiles in patient safety: A 'perfect storm' in the emergency department. Academic Emergency Medicine 2007;14(8):743–9.

85. Croskerry P, Shapiro M, Campbell S et al. Profiles in Patient Safety: Medication Errors in the Emergency Department. Academic Emergency Medicine 2004;11(3):289–99.

86. Croskerry P. To err is human—and let's not forget it. Canadian Medical Association Journal 2010;182(5):524.

87. Australasian College of Emergency Medicine. Policy on the Australasian triage scale. West Melbourne, Australia: Australasian College of Emergency Medicine; 2006.

88. Whitby S, Ieraci S, Johnson D et al. Analysis of the process of triage: the use and outcome of the national triage scale. Liverpool: Liverpool Health Service; 1997.

89. Wuerz R, Fernandes C, Alarcon J. Inconsistency of emergency department triage. Annals of Emergency Medicine 1998;32(4):431–5.

90. LeVasseur SA, Considine J, Charles A et al. Consistency of triage in Victoria's emergency departments: triage consistency report. Monash Institute of Health Services Research. Report to the Victorian Department of Human Services; 2001.

91. Jelinek GA, Little M. Inter-rater reliability of the National Triage Scale over 11,500 simulated occasions of triage. Emergency Medicine 1996;8(4):226–30.

92. Fernandes C, Wuerz R, Clark S, Djurdjev O. How reliable is emergency department triage? Annals of Emergency Medicine 1999;34(2):141–7.

93. Doherty S. Application of the national triage scale is not uniform. Australian Emergency Nursing Journal 1996;1(1):26.

94. Dilley SJ, Standen P. Victorian nurses demonstrate concordance in the application of the National Triage Scale. Emergency Medicine 1998;10(1):12–18.

95. Asplund K, Castren M, Ehrenberg A et al. Emergency department triage scales and their components: A systematic review of the scientific evidence. Scandinavian Journal of Trauma, Resuscitation and Emergency Medicine 2011;19:42.

96. Considine J, Ung L, Thomas S. Triage nurses' decisions using the National Triage Scale for Australian emergency departments. Accident and Emergency Nursing 2000;8(4):201–9.

97. Considine J, Ung L, Thomas S. Clinical decisions using the national triage scale: how important is postgraduate education? Accident and Emergency Nursing 2001;9(2):101–8.

98. Richardson D. No relationship between emergency department activity and triage categorization. Academic Emergency Medicine 1998;5(2):141–5.

99. Hollis G, Sprivulis P. Reliability of the National Triage Scale with changes in emergency department activity level. Emergency Medicine 1996;8(4):231–4.

100. Cameron PA, Kennedy MP, McNeil JJ. The effects of bonus payment on emergency service performance in Victoria. Medical Journal of Australia 1999;171(5):243–6.

101. Crellin DJ, Johnston L. Poor agreement in application of the Australasian triage scale to paediatric emergency department presentations. Contemporary Nurse 2003;15(1–2):48–60.

102. Considine J, LeVasseur SA, Villanueva E. The Australasian Triage Scale: Examining emergency department nurses' performance using computer and paper scenarios. Annals of Emergency Medicine 2004;44(5):516–23.

103. Considine J, Botti M, Thomas S. Do knowledge and experience have specific roles in triage decision-making? Academic Emergency Medicine 2007;14(8):722–6.

104. Smart D, Pollard C, Walpole B. Mental health triage in emergency medicine. Australian & New Zealand Journal of Psychiatry 1999;33(1):57–69.

105. Council of Ambulance Authorities. CAA Annual Report Data Dictionary. 2011–2012.

106. Noon AJ. The cognitive processes underpinning clinical decision in triage assessment: A theoretical conundrum? International Emergency Nursing 2014;22(1):40–6.

107. Dinh MM, Bein KJ, Oliver M et al. Refining the trauma triage algorithm at an Australian major trauma centre: derivation and internal validation of a triage risk score. European Journal of Trauma and Emergency Surgery 2014;40(1):67–74.

108. Smith A. Using a theory to understand triage decision making. International Emergency Nursing 2013;21(2):113–17.

109. Hagiwara MA, Sjöqvist BA, Lundberg L et al. Decision support system in prehospital care: a randomized controlled simulation study. American Journal of Emergency Medicine 2013;31(1):145–53.

110. Ranse J, Zeitz K. Disaster triage. In: Powers R, Daly E, eds. International disaster nursing. Melbourne, Australia: World Association of Disaster and Emergency Medicine: Cambridge University Press; 2010.

111. Marshall S, Harrison J, Flanagan B. The teaching of a structured tool improves the clarity and content of interprofessional clinical communication. Quality and Safety in Health Care 2009;18(2):137–40.

112. Haig KM, Sutton S, Whittington J. SBAR: a shared mental model for improving communication between clinicians. Joint Commission Journal on Quality and Patient Safety 2006;32(3):167–75.

113. Australian Commission on Safety and Quality in Health Care (ACSQHC). National Safety and Quality Health Service Standard for Clinical Handover. Sydney: Commonwealth of Australia; 2014.

114. Gaston C. How an ambulance service can contribute to the health care continuum. In Sight. 2007. http://cpd.org.au/category/publications/insight/.

115. Australian Medical Association. AMA clinical handover guide—safe handover: safe patients. Kingston, ACT: Australian Medical Association; 2006.

116. Wong MC, Yeek KC, Turner P. A structured evidence-based literature review regarding the effectiveness of improvement interventions in clinical handover. Canberra: Australian Commission on Safety and Quality in Health Care; 2008.

117. Bruce K, Suserud B. The handover process and triage of ambulance-borne patients: the experiences of emergency nurses. Nursing in Critical Care 2005;10(4):201–9.

118. Shanley C, Sutherland S, Stott K et al. Increasing the profile of the care of the older person in the ED: A contemporary nursing challenge. International Emergency Nursing 2008;16(3):152–8.

119. Bartlett G, Blais R, Tamblyn R et al. Impact of patient communication problems on the risk of preventable adverse events in acute care settings. Canadian Medical Association Journal 2008;178(12):1555–62.

120. Sutcliffe KM, Lewton E, Rosenthal M. Communication failures: an insidious contributor to medical mishaps. Academic Medicine 2004;79(2):186–94.

121. The Joint Commission. The joint commission's annual report on quality and safety 2007. Washington DC: The Joint Commission; 2007.

122. Witherington EMA, Pirzada OM, Avery AJ. Communication gaps and readmissions to hospital for patients aged 75 years and older: observational study. Quality and Safety in Health Care 2008;17(1):71–5.

123. Fleischer S, Berg A, Zimmermann M et al. Nurse–patient interaction and communication: A systematic literature review. J Public Health 2009;17(5):339–53.

124. Watson WT, Marshall ES, Fosbinder D. Elderly patients' perceptions of care in the emergency department. Journal of Emergency Nursing 1999;25(2):88–92.

125. Engel K. Patient comprehension of emergency department care and instructions: are patients aware of when they do not understand? Annals of Emergency Medicine 2008;53(4):454–61.

126. Kessels P. Patients' memory for medical information. Journal of the Royal Society of Medicine 2003;96(5):219–22.

127. Baker DW. Health literacy and mortality among elderly persons. Archives of Internal Medicine 2007;167(14):1503–9.

128. Agency for Healthcare Research and Quality. Literacy and health outcomes: summary, evidence report/technology assessment No. 87. 2004. http://archive.ahrq.gov/clinic/epcsums/litsum.htm.

129. Barnett R. The idea of higher education. Buckingham: The Society for Research into Higher Education and Open University Press; 1990.

130. Johnstone M, Kanitsaki O. Culture, language, and patient safety: making the link. International Journal for Quality in Health Care 2006;18(5):383–8.

131. Sanders MJ. Mosby's paramedic textbook. 3rd edn. St Louis: Mosby/JEMS; 2007.

132. Iedema R et al. Design and trial of a new ambulance-to-emergency department handover protocol: 'IMIST-AMBO'. BMJ Qual Saf 2012;21:627–33.

CHAPTER 12
MAJOR INCIDENT PREPAREDNESS MANAGEMENT

MARTIN WARD AND DAVID KOOP

Essentials

- When planning for a mass-casualty incident (MCI), all facets of the incident must be considered—namely the prevention, preparedness, response and recovery (PPRR) phases. It is essential that all staff involved in an MCI response are aware of their roles.
- Business continuity plans (BCPs) are extremely important to ensure that adequate systems are in place to allow first-responders, hospital facilities and staff to continue to respond to a MCI in the event of power failures and other possible critical systems failures.
- Communication is the key to any effective MCI response and alternative methods of communication need to be established so as not to compromise information flow.
- Effective MCI triage is 'doing the greatest good for the greatest number of victims'. Therefore, it is important to have knowledge of the various methods of triage.
- Advanced triage is instigated in the pre-hospital and hospital environments when medical staff are required to make decisions about which seriously injured people should or should not receive advanced care, based on the likelihood of survival.
- Advanced triage is instigated when the number of MCI victims overwhelms available resources. Advanced triage should continue once victims are inside receiving hospitals.
- The development of standing operational procedures (SOPs) assists in streamlining MCI victim flow by determining what essential tests and investigations are required in a MCI event. This assists in ensuring a more ordered victim flow.
- Development of agreed key coordinator positions—i.e. imaging, radiology, an operating room surgical director—to assist in prioritising care and assisting flow of MCI victims.
- Ensure pre-numbered MCI record numbers are easily entered into an electronic system and electronic links to key areas in the hospital are tested. Have a robust back-up system that is easily understood.
- Keep all paperwork simple and relevant.
- Negotiate an agreement with hospital blood banks about minimal checking requirements of MCI victim details.
- Practise MCI and CBR responses as often as possible and include MCI updates in regular education session for all staff.
- Ensure the emergency department (ED) and organisation have a critical mass of staff ready to be deployed to an MCI.
- In a chemical–biological–radiological (CBR) MCI it is essential to ensure that staff and facilities are not contaminated. This can be achieved by controlling access to sites including EDs and ensuring that staff treating patients have the appropriate personal protective equipment (PPE) available.
- In an MCI response, it is essential to have highly trained multidisciplinary staff who have received regular training, have current vaccinations and passports and are ready for deployment locally and internationally.
- Staff occupational health and safety issues are a priority when considering the PPRR phases of MCI planning.

INTRODUCTION

This chapter describes the broad categories of MCIs, both natural and man-made. The principles of preparation and management (PPRR) described in this chapter are applicable to all types of MCIs. Australian and New Zealand Government legislation and terminology are outlined, and more recent MCI incidents are cited as examples that incidents can occur at any time and that early consideration towards planning the prevention, preparedness, response and recovery phases of MCIs goes some way to lessening the damage and impact of the incident. The section on CBR is designed to be extensive to enhance the reader's understanding of the three distinct types of CBR MCIs.

What is a mass-casualty incident?

Hirshberg states that: 'In a MCI, a hospital is challenged with a large number of casualties generated within a short period of time. A discrepancy is created between the victim load and available resources.'[1]

A broader and more descriptive definition is offered by the New Zealand Ministry of Health, which describes an MCI as any occurrence that presents a serious threat to the health of the community or disruption to the health services, or causes (or is likely to cause) numbers or types of casualties that require special measures to be implemented by appropriate responding agencies, including ambulance services, District Health Boards (DHBs) e.g. hospitals, primary care and public health and the ministry, in order to maintain an effective, appropriate and sustainable response.[2]

MCI incidents are most commonly classified into two broad categories: natural and generated (Table 12.1). The New Zealand Government defines MCIs as:

- **no-notice incidents:** happen suddenly, with little or no warning. A no-notice incident may occur in isolation, or a series of incidents may occur consecutively or concurrently. A no-notice incident could be caused by an earthquake, an explosion, a serious transport accident, a tsunami or a series of simultaneous incidents, e.g. multiple bomb blasts, and can result in a large and immediate increase in the number of casualties.

- **a rising-tide incident:** sometimes known as a slow-onset incident, produces a surge in the number of casualties over time. It may result from a single event, such as a hazardous material incident, which produces no immediate casualties, but where over time a growing number of people present with health effects resulting from the incident. Some rising-tide incidents may be extremely difficult to detect. Discrete groups of patients presenting with signs and symptoms at a range of health care facilities may only be linked by epidemiological tracking.

  This type of incident is likely to have a greater and more sustained effect on the primary sector in the immediate vicinity, possibly with an increased need for community-based resources (Table 12.1).

There have been some devastating large-scale natural disasters, beginning with the 2004 Boxing Day tsunami in South-East and East Asia, and Hurricane Katrina in New Orleans in 2005. In 2009 the Pacific region was struck by a submarine earthquake

TABLE 12.1 Classification of disasters[102]	
NATURAL DISASTERS	**HUMAN-GENERATED DISASTERS**
Acute onset	
Floods	Transportation/vehicular crashes
Cyclones/hurricanes	
Heatwaves	Structural fires
Bushfires	Structural collapses
Earthquakes	Mining accidents
Landslides	Hazardous material releases
Tornadoes	Radiation accidents
Volcanic eruptions	Terrorism
Epidemics	War/complex humanitarian emergencies
Gradual/chronic onset	
Drought	
Desertification	
Pest infestations (e.g. locusts)	

Reviewed January 2014; no changes to date.

generating a tsunami which caused substantial damage and loss of life in Samoa and Tonga. The earthquake occurred on the same day as earthquakes in Sumatra (Indonesia), which resulted in a large loss of life and property.[3] The 2009 Victorian bush fires resulted in Australia's highest ever loss of life from bush fire. In 2010, the island of Haiti in the Caribbean Sea was devastated by an earthquake, with a huge loss of life and infrastructure such as roads, airports, communications and hospitals.[4]

On 22 February 2011 a 6.3 magnitude earthquake struck Christchurch, New Zealand. Several aftershocks were reported, some registering at 5.6 in magnitude (Fig 12.1). This was the second major earthquake to hit the city. The disaster caused 185 deaths, an estimated 6659 major injuries in the first 24 hours and extensive damage to infrastructure and buildings.[5] The Civil Defence declared a Category 3 emergency, the highest possible for a regional disaster.[6]

Other examples of devastating large-scale natural disasters are:

- In 2013 there was loss of property in the Blue Mountains, NSW, Australia, when severe fires took hold across the area, destroying 210 houses and other buildings. The fires in the Greater Blue Mountains area had burnt out over 65,000 hectares (Fig 12.2).

- In March 2011 an earthquake struck Japan, resulting in a subsequent tsunami and major loss of life.

- In November 2013 Typhoon Haiyan, known in the Philippines as Typhoon Yolanda, was the second-deadliest Philippine typhoon on record, killing at least 3633 people.[7] The cyclone caused catastrophic destruction, and about

11 million people have been affected with many left homeless (Fig 12.3).[8]

- The beginning of 2014 heralded severe flooding in the United Kingdom and extreme freezing conditions in North America (Fig 12.4).

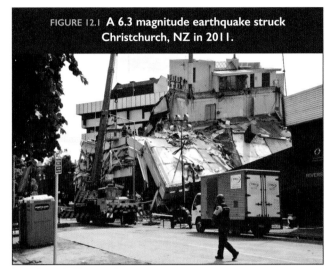

FIGURE 12.1 **A 6.3 magnitude earthquake struck Christchurch, NZ in 2011.**

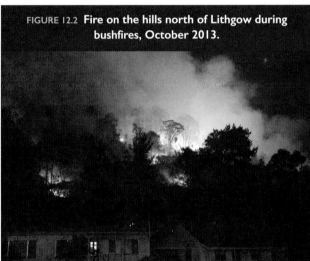

FIGURE 12.2 **Fire on the hills north of Lithgow during bushfires, October 2013.**

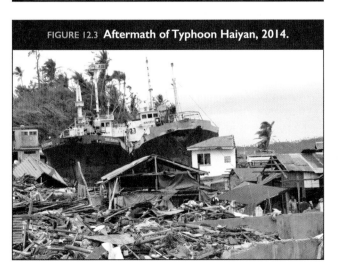

FIGURE 12.3 **Aftermath of Typhoon Haiyan, 2014.**

There have also been an increasing number of terrorist attacks around the world. Terrorism is defined in the *Criminal Code Act 1995* (Australia) which to date remains unchanged, as:

a terrorist act is an act or threat, intended to advance a political, ideological or religious cause by coercing or intimidating an Australian or foreign government or the public, by causing serious harm to people or property, creating a serious risk of health and safety to the public, disrupting trade, critical infrastructure or electronic systems.[9]

For example, the most notable and publicised terrorist attacks were the World Trade Centre attacks in September 2001, the Bali bombings in October 2002 and 2005, and the Madrid (Fig 12.5) and London bombings in March 2004 and July 2005 (Fig 12.6). In 2008 one of India's largest cities, Mumbai, was under siege by a coordinated shooting and bombing attack.[10] In December 2014, a lone gunman held hostages in a cafe at Martin Place in Sydney, Australia. Police treated the event as a terrorist attack. The gunman and two hostages died in the siege.[11,12]

Infectious disease emergencies can cause MCIs. An example of a recent infectious disease emergency was the March 2003 outbreak in Singapore of the highly contagious

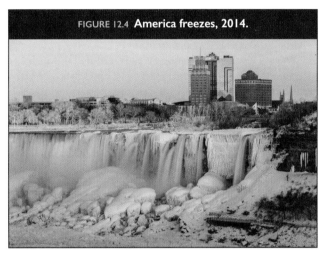

FIGURE 12.4 **America freezes, 2014.**

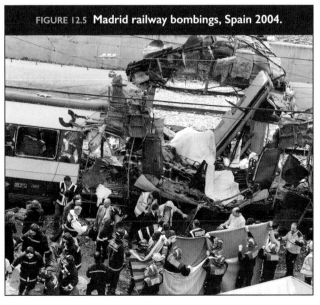

FIGURE 12.5 **Madrid railway bombings, Spain 2004.**

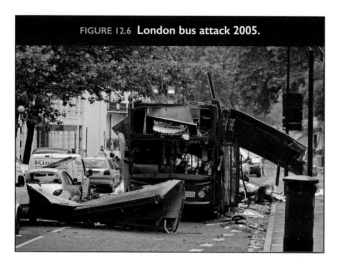

FIGURE 12.6 **London bus attack 2005.**

respiratory disease severe acute respiratory syndrome (SARS). This outbreak required a coordinated health response and the introduction of strict infection-control precautions to protect victims, visitors and people in the surrounding environment. As a result, a national strategy for SARS containment was enacted.[13]

In 2009 an influenza pandemic was declared when there was a global outbreak of a new subtype of influenza A identified by virologists as H1N1[14] and commonly known as 'swine flu'. The World Health Organization (WHO) declared the outbreak to be pandemic on 11 June 2009. In September 2012 the WHO first reported cases of a novel coronavirus, now referred to as Middle East Respiratory syndrome (MERS-CoV). MERS coronavirus is a disease caused by a new virus that causes a rapid onset of severe respiratory disease in people. Most cases have occurred in people with underlying conditions that may make them more likely to suffer respiratory infections.[15] In March 2014, the WHO reported an Ebola outbreak in Guinea, a western African nation. The disease then rapidly spread to the neighbouring countries of Liberia and Sierra Leone. It is the largest Ebola outbreak ever. As of 21 February 2015, 23,574 suspected cases and 9556 deaths had been reported.[16,17]

The response to and effects of pandemic emergencies are discussed extensively in Chapter 28.

It is evident that whatever the cause, MCI events present many varied challenges for governments with regard to search and rescue through to repair of services and recovery from the incident.

Government planning for mass-casualty incidents

Governments in Australia and New Zealand have developed comprehensive plans that cover the main considerations of MCI planning, namely prevention, preparedness, response and recovery. Both governments' plans encompass one of the fundamental principles of disaster management, which is to provide 'the greatest good for the greatest number'; the plans also strive to rapidly rebuild communities to enable them to recover from the MCI and 'to minimise the health impacts to individuals and the community during an emergency'.[18]

A comprehensive approach to MCI management is used, which draws from the expertise of paramedics and healthcare

professionals who, in consultation with local communities, develop strategies which are continually refined for MCI planning. A synopsis of these plans is outlined below. The Australian section is rather large due to the vastness of the continent.

Australian Government plans

Australian Commonwealth Government plans are in place to clearly define roles and responsibilities between the states and territories. The following are a synopsis of such plans.

- **Australian Emergency Management Arrangements (AEMA)**
  These Arrangements provide an overview of how federal, state, territory and local governments collectively approach the management of emergencies, including catastrophic MCI events.

- **Australian Government Disaster Response Plan (COMDISPLAN)**
  The aim of COMDISPLAN is to describe the coordination arrangements for the provision of Australian Government physical assistance to states or territories or offshore territories in the event of a disaster. The plan can be activated for any disaster regardless of the cause.

- **Australian Government Plan for the Reception of Australian Citizens and Approved Foreign Nationals Evacuated from Overseas (COMRECEPLAN)**
  The aim of COMRECEPLAN is to outline the arrangements for the reception into Australia of Australian citizens, permanent residents and their immediate dependants and approved foreign nationals evacuated from overseas.
  The evacuation would normally be coordinated by the Department of Foreign Affairs and Trade (DFAT).

- **Australian Government Aviation Disaster Response Plan (CAVDISPLAN)**
  The aim of CAVDISPLAN is to outline how the Australian Government would assist states and Territories in the event of a state or territory activating its applicable response plan to deal with a major aircraft accident. It also describes how the Australian government would coordinate the response to a major aircraft accident outside a state or territory, such as at sea, or on an Australian offshore territory or in its vicinity.
  CAVDISPLAN addresses the processes associated with rapid deployment of search and rescue facilities and the establishment of the subsequent investigatory processes. COMDISPLAN can be activated to support CAVDISPLAN.

- **Australian Government Maritime Radiological Response Plan (COMARRPLAN)**
  COMARRPLAN is a contingency plan for the provision of Australian Government assistance in the event of a radiological incident involving ships carrying radiological material. COMARRPLAN is a sub-plan of COMDISPLAN.

- **National Response Plan for Mass Casualty Incidents Involving Australians Overseas (OSMASSCASPLAN)**
  OSMASSCASPLAN is the national overseas mass casualty response plan. The plan provides an agreed framework for

agencies in all Australian jurisdictions to assess, repatriate and provide care for Australians and other approved persons injured or killed overseas in numbers that exceed the capacity of normal day-to-day operations of relevant agencies in any incident and is declared a mass casualty event by Ministers.

- **Australian Government Overseas Disaster Assistance Plan (AUSASSISTPLAN)**

  The aim of AUSASSISTPLAN is to detail the coordination arrangements for the provision of Australian emergency assistance, using Commonwealth physical and technical resources, following a disaster or emergency in another country. AusAID may call upon EMA, as AusAID's agent, to prepare contingency plans. AusAID may also request EMA to coordinate the operational aspects of a post-impact (emergency) response to an overseas disaster employing Australian Government physical or technical resources.[19]

Australian Government Emergency Management Plans

Australian state and territory governments

State and territory governments have primary responsibility within their own jurisdictions for emergency management in the interests of community safety and well-being. This involves responsibility for:

- developing, implementing and ensuring compliance with comprehensive emergency mitigation policies and strategies in all relevant areas of government activity, including land use planning, infrastructure provision and building standards compliance
- strengthening partnerships with and encouraging and supporting local governments, and remote and Indigenous communities, to undertake emergency risk assessments and mitigation measures
- ensuring provision of appropriate emergency awareness and education programs and warning systems
- ensuring that the community and emergency management agencies are prepared for and able to respond to emergencies
- maintaining adequate levels of well-equipped and trained career and volunteer disaster response personnel
- ensuring appropriate emergency relief and recovery measures are available, and
- ensuring that post-emergency assessment and analysis is undertaken.

Prevention and preparedness

Prevention measures seek to eliminate or reduce the impact of hazards and/or to reduce the susceptibility and increase the resilience of the community subject to the impact of those hazards. Prevention covers a range of activities and strategies by individuals, communities, businesses and governments. State and territory governments have the primary role in prevention within their respective jurisdictions. This role is supported by legislation and policy; however, government agencies at all levels undertake prevention programs as part of their day-to-day functions within their responsibilities.

Prevention strategies include:

- hazard-specific control programs, such as building flood levees, bushfire mitigation and installation of fire alarms
- land-use planning and building controls in legislation and regulations
- quarantine and border control measures
- public health strategies
- community education and awareness
- hazardous material safety/security initiatives
- critical infrastructure protection programs
- mass gathering safety/protection programs.

Emergency planning

A key element of Australia's arrangements is effective emergency planning for all hazards. The existence of such plans allows all emergency managers and responders to understand the roles, responsibilities, capabilities and capacity of other organisations. These plans are tested through exercises and experiences to ensure they are current and appropriate to the task.

Preparedness

Planning is a key element of being prepared. However, there are many other aspects associated with being prepared, such as training, equipment, public education, public communication arrangements and stockpile of essential items. Australia addresses these issues at several levels with individuals encouraged to make appropriate provision for their own preparedness, as well as at community and multi-government levels. In addition to stockpiling essential items, such as generators and medicines, there are education and training programs; interoperability across the country; testing of procedures through exercise programs; and warning systems for the public. An example of preparedness is the critical infrastructure protection planning and cooperation by all spheres of government in partnership with the private sector.

Response

Emergency response involves actions taken in anticipation of, during and immediately after an emergency to ensure that its effects are minimised, and that people affected are given immediate relief and support. The response to an emergency is managed first at the local level. Assistance from adjacent local areas, across the state or territory, other states or territories or the Commonwealth Government is provided according to the scale of the emergency and requests from the jurisdictions for assistance.

A response may include:

- providing warning messages and public information
- evacuating people or communities
- fire fighting
- hazardous materials containment, neutralisation and containment
- providing medical support
- providing food, water and shelter
- searching and rescuing
- establishing coordination or evacuation centres
- animal/stock welfare, e.g. fodder drops
- assessing damage.

Each state and territory has its own emergency management legislation, structures, plans and procedures that can be used to respond to an impending or actual emergency. All states and Territories have established groups of representatives from emergency agencies that coordinate all available resources, whether at the local or state level. These coordination arrangements are also in place at the Commonwealth Government level and the national level to cover those emergencies that are beyond the resources available from within a state or territory or where the emergency involves another country.

Recovery

It is not possible to prevent all emergencies. Therefore, recovery activities are needed to address reconstruction, rehabilitation and re-establishment demands across physical, social, emotional, psychological, environmental and economic elements. Recovery is, however, more than simply the replacement of what has been destroyed and the rehabilitation of those affected. The aim is to leave the community more resilient than it was before. Planning for recovery is integral to emergency preparation and mitigation actions may often be initiated as part of recovery. Recovery starts with the initial response and may continue for a long period of time, well after the physical damage has been repaired. It requires the collaboration of all spheres of government, the private sector and, most importantly, the community.

Recovery arrangements

Australia has in place coordinated recovery arrangements across all levels of government. Recovery agencies are part of each state and territory's emergency management committees to ensure continuity and consistency between response and recovery. This includes input from the community and non-government agencies. The arrangements in each state and territory are detailed in stand-alone state-wide plans or as sub-plans of broader emergency management plans. Generally these plans:

- outline the arrangements for managing recovery activities at local and state or territory levels
- provide protocols for establishing and managing local evacuation, relief or recovery centres
- provide processes for disaster relief and assistance measures
- suggest arrangements for establishing and managing public appeals
- recommend approaches for providing continuing information to the affected population
- identify the types of activities which rebuild communities
- include the need to capture 'lessons learned' to improve recovery operations in the future.

Recovery principles

Successful recovery management in Australia is based on the following six nationally endorsed principles:

1. Is based on an understanding of the community context.
2. Acknowledges the complex and dynamic nature of emergencies and communities.
3. Is responsive and flexible, engaging communities and empowering them to move forward.
4. Requires a planned, coordinated and adaptive approach based on continuing assessment of impacts and needs.
5. Is built on effective communication with affected communities and other stakeholders.
6. Recognises, supports and builds on community, individual and organisational capacity.

Roles and responsibilities

- States and territories have primary responsibility for the management of emergencies within their jurisdictions.
- When emergencies occur, the Australian Government provides certain forms of physical and financial assistance to states and Territories when requested to do so and may also provide financial and other assistance to individuals directly affected by an emergency.
- The Australian Government also has specific responsibilities in relation to national security and defence, border control, aviation and maritime transport, quarantine and the enforcement of Commonwealth legislation and international relations.
- Each jurisdiction is responsible for determining its own internal coordination mechanisms to give effect to these Arrangements.

New Zealand Government

The New Zealand Government enacts the *Civil Defence Emergency Management Plan (CDEM) Act 2002*, which is now updated to the National Civil Defence Emergency Management Plan Order 2005, pursuant to sections 39(1) and 45(b) of the *Civil Defence Emergency Management Act 2002.*[20]

- **Civil Defence Emergency Management Group (CDEMG)**

A group established under the Civil Defence Emergency Management Act 2002 to assist in coordination and management of the Civil Defence Emergency Management Plan

Co-ordinated Incident Management System (CIMS)

A structure used to systematically manage emergency incidents. The structure allows multiple agencies or units involved in an emergency to work together to systematically manage emergency incidents.

New Zealand has a series of codes issued by the Ministry to District Health Boards (DHB) to alert DHBs about incidents and to trigger a series of actions.

- Code White—Information
- Code Yellow—Standby
- Code Red—Activation
- Code Green—Stand down/recovery

The New Zealand Government uses 'the four Rs' in planning for an MCI:

- **Reduction:** identifying and analysing long-term risks to human life and property from natural or non-natural hazards; taking steps to eliminate these risks if practicable; and, if not, reducing the likelihood and the magnitude of their impact and the likelihood of their occurring.
- **Readiness:** developing operational systems and capabilities before a civil defence emergency happens, including self-help and response programs for the general public, and specific programs for emergency services, lifeline utilities and other agencies.

THREAT	CATEGORY OF THREAT	5-YEAR RISK	IMPACT ON COMMUNITY	DISASTER RESPONSE IMPACT	PRIORITY (1 TO 5)
Biological—small numbers	Biological	2	4	3	5
Biological—large numbers	Biological	1	5	5	5
Chemical or radiological—small numbers	Chemical	3	4	3	3
Chemical or radiological—large numbers	Major community	1	5	5	3
Pandemic infection	Pandemic	2	5	5	1
Bush fire	Fire and flood	4	4	2	4
Major transport incident (e.g. train)	Major community	4	4	3	2
Bomb/terrorist attack off-site	Major community	2	4	3	3
Bomb/terrorist attack on-site	Physical	1	5	5	2
Health facility fire or evacuation	Physical	4	4	4	2
Service interruption	Physical	4	4	3	2
Storm and/or flood	Fire and flood	2	4	5	4

TABLE 12.2 Potential incident risk analysis and prioritisation

- **Response:** actions taken immediately before, during or directly after a civil defence emergency to save lives and property and to help communities recover.
- **Recovery:** the coordinated efforts and processes used to bring about the immediate, medium-term and long-term holistic regeneration of a community following a civil defence emergency.

- **District Health Emergency Plan (DHEP)**

A plan that describes the health emergency functions and capability required by the DHB, which takes an all-hazards approach and provides for both immediate events, short duration events and extended emergencies, on both small and large scales, as relevant to the DHB population.[21]

The challenge for paramedics and other healthcare providers

To date, governments, health services and local communities have responded to a global economic crisis and ever-growing demands on their services, and have had to respond with tighter budget controls in an effort to make the tax dollar go further. This has resulted in a rationalisation of services and staff. Hospitals, for example, have made service delivery changes— e.g. shorter lengths of stay and the introduction of 24-hour wards and day-surgery. Added demands for services, along with these factors, have contributed to the reduction in the number of beds available. An initiative by Australasian Departments of Health is the introduction of the National Emergency Access Target (NEAT), which has a key performance indicator that by 2015, 90% of all patients presenting to a public hospital ED in Australia will either physically leave the ED for admission to hospital, be referred to another hospital for treatment or be discharged home within 4 hours. In New Zealand the target is 95% within 6 hours.[22] These targets are intended to be a 'whole

of hospital approach'. The future may reveal that these targets are an advantage in MCI planning as each day the hospital is geared up to move patients through the organisation at a faster rate. This is good practice for any future MCI events.[22]

Risk analysis in planning by hospitals

In addition to planning for external disasters, hospital emergency planning committees need to consider internal disasters, such as flooding, fire damage and chemical spillage, which may disrupt normal operations.[23] Business continuity plans should be developed to help the organisation get back to normal business, or at least to ensure that organisational capability is either partially or fully restored to ensure continued emergency care.[24]

When assessing risk, planners identify and prioritise major types of threats to an organisation and the surrounding community, and consider what the impact of any response will be on the organisation: staffing requirements, equipment needs and education. It is worthwhile for organisations to engage the services of an expert panel/committee. The membership of the risk analysis committee is best kept to a minimum, but should include public health officials, the chief executive officer, ED and trauma staff and the hospital disaster controller. To make the task manageable, the timespan of predicted events should not exceed five years. Using a scale of 1 to 5, risk is rated from 1 (least likely) to 5 (highly likely). An example is shown in Table 12.2.

After a risk analysis has been done and threats have been identified and prioritised, the next step is to develop response plans. These should incorporate the following:

- Rapid communication to key personnel established, with appropriate back-up.
- A call-in system and designated assembly areas set up for staff, relatives and media.

- Roles and responsibilities of key personnel identified.
- Tabards (identification vests) supplied—essential for identifying personnel in charge of key areas and to permit rapid identification of various responder groups.
- Task cards produced to instruct staff about their roles and responsibilities.
- Consideration given to communication modes and associated problems such as:
  - mobile telephone systems may become overloaded after large sporting events and public gatherings. In cases of extreme public unrest, an MCI or a threatened terrorist attack, authorities might shut the system down to prevent bomb activation[25]
  - faxes can be a useful hard-copy transfer medium for the delivery of situation reports
  - telephones must have 'fail-safe' lines in the event of switchboards being disrupted. These telephones must be clearly marked and listed in disaster communication centres (DCCs)
  - radios do not always work in blackout areas, especially basements and tunnels. It is therefore essential to have adequate repeater stations located throughout the facility
  - pagers are reliable for message transfer. Repeater systems are installed in most regions.

- Contingency plans should be in place in case of a major communications failure. For example, the use of runners and loud-hailers has proven to be effective.
- Decontamination facilities should be readily available.
- Isolation areas should have been identified for use in the event of a pandemic infection.
- Extra supplies are readily accessible.

MCI management pre-hospital phase

In Australasia, the pre-hospital health role remains predominantly the responsibility of the ambulance services. In a protracted MCI, health commanders will be deployed to the disaster site and become part of the incident management team (IMT), working in conjunction with the ambulance commander. Initial reports from the ambulance services are passed on to the ambulance or health services controller, who will make a decision as to whether medical teams are to be deployed to the MCI site.

Communication and authority at the site will have been established, and referred to as command and control (see Fig 12.7).[26] The police have overall responsibility at the scene of a MCI. They coordinate the scene and ensure that there is close communication and cooperation between emergency services. Access to disaster sites is strictly controlled. The police will cordon off areas and control movement in and out of the scene.

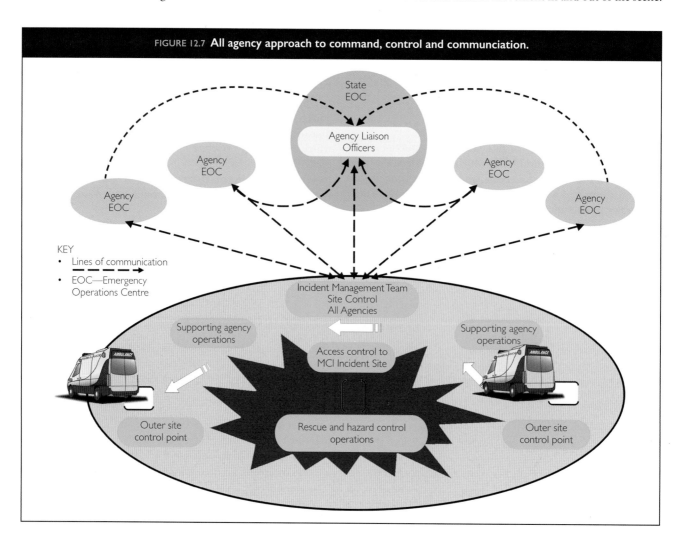

FIGURE 12.7 **All agency approach to command, control and communciation.**

MCI site command and control

The incident site is where the rescue operation is taking place, and is a forensic crime scene for police purposes. It is where the rescue and hazard control operation is situated. The incident site may have no physical boundary, and there may be a number of incident site areas within the overall MCI site—for example, the wreckage of an aircraft, which may have broken on impact into many pieces over a wide area.[24] The incident management and supporting agency operations site surrounds the incident site, and is a safe distance from any hazard, such as a secondary explosive device and positioned upwind from possible contamination. Entry and exit through this area is controlled through a control point. Any healthcare activity within this area is the responsibility of the health commander at the scene. The state emergency operations centre is normally situated some distance from the MCI scene, in an Emergency Operations Centre (EOC) or a DCC.[26]

Mass-casualty incident triage

Triage is a fundamental component of MCI victim management and may well determine the outcome for many MCI victims. Triage is performed by trained first-responders, paramedics and medical and nursing strike teams. The principles of MCI triage must be applied strictly whenever the number of casualties would overwhelm the available resources.

> **PRACTICE TIP**
>
> It is important to follow all training guidelines and not become emotionally involved in the appearance or age of the victim. Maintain the MCI philosophy of do the greatest good for the greatest number. See section on pitfalls in MCI triage in this chapter.

What is triage?

Triage originated during the Napoleonic wars and is credited to Napoleon's surgeon Baron Dominique Jean Larrey (1766–1842), who used a classification system that enabled priority-setting for evacuation of the wounded from the battlefield. Since this time triage has, mainly through military conflicts, been continually refined.[27] To date there has been a broad range of methods used to triage victims, and various approaches to victim labelling and tracking systems have been explored. Following removal of the wounded from the battlefield, the victims have always been divided into three basic categories:

1. Those who are likely to live, regardless of what care they receive.
2. Those who are likely to die, regardless of what care they receive.
3. Those for whom immediate care might make a positive difference in outcome.[28]

The sheer number of casualties will determine if the model above needs to be used, and a strict rule of 'first aid only, don't stop and play' will be the most effective way of doing the 'greatest good for the greatest number'.

Types of MCI triage

Simple MCI triage

Simple triage is usually used at a scene of an MCI to separate victims into two distinctive groups:

1. Victims who need immediate attention and rapid transport to hospital.
2. Victims with less-serious injuries, for whom treatment can be delayed.

To date, however, approaches to triage have become progressively more evidence-based. The triage category of the victim is frequently the result of an alteration in the victim's vital (physiological) signs and physical assessment findings.

The Simple Triage and Rapid Treatment (START) model which has been adopted by Australasian emergency medical services and is taught in the Major Incident Medical Management and Support (MIMMS) training program as devised by Hodgetts in 1998[26] is practised and memorised by responders, and an algorithm system is used. START is a simple triage system that can be performed by trained first-responders, paramedics and emergency personnel in emergencies.[29,30] Treatment and transport decisions are determined by using the Triage Revised Trauma Score (TRTS), a medically validated scoring system incorporated in some triage cards and discussed later in the chapter.[31] Once a triage decision is made, categorisation and identification of victims is aided with the use of printed triage tags (Fig 12.8).

The START triage technique separates MCI victims into four priority groups:

1. The injured who can be helped by immediate transportation.
2. The injured whose transport can be delayed.
3. Those with minor injuries, who may need help less urgently.
4. The deceased.

It should be noted that the 'moribund' label, issued to victims who are not dead but are severely injured and might not survive their injuries if treated and transported, does not exist in this

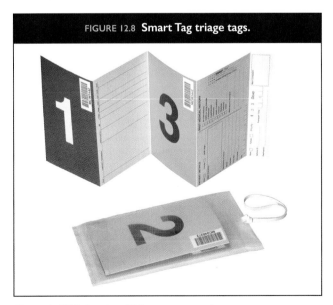

FIGURE 12.8 **Smart Tag triage tags.**

Copyright TSG Associates LLP, www.smartmci.com

triage system. For ethical reasons, a priority 1 label (or an urgent, red, label) is allocated by first-responders, paramedics and nursing teams. Ethical decisions are made by senior medical staff either at the site or in a hospital setting. Further discussion of this type of 'advanced' triage is outlined below.

Advanced MCI triage

In advanced triage, medical staff may decide that some seriously injured people should not receive advanced care because they are unlikely to survive. Therefore, advanced care will be used on victims with less-severe injuries and who are more likely to survive their injuries. Advanced triage is therefore used to divert scarce resources away from victims with little chance of survival in order to increase the chances of others who are more likely to survive. It becomes the task of the MCI medical staff to make such decisions. This process should continue once victims are inside receiving hospitals.

Reverse triage

This is a form of triage that is utilised by the armed forces where the less severely wounded are treated in preference to the more severely wounded. This is normally implemented in wars where the military setting may require soldiers be returned to combat as quickly as possible, or where medical resources are limited.[32]

The MCI triage process used in Australasia

Sieve

First-responders, normally paramedics assisted by health teams if deployed to the incident site, utilise a 'sieve' process. Sieve is the first triage decision and is made at the scene where the victim is found. Sieve is so-called because, as with a sieve, those victims who are standing are able to pass through the sieve mesh while those not standing are trapped; the ones trapped are sorted into one of the five categories described below. Sieve is an instant snapshot, and not a predictor of victim recovery or outcome at a later stage.

PRACTICE TIP

It is important to ensure that senior staff are deployed to the green label reception areas. Many victims that are processed through sieve triage may have covert injuries and deteriorate quickly while awaiting transport.

Triage priorities allocated during the sieve

The system is:

- Immediate (Red)—those victims who require immediate life-saving interventions.
- Urgent (Yellow)—those victims who require urgent and immediate intervention and treatment.
- Delayed (Green)—those victims who have no serious life-threatening injuries, and may wait longer to receive treatment.
- Expectant (various colours)—victims whose injuries are so severe that the resources required to treat them would jeopardise treatment of larger numbers of less severely injured victims. This group is likely to have been initially

triaged to the Red group by first-responders. Treatment decisions are made by senior medical staff, either at the site or in a hospital setting. Emergency Management Australia has suggested physiological parameters which might be used to allocate victims to the Expectant category:[33]
- cardiorespiratory arrest
- a Glasgow Coma Scale (GCS) score of 3
- major burns when the victim is aged >60 years with burns to >50% of the body surface area
- elderly victims with thoracic and central nervous system (CNS) injuries with signs of shock
- Dead (White)—those victims who require no further treatment or intervention.[26]

Some authors[34–36] have debated which physical parameters are the best predictors for those victims requiring urgent care. A decrease in the GCS has been shown to be a predictor of those victims requiring immediate care. The triage tools used most commonly are those devised by Hodgetts et al[24] where the GCS is not formally assessed in the sieve process, but is used extensively in the sort process (discussed below).

The triage sieve process

Triage sieve involves assessment of airway, breathing and circulation (see Fig 12.9). Those victims able to walk—who therefore must be breathing—are allocated a priority 3 Delayed category. Those victims unable to walk have their airway, breathing and circulation assessed. Victims unable to breathe despite airway opening are allocated a Dead label. Those victims able to breathe with a respiratory rate < 10 or > 29 breaths/minute are allocated priority 1 Immediate, and those victims with a respiratory rate between 10 and 29 breaths/minute have their capillary refill assessed. A victim with a capillary refill time below 2 seconds—brisk response—is allocated priority 2 Urgent. A capillary refill time longer than 2 seconds—sluggish response—is allocated a priority 1 Immediate.

The use of capillary refill time as an assessment of circulation is controversial because the ambient temperature may well affect the speed of the capillary refill. However, the pulse is considered a good circulatory assessment tool.[26] A pulse rate > 120 beats/minute receives a priority 1 Immediate. A victim with a pulse rate < 120 beats/minute receives a priority 2 Urgent. Note that taking the pulse only takes 2 seconds: if the pulse beats twice in 1 second then the rate is 120 beats/minute.

PRACTICE TIP

If the pulse does not beat twice in 1 second then it is assumed to be below 120 beats/minute.

Sort

Triage sort occurs once the casualties arrive in a casualty clearing station. There are two useful methods of sorting, as described below.

Physiological triage

Physiological triage is a method that uses the TRTS.[26] Physiological triage is not designed to be descriptive of the casualty's injuries, but is indicative of the physiological consequences of

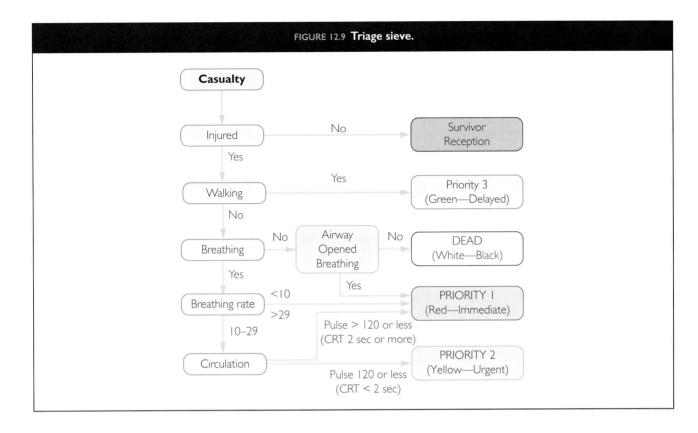

FIGURE 12.9 **Triage sieve.**

injuries sustained, whether the injuries are overt or covert. In the TRTS, a score from 0 to 4 is given to each of the following clinical parameters:

- GCS
- respiratory rate
- systolic blood pressure.

TRTS combines all three clinical parameters and awards a top score of 12 to indicate that all physiological parameters measured are within acceptable limits. A Green (Delayed) label is allocated to such a victim. If any one of the clinical parameters scores 1 point lower, giving a total score of 11, an yellow (Urgent) label is allocated to the victim. If another 1 point or more is lost (a total score of 10 or below), the victim will be allocated a Red (Immediate) label. A zero score indicates death.

Anatomical triage

Anatomical triage does not require the triage officer to refer to a TRTS; however, an extensive knowledge of the consequences of the mechanism of injuries is used as a good predictor of injury patterns. Some would argue that to perform anatomical triage, a secondary assessment would have to be performed.[26] However, some injuries are so overt that a detailed secondary survey is not required. A well-planned education program would develop fast head-to-toe assessment of MCI victims. Naturally, a combination of physiological and anatomical triage would complement each other during the sort phase of triage (Fig 12.10).

Treatment at the scene

Treatment at the scene is initially carried out by members of the public acting as first-aiders. When the ambulance services arrive,

FIGURE 12.10 **Triage sort.**

GLASGOW COMA SCALE

Eye opening	Code	Verbal response	Code
Spontaneous	4	Oriented	5
To voice	3	Confused	4
To pain	2	Inappropriate words	3
None	1	Incomprehensible	2
		None	1

Motor response	Code
Obeys commands	6
Localises to pain	5
Withdraws to pain	4
Flexes to pain	3
Extends to pain	2
None	1

REVISED TRAUMA SCORE

Glasgow Coma Scale	AVPU	Code	Respiratory rate	Code
13–15	Awake	4	10–29	4
9–12	Verbal	3	≥ 29	3
6–8	Pain	2	6–9	2
4–5	Unresponsive	1	1–5	1
3		0	0	0

Systolic blood pressure	Code
≥ 90	4
76–89	3
50–75	2
1–49	1
0	0

they have overall responsibility for victim treatment in the pre-hospital environment and will, if necessary, be supplemented by mobile health teams deployed from hospitals.[26] If health teams have been deployed to the MCI site, a casualty treatment area would be operational. If no health teams are deployed, then only triage and minimal life-saving treatment would be attempted. In most cases, only life-saving manoeuvres should be employed so as not to delay transfer of the majority of victims to definitive care.

Labelling of victims

In an MCI situation, the triage system should facilitate identification of the victim's medical need and encompass a documentation system for treatment given, enabling appropriate medical and nursing resource deployment and management. The use of victim triage labels is part of this process. The issue of multiple triage systems for mass-casualty situations throughout Australasia was resolved by an agreement reached between state and territory governments in Australia and New Zealand's Civil Defence Emergency Management Group (CDEM) in 2011; the resultant changes improved collaborative efforts and uniformity in disaster management within Australasia.

In early 2010, the SMART Triage Tags were approved as an Australian standard mass casualty triage label by the Council of Ambulance Authorities (CAA) following consultation with jurisdictional Health Departments.[37] The Ministry of Health Counter Disaster Unit NSW issued a policy that specifies the use of Mass Casualty Triage Pack—SMART Triage Pack. The SMART Triage Tags are intended to provide a standard tool for mass casualty triage process for both health response teams and ambulance services in an MCI. These tags also provide, for the first time, a national consistency for mass casualty triage tags across Australia and allow inter-operability.

The SMART Triage Tags meet world's best practice and have been tested and evaluated for Australian conditions.

Victim transport

Different modes of victim transport are useful to facilitate an even victim distribution across metropolitan and rural areas. In MCIs, ambulance services are the main mode of victim transport. Large buses are used to transport large numbers of non-critically-ill victims away from the MCI scene to reception centres or definitive care in a non-trauma centre. Air ambulance fixed-wing and rotary-wing craft are used to move critically ill victims rapidly to trauma centres. An example of an incident site flow process and victim transfer is illustrated in Figure 12.11; physiological implications are discussed in Chapter 16.

In an MCI there may be an overwhelming influx of victims who are not critically injured;[36–40] therefore planners need to put in place an effective triage system for Green label victims and those not requiring medical attention. Triage distribution of Green label victims to non-trauma centres will enable

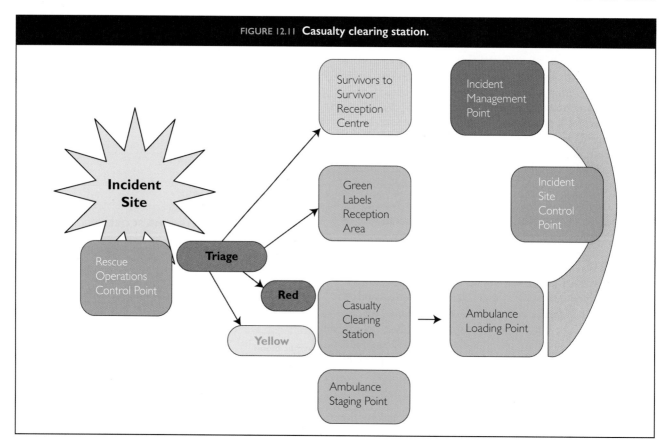

FIGURE 12.11 **Casualty clearing station.**

stretched resources in trauma centres to be concentrated on the Red and Yellow label victims.[39–43] Those people involved in an MCI who do not require medical assistance are triaged to a survivors' reception area where social workers and mental health support responders are deployed. The remaining victims are assessed using sieve and sort.

A well-planned casualty clearing station (Fig 12.11) effectively filters out those who do not require treatment and those with minor injuries who may be best transferred to non-trauma centres. However, experience has proven that despite the intentions of site organisers, a large number of victims will attend the closest or most familiar hospital and potentially overwhelm the ED. Planning for this should be covered in ED MCI plans.

Alternative care facilities

Alternative care facilities are places that can be set up for the care of large numbers of victims; examples include schools and sports stadiums that can be prepared and used for the care, feeding and holding of large numbers of victims of an MCI.[44] During the Pope's visit to Sydney in August 2008, there was an endemic outbreak of influenza and many pilgrims became infected. It became necessary to utilise large 'tent hospitals' pitched in sport stadiums, social clubs and in school grounds. Paramedical and medical strike teams were deployed to these sites. The intention of this strategy was to divert low-acuity victims away from hospitals and prevent EDs from becoming overwhelmed.

Typical casualty mix of a MCI

Several authors have analysed the injuries caused by bombing incidents and note that, apart from those immediately killed, about 10–15% of survivors are severely injured and the remainder have mild to moderate injuries.[10,43–47] For example, in the terrorist attack on a federal building in Oklahoma City in 1995, 88% of people in or near the building were injured and 11% required hospitalisation.[43] In the September 2001 terrorist attack on the World Trade Centre, 15% of victims were admitted to hospital and 85% were walking wounded.[48] It may be possible to extrapolate these figures to non-explosive MCIs where multiple injuries are experienced, for example, bridge collapse, train crash, earthquake and aeroplane crash. The clinical assessment and management of blast injuries is described in Chapter 51.

Hirshberg et al[49] estimate that if a hospital could assemble seven trauma teams to treat the expected 10–15% victim load of injured victims following an MCI, then a realistic victim load presentation to an ED would be 7–10 victims who are severely injured (Red labels) and 60–70 victims in the 'Urgent' and 'Delayed' label categories combined.

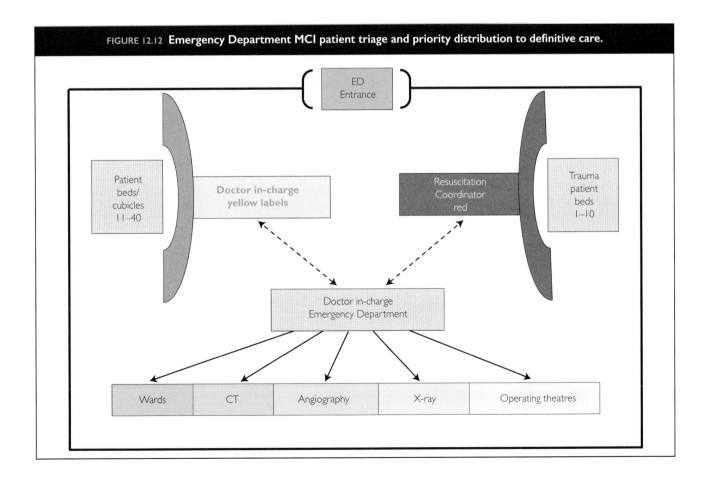

FIGURE 12.12 **Emergency Department MCI patient triage and priority distribution to definitive care.**

The principle of doing 'the greatest good for the greatest number' in an MCI involving multiple injuries that require surgical intervention hinges on the availability of trauma surgical teams. This availability should determine the hospital's capacity to receive and treat victims. To accept victim numbers far in excess of available resources might well be detrimental to victim care and outcome.[48,49]

Hospital phase

Creating surge capacity at hospitals

Receiving hospitals are required to have plans to deal with surge capacity. After a MCI, hospital surge-capacity plans will have to be activated quickly. Surge capacity 'refers to more than just the maximum victim load a hospital can handle during a crisis situation'.[49] Hospitals need to be able to respond rapidly in response to such a surge by creating bed capacity, making operating theatres available, increasing levels of staffing and ensuring supplies and equipment are adequate. Each MCI will make different demands on resources. For example, following terrorist attacks in New York (2001), Bali (2002) and Madrid (2004), there was a great need for burn beds because, in addition to multisystem trauma, many victims suffered burn injuries. In Australia after the Bali bombings, surge capacity was 42.4% into available burn beds.[50]

It is worth noting that not all victims of a MCI need to be in the ED or hospital beds. Following victim assessment it should become apparent that many victims of MCIs can be triaged, treated and discharged (with follow-up) without being processed in the ED or disrupting the main core functions of organisations and hospitals. Examples are influenza clinics and displaced persons requiring minimal medical attention as a result of fire or floods.

The hospital bed state

The capacity to rapidly clear patients out of the ED and prepare for the reception of MCI victims is of paramount importance. It is essential that an MCI-bed state which gives an instant snapshot of available hospital beds is activated. An example of an MCI-bed state is given below:

- *available beds*—beds vacant at the time of the MCI
- *potential beds*—beds which can be created by postponement of surgical operations and movement of patients to other facilities
- *closed-ward beds*—beds which may be opened now, or later, to accommodate the immediate victim surge and to later assist the hospital to return to normal business.

> **PRACTICE TIP**
>
> Incorporate the hospital bed state into daily hand-over practice and embed it into cultural practice.

Emergency department plans

Paramedics and ED staff are quite familiar with the peak patient influx and congestion in the triage area and subsequent congestion in the whole ED. The authors of this chapter advise

larger organisations to adopt a minor and major response to MCI incidents.

Minor MCI: is when small numbers of victims are expected, with mixed injuries, and is deemed manageable within currently available resources and operational systems. On notification of a minor MCI, normally via a direct telephone call from the ambulance service, the nurse in charge of ED puts out a pre-selected pager notifying key staff; for example the bed manager, deputy director of nursing and orderlies. The page also gives the rest of the hospital a 'heads up' about the influx of victims.

A brief meeting is held to ensure all involved are agreed on the plan of action. Beds are rapidly made available so that the less-injured victims may be cohorted in one area of the ED and resources directed to their care. This system is a perfect rehearsal for a major MCI.

Major MCI: is when there are large numbers of victims and injuries of high complexity, requiring a whole organisational response and the establishment of a Command Centre. The MCI paging system is the same as above; however, the response is multi-operational (see Fig 12.11).

Registration and documentation

Documentation has to be streamlined and readily available to all participants in the victim's journey through various departments in the hospital. In hospitals that utilise electronic medical records, a bank of pre-determined MCI medical record numbers need to be preloaded into the electronic medical record system. Electronic records have a huge advantage over paper records as all users are able to view progress notes and management plans. All investigation orders and vital sign observations are readily available. Planned surgical procedures are able to be booked electronically.

The paper system severely limits these opportunities as the record can only be accessed where the paper is located. Pathology results still have to be accessed via a computer. Moreover, the risk of losing the records is multiplied in the busyness of a MCI.

At triage it is a matter of safety to register the MCI victims onto the electronic registration system and attach the pre-numbered armband to the victims before they enter designated areas of the ED. The unique MCI number is readily identifiable throughout the organisation. Previous medical records are merged much later.

In the event of computer failure departmental regular 'down time' papers are to be always readily available. The authors of this chapter recommend the addition of a trauma form (Fig 12.17) on which MCI victim management plans will be concisely documented. A robust manual tracking system is essential to retain control of victim movement and is accessible to members of staff without computer access. It also assists allied health staff and the police in locating victims for worried relatives and friends.

> **PRACTICE TIP**
>
> Develop a manual patient tracking form that is universally understandable and is used throughout the organisation (Fig 12.15).

FIGURE 12.13 **MCI major doctor task card.**

Code Brown Major Task Card
DOCTOR IN CHARGE ED

MAJOR MCI CODE BROWN TASK CARD

Responsible for:	Liaising with medical and nursing staff and organising ED to respond to a Major MCI incident		
Report to:	Hospital disaster controller	Direct Report Contact Number:	XXXX

CONVENE A BRIEF MEETING IN THE NUMS OFFICE WITH KEY ED STAFF TO OUTLINE THE PLAN

WEAR THE SILVER "DOCTOR IN CHARGE EMERGENCY" TABARD.

DO NOT ATTEND THE DCC UNTIL REQUESTED TO DO SO VIA THE PAGING SYSTEM.

DELEGATE THE IDENTIFICATION OF PATIENTS FOR IMMEDIATE WARD ADMISSION OR DISCHARGE TO RED AND YELLOW PRE-MCI MEDICAL TEAM LEADERS. THEY WILL THEN LIAISE WITH THE DOCTOR AND NUM IN CHARGE OF THE ED and ED IMAGING COORDINATOR (IF REQUIRED)

ALLOCATE THE FOLLOWING ROLES (TASK CARDS AND TABARDS KEPT IN TRIAGE CUPBOARD):

• ED Imaging coordinator (Ideally ED SS with an Intern to assist)	Tick when complete ☐
• Surgical coordinator (Ideally surgical Consultant)	☐
• Doctor in charge of Red Area (Ideally ED SS)	☐
• Doctor in charge of Yellow Area (Ideally ED Registrar)	☐
• Doctor in Charge of Green Area (ACC level 3 or Fast Track, Ideally ED Reg)	☐
• Doctor in Charge of TED (Ideally ED Registrar)	☐

These positions have task cards that outline preparation for MCI and the "Rules of MCI Management"

ED LAYOUT
- Admitted patients are to be transferred to ward areas.
- **Resuscitation rooms are not to be used for MCI victims**.
- North End (Beds 1–12) – Red Label Victims
- South End (Beds13–22) +/– Fast Track – Yellow Label victims
- Clinic 8 ACC level 3 – Green Label victims. If ACC is not operational, Green Victims will go to Fast Track
- Green label victims will be triaged, given a pre-allocated MCI MRN, have an ID band attached and then will be escorted to ACC via the ambulance corridor and access the brown lifts in the south corridor. If ACC is not operational (outside working hours 7am to 7pm Mon–Fri), green victims will be directed to fast track, at least in the initial phase of the MCI response.
- Temporary Emergency Department (TED) is in EMU/Resus for NON-MCI patients.
- The moribund are to be nursed in the side rooms in fast track, and if required, there will be two to a room.
- Mortuary arrangements: 15 deceased MCI victims may be placed in the 2H and 2I tutorial rooms.

RULES OF MCI MANAGEMENT
- **Disaster trauma forms** will be used for all MCI victim documentation and management plans
- **Damage control resuscitation** and damage control surgery should be employed if appropriate
- **Radiology requests** are to be made on the "Radiology and Surgical Request Forms". These are sent to the ED Imaging Coordinator who will prioritise and negotiate time slots in the radiology department and their assistant will enter the order on FirstNet®
- **Surgical requests** for OT are to be written on the "Radiology and Surgical Request Forms". These are to be sent to the ED Surgical Coordinator who will prioritise and negotiate time slots in theatre
- **Victim movements** will be recorded by a clerk on the "Code Brown MCI Victim Tracking Form"
- **Admissions**: victims will be admitted under the Upper GI Surgeon of the day
- **Antibiotics** are only prescribed from the preselected list (to be found in the pre-packaged victim folders)
- **Pharmacy** will set up a satellite unit in A.A.A. and A.C.C. for analgesia, ADT and antibiotics
- **Pathology** will send a "Blood Safety Officer" who is responsible for ensuring all blood specimens meet the zero tolerance labelling policy. **Transfusion requests must be witnessed**
- **Documentation** for ALL staff is only to be on the papers provided in the pre-registration packs
- **A management plan** is to be written before the victims leave the ED
- **Victim flow is one way** i.e. MCI victims do not return to the ED once they leave for radiology
- **Non-MCI patients in radiology** will return to the ED for review and management prior to disposition

KEY ROLES AND RESPONSIBILITES
- ED NUM and Doctor in Charge will provide overall coordination of the ED
- ED Surgical Coordinator will determine the priority for all surgical interventions for MCI Victims and liaise with the Operating Theatres Duty Director
- ED Imaging Coordinator will determine the priority and suitability for all radiological interventions for all MCI and non MCI victims and liaise with the Radiology Imaging Coordinator

Sample Task Card Courtesy: Emergency Department, Royal North Shore Hospital, St Leonards NSW 2065 Australia (2014)   Page 1 of 2

Continued

FIGURE 12.13 MCI major doctor task card.—cont'd

- **NURSING POSITIONS TO BE ALLOCATED BY NUM**
  - Nurse in Charge ED
  - Triage all MCI Victims
  - Nurse team leader Yellow Victims
  - Nurse team leader Red Victims
  - Nurse in Charge of Temporary Emergency Department (TED)
  - TED Communication Clerk
  - Triage Clerk assigned to the MCI Triage nurse

- **STAFF TO BE SENT FROM THE DDC**
  - Tracking coordinators Red × 1 Yellow × 2
  - Imaging tracker
  - Surgical tracker
  - Administration assistance to in charge nurse and doctor
  - Tracker in TED

- **TRACKING PAPERWORK**
  The following MCI registration and tracking forms will be used:
  - Triage Code Brown MCI Registration Form
  - Code Brown MCI Victim Tracking Form
  - Radiology and Surgical request Form
  - Surgical Coordinator Tracking Form
  - Radiology Coordinator Tracking Form
  - Green Label Registration and Tracking Form

- **VICTIM PAPERWORK**
  All victims will have a pre-registration MRN and a pre made, pre labelled, paperwork pack containing:

Arm band	Victim ID stickers × 10	Disaster Trauma forms	Adult "BTF" obs charts
Blood request forms	Radiology/Surgical request forms × 4	Antibiotic prescribing guidelines	Victim Admission Summary

- **STAFF CALL-IN**
  - There is a staff call-in book in the triage MCI folder.
  - Telephone numbers are kept with the ED NUMs and department secretary

- **STAND DOWN:**
  - ED will receive notification from the DCC of de-escalation and of final MCI victims being received

- **CONTINUATION OF CORE BUSINESS**
  - **Non MCI** victims will receive a regular MRN via the FirstNet registration system and be directed to TED, AAU or RR.
  - Paediatric patients will be assessed and triaged to EP or RR.
  - Mental health patients will be kept in the ED waiting room and reviewed by the CNC mental health. Patients requiring close observation and monitoring will be admitted directly to the Cummins Unit.
  - Code Blue Emergencies: the ED will continue its usual responses

- **DEBRIEF**
  - The ED will hold a departmental "hot" debrief for ED staff.
  - An operational debrief will be conducted at which the ED along with other departments will provide a documented report on the operational response.

DCC PHONE NUMBERS:	
HDIC	XXXX
COMMUNICATIONS	XXXX
LOGISTICS	XXXX
DCC FAX NUMBER:	XXXX XXXX

FIGURE 12.14 **MCI major nurse task card.**

Code Brown MAJOR Task Card
NURSE IN CHARGE ED

MAJOR MCI CODE BROWN MCI TASK CARD

Responsible for:	Liaising with medical and nursing staff and organising ED to respond to a Major MCI incident		
Report to:	Hospital disaster controller	Direct Report Contact Number:	XXXX

- **IF NOT ALREADY DONE, PUT OUT THE "CODE BROWN MAJOR" PAGE VIA SWITCHBOARD ON XX**

- **ATTEND A BRIEF MEETING IN THE NUMS OFFICE WITH KEY ED STAFF TO OUTLINE THE PLAN**

- **WEAR SILVER "NURSE IN CHARGE EMERGENCY" TABARD**

- **DO NOT ATTEND THE DCC UNTIL REQUESTED TO DO SO VIA THE PAGING SYSTEM**

- **LIAISE WITH NURSE T/LS AND BED MANAGER (LOCATED IN ED) REGARDING PT ADMISSIONS**

- **ALLOCATE THE FOLLOWING ROLES:** (TASK CARDS AND TABARDS KEPT IN TRIAGE CUPBOARD):
  - Triage (all MCI Victims)   Tick when complete   ☐
  - Triage (non MCI Patients)   ☐
  - Nurse team leader Yellow Victims   ☐
  - Nurse team leader Red Victims   ☐
  - Nurse in Charge of Temporary Emergency Department (TED)   ☐
  - TED Communication Clerk   ☐
  - Clerk assigned to the MCI Triage nurse   ☐
  - Nurse in Charge Green label victims (ACC or Fast Track)   ☐

  The above positions have task cards that outline preparation for MCI and the "Rules of MCI Management"

- **ED LAYOUT**
  - Admitted patients are to be transferred to ward areas.
  - **Resuscitation rooms are not to be used for MCI victims.**
  - North End (Beds 1–12) – Red Label Victims
  - South End (Beds 13–22) +/– Fast Track – Yellow Label victims
  - Clinic 8 ACC level 3 – Green Label victims. If ACC is not operational, Green Victims will go to Fast Track
  - Green label victims will be triaged, given a pre-allocated MCI MRN, have an ID band attached and then will be escorted to ACC via the ambulance corridor and access the brown lifts in the south corridor. If ACC is not operational (outside working hours 7am to 7pm Mon–Fri), green victims will be directed to fast track, at least in the initial phase of the MCI response.
  - Temporary Emergency Department (TED) is in EMU/CDU for NON-MCI patients.
  - The moribund are to be nursed in the side rooms in fast track, and if required, there will be two to a room.
  - Mortuary arrangements: 15 deceased MCI victims may be placed in the 2H and 2I tutorial rooms.

- **RULES OF MCI MANAGEMENT**
  - **Disaster trauma forms** will be used for all MCI victim documentation and management plans
  - **Damage control resuscitation** and damage control surgery should be employed if appropriate
  - **Radiology requests** are to be made on the "Radiology and Surgical Request Forms". These are sent to the ED Imaging Coordinator who will prioritise and negotiate time slots in the radiology department and their assistant will enter the order on FirstNet®
  - **Surgical requests** for OT are to be written on the "Radiology and Surgical Request Forms". These are to be sent to the ED Surgical Coordinator who will prioritise and negotiate time slots in theatre
  - **Victim movements** will be recorded by a clerk on the "Code Brown MCI Victim Tracking Form"
  - **Admissions**: victims will be admitted under the Upper GI Surgeon of the day
  - **Antibiotics** are only prescribed from the preselected list (to be found in the pre-packaged victim folders)
  - **Pharmacy** will set up a satellite unit in A.A.A. and A.C.C. for analgesia, ADT and antibiotics
  - **Pathology** will send a "Blood Safety Officer" who is responsible for ensuring all blood specimens meet the zero tolerance labelling policy. **Transfusion requests must be witnessed**
  - **Documentation** for ALL staff is only to be on the papers provided in the pre-registration packs
  - **A management plan** is to be written before the victims leave the ED
  - **Victim flow is one way** i.e. MCI victims do not return to the ED once they leave for radiology
  - **Non-MCI patients** in radiology will return to the ED for review and management prior to disposition

- **KEY ROLES AND RESPONSIBILITES**
  - ED NUM and Doctor in Charge will provide overall coordination of the ED

Continued

FIGURE 12.14 MCI major nurse task card.—cont'd

- ED Surgical Coordinator will determine the priority for all surgical interventions for MCI Victims and liaise with the Operating Theatres Duty Director
- ED Imaging Coordinator will determine the priority and suitability for all radiological interventions for all MCI and non MCI victims and liaise with the Radiology Imaging Coordinator

MEDICAL POSITIONS TO BE ALLOCATED BY DR IN CHARGE ED
- ED Imaging coordinator and Assistant (Intern)
- Surgical coordinator
- Doctor in charge of Red area
- Doctor in charge of Yellow area
- Doctor in Charge of Green area
- Doctor in Charge of TED

STAFF TO BE SENT FROM THE DDC
- Tracking coordinators Red × 1 Yellow × 2
- Imaging tracker
- Surgical tracker
- Administration assistance to in charge nurse and doctor
- Tracker in TED

TRACKING PAPERWORK
The following MCI registration and tracking forms will be used:
- Triage Code Brown MCI Registration Form
- Code Brown MCI Victim Tracking Form
- Radiology and Surgical request Form
- Surgical Coordinator Tracking Form
- Radiology Coordinator Tracking Form
- Green Label Registration and Tracking Form

VICTIM PAPERWORK
All victims will have a pre-registration MRN and a pre made, pre labelled, paperwork pack containing:

Arm band	Victim ID stickers × 10	Disaster Trauma forms	Adult "BTF" obs charts
Blood request forms	Radiology/Surgical request forms × 4	Antibiotic prescribing guidelines	Victim Admission Summary

STAFF CALL-IN
- There is a staff call-in book in the triage MCI folder.
- Telephone numbers are kept with the ED NUM's and department secretary

STAND DOWN:
- ED will receive notification from the DCC of de-escalation and of final MCI victims being received

CONTINUATION OF CORE BUSINESS
- **Non MCI** victims will receive a regular MRN via the FirstNet registration system and be directed to TED, AAU or RR.
- Paediatric patients will be assessed and triaged to EP or RR.
- Mental health patients will be kept in the ED waiting room and reviewed by the CNC mental health. Patients requiring close observation and monitoring will be admitted directly to the Cummins Unit.
- Code Blue Emergencies: the ED will continue its usual responses

DEBRIEF
- The ED will hold a departmental "hot" debrief for ED staff.
- An operational debrief will be conducted at which the ED along with other departments will provide a documented report on the operational response.

DCC PHONE NUMBERS:	
HDIC	XXXX
COMMUNICATIONS	XXXX
LOGISTICS	XXXX
DCC FAX NUMBER:	XXXX XXXX

Sample Task Card Courtesy: Emergency Department, Royal North Shore Hospital, St Leonards NSW 2065 Australia (2014)   Page 2 of 2

FIGURE 12.15 **MCI patient master tracking form.**

EMERGENCY DEPARTMENT
MCI PATIENT MASTER TRACKING FORM (TRIAGE)

THIS FORM MUST REMAIN AT THE TRIAGE AREA AT ALL TIMES

DATE:

MCI No.	Triage Time	SURNAME, First Name (if known)	DOB	Main Injury/ies	Triage To (circle)	LOCATION Time	LOCATION Area	Time	Area	Relative/s Contact No.	Called	Pt Address	SW involved Y/N & name	Hosp. MRN
000-001	0830	Joe Bloggs	23/7/58	Chest Trauma	R Y G	0840	OR			00000000	Y N	22 Bloggs Street	Y BW	777
000__					R Y G						Y N			
000__					R Y G						Y N			
000__					R Y G						Y N			
000__					R Y G						Y N			
000__					R Y G						Y N			
000__					R Y G						Y N			
000__					R Y G						Y N			
000__					R Y G						Y N			
000__					R Y G						Y N			
000__					R Y G						Y N			
000__					R Y G						Y N			

RECORD THE TIME ON THE PHOTOCOPY OF THIS FORM: COPY TIME=   PAGE [ ] of [ ]

Courtesy: Emergency Department, Royal North Shore Hospital, St Leonards NSW 2065 Australia (2014).

FIGURE 12.16 **Radiological and surgical request forms.**

RADIOLOGY AND SURGERY PRIORITY REQUEST

Place Victim/Patient I.D. label here

☐ YELLOW
☐ RED

☐ TEMPORARY ED
☐ AAU
☐ RR

LOCATION/BED NO: _____

INJURIES/OPERATION _____

RADIOLOGY

CT
☐ ABDO
☐ HEAD
☐ OTHER _____

X-RAY
☐ CHEST
☐ LIMB
☐ PELVIS

☐ C-SPINE
☐ OTHER _____

RADIOLOGY PRIORITY (circle)	1	2	3
SURGERY PRIORITY (circle)	1	2	3

PRIORITY KEY	**1 = IMMEDIATE**	**2 = SOON**	**3 = LATER**

RADIOLOGY AND SURGERY PRIORITY REQUEST

Place Patient I.D. label here

☐ YELLOW
☐ RED

☐ TEMPORARY ED
☐ AAU
☐ RR

LOCATION/BED NO: _____

INJURIES/OPERATION _____

RADIOLOGY

CT
☐ ABDO
☐ HEAD
☐ OTHER _____

X-RAY
☐ CHEST
☐ LIMB
☐ PELVIS

☐ C-SPINE
☐ OTHER _____

RADIOLOGY PRIORITY (circle)	1	2	3
SURGERY PRIORITY (circle)	1	2	3

PRIORITY KEY	**1 = IMMEDIATE**	**2 = SOON**	**3 = LATER**

Courtesy: Emergency Department, Royal North Shore Hospital, St Leonards NSW 2065 Australia (2014).

FIGURE 12.17 **MCI trauma form.**

FORM ##

EMERGENCY TRAUMA MAJOR CODE BROWN RECORD

Royal North Shore Hospital Trauma Service

MRN

First Name

Last Name

DOB

Allergies

Injuries

PMHx

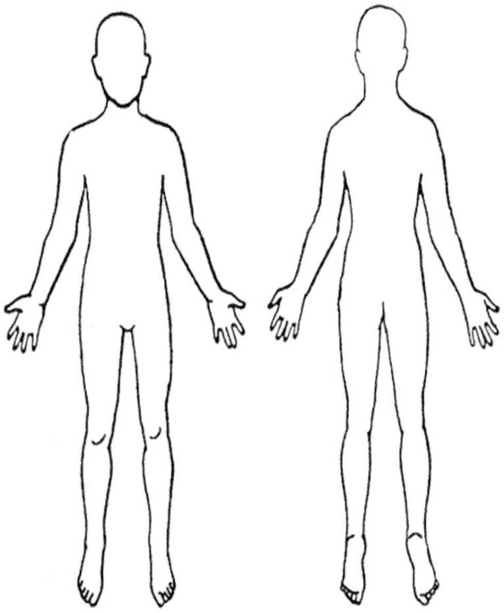

Investigations **Bloods / Crossmatch / XR / CT**

Plan

Transfer to:

PTO FOR FURTHER NOTE SPACE

Disaster Trauma Management Form Code Brown ED Plan and Task Cards Courtesy: Trauma Service Royal North Shore Hospital Page 1 of 2

Courtesy: Emergency Department, Royal North Shore Hospital, St Leonards NSW 2065 Australia (2014).

Is that test necessary?

It is important to resist the temptation to order multiple non-urgent radiological investigations, because such investigations may congest victim flow and jeopardise lives.[39] The development of standing operational procedures (SOPs) involving key stakeholders should be undertaken in the early planning stages to determine what essential tests and investigations are required in an MCI event.

Imaging and radiology coordinators

Ideally an *ED imaging coordinator* is to be appointed during a major MCI. This position receives all radiological requests for the whole department, including non-MCI victims. The imaging coordinator will determine the priority and appropriateness of all radiological interventions requests. A flow sheet is used to document all decisions (Fig 12.18). The imaging coordinator liaises directly with the radiology imaging coordinator in the radiology department. This practice ensures equity in allocation of resources and patient safety.

Radiology requests are entered into an electronic ordering system and are visible to the radiology department. This eliminates paper requests and the loss of requests and repeated phone calls to the radiology department. The imaging coordinator is in direct contact with the radiology co-ordinator. Priorities are discussed and determined and collection of the MCI victim occurs.

The *ED surgical coordinator* will prioritise surgical cases for MCI victims and non-MCI patients in the ED. The same referral form is used. The ED surgical coordinator will communicate with the duty director of operating rooms (OR) and the floor manager OR to arrange OR times and equipment. If a victim has radiological investigations a surgical registrar will be located in the radiology department to be available to discuss surgical interventions with the duty director of OR and assist in decision making and communication with the MCI ward or ICU if a decision is made to delay surgery. All decisions in the ED are documented on the surgical tracking form (Fig 12.19).

To ensure effective victim movement through diagnostic facilities and definitive care, there also needs to be an agreed method of priority setting. Prioritising by category—that is, category 1 (now), category 2 (soon) and category 3 (later)—gives an order of urgency to all involved in the MCI. Experience shows that not all green label victims will have the same degree of injury. In line with this system they will be split into the same MCI categories.

Satellite pharmacy

Accessing analgesia in a major MCI is problematic. Most EDs have electronic medication dispensers that require two nurses to insert a barcode and scan a fingerprint to access scheduled drugs, a stock balance is checked and both nurses have to be present during this procedure. An alternative is to introduce a satellite pharmacy staffed by pharmacy staff. Pharmacy staff only

---

PRACTICE TIP

Delegate a staff member to be responsible for checking that all MCI packs and antibiotic guidelines are current. Engage electronic calendar reminders for managers.

---

require a patient identification label to dispense the scheduled drugs directly to nursing staff. Antibiotics, determined by agreed guidelines, are dispensed in the same manner.

Blood availability

MCI pre-numbered packs have proven to be a challenge for pathology laboratories. With the introduction of correct patient correct procedure, and in most organisations zero tolerance for incorrect or insufficient labelling of blood specimens, pathology departments have insisted on written labels on blood specimens and a pathology form signed by two witnesses.[51,52] In a major MCI the only check will be the pre-registered number on the patient's arm band. Mindful of safety issues, the inclusion of a 'blood control' technician is best deployed to the ED. This position wears a tabard and all blood specimens are directed via this position to pathology. This practice ensures no delays in processing of specimens, or worse, the return of the specimen for clarification labelling; this would cause much chaos as the victim may have left the ED for radiology or surgery.

In the event of a shortage of O−ve blood, O+ve blood may be given to males and females of non-child-bearing age. To assist this process, the pre-numbered electronic labels are coded male and female and issued an approximate age. This second set of labels is taken to the patient and placed in the pre-registration package. This information is invaluable to the blood bank and eliminates too many telephone calls regarding clarification of these details.

Victim flow: it is best practice to have a one-way policy for MCI victims. This differs remarkably from normal practice, where the patient returns to the ED for a definitive diagnosis. The introduction of the position mentioned above allows one-way flow and assists the ED, and organisation returning as quickly as possible to normal functions.

Triage at receiving hospital

MCI triage differs greatly from normal ED triage (Ch 13), where, in a 'normal' working day, severely injured trauma victims are assigned immediate triage categories 1 or 2 using the Australasian Triage Scale (see Ch 13).[43] During an MCI there has to be a mindset change 'from greatest good for each individual' to 'greatest good for the greatest number', so that treatment of the 'masses' supersedes that of the individual.[42] This philosophy permits the allocation of a moribund, not-for-resuscitation (Expectant) category and such victims are directed to palliative care areas adjacent to the ED. A doctor appointed as the surgical coordinator and working in conjunction with the resuscitation coordinator is the best-placed person to determine this category of victim. MCI victims allocated to the Expectant category who have high-acuity injuries raise potential ethical and emotional issues for members of staff who, in normal circumstances, would be able to treat such victims. Therefore, discussion of these concepts in the education and planning phases is essential to minimise staff anxiety.

Hirshberg et al[53] and Kirschenbaum et al[54] attribute the success of appropriate triage to the appointment of a senior ED doctor or trauma surgeon as the triage officer. Common MCI reception practice is to assemble doctors and nurses at the ED entrance, wait for the triage officer to determine a victim triage category and allocation of victims to assembled teams. An alternative method (offered here) is that the triage officer

FIGURE 12.18 **Imaging coordinator tracking form.**

CODE BROWN MAJOR: ED IMAGING COORDINATOR TRACKING FORM

TIME OF REQUEST	VICTIM/PATIENT ID STICKER	Location & Bed No.	CLINICAL DETAILS	TESTS REQUIRED	PRIORITY	
					1 2 3	XR Done (Tick)
					DW CT? (Tick)	Time sent to CT
					1 2 3	XR Done (Tick)
					DW CT? (Tick)	Time sent to CT
					1 2 3	XR Done (Tick)
					DW CT? (Tick)	Time sent to CT

CROSS OUT PATIENTS THAT HAVE LEFT ED

KEY: 1 = Immediate 2 = Soon 3 = Later	CT Coordinator: 59460	Imaging Coordinator: 59208

ISSUES

ED Imaging Coordinator Tracking Form Major MCI Code Brown 11/10/13 S:\Code Brown ED Plan and Task Cards Page 1/1

Courtesy: Emergency Department, Royal North Shore Hospital, St Leonard's NSW 2065 Australia (2014).

FIGURE 12.19 **Surgical coordinator tracking form.**

CODE BROWN MAJOR: ED SURGICAL COORDINATOR TRACKING FORM

TIME OF REQUEST	VICTIM/PATIENT ID STICKER	INJURIES/DAIGNOSIS	Location & Bed No.	Theatre Priority	OPERATION REQUIRED		
				1 2 3		DESTINATION TIME LEFT ED	OT Coordinator contacted? Y / N
				1 2 3		DESTINATION TIME OT READY	OT Coordinator contacted? Y / N
				1 2 3		DESTINATION TIME OT READY	OT Coordinator contacted? Y / N

CROSS OUT PATIENTS THAT HAVE LEFT ED

KEY: 1 = Immediate 2 = Soon 3 = Later	OT Floor Manager: 58386	OT Floor Director: 58385

ISSUES

ED Surgical Coordinator Tracking Form Major MCI Code Brown 11/10/13 S:\Code Brown ED Plan and Task Cards Page 1/1

Courtesy: Emergency Department, Royal North Shore Hospital, St Leonards NSW 2065 Australia (2014).

be a senior ED nurse. ED nurses are consistently rostered into the triage position and have received disaster training. Medical staff, often not conversant with MCI triage concepts, are better deployed in the ED supervising resuscitation teams and prioritising those victims who require immediate radiology, imaging or direct transfer to operating theatres, and determining those victims, as discussed earlier, who are deemed to be Expectant.

Pitfalls in MCI hospital triage

Over-triage may be as life-threatening as under-triage because resources are then not utilised to their best advantage in an MCI situation.[48,53] Over-triage occurs when those victims assigned Red labels (Immediate) do not warrant this triage category. Frykberg et al,[55] Cook et al[56] and Feliciano et al[57] refer to over-triage as an administrative, logistical and economic problem, as person hours are applied unnecessarily to a few.[46]

Over-triage can be avoided by good communication with the MCI site commander and the receiving hospital. By doing so, limited resources and incoming victims are balanced by the hospital triage officer.[53] A debrief paper following the 2004 Madrid bombings acknowledged that 'there was probably an over-triage to the closest hospital'.[58] Some studies suggest that over-triage is less likely to occur when triaging is performed by hospital medical teams rather than by paramedics.[59] Authors of this chapter surmise that this is due to application of 'anatomical' triage at the site by medical teams.

The need for repeated triage surveys of victims during the chaos of the initial surge is stressed, in order to avoid under-triage.[60] There have been no reported cases of under-triage; that is, assigning yellow or green labels to victims who require immediate care.[46–48]

Debriefing

During the MCI or some time later, people directly involved and other members of the community may exhibit psychological symptoms as a result of the catastrophic nature of the MCI.[61] Mental health planning will provide counselling and other ongoing supportive programs.[55] 'Hot' debriefs are usually held immediately after the event to allow for agency and services personnel to voice their thoughts on operational (not emotional) aspects of the MCI response. A cautionary note about debriefs is made by Reid,[61] who states: 'The kind of terse questioning often seen in "debriefing" should be avoided.' Carlier et al[62] cite recent studies which indicate that critical incident stress debriefing (CISD) may in fact increase the symptomatology of those airing their emotional reactions to the event. Therefore, debriefing should be offered to, but not be compulsory for, those members of response services involved in the MCI.

Chemical–biological–radiological MCIs

Chemical–biological–radiological (CBR) MCIs may be the result of accidents (Hazmat incidents) or deliberate incidents. Terrorist incidents can involve the use or threat of the use of chemical, biological and radiological agents with the intent to disrupt infrastructure and maim and kill populations. Australasia's geographical isolation does not reduce the likelihood of CBR attacks in this region.

CBR attacks, despite the perception of the general public, are neither new events nor a product of this century. Historically, biological agents have long been used in warfare. The practice of hurling plague-ridden bodies at the enemy was used in the early 14th century.[63] In World Wars I and II (1914–1918 and 1939–1945), a variety of gases were used with devastating effect. In 1995 the Aum Shinrikyo sect's sarin gas chemical attack on the Tokyo rail system resulted in 5510 people seeking medical treatment. There were 12 deaths, 17 people were critically injured, 1370 sustained mild to moderate injuries and 4000 had no or minimal injury.[63]

On 16 March 1988 during the closing days of the Iran–Iraq war in the city of Halabaja in Southern Kurdistan a chemical attack against the Kurdish people took place. The attack killed between 3200 and 5000 people and injured 7000 to 10,000 more, most of them civilians. The incident was and still remains the largest chemical weapons attack directed against a civilian-populated area in history.[63,64] On 21 August 2013 the worst chemical weapons attack in 25 years took place in eastern Damascus involving specially designed rockets that spread sarin nerve agent over the suburbs of Ghouta. Hundreds of people and animals were killed in the attack. Estimates of the death toll range from 281 to 1729 fatalities.[65]

Likelihood of a CBR attack

Obtaining chemical, biological or radiological ingredients and procuring the technological expertise to manufacture and effectively disperse such agents is difficult for terrorists.[62] Instead, in recent times suicide bombers, such as in Bali (2002 and 2005) and London (2005), and many spasmodic bombing attacks in Africa and the Middle East, have used improvised explosive devices (IEDs) to cause mayhem, multiple injuries and immediate death. The Australian government's Counter-Terrorism White Paper 2010 identifies an increase in a terrorist threat from people born or raised in Australia.[66,67] Suicide bombing is an increasing form of terrorism; therefore, the tendency to use bombs may well lower the probability of a CBR attack. However, complacency because of the belief that a CBR attack, Hazmat incident or pandemic (natural) outbreak of influenza (or other illness) will not happen is foolhardy. Training and education in CBR equipment and use should be maintained. If a CBR event does happen, then a huge amount of ventilator support will be required and may well exceed available resources.[62,68] Therefore, strict triage for access to definitive treatment is essential to 'do the greatest good for the greatest number'.

CBR agents and their effects

CBR agents are divided into chemical, biological and radiological agents. What follows is an overview of these agents and some examples of the use of such agents by terrorist groups.

Chemical agents

Chemical agents fall into five major categories: nerve, blister, choking, blood and riot control (see Table 12.3). Other chemical agents that affect the nerves are organophosphates. Chemical agents are able to penetrate the body via inhalation, dermal absorption, ingestion and injection. Clothing is not a protective barrier and may well, if not removed, provide a continual source of exposure to the chemical agent.[69] Nerve

TABLE 12.3 Muscarinic effects of nerve agents	
Diarrhoea	**S**alivation
Urination	**L**acrimation
Miosis	**U**rination
Bradycardia, bronchorrhoea, bronchospasm	**D**efecation
Emesis	**G**astroenteritis
Lacrimation	**E**mesis
Salivation	
NICOTINIC EFFECTS OF NERVE AGENTS	
Mydriasis, **T**achycardia, **W**eakness, **H**ypertension and **F**asciculation	

Adapted from Advanced Hazmat life Support (AHLS) Instructor manual University of Arizona Emergency Medicine Research Center American Academy of Clinical Toxicology. 2nd edn, 2000:91–2.[81] Reviewed January 2014; no changes.

agents are described more fully here, as they are the most commonly known and have created interest since the Tokyo sarin attacks in 1995.

The list of potential chemical agents resulting in injury is long and, war and terrorist activity aside, for the average Australian ED, chemical injury is more likely to arise from an industrial or a domestic accident. The severity of the injury and the number of people involved will be directly related to the chemical, its concentration, the length of time of exposure and the location of the incident.

Nerve agents

An overview of nerve cell activity will assist the reader in gaining an understanding of the effects of nerve gases on nerve cells. Nerve cells transmit messages through the body via nerve synapses using neurotransmitters. Acetylcholine is a neurotransmitter and is found throughout the central nervous system (CNS) and the peripheral nervous system (PNS).

There are two types of receptors, called muscarinic and nicotinic receptors, which receive the neurochemical messenger acetylcholine via the synaptic junction. Once acetylcholine has transmitted its message, it is broken down into choline and acetic acid by an enzyme called acetylcholinesterase.[70,71] Acetylcholinesterase is only one type of cholinesterase. Cholinesterase is also present in red blood cells (RBCs) and may be used as an inferred measurement of cholinesterase in synaptic junctions. RBC cholinesterase is used as a physiological measurement of the effects of treatment of nerve gas poisoning.[72]

Nerve agents are cholinesterase inhibitors. When nerve agents are present in the body, cholinesterase is unable to break down acetylcholine in the synaptic junction and, as a result, the acetylcholine continues to stimulate the receptors, resulting in the symptoms listed in the mnemonics DUMBELS and SLUDGE given in Table 12.3.

In addition to PNS muscarinic stimulation, nicotinic stimulation occurs in tandem, causing mydriasis, tachycardia, weakness, hypertension and fasciculations (MTWHF) (Table 12.4). These signs and symptoms are often the first clinical presentations of nerve gas poisoning observed by first-responders. The signs and symptoms are normally followed by a combination of muscarinic (DUMBELS) and nicotinic (MTWHF) symptoms. In the latter stages, muscarinic symptoms are the predominant symptoms.[71]

Treatment of victims affected by nerve agents

Nerve gases in the initial stages bind reversibly to acetylcholinesterase. This is an important characteristic of nerve gas that enables antidotes, when administered, to prevent irreversible binding to the acetylcholinesterase. In the case of soman gas there is only a 2-minute window of opportunity from gas absorption to irreversible binding, which can vary depending on toxicity. Other gases (sarin, tabun and VX) take from 5 to 40 hours to become irreversibly bound, thus allowing first-responders time to establish decontamination centres to treat victims and administer antidotes.

The antidote to nerve gases that prevents irreversible binding is pralidoxime. Pralidoxime is an oxime. In Australia the ComboPens (Auto Injectors) used contain Obidoxime 220 mg and Atropine 2 mg, the principal action of which is to reactivate cholinesterase that has been inactivated by phosphorylation due to the nerve-gas poisoning.[72] Once activated, cholinesterase is able to metabolise acetylcholine into choline and acetic acid; thus the acetylcholine is no longer available to transmit messages across the nerve synapse to stimulate the muscarinic and nicotinic receptors. Therefore, symptoms will abate.[70,71] Hypotension associated with pralidoxime administration can be managed with intravenous phentolamine 5 mg in adults and 1 mg in repeat doses in children, or as local policy dictates.

PRACTICE TIP

Pralidoxime-atropine auto-injectors are to be held like a 'baton' to prevent inadvertent self-injection which may prove to be a painful and an unpleasant experience and will compromise the integrity of the PPE.

The administration of atropine will relieve the symptoms of nerve-gas poisoning, i.e. DUMBELS and SLUDGE (see Table 12.3). Atropine is an antimuscarinic agent[72] and acts only at muscarinic receptors. Atropine has no effect on nicotinic receptors; therefore, the symptoms of MTWHF (mydriasis, tachycardia, weakness, hypertension and fasciculations) are not abated. To decrease these symptoms, benzodiazepines are used. For further information about chemical agents refer to Table 12.4.

Blister agents—vesicants

Vesicants are chemical agents which produce blistering on the skin on contact. The usual chemical of choice is mustard gas, infamous for its use in World War I and, more recently, against the Kurds. Mustard gas is faintly garlic in scent, carcinogenic, myelotoxic and teratogenic.[72] Mustard has both liquid and vapour toxicity and is usually deployed in the gaseous form, with

TABLE 12.4 Examples of chemical agents

CHEMICAL AGENT GROUP	NAME	CODE	ONSET	ENTRY MODE	PHYSICAL STATE AT 20°C	SIGNS AND SYMPTOMS	TREATMENT
Nerve	Tabun	GA	Very rapid	All*	Colourless to brown liquid	*Nicotinic* — Mydriasis, Tachycardia, Weakness, Hypertension, Fasciculations; *Muscarinic* — Diarrhoea, Urination, Miosis, Bradycardia, Emesis, Lacrimation, Salivation	Decontamination, Pralidoxime, Atropine, Benzodiazepine
	Sarin	GB	Very rapid	All*	Colourless liquid		
	Soman	GD	Very rapid	All*	Colourless liquid		
	VX	VX	Rapid	All*	Colourless liquid to brown liquid		
Blister	Lewisite	L	Rapid	All*	Dark brown or yellow oily liquid	Immediate pain with blister formation (vesiculations)	Decontamination, British antilewisite (BAL), Supportive care
	Distilled mustard	HD	Delayed	All*	Colourless to pale yellow liquid	Blister formation (vesiculations) chemical burns to skin and mucous membranes	Decontamination, Supportive care
	Nitrogen mustard	HN3	Delayed	All*	Dark liquid		
	Phosgene oxime	CX	Immediate	All*	Colourless solid	Immediate pain with delayed blister formation (vesiculations)	Decontamination, Supportive care
Choking	Phosgene	CG	Rapid	Respiratory	Colourless gas	Short of breath, chest tightness, hypoxaemia, noncardiac pulmonary oedema	Decontamination, Supportive care
Blood	Hydrogen cyanide	AC	Very rapid	Respiratory	Colourless gas	Cyanosis, cellular asphyxia, lactic acidosis, seizures and coma	Decontamination, Amyl nitrate, Sodium nitrate, Sodium thiosulfate
	Cyanogen chloride	CK	Rapid	Respiratory	Colourless gas		
	Arsine	SA	Delayed	Respiratory	Colourless gas		
Riot control	Orthochloro-benzylmalonitrile	CS	Instant	Respiratory	White solid	Mucous membrane and skin irritation, lacrimation (tearing)	Decontamination, Supportive care
	Chloroacetophenone	CN	Instant	Respiratory	Solid		

initial injury occurring within 2 minutes.[73] However, symptom development is delayed for some 4–8 hours. Producing both local and systemic toxicity, mustard damages DNA, resulting in eventual cell death.

Local effects are seen on the skin, eyes and airway. Eye injury includes corneal ulceration and perforation, with a small percentage of victims developing permanent eye damage. Injury to the skin is the cardinal indication of mustard exposure. Within 8 hours of injury the skin will become red, burn and develop blisters resembling partial-thickness burns. Full-thickness burn may occur with liquid mustard exposure, but rarely with the more common vapour contamination. Airway damage is dose dependent and in the mildest cases involves rhinorrhoea and pharyngeal irritation. Moderate injury involves the larynx and trachea, with severe exposure including haemorrhagic necrosis of the bronchioles and pulmonary oedema.[68] Systemic effects are related to bone marrow suppression, with absorbed mustard killing stem cells and producing a drop in the white blood cell (WBC) count 3–5 days after exposure. Fatality from secondary infection usually occurs if the WBC count falls below 2×10^9/L.[73]

Rapid decontamination will reduce the severity of injury, and while delayed decontamination will do little to reduce injury in the victim, it is recommended to prevent injury to staff from exposure to the agent.[73] Airway management may require oxygen, intubation and non-invasive ventilation support; for example, continuous positive airway pressure (CPAP), positive end-expiratory pressure (PEEP) and nebulised bronchodilators. The decision to fluid-resuscitate is based on an assessment of cardiovascular status and the extent of the burn. Immediate irrigation of the eyes may alleviate the severe pain associated with mustard contamination. However, once symptoms develop the primary focus of treatment is on mydriatics, topical antibiotics, analgesia and petroleum jelly on the eyelids to prevent adhesions.[73] Topical steroids may be considered during the first 24 hours. Skin wound management is the same as for other burns, including analgesia and tetanus prophylaxis.

Blood and pulmonary (choking) agents

Cyanide binds to cytochromes in the mitochondria and inhibits oxygen use by cells, thus producing a histotoxic hypoxia.[71] Mild exposure will produce headache, dizziness, vomiting, increased heart rate and anxiousness. Higher doses result in respiratory arrest, seizures and asystole within minutes of exposure. Treatment is focused on removal from the source of contamination, clothing removal and high-flow oxygen. No improvement on oxygen warrants administration of the cyanide antidote, sodium thiosulfate.

Pulmonary or choking agents produce an inflammatory reaction where they come into contact with the eyes and upper airway. Two common pulmonary agents are phosgene and chlorine; phosgene also has nerve-agent properties. Pulmonary agents can be life-threatening if inhaled because of the direct damage they produce. Treatment is primarily supportive, including removal from the source, decontamination, symptomatic treatment of eye irritation, airway management and nebulised bronchodilators.[73]

Biological agents

Biological agents are broken into three main types: viruses, bacteria and toxins. The effectiveness of biological weapons is determined by their ability to disseminate disease, to multiply in the object they target and to spread quickly. Signs and symptoms in all types of biological agent poisoning are delayed for from 1–2 days up to 21 days or longer, and usually present as influenza-like symptoms such as cough, malaise, fever and muscle pains. Specific symptoms, such as rashes, pustules and ulcerations, as noted in cutaneous anthrax, may be visible.

Identifying a terrorist biological attack is difficult during normal influenza seasons. Naturally, out of season cluster identification is easier. Detection of outbreaks is aided by surveillance systems which identify unusual patterns of disease that may indicate deliberate biological agent release. Table 12.5 presents a comprehensive list of biological agents and their physiological effects and treatment.

Unlike chemical and large-dose radiological contamination, the onset of signs and symptoms of biological agents is delayed.[43] Victims are more likely to seek medical care at local facilities and to not present initially to hospitals.[36,74] Those victims referred or self-presenting to hospitals are more likely to be admitted for ongoing treatment and supportive therapy rather than being treated and discharged, as in conventional terrorist attacks.[75]

An example of a bioterrorism attack occurred in the USA in 2001. Letters containing anthrax spores (*Bacillus anthracis*) were mailed to media personnel and two US senators. These were the first cases of bioterrorism-related anthrax in the USA. The contaminated letters, which were delivered through the US mail system, caused 22 cases of anthrax—11 pulmonary and 11 cutaneous. Five of these cases were fatal. The fatalities were all from pulmonary anthrax.[43] The WHO has estimated that 50 kg of anthrax aerosolised above a city with a population of five million would have the potential to result in 100,000 deaths.[75] In addition, 150,000 people would suffer severe infection, overwhelming existing resources.

To assist emergency planners in developing a response to biological agent incidents, the Centers for Disease Control and Prevention (CDC) organisation in the USA categorises biological agents into three categories: A, B and C:

A—ease of agent dissemination or transmission from person to person, with a high mortality rate

B—moderately easy to disseminate with a low mortality rate

C—emerging viruses with the potential to be widely manufactured and made readily available.

In all categories the psychological and social effects of biological agents is high.[62] The USA anthrax incidents had wide-ranging effects. Some examples of the ramifications are as follows:

- Psychological issues—fear of contracting anthrax from personal mail was generated in the community
- Logistical issues—these were encountered in the distribution of prophylaxis to unaffected workers at sites of confirmed contamination
- Ensuring that people took prophylaxis for prescribed period (60 days) was difficult
- Laboratories were overwhelmed by the number of required tests
- Copycat attacks/hoaxes caused frequent emergency responses—over 20,000 in the USA. Copycat hoax attacks also occurred in Australia

TABLE 12.5 Examples of biological agents[103–106]

BIOLOGICAL AGENT GROUP	DISEASE NAME	TIME OF ONSET OF SYMPTOMS	TRANSMISSION (HUMAN TO HUMAN)	MODE OF DISSEMINATION	SIGNS AND SYMPTOMS	TREATMENT
Viruses	Venezuelan equine encephalitis	1–5 days	No	Aerosol/direct	Headaches, pains, fever, malaise, photophobia, myalgia of legs	Supportive
	Smallpox	7–17 days	Yes. High	Aerosol	Severe fever, pox blisters on skin—starts on face and hands	Supportive
Virus (haemorrhagic)	Ebola	2–21 days	Yes. High	Direct	Fever, muscle joint pain, abdominal discomfort, vomiting, bleeding into skin and abdomen	Supportive
	Dengue fever	3–15 days	No	Vector/aerosol		
	Yellow fever	3–6 days	No	Vector/aerosol		
Bacteria	Anthrax (inhalation)	1–7 days	No	Vector/aerosol	Flu-like symptoms, tachycardia, cyanosis and shock	Antibiotics
	Pneumonic plague	2–5 days	Yes. High	Vector/person to person/aerosol	Extreme weakness, glandular swelling, skin haemorrhages	Antibiotics
	Tularaemia	1–10 days	No	Vector/direct/aerosol	Extreme weakness, glandular swelling, skin ulcers	Antibiotics
	Q fever	10–20 days	No	Vector	Headaches, pains, fever, chills, coughs	Antibiotics
Toxins	Botulism	1–12 hours	Non transmissible	Aerosol	Fevers and cough, weakness, respiratory failure	Supportive
	Ricin	4–8 hours				
	Staphylococcal enterotoxin B	1–12 hours				

Reviewed January 2014; no changes.

- Facilities were closed in the USA and cost tens of millions of dollars to decontaminate.
- Ongoing cost to all mail systems in the development of safe methods of detection and identification of biological agents to protect the public.

Anthrax

Infection from anthrax can occur in three forms:

1. cutaneous (skin), usually through a cut or an abrasion
2. gastrointestinal, by ingesting undercooked contaminated meat
3. pulmonary (inhalation), by breathing aerosolised (airborne) anthrax spores into the lungs.

When anthrax is aerosolised and subsequently inhaled, it has a mortality rate of greater than 90%.[73]

Bacillus anthracis was traditionally a zoonosis disease of people working with animals and is usually contracted naturally via contact with spores from infected lesions. The Gram-positive bacilli form spores which are extremely hardy and may be inhaled, ingested or inoculated via the skin.[72,73] The spores germinate into bacilli, producing infection when they release toxins resulting in cell oedema and death.[73] The incubation period is from 2 to 20 days and the usual presentation is with a flu-like illness, rapidly deteriorating within 24–48 hours of initial symptoms to sepsis, shock, haemorrhagic mediastinitis, respiratory distress and supraglottic oedema. Fifty per cent of victims will develop haemorrhagic meningitis.[69] After the 2001 anthrax incidents in the USA, experts found that symptoms typically appear within 4–6 days post exposure; however, some cases may take as long as 43 days after exposure for symptoms to appear.[73]

Cutaneous anthrax is the most common form of natural transmission, with inoculation via open wounds. Untreated cutaneous anthrax has a mortality rate of 20%.[70] Following inoculation, the incubation period is 1–7 days before a papule develops, usually on the head or arms. The papule forms a vesicle over several days, with severe surrounding oedema and regional lymphangitis.[72,73] The lesion ruptures after 1 week and forms a depressed black eschar. Over the following 2–3 weeks the eschar sloughs off and the illness resolves, except in a small percentage of people who develop disseminated illness and die.

Gastrointestinal exposure is possible, although rare, and occurs due to ingestion of infected meat. The incubation period is the same as for cutaneous anthrax and the victim presents with abdominal pain, cramping, haematemesis and rectal bleeding, followed by sepsis and cardiovascular collapse.[72]

Diagnostic confirmation is by blood culture, although treatment should not be delayed by waiting for results. Death will usually occur before results are available, and thus the decision to treat is based on clinical findings and history. Anthrax commonly results in a widened mediastinum (although not dramatically) on chest X-ray, making this an important diagnostic clue in the initial presentation. Pneumonia is rare and lung fields are often clear.

Current treatment guidelines recommend the use of ciprofloxacin and doxycycline.[72,73] Amoxicillin may be used in children or pregnant women, where the organism is penicillin sensitive.[72,73] The severity of the disease and the method by which it was contracted will determine the use of oral or intravenous antibiotics. Systemic toxicity warrants the use of intravenous antibiotics, and all antibiotic regimens must continue for 60 days or until the victim has received three anthrax vaccinations.[74] A course of antibiotics to treat anthrax takes a minimum of 4 weeks to administer. Anthrax is an example of a disease where the initial presentation is vague, although deterioration and death follow rapidly. Symptoms of anthrax infection are outlined in Table 12.5.

Plague

A disease associated with death over the millennia, *Yersinia pestis* (plague) remains naturally prevalent in Asia, the Indian subcontinent and the western half of the USA. Unlike the hardy anthrax spores, plague bacilli usually die quickly in the open, although they will remain viable in sputum, flea faeces and human remains for days. Natural transmission occurs from infected rodents to humans via the bite of a flea or inhalation of the Gram-negative bacillus from animal droppings. The disease exists in three forms: septicaemic, pneumonic and bubonic plague.[70]

Pneumonic plague is the result of inhaling bacilli and is 100% fatal if treatment is not instigated early. Transferable human-to-human, pneumonic plague is the most likely form of the disease for terrorist use, as it is producible with aerosolisation of the bacillus. After an incubation period of 2–3 days the victim develops a highly febrile flu-like illness, followed rapidly by fulminant pneumonia.[70] The pneumonia is usually lobar and associated with chest pain, shortness of breath, haemoptysis, respiratory failure and septicaemia. In addition to a small percentage of victims who will develop meningitis, hepatic injury and coagulation disorders are common. The coagulopathy will lead to production of the coagulase enzyme in areas of the body where the temperature drops below 37°C.[70] This in turn leads to capillary clotting, ischaemia and gangrene of fingers, toes and the nose. Hence the name traditionally associated with the plague, Black Death.

Bubonic plague is a form of the disease resulting from inoculation of the skin with bacilli from an infected flea. The incubation period is the same; however, bacilli migrate to the nearest lymph nodes, multiply and produce inflammation and necrosis of lymphatic tissue. This results in swollen, tender lymph nodes commonly known as *buboes*. The buboes are not fluctuant and rarely rupture.[70] Incision and drainage is not recommended because of the risk of contaminating staff; the buboes will resolve with antibiotic treatment. Fifty per cent of victims with bubonic plague will develop disseminated disease, with subsequent pneumonic or septicaemic illness. Untreated, disseminated illness results in death. While bubonic and septicaemic plague are not directly transmissible from human to human, both forms of the disease can become pulmonary, in turn making it possible to transmit the disease via respiratory secretions. Thus, all victims with suspected plague should be isolated, regardless of the initial form of the disease they have. Victims will remain infective until they have received at least 72 hours of antibiotic therapy.[76]

A chest X-ray will demonstrate bronchopneumonia. Diagnostic confirmation is by sputum culture and fluorescent antibody testing. The bacilli may be found in CSF, blood or lymph node aspirate, although collection of any specimen should be done using full universal precautions and careful transfer of specimens to the laboratory. As all these tests take several days to produce results, treatment is commenced immediately based on clinical presentation and a history of travel to an endemic area. Traditionally, the standard initial treatment for all types of plague is immediate intravenous streptomycin, or more recently gentamicin.[69,76] Chloramphenicol is used for plague meningitis. Doxycycline and ciprofloxacin have been used with success, although some resistant strains have developed.[69,76] Treatment may progress to oral antibiotics once victims improve, so long as the total antibiotic course runs for at least 10 days.

Smallpox

A Variola virus, smallpox was supposedly eradicated in 1980. However, scientists kept repositories of the disease in the USA and Russia in case there was a requirement to reproduce the vaccine and to study the disease. It is believed that unfortunately quantities of the virus have been sold and could potentially be used as a biological weapon.[77] Smallpox is a highly contagious disease spread by contact with respiratory secretions. Most of the world is no longer immune to the disease because vaccination programs ceased over 20 years ago. Repositories of the vaccine are old and the efficacy of the vaccine is questionable, although it remains in use by the US armed forces.

The disease is transmissible via the airborne route human-to-human once the rash appears, and the individual is infective until the scabs fall off. The incubation period is 7–17 days. The classic form of smallpox is known as Variola major and the mortality rate is 30%.[69] Variola minor is a milder disease, producing fewer lesions and with lower toxicity and mortality. A small percentage of victims will develop haemorrhagic smallpox, characterised by a petechial rash as opposed to the classic pox.

The smallpox virus initially migrates to the lymph nodes, replicates, then disseminates to the spleen and other lymphatic tissue. The initial viraemia is characterised by a flu-like illness with fever, headache, malaise and occasional mental state changes. Eventually the virus localises in the skin and pharynx, producing a maculopapular rash, which becomes vesicular and then forms pustules. Starting on the face, the lesions will then appear on any given part of the body. Over 2 weeks the lesions will crust and separate from the skin to leave a pitted scar or 'pox' mark. The difference between smallpox and chickenpox is the area in which the rash commences. A chickenpox rash will begin on the trunk and migrate to the face and peripheries. Smallpox begins on the face, moves to the arms and then invades the trunk and legs. Chickenpox lesions will also develop at different rates in any given area of the body. Death from smallpox is due to multiple-organ failure and the disease is grossly disfiguring. Diagnosis is clinical, with confirmation by electron microscopy.[69,76,78] There is no known effective therapy for victims with smallpox who become symptomatic. Vaccination of populations at risk remains the best way to prevent spread of the disease.

Radiological agents

Before the end of World War II, ionising radiation was considered by most to be rather innocuous. Low-level exposure to radiation occurred from exposure to household goods such as paints and some cosmetics. However, the explosion of nuclear warheads over the cities of Hiroshima and Nagasaki in Japan at the end of World War II and subsequent test explosions in Australia and Pacific atolls in the 1960s rapidly changed the perception that radiation was harmless and a safe thing to be exposed to.[79]

Today many organisations use a variety of radioactive materials as part of normal business: laboratories, universities, the construction industry, hospitals and factories. The risk of radiological accidents occurring and causing industrial contamination from radioactive material release is therefore always present. Radioactive material availability is strictly controlled; however, the probability of unscrupulous people stealing radioactive materials or obtaining 'discarded' radioactive materials is always a possibility. Some examples of radioactive material used in industry are cobalt-60, caesium-137 and strontium-90.

The threat of terrorists trying to use radioactive material in the form of radiological dispersal devices (RDDs) to cause mass contamination is a possibility. An explosive RDD is commonly referred to as a 'dirty bomb'. Dirty bombs can be made containing any radioactive material. The results of a terrorist group using an RDD would not necessarily result in an MCI, but could cause contamination to large areas of cities and cause injuries to those people in the immediate vicinity. The fear created in the community and the economic, political and social consequences would be immeasurable. The clean-up operation would be extremely costly.

What is radiation?

Radiation is feared by many because we cannot see it or smell it. Radiation spillage is depicted in movies as catastrophic; this is not always the case. Radiation surrounds us, is emitted from the atmosphere and is essential to maintain life; for example the rays of the sun, infrared (long waves) and ultraviolet (short waves). Radon is another type of radiation that is emitted from the Earth. However, over-exposure is harmful.

Effect of radiation on human cells

Radiation is emitted from the atoms of elements. Atoms have different-sized nuclei composed of protons (positive charges) and neutrons (negative charges); orbiting the nucleus are electrons. Unstable atoms are referred to as 'isotopes'. Unstable isotopes have excess internal energy and emit radiation in the form of radioisotopes during the process of undergoing spontaneous change to become stable atoms. This change process is called radioactive decay. Uranium is an example of an element that has no stable isotopes.[79]

Radiation affects matter in two primary ways: *non-ionising radiation* is able to break bonds in DNA and produce subsequent damage, which is easily understood in terms of DNA breakdown; *ionising radiation* loses energy as it passes through matter, resulting in the production of ion pairs. This energy loss produces a state of excitation in atomic electrons, raising the level of energy produced above the level of ionisation potential.[79] Therefore, excessive radiation exposure is able to cause irreparable cell damage and cause the cell to malfunction or die.[70,79]

Types of radiation emissions

Radiation emission is classified in the following way.

- *Alpha* radiation has the largest particles, and these do not readily pass through 'dead layers' of skin, paper or clothing.
- *Beta* particles are smaller particles and are able to penetrate a short distance into deeper tissue. If large quantities of beta radiation are present on skin or in tissue, penetration may occur and produce damage to the basal layer of skin. The resulting burn has a similar appearance to thermal burns.
- *Gamma* rays are normally emitted during a nuclear detonation, and the fallout is able to penetrate easily into deep tissues and cause whole-body exposure.[70,79]

Signs and symptoms of radiation exposure

Acute radiation syndrome is a complex series of symptoms resulting from whole-body irradiation over a short period of time. The clinical presentation and severity will depend on the dose of radiation, the speed with which the dose was delivered, the area of dose distribution and individual sensitivity to radiation. As attempting to quantify the dose of radiation is problematic, diagnosis and management is based on an assessment of the signs and symptoms. While all organ systems are affected by radiation exposure, the systems at greatest risk are those with high rates of cellular division. Thus the haematopoietic and gastrointestinal systems account for the greater percentage of signs and symptoms. Granulocytopenia is one of the earliest signs and occurs over a 1-month period. The speed at which the lymphocyte count reaches its maximum level and the level to which it rises are indicative of the severity of exposure. The development and severity of thrombocytopenia and reticulocytopenia are also indicative of radiation exposure and severity. Nausea and vomiting are early signs of gastrointestinal radiation. The length of time gastrointestinal symptoms take to emerge and how long they last for indicates severity of radiation exposure. Both fever and rectal bleeding are ominous signs.[73]

Non-lethal doses of radiation may produce transient sterility; however, the greatest problem is with changes in the DNA of gametocytes and the effect on future generations. CNS changes will occur with very high, lethal doses of radiation. Skin burns may result from radiation exposure. A radiation burn should be suspected in anyone who has been in the presence of radiation and has no memory of coming in contact with a hot object.[79] People exposed to a very high level of radiation will have little chance of survival.[79]

Pre-hospital management of a CBR MCI

The actions to be considered when responding to a CBR MCI should include:

- minimising CBR agent injuries by utilising personal protective equipment (PPE)

- controlling the spread of CBR contamination by setting up incident control systems
- fast and timely response of appropriate services and rapid establishment of good communication pathways
- timely and accurate information dissemination to enable rapid identification of hazards
- rapid set-up of decontamination facilities on-site and at hospitals
- preventing aggravation of traumatic injuries during first-aid and decontamination procedures.

CBR response zone descriptions

Hot zone

The hot zone is the area of known contamination, and is referred to as the incident site (Fig 12.20). This zone is controlled by fire services and is usually only staffed by specially trained fire,

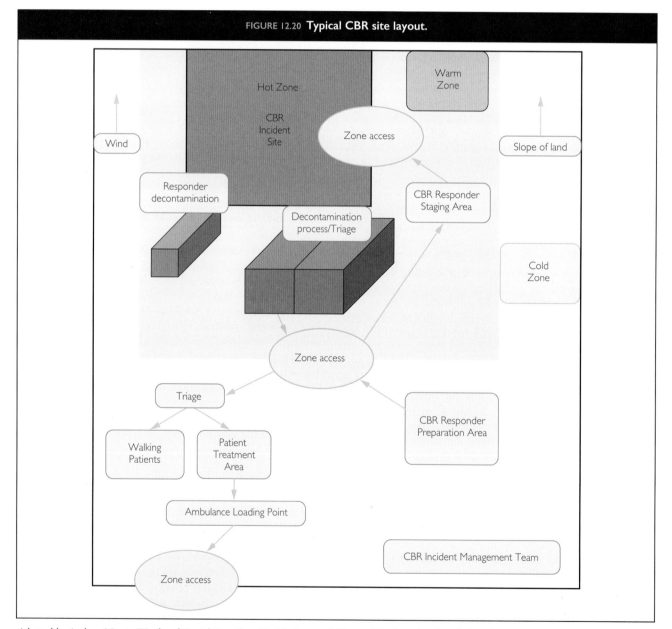

FIGURE 12.20 Typical CBR site layout.

Adapted by Authors Martin Ward and David Koop from Health Aspects of Chemical Biological and Radiological Hazards Australian Emergency Series part 111 Emergency Management Practice Volume 2—specific issues manual 3, 2000.

police and paramedical personnel. For example, paramedics enter this area if rapid victim assessment and treatment is required. In the hot zone, the highest level of PPE, level A, is usually worn unless the fire services have determined that a lesser level of PPE is safe (Fig 12.21A).

Warm zone

The warm zone is the area surrounding the hot zone, where decontamination and triage sieve is begun. Only minimal response staff are deployed into this area. Usually a medium level of PPE is worn, for example, level B (Figs 12.21B and 12.21C).

Cold zone

The cold zone is an area clear of contamination; casualty clearing treatment areas and transport are located in this zone. In this area usually the lowest level of PPE is worn; for example, level C (Fig 12.21D).

Team deployment to a cold zone

If an explosive device to disseminate radioactive matter activates a CBR MCI, then medical teams may be deployed to deliver direct victim care in the cold zone. Consideration of wind direction is also essential for team placement in CBR incidents. Caution must be considered in team deployment to a terrorist CBR MCI because of the likelihood of hazards such as a secondary explosion or building collapse.[48] The World Trade Center attacks on 11 September 2001, where 479 fire-fighters and rescuers were killed by the buildings collapsing, demonstrates this point.[38,42]

Initial presentations to healthcare facilities

What we know from previous CBR MCIs is that victims flee the scene of a CBR incident before on-scene decontamination facilities are able to be erected,[80] and arrive at EDs via private vehicle or on foot and not by ambulance.[81,82] The majority of victims involved in a bomb or chemical attack are seen by EDs,[80,82,83] and the initial surge will overwhelm hospital resources.[82–85] Most victims are seen within the first 6 hours following an attack.[80,82,83] Hospital emergency procedures should detail how, in the event of a surge of CBR-contaminated victims, the facility is quickly locked down to protect it from contamination. The hospital CBR plan should also detail the corralling of large numbers of victims to be decontaminated and their movement to a treatment area, or a reception centre for registration and counselling.

Decontamination process and treatment

Victim decontamination is essential for the removal of the agent from the victim and to ensure that the agent does not enter the hospital facility or leave the incident site. The following six steps are an overview of the decontamination process:

1. Wet down the victim to reduce the likelihood of secondary contamination from radioactive material or

FIGURE 12.21 **Personal protective equipment.**

Level A	Level B	Level C1 & C2
• Fully encapsulated gas-tight suit • Attached boots and gloves • Self-contained breathing apparatus worn inside suit • Highest level of PPE	• Chemical protective suit • Self-contained breathing apparatus • Chemical protective gloves • Chemical resistant boots	• Positive air pressure respirator (PAPR) (C1) • Air purifying respirator (APR) (C2) • Chemical protective gloves • Chemical resistant boots • Chemical protective suit or charcoal suit
Level A	Level B	Level C1	Level C2

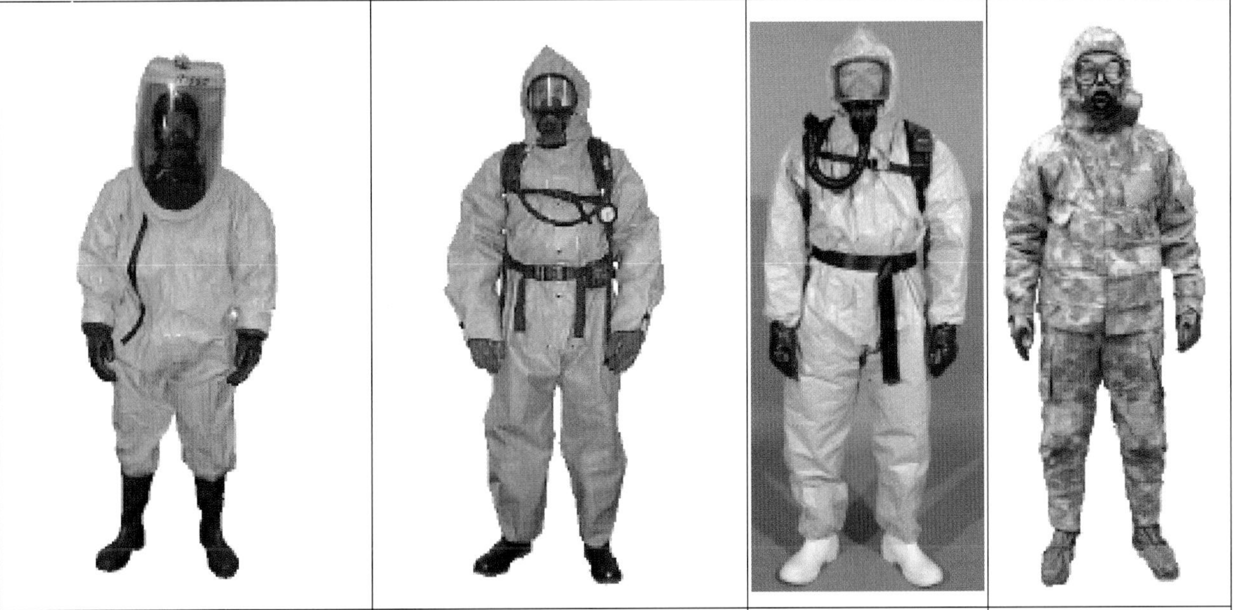

Courtesy NSW Ambulance, Martin Ward and David Koop.

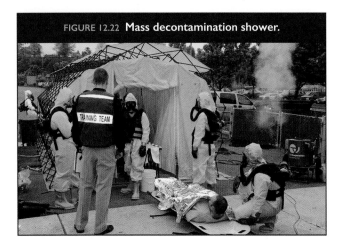

FIGURE 12.22 **Mass decontamination shower.**

other hazardous materials that may be adhering to their clothing and skin.

2. Remove wet contaminated clothing from the victim.

3. Secure the victim's clothing in a large plastic bag. Jewellery and personal items should be secured in a small clear plastic bag which is to stay with the victim. All items are to be taken through the shower process.

4. Shower the victim with warm water and soap (if available) to remove any remaining contamination from skin and hair. Showering is considered to be effective in removing hazardous substances from the victim's body (Fig 12.22).[86]

5. Cover the victim to maintain modesty and to prevent hypothermia. Return personal items such as jewellery to the victim.

6. Register and remove victim from the decontamination area to a safe zone where social and medical services are available if required.

Treatment of internal contamination is similar to acute heavy metal poisoning decontamination and is aimed at reducing the risk of damage.[87] Depending on the carrier of the radioactive isotope, this involves chelation therapy such as desferrioxamine or Prussian blue. As with burns, if the contaminant remains in place, the damage will increase. There is no treatment to reduce the damage caused by radiation once the victim has been irradiated. Management is essentially supportive and irradiation sequelae will usually be a problem for inpatient care because of the time delay in onset of effects. Wound management of radiation burns is the same as for burns of other causes and will involve follow-up surgical assessment.

It is important for all irradiated victims to receive advice on avoiding pregnancy until the degree of damage to DNA can be assessed. This includes both males and females who should be advised to use contraception. The teratogenicity of radiation is very high and DNA damage can bypass generations.[88]

Dangers to first-responders

A clear distinction has been made between the site of the CBR incident and the hospital decontamination facilities.[89] The main hazard to healthcare workers is secondary contamination, such as 'off-gassing' or direct contact with the contaminated victims.[90] Georgopoulos et al[91] and Horton et al[92] determined that when highly volatile substances are sprayed onto victims, they would evaporate within 5 minutes. It is unlikely that victims will arrive seeking medical aid within 5 minutes. A more realistic time-frame for the earliest arrival of contaminated victims to decontamination facilities would be at least 10 minutes from time of exposure. Therefore the possibility of 'off-gassing' affecting treating personnel (not in PPE) outside the hospital and away from the 'incident' site is minimal. This fact will assist in minimising staff fears of becoming contaminated during the initial surge in a chemical MCI.

In the event of a radiation incident, a victim who is critically ill or injured 'cannot be so radiologically contaminated as to present an acute hazard to medical personnel'.[90] Therefore life-saving procedures should never be delayed because the victim has been exposed to radiation. The possibility of other chemical agent contamination should be considered if the victim displays the signs and symptoms shown in Tables 12.3, 12.4.

Reducing the risk of contaminating staff
Removal of the contaminated victim's clothing can reduce the quantity of contaminant by 75–90%.[90] The type of clothing worn at the time of exposure will affect the amount of contaminant adhering to clothing. If personnel wearing protective military uniforms removed their uniforms, this could increase their contaminant removal to as high as 94%.[92]

An example of 'off-gassing' is illustrated in the Tokyo subway sarin gas attack in 1995, where 100 healthcare workers treating victims of the attack experienced symptoms of 'off-gassing'—blurred vision and nausea.[93] A review by Hick et al[94] noted that the sarin gas victims had not been decontaminated and remained fully clothed in a poorly ventilated room. No PPE was used during treatment, and doctors who spent over 40 minutes resuscitating victims were most affected. An inference can be made that worker exposure to the gas would have been reduced by removal of victim clothing and by wearing PPE. If the victims had been kept outside the facility, i.e. by following a lock-down procedure, secondary contamination to responders would have been greatly reduced.

Personal protective equipment

Healthcare professionals in their everyday duties are required to wear PPE. Therefore they already have an understanding of why there is a need for the use of PPE, such as latex-free gloves, eye protection and impervious gowns. The use of PPE is second nature. Standards exist in Australia to determine the appropriate type of PPE to be worn in situations where healthcare professionals are required to treat victims contaminated with hazardous materials.[40,93–97] Levels A and B PPE are required when the nature of the agent has not been determined. PPE for these levels is normally only worn by Hazchem-trained fire services personnel. One marked difference between the everyday PPE and CBR PPE is that the PPE used in CBR incidents is somewhat heavier and more constrictive. The delivery of medical care can be made very difficult when wearing this PPE because of restricted visual fields and loss of dexterity. The higher the level of PPE, the lower the level of care that can be delivered to the victim.

In Australia during preparation for the Olympic Games of 2000, PPE was introduced to health facilities and throughout the pre-hospital environment. Since that time PPE has been supplied and maintained. It is now not unusual for hospital emergency response staff to be trained in the use of level C PPE.

Training staff in the use of PPE

Regular training has enabled clinicians to become more comfortable and confident in wearing PPE. Initial comments and reactions from trainees often include that they feel unable to perform tasks such as intubation and cannulation, or even opening dressing packs. The main concerns are the thickness of the butyl gloves and the bulky, and noisy, protective suits. Full vision is hindered while wearing canister masks in the positive air pressure respirator (PAPR), and some trainees note that the noise generated by the motorised respirators presents another anxiety factor (see Fig 12.23B). But regular training has demonstrated that trainees will learn to adapt and modify procedures to enable successful completion of various tasks. An example of this is where trainees discovered that wearing latex-free gloves over the butyl gloves increased tactile sensation during procedures.

Monitoring issues with PPE

PPE suits are designed not to 'breathe'; therefore the wearer becomes hot and clammy very quickly. Staff should be instructed to hydrate prior to wearing the PPE. Staff need to be monitored for signs of dehydration, heat exhaustion and heat stroke. Symptoms include sweating, clammy skin, a pale or flushed complexion, weakness, dizziness, hypertension, tachycardia and nausea. To minimise these symptoms, rest cycles must be rostered. Psychological effects of claustrophobia and fear need to be addressed prior to the responders being deployed.

Bioethical implications in triage

Bioethical concerns have historically played an important role in triage decisions, such as the allocation of iron lungs during the polio epidemics of the 1940s and of dialysis machines during the 1960s.[98] As many healthcare systems continue to plan for an expected influenza pandemic, bioethical issues regarding the triage of victims and the rationing of care continue to be discussed.

Ventilator rationing

In a potential influenza pandemic or a CBR incident involving victims with respiratory distress, it is anticipated that hospitals may become overwhelmed by victims—and shortages of critical equipment, in particular ventilators, will occur. In addition, medications may be in short supply or rationed. Therefore decisions will have to be made for determining who will receive access to life-saving medications and technologies, and who will not. For example, a concern arises as to whether long-term patients in chronic care facilities should be removed from life-support to provide their ventilators to acutely ill influenza victims.[99] Practitioners, bioethicists and others are debating these questions; at the same time, organisations are establishing medical decision-support models for these types of situations.[99]

Awareness training and education

Because of the immensely difficult task of allocating time to educate various multidisciplinary staff in the pre-hospital and hospital settings, the ideology of 'the perfect disaster course' has to be revisited. One solution is to select enthusiastic super-trained staff who are retained on a register ready for deployment locally and internationally. Courses currently offered can run from days to weeks. To enable MCI education to be provided

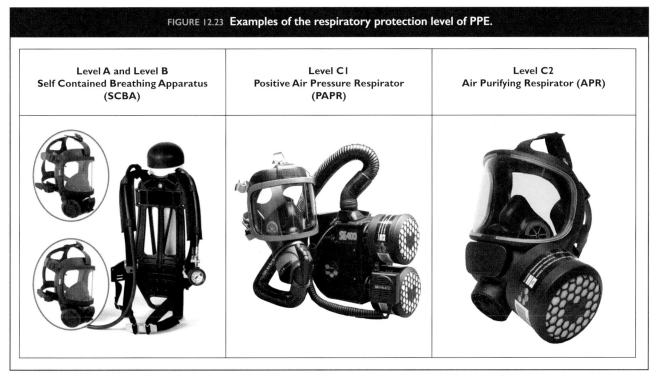

FIGURE 12.23 **Examples of the respiratory protection level of PPE.**

Level A and Level B Self Contained Breathing Apparatus (SCBA)	Level C1 Positive Air Pressure Respirator (PAPR)	Level C2 Air Purifying Respirator (APR)

Courtesy: Safety Equipment Australia

to the maximum number of staff (who are not first-responders) in a reasonable length of time, we suggest that local emergency planning committees be responsible for awareness education. As an example, receiving hospitals could endorse the inclusion of MCI awareness in orientation programs and mandatory update programs. Local training and testing of plans has now been included in hospital accreditation programs.[100]

Table-top exercises are a useful tool to help raise awareness of MCI plans; however, table-top exercises do not test real time-frames for clinical decision-making and application of treatment. A more realistic test of MCI plans is to simulate victims and events with actors and realistic scenarios. This method requires the use of sophisticated equipment and large numbers of personnel. An alternative method is using simulation exercises that do not require so many resources yet is still a realistic test of emergency planning procedures. An example of such a system is the Emergo Train System (ETS). This system was developed in the early 1980s and offers an educational tool to test preparedness for an MCI. The ETS has a training system which is modulated and may commence at the scene of the incident through to definitive care. It is therefore ideal for pre-hospital paramedical, medical, nursing and support service personnel. ETS does not replace clinical decision-making education. The main strength of ETS is that it is interactive and enables decision-making by providing enough clinical information for attending staff to make decisions.

ETS has a large bank of magnetic figures of victims, staff and resources. Each victim is assigned injuries and a set of vital signs.

Unlike a table-top exercise ETS uses 'real time' for all resources. ETS requires a predetermined realistic time that it takes staff to do certain procedures; for example, various surgical operations and local transport times from the ED to ward areas, etc. The 'times' are given to the exercise team instructors prior to the commencement of the exercise. Exercise staff monitor and ensure that the times are adhered to by staff participating in the exercise. Each 'victim' is tracked throughout the exercise and, quite realistically, will 'die' if not given certain interventions or sufficiently early surgery. Evaluation of clinical judgement, staff allocation, communication systems and how MCI plans interlink becomes a powerful tool to future organisational MCI planning.[101]

Points to consider

The following points need to be considered when developing training and education programs:

- recognition of the numbers and types of staff to be trained to enable safe cover during annual leave and sickness
- realistic performance indicators for the staff to be trained need to be established by management
- testing of equipment and rotating stock to be encouraged to increase staff awareness of equipment location and content; regular checking and rotation of stock will prevent stock wastage and re-educate staff about equipment available
- practising MCI and CBR responses requires regular exercises.

SUMMARY

MCIs can occur at any time; therefore authorities and professional groups need to be prepared. The development and frequent rehearsal of MCI plans are the keys to a controlled and effective response. Risk analysis assists planners in exploring inside and outside their organisations for events that may well have catastrophic effects on their organisations. The triage process has some pitfalls, and the initial reception processes of MCI victims into hospitals should be discussed to assist planners in choosing which members of staff are most suitable to perform the various functions of the MCI plan.

Members of staff who may be deployed to the site of a CBR MCI need an overview of the site layout, scene management and knowledge of the CBR agent effects and antidotes required. Staff responding need to be trained in using the appropriate PPE. This chapter gives an overview of the more common CBR agents that may be involved in CBR incidents; note that Table 12.5 only gives examples and is not a definitive information document. Further reading on the subject of CBR is given below.

The associated response to and the initial-surge reception of victims from an MCI can be complex, especially when CBR agents are involved. The training of as many staff as possible to make them familiar and competent in their response to an MCI will assist greatly in any response the institution has to an MCI. Such training cannot be emphasised enough. It is important to offer frequent refresher courses and updates.

USEFUL WEBSITES

Australian Radiation Protection and Nuclear Safety Agency, www.arpansa.gov.au

Centers for Disease Control and Prevention (USA), www.cdc.gov

Emergency Management in Australia, www.em.gov.au

Federal Emergency Management Agency (USA), www.fema.gov

International Atomic Energy Agency, www.iaea.org

Ministry of Civil Defence and Emergency Management (New Zealand), www.civildefence.govt.nz/memwebsite.nsf

US Department of Homeland Security, www.dhs.gov

World Health Organization, www.who.int

FURTHER READING

Arbon P, Cusack L et al. Exploring staff willingness to attend work during a disaster: A study of nurses employed in four Australian emergency departments. Australasian Emergency Nursing Journal 2013;16:103–9.

Australian Radiation Protection and Nuclear Safety Agency. Intervention in emergency situations involving radiation exposure: radiation protection series publication no.7. Canberra: Australian Government Printing; 2004.

Goozner B, Lutwick L, Bourke E. Chemical terrorism: a primer for 2002. J Assoc Acad Minor Phys 2003;13(1):14–18.

Hadden WA, Rutherford WH, Merrett JD. The injuries of terrorist bombing: a study of 1532 consecutive patients. Br J Surg 1978; 65:525–31.

Incident control system. The operating system of AIIMS. 2nd edn. Mooroolbark: Australasian Fire and Emergency Service Authorities Council, Victoria; 1994.

Ranse J, Shaban RZ, Considine J et al. Disaster content in Australian tertiary, postgraduate emergency nursing courses: a survey. Australasian Emergency Nursing Journal 2013;16(2):58–63.

Standards Australia. AS/NZS 4360:1995. Risk management. 3rd edn. 2004 Sydney: Standards Australia; 1995.

Standards SAA HB9-1994. Occupational personal protection. 2nd edn. Sydney: Standards Australia; 1994.

Stein M, Hirshberg A. Medical consequences of terrorism: the conventional weapon threat. Surg Clin North Am 1999;79:1537–52.

Vogt BM, Sorrensen JH. How clean is safe? Improving the effectiveness of decontamination of structures and people following chemical and biological incidents. Final report (ORNL/TM-2002/178). Prepared by Oakridge National Laboratory for the US Department of Energy. Online. http://emc.ornl.gov/publications/PDF/How_Clean_is_Safe.pdf; accessed 25 Feb 2015.

REFERENCES

1. Hirshberg A, Holcomb J, Mattox K. Hospital trauma care in multiple-casualty incidents: a critical review. Ann Emerg Med 2001;37(6):647–52.

2. Ministry of Civil Defence and Emergency Management. Proposed national civil defence emergency management plan 2002. Online. www.mcdem.govt.nz; accessed January 2014.

3. Sagapolutele F. At least 34 dead as tsunami hits Samoas. Los Angeles Times. Online. www.latimes.com/news/nationworld/world/la-fgw-samoa-quake30-2009; accessed 29 Dec 09.

4. Fremson, R The New York Times: A massive earthquake struck Haiti on 12 Jan 2010, levelling capital, Port-au-Prince. Online. www.nytimes.com/info/haiti-earthquake-2010; accessed 02 Feb 10.

5. McSaveney, E. Historic earthquakes—The 2011 Christchurch earthquake and other recent earthquakes, Te Ara—the Encyclopedia of New Zealand, updated 20-Aug-13 URL: www.TeAra.govt.nz/en/historic-earthquakes/page-13Emergency

6. Greater Blue Mountains Press release New South Wales Rural Fire Service. 19 October 2013; accessed 21 October 2013.

7. SitRep No. 22 Effects of Typhoon 'Yolanda' (Haiyan). National Disaster Risk Reduction and Management Council. November 16, 2013; accessed 16 November 2013.

8. 'Tacloban: City at the centre of the storm'. BBC. 12 November 2013; accessed 13 November 2013.

9. National Counter Terrorism Plan. Chapter 2: Legal and administrative framework. 2nd edn. Online. www.nationalsecurity.gov.au/.../national-counter-terrorism-plan-2012; accessed 25 Feb 2015.

10. Ian Black. The Guardian. Attacks draw worldwide condemnation. Online. www.guardian.co.uk/world/2008/nov/28/mumbai terror attacks international response; accessed 08 Dec 09.

11. Ralston N, Partridge, E. Martin Place siege being treated as terrorist attack, police confirm. 15 December 2014. Sydney Morning Herald. http://www.smh.com.au; accessed 25 February 2015.

12. Australian Broadcasting Corporation. Sydney siege: What we do and don't know about hostage situation in Martin Place. ABC News 15 December 2014. www.abc.net.au; acessed 25 Feb 2015.

13. Kum-Ying T. An emergency department response to severe acute respiratory syndrome: a prototype response to bioterrorism. Ann Emerg Med 2004;43(1):15–16.

14. Chan M. World now at the start of 2009 influenza pandemic. Online. icmjournal.esicm.org/Journals/abstract.html feb 2015; accessed 25 Feb 2015.

15. Department of Health. Middle East Respiratory Syndrome Coronavirus (MERS-CoV). Consumer information. www.health.gov.au/internet/main/publishing.nsf/Content/ohp-mers-cov.htm; accessed 20 Feb 2015.

16. Centre for Disease Control and Prevention. 2014 Ebola outbreak in West Africa—case counts. 2014 Ebola Outbreak in West Africa. www.cdc.gov; accessed 25 Feb 2015.

17. CDC. Guidelines for evaluation of us patients suspected of having ebola virus disease. 1 August 2014; accessed 5 August 2014.

18. Ministry of Civil Defence and Emergency Management. Proposed national civil defense emergency management plan 2002. Online. www.mcdem.govt.nz; accessed Oct 2005.

19. Australian Government. Emergency Management. Online. www.em.gov.au/Emergencymanagement/Preparingforemergencies/Plans; accessed 22 May 2015.

20. Ministry of Civil Defence and Emergency Management. www.civildefence.govt.nz/memwebsite.NSF/Files/NatCDEMPlanOrder43191/$file/NatCDEMPlanOrder43191

21. National Health Emergency Plan: Mass Casualty Action Plan. Ministry of Health. September 2011 (Updated Nov 2011) Wellington: Ministry of Health. Online. www.moh.govt.nz

22. The National Emergency Access Target. Online. www.health.nsw.gov.au/Performance/Pages/NEAT

23. Standards Australia. Australian/New Zealand Standard (AS/NZS 4083) infrastructure protection. Sydney: Standards Australia; 2010.

24. Standards Australia/Standards New Zealand. SAA/SNZ HB76: 1997. Dangerous goods—initial emergency response guide (revised edition of SAA/SNZ HB76: 1996 incorporating Amdt 1):4–5, 220. Sydney: Standards Australia; 3rd edn; 2004.

25. Kirschenbaum L, Keene A, O'Neill P et al. The experience at St Vincent's Hospital, Manhattan, on September 11, 2001: preparedness, response, and lessons learned. Crit Care Med 2005;33(suppl 1):s48–52.

26. Hodgetts TJ, Mackaway-Jones K, eds. Major incident medical management and support, the practical approach. Plymouth: BMJ Publishing; 1998.

27. Mitchell GW. A brief history of triage. Disaster Med Public Health Preparedness 2008;2(Suppl 1):S4–7.

28. Chipman M, Hackley BE, Spencer TS. Triage of mass casualties: concepts for coping with mixed battlefield injuries. Mil Med 1980;145(2):99–100.

29. National Research Council of Canada. Transforming Triage Technology. Online. www.nrc-cnrc.gc.ca/eng/news/nrc/2006/06/06/triage.html; accessed 27 Dec 09.

30. Burstein JL, Hogan DE. Disaster medicine. 2nd edn. Philadelphia: Lippincott Williams & Wilkins; 2007.

31. The Field Triage (European Trauma Course). Online. www-cdu.dc.med.unipi.it/ECTC/etria.htm; accessed 25 Feb 2015.

32. Military triage. Online. www.medscape.com/viewarticle/431314_2; accessed 25 Feb 2015.

33. Emergency Management Australia. Australian emergency manuals series. Part III. Vol 1; manual 2:21: Disaster medicine. Canberra: Commonwealth of Australia; 1999. Online. www.em.gov.au/documents/manual09-disastermedicine.pd; accessed 25 Feb 2015.

34. Garner A, Lee A, Schultz CH. Comparative analysis of multiple-casualty incident triage algorithms. Ann Emerg Med 2001;38(5):541–8.

35. Meredith W, Rutledge R, Hansen AR et al. Field triage of trauma patients based upon the ability to follow commands: a study in 29,573 injured patients. J Trauma 1995;38:129–35.

36. Ross S, Leipold C, Terregino C et al. Efficacy of the motor component of the Glasgow Coma score in trauma triage. J Trauma 1998;45(1):42–4.

37. Mass Casualty Triage Pack—SMART Triage Pack Document Number PD2011_044 Ministry of Health NSW Publication date 04-Jul-2011 accessed www.health.nsw.gov.au/policies/; accessed January 2014.

38. Jacobs LM, Ramp JM, Breay JM. An emergency medical system approach to disaster planning. J Trauma 1979;19:157–62.

39. Teague D. Mass casualties in the Oklahoma city bombing. Clin Orthop Rel Res 2004;422:77–81.

40. Australian/New Zealand standard. AS/NZS 1715:1994—selection, use and maintenance of respiratory protective devices. Sydney: Standards Australia; 1994.

41. Ammons MA, Moore EE, Pons PT et al. The role of a regional trauma system in the management of a mass disaster: an analysis of the Keystone, Colorado chairlift accident. J Trauma 1988;28:1468–71.

42. Frykberg ER. Medical management of disasters and mass casualties from terrorist bombings: how can we cope? J Trauma 2002;53(2):201–12.

43. United States Government Accountability Office (GAO–04–239). US Postal Service: better guidance is needed to ensure an appropriate response to anthrax contamination. 2004 report to congressional requesters. Online. Available: www.gao.gov/new.items/d04239.pdf; 28 Dec 2006.

44. Public Health Agency of Canada. Clinical and public health systems issues arising from the outbreak of SARS in Toronto. Chapter 8: Public health agency of Canada. Online. www.phac-aspc.gc.ca/publicat/sars-sras/naylor/8-eng.php; accessed 28 Dec 2009.

45. Australian Health Ministers Conference (AHMC). National burns planning and coordinating committee. AusBurnPlan strategy paper: Australian mass casualty burn disaster plan. Commonwealth Government Printing Australia; 2004. Online. www.health.gov.au/internet/wcms/publishing.nsf/content/phd-health-emergency.htm/$file/ausburn.pdf; accessed 28 Dec 2006.

46. Frykberg ER, Tepas JJ. Terrorist bombings: lessons learned from Belfast to Beirut. Ann Surg 1988;208(5):569–76.

47. Mallonee S, Shariat S, Stennies G et al. Physical injuries and fatalities resulting from the Oklahoma City bombing. JAMA 1996;276(5):382–7.

48. Cushman JG, Pachter HL et al. Two New York city hospitals surgical response to the September 11, 2001 terrorist attack in New York City. J Trauma 2003;54(1):147–55.

49. Hirshberg A, Stein M, Walden R. Surgical resource utilization in urban terrorist bombing: a computer simulation. J Trauma 1999; 47:545–50.

50. Securing Australia/protecting our Community Counter. Terrorism white paper department of the Prime Minister and cabinet 2010. Online. www.ag.gov.au; accessed 1 Mar 2010.

51. Patient Identification Procedure—NSLHD Doc.Num PO2011_301 04/10/13.

52. Correct Patient, Correct Procedure and Correct Site. Document Number PD2007_079 Publication date 30-Oct-2007 NSW

53. Hirshberg A, Holcomb J, Mattox K. Hospital trauma care in multiple-casualty incidents: a critical review. Ann Emerg Med 2001;37(6):647–52.

54. Kirschenbaum L, Keene A, O'Neill P et al. The experience at St Vincent's Hospital, Manhattan, on September 11, 2001: preparedness, response, and lessons learned. Crit Care Med 2005;33(1 suppl):s48–52.

55. Frykberg ER, Hutton PMJ, Balzer RH. Disaster in Beirut: an application of mass casualty principles. Mil Med 1987;152(11):563–6.

56. Cook CH, Muscarella P, Praba AC et al. Reducing over-triage without compromising outcomes in trauma patients. Arch Surg 2001;136:752–6.

57. Feliciano DV, Anderson GV, Rozycki GS et al. Management of casualties from the bombing at the Centennial Olympics. Am J Surg 1998; 176:538–43.

58. Gutierrez de Ceballos JP, Feuentes F, Diaz D et al. Casualties treated at the closest hospital in the Madrid, March 11, terrorist bombings. Crit Care Med 2005;33(1 suppl):s107–12.

59. Fuentes F, Diaz D, Sanz-Sánchez et al. Overall assessment of the response to terrorist bombings in trains, Madrid, 11 Mar 2004. Eur J Trauma Emerg Surg 2008;34(5):433–41.

60. Almogy G, Belzberg H, Mintz Y et al. Suicide bombings attacks: update and modifications to the protocol. Ann Surg 2004; 239(3):295–303.

61. Reid WH. Psychological aspects of terrorism. J Psychiatr Pract 2001;7(6):422–5

62. Carlier Y, Lambert RG, Ulchelen AJ et al. Disaster related post-traumatic stress in police officers: a field study of the impact of debriefing. Stress Med 1998;14:143–8.

63. Karwa M, Currie B, Kvetan V. Bioterrorism: preparing for the impossible or the improbable. Crit Care Med 2005;33(1 suppl):s75–95.

64. 'BBC on this day 16th 1988: thousands die in Halabja gas attack' news.bbc.co.uk/onthis day/hi/dates/stories/march/16/news; accessed 2 July 2014.

65. 'Halabja, the massacre the west tried to ignore' thetimesonline.co.uk/tto/news; accessed 2 July 2014.

66. The Guardian Syrian Chemical Attackonline www.theguardian.com/world/2013/sep/16/syrian-chemical-attack-sarin-says-un; accessed December 2013.

67. Securing Australia/protecting our Community Counter. Terrorism white paper department of the Prime Minister and cabinet 2010. Online. via www.ag.gov.au; accessed 1 Mar 2010.

68. Karwa M, Bronzert P, Kvetan V. Bioterrorism and critical care. Crit Care Clinic 2003;19(2):279–313.

69. Klein R, Walter GW et al. Advanced HAZMAT life support instructor manual. 2nd edn. Tucson: University of Arizona Emergency Medicine Research Center; American Academy for Clinical Toxicology; 2000:290–2.

70. Emergency Management Australia. Australian emergency manuals series. Part III, vol. 2; manual 3: 327: health aspects of chemical, biological and radiological hazards. Canberra: Commonwealth of Australia; 2000. Online. www.em.gov.au/Documents/Manual13-HealthAspects.pdf; accessed 25 Feb 2015.

71. Hall EJ. Radiation and life. 2nd edn. New York: Pergamon; 1984. Online (sections only). Online. www.uic.com.au; accessed 9 Sept 2005.

72. Oh TE, Bersten AD, Soni N, eds. Oh's intensive care manual. 5th edn. Edinburgh: Butterworth–Heinemann; 2003

73. Rosen P, Barkin RS, Hockberger RS et al, eds. Emergency medicine: concepts and clinical practice. 5th edn. St. Louis: Mosby; 2002.

74. Joint Commission on Accreditation Health Organizations. Special issue: emergency management in the new millennium. Joint commission perspectives; 2001. Online. www.jcrinc.com/perspectivesspecialissue; accessed 26 Aug 2005.

75. Dixon TC, Meselson M, Guillemin J et al. Anthrax. N Engl J Med 1999;341(11):815–26

76. Committee on Trauma (ACS). Mass casualties: resources for optimal care of the injured patient. Chicago: American College of Surgeons; 1999:87–91.

77. O'Toole T. Smallpox: an attack scenario. Emerg Infect Dis 1999;5(4):540–6.

78. MIMS. Online. www.mims.com.au; accessed 20 Feb 2015.

79. Military Medical Operations Armed Forces Radiology Research Institute. Medical management of radiological casualties handbook. Bethesda: MMOAFRRI Bethesda; 2003:1–6. Online. www.afrri.usuhs.mil; accessed 28 Dec 2006. Manual+13A.pdf/$file/Manual+13A.pdf; 31 Dec 2006.

80. Okumura T, Suzuki K, Fukuda A et al. The Tokyo subway Sarin attack: disaster management, part 1: community emergency response. Acad Emerg Med 1998;5(6):613–17

81. Okumura T, Suzuki K, Fukuda A et al. The Tokyo subway Sarin attack: disaster management, part 2: hospital response. Acad Emerg Med 1998;5:618–24.

82. Bradt DA. Rapid assessment of injuries among survivors of the terrorist attack on the World Trade Center. New York City, September 2001: MMWR 2002;51(1):1–5.

83. Hogan DE, Waeckerle JF, Dire DJ et al. Emergency department impact of the Oklahoma city terrorist bombing. Ann Emerg Med 1999;34:160–7.

84. Okudera H, Morita H, Iwashita T et al. Unexpected nerve gas exposure in the city of Matsumoto: report of rescue activity in the first sarin gas terrorism. Am J Emerg Med 1997;15:527.

85. Okumura T, Takasu N, Ishimatsu S et al. Report on 640 victims of the Tokyo subway sarin attack. Ann Emerg Med 1996;28:129–35.

86. Macintyre AG, Christopher GW, Eitzen E Jr et al. Weapons of mass destruction events with contaminated casualties: effective planning for health care facilities. JAMA 2000;283(2):242–9.

87. Forster PL, Wu LH. Traumatic stress and natural disasters: implications for psychiatric emergency services. J Am Assoc Emerg Psychiatry 2001;7(3):76–80.

88. Stewart CE. Environmental emergencies. Baltimore: Williams & Wilkins; 1990.

89. OSHA. Best practices for hospital-based first receivers of victims from mass casualty incidents involving the release of hazardous substances. Occupational Safety and Health Administration (OSHA). Online. www.osha.gov/pls/oshaweb/owadisp; accessed Jan 2005.

90. Horton DK, Berkowitz Z, Kaye WE. Secondary contamination of ED personnel from hazardous materials events, 1995–2001. Am J Emerg Med 2003;21:199–204.

91. Georgopoulos PG, Fedele P et al. Hospital response to chemical terrorism: personal protective equipment, training, and operations planning. Am J Ind Med 2004;46(5):432–45.

92. US Army Center for Health Promotion and Preventive Medicine. The medical NBC battlebook, USACHPPM Tech Guide 244. Aberdeen Proving Ground MD. United States Army Center for Health Promotion and Preventive Medicine; 2002.

93. National counter-terrorism plan. Chapter 2: Legal and administrative framework. 2nd edn. Online. www.nationalsecurity.gov.au/agd/WWW/rwpattach.nsf/VAP/(5738DF09EBC4B7EAE52BF217B46ED3DA)~NCTP_Sept_2005.pdf/$file/NCTP_Sept_2005.pdf; accessed 28 Dec 2006.

94. Hick JL, Hanfling D, Burstein JL et al. Protective equipment for healthcare facility decontamination personnel: regulations, risks, and recommendations. Ann Emerg Med 2003;42(3):370–80.

95. Slater MS, Trunkey DD. Terrorism in America: an evolving threat. Arch Surg 1997;132:1059–66.

96. Simon R, Teperman S. The World Trade Center attack: lessons for disaster management. Crit Care 2001;5:318–20.

97. Standards Australia. AS3765.1-1990. Clothing for protection against hazardous chemicals. Part 1: Protection against general or specific chemicals. Sydney: Standards Australia; 1990.

98. The coming ethical crisis: oxygen rationing. Online. www.huffingtonpost.com/jacobm-apppeal/the-coming-ethical-crisis; accessed 28 Dec 2009

99. Who dies, who doesn't: docs decide flu pandemic guidelines (CBC News Item). www.cbc.ca/health/story/2006/11/20/pandemic-triage; accessed 28 Dec 2009.

100. The Australian Council on Health Standards (ACHS). The ACHS EQuIP. 4th edn. Australia: Sydney; 2006.

101. Lennquist S. The emergotrain system for training and testing disaster preparedness: 15 years of experience. Int J Dis Med 2003;1:25–34.

102. Brennan RJ, Bradt DA, Abrahams J. Medical issues in disasters. In: Cameron P, Jelinek G, Kelly A et al. eds. Textbook of adult emergency medicine. 2nd edn. Edinburgh: Churchill Livingstone; 2004:694.

103. Center for Biological Defense WMD agent quick reference guide. Online. www.bt.usf.edu/files/WMD.pdf; accessed 8 Jan 2010 (Biochart).

104. Centers for Disease Control and Prevention. Emergency preparedness and response: bioterrorism agents/diseases. Department of Health and Human Services. Online. www.bt.cdc.gov/agent/agentlist-category.asp; accessed Jan 2010.

105. Klein R, Walter GW et al. Advanced HAZMAT Life support instructor manual. 2nd edn. University of Arizona Emergency Medicine Research Center American Academy for Clinical Toxicology 2000:290–2.

106. Potential biological agent operational data charts. Adapted from FM8–9: NATO handbook the medical aspects of NBC defensive operations. AMedP–6(B). Online. www.cbwinfo.com/biological/FM9Table.html; accessed Jan 2010.

CHAPTER 13
TRIAGE AND EMERGENCY NURSES

MARGARET FRY

Essentials

- Triage is the sorting of patients on arrival at the emergency department (ED).
- There are many validated and reliable triage tools used to determine patient urgency.
- The Australasian Triage Scale comprises five scales, each with a corresponding time-frame.
- The triage nurse requires advanced emergency knowledge, experience and skills to discriminate between life-threatening, urgent and non-urgent conditions.
- The role and responsibilities of the triage nurse require advanced skills to enable the fast-tracking of patients and management of overcrowding.
- The triage nurse requires advanced communication and interpersonal skills to optimise clinical hand-over and the patient's understanding of the ED journey.

INTRODUCTION

This chapter provides an understanding of the background and development of triage nursing practice. With emergency department (ED) patient presentations increasing, formalised triage systems have been developed to identify and prioritise those patients presenting with actual or potentially life-threatening conditions. Australasian triage guidelines were developed to assist the nurse to discriminate between life-threatening, urgent and non-urgent conditions. However, triage involves more than the application of triage guidelines. Triage nurses determine the need for a bed, allocate ED resources, fast-track patient care, deliver first aid and provide a safety net for waiting patients. Today, in order to undertake triage and meet the additional extended role demands requires extensive emergency experience and advanced practice and decision-making skills.

Origin of triage nursing

The origin of the word 'triage' is from the French verb 'trier', a word used in the 18th century to sort farming and agricultural products.[1] The application of this word to the sorting of medical casualties dates back to the Franco-Prussian military campaigns.[2] Prior to this, soldiers were generally cared for according to their rank and often by their families or retainers. It was the surgeon Baron Dominique Jean Larrey who first prioritised the need for medical intervention and hospital transportation for wounded soldiers. The role of military triage at this time was to identify soldiers with non-fatal wounds. This meant that soldiers with minor injuries were medically treated while those mortally wounded were left to die. The main benefit of implementing a triage system was to accelerate the return of soldiers to the battlefield.[3]

While triage remained a process confined to military campaigns, it underwent extensive refinement during sub-sequent wars (World Wars I and II, and the Korean, Vietnam, Falkland and Gulf wars). Evidence was building of mortality-rate reduction by early assessment, prompt resuscitation and fast patient transfer in military hospital settings and battlefields. Soldier mortality rate reduced from 5% during World War II to 1% by the end of the Vietnam War.[4] By the 1970s the patient outcome benefits evident in military triage had captured the interest of governments and hospital service providers resulting in formal triage systems being implemented in some civilian emergency departments.[5]

In Australia, before the introduction of triage into civilian EDs, medical and non-medical personnel, such as clerks and paramedics, performed the initial patient assessment. The need to obtain patient and financial details saw the role commonly performed by clerical staff.[6] Generally, patients were processed on a first-come first-served basis. While this was an efficient system when patient presentation numbers were low, it proved unsafe when large numbers of patients arrived at the same time.

The nurse triage role was introduced to improve the timely recognition of patients with life-threatening conditions, and to ensure the safety of waiting patients, the appropriate allocation of resources and the overall efficiency of ED services.[7] By the late 1980s people presenting to an Australasian ED for care were for the first time met by the triage nurse who assessed their clinical urgency. Since this time, decision-making and activity by triage nurses has been shown to significantly influence the patient's experience of emergency care, mortality, morbidity and satisfaction rates.[8–11]

The Australasian Triage Scale

During the period 1985–1990, there was a significant increase reported in the number of patient presentations to ED.[6] With the increase in the number of patient presentations there was growing concern that the identification of patients with urgent conditions was haphazard. The increase in patient presentations was attributed to an ageing population, improved life expectancy for chronic conditions and increased patient acuity and complexity. In addition, there was a decrease in the number of privately insured patients and increased hospital bed closures.[9,10] Consequently, the first purpose of introducing Australasian national triage guidelines was to assist the nurse in the recognition of patient urgency and enable greater consistency within practice.[12,13]

With the increase in ED patient presentations, governments were seeking ways to regulate, compare and predict the cost of emergency services. To gain some control over the escalating cost of healthcare, financial models made use of ED triage code data.[14] Given that triage codes were being examined to predict costs and that many EDs had developed their own guidelines, clinicians were motivated to establish national triage guidelines to secure greater equity within funding models.[15] While concerns about linking triage codes with ED funding were raised, triage code incentive funding was introduced in 1996.[16]

Therefore, national triage guidelines were developed to assist triage nurse recognition of patient urgency; to achieve greater consistency and uniformity within practice; and to create equity within ED funding models. In 1994 the National Triage Scale (NTS), which in 2002 became known as the Australasian Triage Scale (ATS), was introduced in Australia.[17] The ATS consists of five scales that link patient history, signs and symptoms, and diagnosis to clinical urgency.[12] Each triage scale incorporates a hierarchy of medical and nursing response times for patients (Table 13.1).

To aid the application, veracity and standardisation of ED costing models, governments implemented ED computer information systems. There are now a number of healthcare information systems throughout Australasia. Currently state governments are integrating electronic medical record (eMR) systems, which aim to interface with ED systems. This has replaced the Australian system known as EDIS (Emergency Department Information System). The purpose of the eMR information system is to enable clinicians to view an integrated patient record, order and review investigations and track the patient journey. The eMR enables greater standardisation, consistency, safety and auditing of healthcare data, thus enabling greater surveillance, regulation and prediction of healthcare costs across specialty areas including EDs. With the implementation of the eMR governments can calculate, audit and predict current and future ED funding needs.[18]

By the early 1990s, Australia, New Zealand and Canada had adopted national five-scale triage guidelines.[19–21] Within Australasia the ATS provides nurses with a uniform method to allocate a triage urgency code for a range of adult and paediatric conditions, thereby authorising them to regulate the distribution of emergency care. Modification and review of

---

TABLE 13.1 Australasian Triage Scale[17]

ATS CODE	RESPONSE TIME
Code 1 (resuscitation)	Requires immediate intervention
Code 2 (emergency)	Requires intervention within 10 minutes
Code 3 (urgent)	Should be seen within 30 minutes
Code 4 (semi-urgent)	Should be seen within 1 hour
Code 5 (non-urgent)	Should be seen within 2 hours

TABLE 13.2 Triage performance benchmarks[17,21]

	ACEM*%	NZ‡%
Triage code 1	100	100
Triage code 2	80	80
Triage code 3	75	75
Triage code 4	70	
Triage code 5	70	

‡New Zealand emergency departments (n = 42); these benchmark against only the first three triage codes.[21]

the ATS has occurred to ensure that vulnerable groups are not marginalised and/or disadvantaged.[22]

Throughout Australasia, triage code waiting times are used to measure and compare ED performance. Waiting times provide a quality indicator for the efficiency and timeliness of ED services.[9,11] Hence, with the implementation of the ATS there was increasing expectation that EDs would demonstrate timely service by meeting the agreed-upon triage code benchmarks. Triage code benchmarks are determined by the percentage of patients seen by a medical officer or nurse practitioner (NP) or extended practice emergency nurse within the specified triage code time-frame (Table 13.2).

Reliability and validity of the Australasian Triage Scale

With the introduction of the ATS, researchers began focusing on establishing the reliability and validity of the tool. The majority of studies used hypothetical patient scenarios as their basis for validation. Jelinek and Little[16] assessed the inter-rater reliability of the ATS by having 115 nurses allocate a triage code to 100 hypothetical patient scenarios. The findings from this study demonstrated that between nurses there was high concordance (95% within one category of the modal response) of triage code allocation. The study provided evidence that despite triage experience and hospital type, the ATS appropriately and consistently measured clinical urgency. The results are supported by other researchers who found inter-rater reliability at between 80% and 95%.[22,23] While these studies confirmed that the ATS was a reliable measure of patient urgency, they identified that some patients continued to be over- or under-triaged—accounting for inter-rater disagreement rates of between 5% and 20%.[22,24,25]

Researchers were also interested in identifying the reliability of the ATS when measuring a range of patient outcomes such as admission rates. Hollis and Sprivulis[26] identified that, despite ED activity, admission rates for codes 1, 2 and 3 were consistent with ATS guidelines. Other researchers examined and demonstrated a strong association between triage codes and patient diagnoses, management, admission, morbidity and mortality rate.[11,25,27–30] The Australian studies convincingly established the inter-rater reliability of the ATS and identified that greater consistency and recognition of clinical urgency were present when triage nurses used the guidelines.

However, the triage guidelines initially were not sensitive in identifying the urgency of specific groups, for example acutely ill children.[31] Browne et al[32] provided evidence that the ATS did not consistently identify children with urgent conditions. Similarly, Durojaiye and O'Meara's[31] study confirmed inconsistent application of the guidelines for seriously ill children. This indicated that the guidelines needed to be revised for specific vulnerable population groups, such as acutely ill children and people with mental health disorders. Consequently, in 2002 the ATS was revised to specifically accommodate these vulnerable population groups. However, triage nurses continue to require paediatric experience to assist in application of the ATS. There is Level II,[28,33] Level III[16,22,32] and Level IV[26,34] evidence to support the continued use and acceptance of the five-level ATS guidelines. (See Ch 7 for a more detailed understanding of research evidence levels.)

Now across Australasia the ATS is used to define the urgency of people presenting with a range of injuries and or conditions. Using this tool clinicians allocate an ATS urgency code within a range of environments. In this way emergency services are able to differentiate urgency and need for medical intervention and allocate appropriate resources.

Rural triage

Across Australia and New Zealand, healthcare infrastructure is composed of hospitals that provide different levels of emergency care (see Ch 1). Designated EDs are located largely in urban settings while rural, remote and very remote health centres have designated treatment rooms that provide limited resuscitation practices. Significant challenges face rural and remote healthcare providers, specifically relating to access, staff retention, resources and distances between geographically isolated locations.[35]

Work demands on healthcare workers in rural and regional areas would appear to be different compared with metropolitan areas.[36,37] A recent Australian study examined general practitioner (GP) income, work hours and dependence on Medicare reimbursement in rural settings. The cross-sectional, retrospective analysis of rural and urban doctors demonstrated that GPs in rural and regional areas provided greater after-hour patient contact episodes, worked longer and earned less than metropolitan-based GPs.[35] The trend was also evident within the international literature.[38,39] In addition, non-metropolitan healthcare workers often lacked separation between work and private life.

Across Australia, there are 217 very remote communities and 271 health services, sites or facilities that provide emergency services with limited resuscitation capabilities.[40] Compared with remote, rural or regional communities, Indigenous Australians largely compose the populations which live in very remote communities (18% of the total population). Many of the very remote services (n = 133) are staffed by, and for, Indigenous communities.[41] By contrast, Māori healthcare providers are under-represented in New Zealand rural and semi-rural healthcare communities. In New Zealand, a Māori health provider is an organisation that delivers health services largely for Māori and is managed by Māori.[21,42,43]

Rural, remote and very remote nurses often undertake triage, but then go on to provide first-line emergency care and definitive patient management and/or referral.[44] For emergency services, where medical review is limited, the ATS waiting time benchmark is examined with respect to the 'nurse seen time'. Many rural, remote and very remote communities experience significant healthcare isolation.[45,46] To reduce isolation and improve healthcare access throughout Australasia, initiatives such as HealthDirect, Telehealth, the Bush Crisis Line and Support Services, and Healthline have been developed.[47–52]

In geographically isolated regions, nurses and paramedical staff have extended their scope of practice through successful completion of educational courses. For example, rural New Zealand nurses are able to expand their scope of practice through the PRIME (Primary Response in Medical Emergencies) course. To improve New Zealand rural health, the PRIME course was implemented nationally.[53,54] Equivalent first line emergency care courses are available throughout Australia.[55,56] These educational initiatives aim to meet the needs of healthcare providers working in rural, remote and very remote emergency settings where, as first responder, they must triage, resuscitate and manage the patient.

Triage decision-making

Triage decision-making involves advanced cognitive processes which are used to determine a patient's medical urgency, the allocation of departmental resources (allocation of beds and clinical areas), initiation of interventions and management of incidents and service flow.[57] To this end, the role of triage requires the nurse to undertake primary and secondary triage.

Primary triage decisions

Primary triage decisions are focused on identifying life-threatening conditions and then delivering appropriate interventions and first aid. The initial assessment evaluates the patient's airway, breathing and circulation, and only if the patient is determined stable should the triage nurse then focus on the patient's primary complaint. Using this primary decision, triage nurses determine the appropriate urgency code. In this way triage code allocation regulates the timing of medical and nursing care.

The determination of a patient's clinical urgency must be independent of ED activity, patient behaviour, benchmarking practices and incentive funding.[58,59] The most urgent clinical patient feature should determine triage code selection. This may be identified during the history, physical assessment or when the clinician obtains vital signs. Selection of the correct triage code will avoid incidences of over- or under-triaging and provide for safer patient outcomes. To minimise over- or under-triaging triage nurses need to have emergency experience to become skilful in the recognition of a range of conditions and injuries and develop information gathering skills to be able to determine patient urgency.

Central to achieving this primary outcome is the triage nurse's ability to trawl for information, recognise and discriminate between patterns of clinical urgency, develop a working diagnosis, predict patient care needs and evaluate collected information.[60] In trawling for information, triage nurses collect objective and subjective data which enable clinical urgency to be determined. Mass casualty and trauma triage concepts and guidelines are presented in chapters 12 and 44 respectively.

> **PRACTICE TIP**
>
> If you are unsure in your decision-making the best and safest approach is to triage up and/or seek clarification from senior staff.

Objective data

Triage nurses should begin each patient assessment with a primary survey. This information process begins with inspection (visual observation of the patient). It is important 'just to look at the patient'. Initial observations of a patient should include general appearance and the degree of distress and emotional responses. This information provides an opportunity to form working diagnoses or suppositions. Triage nurses should also use all available information sources. For example, a patient may present with pathology, radiological and/or interventional reports. These information sources can help to solidify triage decision-making. A triage working diagnosis frames impressions of a patient's urgency and the need to allocate a bed. A working diagnosis can be confirmed or refuted during the triage interview and on the collection of physiological data.

Physiological data

Triage nurses should regularly choose to collect haemodynamic observations. Such observations provide a useful reference point for triage decision making when further information is necessary to discriminate between more- or less-urgent cases. The allocation of a triage code and clinical area are more confidently and accurately determined when a triage nurse has access to haemodynamic information.[61–64] However, vital signs may not be required for life-threatening conditions, actual or potential (triage code 1 and 2 patients). For vital sign values see Chapter 14.

> **PRACTICE TIP**
>
> If you are unsure use vital signs to support decision-making and triage code selection to minimise over- or under-triaging.

Subjective data

The triage nurse concurrently collects and collates subjective data. This involves collecting information that provides an understanding of 'why' the patient is presenting (primary complaint). Additional patient information to be elicited and collated includes: the precipitating event, onset of symptoms, medical history and medications and allergies. This information enables more confident triage decision-making to take place.

Triage nurses typically gather information using focused questioning. Triage nurse questioning should target the main reason for a patient presenting to an ED (chief complaint). By using open-ended questioning techniques, triage nurses should be able to gather information that 'funnels down' from the broad complaint to specific signs and symptoms. This funnelling process enables triage nurses to quickly gain insight into the patient's chief complaint.

While in the process of collecting patient information, the triage nurse will be actively ruling in, or out, life-threatening diagnoses such as myocardial infarction.[57]

Working diagnosis

When triage nurses gather patient information, they measure this against clinical templates stored from practical experience and theoretical knowledge. By taking a patient's history, focused physical examination, vital signs and symptoms and comparing with medical templates, triage nurses are able to discriminate between the different levels of urgency. Triage nurses rely on pattern recognition when gathering information to refine decision-making processes, direct choice and accelerate decision-making.[65,66]

While pattern recognition enables triage nurses to discriminate between more or less urgent cases, the prioritisation of a patient's need for care is accelerated through the development of a working diagnosis. A working diagnosis is used by triage nurses as a strategy to confirm or refute life-threatening conditions, patient urgency, determine an appropriate clinical area and predict care interventions. A triage working diagnosis helps to make sense of the act of triage, assists decision-making processes, reduces patient and family anxiety, expands professional confidence and adds an element of personal satisfaction to the role.[59,67]

Secondary triage decisions

Secondary triage decisions involve the appropriate allocation of ED resources and the initiation of nursing extended practices (timekeeping practices). Secondary decisions are based on suppositions or a working diagnosis confirmed during the primary assessment, which frame the need for investigational or extended nurse-initiated activities. Evidence suggests that triage nurses are undertaking or directing a range of investigational activities to assist in decision-making and patient safety.[68,69]

Triage timekeeping processes

Triage nurses initiate extended practices, which modulate a timing of ED care that creates a process of 'timekeeping'. Triage nurses use timekeeping practices to maintain, regulate or restore a normal rhythm of emergency care. Triage timekeeping processes sustain and maintain appropriate patient flow and resource use, while supporting patient assessment and urgency recognition decision-making. The decision to undertake investigational and/or extended activities occurs simultaneously with triage code and clinical area allocation. Evidence suggests that triage nurse pain management[68,70] and radiological investigations[69,71] contribute to improved patient outcomes and more timely, efficient and equitable healthcare services.

Triage gatekeeping processes

Primary and secondary triage decision-making is sustained through a process of gatekeeping. Gatekeeping regulates patient flow, and through this process a patient's clinical need is appropriately matched with a geographical ED workspace 'inside'.[57] For example, a patient requiring urgent medical intervention would be allocated to an appropriate resuscitation workspace where care is optimised and delivered by appropriately qualified nursing and medical staff. Triage nurses know that clinical areas provide different levels of care appropriate for a patient's condition or injury and that this determines a normal pattern of patient movement.

The fragmentation of workspaces into 'place' enables a process of gatekeeping to occur and triage decision-making to be ordered and consistent. Different meanings of time punctuate clinical areas that hierarchically order practice and staff activities. Consequently, each ED clinical area reflects varying levels of urgency, timeliness, efficiency and control, characterising different workspaces into 'places'. Once nurses have learnt the meanings applied to work 'places' and the different patient groups, they are able to make effective triage choices and predict care needs. Triage nurses use gatekeeping processes to accomplish the appropriate allocation of service resources to a patient's medical need, thereby securing flow, order, consistency and patient safety.[3]

Communication

Triage nurses through communication processes act as a cultural broker for patients and family, staff and other healthcare professionals. A patient's first encounter with the acute healthcare system is often with the triage nurse. Professional conduct needs to be conveyed within all communication processes and informed patient consent obtained before undertaking relevant triage activities. Indeed, ineffective or inappropriate communication is often the primary source of patient complaints and dissatisfaction.[72]

Advanced triage nurse communication and interpersonal skills are critical to ensure that information from the patient, primary care sector and/or paramedic is appropriately interpreted and synthesised. In this way triage decision-making can be supported and appropriate. At the same time, nurses must communicate a caring and compassionate professional attitude towards patients, families and relatives.[73] In addition, triage nurses should take the opportunity to explain to patients about activities taking place in the triage area and potentially along the patient journey.

Triage nurses need to be aware that patients, families and carers presenting to the ED are often experiencing anxiety and fear.[74,75] Being a skilful communicator enables the triage nurse to elicit appropriate patient information and to facilitate a patient's understanding of the ED journey.

> **PRACTICE TIP**
>
> To de-escalate negative emotions, triage nurses should inform patients of the waiting times and comfort family, carers and/or patients by explaining the triage process, the technology that is being used and the potential procedures and care interventions that may take place at the bedside.

Through communication and documentation skills, triage nurses are able to convert patient language into an urgency code and allocated clinical area, a useable currency which provides an understanding for emergency clinicians to orientate their practice. In this way the triage nurse is responsible for ensuring ED staff receive an appropriate and relevant hand-over to enable the continuity of care to match the patient's need. This ensures patients receive the appropriate care and intervention in the 'right' clinical area. To achieve effective 'cultural brokering', triage nurses require advanced communication and interpersonal skills. Further discussion on communication is found in Chapter 14.

Triage nurse education

The triage role requires the nurse to have advanced cognitive, communication and decision-making skills and to be able to collate knowledge systems, patterns of knowing and ways of doing with a patient's physiological, interpersonal and communicative signs. Emergency nurses often require up to two years emergency experience to gain the sufficient level of knowledge required to triage safely and appropriately. In addition, the ATS guidelines, well validated and reliable, provide a frame of reference for nurses to determine an appropriate urgency scale for presenting patients.[59]

Triage education programs need to develop strategies, in combination with the ATS Education Kit, that foster advanced skills and provide practical opportunities to develop patterns of 'knowing'.[59] To this end, emergency educators can support triage decision-making by designing local educational initiatives that target high levels of problem-solving and questioning in order to achieve more-thoughtful triage practice responses.[9,76]

> **PRACTICE TIP**
>
> Blended triage educational learning opportunities that comprise mentoring, patient urgency scenario practice, interviewing skills and simulation will better support knowledge translation and build triage skill capacity.

Triage education programs using a framework based on gatekeeping processes can assist nurses to understand the character of the role. Patients, families and carers and triage nurses have established values and expectations of services that are not often aligned. Greater awareness of differing expectations can increase tolerance, particularly when experiencing a clash of expectations in the allocation of beds, resources and the management of incidents, such as with patient overcrowding. Triage educational strategies should provide opportunity for novice triage nurses to work beside an experienced clinician to assist the development of these practical aspects of gatekeeping.[57]

Timekeeping processes are often constrained during incidents such as patient overcrowding. These incidents often induce negative experience patterns.[77-79] By making this dimension of triage practice transparent, conflicting interests and knowledge systems that compete to build 'threatening' or 'blame' environments can be avoided. In addition, novice triage nurses may benefit from an introductory period free of extended-role activities. Once adjustment to the role is complete, extended practices can be introduced into the nurse's craft repertoire. This may result in greater consistency in triage practice.[80]

Triage nurses need to be provided with opportunities to reflect on belief systems, biases, assumptions, expectations and ways of thinking, which are embedded within emergency care. Through reflective practices, nursing independence within the context of triage practice can be secured; and more-responsible decision-making, disciplined and compassionate work practices achieved.[73] This educational process should give triage nurses the wherewithal to extract complex meanings from experiences and analyse practice patterns (see Ch 7).

Educational forums need to be structured whereby experienced and novice triage nurses are brought together as a group. These focus groups provide opportunity for triage nurses to share their experiences and practices for information gathering, managing difficult triage situations and resource allocation, thus improving gatekeeping, timekeeping and decision-making skills. This process would assist nurses to understand what makes practice reasonable and would promote ethical and compassionate patterns of knowing and acting.

To reduce the potential influence of an emotionally charged triage response to a particular situation or event, triage nurses must learn how emotions can hold sway over gatekeeping, timekeeping and decision-making processes.[58] The convergence of different expectations (patient and/or nurse) often precipitates emotionally labile situations that escalate troubling or aggressive behaviour. Triage nurses must be prepared to confront and mediate ethical issues, contradictions, conflict and practical dilemmas in order to foster more tolerant and caring triage practices.

Triage documentation

The documented triage assessment should constitute the first part of the patient's medical notes. The triage nurse should document every triage episode undertaken within their institution. The triage nurse should also enter treatment contemporaneously, as this avoids reliance on personal memory.

> **PRACTICE TIP**
>
> Triage documentation should include the nurse's name, date and time of assessment, presenting complaint, a focused initial patient assessment,[81,82] triage code, treatment area and interventions implemented.[59,83]

The documented patient assessment should be sufficient to explain the allocated triage code, clinical area and interventions instigated by the nurse. The triage nurse should not make an entry on behalf of someone else. The legal implications of documentation are discussed in Chapter 4.

Legal aspects of triage

Triage documentation has the potential to be admitted as legal evidence if it is relevant to a matter being dealt with in a court of law or a coronial inquest. While medical records are not legal documents, they can be submitted as legal evidence. In some instances medical records are used to determine whether a coronial investigation is required to determine the cause of death. High-quality nursing documentation remains part of a nurse's accountability. Good documentation can assist a nurse if called upon to account for their professional actions.

Medical records require explanation of actions. The triage nurse should only document the facts, relevant patient assessment and interventions. Triage nurses should document treatments/procedures and reasons why. Triage assessments must be contemporaneous, and notes and information should never be obliterated (see Ch 4).

If triage nurses take a medical order via the telephone, it is important to try to get another person to listen to and counter-sign the order on the phone. If this is not possible, make sure the medical officer repeats the order and then for confirmation repeat the order back to them. Write the order immediately and have the referring doctor in the triage record and note the date, time, amount, etc, and sign the entry.

Special conditions

Patient overcrowding

Patient overcrowding is a pandemic ED problem. Incidents of overcrowding can jeopardise care practices, patient and staff safety and the overall functioning of the ED.[77,79,84] Within Australasia, overcrowding is commonly blamed on the increase in non-urgent cases; however, this is often not the case. Instead, incidents of ED overcrowding are largely the result of declining hospital bed numbers. This has meant that admitted patients are waiting longer in the ED for a ward bed to become available.[77,79,85] Overcrowding has specific implications for the triage nurse in that their ability to allocate an appropriate clinical area to match the patient's need is significantly reduced. Hence, for triage nurses overcrowding usually results in patients with higher urgency conditions being placed in the waiting room until an appropriate bed (and monitoring) becomes available.

Overcrowding poses a great challenge to triage nurses, as the risk of deterioration for patients in the waiting room escalates. To ensure patient safety during episodes of ED overcrowding, strategies need to be in place that enable regular patient reassessment, communication and evaluation to occur. Additional nursing resources may need to be implemented to enable more-frequent patient re-evaluations to take place until an appropriate clinical area becomes available.

During periods of overcrowding, aggression and troubling behaviour are a common experience for the triage nurse. In this situation, the triage nurse needs to undertake a risk assessment to maintain or restore a safe triage environment for staff, patients, families and/or carers.

> **PRACTICE TIP**
>
> Maintaining or restoring a safe environment can often be achieved by the triage nurse's ability to implement aggression minimisation strategies.[86,87]

Overcrowding impacts heavily on the role of the triage nurse because waiting rooms are often overflowing with acute patients awaiting a bed.[88] In these instances, frequent reassessment is required to minimise the risk of patient deterioration within the waiting room. To date, while EDs may have dedicated nurse–patient ratios for bed areas, the waiting room has never been included in workforce planning. As a result triage nurses may need to seek assistance to better ensure the safety of and early identification of deterioration for those waiting. For ED staff and patient safety, the following hospital resources and equipment should be viewed as standard. Security personnel should be located within the ED to ensure a timely and active security presence and the resolution of troubling behaviour. The triage and clerical areas should have access to direct telephone lines to police and security. Other security features to be considered include personal staff mobile duress alarms, metal detectors and camera surveillance equipment. All ED staff should be required to undertake educational courses in aggression minimisation.[89]

National Emergency Target

Within Australian EDs the introduction of the Australian National Emergency Access Targets (NEAT) have created added pressure on the triage nurse.[90] This performance indicator was introduced to ensure patients presenting to ED are managed and discharged within 4 hours.[90] In part the NEAT was introduced to drive service delivery and reduce overcrowded situations, commonly the result of ED processing patterns and/or hospital admission delays. NEAT is measured from the time of triage (first clinician assessment) to ED discharge. While NEAT is a hospital issue, meeting this performance target should assist to reduce the number of patients within the ED. In meeting this target, the triage role is critical as NEAT commences from the first patient contact experience. First contact in the ED should always be with the triage nurse to optimise patient safety outcomes. Therefore, triage assessments should be undertaken as soon as the person presents to an ED.

Further research is needed to explore the impact of the NEAT policy on the triage role, activities and function. To date there is little evidence to determine whether the intent of the role will remain as relevant, the same or change as a result of this national policy.

Telephone triage

Telephone triage has evolved alongside emergency triage to better manage ED workload. During the late 1990s, the strategy was widely implemented to reduce ED patient over-crowding.[91] The purpose of telephone triage is to reduce the burden on GPs and acute services, particularly after hours, by screening and referring patients to appropriate services.[92–94] In the UK, a national telephone triage centre independent of EDs was initiated, a model that is increasingly being adopted throughout Australasia.[93]

Internationally, telephone triage and advice services have been highly effective in reducing ED utilisation.[95–97] Within the context of healthcare reform, there was already widespread acceptance of nurses providing autonomous, safe, competent and often more-timely care for a range of patient conditions. There was broad engagement with medical staff in the development of agreed protocols and computer software triage programs.[91] Incentives for those calling included the additional provision of screening, health information, secondary urgency triage and a residential care online care service. Telephone triage advice centres enabled quicker access to health information and advice, reducing the need to attend an ED.[95,98–100] Utilisation was better when one contact number was available, and service was timely, national, free and well advertised.

Telephone triage has its own unique difficulties when compared with ED triage. These difficulties include the lack of visual cues for assessment and patient compliance. Given legal and patient safety concerns, many Australian EDs have stopped providing telephone triage. As a result, governments have developed triage centres with specific telephone triage guidelines. Throughout Australasia, telephone triage systems are able to refer patients to local practitioners, EDs or community services.

To date, Australasia has adult and paediatric telephone triage systems. The telephone advice call centres established include PlunketLine (1994) and Healthline (2005) in New Zealand; and in Australia Kidsnet (1997), HealthDirect (1999) and HealthConnect (2000), and Nurse on Call (Victoria, 2006). Bolton et al[92] evaluated HealthConnect and identified that the service received over 12,000 calls, of which about 50% were managed without referral; HealthConnect has since been discontinued. The demand for Kidsnet in NSW increased from 18,327 in 1997–98 to 22,844 in 2001–02, with an average of 1669 callers per month. Most callers were reassured and were referred for a next-day GP appointment.[101] By 2009, Nurse on Call had received its one millionth caller.[102]

In Western Australia in 1999, HealthDirect commenced with experienced nurses to manage telephone calls and provide a range of services, from screening, health information, secondary-urgency triage and a residential care online care service. In July 2007, HealthDirect became part of the National Health Call Centre Network (NHCCN), a nationwide system operating from a single telephone number. A review of the Residential Care Line (part of the service) identified a reduction of ED activity by 15.5%. Patients were redirected to their local GP rather than calling an ambulance. The review noted that service activity had increased by 113% compared with previous results in 2007.[47] New Zealand's equivalent is PlunketLine, which also provides expert advice to healthcare workers, parents and caregivers.[103] PlunketLine is now incorporated into HealthLine, the free 24-hour 7-day-a-week national service and has received over a million calls.[52,104] Evaluation of Healthline reported high consumer satisfaction, a good safety record and reduced demand on health services.

Despite legal and safety concerns, the implementation of telephone triage systems provides evidence of significant positive outcomes for EDs, GPs and consumers.

SUMMARY

Triage nurses must decide within a few minutes the patient's medical urgency, allocate appropriate resources and initiate or direct interventions according to patient need. The development of triage nursing has led to improved patient outcomes and the delivery of safer emergency care. Standardised triage guidelines have assisted the triage nurse to discriminate between more- and less-urgent conditions. In this way, the ATS has contributed towards safer, consistent and more-equitable triage practices.

The increasing complexity and acuity of patient presentations and extended scope of triage practice requires the emergency nurse to be highly experienced and have advanced knowledge, communication and problem-solving skills. The nurse also requires prior understanding of the gatekeeping and time-keeping processes embedded within the triage role. There is overwhelming evidence that triage nurses bring about a quality difference in ED services and patient outcomes. However, it remains unclear how new models of care may impact, change or influence the role of triage nursing in the future.

CASE STUDY

A 36-year-old Caucasian male presents to the ED at 8.30 am with fever, cough, dyspnoea and chest pain over 3 days. He is able to walk to the triage desk unassisted. He was on his way to work but felt too unwell and so decided to come to the ED.

PRACTICE TIP

The aim of the triage assessment is to gain relevant information quickly and efficiently. Your attitude is important and may well govern what type of reply you receive. Always speak with and observe the client yourself.

At triage you begin your assessment and discover:

- he is alert, lucid and well perfused with no evidence of respiratory distress or cyanosis.

- he has no accessory muscle usage and is able to comfortably talk in full sentences.

- his chest pain was pleuritic and worse with coughing (pain 4 out of 10), he had a productive cough with green sputum and felt mildly short of breath only on exertion. He had not sought any medical intervention for the presenting condition.

- on auscultation, he had reduced breath sounds at the right lung base with some coarse inspiratory crepitations and bronchial breathing. He had increased vocal resonance at the right lung base but there was no pleural rub.
- his vital signs were: temperature 38.4°C, Heart rate/min 90; BP 125/75; Respiratory rate/min 22 and oxygen saturation 98%.

Questions

1. What information and observations would you obtain?
2. What potential life-threatening risks are there for this patient?
3. What triage category would you allocate to this patient?
4. Where would you allocate this patient within the ED?
5. What fast-track activities or additional interventions could you provide or initiate at triage?
6. What would have to be different in this scenario for you to change your decision-making?
7. What do you think is the likely diagnosis of this patient?
8. How do you ensure the safety of patients in waiting areas?

 Answers to Case Study Questions can be found on evolve
http://evolve.emergencytrauma.curtis

USEFUL WEBSITES

Australasian College for Emergency Medicine: information relating to emergency medicine policy, education and workforce issues, www.acem.org.au

Bush Crisis Line: information relating to healthcare choices and services for consumers in rural and remote areas, https://crana.org.au/

College of Emergency Nursing Australasia: information relating to emergency medicine policy, education and workforce issues, www.cena.org.au

Commonwealth Department of Health and Ageing: government information publications relating to policy, education and workforce issues, https://www.health.gov.au/internet/main/publishing.nsf/Content/publications-Ageing

New Zealand government information publications relating to policy, education and workforce issues, https://www.health.govt.nz/publications/health?f[0]=im_field_category%3A41

Council of Remote Area Nurses of Australia (including rural triage): policy, education and workforce information relating to nursing and midwifery in rural and remote areas, https://crana.org.au/

Australian Emergency Management: information relating to emergency disaster response at a national policy, education and workforce level, www.em.gov.au/Pages/default.aspx FLEC courses: information for health workers regarding first-line emergency care in rural and remote areas, https://crana.org.au/education

Ministry of Civil Defence and Emergency Management (New Zealand): government information relating to emergency disaster response at a national level, www.civildefence.govt.nz/

PRIME course: information relating to emergency education, www.stjohn.org.nz/What-we-do/Community-programmes/Partnered-programmes/PRIME/

REFERENCES

1. Mitchell G. A brief history of triage. Disaster Medicine and Public Health Preparedness 2008;2:S4–7.
2. Hughes G. Giving emergency advice over the telephone: it can be done safely and consistently. New Zealand Medical Journal 2003;116:493.
3. Fry M. Triage nursing practice in Australian emergency departments 2002–2004: An ethnography [PhD]. University of Sydney; 2005.
4. Kennedy K, Aghababian R, Gans L, Lewis CP. Triage: technique and applications in decision making. Annals of Emergency Medicine 1996;28:136–44.
5. McKay-Ingalls J, Canton M. The emergency department of the future—the challenge is in changing how we operate! Journal of Emergency Nursing 1999;25:480–8.
6. Brentnall E. A history of triage in civilian hospitals in Australia. Emergency Medicine 1997;9:50–4.
7. Lahdet E, Suserud B, Jonnsson A, Lundberg L. Analysis of triage worldwide. Emergency Nursing Journal 2009;17:16–19.
8. Schull M, Morrison L, Vermeulen M, Redelmeier D. Emergency department overcrowding and ambulance transport delays for patients with chest pain. Canadian Medical Association Journal 2003;168:277–83.
9. Gerdtz M, Chu M, Collins M et al. Factors influencing consistency of triage using the Australasian Triage Scale: implications for guideline development. Emergency Medicine Australasia 2009;21:277–85.

10. Elder R, Neal C, Davis B, Almes E. Patient satisfaction with triage nursing in a rural hospital emergency department. Journal of Nursing Care Quality 2004;19:263–7.

11. Ducharme J, Tanabe P, Homel P et al. The influence of triage systems and triage scores on timeliness of ED analgesic administration. American Journal of Emergency Medicine 2008;26:867–73.

12. Australasian College for Emergency Medicine. Policy on the Australasian Triage Scale. Melbourne, 2013.

13. Jelinek G. Triage. Emergency Medicine Australasian 2008;20:196–8.

14. Hindle D. Health care funding in New South Wales: from health care needs to hospital outputs. Australian Health Review 2002;25: 40–71.

15. Fitzgerald G. The National Triage Scale. Emergency Medicine Australasia 1996;8:205–6.

16. Jelinek G, Little M. Inter-rater reliability of the National Triage Scale over 11,500 simulated occasions of triage. Annals of Emergency Medicine 1996;8:226–30.

17. ACEM. The Australasian Triage Scale. Emergency Medicine 2002;14:335–6.

18. NSW Health. Emergency Department System. Sydney: NSW Department of Health, 2008.

19. Travers D, Waller A, Bowling J, Flowers D, Tintinalli J. Five-level triage system more effective than three-level in Tertiary emergency department. Journal of Emergency Nursing 2002;28:395–400.

20. Gerdtz M. National development and validation of the Emergency Triage Education Kit (ETEK), Vol. 10. Commonwealth Department of Health and Ageing: Canberra, 2007.

21. District Health Board. DHB Hospital Benchmark Information. Wellington: New Zealand Ministry of Health, 2010.

22. Creaton A, Liew D, Knott J, Wright M. Interrater reliability of the Australasian Triage Scale for mental health patients. Emerg Med Australas 2008;20:468–74.

23. Westman J, Grafstein E. The interrater reliability of triage in an acute care ED setting. Journal of Emergency Nursing 2003;29:413.

24. Doherty S. Application of the National Triage Scale is not uniform. Australian Emergency Nursing Journal 1996;1:26.

25. Doherty S, Hore CT, Curran SW. Inpatient mortality as related to triage category in three New South Wales regional base hospitals. Emergency Medicine 2003;15:334–40.

26. Hollis G, Sprivulis P. Reliability of the National Triage Scale with changes in emergency department activity level. Emergency Medicine 1996;8:231–4.

27. Whitby S, Ieraci S, Johnson D et al. Analysis of the process of triage: The use and outcomes of the National Triage Scale. Sydney. In: Whitby S, Ieraci S, Johnson D et al. Commonwealth Ambulatory Care reform Package. Report to the Commonwealth Department of Health and Family Services; 1999.

28. Whitby S, Ieraci S, Johnson D, Mohsin M. Analysis of the process of triage: the use and outcomes of the National Triage Scale. Sydney: Commonwealth Ambulatory Care Reform, 1999; 1–117.

29. van der Wulp I, van Stel H. Adjusting weighted kappa for severity of mistriage decreases reported reliability of emergency department triage systems: a comparative study. Journal of Clinical Epidemiology 2009;62:1196–201.

30. Santos A, Freitas P, Martins H. Manchester triage system version II and resource utilisation in the emergency department. Emerg Med J 2014;31:148–52.

31. Durojaiye L, O'Meara M. A study of triage of paediatric patients in Australia. Emergency Medicine 2002;14:67–76.

32. Browne G, Gaudry P, Lam L. A triage observation scale improves the reliability of the National Triage Scale in children. Emergency Medicine 1997;9:283–8.

33. Wuerz R, Travers D, Gilboy N et al. Implementation and refinement of the Emergency Severity Index. Academic Emergency Medicine 2001;8:170–5.

34. Considine J, Ung S, Thomas S. Triage nurses' decisions using the National Triage Scale for Australian emergency departments. Accident & Emergency Nursing 2000;8:201–9.

35. Weeks WB, Wallace A. Rural–urban differences in primary care physicians' practice patterns, characteristics, and incomes. Journal of Rural Health 2008;24:161–70.

36. Mira M, Cooper C, Maandag A. Contrasts between metropolitan and rural general practice in the delivery of after-hours care. Australian Family Physician 1995;24:1064–7.

37. Tolhurst H, Ireland M, Dickinson J. Emergency and after-hours work performed in country hospitals. Medical Journal of Australia 1990;153:458–65.

38. Gunn I, Little A, Payne R. Effects of workload and analysis time on the cost of out-of-hours investigations. Annals of Clinical Biochemistry 1986;23:501–3.

39. Scott A, Simoens S, Heaney D et al. What does GP out of hours care cost? An analysis of different models of out of hours care in Scotland. Scottish Medical Journal 2004;49:61–6.

40. Kelly K. Report on health resource allocation in ARIA classified Very Remote communities. Outback Flyer 2004;61:14–17.

41. AIHW. Expenditure on health for Aboriginal and Torres Strait Islander people 2010–11. Canberra: Australian Institute of Health and Welfare, 2013 Health and welfare expenditure series no. 39.

42. New Zealand Ministry of Health. A Portrait of Health: Key results of the 2006/2007 New Zealand Health Survey. Wellington: NZ Ministry of Health, 2008.

43. New Zealand Ministry of Health. The health of New Zealand adults 2011/12. Auckland: New Zealand Government, 2013.

44. Yuginovich T. A Potted History of 19th-Century Remote-Area Nursing in Australia and, in Particular, Queensland. Australian Journal of Rural Health 2000;8:63–7.

45. Centre for Rural Health. The 2005 Rural Health Workforce Survey. Christchurch: Centre for Rural Health, 2005.

46. New Zealand Ministry of Health. Māori Providers: Primary Health Care delivered by doctors and nurses. Wellington: New Zealand Government, 2004.

47. Western Australian Department of Health. Healthdirect 2nd Quarterly Report 2008 January–March. WA Department of Health, 2008.

48. HealthDirect Australia. Annual Report: Business Highlights 2011–2012. Western Australia: HealthDirect Australia, 2012.

49. Carati C, Margelis G. Towards a National Strategy for Telehealth in Australia 2013–2018. Sydney: International Society for Telehealth and eHealth, 2012.

50. Smith J, Margolis S, Ayton J et al. Defining remote medical practice: A consensus viewpoint of medical practitioners working and teaching in remote practice. MJA 2008;188:159–61.

51. St George I, Cullen M, Gardiner L, Karabatsos G. Universal telenursing triage in Australia and New Zealand – A new primary health service. Australian Family Physician 2008;37.

52. New Zealand Ministry of Health. About Healthline. Wellington: New Zealand Government, 2013.

53. Hore T, Coster G, Bills J. Is the PRIME (Primary Response In Medical Emergencies) scheme acceptable to rural general practitioners in New Zealand? The New Zealand Medical Journal 2003;116.

54. St John. Primary Response in Medical Emergency—Operational Guidelines. Auckland: The Accident Compensation Corporation, 2008.

55. CRANAPlus. First Line Emergency Care Northern Territory: CRANAPlus, 2013.

56. Commonwealth Department of Health and Ageing. Rural Specialist Program. Canberra: Commonwealth Department of Health and Ageing, 2009.

57. Fry M, Stainton C. An educational framework for triage nursing based on gatekeeping, timekeeping and decision-making processes. Accident and Emergency Nursing 2005;13:214–19.

58. Acorn M. Nurses' triage assessment were affected by patients' behaviours and stories and their perceived credibility. Evidence Based Nursing 2009;12:61.

59. Commonwealth Department of Health and Ageing. Emergency Triage Education Kit. Canberra: Commonwealth of Australia, 2007.

60. Victorian Department of Health. Consistency of triage in Victoria's Emergency Department. Melbourne: Monash Institute, 2001.

61. Vatnoy T, Fossum M, Smith N, Slettebo S. Triage assessment of registered nurses in the emergency department. International Emergency Nursing 2013;21:89–96.

62. Cooper R, Schriger D, Flaherty H et al. Effects of vital signs on triage decisions. Annals of Emergency Medicine 2002;39:223–32.

63. Alcock K, Clancy M, Crouch R. Physiological observations of patients from A&E. Nurse Researcher 2002;16:33–7.

64. Salk E, Schriger D, Hubbell K, Schwartz B. Effects of visual cues, vital signs, and protocols on triage: a prospective randomized crossover trial. Annals of Emergency Medicine 1998;32:655–64.

65. Cone K, Murray R. Characteristics, insights, decision making, and preparation of ED triage nurses. Journal of Emergency Nursing 2002;28:401–6.

66. Jeffries D. Should triage nurses trust their intuition? Journal of emergency nursing: JEN: official publication of the Emergency Department Nurses Association 2008;34:86–8.

67. Commonwealth Department of Health and Ageing. Triage Education References. Canberra: Commonwealth of Australia, 2002.

68. Fry M, Ryan J, Alexander N. A prospective study of nurse initiated Panadeine Forte: expanding pain management in the ED. Accident & Emergency Nursing 2004;12:136–40.

69. Fry M. Triage nurses order X-rays for patients with isolated distal limb injuries: A 12 month ED study. Journal of Emergency Nursing 2001;27:17–22.

70. Fry M, Holdgate A. Nurse initiated intravenous morphine in the emergency department: efficacy, rate of adverse events and impact on time to analgesia. Emergency Medicine 2002;14:249–54.

71. Lindley-Jones M, Finlayson B. Triage nurse requested x rays—the results of a national survey. Journal of Accident and Emergency Medicine 2000;17:108–10.

72. Taylor D, Wolfe R, Cameron P. Complaints from emergency department patients largely result from the treatment and communication problems. Emergency Medicine 2002;14:43–9.

73. Fry M, McGregor C, Ruperto K et al. Nursing praxis, compassionate caring and interpersonal relations: an observational study Australasian Emergency Nursing Journal 2013;16:37–44.

74. Fry M, Gallagher R, Chenoweth L, Stein-Parbury J. Nurses' experiences and expectations of family and carers of older patients in the emergency department. International Emergency Nursing 2014;22:31–6.

75. Ekwall A. Acuity and anxiety from the patient's perspective in the emergency department. J Emerg Nurs 2013;39:534–8.

76. Gerdtz M. Scenario development for emergency triage education Kit (EDEK). Melbourne: Commonwealth Department of Health and Ageing, 2007.

77. Richardson D, Mountain D. Myths versus facts in emergency department overcrowding and hospital access block. Medical Journal of Australia 2009;190:369–74.

78. Fatovich D, Hughes G, McCarthy S. Access block: it's all about available beds. Medical Journal of Australia 2009;190:362–3.

79. Forero R, McCarthy S, Hillman K. Access block and emergency department overcrowding. Critical Care 2011;15:216–22.

80. Considine J, Payne R, Williamson S, Currey J. Expanding nurse initiated X-rays in emergency care using team-based learning and decision support. Australas Emerg Nurs J 2013;16:10–20.

81. CENA. Position Statement Triage Nurse. Victoria: College of Emergency Nursing Australasia, 2009.

82. Office of the Assistant Secretary for Preparedness and Reposnse. Primary and secondary survey. Washingtgon: U.S. Department of Health and Human Services, 2011.

83. ACEM. Guidelines for Implementation of the Australasian Triage Scale in Emergency Departments. Melbourne: ACEM, 2000.

84. Forero R, Hillman K. Access block and overcrowding: a literature review. vol 2009, 2008.

85. Cameron P, Joseph A, McCarthy S. Access block can be managed. Medical Journal of Australia 2009;190:364–8.

86. Angland S, Dowling M, Casey D. Nurses' perceptions of the factors which cause violence and aggression in the emergency departments: a qualitative study. International Emergency Nursing 2013; available on-line accessed 7 October 2013.

87. Rippon J. Aggression and violence in health care professions. Journal of Advanced Nursing 2000;31:452–60.

88. Fry M, Ruperto K, Jarrett K et al. Managing the wait: clinical initiative nurses' perceptions of an extended practice role. Australasian Emergency Nursing Journal 2013;15:202–10.

89. Gerdtz M, Daniel C, Dearie V et al. The outcome of a rapid training program on nurses' attitudes regarding the prevention of aggression in emergency departments: a multi-site evaluation. International Journal of Nursing Studies 2013;50:1434–45.

90. COAG Reform Council. National Partnership Agreement on Hospital and Health Workforce Reform. Canberra: Council of Australian Governments (COAG), 2012.

91. Breslin E, Dennison J. The development of telephone triage: historical, professional and personal perspectives. Journal of Orthopaedic Nursing 2002;6:191–7.

92. Bolton P, Gannon S, Aro D. HealthConnect: a trial of an after-hours telephone triage service. Australian Health Review 2002;25:95–103.

93. Boardman J, Steele C. NHS Direct — a telephone helpline for England and Wales Psychiatric Bulletin 2002;26:42–4.

94. New T. Safety and effectiveness of nurse telephone consultation in out of hours primary care: randomised control trial. Nurse Researcher 2000;14:32–9.

95. Giesen P, Ferwerda R, Tijssen R et al. Safety of telephone triage in general practitioner cooperatives: do triage nurses correctly estimate urgency? Quality & Safety in Health Care 2007;16:181–4.

96. Dunt D, Wilson R, Day S, Kelaher M, Gurrin L. Impact of telephone triage on emergency after hours GP Medicare usage: a time-series analysis. Australia and New Zealand Health Policy 2007;4:21.

97. Richards A, Meakins J, Tawfik J et al. Nurse telephone triage for same day appointments in general practice: multiple interrupted time series trial of effect on workload. British Medical Journal 2002;325:1–6.

98. Raftery J. Nurse telephone consultation for out-of-hours primary care can save money through reduced ER admissions, surgery attendance and GP home visits. Evidence-based Healthcare 2000;4:61.

99. Gerard K, Lattimer V, Surridge H et al. The introduction of integrated out-of-hours arrangements in England: a discrete choice experiment of public preferences for alternative models of care. Health Expectations 2006;9:60–9.

100. Lattimer V, George S, Thompson F et al. Safety and effectiveness of nurse telephone consultation in out of hours primary care: randomised controlled trial. The South Wiltshire Out of Hours Project (SWOOP) Group. British Medical Journal 1998;317:1054–9.

101. Hanson R, Exley B, Ngo P et al. Paediatric telephone triage and advice: the demand continues. Medical Journal of Australia 2004;180:333–5.

102. Ministry of Health. Nurse on Call NewsLetter. Melbourne: Victoria Government, 2009.

103. Scheme B. Health: Primary Care. Policy. Wellington: New Zealand Government, 2011;1.

104. St George I, Cullen M. The HealthLine pilot call centre in New Zealand. New Zealand Medical Journal 2001;114:429–30.

105. Maxwell D, McIntosh K, Pulver L, Easton K. Empiric management of Community Acquired Pneumonia in Australian emergency departments. Medical Journal of Australia 2005;183:520–4.

CHAPTER 14
PATIENT ASSESSMENT AND ESSENTIALS OF CARE

LUCY PATEL, BELINDA MUNROE AND KATE CURTIS

Essentials

- Patient assessment should always begin with DRSABCDE (Danger, Response, Send for help, Airway, Breathing, Circulation, Disability and Exposure). Once the patient is secure, a more focused assessment can be completed.
- If a patient deteriorates, then reassessment should always start again at DRSABCDE.
- Use an aid such as the SAMPLE mnemonic to ensure that all relevant history data is obtained.
- 'Red flags' become evident when taking the history, and when performing an assessment these should never be ignored.
- A set of vital signs comprises blood pressure, pulse, respiration rate, temperature and oxygen saturations.
- When performing a physical assessment, remember to inspect, auscultate, percuss and palpate.
- When handing over care of your patient, repeat your GCS score with the paramedic or nurse receiving the patient to maintain consistency.
- Use a structure at hand-over, such as IMIST-AMBO or ISBAR; this ensures that no vital information is forgotten. Double-check your documentation for errors.
- Reposition your patient every 2 hours and ensure they receive adequate fluid and nutrition while in your care.

INTRODUCTION

Assessment is the ability to observe and interpret any situation, thereby influencing any decisions emergency department (ED) nurses or paramedics make. It helps evaluate actions and practices and lies at the core of the professions. How well patients are cared for has a direct effect on their sense of wellbeing and recovery. This chapter also discusses the essential 'back to basic' aspects of nursing care.

Assessment enables ED nurses and paramedics to prioritise care. The triage nurse or first-responder initiates this, but, as every patient's condition has the potential to change, there is a need to recognise the importance of a detailed initial assessment, followed by the ability to recognise how often reassessment should take place. In EDs, access block now has an impact and the importance of reassessment has never been more emphasised.[1]

Different assessment models exist with their own distinct purpose. The triage assessment is brief with the aim to sort patients into order of urgency. The medical model focuses on the underlying cause of the patient's presenting signs and symptoms.[2] The primary survey ensures life-threatening conditions are identified and treated first.[3] Assessment models such as these ensure a structured evidence-based approach to assessment and is imperative to enhance the clinician's performance and optimise patient safety.[4,5]

ED nurses and paramedics make important clinical decisions every day and these decisions have an effect on the patient's healthcare and the actions of healthcare professionals. As care provision is becoming increasingly complex, ED nurses and paramedics have to rely on sound decision-making skills to maintain up-to-date care and positive outcomes.[6]

The assessment process

Assessment starts from the first moment you see your patient. This begins with the primary survey and collection of details about the patient's history, followed by a systematic assessment of relevant body regions and systems. Assessment findings inform the selection and prioritisation of interventions. Diagnostic and laboratory tests also contribute to developing a complete picture of the patient's condition.

The primary survey consists of DRSABCDE (**D**anger, **R**esponse, **S**end for help, **A**irway, **B**reathing, **C**irculation, **D**isability and **E**xposure). (See Box 14.1.) The patient environment should always be checked for danger before commencing patient assessment to ensure it is safe to approach the patient. Any foreseeable risks should be removed to prevent injury prior to commencing the assessment. A scan of the surroundings will inform you of any danger or hazards that need to be negotiated. These can include a patient who has collapsed in the waiting room bathroom and is lying in a pool of water, or at a motor vehicle collision (MVC) where traffic is still passing at speed. As a paramedic arriving on the

scene, assessment can also tell you about the mechanism of injury, how many casualties there are and what resources you may need. You will need to note the position of the casualties and any points of impact, as this is important information to include when handing over your patient. Once the scene has been sized up and any danger removed, then an initial patient assessment of ABCDE can take place. See Chapter 10 for a detailed discussion of scene assessment and management.

The Australian Resuscitation Council recommends the primary survey follows DRSABCD to preserve and restore life when resuscitating the unconscious patient.[3] The Advanced Trauma Life Support guidelines also teach the step called 'exposure', which involves the removal of the patient's clothing to expose and identify any immediate life-threatening injuries and ensure adequate temperature control is achieved.[7] Undressing and exposing all patients is necessary to enable a complete assessment, particularly once the patient has reached the ED where privacy may be maintained. Early measurement of temperature is important to identify hypothermia, hyperthermia and febrile illnesses in both trauma- and non-trauma-related presentations such as sepsis, which requires urgent identification and treatment to reduce morbidity and mortality.[8] See Chapter 15 for patient resuscitation and Chapter 44 for a detailed assessment of the major trauma patient.

During this phase, life-threatening problems are identified and interventions commenced if required. The clinician should ensure each step of the primary survey is complete and any life threatening conditions identified are treated first, before moving onto the next stage of assessment. If nothing imminently life-threatening is detected then a further, more-focused assessment can take place.[3] It is important to have a systematic approach to this assessment to ensure that important information is not missed, particularly when there is uncertainty around the patient's underlying problem.[9]

HIRAID: an emergency nursing assessment framework

The five-step emergency nursing assessment framework HIRAID as adapted from Curtis et al[9] can ensure that a systematic approach is taken when performing an initial nursing assessment.[10] The five steps of the HIRAID assessment process are:

- **H**istory
- **I**dentify **R**ed flags
- **A**ssessment (clinical examination)
- **I**nterventions
- **D**iagnostics.[9,10]

Figure 14.1 illustrates the relationship between the steps. They do not necessarily occur in this order, as in reality they often happen simultaneously. While performing each step the clinician should continue to reassess and communicate.

The history is gained from the patient, relative, carer or significant other. It should include details about the chief complaint and the patient's individual health history, such as past medical history, medications and allergies. Identification of red flags involves recognition and response to clinical indicators of urgency identified during the steps of history and

---

BOX 14.1 Assessment of DRSABCDE

DR—Danger and Responsiveness	Check for danger and patient responsiveness
S—Send for help	If patient unresponsive send for help
A—Airway	Is the airway patent and protected?
	Is there any sign of obstruction?
	Is the cervical spine immobilised (for trauma patients)?
B—Breathing	Is the chest rising and falling?
	Is breathing adequate?
C—Circulation	Is the circulation sufficient to meet the needs of the patient?
	Is there ongoing bleeding?
D—Disability	What is the patient's neurological status? Assess using AVPU (**A**lert, responding to **V**oice, responding to **P**ain or **U**nresponsive) scale
	Check pupil response
	Don't forget the glucose
E—Exposure	Remove clothing and look for immediate threats to life or limb
	What is the patient's temperature?

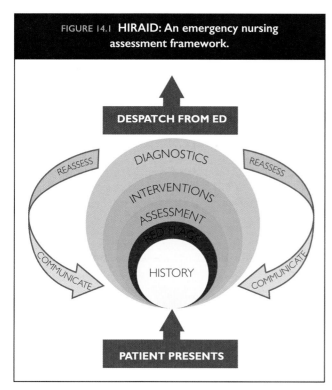

FIGURE 14.1 HIRAID: An emergency nursing assessment framework.

Adapted from Curtis et al.[10]

clinical examination. The ED nurse must respond to red flags and escalate care as required in a timely manner to prevent deterioration and optimise patient recovery. Assessment involves the clinical examination of the patient including skills such as inspection, auscultation, percussion and palpation. Smell can also give clues to certain medical conditions; for example the fruity smell of ketones on the breath of a patient with diabetic ketoacidosis. Smells may also be associated with certain types of infection. Interventions which may be required include giving first aid, applying oxygen and giving analgesia. Once the patient has arrived at an ED and life-threatening conditions are identified and treated, then diagnostic and laboratory testing can take place.

The triage nurse is initially responsible for identifying the chief complaint and the ideal room placement for the patient. If the patient is moved to a cubicle area, then this is where a more thorough and detailed assessment is performed. It ensures that any life-threatening illnesses or injuries not found initially are detected and treatment commenced. In many EDs, patients arriving by ambulance bypass triage and are delivered directly into a cubicle. Therefore it is vital that every nurse working in the ED has the ability to perform an assessment on a patient with a view to determining the chief complaint and not just record a set of vital signs which, taken in isolation, is often meaningless.

History

Taking a history requires collection of subjective data. This is the information that you gather from the patient, relative, carer or significant other. In the pre-hospital setting this may also be a witness to an accident. Developing and maintaining rapport are central to good communication and effective information gathering.[11] It is important to take some time at the beginning

of any assessment to explain who you are and what it is you are planning to do. Ask open-ended questions and let the patient speak for a minute or two without interruption, and the main problem and any concerns should become apparent. Examples of open-ended questions are: 'What's troubling you today?', 'Why have you come to hospital?' or 'Why did you call the ambulance?'. The ED nurse or paramedic should then be able to focus the assessment and gather required additional information, and allay any immediate anxieties. Asking open-ended questions of Indigenous people is very important, as they may not respond well to direct questioning. (See Ch 5 for further discussion of cultural considerations.) When the patient is acutely unwell, the amount of time spent asking open-ended questions should be limited so that the assessment can move promptly to the area of concern, allowing quick evaluation and management.[12]

It is important to also speak to family, carers or witnesses, as they may be able to add pertinent information that the patient considered insignificant or is unable to give due to altered mental state. If the patient has an altered level of consciousness, then the nurse or paramedic has to rely more heavily on other assessment skills, and once the patient has arrived in the ED the nurse may need to obtain old hospital records or contact the general practitioner if friends or relatives are not able to help or are uncontactable. However, such searches can be quite time-consuming. The ED nurse responsible for assessing the patient once they have been allocated to a treatment space should review the ambulance case sheet and triage form to ensure information has not been omitted during the hand-over process.

When taking a history, it is useful to develop a systematic approach to ensure that all the important questions are asked. A mnemonic for paramedics to use is SAMPLE (see Box 14.2). This is described by Elling and Elling[13] as being an effective way to structure history-taking in a pre-hospital environment. It should not delay transport to a facility and can be conducted while en route.

Once the patient has arrived at an ED, these details can be handed over to the accepting nurse. The patient's condition may have changed during transportation, so conducting a thorough assessment on arrival in a more controlled environment is important. See Box 14.3 for the questions that should be asked and the rationale for these.[11,12]

When assessing a patient's pain, the mnemonic PQRST can be very useful. It helps determine the **P**rovoking factors, **Q**uality, **R**adiation, **S**everity and **T**iming of the pain, and is a useful tool to assist in exploring all realms of the pain. (See Box 14.4 for full explanation of terms, and Ch 19 for

---

BOX 14.2 The SAMPLE mnemonic for history-taking

S	Signs and symptoms
A	Allergies
M	Medications
P	Pertinent past history
L	Last oral intake
E	Events leading up to the illness/injury

BOX 14.3 Pertinent questions to obtain history

History of presenting complaint
It is advisable to document this using the patient's own words. It is then very clear what the patient complained of on presentation, as symptoms can change.

Aggravating causes and relieving factors
What exacerbates or relieves the symptoms? This can provide clues as to the cause. For example, cough started after being commenced on new medication.

Duration of onset
You need to explore when the symptoms started, and whether they are continuous or intermittent. How long do they last?

Pain history
This can be explored using PQRST (see Box 14.4).

Medications taken to relieve symptoms and effectiveness
Some patients take multiple pain medications when pain is severe. If one type over another is more effective, this can also offer clues.

Past medical history
This is an essential component of your assessment. Patients may not realise the significance of prior problems and may not think them relevant. You should prompt your patient to divulge all past medical history, however irrelevant it may seem to them.

Current medications (including smoking, alcohol, illicit drugs)
It is important to elicit details of current medications as they may be linked to the problem. Not only prescription medications, but also over-the-counter and herbal or homeopathic ones.

Allergies
Information about allergies is important. However, many patients attribute adverse reactions or intolerance to allergies. Therefore the reaction to any drug should be noted; e.g. 'Patient states they are allergic to morphine but the reaction they suffered was nausea and vomiting. This is a common side effect and not a true allergy.'

Relevant family and social history
The patient's problem may be hereditary or genetic. Important diseases to ask about are cardiovascular, respiratory, cancer, diabetes, renal disease, allergies and mental health problems. Although family history is not diagnostic, it allows risk stratification. The social history should be tailored to the individual, but an understanding of the patient's social habits helps to determine further risk factors.

Tetanus status; last menstrual period
These are asked about only if relevant to the presenting problem.

BOX 14.4 Pain assessment using PQRST

P—Provoking factors	What factors precipitated the patient's discomfort?
	What were they doing at the onset of pain?
Q—Quality	Get the patient to describe the pain/ache/dullness.
	Ask them to tell you its characteristics: 'Describe the pain and how it feels.'
R—Region/radiation	Ask the patient to show you where the pain is and where it radiates to, if applicable.
	Ask if there is pain anywhere else.
S—Severity	Get the patient to rate their pain/ache/dullness on a pain scale.
T—Time	How long has the patient had the pain; or, if it is gone, how long did it last?
	Does anything make it worse or better?

---

it is important not to make assumptions about the patient's clinical presentation until a comprehensive assessment is completed. For example, underlying cardiac pathology cannot be dismissed in the patient with pleuritic chest pain without conducting a thorough assessment. The pleuritic chest pain may be masking other symptoms, or the patient may have two clinical conditions.

PRACTICE TIP

When taking a history, it is useful to develop a systematic approach to ensure that all the important questions are asked.

Red flags

In determining the severity of the patient's illness and how urgent the need for intervention is, the ED nurse or paramedic relies on a combination of clinical signs and historical data. These may be actual or potential cues that indicate presence or risk of serious illness or injury including abnormal vital signs, a history of pre-existing illness or time-sensitive presentations (such as chest pain or the onset of acute neurological signs). These can be referred to as clinical or historical indicators of urgency, also termed 'red flags'. They can be identified when listening to the patient's history or conducting a clinical assessment. See Table 14.1 for examples. Each patient should be assessed using the 'worst first' approach, and no assumptions should be made until all high-morbidity and high-mortality conditions have been ruled out.[9]

PRACTICE TIP

Red flags can be found at any stage of the assessment process, when listening to the patient's history or conducting a clinical assessment.

---

discussion of pain management.) The information gathered while taking the history will guide the nurse or paramedic as to which body systems need to be examined, as well as the extent of the investigation.[14] However, during history taking

TABLE 14.1 Historical and clinical red flags		
PRESENTING COMPLAINT	HISTORICAL RED FLAG	CLINICAL RED FLAG
Chest pain	History of ischaemic heart disease	Abnormal ECG
	Prolonged chest pain	Pale and diaphoretic
	Diabetes or chronic renal failure	Abnormal vital signs
Abdominal pain	Recent abdominal surgery	Pregnancy
	Vascular disease	Rigid abdomen
	Haematemesis or malaena	Abnormal vital signs
Fever	Prolonged fever	Infected wound
	Recent surgery	Elevated white blood cell count
	Immunosuppresed	Abnormal vital signs
Vomiting	Elderly or paediatrics	Hypo/hyperglycaemia
	History of diabetes	Haematemesis
	Pregnancy	Abnormal vital signs
Shortness of breath	Sudden onset	Abnormal CXR
	History of COPD	Use of accessory muscles
	Productive cough	Abnormal vital signs

ECG: electrocardiogram; COPD: Chronic Obstructive Pulmonary Disease; CXR: Chest X-ray.

Assessment (clinical examination)

The next step of the assessment process is the clinical examination. It is advisable to use the ABCDE approach and reassess for potential or actual threats to the airway, breathing, circulation, disability (neurological status) and exposure before moving on to a focused assessment. If any of the ABCs are compromised, then interventions will need to be performed before moving on with the assessment. In airway management this could be as simple as performing a jaw thrust or chin lift (while maintaining cervical spine precautions), through to intubating the patient and securing the airway for transportation. If at any stage during the assessment the patient appears to deteriorate, you must return to ABC and reassess these again, stopping if any interventions are required and only moving forward once the patient is stable. A focused assessment can then be initiated.

Once life-threatening problems have been identified and stabilised the general survey of the patient and collection of vital signs should be performed. The examination sequence is then inspection, auscultation, percussion and palpation. A head-to-toe review of the relevant body regions and systems should follow.

General survey

Your general survey commences the moment you first see your patient. This may be as you approach them in their house or at the scene of an accident, or as they approach you at the triage window. Posture and gait should be noted. Listening to the patient speak will reveal clues to neurological and respiratory function. The overall appearance of the patient can also give clues to mood, altered conscious level and signs of pain and distress.[14,15]

> **PRACTICE TIP**
>
> The overall appearance of the patient can give clues to mood, altered conscious level and signs of pain and distress.[14,15]

Vital signs

A set of vital signs should be recorded, remembering that red flags may appear at any stage of the assessment process and there needs to be flexibility to move about the five-step framework.[9]

Stevenson[16] states that monitoring patients' observations and acting on abnormal results could potentially prevent admissions to intensive care and high-dependency units. This is supported by research into cardiopulmonary arrest in hospital, which has shown that 60% of cardiac arrests, deaths and unplanned admissions to intensive care had a detectable deterioration in vital signs.[17] Monitoring of vital signs, in addition to other objective data including neurological status, urine output and blood gas results, have been shown to assist in the early detection of deterioration and to prevent loss of life.[18] Taking vital signs and identifying deterioration are an essential part of the nurse's or paramedic's role, and they must know the normal limits and perform repeat observations to observe for trends. The frequency should be determined by patient condition and individual department protocols. There are times when seriously ill patients are not recognised because of the staff's busy, unpredictable workload. Their condition can quickly become critical.[19]

Taking observations or measuring vital signs is increasingly being seen as a task-orientated activity rather than the gathering of clinical information. This can pose a threat to patients, as there is the potential for observations to not be seen as a serious responsibility.[17] A set of vital signs is considered to consist of:

- blood pressure (BP)
- pulse (P)
- respirations (R)
- temperature (T) and
- oxygen saturations (SpO$_2$).

The challenge is in meeting patients for the first time and determining if the vital signs are within normal limits for them (see Table 14.2 for normal values). Once the patient has arrived in hospital, obtaining hospital records may assist with this. It should also be noted that having normal vital signs does not necessarily guarantee a stable physiological status. Examples of this include: failure to detect large blood losses in a fit healthy person, failure to identify serious illness in infants and inability to detect an inadequate plasma volume in burn injury patients or a patient taking beta-blockers who cannot mount a tachycardic response to correct hypotension. Therefore it should be remembered that although the vital signs may appear within normal limits, this may be due to compensatory mechanisms and/or may be masked by medications; the patient may in fact be compromised.[22]

PRACTICE TIP

Vital signs may appear within normal limits, however this may be due to compensatory mechanisms and/or may be masked by medications; the patient may in fact be compromised.[22]

Blood pressure

This assesses the efficiency of the circulatory system. Blood pressure (BP) measurement reflects: (1) the ability of the arteries to stretch; (2) the volume of the circulating blood; and (3) the amount of resistance the heart must overcome when it pumps blood.[23] The systolic pressure is the pressure within the arterial system when the ventricles contract. The diastolic pressure is the pressure within the arterial system when the ventricles relax and fill with blood. The pulse pressure is the difference between the two; a pulse pressure of between 30 and 50 mmHg is considered a normal range.

There are several factors that can influence BP, and these need to be taken into account. These include the patient's age, gender, fitness, emotional state and medications (see Box 14.5). It is important to remember that a fit, healthy person has compensatory mechanisms and may not display signs of depleted circulating volume until late.

Other factors to consider include BP cuff size and equipment. If the BP cuff is too large, then the result will be a false low reading. If the cuff is too small, the result will be falsely elevated. If a patient has poor peripheral circulation or cardiac dysrhythmias, then electronic BP machines become inaccurate and may not be able to record a reading at all. In this instance, and with any resuscitation or clinically unwell patient, a manual reading should be obtained. It is also good practice to double-check any high or low reading obtained from an electronic BP machine manually.

To obtain the most accurate BP reading, the patient should be seated, with back supported and both feet rested on the ground and have rested in this position for 5 minutes.[24] The arm should be supported at heart level as the position of the arm effects the pressure observed. For every 2.5 cm that the arm is above the level of the heart, the pressure reading will be 1 mmHg lower; similarly, if the arm is lower than the level of the heart the reading will be too high.[25] It may not always be possible to position the patient in a seated position, the ED nurse or paramedic should therefore consider the effects the position of the patient has on the blood pressure reading.

While most healthy patients will demonstrate little difference in their lying and standing blood pressure, a significant fall (20 mmHg) can occur in older people, patients with diabetes and those with symptoms suggestive of postural hypotension

TABLE 14.2 Normal values for blood pressure (BP), pulse (P) and respirations (R)[20,21]

AGE	SYSTOLIC BP*	P†	R‡
< 3 months	60–100	110–160	30–55
3–12 months	70–110	100–160	30–45
1–4 years	90–110	90–140	20–40
5–11 years	90–110	80–120	20–30
12–16 years	90–120	60–100	15–20
Adult (>16 years)	100–160	50–100	10–20

*mmHg
† beats per minute
‡ breaths per minute

BOX 14.5 Factors affecting blood pressure

Age
BP tends to rise with age—attributed to arteriosclerosis, a process whereby the arteries become rigid and lose elasticity, and atherosclerosis, a narrowing of the arteries caused by cholesterol deposits.

Gender
Women generally have lower BP than men of a similar age.

Fitness
Athletes tend to have BP in the lower ranges.

Emotional state
Strong emotions and pain can cause the BP to rise as a result of sympathetic nervous system stimulation.

Medications
Consider if the patient is taking antihypertensives. Also drugs such as nicotine, caffeine and cocaine tend to constrict arteries and raise BP.

such as dizziness, syncope and falls on changing position.[26] A lying and standing blood pressure should be recorded for these groups. First, the patient should have been lying down for 5 minutes, and have their arm supported at heart level. Record the blood pressure and then get the patient to stand, keeping the cuff in place. Allow the patient to stand for 3–5 minutes to allow for delayed orthostatic hypotension which usually occurs in the first 5 minutes of standing.[27] Support the arm at heart level and repeat the reading. If on standing the patient reports dizziness, faintness or lightheadedness, the procedure should be aborted for the safety reasons. For patients with a side affected by stroke, mastectomy or renal fistula, the BP should be taken on the opposite arm.[28] It is important to remove the BP cuff for all patients between readings to prevent injury from prolonged pressure in one area.

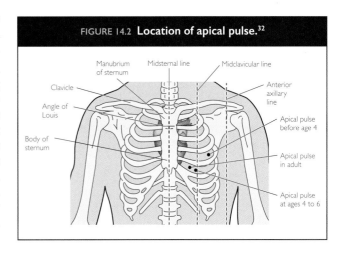

FIGURE 14.2 **Location of apical pulse.**[32]

PRACTICE TIP

Patients with diabetes and those with symptoms suggestive of postural hypotension such as dizziness, syncope and falls on changing position, should have a lying and standing blood pressure taken.

Pulse

There is more to a pulse than its rate. Its rhythm and character should also be noted. These are best detected by palpation rather than by electronic equipment. In healthy adults the normal pulse rate is between 50–100 beats/minute, but this is higher for children and babies. Tachycardia is defined as a pulse rate greater than 100 beats/minute while bradycardia is a pulse rate less than 50 beats/minute.[29] Factors which can affect the pulse rate need to be considered when obtaining the patient history. A slow pulse rate may be normal for a fit athlete, but it may also indicate a cardiac dysrhythmia, metabolic disturbance, hypothermia, hypoxia or neurological issue, or be caused by certain medications such as beta-blockers. A fast pulse rate can be triggered by emotion, exercise, drugs, infection/inflammation, cardiac dysrhythmias, hypovolaemia or haemorrhage and hypoxia.[29,30] A pulse may be described as bounding, normal, weak, thready or absent. A bounding pulse may indicate sepsis, carbon dioxide retention or liver failure, and a thready pulse is indicative of shock. In general the pulse is taken over the radial artery but in a patient in shock it may be difficult to assess the pulse at this site; the carotid or femoral artery can be used instead. In patients with atrial fibrillation, an apical measurement for 1 minute has been shown to be the most accurate. It is also recommended for monitoring the pulse in babies[31] (see Fig 14.2). In young children the brachial pulse is the preferred site.[29] If a patient is found to have an irregular pulse, cardiac monitoring should be considered (see Ch 36).

PRACTICE TIP

The rate, regularity and characteristic of the pulse should be assessed through palpation.

Respirations

Abnormal respiratory rate is a significant predictor of deterioration, cardiac arrest and/or need for admission to the intensive care unit (ICU).[33] The rate, depth, rhythm and effort of respiration should be recorded. A respiratory rate of less than 8 breaths per minute indicates severe respiratory depression.[34] It is recommended that respirations be counted for a full 60 seconds and for infants should be counted using a stethoscope.[31] The depth of respiration can be established by watching the person's chest rise and fall, and is best done at a distance so that the patient is not aware of what you are counting. It can be described as shallow, normal or deep. The chest wall should expand symmetrically. The rhythm of breathing should be regular. Normal effort of breathing should not display signs of tracheal tugging, nasal flaring, use of accessory muscles or signs of intercostal, substernal or suprasternal recession. It should be quiet with no audible sounds such as wheezes. Peak flow and spirometry can be measured as an indicator to lung function.

PRACTICE TIP

The depth of respiration can be established by watching the person's chest rise and fall, and is best done at a distance so that the patient is not aware of what you are counting.

Peak flow

Peak flow meters are relatively inexpensive hand-held devices that measure the peak expiratory flow rate (PEFR). To obtain a valid peak flow reading, the technique should be as good as possible. This includes getting the patient to stand (preferably) or to sit as upright as possible and to hold the peak flow meter horizontally to the mouth, keeping fingers free of the scale. The patient should be instructed to take in the biggest breath possible then blow out as quickly as possible, ensuring their lips are tightly sealed around the mouthpiece. Children under the age of 5 years cannot adequately use a peak flow meter, so PEFR is not recommended for this age group.[35]

Spirometry

Spirometry can be used to measure lung volumes and airflow limitations to diagnose diseases such as asthma and chronic obstructive pulmonary disease (COPD). It is often performed to monitor the patient's progress, before and after treatment, and to see if the patient's respiratory condition is improving or getting worse. It is a relatively easy measurement, but it does require effort and cooperation from the patient. If the patient is unable to talk due to laboured breathing, it is unlikely they will be able to perform the test and attempting it may increase respiratory fatigue. It is also essential that the healthcare professional taking the measurement is trained in the technique and able to recognise technically acceptable results and correct technique errors.[36]

Temperature

Temperature has been referred to as the forgotten vital sign, particularly in critical patient situations, yet is extremely important.[37] Temperature measurement is indicated in all patients to identify hypothermia, hyperthermia and other febrile illnesses.

- A normal temperature range is 36–37.5°C.
- Hypothermia is defined as a core temperature below 35°C.
- There are three grades of pyrexia:[38]
  - low grade (normal to 38°C) indicates an inflammatory response that may be due to a mild infection or allergy
  - moderate to high grade (38–40°C) could be due to an infection
  - hyperpyrexia (40°C plus) is caused by bacteraemia, damage to the hypothalamus, adverse drug reaction or high environmental temperatures.[38]

There are a variety of thermometers that can be used at various sites. The most common types of thermometer found are tympanic thermometers, digital electronic and single-use chemical-dot thermometers.

Oral temperature measurement devices are reported to be the most accurate out of the non-invasive thermometers in measuring core body temperatures, followed by temporal artery thermometers.[39]

Both digital electronic and single-use chemical dots can be used in the oral or axillary site. However, chemical thermometers have been found to be less precise than digital thermometers.[40] The single-use chemical-dot thermometer only has a range between 35.5 and 40.4°C, so in patients suspected of having a temperature outside this range an alternative thermometer should be used. Temperature strips, which are liquid-crystal strips applied to the forehead, have been found to be inaccurate and can miss fevers in children.

When taking an oral temperature, it is vital to ensure the thermometer is placed correctly—it needs to sit in the posterior sublingual pocket of the mouth. This method should not be used in children under the age of 5 years due to the difficulty they experience in holding the thermometer in the correct position. A digital electronic thermometer will beep when ready; a single-use chemical-dot thermometer should be left in place for 3 minutes.[41] Factors that can influence the reading are a respiratory rate of greater than 18 breaths/minute and eating, drinking or smoking prior to the reading being taken.[38,42]

Tympanic thermometers measure the body heat given off by the tympanic membrane. They are quick and easy to use, and in some studies it has been reported that they are as accurate as oral thermometers in adult patients.[43] However, the accuracy of tympanic thermometers can vary significantly.[40] The ear canal must be straightened by pulling the pinna slightly up and back in an adult. It can be inaccurate in people with a small ear canal, a build-up of cerumen, otitis media and incorrect placement. These should be taken into consideration when using this method.[38,42]

The axillary site is also considered similar to the oral site when measuring temperature in adults; however lack of precision may result in failure to detect low grade fevers in paediatric patients.[40]

Rectal temperatures are considered the 'gold standard' when an accurate core temperature is required. Due to its invasive nature, this tends to be only done on trauma or critically unwell patients when ongoing monitoring is required. The thermometer needs to be placed to a depth of 4 cm to obtain an accurate reading.[42] It is not recommended that temperatures in children be acquired rectally because of the risk of perforating the bowel.

It should be carefully noted on the patient's documentation which kind of thermometer and which site was used to record the temperature. It is not possible to accurately convert the temperature taken at one site to compare it with a temperature taken at a different site, with or without using a different kind of thermometer.[42] This is also an important consideration when the paramedic hands over a patient to the accepting nurse.

PRACTICE TIP

Rectal temperatures are considered the 'gold standard' when an accurate core temperature is required. However, due to its invasive nature it should not be performed in children and only used in adults who are critically unwell.

Oxygen saturations

Oxygen saturations (SpO_2) are measured using a pulse oximetry monitor, which detects a pulse in the peripheral circulation. Oxygen saturation readings tell the ED nurse or paramedic the amount of haemoglobin that is bound to oxygen or another substance, and is used as an adjunct to assessing respiratory function. However, the monitor does have limitations. The probe will not work through nail varnish, dirt or dried blood. Dysrhythmias or poor peripheral circulation may also cause low readings because of inadequate and irregular perfusion. Anaemic patients will have a normal SpO_2 reading, but may be hypoxic. The SpO_2 tells how much haemoglobin is saturated, but the patient may have insufficient haemoglobin to attain tissue perfusion. Following smoke or exhaust inhalation, SpO_2 readings may also be useless. Carbon monoxide has a greater affinity to haemoglobin than to oxygen, so saturation levels could be 99%—but of carbon monoxide, not oxygen. A blood gas should be performed in these patients to accurately measure the blood oxygen content and saturation levels. With elderly patients and infants, the probe can also cause pressure areas on the skin if left in one position for an extended period of time, so it is recommended to change and document probe placement regularly, and place a light source over nails.[44]

The SpO$_2$ tells how much haemoglobin is saturated, but the patient may have insufficient haemoglobin to attain tissue perfusion.

Inspection

It is important to look at the patient as a whole before undertaking a more focused assessment. Inspection commences when you first see the patient either at the scene or when receiving clinical hand-over in view of the patient. Questions to consider are: Does the patient appear unwell or in pain? Are they unkempt, inappropriately dressed, under- or overweight? Once a general view of the patient has been obtained, observations should become specific, focusing on the chief complaint and affected system. When inspecting as part of your focused assessment you are looking for discharge, skin integrity, swelling, redness and other abnormalities. You should also take note of any diaphoresis, and document pallor.

PRACTICE TIP

Inspection commences when you first see the patient, either at the scene or when receiving clinical hand-over in view of the patient.

Auscultation

Auscultation is the process of listening, usually with a stethoscope, to sounds produced by the movement of gas or liquid within the body. The heart, lungs and abdomen are the areas most often auscultated. The diaphragm of the stethoscope is used to hear high-pitched sounds such as bronchial sounds, and the bell is used for low-pitched sounds such as heart sounds. If too much pressure is applied with the bell, then it tightens the skin and acts as a diaphragm. It is important to auscultate before percussing or palpating as these techniques may change sounds that are heard. Discussions of normal and abnormal findings are found below in the section on head-to-toe assessment.

PRACTICE TIP

It is important to auscultate before percussing or palpating as these techniques may change sounds that are heard.

Percussion

Percussion is the technique of examining part of the body by tapping it with the fingertips and hearing the resultant vibratory sounds. The quality of the sound aids in determining the location, size and density of underlying structures. The sound can be described as flat, dull, resonant, tympanic or hyperresonant. See Table 14.3 for sound characteristics and examples of where they can be heard.

Palpation

Palpation is the process of examining parts of the body by careful feeling with the hands and fingertips. Light palpation is used for feeling the surface of the skin, structures that lie just beneath the skin, vibrations in the chest and for the pulsation of peripheral arteries. The examiner uses the fingertips, or the back or palm of one hand. When examining the abdomen, deep palpation may also be used to identify organ structures. This is performed by placing one hand on the other and using the top hand to apply pressure to depress the abdomen by 2.5 cm. The bottom hand remains relaxed. Palpation provides information about the temperature and moisture of the skin, the presence of tenderness, unusual vibrations, distension and the size, shape, consistency and mobility of organs or masses.

Analgesia should be administered if required before palpation is performed to provide comfort during examination. While many patients have concerns that the use of pain relief before seeing a doctor may mask important physical symptoms, the early provision of analgesics has been reported to have no effect on the accuracy of diagnosis[45] and should not be withheld.

PRACTICE TIP

Analgesia should be administered before palpation is performed to provide comfort during physical examination.

Head-to-toe assessment

In the ED and pre-hospital setting, the history taken will assist you in determining which systems you should review. For a more indepth review of trauma patient assessment using the primary and secondary survey, refer to Chapter 44.

HEENT (Head, Ears, Eyes, Nose and Throat)

Inspection of the external surfaces of the head will reveal the presence of discharge, redness, abrasions, contusions and bleeding. Palpation can be performed to feel for any unusual lumps or bumps at the same time.

TABLE 14.3 Percussion sounds			
SOUND	INTENSITY	QUALITY	COMMON LOCATION
Flat	Soft	Muted	Muscle, bone
Dull	Medium	Thud-like	Liver, heart, full bladder
Resonant	Loud	Hollow	Normal lung
Tympanic	Loud	Cavernous	Intestine filled with air
Hyperresonant	Very loud	Booming	Emphysematous lung

Inspect the face for asymmetry or swelling, as abnormalities could indicate facial nerve problems, or an allergic reaction. Palpation will reveal step-offs, deformity and tenderness. (See Ch 46.)

Ears are inspected for discharge, foreign bodies, deformities and lumps. If infection is suspected, the tympanic membrane (TM) and external auditory canal are viewed with an auroscope. The pinna is pulled up and back to straighten the ear canal in an adult, and down and back in a child. The TM should appear pearly-grey; redness is a sign of infection. In head injury, blood may be seen in the canal or behind the TM.

Common presentations for eyes include foreign bodies, infection and trauma. The standard examination for eyes is to perform visual acuity using a Snellen chart. If the patient wears glasses for reading, then these should be worn during testing if available; otherwise, the use of a pinhole is advised. The smallest line the patient can read with each eye individually and then together is noted. Acuity is written as a fraction, with the numerator indicating the distance from the chart (usually 6 m, but a 3 m modified chart can also be used) and the denominator describing the distance at which a person with normal vision could read the line. Therefore, 6/6 is a normal finding.[37] The eye should be examined for obvious foreign bodies. Inflammation, pain, discharge, tearing and changes in appearance should be noted. Further eye assessment is discussed in Chapter 33.

The mouth can offer several clues as to the wellbeing of the patient. Assess the tongue for dryness and colour. A dry tongue can mean dehydration. Do the gums show evidence of bleeding or swelling? If the patient complains of a sore throat, check for swelling, redness and ulceration.

Neurological examination

Assessing a patient's level of consciousness is an essential component of a neurological examination, which is usually performed alongside an assessment of pupil size and reaction, vital signs and focal neurological signs in the limbs.[46] In the pre-hospital setting and at triage, the AVPU scale is often used when assessing disability to quickly determine a patient's level of consciousness. It crudely measures response: are they Alert, responding to Voice, responding to Pain or Unresponsive? This should be followed up with a formal assessment of the patient's score on the Glasgow Coma Scale (see below).

Glasgow Coma Scale

When performing a more focused assessment, a neurological observation chart incorporating a Glasgow Coma Scale (GCS) is used. The GCS was first described in the early 1970s as an objective and reliable measure of conscious state in patients with head injury.[47–49] The GCS is an internationally accepted measure of conscious state in victims with head trauma[50–52] and is now used extensively in non-trauma populations.[50,52,53]

The GCS evaluates three key categories of behaviour that most closely reflect activity in the higher centres of the brain: eye opening, verbal response and motor response. These behaviours enable us to determine whether the patient has cerebral dysfunction.[54] There are separate scoring criteria for adults, children and babies, and the appropriate chart should be selected. The GCS evaluates each of these parameters by allocating a numerical score (see Tables 14.4 and 14.5). The scores for each parameter are then added up to give a total out

TABLE 14.4 Glasgow Coma Scale[47]

	SCORE
Eye opening	
Spontaneously	4
To verbal stimulus	3
To painful stimulus	2
None	1
Verbal response	
Orientated	5
Confused	4
Inappropriate words	3
Incomprehensible sounds	2
None	1
Motor response	
Obeys command	6
Localises to pain	5
Flexion—withdrawal	4
Flexion—abnormal	3
Extension	2
None	1

of 15.[48] Because the lowest number that can be given for each part of the assessment is 1, the lowest score that can be given is a GCS of 3. 'Coma' is arbitrarily defined as a GCS score of <8, and a GCS score ≤8 has been used to indicate the need for endotracheal intubation.[50,52,53]

Although widely used in emergency care, research has shown variability in the reliability of the GCS,[49,51,52,56] making consistency of its application an important aspect of the nursing management of patients with a neurological emergency.[51] It is best if the same nurse or paramedic does the assessment each time so that if there is a drop in score it can be attributed to the patient and not the evaluator. At change of shift or transfer of the patient, the nurse escort or paramedic and receiving nurses should perform the evaluation together in order to avoid misinterpretation and to ensure continuity. Sleeping patients must be woken before commencing the evaluation. A deterioration of one point in the 'motor response' or one point in the 'verbal response' or an overall deterioration of two points is clinically significant and must be reported to medical staff.[46,57]

The Paediatric Glasgow Coma Scale is a modification of the GCS. Assessment of conscious state in infants and young children is difficult due to developmental issues and lack of verbal response in young children.[47] Well children may have decreased responses because of fear, and crying may be misinterpreted as a normal response in the context of significant

TABLE 14.5 Paediatric Glasgow Coma Scale[55]

	SCORE
Eye opening	
Spontaneously	4
To speech	3
To pain	2
None	1
Verbal response	
Coos, babbles	5
Irritable, cries	4
Cries to pain	3
Moans to pain	2
None	1
Motor response	
Normal spontaneous movement	6
Withdraws to touch	5
Withdraws to pain	4
Abnormal flexion	3
Abnormal extension	2
None	1

neurological pathology.[47] If using the adult GCS, it is expected that a child will have a reduced score. Refer to Chapter 36 for further details.

Conducting the GCS

Assessment of eye opening tests the function of the arousal mechanisms in the brain stem. There are four possible responses when assessing eye opening: spontaneous, to voice, to pain and none. If the patient is unable to open their eyes due to paralysis, this should be documented as a 'P', and if the patient's eye is swollen shut an 'S' should be documented.[51]

Verbal response may be assessed as: orientated (5), confused (4), inappropriate (3), incomprehensible (2) and no response (1). To be assessed as orientated, the patient must *correctly* tell the nurse their name, location, day, month and year.[51] Do not assume that a patient is orientated because they are conversing with you in a normal manner; they need to be able to correctly answer the above questions to be assessed as orientated. If verbal response is altered by other processes, for example dysphasia, aphasia or facial fractures, this should be documented; and if the patient is intubated, a 'T' should be documented.[51]

Motor response may be assessed as: obeys command (6), localises to pain (5), normal flexion/withdraws from pain (4), abnormal flexion to pain (3), extension to pain (2) and no response (1). Although responses of all limbs should be documented as part of neurological observations, only the *best* response counts towards GCS.[51] To be assessed as 'obeys

commands', the patient needs to squeeze *and let go* of the nurse's hands on command. The nurse should take care not to place their hands into the patient's hands: this may elicit a reflex response that may be misinterpreted as obeying command. If the patient is paralysed, a 'P' should be recorded.[51]

There are two types of painful stimuli: central and peripheral painful stimuli. Use caution when applying stimuli and do not cause injury such as bruising. It is recommended that when eliciting a response using pain that supraorbital pressure be used, but this carries a risk of damage to the eye, so should be used with caution and not if facial fractures are suspected. Other recommended methods include jaw margin pressure (the flat of the thumb is applied to the corner of the maxillary and mandibular junction and pressure is increasingly applied for up to 60 seconds), squeezing the trapezius muscle or applying pressure to the earlobe.[56]

Assessing pupils is not necessarily effective in the sedated or paralysed patient; however, any changes in pupil reaction, shape or size are a late sign of raised intracranial pressure. Very small pupils may be a result of opiates or barbiturate use. Each limb should be assessed. A peripheral painful stimulus needs to be applied if the patient does not appear to be able to voluntarily move the limb. This can be done by applying pressure to the nail bed of a patient's finger. Bilateral responses should be assessed. A more detailed assessment of the patient with altered consciousness is discussed in Chapter 23.

PRACTICE TIP

When recording the GCS in your documentation—note what the patient scored for each response being tested, i.e. eye opening, motor response and verbal response.

Cervical spine and neck

Examine the external neck for swelling and symmetry. Both the front and the back should be inspected for injuries. Look for enlargement of the parotid or submandibular glands and note any visible lymph glands. Palpate for lumps or enlarged lymph nodes. All trauma patients should be presumed to have a cervical spine injury until proven otherwise; clearance of the cervical spine is discussed in Chapter 49.

PRACTICE TIP

All trauma patients should be presumed to have a cervical spine injury until proven otherwise.

Thorax

When examining the thorax, both the respiratory and the cardiovascular systems will be assessed. The respiratory assessment focuses on the function of the respiratory system to exchange oxygen and carbon dioxide in the lungs and its role in regulation of the acid–base balance.

Start by looking for signs of respiratory distress such as tachy/bradypnoea, dyspnoea, nasal flaring, use of accessory muscles and cyanosis. Patient's speech, change in voice and drooling are also important signs. Examine the hands for clubbing indicative of chronic illness such as bronchiectasis, endocarditis and empyema. Observe for evidence of respiratory failure, for example, hypoxia (central cyanosis), or hypercarbia (drowsiness, confusion, warm hands, bounding pulse, dilated veins and a coarse tremor). Observe the pattern of breathing—see Table 14.6.

Inspect the shape of the chest, and look for deformities or asymmetry. The posterior and anterior surfaces should both be inspected, most easily done with the patient sitting on the edge of the bed. Note the position of the trachea and watch for unequal movement of the chest. This is more easily ascertained by placing both hands on the chest wall and feeling for movement. Palpation of the chest should identify any tender areas or crepitus. The clavicles, sternum, ribs, spine and shoulder blades should be palpated for any abnormalities and to determine if there are any factors that will restrict the patient's ability to breathe.[14] Respiratory excursion (thoracic expansion) should be measured. This is best assessed by standing behind the seated patient and placing the thumbs next to each other along the spinal processes at the level of the tenth rib. As the patient breathes in, the thumbs will separate. You should watch for a loss of symmetry, absence or delay in movement. These could indicate complete or partial obstruction of the airway, or underlying lung or diaphragmatic dysfunction on the affected side.[58]

Percuss the chest bilaterally for resonance. Dullness or hyperresonance indicates an abnormality. Dullness to the anterior lower lung fields is not conclusive, as the heart is on the left side and the liver on the right.[14] Then auscultate the chest. It is recommended that the patient cough first to remove sputum that could create adventitious sounds.

Use the sequence shown in Figure 14.3 and always compare one side with the other. Listen for normal breath sounds first, summarised in Table 14.7, then listen for added sounds (Table 14.8) and note if they are inspiratory or expiratory. Inspect any sputum produced for colour, consistency, quantity and presence of blood. Figure 14.4 summarises the clinical findings for certain respiratory pathologies. See Chapter 21 for a more detailed description of respiratory assessment.

The purpose of examining the cardiovascular system is to assess the function of the heart as a pump and of the arteries and veins throughout the body in transporting oxygen and nutrients to the tissues and in transporting waste products and carbon dioxide from the tissues.[15] Refer to Chapter 22 for the anatomy and physiology of these processes.

Sit the patient at 45° and observe the jugular veins. Distension is suggestive of cardiac failure. Auscultate over the main areas of the heart (see Fig 14.5), listening for normal heart sounds followed by added sounds and then murmurs. Normal heart sounds consist of two distinct parts. The first, named S1, is due to the mitral and tricuspid valves closing at the start of ventricular contraction or systole. It is best heard over the mitral and tricuspid areas (Fig 14.5). The second sound, S2,

TABLE 14.6 Patterns of breathing

NAME	PATTERN OF RESPIRATION	AETIOLOGY
Eupnoea	Normal respiration	
Tachypnoea	Rapid respiration > 24 breaths/minute	Fever, pneumonia, pleuritic chest pain
Bradypnoea	Slow and regular	Drug intoxication, tumour
Cheyne-Stokes	Hyperventilation alternating with apnoea	Left ventricular failure, raised intracranial pressure, high altitude
Biot's or ataxic	Irregular in depth and rate, with periods of apnoea	Neurological disorders/disease
Kussmaul	Deep, rapid respiration	Metabolic acidosis
Pursed-lip breathing	Expiration against partially closed lips	Chronic obstructive pulmonary disease

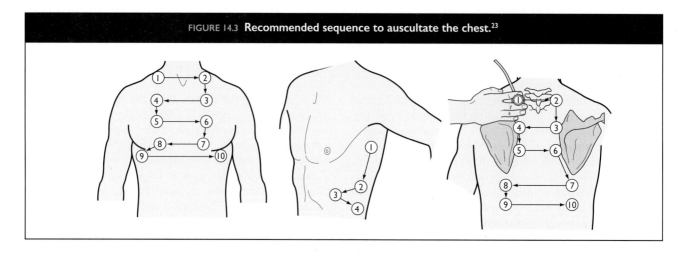

FIGURE 14.3 **Recommended sequence to auscultate the chest.**[23]

TABLE 14.7 Normal breath sounds	
SOUND	LOCATION
Vesicular	Lung tissue
Bronchovesicular	Near the bronchi
Bronchial	Lower part of trachea
Tracheal	Upper part of trachea

is the closing of the aortic and pulmonary valves at the end of systole. It is best heard over the aortic and pulmonary areas (Fig 14.5).

Added sounds are S3 and S4. S3 is the rapid ventricular filling as soon as the mitral and tricuspid valves open. It is common in children and young adults, but in the older adult is a sign of left ventricular failure, a fibrosed ventricle or constrictive pericarditis. S4 is an atrial contraction (also known as atrial kick) which induces ventricular filling towards the end of diastole. It may be normal in middle age, but in an older adult suspect hypertensive cardiovascular disease, coronary artery disease, aortic stenosis, myocardial ischaemia, infarction and congestive heart failure.[15]

Murmurs are produced by turbulent blood flow. Turbulence occurs when there is high blood flow through a normal valve or normal blood flow through an abnormal valve or into a dilated chamber. It is also caused by regurgitation of blood through a leaking valve. A pericardial friction rub is a high-pitched noise heard most loudly in systole and is due to inflammation of the pericardial sac. Identifying abnormal heart sounds is a skill that is generally mastered after the practioner becomes proficient at distinguishing between S1 and S2.[23]

Abdomen

The abdomen can be divided into four quadrants (see Fig 14.6). It is useful to consider this when examining the abdomen, as the area of pain or injury can give clues to the cause and help give consideration to which structures may have been injured in a trauma patient.

The patient is best examined while lying flat with one pillow under the head and knees slightly bent. This allows the abdomen to become as relaxed as possible. Inspect the abdomen for scars, bruising, distension, symmetry, pulsation and masses. Auscultate over each of the four quadrants. It is important to listen before touching, as palpating can alter the frequency of bowel sounds. Listen for 10–15 seconds, but for up to 7 minutes if sounds are difficult to hear.[59] Normal bowel sounds occur every 5–20 seconds. Hyperactive sounds indicate increased peristalsis. They have a loud tinkling sound and can indicate diarrhoea or an early bowel obstruction. Hypoactive sounds occur infrequently and signify decreased motility of the bowel, and can indicate inflammation or late bowel obstruction. Absent bowel sounds indicate paralytic ileus.

Before palpating the abdomen, allow the patient to empty their bladder as this makes examination more comfortable. Start away from the pain. Look for tenderness, rebound tenderness,

TABLE 14.8 Added breath sounds		
SOUND	DESCRIPTION	POSSIBLE CAUSE
Tracheal/tubular or bronchial	Heard outside the upper or lower trachea	Consolidation (pneumonia)
		Neoplasm
		Fibrosis
		Abscess
Diminution	Either no air movement or air or fluid preventing sound conduction	Effusion
		Pneumothorax
		Emphysema
		Collapse—obstruction
Crackle	Caused by either alveoli opening during inspiration or air bubbling through fluid	Fine—heart failure
		Medium—infection
		Coarse—pulmonary oedema or bronchiectasis
Wheeze	Rapid airflow through constricted airway	Asthma
		Bronchitis
		Pulmonary oedema
		Congestive heart failure
Pleural rub	Inflammation of pleura	Pleurisy

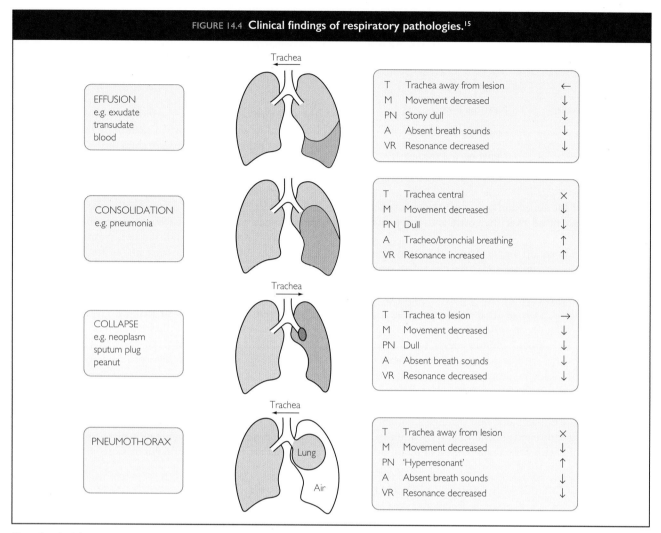

FIGURE 14.4 **Clinical findings of respiratory pathologies.**[15]

EFFUSION e.g. exudate transudate blood		T	Trachea away from lesion	←
		M	Movement decreased	↓
		PN	Stony dull	↓
		A	Absent breath sounds	↓
		VR	Resonance decreased	↓
CONSOLIDATION e.g. pneumonia		T	Trachea central	×
		M	Movement decreased	↓
		PN	Dull	↓
		A	Tracheo/bronchial breathing	↑
		VR	Resonance increased	↑
COLLAPSE e.g. neoplasm sputum plug peanut		T	Trachea to lesion	→
		M	Movement decreased	↓
		PN	Dull	↓
		A	Absent breath sounds	↓
		VR	Resonance decreased	↓
PNEUMOTHORAX		T	Trachea away from lesion	×
		M	Movement decreased	↓
		PN	'Hyperresonant'	↑
		A	Absent breath sounds	↓
		VR	Resonance decreased	↓

Reproduced with permission.

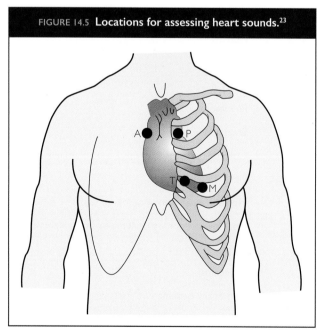

FIGURE 14.5 **Locations for assessing heart sounds.**[23]

M = mitral area, T = tricuspid area,
P = pulmonary area, A = aortic area.

guarding and rigidity. Rebound tenderness is identified by pressing slowly and deeply over the painful area and then quickly releasing. Sharp pain is felt on release. Percussion of the abdomen should reveal a hollow, tympanic sound due to the presence of gas. Fluid masses or organs result in an abnormal dull sound.[13]

Pelvis

The presence of a genitourinary problem is usually elicited when taking a history. The patient might complain of difficulty passing urine, urgency, burning on micturition, altered volume and flank pain. A mid-stream urine sample is obtained for analysis (see Ch 25). In addition to performing a urinalysis, colour, clarity and any offensive odour should be noted.

A menstrual history should be taken in female patients. It should include date of last menstrual period, contraceptive use and past pregnancy history. In women of childbearing age, a pregnancy test is indicated if any doubt is present. Males should be assessed for problems specific to their genitourinary anatomy. A slow stream or inability to void may be indicative of a prostate problem. Painful swelling of the testes could mean a testicular torsion. Presence of any discharge (penile/vaginal) or lesions may be indicative of a sexually transmitted infection (STI) and should prompt an inquiry about the patient's sexual

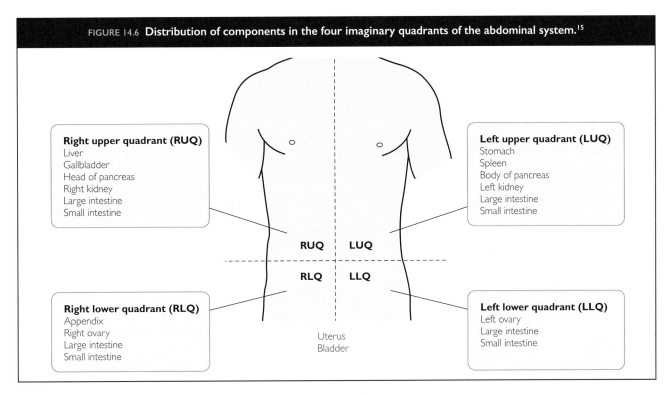

FIGURE 14.6 **Distribution of components in the four imaginary quadrants of the abdominal system.[15]**

history. This should include asking about sexual partners and their health, contraception methods used, previous history of STI or high-risk behaviour. It may be difficult to get a full history in the presence of a partner or parents, and so the emergency nurse should attempt to speak to the patient alone. This may feel awkward, but most patients understand the necessity of acquiring a full history. Ascertaining sexual practices can provide a valuable arena for safe-sex education and referral, if appropriate.

Genitourinary trauma (saddle injuries) in children can be caused by non-accidental injury and the nurse should be alert for this possibility when taking a history (see Ch 40).

Musculoskeletal and skin

Most presentations concerned with the musculoskeletal system are due to pain. This can be caused by trauma, infection and vascular, autoimmune or degenerative disease. Observation and palpation are done simultaneously and should start on the unaffected side to give a base for comparison. Inspect for size, symmetry, deformities, swelling and colour. Palpate for pain, tenderness, swelling and warmth. Compare range of movement to the unaffected side. Assess active range of movement before passive movement. A dislocated limb is considered an emergency if distal circulation and sensation is affected. See Chapter 18 and 50 for more information.

Assessment of the skin comprises observation for colour, integrity, rashes, lesions and perspiration and palpation to feel temperature and turgor. Skin colour can also give clues to the underlying pathology; for example, cherry red lips in carbon monoxide poisoning, generalised yellowness in jaundice or the pallor of anaemia.

The hands and feet should also be inspected for colour, warmth, movement and sensation. Adequate peripheral perfusion is established by feeling a strong radial pulse and a capillary refill time of under 3 seconds. Observe the peripheral limbs for pitting oedema, as this can be an indication of heart failure.

PRACTICE TIP

Observation and palpation of both sides/limbs are done simultaneously and should start on the unaffected side to give a base for comparison.

Other considerations

Signs of an endocrine or haematological condition may become obvious during history taking. Areas to focus on in the clinical examination are discussed in brief here.

Symptoms of an endocrine disorder can include changes in weight, appetite, bowel habit, hair distribution, pigmentation, sweating or alteration in menstruation, as well as lethargy, weakness, polyuria, polydipsia, headaches and impotence. Therefore it is best to focus on the specific presenting complaint (see Ch 26).

A haematological disease can affect red blood cells, white blood cells, platelets and haemostatic mechanisms. Patients may present with anaemia characterised by weakness, tiredness, dyspnoea, fatigue or postural dizziness. Platelet or blood clotting disorders may present with easy bruising or bleeding problems. Recurrent infections could be an indication of a disorder of the immune system. Laboratory testing of blood confirms the diagnosis. See Chapters 27 and 29 for further discussion.

Mental health assessment

A mental health assessment should consist of gathering general information, then following with more specific questions to clarify ambiguities and confirm or refute initial impressions. The main areas looked at are: appearance (cleanliness, posture, gait), behaviour (facial expression, cooperation, aggression, agitation, activity levels), speech (form and pattern, coherent, logical), mood (apathetic, irritable, optimistic or pessimistic, suicidal), thought (preoccupied, delusional, safety of patient and others), perception (hallucinations, auditory, visual, smell, taste, touch), cognition (orientation to time, place, person) and insight (understanding of their condition). For further information on mental health emergencies see Chapter 37.

PRACTICE TIP

The main areas looked at when performing a mental health assessment are: appearance, behaviour, speech, mood, thought, perception, cognition and insight.

Interventions

During the assessment process, interventions will be initiated. They will occur simultaneously with other aspects of the assessment. While helping the patient to get onto the trolley you will already have started to gather historical data, taking note of how the patient moves and signs of pain. You might note they have some difficulty breathing, so commence oxygen therapy, or they might appear to have severe pain so analgesia is given. An intravenous cannula may need to be sited. In the pre-hospital setting, this may be used to administer fluid resuscitation or drugs. In the ED setting it could be used to administer analgesia and to collect blood for laboratory testing.

PRACTICE TIP

All patients need to be re-evaluated for a response to these interventions and for any deterioration in general condition.

All patients need to be re-evaluated for a response to these interventions and for any deterioration in general condition. Based on the findings of the re-evaluation, more interventions may be required or, in an ED setting, medical review sought earlier.

Diagnostics/Investigations

Diagnostic tests may commence in the pre-hospital setting, such as the performance of 12-lead ECGs which in some settings are sent to the local hospital during transport to expedite transfer to the angiogram suite on arrival to hospital of patients requiring rapid reperfusion. When a patient arrives in the ED there is then an opportunity to obtain more extensive diagnostic and laboratory tests. The availability of this will depend on the facility. Most major metropolitan hospitals will have access to 24-hour facilities; however, in more rural and remote areas access may be restricted, particularly after hours.[9]

While the primary responsibility for determining which diagnostic and laboratory tests are required remains that of the medical practitioner, paramedics and ED nurses need to understand why particular tests might be required and the significance of the results. This will help with the early identification of sick or complex patients, initiating investigations and their subsequent reporting to medical staff. Rather than ordering standard groups of tests for particular sets of presenting symptoms, clinicians need to consider whether the tests they order are relevant to the patient's current condition. For example, ordering thyroid function tests can be fairly common practice for many presentations, yet it is important to think critically about whether this is clinically indicated. If it *is* indicated, findings may not result in clinical intervention in the acute ED setting, for reasons such as time delays in receiving results. However, results can be followed up by the general practitioner if the patient is discharged, or can prevent delay in inpatient treatment; for example, if blood collection did not occur until the following day.

There are certain other tests that are performed during an assessment to either confirm or rule out a diagnosis. Electro-cardiograms (ECGs) are usually performed on any patient presenting with chest pain, jaw pain, difficulty breathing, nausea and vomiting or collapse. Falls in the elderly that are not witnessed could be a result of a cardiac cause, and an ECG should also be recorded in this group. All patients with a suspected cardiac problem should have continuous cardiac monitoring according to department protocol. (See Ch 22 for more detail on ECGs.) Blood glucose levels (BGLs) should be obtained and recorded for all patients with diabetes and in patients who present with collapse, altered consciousness level, multiple abscesses or non-healing wounds, dizziness and nausea and vomiting, and in neonates. (See Ch 17, p. 332, for more details on BGL.) Nurse-initiated X-rays are also a consideration when a patient presents with pain over a distal limb from trauma. Nurses will have to have completed additional training before being assessed as competent to perform this skill, and it will depend on whether the facility has a policy or procedure in place to support this practice. See Chapter 17.

PRACTICE TIP

Rather than ordering standard groups of tests for particular sets of presenting symptoms, clinicians need to consider whether the tests they order are relevant to the patient's current condition.

Age-specific assessment

The familiar adage in paediatrics that 'children are not just small adults' could be adapted to the care of geriatric patients.[60] Considerations of the patient's age must be taken into account when performing an assessment.

PRACTICE TIP

Considerations of the patient's age must be taken into account when performing an assessment.

Developmental milestones

Developmental milestones can be divided into four major areas: gross motor, fine motor, speech and language, and social. A delay in one area is not uncommon. When assessing a child, it is important to know developmental milestones.

- *Gross motor*—by 4 months of age the child should be able to lift their head and shoulders off the bed. By 6 months, the arms are extended lifting the chest off the bed. By

6–7 months the child will stay in sitting position if pulled up, but by 9 months they are able to get themselves into sitting position. At 9–12 months the child is able to pull themself to a standing position, and by 12–16 months they should be able to walk independently.

- *Fine motor*—by 3 months, the grasp reflex will disappear and the baby will be able to hold and shake a rattle purposefully. At 5 months they will reach for objects and at 6 months pass the object from one hand to the other. By 7 months they should be able to finger-feed. By 10 months, they should have developed a pincer grip

enabling them to hold an object using index finger and thumb apposition. Also at this age, the child will be able to give the examiner 1 building block; by 12 months they will be able to build a tower with 2 blocks; and by 18 months the tower will be 3–4 blocks high.

- *Speech and language*—by 3 months they are vocalising, squealing aloud to show pleasure. By 7 months the child starts making consonant sounds such as 'da', 'ma', and by 8 months should be producing double syllables such as 'mama', 'dada'. By 12 months the child is saying 2–3 words with meaning; by 18 months they have 10 words. By 24 months they can make 2-word sentences, and by 3 years can make full sentences.

- *Social*—at 6 weeks the baby will smile responsively and by 16 weeks will laugh out loud. At 7 months they show stranger anxiety and don't like being picked up by people they don't know. By 9 months the child should play 'peek-a-boo' and wave goodbye, and by 10 months should understand the word 'no'. At 12–16 months they should be drinking from a cup and at 18 months attempting to eat from a spoon. Toilet training in the daytime is usually achieved by 2 years, and the child should be able to fully dress by 3 years (except buttons).

To make assessment easier, memorise the important milestones summarised in Table 14.9.

Age-specific commonalities

In the paediatric or elderly patient, considerations have to be made for their different anatomy or physiology (see Table 14.10). For more specific information on paediatric emergencies and on older people, see Chapters 36 and 39 respectively.

TABLE 14.9 Important milestones to remember[61]

AGE	MILESTONE
4–6 weeks	Smiles responsively
6–7 months	Sits unsupported
9 months	Gets to a sitting position
10 months	Pincer grip
12 months	Walks unsupported
	2 or 3 words
	Tower of 2 cubes
18 months	Tower of 3 or 4 cubes
24 months	2- or 3-word sentences

TABLE 14.10 Age-specific commonalities

SYSTEM	PAEDIATRICS		GERIATRICS	
Cardiovascular	S3	Is heard in up to a quarter of children	Coronary artery disease	A high incidence over age 60
	Murmurs	Heard in up to 50% of 3- to 7-year-olds		
Respiratory	Inhaled foreign object	At risk of obstruction due to small airway	Lung function	Declines with age
			Pneumonia	Increased risk of death with age
Gastrointestinal	Abdominal pain	Appendicitis, intussusception	Gastric and duodenal ulcers	At greater risk and mortality 4–10 times greater from GI bleeding
	Vomiting and diarrhoea	Caused by viral infection. Give fluids to prevent dehydration	Constipation	Due to decreased mobility and fluid intake or as side effect of medications
Genitourinary	Scrotal swelling	Generally caused by hernia but if acutely painful consider torsion	Prostatism	Enlarged prostate causing micturition problems
	UTI	Requires follow-up due to risk of renal scarring	Acute renal failure	Function declines with age, side effects from medications
			UTI	Due to increased urinary stasis, obstruction or presence of IDC

Continued

TABLE 14.10 Age-specific commonalities—cont'd

SYSTEM	PAEDIATRICS		GERIATRICS	
Neurological	Meningitis	Common in childhood during neonatal period	Dementia	
	Convulsions	Occur in 20% of children under 5 years. Commonly due to fever	Acute confusional state secondary to infection	May be the only sign of infection
			Head injury	Minor trauma can result in significant head injury
Head, ears, eyes, nose and throat	Tonsillitis	If chronic may cause upper airway obstruction, sleep apnoea	Decreased vision	Physiological changes occur in aged eye
	Otitis media	Common until age 7	Ulceration of cornea	Eyelids lose elasticity and turn inwards
			Epistaxis	Due to anticoagulants, hypertension
Integumentary	Jaundice	Common in neonates but in older children viral hepatitis is the commonest cause	Paper-thin skin	Easily damaged and difficult to heal
	Rashes	Most likely due to measles, chickenpox with fever	Hypothermia	Increased risk due to fat loss
Musculoskeletal	Painful limb in absence of trauma	Septic arthritis. Present with fever and hot, swollen joint	Osteoporosis	Makes bones more fragile and can sustain fractures from minor trauma
Mental health	Depression and mood swings	Common in adolescence	Depression	Due to social isolation or loss of independence

Essentials of care

How well patients are cared for has a direct effect on their sense of wellbeing and their recovery. Effective communication is essential to good patient care and their subsequent outcomes. The time for an ambulance patient to be offloaded may be delayed until a treatment space becomes available. The length of stay of the patient in the ED may be extended at times by the use of holding wards while waiting for results for patients for probable discharge. This means that paramedics and ED nurses need to consider other essential aspects of patient care. Paramedics and ED nurses are expected to work under pressure to many standards, guidelines and protocols related to patient care. However, posing the question 'How would I want this patient to be cared for if they were my grandmother/father/child?' provides an answer that sets a benchmark for nursing practice.[41] A similar approach should be taken when interacting with the patient's relatives. Aspects of care, such as culture, pain and infection control, are discussed in detail elsewhere (Chs 5, 19 and 27 respectively).

Two key areas of care—reducing risk and providing high-quality care—are served by a series of principles (see Table 14.11) and are closely related. Good risk management is an important component of high-quality care; if patients are assessed thoroughly and on a continuing basis then problems may be detected and treated early, thus preventing the development of unnecessary complications.[62]

Communication

Working with others effectively in healthcare is a challenge, and communication and human relationships with all those involved in the patient's care have an impact on nursing practice, patient care and how nurses feel about themselves.[63–65] As paramedics and nurses, we have a responsibility to provide safe and high-quality care. As a component of this, throughout the assessment process it is essential that communication occurs on several levels: paramedic to paramedic, paramedic to nurse, paramedic/nurse to patient and family/carers, nurse to nurse, and nurse to medical staff. Harmonious relationships with patients, between healthcare providers/team members, the organisation and the community are dependent on effective communication.[50] Although paramedics and ED nurses are extremely busy, a large proportion of their time is spent communicating, so good communication is an essential aspect of care. On this score, public surveys, practitioner accounts, emerging policy and practice-based research are unanimous: communication determines clinical quality, patients' safety, clinicians' wellbeing and public satisfaction.[66]

Principles of communication

Communication is made up of a sender, a receiver and a message sent within a particular context. The sender intends to convey a particular message; however, the ways in which the message is sent and/or received may be numerous as a result

TABLE 14.11 Principles of practice[62]	
REDUCING RISKS TO PATIENTS	PROVISION OF HIGH-QUALITY CARE
Recognition of the specific needs of critically ill patients, particularly those who are unconscious, sedated or immobile	Development of knowledge and skills for practice
	Evidence-based practice
Recognition of specific complications that may require special observation or treatment	Optimal use of protocol-driven therapy
	Competent practice
Vigilant monitoring and early recognition of signs of deterioration	Efficient and safe practice
Selection, implementation and evaluation of specific preventive measures	Selection and application of appropriate nursing interventions
Management of potentially detrimental environmental factors that may affect the patient	Monitoring the effects of nursing interventions
	Evaluation of nursing practice

of paralinguistic features, body language and psychological factors. Factors which have an impact on communication, both sending and receiving messages, are listed in Box 14.6, and it is important that the clinician is familiar with these to avoid hidden messages, misunderstandings and misinterpretations.[67] There are four basic principles of communication:

1. It is impossible not to communicate. All behaviour has a message of some sort. As well as the more obvious carriers of messages like words or gestures, saying or doing nothing is in itself a message. Once a message has been sent it cannot be retracted.

2. Every communication has a context and relationship aspect.

3. A series of communications can be viewed as an uninterrupted series of interchanges. There is no clear beginning or ending to a series of interchanges—communication between two individuals has a history and a future in itself and is affected by the past experiences of each individual.

4. All communication relationships are either symmetrical or complementary, depending on whether they are

based on equality or inequality. With a status or power differential between two people, such as between a nurse and a doctor, the complementary relationship will affect any communication between them. In general, how communication is interpreted depends on the relationship the sender has with the receiver.[68]

There is an extensive body of work on cognitive science and ideology in the context of an organisation, which supports the statement that the organisation has a responsibility to implement and support clinicians with a shared mental model in relation to fostering communication, especially in the context of uncertainty.[69]

Communication in the ED

Studies of human cognition and analysis of high-reliability organisations all predict that, despite excellent training, human error is unavoidable.[70] A British study[71] examined the communication load for a head nurse in an ED and documented over 1000 separate events over a 10-hour shift. 14% of these were simultaneous, and 30% were interruptions to a task already at hand.[71] An error rate of only 1% could potentially lead to 10 errors relating to patient management over the course of a typical shift.

However, the high rate of poor communication causing error can be improved. Communication in the ED occurs verbally, physically and using written or computerised documentation. Brereton[64] explains that there are several basic principles to effective communication in the workplace. These include:

- an appropriate knowledge base
- a range of behavioural skills which are essential to effective performance, such as authenticity, empathy, active listening and respect for others
- a positive attitude towards communicating
- the availability of opportunities to communicate.

A positive attitude towards communicating can be hindered by aspects of organisational behaviours, and opportunities to communicate can be thwarted by lack of resources and heavy workloads. ED nursing and medical staff experience barriers to communication such as stress and interruptions. Senior medical and nursing staff experience higher rates of interruption than

---

BOX 14.6 Factors that have an impact on communication[67]

Type of language used	Jargon, dialect, social linguistics
Paralinguistic features	Pitch, tone, pace, emphasis and volume
Body language	Posture, touch, eye contact, proximity, facial expression, gestures
Social	Age, gender, ethnicity, power, social status, relationship
Psychological	Attitudes and beliefs, prejudices, perceptual distortions, defence mechanisms, frame of mind/mood, stress, trust
Environmental	Privacy, layout of room, odours, lighting, colour

do junior medical staff and registered nurses with an allocated patient load.[72]

Documentation in the patient record should be continual—with each intervention—rather than once at the end of a shift. Treating clinicians should be able to read the patient notes and determine the patient status (waiting for review, ward bed), condition, interventions that have been performed and response to those interventions. Up-to-date documentation also allows the patient to be transferred without delay.

Clinical hand-over

Paramedics, nurses and doctors undertake segregated and distinct preparation for clinical practice, yet are expected to communicate effectively with each other in the workplace and ensure excellent and accurate clinical hand-over. There are three distinct times when hand-over occurs: the paramedic handing over to the triage nurse or resuscitation team on arrival at the ED; nurse-to-nurse hand-over at change of shift; and hand-over by the ED nurse to the ward nurse (Ch 11). Often the patients are critically unwell and may be unstable at this time. The aim of hand-over in all circumstances is to ensure a seamless exchange of information between care providers.[73] It is acknowledged that without a proper structure to the hand-over, vital information is likely to be forgotten and this can lead to adverse outcomes.[74–77] There is much work currently being conducted in the clinical hand-over forum; with different tools suited to different practice environments.[78] The mnemonic IMIST-AMBO (**I**dentification of the patient, **M**echanism/Medical complaint, **I**njuries/information relative to the complaint, **S**igns vitals and GCS, **T**reatment and trends/response to treatment – **A**llergies, **M**edications, **B**ackground history and **O**ther (social) information)[79] is a recommended structure used for hand-overs from paramedics to emergency staff, and is discussed in detail in Chapter 44. ISBAR (**I**ntroduction, **S**ituation, **B**ackground, **A**ssessment/Agreed plan and **R**ecommendations/**R**ead back) is a demonstrated effective strategy that can be employed to promote good communication with other in-hospital staff (Box 14.7).[80]

Using a communication tool allows accurate and relevant information to be shared in a structured format. This leads to a better patient experience, increases the credibility of the hand-over and allows the person receiving the information to be in possession of all the facts.[76] This will lead to them being able to quickly prioritise what they need to do first when taking over the care of the patient.

Communication with patients

Dialogue is more than sending and receiving messages verbally and non-verbally, and each patient should be treated as a unique individual.[81] Inability of the patient to communicate causes anxiety, frustration and stress as they lose control over their life and decisions. Critically ill patients commonly have communication difficulties due to mechanical devices (e.g. endotracheal tubes), cognitive impairment from the disease and/or pharmacological medications or language difficulties.[82]

The AIDET™ (**A**cknowledge the patient, **I**ntroduce yourself, **D**uration of procedures/test/interaction, **E**xplanation of procedure/test/procedure, **T**hank the patient for their cooperation) mnemonic, developed by the Studer Group, encapsulates five principles of communication identified to

---

BOX 14.7 The ISBAR communication tool

I Introduction: identify yourself and introduce the patient

S Situation: what is the main problem? What are your observations?

B Background: pertinent information, including past medical history

A Assessment/Agreed plan: include the clinical assessment and the plan of the care

R Recommendation/Read back: outline any outstanding items that need attending to and clarify and check for understanding.

BOX 14.8 The AIDET™ communication principles[83]

A—Acknowledge the patient
Greet the patient and other visitors with a smile, maintaining appropriate eye contact. Demonstrate warm, receptive attitude. Address the patient by their name. Ask them what they would like to be called. Acknowledge others present.

I—Introduce yourself and your role
Introduce yourself by name and role. Indicate your desire to help the patient by providing them with your full attention.

D—Duration of the procedure/test/interaction
Provide a brief explanation of how long any procedures/tests will take to perform or for results to come back. Let them know who they are waiting for and possible time-frames. Inform them of any delays.

E—Explanation of procedure/test/interaction
Keep the patient informed to enable them to make informed decisions and reduce any anxieties they have about the care of their condition. Provide details about tests and procedures, such as why it is being performed, who will perform it, whether there is pain or discomfort associated with the test and what will happen afterwards. Provide them an opportunity to ask questions.

T—Thank the patient for their cooperation
Thank the patient for their cooperation and patience. Ask if there is anything else you can do.

---

promote patient satisfaction.[83] (See Box 14.8 for explanation of each principle.) These communication strategies assist clinicians in making patients feel safe and calm, and to gather the key pieces of information needed to treat patients safely.[83]

Communication can also occur through physical contact: touch often communicates empathy and provides spiritual comfort.[84] Spiritual needs may further be met by providing comfort, reassurance and respect for privacy, and by helping patients relate to others.[85] Language barriers may necessitate the assistance of an interpreter with knowledge of healthcare terminology to ensure the content is adequately translated. An independent person ensures that the patient receives the message in its entirety from the healthcare professional.[86]

As a result of greater than ever access to medical information through superior communication systems and technology, patients and families recognise and may understand the basic definition of many medical terms and jargon. However, there are large variations of comprehension which may be of clinical significance. Healthcare providers should not assume that the patient or family is using the medical jargon in the same manner as a medical professional.[87]

Communication and patient outcomes

It is important to discuss the relationship between communication, sub-optimal care and patient outcomes, as there is a direct correlation.[88,89] The most common characteristics of international crisis-prompted healthcare inquiries are: care is not delivered in multidisciplinary teams; people do not communicate well across the clinical divides; and care is not delivered in a coordinated, organised way. The variety of healthcare areas investigated demonstrates that no one specialty is immune from error if poor communication exists.[88]

While patients may be satisfied with each individual healthcare professional, they recognise that the overall episode of care is often poorly coordinated or managed, and potential distortions of information regarding patient care lead to patients believing that care could be suboptimal.[90,91] In addition, poor communication can lead to delays in transfer from the ED, and there is a correlation between increased hospital length of stay (LOS) and increased LOS in the ED, especially on weekend shifts when patients are not reviewed by specialist teams and are often placed on outlying wards, or wards that are not related to the condition of the patient, because of the unavailability of appropriate beds.[92,93]

Poor communication is also one of the most common elements of frustration and stress among healthcare professionals.[94–96] Stress placed on critical care nurses decreases enthusiasm and impairs problem-solving capabilities.[97] In our current healthcare system where most media portrayals of EDs are negative,[98] and the availability and retention of nursing staff is of great concern, this remains a problem.

Patient satisfaction

Common public expectations of emergency care include staff communication with patients, appropriate waiting times, the triage process, information management and good quality of care.[99] While the paramedic and ED nurse cannot control all of these elements, effective communication is achievable. The way in which communication is conducted is closely related to ED patient satisfaction,[100] and is particularly related to the interpersonal skills and attitudes of staff.[101] Patients and their families need provision of information/explanation on a consistent basis, especially on arrival.[71] Areas in which communication is particularly important are: the cause of delays, patient management plans, and how to get to other locations within the hospital.[100] Studies on the psychology of waiting show that experiencing uncertain and unexplained waits makes the wait seem longer.[102] Regular communication with patients in the waiting room, explaining the reasons for any delays, improves satisfaction levels.[103,104]

Open disclosure

Open disclosure is providing an open, consistent approach to communicating with patients following an adverse event. This includes expressing regret for what has happened, keeping the patient informed and providing feedback on investigations, including the steps taken to prevent an event from recurring. It is also about providing information that will enable systems of care to be changed to improve patient safety. The Australian Open Disclosure Framework provides a nationally consistent basis for open disclosure in Australian healthcare. It was endorsed in 2013 and replaces the former Open Disclosure Standard.[105]

Improving healthcare safety begins with ensuring that communication is open and honest, and immediate. This includes communication between healthcare professionals and patients and their carers. It also includes communication between healthcare professionals, healthcare managers and all staff. It is important when this framework is put in place that people feel supported and are encouraged to identify and report adverse events so that system improvements can be identified and acted on. This should include the following:

- Provide an environment where patients, their family and carers:
  - Receive the information they need to understand what happened
  - Can contribute about the adverse event and, where possible and appropriate, participate in the incident review, creating a culture where patients, their family and carers, clinicians and managers all feel supported.
- Integrating open disclosure with investigative processes to identify why adverse events occur.
- Implementing the necessary changes in systems of clinical care based on the lessons learned.[105]

Disclosure is required where a patient has suffered some harm (physical or psychological) as a result of treatment. This may be a recognised complication or a result of human or systems error. As soon as an event is noticed, you should ensure patient safety, perform any immediate care interventions required and inform your manager. If the paramedic or ED notices harm caused under the care of another clinician, they should always speak first to their manager and the senior clinician of the team involved. If these members of staff are unwilling to initiate the disclosure process, refer the matter to the person responsible for clinical risk or medical administration.

Disclosure with the patient and family

The individual making the disclosure should be the most senior healthcare professional involved; for example, the nurse manager, and someone with experience or training in communication and open disclosure. Effective communication is pivotal to the open-disclosure process. Patients, their families and carers may become upset or angry when they have suffered an adverse event. This is a natural response, so it is important not to become angry or react defensively in this situation. An adverse incident is an emotionally-charged event for all parties. Guidelines for communicating with the patient and family can be found on the Australian Commission on Safety and Quality in Health Care website (www.safetyandquality.gov.au), and include the following:

- Arrange a face-to-face meeting that allows adequate time for detailed discussion as soon as possible after an adverse outcome has occurred.
- Listen actively and respectfully to the patient.

- Use plain language and avoid jargon.
- Acknowledge the validity of the emotions the patient and/or carer may feel.
- Where a family member is present, include them in your dialogue where appropriate.
- In all discussions, avoid defensiveness and laying blame. Avoid statements that include terms such as 'fault', 'blame' or 'feel responsible'.[105]

Support for staff involved

If directly involved in an adverse event, staff have the right to seek appropriate legal advice and to disclose information to legal advisers in a manner that ensures that it attracts legal professional privilege. The breaking of bad news can be extremely stressful on a staff member.[105] They have the right to be treated fairly by the institution and to receive natural justice and procedural fairness, and the right not to be defamed.[105] Avoid statements such as:

- 'I'm sorry—I appear to have made an error in judgement.'
- 'I apologise for this mistake.'
- 'It is my fault that this has happened.'

The best approach is to give an honest and factual account of what happened.

Healthcare professionals who have been involved in an adverse event may be angry with themselves or someone else for what occurred. They may feel that they have let the patient down. It is important to make sure they receive emotional support and advice after the incident.[94]

Needs of the family

In light of the various definitions of family and the regulations regarding the release of information, how people define themselves has implications for clinicians (see Ch 4). It is important to ask the patient who is to be considered family, receive information and be allowed in the treatment area. When that is not possible, the clinician must be guided by good judgement, policy and regulations and ethics.[107] Although ED nurses are usually very busy, it can be crucial to conduct a brief family assessment, and determine if social work intervention may be required. There are several ways to develop a dialogue with families and conduct a quick assessment of family strengths and potential resources.[108]

- Introduce yourself to the patient and the family.
- Ask about people at the bedside and determine their relationship to the patient.
- Call patients by name, after having asked how they wish to be addressed.
- Explain procedures and equipment, and be honest about the anticipated length of the wait.
- Repeat information; the anxiety of being in the ED, even in non-urgent situations, decreases the ability to remember what is said.
- Stop in the patient's doorway or at the foot of the bed to update them and their family whenever the situation in the ED changes.
- After any explanation, always ask if anyone has questions. If the answer is not known, say so, then find out the answer.[107]

When encountering a family in the initial stages of a life-changing event, paramedics and ED nurses often interact with and provide support for family members who feel despair, fear, anger, guilt or helplessness, or who are in a state of disbelief or denial. Family members present at the scene or who come to the ED with a loved one nearing the end of a long and debilitating illness may be fatigued, frustrated or ambivalent. The paramedics or ED nurse may be the first to recognise a family that is bordering on crisis because of the drain on their emotional and physical resources. Further assessment would determine whether the family needs a referral for services such as home care, hospice or counselling.[107]

Family needs have been extensively researched, and include the need for information, reassurance, closeness, support and comfort.[109] Practical ways to meet these are given in Box 14.9.

The Institute For Patient and Family-Centered Care (IPFCC) promotes the relationship between the patient, their family members and the healthcare professional. The core concepts of patient and family-centered care are:[110]

- *Respect and dignity.* Healthcare practitioners listen to and honour patient and family perspectives and choices. Patient and family knowledge, values, beliefs and cultural backgrounds are incorporated into the planning and delivery of care.
- *Information sharing.* Healthcare practitioners communicate and share complete and unbiased information with patients and families in ways that are affirming and useful. Patients and families receive timely, complete and accurate information in order to effectively participate in care and decision-making.
- *Participation.* Patients and families are encouraged and supported in participating in care and decision-making at the level they choose.
- *Collaboration.* Patients and families are also included on an institution-wide basis. Healthcare leaders collaborate with patients and families in policy and program development, implementation and evaluation; in healthcare facility design; and in professional education, as well as in the delivery of care.

BOX 14.9 Family needs[82,109,111,112]

Ways to meet families' needs include the following:
- listen compassionately
- compliment the family on how well members are coping
- involve the family early
- communicate regularly
- praise family strengths
- acknowledge how difficult the experience is
- commend patience
- update them on relative progress and prognosis
- answer questions honestly
- give consistent information
- demonstrate caring (offer a chair and a cup of tea/coffee)
- call them at home to update on patient condition or any change
- inform about transfer plans as they are being made.

Caring

Caring is a core characteristic of healthcare. In emergencies, life-saving procedures are, of course, the priority, but it is important not to forget to meet the patient's psychological needs as well.[81,82,113] Professional caring consists of three essential elements: competence, caring and connection. *Competence* involves empowering, connecting and educating people, making clinical judgements and being able to do tasks and take action on behalf of people. Aspects of *caring* are outlined below and involve being dedicated and having the courage to be appropriately involved as a professional paramedic and nurse. The *connection* aspects of professional caring involve initiating professional connection, which requires both the patient and the clinician to reach out and respond. A bridge is built when patients realise the connection and feel free to ask for help. Professional intimacy then occurs when patients begin to trust the clinician. As a result of the connection and professional intimacy, paramedics and nurses work with patients towards their common goal. Professional boundaries are discussed in Chapter 3.

An uncaring encounter can consist of incompetence and indifference, lack of trust, mutual avoidance and disconnection between the nurse and the patient. The clinician may be perceived as inconsiderate, insensitive, disrespectful and disinterested.

Aspects of caring in emergencies

- *Being open to and perceptive of others:* patients are often affected by the acute event, as they have abruptly lost control of their own situation and are in a position of dependence. A caring paramedic or ED nurse has to be sensitive to such patients and capable of interpreting or predicting their needs. The caring clinician needs an open attitude and should communicate openly with the patient.
- *Being genuinely concerned for the patient:* paramedics and nurses with this caring quality display genuine feelings of goodwill towards patients and a holistic view of caring.
- *Being morally responsible:* from the patient's perspective, calling an ambulance and visits to the ED are not planned. Suddenly, they become dependent on others to fulfil their needs. Clinicians have to act to maintain and strengthen the patient's dignity in this serious situation.
- *Being truly present:* this means that clinicians have to be attentive to the present moment, and be present in dialogue, in listening and responding. They should be present in the situation, physically and emotionally. In order to be truly present in the dialogue, nurses require good communication skills.[81]
- *Meeting the patient's psychological needs* could reduce the risk of developing post-traumatic stress syndrome. To create an authentic encounter, paramedics and nurses need to display several aspects of sensitive and effective communication, be dedicated and have the courage to be appropriately involved.[81]

Care of paramedics

Just as patients require care, so do paramedics. The role of the paramedic has moved away from its focus of giving first aid and transporting patients to hospital, to a more dynamic role that encompasses higher levels of patient care and instigating interventions based on a thorough patient assessment.[114] Furthermore, they are exposed to increasing levels of physical and verbal aggression. As part of their role, paramedics are exposed to a range of highly stressful incidents;[115] on top of which the service is getting busier and busier with no real downtime between calls in which to relax or socialise at the station.[114] It has been reported that this is a cause of increasing stress-related illnesses and work dissatisfaction.[116] It is an accepted belief that to do their job well paramedics should appear 'tough', but by failing to talk about a traumatic incident the likelihood of suffering stress is increased. The value of social support from colleagues cannot be underestimated as it can help mitigate the impact of traumatic events.[115] Managers in the profession should be aware of the value of debriefing or offering counselling, and encompass this into the role where able. One way to achieve this is to promote the use of an employee assistance program that offers free, confidential counselling to employees.

Care of emergency nurses

ED nurses also require care. Providing thorough and effective care for emergency patients is emotionally draining and highly demanding of busy emergency nurses, who often fail to notice or acknowledge their own needs.[117] A certain amount of stress at work can be a motivator, but repeated exposure to stressful events can have adverse outcomes.[118] Nurses have been extensively studied as groups experiencing high levels of stress, burnout and fatigue.[119] Critical care nurses may feel they are acting unprofessionally if they show overt signs of grief. Being aware of the signs of stress and developing and implementing coping mechanisms is essential.[120] Also, nurses depend on colleagues and friends for support and value debriefing sessions, whether it be an opportunity to share feelings or a procedural clinical review of events. The effectiveness of sessions should be evaluated and staff health and welfare monitored by ED managers and colleagues. An awareness of colleagues' needs is a key to providing the support they require.[82]

Privacy and dignity

Respect, autonomy, empowerment and communication have been identified within the literature as being the defining attributes of dignity. In the busy ED, maintenance of dignity may be unintentionally overlooked. Patients can be nursed in a corridor, or other patients and relatives may overhear the hand-over, which does not lend itself to upholding the dignity, privacy and confidentiality of the patient.[121] Discretion should be used if updating relatives in a crowded waiting room, triage assessment should be conducted in a safe and private location and the patient's dignity should be maintained at all times.[122]

Personal hygiene

Patients presenting to the ED can be in various states of hygiene as a result of injury, vomiting, incontinence or neglect. Also, despite the 4-hour National Emergency Access Target, patients may remain in the ED for an extended period of time and desire to maintain their regular hygiene routine. Personal hygiene is closely related to individual esteem and sense of wellbeing, and is an important sensory determinant by family members that influences their perception of the quality of care the patient is receiving and the confidence they have in the staff. But while personal hygiene is a basic right for all patients, it should not be placed above the need for other therapies, forensic requirements and rest.[62]

As with all aspects of care and treatment, the patient has the right to refuse personal hygiene measures. Bathing or washing patients provides opportunities for the ED nurse to assess the patient's skin and tissue. Often this enables the nurse to identify tissue damage that requires treatment, and to identify dressings or wounds that require attention. Some patients who are sweating, incontinent or bleeding need to be washed and their linen changed as often as necessary. Wet, creased sheets alter skin integrity and may cause pressure on dependent areas, increasing the risk of pressure-ulcer development. A bed bath can be a major and painful undertaking, which often requires at least two people to support and move the patient and prophylactic pain relief before commencing.[62] The length of time taken to wash a patient and the environmental temperature are factors that affect cooling. Water on exposed skin causes rapid heat loss and shivering increases metabolism and oxygen consumption, which is detrimental in a compromised patient (see Ch 28).

It is essential to maintain patient privacy and avoid interruptions that affect the dignity of the patient. Careful handling of patients to reduce skin friction and shear during repositioning and transfers can prevent skin tears. Padded bed rails, pillows and blankets can be used to protect and support arms and legs. Paper-type or non-adherent dressings should be used on frail skin, and should be removed gently and slowly. Wraps or nets can be used instead of surgical tape to secure dressings and drains in place.[62] The management of skin tears is discussed in Chapter 18.

> **PRACTICE TIP**
>
> Consider the length of time a patient has spent, or will spend, in the ED and ensure opportunities are given for attending to their personal hygiene needs, which will differ from person to person.

Eye care

Eye care involves the cleansing of the eyes, as well as the prevention of dry eyes and corneal abrasions by the use of artificial tears and measures to maintain eyelid closure. It is an important aspect of caring for the sedated or unconscious patient.[62] There are a number of physiological processes that protect the eye. The eye is protected from dryness by frequent lubrication facilitated by blinking. Antimicrobial substances in tears help prevent infection, and the tear ducts provide drainage. When the eye is unable to close properly, tear film evaporates more quickly.[123] The blink response may be slowed or absent in some patients, such as individuals receiving sedatives and muscle relaxants, which can potentially cause keratopathy, corneal ulceration and viral or bacterial conjunctivitis.[124] Patients who are exposed to high flows of air/oxygen may be vulnerable to its drying effects. (See Ch 33 for assessment and management of eye injury.)

Eye care and the administration of artificial tears should be provided if required, if the patient complains of sore or dry eyes or if there is visible evidence of encrustation. If a patient

is receiving high-flow oxygen therapy via a mask, they may benefit from regular 4-hourly administration of artificial tears to lubricate the eyes and prevent the drying effect of oxygen.[123] Conjunctival oedema is a common problem associated with positive-pressure ventilation with high positive end-expiratory pressure (PEEP) (above 5 cmH$_2$O), and prone positioning[124] often results in the patient's inability to maintain eye closure. Eye closure may be maintained by applying a wide piece of adhesive tape horizontally to the upper part of the eyelid. This usually anchors the lid in the closed position, allowing the eyelid to be opened for pupil assessment and access for eye care.[62]

> **PRACTICE TIP**
>
> Apply 4-hourly artificial tears to lubricate the eyes to prevent the drying effect of high flow oxygen therapy.

Oral hygiene

Mouth care is one of the most basic nursing activities.[125] Oral care aims to ensure a healthy oral mucosa, prevent halitosis, maintain a clean and moist oral cavity, prevent pressure ulcers from devices such as endotracheal tubes (ETTs), prevent trauma caused by grinding of teeth or biting of the tongue, and reduce bacterial activity that leads to local and systemic infection.[125,126]

If the ED patient has had an extended stay, a toothbrush and toothpaste and assistance to clean teeth should be provided. The use of mouth swabs only for oral hygiene is ineffective.[127] Many oncology and immunology patients suffer from mouth ulcers and are on oral care regimens at home. The maintenance of such a regimen is essential for patient comfort and may require the ED nurse organising and obtaining prescribed mouthwashes from the pharmacy department. Regular sips of fluid or mouthwashes with water for those patients who are required to have no oral intake prevents drying, coating and subsequent oral discomfort. If the patient is able to suck and swallow, small pieces of ice are very refreshing.[62] The application of lanolin or petroleum jelly eases the discomfort of dry lips and maintains the integrity of lips.

For patients with crusty build-up on their teeth, common in the elderly, dehydrated patient, a single application of warm dilute solution of sodium bicarbonate powder with a toothbrush is effective in removing debris and causes mucous to become less sticky, although its use is sometimes contested as it can cause superficial burns. Its use should be followed immediately by a thorough water rinse of the mouth to return the oral pH to normal.[128,129]

In the sedated, intubated or unconscious patient, absence of mastication leads to a reduction in saliva production. Saliva produces protective enzymes. An endotracheal tube can cause pressure areas in the mouth (which may be exacerbated if the patient is oedematous). Once the patient is in the intensive care unit, an oral care program will be commenced.

> **PRACTICE TIP**
>
> Ensure patients who have an extended stay in ED have access to a toothbrush and toothpaste as using mouth swabs alone is ineffective.

Patient positioning

Positioning patients correctly and as soon as possible in the ED, while considering cardiovascular stability, respiratory function and cerebral or spinal injury, is important to contribute to the prevention of common short- and long-term complications of immobility. These include pressure ulcers, venous thromboembolism and pulmonary dysfunction, atelectasis, retained secretions, pneumonia, dysoxia and aspiration, each of which carries a significant co-morbidity.[130] Good body alignment helps prevent pressure points, contractures and unnecessary pain or discomfort for the patient. In addition, lying in bed for long periods can be a painful experience.[131] It is also important to remember that Australian healthcare organisations are required to be accredited for Standard 8: Preventing and Managing Pressure Injuries.[132]

Patients at the highest risk of complications related to their position are those who are unable to move for long periods, for whatever reason.[131] For example, unstable patients whose status is compromised when they are moved, elderly and frail or malnourished patients, and patients who are unable to move themselves (e.g. due to sedation, trauma, surgery or obesity) are all at risk. The risk of hospital-acquired pneumonia is heightened when patients are in the supine position.[133] Provided there are no contraindications, the immobile patient should be positioned with the head raised by 30° or more, as research has demonstrated that this improves mortality outcomes.[134]

Provided there are no contraindications, function should be stimulated by regular passive movements of all limbs and joints to maintain both flexibility and comfort, as it takes only 7 days of bed rest to reduce muscle mass by up to 30%.[135] Movement of the lower legs, ankles and feet can be achieved in conjunction with a gentle massage or application of moisturiser. Family members may wish to undertake this, giving them an opportunity to provide the patient with care and touch. The ED nurse should encourage the able patient to perform exercises, and conduct an early physiotherapy referral for patients who may have an extended ED stay awaiting a ward bed.

The standard for immobile patients is 2-hourly body repositioning, although this does not always happen.[130] It may also be required more frequently than this and this is determined by the nurse based on patient factors and clinical situation.[132] The nurse caring for the immobile patient is most often responsible for determining position. It is important to fully consider the individual needs of patients: they may have a history of back or neck problems, and the selective use of soft or firm pillows and mattresses may be relevant. Pillows can optimise the patient's position so that the shoulders and chest are squared, and may reduce the work of breathing for patients with chronic airways disease. Some pressure-relieving mattresses have an adjustable pressure control, which can be changed according to pressure-relief assessment and patient comfort. When patients are positioned lying on one side, consideration should be given to their feeling of security— for example, ensuring that they are well supported by pillows and the bed rails are raised. When planning to reposition the patient, ensure that there are enough staff to give the patient a feeling of security during the positioning; also that all the patient devices (e.g. intravenous lines) are managed. Check that all devices are placed to accommodate the repositioning before you begin to move the patient.

Pressure-area care

Pressure-area risk for critically ill and/or immobile patients can be attributed to their lack of sensory protective mechanisms, the length of time pressure is exerted on the skin, excessive moisture, suboptimal tissue perfusion and friction (two surfaces rubbing against each other, such as sliding against sheets on lifting, or rubbing). The most common locations for pressure ulcers are the sacrum, the heels and the head.[136,137] Significant risk factors include the age of the patient, malnutrition and delays in the use of pressure-relieving mattresses (see Box 14.10).[137,139,140] Pressure-ulcer risk-assessment tools, such as the Braden and Waterlow Scales,[141] can help nurses identify at-risk patients early.

Any pressure ulcers should be documented and described in relation to size, grade/stage and treatment and monitored closely. If a patient develops one pressure ulcer, there is a good chance they could develop another. While the pressure ulcer may not be evident in the ED, the initial reddened areas give clues to potential locations for development, and any preventative measures implemented in the ED contribute greatly to prevention.

Simple preventative measures include water-filled gloves under the heels, removing additional bed linen from under the patient which may have been transferred from the ambulance trolley, ensuring the patient is kept clean and dry (particularly those under stiff neck collars and incontinent patients), the use of foam boots and alternating pressure-relief mattresses and foam mattresses with adequate thickness and stiffness. However, none of these are a substitute for regular repositioning and avoiding pressure on any affected areas.[137] It is also important to document the details of position each time the patient is repositioned and communicate this on hand-over, as well as to maintain the patient's hydration and nutrition to improve tissue perfusion and integrity.

Patients are also at risk of developing pressure ulcers and injury from a number of devices in everyday use, such

---

BOX 14.10 Risk factors for pressure ulcers[138]

- Advanced age
- Anaemia
- Contractures
- Diabetes mellitus
- Elevated body temperature
- Immobility
- Impaired circulation
- Incontinence
- Low diastolic blood pressure (< 60 mmHg)
- Mental deterioration
- Neurological disorders
- Obesity
- Pain
- Prolonged surgery
- Vascular disease

as endotracheal tubes, backboards and blood-pressure cuffs (Table 14.12). Close attention to detail with frequent observation of the patient, the patient's position and the presence and location of equipment is required to prevent skin damage.[62]

Nutrition

The impact of adequate nutrition on patient outcome is well documented. The intake of nutrients, such as protein, calories, vitamins, minerals and fluids, provides the energy source required for growth of all body structures and maintenance of body functions, as well as supporting the immune function of the bowel.[143,144] Patients presenting to the ED are often in an altered metabolic state due to the stress response to illness, injury or starvation (when nutrient intake is unable to meet the body's energy demands). Wounds place increased metabolic and hence oxygen and nutritional demands on patients.[145,146] Critically ill patients are usually in a hypermetabolic state, characterised by rises in oxygen consumption and use of nutritional substitutes such as amino acids. The effects of the hypermetabolic state on homeostasis are discussed in depth in Chapter 20. Malnutrition and starvation increase electrolyte imbalances, muscle wasting, morbidity and mortality; delay recovery; impede healing of acute and chronic wounds; interfere with the body's ability to fight infection; and increase the cost of hospitalisation.[147–149] Knowledge of nutrition's effect in the patient is integral for nurses to predict and promote successful outcomes and is a priority of care.[149]

About 25–40% of hospital patients are malnourished,[150,151] and nursing staff play a key role in identification and prevention of this.[152–155] Screening tools and early, standardised nutritional care improves the recognition of malnourished patients and provides the opportunity to start treatment at an early stage of hospitalisation. Older people are at higher risk of malnutrition if they are ill, live alone or have difficulty in eating, and are often in a state of malnutrition or starvation prior to the cause of admission, adding further insult.[151] They should have their nutritional status and nutritional intake assessed on admission. For the ED nurse this may involve referral to the dietetics department, who will assess and monitor the patient regularly to ensure they are receiving adequate nutrition.[156] If the patient is going to be discharged, referral to community services should occur.

While it is often inappropriate for the ED patient to have oral intake as they have the potential to require emergency surgery, or they may have suffered cerebral insult that compromises swallowing and gag reflexes, or have an altered level of consciousness, it is essential to establish nutritional status

---

TABLE 14.12 Risk of pressure sores from commonly used equipment[142]

EQUIPMENT	RISKS
Endotracheal (ETT) tubes	Care should be taken when positioning and tying ETT tapes: friction burns may be caused if they are not secure; pressure ulcers may be caused if they are too tight (particularly above the ears and in the nape of the neck).
	Moist tapes exacerbate problems and harbour bacteria.
Oxygen saturation probes	Repositioning of oxygen saturation probes 1–2 hourly prevents pressure on potentially poorly perfused skin.
	If using ear probes, these must be positioned on the lobe of the ear and not on the cartilage, as this area is very vulnerable to pressure and heat injury.
Blood-pressure cuffs	Non-invasive blood-pressure cuffs should be regularly reattached and repositioned. If left in position without reattachment for long periods of time, they can cause friction and pressure damage to skin.
	Care should be taken to ensure that tubing is not caught under the patient, especially after repositioning.
Urinary catheters, central lines and wound drainage	The patient should be checked often to ensure that invasive lines are not trapped under the patient. In addition to causing skin injury, they may function ineffectively.
Bed rails	Limbs should not press against bed rails; pillows should be used if the patient's position or size makes this likely.
Oxygen masks	Use correct-size mask and a hydrocolloid protective dressing on the bridge of the nose to assist with prevention of pressure from non-invasive or CPAP masks, especially when these are in constant or frequent use.
Splints and cervical collars	Devices such as leg/foot splints and cervical collars can all cause direct pressure when in constant use and friction injury if they are not fitted properly.
Hard backboards	Hard backboards or spine-boards used by ambulance personnel for patient extrication cause pressure areas and should be removed on patient arrival to the ED or on initial log roll.

CPAP: continuous positive airway pressure

as soon as possible. Nutritional status should be documented clearly and handed over to ward nursing staff. The dietetics department should be notified of special requirements and speech pathology referral and assessment conducted promptly. Those ED patients who are clinically able to tolerate some form of diet should be encouraged to eat and drink and should be assisted if necessary, enlisting the aid of family members, if present. Particular consideration should be given to the diabetic patient and monitoring of their BGLs. This will help prevent the development of a compromised nutritional state.

Elimination

Effective urine and bowel elimination is a basic human need, and adequate privacy, discretion and dignity is essential. While it can be difficult in a busy ED, it is important to facilitate prompt toileting and maximise access to toilets.

More than one million people living in Australia and New Zealand suffer from urinary incontinence from causes such as poor pelvic floor tone, central nervous system disorders, spinal cord injury, fistulas and bladder disorders.[157] Also, the normally continent patient may present having been incontinent following a seizure or traumatic event. The paramedic and ED nurse must recognise the physical and emotional problems associated with urinary incontinence and frequency. The patient's dignity, privacy and feelings of self-worth must be maintained. The discreet disposal of soiled pads, patient sponging (wet skin contributes to pressure-ulcer development), cleansing of the perineum, provision of clean incontinence pads and referral to appropriate continence services should be done if required. If urinary catheter insertion is needed, thorough cleansing and aseptic techniques are essential to prevent the development of urinary tract infections.

Bowel management

The prevention of constipation is important as it may contribute to the exacerbation of other conditions, such as myocardial infarction, congestive cardiac failure, stroke and head injury,[158,159] as well as considerable discomfort, nausea and loss of dignity. Risk factors include immobility, medications such as opiates, anticonvulsants, diuretics and calcium channel blockers, reduced gut motility, a poor dietary intake, dehydration and older age.

Interventions that can be commenced in the ED include exercise—even in the bed-bound patient—as peristaltic movement of the gut is stimulated. Diet and fluids are also important considerations in maintaining normal bowel function, ensuring, if clinically appropriate, that the patient receives adequate administration of fluid and diet in the ED. Prior to patient transfer to the ward from the ED, if the patient is at risk of constipation, ensure that oral aperients have been charted, if clinically appropriate, the risk has been handed over to the ward nursing staff and the patient has been educated on prevention techniques.

SUMMARY

This chapter has discussed a 'head-to-toe' approach to assessment. The ED nurse or paramedic should consider the assessment process as more than just recording a set of vital signs. Although the process appears to be time-consuming, with practice and experience the ED nurse or paramedic is able to automatically and quickly proceed through the process. This is made easier by adopting an assessment template such as HIRAID. Reassessment has been highlighted in monitoring dynamic changes in a patient's condition and comparing them with the baseline. This can help initiate timely and appropriate measures to maximise patient care and outcomes.

Effective communication between healthcare providers and the patient and their family is instrumental in patient outcomes and satisfaction. The paramedic or ED nurse conducting or commencing the discussed aspects of essential nursing care contributes greatly to reducing the risk of the patient developing complications during their hospital stay. Simple measures, such as timely toileting of patients, will assist to maintain comfort and dignity; documentation of nutritional status will help avoid malnutrition; regular pressure-area and skin care will prevent pressure ulcer development. While it is easy to be distracted by performing advance procedures, it is vital that these basic but essential elements of patient care are provided for the health, comfort and dignity of the patient.

CASE STUDY

Part A: Pre-hospital

You are the treating paramedic of a morbidly obese man in his forties complaining of shortness of breath. On arrival to his home the patient is sitting upright in a chair talking in short phrases, but complaining primarily of severe left leg pain.

1. Where would you start your assessment?

   A. Inspect his leg.

   B. Record a set of vital signs.

   C. Check his BGL.

   D. Assess DRSABCD

You assess the scene and identify no immediate dangers to yourself so you approach the patient. He responds appropriately and you commence taking a history while performing your physical assessment.

2. What mnemonic could you use to structure taking the patient's history?

The patient's wife informs you that she called the ambulance service, worried as she felt his breathing had become more laboured over the course of the day. You also learn that the patient has a known history of type I diabetes and a chronic ulcer on his left leg, which has become malodourous.

3. What 'red flags' have you already identified in this patient?

While undertaking your physical assessment you identify that the patient has a respiratory rate of 28 breaths per minute with some mild accessory muscle use. Oxygen saturations are adequate. On auscultation air entry is equal. You inspect the left leg ulcer and find a red sloughy, odourous wound. There is decreased sensation to the affected limb but strong pedal pulses present. You dress the wound to absorb the exudate and transport the patient to hospital.

4. How would you (the paramedic) structure your hand-over to the receiving ED nurse on arrival to hospital?

Part B: At the ED

You are the ED nurse receiving care of this patient in the acute treatment area.

5. How would you start your assessment?
   A. Collect the patient's history
   B. Identify Red flags

C. Perform a set of vital signs
D. Apply oxygen.

6. You commence your physical assessment. When attempting to check his blood pressure the cuff keeps popping off. What do you do?
   A. Tape it on with micropore.
   B. Not bother, he has just presented with a leg ulcer.
   C. Find an appropriate-size cuff.
   D. Use the manual syphygmomanometer as you can stop inflating before the cuff pops open.

After completing the primary survey you perform a head-to-toe examination including a focused respiratory assessment. You identify that the patient is still only able to speak in short sentences and has moderate accessory muscle use. The respiratory rate is counted at 32 breaths per minute, oxygen saturations measure 92% on room air and temperature 38.7°C. The patient denies any history of lung disease.

7. What new 'red flags' have been identified and how should you respond to these?

8. What diagnostic test is this patient likely to require?

9. Your patient suddenly becomes very sweaty and disorientated. What do you do next?

10. After medical review and initial treatment the patient is admitted into hospital. There is no access to a bed for several hours. What factors do you need to consider for his ongoing care?

Answers to Case Study Questions can be found on evolve
http://evolve.emergencytrauma.curtis

REFERENCES

1. Alcock K, Clancy M, Crouch R. Physiological observations of patients admitted from A&E. Nurs Stand 2002;16(34):33–7.
2. Fennessey A, Wittmann-Price RA. Physical assessment: a continuing need for clarification. Nursing Forum, 2011. 46(1):45–50.
3. Australian Resuscitation Council. ARC guidelines. 2011 Online. www.resus.org.au/; accessed January 2014.
4. Munroe B et al. The impact structured patient assessment frameworks have on patient care: An integrative review. Journal of Clinical Nursing 2013;22(21–22):2991–3005.
5. Considine J, Currey J. Ensuring a proactive, evidence-based, patient safety approach to patient assessment. J Clin Nurs. 2015; 24(1–2):300–7.
6. Muir N. Clinical decision-making: theory and practice. Nurs Stand 2004;18(36):47–52.
7. American College of Surgeons. Initial assessment and management. Advanced Trauma Life Support for doctors (ATLS): student course manual. Chicago, USA; 2012.
8. Society of Critical Care Medicine. Surviving Sepsis Campaign Responds to ProCESS Trial. 2014. Online. www.survivingsepsis.org/ SiteCollectionDocuments/SSC-Responds-Process-Trial.pdf; accessed 25 Feb 2015.
9. Curtis K, Murphy M, Lewis MJ. The emergency nursing assessment process—a structured framework for a systematic approach. Australas Emerg Nurs J 2009;12:130–6.
10. Munroe B, Curtis K, Murphy M et al. HIRAID: An evidence informed emergency nursing assessment framework. Australasian J Emerg Nurs 2015 (in press).
11. Kaufman G. Patient assessment: effective consultation and history taking. Nurs Stand 2008;23(4):50–6.

12. Semil DL. Approach to the patient: history and physical examination. In: Goldman L, ed. Cecil medicine. 23rd edn. Philadelphia: Elsevier; 2007.

13. Elling B, Elling K. Principles of patient assessment in EMS. 1st edn. Delmar Cengage Learning; 2003.

14. Baid H. The process of conducting a physical assessment: a nursing perspective. Br J Nurs 2006;15(13):710–14.

15. Cox C. Examination of the cardiovascular system. Physical assessment for nurses. Oxford: Blackwell Publishing; 2004: 46–72.

16. Stevenson T. Achieving best practice in routine observation of hospital patients. Nurs Times 2004;100(30):34–5.

17. Boulanger C, Toghill M. How to measure and record vital signs to ensure detection of deteriorating pateints. Nurs Times 2009;105(47):10–12.

18. Harrison G et al. Combinations of early signs of critical illness predict in-hospital death—The SOCCER Study (signs of critical conditions and emergency responses). Resuscitation, 2006. 71(3):327–34.

19. O'Neill D, Le Grove A. Monitoring critically ill patients in accident and emergency. Nurs Times 2003;99(45):32–5. Online. www.nursingtimes.net.

20. Horswill MS et al. Detecting abnormal vital signs on six observation charts: An experimental comparison. 2010. Online. www.safetyandquality.gov.au/wp-content/uploads/2012/01/35983-DetectingAVS.pdf; accessed 25 Feb 2015.

21. NSW Health, Child Health Networks. Paediatric resuscitation reference chart 2012.

22. Joanna Briggs Institute. Vital signs—evidence-based practice information sheets for health professionals. Bad Practice 1999;3(3):1–6.

23. Timby B. Fundamental skills and concepts in patient care. 7th edn. Philadelphia: Lippincott Williams & Wilkins; 2002.

24. Padwal RS et al. The 2008 Canadian Hypertension Education Program recommendations for the management of hypertension: Part 1 – blood pressure measurement, diagnosis and assessment of risk. Can J Cardiol, 2008;24(6):455–63.

25. Frese EM, Fick A, Sadowsky HS. Blood pressure measurement guidelines for physical therapists. Cardiopul Phys Ther J, 2011;22(2):5–12.

26. Jevon P, Holmes J. Blood pressure measurement—part 3: lying and standing blood pressure. Nurs Times 2007;103(20):24. Online. www.nursingtimes.net.

27. Naschitz JE, Rosner I. Orthostatic hypotension: framework of the syndrome. Postgrad Med J, 2007;83(983):568–74.

28. Trim J. Blood pressure. Nurs Times 2005;101(2):32–3. Online. www.nursingtimes.net.

29. Higgins D. Patient assessment—part 5: measuring pulse. Nurs Times 2008;104(11):24–5. Online. www.nursingtimes.net.

30. Docherty B, Coote S. Monitoring the pulse as part of track and trigger. Nurs Times 2006;102(43):28–9. Online. www.nursingtimes.net.

31. Evans D, Hodgkinson B, Berry J. Vital signs in hospital patients: a systematic review. Int J Nurs Studies 2001;38(6):643–50.

32. Berman A, Snyder S, Kozier B et al. Kozier and Erb's techniques in clinical nursing. 5th edn. Prentice Hall; 2003.

33. Hodgetts TJ, Kenward G, Vlachonikolis IG et al. The identification of risk factors for cardiac arrest and formulation of activation criteria to alert a medical emergency team. Resuscitation 2002;54(2):125–31.

34. Benham L, Benbow H, Hansen C. The development of a respiratory assessment tool. Nurs Times 2003;99(23):52–5.

35. Scullion J. A proactive approach to asthma. Nurs Stand 2005;20(9):57–65.

36. Booker R. Best practice in the use of spirometry. Nurs Stand 2005;19(48):49–54.

37. Kay Sedlak S. Patient assessment. In: Newberry L, ed. Sheehy's emergency nursing. 5th edn. St Louis: Mosby; 2003:84–97.

38. Trim J. Monitoring temperature. Nurs Times 2005;101(20):30–1.

39. Barnason S, Williams J, Proehl J et al. Clinical practice guideline: Non-invasive temperature measurement in the emergency department, 2011, Emergency Nurses Association. Online. www.ena.org/practice-research/research/CPG/Documents/TemperatureMeasurementCPG.pdf; accessed 25 Feb 2015.

40. Fadzil FM, Choon D, Arumugam K. A comparative study on the accuracy of noninvasive thermometers. Aust Fam Phys, 2010; 39(4):237–9.

41. Rajee M, Sultana RV. NexTemp thermometer can be used interchangeably with tympanic or mercury thermometers for emergency department use. Emerg Med Australas 2006;18(3):245–51.

42. Sund-Levander M, Grodzinsky E. What is the evidence base for the assessment and evaluation of body temperature? Nurs Times 2010;106(1):10–13. Online. www.nursingtimes.net.

43. Onur OE, Guneysel H, Akoglu H et al. Oral, axillary, and tympanic temperature measurements in older and younger adults with or without fever. Euro J Emerg Med 2008;15(6):334–7.

44. Woodrow P. Pulse oximetry. Emerg Nurse 1999;7(5):34–9.

45. Thomas S, Silen W, Cheema F et al. Effects of morphine analgesia on diagnostic accuracy in Emergency Department patients with abdominal pain: a prospective, randomized trial. J Am Coll Surg, 2003;196(1):18–31.

46. Fairley D, Timothy J, Donaldson-Hugh M et al. Using a coma scale to assess patient consciousness levels. Nurs Times 2005; 101(25):38–41.

47. Teasdale G, Maas A. Lecky F et al. The Glasgow Coma Scale at 40 years: standing the test of time, The Lancet 2014;13(8):844–54.

48. Teasdale G, Jennett B. Assessment of coma and impaired consciousness: a practical scale. Lancet 1974;2(7872):81–4.

49. Middleton, P. M. (2012). Practical use of the Glasgow Coma Scale; a comprehensive narrative review of GCS methodology. Australasian Emergency Nursing Journal. 15;170–83.

50. Kelly AE. Relationships in emergency care: communication and impact. Top Emerg Med 2005;27(3):192–7.

51. Proehl JA. The Glasgow Coma Scale: do it and do it right. J Emerg Nurs 1992;18(5):421–3.

52. Gill MR, Reiley DG, Green SM. Interrater reliability of Glasgow Coma Scale scores in the emergency department. Ann Emerg Med 2004;43(2):215–23.

53. Hew R. Altered conscious state. In: Cameron P, Jelinek G, Kelly A et al. eds. Textbook of adult emergency medicine. 3rd edn. Sydney: Churchill Livingstone; 2009;386–91.

54. Waterhouse C. The Glasgow coma scale and other neurological observations. Nurs Stand 2005;19(33):56–64.

55. James HE, Ana NG, Perkins RM. Brain insults in infants and children: pathophysiology and management. Elsevier; 1985.

56. Waterhouse C. The use of painful stimulus in relation to Glasgow Coma Scale observations. British Journal of Neuroscience Nursing, 2009;5(5):209–15.

57. Jacques T et al. Signs of critical conditions and emergency responses (SOCCER): A model for predicting adverse events in the inpatient setting. Resuscitation, 2006. 69(2):175–83.

58. Cox CL. Respiratory assessment. In: Esmond G, ed. Respiratory nursing. London: Elsevier; 2003.

59. McGrath AN. Examination of the abdomen. In: Cox C (ed.), Physical assessment for nurses. Oxford: Blackwell Publishing; 2004:91–103.

60. Meldon S, Ma OJ, Woolard R. Geriatric emergency medicine. New York: McGraw-Hill; 2004.

61. Rudolf M, Malcolm I. Milestones that it is essential to memorise. In: Paediatrics and child health. London: Blackwell Science; 1999:42.

62. Grealy B, Chaboyer W. Essential nursing care of the critically ill patient. In: Elliot D, Aitken L, Chaboyer W, ACCCN's Critical care nursing. 2nd edn. Chatswood Australia. 2012.

63. O'Mara A. Communicating with other health care professionals in interpersonal relationships. In: Arnold E, Boggs K, eds. Interpersonal relationships. Philadelphia: WB Saunders; 1995.

64. Brereton ML. Communication in nursing: in theory–practice relationship. J Adv Nurs 1995;21(2):314–24.

65. Curtis K, Tzannes A, Rudge T. How to talk to doctors—A guide for effective communication. International Nursing Review 2011;58(1):13–20.

66. Iedema R. Communication, quality and safety. Health Care Advisory Council (HCAC) Newsletter issue 8, NSW Health 2009. Online. www.safetyandquality.gov.au/wp-content/uploads/2012/02/Final-Report-Patient-Clinician-Communication-Literature-Review-Feb-2013. pdf; accessed 25 Feb 2015.

67. Ellis RB, Gates RJ, Kenworthy N, eds. Interpersonal communication. In Nursing: theory and practice. 2nd edn. New York: Churchill Livingstone; 2003.

68. Watzlawick P, Beavin J, Jackson D. Pragmatics of human communication. New York: Norton; 1967.

69. Denzau AT, North DC. Shared mental models: ideologies and institutions. In: Lupia A, McCubbins MD, Popkin SL, eds. Elements of reason: cognition, choice, and the bounds of rationality. 1st edn. Cambridge: Cambridge University Press; 2000.

70. Hobgood C, Hevia A, Hinchey P. Profiles in patient safety: when an error occurs. Acad Emerg Med 2004;11(7):766–70.

71. Woloshynowych M, Davis R, Brown R et al. Communication patterns in a UK emergency department. Ann Emerg Med 2007;50(4):407–13.

72. Spencer R, Coiera E, Logan P. Variation in communication loads on clinical staff in the emergency department. Ann Emerg Med 2004;44(3):268–73.

73. Evans SM, Murray A, Patrick I et al. Assessing clinical handover between paramedics and the trauma team. Injury 2010;41(5):460–4.

74. Bost N, Crilly J, Wallis M et al. Clinical handover of patients arriving by ambulance to the emergency department—a literature review. Int Emerg Nurs 2010;18(4):210–20.

75. Porteous J, Stewart-Wynne EG, Connolly M et al. iSoBAR—a concept and handover checklist: the national clinical handover initiative. Med J Aust 2009;190(11):S152–6.

76. Christie P, Robinson H. Using a communication framework at handover to boost patient outcomes. Nurs Times 2009;105(47):13–15. Online. www.nursingtimes.net.

77. Owen C, Hemmings L, Brown T. Lost in translation: maximizing handover effectiveness between paramedics and receiving staff in the emergency department—original research. Emerg Med Australas 2009;21(2):102–7.

78. Cohen M, Hilligoss B. Handoffs in hospitals: a review of the literature on information exchange while transferring patient responsibility or control. Ann Arbor: University of Michigan, 2009.

79. Iedema R et al. Design and trial of a new ambulance-to-emergency department handover protocol: IMIST-AMBO. BMJ Qual Saf 2012;21:627–33.

80. Hunter New England NSW Health. ISBAR revisited: Identifying and Solving BARriers to effective clinical handover in inter-hospital transfer. Public report on pilot study for Australian Commission on Safety and Quality in Healthcare as part of the National Clinical Handover Initiative 2009. www.safetyandquality.gov.au/wp-content/uploads/2012/01/ISBAR-PSPR.pdf; acccessed 25 Feb 2015.

81. Wiman E, Wikblad K. Caring and uncaring encounters in nursing in an emergency department. J Clin Nurs 2004;13(4):422–9.

82. Mitchell M, Wilson D, Wade V. Psychosocial and cultural care of the critically ill. In: Elliot D, Aitken L, Cheboyer W eds. Critial care nursing. Sydney: Elsevier; 2006.

83. Studer Group. AIDET guidelines and keywords. 2013. https://az414866.vo.msecnd.net/cmsroot/studergroup/media/studergroup/pages/ what-we-do/learning-lab/aligned-behavior/must-haves/aidet/aidet_guidelines_and_key_words_aidet1.pdf?ext=.pdf'; accessed 25 Feb 2015.

84. Nussbaum GB. Spirituality in critical care: patient comfort and satisfaction. Crit Care Nurs Q 2003;26(3):214–20.

85. Narayanasamy A, Clissett P, Parumal L et al. Responses to the spiritual needs of older people. J Adv Nurs 2004;48(1):6–16.

86. Travaline JM. Communication in the ICU: an essential component of patient care; strategies for communicating with patients and their families. J Crit Illness 2002;17(11):451–6.

87. Gittelman MA, Mahabee-Gittens EM, Gonzalez-del-Rey J. Common medical terms defined by parents: are we speaking the same language? Pediatr Emerg Care 2004;20(11):754–8.

88. Hindle D, Braithwaite J, Iedema R et al. Patient safety: a review of key international enquiries. Sydney: NSW Clinical Excellence Commission; 2005.

89. Menadue J. Reforms in NSW to include case mix, three-year budgets and a metropolitan plan. Healthcover 2000;10(5):11–14.

90. Anderson MA, Tredway CA. Communication: an outcome of case management. Nurs Case Manag 1999;4(3):104–11.

91. Schoenbaum S. Implementation: it's the way care is organised that counts. J Qual Improv 2000;26(9):550–1.

92. Richardson DB. The access-block effect: relationship between delay to reaching an inpatient bed and inpatient length of stay. Med J Aust 2002;177(9):492–5.

93. Sprivulis PC, Da Silva JA, Jacobs IG et al. The association between hospital overcrowding and mortality among patients admitted via West Australian emergency departments. Med J Aust 2006;184(5):208–12.

94. Perry L. Critical incidents, crucial issues: insights into the working lives of registered nurses. J Clin Nurs 1997;6(2):131–7.

95. Curtis K. Current issues in trauma nursing, an Australian perspective. Nurs Stand 2001;16(9):33–8.

96. Sutton K. Registered nurse turnover. J Emerg Nurs 1999;25(4):313.

97. Erlen JA, Sereika SM. Critical care nurses, ethical decision-making and stress. J Adv Nurs 1997;26(5):953–61.

98. Kennedy JF, Trethewy C, Anderson K. Content analysis of Australian newspaper portrayals of emergency medicine. Emerg Med Australas 2006;18(2):118–24.

99. Watt D, Wertzler W, Brannan G. Patient expectations of emergency department care: phase I—a focus group study. CJEM 2005;7(1):12–16.

100. Saunders K. A creative new approach to patient satisfaction. Top Emerg Med 2005;27(4):256–7.

101. Taylor C, Benger JR. Patient satisfaction in emergency medicine. Emerg Med J 2004;21(5):528–32.

102. Maister, D.H. Psychology of waiting lines. 1985 http://davidmaister.com/wp-content/themes/davidmaister/pdf/PsycholgyofWaitingLines751.pdf; accessed 25 Feb 2015.

103. Nielsen D. Improving ED patient satisfaction when triage nurses routinely communicate with patients as to reasons for waits: one rural hospital's experience. J Emerg Nurs 2004;30(4):336–8.

104. Lee G, Endacott R, Flett K et al. Characteristics of patients who did not wait for treatment in the emergency department: a follow up survey. Accid Emerg Nurs 2006;14(1):56–62.

105. Clinical Practice Improvement Unit, Northern Sydney Health. Open Disclosure: Health Care Professional Handbook. Commonwealth of Australia. Online. www.safetyandquality.health.wa.gov.au/docs/open_disclosure/Open%20Disclosure%20Health%20Professionals%20Handbook.pdf; accessed 25 Feb 2015.

106. Brown R, Dunn S, Byrnes K et al. Doctors' stress responses and poor communication performance in simulated bad-news consultations. Acad Med 2009;84(11):1595–602.

107. Kamienski MC. Emergency: family-centered care in the ED. Am J Nurs 2004;104(1):59–62.

108. Leahey M, Wright L. Maximizing time, minimizing suffering: the 15-minute (or less) family interview. J Fam Nurs 1999;5(3):259–74.

109. Lee LY, Lau YL. Immediate needs of adult family members of adult intensive care patients in Hong Kong. J Clin Nurs 2003;12(4):490–500.

110. Institute for Family and Family-Centred Care. Frequently asked questions. What are the core concepts of family centered care? Online. www.ipfcc.org/faq.html: 25 Feb 2015.

111. Frank AW. Just listening: narrative and deep illness. Families, Systems and Health 1998;16(3):197–212.

112. Saunders K. A creative new approach to patient satisfaction. Top Emerg Med 2005, Oct–Dec;27(4):256–7.

113. NSW Health. NSW Health patient study 2008 statewide report. Sydney NSW Health; 2009.

114. Ball L. Setting the scene for the paramedic in primary care: a review of the literature. Emerg Med J 2005;22(12):896–900.

115. Lowery K, Stokes MA. Role of peer support and emotional expression on posttraumatic stress disorder in student paramedics. J Trauma Stress 2005;18(2):171–9.

116. Bennett P, Williams Y, Page N et al. Levels of mental health problems amongst UK emergency ambulance workers. Emerg Med J 2004;21(2):235–6.

117. Stockbridge J. Care for the carers. Emerg Nurse 2004;12(7):10–11.

118. Healy S, Tyrrell M. Stress in emergency departments: experiences of nurses and doctors. Emergency Nurse 2011;19(4):31–7.

119. Duffield CM, Roche MA, O'Brien-Pallas L et al. Glueing it together: nurses, their work environment and patient safety. Sydney: Centre for Health Services Management, UTS; 2007:1–243.

120. Barkway P. Stress and adaptation. In: Brown H, Edwards D, eds. Lewis's medical-surgical nursing. Sydney: Elsevier; 2005.

121. Ball J, Dixon M, Dolan B et al. Why are we waiting? Emerg Nurse 2000;8(1):22–7, 173–80.

122. Griffin-Heslin VL. An analysis of the concept dignity. Accid Emerg Nurs 2005;13(4):251–7.

123. Hernandez EV, Mannis MJ. Superficial keratopathy in intensive care unit patients. Am J Ophthalmol 1997;124(2):212–16.

124. Joyce N. Eye care for the intensive care patient. Adelaide: Joanna Briggs Institute for Evidence Based Nursing and Midwifery; 2002.

125. Miller M, Kearney N. Oral care of patients with cancer: a review of the literature. Cancer Nurs 2001;24(4):241–54.

126. Buglass EA. Oral hygiene. Br J Nurs 1995;4(9):516–19.

127. Grap MJ, Munro CL, Ashtiani B et al. Oral care interventions in critical care: frequency and documentation. Am J Crit Care 2003;12(2):113–18.

128. Kite K, Pearson L. A rationale for mouth care: the integration of theory with practice. Intensive Crit Care Nurs 1995;11(2):71–6.

129. O'Reilly M. Oral care of the critically ill: a review of the literature and guidelines for practice. Aust Crit Care 2003;16(3):101–10.

130. Krishnagopalan S, Johnson EW, Low LL et al. Body positioning of intensive care patients: clinical practice versus standards. Crit Care Med 2002;30(11):2588–92.

131. Drakulovic MB, Torres A, Bauer TT et al. Supine body position as a risk factor for nosocomial pneumonia in mechanically ventilated patients: a randomised trial. Lancet 1999;354(9193):1851–8.

132. Miles S, Nowicki T et al. Repositioning to prevent pressure injuries: evidence for procatice. Aust Nurs Midw J 2013;21(6):32–33.

133. Todres L, Fulbrook P, Albarran J. On the receiving end: a hermeneutic-phenomenological analysis of a patient's struggle to cope while going through intensive care. Nurs Crit Care 2000;5(6):277–87.

134. Berenholtz SM, Dorman T, Ngo K et al. Qualitative review of intensive care unit quality indicators. J Crit Care 2002;17(1):12–15.

135. Adam S, Forrest S. ABC of intensive care: other supportive care. Br Med J 1999;319(7203):175–8.

136. Boyle M, Green M. Pressure sores in intensive care: defining their incidence and associated factors and assessing the utility of two pressure sore risk assessment tools. Aust Crit Care 2001;14(1):24–30.

137. Yates P. Inflammation, infection and healing. In: Brown H, Edwards D, eds. Lewis's medical-surgical nursing. Sydney: Elsevier; 2005.

138. Lewis SM, Collier IC, Heitkemper MM et al, eds. Medical-surgical nursing: assessment and management of clinical problems. 7th edn. St Louis: Mosby; 2007.

139. Weststrate J, Heule F. Prevalence of PU, risk factors and use of pressure-relieving mattresses in ICU patients. Connect Crit Care Nurs Eur 2001;1(3):77–82.

140. Carlson EV, Kemp MG, Shott S. Predicting the risk of pressure ulcers in critically ill patients. Am J Crit Care 1999;8(4):262–9.

141. Tannen A, Balzer K et al. Diagnostic accuracy of two pressure ulcer risk scales and a generic nursing assessment tool. A psychometric comparison. J Clin Nurs 2010;19(11–12):1510–18.

142. Fulbrook P, Grealy B. Essential nursing care of the critically ill patient. In: Elliot D, Aitken L, Cheboyer W, eds. ACCCN Critical care nursing. Sydney: Elsevier; 2006.

143. Loan T. Metabolic responses. In: Kidd PS, Wagner KD, eds. High acuity nursing. 2nd edn. Stamford: Appleton & Lange; 1997.

144. Brogden BJ. Clinical skills: importance of nutrition for acutely ill hospital patients. Br J Nurs 2004;13(15):914–20.

145. Casey G. Nutritional support in wound healing. Nurs Stand 2003;17(23):55–8.

146. Fox VJ, Miller J, McClung M. Nutritional support in the critically injured. Crit Care Nurs Clin North Am 2004;16(4):559–69.

147. Heersink, JT, Brown CJ, Dimaria-Ghalili RA et al. Undernutrition in hospitalized older adults: patterns and correlates, outcomes, and opportunities for intervention with a focus on processes of care. J Nutr Elder 2010;29(1):4–41.

148. Posthauer ME. The role of nutrition in wound care. Adv Skin Wound Care 2006;19(1):43–52.

149. Holmes S. Undernutrition in hospital patients. Nurs Stand 2003;17(19):45–52.

150. Young A. Hospital food trial addresses malnutrition in patients. ABC AM radio transcript, 27 May 2010, 09:18:54. Online. www.abc.net.au/am/content/2010/s2910630.htm; accessed 25 Feb 2015.

151. Kruizenga HM, Van Tulder MW, Seidell JC et al. Effectiveness and cost-effectiveness of early screening and treatment of malnourished patients. Am J Clin Nutr 2005;82(5):1082–9.

152. Genton L, Romand JA, Pichard C. Basics in clinical nutrition: nutritional support in trauma. e-SPEN J 2010;5(2).

153. Banks M, Bauer J, Graves N et al. Malnutrition and pressure ulcer risk in adults in Australian health care facilities. Nutrition 2010;26(9):896–901.

154. Rodriguez L. Nutritional status: assessing and understanding its value in the critical care setting. Crit Care Nurs Clin North Am 2004;16(4):509–14.

155. Beck AM, Balknas UN, Furst P et al. Council of Europe (the committee of experts on nutrition, food safety and consumer health of the partial agreement in the social and public health field). Food and nutritional care in hospitals: how to prevent undernutrition—report and guidelines from the Council of Europe. Clin Nutr 2001;20(5):455–60.

156. Devlin M. The nutritional needs of the older person. Prof Nurse 2000;16(3):951–5.

157. Bonner A. Renal and urological problems. In: Brown H, Edwards D, editors. Lewis's medical-surgical nursing. Sydney: Elsevier; 2005.

158. Thorpe D, Harrison L. Bowel management: development of guidelines. Connect Crit Care Nurs Eur 2002;2(2):61–6.

159. Hill S, Anderson J, Baker K et al. Management of constipation in the critically ill patient. Nurs Crit Care 1998;3(3):134–7.

CHAPTER 15
RESUSCITATION

JULIE CONSIDINE AND RAMON Z SHABAN

Essentials

- Prevention of cardiac arrest will save more lives than even the best resuscitation: early recognition and treatment of the deteriorating patient is vital.
- Coronary perfusion pressure has a direct relationship with successful resuscitation; the best way to optimise coronary perfusion pressure and therefore chance of survival is to provide effective, uninterrupted chest compressions.
- Attempts at endotracheal intubation should not interrupt chest compressions for more than 15–20 seconds.
- The time between stopping chest compressions and starting defibrillation should be as short as possible; compressions should continue until the time of defibrillation.
- Chest compressions should recommence immediately following defibrillation, irrespective of electrical success.
- Inadequate compression depth, overventilation and excessive interruptions to chest compressions are ongoing problems in resuscitation, even for experienced healthcare professionals.
- There is no evidence that medications improve long-term survival following cardiac arrest: defibrillation, oxygenation and ventilation always take priority over drug administration.
- There is good evidence that therapeutic hypothermia following successful resuscitation improves neurological outcomes of survivors; therapeutic hypothermia should be a routine part of post-arrest care.

INTRODUCTION

In this chapter, an overview of the principles of the resuscitation of adults and children will be discussed However, resuscitation of the newly born infant is beyond the scope of this chapter; sepsis, respiratory and cardiac illness are discussed in Chapter 36. The importance of effective recognition of, and response to, deteriorating patients will be highlighted and a summary of the evidence related to predictors of mortality is provided. Non-clinical issues, such as communication, teamwork and leadership are considered, before the major chapter content on Basic and Advanced Life Support (ALS).

It is important to consider different causes of cardiac arrests. Ventricular fibrillation (VF) is the most common primary rhythm in sudden cardiac arrest in adults and the majority of patients who survive have had a primary VF arrest.[1] This means that the focus of resuscitation in adults is early defibrillation.[1] In children, the primary cause of cardiac arrest is hypoxaemia or hypotension (or a combination of both), and the most common cardiac rhythm is a severe bradycardia or asystole.[2] This means that the focus of ALS in paediatric patients is to restore oxygenation and circulating volume. VF is uncommon in children but may be seen in children with congenital cardiac conditions or as a consequence of poisonings.[2] The anatomy and physiology relevant to cardiac arrest and resuscitation in adults are given in Chapter 22. The major anatomical and physiological considerations for resuscitation in children are detailed in Chapter 36, and those for resuscitation of the elderly are detailed in Chapter 39.

Basic Life Support (BLS) is the preservation or restoration of life by establishing and maintaining airway, breathing and circulation without the need for adjunctive equipment (although use of an Automated External Defibrillator (AED) is commonly accepted as part of BLS in many protocols).[3] Effective BLS may increase the likelihood of successful defibrillation and may enable time to detect and correct reversible causes of cardiac arrest.[3] Advanced Life Support (ALS) is BLS with the addition of invasive techniques, such as emergency defibrillation, advanced airway management, vascular access and administration of drugs.[3] In this chapter, both BLS and ALS are detailed, primarily referenced to the Australian Resuscitation Council guidelines, which are freely available at www.resus.org.au. In addition, an evidence-based approach to prevention of cardiac arrest, post-arrest care and care of families of patients suffering cardiac arrest is also provided.

Identification of and response to the deteriorating patient

It is well documented that if the deteriorating patient is allowed to progress to cardiac arrest, mortality rates increase dramatically. Patient assessment is one of the most important elements of emergency nursing and pre-hospital care as decisions are based on patient assessment findings. Research supports the use of physiological criteria as a basis for clinical decisions. There is clear evidence that the majority of patients exhibit physiological abnormalities in the hours preceding cardiac arrest.[4–11] The primary survey approach is advocated by emergency care personnel as a structured approach to patient assessment, particularly in the critically ill or injured patient.[12,13] The primary survey is defined as the systematic assessment of airway, breathing, circulation and conscious state, and aims to identify and correct life-threatening conditions.[14] A more detailed discussion of patient assessment is given in Chapter 14.

Predictors of mortality

It has been well documented for over 20 years that early recognition and appropriate management of physiological abnormalities or clinical instability is a major factor in preventing mortality and morbidity,[6,7,15–22] and that most adverse events in healthcare (cardiac arrest, unplanned intensive care unit (ICU) admission and mortality) are predictable.[13,23] There is a known association between abnormal vital signs and mortality,[24,25] and over 60% of patients who suffer an in-hospital cardiac arrest have documentation of physiological abnormalities, biochemical deterioration or new symptoms.[26]

There is a clear relationship between respiratory dysfunction and in-hospital adverse events,[27–29] and respiratory rate abnormalities have been linked with increased in-hospital mortality rates and an increased risk of unplanned ICU admission in ED patients.[23,30,31] Respiratory rate abnormality is a more accurate predictor of serious illness than any other vital sign change,[29,31] and tachypnoea is highly predictive of serious adverse events.[25,27,29,31–33] Respiratory rate abnormalities have been found to increase the odds of in-patient death in non-surgical ED patients by a factor of 5,[30] and in emergency department (ED) patients, respiratory rate abnormality at first ED nursing assessment increased the odds of critical care admission by a factor of 1.6.[23] It is important to note that a respiratory rate of > 27/minute was shown to be an *independent predictor* of cardiac arrest (OR = 5.6) while in the same study, pulse rate and blood pressure were *not predictive* of cardiac arrest.[32] Tachypnoea has a 95% specificity for adverse events, such as cardiac arrest or unplanned ICU admission,[28,29] and numerous studies have shown that there is an increased risk of serious illness in adults with a respiratory rate > 24/min.[25,29,33,34]

Heart rate abnormalities have been implicated in adverse events by a number of researchers. Abnormal pulse rate was a significant risk factor for cardiac arrest (present in 79.1% of cardiac arrest patients versus 38.6% of controls, $p<0.001$) and abnormal pulse rate increased the odds of cardiac arrest by a factor of 4.07 (95% CI: 2.0–8.31).[33] In the ED context, heart rate abnormalities at triage and first nursing assessment were also associated with increased odds of critical care admission,[23] and abnormal heart rate in ED patients increased odds of in-hospital mortality in ED patients by a factor of 2.5.[30]

Hypotension has a well-known association with poor outcomes. Reduced systolic blood pressure (SBP) was found to be a significant risk factor for cardiac arrest (present in 86.0% of cardiac arrest patients versus 22.7% of controls, $p<0.001$) and increased the odds of cardiac arrest by a factor of 19.9 (95% CI: 9.5–41.8).[33] In addition, as many as 52% of patients with abnormal vital signs prior to cardiac arrest had SBP < 90 mmHg.[35] Episode(s) of hypotension (SBP < 100 mmHg) in a pre-hospital environment increased in-hospital mortality by more than 25%.[36] Patients who had experienced hypotension (SBP < 100 mmHg) in the ED accounted for more than 2.5 times in-hospital mortality and ten times higher incidence of sudden and unexpected death.[37] Hypotension is a predictor of in-hospital mortality in patients successfully resuscitated from cardiac arrest.[38]

Altered conscious state is a recurrent finding preceding adverse events: as many as 42% of patients have a decreased conscious state prior to cardiac arrest and the mortality rate in patients with altered conscious state prior to adverse events is greater than 50%.[26] Abnormal temperature was found to be a significant risk factor for cardiac arrest (present in 47.2% of cardiac arrest patients versus 23.1% of controls, $p<0.001$) and increased the odds of cardiac arrest by a factor of 3.00 (95% CI: 1.6–5.5).[33] In ED patients, abnormal temperature on ED arrival (at triage) increased the odds of critical care admission almost three-fold.[23] In non-surgical ED patients, temperature abnormalities increased the odds of in-hospital mortality by a factor of 2.5,[39] and ED patients admitted to ICU had significantly lower mean temperatures than those admitted to the general wards.[40]

Systems approach to deteriorating patients

There is clear evidence that early recognition of, and response to, deteriorating patients, prevention of cardiac arrest and ensuring critically ill patients have access to expert care saves lives.[41,42] The decisions that paramedics and emergency nurses make when faced with a patient suffering cardiac arrest or critical illness impact on patient outcomes. The notion of cardiac arrest centres which specialise in evidence-based post cardiac arrest care is gaining momentum both in Australia and overseas.[43] It is well known that regional systems of care have improved outcomes for patients suffering major trauma, stroke and acute coronary syndrome, and there is clear evidence that hospital factors, such as hospital size and interventional cardiac care capabilities, influence patient outcomes, specifically mortality.[43] The Australian Resuscitation Council recognises that it may be reasonable for patients suffering cardiac arrest or ST elevation myocardial infarction to be transferred directly to centres with primary percutaneous coronary intervention capability, even if that means bypassing other hospitals with less cardiac care capability.[44]

In the hospital setting, rapid response teams (RRTs) facilitate early recognition of, and response to, deteriorating ward patients.[41] Any member of hospital staff can activate RRS, guided by objective calling criteria and, once activated, an organisational response is triggered where a team of experts in the management of critically ill patients provides assessment and management at the point of care.[41,45] RRS evolved from cardiac arrest teams where an organisational response was triggered by cardiac arrest (unresponsiveness, apnoea or pulselessness).[41] In Australia, the most common model of RRS is the Medical Emergency Team (MET), which functions in parallel with the cardiac arrest team and is activated for patients who have not yet suffered cardiac arrest but have respiratory, cardiovascular or neurological deterioration.[41]

Despite decades of research showing positive outcomes of RRTs in general ward areas,[46–49] there has not been widespread use of RRT in Australian EDs,[45,50] and recognising and responding to deteriorating patients in the ED remains largely clinician dependent.[51,52] Based on the small amount of ED-specific literature regarding deteriorating patients published to date, two simple but important strategies should be considered by emergency nurses to improve the recognition of, and response to, deteriorating ED patients. First, there should be a clear and objective definition of clinical deterioration to enable increased recognition of physiological abnormalities, minimise decision bias and assist clinicians to differentiate between normal and abnormal clinical signs in a busy environment and in specific patient populations such as children.[45,50,51] Second, escalation protocols will enable a consistent response to patients with abnormal physiological parameters, ensure early involvement of senior decision makers and minimise failure of reporting which may result from decision error, authority gradients, decision biases or communication failures.[45,53,54]

There are specific features of the ED context that increase the risk of unrecognised and unreported deterioration and the ideal response to deteriorating ED patients is unknown. For many deteriorating patients, the ED response will be appropriate, albeit ad hoc. However, the advantages of a structured and consistent approach to escalation of care include further development of already positive multidisciplinary relationships, enhanced inter-professional communication and increased patient safety.[45] A systematic approach to recognising

and responding to deterioration has improved outcomes in hospitalised ward patients and there is emerging evidence that mortality in ED patients can be predicted. A organised approach to recognising and responding to deteriorating ED patients is a logical progression and builds on other patient safety systems, such as triage and systematic approaches to ED care of critically ill or injured patients.[45]

> **PRACTICE TIP**
> ## RECOGNISING AND RESPONDING TO DETERIORATING PATIENTS
>
> One of the key strategies to improving patient outcomes from cardiac arrest is to prevent cardiac arrest by timely recognition of, and response to, clinical deterioration. All clinicians should understand the mechanisms and processes for escalating care of a deteriorating patient related to their specific area of practice and work environment.

Shock states

In general terms, shock is defined as failure of the circulatory system to adequately perfuse organs and peripheral tissue.[55] It is a condition of severe haemodynamic and metabolic disturbance resulting in an imbalance between the supply and demand of oxygen at the cellular level.[56] At the cellular level, shock is a secondary physiological response to injury, resulting in an imbalance between the supply and demand of oxygen. It precipitates anaerobic respiration and cellular hypoxia. Injury may take many forms, such as trauma, blood loss, heart disease, burns, poisoning and infection, all of which have particular consequence for physiology of the body at the cellular level. They may be acute or chronic, communicable or non-communicable, or a combination of any of these. As these injuries events unfold, compensatory mechanisms are implemented to ameliorate the effect, which are the first indicators or sign of the need for resuscitation.

There are four broad categories and types of shock:[56]

- *Cardiogenic shock* is associated with cellular injury of the heart and its related structures, and results in a failure of cardiac function. Common causes of cardiogenic shock include myocardial infarction, cardiomyopathy, valve disease or trauma of anatomical rupture. If unmanaged, the heart progressively decompensates, leading to cardiac failure.

- *Hypovolaemic shock*, as the name implies, results from a loss of blood or extracellular fluid, typically from haemorrhage, burns or, in extreme cases, vomiting and diarrhoea.

- *Obstructive shock* occurs when blockages or disruptions of systemic, pulmonary or coronary circulation interfere with cardiac output, as would occur during cardiac tamponade, pulmonary embolism or dissecting aortic aneurysm.

- The fourth category, *distributive shock*, occurs because of a shift of fluid into the peripheral vasculature, where an increase in extravascular spaces results in pooling of fluid, resulting in hypotension and poor tissue perfusion.

Distributive shock may be anaphylactic, septic or neurogenic in nature.[56,57]

Collectively, all types of shock result in a cellular hypoxia, anaerobic metabolism and respiration, an ultimately irreversible cell injury.[57] For resuscitation to be successful, it is imperative to treat the precipitating injury. Failure to stop uncontrolled haemorrhage in haemorrhagic shock, or untreated anaphylaxis in distributive shock, will render resuscitative efforts futile. Preventing deterioration of the patient which would otherwise result in aggressive resuscitation is the priority in emergency trauma and care.

PRACTICE TIP
EARLY RECOGNITION OF SHOCK

- Tachycardia[58]
  - <1 yr >160
  - 1–2 yr >150
  - 2–5 yr >140
  - 5–12 yr >120
  - >12 yr >100
- Diminished capillary refill
- Cool, clammy skin
- Cutaneous vasoconstriction
- Tachypnoea
- Thirst, nausea, abdominal pain
- Altered levels of consciousness
- Decreased urine output
- Dilated pupils (late sign)
- Decreased heart rate (late sign)

Effective communication

One of the most important elements of communication in healthcare is clinical deterioration prior to cardiac arrest and should include information about the patient's current state and perceived future events.[59] A possible strategy for improving information transfer is the use of standardised systems for communication.[59] Advantages of standardised communication systems and using a predetermined structure are a decrease in omission of important information and also clear expectations about the order in which information will be conveyed.[59]

PRACTICE TIP
EFFECTIVE COMMUNICATION

An example of a structured approach to communication is the situational briefing tool ISBAR, which stands for:[59,60]

Identify
Situation
Background
Assessment
Recommendation.

Studies of interprofessional communication comparing standard information transfer with communication using ISBAR showed that the content and clarity of communication was higher when ISBAR was used, and that use of a structured method improved communication during telephone referral in a simulated clinical setting.[60]

Another effective communication strategy for when crises are evolving or when there is a need to rapidly communicate concern is *critical assertiveness*, also known as *graded assertiveness*. Critical assertiveness is assertive communication aimed at preventing adverse events, and encourages challenge and then escalation or assertion.[54] The initial challenge may be framed as a question: 'Are you sure we should be …?', and this is a particularly useful strategy when questioning figures of authority. Escalation and assertion should be polite and professional but also draw attention to concern, using phrases such as 'I'm uncomfortable', 'I'm worried', 'I'm concerned'.[54] Critical assertiveness focuses on patient wellbeing as a central common interest rather than the merit of individual judgements or actions.[54]

ED and pre-hospital environments are complex and dynamic working environments prone to crises. A crisis is a situation that engenders a serious threat to patient safety and which is unable to be solved by knowledge alone.[61] The need for a standardised approach to communication has been long recognised by other high-risk industries, particularly the aviation industry. Many years of research into airline disasters demonstrated a lack of skills in managing rapidly developing complex situations, so the simulation-based curriculum to teach teamwork and leadership skills called Crew Resource Management (CRM) was developed. It is now a standard requirement in the airline industry. In the late 1980s the principles of CRM were adapted for use in anaesthetics and have since also been applied in emergency medicine.

These are the principles of emergency medicine CRM:[61]

- Know your team and your environment.
- Anticipate and plan.
- Allocate attention wisely.
- Use all available information and confirm it.
- Use cognitive aids (e.g. checklists).
- Take a leadership role.
- Call for help early.
- Communicate effectively.
- Distribute the workload.
- Mobilise and use all available resources.

Teamwork and leadership

Resuscitation in both pre-hospital and hospital environments can involve a single responder or a large team. The effectiveness of resuscitation is often determined, to some degree, by the effectiveness of team functioning. The identification of a team leader is regarded as one of the most important determinants of successful resuscitation; often the team leader will, by default, be the first member of staff who discovers the patient in cardiac arrest. The team leader role may be passed on as more-experienced staff arrive, but it is important to make sure that there is *one* person clearly identified as the team leader at all times. All orders/requests coming from other personnel should be directed to the team leader, and staff involved in the resuscitation should only accept orders/requests from the team leader.

It is also important that the team leader communicates effectively with the team. Orders should be stated loudly and clearly and should be directed to the individual expected to carry out the order, not simply announced into the room. As tasks are completed they should be announced loudly and clearly, for example, '1 mg adrenaline given IV' to ensure that all members of the team are aware of what is happening, duplication of tasks is avoided and the 'scribe' or note-taker is assisted in keeping accurate records.

Basic life support

There are varying statistics relating to survival following cardiac arrest as different states have published varying degrees of detail. In Australia, Ambulance Victoria data suggests that survival to hospital following out-of-hospital cardiac arrest is 36% and survival to hospital discharge is 11.8%.[62] Cardiac arrest from shockable rhythm was associated with higher survival-to-hospital rates (57% vs 24%) and survival-to-hospital discharge rates (28% vs 3.1%) than cardiac arrests caused by non-shockable rhythms.[62] Australian data from Brisbane regarding outcomes from in-hospital cardiac arrest suggest approximately 58% of patients achieve return of spontaneous circulation (ROSC) and 36% survive to hospital discharge however, the neurological status of survivors is not well documented.[63] Analysis of in-hospital cardiac arrest outcomes (2000–09) in the US has shown significant improvement in ROSC (42.7% vs 54.1%, $p<0.001$) and survival to hospital discharge rates (13.7% vs 22.3%) after adjustment for trends in patient and hospital characteristics.[64] Further, rates of clinically significant disability in cardiac arrest survivors have decreased from 32.9% in 2000 to 28.1% in 2009 ($p=0.02$).[64]

In all emergency situations, irrespective of whether the event occurs in the pre-hospital setting or hospital environment, the priorities in an emergency are to:[65]

- quickly assess the situation
- ensure safety for personnel, patient and bystanders
- send for help
- commence BLS.

PRACTICE TIP

PRIORITIES IN RESUSCITATION

During any resuscitation it is important that:[66–68]

- interruptions to cardiopulmonary resuscitation (CPR) are minimised
- hyperventilation and overventilation are avoided
- attempts to secure the airway should not delay CPR for more than 20 seconds
- intravenous (IV) access should be obtained.

It is also important to consider reversible causes of cardiac arrest; and if present, attempts should be made to correct these causes. To remember these causes, think of the '4 Hs' and '4 Ts' (Box 15.1).[68]

Patients who are most likely to survive a cardiac arrest with intact neurological function are patients who:[3]

- have a witnessed arrest

BOX 15.1 Reversible causes of cardiac arrest—the '4 Hs' and the '4 Ts'

- Hypoxaemia
- Hypovolaemia
- Hypo- or hyperthermia
- Hypo- or hyperkalaemia
- Tamponade: pericardial
- Tension pneumothorax
- Toxins/poisons/drugs
- Thrombosis: pulmonary or coronary

- receive immediate BLS
- whose cardiac rhythm is VF or VT (ventricular tachycardia)
- receive early defibrillation.

Danger

There are many actual and potential sources of danger, both for you and for your patient. Your safety is paramount; there is absolutely no point in putting your safety at risk. Sources of danger may include patients who have suffered cardiac arrest as a result of electrocution, so the power should be turned off before touching the patient.[69] In the context of road trauma, both the patient and health care personnel should be safe from other vehicles, fire and fuel spills.[65] When working in confined spaces, toxic fumes, exposure to carbon monoxide gas and risk of a low oxygen environment should be considered.[69] In mass casualty incidents or events with possibility of terrorism, second wave attacks should be considered.[69]

Response

Unconsciousness or unresponsiveness may be caused by lack of cerebral circulation, lack of cerebral oxygenation, metabolic problems (such as hypoglycaemia, diabetic emergencies) or central nervous system problems (such as head injury, stroke and tumour). When assessing response, clinicians should assess for responsiveness and breathing. If the patient is unresponsive and not breathing normally, resuscitation is required.

Send for help

Calling for help will be different depending on the context of practice, but examples of common methods of requesting assistance include calling for colleagues with additional training or more experience, calling an ambulance via 000, using emergency buzzers, or activation of a Medical Emergency or Cardiac Arrest (Code Blue) team. In the pre-hospital setting, a 'phone first' approach is recommended because the majority of cardiac arrests are due to ventricular fibrillation and outcomes are improved when time to defibrillation is minimised.[65,66] In children or cardiac arrest due to airway or ventilation issues (drug overdose, drowning), there may be some benefit in commencing resuscitation prior to calling for help, so the 'phone fast' approach is recommended.

Airway

In an unconscious patient there is a major risk of death from airway obstruction as the tongue falls against the back of the throat when in a supine position. Airway obstruction may also occur from aspiration of foreign material in the airway, such as blood, vomit or food.[70]

In unconscious patients the airway always takes precedence over other injuries, including potential spinal injuries.[65,71] Risk factors for cervical spine injury and cervical spine immobilisation are detailed in Chapter 49. Chapter 17 details procedures for cervical spine immobilisation (pp. 323–325).

When assessing the airway, there is no need to routinely roll the patient on their side.[70] Loose dentures should be removed, but well-fitting dentures can be left in place.[70] The mouth should be opened and inspected for obvious foreign material:[70] if foreign material is clearly visible, suction should be used to clear the oral cavity and oropharynx. If breathing commences, the patient should be placed on their side and monitored.[70]

Airway management is required when the patient is unconscious, has an obstructed airway or needs rescue breathing. The most common technique to establish/ensure a patent airway in adults is the backward head tilt with chin lift.[70] When using head tilt, do not use excessive force, particularly if neck injury is suspected. Chin lift facilitates airway patency by opening the mouth and pulling the tongue and soft tissues away from the back of the throat.[70]

Children should be managed in a similar manner to adults (as above).[70] In infants, the airway is easily obstructed because of the narrow diameters of nasal passages, vocal cords and trachea, and also their soft and pliable trachea may be compressed by excessive backwards head tilt.[70] In infants under 1 year,[72] a neutral head position should be used and the lower jaw should be supported at the chin with the mouth open. If these manoeuvres do not provide a clear airway, slight backwards tilt to the head may be applied.[70]

In patients with suspected cervical spine injury, jaw thrust is a preferable method of opening the airway.[70]

Foreign-body airway obstruction (choking)

Foreign body airway obstruction is a life-threatening condition.[70] Foreign body airway obstruction may be caused by relaxation of airway muscles in an unconscious patient, inhalation of a foreign body, trauma or injury involving the face/airway or anaphylaxis.[70]

Signs and symptoms will depend on the cause and severity of obstruction (partial or complete). Table 15.1 shows the signs of partial and complete airway obstruction. Airway obstruction may not be obvious until you attempt rescue breathing or bag–valve–mask ventilation.

TABLE 15.1 Signs of airway obstruction

PARTIAL AIRWAY OBSTRUCTION	COMPLETE AIRWAY OBSTRUCTION
Laboured breathing	There may be efforts at breathing
Noisy breathing, e.g. stridor, snoring	There are no sounds associated with breathing
Some escape of air felt at the mouth	There is no escape of air from the nose or mouth

Assessment of a cough is a useful way to assess severity of airway obstruction.[70] In mild airway obstruction with an effective cough, the patient should be encouraged to cough and be monitored for recovery or deterioration. If the patient has severe airway obstruction with an ineffective cough, then management will depend on whether the patient is conscious or unconscious. The conscious patient should be given up to five back blows and if that is not effective then up to five chest thrusts may be attempted. Abdominal compression (e.g. Heimlich Manoeuvre) is not recommended as there have been a number of reports of life-threatening complications from this procedure.[70] BLS should be commenced in the unconscious patient. Figure 15.1 shows the ARC flow chart for management of foreign body airway obstruction.[70]

Breathing

Breathing may be absent or ineffective due to upper airway obstruction, damage to the respiratory centre in the brain, paralysis of nerves and/or muscles of respiration, lung dysfunction or immersion.[73] Breathing may be assessed by the 'look, listen, feel' approach: look for chest rise and fall, listen for breath sounds and feel for movement of the chest and upper abdomen: chest movement does not necessarily guarantee a patent airway.[73] It is important to remember that complete absence of breathing is no longer a prerequisite for cardiac arrest and the need for BLS.

Cardiopulmonary resuscitation is indicated in patients who are unresponsive and not breathing normally after the airway has been opened and cleared. Chest compressions should be commenced, followed by rescue breathing.[73] Options for rescue breathing in the pre-hospital environment are mouth-to-mouth, mouth-to-nose or mouth-to-mask rescue breathing.[73] If the chest does not rise, consider airway obstruction, insufficient tidal volume, inadequate seal or air leak. It is important to promote to lay rescuers that if they are unwilling or unable to perform rescue breaths, they should do continuous chest compressions.[66,73,74]

Compressions

Resuscitation should be commenced if the patient is unresponsive and not breathing normally.[74] Palpation of a pulse is unreliable, and should not be performed to confirm the need for resuscitation by either lay rescuers or care professionals.[74,75]

To commence chest compressions in all age groups, the lower half of the sternum should be located visually (this generally equates to the centre of the chest).[74] There is no need to measure using methods such as the caliper method, as this delays chest compression. The chest should be compressed one-third of the depth of the chest[74] (in most adults this will be 4–5 cm). The compression rate is 100 per minute for all ages (almost 2 compressions/second), but it is important to note that 100 compressions will not be delivered in 1 minute because of interruptions for breaths. In adults and children, the heels of both hands should be used; in infants, a two-finger/two-thumb technique is recommended. It is vital that personnel performing chest compressions allow complete recoil of the chest after each compression.[74]

Cardiopulmonary resuscitation

The fundamental aim of CPR (chest compressions combined with rescue breathing) is to preserve brain function until

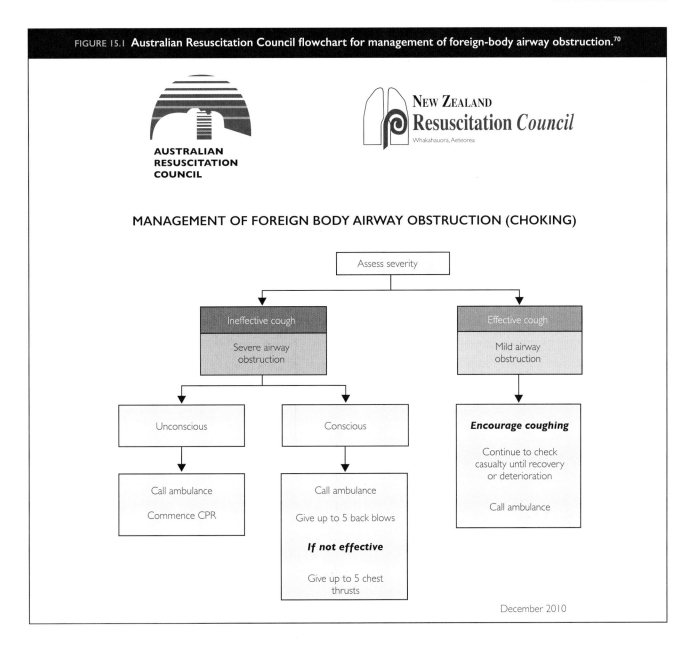

FIGURE 15.1 Australian Resuscitation Council flowchart for management of foreign-body airway obstruction.[70]

definitive treatment of cardiac arrest. CPR should be commenced in patients who are unresponsive and not breathing normally.[66] There is no evidence about optimal compression–ventilation ratios from human studies; however, current guidelines recommend a compression to ventilation ratio of 30:2 in all age groups and irrespective of the number of rescuers, and that compressions are paused for ventilation.[66] The 30:2 compression to ventilation ratio was selected to increase the number of compressions, minimise interruptions to compressions, prevent excessive ventilation, simplify teaching, maximise skill retention and maintain consistency with other international guidelines.[66]

Although many healthcare professionals regard themselves as skilled in BLS, research has consistently shown that even in healthcare professionals, inadequate compression depth, overventilation and excessive interruptions to chest compressions are ongoing problems.[3]

PRACTICE TIP

BASIC LIFE SUPPORT

The ARC recommends using a DRS-ABCD sequence for resuscitation:[3]

- check for **D**anger
- assess **R**esponse: is the patient unresponsive?
- **S**end for help
- open the **A**irway
- check **B**reathing: is the patient not breathing normally?
- commence 30 chest **C**ompressions followed by 2 breaths
- attach an Automatic External Defibrillator (AED) and provide **D**efibrillation if indicated.

Figure 15.2 shows the ARC flowchart for BLS.

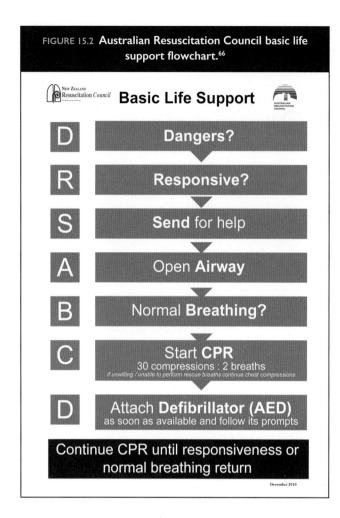

FIGURE 15.2 Australian Resuscitation Council basic life support flowchart.[66]

Resuscitation science: rationale for current recommendations

Current evidence suggests that ventilation is less important in the first 5 minutes of cardiac arrest because during this time, uninterrupted chest compressions are of paramount importance. In adults with primary cardiac arrest, arterial blood oxygenation is usually normal at the time of cardiac arrest.[76] Therefore, the blood flowing through the pulmonary circulation during CPR will have some oxygen content.[76,77]

Overventilation is common, even by trained healthcare professionals, and is detrimental; hyperventilation/excessive tidal volumes are detrimental during cardiac arrest.[78,79] High intra-thoracic pressure or prolonged time with positive intra-thoracic pressure results in failure to develop negative pressure between chest compressions.[79] Failure to develop negative pressure between chest compressions results in decreased venous return (preload), decreased cardiac output, decreased cerebral and coronary perfusion and ultimately decreased survival. When ventilation rates are greater than 30 breaths per minute, intra-thoracic pressure *never* goes below zero. As a result of these physiological processes, there is decreased emphasis on ventilation during CPR.

In recent years there has been increased focus on decreasing interruptions to chest compressions during CPR.[80-84] The optimal rate of compression is unknown; however, one study has shown that compression rates of less than 87 per minute were associated with a lower likelihood of return of spontaneous

circulation and that rates greater than 120 per minute had no additional benefit when compared with compression rates of 100–120 per minute.[85] While allowing complete recoil of the chest after each compression may improve circulation, there is insufficient evidence to determine the optimal method to achieve the goal without compromising other aspects of chest compression technique.[67]

Interruption of chest compressions is associated with lower survival rates, decreased probability of successful defibrillation and higher incidence of myocardial dysfunction following resuscitation. The heart needs a continuous supply of energy (adenosine triphosphate: ATP): increased chest compressions result in increased myocardial blood flow, increased probability that ventricular fibrillation will become more coarse and increased likelihood of successful defibrillation. There is a direct and important relationship between coronary perfusion pressure and survival: coronary perfusion pressure increases during chest compressions and decreases when compressions are stopped (e.g. for ventilation). When chest compressions resume, it takes 8–10 compressions before coronary perfusion pressure increases to acceptable levels, so all interruptions to chest compressions should be mimimised. In particular, the time between stopping chest compressions and starting defibrillation should be as short as possible; compressions should continue until the time of defibrillation and compressions should recommence immediately following defibrillation *irrespective of electrical success*.[67,80-84] (See the following section on defibrillation.)

In the first minute following defibrillation, the likelihood of developing a rhythm that results in cardiac output is low.[67] Commencing CPR immediately following defibrillation increases the likelihood of return of spontaneous circulation as cerebral and coronary perfusion are restored.[67] In addition, effective CPR for a period of 1–3 minutes is associated with an increased likelihood of successful subsequent attempts at defibrillation.[67]

There is still debate over the exact mechanism by which chest compressions generate blood flow.

- The *thoracic pump* theory is that changes in intrathoracic pressure during CPR cause forward blood flow with venous valves preventing backward flow.[69] Research has provided some support for the thoracic pump theory, as transthoracic echocardiography during CPR shows that cardiac valves remain open during the relaxation phase of chest compressions.[69]

- The *cardiac pump* theory suggests that the left ventricle is compressed between the sternum and the thoracic spine during chest compressions and is dependent on intact heart valves.[86] Although the cardiac pump mechanism is effective while the heart valves function normally during early CPR, it may become less effective as valves lose competence after prolonged CPR.

Defibrillation using an AED

The time to defibrillation is a key factor that influences survival. For every minute defibrillation is delayed, there is approximately a 10% reduction in survival if the victim is in cardiac arrest due to VF.[87] As a result, defibrillation using AEDs has become a valuable adjunct to BLS, particularly in the out-of-hospital environment.

Most adults who are salvageable from cardiac arrest are in VF or pulseless VT, making defibrillation the single most important intervention for these patients.[78,88] AED use should not be restricted to trained personnel: allowing AED use by lay people with no formal training may be life-saving.

The chance of successful resuscitation increases as the time to defibrillation decreases in patients who are in VF.[78] Chances of survival decrease by approximately 10% for every minute that defibrillation is delayed.[88] The advantage with using an AED is that you do not need to be able to recognise and interpret cardiac rhythms.[88] Numerous studies have shown that CPR prior to defibrillation increases the likelihood of successful defibrillation.[1] It is also important to minimise the time between ceasing CPR and defibrillating and to recommence CPR immediately following defibrillation.[67,89,90]

Emergency nurses and paramedics should be familiar with the AED that is available in their clinical environment and the manufacturer's recommendations in terms of its operation. In general, the principles of operation of AED are:

- locate the AED as soon as it is available and turn it on
- apply pads as per manufacturer's recommendations, while minimising interruptions to chest compressions
- follow the verbal prompts.

If shock is advised, ensure safe defibrillation by ensuring the pads are applied correctly and are not touching, following the AED prompts and not touching the patient during shock delivery.[88] If shock is not advised, continue BLS and seek assistance from ALS personnel.

Advanced life support

The techniques and rationales discussed so far in this chapter from a BLS perspective are equally applicable to ALS. Like BLS, ALS should be commenced in patients who are unresponsive and not breathing normally.

Palpation of a pulse is unreliable and should not be performed to confirm cardiac arrest.[74] For healthcare professionals, it is reasonable to check a pulse if an organised rhythm is visible on the monitor at the next rhythm check. Planned pauses in cardiac compressions for rhythm analysis (and/or pulse check) should not take more than 10 seconds.[67]

Given that ALS involves the addition of invasive techniques such as emergency defibrillation, advanced airway management, vascular access and administration of drugs,[67] it is imperative that these additional therapies do not result in interruptions to chest compressions. Ideally, chest compressions should continue during attempts at intubation and, at worst, interruption to compressions for intubation should be 20 seconds or less.[91] Planned pauses for rhythm analysis and/or pulse check should take no more than 10 seconds.[67,68]

The cardiac rhythm should be checked after 2 minutes of CPR or if the patient becomes responsive and starts breathing; if the rhythm appears compatible with return of spontaneous circulation (ROSC), then the pulse should be checked.[74] After ROSC, the ventilation rate should be approximately 12 breaths/minute until the arterial partial pressure of carbon dioxide ($PaCO_2$) is confirmed by blood gases;[67] after which time, ventilation rates may be adjusted accordingly.

Life-threatening dysrhythmias

Life-threatening dysrhythmias can generally be considered in two categories: shockable and non-shockable rhythms. The shockable life rhythms covered in detail in this chapter are ventricular fibrillation (VF) and unconscious, pulseless ventricular tachycardia (VT); as the term suggests, these rhythms are responsive to defibrillation. The non-shockable rhythms covered here are asystole and pulseless electrical activity (PEA), also called electromechanical dissociation (EMD); these rhythms are *not* responsive to defibrillation. In addition, there is a section discussing symptomatic bradycardia.

Shockable rhythms: VF and pulseless VT

The major characteristics of VF and VT are summarised in Table 15.2.

Non-shockable asystole and PEA/EMD

The major characteristics of asystole and PEA are summarised in Table 15.3.

ALS—adult

The current ARC protocol for adult ALS is shown in Figure 15.3.

ALS—paediatric

Paediatric ALS presents additional challenges to ED clinicians as the size and weight of children of various ages is different, and almost all paediatric ALS interventions are weight-based (medication doses, ETT size, defibrillation energy). There are a number of methods which can be used to calculate weight in children and assist with decision-making regarding weight-related interventions (see below). The current ARC protocol for paediatric ALS is shown in Figure 15.4.

Length-based resuscitation tapes

Length-based resuscitation tapes, such as Broselow tape (Fig 15.5), were developed to provide a length-based estimate of bodyweight and equipment size during resuscitation. The tape is laid on the trolley with the top end level with the child's head, and the coloured section that corresponds with the level of the child's feet is the section to be used for that child. There are studies that suggest these tapes do have limitations, including underestimating weight in young obese children, older children and adolescents.[92,93] In addition, studies of the Broselow tape in different cultural groups have shown it to overestimate weight by more than 10% in Indian children weighing over 10 kg.[94] It is very accurate in estimating endotracheal tube (ETT) size.[95]

Weight estimation

All drugs in a paediatric ALS context are given in weight-related doses. There are numerous methods of weight calculation in children, including parental/clinician estimation, Broselow tape and a range of formulae based on age (Table 15.4). Despite longstanding use of age-based formulae, a recent Australian study of 410 children in the ED showed that parental estimation of children's weight is more accurate than the other weight-estimation methods studied (Advanced Paediatric Life Support (APLS), Broselow tape and Best Guess formulae).[96] For 75% of cases, parent estimate of weight was within 10% of measured weight.[96] The Broselow tape was the most accurate of the other methods, with 61% of estimations within 10% of measured weight.[96]

TABLE 15.2 Characteristics of ventricular fibrillation (VF) and ventricular tachycardia (VT)[1,68,141]

	VENTRICULAR FIBRILLATION	VENTRICULAR TACHYCARDIA
Rate	Rapid, disorganised	150–250 beats/minute
Rhythm	Irregular	Regular most of the time May occasionally be slightly irregular
ECG trace		
Pacemaker	Disorganised electrical activity in the ventricles makes ventricular muscle fibres contract independently. This causes 'quivering' of ventricular myocardium and makes the ventricles incapable of pumping blood	Ventricular pacemaker fires rapidly Impulse spreads through the ventricles via an abnormal pathway
P waves	Not seen	Not seen
QRS complex	Absent Fibrillation waves of various sizes and shapes present	Wide and bizarre Width > 0.12 seconds
P–QRS relationship	—	—
PR interval	—	—
Clinical significance	The cause of VF is still not completely understood. VF is the most common cause of sudden cardiac death and may be preceded by VT Results in no cardiac output Often associated with acute myocardial ischaemia (AMI) and occurs in up to half of cardiac arrest survivors Begins as a coarse, irregular rhythm and then degenerates to a fine irregular rhythm and eventually asystole; the likelihood of successful defibrillation decreases as these changes occur	VT is usually defined as greater than 4 consecutive ventricular beats VT that lasts for longer than 30 seconds is considered sustained Causes significant reduction in cardiac output as ventricular filling time is severely reduced, so cannot be tolerated for long periods of time Can deteriorate into VF then asystole Re-entry (or a single circular pathway of electrical impulse) is the most common mechanism responsible for VT
Intervention	The mainstay of resuscitation for VF is early defibrillation	Pulseless VT → treat as VF → defibrillation VT with pulse → antiarrhythmic drugs

ECG: electrocardiogram

Defibrillation

Early defibrillation provides the best chance of survival for patients (adult and paediatric) with VF or pulseless VT.[1,88] Defibrillation is the only proven definitive treatment for VF.[97,98]

Defibrillation is the application of an electric shock through the chest with the aim of producing simultaneous depolarisation of myocardial cells and restoring organised electrical activity.[1] The discussion in this chapter is focused on emergency defibrillation rather than synchronised cardioversion. Current ALS protocols recommend that defibrillation be indicated for VF and pulseless VT. The chance of successful defibrillation decreases as time to defibrillation increases.[1] As time increases,

the high-energy phosphate stores in the myocardium decrease, resulting in deterioration of VF amplitude and waveform.[97] Effective CPR will slow the rate of deterioration of VF, but will not stop it from occurring.[97] One of the ongoing debates in ALS is whether CPR should be performed prior to defibrillation. Research studies comparing CPR prior to defibrillation versus immediate defibrillation have had inconsistent findings.[1]

There is some evidence that good CPR increases the chance of successful defibrillation during out-of-hospital arrest. International studies of 1.5–3 minutes of CPR by paramedics prior to defibrillation have shown higher rates of return of spontaneous circulation and survival in adults with VT or VT

TABLE 15.3 Characteristics of asystole and pulseless electrical activity (PEA)[1,68,141]

	ASYSTOLE	PEA
Rate	None	Variable
Rhythm	None	Variable (remember, can be sinus rhythm)
ECG trace		
Pacemaker	No electrical activity	Variable
P waves	None	Variable
QRS complex	None	Variable
P–QRS relationship	–	Variable
PR interval	–	Variable
Clinical significance	Asystole carries the poorest prognosis of all the ALS-requiring rhythms Asystole has an extremely high mortality rate (> 95%) As asystole is often preceded by VT/VF, the presence of asystole indicates a prolonged state of arrest It is important to confirm the diagnosis of asystole by checking for electrical activity in more than one monitor lead to make sure that it is not a technical problem or fine VF	PEA occurs when there is electrical myocardial activity but no cardiac output. This can occur because of: —no cardiac contractions ('pump failure') —cardiac contractions that are too weak to generate adequate cardiac output —cardiac contractions with no blood flow due to hypovolaemia or obstruction to flow
Intervention [66,68]	BLS and adrenaline	BLS and adrenaline Correct underlying cause of PEA

ALS: advanced life support; BLS: basic life support; ECG: electrocardiogram; VT: ventricular tachycardia; VF: ventricular fibrillation

where time to defibrillation was greater than 4–5 minutes.[99,100] However, an Australian study of out-of-hospital arrest has shown that 1.5 minutes of CPR by paramedics prior to defibrillation did not improve return of spontaneous circulation or survival to hospital discharge.[101] In terms of in-hospital cardiac arrest, there is currently no evidence to support or refute the use of CPR prior to defibrillation in the hospital setting. 1.5–3 minutes of CPR prior to defibrillation may be considered if emergency response time is greater than 4–5 minutes. In a hospital context, if a defibrillator is not immediately available, CPR should be commenced as per BLS protocol earlier in this chapter. Chapter 17 contains information on using a defibrillator, p. 337.

Pad placement

The aim of defibrillator pad placement is to place the heart directly in the current pathway and maximise current flow through the myocardium. Pad placement may be anterolateral or anteroposterior. Anterolateral is the most common placement, as the anterior chest is usually more accessible.[1] However, both methods are effective as long as pads are positioned correctly; currently there is no evidence to support one pad placement method over another.[1]

- If using anterolateral placement, the sternal pad/paddle should be placed to the right of sternum over the 2nd intercostal space and the apical pad/paddle should be placed on the left mid-axillary line over the 6th intercostal space.[1]
- For anteroposterior placement, the anterior pad should be placed over the apex of the heart just to the left of the sternal border and the posterior pad should be placed on the left side of the patient's back, just below the left scapula.
- In patients with large breasts, it is acceptable to place the apical pad/paddle lateral to or underneath the breast.[1]
- Irrespective of the pad/paddle placement method chosen, defibrillator pads/paddles should not be placed over electrocardiogram (ECG) electrodes/leads, implanted pacemakers, central venous catheter insertion sites and glyceryl trinitrate (GTN) or other medication patches.[1]

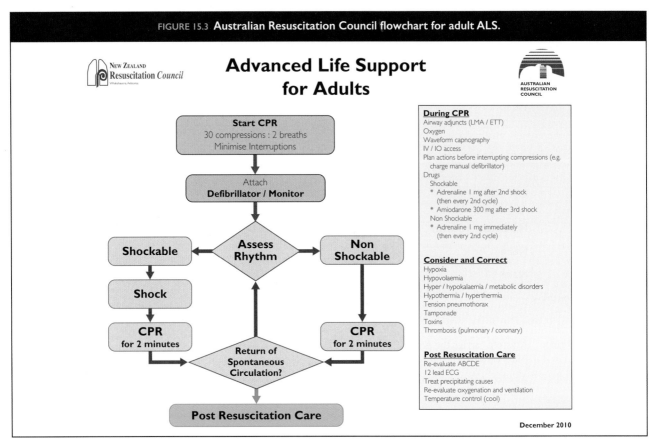

FIGURE 15.3 **Australian Resuscitation Council flowchart for adult ALS.**

Reproduced with permission of the Australian Resuscitation Council.

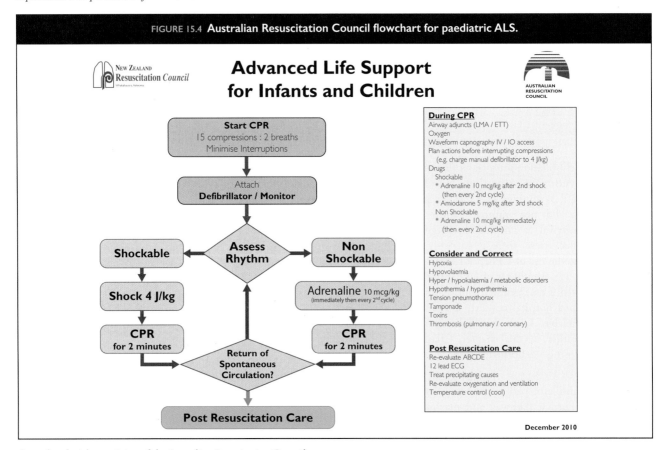

FIGURE 15.4 **Australian Resuscitation Council flowchart for paediatric ALS.**

Reproduced with permission of the Australian Resuscitation Council.

FIGURE 15.5 **Broselow tape.**

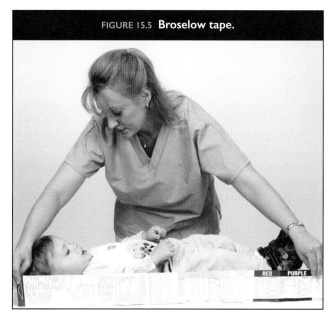

Photo courtesy of Armstrong Medical Industries, Inc.

TABLE 15.4 Formulae for determining children's weight[96]

METHOD	AGE GROUP	FORMULA (AGE IN YEARS)
Argall	1–10 years	Weight (kg) = (age + 2) × 3
Advanced Paediatric Life Support	1–10 years	Weight (kg) = (age + 4) × 2
Best guess	1–4 years	Weight (kg) = (age × 2) + 10
	5–14 years	Weight (kg) = age × 4

BOX 15.2 **Strategies to minimise transthoracic impedance**[1,97]

- Drying the skin prior to application of pads
- Increased pad size—as pad size is increased:
  - resistance to current flow decreases
  - chance of successful defibrillation increases
  - risk of myocardial damage secondary to defibrillation decreases.
- Optimal contact between the skin and pad and use of conductive pads
  - skin is a poor conductor of electricity, so a conductive interface between the skin and defibrillator pads is required for effective defibrillation (this is why defibrillator pads use conductive gels in their design)
  - lack of conductive interface increases impedance, decreases effectiveness of defibrillation and increases likelihood of burns from defibrillation.
- Delivery of defibrillation shock during expiration
  - air is a poor conductor of electricity, so the more air in the patient's lungs at the time of defibrillation, the higher the resistance to current flow.

Transthoracic impedance

Transthoracic impedance is the resistance to flow of electrical current by the chest wall, lungs and myocardium.[97] Decreased transthoracic impedance results in increased effectiveness of defibrillation. Transthoracic impedance may be minimised by a number of strategies (Box 15.2).[97]

Shock protocols

Current recommendations are that single shocks be used for patients in VF or pulseless VT and that CPR should be commenced immediately following shock delivery.[1]

Energy levels in adult patients should be set at 200 J when using a biphasic defibrillator unless there is clinical data for the specific defibrillator which suggests an alternative energy level that provides greater than 90% shock success.[1] For monophasic defibrillators, energy levels for adult patients should be set at 360 J.[1] In children, the optimal energy dose for VF or pulseless VT is unknown. Current recommendations are that 4 J/kg should be used irrespective of whether the defibrillator is monophasic or biphasic.[102]

A praecordial thump (a single, sharp blow to the patient's mid sternum using the rescuer's fist) may be considered in the first 15 seconds of a monitored VF/VT arrest if a defibrillator is not immediately available.[103] Praecordial thump should not be used in patients who have had recent sternotomy or chest trauma.[103]

Defibrillation safety

The operator of the defibrillator is ultimately responsible for defibrillator safety. In terms of patient safety, ensure that the rhythm is a shockable rhythm (VF/pulseless VT), that the patient is not touching any metal objects and that there is proper application of pads to the patient's chest (air pockets increase the risk of burns/arcing). Risk of oxygen-related fire is minimised by correct application of defibrillator pads to prevent arcing and removal of oxygen sources from the patient's chest and immediate bed area. Never place defibrillator pads over transdermal medication patches such as glyceryl trinitrate (GTN) patches, as there is a risk of burns and/or explosion.

To ensure safety of personnel and bystanders, announce loudly and clearly 'CHARGING' as the defibrillator is being charged. Then announce loudly and clearly 'STAND CLEAR' and perform a visual check of the area surrounding the patient before pressing 'SHOCK'.

Troubleshooting

If the defibrillator fails to defibrillate, common reasons that need to be excluded are shown in Box 15.3.

External (trancutaneous/non-invasive) pacing

External pacing delivers an electrical current via the chest with the aim of stimulating myocardial depolarisation and cardiac contraction.[104] Although it has been used successfully for the management of bradycardia with associated haemodynamic instability, external pacing does cause skeletal muscle and cutaneous nerve stimulation, which results in considerable pain and discomfort for the patient.[104] External pacing has not been shown to be effective in the routine management of asystole.[78]

BOX 15.3 Troubleshooting defibrillator failures

- Poor contact between defibrillator pads and patient:
  - defibrillator may have a display prompt or voice alert that indicates pads are ill-applied or missing
  - check that pads are applied to patient's bare chest
  - if the problem continues, replace defibrillator pads.
- Pad cable is not connected to the defibrillator:
  - defibrillator may have a display prompt or voice alert indicating cable disconnection or pads missing
  - check cable connection
- Defibrillator charge automatically discharged:
  - defibrillator may have a prompt that indicates shock cancelled
  - after 30 seconds the defibrillator automatically discharges itself if the 'SHOCK' button is not pressed; if this occurs, recharge defibrillator and deliver shock within 30 seconds.
- Battery failure
- Synchronised mode engaged:
  - defibrillator may have a prompt that indicates synchronised mode or 'SYNC' is engaged, and a highlighted R wave on the monitor display
  - synchronised cardioversion is different to emergency defibrillation, as during emergency defibrillation the shock is delivered at random during the cardiac cycle[82]
  - synchronised cardioversion is used to treat cardiac arrhythmias such as conscious VT, SVT, AF or atrial flutter when drugs have failed to revert the arrhythmia or if the patient becomes haemodynamically unstable
  - during synchronised cardioversion, the shock is delivered during the absolute refractory period after ventricular depolarisation (just after the QRS complex on ECG), thus decreasing the potential for the shock to be delivered during the vulnerable period of repolarisation (upslope of the T wave on ECG)
  - 'R on T phenomenon' occurs when a shock is delivered during the vulnerable period—this is dangerous and can result in VF
  - if the 'SYNC' button is activated during emergency defibrillation and the cardiac rhythm is VF, the defibrillator will still attempt to sense an R wave and deliver the shock just after the QRS complex; as there are no R waves in VF, the defibrillator will not discharge
  - if the rhythm is pulseless VT (rapid rate and wide and bizarre QRS complexes), it may be difficult for the defibrillator to sense the R wave or to distinguish the R wave from the T wave; therefore it is recommended that emergency defibrillation is a safer option for pulseless VT.

AF: atrial fibrillation; ECG: electrocardiogram; SVT: supraventricular tachycardia; VT: ventricular tachycardia; VF: ventricular fibrillation

---

External pacing increases heart rate, increases mean arterial pressure, increases cardiac output and decreases systemic vascular resistance.[104] Many defibrillators also have an external pacing capacity: clinicians should have a sound understanding of the equipment available in their clinical area and how to operate their equipment according to the manufacturer's recommendations. Most pads and cables are multifunctional and can be used to monitor cardiac rhythm, defibrillate and pace. *However*, the pads cannot monitor and pace simultaneously— so if the patient requires external pacing, standard chest leads will need to be used to monitor the cardiac rhythm.

In general, most external pacing devices will have fixed or demand modes. In fixed mode, the pacer will deliver pacing impulses at the rate selected on the pacer irrespective of the patient's intrinsic cardiac activity.[105,106] In demand mode (the preferred mode of pacing), the pacer will deliver pacing impulses only when the patient's heart rate falls below the rate selected on the pacer and will attempt to time 'paced' beats with the intrinsic cardiac activity.[105,106]

Again, clinicians should be aware of their organisational policies and the recommendations related to their specific equipment, but the following paragraph will briefly outline the general principles of external pacing. Continuous ECG monitoring should be in place and once the pads are applied to the patient's chest and the cable connected to the pacer, the pacer should be switched on and the appropriate mode of pacing (fixed or demand) selected. The desired rate at which the patient is to be paced should be selected (should resemble usual heart rate of approximately 70–80 beats/minute). To commence pacing, the output should be increased until capture is achieved, bearing in mind that the patient will require analgesia and/or sedation. Capture may be electrical or mechanical.

Electrical capture occurs when a pacing impulse leads to depolarisation of the ventricle and is confirmed by a pacing spike followed by a wide QRS complex and tall, broad T wave on the ECG monitor.[105,106]

Mechanical capture is the contraction of the myocardium in response to the paced impulse, and is confirmed by the following signs of improved cardiac output: presence of palpable peripheral pulses, increased blood pressure, improved level of consciousness and improved skin colour.[105,106]

If the patient requires defibrillation during pacing, the pacer will automatically turn off when the defibrillator is discharged. Be aware that the pacer will remain switched off after defibrillation, so to resume pacing you will need to go through the above process again.

Troubleshooting

Common general troubleshooting issues that may arise during external pacing are shown in Box 15.4.

Advanced airway management

There is still no evidence to support the routine use of any specific advanced airway management during cardiac arrest,[78] or to determine the optimal timing of advanced airway placement during cardiac arrest.[78] Decisions about airway management will depend on the availability of devices and the skills and experience of resuscitation team members.[78] Options for advanced airway management during cardiac arrest include:

- manual airway manoeuvres (see BLS section earlier in the chapter)
- oropharyngeal airway

BOX 15.4 **Troubleshooting external pacing**[105,106]

Patient discomfort
- Most patients will have difficulty tolerating external pacing when the current is greater than 50 mA; however, patient thresholds for tolerating external pacing are variable
- Sedation and analgesia should be offered to all patients undergoing external pacing.

Failure to capture
- The most common reason for failure to capture is failure to increase the current high enough to achieve capture
- Capture thresholds are variable and may change in the same patient at different times, but most patients achieve capture at 50–90 mA
- The following factors may increase the capture threshold and these patients may require higher current to achieve capture: hypoxia, acidosis, recent thoracic surgery, pericardial effusion, pericardial tamponade
- The most common error in external pacing is failure to increase the current high enough to achieve capture.[85]

Electrical capture, but no mechanical capture
- Increase the current
- Ensure that artifact is not being misinterpreted as electrical capture
- Consider the cause of the bradycardia and patient viability.

Under-sensing
- Sensing is the ability of the pacer to identify the patient's intrinsic beats; under-sensing occurs when the pacer does not sense the patient's intrinsic beats and there is asynchrony between the paced impulses and patient's intrinsic beats
- To correct under-sensing, try the following: increase the ECG size on the ECG machine or monitor, select a different lead, reposition monitoring leads, ensure adequate contact between monitoring electrodes and patient's skin.

Over-sensing
- Over-sensing is inappropriate inhibition of a demand pacemaker due to detection of signals other than R waves, such as muscle artefact or T waves
- When over-sensing occurs, the pacemaker will not maintain the specified rate; this can usually be corrected by decreasing the ECG size or selecting a different lead.

ECG: electrocardiogram

- nasopharyngeal airway
- laryngeal mask airway (LMA)
- oesophageal-tracheal combitube
- endotracheal intubation.

Once an advanced airway is inserted (LMA or endotracheal tube), the ventilation rate should be 8–10 per minute and chest compressions should be continuous without pausing for ventilations.[78] One strategy is to deliver 1 ventilation after 15 compressions in order to deliver consistent ventilation and adequate tidal volume.[78] Refer to Chapter 17, pp. 314–322, for further information on airway management.

Oro- or nasopharyngeal airways

An oropharyngeal airway or nasopharyngeal airway may be used to maintain a patent airway. Oropharyngeal airways should be of an appropriate size and not forcibly inserted.

- To determine the correct-size oropharyngeal airway, the airway should reach from the centre of the incisors to the angle of the jaw.[106,107]
- To determine the correct-size nasopharyngeal airway, the correct size should reach from tip of the nose to the tragus of the ear.

Insertion of an oropharyngeal airway in children is different to that in adults.[106,107] In adults, the oropharyngeal airway is inserted upside down until it reaches the soft palate, then is rotated 180° so it is 'right way up' and slid over the tongue. In infants and small children, the airway is inserted 'right way up' using a tongue depressor to aid insertion. In large children, the same technique as adults may be used.[106,107] Oropharyngeal airway is preferred in the context of head trauma with potential for a fractured base of skull.[78]

Laryngeal mask airways

Laryngeal mask airways or supraglottic airways were developed to bridge the gap between bag–valve–mask ventilation and endotracheal intubation.[78] The advantage of LMA over bag–valve–mask ventilation is that ventilation can be commenced in similar timeframes and regurgitation is lower with the use of LMA.[78] Studies comparing use of LMA with endotracheal intubation have shown that both experienced and inexperienced personnel can successfully insert and ventilate the patient using an LMA with low complication rates.[78] LMAs should not be used in patients with a gag reflex.[78] See Chapter 17, p. 327, for details on laryngeal mask airway insertion.

Endotracheal intubation

Endotracheal intubation remains the gold standard for airway maintenance and protection during CPR; however, there is no evidence to support endotracheal intubation over other airway management options *during cardiac arrest*.[78] The disadvantages of endotracheal intubation during cardiac arrest include a 6–14% incidence of unrecognised oesophageal intubation and interruption to chest compressions.[78] The advantages of endotracheal intubation during cardiac arrest include no need to interrupt chest compressions for ventilation once the endotracheal tube (ETT) is in place; can provide 100% oxygen; and provides alternative route for medication administration.[78]

Decisions about endotracheal intubation should be informed by assessing the benefit of intubation versus consequences of interrupted chest compressions, and the skills and availability of personnel.[78] In some cases, it may be more appropriate to intubate the patient following return of spontaneous circulation.

Attempts at endotracheal intubation *should not* interrupt chest compressions for more than 20 seconds.[67,68] Once the ETT has been inserted, the cuff should be inflated using a manometer to ensure the minimum amount of inflation to prevent air leaks. ETT placement should be confirmed by chest inflation, auscultation and direct observation.[78] Waveform capnography is also recommended to confirm and continuously monitor the ETT position and to protect against unrecognised oesophageal intubation.[78]

For all patients, selection of the correct-size ETT is dependent on the size of the patient. In prepubescent children or children under the age of 12 years, uncuffed ETTs are used because the cricoid cartilage is the narrowest part of a paediatric airway and provides a physiological cuff. The cricoid cartilage is susceptible to oedema, so use of an uncuffed ETT will decrease oedema at the cricoid ring and will allow the use of an ETT with maximal diameter and therefore decrease resistance to airflow.[108] To estimate the tube size for a child over 1 year of age, the following formula may be used:[108] ETT (mm) = (age (years)/4) + 4. Neonates generally require a size 3–3.5 ETT. A useful guide to ETT size is to select an ETT that is approximately the same diameter as the child's little finger.[108]

Monitoring during resuscitation

There are few high-level studies related to monitoring the adequacy of CPR.

End-tidal carbon dioxide

There is some evidence that end-tidal carbon dioxide ($EtCO_2$) is a safe, effective and non-invasive indicator of cardiac output during CPR, and may be an early indicator of return of spontaneous circulation (ROSC) in intubated patients.[78] Although research to date suggests that low $EtCO_2$ values are associated with lower survival rates, there is insufficient evidence to support or refute a specific $EtCO_2$ value as a prognostic indicator of outcome in adult cardiac arrest.[78] It is important to note, however, that $EtCO_2$ should not be used to guide ventilation during cardiac arrest because there is decreased CO_2 returning to the lungs as a result of low blood flow. Refer to Chapter 17, p. 323, for further information on its use.

Arterial blood gases

Arterial blood gases (ABGs) provide an indication of degree of hypoxaemia and metabolic acidosis.[78] Arterial blood gases are only an approximate indicator of adequacy of ventilation during CPR and may be improved by better ventilation or increased cardiac output.[67] If ventilation is constant, an increase in $PaCO_2$ is a potential marker of improved perfusion.[67] Low $PaCO_2$ levels may indicate that a decreased ventilation rate is warranted, and high $PaCO_2$ levels may need to be tolerated during resuscitation as the $PaCO_2$ benefit of increasing the ventilation rate is outweighed by the detrimental effects of overventilation (increased intrathoracic pressure, decreased coronary perfusion pressure).[67]

ABG sampling also enables rapid determination of electrolyte levels, including potassium, calcium and magnesium.[67] ABG sampling should not interfere with provision of effective CPR, nor should it interrupt chest compressions. Refer to Chapter 17, p. 329, for information on ABG collection and sampling.

Medications/fluids used in cardiac arrest

It is important to remember that no drug has been shown to improve long-term survival following cardiac arrest.[91] Defibrillation, oxygenation and ventilation will always have priority over drug administration.[91] Despite this knowledge, drugs continue to be used based on historical precedents and theoretical or anecdotal reports of efficacy.[97]

Methods of administration

It is always preferable in a resuscitation situation to give drugs via the intravenous route using a large-bore peripheral IV cannula inserted into a large peripheral vein;[91] for example, the cubital fossa. Placement of IV cannulae in lower limbs should be avoided because in the arrested patient there is decreased venous return. IV drug administration should always be followed by a Normal saline flush of at least 20 mL in adults; in children the flush should be appropriate to the age/size of the child and the length of extension tubing if present. Drug administration in cardiac arrest should also be followed by a full 2-minute cycle of CPR.

Intraosseous (IO) administration is also a good alternative to IV administration, particularly in children; the IO route can be used in infants and adults as well.[109] The bone marrow has a rich blood supply and is part of the peripheral circulation, so drugs and fluids administered via the IO route are absorbed and distributed as quickly and in the same concentrations as they would be if they were administered using the IV route.[109] Any drug that can be given via the IV route can also be given using the IO route[109] and the dose is the same as the dose that would be used for IV administration.[109] The most common place for insertion of an IO needle is the anterior surface of the tibia 2–3 cm below the tibial tuberosity.[110]

Bone marrow may also be aspirated for biochemistry and haematology (excluding white cell count). When giving drugs and/or fluids via the IO route, usually they will not run using gravity alone. A common method of fluid administration via the IO route is to place a three-way tap between the IO needle and the fluid line, turn the three-way tap off to the patient, use an appropriate-size syringe to draw up the required amount of fluid from the flask, turn the three-way tap off to the flask and then inject the fluid into the IO needle.

If IV or IO access cannot be established, drugs may be administered via an ETT, although absorption may be variable.[91] The drugs that can be administered via ETT are adrenaline, atropine and lignocaine.[91] Other cardiac arrest drugs should not be given via an ETT as they may cause mucosal and/or alveolar damage.[91] In adults, the ETT dose should be increased (3 to 10 times the IV dose); there is some evidence that dilution with water increases drug absorption.[91]

Classical pharmacology

Tables 15.5 and 15.6 outline classical pharmacology indicated during resuscitation.

Fluid resuscitation

There is insufficient evidence to recommend for or against routine use of IV fluids during cardiac arrest.[91] If hypovolaemia is suspected as a cause of cardiac arrest, either IV colloid or IV crystalloid may be given during resuscitation. In both adults and children, an initial bolus of 20 mL/kg should be given via either the IV or the IO route and additional boluses titrated against response.[91,102]

Additional procedures—pericardiocentesis and chest decompression

There are a number of procedures that may be undertaken during resuscitation in an attempt to correct reversible causes of cardiac arrest or to increase the effectiveness of resuscitation. Pericardial tamponade, where impairment of diastolic filling of the right ventricle due to significant amounts of fluid in the sac surrounding the heart results in decreased cardiac output, is a major cause of obstructive shock.[111] It has predicable

	ADRENALINE[97,102]	AMIODARONE[91,97,102,142]	ATROPINE[91]	SODIUM BICARBONATE[102]
Presentation	β	150 mg/3 mL ampoules	600 µg/1 mL ampoules 1 mg/10 mL 'mini-jet'	8.4 g (100 mmol)/100 mL vials (each mL contains 1 mmol each of sodium and bicarbonate)
Actions	Naturally occurring catecholamine with alpha (α) and beta (β) adrenergic effects Causes peripheral vasoconstriction (α effects) directing cardiac output to the brain and myocardium Is thought to facilitate defibrillation by improving myocardial blood flow during CPR	Class III antiarrhythmic drug Has effects on sodium, potassium and calcium channels as well as alpha (α) and beta (β) adrenergic blocking effects Lowers defibrillation threshold and has antifibrillation effects	Parasympathetic antagonist that blocks the action of the vagus nerve on the heart Increases automaticity and rate of conduction at SA and AV nodes	An alkalising solution which combines with H^+ ions to form carbonic acid (H_2CO_3) which then breaks down to CO_2 and H_2O Theoretically reverses metabolic acidosis that is associated with profound or prolonged ischaemia The need for sodium bicarbonate in cardiac arrest should be avoided by early and effective basic life support
Evidence review	Currently there is no evidence that high-dose adrenaline improves long-term outcomes following cardiac arrest or that ETT-administered adrenaline is effective	There is no conclusive evidence that antiarrhythmic medications during cardiac arrest improve survival-to-discharge rates	There is insufficient evidence to support or refute the use of atropine in cardiac arrest to improve survival to hospital discharge	Currently there is no strong evidence that supports the use of alkalinising agents in cardiac arrest Routine use of sodium bicarbonate in cardiac arrest is not recommended
Indications	VF/pulseless VT in conjunction with defibrillation Asystole/PEA as initial treatment	VF/pulseless VT when defibrillation and adrenaline have failed to revert arrhythmia Prophylaxis of recurrent VF/VT	Asystole Severe symptomatic bradycardia	Hyperkalaemia Documented metabolic acidosis Overdose of tricyclic antidepressants Prolonged arrest (> 15 minutes) as the likelihood of acidosis is increased
Adverse effects	Tachyarrhythmias Increased oxygen requirements Severe hypertension post resuscitation Tissue necrosis if extravasation occurs	Hypotension Bradycardia Heart block	Tachycardia Delirium, hyperthermia in large doses	Alkalosis Hypernatraemia Hyperosmolarity Risk of intracellular acidosis as CO_2 liberated from sodium bicarbonate enters cells If sodium bicarbonate is mixed with adrenaline or calcium, precipitation occurs causing both drugs to be inactivated and block IV lines

TABLE 15.5 Drugs used in resuscitation

Continued

TABLE 15.5 Drugs used in resuscitation—cont'd

	ADRENALINE[97,102]	AMIODARONE[91,97,102,142]	ATROPINE[91]	SODIUM BICARBONATE[102]
Dose	**Adult** IV dose: 1.0 mg repeated at regular intervals (every 2nd cycle)	**Adult** 300 mg IV; an additional dose of 150 mg may be considered May be followed by an infusion once return of spontaneous circulation is achieved	**Adult** IV dose (asystole): 1 mg repeated to a maximum of 3 mg	**Adult** IV dose: 1 mmol/kg given over 2–3 minutes; should be guided by arterial blood gases
	Paediatric IV or IO: 10 µg/kg	**Paediatric** 5 mg/kg Amiodarone is incompatible with Normal saline, so needs to be diluted in 10–20 mL 5% dextrose	**Paediatric** IV or IO dose: 20 µg/kg	**Paediatric** IV or IO dose: 1.0 mmol/kg

AV: atrioventricular; CPR: cardiopulmonary resuscitation; ETT: endotracheal tube; H⁺: hydrogen ion; IO: intraosseous; IV: intravenous; SA: sinoatrial; VF: ventricular fibrillation; VT: ventricular tachycardia

clinical features that are not dissimilar to other cardiac-related conditions, such as tension pneumothorax. Patients present with Beck's triad (venous pressure elevation, decline in arterial pressure and muffled heart tones), pulsus paradoxus, Kussmaul's sign and ultimately PEA (see Table 15.7). The definitive treatment for this form of shock is pericardiocentesis, coupled with hyperoxygenation. Without this intervention, resuscitation is largely futile.

Needle decompression, or needle thoracocentesis, is a life-saving procedure used to treat tension pneumothorax (Box 15.5).

Post-resuscitation care

It is important to recognise that resuscitation is an ongoing process that does not stop when the patient exhibits return of spontaneous circulation.[42] The majority of deaths following resuscitation are due to hypoxic brain injury or myocardial injury:[42] the risk of these adverse events can be minimised by the delivery of structured, evidence-based post-resuscitation care.

In recent years it has become apparent that there is a post-cardiac arrest syndrome, which is a unique and complex combination of the following pathophysiological processes: i) brain injury, ii) myocardial dysfunction, iii) systemic response to reperfusion and iv) residual issues related to the cause of cardiac arrest.[112] There is a growing body of evidence that shows that post-cardiac arrest syndrome has a significant impact on mortality and morbidity.[112] Protocols for the structured and standardised management of patients who have suffered cardiac arrest have been shown to improve outcomes.[113,114]

Factors known to reduce the impact of post cardiac arrest syndrome include:

- targeted temperature management/therapeutic hypothermia, blood pressure control, airway protection and ventilation, oxygenation and seizure control to limit brain injury[115–119]

- blood pressure control, intravenous fluids, inotropic support and in some cases Intra-Aortic Balloon Pump (IBP) or Extra Corporeal Membrane Oxygenation (ECMO) to minimise myocardial dysfunction[118,120]

- blood pressure control, vasopressors, temperature control, glucose control and early administration of antibiotics if evidence of infection to limit the systemic response to reperfusion[42,121]

- strategies such as early reperfusion, percutaneous coronary intervention (PCI), fibrinolysis, management of traumatic injury and antidote therapy to address residual issues related to the cause of cardiac arrest.[42]

PRACTICE TIP

POST RESUSCITATION CARE

The aims of post-resuscitation care are to:[42]

- continue respiratory support and maintain adequate oxygenation
- maintain cerebral perfusion by restoration and maintenance of adequate blood pressure
- prevent and treat cardiac arrhythmias
- identify and treat the cause of cardiac arrest:
  - hypoxaemia
  - hypovolaemia
  - hypo- or hyperkalaemia
  - hypo- or hyperthermia
  - pericardial tamponade
  - tension pneumothorax
  - toxins/poisons/drugs
  - thrombosis: pulmonary embolism or acute myocardial infarction.

TABLE 15.6 Electrolytes used in resuscitation[78,102]

	POTASSIUM	MAGNESIUM	CALCIUM
Presentation	10 mmol/100 mL bags potassium chloride (KCl)	10 mmol/5 mL ampoules magnesium sulfate ($MgSO_4$)	2.2 mmol/10 mL ampoules calcium gluconate 5 mmol/5 mL ampoules calcium chloride
Actions	An electrolyte essential for membrane stability ↓ K^+ causes ventricular arrhythmias especially in the presence of ↓ Mg^{2+} and digoxin	An electrolyte essential for membrane stability ↓ Mg^{2+} causes myocardial hyperexcitability, especially in the presence of ↓ K^+ and digoxin	Essential for normal muscle and nerve activity Causes a transient increase in myocardial excitability, contractility and peripheral resistance
Evidence review	Not available	Several studies into the effect of magnesium on cardiac arrest have had contradictory results, so currently there is little evidence to support the routine use of magnesium in cardiac arrest	Routine administration of calcium in cardiac arrest is not recommended Calcium is seldom indicated in the management of cardiac arrest *unless* there is evidence that cardiac arrest is associated with hyperkalaemia, hypocalcaemia or calcium channel blocker toxicity
Indications	Persistent VF Documented hypokalaemia	Torsades de pointes Cardiac arrest associated with digoxin toxicity VF/pulseless VT when defibrillation and adrenaline have failed to revert arrhythmia Documented hypokalaemia Documented hypomagnesaemia	Hyperkalaemia Hypocalcaemia Overdose of calcium channel blockers
Adverse effects	Inappropriate or excessive use may cause hyperkalaemia which may result in bradycardia, hypotension and asystole Tissue necrosis if extravasation occurs	Hypotension Heart block Muscle weakness and respiratory failure	May mediate cell damage causing possible increase in myocardial and cerebral injury Digoxin causes an increase in intracellular calcium, so calcium should be given with caution in the setting of known or suspected digoxin toxicity Tissue necrosis if extravasation occurs
Dose	**Adult** IV dose: 5 mmol KCl **Paediatric** IV or IO dose: 0.03–0.07 mmol/kg KCl	**Adult** IV dose: 5 mmol $MgSO_4$ **Paediatric** IV or IO dose: 0.1–0.2 mmol/kg $MgSO_4$	**Adult** IV dose: 5–10 mL calcium chloride IV dose: 10 mL calcium gluconate **Paediatric** IV or IO dose: 0.2 mL/kg 10% calcium chloride[102] IV or IO dose: 0.7 mL/kg 10% calcium gluconate (20 mg/kg)[102]

IO: intraosseous; IV: intravenous; K^+: potassium ions; Mg^{2+}: magnesium ions; VF: ventricular fibrillation

Ventilation should continue via an ETT in the immediate post-arrest period. Arterial blood gases should be taken as a guide to pH, PaO_2 and $PaCO_2$. $PaCO_2$ should be maintained at normal levels (35–45 mmHg), as decreased CO_2 levels cause cerebral vasoconstriction and reduce cerebral perfusion. A nasogastric tube (NGT) should be inserted for all intubated patients, as

TABLE 15.7 Comparison of pericardial tamponade and tension pneumothorax[111]

CLINICAL FEATURE	PERICARDIAL TAMPONADE	TENSION PNEUMOTHORAX
Presenting condition	Shock	Respiratory distress
Neck veins	Distended	Distended
Trachea	Midline	Deviated
Breath sounds	Bilaterally equal	Diminished on the side of the injury
Chest percussion	Normal	Hyperresonant on the side of injury
Heart sounds	Muffled	Normal

BOX 15.5 Needle decompression/thoracocentesis in tension pneumothorax

Needle decompression/thoracocentesis
1. Confirm definitive diagnosis of tension pneumothorax and clinical indication for procedure.
2. High-flow oxygenation of the patient (12–15 L/min non-rebreathing mask or bag–valve–mask or LMA or ETT).
3. Prepare equipment:
   a) thoracocentesis needle (or large-bore IV cannula (10–14 gauge) and a sterile glove)
   b) surgical skin preparation (povidine–iodine or similar)
   c) adhesive tape.
4. Locate insertion point: the intercostal space between the 2nd and 3rd ribs down the mid-axillary line.
5. Apply topical skin preparation, and allow to dry.
6. Insert the needle at 90° to the chest and listen for the release of air.
7. Advance the catheter over the needle and secure.
8. Monitor the patient.

Indications
- Tension pneumothorax.
- Trauma CPR patients may require bilateral chest decompression.

Detailed procedure
- Assess chest and respiratory excursion.
- Apply oxygen per non-rebreather mask or with 100% with bag–valve–mask.
- Identify 2nd intercostal space, on the mid-clavicular line on the affected side.
- Prepare the area.
- Locally anaesthetise the area if patient is conscious or if time permits.
- Snugly attach a 14 or 16 gauge angiocath to a 10 mL syringe or use arrow kit.
- Insert the needle into the skin and over the rib into the 2nd or 3rd intercostal space on the mid-clavicular line.
- Puncture the parietal pleura.
- Aspirate air as necessary to relieve the patient's symptoms.
- Leave the plastic catheter remaining but remove the stylet.
- Secure the catheter to the chest.
- Connect the catheter to a one-way valve such as a Heimlich valve.
- Re-assess ventilatory status, jugular veins, tracheal position, pulse and blood pressure.
- Document procedure and responses.

Complications
- Pneumothorax.

CPR: cardiopulmonary resuscitation; ETT: endotracheal tube; LMA: laryngeal mask airway

gastric decompression will facilitate ventilation and decrease the risk of vomiting. In patients with facial or head trauma, an orogastric tube should be used.

Systolic blood pressure should be at least 100 mmHg and hypotension should be treated with inotropes, vasopressors and/or restoration of circulating volume.[42] Cardiac monitoring should continue and a 12-lead ECG should be performed to determine if any time-critical re-perfusion is warranted: if there is evidence of ST-segment elevation myocardial infarction (STEMI) or new left bundle branch block (LBBB), PCI is the preferred re-perfusion strategy if primary PCI can be achieved in less than 90 minutes.[44] (Refer to Ch 17, p. 336, for further information on cardiac monitoring and how to perform ECGs.) Fibrinolytic therapy is an alternative if there is limited access to primary PCI.[44] Thrombolysis may be indicated for pulmonary embolism. Although there are no studies of the prophylactic use of antiarrhythmics, if antiarrhythmic drugs have been given during the resuscitation, it is reasonable to continue those drugs as an infusion.[42]

Hyperglycaemia has been associated with poor neurological outcomes following cardiac arrest.[42] Evidence about the optimal blood glucose level following cardiac arrest is lacking; however, blood glucose should be frequently monitored following cardiac arrest, hypoglycaemia should be avoided and hyperglycaemia (blood glucose > 10 mmol/L) should be treated with insulin.[42] Blood should be taken for serum electrolytes; anticonvulsant drugs may be considered if fitting occurs; and analgesia and/or sedation should be given as required.[42]

Complications of resuscitation such as rib fractures or other injuries should be assessed and treated, and the location of all tubes and lines placed during resuscitation should be confirmed.[42] It may also be necessary to replace IV lines inserted under emergency conditions.[42] If in a rural or remote location, preparation for transfer will also be required.

Targeted temperature management following cardiac arrest

Targeted temperature management following ROSC has been recommended in national and international guidelines for more than a decade.[122] Two landmark randomised controlled trials

showing improved neurological outcomes in patients cooled to a target temperature of 33°C[116,117] prompted therapeutic hypothermia to be included as a standard of care in national and international resuscitation guidelines.[122,123] A more recent study comparing targeted temperature management at either

33°C or 36°C for 28 hours showed no significant differences between the two groups in overall mortality or neurological function or death at 180 days.[119] It is important to note that both groups of patients in this study had active target temperature management, which prevented fever, and was part of intensive post-resuscitation care; the mean temperature of patients in both groups at time of recruitment was 35°C; and that the study included patients with both shockable and non-shockable arrest rhythms.[124] As research continues regarding targeted temperature managment, the position of the ARC at the time of writing is that targeted temperature management remains an important treatment strategy in the post resuscitation care of unconscious cardiac arrest patients. The Australian Resuscitation Council guidelines recommend that unconscious adult patients who have ROSC after VF arrest should be cooled to 32–34°C for 12–24 hours and that induced hypothermia may also be of benefit in patients whose initial rhythm was not VF.[122] If clinicians are not cooling to 32–34°C, they should aim for a target temperature of 36°C and fever should be avoided.[124]

Care of families and family presence during resuscitation

Traditionally, families of patients who are undergoing active resuscitation have been excluded from the resuscitation room on the premise that invasive procedures and active resuscitative efforts would be distressing to families and distracting to staff.[125] Over recent years, research findings[126–135] suggest that, in fact, witnessing resuscitation is beneficial for families, patients and staff. The routine exclusion of families by staff is not supported by evidence.[125,136] Rather, families should be offered the choice of being present during the resuscitation of their family member.[125,136,137] The decision of family members who choose not to witness resuscitation should be respected and these family members supported.[125,137] Family members who choose to be present during resuscitation should be accompanied at all times by an experienced member of staff, who should:[137]

- prepare the family prior to entering the resuscitation area (this includes the patient's appearance, number of people in the room and their roles, resuscitative efforts in progress)
- make it clear that resuscitation of the patient is the first priority and that the family will be removed from the room if they are disruptive or combative
- explain interventions and the patient's response to those interventions
- interpret medical and nursing jargon
- provide comfort measures such as tissues or chairs
- give the opportunity for the family to ask questions
- facilitate touching and talking to the patient if possible.

Research findings have demonstrated that, of family members who were present during resuscitation:

- 100% felt that it was important that they were with the patient[137]
- 64% felt that their presence had helped the patient who was dying[136]
- 95–100% felt that it helped them to comprehend the seriousness of the situation and to know that everything possible was done for the patient[136,137]
- 95% felt that their presence helped the patient even when the patient was unconscious[137]
- family members (no percentage given) felt that it provided factual knowledge about what was happening to the patient and relief from wondering what was going on[137]
- family members (no percentage given) felt that it gave a sense of closure when the outcome was that the patient died[137]
- 76% felt that adjustment to death had been made easier and that their grieving had been facilitated[136]
- 94% reported that they would be present during resuscitation again if given the opportunity.[136]

The experience of witnessing procedures such as defibrillation, intubation, central line insertion, thoracocentesis and pericardiocentesis have been examined in research. In these studies,[125,136,137] it was found that no family member was frightened by the process of witnessing resuscitation and no family member had to leave the resuscitation room because of distress.[125] While families were greatly concerned about the patient's fear, pain and survival,[137] they had a good understanding of the need for appropriate behaviour while in the resuscitation room (irrespective of age, gender, education or ethnicity),[137] appreciated that their presence did not impede the efforts of the resuscitation team or harm the patient[136,137] and were not concerned about what they might see or hear.[136] From the perspective of staff, although 38% of staff were concerned that families would be disruptive, no disruptions occurred and 97% of staff felt that families behaved appropriately.[137] Nurses have reported greater levels of comfort with family prescence during resuscitation than medical staff (95% vs 64%), although 84% of staff felt that their performance and the patient outcome were unchanged by the presence of families.[137]

Recent research has compared families who witnessed the resuscitation of their family member in the ED with families who were not permitted in the resuscitation area. Studies suggest that while there was no difference in levels of general distress 3 months post resuscitation, those who had witnessed it reported lower levels of anxiety, depression, intrusive imagery, post-traumatic avoidance behaviour and symptoms of grief.[125] One-third of families were with the patient when they collapsed and assisted in getting help and providing first aid, so for these families, presence during resuscitation was simply the continuation of an incident that they were already a part of.[137] Future research[138,139] will continue to examine the safety of family presence during resuscitation.

CASE STUDY

Abe is a 3-year-old boy found by his mother floating face-down in a home swimming pool. It is not known how long he had been in the water; he was last seen playing with siblings approximately 20 minutes earlier. When his mother pulled him from the water, he was pale, floppy, unconscious and did not appear to be breathing. A neighbour heard Abe's mother screaming and called an ambulance.

When paramedics arrive, Abe's mother is performing cardiopulmonary respiration with both chest compressions and mouth-to-mouth ventilation.

Paramedics suction Abe's airway, apply a cervical collar and continue with bag–valve–mask ventilation and chest compressions. Application of a cardiac monitor showed a sinus tachcardia of 160 beats/minute; however, Abe has no palpable pulse.

Paramedics achieve return of spontaneous circulation and transport Abe to the emergency department (ED). On arrival, Abe has poor blood pressure and poor peripheral perfusion so an adrenaline infusion is commenced. He is hypothermic at 29°C so is re-warmed to 33°C. Abe then has a ventricular fibrillation arrest. The ED staff achieve return of spontaneous circulation after administration of adrenaline, amiodarone and defibrillation.

Questions

1. While the ambulance is en route, what is the best thing that Abe's mother can do to improve the chance of her child's survival?

2. What are the priorities for paramedics in this case?

3. How should paramedics treat Abe?

4. How should ED staff treat Abe?

5. What are the management priorities for Abe now he is in a post-arrest state?

 Answers to Case Study Questions can be found on evolve
http://evolve.emergencytrauma.curtis

REFERENCES

1. Australian Resuscitation Council. Guideline 11.4: Electrical Therapy for Adult Advanced Life Support. Melbourne: Australian Resuscitation Council. 2011. Online. www.resus.org.au; accessed 28 Jan 2014.

2. Australian Resuscitation Council. Guideline 12.1: Introduction to Paediatric Advanced Life Support. Melbourne: Australian Resuscitation Council. 2011. Online. www.resus.org.au; accessed 28 Jan 2014.

3. Australian Resuscitation Council. Guideline 11.1: Introduction to Adult Advanced Life Support. Melbourne: Australian Resuscitation Council. 2011. Online. www.resus.org.au; 2011; accessed 28 Jan 2014.

4. Knaus W, Draper E, Wagner D, Zimmerman J. APACHE II: a severity of disease classification system. Critical Care Medicine 1985;13:818–22.

5. Franklin C, Mamdani B, Burke G. Prediction of hospital arrests: toward a preventative strategy. Clinical Research 1986;34:954A.

6. Franklin C, Matthew J. Developing strategies to prevent in hospital cardiac arrest: analyzing responses of physicians and nurses in the hours before the event. Critical Care Medicine 1994;22:244–7.

7. Hourihan F, Bishop G, Hillman K et al. The Medical Emergency Team: a new strategy to identify and intervene in high risk patients. Clinical Intensive Care 1995;6:269–72.

8. Buist MD, Jarmolowski E, Burton PR et al. Recognising clinical instability in hospital patients before cardiac arrest or unplanned admission to intensive care. A pilot study in a tertiary-care hospital. Medical Journal of Australia 1999;171:22–5.

9. Ferraris VA, Propp ME. Outcome in critical care patients: a multivariate study. Critical Care Medicine 1992;20:967–76.

10. Dubois RW, Brook RH. Preventable deaths: who, how often, and why? Annals of Internal Medicine 1988;109:582–9.

11. Sax F, Charlson M. Medical patients at high risk for catastrophic deterioration. Critical Care Medicine 1987;15:10–15.

12. Curtis K, Hoy S, Murphy M, Lewis MJ. The emergency nursing assessment process: A structured framework for a systematic approach. Australasian Emergency Nursing Journal 2009;12:130–6.

13. Considine J, Botti M. Who, when and where? Identification of patients at risk of an in-hospital adverse event: implications for nursing practice. International Journal of Nursing Practice 2004;10:21–31.

14. Gumm K. Emergency department trauma management. In: Curtis K, Ramsden C, Friendship J, eds. Emergency and Trauma Nursing. Sydney: Elsevier; 2007:706–32.

15. Buist M, Jarmolowski E, Burton PR et al. Recognising clinical instability in hospital patients before cardiac arrest or unplanned admission to intensive care. A pilot study in a tertiary-care hospital. Med J Aust 1999;171:22–5.

16. McGloin H, Adam SK, Singer M. Unexpected deaths and referrals to intensive care of patients on general wards. Are some cases potentially avoidable? Journal of the Royal College of Physicians: London 1999;33:255–9.

17. Buist M, Moore G. A risk reduction strategy: The prevention of adverse clinical events by the implementation of a hospital based emergency team and retrospective audit process. Report to the Victorian Department of Human Services. Dandenong: Dandenong Hospital; 2000.

18. Camarata SJ, Weil MH, Hanashiro PK, Shubin H. Cardiac arrest in the critically ill. I: A study of predisposing causes in 132 patients. Circulation 1971;44:688–95.

19. Bedell SE, Delbanco TL, Cook EF, Epstein FH. Survival after cardiopulmonary resuscitation in the hospital. New England Journal of Medicine 1983;309:569–76.

20. Suljaga Pechtel K, Goldberg E, Strickon P et al. Cardiopulmonary resuscitation in a hospitalized population: prospective study of factors associated with outcome. Resuscitation 1984;12:77–95.

21. George A, Folk B, Crecelius D, Barton Campbell W. Pre-arrest morbidity and other correlates of survival after in-hospital cardiopulmonary arrest. American Journal of Medicine 1989;87:28–34.

22. Bedell SE, Deitz DC, Leeman D, Delbanco TL. Incidence and characteristics of preventable iatrogenic cardiac arrests. JAMA 1991;265:2815–20.

23. Considine J, Thomas S, Potter R. Predictors of critical care admission in emergency department patients triaged as low to moderate urgency. Journal of Advanced Nursing 2009;65:818–27.

24. Ashworth S. A prelude to outreach: prevalence and mortality of ward patients with abnormal vital signs. 15th Annual Congress of the European Society of Intensive Care Medicine; 2002; Barcelona, Spain Intensive Care Medicine; Adverse events. p. S21.

25. Goldhill DR, McNarry AF. Physiological abnormalities in early warning scores are related to mortality in adult inpatients. British Journal of Anaesthesia 2004;92:822–4.

26. Berlot G, Pangher A, Pettrucci L et al. Anticipating events of in-hospital cardiac arrests. European Journal of Emergency Medicine 2004;11:24–8.

27. Considine J. The role of nurses in preventing adverse events related to respiratory dysfunction: literature review. Journal of Advanced Nursing 2005;49:624–33.

28. Cretikos MA, Bellomo R, Hillman K et al. Respiratory rate: the neglected vital sign. Med J Aust 2008;188:657–9.

29. Subbe CP, Davies RG, Williams E et al. Effect of introducing the Modified Early Warning score on clinical outcomes, cardio-pulmonary arrests and intensive care utilisation in acute medical admissions. Anaesth 2003;58:797–802.

30. Olsson T, Lind L. Comparison of the Rapid Emergency Medicine Score and APACHE II in nonsurgical emergency department patients. Academic Emergency Medicine Journal 2003;10:1040–8.

31. Cretikos M, Chen J, Hillman K et al. The objective medical emergency team activation criteria: A case-control study. Resuscitation 2007;73:62–72.

32. Fieselmann J, Hendryx M, Helms C, Wakefield D. Respiratory rate predicts cardiopulmonary arrest for internal medicine inpatients. J Gen Int Med 1993;8:354–60.

33. Hodgetts TJ, Kenward G, Vlachonikolis IG et al. The identification of risk factors for cardiac arrest and formulation of activation criteria to alert a medical emergency team. Resuscitation 2002;54:125–31.

34. Harrison GA, Jacques TC, Kilborn G et al. The prevalence of recordings of the signs of critical conditions and emergency responses in hospital wards—the SOCCER study. Resuscitation 2005;65:149–57.

35. Skrifvars M, Nurmi J, Ikola K et al. Reduced survival following resuscitation in patients with documented clinically abnormal observations prior to in-hospital cardiac arrest. Resuscitation 2006;70:215–22.

36. Jones AE, Stiell IG, Nesbitt LP et al. Nontraumatic out-of-hospital hypotension predicts inhospital mortality. Annals of Emergency Medicine 2004;43:106–13.

37. Jones AE, Yiannibas V, Johnson C, Kline JA. Emergency Department hypotension predicts sudden unexpected in-hospital mortality: A prospective cohort study. Chest 2006;130:941–6.

38. Kilgannon JH, Roberts BW, Reihl LR et al. Early arterial hypotension is common in the post-cardiac arrest syndrome and associated with increased in-hospital mortality. Resuscitation 2008;79:410–16.

39. Olsson T, Terent A, Lind L. Rapid Emergency Medicine score: a new prognostic tool for in-patient mortality in non-surgical emergency department patients. Journal of Internal Medicine 2004;255:579–87.

40. Subbe CP, Slater A, Menon D, Gemmell L. Validation of physiological scoring systems in the accident and emergency department. Emerg Med J 2006;23:841–5.

41. Jones DA, DeVita MA, Bellomo R. Rapid-Response Teams. New England Journal of Medicine 2011;365:139–46.

42. Australian Resuscitation Council. Guideline 11.7: Post-Resuscitation Therapy in Adult Advanced Life Support. Melbourne: Australian Resuscitation Council. 2011. Online. www.resus.org.au; 2011; accessed 28 Jan 2014.

43. Stub D, Bernard S, Smith K et al. Do we need cardiac arrest centres in Australia? Internal medicine journal 2012;42:1173–9.

44. Australian Resuscitation Council. Guideline 14.3: Acute Coronary Syndromes: Reperfusion Strategy. Melbourne: Australian Resuscitation Council. 2011. Online. www.resus.org.au; 2011; accessed 28 Jan 2014.

45. Considine J, Jones D, Bellomo R. Emergency department rapid response systems: the case for a standardized approach to deteriorating patients. European Journal of Emergency Medicine 2013;20:375–81.

46. Bristow P, Hillman K, Chey T et al. Rates of in-hospital arrests, deaths and intensive care admissions: The effect of a medical emergency team. Med J Aust 2000;173:236–40.

47. Buist M, Moore GE, Bernard SA et al. Effects of a medical emergency team on reduction of incidence of and mortality from unexpected cardiac arrests in hospital: preliminary study. British Medical Journal 2002;324:387–90.

48. Bellomo R, Goldsmith D, Uchino S et al. A prospective before-and-after trial of a medical emergency team. Med J Aust 2003;179:283–7.

49. DeVita MA, Braithwaite RS, Mahidhara R et al. Use of the medical emergency team responses to reduce hospital cardiopulmonary arrests. Quality and Safety in Health Care 2004;13:251–4.

50. Considine J, Lucas E, Wunderlich B. The uptake of an early warning system in one Australian Emergency Department: a pilot study. Critical Care and Resuscitation 2012;14:135–41.

51. Hosking J, Considine J, Sands N. Recognising clinical deterioration in Emergency Department patients. Australasian Emergency Nursing Journal 2014;17:59–67.

52. Jones D, Considine J. Rapid response systems and the emergency department. In: Cameron P, Jelinek G, Kelly A et al. (eds) Adult Textbook of Emergency Medicine. 4th ed. Sydney: Churchill Livingstone; 2014.

53. Cosby K, Croskerry P. Profiles in patient safety: Authority gradients in medical error. Acad Emerg Med 2004;11:1341–5.

54. Dayton E, Henriksen K. Communication failure: Basic components, contributing factors, and the call for structure. Jt Comm J Qual Patient Saf 2007;33:34–47.

55. Barkmann A, Pooler C. Heart failure and circulatory shock. In: Porth CM, Matfin G, eds. Pathophysiology: Concepts of Altered Health States. 8th ed. Philadelphia: J. B. Lippincott Company; 2009:606–37.

56. Banasik JL. Shock. In: Banasik JL, Copstead LC, eds. Pathophysiology. St Louis, Missouri: Elsevier Saunders; 2005.

57. Caroline N. Emergency care in the streets. Sudbury, MA: Jones and Bartlett Publishers; 2007.

58. O'Meara M, Watton DJ, for the Advanced Life Support Group. Advanced Paediatric Life Support, Australia and New Zealand: The Practical Approach 5th edn. West Sussex: Wiley Blackwell BMJ Books; 2012.

59. Marshall S, Harrison J, Flanagan B. The teaching of a structured tool improves the clarity and content of interprofessional clinical communication. Quality and Safety in Health Care 2009;18:137–40.

60. Haig KM, Sutton S, Whittington J. SBAR: a shared mental model for improving communication between clinicians. Jt Comm J Qual Patient Saf 2006;32:167–75.

61. Reznek M, Smith-Coggins R, Howard S et al. Emergency medicine crisis resource management (EMCRM): pilot study of a simulation-based crisis management course for emergency medicine. Acad Emerg Med 2003;10:386–9.

62. Deasy C, Bray JE, Smith K et al. Cardiac arrest outcomes before and after the 2005 resuscitation guidelines implementation: Evidence of improvement? Resuscitation 2011;82:984–8.

63. Boyde MS, Padget M, Burmeister E, Aitken LM. In-hospital cardiac arrests: effect of amended Australian Resuscitation Council 2006 guidelines. Australian Health Review 2013;37:178–84.

64. Girotra S, Nallamothu BK, Spertus JA et al. Trends in survival after in-hospital cardiac arrest. New England Journal of Medicine 2012;367:1912–20.

65. Australian Resuscitation Council. Guideline 2: Priorities in an Emergency. Melbourne: Australian Resuscitation Council. Retrieved 28 January 2014 www.resus.org.au; 2011; accessed 28 Jan 2014.

66. Australian Resuscitation Council. Guideline 8: Cardiopulmonary Resuscitation. Melbourne: Australian Resuscitation Council. 2011. Online. www.resus.org.au; 2011; accessed 28 Jan 2014.

67. Australian Resuscitation Council. Guideline 11.1.1: Cardiopulmonary Resuscitation for Advanced Life Support Providers. Melbourne: Australian Resuscitation Council. 2011. Online. www.resus.org.au; accessed 28 Jan 2014.

68. Australian Resuscitation Council. Guideline 11.2: Protocols for Adult Advanced Life Support. Melbourne: Australian Resuscitation Council. 2011. Online. www.resus.org.au; accessed 28 Jan 2014.

69. Bernard S. Basic life support. In: Cameron P, Jelinek G, Kelly A et al. eds. Adult Textbook of Emergency Medicine. 3rd ed. Sydney: Churchill Livingstone; 2009:1–5.

70. Australian Resuscitation Council. Guideline 4: Airway. Melbourne: Australian Resuscitation Council. 2011. Online. www.resus.org.au; accessed 28 Jan 2014.

71. Australian Resuscitation Council. Guideline 3: Unconciousness. Melbourne: Australian Resuscitation Council. 2011. Online. www.resus.org.au; accessed 28 Jan 2014.

72. Australian Resuscitation Council. Glossary of Terms. Melbourne: Australian Resuscitation Council. 2012. Online. www.resus.org.au; accessed 28 Jan 2014.

73. Australian Resuscitation Council. Guideline 5: Breathing. Melbourne: Australian Resuscitation Council. 2011. Online. www.resus.org.au; accessed 28 Jan 2014.

74. Australian Resuscitation Council. Guideline 6: Compressions. Melbourne: Australian Resuscitation Council. 2011. Online. www.resus.org.au; accessed 28 Jan 2014.

75. Koster RW, Baubin MA, Bossaert LL et al. European Resuscitation Council Guidelines for Resuscitation 2010 Section 2. Adult basic life support and use of automated external defibrillators. Resuscitation 2010;81:1277–92.

76. Bobrow BJ, Ewy GA. Ventilation during resuscitation efforts for out-of-hospital primary cardiac arrest. Current opinion in Critical Care 2009;15:228–33.

77. Ewy GA, Kern KB, Sanders AB et al. Cardiocerebral resuscitation for cardiac arrest. The American Journal of Medicine 2006;119:6–9.

78. Australian Resuscitation Council. Guideline 11.6: Equipment and Techniques in Adult Advanced Life Support. Melbourne: Australian Resuscitation Council. 2011. Online. www.resus.org.au; accessed 28 Jan 2014.

79. Aufderheide TP, Lurie KG. Death by hyperventilation: a common and life-threatening problem during cardiopulmonary resuscitation. Critical Care Medicine 2004;32:S345–51.

80. Kern KB, Hilwig RW, Berg RA et al. Importance of continuous chest compression during cardiopulmonary resuscitation: improved outcome during a simulated single lay-rescuer scenario. Circulation 2002;105:645–9.

81. Dorph E, Wik L, Stromme TA et al. Quality of CPR with three different ventilation:compression ratios. Resuscitation 2003;58:193–201.

82. Sanders AB, Kern KB, Berg RA et al. Survival and neurologic outcome after cardiopulmonary resuscitation with four different chest compression-ventilation ratios. Annals of Emergency Medicine 2002;40:553–62.

83. Hallstrom AP. Dispatcher-assisted 'phone' cardiopulmonary resuscitation by chest compression alone or with mouth-to-mouth ventilation. Critical care medicine 2000;28:N190–2.

84. Paradis NA, Martin GB, Rivers EP et al. Coronary perfusion pressure and the return of spontaneous circulation in human cardiopulmonary resuscitation. JAMA 1990;263:1106–13.

85. Abella BS, Sandbo N, Vassilatos P et al. Chest compression rates during cardiopulmonary resuscitation are suboptimal: a prospective study during in-hospital cardiac arrest. Circulation 2005;111:428–34.

86. Haas T, Voelckel WG, Wenzel V et al. Revisiting the cardiac versus thoracic pump mechanism during cardiopulmonary resuscitation. Resuscitation 2003;58:113–16.

87. Sunde K, Jacobs I, Deakin CD et al. Part 6: Defibrillation: 2010 International Consensus on Cardiopulmonary Resuscitation and Emergency Cardiovascular Care Science with Treatment Recommendations. Resuscitation 2010;81:e71–85.

88. Australian Resuscitation Council. Guideline 7: External Automated Defibrillation (AED) in Basic Life Support (BLS). Melbourne: Australian Resuscitation Council. 2011. Online. www.resus.org.au; accessed 28 Jan 2014.

89. Steen S, Liao Q, Pierre L et al. The critical importance of minimal delay between chest compressions and subsequent defibrillation: a haemodynamic explanation. Resuscitation 2003;58:249–58.

90. Yu T, Weil MH, Tang W et al. Adverse outcomes of interrupted precordial compression during automated defibrillation. Circulation 2002;106:368–72.

91. Australian Resuscitation Council. Guideline 11.5: Medications in Adult Cardiac Arrest. Melbourne: Australian Resuscitation Council. 2011. Online. www.resus.org.au; accessed 28 Jan 2014.

92. Hofer C, Ganter M, Tucci M et al. How reliable is length-based determination of body weight and tracheal tube size in the paediatric age group? The Broselow tape reconsidered. British Journal of Anaesthesia 2002;88:283–5.

93. Hashikawa A, Juhn Y, Homme J et al. Does length-based resuscitation tape accurately place pediatric patients into appropriate color-coded zones? Pediatric Emergency Care 2007;23:856–61.

94. Ramarajan N, Krishnamoorthi R, Strehlow M et al. Internationalizing the Broselow Tape: How reliable is weight estimation in Indian children? Acad Emerg Med 2008;15:431–6.

95. Sanders J. Simple height-based method of choosing the correct tracheal tube size in children. British Journal of Anaesthesia 2002;88:457–8.

96. Krieser D, Nguyen K, Kerr D et al. Parental weight estimation of their child's weight is more accurate than other weight estimation methods for determining children's weight in an emergency department? Emergency Medicine Journal 2007;24:756–9.

97. Maguire J. Advanced life support. In: Cameron P, Jelinek G, Kelly A et al. eds. Adult textbook of emergency medicine. 3rd edn. Sydney: Churchill Livingstone; 2009:5–13.

98. Australian Resuscitation Council. Guideline 11.5: Electrical therapy for adult advanced life support. Melbourne: Australian Resuscitation Council; 2006.

99. Wik L, Hansen TB, Fylling F et al. Delaying defibrillation to give basic cardiopulmonary resuscitation to patients with out-of-hospital ventricular fibrillation: a randomized trial. JAMA 2003;289:1389–95.

100. Cobb LA, Fahrenbruch CE, Walsh TR et al. Influence of cardiopulmonary resuscitation prior to defibrillation in patients with out-of-hospital ventricular fibrillation. JAMA 1999;281:1182–8.

101. Jacobs I, Finn JC, Oxer HF, Jelinek GA. CPR before defibrillation in out-of-hospital cardiac arrest: A randomized trial. Emergency Medicine Australasia 2005;17:39–45.

102. Australian Resuscitation Council. Guideline 12.4: Medications & Fluids in Paediatric Advanced Life Support. Melbourne: Australian Resuscitation Council. 2011. Online. www.resus.org.au; accessed 28 Jan 2014.

103. Australian Resuscitation Council. Guideline 11.3: Precordial Thump & Fist Pacing. Melbourne: Australian Resuscitation Council. 2011. Online. www.resus.org.au; 2011.

104. Feldman MD, Zoll PM, Aroesty JM et al. Hemodynamic responses to noninvasive external cardiac pacing. The American Journal of Medicine 1988;84:395–400.

105. Bessman ES. Emergency cardiac pacing. In: Roberts JR, Hedges JR, eds. Clinical procedures in emergency medicine. 4th ed. Philadephia: Sanders; 2004:283–304.

106. Colquhoun M, Handley A, Evans T, eds. ABC of resuscitation. 5th ed. Bristol: BMJ Publishing Group; 2004.

107. Vrocher D, Hopson LR. Basic airway management and decision making. In: Roberts JR, Hedges JR, eds. Clinical procedures in emergency medicine. 4th ed. Philadelphia: Sanders; 2004:53–68.

108. Mackway-Jones K, Molyneux E, Phillips B, Wieteska S, for Advanced Life Support Group. Advanced Paediatric Life Support: The Practical Approach 4th ed. Oxford, UK: Blackwell Publishing Ltd; 2008.

109. Australian Resuscitation Council. Guideline 12.6: Techniques in Paediatric Advanced Life Support. Melbourne: Australian Resuscitation Council. 2011. Online. www.resus.org.au; accessed 28 Jan 2014.

110. Zideman DA, Spearpoint K. Resuscitation of infants and children. In: Colquhoun M, Handley A, Evans T, eds. ABC of resuscitation. 5th ed. Bristol: BMJ Publishing Group; 2004:43–9.

111. British Paramedic Association. Nancy Caroline's Emergency Care in the Streets. Sudbury/US: Jones and Bartlett Publishers, Inc; 2009.

112. Nolan JP, Neumar RW, Adrie C et al. Post-cardiac arrest syndrome: Epidemiology, pathophysiology, treatment, and prognostication. A Scientific Statement from the International Liaison Committee on Resuscitation; the American Heart Association Emergency Cardiovascular Care Committee; the Council on Cardiovascular Surgery and Anesthesia the Council on Cardiopulmonary, Perioperative, and Critical Care the Council on Clinical Cardiology. Resuscitation 2008;79:350–79.

113. Cokkinos P. Post-resuscitation care: current therapeutic concepts. Acute cardiac care 2009;11:131–7.

114. Reynolds JC, Lawner BJ. Management of the post-cardiac arrest syndrome. Journal of Emergency Medicine 2012;42:440–9.

115. Langhelle A, Tyvold S, Lexow K et al. In-hospital factors associated with improved outcome after out-of-hospital cardiac arrest. A comparison between four regions in Norway. Resuscitation 2003;56:247–63.

116. Bernard SA, Gray TW, Buist MD et al. Treatment of comatose survivors of out-of-hospital cardiac arrest with induced hypothermia. New England Journal of Medicine 2002;346:557–63.

117. The Hypothermia after Cardiac Arrest Study Group. Mild Therapeutic Hypothermia to Improve the Neurologic Outcome after Cardiac Arrest. New England Journal of Medicine 2002;346:549–56.

118. Hovdenes J, Laake J, Aaberge L et al. Therapeutic hypothermia after out-of-hospital cardiac arrest: experiences with patients treated with percutaneous coronary intervention and cardiogenic shock. Acta anaesthesiologica scandinavica 2007;51:137–42.

119. Nielsen N, Wetterslev J, Cronberg T et al. Targeted temperature management at 33 C versus 36 C after cardiac arrest. New England Journal of Medicine 2013;369:2197–206.

120. Morris MC, Wernovsky G, Nadkarni VM. Survival outcomes after extracorporeal cardiopulmonary resuscitation instituted during active chest compressions following refractory in-hospital pediatric cardiac arrest. Pediatric Critical Care Medicine 2004;5:440–6.

121. Van Den Berghe G, Wouters P, Weekers F et al. Intensive insulin therapy in critically ill patients. New England journal of medicine 2001;345:1359–67.

122. Australian Resuscitation Council. Guideline 11.8: Therapeutic Hypothermia after Cardiac Arrest. Melbourne: Australian Resuscitation Council. 2011. Online. www.resus.org.au; accessed 28 Jan 2014.

123. Deakin CD, Morrison LJ, Morley PT et al. Part 8: Advanced life support: 2010 International Consensus on Cardiopulmonary Resuscitation and Emergency Cardiovascular Care Science with Treatment Recommendations. Resuscitation 2010;81:e93–174.

124. Australian Resuscitation Council. Therapeutic Hypothermia in Cardiac Arrest: An information update. Melbourne: Australian Resuscitation Council. 2014. Online. www.resus.org.au; accessed 28 Jan 2014.

125. Robinson S, Mackenzie-Ross S, Hewson G et al. Psychological effect of witnessed resuscitation on bereaved relatives. The Lancet 1998;352:614–17.

126. Hodge AN, Marshall AP. Family presence during resuscitation and invasive procedures. Collegian 2009;16:101–18.

127. Miller JH, Stiles A. Family presence during resuscitation and invasive procedures: the nurse experience. Qualitative Health Research 2009;19:1431–42.

128. Fell OP. Family presence during resuscitation efforts. Nursing Forum 2009;44:144–50.

129. Fallis W. Family presence during resuscitation: bereaved family members' perspectives ... Canadian Hospice Palliative Care Conference, Voyages in Care and Understanding, 18–21 October 2009, Winnipeg, Manitoba, Canada. Journal of Palliative Care 2009;25:237–47.

130. McClement SE, Fallis WM, Pereira A. Family presence during resuscitation: Canadian critical care nurses' perspectives. Journal of Nursing Scholarship 2009;41:233–40.

131. Riwitis C, Twibell RS. Family presence during resuscitation: the in's and out's. American Nurse Today 2006;1:12–15.

132. Twibell R, Siela D, Riwitis C et al. Family presence during resuscitation: who decides? Creating a consensus to honor the family's wishes. American Nurse Today 2009;4:8–10.

133. Albarran J. Family witnessed resuscitation: an invitation to share your experiences. Journal of Perioperative Practice 2009;19:198.

134. Scheans P. Family-witnessed resuscitation in the perinatal arena: strategies to develop and implement a policy. Nursing for Women's Health 2009;13:208–24.

135. Meusling F. Family-witnessed resuscitation ... Scheans P. Family-witnessed resuscitation in the perinatal arena: strategies to develop and implement a policy. Nurs Womens Health. 2009;13(3):208–15.

136. Meyers T, Eichhorn D, Guzzetta C. Do families want to be present during CPR? A retrospective survey. Journal of Emergency Nursing 1998;24:400–5.

137. Meyers T, Eichhorn D, Guzzetta C et al. Family presence during invasive procedures and resuscitation: the experience of family members, nurses and physicans. American Journal of Nursing 2000;100:32–43.

138. Albarran J. Call to readership. Family witnessed resuscitation: an invitation to share your experiences. Journal of Advanced Perioperative Care 2009;4:55.

139. Albarran J. Seeking experiences of family witnessed resuscitation. Nursing Standard 2009;23:33.

140. Australian Resuscitation Council. Guideline 12.7: Management after Resuscitation in Paediatric Advanced Life Support. Melbourne: Australian Resuscitation Council. 2011. Online. www.resus.org.au; accessed 28 Jan 2014.

141. Aehert B. ECGs made easy. 4th edn. Elsevier Science; 2009.

142. MIMS. Amiodarone Hydrochloride Injection Concentrate. November 2003–January 2004.

CHAPTER 16
STABILISATION AND TRANSFER
DANIEL MARTIN AND ANDREW PEARCE

Essentials

- Taking time to appropriately expose and package the patient prior to transport increases patient comfort and safety, and also decreases the risk of missed injury. All anticipated interventions and procedures must be completed prior to moving the patient.

- High-risk and complex procedures should be trained for and based on rigorous, evidence-based standard operating procedures.

- Talking through the plan for any attempt at intubation, allocating roles and preparing the patient increases the likelihood of a successful first attempt at endotracheal intubation.

- Transport staff must be able to weigh up the risks versus benefits for all patient transport, whether within a hospital or between locations.

- Internationally recognised minimum standards for the transport of the critically ill patient should be adhered to.[1]

- The transport environment places specific stressors on both the patient and the team.

- The effects and risks of each transport mode must be fully appreciated and understood by all transport staff.

- Centralised clinical coordination provides advice to both metropolitan and rural healthcare teams, and also allows for effective and safe movement of teams and asset tracking.

- A formalised hand-over tool increases the opportunity for a complete and brief hand-over of all patient details.

- Monitoring equipment must be lightweight, robust and easy to use. All staff must be completely familiar with the workings of all equipment and how to troubleshoot during the transport.

- Each member of the team, and the organisation on the broader scale, facilitates and undertakes regular debriefing, auditing and quality improvements for all retrieval activites.

INTRODUCTION

The critically ill patient will often require transport, both within (intrafacility) and between (interfacility) facilities. These tasks require the nurse and/or paramedic to be highly trained, current in their practice and able to be flexible and adaptive to the environment and the circumstances they are placed in. The transport environment places specific demands on both the patient and the team caring for them, and these must be keenly understood and appreciated. These may include, but are not limited to, noise, vibration, temperature and barometric pressure changes, and any intervention may need to be undertaken under extreme circumstances where access to the patient is limited or taking place while on the move.

Even the most closely attended and organised transfer can be subject to delays due to external factors. Ambulances arrive late, weather can ground aircraft, and taxis for team transport may never arrive. Time can be of the essence and treatment may be time-critical; these factors must be considered and accounted for when organising the retrieval.

The key to good transport practice is to bring definitive or optimal care to the patient as soon as possible. For example, definitive care can be maximised through inotrope support, securing an airway, intubation and mechanical ventilation or life-saving surgical procedures. Fundamentally, the care that is provided by the transport team should be at least equal to if not exceed that which is offered at the referring facility.[2] Teamwork, leadership and good communication are paramount to successful integration of teams and missions in potentially austere and stressful circumstances.

Transport teams are staffed with a variety of skill sets and healthcare professionals. The team composition should suit the patient's condition and treatment requirements. Whichever combination of doctor, nurse or paramedic, each has its advantages and disadvantages. In deciding on which team to task, there needs to be a risk–benefit analysis in deciding which skill mix is the most appropriate. The ultimate goal of the mission is to get the patient to the right place, by the right means, in a timely fashion, at the right cost and—most importantly—safely.

Transport platforms include road ambulances, rotor-wing aircraft, fixed-wing aircraft and, for long-haul missions, commercial and Lear jet aircraft and in special circumstances Australian Defence Force (ADF) assets. Selection is dependent on distance travelled, landing options, the patient's clinical status, availability, weather and cost. The focus of this chapter is on team preparation; retrieval/transport types; patient assessment and preparation; stabilisation and transfer of critically ill patients; and the factors that influence the mission.

The following list broadly outlines the types of missions that transport teams are likely to be tasked with in Australasia:
- Metropolitan interfacility transfer of patients
- Rural/remote medical centre/hospital transfer to tertiary centres
- Ambulance service activation for roadside trauma
- International repatriation of patients back to their country of origin
- Major incident (local or international) activation and field medical team response.

Intra- and interfacility patient transport

Incumbent in the treatment of the critically ill patient is a transport phase of care, either intra- or interfacility. Moving a critically unwell patient takes great consideration, planning and execution. Patients are regularly moved for a variety of reasons. Movement may be as simple as to radiology for simple imaging, or as complex as a decompensating patient being moved rapidly to theatre for definitive surgical intervention. The mode or urgency may differ, but the fundamentals remain the same.

Staffing and preparation

The staff transferring the critically ill patient should be senior, experienced clinicians who are familiar with the equipment and travel times, whether between the emergency department

(ED) and intensive care unit (ICU) or between a rural hospital and the tertiary facility. Intrafacility transport requires the same level of planning and preparation as does transport over longer distances—the team should be able to provide the equivalent standard of care during the transport as is available in the ED or ICU, and should therefore be ALS (advanced life support) accredited with consummate knowledge of the necessary interventions and equipment. The transport team should be self-sufficient during patient transfer, prepared for any eventuality, and able to perform independently. They often do not have at-hand support, so need to be able to respond to any emergency or change in patient condition. However, they are not isolated, as good two-way communication ensures that advice and coordination is available.

Preparation for transfer should be carefully completed for every movement and the risk of movement should be weighed against the potential benefit for the patient. The team should re-assess the patient prior to movement, ensure that the receiving facility/unit is aware of the impending arrival, consider the route, agree on plans to address patient deterioration, and ensure that communication devices are working and at hand.[3]

Preparation tips to remember prior to patient transport include, but are not limited to, the following:
- Staff doing the transferring should be experienced and accredited.
- Plans for worse-case scenarios should be discussed and formulated, to ensure mutual understanding.
- Re-assess the patient (primary survey) prior to movement.
- The number and type of infusions should be rationalised; be prepared to discontinue those not deemed necessary.
- Ensure all intravenous, arterial or other, i.e. indwelling urinary catheter lines, are secure, and equipment or monitor cables are accessible to aid in troubleshooting or manipulation.
- Ensure the patient is secure and kept warm to minimise hypothermia.
- Check that monitoring is attached correctly, working with sufficient battery life for duration of mission, and with maximal visibility around the patient.
- Communicate the plan for movement with patient and family where possible.
- Communicate with receiving facility regarding the patient's impending arrival and any pertinent clinical information.
- Ensure all documentation, X-rays, blood results etc, are up to date and available.
- Devise hand-over strategy prior to arrival.

Every effort should be made to minimise the effects of hypothermia when travelling through air-conditioned corridors or in the elements. At a minimum, monitoring should include electrocardiogram, pulse oximetry and non-invasive blood-pressure monitoring. The equipment must be safely secured to either the bed or a stretcher bridge. A capacity to increase the level and complexity of monitoring must be readily available. There must be enough power, whether this be from an internal battery or an ability to plug-in to an external power source to ensure full functionality throughout the transfer, and ideally there should be back-up means such as spare 'hot swappable' batteries or mains power access in the transport platform. The monitor, and indeed any infusion devices, must be able to withstand accidental damage and be lightweight enough to be carried with ease by any member of the retrieval team. Knowing the inherent limits of the equipment being used in retrieval medicine ensures that the team does not expect the equipment to perform beyond its limits. All equipment must be rigorously tested prior to the introduction and use on any aircraft, with special attention paid to electro-magnetic interference.

Interfacility transfer is necessary when a critically ill patient requires movement from a a referring facility to a receiving one. This may be from a regional or country setting to a metropolitan location or between two city-based facilities for specialist therapy. In the UK, 90% of patients are transported by staff from the referring hospital.[4] This practice removes valuable staff from rural/district facilities, leaving those hospitals with inadequate staffing and resources. Ideally, the retrieval service should be a stand-alone source so as to not draw valuable staff from the ED or ICU, and these staff should be specifically trained in retrieval or transport medicine. Transport teams are at times required to move patients who are undergoing very complex and highly sophisticated treatment. Common examples of these include intra-aortic balloon pump (IABP) and extra-corporeal membrane oxygenation (ECMO) therapies. In such circumstances the coordination and logistical issues are compounded by the size and weight of the equipment and the need for specifically trained personnel to manage them. These extra staff may not be familiar with the transport environment, so it is important that they are well briefed and advised throughout the entirety of the transport.

Oxygen consumption, calculation and sourcing are paramount when in transit, and this is especially important for intubated and non-invasively ventilated patients. A careful calculation of anticipated oxygen requirements must be carried out prior to the commencement of the mission. Box 16.1 shows a suggested formula for calculating oxygen requirements.[3] Oxygen cylinders are heavy and expensive and on commercial airlines and military aircraft are considered dangerous goods. Knowing if the ventilator in use is gas- or power/turbine-driven and having a contingency back-up in the form of a bag-valve-mask assembly is part of the planning and preparation needed prior to commencing the mission. See Table 16.4 for oxygen bottle capacity and approximate life at varying flow rates.

Central coordination and communication are vital to the success of an organised transfer—continual downstream communication to the destination via a centralised clinical coordination centre is a must. Providing the receiving facility with an estimated time of arrival and by which means, and with up-to-date clinical detail will give the receiving facility enough time to have appropriate staff ready to accept the patient, and any infusions or equipment ready to go immediately.

The Joint Faculty of Intensive Care Medicine, the Australian and New Zealand College of Anaesthetists and the Australasian College for Emergency Medicine have developed minimum standards for the transfer of the critically unwell. They make recommendations as to the basic essential standards for equipment, monitoring capability and minimum training requirements for staff, among other items; these are currently undergoing review.[1]

En route to transfer

The en route time to the referring facility for an interhospital transfer is time that can be well used to plan for the upcoming mission. Detailed plans can be agreed upon by all team members to deal with any potential deterioration in patient condition, or indeed any threats to safety while travelling. Relevent drugs can be pre-drawn-up and labelled to facilitate quicker administration and a reduction in workload at the scene or hospital; these must remain the responsibility of the team until they are administered or correctly disposed of. Further, calculations can be checked by the team to reduce errors, equipment can be identified as priority for attachment to the patient and building team cohesion can also be achieved.

A mental rehearsal and checklist of how to assess, treat and package the patient is a cheap, reproducible and effective method of preparation. It is useful to try to anticipate any problems before being faced with them, and the time without the patient on the way is the perfect opportunity to do this.

Types of transport

The type of transport frame used for each mission will be dependent on a variety of factors. Some are directly patient-focused, and others are environmental or logistical in nature. Transfer generally takes place in two very distinct environments: on the ground or by air via fixed- or rotary-wing aircraft. Each has its advantages and disadvantages, and these must be appreciated when determining the type of transport platform to be used. Table 16.1 highlights the strengths and weaknesses of the various transport platforms.

Regardless of transport platform, all staff require significant training and orientation in terms (where relevant) of flight safety, loading and unloading patients, hazardous materials, emergency exits, fire procedures, seat belts, life jacket operation and location of emergency oxygen and masks for rapid decompression. All flight teams should receive a pre-flight brief before departure to familiarise themselves with the unique safety aspects of each aircraft, and be briefed on patient oxygen

---

BOX 16.1 Suggested formula for calculating in-transit oxygen requirements[3]

Oxygen requirements during transfer

$2 \times$ Transport time in minutes $\times$ [(MV $\times$ FiO$_2$) + ventilator driving gas]

where:

MV = minute volume

FiO$_2$ = inspired oxygen fraction.

Ventilator driving gas is dependent on ventilator make (e.g. an Oxylog 3000 uses 0.5 litres per minute)

Note that transport time is doubled, for safety.

Sample calculation for a 1-hour transport

MV = 6 litres per minute

FiO$_2$ = 0.6

Ventilator driving gas = 0.5 litres per minute

Requirements

$2 \times 60 \times [(6 \times 0.6) + 0.5]$

$= 120 \times 4.1 = 492$ litres of oxygen

	FIXED-WING	ROTARY-WING	ROAD
TABLE 16.1 Comparison of transport platforms[5]			
Speed	450 kph approximately	240 kph approximately	140 kph maximum
Landing	Requires landing strip	Versatile landing options	Not required
Altitude	0–35,000 ft, pressurised	5000–6000 ft, non-pressurised	Ground level
Cost	A$3000–$5000 approximately	$5000/h approximately	Dependent on crew wage level
Patient capacity	1–2 only	1 as standard; 4 at maximum	Single patient only
Activation time	40 minutes minimum needed before take-off	Rapid activation possible	Immediate activation possible
Gas laws	Can be pressurised	Nil pressurisation ability	Not affected, aside from alpine services
Range	3300 km	760 km	Limitless, though dependent on resource availability
Weather	Able to fly above weather	Can be affected by poor weather	Unaffected by weather, unless flood or road damage present

outlets, suction operation, power outlets and ALS equipment. Further, a mental rehearsal of Helicopter Underwater Escape Training (HUET) drills is advised whenever the flight path takes the aircraft and team over a body of water.

The Civil Aviation Safety Authority (CASA) have orders in place (specifically 20.11) that stipulate requirements with regards to emergency and life-saving equipment. These orders apply to all Australian registered aircraft and all team members who board an aircraft must have a current safety brief in place.

For all missions in the aviation environment, the pilot in command has ultimate responsibility for the safety of all those on board their aircraft. As such, they have the final say if they perceive a significant risk to the mission, therefore it is vital that the pilot is aware of the patient's condition and any requirements for the transport phase. It is therefore incumbent on the retrieval team to voice any of these prior to take-off. This should not be confused with trying to rush the pilot (i.e. potential or actual patient deterioration).

Ground transport

Ground transport of patients is the mainstay of ambulance services throughout Australasia. The vast majority of patient transports in the metropolitan environment are performed by road and over short distances. Long distances in the rural setting compound the issue of timely patient transport, and here it may be necessary to use rotary- or fixed-wing aircraft.

Adverse weather conditions may influence the decision of transport medium, and on occasion, ground transport may be the only option. Conversely, when traffic is heavy, roads are impassable or the topography contains mountains, winding roads etc, air transport may be a better option. Other considerations are transport time and the number of casualties/patients requiring transport.

Specialised options including bariatric transport platforms and teams are now standard in our society. Obtaining a clear and current weight of the patient is important fact-finding; once over 130 kg, transport becomes difficult. As with the transport of

patients undergoing complicated, specialist therapies, the bariatric patient also requires specialised teams and lifting equipment. This further increases the workload of the coordinating team who need to ensure that the patient destination is aware of any special needs (i.e. bariatric bed and lifting team made available on arrival). This can at times pose delays for the movement of the patient and access to definitive care.

The bariatric patient is subject to all of the stressors of flight or transport the same way as any other patient; however, consideration must be made for vibration (increased potential for pressure areas), temperature and hypoxia. Time spent for close attention to patient positioning to maximise chest excursion and ventilation is worthwhile, utilising a low threshold for supplemental oxygen delivery.

Rotary-wing aircraft

Rotary-wing aircraft provide rapid transport from point to point or from accident scene direct to a trauma centre. Helicopters can bypass traffic conditions in urban areas and rapidly transfer a critically ill patient to a tertiary hospital. In addition to those at major metropolitan hospitals, there are helipads at many rural and regional centres, and teams can be mobilised quickly to provide an increase in the level of care. Alternative landing zones can be created quickly at trauma scenes; for example, country sporting fields can be used as temporary helicopter landing zones easily by ground staff (i.e. local ambulance and/or fire services). However, the final decision of where the helicopter will land always sits with the Captain in charge of the aircraft. Helicopter transport is also beneficial across water or mountains, thus decreasing transit time.

Most Australasian helicopters operate up to 250 km from their base station without refuelling, with an average cruising speed of about 120 knots (220 kph). Operating from helipad to helipad negates the need for ground transport, preventing further delays in transport.

Although in some regions there is a survival benefit for major trauma patients when treated by a helicopter medical retrieval team,[9] helicopter transport is expensive,[5] and can expose the patient and crew to significant risks. Safety of helicopter aeromedical transport in Australia has been reviewed by Holland and Cooksley,[6] who reported that from 1992 to 2002, the accident rate was 4.38 per 100,000 flying hours, with one patient fatality as a result of a helicopter accident in 50,164 journeys. Helicopter operations can be restricted by adverse weather conditions, resulting delays, cancellations or alternative transport methods found. The Captain has the overarching authority to base the decision for flight on safe conditions regardless of clinical urgency. Coordinating staff must always consider alternative transport means and have them readily available should the team be unable to fly (grounded by potentially unsafe circumstances).

Fixed-wing aircraft

In 1928 the Royal Flying Doctor Service (RFDS) was the first comprehensive aero-medical organisation in the world and remains unique for the range of primary healthcare and emergency services it provides to the rural population of Australia.[7] With an average cruising speed of 240 knots (450 kph), the fixed-wing aircraft has the ability to cover vast distances in a relatively short time period, but is dependent on runways. The pressurised cabin provides the pilot with flight options regarding cruising altitude, as this can have negative effects on the patient and flight crew (see the section below on stresses of transport). When clinically indicated, the pilot can pressurise the cabin to ground-level pressure, but this can restrict flight options and increases fuel consumption and slow the journey. However, this must be articulated to the pilot prior to take-off.

Most aeromedical fixed-wing aircraft in Australasia can carry two patients and up to five crew (depending on aircraft and configuration), giving flight crew the flexibility of allowing family members to accompany the patient (if appropriate). All-weather navigational equipment allows the fixed-wing aircraft to fly in adverse weather conditions which may not be possible for rotary-wing aircraft. Once again, the fixed-wing captain needs to make an autonomous decision regarding flight safety. The mission is *never* more important than the safety of the crew.

The destination of fixed-wing aircraft is limited to the location of the nearest airstrip, so transport teams still rely on ground transport at both ends of the mission, adding time and increasing the clinical risk to the patient. All equipment must be secured in the aircraft in accordance with CASA regulations. All mounting brackets must comply with CASA regulations. This requirement ensures that flight crew and patients are not subjected to flying objects or missiles in the cabin during turbulence or in the event of a crash.

Commercial transport

For patient transport beyond the range of turbo-prop, fixed-wing aircraft, commercial aircraft can be used in two distinct environments: commercial passenger aircraft and medically configured jet aircraft.

With notice, the major commercial airliners can install a stretcher over 9–12 seats of domestic and international passenger aircraft. This would be at an additional cost, both in terms of a dollar value as well as space. This allows transport teams to transfer patients over long distances in relative comfort in a relatively larger working environment. With passengers surrounding the stretcher, interventions should be kept to a minimum and privacy needs to be maintained for the patient. Similar to an in-hospital ward environment, patient care requirements such as hygiene, toileting and nutrition must be attended to with discretion. There is always a risk of patient deterioration in any patient transport; however, when using commercial national or international aircraft, the risk of diversion or delays due to patient need is ever-present and must be considered.

Oxygen supply should be pre-organised and approved and must be able to be secured at all times. Patient monitoring can be difficult, as access to onboard power supplies may be

TABLE 16.2 Body cavities, symptoms and treatment for the effects of altitude[14]

CAVITY (CONDITION)	SYMPTOMS (CAUSES)	TREATMENT
Middle ear (barotitis media)	Pain on descent due to blocked eustachian tube (viral illness, infection)	Moving jaw, Valsalva manoeuvre, swallowing
Sinuses (barosinusitis)	Pain on descent due to cough/cold, sinus infection	Decongestants, avoiding flying
Teeth (barodentalgia)	Pain on descent in dental decay/abscesses	Avoiding flying when affected, and good dental care
Gastrointestinal tract	Abdominal bloating and pain, respiratory distress Post-operative free gas	Nasogastric tube insertion
Thoracic cage (pneumothorax)	Respiratory distress, chest pain, hypoxia, hypotension	Chest drain insertion, needle thoracocentesis
Cranium (pneumocephalus)	Headache, altered conscious state	Cranial decompression, intraventricular drain, sea-level cabin (or as close as possible)
Endotracheal tube	Gas leak on descent	Cuff check and addition of air to tube, using saline in cuff instead of air

difficult due to incompatibility, and few biomedical devices have a battery life that will last the length of a long flight. Back-up power supplies, i.e. spare batteries, must be accounted for during the planning phase of this type of transport.

Using a roster system to manage fatigue in the team is vital in these long-haul missions and simple down time will go a long way to ensuring the team is able to care for and respond to any patient need. Further, hydration and nutrition will also enable the team members to stay vigilant over long periods.

In Australasia, there are a number of medically configured jets which are used for patient transport. Commercial transport costs are expensive, with most funded by the patient's travel insurance company or by outright payment. The jet provides similar challenges in patient management to the fixed-wing aircraft in terms of stressors of transport. These aircraft have ranges of 3300 km or more and can fly at speeds exceeding 800 km/hr, making them a swift option for flight. For example, Adelaide to Darwin (approximately 2600 km flight distance) via propeller fixed-wing aircraft takes approximately 6 hours, while a Lear jet takes approximately 3.5 hours.

Australian Defence Force assets

At times, special needs, such as a natural disaster (Bundaberg floods, the evacuation of Cairns Base Hospital) or patient need (a bariatric patient who exceeds the size and weight limits for civilian ambulance services), require the assistance of the Australian Defence Force through the Defence Aid to the Civil Community (DACC) system. The Royal Australian Air Force (RAAF) provides the aeromedical evacuation capability Defence-wide, and this mature, responsive system can be provided to the civilian community. The RAAF has highly trained and experienced personnel, as well as airframes with a large patient load capacity.

Clinical coordination and communication

A single point of contact, attended 24 hours a day, 7 days a week, answered by clinically experienced staff, provides invaluable support to rural/regional referring facilities. Medical coordination staff provide clear advice for all types of presentations and for numerous and, at times, simultaneous requests for assistance. Clinical coordinators benefit from a background in aeromedical retrievals, giving them an inherent awareness of tasking, teams, platforms and resources.

The National Clinical Handover Initiative of the Australian Commission on Safety and Quality in Health Care has identified a need for a standardised hand-over checklist.[8] The failure of effective communication is a recurring theme in the patient safety literature, specifically as it relates to hand-over. A review of local clinical incidents confirmed that this pattern was particularly evident for acutely ill, deteriorating patients who require transfer to a higher level of care.[8]

The ISBAR hand-over tool has been suggested as one appropriate tool for safe and effective hand-over.[16] Like the primary survey, there is safety in following a process to make it easier to communicate all the relevant detail and information. The hand-over should be short, concise and practised prior to delivering the patient to the destination facility (see also Ch 11).

I **Identify**. This is the time to introduce both yourself and the patient.
  • Who are you and what is your role?
  • Patient identifiers (at least three).

S **Situation**. This is where you can provide information regarding where the patient has come from, a presenting complaint or provisional diagnosis and/or the mechanism of injury in the presence of trauma.
  • What is going on with the patient?
  • Patient stability/level of concern?

B **Background**. Any pertinent treatment and medical history must be relayed to the receiving facility.
  • What is the clinical background/context?
  • History of presentation

A **Assessment**. Providing physiological data is a place from which the primary assessment can take place. It is useful to provide the observations at the time or referral, in transit and when you arrive at the receiving facility.
  • What do you think the problem is?
  • What have you done so far?

R **Recommendation/Response/Rationale**. This may be the most important phase of the hand-over, as it confirms a shared understanding of patient care priorities. Any questions or concerns can be discussed at this stage.
  • What would you recommend or want done?
  • Risk—patient/occupational health and safety?
  • Assign and accept responsibility/accountability.
  • What is the plan from here?

This is just a suggested tool for hand-over; the facility you work in may have a process in place. It merely highlights the need for a structured, reproducible hand-over tool which is easy to remember and use. In the electronic age there are many additional resources such as the ISBAR smart phone application produced by New South Wales Health and South Australian Health as a handy guide and prompt when formulating a hand-over (see https://itunes.apple.com/au/app/isbar/id465890292?mt=8).

Telemedicine is a useful means of communication between the regional setting and central clinical coordination services. A combination of digital photography, real-time vision and the internet has made it possible for doctors to provide accurate advice, and interpret radiographs and monitoring to directly influence patient care. Studies have found that 75% of coordinators felt that telemedicine improved patient care, and, further, that both the referring doctors and the medical coordinators felt that telemedicine improved communication and patient assessment.[10] It should be understood that time spent organising and utilising telemedicine must not be at the expense of clinical care to the patient, or cause delay. In reality it can occur simultaneously and will influence decisions, i.e. active resuscitation of the patient while the team is en route, high fidelity patient information could dictate the urgency, speed of activation or determine the need for retrieval at all.

Team preparation

Training

Team members who are to be involved in the transfer of the critically ill must have appropriate situational awareness, experience and training. Each organisation will have specific training and experience requirements for their own services, but in general terms these should include:

- entry level nursing or paramedic qualifications
- a critical care specialty:
  - emergency
  - intensive care (neonate, paediatric and adult, specific to service)
  - intensive care paramedicine
- postgraduate aeromedical/retrieval qualifications
- Emergency Management Severe Trauma (EMST)
- Advanced Paediatric Life Support (APLS)
- Major Incident Medical Management Support (MIMMS)
- Helicopter Underwater Escape Training (HUET)

Keen patient assessment skills and the ability to diagnose and treat independently are ideal. Teamwork and excellent communication skills are also vital for safe and efficient transport of patients. Service-specific standing operating procedures (SOPs), clinical guideline and work instructions are site-specific and should be evidence-based.

Accreditation

Continual service accreditation and currency maintenance are a prerequisite for the transport environment. The level of skill required to safely practise in these circumstances is high, and team members are expected to be able to think and react very quickly and in difficult scenarios. Each team member has their own specialisation or craft mix, requiring ongoing registration, maintenance of professional standards and continual professional education.

Simulation training and mock scenarios are methods of introducing new theoretical and practical skills to those starting in retrieval medicine, and also a way to hone existing skills and maintain currency for the experienced practitioner. Consistent re-orientation of all transport modes must be adhered to, to maintain currency and familiarisation. Retrieval and transfer of the critically ill is a dynamic and evolving industry. New safety upgrades and technological improvements are continual, so the team must be current and up to date with these issues.

Helicopter Underwater Escape Training

Helicopters are noisy, distracting and generate an enormous amount of down-force from rotor wash, with almost invisible tail rotors located at head height in some models. Training and orientation are key to providing the safest working environment and reducing the opportunity for adverse outcomes when involved in rotary-wing aircraft emergencies or ditching over water. HUET has been made mandatory across many rotary-wing services, and is at times a service standard for all flight crew. The training involves

the demonstration and actual participation in how to exit an underwater rotary-wing aircraft in any orientation i.e. upside down or right way up (Figs 16.1 and 16.2). This training improves the chances of survival for the aircraft passengers, flight crews, patients and passengers.[11]

PRACTICE TIP

On every entry into the rotor wing aircraft, identify primary and secondary exits and undertake a personal rehearsal of escape drill.

Personal Protective Equipment (PPE) and uniforms

A properly sized and fitted uniform is essential as personal protective equipment and for identifying team members and roles. It should contain multiple pockets in which items such as gloves, a notebook, pens, food etc. can be carried, and form part of a safety standard. A brightly coloured uniform, complete with reflective tape, offers increased safety and visibility, especially after dark where ambient light will be low and provided by

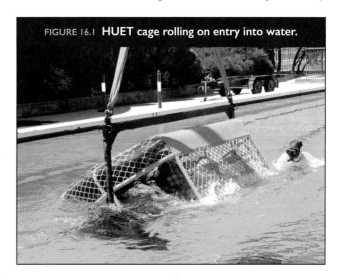

FIGURE 16.1 **HUET cage rolling on entry into water.**

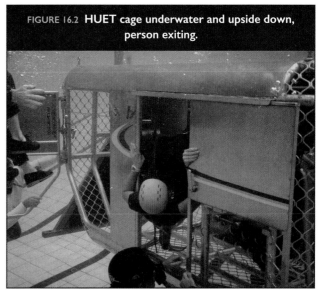

FIGURE 16.2 **HUET cage underwater and upside down, person exiting.**

electrical means. A fire-resistant Kevlar fabric is a standard in the aeromedical environment to reduce the effects of fire and the potential for burns to the team members. Helmets, rigger's gloves, eye and ear protection, hard-soled boots and life jackets with specific survival equipment when flying in rotary-wing aircraft are also essential in the out-of-hospital transport environment. When responding to roadside trauma scenes, high visibility tabards and safety helmets provide further safety in this, at times, austere environment. See Chapter 10 for scene assessment and management and Chapter 12 for information on different types of PPE.

Fitness

Fitness among aeromedical crew is a controversial topic; however, team members should have a reasonable level of fitness in order to be able to perform clinical duties in the relevant transport platform. A fit-for-task assessment prior to inclusion in the team is a method of identifying areas of need and will reduce the opportunity for adverse events and injury. A combination of aerobic fitness and strength will enable the team to adapt to any circumstances, such as carrying packs over great distances, handling stretchers over uneven surfaces or working in confined spaces.

Principles of transport

Pre-departure pack checking

Key to mission success is gear that is complete and regularly checked. Checking the packs can be carried out by both team members at the beginning of the shift, in a challenge and response format.[17] This will reduce the chance of discovering equipment is missing from the pack and therefore ensure that all necessary equipment is available for use on all missions. It places the responsibility of mission readiness squarely on the team, as well as keeping them familiar with the contents of the pack sets. Resources such as smart phone applications can hold all checklists and provide an easy-to-use method of checking and refamiliarisation. Case cards or patients' records can also contain specific areas for documenting or pre-planning the handover in readiness for delivery to the receiving facility.

Patient packaging

Taking the time to adequately package the patient is time well spent. The benefits include, but are not limited to:

- temperature management
- return of 'as-close-to' anatomically correct alignment of fractures, both obvious and suspected
- pain reduction and patient comfort
- reduction of undue handling
- reduction of unnecessary intervention or replacement of therapy at the receiving facility
- ease of access to intravenous lines during transport or in an emergency.

The patient should be totally exposed for a thorough examination, after which they must be kept warm to alleviate the effects of hypothermia. A skin-to-sheet or skin-to-device approach is an effective way to prepare the patient for transport. It is also a challenge to minimise the amount of times that the patient needs to be moved. Undue rough or multiple movements may disrupt any haemostatic clots about long bone

or pelvic fractures, increase pain and expose the patient to unnecessary environmental factors.

Where the index of suspicion for pelvic fractures is high, the pelvic splint is a device that is wrapped around the pelvic girdle of the traumatically injured patient. When applied correctly and directly to the skin, it can close previously separated or acutely fractured pelvic rings to reduce the haemorrhage and pain experienced by the patient. Likewise, the femoral traction splint is able to re-align femur fractures and thereby reduce pain and the potential for uncontrolled bleeding into the femoral space. The limb extremity must be assessed for perfusion and sensitivity, both pre- and post-application and during movement. It is useful to mark the site where a pulse is found and also to ensure the site is accessible during the transport phase for continual reassessment.

Figure 16.3 shows an example of a patient packaging technique. Note the use of a stretcher bridge for the securing of medical equipment, vacuum mattress, vital signs monitoring and ventilator. Challenges and considerations include reducing hypothermia (in this instance the patient has been kept exposed to show pelvic binder and monitoring leads), securing the ventilator circuit and maintaining stability of the stretcher as the centre of gravity is relatively higher and, as such, poses a tipping risk on uneven surfaces.

> **PRACTICE TIP**
>
> Good patient packaging promotes comfort, can reduce pain and allows for rapid access to the patient in the event of an emergency.

Aeromedical retrieval services have different methods for securing equipment onto the patient stretcher for transport. Often they will be in the form of stretcher bridges which are specifically designed to hold all monitoring and ventilation equipment. They are engineered and rated to cope with acceleration and deceleration forces in the event of a collision and make the equipment easily viewable and adjustable throughout the mission.

Providing in-transit care is challenging at best. The vehicle or aircraft can be subject to noise, movement and vibration and is a

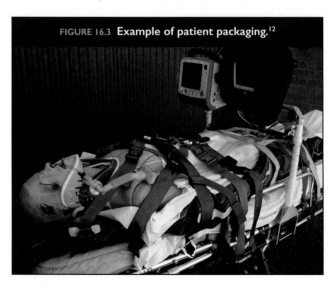

FIGURE 16.3 **Example of patient packaging.**[12]

cramped environment. This may hinder any access to the patient and can put the team at risk if they are out of safety harness, moving around in the cabin. Attempts must be made to package the patient in such a way as to optimise the access and anticipate any change in clinical state and to remain in a seated position throughout the critical phases of flight (i.e. take-off and landing).

Airway

The protection of any potentially unstable airway is of paramount importance, and plans should be put in place to make sure the first attempt at intubation is successful. A failed attempt at intubating a deteriorating patient in the rear of an aircraft or ambulance adds unnecessary stress to team members.

Methods to improve intubation success rate include, but are not limited to:

- *talking through the plan for an intubation.* This enables the practitioner to allocate roles to assistants, advise and educate those who may not be as familiar with the process and properly prepare the patient. This also ensures that all team members are attentive and concentrating on the task at hand.
- *using a 'kit dump' bag* (Fig 16.4). This is a suggested method for making the first attempt as easy as possible. Essentially, it is a yellow plastic bag (these may differ depending on the service preference) with outlines representing all equipment that is needed to carry out an intubation. It is placed at the right-hand side of the practitioner and is managed by the assistant, and allows for easy recognition and access to all equipment including secondary devices.

Once the patient has been successfully intubated, the team must spend time securing the tube, confirm cuff integrity and document the intervention. Vital information to be recorded should include: tube postion at teeth or lips, size of tube, position of patient, whether in-line immobilisation was utilised, drugs used for induction and doses.

Tying the tube in with tape does not guarantee security. Unexpected extubation, especially in-flight, is a challenging circumstance and all care must be taken to avoid this on all patient movement; a team member must therefore take control of the tube and be responsible for the coordination of the rest of the team.

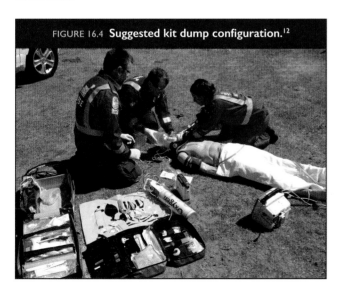

FIGURE 16.4 **Suggested kit dump configuration.**[12]

Breathing

Assessment of the patient's respiratory state forms part of the continuous assessment and should be carried out throughout the entirety of the patient transport. Subtle pathology has the potential to increase markedly on patient movement, especially at altitude. Close monitoring of arterial oxygen saturation (SaO_2) ± end-tidal carbon dioxide levels ($EtCO_2$) helps with recognising changes in respiratory state, but these must not be relied on in lieu of clinical assessment. The patient's respiration rate, work of breathing equality and depth of chest excursion must be continually monitored, all of which can be difficult in different circumstances such as at night or when the patient's chest is covered by blankets or monitoring equipment leads.

Hypoxia at altitude is of concern; therefore, all patients transferred by aircraft must have supplemental oxygen delivered to mitigate its effects (see sections below on gas laws and stressors of transport).

The assessment, diagnosis and treatment of a pneumothorax in flight or in the rear of an ambulance is almost impossible due to ambient noise and vibration (see below), and therefore in the presence of trauma, either blunt or penetrating, the transport team should have a low threshold for the insertion of chest drains. Ultrasound in the hands of an experienced practitioner can help with diagnosis of intra-thoracic pathology and can be performed prior to, during and post transport.

> **PRACTICE TIP**
>
> Keep basic airway adjunct and bag–valve–mask assemblies close at hand during the transport phase in case of an unexpected airway emergency.

Circulation

Before transporting the patient, two peripheral, well-secured and working intravenous (IV) cannula should be present and patent. Having a second line in situ offers redundancy if the first one should be dislodged during transfer. Monitoring should include electrocardiography (ECG), pulse oximetry and non-invasive blood pressure, as a minimum. Refer to Chapter 17, p. 339, for information on inserting an IV cannula and p. 336 for cardiac monitoring. For patients requiring inotropic support the discussion regarding central access should be considered and discussed by the referring and receiving facilities/units. Inotrope support should not be provided for via peripheral intravenous access for extended periods of time.

If the team is experiencing difficulty in gaining peripheral IV access, intra-osseous access should be the next step. Sites for insertion include the tibial plateau and the humeral head. Both sites are easily accessible and offer quick and effective access to the venous circulation. Any medication and fluid can be infused through these access points; however, they do need supplementary pressure as gravity alone is not strong enough to overcome the intra-osseous tissue.

> **PRACTICE TIP**
>
> If done correctly, intra-osseous access is quick, easy and in some cases may be the first choice for intra-vascular access.

Serial observations of the patient's haemodynamic state, including pulse rate and blood pressure, must be taken. The timing of these is determined by the patient's clinical state, but should be documented at least every 30 minutes. Once again, reliance on electronic equipment alone to monitor the patient's haemodynamic state can be difficult. At extremes of blood pressure, portable non-invasive blood-pressure (NIBP) monitors are inaccurate so observe for clinical signs of hypovolaemia and hypoperfusion. Observing skin colour, conscious state and palpating for peripheral pulses are useful techniques to monitor blood pressure. All efforts must be made to halt or reduce the amount of external blood loss with direct pressure being the most effective method.

Invasive monitoring, i.e. arterial lines, are a useful tool for continuous haemodynamic monitoring. A decrease or loss of cardiac output can be observed in the sometimes cramped and noisy transport environment. However, lengthy or troublesome insertions should not unduly delay the transport of the patient, especially in a time-critical scenario.

Disability

Assessing the patient's neurological state can be done quickly using AVPU (**A**lert, **V**erbalising, responding to **P**ain or **U**nresponsive) or using a formal Glasgow Coma Scale (see Ch 14). AVPU allows a quick assessment, and the GCS allows for a more detailed and thorough examination. Pupillary response to light must also be included in any neurological examination, and changes in response acted upon.

The agitated patient with an altered conscious state represents a danger to all team members, whether they are flying in an aircraft or travelling by road to the destination. Consideration must be given to sedation techniques, securing devices or, as a last resort, elective intubation of the patient, and also the exploration of alternative methods of transport. Likewise, the patient who has a labile conscious state may require intubation to secure the airway and avoid potential intubation in the cramped transport environment.

Monitoring and equipment

The ideal vital signs monitor needs a number of key features to satisfy all the requirements of the transport team. It must:

- be light and easy to carry
- be 'user friendly' and intuitive in its operations, both basic and advanced
- have a large, easy-to-read screen that can be read in bright sunlight and backlit when working in the dark or low light
- be robust and able to withstand rough handling and potential dropping
- have a long battery life with all parameters functioning
- have a short recharge time
- be able to measure ECG, SpO_2, NIBP, two invasive pressure lines, $EtCO_2$, temperature
- have consumables and biomedical engineering support readily available
- have an ease of interchangeability between services
- be safe for use in an aircraft, especially when defibrillating or pacing.

Not all monitoring devices are able to provide all of the attributes listed above, and sound understanding of the monitor's capabilities and limitations is imperative. The equipment and consumables carried by the retrieval team should be capable of responding to a variety of patient presentations, i.e. extremes of age, size and physiology. Care must be given to the overall weight and design of the pack sets, with special consideration as to the contents. A certain amount of redundancy in the packs offers a 'plan B' in the event of a failed procedure attempt or multiple patients. Table 16.3 shows a suggested contents list for a single-team pack set. It is completed by a transport 'suite' of monitor/defibrillator, stretcher bridge and ventilator.

Stressors of transport

The transport environment has specific stressors that must be understood, as they have the potential to have adverse effects on the patient who often already has altered physiology, as well on as the team caring for the patient. Once appreciated, the team can anticipate and plan for these. The effects are predictable and some are specific to the aviation environment, but they are also considered of importance in the road-transport platforms.

Hypoxia

Hypoxia is of concern in the aeromedical environment due to changes of the partial pressure of oxygen at altitude and can be defined as an oxygen deficiency in body tissues which, when sufficient, will cause impairment, either transient or permanent, of physiological function.[13] Oxygen comprises approximately 21% of inspired gas at sea level (760 mmHg) and its partial pressure is 159 mmHg. As the aircraft ascends in altitude, the atmospheric pressure decreases exponentially, therefore decreasing the partial pressure of oxygen. At 10,000 ft (3000 metres) oxygen is still at 21%; however, the barometric pressure falls to 523 mmHg resulting in a drop in partial pressure of oxygen to 110 mmHg. With this in mind, all patients transported by air should have supplemental oxygen delivered by the most appropriate device, dependent on clinical state.

Barometric pressure

The effects of altitude have direct consequences on the human body and equipment utilised for patient transport missions. Specifically, the effects of Boyle's Law must be understood. Boyle's Law relates to the expansion of gases and states that when temperature remains constant, the volume of a given mass of gas is inversely proportional to its pressure (see Ch 28). So as an aircraft increases its altitude, the barometric pressure decreases and the volume of gas in an enclosed space will expand. Therefore, any gas trapped in any enclosed space—whether it is a human or equipment space—is subject to this law.

Noise

Continuous noise has an insidious effect on the retrieval team, and levels vary depending on the type of transport frame utilised. The inability to clearly communicate with your team and hear any audible alarms on monitoring equipment places the patient at risk. Regular visual assessment of the monitor is essential, coupled with notifying any non-verbal cues provided by the patient. Grimacing, agitation, alteration in perfusion and skin colour are some of the signs to watch out for.

TABLE 16.3 Suggested transport pack contents list[12]

RESUSCITATION PACK		INSIDE MIDDLE POCKET	
Green Folder		Crepe bandage—5 cm	2
Patient records	2	Combine dressing—20 × 75 cm	1
MedSTAR Airway Register (inside patient record)	2	Combine dressing—10 × 20 cm	2
Cooksley Paediatric Card	2	Windlass bandage—6"	1
Mass Casualty recording sheet	1	1 Mersilk suture	1
RAH Helipad Lift Key work instruction	1	Spencer wells forceps	1 pr
RAH swipe card	1	Arterial tourniquet	2
FMC swipe card	1	Indwelling Foley catheter—18 fr	1
LMH swipe card	1	INSIDE BOTTOM POCKET	
Sharps container	1	500 mL normal saline bag	1
Yellow securing strap	1	Pressure bag	1
BAG/MASK MODULE—ADULT		IV giving set	1
Adult resuscitation bag with hose	1	Lever lock cannula	1
Resuscitation mask—size 4 & 5	1 ea	50 mL syringe	1
OPA—size 8, 9, 10	1 ea	Permanent marker	1
NPA—size 6, 7, 8	1 ea	Plastic bag	1
PEEP valve	1	AIRWAY MODULE	
KY jelly sachet	1	PANEL 1	
Safety pin	1	Laryngoscope handle	2
BAG/MASK MODULE—PAEDIATRIC		Laryngoscope blade, Mackintosh—size 3, 4	1 ea
Paediatric resuscitation bag with hose	1	Laryngoscope blade, Miller—size 1, 2	1 ea
Resuscitation mask—size 0/1, 2, 3	1 ea	10 mL syringe	1
OPA—size 5, 6, 7	1 ea	ETT mount	1
NPA—size 4, 5	1 ea	KY lube sachet	2
PEEP valve	1	PANEL 2	
KY jelly sachet	1	Intubating stylet—size S, M, L	1 ea
Safety pin	1	Cloth tube tie—1 m	2
INSIDE TOP POCKET		Bougie	1
Howard Kelly's forceps	2 pr	Magill forceps, adult & child	1 ea
No. 20 scalpel blade	2 ea	LMA fast trach armoured tube	1
Maxiswabs	2 ea	Dump bag	1
Sterile gloves—size 6, 7, 7.5, 8	1 pr ea	ETT, uncuffed—size 3	1
Sterile shears	1 pr	ETT, cuffed—size 3.5, 4, 4.5, 5, 6, 7, 8	1 ea
Gigli saw	1	Needle cric kit	1
Gigli saw handle	1 pr	Nasal prongs—adult, paediatric	1 pr ea

Continued

TABLE 16.3 Suggested transport pack contents list[12]—cont'd

PANEL 3	
Easi-cap	1
Paedi-cap	1
Persist plus swabs	1
No. 20 scalpel blade	1
Tracheal dilator forceps	1 pr
50 mL catheter tip syringe	1
Dental props—adult & child	1 pr ea
Nasogastric tube—10 g, 14 g	1 ea
Drainage bag	1
Epistat nasal catheter	2
25 mm durapore tape	1 roll
PANEL 4	
LMA—size 2, 3, 5	1 ea
LMA fast-trach—size 4	1
Tracheostomy tube—size 6 mm	1
Pre-RSI checklist	1
INTRAOSSEOUS/VASCULAR ACCESS MODULE	
Intraosseous insertion device	1
IO needle—adult, paediatric, obese	2 ea
3-way tap	2
10 mL syringe	1
10 mL normal saline ampoule	2
Persist plus swabs	2
IV cannula—14 g, 16 g, 18 g, 20 g	1 ea
IV bungs	2
Tegaderm	2
25 mm transpore tape	1 roll
Tourniquet	1
IV PACK	
500 mL normal saline bag	1
IV giving set	1
Pressure bag	1
IV cannula—14 g, 16 g, 18 g, 20 g	1 ea
Lever lock cannula	1
IV bungs	2

Tourniquet	1
25 mm transpore tape	1 roll
Persist plus swabs	2
Tegaderm	2
MAIN COMPARTMENT	
Limb splints	2
Pelvic binder, standard	1
Triangular bandage	1
Femoral traction device	1
PROCEDURE AND DRUG PACK	
IV/DRUG MODULE	
PANEL 1	
Tourniquet	1
Persist plus swabs	4
Alcohol swabs	10
IV cannula—14 g, 16 g, 18 g, 20 g, 22 g, 24 g	2 ea
Angiocath cannula—14 g, 16 g	1 ea
3-way tap	2
Lever lock cannula	2
IV bung	4
Drug added labels	4
Tegaderm	6
Rapid Infusor Catheter (RIC)	2
PANEL 2	
50 mL syringe	1
30 mL syringe	2
10 mL syringe	5
50 mm short bevel needle	1
Minimum volume extension set	2
Mucosal Atomising Device (MAD)	1
5 mL syringe	3
2 mL syringe	2
1 mL Leur Lock syringe	2
0.5 mL insulin syringe	1
18 g drawing up needle (red)	5
Vial access cannula (purple)	5

TABLE 16.3 Suggested transport pack contents list[12]—cont'd

Blunt access cannula (pink/green)	5	Monthly drug and consumables expiry matrix	1
21 g needle (green)	5	Glucometer pouch:	
25 g needle (orange)	5	Glucometer	1
25 mm durapore tape	1 roll	Test strips—individual	10 ea
PANEL 3		Lancets	10
Row 1:		**PANEL 5**	
Salbutamol metered dose inhaler (MDI)	1	Syringe roll containing:	
MDI ET tube mount	1	• 30 mL syringe	1
Ipratropium 500 mcg/1 mL	2	• 10 mL syringe	1
Salbutamol IV 5 mg/5 mL	2	• 5 mL syringe red plunger	3
Salbutamol nebules 5 mg/2.5 mL	5	Blunt access cannula (pink/green)	5
Row 2:		Vial access cannula (purple)	5
Meropenem 1 g	2	Blank medication labels	10
Vancomycin 1 g	2	Rocuronium 50 mg/5 mL (expires after 3 months out of fridge)	2
Aciclovir 500 mg/20 mL	2	Suxamethonium 100 mg/2 mL (expires after 3 months out of fridge)	2
Row 3:		Alcohol swabs	5
Cephazolin 1 g	1	Red bungs	5
0.5% Bupivacaine 50 mg/10 mL	2	10 mL normal saline ampoule	2
2% Lignocaine 100 mg/5 mL	2	On flap:	
Ondansetron 4 mg/2 mL	2	• 10 mL water for injection ampoule	4
Actrapid insulin 100 IU (expires after 3 months out of fridge)	1	• 10 mL normal saline ampoule	4
Row 4:		• 5% Glucose 100 mL	2
Hydrocortisone 100 mg	2	**PANEL 6**	
Naloxone 400 mcg/1 mL	2	Row 1:	
Phenytoin 250 mg/5 mL	4	Propofol 500 mg/50 mL	2
Tranexamic Acid 1000 mg/10 mL	2	Thiopentone 500 mg	2
Row 5:		Row 2:	
8.4% Sodium Bicarb 100 mL & hanger (in clear pouch)	1	Suxamethonium 100 mg/2 mL (expires after 3 months out of fridge)	2
50% Glucose 50 mL (in clear pouch)	1	Rocuronium 50 mg/10 mL (expires after 3 months out of fridge)	4
Potassium Chloride 10 mmol (in clear pouch)	2	Row 3:	
PANEL 4		Metaraminol 10 mg/1 mL	1
Medi-Wheel calculator	1	Amiodarone 150 mg/3 mL	3
Ziplock rubbish bag	1	GTN infusion 50 mg/10 mL	1
Drug infusion chart	1	SNP 50 mg/2 mL—shroud in box, behind clear plastic	1
Frank Shann drug book	1	Atropine 600 mcg/1 mL	5
Intra-nasal Fentanyl dosing guideline	1		

Continued

TABLE 16.3 Suggested transport pack contents list[12]—cont'd

Row 4:			Spencer Wells forceps	2 pr
GTN spray	1		**PANEL 3**	
Adrenaline 1 mg/1 mL	6		Sterile plastic drape	2
Metoprolol 5 mg/5 mL	2		Sterile regional adhesive drape	2
Noradrenaline 2 mg/2 mL	6		Maxi-swab	4
Row 5:			**PANEL 4**	
Calcium Chloride 1 g/10 mL	1		Sterile glove—size 6, 6.5, 7, 7.5, 8, 8.5	1 pr ea
Hydralazine 20 mg	2		Sterile hypafix dressing—10 cm × 25 cm	8
Adenosine 6 mg/2 mL	5		Dressing pack	1
Magnesium Sulphate 10 mmol/5 mL	2		**ARTERIAL LINE MODULE**	
INSIDE TOP POCKET			**PANEL 1**	
Adult manual BP cuff set—complete	1		Pressure cable	1
Stethoscope	1		10 mL normal saline ampoule	5
NIBP cuff, child, obese/thigh	1 ea		10 mL syringe	2
INSIDE MIDDLE POCKET			10 mL springfusor	1
50 mL syringe	4		Velcro support strap	1
Minimum volume extension set	4		Red bungs	4
Lever lock cannula	4		Stitch cutter	1
3-way tap	4		2.0 silk suture	1
INSIDE BOTTOM POCKET			Steri strip	1 pkt
Disposable gowns	2		Spencer Wells forceps	1 pr
Safety glasses	2		Gauze swab—10 cm × 10 cm	1 pkt
N95 mask—S, M	2 pr ea		Tegaderm	2
3M protector mask	2 pr		Sterile plastic drape	1
MINOR SURGICAL MODULE			**PANEL 2**	
PANEL 1			20 g radial artery catheter	2
Portex drainage bag	2		Persist plus swabs	2
Atrium connector	2		0.5 mL insulin syringe	1
PANEL 2			2% lignocaine	1
Tegaderm	2		20 g IV cannula	2
Gauze swab—10 cm × 10 cm	4		Pressure transducer set	2
1 mersilk suture	2		**CENTRAL ACCESS MODULE**	
2.0 silk suture	2		7 fr/20 cm triple lumen CVC	1
Stitch cutter	1		16 g/20 cm single lumen CVC	1
No. 11 scalpel	1		9 fr swann sheath	1
Scissors	1 pr		Spare guide wire	1

TABLE 16.3 Suggested transport pack contents list[12]—cont'd			
18 g spare access needle	1	INTERCOSTAL CATHETERS	
HYPERTONIC SALINE		ICC—12 fr, 20 fr, 28 fr	1 ea
250 mL 7.5% saline bag	1	ICC—32 fr	2
IV giving set	1	MAIN COMPARTMENT	
Lever lock cannula	1	NIV mask—S, M, L—in zip-lock bag	1 ea
Laminated dosing guideline	1	Syringe driver (>80% charge)	2

TABLE 16.4 Oxygen cylinder size, contents and duration at varying flow rates (duration is approximate only)[18]

CYLINDER SIZE	400 C	400 CD	400 ND	400 NE	400 NG
CONTENTS (LITRES)	490	630	1,600	4,000	8,075
1 Litre/min	8:10	10:30	26:40	66:40	134:35
2 Litre/min	4:05	5:15	13:20	33:20	67:17
3 Litre/min	2:43	3:30	8:53	22:13	44:51
4 Litre/min	2:03	2:37	6:40	16:40	33:38
5 Litre/min	1:38	2:06	5:20	13:20	26:55
6 Litre/min	1:21	1:45	4:26	11:06	22:25
7 Litre/min	1:10	1:30	3:48	9:31	19:13
8 Litre/min	1:01	1:18	3:20	8:20	16:49
10 Litre/min	0:49	1:03	2:40	6:40	13:27
15 Litre/min	0:32	0:42	1:46	4:26	8:58

In the self-ventilating patient, predetermined hand signals may be useful to alert the team of any increasing symptoms, nausea or anxieties. Patient education of what to expect is important to allay any fears they may have and potentially decrease the workload for the team.

Classic assessment techniques such as chest auscultation, manual blood pressure measurement and percussion can be rendered useless in the transport environment; subtle changes or notes will be affected by the ambient noise.

To protect the hearing of both the team and the patient, hearing protection is mandatory in the form of mouldable ear plugs or rigid external muffs. This is still the case for intubated and ventilated patients who are sedated; they are still at risk of hearing damage. The longer the exposure and the more intense the noise, the greater the potential damage.[16]

Vibration

Vibration affects the management of the critically ill patient in transit, and is present in all forms and all transport platforms. The body's responses to vibration include increased muscle activity, increased metabolic rate, vasoconstriction, disturbed visual acuity and increased respiratory rate.[14] The already compromised patient may be further destabilised by these physiological changes.

It is difficult to minimise the effects of vibration on both the patient and the team alike. Reducing the amount of body contact with the airframe by sitting on cushioned seats for the team and effective packaging of the patient will serve to alleviate the effects. However, it should be relayed to the patient that they will experience vibration and shudder, especially on take-off and landing.

Transport equipment, particularly monitoring, is susceptible to interference. ECG and SaO_2 waveforms can become unrecognisable, even being interpreted as VT/VF. It is therefore required of the team member to visually assess the patient, elicit a response or feel for a pulse. It should be understood that clear visualisation of all patients at all times is imperative.

Temperature

During transport, both the team and the patients are exposed to variations in temperature. As the altitude of the aircraft increases, the internal ambient temperature will decrease at a rate of approximately 2°C every 1000 ft (300 metres). In fixed-wing aircraft, temperature is more controlled; however, special consideration must be given to any patient contact with the fuselage of the aircraft as the walls will be cooler than the ambient temperature. In rotary-wing aircraft, the change in temperature is more important. Depending on helicopter model, there are varying levels of in-cabin temperature control, ranging from climate control to exhaust-driven piped heating only.

Both hyperthermia and hypothermia create an increase in metabolic rate and subsequent increased oxygen demand and consumption. This additional stress may compound problems for the already compromised patient. Prolonged exposure to extremes of temperature may cause irritability, impaired performance of the team, motion sickness, fatigue, headache and a reduction in any stress-coping mechanisms the patient or team may have.

Strategies to reduce the effect of temperature on the patient include: reducing exposure to the elements when transiting between aircraft, ambulance and hospital and accessing the patient; warm blankets, including space (thermal) blankets; removing any wet clothes from the skin; covering the head; and the use of warmed IV fluids when possible.

Fatigue

Fatigue is the cumulative end-product of all the stressors combined. The fatigue management of staff must always be considered a high priority for any tasking and coordination. It is important to minimise the effects of fatigue on the team by ensuring appropriate downtime, satisfactory time off between shifts and the provision of good teamwork in monitoring each other for signs of exhaustion and off-lining those who are fatigued. A culture where team members feel empowered to speak up and advise others of their fatigue is important, and this also must be supported by policy.

Debrief and post-mission review

Discussing every mission should be standard procedure for all team members involved in the retrieval of the critically unwell. All attempts should be made to have this discussion as close to the date of the mission as possible. The case details, good and bad, will be fresh in the team members' minds and will offer useful insights for other staff to reflect upon. This can be done in two ways: either a formal audit or an informal debriefing process directly post mission. Working from a template will offer prompts for detailed conversation. See Table 16.5 for a suggested post-mission debrief form. The audit forum will often take place the next day, and provides the opportunity for staff to discuss the case, identify areas for improvement and make innovative suggestions for treatment. It is of value to discuss the case post-mission, when returning to base or to the home unit. Informally debriefing case details while they are fresh in your mind and all team members are available will provide valuable discussion points and an opportunity to acknowledge the team's efforts.

Further, it is just as important to provide the referring hospital with feedback on the patient's treatment and condition post transfer. Often the sick patient will represent the biggest source of stress and anxiety for these referring staff, and it is important from both a patient safety and a staff morale point of view to provide constructive feedback on the case.

Feedback can be sought from a senior team member who ensures impartiality and a useful opportunity to discuss the case in full, without any prejudice or preconceived ideas.

Psychological considerations

Open and transparent communication with both the patient and the family cannot be overlooked. The family have been exposed to an increased level of stress already, seeing their loved one acutely ill or injured, and on top of that the patient is to be moved from the local community to a larger, foreign and often city-based receiving facility far away. Clear explanations of procedures (time permitting), plans for movement, destination and expectations during transport will go a long way to reducing anxieties and provide important information that can be disseminated to extended family and friends. Providing phone numbers for the patient's destination is also useful. If the patient survives, they will be returning to the home community and will be cared for by the referring hospital in the future.

The team must demonstrate a cohesive and professional demeanour with the family and patient to instil confidence that the patient will be taken care of in the best possible fashion. The augmentation of care that the transport team provides will help with this; however, a disjointed and abrupt approach to the patient will not only put them in jeopardy but will also serve as another source of stress and anxiety. This confidence from the patient cannot be underestimated.

At times a family member will request that they accompany the patient while in transit. In fixed- and rotary-wing environments this request often cannot be granted due to weight and space limitations. However, the request should not be flatly refused and should be discussed with the team at large, including the pilot and crewperson. The patient's condition should also be factored in to the decision-making process, as an unstable patient in transit who may require continual care could represent further opportunities for stress reactions and the family member may in fact cause a hindrance or block to adequate and safe patient access. Alternatively, the family member's presence may alleviate some of the patient's anxiety, especially when the patient is a child. The decision should not be made until the time of the transport, because the patient's condition may change and promises cannot always be kept. The final decision as to whether the family member accompanies the patient always rests with the aircraft captain.

Providing as much information as possible to the family about the relieving facility is also important. The actual destination (ED, ICU or ward number) gives a clear picture of a first port of call for the family, as well as maps and current contact phone numbers. The family should be informed of the estimated length of transport and expected time of arrival at the receiving hospital. Ensuring that the family has time with the patient before departure will prove to be a very valuable part of the transport. This may indeed be the last time they have with their loved one, and the importance of goodbyes and farewells cannot be trivialised. Overestimation of time is always best—if the transport is completed sooner than anticipated, the family will feel relief.

> **PRACTICE TIP**
>
> The stressors of flight and transport are experienced by the team as well. Keep an eye on your team mate and do not be afraid to voice any issues you may identify or are experiencing yourself.

TABLE 16.5 Suggested post-mission, team debrief template[12]		
Crew names:	Date and shift:	Mission outline:
Coordination and tasking (involve coordination staff where able)		Action points
En route to scene (including driving, enplaning, in-flight, deplaning etc.)		Action points
Scene safety		Action points
Team organisation and interaction with local team/crew/staff		Action points
Clinical plan		Action points
Interventions, SOP compliance and knowledge		Action points
Communications		Action points
Departing scene, loading into aircraft or vehicle		Action points
En route to destination care		Action points
Hand-over and documentation		Action points
What if …?		Action points

SUMMARY

The successful transfer of the critically unwell patient can have far-reaching consequences for the patient, as there is a large portion of the community who have limited access to an increased scope of care. The transport environment is an emerging specialist role and cannot be considered a part-time job. It is a constantly evolving specialty, with significant improvements and changes occurring on an international scale.

It takes dedicated and motivated retrieval team members to prepare, respond and deliver patient care in challenging circumstances while maintaining perspective on the safety of teams and patients. At times the team will be expected to work in austere and potentially dangerous environments, so they must be supported by a framework of training, education, teamwork and clinical governance.

CASE STUDY

Three young female occupants of a car were involved in a high-speed rollover on a highway in a distant rural location. Pre-hospital, they were attended to by paramedic staff and taken to the local hospital. This hospital has a three-bed emergency department and telemedicine facilities.

Patient 1

20-year-old female
- Injuries etc include:
  - severe maxillo-facial and head injuries with altered conscious state
  - traumatic above-elbow amputation of the right arm
  - multiple abrasions and contusions to chest, abdomen and lower limbs
- no IV access
- patient receiving assisted bag-and-mask ventilation with upper airway noises
- stiff neck collar applied
- nil obvious haemorrhage from amputation site
- patient fully exposed and not covered by a blanket.

Patient 2

19-year-old female

- Injuries etc include:
  - mid-thigh swelling and deformity of right lower limb
  - multiple contusions and abrasions
  - screaming with pain, though orientated
- stiff neck collar applied, though not compliant with request to lie still.

Patient 3

20-year-old female

- Injuries etc include:
  - multiple abrasions and contusions–
  - left arm pain
  - closed head injury with ? no loss of consciousness
  - awake and aware of surroundings
- stiff neck collar in situ
- crying with repetitive questioning regarding her friends' welfare.

Two aircraft have been tasked to this hospital, and each has the ability to carry two patients. The transport team includes two senior doctors, a retrieval nurse, two flight nurses and local resources such as the GP, paramedic and nursing staff. Flight time via a fixed-wing aircraft back to the trauma centre is approximately 2 hours (including ambulance legs from airport to hospital).

Questions

1. What are the priorities of the retrieval team?
2. How would you allocate the available resources?
3. How would you assess the patients and what would your treatment priorities be?
4. What should the retrieval team expect in terms of patient condition and potential complications in-flight?
5. What configuration of transport teams would you choose?
6. How would you prepare the patients for transport?
7. What methods would you use to integrate with the local healthcare team?
8. What communication needs to occur, and at what time?

 Answers to Case Study Questions can be found on evolve
http://evolve.emergencytrauma.curtis

REFERENCES

1. Australian and New Zealand College of Anaesthetists, Joint Faculty of Intensive Care Medicine, Australasian College for Emergency Medicine. Minimum standards for transport of critically ill patients. Updated 2013. Online. www.anzca.edu.au/resources/professional-documents/pdfs/ps52-2010-minimum-standards-for-transport-of-critically-ill-patients.pdf; accessed May 2014.
2. Shirley PJ, Hearns S. Retrieval medicine: a review and guide for UK practitioners. Part 1: clinical guidelines and evidence base. Emerg Med J 2006;23(12):937–42.
3. Ellis D, Hooper M. Cases in pre-hospital and retrieval medicine. Sydney: Churchill Livingstone; 2010.
4. Wallace PG, Ridley SA. ABC of intensive care: transport of critically ill patients. Br Med J 1999;319(7206):368–71.
5. Taylor CB, Stevenson M, Jan S et al. A systematic review of the costs and benefits of helicopter emergency medical services. Injury 2010;41(1):10–20.
6. Holland J, Cooksley DG. Safety of helicopter aeromedical transport in Australia: a retrospective study. Med J Aust 2005;182(1):17–19.
7. O'Connor J. The Royal Flying Doctor service of Australia: the world's first air medical organization. Air Med J 2001;20(2):10–12.
8. Porteous JM, Stewart-Wynne EG, Connolly M et al. ISoBAR—a concept and handover checklist: the national clinical handover initiative. Med J Aust 2009;190(11 suppl): S152–6.
9. Saffle JR, Edelman L, Morris SE. Regional air transport of burns patients: a case for telemedicine? J Trauma 2004;57(1):57–64.
10. Mathews KA, Elcock MS, Furyk JS. The use of telemedicine to aid in assessing patients prior to aeromedical retrieval to a tertiary referral centre. J Telemed Telecare 2008;14(6):309–14.
11. CareFlight Safety Services. Helicopter underwater escape training-training manual. 1st edn. 2005.
12. MedSTAR Emergency Medical Retrieval Services. Agency overview. SA Health: SA Ambulance Service. South Australia: Government of South Australia; 2007.
13. Martin TE. Clinical aspects of aeromedical transport. Curr Anaesth Crit Care 2003;14:131–40.
14. Harding J, Goode D. Physical stresses related to the transport of the critically ill: optimal nursing management. Aust Crit Care 2003;16(3):93–100.
15. Blumen IJ. Altitude and flight physiology: a reference for air medical physicians. Air Medical Physician Association 1994.
16. Thompson JE, Collett LW, Langbart MJ et al. Using the ISBAR handover tool in junior medical officer handover: a study in an Australian tertiary hospital. Postgrad Med J 2011;87:340–4.
17. Degani, A, Wiener E. Human Factors of Flight-Deck Checklists: The Normal Checklist. National Aeronautics and Space Administration 1990.
18. BOC Healthcare Australia website. www.boc-healthcare.com.au/en/quality-safety/download-centre/index.html; accessed 26 May 2015.

CHAPTER 17
CLINICAL SKILLS

JAMES BRINTON AND WENDY FENTON

Essentials

- Clinical skills range from those skills performed frequently on a day-to-day basis to skills which will only be encountered on a very infrequent basis.
- Skills will range from the complex to the simple. It is of course beyond the scope of this text to present all the clinical skills that the emergency clinician would require; rather, a broad range of specifically selected skills is presented.
- The skills outlined are presented in association with the relevant anatomy and physiological considerations and based upon the latest available evidence.
- The emergency clinician requires the skills outlined, as they are a valuable resource in order to (1) refresh previously learnt skills and (2) acquire knowledge to develop new and more advanced skills to deliver patient care.

QUICK REFERENCE TO SKILLS IN THIS CHAPTER:

INTRODUCTION

The emergency clinician requires a vast repertoire of clinical skills in order to provide care. This repertoire of skills increases with time and experience. Some skills are utilised daily, while others may be learnt but never used. It is essential that the emergency clinician has a solid theoretical and practical knowledge base in order to perform these skills competently. Many of these skills may be utilised outside the emergency environment in the pre-hospital setting or in the general ward environment; or by clinicians not normally involved in the provision of emergency care, for example, in outpatient clinics, local doctors' rooms or medical centres.

The procedures outlined in this chapter should only be performed by clinicians who have the necessary knowledge, skill development and demonstrated competency. These skills should be performed in accordance with any professional licensing requirements and in accordance with the employing institutions' policy and procedures.

Airway management

Assessment of the adequacy of a patient's airway is a priority in any patient's initial assessment and management. Assessment and management of the airway in any critically ill patient is of particular importance, especially for those patients with an altered level of consciousness. Any patient identified as having an inadequate airway will require immediate interventions. Interventions utilised in airway management generally begin simply and move to the more complex, and are described here.

Basic airway management

Basic airway management involves the assessment of the patient and the implementation of a variety of simple interventions aimed at opening and maintaining the patency of the patient's airway. This often involves suctioning of the airway where required and the administration of oxygen, both of which are described later in this chapter (p. 327 and p. 316, respectively). These simple interventions, while providing a patent airway to assist with ventilation, do not provide airway protection against aspiration. Airway protection is achieved through the more-complex interventions described below, such as intubation.[1]

Upper airway obstruction can occur by the tongue, substances retained in the mouth such as saliva, vomitus, blood or foreign bodies, or by laryngospasm, leading to ineffective ventilation. Obstruction may be *complete* or *partial*. Complete obstruction results in the absence of air exchange. Signs of partial upper airway obstruction include snoring, inspiratory stridor and retractions of the neck and intercostal muscles. The most common cause of upper airway obstruction is by the relaxation of the tongue and jaw which causes the base of the tongue to fall backwards against the posterior pharyngeal wall in the supine patient.[2] Upper airway obstruction caused by the tongue can be relieved by head tilt/chin lift or jaw thrust manoeuvres and by the insertion of either nasopharyngeal or oropharyngeal airways.[1]

Head tilt/chin lift manoeuvre

To perform the head tilt/chin lift manoeuvre, the palm of one hand is placed on the patient's forehead while the tips of the fingers of the other hand are placed under the patient's

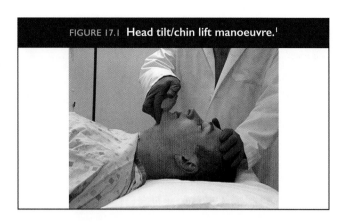

FIGURE 17.1 Head tilt/chin lift manoeuvre.[1]

chin, avoiding the soft tissues of the submandibular region. The chin is then lifted up and back towards the back of the patient's head and upwards to the ceiling (Fig 17.1). The upper neck will naturally extend when the head tilts backwards and therefore this manoeuvre is not preferred in the patient with a possible cervical spine injury. An additional step which may be considered with this manoeuvre is to use the thumb to open the patient's mouth.[1,2]

Jaw thrust manoeuvre

To perform the jaw thrust manoeuvre, the hands are placed on the patient's face with the middle or index fingers behind the angle of the mandible. The mandible is then lifted vertically towards the ceiling (see Fig 17.2). This manoeuvre may also be performed in combination with a head tilt; however, the head tilt should not be performed if there is suspected cervical spine injury.[1,2] The preferred airway manoeuvre in suspected cervical spine injury is the jaw thrust without head tilt performed with the neck in the neutral position and supported by in-line stabilisation.[1]

> **PRACTICE TIP**
>
> The preferred airway manoeuvre in suspected cervical spine injury is the jaw thrust without head tilt performed with the neck in the neutral position and supported by in-line stabilisation.

Airway adjuncts

Airway adjuncts are used in addition to initial airway manoeuvres and suctioning in order to maintain airway patency,

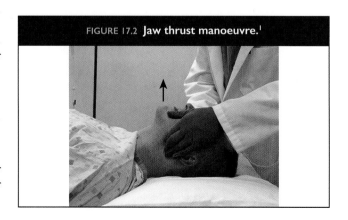

FIGURE 17.2 Jaw thrust manoeuvre.[1]

facilitating either spontaneous respirations or assisted bag–mask ventilation. Two types of airway adjuncts are available: the *oropharyngeal airway* and the *nasopharyngeal airway*.

Oropharyngeal airway

The oropharyngeal airway (Fig 17.3) is a semicircular-shaped airway made of hard plastic. The airway is inserted through the open mouth, over the tongue, with the tip positioned in the patient's pharynx. The airway displaces the tongue forwards off the posterior pharyngeal wall. The airway has four parts: flange, body, tip and channel. The flange protrudes from the patient's mouth, resting against the lips. The body of the airway covers the tongue. The channel allows the passage of a suction catheter.[3]

The oropharyngeal airway is indicated only in unconscious patients; otherwise it is likely to initiate gagging and vomiting. Due to its hard plastic construction it also prevents teeth clenching and is often used in conjunction with an oral endotracheal tube. Care must be taken on insertion not to push the tongue backwards into the posterior pharyngeal wall, causing obstruction.[1,3]

Procedure for oropharyngeal airway insertion

1. Wash hands and don personal protective equipment (PPE).
2. Select the correct-sized airway by selecting an airway measuring the same distance from the patient's lips to the angle of the jaw (see Fig 17.4).
3. Suction the mouth and pharynx if required.
4. Open the patient's mouth and remove dentures if present.
5a. Insert the oral airway—method 1 (see Fig 17.5):
   - Hold the oral airway with the curve facing upwards.
   - Advance the airway towards the hard palate and into the back of the mouth
   - Rotate the airway 180 degrees over the base of the tongue and into the oropharynx.
5b. Insert the oral airway—method 2; this method is recommended in paediatric patients due to the size of their tongue and the softness of their hard palate:
   - Hold the oral airway with the curve facing downwards.

   - With a tongue depressor, displace the tongue down and forwards.
   - Insert the airway directly over the tongue into the oropharynx.
6. Recheck the size and position of the airway.
7. Verify patency of the airway.

Nasopharyngeal airway

The nasopharyngeal airway is a soft, flexible tube consisting of three parts: flange, cannula and bevel or tip. The flange, at the proximal end, is trumpet-shaped to prevent the airway slipping into the nasal cavity. A hollow cannula allows airflow into the hypopharynx and also allows the passage of a suction catheter. The bevelled tip assists with insertion and when inserted correctly sits posterior to the base of the tongue (see Fig 17.6).[4]

The nasopharyngeal airway has advantages over the oropharyngeal airway as it is much better tolerated in semiconscious patients and is less likely to induce vomiting in patients with an intact gag reflex.[1] Other benefits over the oropharyngeal airway include its use in patients with trismus and dental trauma.[5] The nasopharyngeal airway may cause epistaxis and the use of this airway is contraindicated in patients with suspected facial fractures and basilar skull fractures.[1,2]

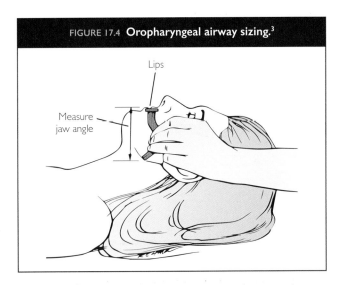

FIGURE 17.4 **Oropharyngeal airway sizing.**[3]

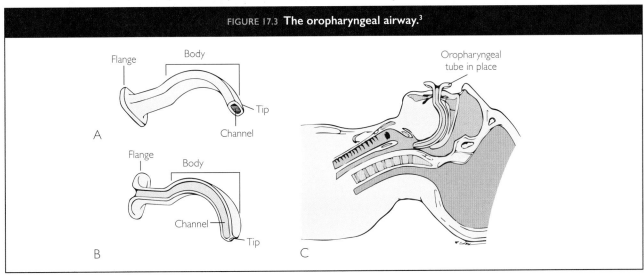

FIGURE 17.3 **The oropharyngeal airway.**[3]

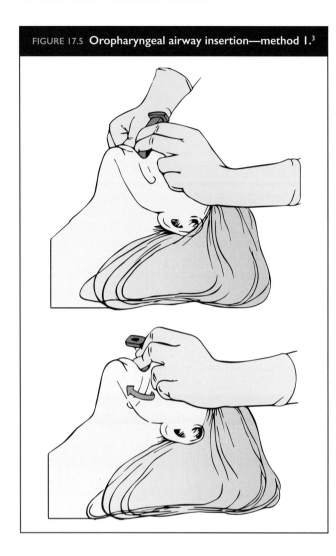

FIGURE 17.5 **Oropharyngeal airway insertion—method 1.**[3]

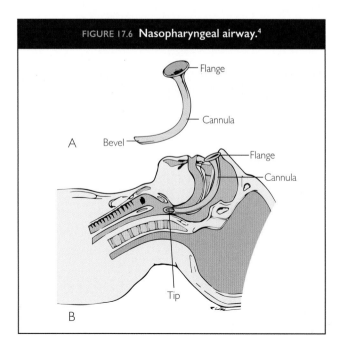

FIGURE 17.6 **Nasopharyngeal airway.**[4]

Procedure for nasopharyngeal airway insertion

1. Wash hands and don PPE.
2. Select the correct-sized airway by selecting an airway measuring the same distance from the tip of the patient's nose to the tip of the earlobe (see Fig 17.7A).
3. Identify the nasal passage with the largest diameter.
4. Generously lubricate the tip and outer surface of the airway with a water-based lubricant.
5. Gently slide the airway into the nostril and direct the airway medially and downwards along the nasal floor.
6. Advance the airway into the nasal passage until the flanged end sits comfortably at the nostril (Fig 17.7B).
7. Verify patency of the airway.
8. Suction secretions as required.

Bag–mask ventilation

Bag–mask ventilation is the single most important skill in airway management. Although it appears simple, it is one of the most difficult procedures to perform correctly. Performed correctly, bag–mask ventilation provides effective oxygenation and ventilation, reduces the urgency for intubation and also reduces anxiety associated with failed intubation attempts. Proficient use of bag–mask ventilation is a prerequisite for more advanced methods of airway management.[1,6]

Successful bag–mask ventilation is dependent on a patent airway, adequate mask seal and proper ventilation.[6] Bag–mask ventilation may be achieved by one or two operators, however the two operator technique is the most effective, and should be used whenever resources allow.[1,6]

With *single-operator bag–mask ventilation*, one hand is used to seal the mask on the face while the other is used to squeeze the bag in order to ventilate the patient. An E–C clamp technique is often effective in providing a mask seal. The thumb and index finger form a 'C' over the mask and apply pressure anteriorly to form a seal, while the third, fourth and fifth fingers form an 'E' to lift the jaw forwards into the mask (see Fig 17.8). Single-operator success is often dependent on the operator's hand size and on their ability to achieve an adequate seal of the face mask and lift the lower jaw into the mask while providing adequate ventilations with the other hand.

The *two-operator technique* has the more experienced person controlling the mask with their thenar eminences and thumbs on top of the mask, to maintain an adequate facemask seal[6] and their second through to fifth fingers performing a jaw thrust, lifting the mandible up into the mask. The other operator controls the bag, providing ventilations (see Fig 17.9).

To provide ventilation using the bag–mask approach, the ventilation bag must be connected to an oxygen supply with a flow rate of 15 L/min. Ventilations must be delivered in such a way as to provide effective oxygenation while avoiding generating large tidal volumes, high peak airway pressures and gastric inflation. It is recommended that bag–mask ventilations in adults be administered to provide a tidal volume of approximately 500 mL at a rate of 10–12 ventilations/ minute, with each ventilation delivered over 1–1.5 seconds. In children and infants, care must be taken to deliver only the volume necessary to achieve effective ventilation. Effectiveness of ventilation can be assessed by rise of the chest, breath sound, oxygen saturation and capnography.[1,6]

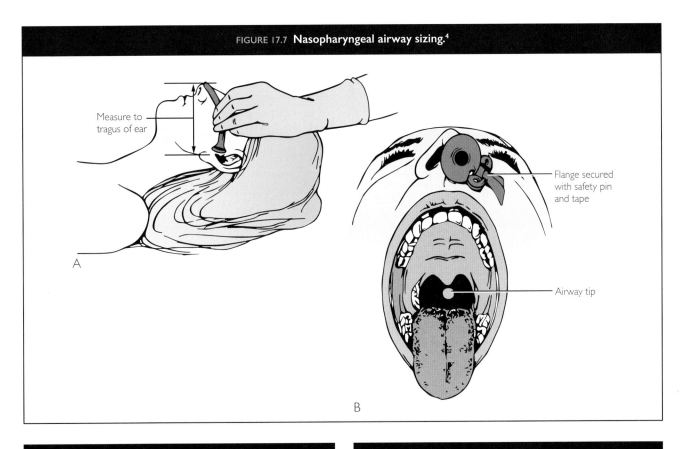

FIGURE 17.7 **Nasopharyngeal airway sizing.**[4]

Measure to tragus of ear

A

Flange secured with safety pin and tape

Airway tip

B

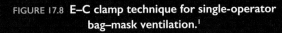

FIGURE 17.8 **E–C clamp technique for single-operator bag–mask ventilation.**[1]

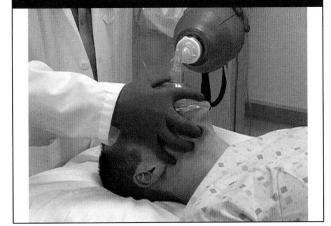

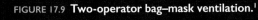

FIGURE 17.9 **Two-operator bag–mask ventilation.**[1]

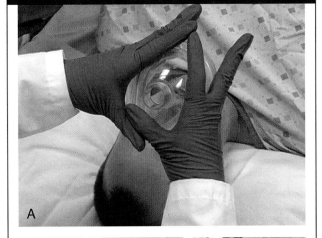

A

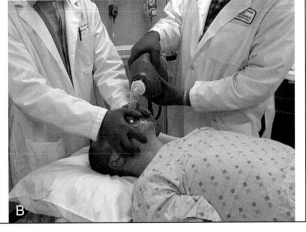

B

PRACTICE TIP

It is recommended that bag–mask ventilations in adults be administered to provide a tidal volume of approximately 500 mL at a rate of 10–12 ventilations/minute, with each ventilation delivered over 1–1.5 seconds.

Cricoid pressure (Sellick's manoeuvre)

While a manoeuvre recommended during rapid-sequence intubation (RSI), cricoid pressure may be considered during bag–mask ventilation if resources allow. Sellick's manoeuvre is performed by placing the thumb and middle finger over

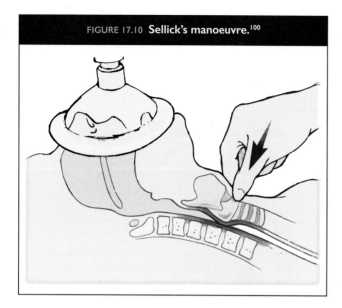

FIGURE 17.10 **Sellick's manoeuvre.**[100]

BOX 17.1 **The seven steps of RSI**[10]

1. Preparation
2. Preoxygenation
3. Pretreatment
4. Paralysis with induction
5. Positioning
6. Placement with proof
7. Postintubation management

the cricoid cartilage and applying downward pressure (see Fig 17.10). The cricoid cartilage is displaced posteriorly, occluding the oesophagus against the spinal column. The airway is not compressed due to the rigid nature of the cricoid ring.

Cricoid pressure attempts to prevent gastric inflation and passive regurgitation of gastric contents. The manoeuvre should only be used in the unconscious patient.[6] Care should be taken in children whose airways are more pliable, to avoid airway obstruction with excessive pressure.[1] The use of cricoid pressure is controversial, as good evidence has not been found to support its efficacy; however, if resources allow it should continue to be utilised.[1,6,7]

Intubation

Rapid-sequence intubation (RSI) is a technique used for the emergency management of the airway. The basic theory behind RSI is that all patients presenting to the emergency department (ED) have a full stomach and therefore pose a significant aspiration risk during intubation.[8] To minimise the risks of aspiration, intubation must be performed in a rapid, safe and controlled manner to stabilise and maintain the airway. RSI is the almost simultaneous administration of an anaesthetic induction agent with a paralysing dose of a neuromuscular blocking agent followed by the insertion of an endotracheal tube (ETT).[8,9] Preoxygenation is provided for a few minutes prior to the administration of the induction agents and paralysing agents. Cricoid pressure is applied during intubation and is maintained until the patient is successfully intubated, the ETT cuff is inflated and the emergency doctor is happy with the ETT placement.[8,9]

RSI can be broken down into a series of seven steps (see Box 17.1).[10]

Preparation

Prior to commencing RSI it is important that any available time has been spent in preparation. This step should involve preparation of both the patient and the necessary equipment.

The patient should have at least one well-functioning intravenous (IV) line and be in an area with readily available resuscitation equipment. The patient should be attached to available monitoring: cardiac, non-invasive blood pressure and oxygen saturation as a minimum. If available, capnography should also be available.

The equipment should be assembled and checked. An appropriate-size ETT is opened, lubricated and the cuff checked. Alternative-sized ETTs should also be readily available. A laryngoscope with appropriate-size blade and the light source are checked. Spare laryngoscopes and blades should be at hand. Suction equipment must be available and functioning. RSI drugs being used should be drawn up and doses calculated. Additional airway equipment should also be readily available, including (for example) intubating stylets, bougies and Magill forceps. Preferably, difficult-intubation equipment should also be close at hand. The staff involved should also be adequately prepared in terms of appropriate PPE, and familiarity with the RSI procedure and the equipment being used.[10,11]

The use of a pre-intubation checklist is recommended as a way to improve communication between the resuscitation team and improve the outcomes of the emergency procedure (Box 17.2).[12]

Preoxygenation

Wherever possible, the patient should be preoxygenated prior to commencing RSI, in order to maximise the period of apnoea while maintaining acceptable oxygen saturations during intubation attempts. In order to achieve optimum preoxygenation, the patient should receive 100% oxygen and breathe at normal tidal volume for 3 minutes or take eight maximal breaths over 60 seconds. In reasonably healthy patients this may maintain acceptable oxygen saturations > 90% for up to 8 minutes of apnoea. However, in the critically ill and a number of specific patient groups, i.e. paediatric patients, obese patients and pregnant patients, this time is likely to be considerably less.[10,11]

Preoxygenation can be delivered via a non-rebreather mask on maximum oxygen flow rate if the patient is awake and breathing. In a critically ill patient bag–valve–mask ventilation will be required. This should be delivered with the FiO_2 on the maximum flow rate using a two-operator technique to obtain a tight face mask seal. Placing a PEEP valve on the bag–valve–mask should be considered in patients with low oxygen saturations.

To prevent desaturation during intubation, particularly during the apnoeic period after the administration of sedation and muscle relaxants, apnoeic oxygenation should occur. In the apnoeic patient high-flow oxygen will cause oxygen to move from the alveoli into the bloodstream, thus preventing significant desaturation.[13] Nasal cannula on 15 L/min oxygen

Example of items for a pre-intubation checklist[12]

Team
- Is ED staff specialist or anaethetist aware of proposed RSI? Consider the difficulty out-of-hours airway.
- Are all members of the resuscitation team aware of their and each other's roles?
- Who is the team leader?
- Plan for difficult intubation?
- Are all team members briefed?
- Difficult airway tray or trolley ready?
- Any team concerns or questions?

Patient
- Preoxygenation performed—nasal cannula ± NIV?
- Best patient position achieved?
- Haemodynamics optimal? Fluid bolus?
- Will it be difficult—BVM, larynscopy, supraglottic airway, cricothyroidotomy?

Equipment and drugs
- IVC patent, fluids connected and running easily?
- Second IVC?
- Monitoring: ECG, BP, SaO_2 monitoring?
- RSI drugs drawn up? Doses calculated?
- Post intubation sedation ready?
- Suction working?
- BVM working? Capnography ready?
- X2 laryngoscopes checked, blade sizes, bulbs working?
- ETT sizes checked, cuffs checked?
- Boogie or stylet in ETT?
- Tube ties or tapes ready?
- Ventilator ready?
- LMA sizes and cuffs checked?
- Surgical airway equipment available?

flow rate will deliver near 100% FiO_2 in the apnoeic patient. These can be placed on the patient under any face masks and left in place until successful tracheal intubations or safe airway has been achieved.

PRACTICE TIP

In order to achieve optimum preoxygenation the healthy patient should receive 100% oxygen and breathe at normal tidal volume for 3 minutes or take eight maximal breaths over 60 seconds.

Pretreatment

This stage involves the administration of drugs in order to counteract any anticipated adverse effects associated with the intubation or the patient's underlying condition.[10] Pretreatment medications may be given during preoxygenation.

Paralysis with induction

This stage involves the administration of a rapid-acting induction agent to produce unconsciousness followed by the administration of a neuromuscular blocking agent leading to paralysis. The induction agents utilised will often be determined by the clinical situation, the experience and training of the medical staff and the institutional policies.[10,14] Commonly used induction agents include: thiopentone, propofol, ketamine and fentanyl. Neuromuscular blocking agents may be depolarising or non-depolarising. Suxamethonium is a depolarising muscle relaxant that is commonly used during RSI and is characterised by muscle fasciculations at the time of onset. Its duration of action is relatively short, 3–5 minutes, compared with other agents. This is beneficial in failed intubations, providing a return of muscle function within a short period. Other longer-acting non-depolarising agents may on occasions be used during RSI; however, these are generally used following successful intubation for ongoing paralysis (see post-intubation management on next page). These agents may include: rocuronium, vecuronium, cisatracurium and pancuronium. Cricoid pressure is applied during this stage at the onset of unconsciousness.

Positioning

The ideal position of the adult patient is a 'sniffing' position with the head extended and neck flexed slightly. This may be facilitated by placing a small towel under the patient's head, raising it 7–10 cm.[11] Ideal positioning will not be possible in any situation where there is potential for cervical spine injury. In these circumstances, in-line immobilisation of the neck/cervical spine is provided by a separate staff member, also positioned at the head of the bed. The staff member providing in-line stabilisation is often required to crouch down, allowing the person intubating room to visualise the airway and intubate the patient.

The 'sniffing' position is, however, not ideal for the obese patient. Increased fat in the chest and abdominal wall have a mechanical effect on the thoracic cage, diaphragm and lungs. This decreases functional residual capacity, increases airway resistance and worsens ventilation perfusion mismatch. The recommended position for obese patients is one where the external auditory canal meatus and the sternal notch are aligned, with the head up and the head and shoulders supported by pillows or blankets. This is called the 'ramp' position (Fig 17.11).[15]

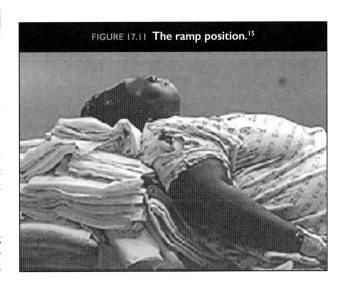

FIGURE 17.11 **The ramp position.**[15]

Placement

Following intubation, the ETT cuff is inflated and placement of the ETT in the trachea must be confirmed. This can be achieved reliably with capnography (caution during cardiac arrest). Other methods to confirm ETT placement include: visualisation of the ETT passing through the cords (by the intubator); auscultation of breath sounds; absence of breath sounds over epigastrium; condensation within the ETT with each breath; rise and fall of the chest with ventilation; and chest X-ray.[11]

Post-intubation management

Following confirmation of placement, the ETT must be secured in place. A number of taping and tying methods and devices are available for securing the ETT, and institutional/departmental policy and procedure should be followed.

Hypotension is common following RSI and the commencement of positive-pressure ventilation, although this is often self-limiting and responds to IV fluids. Persistent hypotension should prompt evaluation of other, more ominous causes.[10]

Patients will require ongoing sedation and analgesia while intubated and ventilated. This is often achieved by continuous IV infusion of various agents, which commonly include morphine, midazolam and propofol. If ongoing paralysis is required, this must always be given in conjunction with sedation. Ongoing paralysis is achieved with intermittent boluses of non-depolarising muscle relaxants, such as rocuronium, vecuronium, cisatracurium and pancuronium.

Laryngeal mask airway insertion

The laryngeal mask airway (LMA) may be used in the profoundly unconscious patient who requires artificial ventilation and when intubation is not readily available or has failed to establish an airway successfully.[16] The LMA may also be the first-line airway choice in patients with known difficult airways or severe facial trauma.[1] The LMA (Fig 17.12) is a wide-bore tube with an oval cuff and when inflated conforms to the contours of the hypopharynx, positioning the opening directly over the laryngeal opening to provide an avenue for ventilation. The seal attained by the LMA provides protection from oral and nasal secretions but does not necessarily protect the airway from aspiration of gastric contents.[1] The LMA is relatively easy to insert and has been successfully used by novice nurses and other healthcare professionals following minimal training.[17] The LMA has also been widely used by pre-hospital personnel.

Several types of LMA devices are available, including an intubating laryngeal mask airway (ILMA) which is specifically designed in order to facilitate intubation of the trachea.

Procedure for laryngeal mask airway insertion[1,16]

1. Wash hands and don PPE.
2. Obtain the correctly sized LMA for the patient (Table 17.1).[18]
3. Perform the deflation and inflation tests according to the manufacturer's instructions.
4. Deflate the cuff by placing it, aperture side down, on a hard, flat surface, and smoothing out any wrinkles as air is withdrawn from the cuff with the syringe (Fig 17.13).
5. Lubricate the posterior tip of the cuff with water-based lubricant.
6. Place the patient's head in the sniffing position.
7. Position yourself at the patient's head and slightly lift the patient's head with your non-dominant hand.
8. Hold the LMA behind the cuff with the index finger and thumb of the dominant hand (Fig 17.14A).
9. Insert the LMA into the patient's mouth, directing upwards towards the hard palate (Fig 17.14B).

TABLE 17.1 Laryngeal Mask Airway (LMA) Classic™, Flexible™ and Unique™ sizing guide 15[18]

LMA SIZE	PATIENT SELECTION INFORMATION	MAXIMUM CUFF INFLATION VOLUME
1	Neonates < 5 kg	4 mL
1½	Infants 5–10 kg	7 mL
2	Infants 10–20 kg	10 mL
2½	Children 20–30 kg	14 mL
3	Children 30–50 kg	20 mL
4	Adults 50–70 kg	30 mL
5	Adults 70–100 kg	40 mL
6	Adults > 100 kg	50 mL

Warning: NEVER OVERINFLATE THE CUFF.

FIGURE 17.12 **Laryngeal mask airway.**[142]

Ambu   Solus   SoftSeal   Unique

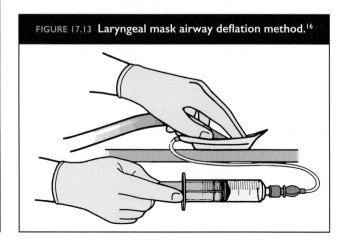

FIGURE 17.13 **Laryngeal mask airway deflation method.**[16]

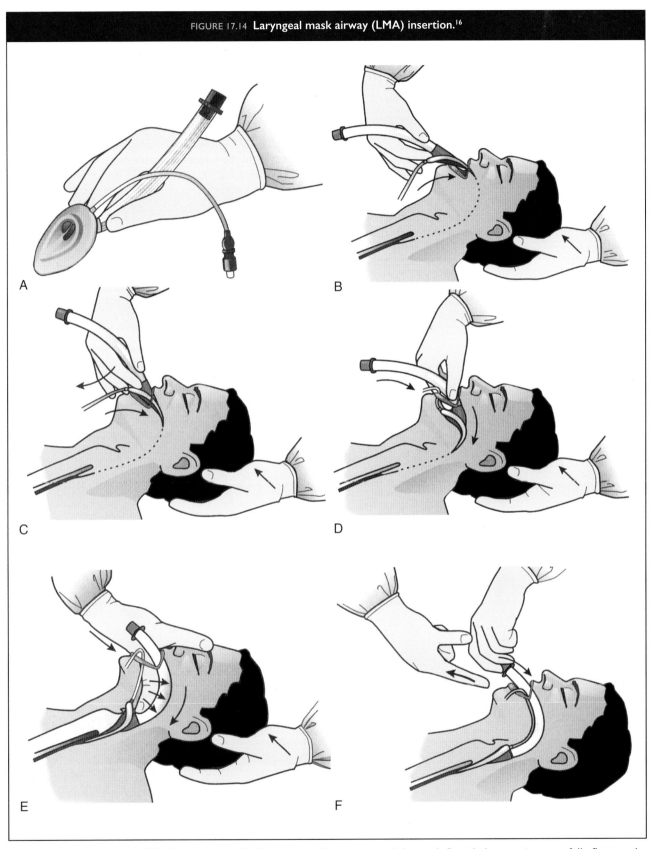

FIGURE 17.14 **Laryngeal mask airway (LMA) insertion.**[16]

A, Method for holding the LMA for insertion. **B**, With the head extended and the neck flexed, the caregiver carefully flattens the LMA tip against the hard palate. **C**, To facilitate LMA introduction into the oral cavity, the caregiver gently presses the middle finger down on the jaw. **D**, The index finger pushes the LMA in the cranial direction following the contours of the hard and soft palates. **E**, Maintaining pressure with the finger in the tube in the cranial direction, the caregiver advances the LMA until definite resistance is felt at the base of the hypopharynx. Note the flexion of the wrist.

10. Using the middle finger, open the patient's jaw and look into the mouth to ensure that the cuff is flattened against the hard palate (Fig 17.14C).

11. Using the index finger, advance the LMA into the hypopharynx in one smooth action (see Fig 17.14D).

12. Continue to advance until resistance is felt (see Fig 17.14E).

13. Remove the non-dominant hand from behind the patient's head and use it to stabilise the LMA and remove the dominant hand index finger from the patient's mouth (see Fig 17.14F).

14. Inflate the cuff the required volume to create a seal.

15. Observe for signs of correct placement and inflation.

16. Connect a resuscitation bag and gently ventilate, looking for chest rise and fall, breath sounds on auscultation and capnography confirmation.

17. Secure the LMA.

Cricothyroidotomy

Cricothyroidotomy is the establishment of a surgical opening in the airway through the cricothyroid membrane and the insertion of a cuffed tracheostomy tube or ETT, providing an avenue for ventilation (see Fig 17.15). The indication for cricothyroidotomy occurs in the 'can't intubate, can't oxygenate' scenario. Where there have been failed attempts at intubation and the patient is unable to be ventilated adequately using bag and mask, cricothyroidotomy should be considered. Alternatively, if the patient is unable to be intubated but able to be ventilated but there is no other device available that is likely to be successful in securing the airway (e.g. LMA), then cricothyroidotomy should also be considered. Additional and persistent attempts at laryngoscopy and intubation are likely to result in significant hypoxia. The final scenario in which cricothyroidotomy is indicated is in the trauma patient with significant lower facial trauma where airway access through the

FIGURE 17.15

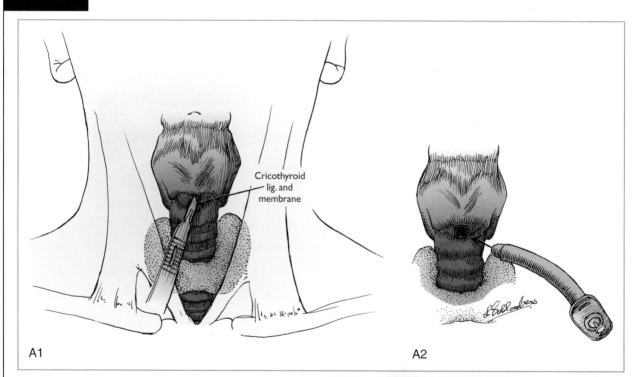

Cricothyroid lig. and membrane

A1   A2

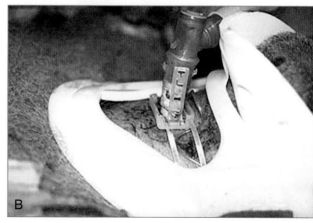

B

A, Cricothyroidotomy technique.[20]
B, Completed cricothyroidotomy.
B Courtesy Liverpool Hospital Trauma Service, Sydney, NSW.

mouth or nose would be considered too time-consuming or impossible.[19]

Cricothyroidotomy is generally contraindicated in children less than 12 years of age. Children have a small, pliable, mobile larynx and cricoid cartilage, making cricothyroidotomy extremely difficult. Children who require an emergency surgical airway require needle cricothyroidotomy with trans-tracheal jet ventilation. In this technique, a 12- to 14-gauge angiocath or IV cannula is inserted through the cricothyroid cartilage into the trachea. The catheter is left in place, providing an avenue for ventilation. Ventilation is provided by jet ventilation (not described here) or via a ventilation bag attached via a suitable adaptor. Needle cricothyroidotomy should be seen as a rescue technique and is not considered a definitive airway. Needle cricothyroidotomy is a temporary measure in order to provide oxygenation until a more definitive airway can be secured.[19,21]

The role of the emergency nurse or paramedic in the situation in which cricothyroidotomy is required is to provide assistance to the person performing the procedure. In order to provide assistance, it is important that the emergency nurse or paramedic is familiar with the indication for cricothyroidotomy, the equipment, particularly its location within their department, and also the techniques for performing this very seldom-occurring procedure.

Capnography/end-tidal carbon dioxide monitoring

Carbon dioxide (CO_2) is produced as an end-product of cellular metabolism and is transported in the venous blood back to the lungs where it is eliminated during the expiratory phase of breathing. During inspiration minimal amounts of CO_2 are drawn into the lungs, and during alveolar ventilation the high concentrations of CO_2 returning via the pulmonary circulation diffuse down a concentration gradient into the alveoli and are expelled during expiration. In healthy lungs where ventilation matches perfusion, exhaled CO_2 levels closely approximate $PaCO_2$ (arterial partial pressure of CO_2) levels, with expired end-tidal carbon dioxide ($EtCO_2$) levels being approximately 2–5 mmHg below the level of arterial CO_2. This gradient may be increased when there is diminished pulmonary perfusion to regions of the lung, resulting in dead-space ventilation.[22]

Uses in emergency care

The assessment and monitoring of $EtCO_2$ has a number of uses in the emergency and pre-hospital environments. These include the following.

Confirmation and monitoring of endotracheal tube placement

The measurement of $EtCO_2$ is an effective way to confirm ETT placement. During intubation, when an ETT is placed in the trachea the CO_2 present is readily detected during expiration by means of capnography, confirming correct ETT positioning. In the event of an oesophageal intubation, no CO_2 is detected and corrective actions can be rapidly undertaken. $EtCO_2$ is also useful in the monitoring of ETT placement especially during transportation or movement of the patient. Due to the continuous monitoring of CO_2 levels on a breath-by-breath basis by capnography, ETT dislodgement, displacement, disconnection or obstruction is rapidly identifiable.[22,23]

Use of capnography during cardiac arrest

During cardiac arrest situations, capnography may be less sensitive due to decreased cardiac output. During cardiac arrest, cardiac output falls resulting in decreased pulmonary blood flow and a decrease in CO_2 elimination. As cardiac output improves with either cardiopulmonary resuscitation (CPR) or return of spontaneous circulation (ROSC), pulmonary blood flow is restored in conjunction with elimination of CO_2. Therefore, capnography is useful in assessing the effectiveness of CPR and also in the recognition of the return or loss of spontaneous circulation.[22,23]

Cervical spine immobilisation

Cervical spine immobilisation is used for suspected acute cervical injury to prevent potential spinal cord damage. The spine should be protected at all times during the management of the patient with multiple injuries. There are a number of different cervical collars available that can be used to stabilise the cervical spine. Most collars are made from rigid plastic or semi-rigid foam reinforced by plastic struts with Velcro straps. The primary function of these collars is to restrict flexion and extension of the middle and lower cervical spine. The most common complication of cervical spine immobilisation is skin breakdown.[24]

Fitting a cervical hard collar

1. Life-saving procedures always take precedence over fitting of a collar.
2. Begin by ensuring that the skin is clean and dry and any wounds are covered. Remove jewellery such as necklaces and earrings.
3. Administer adequate analgesia where possible.
4. Measure the distance from the top of the shoulder to the angle of the jaw using your fingers (Fig 17.16).
5. Find the correct Stifneck or hard collar by sizing the same number of fingers on the collar's measuring bar found on the side. Select the tallest collar that does not cause hyperflexion (Fig 17.17).
6. Immobilise the patient's head in a neutral position with manual in-line stabilisation.
7. Slide the back part of the collar around the back of the neck.
8. Fold the front of the collar under the chin and secure the Velcro strap in place. Ensure the chin is well supported.

Philadelphia collar

The Philadelphia tracheotomy collar is a semi-rigid foam collar used to support the cervical spine. It is often used to replace the rigid cervical spine extrication collars that are applied in the field; spinal column injury should be presumed until it is excluded, although application of definitive immobilisation devices should not take precedence over life-saving procedures.

The Philadelphia collar is more comfortable, softer and can remain in place longer than a rigid extrication collar. Rigid cervical spine immobilisation collars should be removed and refitted every 2 hours for pressure-area care over the bony prominences, but the Philadelphia collar can remain in place for up to 48 hours without the need for removal (Fig 17.18).

FIGURE 17.16 **Cervical collar sizing.**

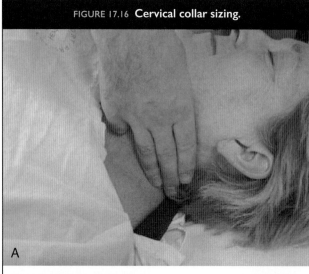

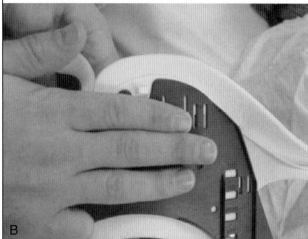

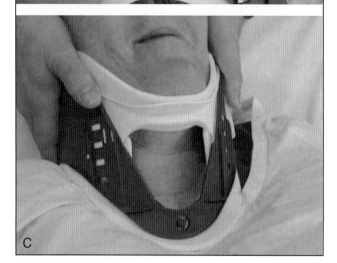

Courtesy Emergency Department, Prince of Wales Hospital, Sydney.

Fitting a Philadephia collar

1. Life-saving procedures always take precedence over fitting of a collar.
2. Begin by ensuring that the skin is clean and dry and any wounds are covered. Remove jewellery such as necklaces and earrings.

FIGURE 17.17 **Stifneck collar made of high-density polyethylene padded with semi-flexible foam margins.**

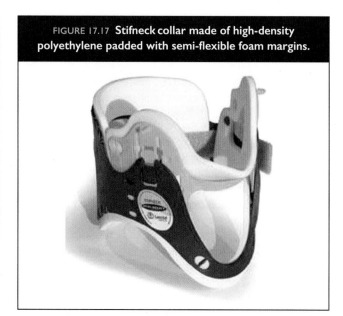

The low-reaching anterior panel contacts the sternum for additional support.[124]

FIGURE 17.18 **Philadelphia collar.**

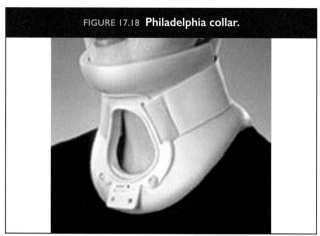

The collar supports the head in a dish-shaped contour formed by the two halves when joined with the Velcro fasteners. When properly sized, it provides excellent support; if too tight, it tends to force the mandible backwards and can cause thyroid compression in some patients.[124]

3. Administer adequate analgesia where possible.
4. Measure the vertical distance from the top of the shoulder to the tip of the chin to give the height of the collar.
5. Measure the circumference of the neck for the second size.
6. Select the correctly sized collar that corresponds with the two measurements. The collar comes in two pieces—do not mix and match sizes.
7. Immobilise the patient's head in a neutral position with manual in-line stabilisation.
8. Fit and centre the back piece of the collar with the black arrow pointing towards the top of the head.
9. Fit the front piece of the collar with the black arrow pointing towards the top of the head.

10. Secure the chin in the cup recess. The front piece of the collar overlaps the back piece and is secured with Velcro straps.

PRACTICE TIP

The Philadelphia tracheotomy collar is more comfortable than a Stifneck extrication collar, but is more difficult to measure and fit.

The Philadelphia collar comes in two pieces and 20 different adult sizes, and can remain on for up to 48 hours. In order to prevent pressure areas, extrication hard collars need to be removed and pressure-area care attended to after 2 hours.

Both collars are X-ray-lucent and safe to use in magnetic resonance imaging scanners.

Head control

Manual in-line cervical spine stabilisation
Manual in-line cervical spine stabilisation involves holding the head and neck in a neutral position, and is often used during life-saving procedures when a hard collar cannot be fitted. Some evidence suggests that manual in-line stabilisation does not effectively immobilise an injured cervical spine, and may retard the view of the airway during intubation.[25]

Procedure
1. Life-saving procedures always take precedence over in-line cervical spine stabilisation.
2. Begin by ensuring that the skin is clean and dry and any wounds are covered. Remove jewellery such as necklaces and earrings.
3. Administer adequate analgesia where possible.
4. Stand at the head of the bed.
5. Place both arms either side of the patient's head down to the top of the shoulder and grip the head and neck with your hands and forearms to prevent movement.
6. Hold the top of the shoulders for additional support.
7. Continue in-line stabilisation until a hard collar or Philadelphia collar can be fitted, or until it is no longer deemed necessary.

PRACTICE TIPS

When providing manual in-line stabilisation of the cervical spine during intubation, hold the head and neck and crouch down below and to the side of the back of the bed. This will allow the proceduralist a good view during intubation.

Manual in-line stabilisation may be useful in paediatric patients, or in patients to whom a cervical collar cannot be fitted, such as the morbidly obese.

Assisting with a spinal immobilisation collar application
If providing manual in-line cervical spine stabilisation so that a spinal immobilisation collar can be fitted, proceed as above for the first 6 steps. Then:

1. Maintain in-line stabilisation while the hard collar or Philadelphia collar is fitted. Usually the back section of the Philadelphia collar is fitted first.
2. Move hands and forearms up to the patient's ears and grip their head in the palm of the hands as the front section of the collar is applied.
3. Check that the collar is in correct alignment and that the head remains in a neutral position throughout.
4. Release manual in-line stabilisation only when the collar is correctly secured.

Sandbags in head control
Sandbags can be used to assist with immobilisation of the head and neck following trauma. In the field, rolled towels, full 1-litre IV fluid bags, foam blocks or pillows can be substituted.[26] Sandbags or rolled towels may play a role in the immobilisation of children or of patients to whom a hard collar cannot be adequately fitted.

Procedure
1. Life-saving procedures always take precedence over placing of sandbags.
2. Begin by ensuring that the skin is clean and dry and any wounds are covered. Remove jewellery such as necklaces and earrings.
3. Administer adequate analgesia where possible. Consider antiemetic use.
4. Place the patient on a spinal board.
5. Restrain the patient's body by strapping or taping it to the spinal board.
6. Place bilateral sandbags along the side of the head and neck. The sandbags should rest at the top of the shoulder and extend in line with the forehead.
7. Apply wide non-elastic adhesive tape across the forehead and chin to tape the sandbags to the spinal board.
8. Sandbags can be used in conjunction with a rigid spinal immobilisation collar with tape applied across the forehead and the body of the collar.

PRACTICE TIP

Pay particular attention to the risk of vomiting and aspiration in any patient who has the cervical spine immobilised. If the patient's head is taped to a spinal board using sandbags or rolled towels, someone should remain with the patient at all times.

Helmet removal

Refer to Figure 17.19 for in-line removal of various types of motorcycle and sports helmets.

Assessment of respiratory function
Due to the correlation of $EtCO_2$ and $PaCO_2$, the clinician is able to evaluate alterations in pulmonary perfusion, in particular dead-space ventilation.[22]

FIGURE 17.19 Motorcycle helmet removal.[153]

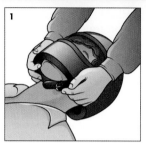

One rescuer maintains in-line immobilisation by placing his or her hands on each side of the helmet with the fingers on the victim's mandible. This position prevents slippage if the strap is loose.

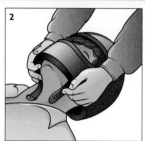

A second rescuer cuts or loosens the strap at the D-ring.

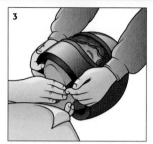

The second rescuer places one hand on the mandible at the angle, the thumb on one side and the long and index fingers on the other. With the other hand the rescuer applies pressure from the occipital region. This manoeuvre transfers the in-line immobilisation responsibility to the second rescuer.

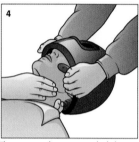

The rescuer at the top moves the helmet. Three factors should be kept in mind:
• The helmet is egg-shaped and therefore must be expanded laterally to clear the ears.
• If the helmet provides full facial coverage, glasses must be removed first.
• If the helmet provides full facial coverage, the nose may impede removal. To clear the nose, the helmet must be tilted backwards and raised over it.

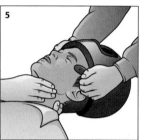

Throughout the removal process the second rescuer maintains in-line immobilisation from below to prevent unnecessary neck motion.

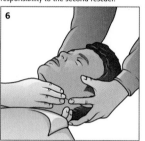

After the helmet has been removed, the rescuer at the top replaces his or her hands on either side of the victim's head with the palms over the ears.

Monitoring of mechanical ventilation

Capnography is today a standard monitoring tool for the ventilated patient. Capnography allows the caring clinician to readily identify changes in ventilation such as ventilator disconnection, apnoea, patient asynchrony with the ventilator and the depth of neuromuscular blockade.[19] Capnography also assists in identifying hypoventilation and hyperventilation in mechanically ventilated patients. This has been shown to be of significant benefit in patients where the tight control of CO_2 is clinically important, such as the head-injured patient with raised intracranial pressure.[27]

End-tidal carbon dioxide detection devices

The majority of $EtCO_2$ detection devices use infrared radiation technology to calculate CO_2 concentrations in a gas sample. This is achieved through the use of photodetectors that identify the amount of infrared radiation that is absorbed by CO_2 present within a given breath sample. This allows for the calculation of concentration or partial pressure of the CO_2. Depending on the location of the photodetector sensor, this is achieved through either sidestream or mainstream devices.

Mainstream devices have the detector located on the endotracheal tube and directly measure gas from the airway. Mainstream devices are primarily designed for intubated patients as the detector forms part of the ventilation circuit.

Sidestream devices aspirate small samples of gas from within the airway and pump the gas through tubing to a sensor located within the machine. Sidestream devices may be configured to be used in either ventilated or non-ventilated patients. Use in non-ventilated patients is for spontaneously breathing patients where a nasal–oral cannula is used, allowing both the sampling of exhaled CO_2 and the administration of oxygen.[27]

$EtCO_2$ detection devices may be *quantitative* or *qualitative*. Quantitative devices measure and display the exact $EtCO_2$ as either a number (capnometry) or as a number and a waveform (capnography). The capnography devices display a continuous waveform depicting the breath-by-breath rise and fall of the $EtCO_2$; this waveform is known as the *capnogram* (see Fig 17.20). The capnography device has become a standard of care for the ventilated patient and is widely used in a number of clinical settings, including the ED. The capnography devices require some form of calibration prior to use in order to ensure their accuracy. This calibration often involves allowing the sensor to warm to its operating temperature, then zeroing the sensor before calibrating it to a predetermined reference value. In addition to this, the sensor may also need to be calibrated to room air outside the patient circuit and away from any exhaled CO_2.[28] While these calibrations routinely do not take more than a few minutes, this may be difficult to achieve in an unanticipated emergency situation. In these instances it would be recommended to utilise a qualitative $EtCO_2$ detection device (*colourimetric device*—see below) to confirm ETT placement, and, when time permits, calibrate and utilise the capnograph.

Qualitative devices measure a range in which $EtCO_2$ falls, rather than a precise number. The most commonly used devices are the colourimetric $EtCO_2$ detection devices.

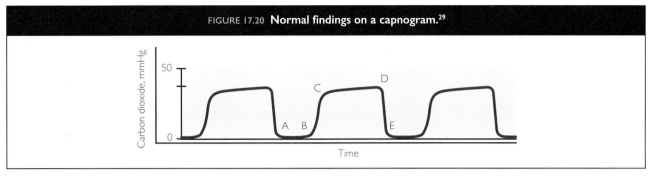

FIGURE 17.20 **Normal findings on a capnogram.**[29]

A → B indicates the baseline; B → C, expiratory upstroke; C → D, alveolar plateau; D, partial pressure of end-tidal carbon dioxide; D → E, inspiratory downstroke.

FIGURE 17.21 **Colourimetric end-tidal carbon dioxide detection device.**[148]

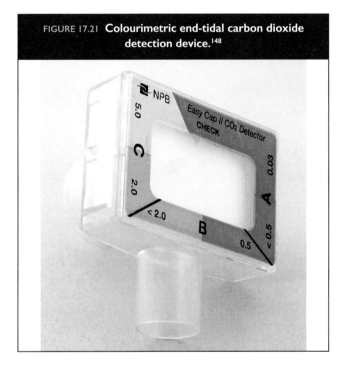

FIGURE 17.22 **Yankauer suction device.**[151]

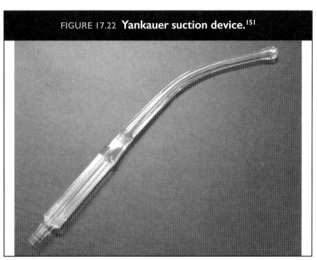

Colourimetric EtCO$_2$ detection devices

Colourimetric devices (Fig 17.21) change colour in the presence of exhaled CO_2 through the use of a specially treated piece of litmus paper. These devices are small, portable and disposable, making them ideal in the pre-hospital setting where they are commonly used. These devices are primarily used to confirm ETT placement within the trachea. The device is placed between the ETT and the resuscitation bag immediately following intubation; the device is then observed for a change in colour in order to confirm the presence of CO_2. It is important to allow adequate exhalation time so that the device can change colour. This may require checking the device for a definitive colour change after up to six ventilations.

If there is an oesophageal intubation the device will fail to change colour, indicating the absence of CO_2 and prompting the need for re-intubation. Failure of the device to change colour may also be seen in cardiac arrest (as discussed above); therefore, in these situations the user should confirm correct ETT placement by other acceptable means. A colour change may be subsequently seen with the ROSC or effective CPR.

These devices are available for patients of all ages and sizes. Some devices have a variable colour change and a numerical

scale showing the $EtCO_2$. These devices may be accurate for up to 2 hours of continuous use or 24 hours of intermittent use (the exact characteristics of individual devices should be confirmed with the product literature). Those devices that are able to be used for an extended period provide an additional benefit that they can be used to monitor ETT placement during transport or movement of the patient, assisting in the early identification of ETT dislodgement. Devices which may become contaminated with fluid, such as respiratory secretions, vomitus or blood, should be replaced to ensure their reliability.[23,27]

Suctioning techniques

Many patients who are critically unwell or who have an alteration in their respiratory function may be unable to cough and remove respiratory secretions. These patients require assistance in removing these respiratory secretions by way of suctioning in order to reduce the risk of consolidation, infection and atelectasis.[30,31]

Routes of suctioning

Suctioning can be performed via a number of routes. Selection of the most appropriate route will be determined by the requirements of the patient and the clinical setting.

Oral

Oral suctioning involves the removal of secretions in the mouth. These secretions may include sputum, saliva, vomitus and/or blood. Suctioning of the oral cavity is usually performed using a Yankauer suction catheter (see Fig 17.22).[30] Solid objects that are not able to be removed with the aid of the Yankauer suction device, for example dislodged teeth or vomitus, may require removal manually with a gloved hand or (Magill) forceps.

Oropharyngeal

The oropharynx extends from the lips to the pharynx. Oropharyngeal suctioning requires the insertion of a suction catheter through the mouth and into the pharynx and/or trachea in order to remove respiratory secretions. Patients who need this form of suctioning may often be unable to maintain an open airway and require the insertion of an oropharyngeal airway (see insertion of oropharyngeal airways, p. 314).[30] The oropharyngeal airway may assist in suctioning by allowing the suction catheter to be passed through the airway to provide suctioning deep in the oropharynx and into the trachea.

Nasopharyngeal

Suctioning of the nasopharynx is performed to remove secretions from within the nasopharynx. This route may also be used for the collection of specific specimen samples such as a nasopharyngeal aspirate. Nasopharyngeal suctioning is commonly performed on patients with an altered level of consciousness and is best performed with the aid of a nasopharyngeal airway. When a nasopharyngeal airway is utilised, the suction catheter is passed through the airway.

Tracheal

Suctioning of the trachea occurs through an artificial opening in the trachea. Suctioning may be performed directly through a tracheal stoma or via an airway adjunct such as a tracheostomy tube.

Endotracheal

This form of tracheal suctioning occurs through an ETT in either spontaneously breathing or ventilated patients in order to remove respiratory secretions.

Indications for suctioning

The common indications for suctioning are outlined in Box 17.3.

BOX 17.3 Common indications for suctioning[30]

- Visible or audible secretions—'rattling' or 'bubbling' sounds, audible with or without a stethoscope
- Sensation of secretions in the chest reported by patient
- Increased airway pressure in the ventilated patient or pre-set tidal volume not being delivered
- Deteriorating arterial blood gases
- Altered chest movement
- Restlessness
- Decreased oxygen saturation
- Altered haemodynamics (increased blood pressure, heart rate)
- Decreased air entry on auscultation
- Tachypnoea
- Colour change in patient (e.g. cyanosis, redness, pallor)
- Specimen collection
- Assessment of airway patency
- Evaluation of cough reflex

Considerations for suctioning

Frequency of suctioning

Suctioning should be performed only when necessary (see indications for suctioning, above). In intubated patients it may be advisable to perform suctioning at least every 8 hours to reduce the risk of secretion accumulation and partial tube occlusion.[31]

Catheter size

In general, suction catheters should be as small as possible yet large enough to facilitate secretion removal. This allows air to enter around the catheter during suctioning, preventing a sudden drop in functional residual capacity and thus reducing the risk of atelectasis. For ETT suctioning, the catheter should occlude less than half of the internal lumen of the ETT[31] (see Box 17.4).

Suction pressure

It is recommended to use the lowest possible suction pressure. For ETT suctioning this pressure is usually 80–120 mmHg. A negative pressure of 200 mmHg may be applied, provided that the appropriate suction-catheter size is used.[31]

Insertion depth

For ETT suctioning, a minimally invasive technique should be used where the suction catheter is inserted to the length of the ET tube only. The suction catheter can be inserted to the carina and withdrawn 1–2 cm before suction is applied, or the catheter length can be estimated against an identical tube.[31]

Suction duration and method

It is recommended that each suction procedure should last no longer than 15 seconds and the suction should be applied continuously rather than intermittently.[31]

Use of saline

The routine instillation of Normal saline prior to ETT suctioning is not recommended. There are no reliable positive effects demonstrated in terms of secretion removal, saturation or ventilation.[31]

Preoxygenation

It is recommended that preoxygenation with 100% oxygen is provided for at least 30 seconds prior to and after ETT suctioning to prevent decreases in oxygen saturation.[31]

Closed suction systems

The closed suction system consists of a reusable sterile suction catheter protected by a flexible, clear plastic sleeve that prevents contact between the catheter and the environment (see Fig 17.23). The closed suction system attaches to the end of the ETT via an adaptor, becoming an integrated part of the ventilator circuit. The closed suction system allows suctioning of the ETT without disconnecting the ventilator circuit. This maintains positive end-expiratory pressure and an uninterrupted oxygen supply, and minimises loss of pulmonary

---

BOX 17.4 Calculation of suction catheter for endotracheal tube (ETT) suctioning[31]

- Suction catheter size [Fr] = (ETT size [mm] − 1) × 2

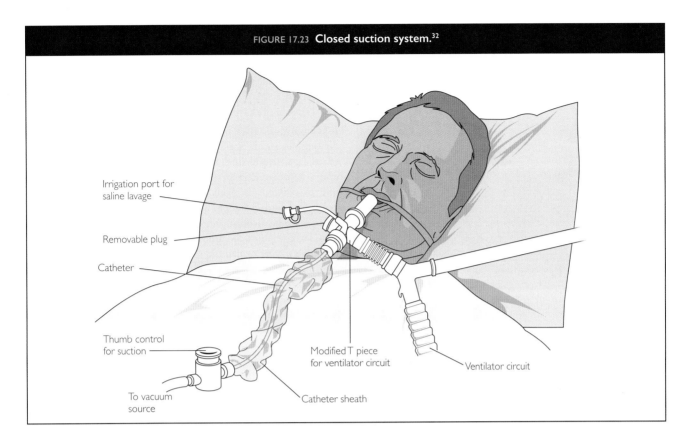

FIGURE 17.23 **Closed suction system.**[32]

Irrigation port for
saline lavage

Removable plug

Catheter

Thumb control
for suction

To vacuum
source

Modified T piece
for ventilator circuit

Catheter sheath

Ventilator circuit

volume (in volume-control ventilated patients). These systems often contain an irrigation port for rinsing the catheter or instilling saline. There is little evidence to support closed suction systems over open suction systems and the use of either system is recommended.[30,31]

Suctioning procedure (open)[20–32]

1. Explain procedure to patient.
2. Obtain consent (verbal).
3. Calculate correct catheter size.
4. Organise equipment.
5. Turn on suction to required pressure (80–120 mmHg).
6. If possible, patient should be sitting upright.
7. Wash hands.
8. Hyperoxygenate for 30 seconds and/or apply hyperinflation before suctioning (if required).
9. Use a sterile, disposable glove on the hand manipulating the catheter and a clean disposable glove on the other.
10. With the clean disposable gloved hand, withdraw catheter from sleeve.
11. Disconnect oxygen supply/ventilator circuit.
12. Introduce the suction catheter gently to the correct length. Do not apply suction on insertion.
13. Apply suction and withdraw catheter slowly (< 15 seconds) in one continuous motion.
14. Reconnect oxygen supply/ventilator circuit.
15. Monitor oxygen saturation levels and heart rate throughout procedure.
16. Wrap the catheter around the sterile-gloved hand and pull the glove back over the soiled catheter and discard.
17. Rinse connection with sterile water and discard other glove.
18. Wash hands.
19. Assess the patient, and if further suctioning is required start the procedure again with another sterile catheter and glove.
20. Repeat until airway is clear, allowing patient to rest between each suction pass.
21. Clean patient's oral cavity.
22. Wash hands.
23. Document procedure and findings.

Arterial blood gases
Collection

Arterial blood samples are usually obtained to perform an arterial blood gas (ABG) analysis. There are a number of possible arterial puncture sites, including the radial, brachial, femoral or dorsalis pedis arteries. Despite these options, the radial artery is the most preferred site for arterial blood gas sampling, as in the majority of people the hand has collateral circulation supplied by both the radial and the ulnar arteries (see Fig 17.24). This means that there is another supply of circulation should the radial artery become blocked distal to the puncture site due to spasm or thrombosis. Before a radial ABG can be taken, collateral circulation must be assessed, by either using a Doppler or the Allen's test (see following page).[33]

If the patient is receiving oxygen, the oxygen concentration must remain the same for 20 minutes before the ABG is taken; if the test is to be taken without oxygen, the oxygen must be turned off for 20 minutes before the test is taken. Blood gas analyser machines measure samples at 37°C. Dissociation of

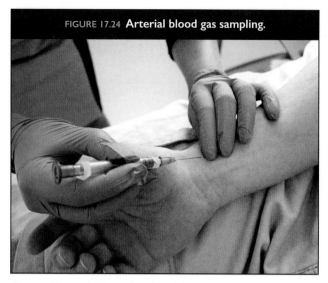

FIGURE 17.24 **Arterial blood gas sampling.**

Courtesy Fremantle Hospital and Health Service Pathology Department, WA.

gases is affected by temperature, so it is important to follow hospital policy and either enter the patient's temperature into the analyser or let it default and measure all samples at 37°C.[34]

Samples can be tested at the point-of-care (in the ward) or in the pathology laboratory. Blood gas analysers require frequent specialised calibration, testing, cleaning and maintenance that is usually performed by pathology laboratory technicians.

Procedure for arterial blood gas sampling

1. Gather all equipment that will be needed:
   - laboratory request form
   - arterial blood gas needle and syringe
   - gloves
   - alcohol swab
   - patient identification sticker to label blood gas syringe
   - specimen bag with ice.
2. Position patient comfortably (lying down if possible).
3. Explain procedure to patient and gain verbal consent.
4. Wash hands.
5. Apply gloves.
6. Position arm appropriately on a pillow with wrist extended.
7. Perform Allen's test (see next section).
8. Palpate pulse and assess position of artery.
9. Clean site with 70% alcohol solution and allow to dry.
10. Immobilise artery between fingers, being careful not to contaminate puncture site.
11. Insert needle at a 45° to 90° angle with bevel up.
12. The syringe will begin to fill spontaneously when inside artery. (This may not occur if the patient's blood pressure is low or the needle is not fully inside the artery; it may be necessary to reposition the needle slightly and pull back on the plunger to aspirate the blood.)
13. Obtain 3–5 mL of blood. Some blood gas analysis machines are able to perform testing on smaller samples of 1 mL or less.
14. Remove needle.

15. Apply gauze square and pressure for 5 minutes.
16. Label specimen and place in ice-filled bag. Ice is not required if the sample will be tested at the point of care.
17. Send to laboratory immediately, or perform point-of-care testing
18. Dispose of sharps safely.

It is important after taking the arterial sample to remove any air bubbles inside the syringe, as they can alter PaO_2 (arterial oxygen partial pressure) results. The needle needs to be removed and a cap placed over the end of the syringe to stop leaking and to prevent air from entering the syringe. The specimen is labelled with a patient identification sticker. Arterial blood gas specimens need to be placed in ice and sent to the lab or tested at the point-of-care immediately. Blood is a living tissue in which oxygen continues to be consumed and carbon dioxide continues to be produced, even after the blood is drawn into the syringe. Placing the blood gas specimen in ice should reduce the specimen temperature to approximately 4°C, which will decrease the metabolic rate to such an extent that the sample may undergo little change over several hours. As a general rule, ABG samples should be analysed within 10 minutes or cooled immediately. Specimens left at room temperature lose 0.01 pH units every 15 minutes.[35]

Allen's test

The Allen's test determines the patency of the ulnar and radial artery (Fig 17.25 and Box 17.5). It involves raising the patient's hand and asking them to make a fist, then occluding the radial

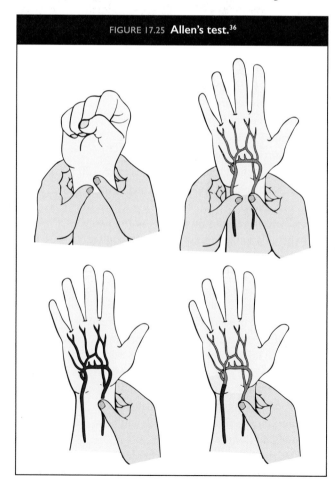

FIGURE 17.25 **Allen's test.**[36]

- Flex patient's arm with hand above level of the elbow.
- Have patient clench fist to force blood from the hand.
- Place pressure on both arteries simultaneously, then ask the patient to open the hand. The hand should appear blanched.
- Remove pressure from the ulnar artery. The blanched area flushes within seconds if collateral circulation is adequate.
- If the area flushes quickly, this is recorded as a positive Allen's test. The test is negative if the blanched area does not flush quickly.
- A negative Allen's test means collateral circulation is inadequate to support circulation to the hand; therefore, an alternative site should be selected.

and ulnar arteries. Observe the hand for blanching. Then release the pressure from the ulnar artery, lower the arm and ask the patient to unclench their fist. Observe the hand for return of colour (usually within 6 seconds). Return of colour within this time indicates ulnar artery patency. Repeat, testing the radial artery.[11]

Arterial blood gases interpretation

ABG sampling and analysis is the gold-standard assessment of the patient's oxygenation and acid–base balance. It is commonly used in EDs and is vital to the management of the patient's condition. Knowledge of normal values for each patient is paramount. Interpretation of these results should follow five simple steps (see Box 17.6).[8,37–39]

Step 1

PaO_2 refers to the measurement of the partial pressure of oxygen dissolved in arterial blood. The normal range should be 80–100 mmHg for a person breathing room air at sea level. Normal levels vary in infants and in people over 60 years of age. For older people, normal levels decrease as a result of a ventilation/perfusion (V/Q) mismatch and the normal ageing of the lung.[37–39] A PaO_2 of less than the normal value is indicative of hypoxaemia, which means the amount of oxygen dissolved in the plasma is lower than normal. A PaO_2 level of 40 mmHg or below, at any age, indicates a life-threatening situation. The patient needs immediate administration of oxygen and/or mechanical ventilation as oxygenation of the tissues is severely compromised.[8,35,37–39]

Step 2

pH refers to the acidity or alkalinity of the blood and the hydrogen ion (H^+) concentration of the plasma. The normal values for arterial blood pH are 7.35–7.45. The mean value for arterial blood pH is 7.40. Any result below this value is on the acidic side of average, and any result above this value is on the alkaline side of average. An arterial blood pH of less than 7.35 is referred to as acidosis and a result of greater than 7.45 is referred to as alkalosis.[8,35,37–39]

Step 3

$PaCO_2$ refers to the measurement of the partial pressure of carbon dioxide dissolved in arterial blood. The normal range should be 35–45 mmHg and does not change as a person ages. The body produces carbon dioxide during normal metabolism. The $PaCO_2$ values indicate the ability of the patient to effectively ventilate to rid the body of carbon dioxide.

The definition of respiratory acidosis is a $PaCO_2$ value above 45 mmHg. This is due to hypoventilation and can be the result of a number of conditions including chronic obstructive pulmonary disease (COPD), over-sedation, head trauma or drug overdose. When the levels of $PaCO_2$ are greater than 50 mmHg, ventilatory failure occurs.[8,35,37–39] Acute ventilatory failure will have abnormal pH values of 7.30; this is because the body has not had enough time to compensate by attempting to bring the pH value back towards the normal value. Chronic ventilatory failure has near-normal pH values of greater than 7.30.

The definition of respiratory alkalosis is a $PaCO_2$ value of < 35 mmHg. Respiratory alkalosis is due to hyperventilation and can be the result of a number of conditions including hypoxia, pulmonary embolus, hyperventilation and pregnancy. It can also be the result of a compensatory mechanism to a metabolic acidosis.[8,35,37–39]

Step 4

The bicarbonate (HCO_3^-) result is a reflection of the renal function. The normal range is 22–26 mEq/L. The definition of a metabolic acidosis is a level below 22 mEq/L. This can be a result of renal failure, lactic acidosis, ketoacidosis or diarrhoea. The definition of a metabolic alkalosis is a level above 26 mEq/L and can be the result of loss of fluid and diuretic therapy.[8,35,37–39]

Step 5

In an *uncompensated* condition (respiratory or metabolic)—if the pH is abnormal, then the $PaCO_2$, HCO_3^-, or both, will also be abnormal, because the body has not had enough time to return the pH value back to the normal range.

In a *compensated* condition (respiratory or metabolic)—if the pH is normal and both the $PaCO_2$ and HCO_3^- values are abnormal, then the body has had time to return the pH values back to the normal range (Tables 17.2 and 17.3).[8,35,37–40]

Step 1
Look at the PaO_2 level and answer the question, 'Does the PaO_2 level show hypoxaemia?'

Step 2
Look at the pH level and answer the question, 'Is the pH level on the acid or alkaline side of 7.40?'

Step 3
Look at the $PaCO_2$ level and answer the question, 'Does the $PaCO_2$ level show metabolic acidosis, alkalosis or normalcy?'

Step 4
Look at the HCO_3^- level and answer the question, 'Does the HCO_3^- level show metabolic acidosis, alkalosis or normalcy?'

Step 5
Look back at the pH level, and answer the question, 'Does the pH show a compensated or an uncompensated condition?'

TABLE 17.2 Arterial blood gases with various stages of compensation

STAGE OF COMPENSATION	CAUSE	PaCO$_2$	UNCOMPENSATED		PARTIALLY COMPENSATED		FULLY COMPENSATED	
			pH	HCO$_3^-$	pH	HCO$_3^-$	pH	HCO$_3^-$
Respiratory alkalosis	Hyperventilation	↓	↑	Normal	↑	↓	Normal	↓
Respiratory acidosis	Drug ingestion (hypoventilation)	↑	↓	Normal	↓	↑	Normal	↑

	CAUSE	HCO$_3^-$	UNCOMPENSATED		PARTIALLY COMPENSATED		FULLY COMPENSATED	
			pH	PaCO$_2$	pH	PaCO$_2$	pH	PaCO$_2$
Metabolic alkalosis	Severe vomiting	↑	↑	Normal	↑	↑	*	↑
Metabolic acidosis	Diabetic ketoacidosis	↓	↓	Normal	↓	↓	*	↓

HCO$_3^-$: bicarbonate; PaCO$_2$: partial arterial carbon dioxide pressure

*Metabolic cannot be fully compensated to a normal pH by the respiratory system.

TABLE 17.3 Normal values of an arterial blood gas sample[40]

NAME	NORMAL VALUE OR RANGE
pH	7.35–7.45
PaO$_2$ (mmHg)	85–90
PaCO$_2$ (mmHg)	35–45
HCO$_3^-$ (meq/L)	22–26

Venous blood gases interpretation

With the increasing availability of point of care (POC) blood-testing devices, it is becoming increasingly common for the emergency clinician to perform venous blood gas (VBG) analysis as a first-line investigation as part of the initial evaluation of the patient. VBGs have several advantages over ABGs, including ease of collection, less pain for the patient and less-significant complications. VBGs will provide results for all the parameters reported on a standard ABG and may also include a number of additional biochemical parameters (depending on the capability of the testing device). These may include such parameters as potassium (K$^+$), sodium (Na$^+$), haemoglobin (Hb) and creatinine. The results for many of the POC devices tend to be quicker than routine pathology testing, providing valuable clinical information in a timely manner. ABG values acceptably compare with the same values collected via venous sampling. Venous values for pH, PvCO$_2$ and bicarbonate have been shown to correlate closely with the values obtained via arterial sampling and are therefore an acceptable alternative to ABG-acquired results.[42–44] There is no acceptable comparison between venous PO$_2$ and arterial PO$_2$; therefore, evaluations of oxygenation continue to require ABG analysis.

Blood glucose level sampling

Blood glucose level (BGL) is the measurable amount of glucose in the blood, and is normally between 3 and 8 mmol/L. A bedside BGL is available as quickly as within 5 seconds with portable glucose meters. As part of a comprehensive assessment of the emergency patient, a finger-prick blood glucose measure should be collected.[39] Maintaining normal serum glucose levels in critically ill patients improves outcomes by reducing infection rates.[44] BGL should be obtained and recorded for all patients with diabetes and in patients who present with collapse, multiple abscesses or non-healing wounds, dizziness and nausea and vomiting and in neonates. Hypoglycaemia should be considered a factor in any unresponsive patient until proven otherwise.

Procedure

1. Select a finger of the non-dominant hand.
2. Begin by ensuring the skin is clean and dry.
3. Ready the glucometer by turning it on and inserting a testing strip.
4. Place the lancet firmly on the side of the distal end of the selected finger and press to trigger the lancet.
5. Gently bleed the wound and wipe away the first drop of blood.[26]
6. Gently bleed the wound to collect sufficient blood by milking the finger from the proximal to the distal end.
7. Touch the testing strip to the blood. Capillary action will draw the sample.
8. Cover the finger wound with a dry dressing and apply momentary pressure.

Underwater-seal drains

Trauma to the chest can produce life-threatening collection of blood or air between the chest wall and the lung. An underwater-seal drain (UWSD) or chest drain is designed to provide a closed system for the one-way removal of air or blood from the pleural space. The water acts to prevent air returning to the pleural space.[26] A pneumothorax with greater than 15% collapse requires the placement of a chest tube or intercostal catheter (ICC). ICCs are inserted in the pleural space to remove air or blood and allow the lung to re-expand under normal negative intrapleural pressures.[45] A UWSD, or more-simple Heimlich valve, is connected to an intercostal catheter or chest drain that is inserted between the ribs into the pleural space.

Assisting with the insertion of an intercostal catheter

1. Set up a sterile procedure tray containing kidney dishes, clamps, needle holders and bowls. Commonly, a large general sterile procedure set-up is used.
2. Add four large sterile drapes if not included in the procedure tray.
3. Open sterile gloves and gowns.
4. Fill a sterile bowl with a skin-cleaning solution such as chlorhexidine with alcohol.
5. Open and place on the tray a 10 mL syringe for local anaesthetic.
6. Open and place a large-bore blunt drawing-up needle to draw up local anaesthetic.
7. Open and place out a 22-gauge injecting needle for the injection of local anaesthetic.
8. Put out a large, long, straight needle with a 2/0 suture to secure the drain.
9. Put out a scalpel for cutting the space between the ribs where the catheter will be pushed.
10. Have ready two large clear dressings to cover the drain insertion site.
11. Have ready two rubber-tipped forceps to clamp the catheter. Often these are left at the bedside during the entire time the drain is in place.
12. Open the intercostal catheter.
13. Open and prepare the UWSD. Different products are prepared using different methods, but most have a water reservoir within the drain that needs filling before use.
14. Administer adequate analgesia where possible.
15. Continue cardiorespiratory monitoring throughout the insertion procedure for signs of immediate deterioration or lethal dysrhythmia.
16. When the ICC is inserted, assist with the connection of the UWSD tubing and secure the two with long lengths of Elastoplast tape. Often these are applied in a spiral or trouser-leg fashion.
17. When the catheter is sutured in place, cover the insertion site with occlusive dressings.
18. Check the UWSD is functioning. This will be indicated by bubbling of air through the water within the drain and oscillation or swinging of any blood in the tube on inspiration.
19. Apply low-pressure suction to the UWSD if indicated.
20. Prepare the patient for X-ray to confirm the placement of the ICC.

- The insertion of a chest drain with underwater-seal drain is an immediate priority in chest trauma, as tension pneumothorax can cause life-threatening complications. As the air collects within the pleura, this alters the inter-pleural pressure and can cause the lung to collapse, putting pressure on the heart and affecting stroke volumes.[46]
- If pre-warning is given about the arrival of a trauma patient, set up bilateral chest drains for immediate insertion.

Caring for the underwater-seal drain and intercostal catheter

1. Keep a pair of rubber-tipped artery forceps at the bedside. If there are complications with the drain, these can be used to clamp the ICC close to the insertion site for a short period of time.
2. Keep the UWSD unit at the patient's bedside and below the level of the insertion site. This is to prevent the return of air or fluid to the chest cavity.
3. Maintain the water level within the drain. The drain should bubble gently rather than vigorously, as the latter can increase evaporation.[26]
4. Continue the required amount of low-pressure suction if ordered.
5. Check the ICC and UWSD from the point of insertion down to the drain.
6. Check the dressing at the point of insertion. Confirm there is an occlusive dressing covering the whole insertion point.
7. Check for air leaks and check all tubes are well secured with long lengths of spiral or trouser-leg tape.
8. Confirm there are no kinks in the tubing (Fig 17.26).[48]

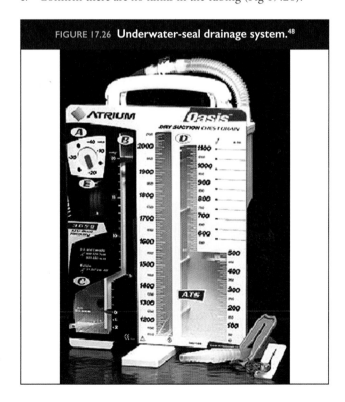

FIGURE 17.26 Underwater-seal drainage system.[48]

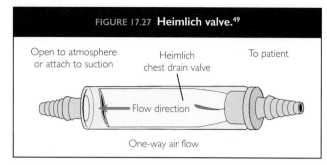

FIGURE 17.27 **Heimlich valve.**[49]

Open to atmosphere or attach to suction

Heimlich chest drain valve

To patient

Flow direction

One-way air flow

A one-way Heimlich valve alone is often sufficient to treat a pneumothorax, but it cannot be used to treat a haemothorax.

Heimlich chest drain valve

The Heimlich chest drain valve or flutter valve (Fig 17.27) is a simple device used to prevent the return of air into the ICC. The Heimlich valve works without suction but can only be used to remove air, not blood, from the pleural space. Normal respiration and cough creates enough intrathoracic pressure to expel air through the valve.[49] The Heimlich valve is commonly used to transport patients with ICC as it reduces the need for bulky UWSD. Heimlich is generally used in the pre-hospital setting for suspected pneumothorax, or in patient transport and less commonly used in the admitted in-hospital patient.

To fit a Heimlich chest drain valve

1. Confirm the ICC is secured in place.
2. Attach the blue end of the Heimlich valve to the distal end of the ICC and tape it in place using lengths of spiral-wrapped tape. There is an arrow on the valve to confirm that it is inserted correctly.
3. Attach the clear end of the valve to a drainage bag. There is no need to secure this with lengths of tubing as the one-way valve prevents back-flow of air.
4. Observe fluttering of the valve on cough and respiration. The collection bag may also fill with air and require venting.
5. Low-pressure suction can be applied to the distal end of the Heimlich valve if required.
6. Beware that the valve will clog with fluids and should be observed closely to ensure it continues to function. To change a blocked valve, clamp the ICC proximally with two rubber-tipped forceps, remove the old valve and replace with a new one.

PRACTICE TIP

A modified Heimlich valve can made by using the fingers of a glove to allow air to escape but prevent its return to the chest cavity. Make a small slit in the glove finger and tape it securely over the end of the ICC.

Removal of underwater-seal drain and intercostal catheter

1. Ensure that the UWSD is no longer bubbling continuously. Confirm on X-ray that the amount of air or blood in the pleural space is adequately reduced and the drain is ready for removal.
2. Have emergency equipment ready for the re-insertion of a new ICC if urgently required.
3. Administer adequate analgesia where possible.
4. Clamp the ICC proximally above the join of the UWSD with two rubber-tipped clamps.
5. Disconnect the UWSD from the chest tube.
6. Remove the occlusive dressings and cut the sutures at the point of insertion.
7. Instruct the patient to inhale completely and perform a Valsalva manoeuvre, and pull the drain out quickly and continuously.[49]
8. Apply an occlusive dressing immediately over the insertion site to prevent air returning to the pleural space. The wound may also be sutured closed, in some cases using a purse-string suture that may have held the drain in place initially.
9. Monitor the patient for signs of pneumothorax by auscultation of lung fields for normal air entry and observing normal vital signs.

Respiratory function testing

Peak expiratory flow rate (PEFR) measurement

Measurement of peak flow in the ED is performed using a simple assessment device that measures airflow, or peak expiratory flow (PEF). Patients blow into the device quickly and forcefully, and the resulting peak flow reading indicates how open the airways are, or how difficult it is for the patient to breathe.[35,50] Peak flow meters have limited accuracy and provide only a single-effort-dependent assessment of ventilatory function. They are also dependent on patient technique. PEF is reduced in diseases causing airway obstruction and for asthmatics. The meter is a very useful tool in the home for patients to assess changes in condition and prevent unnecessary attendance at the ED.[8,35,39,50]

Spirometry

Spirometry is a physiological test to measure lung function; it is the broadest non-invasive test of ventilatory function. Spirometry is used to detect and assess diseases which limit ventilatory capacity and affect the mechanics of the chest wall and lungs, and it assesses the function of the airways. Spirometry is used to measure timed expired and inspired volumes and, from this, calculation of how readily the lungs can be emptied and filled is possible.[35,50] This assessment provides information on whether the lung disease is of an obstructive or a restrictive nature. Acceptable spirometry measurement requires cooperation by the patient and knowledge of the technique by the operator. Constant verbal reinforcement of patient technique throughout the spirometry test will help to produce favourable results (Fig 17.28).[8,35,38,39,50]

PRACTICE TIP

Constant verbal reinforcement of patient technique throughout the spirometry test will help to produce favourable results.

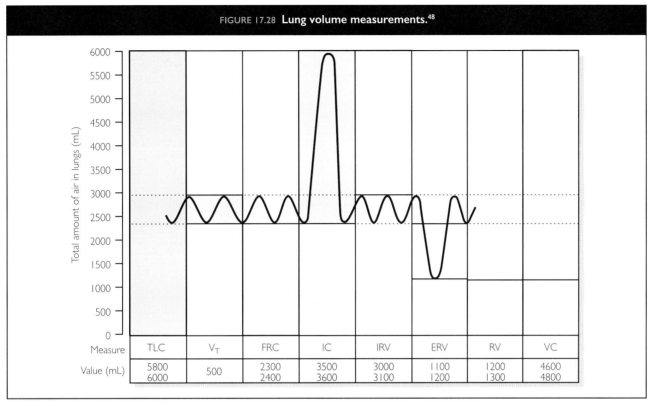

FIGURE 17.28 **Lung volume measurements.**[48]

All values are approximately 25% less in women. *TLC: total lung capacity; V_T: tidal volume; FRC: functional residual capacity; IC: inspiratory capacity; IRV: inspiratory reserve volume; ERV: expiratory reserve volume; RV: residual volume; VC: vital capacity.*

Measure	TLC	V_T	FRC	IC	IRV	ERV	RV	VC
Value (mL)	5800 6000	500	2300 2400	3500 3600	3000 3100	1100 1200	1200 1300	4600 4800

Measurements obtained from spirometry

The data obtained following spirometry is interpreted against predicted normal values and within the clinical context of the patient. The measurements commonly obtained from performing spirometry are outlined below.[51]

- **Vital capacity (VC)** is the maximum volume of air which can be exhaled or inspired during either a maximally forced (FVC) or a slow (SVC) manoeuvre.
- **Forced expired volume in one second (FEV_1)** is the volume expired in the first second of maximal expiration after a maximal inspiration and is a useful measure of how quickly full lungs can be emptied.
- **FEV_1/VC (or FEV_1/FVC)** is the FEV_1 expressed as a percentage of the VC or FVC (whichever volume is larger), and gives a clinically useful index of airflow limitation.
- **$FEF_{25-75\%}$** is the average expired flow over the middle half of the FVC manoeuvre and is regarded as a more sensitive measure of small airways narrowing than FEV_1.
- **Peak expiratory flow (PEF)** is the maximal expiratory flow rate achieved; this occurs very early in the forced expiratory manoeuvre.
- **$FEF_{50\%}$ and $FEF_{75\%}$** (forced expiratory flow at 50% or 75% FVC) is the maximal expiratory flow measured at the point where 50% of the FVC has been expired ($FEF_{50\%}$) and after 75% has been expired ($FEF_{75\%}$).
- **FVC_6** is the forced expiratory volume during the first 6 seconds and is a surrogate of the FVC. The FVC_6 (and FEV_1/FVC_6) is gaining popularity because

stopping the expiratory manoeuvre after 6 seconds is less demanding and easier to perform for patients with airflow obstruction and the elderly, yet is similar to conventional FVC and FEV_1/FVC for diagnosing and grading airflow obstruction.

Performing a spirometry measurement

The procedure for performing a spirometry measurement is given in Box 17.7.

BOX 17.7 Procedure for performing a spirometry measurement (forced expiratory manoeuvre)[51,61]

1. Obtain spirometer and any disposable equipment required (e.g. mouth piece, filter or nose clip).
2. Ensure the spirometer has been calibrated in accordance with the manufacturer's recommendations.
3. Measure the patient's weight and height. For patients who are unable to stand, height can be calculated by measuring from the patient's mid-sternum along their outstretched arm to the tip of the middle finger (demispan, in cm) and using the following equations to calculate height:[42]
   - females: height (cm) = (1.35 × demispan) + 60.1
   - males: height (cm) = (1.40 × demispan) + 57.8
4. Explain the procedure to the patient, stressing the following points:
   - Take a full breath in (must be absolutely full).

Continued

BOX 17.7 Procedure for performing a spirometry measurement (forced expiratory manoeuvre)[51,61]—cont'd

– Place the mouthpiece in your mouth and ensure a good, tight seal.
– Immediately blast air out as hard and as fast for as long as possible.
– Do not lean forwards during the test.

5. Position the patient, preferably in a seated position with feet flat on the floor (adults). Children may stand.

6. Turn on the spirometer and enter the required test details. This may include such information as name, age, gender, height, ethnicity, temperature, weight or smoking history.

7. Apply the nose clip.

8. Instruct the patient to take a full deep breath in and start the test.

9. Provide encouragement throughout the test. 'Blow … blow … good … keep going … keep going'—the importance of active encouragement cannot be overstated.

10. Allow the patient to rest following each forced expiration.

11. Repeat the test to ensure that at least three technically acceptable manoeuvres are obtained to ensure reproducibility. Reproducibility is achieved when the best two results are within 5% or 100 mL of each other. The patient should perform no more than 8 tests in a single session; however, if reproducibility cannot be achieved within 4 attempts with proper instruction and active encouragement, it is unlikely that additional testing will be helpful.

12. Terminate procedure and dispose of equipment.

13. Collect data—generally this is provided in a printed format; however, on older manual-style machines data may have to be obtained from the graphed results.

14. Interpret data (see the section 'Measurements obtained from spirometry').

Cardiac monitoring

The following section contains information on the skill of performing electrocardiograph (ECG) and continuous cardiac monitoring.

Performing an electrocardiograph

Performing an electrocardiograph (ECG) is an essential skill for all emergency clinicians. An ECG can provide timely and important information about the electrical activity of the heart. ECG should be performed promptly:

- in patients with chest pain
- following a life-threatening dysrhythmia (ventricular tachycardia, ventricular fibrillation, asystole, atrioventricular blocks or symptomatic bradydysrhythmias)
- in haemodynamically compromised patients

- routinely after cardiac surgery
- following the ingestion of pro-dysrhythmic drugs
- peri-operatively.

Figure 17.29 below shows placement of the leads on the chest for performing an ECG.

Heavy vertical lines represent the midclavicular, anterior, axillary and midaxillary lines (from left to right). V1 and V2 are referenced to the fourth intercostal space and V4 to the fifth space. V3 lies on a line between V2 and V4. V5 and V6 lie on a horizontal line from V4. Additional praecordial leads can be obtained on the right side (V3 R, V4 R), as well as extending further left from V6 (V7).[52]

Procedure:

1. Inform the patient of the steps and gain consent.
2. The patient should be supine.
3. Shave the hair at electrode placement if required.
4. Anatomically position the leads.
   Electrode position
   - RA (Right arm) Right forearm, proximal to the wrist
   - LA (Left arm) Left forearm, proximal to the wrist
   - LL (Left leg) Left lower leg, proximal to the ankle
   - RL (Right leg) Right lower leg, proximal to the ankle
   - V1 Fourth intercostal space at the right sternal edge
   - V2 Fourth intercostal space at the left sternal edge
   - V3 Midway between V2 and V4
   - V4 Fifth intercostal space in the mid-clavicular line
   - V5 Left anterior axillary line at same horizontal level as V4
   - V6 Left mid-axillary line at same horizontal level as V4 and V5.

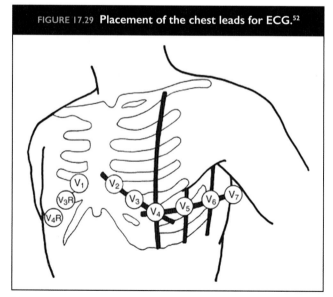

FIGURE 17.29 Placement of the chest leads for ECG.[52]

The locations of the praecordial leads. Heavy vertical lines represent the midclavicular, anterior, axillary and midaxillary lines (from left to right). V1 and V2 are referenced to the fourth intercostal space and V4 to the fifth space. V3 lies on a line between V2 and V4. V5 and V6 lie on a horizontal line from V4. Additional praecordial leads can be obtained on the right side (V3 R, V4 R), as well as extending further left from V6 (V7).

5. Ensure the patient is still and relaxed.

6. Record and print a 12-lead ECG at 25 mm/sec with a gain setting of 10 mm/mV.

7. Label the ECG with the patient demographic details, and clinical information such as current and past medical history.

8. Clean the equipment after the procedure.

9. Most emergency services have policies about the interpretation and review of an ECG, but in general, most ECGs should be reviewed within 10 minutes.

Continuous cardiac monitoring

Continuous cardiac monitoring should be performed:[53,54]

- in patients with acute coronary syndromes
- post cardiac arrest
- following a life-threatening dysrhythmia (ventricular tachycardia, ventricular fibrillation, asystole, atrioventricular blocks or symptomatic bradydysrhythmias)
- in haemodynamically compromised patients
- for 48 hours after cardiac surgery
- following the ingestion of pro-dysrhythmic drugs.

Patients should be regularly assessed by the medical team for the need for continuous electrocardiogram monitoring.

Procedure

1. Inform the patient of the procedure and gain consent.

2. The patient should initially be supine.

3. Shave the hair at electrode placement if required.

4. Anatomically position the leads.

Electrode position for the 5-electrode monitor (see Fig 17.30)
- RA (Right arm) Right shoulder

- LA (Left arm) Left shoulder
- LL (Left leg) Left side torso
- RL (Right leg) Right side torso
- V Fourth intercostal space at the right sternal edge

Electrode position for the 3-electrode monitor (see Fig 17.31)
- RA (Right arm) Right shoulder
- LA (Left arm) Left shoulder
- LL (Left leg) Left side torso

5. Confirm continuous electrocardiogram monitoring.

6. Electronically label the cardiac monitor with the patient demographic details (if required).

Temporary cardiac pacing

The following section contains information on the use of temporary cardiac pacing for cardiac dysrhythmia.

Transcutaneous (external) pacing

Transcutaneous or external cardiac pacing is the most readily available form of cardiac pacing in the ED. Many defibrillators have the ability to provide transcutaneous cardiac pacing through self-adhesive multifunctional pads which are able to monitor, defibrillate and pace. This method is non-invasive and relatively fast to initiate, and is therefore the preferred method of pacing in an emergency situation. Pads are placed on the chest in either a left anterior/posterior position or an anterior/lateral position. The pacemaker generates an electrical impulse which is delivered through the pads, causing depolarisation of myocardial tissue as the current travels though the chest wall and heart muscle. External cardiac pacing is generally a temporary measure providing time to make arrangements and decisions regarding transvenous pacing.[55]

External pacing is indicated in haemodynamically compromising bradydysrhythmias (such as complete heart block and second-degree heart block Mobitz type II) if the patient has not responded to medical therapies (e.g. drug therapy, IV fluids).[55] Pacing is not recommended for patients in asystolic cardiac

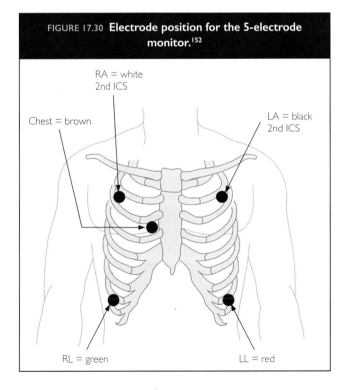

FIGURE 17.30 **Electrode position for the 5-electrode monitor.**[152]

RA = white
2nd ICS

LA = black
2nd ICS

Chest = brown

RL = green   LL = red

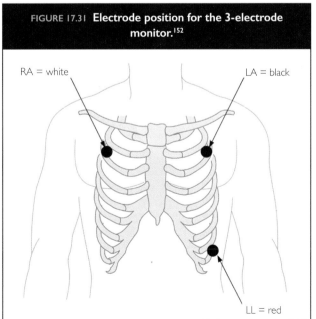

FIGURE 17.31 **Electrode position for the 3-electrode monitor.**[152]

RA = white   LA = black

LL = red

arrest. There is no proven improvement in the rate of admission to hospital or survival to hospital discharge when pacing is initiated in asystolic patients in the pre-hospital or ED settings.[56]

Procedure

1. Explain the procedure to the patient, where possible.
2. Prepare the patient's skin over which the external pacing pads are to be placed. The skin should be clean and dry to promote good adhesion and contact of pacing electrodes. Any transdermal drug delivery patches should be removed. If time permits, excessive body hair should be removed.[55,57]
3. Apply the electrocardiograph (ECG) electrodes attached to the pacing unit. If using multifunctional pads, an ECG tracing may be obtainable through these; however, if the ECG trace is inadequate the separate ECG electrodes should also be used.
4. Apply the pacing pads in the desired position. Many pads come with an image of the correct position. Avoid positioning the pads over bone as this is likely to increase transthoracic resistance, increasing the amount of energy required. In females the pad should be placed under the breast.
   - Anterior/posterior positioning—generally the preferred position. The anterior pad is placed on the left anterior chest at the point of maximal impulse (approximately V_3 position) and the posterior pad is placed on the patient's back immediately opposite the anterior pad, to the left of the spinal column and below the scapula[58–60] (see Fig 17.32A).
   - Anterior/lateral positioning—alternative position. One pad is positioned on the right side of the chest at the sternal border and the other pad is placed on the left lateral chest wall[74] (see Fig 17.32B).
5. Provide the patient with analgesia and/or sedation. External pacing can be uncomfortable and wherever possible this should be mitigated.
6. Select the mode of pacing:
   - Demand (synchronous) mode—the pacer senses the patient's own QRS complexes and only generates an

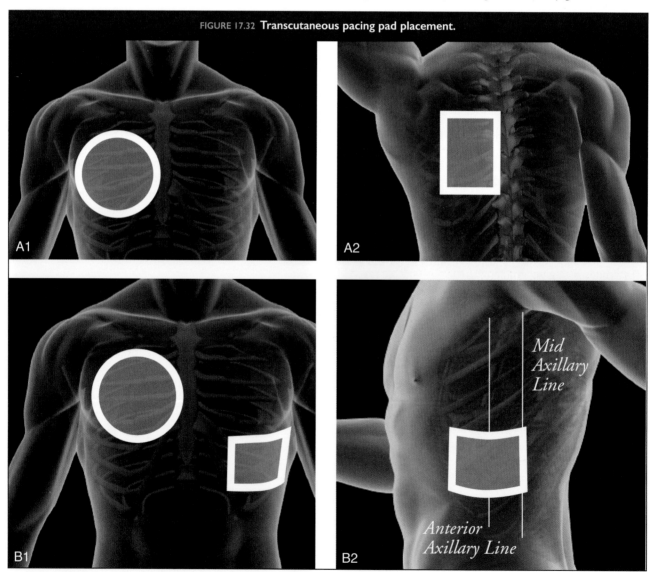

FIGURE 17.32 **Transcutaneous pacing pad placement.**

A1

A2

B1

B2

Mid Axillary Line

Anterior Axillary Line

A, Anterior/posterior positioning, **B,** Anterior/lateral positioning.
Courtesy ZOLL Medical Corporation.

impulse to achieve the set rate when the heart does not produce its own intrinsic QRS complex.[59,60] This is the preferred mode of pacing and the most commonly used.

- Non-demand (asynchronous) mode—a fixed-rate mode where impulses are delivered at the set rate regardless of the patient's own intrinsic heart rate. Non-demand or fixed-rate pacing is rarely used as it can have potential complications by delivering an impulse on the T wave and precipitating ventricular fibrillation.[59,60]

7. Select the pacing rate—this is generally set at 60–70 beats/minute in order to achieve an adequate blood pressure and cerebral perfusion.

8. Slowly increase the energy output level.

9. Observe the ECG tracing for pacing spikes and signs of electrical capture. Electrical capture occurs when every pacing spike is followed by a wide QRS complex.

10. Slightly increase the energy output after the point of electrical capture. Ideally, pacing should be continued at an output level just above the threshold of electrical capture so as to minimise discomfort.[55]

11. Assess the patient for mechanical capture—this is assessed by palpating the pulse. The femoral pulse is preferred, as the muscle contractions associated with external pacing may make the carotid pulse difficult to assess.[55]

12. Assess the patient's haemodynamic response.

Maintain close observation and adequate analgesia/sedation. Patients should be continually observed and assessed. In particular, the patient should be observed for loss of electrical capture which may result from pad dislodgement or patient movement. Patients require ongoing analgesia/sedation as they may become increasingly aware of and distressed with the discomfort associated with external pacing, especially patients who have an improved level of consciousness with external pacing.

Transvenous pacing

Transvenous pacing involves the insertion of a pacing electrode into the right ventricle via the subclavian or external jugular venous route under fluoroscopy or with a flotation-pacing catheter under guidance by the ECG. The electrodes are connected to an external pulse generator where the output can be selected in milliamps along with the rate.[59,60] This type of pacemaker also has a fixed-rate mode or a demand mode.

Vascular access

Inserting peripheral intravenous catheters is an essential skill for paramedics and emergency nurses. The decision to insert should be made in consultation with the patient, who should also be informed of the reasons for insertion.[63] The traditional sites chosen for peripheral intravenous catheter in both an emergency and an acute situation are the cephalic and basilic veins in the lower arm and the vein in the dorsum of the hand, as they are large, constant and straight, making venous access easy (see Figs 17.33 and 17.34).

In some clinical environments the insertion of central catheters may also be required (see p. 346), but this is not a basic skill for the majority of emergency nurses or paramedics, and reference to local organisational and departmental policy

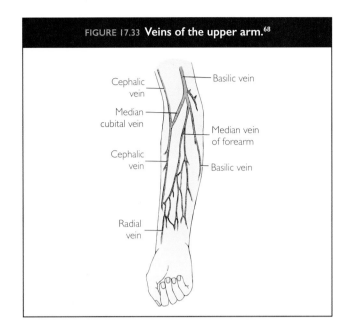
FIGURE 17.33 **Veins of the upper arm.**[68]

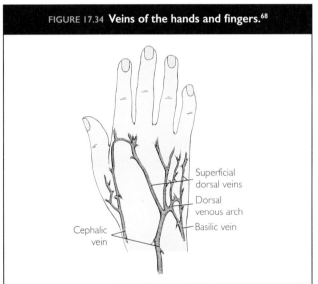
FIGURE 17.34 **Veins of the hands and fingers.**[68]

and procedure is required. Nurses and paramedics have certain responsibilities to use and maintain established vascular access points. Catheters are usually inserted into peripheral veins of the hand and arm. Other sites include veins of the lower extremities, or the external jugular, internal jugular and femoral veins. Cannulation of the lower extremities, such as the foot and leg, are usually avoided due to the risk of complications such as thrombophlebitis and pulmonary embolism.[64]

Vascular access is obtained using aseptic technique. Initial insertion attempts should begin with distal veins and progress up the extremity. Proximal veins are not routinely used unless patients need immediate fluid replacement, such as in trauma patients or patients in hypovolaemic shock. These veins are also used for patients receiving drugs that have an extremely short half-life (e.g. adenosine). Scalp veins have no valves, so fluid can be infused in either direction; they are also easily visualised, making them an ideal alternative in infants.

Insertion of intravenous catheters is not without risk to the patient and the emergency clinician. In the era of HIV and

> **BOX 17.8 Complications of intravenous catheters**
>
> • Haematoma at insertion site
> • Fluid infiltration
> • Phlebitis
> • Embolism of blood, air or catheter fragments
> • Infection
> • Cellulitis

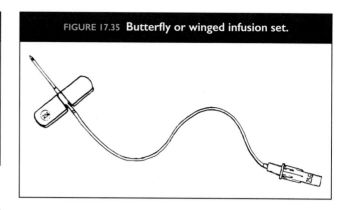

FIGURE 17.35 **Butterfly or winged infusion set.**

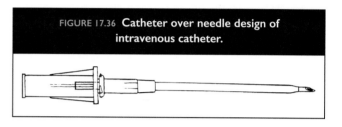

FIGURE 17.36 **Catheter over needle design of intravenous catheter.**

hepatitis, safety in placing IVs cannot be overemphasised. Standard precautions must be applied to all patients, especially in emergency care settings where the risk of blood exposure is increased and the infection status of patients is largely unknown. Potential complications for the patient include infection and haematoma (Box 17.8). Hand-washing and aseptic technique remain major prevention strategies for catheter-related infections.[63] The emergency nurse or paramedic risks exposure to potentially infectious blood through a needle-stick or direct contact with blood or body fluids. Extreme care should be taken to minimise risks through use of standard precautions and appropriate disposal of needles. Intravenous catheters with safety features such as self-capping needles and retracting needles are readily available.[65]

Catheter selection

The size and type of catheter are determined by the clinical scenario, urgency of need, patient size, age and vasculature. The general rule when choosing a cannula is the smallest gauge and the shortest length to meet the needs of the client. Cannula selection is also determined by the purpose of the IV, the type of fluid to be administered, the location of the insertion site, the duration of the IV therapy and the condition of the vein.[66]

The chosen vein should be larger than the cannula so that blood can flow easily around the catheter after insertion. This allows haemodilution to occur, therefore reducing venous wall trauma and distal oedema.[66] The rate of infusion flow is not determined by the vein itself but by the diameter of the cannula, and is inversely affected by the cannula length.[67] Larger-diameter catheters are used for administering significant volume, colloid solutions, blood or blood products, whereas smaller-diameter catheters are used for routine vascular access.

A guide for catheter selection[66]

• 22–24 gauge—children/adults with extremely small and/or fragile veins, e.g. the elderly. Infusion rate will be slow.

• 18–20 gauge—medical and surgical patients (depending on purpose of infusion).

• 16–20 gauge—blood product administration, surgical admissions and trauma.

• 14–16 gauge—life-threatening situations.

All intravenous catheters now use a catheter-over-needle design. Catheters used for peripheral access include a butterfly or winged catheter (Fig 17.35) and straight catheter-over-needle design (Fig 17.36). Winged catheters are easily inserted and can be stabilised with minimal effort; however, these catheters are not ideal for rapid fluid replacement. Catheters over needles are ideal for aggressive fluid replacement, but can present problems with stabilisation, particularly in distal veins of the hand.

Insertion

Aseptic technique is essential to protect the patient from infection during intravenous catheter insertion. Gloves should be worn for site preparation and catheter insertion. The selected insertion site should have adequate circulation and be free of infection. In general, IV cannulation should be performed on the most distal part of the client's arm, but proximal to previous attempts.[66] Peripheral veins in hands and arms are the first choice for intravenous access. The hand veins are appropriate for 22- to 20-gauge IV cannulas. Cephalic, accessory or basilic veins are ideal for larger-bore cannulas. The femoral vein is an excellent choice in cardiac arrest because cardiac compressions can continue. Femoral access also provides an opportunity for haemodynamic pressure monitoring.

Veins should be avoided if they are below previous IV infiltration, close to arteries at points of flexion or show signs of skin inflammation, bruising or infection. If patients have undergone radical mastectomy, avoid the arm on the same side as the surgery because circulation may be impaired, affecting flow, causing oedema and other complications like thrombosis. In renal dialysis patients who have an arteriovenous (AV) fistula in place, this arm should be avoided to prevent damage above and below the fistula. Deep percutaneous antecubital or external jugular vein cannulation are also options in the patient with difficult veins or those who need IV access in a hurry.[65]

After a site is selected, palpation is the next crucial step in successful cannulation.[65] A tourniquet is placed proximally to distend vessels for easy insertion (see Fig 17.37A). Because veins may be more prominent in elderly patients, a tourniquet may not be required. Tourniquets may actually rupture vessels because of increased pressure in fragile veins. Gently tapping or rubbing vessels below the tourniquet increases vessel size

FIGURE 17.37[68]

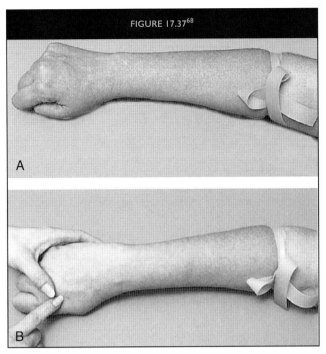

A, Placement of tourniquet. **B**, Technique for increasing vein size by dilation.

FIGURE 17.38 **Venepuncture.**[68]

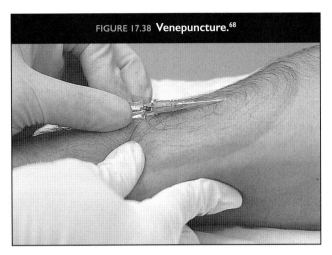

by dilation. When vessels are not easily visualised or palpated, applying warm towels over the vein for 5 minutes causes vasodilation and can facilitate catheter insertion (Fig 17.37B).

Skin preparation begins with initial cleansing using an antiseptic solution such as alcohol 75% with chlorhexidine gluconate or some other form of alcohol wipe. The solution is applied directly over the insertion site in a circular pattern moving slowly outwards. The ideal bactericidal effect requires that the solution remain on the skin for 30 seconds. The cleansed area should not be re-palpated.[66]

Local anaesthesia is not routinely used for catheter insertion. If local anaesthetic is required, lignocaine 1% may be injected at the insertion site for immediate anaesthetic effect. EMLA cream (Eutectic Mixture of Local Anaesthetics), 2.5% lignocaine or 2.5% prilocaine should be applied topically prior to skin preparation.[69] EMLA is particularly useful in children.[70]

After the site is prepared, the catheter is inserted by stabilising the vein to prevent movement during puncture. With the needle bevel up, skin is punctured using the smallest angle possible between skin and needle (Fig 17.38). Veins may be entered on the top or side. The catheter is advanced slowly until blood flashes into the catheter, then the catheter is advanced over the needle into the vein and the needle removed. The tourniquet is removed; fingertip pressure is applied at the distal end of the catheter tip to prevent extravasation of blood. The injection port is attached and catheter flushed with 0.9% Normal saline or connected to primed IV tubing. The catheter and tubing should be secured with tape according to hospital policy; however, tape should never be applied directly over the insertion site. The evidence regarding the nature of site dressings is debated.[63] However, clear, occlusive dressings such as Opsite, Tegaderm or Bioclusive should be applied over the insertion site. Sites should be labelled with the date, time,

catheter size and initials of the person inserting to facilitate monitoring and evaluation.[63]

For patients remaining in the ED longer than 6 hours, care must be taken to maintain patency with frequent saline flushes. IV lines and the cannula itself should be changed according to hospital policy, although some hospitals now differentiate out-of-hospital (paramedic-inserted) and in-hospital-inserted cannulae. The Joanna Briggs Institute (JBI) systematic review[63] conducted in 1998 advises replacement of IV cannulae between 48 and 72 hours post-insertion and replacement of giving sets every 72 hours.

The JBI website provides some significant resources that may be of some use to paramedics and emergency nurses. As the JBI is an international organisation which promotes evidence-based practice and fosters knowledge translation, many public and some private hospitals have membership status that allows employees to access up-to-date materials for their practice.

Paediatric considerations

Paediatric IV cannulations can be very traumatic for both the child and the parents, and therefore consideration should be given first to the need for the procedure and second to the urgency with which the procedure needs to be performed. Once the need for IV cannulation has been determined it is important to plan and prepare for the procedure adequately, if the clinical situation allows, ensuring the best chance at success.

The anxiety and pain associated with cannulation may be limited with the use of topical anaesthetic creams such as EMLA and/or the use of nitrous oxide during the procedure. Topical anaesthetic creams need to be applied 45–60 min prior to performing the procedure for them to successfully anaesthetise the area, an effect which persists for at least 2 hours after removal of the patch.[71] Therefore the procedure time needs to be planned in conjunction with the action of the anaesthetic cream. It is also important to apply the patch to a site that has a potentially suitable vein, as the maximum number of patches that can be applied is limited by age.

The need to provide appropriate psychosocial support to a child cannot be over-emphasised. Anxiety is a significant factor in a child's perception of pain and thereby influences the level of pain experienced during cannulation. Moreover, this may also affect the degree of cooperation by the child. Previous experience may also influence the degree to which the child will cooperate during the cannulation procedure, and may even flow onto future procedures and healthcare.[72] It is therefore important to have an adequate understanding of the perception of children of various age groups in terms of how they may react to IV cannulation.

Parental support can also be very beneficial. Most parents prefer to be present during the procedure and almost all children perceive that parental presence 'helps the most'.[73] Parents need to have an active role in the procedure—providing distraction, encouragement and comfort. Caution should be taken with parental involvement where the parents themselves have a needle phobia or show high levels of distress, and this needs to be discussed openly to avoid causing blame or guilt.[73]

Where practical, the procedural steps and what they may feel should be explained to the child in terms that they understand. During the procedure diversional tactics can be beneficial in reducing anxiety and distracting the child from the procedure. Many departments have a range of distraction equipment. Where possible, it may be of some benefit to develop some more-positive reinforcement for cooperation, for example, a sticker, special toy, cuddles from mum or playing their favourite DVD after the procedure. This can often assist with cooperation in patients who may be having this procedure on a regular basis, or for future hospital presentations.[74]

In some instances the child may become very objectionable, uncooperative and physical, in an attempt to gain some control over what is happening to them. This may make the procedure very difficult to perform and physical restraint may be required in order to continue. The restraint should be at the least restrictive level in order to perform the procedure. The child should be given some reassurance that the pain and restraint they are experiencing is not punishment for any wrong-doings. Parents where possible should not be involved in restraint as their presence is as a resource for the child.[73]

Intraosseous access

Intraosseous (IO) access involves the insertion of specifically designed IO devices into the IO space of the bone matrix. The IO space refers to the spongy cancellous bone of the epiphysis and the medullary cavity of the diaphysis. The medullary cavity consists of a vast non-collapsible vascular structure which connects to the central circulation by a series of longitudinal canals which contain an artery and a vein. Volkmann's canals connect the IO vasculature with the major arteries and veins of the central circulation (Fig 17.39).[75,76] IO access provides a safe, rapid and reliable route for administration of drugs, crystalloids, colloids and blood. Medications and fluids administered via the IO route enter the central circulation in comparable concentrations and time as the IV route.[75,77]

IO access is indicated in both children and adults requiring immediate resuscitation and in whom peripheral intravascular access cannot be achieved in a timely or reliable manner.[77] IO access can be achieved quickly and is as fast as IV access. Successful insertions rates have been shown to be high following failed IV attempts.[77] Contraindications include fracture of the bone, previous IO attempts in the same bone, osteoporosis, osteogenesis imperfecta, infection of the overlying insertion site and inability to identify insertion landmarks.[75,77] Complications related to IO access include extravasation, fat

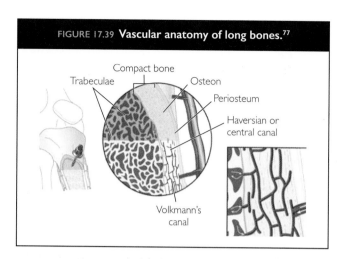

FIGURE 17.39 Vascular anatomy of long bones.[77]

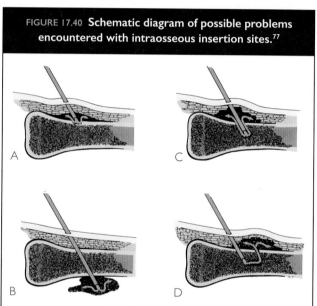

FIGURE 17.40 Schematic diagram of possible problems encountered with intraosseous insertion sites.[77]

A, Incomplete penetration; **B**, Penetration of posterior cortex; **C**, Fluid escaping around needle; **D**, Fluid leaking through nearby cortical puncture.

emboli, osteomyelitis and subcutaneous abscess (Fig 17.40). Epiphyseal damage can occur in children.[78]

PRACTICE TIP

IO access is indicated in both children and adults requiring immediate resuscitation and in whom peripheral intravascular access cannot be achieved in a timely or reliable manner.

Various IO devices are available and generally fall into one of three categories: manual, impact-driven or powered drill devices. Manual devices (see Fig 17.41) consist of hollow steel needles with a removable trocar that prevents plugging of the needle with bone during insertion. Manual devices are inserted using the hand-delivered force of the clinician. Impact-driven devices (Fig 17.42) contain a spring-loaded mechanism designed to penetrate through the bone cortex

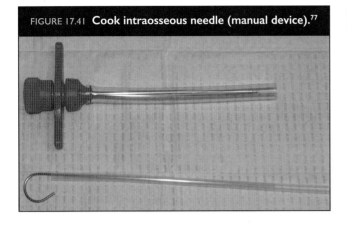

FIGURE 17.41 **Cook intraosseous needle (manual device).**[77]

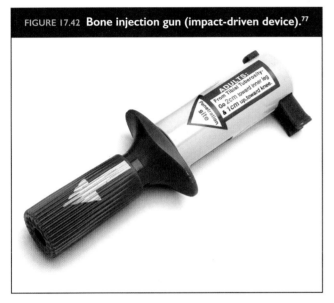

FIGURE 17.42 **Bone injection gun (impact-driven device).**[77]

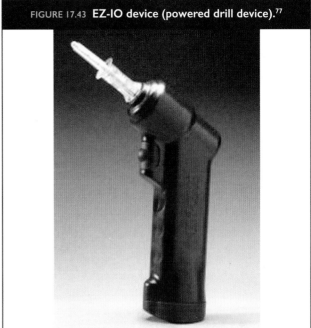

FIGURE 17.43 **EZ-IO device (powered drill device).**[77]

7. Penetrate the bone cortex. A sudden decrease in resistance is felt along with a 'pop' or 'crunch' sensation.

8. Remove the stylet from the IO needle. The IO needle should feel secure and stable in position.

9. Attach a syringe to the IO needle and aspirate bone marrow or blood to confirm correct position. Aspirate may be used for blood typing, cross-matching and blood chemistry testing.[57]

10. Connect a primed extension set to the hub of the IO needle and flush with 10 mL of Normal saline to confirm patency.

11. Secure the extension set to the patient's skin to avoid movement and/or dislodgement of the IO needle. All fluids and medication should be given through the extension set and not directly into the hub of the IO needle as this is likely to cause movement and loss of stability at the insertion site.[79]

12. Dress as appropriate. Avoid covering the insertion site as this may hide evidence of extravasation. Splinting of the limb may also be considered.

Venous cutdown

Vascular access may be obtained surgically when a large volume of fluid is required or when peripheral access cannot be obtained. The procedure is used more often in children than in adults, but has lost favour with increased use of intraosseous needles. Venous cutdown involves surgical isolation of the basilic vein or saphenous vein (Fig 17.45A) followed by insertion of a large-bore catheter, intravenous tubing or feeding tube (5 Fr or 8 Fr), which is sutured in place (Figs 17.45B and C).[80] Disadvantages of this technique include time and skill required to complete the procedure. This implies that cutdown should be resorted to only when percutaneous access has failed or is deemed likely to be unsuccessful.[81]

It is more common, and preferential, to attempt central venous access over venous cutdown.

into the IO space. These devices do not use a drill motion but instead use the force from the spring-loaded mechanism to drive the sharpened IO needle into the IO space. Powered drill devices (Fig 17.43) are battery powered, handheld drills that insert the IO needle into the IO space with a high-speed rotary motion.[76]

Sites commonly used for insertion include proximal tibia, distal tibia and distal femur (Fig 17.44). In infants and children younger than 6 years, the proximal tibia is the preferred site followed by the distal tibia and distal femur. In adults the most common site is the distal tibia.[77] Other sites include the sternum, proximal humerus, calcaneus and clavicle; however, these sites are far less popular, have difficult-to-locate landmarks (humerus) or require specific insertion devices (sternum).[75,77]

Intraosseous device insertion method

1. Gather equipment.
2. Wash hands and don PPE.
3. Locate insertion site.
4. Prepare insertion site—sterile technique.[76]
5. Prepare IO device.
6. Insert IO device in accordance with manufacturer's instructions.

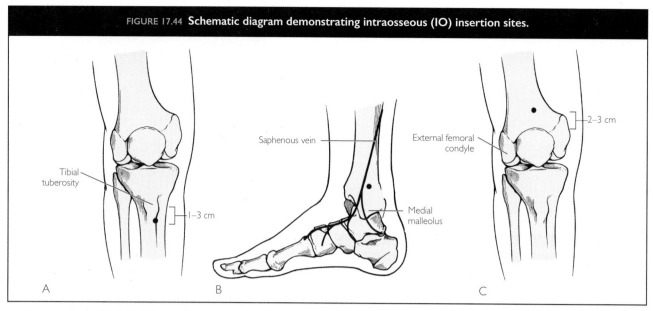

FIGURE 17.44 Schematic diagram demonstrating intraosseous (IO) insertion sites.

Saphenous vein

External femoral
condyle

2–3 cm

Tibial
tuberosity

Medial
malleolus

1–3 cm

A

B

C

A, The proximal tibia. The IO needle is inserted 1–2 cm distal to the tibial tuberosity and over the medial aspect of the tibia. The bevel of the needle is directed away from the joint space. **B,** The distal tibia. The IO needle is inserted on the medial surface of the distal tibia at the junction of the medial malleolus and the shaft of the tibia, posterior to the greater saphenous vein. The needle is directed cephalad, away from the growth plate. **C,** The distal femur. The IO needle is inserted 2–3 cm above the external condyles in the midline and directed cephalad, away from the growth-plate.

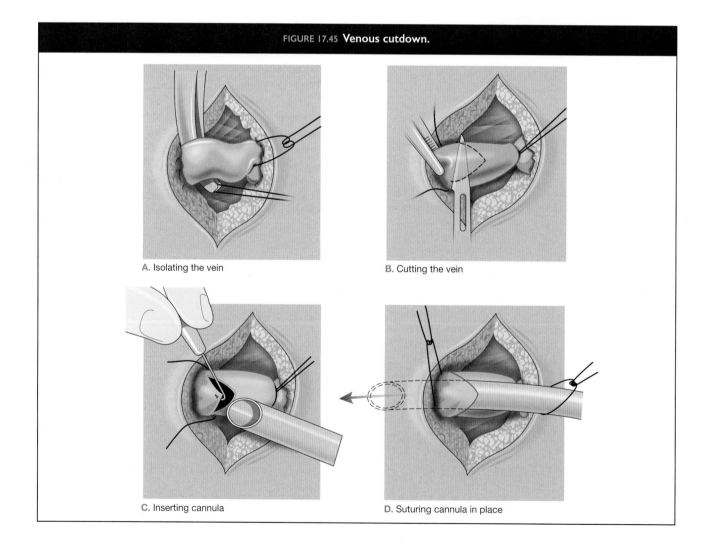

FIGURE 17.45 Venous cutdown.

A. Isolating the vein

B. Cutting the vein

C. Inserting cannula

D. Suturing cannula in place

Haemodynamic monitoring

Haemodynamic monitoring is utilised in critically ill patients to allow prompt recognition and accurate assessment of circulatory characteristics and dynamics. Haemodynamic monitoring involves the placement of invasive catheters into the vascular system for the purpose of either continuous or intermittent measurement of haemodynamic parameters. In the emergency environment these parameters are generally limited to the measurement of arterial blood pressure (ABP) and central venous pressure (CVP).

For nurses caring for patients where haemodynamic monitoring is being utilised, it is important to have an understanding of the underlying physiology of arterial and venous pressure and the relationship of these pressures to the production of the waveforms and values which are monitored at the bedside. This knowledge is important when relating and interpreting these waveforms and values to the nursing care and management of these patients.

Production of visual pressure waveforms

The production of a pressure waveform occurs through the insertion of an intravascular (arterial or venous) catheter which is connected via fluid-filled rigid plastic tubing to a transducer. The fluid-filled system beyond the transducer is pressurised to 300 mmHg. Changes in pressure are transferred through the tubing to the transducer. These changes in pressure are converted to an electrical signal by the transducer. These signals are then amplified and converted by a monitoring device into graphical and numerical displays.

Arterial lines

Indications

The indications for ABP monitoring include:
1. Conditions requiring continuous arterial pressure monitoring. These may include:
   - uncontrolled hypertension
   - hypovolaemia
   - shock of all aetiology
   - patients receiving vasoactive drugs (e.g. adrenaline, dopamine, dobutamine, aramine, sodium nitroprosside).
2. Patients requiring frequent blood samples without venepuncture (e.g. in diabetic ketoacidosis and severe respiratory illnesses).

Sites

The following sites may be used for arterial cannulation and arterial blood pressure monitoring.
- Radial artery—this site is the most common site chosen due to the fact that it is easy to access and the site is easy to maintain and manipulate if required. It is important to perform an Allen's test prior to cannulation of the radial artery (see Fig 17.25).
- Femoral artery—recommended for use in long-term critically ill patients as it is associated with a lower complication rate.
- Axillary artery—again, this site is also recommended for long-term use.
- Brachial artery—not a commonly used site due to concerns regarding lack of effective collateral

circulation and also the close proximity of the median nerve.
- Dorsalis pedis artery—also not commonly used. The anatomy is less predictable and success rates are lower. This site should also be avoided in patients with peripheral vascular disease and diabetes.[82,83]

Equipment

Equipment required for arterial line insertion is given in Box 17.9.

Care of arterial catheter

The care of the arterial catheter and line should include the following:
- The site (e.g. arm) should be immobilised (on an arm board) to prevent movement which may result in catheter displacement.
- Ensure that lines are secured and connections are tight, to avoid haemorrhage from accidental dislodgement.
- **The site and all connections should be always left exposed**. An unexposed disconnected arterial line can result in significant blood loss before being noticed.
- Check distal circulation (colour, warmth, movement and sensation) hourly and report any abnormalities.
- Label the arterial catheter and/or tubing of the arterial line as 'arterial'; labels are generally available in the packaging.
- **Never inject anything into the arterial line**. Anything injected into the line may cause significant effects distal to the site of the catheter.
- Maintain the pressure bag at 300 mmHg. This ensures that a fluid administration rate of 3 mL/h will be maintained and that no blood will flow back into the tubing.
- Zero the transducer at the beginning of each shift or when the patient has been repositioned.

Zeroing

Following insertion and care of the arterial catheter, the arterial line needs to be zeroed in order to ensure accuracy of the recorded values. Zeroing is the process of eliminating the weight of the air or the atmospheric pressure (usually about 760 mmHg) from the pressure measurements. This is achieved by opening the transducer to air and adjusting the display system (monitor) to read zero. This will eliminate all the pressure contributions from the atmosphere and only the pressure values that exist within the vessel being monitored will be displayed.[85] The procedure is:

1. Prime the transducer giving set and insert into a pressure bag.
2. Pump the pressure bag to 300 mmHg.
3. Connect transducer IV line to arterial cannula and secure.
4. Plug pressure cable into monitor.
5. Connect pressure cable from monitor to transducer set.
6. Adjust transducer to the height of the phlebostatic axis. The phlebostatic axis is found at the intersection of a vertical line from the fourth intercostal space and midway between the anterior and posterior surfaces of the patient's chest, in the supine position. This position correlates to the level of the patient's right atrium.[86]
7. Switch the transducer 'off' to the patient (open to sampling port) by turning the three-way stopcock.
8. Remove the cap from the sampling port, opening the transducer to the atmosphere.
9. Press 'Zero' on the monitoring device.

Blood sampling—arterial lines

Blood sampling from an arterial line is performed to obtain blood samples for ABG analysis and other pathology testing. Blood sampling from the arterial line may be required frequently, for example in unstable patients who require frequent ABGs.

The procedure for blood sampling from an arterial line[87,88] is given below.

1. Assemble equipment:
   - clean (non-sterile) gloves
   - goggles/face shield
   - syringe for discarding
   - sampling syringe
   - sterile bung/cap for the access/sampling port
   - sterile gauze.
2. Silence alarm on monitor.
3. Explain procedure to patient.
4. Remove the cap from the sampling port and attach spare syringe.
5. Turn the three-way stopcock off to the transducer and open to the sampling port.
6. Allow sufficient 'dead-space' fluid to enter the syringe until undiluted blood reaches the syringe.
7. Turn the three-way stopcock off to the patient (open to the transducer).
8. Remove the syringe and discard.
9. Attach the sampling syringe.
10. Turn the three-way stopcock off to the transducer and open to the sampling port.
11. Collect sample volume required by allowing blood to flow into the syringe; assist aspiration gently if required.
12. Turn the three-way stopcock off to the patient (open to the transducer).
13. Remove sampling syringe.
14. Flush the sampling port into sterile gauze to remove blood from port.
15. Place a new sterile cap on the sampling port.
16. Turn the three-way stopcock off to the sampling port.
17. Use the fast-flush device to clear the line of blood.
18. Reactivate alarms and ensure arterial waveform is present.
19. Prepare and send collected samples.
20. Discard used supplies.
21. Wash hands.

Some haemodynamic monitoring line systems contain a reservoir into which fluid from between the catheter and the sampling port can be moved, allowing undiluted blood to be accessible without having to discard a sample prior to collection of the true sample. The reservoir is then emptied at the completion of the sample collection to flush the line of blood.

Central venous catheters

Central venous access plays an important role in the management of critically ill patients, as it affords staff the ability to draw blood samples, instil high doses of multiple medications while simultaneously measuring pressures within the vascular system. Central venous access is commonly used in traumatically injured patients for the restoration of blood volume, and in septic patients who require inotropic support and multiple antibiotics to stabilise circulation. In patients with vascular compromise or circulatory collapse, central venous access may be the only way to access the venous system.

Indications

The indications for insertion of a central venous catheter (CVC) include:

- administration of drugs and fluid
- administration of total parenteral nutrition (TPN)
- insertion of a temporary cardiac pacing wire
- to monitor CVP in order to:
  - assist in the estimation of a patient's hydration status as a guide to fluid replacement
  - assess the extent of heart failure (right-sided).

Sites

Commonly the following sites are chosen for CVC insertion:

- internal jugular
- subclavian vein
- femoral vein
- brachial vein. The brachial vein is usually used for peripherally inserted central catheters (PICCs).

The advantages and disadvantages of these sites are outlined in Table 17.4.

Equipment

The equipment commonly used for CVC insertion is outlined in Box 17.10. The nurse needs to be familiar with the equipment required and the main steps in CVC insertion in order to be able to assist with preparation and insertion. Insertion of CVCs

TABLE 17.4 Advantages and disadvantages of commonly used CVC insertion sites[89,90]

SITE	ADVANTAGES	DISADVANTAGES
Internal jugular	Large vessel	Uncomfortable for patient
	Easy to locate, good external landmarks	Hard to maintain dressing
	Easy access	Close proximity to carotid artery
	Short, straight path to vena cava (right side)	High infection rate
	Low rate of complications	Problematic in patients with tracheostomies
Subclavian	Large vessel with high flow rate	Lies close to lung apex (pneumothorax risk)
	Lowest infection rates	Close proximity to subclavian artery
	Easy to dress and maintain	Difficult to control bleeding (non-compressible site)
	Supra to infraclavicular approaches	
	Less restrictive for patient	
Femoral	Easy access, good external landmarks	Decreased patient mobility
	Large vessel	Increased rate of thrombosis and phlebitis
	Advantageous during resuscitation	High rates of infection
		Risk of femoral artery puncture
		Dressing may be problematic
Brachial	Easy access	Large incidence of phlebitis
	Advantageous during resuscitation	Longer time for drugs to access central circulation
		Catheter tip movement related to arm movement

BOX 17.10 Equipment commonly used for CVC insertion[91]

- CVC—single/triple lumen/size
- Procedure tray
- Moisture-proof underpad
- Personal protective equipment
- Sterile gown/gloves
- Sterile drapes
- Antiseptic solution
- 2 mL, 10 mL syringes
- 10–20 mL Normal saline for injection
- 25, 23 and 19 gauge needles
- 1% lignocaine
- Gauze
- Scalpel—11 or 12 gauge
- 2/0 silk suture—straight needle
- Transparent occlusive dressing (sterile)
- Additional equipment may be required based upon local policy/procedures

and PICCs by specialised registered nurses is also becoming increasingly common throughout Australasia.

Insertion

The most common insertion method for CVCs is the use of the Seldinger (guidewire) technique. This technique is performed under sterile conditions and involves the insertion of a small needle into the intended vessel, through which a guidewire is passed into the lumen of the vessel. The needle is then withdrawn, leaving the guidewire within the vessel. The insertion site is often enlarged with a scalpel and a dilator is used over the guidewire to widen the intended path of the catheter. The dilator is then removed and the catheter inserted into the vessel over the guidewire. The guidewire is then removed and the catheter secured in place with a suture, and a transparent dressing is applied. Although this approach has several steps, once mastered the procedure can be performed quickly.[89]

Following insertion involving puncture of the neck or thorax, a chest X-ray (CXR) should be obtained. The X-ray is assessed to identify any complications associated with insertion, such as haemothorax or pneumothorax, and to confirm the correct position of the catheter tip. Where possible the CXR should be performed in the upright or semi-upright position as small amounts of air or blood within the intrapleural space may not be seen in the supine patient. The catheter tip should sit in the lower third of the superior vena cava outside the right atrium[86] (Fig 17.46). Correct position of the catheter tip should be confirmed prior to the commencement of any infusions. A post-procedure CXR is not indicated for CVCs inserted into the femoral vein because, due to the distance away from the heart, there is less risk of misplacement.

Central venous pressure measurement

There are two methods of measuring CVP: these include the water manometer method and more commonly the use of a

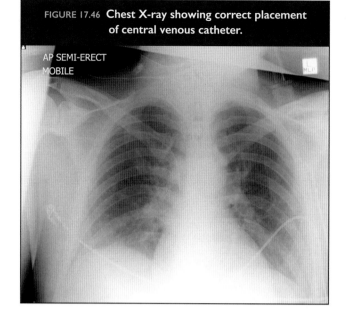

FIGURE 17.46 **Chest X-ray showing correct placement of central venous catheter.**

AP SEMI-ERECT
MOBILE

haemodynamic monitoring system. With either system the measurement is taken at the level of the phlebostatic axis. Once the phlebostatic axis point has been determined, a small ink mark may be made on the patient's skin for future reference. It is important that all measurements are taken from the same location to ensure accuracy.

The water manometer measures CVP in centimetres of water (cmH₂O), while haemodynamic monitoring records the CVP in millimetres of mercury (mmHg). This makes it more difficult to compare readings from one system against the other, although conversion formulae are available if required. The water manometer readings are performed intermittently while the haemodynamic monitoring records the CVP continuously, improving its accuracy over the water manometer method.[86,92]

Water manometer method

Box 17.11 shows the recommended procedure for CVP measurement using a water thermometer.

Haemodynamic monitoring method

Box 17.12 shows the recommended procedure for CVP measurement using a haemodynamic monitor.

Soft tissue injuries

Soft tissue injures are a common reason that patients will seek help.

An assessment of the affected area should include: noting the colour of the skin and surrounding tissue, feeling the warmth of the area, assessing range of motion and strength and testing for sensation. A measure of the pulses in the affected area should also be included in the assessment of soft tissue injuries. It is important to consider the mechanism of injury and potential underlying structures involved.

RICE principle for soft-tissue injury management

Simple, cheap and non-invasive measures of the rest, ice, compression and elevation (RICE) principle can improve the patient's outcome by improving vascular flow.

BOX 17.11 Procedure for central venous pressure (CVP) measurement—water manometer[92,93]

1. Explain the procedure to the patient.
2. Locate the phlebostatic axis.
3. Position the patient in the supine position (preferred) or semi-recumbent position.
4. Ensure all intravenous fusions running through the manometer line are stopped.
5. Zero the manometer by placing the zero of the water manometer at the level of the phlebostatic axis. To ensure the level is accurate, a spirit or laser level should be used.
6. Close the three-way stopcock off to the patient and allow the manometer to fill with fluid to a level beyond the expected pressure.
7. Close the three-way stopcock off to the fluid supply and open to the patient.
8. Observe the column of water in the manometer. It should fall until gravity pressure equals the CVP. The water level will fluctuate gently with the patient's respiratory cycle.
9. Record the CVP measurement at end expiration.
10. Turn the three-way stopcock open to the flush system and the patient (off to the manometer) and re-establish the IV fluid infusion.

BOX 17.12 Procedure for central venous pressure (CVP) measurement—haemodynamic monitor[86,93]

1. Explain procedure to patient.
2. Locate the phlebostatic axis.
3. Position patient in the supine or semi-recumbent position.
4. Adjust the height of the transducer to the level of the phlebostatic axis using a spirit or laser level.
5. Zero the transducer to atmospheric pressure (as described in the text).
6. Ensure all IV fusions running through the same access port are switched off.
7. Flush the device to ensure good flow within the system and that the catheter is not obstructed.
8. Observe the waveform on the monitor to ensure that the key features are visible.
9. Record CVP measurement.
10. Recommence any infusions that were stopped.

Rest

Resting a sprain or strained limb by not weight-bearing and by using crutches will allow strained ligaments time to heal.

Ice

Cold therapy should be initiated from the time of injury and aggressively for the first 48 hours.[94] It decreases blood flow by causing vasoconstriction and increasing blood viscosity. By slowing tissue metabolism, oxygen consumption is reduced.

Ice decreases inflammation and swelling and can cause some local anaesthetic effects.[26] Ice packs or bags of ice wrapped in a towel should be applied for 20 minutes, with 20 minutes between applications. Ice should not be applied directly to the skin because it can cause frostbite by freezing the surface of the skin.[95] For cost-effective ice therapy, patients can purchase a bag of party ice and separate out the required amounts. If using reusable cold packs, these will need to be continually rotated as they warm up. Disposable cold packs are activated when squeezed but cannot be used again.

Compression

Compression bandaging helps to reduce swelling; swelling causes pain. The application of a tubular compression bandage until pain improves and swelling subsides reduces compression on nerve endings and improves venous return.

Elevation

Elevating the affected limb helps to reduce swelling and improves venous return. The limb needs to be elevated above the level of the heart for the first 24 hours. Elevation methods include placing injured feet on pillows, resting injured hands in elevated hanging slings or wearing broad arm slings following splint application.

> **PRACTICE TIPS**
>
> - Ice should be applied from the time of the injury—on for 20 minutes, off for 20 minutes—for the first 48 hours.
> - Applying a compression bandage and elevating the limb on pillows reduces swelling that causes pain.

Bandaging

Bandages are strips of gauze, crepe or elastic material used to cover wounds, compress swollen limbs and hold dressings in place.[26] It is important to select the correct type, size and method of bandaging as each provides different levels of compression, immobilisation and support.

Figure of eight bandage

The figure of eight bandage is used to provide support to joints and may be used in combination with RICE. The figure of eight bandage encircles below the joint and crosses over to immobilise above the joint like a figure 8. The bandage ascends obliquely in a circular motion in a figure-8 fashion, overlapping, until immobilisation is achieved.[26] To fit:

1. Begin by ensuring that the skin is clean and dry and any wounds are covered.
2. Start by wrapping twice around the limb to stabilise the bandage.[26]
3. Wrap a single layer distally and cross up like a figure 8 over the joint proximally.
4. Continue to wrap proximally and then cross back down over the joint distally, like a figure 8.
5. Continue the figure-8 wrap until immobilisation is attained.
6. Ensure there are no wrinkles or creases which could cause tissue injury.

7. Secure the end of the bandage well with tape.
8. Apply an elasticised tubular compression bandage and RICE over the figure-8 for additional compression and pain relief.

> **PRACTICE TIP**
>
> Use a figure of eight dressing in combination with RICE and elasticised tubular compression bandage on ankle injuries to provide immobilisation, compression and pain relief.

Elasticised tubular compression bandages

Elasticised tubular compression bandages such as the Tubigrip brand are strands of cotton-covered elastic and are used to provide support and reduce swelling. The bandage will provide compression but does not immobilise the limb. Acute ankle sprains and strains are a common ED orthopaedic presentation that can be effectively treated with elastic compression bandages.[96] Scarring from burns can be controlled with the use of tubular compression bandaging in the weeks after injury.[42] Patients can wash and reuse Tubigrip without it losing its effectiveness. Elastic compression bandages can be worn for 2–3 days. To apply:

1. Begin by ensuring the skin is clean and dry and any wounds are covered.
2. Cut the elasticated tubular bandage to twice the length of the patient's limb.
3. Pull the bandage onto the limb like a sock and then double it over by pulling the second layer up.
4. Ensure the bottom layer is 2–3 cm higher on the limb than the top layer.
5. Ensure there are no wrinkles or creases which can cause tissue injury.

> **PRACTICE TIPS**
>
> - Use elasticised tubular compression bandages (e.g. Tubigrip) to provide compression in combination with RICE where immobilisation of the injury is not required, such as soft-tissue ankle injuries.
> - Patients can wash and reuse tubular compression bandages.

Spica bandage

The finished spica bandage resembles a spike of wheat with overlapping V-like layers, providing compression, support or retention of wound dressings. The term 'spica cast' is sometimes used to describe a plaster cast that involves the limb and the trunk of the body.

Procedure:

1. Begin by ensuring that the skin is clean and dry and any wounds are covered.
2. Start by wrapping twice around the limb, above the joint, to stabilise the bandage.[81]
3. Wrap the first layer down distally across the joint and around, bringing it back up to the beginning point.

4. Repeat the layers overlapping two-thirds ascending and descending until the final bandaging represents a series of V-like shapes down the limb.

5. Ensure there are no wrinkles or creases which can cause tissue injury.

6. Secure the end of the bandage well with tape.

7. Check for distal pulse to ensure adequate blood flow.

Robert-Jones bandage

A Robert-Jones bandage is a heavy multilayered application consisting of alternate layers of bandage and padding or wadding. The purpose of the Robert-Jones bandage is to immobilise and support.

Procedure:

1. Begin by ensuring that the skin is clean and dry and any wounds are covered.

2. Wrap from distal to proximal with an overlapping layer of wadding or soft, absorbent orthopaedic padding (e.g. Velband).

3. Ensure there are no wrinkles or creases which can cause tissue injury.

4. Wrap an alternate layer of wide elastic compression or crepe bandage firmly enough to allow distal blood flow. Select a bandage that is at least 15 cm wide.

5. Repeat with alternate layers of orthopaedic padding and bandaging for up to six layers in total, with the final layer being bandage.

6. Secure the end of the final bandage well with tape.

7. Check for distal pulse to ensure adequate blood flow.

Pressure-immobilisation or compression bandage

A compression bandage is an elasticised, stretchable bandage that applies pressure to prevent or relieve swelling. Compression or pressure-immobilisation bandaging (PIB) is commonly used to prevent limb swelling, but can be used pre-hospital for the management of envenomation. The PIB compresses the lymphatic vessels and inhibits limb muscle movement, thus retarding venom transport and slowing venom entering the systemic circulation.[97] To be effective, a PIB should have a final pressure of 50–75 mmHg.[98] Crepe bandages are less effective than elasticised bandages in maintaining this pressure.

Procedure:

1. Ensure that the skin is clean and dry and any wounds are covered.

2. In cases of suspected envenomation the bite area can be circled with pen for later reference; do not wash the area to allow easier venom identification.

3. Begin by wrapping at the point of injury down the limb, overlapping the bandage one-third each time. Select an elastic bandage that is at least 15 cm wide.

4. Wrap to the end of the limb, including fingers or toes, and then continue proximally until the entire limb is covered.

5. Use firm pressure to occlude lymphatic flow but preserve blood flow. Check for distal pulse to ensure adequate blood flow.

6. Ensure there are no wrinkles or creases which can cause tissue injury.

7. Secure the end of the bandage well with tape.

8. Splint the limb to further restrict movement.

PRACTICE TIPS

- Compression bandaging is an effective first-aid measure in snake bite and where reduction of swelling is desired.
- Compression or pressure-immobilisation bandaging (PBI) can be used in combination with splinting to achieve limb immobilisation.
- A correctly fitted PBI for use in snakebite requires between 50 and 70 mmHg pressure. To determine how tightly to fit a bandage, apply a blood pressure cuff to your own arm and inflate it to this pressure.

Tourniquet

A tourniquet is a tight cuff, bandage or purpose-made device to control haemorrhage in the pre-hospital or early resuscitation stage of trauma. The use of a tourniquet can prevent exsanguinating haemorrhage that accounts for half of the deaths in the first 24 hours of trauma.[99] In the field the control of life-threatening haemorrhage may even become a priority over the management of airway and breathing assessments, particularly in combat situations[100] as uncontrolled haemorrhage is a leading cause of battlefield death.[101]

A cuff tourniquet is applied using a sphygmomanometer cuff inflated to 250 mmHg or 300 mmHg or 70–100 mmHg above the systolic pressure, to stop venous and arterial bleeding without crushing underlying tissues (Fig 17.47).

Direct damage to underlying vessels and nerves and limb ischaemia remain the risks of tourniquet application. Limiting the time a tourniquet is on for and avoiding excessive pressures will reduce the risks.

Tourniquets can be used on fingers, arms and legs for haemorrhage control and facilitating a bloodless field for wound care. Because of the risk of nerve and vessel injury, tourniquet use should be limited to 1 hour[103] and conversion to PIB should be considered.[102] There is no evidence that tourniquet use plays a role in the treatment of envenomation.[104]

Correct bandaging can effectively immobilise injuries and reduce pain. It is important to select the correct type of bandage, as each has different properties. It is also important to select the correct method of bandaging to suit the injury, as each provides different levels of compression and immobilisation.

Casts

Plaster of Paris (POP) is still widely used as a splint. Casts are used for three main reasons: to relieve pain, to stabilise a fracture and to immobilise a fracture to promote healing.[105,106]

Analgesia is essential in the reduction of fractures and the application of a POP cast. Reduction of fractures should only be performed by a trained clinician. A regional block provides good anaesthesia to the limb and can be used safely in the ED.[106]

FIGURE 17.47 **Haemorrhage control A-D, Haemorrhage control: use of tourniquets.**[102]

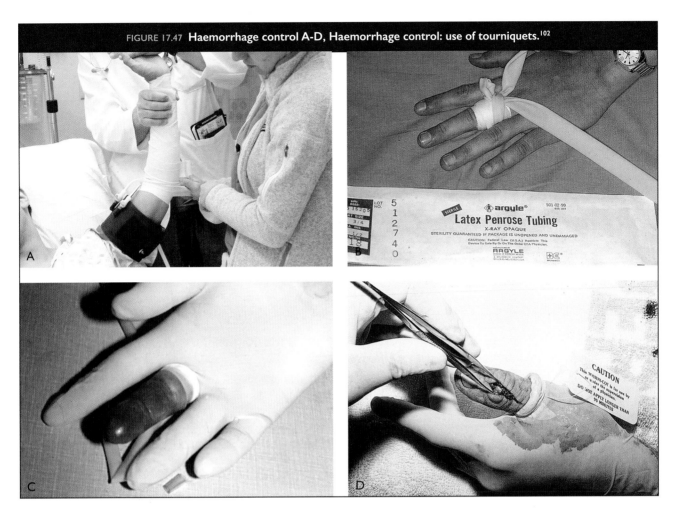

When applying POP, first apply wadding from the distal end to the proximal end of the limb, ensuring that padding extends beyond the planned margins of the cast. To prepare the POP roll, water must be added, which causes a chemical reaction that releases heat. Patients should be warned that they might feel heat on application. Place the plaster roll in a bowl of water (the colder the water, the longer the plaster takes to set). Squeeze out excess water by squeezing the ends together. The POP bandage should be rolled in the same direction as the wadding, overlapping at each turn. Each roll should be smoothed by the palms. The strength of the cast relies on the overlapping and linking together of each individual layer.[106]

Complications are commonly caused by tight or ill-fitting casts. When casts are applied too tightly, neurovascular compromise can occur, producing symptoms such as pins and needles, numbness and changes in skin colour. Swelling should be anticipated in all acute fractures and therefore these should always be managed in a POP backslab/half-cast, during the acute phase. The exception to this rule is any fracture that has been closed-reduced. Such fracture reductions may require two backslabs or a full POP cast to support the reduction in the initial phase. These can be reinforced during the subacute phase to improve strength of the cast for the long term, but should not be removed and changed to a full cast as the reduction will be lost.

Pressure sores can develop from ill-fitting casts; common sites for increased pressure include bony prominences such as the patella, elbow, head of the ulna and the heel. Padding all bony prominences prior to POP application may prevent these pressure sores. Once swelling has subsided the patient may complain that the cast is too loose; in these cases the cast should be replaced.[105,106]

Advanced practice emergency nurses and extended care paramedics should be able to apply backslabs and full casts after education and assessment. The emergency nurse or paramedic must explain to the patient the purpose of the cast, the margins of the cast, the process and equipment used and the need to maintain correct alignment of specific joints during application. Neurovascular observations are essential for at least the first 4 hours after POP application. The clinician must educate the patient regarding warning signs and cast care. The patient should be made aware that the POP cast is not waterproof and they should be alerted to symptoms of increased pain and swelling, and changes in skin colour and sensation; they should be instructed to seek medical attention immediately as this may indicate ischaemia. Some full POP casts take 24–48 hours to dry completely. The patient should not bear weight on the cast until it is completely dry.[107,108]

The application of a cast may seem a minor procedure; however, if the cast is ill-fitting, the fracture is not aligned or the assessment and care is inadequate, the patient may suffer significant complications, such as lifelong deformity or even amputation of the extremity.[109]

Splinting

Splinting plays an important role in combination with bandaging to ensure effective limb immobilisation. Early splinting and limb immobilisation can reduce pain and minimise the risk of further injury from bony fragments in fracture or neurovascular injury in sprain. Splinting is important in controlling blood loss and facilitates healing.[26] The basic splints include soft splints, hard splints, inflatable air splints and traction splints.[110]

> **PRACTICE TIPS**
>
> - Pad all splints, particularly over the site of injury.
> - Immobilise the joints above and below the injury.
> - Gentle traction can be applied while fitting a splint.
> - Assess neurovascular status before and after splinting.

Splints for minor injuries

Finger splint

A finger splint is used to immobilise carpal and metacarpal injuries. A simple field finger splint can be made using tongue depressors and tape. Commercial finger splints, such as the Zimmer finger splint, are usually made from padded aluminium that can be conformed to the required shape.

To fit an aluminium finger splint

1. Begin by ensuring that the skin is clean and dry and any wounds are covered.
2. Use a finger on the uninjured hand to measure and mould the splint to the desired shape and size.
3. Slide the splint in place on the injured finger.
4. Secure the splint in place with tape.
5. Check for capillary refill to ensure adequate blood flow.
6. Apply RICE to the hand.

Knee immobiliser

A knee immobiliser (Fig 17.48) or Zimmer knee splint is a three-panelled soft splint with fibreglass or aluminium inserts.

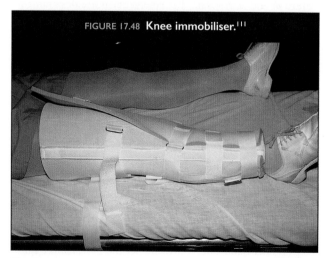

FIGURE 17.48 **Knee immobiliser.**[111]

Can be worn over clothes and be easily removed and applied by the patient.

They are used in mild to moderate knee injuries that don't require complete knee immobilisation, such as ligament or soft-tissue injuries.[111]

To fit a knee immobiliser

1. Begin by ensuring that the skin is clean and dry and any wounds are covered.
2. Check for distal pulse to ensure adequate blood flow.
3. Administer adequate analgesia where possible.
4. Select the correct size of immobiliser by laying it next to the leg. The proximal end should be just below the buttocks crease and the tapered distal end should be just above the ankle.
5. Place the splint behind the leg. Align the splint so that when closed, the patella sits within the patella opening.
6. Adjust the two side panels so that when they are closed on the leg, they touch the midline.
7. Close the Velcro straps from bottom to top.
8. Check for distal pulse to ensure adequate blood flow.

Splints for major injuries/trauma

Femoral traction splint

Femoral traction splints apply traction to the femur to reduce blood loss and relieve pain.[95] The splints are generally divided into two categories: ring splints, which include Donway, Hare (Fig 17.49) and Thomas; and non-ring splints, which include Sager, Kendrick Traction Device, CT-6 and the Slishman splint.

Fitting a Hare traction femoral splint

1. Begin by ensuring that the skin is clean and dry and any wounds are covered.
2. Check for distal pulse to ensure adequate blood flow.
3. Administer adequate analgesia where possible.
4. Place the ischial pad against the iliac crest.
5. Adjust the splint so that the bend is in line with the heel, and tighten the locking collars.
6. Fit the proximal ring on the splint to the ischial tuberosity on the affected leg. This will apply counter-traction.
7. Apply the pubic strap over the groin and high on the femur.
8. Apply the ankle strap. This will apply longitudinal traction.
9. Apply traction using the ratchet until the legs are approximately the same length.
10. Check for distal pulse to ensure adequate blood flow.

> **PRACTICE TIP**
>
> The disadvantage of the Hare traction splint is that it is bulky, and makes transport of the patient difficult as it extends past the foot. The Hare traction splint can only provide unilateral leg traction and different-sized splints are required for paediatric and adult patients.

FIGURE 17.49

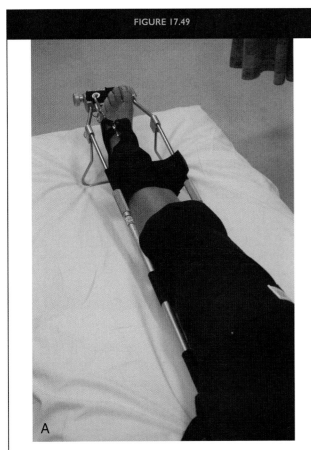

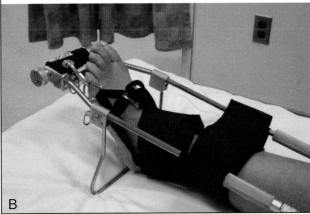

A, Hare traction splint. **B**, Commercial hitch designed to protect the ankle and heel during traction.[95]

Fitting a Donway femoral splint

1. Begin by ensuring that the skin is clean and dry and any wounds are covered.
2. Check for distal pulse to ensure adequate blood flow.
3. Administer adequate analgesia where possible.
4. Fit the ischial ring by sliding it under the top of the leg and tightening.
5. Unlock the side arms of the splint.
6. Fit the metal frame over the leg so that the foot rests on the footplate, and lock the side arms of the splint.
7. Fit and tighten the ankle and foot straps.
8. Apply traction by using the hand pump to apply pneumatic pressure of 10 lb (4.5 kg) and tighten the side arms.
9. Secure the leg straps.
10. With the side arms locked in position and traction applied, release the pneumatic pressure by depressing the air-release valve.

> **PRACTICE TIP**
>
> The Donway femoral splint provides pneumatic traction and no lifting of the limb is required. The disadvantage is that different-sized splints are required for adult and paediatric patients. The splint is cumbersome, requires a hand pump to function and can only provide unilateral traction.

Fitting a Sager femoral splint

The Sager splint allows simultaneous bilateral leg traction from a single splint.

1. Begin by ensuring that the skin is clean and dry and any wounds are covered.
2. Check for distal pulse to ensure adequate blood flow.
3. Administer adequate analgesia where possible.
4. Position the ischial perineal cushion against the ischial tuberosity between the patient's legs on the side of the injury.
5. Apply the proximal thigh strap.
6. Apply the ankle harness above the ankle and below the heel.
7. Apply traction using the traction handle. The manufacturer recommends 10% of the patient's body weight up to a maximum of 7 kg for each leg. In the case of bilateral fracture, a maximum of 14 kg of traction would be applied. There is a scale on the traction handle.
8. Check for distal pulse to ensure adequate blood flow.

> **PRACTICE TIP**
>
> The advantage of the Sager splint is that a single splint can provide bilateral leg traction. It comes as a single piece with no assembly required, has a numbered gradient for applying the correct amount of traction and doesn't extend past the foot. The disadvantage is that different-sized splints are required for adult and paediatric patients.

Fitting a FareTec CT-6 femoral splint (Fig 17.50)[95,112]

1. Begin by ensuring that the skin is clean and dry and any wounds are covered.
2. Check for distal pulse to ensure adequate blood flow.
3. Administer adequate analgesia where possible.
4. Lay the unfurled splint alongside the injured leg and fit the ischeal strap.
5. Apply the ankle hitch.
6. Apply tension by pulling the cord and lock it into the V-lock.

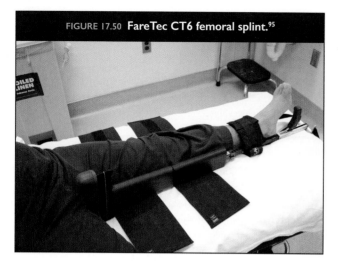

FIGURE 17.50 **FareTec CT6 femoral splint.**[95]

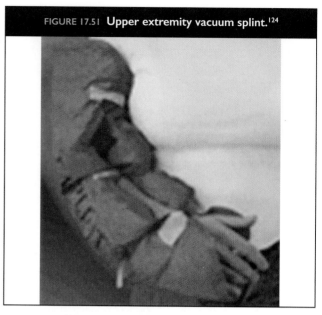

FIGURE 17.51 **Upper extremity vacuum splint.**[124]

7. Fit the leg straps.
8. Apply further tension until the patient is comfortable.
9. Check for distal pulse to ensure adequate blood flow.

Fitting a Kendrick Traction Device

1. Begin by ensuring that the skin is clean and dry and any wounds are covered.
2. Check for distal pulse to ensure adequate blood flow.
3. Administer adequate analgesia where possible.
4. Apply the ankle strap and tighten the stirrup.
5. Apply the upper thigh strap and fasten the buckle.
6. Place the traction pole alongside the injured leg so that it extends 20 cm past the bottom of the foot.
7. Apply traction. The manufacturer recommends 10% of the patient's body weight up to a maximum of 7 kg.
8. Fit the remaining leg straps.
9. Check for distal pulse to ensure adequate blood flow.

Fitting a Slishman splint

1. Begin by ensuring that the skin is clean and dry and any wounds are covered.
2. Check for distal pulse to ensure adequate blood flow.
3. Administer adequate analgesia where possible.
4. Apply the ankle strap.
5. Apply the groin strap.
6. Lock in the coarse adjustment with tension on the leg.
7. Apply traction by pulling the cord and locking it in place.
8. Check for distal pulse to ensure adequate blood flow.

PRACTICE TIP

The advantage of folding leg traction devices is that a single size of splint can be used for both adult and paediatric patients. They are more compact and lightweight than other femoral traction splints, folding into a small bag and weighing less than 0.5 kg. They are also advantageous in the transportation of patients, as they are much smaller than ring splints. The disadvantage of folding traction devices is that they can only provide single-leg traction and some assembly is required before using them.

Vacuum splints

Vacuum splints such as the Evac U Splint can be used to splint all limb fractures. They are applied to the affected limb and air is evacuated so the splint conforms around the fracture (Fig 17.51). Whole-body vacuum splint mattresses are used to immobilise and transport patients with suspected spinal injuries.

Vacuum splints have the advantage of being able to conform to the exact shape of the wearer. They are much more bulky than other types of splint, require a pump to evacuate air and there may be changes in the conformity in altitude retrieval, requiring adjustment. Vacuum splints are available in multiple sizes and they do not apply any traction to fractures.

Fitting an Evac U Splint

1. Begin by ensuring that the skin is clean and dry and any wounds are covered.
2. Check for distal pulse to ensure adequate blood flow.
3. Administer adequate analgesia where possible.
4. Slide the splint into place.
5. Conform the splint and hold it in place.
6. Attach the hand pump and evacuate the air from the splint.
7. Secure any straps.
8. Check for distal pulse to ensure adequate blood flow.

Pelvic splint

The purpose of a pelvic splint is to reduce the pelvic volume, which in turn reduces potential space for bleeding that may aid in the formation of blood clots. Aligning fracture surfaces may reduce bleeding from bones. Attention is then given to stabilisation of the pelvis by initially using a sheet or a commercially available pelvic binder such as a SAM Pelvic Sling II or T-POD splint.

Fitting a SAM pelvic sling (Fig 17.52)

1. Begin by ensuring that the skin is clean and dry and any wounds are covered.
2. Administer adequate analgesia where possible.

FIGURE 17.52 **Application of the SAM pelvic sling.**[124]

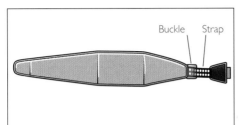

1. Remove objects from patient's pocket or pelvic area. Unfold SAM Pelvic Sling with non printed side facing up. *Keep strap attached to buckle.*

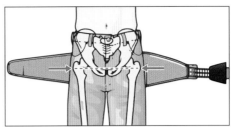

2. Place non-printed side of SAM Pelvic Sling beneath patient at level of buttocks (greater trochanters).
CORRECT PLACEMENT. The correct level of application is at the greater trochanters.

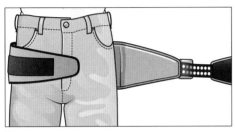

3. Wrap non-buckle side of SAM Pelvic Sling around patient.

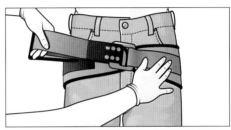

4. FIRMLY WRAP buckle side of sling around patient, positioning buckle in midline. Secure by pressing flap to sling.

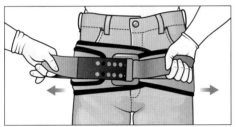

5. Lift the BLACK STRAP away from Sling by pulling upwards.

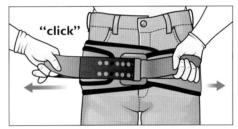

6. With or without assistance firmly pull orange and black straps in opposite directions until you hear and feel the buckle click.
MAINTAIN TENSION!

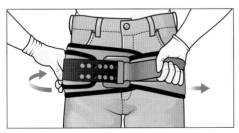

7. IMMEDIATELY press black strap on to surface of SAM Pelvic Sling to secure.
Note: do not be concerned if you hear a second 'click' after sling is secured.

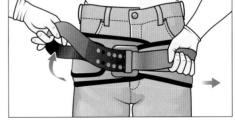

8. To remove lift black strap by pulling upwards. Maintain tension and slowly allow SAM Pelvic Sling to loosen.

3. Slide the sling posteriorly or lay it on the bed before transferring the patient onto it.

4. Position the SAM sling with the midline of the sling at the greater trochanters.

5. Wrap and buckle the sling around the pelvis.

6. Apply tension equally in both directions until a click is heard.

7. Secure the straps.

Fitting a Trauma Pelvic Orthotic Device T-POD pelvic splint

1. Begin by ensuring that the skin is clean and dry and any wounds are covered.
2. Administer adequate analgesia where possible.
3. Slide the splint posteriorly or lay it on the bed before transferring the patient onto it.
4. Position the T-POD splint with the midline of the splint at the greater trochanters.
5. Cut the belt to allow a 15 cm gap between the ends at the front.
6. Apply the Velcro pulley system to the front.
7. Pull the tab to apply tension equally in both directions on the pulley system.
8. Maintain a 15 cm gap between the two ends of the strap and ensure that two fingers can be fitted under the splint when tension is applied.
9. Secure the pull tab.
10. The T-POD device is wide and does not allow complete access for laparotomy or angiography. Different devices are required for adults and children, although two devices can be combined for obese patients. The manufacturer suggests that the device provides stabilisation equivalent to a surgical stabilisation.

Rigid limb splint

The purpose of a fixed or rigid splint is to prevent the movement of fractured bones which can cause bleeding and pain. Rigid splints can be made from a variety of materials, including cardboard, aluminium or wood; some come pre-padded. (See Figs 17.53, 17.54.)

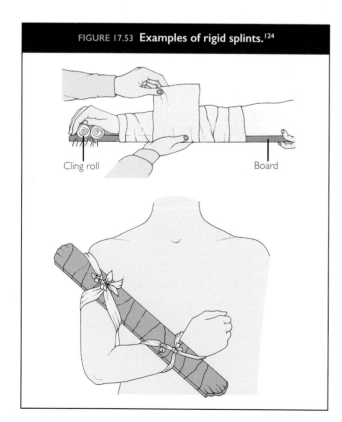

FIGURE 17.53 **Examples of rigid splints.**[124]

Cling roll   Board

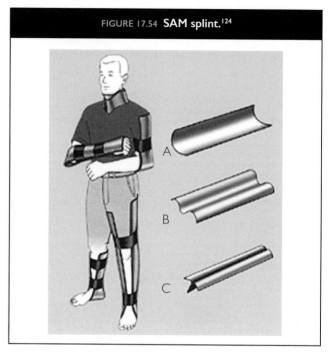

FIGURE 17.54 **SAM splint.**[124]

Bent into any of three simple curves (**A**, **B** and **C** in the figure), the SAM splint provides support for any fractured or injured extremity.

To fit:

1. Begin by ensuring that the skin is clean and dry and any wounds are covered.
2. Check for distal pulse to ensure adequate blood flow.
3. Administer adequate analgesia where possible.
4. Apply gentle traction to deformed and neurovascularly compromised limbs.
5. Apply the rigid splint with additional padding where required.
6. Fix the splint with bandages or tape.
7. Check for distal pulse to ensure adequate blood flow.

Crutches and walking sticks

Crutches are used to aid walking where there is a lower limb injury, to prevent weightbearing on the injured leg or to aid in mobility; however, note that patients should be admitted for further gait retraining if they are unable to use them safely or are at risk of falling. The most common type of crutch used in emergency injury is the underarm or axilla crutch.

Underarm crutches

Underarm crutches are the most common type of crutches. They sit under the axilla and are also called axillary crutches.[109] The appropriate height of axillary crutches can be measured with the patient lying supine in bed or standing. To fit (instructions given for standing):

1. Stand the patient straight.
2. Place the base of the crutch 15 cm to the side of and 15 cm in front of the foot. This will allow room for the hips to swing through.
3. There should be 2–3 fingers width, or about 5 cm, between the top of the crutch and the armpit.

4. The hand piece should be at wrist height allowing the elbow to bend at 30°. This is called the tripod position and provides the most stability.

The patient should be provided with information about how to ambulate using the crutches (Fig 17.55).

The patient should have a pair of well-fitting, flat shoes to prevent slipping. The patient should be instructed not to bear weight through the axilla, as this may cause axillary nerve palsy; they should instead use their hands to support their bodyweight. There should be clear instructions in the medical records from the orthopaedic surgeon regarding weightbearing status prior to mobilisation, such as non-weightbearing (NWB), partial weightbearing (PWB), touch weightbearing (TWB) or full weightbearing/weightbear as tolerated (FWB/WBAT).

The usual gait that is taught to patients who are NWB is the swing-through gait; this involves moving the crutches forwards and swinging the legs past the crutches, before regaining balance and continuing forwards. For weight-bearing patients, use the step-to or swing-to gait, as it is steadier: step up to the crutches with injured leg, putting weight through the hands, and step up to the crutches with the uninjured leg.

Patients should be taught how to go up and down stairs (Fig 17.56).

When mobilising down stairs, the patient should place the crutches down onto the lower step, followed by the uninjured limb and then the injured limb. This ensures that the patient's stronger limb is used to lower bodyweight onto the lower step and enables the crutches to support the injured limb.

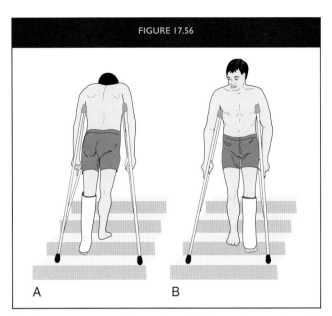

A, Going up stairs with crutches. **B,** Going down stairs with crutches.

When mobilising up stairs, the patient places the uninjured limb onto the upper step, pushes through the crutches to raise the injured limb up onto the same step, followed by the crutches.

The patient should always have a 'support' person with them in the initial stages when going up and down stairs.

Forearm crutches

Forearm crutches are used to prevent compressive radial neuropathy caused by excessive underarm pressure rarely caused by axillary crutches. They have a forearm and hand piece but provide less support and require a greater level of skill to use.[113] They are more commonly used in patients requiring long term crutches or where partial weightbearing is allowed. To fit:

1. Stand the patient straight.
2. Fit the forearm piece 2.5 cm below the elbow crease. The forearm piece should be firm-fitting enough to prevent the crutch from falling when the wearer opens a door.
3. The hand piece should be at wrist height allowing the elbow to bend at 30°.
4. The patient should be provided with information about how to ambulate using the crutches.

Walking sticks

A walking stick is used to assist with balance where weightbearing on the affected leg is still possible. To fit:

1. Stand the patient straight.
2. Place the base of the walking stick next to the heel.

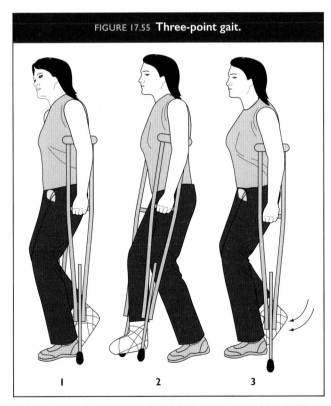

FIGURE 17.55 **Three-point gait.**

1, Standing with crutches, all weight is on the good leg. **2,** Move crutches and injured leg forward simultaneously. **3,** Bearing weight on the palms of the hands, step forward onto the good leg.

3. The hand piece of the walking stick should be at wrist height allowing the elbow to bend at 30°.
4. A walking stick should be used on the side opposite to the injury. The patient is provided with information about how to ambulate using a walking stick.

Regional anaesthesia and nerve blocks

Regional anaesthesia and regional nerve blocks are simple, convenient and provide effective pain relief for patients in the ED.

Regional nerve blocks may prove superior to local anaesthetic infiltration or systemic delivery of analgesia in providing pain relief in specific scenarios in the ED. Emergency clinicians should be aware of the indications for using regional nerve blocks. Advanced practice emergency clinicians may be able to perform these procedures after appropriate education and assessment. Scenarios in which regional nerve blocks may be appropriate include:

- reduction of pain to digits during procedures, e.g. reduction of dislocations or fractures, repair of wounds
- procedures such as wound repair or foreign body removal in areas where local infiltration is particularly painful, such as the plantar surface of the foot or the palm of the hand
- for manipulation/reduction of fractures, e.g. a Colles fracture
- to reduce the need for systemic analgesia and improve pain relief in the elderly with a fractured femur.

Nerve block in hip fracture

A particular consideration is analgesia in hip fracture and the elderly. Pain management for this vulnerable group of patients is particularly challenging.[114] Multiple co-morbidities, polypharmacy and altered pharmacokinetics can limit the range of suitable analgesics. Furthermore, anecdotal evidence from emergency clinicians suggests that time in cannulating, performing frequent observation of blood pressure, drawing-up and administering (in the presence of two nurses) aliquots of intravenous (IV) opioids is a boundary to treatment. An alarming overseas study[115] showed some patients with hip fracture were receiving no analgesia.

A proportion of elderly hip fracture patients have cognitive impairment from dementia. Some may suffer acute confusion from comorbidities, their injury or as a result of admission into hospital. This cognitive impairment may prevent them from asking for, or accepting, analgesia.[116]

Older patients often have preconceived ideas about the addictive properties of opioids. Staff may also have misconceptions regarding pain perception and ageing. Together this can contribute to inadequate prescribing or administration of pain relief in the elderly.[117]

A number of studies support the use of femoral nerve block in emergency departments, for effective pain relief following hip fractures.[118,119]

Femoral nerve block can provide rapid and effective analgesia for most patients, with a reduction in opioid consumption when compared with controls.[120–122] The result is faster, longer lasting pain relief without the associated side effects of opioids. Undesirable opioid side effects can include sedation and respiratory depression. The 2011 NICE Clinical

Guideline on Management of Hip Fracture suggests 'Consider adding nerve blocks if paracetamol and opioids do not provide sufficient preoperative pain relief, or to limit opioid dosage'.[123]

> **PRACTICE TIP**
>
> Femoral nerve block provides rapid and effective pain relief for patients with hip fractures. A nerve block should be considered in all hip fracture patients

Anatomy of the fascia iliaca block[53]

The iliacus muscle is a large, flat, triangular muscle that lines and fills the ilium. It originates from all along the upper portions of the ilium and iliac crest, sacrum and iliolumbar ligaments. The iliacus muscle joins with the lateral side of the psoas major muscle. Together they are referred to as the iliopsoas. The iliopsoas exits the pelvis from beneath the inguinal ligament, wraps around the proximal neck and inserts into the lesser trochanter, acting as a powerful hip flexor.

The fascial covering of the iliopsoas is thin superiorly, becoming significantly thicker as it reaches the level of the inguinal ligament. This thickness provides a great deal of resistance and a large 'pop' as a needle tip is passed through the fascia.

The lumbar plexus is made up of the nerve roots from the T12 through L5 vertebrae. The largest branch of the lumbar plexus is the femoral nerve, arising from the L2, L3 and L4 roots. The femoral nerve descends through the fibres of the psoas major and exits at the lower portion of the psoas's lateral border, passing downwards between the psoas and iliacus muscle, deep to the iliacus fascia. The femoral nerve exits the pelvis into the upper thigh, lateral to the common femoral artery and vein.

The lateral femoral cutaneous nerve is a purely sensory nerve arising from the L2 and L3 nerve roots that provides sensation from the iliac crest down the lateral portion of the thigh to the area of the lateral femoral condyle. The lateral femoral cutaneous nerve emerges from the lumbar plexus and travels downwards lateral to the psoas muscle and crosses the iliacus muscle deep to the iliacus fascia.

The anterior and posterior obturator nerves innervate a portion of the distal, medial thigh. They arise from the L2, L3 and L4 nerve roots and cross the iliacus muscle, deep to the fascia, to the medial thigh. The obturator nerves are sometimes involved in the FICB, but probably plays little role in postoperative pain relief for most surgeries of the hip and proximal femur.

Complications

All complications identified during the procedure should be discussed with the patient and their family, discussed with the treating clinicians and documented in the patient record.

Potential complications include inadvertent intravascular injection, haematoma and nerve injury. Complications relating to the local anaesthetic include hypotension and toxicity. Motor block of the affected limb is common.

Block failure

There is a potential that the nerve block with be only partially successful or unsuccessful in relieving pain.

Infection

There is a risk of infection with all invasive procedures that can be reduced with good hand-washing, skin-cleaning and a sterile technique for needle insertion.

Accidental vascular puncture and haematoma formation

An accidental vascular (venous or arterial) puncture can result in haematoma formation. A blunt-ended brachial plexus needle set reduces the risk of accidental vascular puncture. A blunt-ended or short bevelled needle pushes fibres away. Needles such as the B Braun Brachial Plexus Plexufix 45° short bevel needle are used to avoid nerve injury and accidental vascular puncture.

Anaphylaxis

Anaphylaxis remains an unavoidable complication of any medication administration. Airway management, oxygenation, ventilation and good basic life support are the necessity of successful resuscitation.

Local anaesthetic systemic toxicity (LAST)

LAST remains an unavoidable complication of regional anaesthesia administration. LAST can result from intravascular injection, absorption from a tissue depot, accumulation of active metabolites, or a combination of these. Attentiveness during the procedure and timely intervention at the earliest signs of toxicity are most important for successful treatment.

The classic description of LAST includes a series of progressively worsening neurological symptoms and signs occurring shortly after the injection of local anaesthetic and mirroring a progressive increases in blood local anaesthetic concentration, climaxing in seizures and coma. In severe cases of LAST, hypotension, bradycardia, confusion, dizziness, agitation, loss of consciousness, followed by seizure, ventricular dysrhythmia or asystole, can occur. Systemic toxic reactions occur in only 0.1% to 0.4% of local anaesthetic administrations. Vagal reactions, anxiety and sensitivity to preservatives have also been incorrectly attributed to LAST.[124]

LAST is usually very rapid, following a single injection by 50 seconds or less, and occurring before 5 minutes in 75% of cases. Peak blood levels are usually within 30 minutes.[124] Rapid onset of symptoms after a single local anaesthetic injection suggests that most systemic toxic reactions are as a result of inadvertent intravascular injection.

Patients with liver disease may not be able to adequately metabolise local anaesthetics such as bupivacaine for excretion, increasing the risk for toxic plasma concentrations. Additionally, patients with cardiovascular disease may not be able to compensate for the functional changes associated with the prolongation of atrioventricular conduction induced by amide-type local anaesthetics.

Adverse reactions to bupivacaine are rare in the absence of overdosage, exceptionally rapid absorption or inadvertent intravascular injection.

PRACTICE TIP

The rapid injection of a large volume of local anaesthetic solution should be avoided. Always calculate a weight-based dose and consider comorbidities that might lead to systemic toxicity.

MIMS Online[125] states:

> Tolerability varies widely between patients and toxic effects may occur after any local anaesthetic procedure. Careful observation of the patient must therefore be maintained. It is recommended that the dose of bupivacaine (Marcain), an anaesthetic used for FICB, at any time should not exceed 2 mg/kg (both plain and adrenaline containing solutions). However, the dose administered must be tailored to the individual patient and procedure.

Injection of repeated doses of bupivacaine may cause significant increase in blood levels with each repeated dose, due to accumulation of the drug or its metabolites, or due to slow metabolic degradation.

The rapid injection of a large volume of local anaesthetic solution should be avoided and fractional doses should be used when feasible. For most indications the duration of Marcain is such that a single dose is sufficient.

Airway management, oxygenation, ventilation and good basic life support are the necessity of successful resuscitation. Seizure suppression is important. Lipid infusion should be considered early, and most EDs have the capability to perform rapid lipid infusion. Literature suggests 'Vigilance, preparedness, and quick action will improve outcomes of this dreaded complication'.[126]

Procedure for femoral nerve block

1. Review the X-ray to confirm hip fracture after discussion with the treating clinicians.
2. Consult the relevant medical officer before nerve block to ensure that:
   - a nerve block is required
   - alternatives have been considered
   - the benefits outweigh the risks.
3. Check for allergies to any of the cleaning solutions or anaesthetics used.
4. Identify any transmission-based precautions such as multi-resistant organisms (MRO), so that appropriate precautions can be taken.
5. Identify comorbidities that may pose a problem with the procedure or the anaesthetic, including partial or complete heart block, advanced liver disease or severe renal dysfunction.
6. Discuss the procedure with the patient and their family/carers, outlining the steps involved, the benefits and the potential complications and risks. Treatment and care, and the information patients are given about it, should be culturally appropriate. It should also be accessible to people with additional needs such as physical, sensory or learning disabilities, and to people who do not speak or read English; use an interpreter if required.
7. Obtain verbal consent from the patient or their family/carers.
   Absolute contraindications to the procedure include:
   - infection or haematoma in the vicinity of the puncture site
   - refusal of the procedure by the patient.
8. View the baseline observations.
9. Estimate the patient's weight for drug dose calculation. Calculate the drug dose and volume required. Estimation

of weight is required if the patient is unable to provide a recent accurate weight, remembering the patient will not be able to sit or stand to be weighed.

10. Bupivacaine (Marcaine/Marcain) without adrenaline is the anaesthetic of choice. Dose is calculated dependent on the patient's weight, but generally 20–30 mL is used in 70 kg adults. The lowest effective dose must be used.

    Bupivacaine preparations come as: 0.125%, 0.25% with or without adrenaline, 0.375% and 0.5% with or without adrenaline.

    Debilitated or elderly patients, including those with partial or complete heart block, advanced liver disease or severe renal dysfunction, should be given a reduced dosage commensurate with their physical condition and according to their estimated weight.

11. Collect and open onto a dressing tray all equipment required (Box 17.13).

12. Expose the site without unnecessarily exposing the patient. The patient lies on his or her back with legs spread slightly apart. Clean the skin with neutral soap and water if the insertion site is visibly dirty. Infection in the vicinity of the puncture site is a contraindication to the procedure.

13. Perform hand hygiene as set out in the Hand Hygiene Policy and identify the landmarks by palpating the anterior superior iliac crest and pubic tubercle. Feel for the femoral artery.

14. Mark the site/side of injury with an arrow denoting the affected hip.

15. Clinicians should wear protective eyewear when performing the procedure due to the low risk of a splash injury occurring.

16. **No touch technique**

    Touching the insertion site, the shaft or tip of the needle or other sterile equipment breaches aseptic technique. To follow aseptic technique, clinicians should avoid touching:
    - the insertion site after decontamination
    - sterile parts of the brachial plexus set
    - other sterile equipment.

17. Perform hand hygiene (see Ch 27). Put on sterile gloves.

18. Draw up the calculated dose of bupivacaine with the drawing-up needle and attach the brachial plexus set.

19. Decontaminate the skin using a single-use swab. Apply antiseptic to cover an area of approximately 5 × 5 cm in a side-to-side or up-and-down motion with light friction. Repeat with a second swab and allow the skin to air-dry (do not wipe, fan or blot dry the area) for at least 1 minute.

    Alcohol-based chlorhexidine gluconate swabs (>0.5% chlorhexidine in >70% isopropyl alcohol) should be used.

    For patients with a history of chlorhexidine sensitivity/allergy, use:
    - 5% alcohol-based povidone-iodine swab
    - ≥70% alcohol
    - 10% aqueous povidone-iodine (suitable for patients in whom alcohol is contraindicated).

    Do not use antimicrobial creams/ointment at the insertion site.

    If the site or equipment is contaminated at any stage during the procedure discard it and start again.

20. Identify the landmarks of the anterior superior iliac crest and pubic tubercle. The foot of the leg to be anaesthetised should be turned loosely to the outside, although it may already be rotated due to fracture (Fig 17.57).

21. The puncture site is located approximately in the region of the inguinal fold, 1.5 cm lateral of the femoral artery, approximately 2–3 cm below the inguinal ligament (IVAN = inner vein artery nerve) (Fig 17.58).

22. Palpate the femoral artery. Insert the needle at 30 degrees to the skin and advance in a cranial direction. After reaching a depth of around 2–4 cm, the femoral nerve is encountered. Progress the needle downwards.

23. Feel for the 'pop' as the needle passes through the fascia lata and then again as the needle passes into the fascia iliaca.

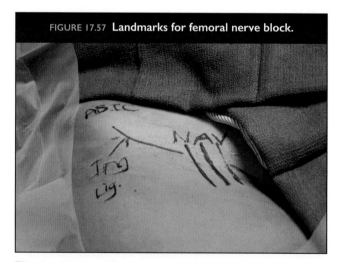

FIGURE 17.57 **Landmarks for femoral nerve block.**

The drawing identifies the anterior superior iliac spine (ASIC), the inguinal ligament ('Ing lig'), and the approximate locations of the femoral nerve (N), femoral artery (A) and femoral vein (V). A good way to remember the relationships is 'NAVEL': going towards the navel, i.e., Nerve, Artery, Vein, Empty, Lymphatics, going from lateral to medial (towards the navel).[143]

BOX 17.13 **Equipment commonly used for Femoral Nerve Block insertion**

- Bupivacaine (Marcain) 0.5% without adrenaline
- 20 mL syringe
- Drawing-up needle
- Blunt-ended brachial plexus needle set
- Alcohol-based chlorhexidine gluconate swabs (>0.5% chlorhexidine in >70% isopropyl alcohol) × 2
- Sterile gloves

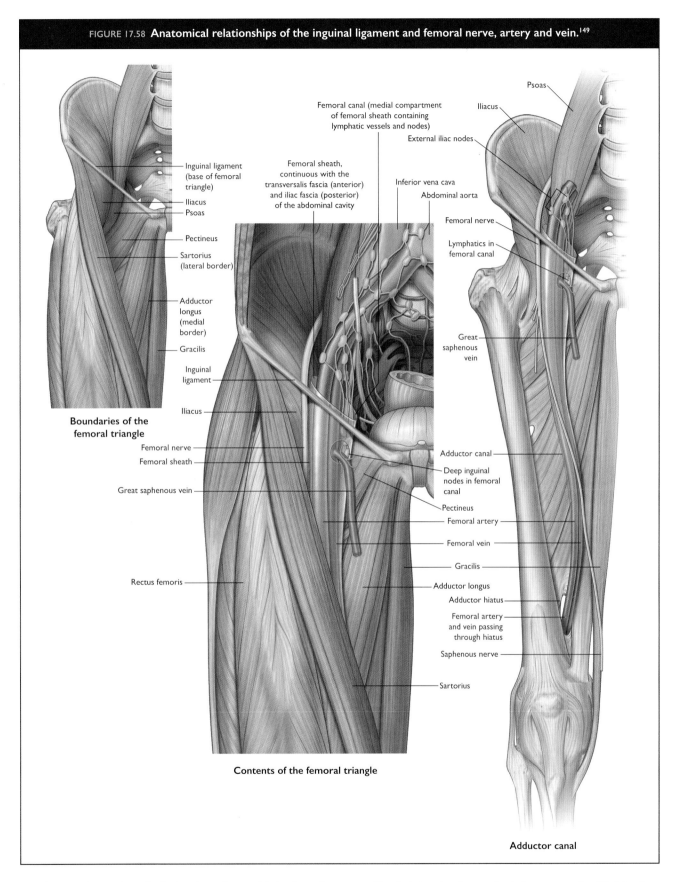

FIGURE 17.58 Anatomical relationships of the inguinal ligament and femoral nerve, artery and vein.[149]

Inguinal ligament (base of femoral triangle)

Iliacus

Psoas

Pectineus

Sartorius (lateral border)

Adductor longus (medial border)

Gracilis

Boundaries of the femoral triangle

Femoral canal (medial compartment of femoral sheath containing lymphatic vessels and nodes)

Femoral sheath, continuous with the transversalis fascia (anterior) and iliac fascia (posterior) of the abdominal cavity

Inferior vena cava

Abdominal aorta

Psoas

Iliacus

External iliac nodes

Femoral nerve

Lymphatics in femoral canal

Great saphenous vein

Inguinal ligament

Iliacus

Femoral nerve

Femoral sheath

Great saphenous vein

Rectus femoris

Adductor canal

Deep inguinal nodes in femoral canal

Pectineus

Femoral artery

Femoral vein

Gracilis

Adductor longus

Adductor hiatus

Femoral artery and vein passing through hiatus

Saphenous nerve

Sartorius

Contents of the femoral triangle

Adductor canal

24. Aspirate intermittently during insertion and injection of anaesthetic to reduce the risk of inadvertent arterial or venous infiltration (Fig 17.59).

25. Slowly inject local anaesthetic incrementally, 10–15 mL after needle placement. Advance the needle into the space created by the volume, and inject the remainder of the

FIGURE 17.59 Needle insertion.[144]

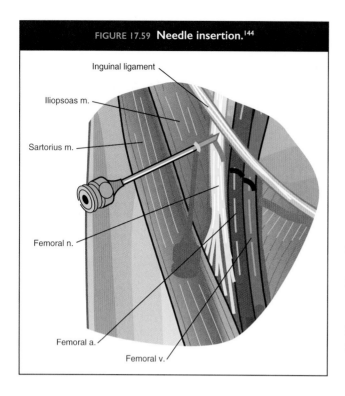

Labels: Inguinal ligament; Iliopsoas m.; Sartorius m.; Femoral n.; Femoral a.; Femoral v.

anaesthetic slowly. Do not continue to inject if excessive resistance is felt (Fig 17.60).

26. Aspirate intermittently during insertion and injection of anaesthetic to reduce the risk of inadvertent arterial or venous infiltration.

27. Remove the needle and dispose of all sharps.

28. Placing pressure over the injection site for 10 seconds after completing the injection may speed up the onset of the block by spreading the local solution with external pressure. This is also a common way of trying to enhance the block's effect. Place pressure below the puncture site to prevent the local anaesthetic from flowing in the distal direction and to promote its dissemination in the cranial direction.

29. Dispose of all sharps. Dispose of all contaminated waste. Cover the patient. Remove gloves and wash hands.

30. Evaluate the occurrence of complete loss of pinprick sensation in the femoral nerve distribution; a sign of nerve block effectiveness.

31. Record a pain score 1 hour after the procedure.

32. Watch for signs of complications. Adverse reactions to bupivacaine are rare in the absence of overdosage, exceptionally rapid absorption or inadvertent intravascular injection.

33. Document the procedure in the clinical record. Record or sign all local anaesthetic doses on the medication chart.

FIGURE 17.60 The femoral nerve/'three-in-one' block.[127]

Anatomy

Labels: Psoas muscle; Lateral femoral cutaneous nerve; Femoral nerve; Obturator nerve; L2; L3; L4; L5

A

The lumbar plexus lies in the psoas compartment between the psoas major and quadratus lumborum muscles. The femoral nerve is formed from the posterior branches of L2–L4 and is the largest branch of the lumbar plexus. The lateral femoral cutaneous and obturator nerves arise from L2–L3 and L2–L4, respectively.

Technique

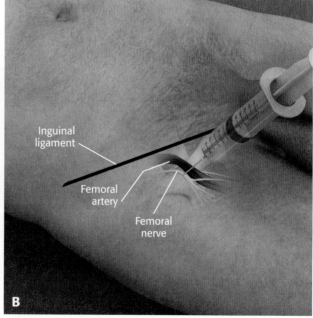

Labels: Inguinal ligament; Femoral artery; Femoral nerve

B

Palpate the femoral artery 2 cm distal to the inguinal ligament. Inject a wheal of lignocaine 1 to 2 cm lateral to this point. Advance the needle at a 45° to 60° angle to the skin until (1) a 'pop' and sudden loss of resistance are felt, (2) paraesthesia is elicited, or (3) the needle pulsates laterally. Inject 25 to 30 mL of anaesthetic. If proximity to the nerve is uncertain, inject in a fanlike distribution lateral to the femoral artery.

CASE STUDY 1

Mrs Lily is a 91-year-old woman who presents at 0800 hours following a trip and fall. She has an extensive medical history that includes ischaemic heart disease, dementia, osteoporosis and falls.

She has pain to the left hip with shortening of the leg and outward rotation of the foot. Her toes are cool with a 3-second capillary return. She has impaired motor function due to severe pain. She looks unsettled and is agitated in bed.

An X-ray reveals a fracture of the left neck of the femur.

Questions

1. Describe the initial assessment of Mrs Lily.
2. What are the options for management of the patient's pain?
3. What are the advantages and disadvantages of using intravenous opioids for pain relief?
4. What are the advantages and disadvantages of using regional anaesthesia for pain relief?

 Answers to Case Study Questions can be found on evolve http://evolve.emergencytrauma.curtis

Digital nerve block

Indications for using a digital nerve block include reduction of dislocations or fractures of phalanges, repair of injuries to nailbeds and nails, assessment and repair of wounds including lacerations, burns and amputations and drainage of infections.[127]

Each finger is supplied by two sets of nerves—the dorsal and palmar digital nerves—and these run in a 2, 4, 8 and 10 o'clock position around the digit (Fig 17.61). There are a variety of approaches to blocking these nerves, the most common being the dorsal proximal-most aspect of the finger or toe (Fig 17.62).[128] An aseptic injection technique is used and the skin is prepped with alcohol preparation. The equipment required is minimal: alcohol wipes, examination gloves, local anaesthetic of choice, 5 mL syringe, drawing-up needle, 25 g needle. The onset and duration of anaesthesia to the digit is dependent on the choice of anaesthetic (see Table 17.5).[129]

> **PRACTICE TIP**
>
> The clinicians involved in administration of regional nerve blocks must ensure a neurovascular assessment of the digit or limb has been performed prior to administration and regularly post administration.

Haematoma block for the reduction of distal radius fractures

A haematoma block is used to anaesthetise the wrist and manipulate deformed distal radius fractures (such as Colles' fracture) in emergency. Haematoma blocks are a safe method of obtaining analgesia without increased post-procedural infections when compared to other regional blocks.[130]

They are equally effective as conscious intravenous sedation in terms of both quality of fracture reduction and pain control before, during and after the procedure, but without the prolonged recovery time.

There is some evidence that haematoma blocks provide slightly inferior anaesthesia and reductions when compared to intravenous regional anaesthesia such as Bier block, though they are quicker, easier and less resource intensive.[130] Adequate pain control will assist with adequate fracture reduction (Box 17.14).[131]

> **PRACTICE TIP**
>
> The rapid injection of a large volume of local anaesthetic solution should be avoided. Always calculate a weight-based dose and consider comorbidities that might lead to systemic toxicity.

Procedure for haematoma block for the reduction of distal radius fractures

1. Review the X-ray to confirm the wrist fracture after discussion with the treating clinicians.
2. Consult the relevant medical officer before haematoma block to ensure that:
   - a haematoma block is required to reduce the fracture
   - alternatives have been considered
   - the benefits outweigh the risks.
3. Check for allergies to any of the cleaning solutions or anaesthetics used.
4. Identify any transmission-based precautions such as MRO so that appropriate precautions can be taken.
5. Identify comorbidities that may pose a problem with the procedure or the anaesthetic, including partial or complete heart block, advanced liver disease or severe renal dysfunction.
6. Ensure all rings have been removed from the affected limb.
7. Discuss the procedure with the patient and their family/carers, outlining the steps involved, the benefits and the potential complications and risks. Treatment and care, and the information patients are given about it, should be culturally appropriate. It should also be accessible to people with additional needs such as physical, sensory or learning disabilities, and to people who do not speak or read English: use an interpreter if required.
8. Obtain verbal consent from the patient or their family/carers.
9. Absolute contraindications to the procedure include:
   - infection in the vicinity of the puncture site
   - refusal of the procedure by the patient

FIGURE 17.61 **Confirmation of needle location within the fracture haematoma site can be obtained by drawing back on the syringe plunger and aspiring haematoma.**[127]

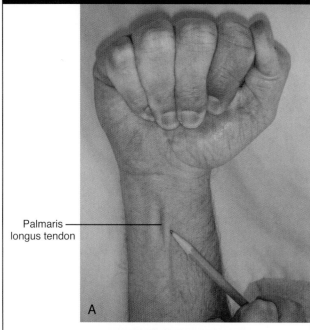

Palmaris
longus tendon

A

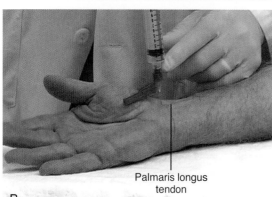

Palmaris longus
tendon

B

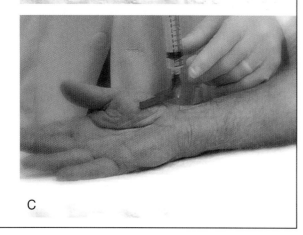

C

10. View the baseline observations.

11. Estimate the patient's weight for drug-dose calculation. Calculate the drug dose and volume required. Estimation of weight is required if the patient is unable to provide a recent accurate weight, remembering the patient may not be able to sit or stand to be weighed if there are comorbidities.

12. Bupivacaine (Marcaine/Marcain) without adrenaline is the anaesthetic of choice. Dose is calculated dependent on the patient's weight, but generally 10 mL is used. The lowest effective dose must be used.

13. Bupivacaine preparations come as: 0.125%, 0.25% with or without adrenaline, 0.375% and 0.5% with or without adrenaline.

14. Debilitated or elderly patients, including those with partial or complete heart block, advanced liver disease or severe renal dysfunction, should be given a reduced dosage commensurate with their physical condition.

15. Collect and open onto a dressing tray all equipment required (Box 17.15).

16. Set up a plaster trolley with all equipment required for a plaster of Paris (POP) backslab (Box 17.16).

17. Expose the arm without unnecessarily exposing the patient. Clean the skin with neutral soap and water if the insertion site is visibly dirty.

18. Perform hand hygiene as set out in the Hand Hygiene Policy.

19. Identify the landmarks by palpating the landmark of the dorsal aspect of the deformity.

20. Mark the site/side of injury with an arrow denoting the affected wrist.

21. Perform hand hygiene as set out in the Hand Hygiene Policy (see Ch 27). Clinicians should wear protective eyewear when performing the procedure due to the low risk of a splash injury occurring.

22. **No touch technique**

Touching the insertion site, the shaft or tip of the needle or other sterile equipment breaches aseptic technique. To follow aseptic technique, clinicians should avoid touching:
- the insertion site after decontamination
- sterile parts of the needle
- other sterile equipment.

23. Put on sterile gloves.

24. Draw up the calculated dose of bupivacaine with the drawing-up needle and attach the 22 g needle.

25. Decontaminate the skin using a single-use swab.

26. Apply antiseptic to cover the area of injection in a side-to-side or up-and-down motion with light friction. Repeat with a second swab and allow the skin to air-dry (do not wipe, fan or blot dry the area) for at least 1 minute.

Alcohol-based chlorhexidine gluconate swabs (>0.5% chlorhexidine in >70% isopropyl alcohol) should be used.

For patients with a history of chlorhexidine sensitivity/allergy, use:
- 5% alcohol-based povidone-iodine swab
- ≥70% alcohol
- 10% aqueous povidone-iodine (suitable for patients in whom alcohol is contraindicated).

Do not use antimicrobial creams/ointment at the insertion site.

If the site or equipment is contaminated at any stage during the procedure discard it and start again.

FIGURE 17.62 **Anatomy of digital nerves. Schematic cross-section of the phalanx demonstrating the relationship of the nerves to the bone.**[127]

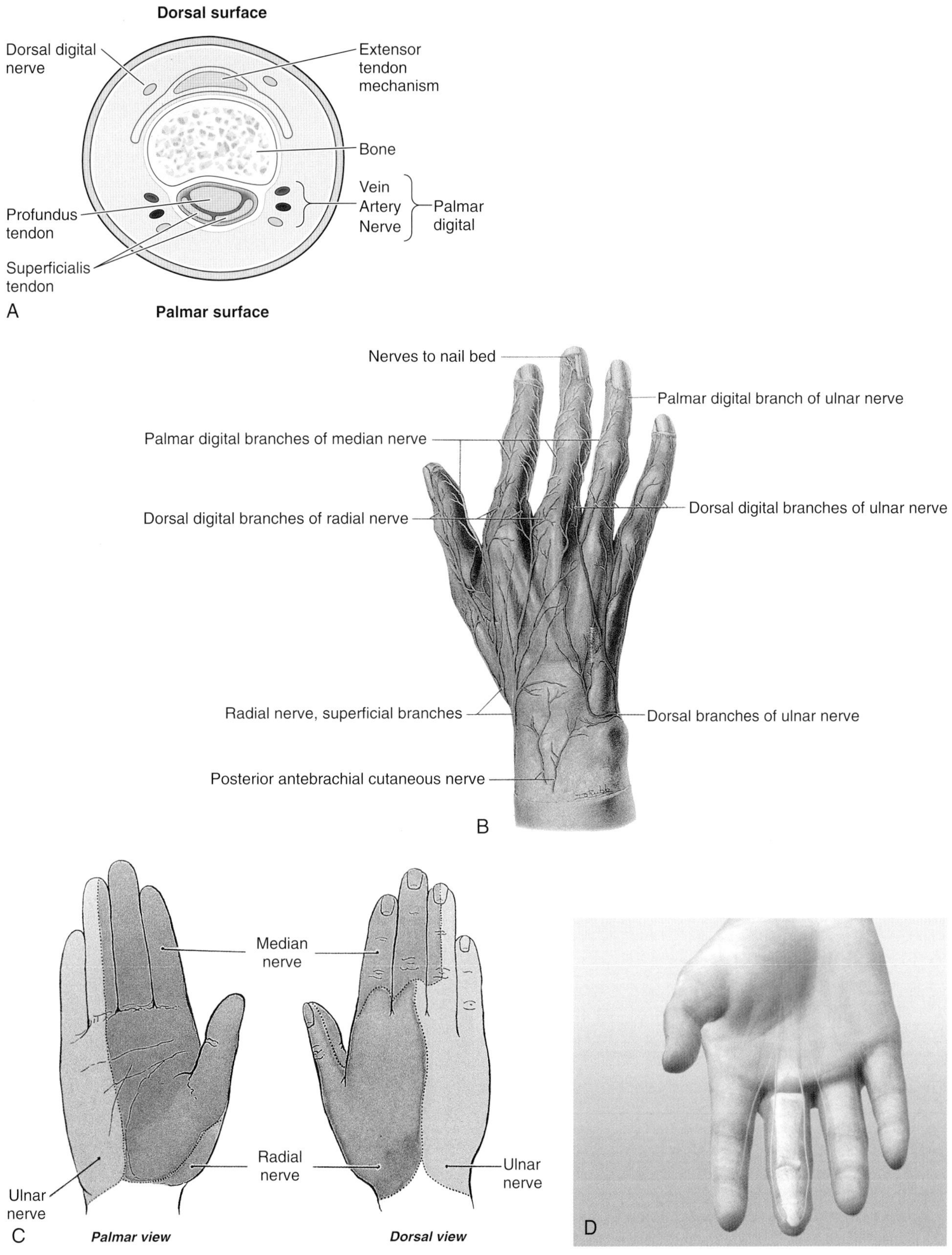

Note that each finger has four digital nerves and that the digital artery and vein run parallel to and near the palmar branches.

TABLE 17.5 Comparison of local anaesthetics[129]

DRUG	MAXIMUM DOSE[1]		AVERAGE ONSET OF ACTION (MINUTES)		AVERAGE DURATION OF ACTION (HOURS)			
	Without adrenaline	With adrenaline	Topical and/or infiltration	Nerve blockade[2]	Topical	Infiltration	Minor nerve block	Major nerve block
Amethocaine	1 mg/kg		30–60		4–6			
Bupivacaine	2 mg/kg	2 mg/kg	10–15	15–30		3–4	2–6	7–14
Cocaine	1.5 mg/kg		1–5		0.3–0.5			
Levobupivacaine	2 mg/kg		10–15	15–30	0.5–1	3–4	2–6	7–14
Lignocaine	3 mg/kg	7 mg/kg	5–10	5–15	0.5–1	1–2.5	1–2	3–4
Mepivacaine[3]	5–7 mg/kg		5–10	5–15		1–25	1–2	
Prilocaine	6 mg/kg	8 mg/kg	5–10	5–15	0.5–1	1–2.5	1–2	3–4
Ropivocaine	3 mg/kg		10–15	15–30	0.5–1	3–4	2–6	7–14

1 When given as a single dose; doses given are guidelines only.
2 Onset of action of nerve blockade also depends on size of nerve; complete blockade takes longer with larger nerves.
3 Only available as dental cartridge.

Adapted from Table 2-3 Comparison of local anaesthetics. Australian Medicines Handbook Pty Ltd, Adelaide; 2015:33.

BOX 17.14 Potential complications of haematoma block

All complications identified during the procedure should be discussed with the patient and their family, discussed with the treating clinicians and documented in the patient record.

- Inadvertent intravascular injection
- Nerve injury
- Motor block of the affected limb is common
- Block failure
- Infection
- Accidental vascular puncture
- Anaphylaxis or adverse reactions
- Local anaesthetic systemic toxicity (LAST)

BOX 17.15 Equipment commonly used for Haematoma Block insertion

- Bupivacaine (Marcain)
- 10 mL syringe
- Drawing-up needle
- 22 g needle
- Alcohol-based chlorhexidine gluconate swabs (>0.5% chlorhexidine in >70% isopropyl alcohol) × 2
- Sterile gloves

27. Identify the landmark of the dorsal aspect of the deformity. Insert the needle into the fracture site with adjustments until the needle progresses into the fracture with loss of resistance felt. Confirmation of needle location within the fracture haematoma site can be obtained by drawing back on the syringe plunger and aspirating haematoma (Fig 17.63).

BOX 17.16 Equipment commonly required for POP backslab application

- Under cast padding
- Warm water
- Bandages 7.5 cm wide × 3
- Plaster 15–20 cm wide (dependent on the patient size) cut to length with 6–8 layers
- Scissors
- Tape
- Sling

28. Inject local anaesthetic incrementally: 5–7 mL after needle placement, advance the needle into the space created by the volume and inject the remainder of the anaesthetic. Do not continue to inject if excessive resistance is felt.

29. Aspirate intermittently during insertion and injection of anaesthetic to reduce the risk of inadvertent arterial or venous infiltration. Some dark blood may be seen as the haematoma is infiltrated. If the ulnar styloid is also fractured, 2–3 mL is also injected into this area.

30. Placing pressure over the injection site for 10 seconds after completing the injection may speed up the onset of the block by spreading the local solution with external pressure. This manoeuvre is also a common way of trying to enhance the block's effect.

31. Dispose of all sharps. Dispose of all contaminated waste.

32. Wait for the haematoma block to take effect. This may take 10–15 minutes. Evaluate the occurrence of complete loss of pinprick sensation in the forearm nerve distribution; a sign of nerve block effectiveness.

33. Reduce the fracture by pulling the arm and manipulating the displaced portion towards normal (Figs 17.64 and 17.65).

FIGURE 17.63 Intravenous regional anaesthesia. A double cuff tourniquet is depicted.[102]

1

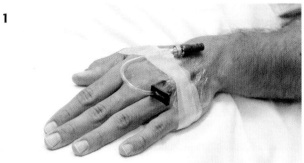

Place an IV catheter or butterfly needle as close to the pathological site as possible. The site should be at least 10 cm distal to the tourniquet. A dorsal hand vein is ideal.

2

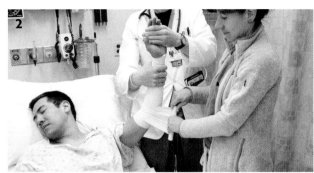

Exsanguinate the extremity by elevating and wrapping it in a distal-to-proximal fashion. Here, an Esmarch bandage is being used.

3

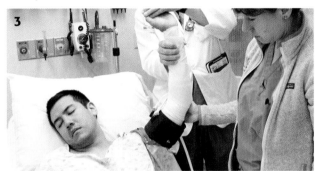

Apply the tourniquet to the patient's arm.

4

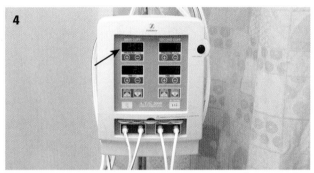

Inflate the tourniquet to 250 mmHg or 100 mmHg above systolic pressure. In the leg, inflate the cuff to 300 mmHg or twice the systolic pressure measured in the arm.

5

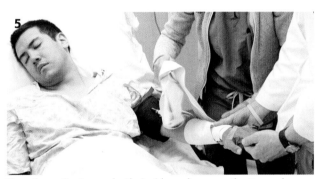

Place the patient's arm by their side and remove the Esmarch bandage. The tourniquet remains inflated.

6

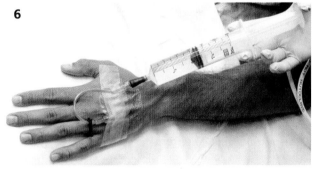

Slowly inject the 0.5% lignocaine solution into the infusion catheter at the calculated dose. See text for details and dosing information.

7

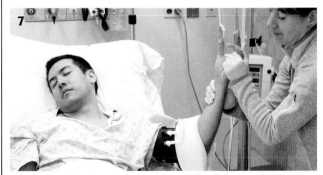

Remove the infusing needle/catheter, and tightly tape the puncture site to prevent extravasation of the anaesthetic agent. Perform the procedure, including postreduction films and casting.

8

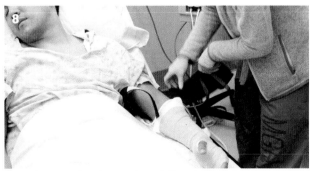

Once the procedure is complete, deflate the tourniquet in a cycling fashion (deflate for 5 seconds, reinflate for 1 to 2 minutes) 2 or 3 times. Then remove the tourniquet.

34. Apply the under cast padding 3 cm beyond the extent of the plaster slab with extra layers around bony prominences. Apply the POP backslab and bandage while continuing to manipulate the wrist to normal position. Consider a short arm sandwich POP for unstable fractures.

35. The wrist may need to be held to a normal position until the POP is dry.

36. Watch for signs of complications. Adverse reactions to bupivacaine are rare in the absence of overdosage, exceptionally rapid absorption or inadvertent intravascular injection.

37. Document the procedure in the clinical record. Record or sign all local anaesthetic doses on the medication chart.

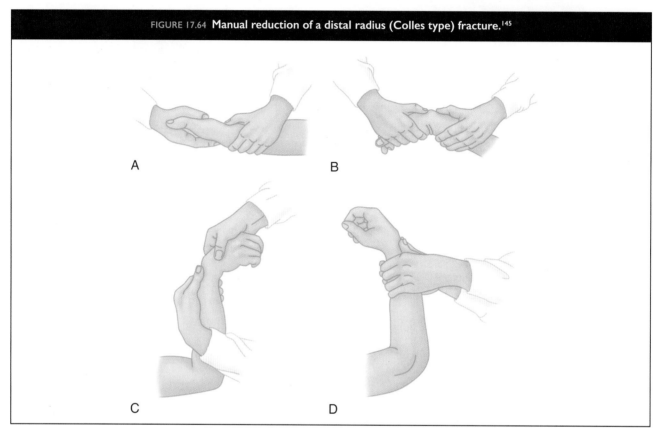

FIGURE 17.64 **Manual reduction of a distal radius (Colles type) fracture.**[145]

A, Disimpaction with longitudinal traction and extension of the wrist. **B,** Reduction with flexion of the wrist to restore palmar tilt and ulnar deviation to restore radial inclination. **C, D,** Stabilisation with double-thumb pressure on the distal fracture fragment in neutral forearm rotation, with slight wrist flexion and ulnar deviation. Extreme pronation, flexion and ulnar deviation (Cotton-Loder position) should be avoided because of problems encountered with median nerve compression.

CASE STUDY

Mrs Lucy is an 86-year-old woman who presents at 0300 hours following a trip and fall onto her outstretched hand. She has pain with an obvious deformity to the right wrist. Her fingers are cool with a 3-second capillary return. The wrist is swollen but a radial pulse is present. She has impaired motor function due to severe pain. An X-ray reveals a transverse fracture of the distal radius with dorsal displacement and angulation. You recognise this as a Colles' fracture that will need reduction.

Questions
1. Describe the initial assessment of Mrs Lucy.
2. What are the options for management of the patient's pain?
3. What are the advantages and disadvantages of using sedation or regional anaesthetic to reduce the fracture?
4. How will you reduce the fracture?
5. What type of splint will you apply?

 Answers to Case Study Questions can be found on evolve
http://evolve.emergencytrauma.curtis

FIGURE 17.65

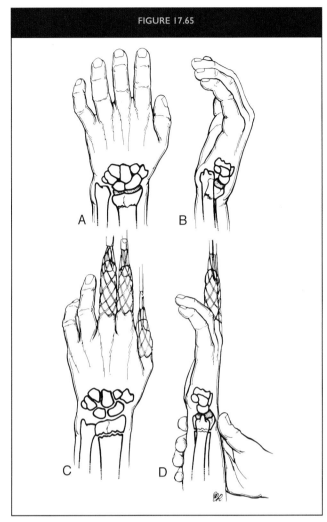

A and B, Distal radius (Colles') fracture. C and D, recommended reduction of this fracture. After suspending the arm from finger traps and allowing disimpaction of the fracture, pressure is applied with the thumb over the distal fragment.[146,147]

Bier Block: intravenous regional anaesthesia

A Bier Block is a type of intravenous regional anaesthesia most commonly used in the ED for manipulation and reduction of fractures and dislocations below the elbow (Fig 17.66). A cooperative patient facilitates the procedure, sedation is generally not needed, and minimal haemodynamic monitoring is required, though ready access to resuscitation equipment should be available. Absolute contraindication for the procedure is an allergy to the anaesthetic agent and relative contraindications include Raynaud's disease, Buerger's disease or a vascularly compromised limb.[132]

Equipment includes: 1% lignocaine, sterile saline solution as diluents, 50 mL syringe/drawing-up needle, pneumatic tourniquet, elastic bandage/padding/splinting or plastering materials; the patient should have two IV cannulas, one on the side of injury distal to injury site and one on the other arm for resuscitation. The lignocaine should be prepared as a 0.5% solution (1% lignocaine mixed with equal parts of saline in the 50 mL syringe). The initial dose is 1.5 mg/kg, and usually results in adequate analgesia; the maximum dose is 3 mg/kg.

FIGURE 17.66 **Administering a Bier Block.**[143]

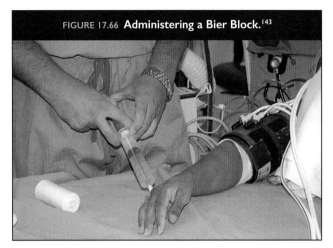

After careful removal of the Esmarch bandage, slowly inject the anesthetic agent in the distal IV cannula.

BOX 17.17 Intravenous regional anaesthesia[102]

1. Begin an intravenous (IV) line in the uninvolved extremity (optional).
2. Draw up and dilute 1% plain lignocaine (1.5 to 3 mg/kg total lignocaine dose) for a final concentration of 0.5% lignocaine.*
3. Place a padded tourniquet and inflate the upper cuff.
4. Insert a small plastic IV cannula near the pathological lesion and secure it.
5. Deflate the tourniquet.
6. Elevate and exsanguinate the extremity.
7. Inflate the tourniquet (250 mmHg), lower the extremity and remove the exsanguination device. Inflate the proximal cuff only if a double-cuff system is used.
8. Infuse the anaesthetic solution.
9. Remove the infusion needle and tape the site.
10. Perform the procedure.
11. If pain is produced by the tourniquet, inflate the distal cuff first, and then deflate the proximal cuff.
12. After the procedure has been carried out, deflate the cuff for 5 seconds and then reinflate it for 1 to 2 minutes. Repeat this step three times. Do not deflate the cuff if total tourniquet time is less than 20 to 30 minutes.
13. Observe 45 to 60 minutes for possible reactions.

See Box 17.17 for procedural steps. Note that the lignocaine is administered in the injured arm in which the circulation has been blocked, not in the IV cannula on the unaffected side. As the lignocaine takes effect the arm will appear blotchy as a result of the residual blood being displaced from the vascular compartment.[124] Complete anaesthesia occurs in 10–20 minutes, though the patient may still sense touch and movement.

Removal of objects

Patients with foreign bodies that require removal are a not too uncommon emergency. It is important to assess the patient and the affected area, consider the type of object and the risks, such as ischaemia or infection, or benefits of removal.

Rings

Rings must be removed to prevent vascular compromise in hand and arm injuries.[81] All rings should be removed on the affected limb.

String-wrap method

The string-wrap method of removing a ring is best attempted when there is no finger laceration or underlying fracture. If there is extensive distal swelling or severe pain, a ring cutter may be required.

1. Begin by wrapping the finger distally to proximally with a Penrose drain or compression bandage to reduce oedema. Leave this in place for up to 5 minutes.
2. Unwrap the compression bandage.
3. Using a long piece of tracheoestomy tape or thick suture, pull a short section from the distal side under the ring.
4. Wind the long end of the tape from the edge of the ring down to the tip of the finger to provide very firm compression with even rows and no skin bulges.
5. Use the short end that was initially pulled through the ring to pull distally and slowly unwrap it, bringing the ring down the finger over the tightly wrapped area.
6. Apply RICE to the finger once the ring is removed (Fig 17.67).[150]

Ring cutter method

Using a ring cutter is best attempted when there is finger laceration or suspected underlying fracture. Manual ring cutters require patience, as the cutting process is slow. Some EDs use electric or battery-operated ring cutters. Some rings are made of tungsten carbide, stainless steel or titanium and cannot be cut by conventional hospital ring cutters. In these cases the assistance of the local fire brigade or police rescue using specialised saws will be required.

1. Fit the small ring cutter hook under the ring. This acts as a guide for the cutting wheel.
2. Turn the cutting wheel slowly, applying firm but not excessive pressure.
3. Continue cutting until there is a break in the ring.
4. Use two large artery forceps or haemostats on either side of the cut to spread the ring (Fig 17.68).

In some cases of severe swelling, the ring may need to be cut again into two pieces.

PRACTICE TIPS

- The string-wrap method of ring removal can be uncomfortable as a high degree of compression is required. The advantage is that this method can be used for rings that cannot be cut. Because it preserves the integrity of the ring, it also has some psychological benefits to those people reluctant to cut a wedding ring because of the superstition that cutting a wedding ring will result in the end of the marriage.
- Using a ring cutter requires patience and is not always possible with modern ring metals. Cutting a ring may be the only technique possible in the case of laceration, fracture or severe swelling.

Body piercings

Body piercings may need to be removed in the case of infection, localised swelling or to permit intubation. Care should be taken when removing any piercing near the mouth or nose so as to prevent aspiration of the separated pieces. Body piercing can involve the nose, ear, tongue, nipple, genitals, navel and eyebrow, including piercings that involve stretching of the skin of the ears or lips. Extreme piercings include piercing of the uvula or multiple facial piercings.

1. If possible, ask the patient how the piercing comes apart. The types of piercings include clip-on ends, screw-on balls, fixed ends with screw-on balls and balls held on with tension.
2. Apply RICE in the presence of swelling to reduce localised oedema.
3. Ensure that the area is clean and dry.
4. Grip each end of the piercing with artery forceps and unscrew counter-clockwise or pull apart the ring.
5. Remove the piercing and apply RICE if required.

Fishhooks

The method of removing a fishhook depends on the location and the depth of the hook.[133]

String-yank technique

This method is used when the hook lies too deep to be passed out through a second wound. It can be used with or without local anaesthesia and is best attempted in the compliant patient.

1. Begin by ensuring that the skin is clean and dry.
2. Loop a long piece of tracheosteomy string or thick suture material around the hook close to the insertion point of the skin (Fig 17.69).
3. Press the long shaft of the hook against the skin while applying downward pressure on the curve of the hook where it enters the skin. This will disengage the embedded barb.
4. Yank or pull sharply on the string with the other hand to remove the hook.
5. Beware of the hook as it flies out of the patient.

Advance and cut technique

This method is best used for superficially embedded hooks as it requires the hook to be advanced through a second wound.[150] Local anaesthesia is required.

1. Begin by ensuring that the skin is clean and dry.
2. Inject local anaesthetic into the tissue overlying the barb.
3. Force the barb through the skin.
4. Cut off the barb using pliers.
5. Remove the remaining hook by passing it back through the entry wound.

PRACTICE TIPS

The string-yank technique of fishhook removal can be used to remove deeply embedded hooks where a secondary wound would be unfavourable. It can performed without local anaesthetic but requires the patient to remain still as the hook is yanked from the skin. There is a chance this technique will be unsuccessful.

The advance and cut technique can be used for superficially embedded hooks but requires local anaesthetic and the creation of a second wound. This method is always successful.

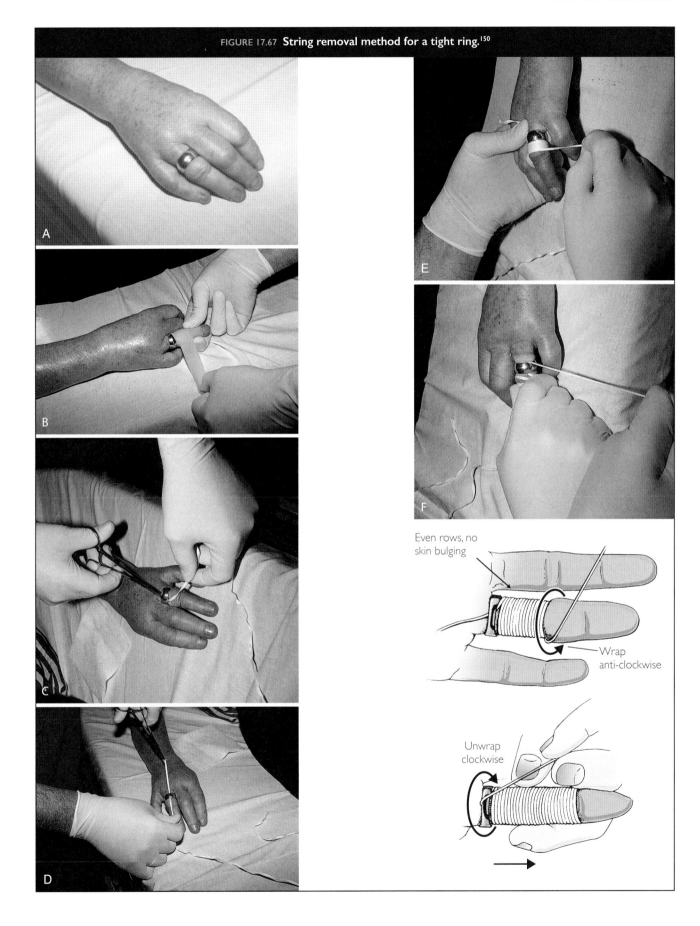

FIGURE 17.67 **String removal method for a tight ring.**[150]

Even rows, no
skin bulging

Wrap
anti-clockwise

Unwrap
clockwise

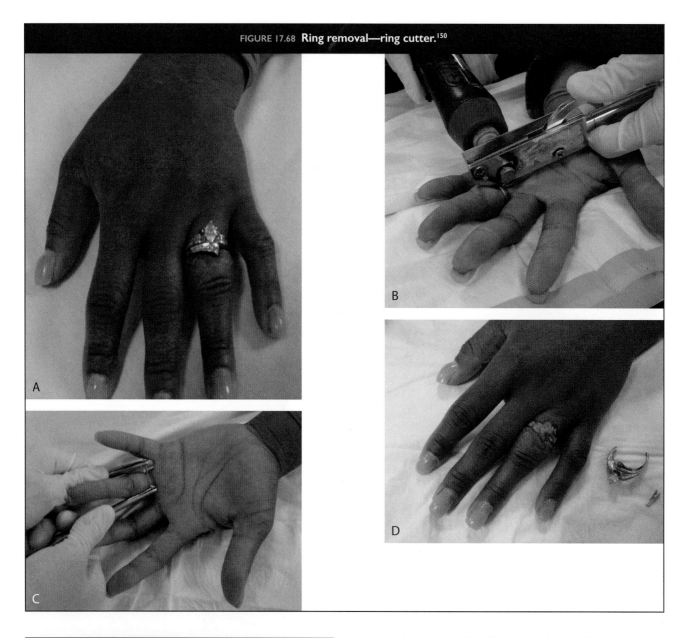

FIGURE 17.68 **Ring removal—ring cutter.**[150]

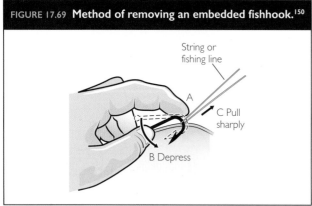

FIGURE 17.69 **Method of removing an embedded fishhook.**[150]

String or
fishing line

A

C Pull
sharply

B Depress

Ticks

Ticks should be removed early to reduce the risk of disease transmission. Removal becomes more difficult the longer the tick has been embedded.

1. Begin by ensuring that the skin is clean and dry.
2. Do not apply alcohol or petroleum jelly to force the tick to disengage as this can cause the tick to regurgitate, increasing the risk of infection. Manual removal is the best method.
3. Using a pair of straight tweezers, grasp the tick at the head as close to the skin as possible.
4. Slowly pull, taking care not to squeeze the body of the tick.
5. Ensure the tick is removed whole or use fine tweezers to remove any remaining parts of the head.

Wound closure

The time of injury and time to repair are crucial for optimal wound healing. The potential for wound infection increases as the time increases between injury and repair. Six to eight hours is considered a safe time interval from injury to primary closure. This is not exact, as factors such as clean lacerations on the face can extend the time, whereas diabetes and steroid use may place the patient at risk for delayed healing.[133] Emergency nurses and Extended Care Paramedics are excellent providers of wound management. Many programs exist in Australia which provide the necessary education and accreditation for primary wound closure by suturing. Nurse practitioners and Extended Care Paramedics may also be skilled in suturing. Studies have demonstrated that advanced practice nurses can provide a high level of patient satisfaction.[134]

Primary wound closure uses a tape closure (e.g. Steri-Strips), sutures or staples. The technique chosen depends on wound size, depth and location.

Tape closure

Tape closure is used for superficial linear wounds under minimal tension or as an adjunct after suture removal in patients with thin, frail skin, such as the elderly or steroid-dependent patients (Fig 17.70). Pretibial lacerations are common in the elderly following minor trauma. The skin is thin and can easily tear, making suturing unsatisfactory.

In tertiary and metropolitan hospitals, pretibial lacerations should be referred to a plastic surgeon for surgical repair. In rural and remote settings, tape closure is appropriate until plastic surgeon review.

Tincture of benzoin should be applied to skin before tape application to ensure adherence. Care must be taken to ensure that the tincture does not contact the open wound or injured skin—it will cause pain. A tape closure may also be used after deeper layers are closed with sutures. Dressings may or may not be applied over the tape closure. An anaesthetic is not necessary, and a lower risk of infection and skin necrosis is associated with tape closure.[95] Tape strips remain in place until they fall off. Figure 17.71 illustrates tape closure.

Suturing

Sutures approximate and attach wound edges, which decreases infection, promotes wound healing and minimises scar formation. A local anaesthetic applied by infiltration or topically is required for suturing. Different suture materials are used to close various wounds depending on depth, location and tension of the wound. Figure 17.72 shows various stitches and their uses. Sutures may be absorbable or non-absorbable, which means they are generally composed of natural or synthetic material, respectively. Essential qualities of suture material are security, strength, reaction, workability and infection potential. Table 17.6 describes these qualities for various suture materials.[137] Ideal suture materials are strong, easily secured, resistant to infection and cause minimal local reaction.

In suturing, absorbable sutures are for dermal and sub-cutaneous layers; non-absorbable sutures are used externally. Sutures cause minimal discomfort after insertion; however, they also act as a foreign body and can cause local inflammation. An initial cover with a non-adherent dressing protects the wound and absorbs fluid.

Staples

Staples are a fast, economic alternative for closure of linear lacerations of the scalp, trunk and extremities (Fig 17.73). Wounds closed with staples have a lower incidence of infection and tissue reactivity but do not provide the same quality of closure as sutures. Scars are more pronounced; therefore, staples are only recommended for areas where a scar is not apparent (i.e. scalp). Staples should not be used in areas of the scalp with permanent hair loss because of poor aesthetic results. Consider the likelihood of the patient attending imaging; for example, head computed tomography (CT) scans, which may be affected by steel staples. If this is a possibility, then suturing using non-absorbable material may be a better option. Local anaesthesia is optional when only one or two staples are required because pain from infiltration of anaesthetic agents may be greater than pain associated with insertion of one or two staples.

Staples usually remain in place for 7–10 days, and they can only be removed using a specialised skin staple remover.

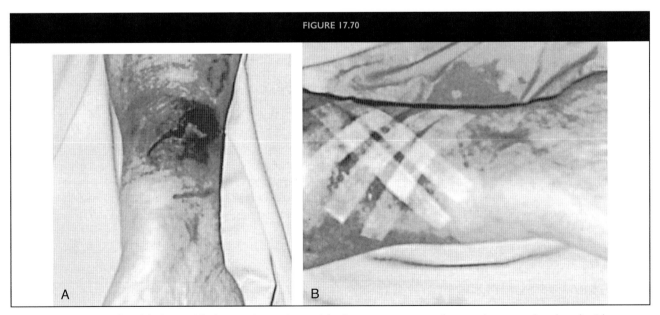

FIGURE 17.70

A, Skin avulsions in the elderly are ideal wounds to close with closure tapes, as such wounds cannot be closed with sutures. The goal is to provide approximation of the avulsed skin and apply skin-flap pressure to avoid movement or fluid accumulation under the avulsion. **B,** The edges of the skin are uncurled, stretched and anatomically replaced.[124]

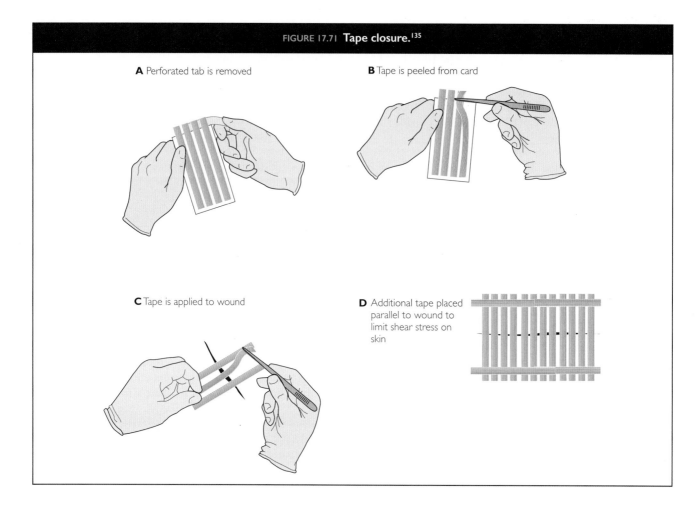

FIGURE 17.71 **Tape closure.**[135]

A Perforated tab is removed

B Tape is peeled from card

C Tape is applied to wound

D Additional tape placed parallel to wound to limit shear stress on skin

Skin adhesives

A topical skin adhesive is another method of non-invasive wound management used to close skin edges that are easily approximated. Studies have demonstrated that adhesive is the preferred wound closure method in small and recent facial wounds.[138] This type of wound closure should not be used in areas of high skin tension or across areas of increased skin tension. Wounds should be less than 5 cm long. Application of three thin layers of adhesive is more effective than a single thick layer: the skin adhesive dries within 2.5 minutes.

Discharge education should stress not applying liquid or ointment to the closed wound because these substances can weaken the adhesive, leading to dehiscence. Patients should also be instructed that the adhesive will slough naturally, usually within 5–10 days. If removal of skin adhesive is necessary, use petroleum jelly or acetone.

Instruct the patient to keep the wound clean and dry. If washing of the wound is required, mild soap and water is all that is required and drying is important. Soaking of the wound and swimming is not advised. Elevation of an affected limb reduces swelling and subsequent pain. Educate about the signs and symptoms of inflammation and early infection. Pain is usually the initial symptom, followed by redness, swelling and discharge. Instruct the patient to seek professional advice from their general practitioner or return to the ED.

Removal of wound closures

Suture removal

Recommendations for suture removal vary with wound location. For wounds in areas of movement or increased surface tension, sutures should remain longer. Table 17.7 provides guidelines for suture removal. To reduce scarring further, sutures in highly visible areas such as the face may be removed earlier than those in other areas, and surgical skin tape (e.g. Steri-Strips) applied to reinforce the wound.

Method (Fig 17.74):

1. Begin by ensuring that the skin is clean and dry.
2. Grasp the suture using fine tweezers and lift the suture.
3. Cut the suture as close to the skin as possible using a suture cutter or scissors.
4. Pull the suture out. Never pull a knot through the skin.
5. Apply surgical skin tape to maintain wound repair after suture removal.

Staple removal

Wound staples should be removed after the same interval as sutures, and require a specialised staple-removal device (Fig 17.75).

1. Begin by ensuring that the skin is clean and dry.
2. Slide the lower jaw of the staple remover under the staple.
3. Squeeze or close the handle to compress the staple.

FIGURE 17.72 **Stitches for suturing.**

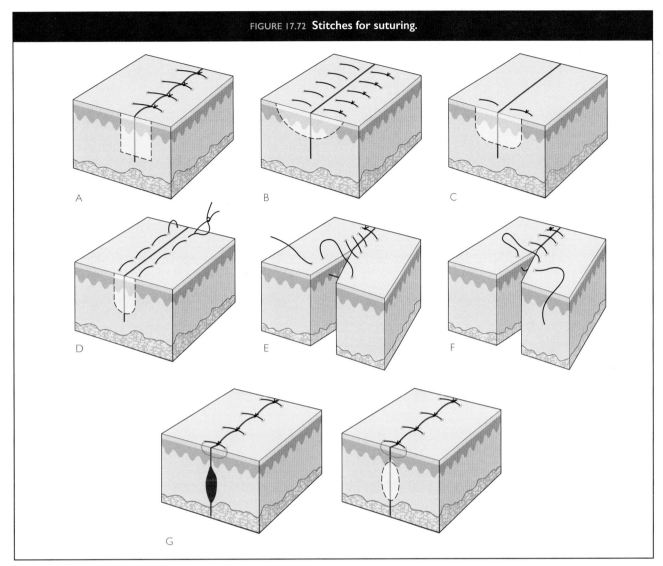

A, Simple interrupted suture: pairing skin edges together evenly; edges are slightly elevated but flatten with healing. **B**, Vertical mattress suture: assures eversion on healing. **C**, Horizontal mattress suture: closely approximates skin edges and has slight amount of eversion, especially in areas under tension. **D**, Half-buried horizontal mattress suture: good with flaps, V-spaced and parallel lacerations. **E**, Subcuticular suture (continuous intradermal suture): good for wounds where sutures should be left in place for longer periods, as in wounds under a great deal of tension. **F**, Continuous suture: good when suture marks will not show, as in scalp. **G**, Buried suture: reduces dead space and reduces surface tension in wound.

4. Ensure the staple is fully compressed to decrease patient discomfort.
5. Lift the staple from the wound.
6. Apply surgical skin tape (e.g. Steri-Strips) to maintain wound repair after staple removal.

Most staple-removal devices are disposable. It is important that the patient has access to a staple-removal device; not all local doctors have them in stock.

Eye emergencies

Most ocular emergencies do not represent a threat to the patient's life; however, these conditions represent a great threat to the patient's wellbeing. Once lost, vision cannot be replaced. The emergency nurse should assess patients who present with ocular problems and identify those with actual or potential threats to vision. Early recognition of true ocular emergencies and preventing further damage is critical for the patient's optimal visual outcome.

Immediate and copious irrigation of chemical burn injuries is essential, because the area and time of exposure determines the injury and overall outcome.[139] Irrigation can be performed using a normal IV giving set or a commercial Morgan lens. The Morgan lens is a moulded plastic lens with tubing that attaches to the end of an IV giving set to run continuous irrigation. It allows hands-free irrigation of unilateral or bilateral eyes. Correct eye irrigation is time-consuming and labour-intensive.

Procedures

Everting an eyelid

1. Ask the patient to look downwards with both eyes gently closed.

TABLE 17.6 Suture materials for wound closure[136]

TYPE	DESCRIPTION	SECURITY	STRENGTH	REACTION	WORKABILITY	INFECTION	COMMENT
Nonabsorbables							
Silk		|||			|||	|||	||	Nice around mouth, nose or nipples; too reactive and weak to be used universally
Mersilene	Braided synthetic	||||	||	|||	||||		Good tensile strength; some prefer for fascia repairs
Nylon	Monofilament	||	|||	||	||	|||	Good strength; decreased infection rate; knots tend to slip, especially the first throw
Prolene Polypropylene	Monofilament	||||	||||					||||	Good resistance to infection; often difficult to work with; requires an extra throw
Ethibond	Braided coated polyester	|||	||||	||½	|||	|||	Costly
Stainless steel wire	Monofilament	||||	||||							Hard to use; painful to patient; some prefer for tendons
Absorbables							
Gut (plain)	From sheep intima			||	|||				Loses strength rapidly and quickly absorbed; rarely used today
Chromic (gut)	Plain gut treated with chromic salts	||	||	|||				Similar to plain gut; often used to close intraoral lacerations
Dexon	Braided copolymer of glycolic acid	||||	||||				||||	Braiding may cause it to 'hang up' when tying knots
Vicryl	Braided polymer of lactide and glycolide	|||	||||				|||	Low reactivity with good strength; therefore, nice for subcutaneous healing; good in mucous membranes
Polydioxanone	Monofilament	||||	||||			Excellent	Unavailable	First available monofilament synthetic absorbable sutures; appears to be excellent

Scale: ||||, high → |, low

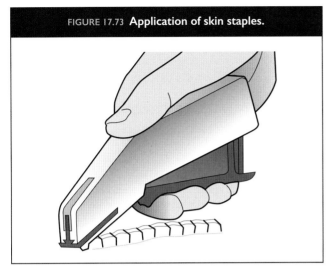

FIGURE 17.73 **Application of skin staples.**

Staples are centred over the incision line using locating arrows or a guideline and placed approximately 10 mm apart.

TABLE 17.7 Guidelines for suture removal

LOCATION	REMOVAL DATE
Eyelids	3–5 days
Eyebrows	4–5 days
Ear	4–6 days
Lip	3–5 days
Face	3–5 days
Scalp	7–10 days
Trunk	7–10 days
Hands and feet	7–10 days
Arms and legs	10–14 days
Over joints	14 days

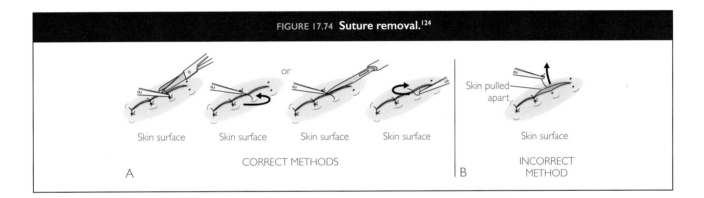

FIGURE 17.74 **Suture removal.**[124]

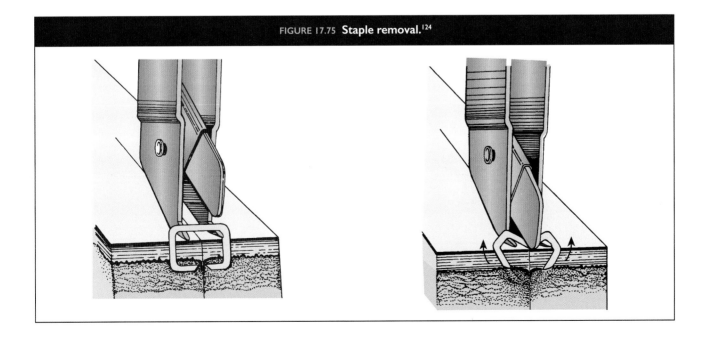

FIGURE 17.75 **Staple removal.**[124]

2. Use your right hand to hold a cotton bud and left hand to open the lid of the patient's left eye; and the other way round for the right eye.

3. Place the cotton bud horizontally so that the soft tip rests on the top eyelid crease.

4. With the other hand, grip the eye lashes.

5. Apply gentle pressure to the cotton tip and lift the lashes to fold the eye lid over the cotton tip (Fig 17.76).

6. Hold the lid in place and slide the cotton bud out.

7. Examine, sweep or irrigate under the lid as required.

8. When finished, ask the patient to blink and look up to return the lid to normal.

Double-everting the top eyelid

1. Life-saving procedures always take precedence over eye emergencies.

2. Apply topical anaesthetic to the eye and wait 3–5 minutes.

3. Ask the patient to look downwards with both eyes gently closed.

4. Use your right hand to hold a cotton bud and left hand to open the lid for the patient's left eye; and the other way round for the right eye.

5. Place the cotton bud horizontally so that the soft tip rests on the top eyelid crease.

6. With the other hand, grip the eye lashes.

7. Apply gentle pressure to the cotton tip and lift the lashes to fold the eyelid over the cotton tip.

8. Hold the lid in place and slide the cotton bud out.

9. Moisten a second sterile cotton tip with anaesthetic or Normal saline.

10. Place this on the everted eye lid and apply pressure to view the upper conjunctival fornix deep under the lid.

11. Examine, sweep or irrigate under the lid as required.

12. When finished, ask the patient to blink and look up to return the lid to normal.

13. Hold the lid in place and slide the cotton bud out.

Irrigating an eye using an IV giving set

Life-saving procedures always take precedence over eye emergencies, but early irrigation can be vital in saving vision.

1. Apply topical anaesthetic to the eye and wait.

2. Begin irrigation with 1 litre of Normal saline or Hartmann's IV solution via an IV giving line, following the steps below.

3. Evert the upper lid and irrigate. Sweep and remove any foreign bodies seen.

4. Open the IV giving set and continue to instil the irrigation into the open eye.

5. Use eyelid retractors or hold the eye open with a gloved hand or gauze.

6. Direct the stream of fluid medially onto the conjunctiva then across the cornea so that the fluid flows laterally down the side of the head.[140]

7. Begin by rapidly flushing the first 500 mL of solution, then slow the infusion to a continuous trickle.

8. Repeat topical anaesthetic every 10 minutes as required.

9. Infuse at least 1 litre of irrigation. Alkali burns (e.g. caustic soda, lime-plaster/cement and ammonia) penetrate the cornea rapidly because of their ability to lyse with the cell membranes, and prolonged irrigation may be required.

10. Wait 5 minutes after the completion of irrigation before checking the pH at the conjunctival fornices. The average pH of tears is 7.35 but a wide normal variation exists from 5.20 to 8.35.[141]

Irrigating an eye using a Morgan lens

The Morgan lens (Fig 17.77) allows the medical team to irrigate the eye without the use of eyelid retractors, which can cause abrasions to the eye, or without a dedicated person holding the eyelids open; it is the hands-free option for eye irrigation. The Morgan lens is relatively expensive, and may not adequately irrigate under the lids. Particulate may be trapped under the lens, causing corneal abrasion. New users may find the lens difficult to fit.

1. Life-saving procedures always take precedence over eye emergencies, but early irrigation can be vital in saving vision.

2. Apply topical anaesthetic to the eye and wait.

3. Begin irrigation with 1 litre of Normal saline or Hartmann's IV solution via an IV giving line before fitting the lens, following the steps below.

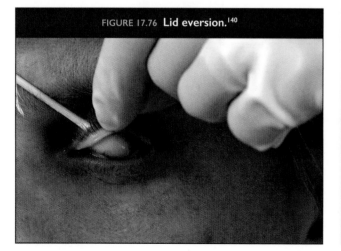

FIGURE 17.76 **Lid eversion.**[140]

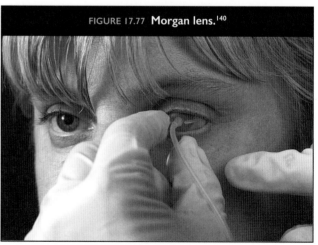

FIGURE 17.77 **Morgan lens.**[140]

4. Evert the upper lid and irrigate. Sweep and remove any foreign bodies seen.

5. Prime an IV giving set with a Morgan lens attached with Normal saline or Hartmann's IV solution.

6. Ask the patient to look down, and place the top half of the lens under the top eyelid by grasping and lifting the eye lashes.

7. Ask the patient to look up, and place the bottom of the lens under the bottom eyelid so that it sits on the eye like a contact lens.

8. Instruct the patient to close their eyes.

9. Begin by rapidly flushing the first 500 mL of solution, and then slow the infusion to a continuous trickle.

10. Repeat topical anaesthetic every 10 minutes as required.

11. Infuse at least 1 litre of irrigation. Alkali burns (e.g. caustic soda, lime-plaster/cement and ammonia) penetrate the cornea rapidly because of their ability to lyse with the cell membranes, and prolonged irrigation may be required.

12. Wait 5 minutes after the completion of irrigation and remove the Morgan lens before checking the pH at the conjunctival fornices.

Checking the pH of an eye

1. Do not wait to check the pH of the eye following chemical burns. Irrigation (see above) must start immediately.

2. Wait 5 minutes after the completion of irrigation, and remove the Morgan lens if used, before checking the pH.

3. Use a strip of universal indicator paper. If none is available, the pH section of a urine analysis dipstick may be used, but beware of the risk of corneal abrasion from the sharp plastic.

4. Ask the patient to look up, and pull down the bottom lid.

5. Hold the universal indicator paper on the bottom conjunctival fornices until it is wet with tears (Fig 17.78A).

6. Compare the reading against the scale. An acceptable eye pH is 6.5–8.5 (Fig 17.78B).

7. Recheck the pH after 30 minutes.

Padding an eye

Eye padding is not commonly used, because a padded eye cannot be frequently examined. It is important to leave eye padding on for no longer than 24 hours as there is an increased risk of infection. Correct eye padding must be firm enough not to allow the padded eye to open. Doing so can cause irritation and abrasion to the cornea. Patients must be aware that padding an eye will result in the loss of binocular vision—they must not drive and should take care when walking.

1. Apply topical anaesthetic to the eye and wait.

2. Ask the patient to close both eyes.

3. Apply a generous amount of antibiotic ointment to the conjunctival fornices and the outer lids.

4. Fold an eye pad in half and place it on the closed eye.

5. Secure this with three pieces of tape, taking care not to apply pressure to the centre of the pad.

6. Tape from above the eyebrow medially diagonally down to the cheek.

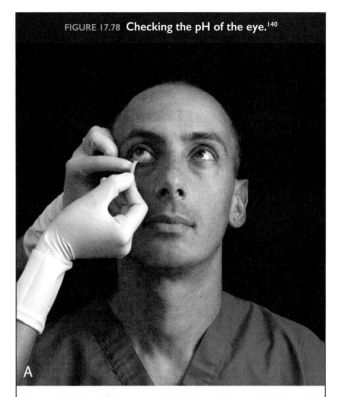

FIGURE 17.78 **Checking the pH of the eye.**[140]

A

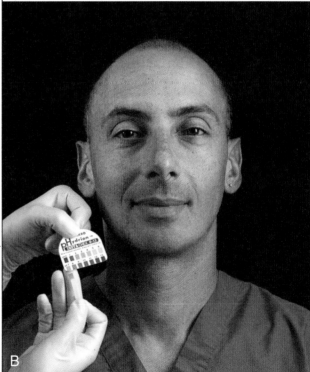

B

7. Place a second eye pad on top of the first and tape with three pieces of tape, taking care not to apply pressure to the centre of the pad. The taping should be firm and even, and on completion the patient should not be able to open the padded eye.

Fitting a protective eye shield

A protective eye shield should be used to prevent further compression to an injured eye and where an eye perforation or penetrating eye injury is suspected. A shield prevents secondary injury.[104]

1. Apply topical anaesthetic to the eye if required. Systemic analgesia may also be required for penetrating eye injuries.
2. Ask the awake patient to close both eyes.
3. Apply a generous amount of antibiotic ointment to the conjunctival fornices and the outer lids.
4. Use a commercial eye shield and secure this with three pieces of tape, taking care not to apply pressure to the centre of the shield.
5. Tape from above the eyebrow medially diagonally down to the cheek.
6. A modified eye shield can be made using a polystyrene or paper cup (Fig 17.79).

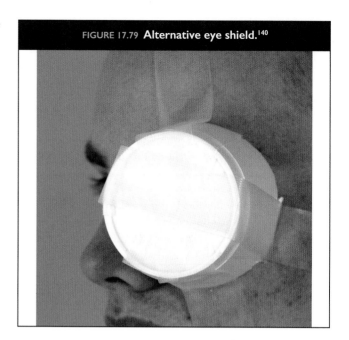

FIGURE 17.79 **Alternative eye shield.**[140]

SUMMARY

This chapter has outlined a broad range of clinical skills relevant to the emergency clinician. The relevant theoretical and practical aspects of the procedures have been included in conjunction with the latest available research. The contents of this chapter can be utilised by the emergency clinician to refresh previously acquired skills and to provide a basis to the attainment of new skills.

ACKNOWLEDGEMENT

The authors acknowledge the work of Mark Wilson, the first edition author.

USEFUL WEBSITES

AirwayRegistry: a multi-centre database to evaluate what is current practice and to assess future developments in techniques and technology in ED airway management; www.airwayregistry.org.au/

Australian Resuscitation Council: useful guidelines for management of emergency presentations, www.resus.org.au

AO Online: the surgical management of trauma and disorders of the musculoskeletal system, www.aofoundation.org/

Australian Wound Management Association. http://www.awma.com.au/nsw/about_nsw.php

BestBETs (Best Evidence Topics), www.bestbets.org

Company resources from Molnlycke, www.molnlycke.com/com/Wound-Care-Products

Company resources from Smith&Nephew, http://wound.smith-nephew.com/

Emergency Eye Manual (an illustrated guide) written by the Statewide Ophthalmology Service NSW, www.cena.org.au/wp-content/uploads/2014/10/eye_manual.pdf

Intraosseous access devices information (e.g. EZ-IO), www.vidacare.com

Joanna Briggs Institute, www.joannabriggs.org

Life in the Fast Lane: LITFL is a medical blog and website dedicated to providing online emergency medicine and critical care insights and education for everyone, everywhere, www.lifeinthefastlane.com/

MIMS Online: Monthly Index of Medical Specialties pharmaceutical prescribing reference guide, www.mimsonline.com.au

Neuraxiom: ultrasound guided regional nerve blocks, www.neuraxiom.com/html/ficb.html

Useful information and user guides for fitting Hare traction splints, www.haretractionsplint.com/

REFERENCES

1. Reardon RF, Mason PE, Clinton JE. Basic airway management and decision-making. In: Roberts JR, Hedges JR, eds. Clinical procedures in emergency medicine. 6th edn. Philadelphia: WB Saunders; 2014:37–57.
2. Heard SO, Kaur S. Airway management and endotracheal intubation. In: Irwin RS, Rippe JM, Lisbon A et al, eds. Procedures, techniques and minimally invasive monitoring in intensive care medicine. 4th edn. Philadelphia: Lippincott Williams & Wilkins; 2008. pp. 3–18.
3. Skillings KN, Curtis BL. Oropharyngeal airway insertion. In: Wiegand DJ, Carlson KK, eds. AACN procedure manual for critical care. 5th edn. St Louis: WB Saunders; 2005:57–61.
4. Skillings KN, Curtis BL. Nasopharyngeal airway insertion. In: Wiegand DJ, Carlson KK, eds. AACN procedure manual for critical care. 5th edn. St Louis: WB Saunders; 2005:53–6.
5. Roberts K, Whalley H, Bleetman A. The nasopharyngeal airway: dispelling myths and establishing the facts. Emerg Med J 2005; 22(6):394–6.
6. Barker TD, Schneider RE. Supplemental oxygen and bag-mask ventilation. In: Walls RM, Murphy MF, eds. Manual of emergency airway management. 3rd edn. Philadelphia: Lippincott Williams & Wilkins; 2008:47–61.
7. Brimacombe JR, Berry AM. Cricoid pressure. Can J Anaesth 1997;44(4):414–25.
8. Wilkins RL, Stoller JK, Scanlan CL. Egan's Fundamentals of respiratory care. 8th edn. St Louis: Mosby; 2003.
9. Reynolds SF, Heffner J. Airway management of the critically ill patient: rapid-sequence intubation. Chest 2005;127(4):1397–412.
10. Walls RM. Rapid sequence intubation. In: Walls RM, Murphy MF, eds. Manual of emergency airway management. 3rd edn. Philadelphia: Lippincott Williams & Wilkins; 2008:23–35.
11. McGill JW, Reardon RF. Tracheal intubation. In: Roberts JR, Hedges JR, eds. Clinical procedures in emergency medicine. 5th edn. Philadelphia: WB Saunders; 2010:58–98.
12. AirwayRegistry.com.au. RSI checklist. http://www.airwayregistry.org.au/the-following-are-links-to-.html; accessed 6 March 2015.
13. Weingart SD, Levitan RM. Preoxygenation and prevention of desaturation during emergency airway management. Annals of Emergency Medicine 2012; 59(3):165–75.
14. Hopson LR, Schwartz RB. Pharmacological adjuncts to intubation. In: Roberts JR, Hedges JR, eds. Clinical procedures in emergency medicine. 5th edn. Philadelphia: WB Saunders; 2010:99–109.
15. Dargin J, Medzon R. Emergency department management of the airway of obese adults. Annals of Emergency Medicine 2010; 56(2);95–104.
16. Day MW. Laryngeal mask airway. In: Wiegand DJ, Carlson KK, eds. AACN procedure manual for critical care. 5th edn. St Louis: Saunders; 2005:42–52.
17. Howes BW, Wharton NM, Gibbison B et al. LMA supreme insertion by novices in manikins and patients. Anaesthesia 2010;65(4):343–7.
18. The Laryngeal Mask Company. LMA instruction manual. Online. www.lmaco.com/products/LMA%20Airway%20Management™; accessed 27 May 2015.
19. Vissers RJ, Bair AE. Surgical airway techniques. In: Walls RM, Murphy MF, eds. Manual of emergency airway management. 3rd edn. Philadelphia: Lippincott Williams & Wilkins; 2008:192–220.
20. Zuidema GD, Rutherford RB, Ballinger WF. Management of trauma. 4th edn. Philadelphia: WB Saunders; 1996.
21. Hebert RB, Bose S, Mace SE. Cricothyrotomy and transtracheal jet ventilation. In: Roberts JR, Hedges JR, eds. Clinical procedures in emergency medicine. 5th edn. Philadelphia: WB Saunders; 2010:110–23.
22. Zwerneman K. End-tidal carbon dioxide monitoring: a VITAL sign worth watching. Crit Care Nurs Clin North Am 2006;18(2):217–25.
23. DeBoer S, Seaver M, Arndt K. Verification of endotracheal tube placement: a comparison of confirmation techniques and devices. J Emerg Nurs 2003;29(5):444–50.
24. Powers J, Daniels D, McGuire C et al. The incidence of skin breakdown associated with use of cervical collars. J Trauma Nurs 2006;13(4):198–200.
25. Manoach S, Paladino L. Manual in-line stabilization for acute airway management of suspected cervical spine injury: historical review and current questions. Ann Emerg Med 2007;50(3):236–45.
26. Altman GB, Kerestzes P, Wcisel MA. Fundamental and advanced nursing skills. 3rd edn. New York: Delmar; 2010.
27. Nagler J, Krauss B. Devices for assessing oxygenation and ventilation. In: Roberts JR, Hedges JR, eds. Clinical procedures in emergency medicine. 6th edn. Philadelphia: WB Saunders; 2014:23–38.
28. Kent B, Dowd B. Assessment, monitoring and diagnostics. In: Elliot D, Aitken LM, Chaboyer W, eds. ACCCN's critical care nursing. Sydney: Mosby; 2007:109–52.
29. Frakes M. Measuring end-tidal carbon dioxide: clinical applications and usefulness. Crit Care Nurse 2001;21(5):23.
30. Moore T. Suctioning techniques for the removal of respiratory secretions. Nurs Stand 2003;18(9):47–53.
31. Pedersen CM, Rosendahl-Nielsen M, Hjermind J et al. Endotracheal suctioning of the adult intubated patient—what is the evidence? Intensive Crit Care Nurs 2009;25(1):21–30.
32. Chulay M. Suctioning: endotracheal or tracheostomy tube. In: Wiegand DJ, Carlson KK, eds. AACN procedure manual for critical care. 5th edn. St Louis: WB Saunders; 2005:62–70.
33. Darovic G. Hemodynamic monitoring: invasive and noninvasive clinical application. 3rd edn. Philadelphia: WB Saunders; 2002.
34. Woodrow P. Arterial blood gas analysis. Nurs Stand 2004;18(21):45–52.

35. Edwards G. Respiratory emergencies. In: Newberry L, ed. Sheehy's Manual of emergency care. 6th edn. St Louis: Mosby; 2005.

36. May JL. Emergency medical procedures. New York: John Wiley and Sons; 1984.

37. Ahern J, Fildes S, Peters R. A guide to blood gases. Nurs Stand 1995;9(49):50–2.

38. Koran Z, Howard PK. Respiratory emergencies. In: Newberry L, ed. Sheehy's Emergency nursing: principles and practice. 5th edn. St Louis: Mosby; 2003:421–49.

39. Urden LD, Stacy KM, Lough ME, eds. Thelan's Critical care nursing: diagnosis and management. 4th edn. St Louis: Mosby; 2003.

40. Vincent, JL, Abraham, E, Moore FA et al. Textbook of critical care, 6th edn, Philadelphia: WB Saunders; 2011:296–302.

41. Tortora G, Grabowski S. Principles of anatomy and physiology. 8th edn. New York: HarperCollins College Publishers; 1994.

42. Kelly AM, McAlpine R, Kyle E. Venous pH can safely replace arterial pH in the initial evaluation of patients in the emergency department. Emerg Med J 2001;18(5):340–2.

43. Malatesha G, Singh NK, Bharija A et al. Comparison of arterial and venous pH, bicarbonate, PCO2 and PO2 in initial emergency department assessment. Emerg Med J 2007;24(8):569–71.

44. Bochicchio GV, Joshi M, Bochicchio KM et al. Early hyperglycemic control is important in critically injured trauma patients. J Trauma 2007;63(6):1353–8.

45. Urden LD, Stacy KM, Lough ME. Urden: Critical care nursing: diagnosis and management. 6th edn. St Louis: Mosby; 2009.

46. Allen DA, Baranoski S, Barron VE et al, eds. Lippincott's Nursing procedures. 5th edn. Philadelphia: Lippincott Williams & Wilkins; 2008.

47. Kelly AM, McAlpine R, Kyle E. Agreement between bicarbonate measured on arterial and venous blood gases. Emerg Med Australas 2004;16(5–6):407–9.

48. Urden LD, Stacy KM, Lough ME. Thelan's Critical care nursing: diagnosis and management. 5th edn. St Louis: Mosby; 2006.

49. Kirsch TD, Sax J. Tube thoracostomy. In: Roberts JR, Hedges JR, eds. Clinical procedures in emergency medicine. 6th edn. Philadelphia: WB Saunders; 2014:189–211.

50. Johns DP, Pierce R. Pocket guide to spirometry. Sydney: McGraw-Hill; 2005.

51. Johns DP, Pierce R. Spirometry: the measure and interpretation of ventilatory function in clinical practice. Online. www.nationalasthma.org.au; 2008.

52. Friedman HH: Diagnostic electrocardiography and vectorcardiography. In: Reich et al. Essentials of cardiac anesthesia. Elsevier; 2008:41.

53. Neuraxiom: ultrasound guided regional nerve blocks, www.neuraxiom.com/html/ficb.html; accessed 6 March 2015.

54. American Heart Association Scientific Statement. Practice standards for electrocardiographic monitoring in hospital settings, Circulation 2004;110:2721–46.

55. Besseman ES. Emergency cardiac pacing. In: Roberts JR, Hedges JR, eds. Clinical procedures in emergency medicine. 6th edn. Philadelphia: WB Saunders; 2014:277–97.

56. Link MS, Atkins DL, Passman RS et al. Part 6: electrical therapies: automated external defibrillators, defibrillation, cardioversion and pacing. 2010 American Heart Association guidelines for cardiopulmonary resuscitation and emergency cardiovascular care. Circulation 2010;122(18 suppl 3):S706–19.

57. Kelly EM. Temporary transcutaneous (external) pacing. In: Wiegand DJ, Carlson KK, eds. AACN procedure manual for critical care. 5th edn. Philadelphia: WB Saunders; 2005:333–9.

58. Gibson T. A practical guide to external cardiac pacing. Nurs Stand 2008;22(20):45–8.

59. Hatchett R, Thompson D, eds. Cardiac nursing: a comprehensive guide. Edinburgh: Churchill Livingstone; 2002.

60. Woods SL, Sivarajan-Froelicher ES, Halpenny CJ et al. Cardiac nursing. 4th edn. Philadelphia: Lippincott; 2000.

61. Booker R. Simple spirometry measurement. Nurs Stand 2008;22(32):35–9.

62. RxKinetics. Estimating height in bedridden patients. Online. www.rxkinetics.com/height_estimate.html; 6 March 2015.

63. The Joanna Briggs Institute. Management of peripheral intravascular devices. Best practice: evidence-based practice information sheets for the health professionals 1998;2(1):1–6. Online. http://connect.jbiconnectplus.org/ViewSourceFile.aspx?0=439; 1998.

64. Tintinalli JE, Kelen GD, Stapczynski JS, eds. Emergency medicine: a comprehensive study guide. 6th edn. New York: McGraw-Hill; 2004.

65. Liu SW, Zane R. Peripheral intravenous access. In: Roberts JR, Hedges JR, eds. Clinical procedures in emergency medicine. 6th edn. Philadelphia: WB Saunders; 2014:385–6.

66. Queensland Health Central Zone. Venepuncture and peripheral intravenous cannulation. Queensland: Queensland Government; 2004.

67. Dolan B, Holt L. Accident and emergency theory into practice. Edinburgh: Baillière Tindall; 2000.

68. Potter PA, Perry AG. Fundamentals of nursing. 5th edn. St Louis: Mosby; 2001.

69. Dutta A, Puri GD, Wig J. Piroxicam gel, compared to EMLA cream is associated with less pain after venous cannulation in volunteers. Can J Anaesth 2003;50(8):775–8.

70. Lander JA, Weltman BJ. Topical anaesthetics (EMLA and AMETOP creams) for reduction of pain during needle insertion in children (Protocol). Cochrane Database Syst Rev 2002;(4).

71. MIMS Online. http://proxy36.use.hcn.com.au/Search/Search.aspx; accessed 22 Oct 2010.

72. Andreoni C. Pediatric emergencies. In: Sheehy SB, ed. Sheehy's Manual of emergency care. 6th edn. St. Louis: Mosby; 2005.

73. Duff AJ. Incorporating psychological approaches into routine paediatric venepuncture. Arch Dis Child 2003;88(10):931–7.

74. Couttie T. Southern health network emergency department. Paediatric Intravenous Cannulation Package. South Eastern Sydney Illawarra Area Health Service; 2009.

75. Fenwick R. Intraosseous approach to vascular access in adult resuscitation. Emerg Nurse 2010;18(4):22–5.
76. Infusion Nurses Society. The role of the registered nurse in the insertion of intraosseous access devices. J Infus Nurs 2009;32(4):187–8.
77. Deitch K. Intraosseous infusion. In: Roberts JR, Hedges JR, eds. Clinical procedures in emergency medicine. 6th edn. Philadelphia: WB Saunders; 2014:455–68.
78. McCarthy G, O'Donnell C, O'Brien M. Successful intraosseous infusion in the critically ill patient does not require a medullary cavity. Resuscitation 2003;56(2):183–6.
79. Vidacare. EZ-IO needle sets. Directions for use. Online. www.vidacare.com/corporate/index.html; 2009.
80. Proehl J. Adult emergency nursing procedures. Boston: WB Saunders; 1999.
81. Lewis SM, Heitkemper MM, Dirksen SR. Medical–surgical nursing: assessment and management of clinical problems. 5th edn. St Louis: Mosby; 2000.
82. Celinski SA, Seneff MG. Arterial line placement and care. In: Irwin RS, Rippe JM, eds. Intensive care medicine. 6th edn. Philadelphia: Lippincott Williams & Wilkins; 2008:38–47.
83. Garretson S. Haemodynamic monitoring: arterial catheters. Nurs Stand 2005;19(31):55–64.
84. Becker DE. Arterial catheter insertion (perform) AP. In: Wiegand DJ, Carlson KK, eds. AACN procedure manual for critical care. 5th edn. St Louis: WB Saunders; 2005:445–50.
85. Daily EK, Schroeder JS, eds. Techniques in bedside hemodynamic monitoring. 5th edn. St Louis: Mosby; 1994.
86. Scales K. Central venous pressure monitoring in clinical practice. Nurs Stand 2010;24(29):49–55.
87. Shaffer RB. Blood sampling from an arterial catheter. In: Wiegand DJ, Carlson KK, eds. AACN procedure manual for critical care. 5th edn. St Louis: WB Saunders; 2005:465–71.
88. Woodrow P. Arterial catheters: promoting safe clinical practice. Nurs Stand 2009;24(4):35–40.
89. McNeil C, Rezaie S, Adams BD. Central venous catheterization and central venous pressure monitoring. In: Roberts JR, Hedges JR, eds. Clinical procedures in emergency medicine. 6th edn. Philadelphia: WB Saunders; 2014:397–431.
90. Arrow International. Central venous catheter: nursing care. Guideline 1996.
91. Munro N. Central venous catheter insertion (assist). In: Wiegand DJ, Carlson KK, eds. AACN procedure manual for critical care. 5th edn. St Louis: WB Saunders; 2005:651–8.
92. Woodrow P. Central venous catheters and central venous pressure. Nurs Stand 2002;16(26):45–51.
93. Munro N. Central venous/right atrial pressure monitoring. In: Wiegand DJ, Carlson KK, eds. AACN procedure manual for critical care. 5th edn. St Louis: WB Saunders; 2005:506–13.
94. Barry ME. Emergency: ankle sprains. Prompt and accurate diagnosis is crucial to proper healing. Am J Nurs 2001;101(10):40–2.
95. Marx JA, ed. Rosen's Emergency medicine: concepts and clinical practice. 7th edn. Philadelphia: Mosby; 2009.
96. Assal M, Crevoisier X. [Entorse aigue de la cheville: quelle immobilisation?] Acute ankle sprain: which immobilization? Rev Med Suisse 2009;5(212):1551–4.
97. Australian Resuscitation Council. Envenomation: pressure immobilisation technique. Revised policy statement: guideline 8.9.1. ARC; 2005.
98. Canale E, Isbister GK, Currie BJ. Investigating pressure bandaging for snakebite in a simulated setting: bandage type, training and the effect of transport. Emerg Med Australas 2009;21(3):184–90.
99. Engels P T, Passos E, Beckett AN et al. IV access in bleeding trauma patients: A performance review. Injury, Elsevier 2013;45(1):77–82.
100. Auerbach Paul S. Wilderness Medicine, 6th edn. St Louis: Mosby; 2012:488–506.
101. Marx JA, Hockberger RS, Walls RM. Rosen's Emergency Medicine, 8th edn. Philadelphia: Saunders. 2014:2449–56.
102. Roberts JR. Intravenous regional anesthesia. In: Roberts JR, Hedges JR, eds. Clinical procedures in emergency medicine. 6th edn. Philadelphia: WB Saunders; 2014:580–5.
103. Geeraedts LM, Kaasjager, HA, van Vugt AB, Frölke JP. Exsanguination in trauma: A review of diagnostics and treatment options. Injury, Elsevier 2008;40(1):11–20.
104. Australian Resuscitation Council. Envenomation: pressure immobilisation technique. Revised policy statement: guideline 8.9.1. ARC; 2005.
105. Solomon L, Warwick D, Nayagam S. Apley's Concise system of orthopaedics and fractures. 3rd edn. London: Arnold; 2005.
106. Simon RR, Sherman SC, Koenigsknecht SJ. Emergency orthopedics: the extremities. 5th edn. New York: McGraw-Hill; 2006.
107. Olson SA. An instructional course lecture, the American Academy of Orthopedic Surgeons. J Bone Joint Surg Am 1996;78(9):1428–37.
108. Landry PS, Marino AA, Sadasivan KK et al. Effect of soft tissue trauma on the early periosteal response of bone to injury. J Trauma 2000;48(3):479–83.
109. Altizer L. Casting for immobilization. Orthop Nurs 2004;23(2):136–41.
110. Howard PK, Steinmann RA. Sheehy's Emergency nursing: principles and practice. 6th edn. St Louis: Mosby; 2009.
111. Chudnofsky CR. Splinting techniques. In: Roberts JR, Hedges JR, eds. Clinical procedures in emergency medicine. 6th edn. Philadelphia: WB Saunders; 2014:999–1027.
112. Peck R, ed. Advanced emergency care manual—8th edn. Australian Ski Patrol Association. Online. www.skipatrol.org.au/training/AECManual10thEditionfeb2012_-_Ch1_to_9.pdf
113. Walsh D, Caraceni AT, Fainsinger R et al. Palliative medicine. Philadelphia: WB Saunders; 2008.
114. Cole A. Nurse-administered femoral nerve block after hip fracture. Nursing Times 2005;101(37):34–6.
115. Ardery G et al. Lack of opioid administration in older hip fracture patients. Mosby, 2003.

116. Wong J et al. A study of hospital recovery pattern of acutely confused older patients following hip surgery. Journal of Orthopaedic Nursing 2002; 6:68–78.

117. Wilson H. Factors affecting the administration of analgesia to patients following repair of a fractured hip. Journal of Advanced Nursing 2000;31(5):1145–54.

118. Finlayson BJ, Underhill TJ. Femoral nerve block for analgesia in fractures of the femoral neck. Archives of Emergency Medicine 1988; 5:173–6.

119. Stella J et al. Nerve stimulator-assisted femoral nerve block in the emergency department. Emergency Medicine 2000;12:322–5.

120. Fernandez DL, Palmer AK. Fractures of the distal radius. In Green DP, Hotchkiss RN, Pederson WC, Wolfe SW, eds. Green's Operative Hand Surgery, 5th edn. Philadelphia: Churchill Livingstone, 2005.

121. Fletcher AK et al. Three-in-one femoral nerve block as analgesia for fractured neck of femur in the emergency department: a randomized controlled trial. Annals of Emergency Medicine 2003;41(2):227–33.

122. Foss NB et al. Fascia iliaca compartment blockade for acute pain control in hip fracture patients: a randomized, placebo-controlled trial. Anesthesiology 2007;106(4):773–8.

123. NICE Clinical Guidelines, No. 124 The Management of Hip Fracture in Adults. National Clinical Guideline Centre (UK). London: Royal College of Physicians (UK). 2011.

124. Roberts JR. Chapter 34, Roberts and Hedges' clinical procedures in emergency medicine. 6th edn. Philadelphia: Saunders 2014; 611–43.

125. MIMs Online https://www.mimsonline.com.au/Search/FullPI.aspx?ModuleName=Product Info&searchKeyword=Marcain+0.25%25+Injection&PreviousPage=~/Search/QuickSearch.aspx&SearchType=&ID=19110008_2; accessed 5 March 2015.

126. Weinberg GL. Treatment of local anesthetic systemic toxicity (LAST). Reg Anesth Pain Med 2010;35(2):188–93.

127. Kelly JJ, Spektor M. Nerve blocks of the thorax and extremities. In: Roberts JR, Hedges JR, eds. Clinical procedures in emergency medicine. 5th edn. Philadelphia: WB Saunders; 2010:554–79.

128. Murphy-Lavoie H, Legros TL. Local and regional anaesthesia. In: Adams JG eds. Emergency medicine. 2nd edn. Philadelphia: Saunders; 2008:1578–86.

129. Australian Medicines Handbook. Adapted from Table 2-3 Comparison of local anaesthetics. Richmond: Hyde Park Press; 2015; 33.

130. Emiley P, Schreier S, Pryor P. Hematoma blocks for reduction of distal radius fractures. www.epmonthly.com/features/current-features/hematoma-blocks-for-reduction-of-distal-radius-fractures-/ Accessed 6 March 2015.

131. Miller M, Hart J, MacKnight J. Essential Orthopaedics, III-III Philadelphia: Saunders. 2010.

132. Roberts J. Nerve blocks of the thorax and extremities in Roberts and Hedges' clinical procedures in emergency medicine, 6th edn, Philadelphia: Saunders 2014;554–79.

133. Brinker D, Hancox JD, Bernardon SO. Assessment and initial treatment of lacerations, mammalian bites, and insect stings. AACN Clin Issues 2003;14(4):401–10.

134. Cooper MA, Lindsay GM, Kinn S et al. Evaluating emergency nurse practitioner services: a randomized controlled trial. J Adv Nurs 2002;40(6):721–30.

135. Meeker MH, Rothrock JC. Alexander's care of the patient in surgery. 11th edn. St Louis: Mosby; 1999.

136. Swanson NA, Tromovitch TA. Suture materials 1980s: properties, uses and abuses. Int J Dermatol 1982;21:373–8.

137. Feliciano DV, Moore EE, Mattox KL, eds. Trauma. 3rd edn. Stamford: Appleton & Lange; 1996.

138. Carley S. Glue is better than sutures for facial lacerations in children. (2001) BestBETs: Best evidence topics. Online. Available: www.bestbets.org/cgi-bin/bets.pl?record=00022; accessed 20 Dec 2006.

139. Yanoff M, Duker JS. Ophthalmology. 3rd edn. St Louis: Mosby; 2008.

140. Knoop KJ, Dennis WR. Opthalmologic procedures. In: Roberts JR, Hedges JR, eds. Clinical procedures in emergency medicine. 6th edn. Philadelphia: WB Saunders; 2014.

141. Riordan-Eva P, Whitcher JP, eds. Vaughan & Asbury's General opthalmology. 17th edn. New York: McGraw-Hill; 2007.

142. López AM, Valero R, Bovaira P et al. A critical evaluation of four disposable laryngeal face masks in adult patients. Journal of Clinical Anesthesia. 2008;20(7):514–20.

143. Fleisher LA, Gaiser R, eds. 2008 Anesthesia procedures consult. Elsevier, Philadelphia, PA. Online. www.proceduresconsult.com/medical-procedures/anesthesia-specialty.aspx; accessed 12 March 2015.

144. Waldman SD. Atlas of interventional pain management. 4th edn. Philadelphia: WB Saunders; 2015.

145. Browner B, Fuller R. Musculoskeletal emergencies, Elsevier; 2012:i–iii.

146. Green DP, Hotchkiss RN, Pederson WC, Wolfe SW, eds: Green's Operative hand surgery, 5th edn. Philadelphia: Churchill Livingstone, 2005.

147. Miller M, Hart J, MacKnight J. Essential Orthopaedics. Philadelphia: Saunders; 2010:424–7.

148. Aehlert BJ. Airway management. Paramedic practice today. Mosby, Elsevier 2010.

149. Drake R, Vogl AW, Mitchell AWM et al. Gray's Atlas of Anatomy. Philadelphia, Churchill Livingstone/Elsevier, 2008:290.

150. Stone DB, Scordino D. Foreign body removal. In Roberts JR, Hedges JR, eds. Clinical procedures in emergency medicine. 6th edn. Philadelphia: WB Saunders; 2014:690–718.

151. Davey AJ. Chapter 20: Medical suction apparatus. In: Ward's Anaesthetic Equipment. Elsevier 2012:425.

152. Life in the Fast Lane. website. http://lifeinthefastlane.com/education/lead-positioning; accessed 29 June 2015.

153. Klimke A, Furin M. Fig 46-35 In: Roberts and Hedges' clinical procedures in emergency medicine. Philadelphia: WB Saunders; 2014: pp. 893–922.e2. Reproduced with permission from Norman E. McSwain, Jr., MD, FACS, and Richard L. Garrnelli, MD, FACS—American College of Surgeons Committee on Trauma, April 1997).

CHAPTER 18
MINOR INJURY AND MANAGEMENT

TESSA ROGERS AND KERYN JONES

Essentials

- Practise a systematic approach to patient assessment to avoid missing injuries. Always look for the second injury.
- Proper wound cleansing is the key to minimising infection. Antibiotic prophylaxis should be the exception rather than the rule.
- Listen to the patient as they describe the mechanism of injury, as this will lead you to the likely diagnosis.

INTRODUCTION

Patients with minor injuries comprise a reasonable portion of workload for clinicians in various clinical settings, ranging from remote and rural clinics to emergency departments (EDs), although the exact percentage they represent is not well documented in Australasia.

The definition of 'minor injury' is also not clear-cut. However, those patients with less-urgent complaints have traditionally waited the longest time for treatment, when often, with a clear diagnostic pathway, their total treatment time could indeed be very short. Many EDs have recognised this and have implemented additional fast-tracking measures[1-3] to expedite and facilitate patient management, often by filtering minor injury and illness patients into a separate queue and area of the department after triage. Many EDs now use specifically trained, extended-practice nurses for this purpose,[4,5] who are able to undertake a focused examination, request X-rays and provide analgesia. A growing number of EDs now employ nurse practitioners who have a major role in the autonomous care of patients falling into this category.[6,7] Controversies regarding the quality and expertise of the nurse practitioner role are now being lifted since many studies have evaluated care as comparable to that of a medical officer. They are cost-effective, have reduced the percentage of patients who do not wait to be seen and generate a high level of patient satisfaction.[8-11]

Pre-hospital care

Initial out-of-hospital care for people with minor injuries follows the same principles of primary and secondary assessment. As for all patients, assessment should be guided by the systematic process of assessing for danger and patient responsiveness, and shouting for assistance where indicated. Assessment then of airway, breathing and circulation (DRSABC), identifying and stabilising the patient before secondary assessment begins. Be mindful of the tendency to focus on a single obvious injury.

A systematic approach from 'head to toe' ensures all injuries are identified, and need not be time-consuming. Minor injuries can often occur concurrently with other, more significant injury and risk being overlooked. Patient history should be used to guide assessment; some injuries are clearly isolated, e.g. crush injury to a digit. A mechanical fall onto an outstretched hand may injure any structure of the upper limb and can potentially cause injury elsewhere.

Some patients with an isolated minor injury may not present to a hospital setting, depending on patient preference for care or geographical location. If a suitably qualified and experienced clinician is available, some injuries may be managed in the field and hospital care may not be required.

Initial assessment

After obtaining a brief history of the injury, use of the simple structure of 'inspect', 'palpate' and 'move' provides a systematic formula for a brief focused assessment (Box 18.1). Remove clothes, cutting them off if necessary to expose the whole limb. If a fracture is suspected, moving the injured limb may not be appropriate; however, it may be diagnostic to do so, e.g. pain on elbow pronation and inability to fully extend the joint helping to diagnose a fracture of the radial head, prior to X-ray.

This structure can be implemented in the pre-hospital, triage or full clinician assessment.

Practical care

The following measures should be implemented to prevent further damage to musculoskeletal structures and enhance comfort while the patient is transported to another care facility.

Cover all wounds with a clean or ideally sterile dressing and apply pressure if the wound is bleeding. Grossly contaminated wounds can be irrigated with clean tap water, if available and time allows, by simply pouring copious amounts of water onto the wound. In the pre-hospital setting, mechanical irrigation with clean drinking water will aid in the removal of debris and contaminants, reduce microbial contamination and serve to reduce infection risk. Bacteria begin multiplying in as little as 6 hours in contaminated wounds. If the wound is left contaminated, an infection can establish itself within 24 hours.[12] Interestingly, more recent studies have challenged the need to irrigate simple, non-contaminated wounds in highly vascular areas, such as the scalp and face.[13]

Consider splinting, particularly if a fracture is suspected (see Chapter 17, p. 352, for splinting techniques). By minimising movement, the bone ends are less likely to cause further damage to nerves, vessels and other soft tissues and will prevent a closed fracture from becoming compound.[14] Chapter 17, p. 348, contains further information on dealing with soft tissue injuries. Obvious deformity can be gently corrected to as normal anatomical positioning as possible. The distal pulses should be checked before and after reduction or splinting, and regularly until definitive care is provided.

Elevate the limb to reduce swelling, which may compromise neurovascular status and increase pain. A sling may be useful for upper limb trauma.

Applying ice for a period of 20 minutes every 1–2 hours has been demonstrated to reduce pain, but it is debatable whether it speeds ultimate recovery.[15] An ice pack can be simply made by wrapping a pack of frozen peas or corn kernels in a damp towel; this conforms to the joint shape.

Provision of oral, inhalational or intravenous analgesia from qualified personnel will aid comfort, and the reduction in pain may reduce anxiety.[16]

Ensure ongoing information and reassurance to the patient and relatives.

Hospital/health facility care

Initial in-hospital care would include several elements of the measures as outlined above and ongoing management will depend on the available facilities and expertise on site. In the ED/hospital/clinic setting, a more thorough examination would assess for changes in motor function or mobility, and neurological or vascular compromise with a view to planning definitive care. After clinician examination, further care should include ongoing pain relief, radiological imaging as indicated, and manipulation, or reduction of displaced fractures or dislocations. Any wounds would require definitive cleansing and dressing, and splints, plaster casts or other immobilisation devices can be applied.

Less complicated injuries may be managed in their entirety by the treating clinician, with more complex injuries requiring referral for specialist consultation, further urgent or elective operative or non-operative management. This may require transferring the patient to another facility. Consideration can also be given to judicious antibiotic use and ensuring adequate tetanus immunity.

A systematic approach to injury assessment

Minor injury assessment may take place as part of a secondary survey, or in some cases as a focused examination isolated to a

---

BOX 18.1 Assessment of musculoskeletal injuries

Inspect
- Deformity
- Swelling
- Bruising
- Skin perfusion at the site and distal to the injury
- Location and type of any wounds
- Comparison with the other limb

Palpate
- Crepitus
- Bony tenderness
- Skin temperature
- Distal pulses
- Altered sensation distal to injury

Move
- *If appropriate*: gentle active range of movement

single limb, for example, a hand laceration, or crush injury to a foot. It is valuable to adopt a methodical examination process, which in due course becomes routine. Remember, a clear history and mechanism of injury will often aid in the process. A systematic approach is suggested below.

Inspection—'LOOK'

Observe for deformity and asymmetry (comparison to the other limb where possible), local swelling, joint effusion, contusions (bruising), open wounds and their location over underlying structures, likely and actual foreign bodies and contamination of wounds. Assess distal perfusion.

Palpation—'FEEL'

Is there generalised tenderness from local inflammation, or a maximal point tenderness indicating possible underlying structural injury? Assess for bony crepitus, palpable mal-alignment, soft tissue swelling, joint instability. Assess for normal distal sensation.

Movement—'MOVE'

Consider testing movement of a limb or joint gently prior to X-ray if it will help with possible diagnosis.

Be cautious where there is significant swelling, deformity, or where movement exacerbates pain considerably. Assess for normal distal nerve motor function. Range of movement may be best tested after radiological examination results are known and may yield better results, particularly once a fracture has been excluded.

Anatomical terms of motion

Flexion: a reduction in angle between two body parts

Extension: an increase in angle between two body parts

Internal rotation: rotation of body part towards the midline axis of body

External rotation: rotation of body part away from the midline axis of body

Abduction: moving of body part away from midline axis of body, spreading the fingers

Adduction: moving of body part towards the midline axis of body, or closing the fingers together

Supination: rotation of forearm or ankle inwards, so that palms of hand/soles of feet turn upwards

Pronation: rotation of forearm or ankle outwards, so that palms of hand/soles of feet turn downwards

Inversion: (ankle/foot) tilting of the foot towards the midline of body

Eversion (ankle/foot) tilting of the foot away from the midline of body

Dorsiflexion: where the foot is moved towards the shin

Plantarflexion: where the foot is moved away from the shin, i.e. standing on tip toes

Opposition: touching the tip of the index and thumb together to form a circle shape

Documenting the patient's range of motion in degrees for a particular body area is a useful way of recording current joint movement. This can be used to judge improvement or deterioration in condition. For example, a knee is considered to be at 0° when it is fully extended and at approximately 135° at full flexion.

Injuries around the shoulder

Anatomy and function

The humerus, clavicle, acromion, scapula and sternum form the articulating bony structure of the shoulder complex. It comprises the sternoclavicular, the acromioclavicular and the 'ball and socket' glenohumeral joints, which in combination attach the upper limb to the scapula and sternum. The shoulder has a wide range of movement and is stabilised by many muscles, ligaments and tendons. The humeral head is held into the glenoid by the four rotator cuff muscles. Blood is supplied to the arm via two branches from the axillary artery, the anterior and posterior circumflex arteries. The axillary nerve curls around the humeral neck, clinically important in injuries to this area, and the three main nerves of the arm, the median, radial and ulnar, all pass through the axilla (Fig 18.1).

Patient assessment

Most shoulder injuries occur following a direct blow to the shoulder girdle or a fall onto the outstretched hand.

Significant injuries to the shoulder will be accompanied by likely swelling, deformity and focal tenderness. Compare the appearance with that of the other shoulder. A patient with an empty glenoid on clinical examination, a slightly externally rotated arm and severe pain is likely to have a shoulder dislocation and should be managed as soon as possible (see Ch 50). The best pain relief for a dislocation is relocation.

There may be bruising if the presentation is delayed. Palpation should begin with the cervical spine and then include the entire clavicle, acromioclavicular joint, humeral head, neck and shaft to the elbow and wrist. Fractures to the scapula, which usually require a significant mechanism, should be excluded by palpating for bony tenderness. Axillary nerve function should be checked specifically by testing sensation over the deltoid muscle in comparison with the other arm. A palpable radial

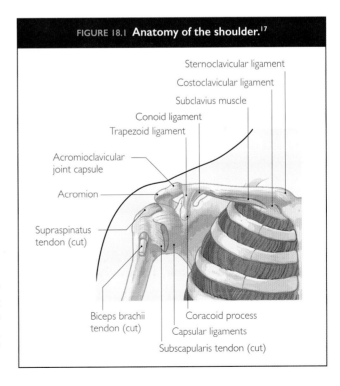

FIGURE 18.1 **Anatomy of the shoulder.**[17]

Sternoclavicular ligament
Costoclavicular ligament
Subclavius muscle
Conoid ligament
Trapezoid ligament
Acromioclavicular joint capsule
Acromion
Supraspinatus tendon (cut)
Biceps brachii tendon (cut)
Coracoid process
Capsular ligaments
Subscapularis tendon (cut)

pulse should also be recorded. If the patient is able, they can be asked to perform gentle passive shoulder movements to assess range of movement.

Clavicle

Clavicular fractures constitute 5% of all fractures; they comprise more than 10–15% of all childhood fractures,[18] and are more common in males.[19] There is focal tenderness, swelling and sometimes bruising over the site and pain on movement of the arm. The skin over the fracture site should be checked and a referral made to an orthopaedic specialist if skin integrity is at risk, or the fracture is compound. Fractures are generally easily identified on X-ray and although there is controversy regarding the value of surgical fixation of displaced mid-clavicular fractures, in Australia most are treated conservatively in a broad arm sling and mobilised as pain allows.[20,21]

There is no evidence that figure-of-eight bandaging aids fracture alignment or healing (see Ch 17, p. 349, for instructions on this technique).[22]

Proximal humerus

Some 70% of fractures to the humeral head and neck are seen in the over-60-years age group, usually following a fall onto an outstretched hand. Like fractures of the hip, they are a major cause of morbidity in the older person,[23] and osteoporosis may be a contributing factor. As in all falls, particularly in the older person, the cause must be established and other injuries excluded. The patient will have pain around the shoulder and restricted range of movement. If the presentation is delayed, there is often marked bruising around the upper arm and sometimes chest wall. Axillary nerve function should be assessed. Extra-articular fractures that are relatively undisplaced can be treated conservatively in a close-fitting support sling that minimises movement. Fracture/dislocations of the humeral head should be referred on for an orthopaedic opinion. Humeral shaft fractures are again treated conservatively unless they are open or there are multiple fractures present elsewhere.

Acromioclavicular joint

The acromioclavicular joint (ACJ) can be sprained or dislocated after a blow or fall onto the shoulder. There will be focal tenderness and swelling over the ACJ. Do not confuse a prominent ACJ with a shoulder dislocation, as the deformity seen can occasionally be quite striking. X-rays should be requested specifically of the ACJ, and comparative views of the other shoulder may be provided. The diagnosis is both clinical and radiological. A sprain may damage the ACJ ligaments, but the clavicle remains in contact with the acromion. Treatment consists of a broad arm sling and rest for 4–6 weeks. In more severe injuries, there is separation of the clavicle from the acromion as the trapezoid and coracoid ligaments are torn. These injuries are more likely to be unstable and the patient should be referred for a specialist orthopaedic opinion.

Injuries to the elbow, forearm and wrist

Anatomy and function

The hinge joint of the elbow consists of the distal humerus, proximal radius and proximal ulna. They are held in position by ligaments and the associated musculature. The elbow can be flexed and extended and the forearm pronated and supinated (a rotational movement of the forearm at the radioulnar joint). The wrist is comprised of a series of joints that are very mobile, particularly between the proximal and distal rows of the carpal bones, allowing a wide range of movement in several planes. The complex ligamentous structure can be easily injured during trauma, particularly in a fall onto the hand. The median, radial and ulnar nerves all travel through the wrist (the median nerve passing through the carpal tunnel) and allow hand and wrist function and skin innervation. The radial and ulnar arteries provide the hand with blood and are both palpable on the volar aspect of the wrist (Fig 18.2).

Patient assessment

Again, mechanism of injury is of particular importance and requires a focused examination. Falls onto the outstretched hand can provide forces that may damage any part of the upper limb. Look for general evidence of injury: swelling, deformity, bruising. Examination should begin with palpation and gross movement of the shoulder to exclude injury here. The humerus can then be palpated down to the elbow region, examining for bony tenderness over the medial and lateral epicondyles, the olecranon and the radial head. It is unusual for the elbow or wrist to be swollen without a fracture being present, in contrast to the ankle, for example.

In the absence of deformity, and if pain allows, gentle active range of movement at the elbow can be assessed. The 'elbow extension test' can be utilised. The patient is asked to extend both arms with the hands supinated. A UK study in 2008[24] found that if patients could fully extend both elbows, the negative prediction for fracture was 98% in adults and 96% for children. Pain on gentle supination and pronation of the forearm is also a common finding in fractures of the radial head and neck.

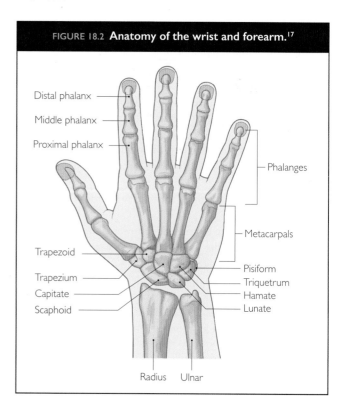

FIGURE 18.2 Anatomy of the wrist and forearm.[17]

Distal phalanx
Middle phalanx
Proximal phalanx
Phalanges
Metacarpals
Trapezoid
Pisiform
Trapezium
Triquetrum
Capitate
Hamate
Scaphoid
Lunate
Radius Ulnar

Palpation should continue to the wrist and hand. Identify and palpate the distal radius, ulnar styloid and the scaphoid bone (Fig 18.3). Be alert not to miss a scaphoid fracture in a patient with a swollen wrist after a fall onto the hand with normal X-rays, and take care to differentiate between a scaphoid facture, a Bennett's fracture and a fracture of the distal radius by careful methodical palpation of each.

X-ray requests depend on the area of tenderness. If there is only elbow tenderness, elbow X-rays alone will suffice. Look carefully for a positive anterior and/or posterior fat pad or 'sail sign' (Fig 18.4) on the lateral elbow radiograph demonstrating a joint effusion. A posterior fat pad is indicative of a fracture in 90% of elbow injuries radiologically investigated,[25] even if the bony anatomy and cortex appear normal.[26,27] Forearm views include the elbow and forearm, while scaphoid views include the wrist so this does not need to be requested separately.

Common injuries around the elbow

Distal humerus

A fracture of the distal third of the humerus or supracondylar fracture is a common injury in childhood and occurs more infrequently in adults, following a fall onto the hand. Significantly displaced fractures pose a risk to neurovascular integrity and should be referred urgently. Excessive swelling may occlude the brachial artery and the radial pulse should be monitored frequently. However, many supracondylar fractures are undisplaced or only identifiable on X-rays by a positive fat pad sign. These are generally treated in a plaster of Paris (POP) above-elbow cast or a 'collar and cuff' sling with hyperflexion of the elbow, depending on local practice.

Proximal radius and ulna

The radial head and neck can both be fractured, causing pain and swelling around the elbow. The patient will generally find pronation and supination painful and will have a limited ability to fully extend the elbow. X-rays may show a fracture and/or a positive fat pad sign. Treatment consists of a broad arm sling, ice and analgesia. Some patients may be unable to pronate and supinate, and this may indicate a significant displacement of the radial head fracture fragment and warrant orthopaedic review.

Olecranon

The olecranon can be fractured from a fall directly onto the point of the elbow, and treatment is dependent on the degree of displacement. Undisplaced fractures can be treated again with a broad arm sling, ice and analgesia. Triceps contraction may displace the fracture, which then needs surgical fixation.

Elbow dislocation is seen in both the adult and the paediatric population and is generally identified clinically by significant pain and deformity at the elbow following a fall onto the hand. Careful neurovascular assessment should be made before and after relocation, which usually requires a general anaesthetic. Post-reduction X-rays should be checked to identify associated fractures, such as a medial epicondyle avulsion in a child.

Pulled elbow

Toddlers may present with a sudden onset of pain and reluctance to move an arm after a traction or pulling type mechanism. The child has no swelling or no bony tenderness, but forearm pronation is painful. In this injury, known as a 'pulled elbow', the radial head becomes subluxed and can be relocated by the simple manoeuvre of either extending the elbow and supinating the forearm or flexing the elbow and pronating the forearm. If the clinician's thumb is placed over the radial head, a click is usually felt with successful relocation. Relocation is usually painful but instantly relieving for the child, who quickly starts using the arm again. Neither method has been shown to be less painful or more successful than the other.[28] X-rays are not normally indicated where there is a good history of mechanism.

The injured forearm and wrist

Distal radius and ulna

The ulna and radius can be fractured in isolation, especially if there is a direct blow to the forearm. However, the bones

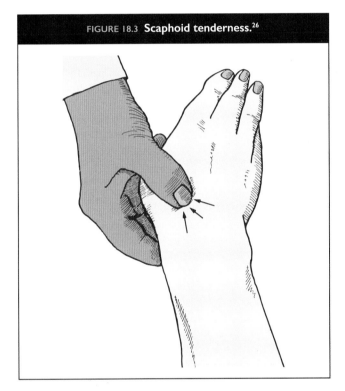

FIGURE 18.3 **Scaphoid tenderness.**[26]

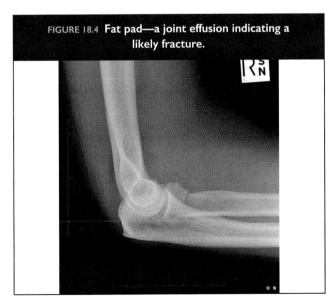

FIGURE 18.4 **Fat pad—a joint effusion indicating a likely fracture.**

are bound together at both ends by ligaments forming a type of linked parallelogram[26] and therefore it is most common for both bones to break. If there is an angulated fracture of either the radius or the ulna, the bone must become shorter in length and it is vital to exclude dislocation at one end of the other forearm bone. It is imperative, as previously discussed, for both the joint above and that below an injury to be examined. A Monteggia injury involves a fracture of the ulna with dislocation of the radial head. Conversely, a Galleazzi fracture–dislocation involves a fracture of the radius with dislocation of the radioulnar joint at the wrist. Both require surgical reduction.

One-third of all fractures in the elderly will involve the wrist, particularly elderly osteoporotic women.[29] It is also the most common fracture site in children, with the incidence increasing with age and in boys.[30]

A Colles' fracture is a fracture of the distal radius within 2.5 cm of the wrist[31] (Fig 18.5). With greater force the distal fragment becomes dorsally angulated, leading to the clinical deformity typical of the fracture, which is likened to a dinner fork. There may be an associated fracture of the ulnar styloid. The forearm can be immobilised with a POP splint for comfort while X-rays are taken.

The need for reduction depends on the degree of angulation and the age, frailness and usual activities of the patient. Methods of anaesthesia for reduction of the fracture vary depending on the facilities available, and include general anaesthetic, Bier block and haematoma block. Bier block, which provides regional anaesthesia, has been well validated for safety and effect;[32] however, resuscitation facilities should be available. Haematoma block effectiveness may vary with individual patients and the technique and expertise of the clinician, but is a technically easy and relatively safe procedure in areas where facilities are limited.

A reverse Colles', known as a Smith's fracture, is occasionally seen after a fall onto the back of the hand. Here the distal fragment is displaced anteriorly and usually requires surgical manipulation to correct it.

Wrist fractures in children

Children's fracture patterns vary from those of adults due to increased bone compliance and lower bone density. The bone frequently bends or wrinkles and a pattern of incomplete fractures is seen. A greenstick fracture involves a break in one bone cortex while the opposite cortex remains intact. They can vary from obvious clinical deformity and radiological angulation to subtle injuries where the child has few clinical signs of injury and mild pain which restricts use of the arm. Some greenstick fractures are so slight that parents may only seek advice after a few days of subtle symptoms. A torus fracture is also a frequently seen paediatric injury where X-rays show a compression deformity to the bone surface with the appearance of a bump or ripple to the cortex. Management in a correctly sized wrist splint for 3 weeks is adequate for torus injuries.[33] Both greenstick and torus fractures heal rapidly.

The young skeleton contains many physes, or 'growth plates' at one or both ends of the bone, where proliferation of cartilage cell growth with eventual differentiation into osteocytes occurs. Simply, bone manufacture occurs here and injuries involving the physis, if not managed correctly, can affect subsequent bone growth. These are known as Salter Harris injuries, named by Robert B Salter and W Robert Harris in 1963.[34] The management varies and depends on ensuring the epiphyseal surface is restored to promote ongoing cell manufacture. All Salter Harris fractures should be reviewed by an orthopaedic specialist.

Scaphoid

The scaphoid bone is the largest carpal bone and has a blood supply that enters from the distal end. A fracture can lead to avascular necrosis causing significant morbidity through hand disability; hence scaphoid injuries should not be overlooked. Clinically the patient will have scaphoid tenderness and often subtle swelling over the anatomical snuff box when compared with the other hand.

FIGURE 18.5 **Colles' fracture.**[31]

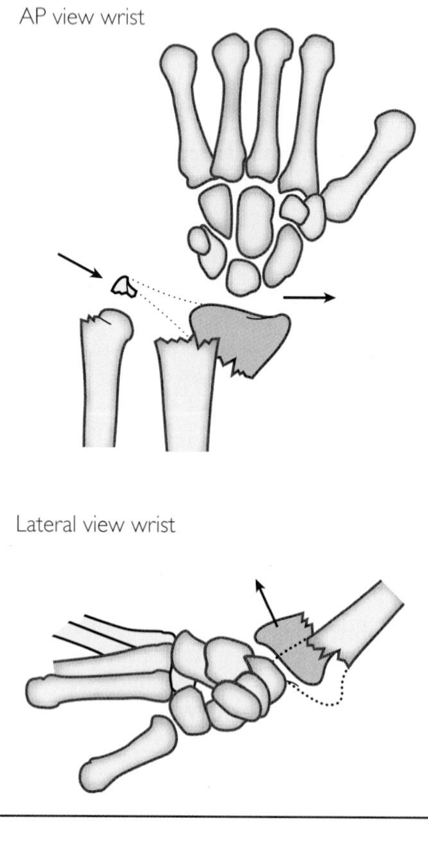

AP view wrist

Lateral view wrist

PRACTICE TIP

To locate the scaphoid bone, first locate the radial styloid and the base of the thumb. The anatomical snuff box, which overlies the scaphoid, is between these two points. Palpate over the scaphoid of both hands simultaneously and push the thumb up towards the wrist (telescoping) to identify tenderness.

Scaphoid fractures are one of the most commonly missed fractures.[35] This may be partially attributed to clinicians not identifying the exact location of the scaphoid on examination, and also to the difficulty of absolute diagnosis of a fracture at the initial consultation as X-rays are often normal. Up to 33% of patients with a proven scaphoid fracture will have normal preliminary X-rays, and of all patients immobilised in a cast or splint for suspected fractures only up to 10% will have a confirmed fracture.[36]

For suspected scaphoid fractures the review process varies greatly, with options varying between MRI (magnetic resonance imaging), computed tomography (CT), repeat X-rays in 7–10 days or bone scan after 4–5 days. A CT exam is likely to be cheaper and more sensitive than a bone scan and involves less radiation. Bone scan is 100% sensitive for excluding a fracture, but a positive bone scan may highlight other fractures and non-bony injuries, which are difficult to distinguish from a scaphoid fracture. MRI is currently the most expensive option in Australia and has to be ordered by a specialist. It is more specific than a bone scan and can be better at diagnosing soft tissue injuries.[37] Whichever mode is chosen, excluding a scaphoid fracture as soon as possible results in less time spent immobilised in a cast, less impact on daily activities and, for patients in employment, less time off work. Generally, local protocol and availability will guide practice. Confirmed scaphoid fractures are placed in a scaphoid cast for immobilisation, which should allow full movement of the finger metacarpophalangeal joints. Displaced fractures may be managed with surgical fixation.

Injuries of the hand and digits

Anatomy and function
The hand is an intricate structure with complex motor and sensory functions. An injury to the hand may interrupt any number of structures, which could in turn affect ability to perform basic functions and potentially affect a patient's livelihood.

The eight carpal bones, which facilitate movement of the hand and wrist, form two rows that articulate proximally with the distal radius and ulna and distally with the metacarpals. The largest carpal bone is the medially situated scaphoid. There are five metacarpals corresponding respectively with each finger and the thumb. The fingers should be correctly termed index, middle, ring and little. Movement of the fingers is controlled by four muscle groups which flex and extend the metacarpal joints and the interphalangeal joints. The back of the hand is known as the dorsal surface and the front as the palmar or volar surface. Sensation is supplied by the median, radial and ulnar nerves leading to the digital nerves in each digit.

Patient assessment
Ascertain the mechanism first. A fall onto an outstretched hand will involve a different injury pattern to that of direct trauma, such as a crush or punch injury. Observe for swelling, deformity and distal perfusion of the fingers. Bruising, especially on the palm, often suggests a metacarpal fracture, and bruising over the volar surface of a finger joint is common after an avulsion fracture. Note the location of any wounds and their cause; for example, a bite injury which may be associated with a tendon injury (see the section on hand and digit wounds later in the chapter).

Palpate systematically, from the clavicle if indicated and ending with the digits. Gently test active movement of the hand by asking the patient to make a fist. Watch for finger rotation,

where the nail orientation appears to be different to that of other fingers, as the fingers are gently flexed into a fist; this clinically identifies a displaced fracture. A fixed interphalangeal joint with obvious deformity is probably dislocated.

X-ray requests should be specific and based on careful clinical evaluation. Carpal and metacarpal tenderness warrants hand X-rays. Remember that a suspected scaphoid X-ray includes wrist and scaphoid views, but not the hand. For suspected finger fractures and dislocations, ask for views of the finger specifically, and ensure a lateral X-ray of the digit(s) is included. Dislocations and, in particular, small avulsion injuries may be seen on the volar surface of an interphalangeal joint, can be overlooked if the lateral is not studied carefully and can cause significant disability if missed.

PRACTICE TIP

If a patient is to be transported to another facility for X-ray or specialist review, the injured hand should be immobilised in a cast in the 'position of safety'. The cast should hold the wrist in extension, the metacarpal joints in flexion at 90° and the fingers extended straight (Fig 18.6).

Fractures and ligamentous injuries of the hand
All hand injuries should be considered significant; incorrect treatment may cause ongoing pain and limitation of future hand use. It is prudent to refer all patients with fractures of the hand and fingers to a hand or orthopaedic specialist, but this will depend on the patient's location, the services available and the experience of the clinician managing the patient.

Metacarpals
Metacarpal fractures are common and may be sustained following a fall onto the hand, crush mechanisms and punch injuries. Check for finger rotation, as this indicates an angulated fracture which may need reduction and fixation. As with all fractures, but of particular importance in the hand, the clinician should observe for corresponding wounds rendering the fracture open and any potential damage to nerves and tendons.

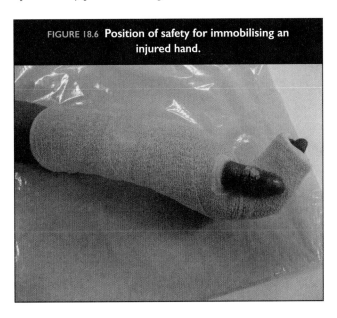

FIGURE 18.6 **Position of safety for immobilising an injured hand.**

The boxer's fracture is one that occurs to the base of the fifth metacarpal, usually following a blow to the knuckles with a clenched fist. Patients may be reluctant to admit the exact mechanism. Unless the fracture is significantly angulated, or there is finger rotation, treatment with a cast or neighbour strapping, depending on local policy, is satisfactory.

A Bennett's fracture occurs at the base of the thumb metacarpal after a fall onto the fist or the hand with the thumb abducted or outstretched, such as a skier falling while holding a ski pole. There is tenderness over the base of the thumb which should not be confused with scaphoid tenderness. The base of the metacarpal becomes subluxed and needs surgical fixation. The ligaments that secure the thumb metacarpal at the first metacarpal-phalangeal joint can also be damaged by a similar mechanism; particularly the ulnar collateral ligament on the medial aspect of the joint can be sprained or torn. There may also be a fracture. Test for instability by passive stressing of the joint with the MCP flexed to 30 degrees. Any instability requires plaster immobilisation and a surgical opinion from a hand specialist.

Phalanges

A mallet finger occurs when a straight finger sustains a blow to the end, flexing the distal interphalangeal joint. The extensor tendon is torn from its attachment and the patient presents with a flexion deformity at the distal interphalangeal joint and is unable to actively extend or straighten the fingertip. There is sometimes an associated fracture. Treatment involves a mallet splint for 6–8 weeks which holds the finger extended. The patient can remove the splint for washing the finger only if the finger is held strictly in extension by pressing the fingertip against a hard surface.

The fingers and thumb joints can become dislocated following a hyperextension type injury, which can be easily identified by clinical deformity (Fig 18.7). The injury may be open if the skin is lacerated over the joint, and good wound cleansing is essential.

Reduction after X-ray can be performed using an inhalational anxiolytic such as nitrous oxide (e.g. Entonox), a digital block or with no additional pain relief at the patient's discretion. Care should be taken to identify any fractures, particularly

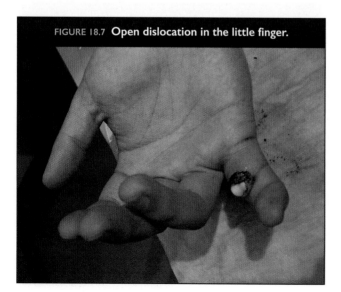

FIGURE 18.7 **Open dislocation in the little finger.**

small avulsion fractures, with a post-reduction X-ray. Fingers should be buddy-strapped to the adjacent digit for 2 weeks and the thumb post dislocation should be splinted with POP, metal splinting material or fibreglass.

Hand and digit lacerations

Wounds involving only the skin layers may be cleaned and closed by primary or secondary intention. Care should be taken to ascertain a thorough history of the injury. Wounds sustained on glass or knives, for example, may appear superficial, but may have penetrated deeply.

> **PRACTICE TIP**
>
> Good hand anatomy knowledge is essential to proper hand laceration assessment. Ask yourself which structures lie beneath the laceration and be thorough in your assessment of them to avoid missing an important injury. If in doubt ask for advice or send the patient for a specialist opinion.

Lacerations of the hand and digits should be explored through a full range of motion, as the deeper structures move below the laceration. A tendon injury sustained with a clenched fist and flexed digits may not be visible on examination when the digits are extended, as the tendon retracts away from the wound site. Complete lacerations of tendons will result in loss of motor function and a loss to the normal finger cascade. Hand cascade can be assessed with the dorsal surface of the hand resting on the examination table. The fingers should normally lie uniformly with a natural curve in slight flexion. An abnormally extended finger in comparison to the other digits has most likely been caused by a complete flexor tendon laceration. Likewise, a drooping finger, when all other fingers are extended, shows an extensor tendon laceration. Partial lacerations of tendons controlling flexion or extension of the digit may not affect the motor function of the hand initially, but may weaken the tendon and completely rupture at a later stage under ongoing tension. Surgery to repair complete tendon rupture can be extensive. Assess for pain at the wound site as the digits are moved against resistance, which is diagnostic of a partial tendon laceration. If a partial or complete laceration is suspected, the patient should be referred for surgical exploration.

Lacerations occurring over a joint may penetrate the joint capsule, risking joint-space infection, or may sever supporting ligaments leaving the joint unstable. Lacerations resulting in changes or loss of distal sensation may have caused injury to nerve fibres or vasculature, and will require surgical repair. Compare the sensation distal to the injury against the same area on the unaffected hand. Remember that different digits are supplied by different nerves, so adjacent digits on the same hand should not be compared with each other. Lacerations with significant blood loss may involve damage to larger vessels.

Where underlying structures are involved and referral is made, the wound should be thoroughly irrigated, under local anaesthesia if needed. A moist primary dressing and non-adherent secondary dressing is normally sufficient, unless an alternative dressing has been advised. If there is to be a delay in review, the injured hand should be splinted in a 'position of safety' and elevated to reduce swelling.

Minor lacerations not involving deeper structures, nor resulting in motor or neurovascular compromise, can be repaired. Lacerations involving underlying structures will require referral for surgical exploration, washout and repair. Ongoing observation and scar management may be required for significant wounds that occur over highly mobile areas, as scar contracture can inhibit mobility.

Antibiotic prophylaxis should be considered for high-risk wounds according to mechanism of injury, compound fractures, involvement of underlying structures, contamination and the patient's co-morbidities.

Primary tetanus vaccination or update may also be required in the instance of an open wound. Indications for tetanus vaccination are discussed later in the chapter under tetanus immunisation.

Crush injuries of the digits

A crush injury of a digit is a common injury, resulting from compression between two hard objects. The resulting injury can be any combination of phalangeal fractures, avulsion or laceration of the nail or digit pulp, subungual haematoma, nail bed laceration or partial or complete amputation of the digit. Sudden soft-tissue swelling can also result in a burst injury of the pulp, where there is an open wound overlying the pulp and the underlying soft tissue protrudes through the breach.

Hands and fingers have a complex nerve supply, and so when injured can result in significant pain. Examination, debridement and wound preparation often requires analgesia and local or regional anaesthesia. A digital block, using plain lignocaine, is an effective form of anaesthesia to manage digit injuries.

Digit injuries should be managed according to the severity and nature of the injury. An X-ray of the digit is indicated to exclude a fracture or foreign body, which may indicate antibiotic prophylaxis and referral. Injuries should be elevated and ice applied to reduce inflammation and pain. Advice should be provided on ongoing analgesia, rest and elevation, as crush injuries can continue to be painful for several days.

Avulsion of digit pulp

Avulsion of digit pulp can occur as a result of a shearing force applied to the finger or thumb, or by direct laceration from a sharp edge with complete removal of overlying skin (Fig 18.8).

Nerve fibres beyond the level of the distal interphalangeal joint are generally not repaired, due to their minute size. Haemostasis is difficult to achieve with avulsions of the pulp as the digit is highly vascular. After thorough irrigation, initial management is elevation and pressure. If this is unsuccessful, a compression dressing can be applied for 1–2 hours, taking care not to apply too much pressure. Excessive pressure will cause a rebound re-bleed when the dressing is removed. Highly compressive digit dressings left in place for an extended period can also reduce tissue perfusion at the injury site and potentially result in tissue necrosis. When haemostasis is achieved, a dressing can be applied to encourage healing by secondary intention. These injuries in many circumstances can be successfully healed with ongoing meticulous wound care. For extensive wounds, or wounds slow to heal, referral to a surgeon may be required to consider skin grafting.

FIGURE 18.8 **Avulsion of digit pulp before (A) and after (B, C) healing.**[107]

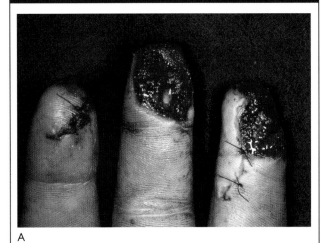

A

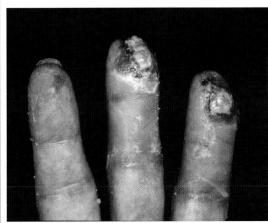

B

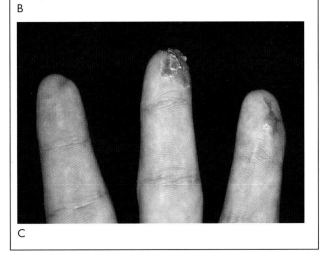

C

Nail avulsions and nail bed lacerations

Nail avulsions and partial nail avulsions result from a shearing force applied to the distal digit, tearing the nail away from the nail bed or nail fold. Nail avulsions can often occur as a result of a crush injury, where the nail is avulsed and the nail bed is also lacerated. Nail avulsions rarely occur in isolation of a nail bed laceration. Where there are lacerations of the onychal folds (see Fig 18.9), and if the digit tip appears torn away, suspect a

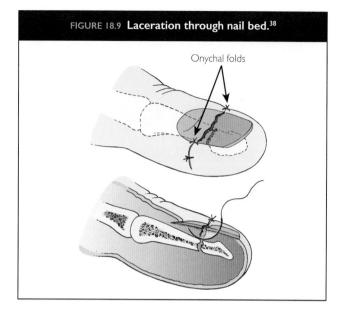

FIGURE 18.9 **Laceration through nail bed.**[38]

Onychal folds

nail bed laceration beneath the nail. Nail bed lacerations should be repaired to avoid infection and abnormal and problematic subsequent nail growth.

If the original nail is intact but damaged, the patient should be advised of possible nail loss. New nail growth is very slow, taking a period of months, and the new nail is often ridged and not as cosmetically acceptable as the original nail.

If the nail is avulsed, the distal digit should be thoroughly irrigated and the nail returned to the nail fold. To repair the nail bed, the nail will require complete removal via blunt dissection, the nail bed should be irrigated and the laceration closed with fine, absorbable sutures. The nail, if salvageable, can then be returned to the nail fold to splint the fold open and

provide protection to the nail bed. If the nail is missing or not salvageable, paraffin-based gauze can be applied into the nail fold and over the nail bed.[38]

Subungual haematoma

A subungual haematoma is a collection of blood between the nail and nail bed, the result of a crush injury or significant blunt trauma to the distal end of the digit (Fig 18.10). Such patients usually present with significant throbbing pain secondary to pressure beneath the nail. Associated injuries include nail bed lacerations and distal tuft fractures.

If the nail and the nail fold remain intact, the haematoma can be drained by trephining the nail. A 22-gauge needle can be rotated against the nail plate at the centre of the haematoma until blood drains. More than one hole can be made, providing immediate relief when the pressure beneath the nail is relieved. Where there is an underlying fracture of the distal phalanx and the nail has been trephined, antibiotics have not shown to be of value in preventing infection.[39]

Digit amputation

In instances where a digit is amputated, the wound should be thoroughly irrigated and a dressing applied. The amputated digit should be wrapped in a sterile gauze moistened in Normal saline, placed in a watertight bag, and then placed in an ice-and-water slush and urgent surgical referral arranged for re-implantation. Antibiotic prophylaxis is indicated for digit amputations.

Injuries around the knee

Anatomy and function

The knee is a large weightbearing joint where stability of the distal femur, proximal tibia, fibula and the patella is provided by a complex of tendons, ligaments, muscles and the menisci.

FIGURE 18.10

A, Subungual haematoma (with trephine hole).
B, Position for trephining nail. **C**, Trephining nail.[38]

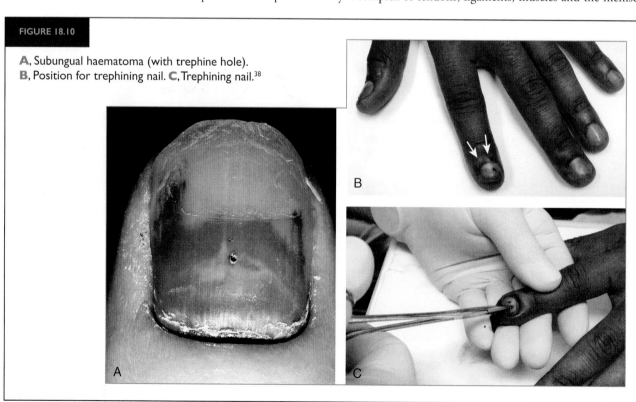

The patella is attached proximally to the quadriceps tendon and distally by the patella tendon, which inserts into the tibial tuberosity. The strong medial and lateral collateral ligaments (MCL and LCL) are situated along the inside and outside of the knee and provide stability from lateral stresses. The anterior (ACL) and posterior (PCL) cruciate ligaments provide stability to the knee from rotational forces and run from the femoral condyles to the tibial spines. The menisci lie between the tibial and femoral condyles and function as cushions during articulation (Fig 18.11). Blood supply to the knee is complex, provided by the popliteal artery, among others.

Patient assessment

Often the injured knee is too painful for a complete systematic examination. In these cases careful consideration of the exact mechanism of injury described by the patient can be of great value in possible diagnosis. Immediate inability to weightbear usually signifies a more serious injury.

Observation and the speed of onset of any effusion (swelling over the entire knee joint) may help to distinguish a significant ligamentous or bony injury. Be certain to distinguish local swelling over a particular structure from an effusion. Note any deformity, particularly to the patella. Use the other knee for comparison. Palpate all bony landmarks, including the fibula head and the medial and collateral ligaments, for tenderness. The extensor mechanism should be tested by asking the patient to lift the leg with a straight knee (straight leg raise).

Examine for active range of movement and combine this with the Ottawa knee rules[40] (Box 18.2) to assist in the decision

to X-ray. The Ottawa study found over a 10-month period that the rules had a sensitivity of 100% and a specificity of 73% for knee fracture.

Ligamentous injuries of the knee

A force striking the side of the knee while weightbearing can cause injury to the MCL or LCL on the opposite side to the blow, causing pain and difficulty weightbearing. On examination the patient may have some local swelling, focal tenderness over the area of injury and pain on passive stressing of the injured tendon. There should be an obvious endpoint at full stretch of the ligament; if not, assume a complete tear. In acute injuries this may be difficult to ascertain. If the patient fulfils Ottawa criteria, an X-ray should be arranged. Stable injuries can be treated conservatively with crutches for mobilisation as needed. If the knee is unstable on examination, surgery for repair may be indicated.

Rotational forces, such as twisting the knee with a stationary foot, can tear the cruciate ligaments, most commonly the ACL. A haemarthrosis may be seen clinically as a sudden effusion within 2–6 hours of the injury, which should lead the clinician to suspect significant damage. In a prospective study of 106 cases of haemarthrosis caused by sporting injury, 71 patients (67%) had complete or partial disruption of the ACL.[41] The haemarthrosis can be drained using a strict aseptic technique to provide pain relief and is diagnostic of significant injury if blood is present. A compression bandage should be applied after drainage to prevent re-accumulation. An avulsion fracture of the anterior tibial spine, the attachment point of the ACL and other fractures should be excluded by X-ray. All haemarthroses warrant a specialist orthopaedic opinion.

Patella dislocation may occur following sudden muscle contraction or a blow to the medial side of the knee[26] (Fig 18.12). Dislocation may be recurrent, particularly in young

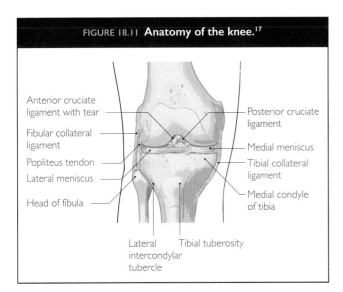

FIGURE 18.11 Anatomy of the knee.[17]

Anterior cruciate ligament with tear

Fibular collateral ligament

Popliteus tendon

Lateral meniscus

Head of fibula

Posterior cruciate ligament

Medial meniscus

Tibial collateral ligament

Medial condyle of tibia

Lateral intercondylar tubercle

Tibial tuberosity

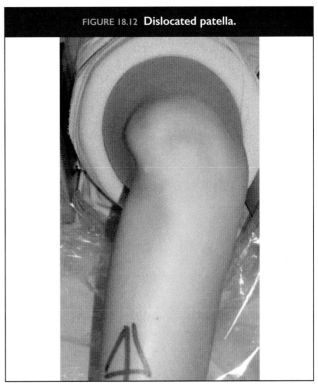

FIGURE 18.12 Dislocated patella.

BOX 18.2 The Ottawa knee rules

- Age 55 years or older
- Tenderness at head of fibula
- Isolated tenderness of patella
- Inability to flex knee to 90°
- Inability to walk four weightbearing steps immediately after the injury and in the emergency department

teenage girls who have ligamentous laxity. Relocation is usually reasonably easy using lateral pressure to the patella with the knee extended. Inhalational anaesthesia, such as nitrous oxide, is useful for this procedure. The knee should be splinted post reduction and the patient referred for orthopaedic follow-up.

Both the quadriceps and the patella tendons can be ruptured by forcible contraction of the quadriceps; check for a more proximal patella than usual indicating a quadriceps tendon rupture, common in the more elderly patient. There may be a palpable defect. Patella tendon rupture is common in the young athlete. These both need surgical repair.

Seen most commonly in male adolescents, a sudden contraction of the quadriceps tendon can avulse the tibial tuberosity, often causing an inability to straighten the knee as the fragment sits in the joint space. This injury requires surgical fixation.

Fractures around the knee

The patella may be fractured by a direct fall or blow to the knee. There will be local swelling and tenderness and the patient will find it difficult to mobilise. Always check ability to straight-leg raise. Transverse fractures which affect the ability to straight-leg raise will need surgical fixation. Longitudinal fractures can be treated conservatively.

The tibial plateau may also be fractured by a direct blow or fall onto the knee. The patient will have great difficulty weight-bearing and there will be considerable swelling and localised bony tenderness. Following X-ray, a CT scan is often required to identify the extent of the injury. Surgery is often required to restore bony alignment of the articulating surface.

The lower leg, ankle and foot

Anatomy and function

The tibia and fibula provide the bony structure to the lower leg for movement and weightbearing. The fibula head can be palpated just distal to the lateral aspect of the knee joint, ending distally at the lateral malleolus. The tibia extends close to the skin at the shin, ending at the medial malleolus at the medial aspect of the ankle. Here the articulation with the talus forms the mortise of the ankle joint with stability and articulation provided by the medial deltoid ligament and lateral anterior talofibular, calcaneal fibular and posterior talofibular ligaments. The anatomical landmarks provided by the medial and lateral malleoli are important for assessing bony tenderness and deciding on X-ray imaging.

The foot creates a surface for weightbearing and is composed of the hind foot, including the calcaneus and talus, the mid foot and its complex ligamentous structure, the metatarsal bones and the toe phalanges, known as the forefoot.

The muscles of the lower leg are contained in individual fascial compartments along with the tibial and common peroneal nerves, and are susceptible to increasing pressure from swelling and bleeding after injury.

Patient assessment

Ask the patient to describe the injury to elicit the likely injury mechanism. Observe for deformity and other signs of injury. Deformity with weak or absent distal pulses may need reduction and splintage in the field, using intravenous

pain relief if available. The aim is to restore as normal anatomy as possible to relieve vascular pressure. Possible compound fractures should be covered.

Regularly assess distal circulation by palpation of the dorsalis pedis, palpated over the dorsum of the foot, and/or the tibialis posterior, found just behind the medial malleolus. Observe the colour of the foot for pallor and warmth.

Systematically palpate the lower leg for bony tenderness, using the mechanism as a guide for potential injury. Also palpate over the ankle ligaments to diagnose ligamentous injury, not forgetting the calcaneum, mid and forefoot and Achilles as indicated.

Depending on the site of tenderness and suspected injury, X-ray examination can be undertaken. X-rays of the tibia and fibula will include the ankle; if an isolated ankle fracture is suspected, request an ankle X-ray alone. It is unusual in a simple inversion injury to need to image the foot and ankle together and a systematic, thorough examination should elicit the area of focal tenderness.

The Ottawa ankle rules

In isolated inversion-type ankle injuries in adults, a decision whether to X-ray the ankle or foot to determine the presence of a fracture may be based on the Ottawa ankle and foot rules[42] (Boxes 18.3 and 18.4; Fig 18.13).

These rules have an accuracy of nearly 100% for excluding a fracture and have reduced the number of ankle X-rays requested by 30–40%,[43] reducing patient and clinician time and saving hospital resources. Several studies have also positively evaluated the Ottawa ankle and foot rules in children over 6 years of age, with a sensitivity of 98.5%.[44]

BOX 18.3 The Ottawa ankle rules

X-rays are only required if there is any pain in the malleolar zone and *any one* of the following:

- bone tenderness along the distal 6 cm of the posterior edge of the tibia or the tip of the medial malleolus
- bone tenderness along the distal 6 cm of the posterior edge of the fibula or tip of the lateral malleolus
- an inability to bear weight both immediately and in the emergency department for four steps.

BOX 18.4 The Ottawa foot rules

X-rays are only required if there is any pain in the midfoot zone and *any one* of the following:

- bone tenderness at the base of the fifth metatarsal (for foot injuries)
- bone tenderness at the navicular bone (for foot injuries)
- an inability to bear weight both immediately and in the emergency department for four steps.

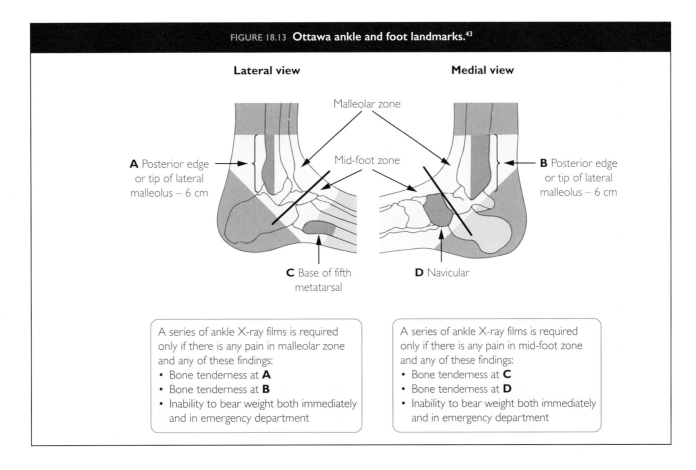

FIGURE 18.13 **Ottawa ankle and foot landmarks.**[43]

Lateral view   **Medial view**

Malleolar zone

Mid-foot zone

A Posterior edge or tip of lateral malleolus – 6 cm

B Posterior edge or tip of lateral malleolus – 6 cm

C Base of fifth metatarsal

D Navicular

A series of ankle X-ray films is required only if there is any pain in malleolar zone and any of these findings:
- Bone tenderness at **A**
- Bone tenderness at **B**
- Inability to bear weight both immediately and in emergency department

A series of ankle X-ray films is required only if there is any pain in mid-foot zone and any of these findings:
- Bone tenderness at **C**
- Bone tenderness at **D**
- Inability to bear weight both immediately and in emergency department

Injuries to the lower leg

Tibia and fibula fractures

These are commonly encountered injuries, and often sports-related. A blow or rotational-type force to the leg may cause an isolated tibia or fibula fracture. Shaft fractures are often compound, as the bone is near to the skin surface at the shin. There may be clinical deformity. Always obtain X-rays of the whole length of the tibia and fibula to exclude an accompanying distal injury and a proximal fracture.[26] Minimally displaced isolated shaft fractures may be treated in an above-knee cast. Any angulation will need to be corrected to avoid long-term stress at the knee and ankle after healing.

Always consider a toddler's fracture (Fig 18.14) in small children who are reluctant to weightbear following a relatively minor fall. These children may sustain a subtle undisplaced fracture of the tibia, or a greenstick fracture that can usually be managed in a long leg cast.

Compartment syndrome is a serious potential risk following fractures of the tibia and fibula and should be considered in patients with increasing pain and a tense, swollen limb; this is discussed further in Chapter 50.

Torn calf muscle

The gastrocnemius, the medial head of the calf muscle, can also be torn during weightbearing activity, often sports-related. The patient reports sudden severe pain in the calf, often likening it to being hit or shot in the leg. There is tenderness over the upper medial calf and walking is very painful. A history of sudden pain should aid in ruling out other causes such as deep

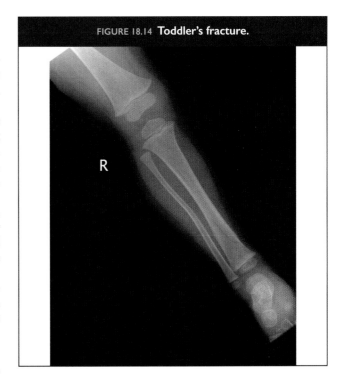

FIGURE 18.14 **Toddler's fracture.**

R

vein thrombosis or a Baker's cyst. Always check the Achilles tendon is intact. Treatment consists of ice, elevation and early mobilisation, where a heeled shoe to raise the heel may be helpful.

Pre-tibial lacerations

Pre-tibial lacerations are common, particularly in the elderly population. They are often the result of a fall and a thorough assessment should be conducted to exclude other injuries and establish the underlying cause of the fall. The anterior aspect of the tibia has minimal subcutaneous tissue, and as a result pre-tibial lacerations have limited vascular supply and can often expose the surface of the tibia. These wounds are commonly managed conservatively with dressings, and referred for skin grafting if the wound fails to heal. Some recent studies have found that early intervention using a split skin graft can significantly reduce healing time of pre-tibial wounds, although this is not yet common practice.[44] For elderly or diabetic patients with poor healing capacity, potentially two wounds subsequently have to be managed and healed.

Wounds of the lower limb are often slower to heal due to the nature of their vascular supply. For the elderly, the normal physiological changes of ageing, including changes in skin integrity and lower limb vasculature, prolonged healing, co-morbidities and often immobility, further exacerbate poor healing. Pre-tibial lacerations in the elderly are often slow to heal and may not completely heal, resulting in ulcers and chronic lower limb wounds.

Management includes thorough irrigation. Where possible, the flap of skin should be softened with gauze soaked in Normal saline and stretched back over the wound to provide wound coverage. If the flap involves dermis and subcutaneous tissue, it can be closed using a half-buried suture to approximate the flap corner, providing the surrounding skin is of good quality and is unlikely to tear under the tension of a suture. A moist dressing should be applied to the wound. Due to the fragility of the surrounding skin in the elderly, topical sticking closure strips should be used minimally and with caution. Integral to optimal healing is the application of compression bandaging to the entire lower limb in appropriate patients with no arterial vascular disease to maximise venous return (see Ch 17, p. 349, for compression bandaging techniques). These wounds require frequent observation, so that specialist referral can be made if wound healing fails. Antibiotics are only indicated for patients with high-risk wounds or a high risk of infection.

Injuries around the ankle and foot

Most commonly the ankle is injured by an inversion mechanism, where the foot is inverted inwards towards the midline. The injury is likely to be on the lateral aspect, injuring the lateral ankle ligaments and sometimes causing a fracture of the distal fibula, the fibular head or the base of the fifth metatarsal of the foot. Ankle injury can also be sustained more infrequently by eversion, where the foot turns outwards and ligamentous and possible bony injury occurs on the medial aspect. Greater force will cause more severe ligamentous and bony injury bilaterally.

Fractures of the ankle

Ankle fractures may involve one, two or three malleoli. Single, relatively undisplaced fractures of the distal fibula below the level of the ankle mortise may be treated in a non-weightbearing cast or, increasingly commonly, in a walking cast boot. Distal fibula fractures that extend from the level of the mortise or above the mortise are often more unstable and may need internal fixation. This is particularly likely if there is tenderness around the medial malleolus, or a medial malleolar facture is present. Talar tilt or shift, where the normal alignment of the talar mortise is displaced, must be corrected, usually under general anaesthetic, and signifies significant disruption to the ligamentous and bony stability of the ankle.

Ankle dislocation

Where there is obvious deformity to the ankle and a mal-positioned foot, relocation is urgently required. There is often critical skin and the injury may be open. X-rays should not delay the procedure and the lower leg should be placed in a below-knee POP cast for stabilisation post reduction. X-rays should then be ordered and will mostly, but not always, demonstrate bi-malleolar ankle fractures, with talar shift. There will always be significant ligamentous rupture. Further operative management is usually required.

Ankle sprains

More than 23,000 people per day in the USA require medical care, sports- and non-sports-related, for ankle sprains.[46] Localised swelling and focal tenderness over the anterior talofibular ligament and no bony tenderness (see Ottawa ankle rules) is diagnostic of a ligamentous injury, comprising 85% of all ankle injuries.[46]

Treatment for ankle sprains remains a wide-ranging topic, based on the severity of the sprain, the functional needs of the patient and the resources available. All ankle sprains should be elevated, and iced regularly. Sprains to the ankle can be graded depending on severity and treatment based around this.[47]

- *Simple sprain, grade 1*—simple inversion injury, tenderness and swelling over anterior talofibular ligament; patient can weightbear.

  Treat with 2 days of rest, then gradual return to mobilisation. Compression with ankle tape-strapping is beneficial and, as some ED teams now include physiotherapists, this is becoming a more commonplace treatment. Simple double-layer bandaging is often used and although patients advocate its comfort, actual benefits in speeding recovery are not proven.[48,49]

- *Moderate sprain, grade 2*—inability to weightbear, marked swelling, tenderness over both the lateral and the medial ligaments.

  Treat as for grade 1; however, patients may require crutches for a short period of time. A review by a physiotherapist should be recommended.

- *Severe sprain, grade 3*—severe mechanism, inability to weightbear, marked bilateral swelling, clinical or radiological effusion, signs of ankle instability (although instability is difficult to establish after an acute injury).

  These injuries are very painful and there is evidence that a short period of immobilisation, either in a POP below-knee cast or a more practical air-cast brace, leads to a more rapid recovery at 3 months post injury.[50] These injuries should be reviewed, depending on the resources available, by the original clinician, an orthopaedic specialist or a physiotherapist to further assess stability.

Considering up to 40% of people will develop some degree of instability after lateral ankle sprain,[51] early referral to a physio-therapist, where available, may be prudent, especially in sports people.

Achilles tendon rupture

Achilles tendon rupture often occurs during sport when there is a sudden dorsiflexion of the foot. The patient recalls a sudden snapping sensation, pain in the back of the heel and difficulty walking normally. They will be unable to stand on tiptoes. There is a palpable gap on palpation of the tendon. Simmonds, an English orthopaedist, devised the Simmonds' test[51,52] to simply diagnose the injury. The patient lies face down with their feet hanging off the edge of the bed and the calf is squeezed. If the test is positive, i.e. the Achilles tendon is ruptured, there is no plantar flexion of the foot. Options to manage these injuries surgically or conservatively are still controversial, with various advantages and disadvantages of both, including re-rupture, and wound infection.

Injuries of the foot

The foot can be injured following an inversion or hyperextension mechanism; for example, landing from a jump or from a crushing force. The toes are often crushed or knocked against a solid object causing dislocation, fracture or a skin or nail injury.

Fractures of the calcaneum

The commonest cause of calcaneal fractures is a fall or jump from a height, and they may be bilateral. Fracture of the lumbar spines occur in 5% of patients with a calcaneal fracture[24] and should be carefully excluded. There is marked swelling around the heel and it will be tender on palpation. The patient will be unable to walk. Calcaneal X-rays will include an axial view where the foot is viewed from behind. Operative and non-operative management options depend on the type of fracture and the degree of displacement, and may need to be confirmed with CT scan.

Lisfranc injuries of the mid foot

The Lisfranc ligament provides bony stability to the tarsal–metatarsal area of the foot. A Lisfranc fracture dislocation is an easily missed, significant but uncommon foot injury sustained after a fall, a crush or a simple inversion mechanism. The patient has significant swelling and tenderness over the mid foot and will be unable to walk. The dorsalis pedis may be minimal or absent. The abnormality on X-ray can be subtle; check for normal alignment of the second metatarsal base with the intermediate cuneiform on the anteroposterior foot X-ray and for displacement on the lateral films. There may also be accompanying metatarsal fractures. Beware of the non-weightbearing patient with significant clinical signs of a mid foot injury and seemingly normal X-rays. Many need operative fixation.

Metatarsal fractures

An avulsion fracture to the base of the fifth metatarsal commonly follows an inversion injury, as the insertion of the peroneus brevis tendon avulses the bone after sudden contraction. Palpation of the base of the fifth metatarsal is included in the Ottawa foot rules; clinically there will be swelling, tenderness and, later, bruising over the site. Treatment is symptomatic only, with supportive bandaging, weightbearing as able, ice and elevation. See Chapter 17, p. 348, for RICE principles and p. 349 for bandaging techniques. Note that fifth metatarsal epiphysis in children may mimic a fracture. Generally, single second to fifth metatarsal shaft fractures are treated conservatively. First metatarsal and multiple fractures may be unstable and will require orthopaedic review.

Stress fractures of the foot are sometimes encountered in patients with a history of insidious foot pain, often related to a repetitive impact such as running. X-ray may demonstrate a calcification at the site of injury, often the second metatarsal. Where X-rays are normal, a bone scan may identify a fracture. The patient will need to rest from the aggravating activity for 6–8 weeks and then gradually progress to full activity again. A firm shoe may aid comfort.

Injury to the toes

The toes are frequently damaged by crushing forces or caught against objects such as furniture. Injury to the nail and skin lacerations may be seen. Suspected fractures of the big toe should be X-rayed, as the big toe has a role in balance. A walking POP cast with a toe platform or an air-cast boot may make mobilisation easier. Suspected fractures to the other phalanges where there is no clinical deformity and the skin is intact do not require X-ray, as management will be unchanged, even if a fracture is present. Fractures can be supported with strapping to the adjacent toe for 3–4 weeks.

Nail and skin wounds involving the toes can be treated similarly to the finger and thumb, covered earlier in the chapter.

Injuries of the skin: wounds

Anatomy and function of the skin

The skin is the largest organ of the body, and consists of three distinct layers: the epidermis, the dermis and the subcutaneous layer, often referred to as the hypodermis (Fig 18.15).

The epidermis is the outermost layer of the skin. It consists of keratinised epithelium consisting of between four and five layers or strata. The thickness of the epithelium varies on the region and on the demands placed upon the skin. The soles of the feet and palms of the hands are the thickest, measuring 1.5 mm thick, compared with the epidermis of the eyelid which is 0.5 mm thick.[53,54] The epidermis has pores to allow for release of sweat. Hair follicles protrude through the epidermis, depending on the region, and also allow for sebum release from the deeper layers of the skin. The epidermis is avascular, and so receives nourishment via diffusion from the deeper dermis.

The dermis is a strong yet flexible layer of the skin. It contains collagen, reticular and elastin fibres which provide strength and elasticity and is the thickest of the skin layers. The dermis is highly vascular and is also rich in lymphatic vessels and nerve fibres. Directly beneath the dermis lies the subcutaneous layer.

The subcutaneous layer is loosely arranged connective tissue containing fat, fibrous bands of tissue, blood and lymphatic vessels, nerves and, in the scalp, hair follicles. Subcutaneous tissue anchors the dermis and epidermis to the underlying structures and organs, and provides insulation and cushioning.

The appendages of the skin, such as eccrine and apocrine glands secreting sweat, sebaceous glands secreting sebum and the hair follicles and roots, arise from the dermis and subcutaneous layers.

The skin has multiple physiological functions:

- it serves as an anatomical barrier between the internal and external environment, protecting from mechanical injury and pathogens

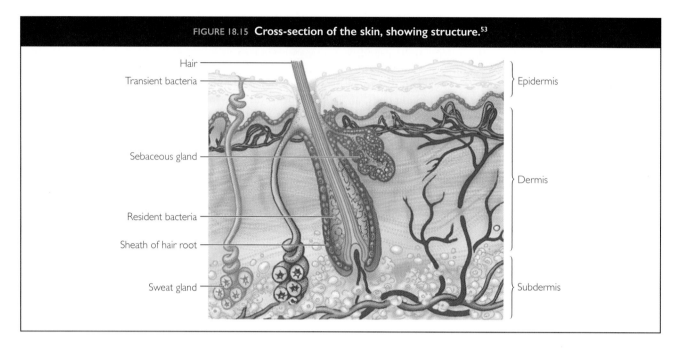

FIGURE 18.15 **Cross-section of the skin, showing structure.**[53]

- it contains an abundance of various nerve endings that respond to heat and cold, touch, pressure, vibration and tissue injury
- it regulates body temperature though vasodilation and vasoconstriction, convection, conduction and evaporation
- it synthesises vitamin D, which is an active component of calcium and phosphate metabolism in the body.

The skin plays an integral role in a person's overall emotional and psychological wellbeing. Disruptions to the skin integrity, such as discolourations, wounds or scarring, can affect a person's self-esteem and psychological wellbeing, particularly where they involve cosmetically significant areas such as the face.

Wound assessment

Wound assessment forms part of the systematic primary and secondary physical assessment processes. Life-threatening wounds or wounds resulting in uncontrolled haemorrhage should be identified during the primary survey and steps taken to promote and obtain haemostasis, which may include the definitive management of the wound at that time. All other wounds, including those only temporarily managed in the primary assessment, should be reviewed in the secondary survey.

The location of wounds should be considered in relation to the mechanism of injury, particularly those where there may have been substantial impact, such as those following a fall or another type of blunt trauma. Once any significant injury has been diagnosed, treated or excluded, wound care will follow the same principles. Before examination of the wound itself, use the mechanism of injury to anticipate the likelihood of complications such as involvement and injury of deeper structures such as bone, tendon, ligament, muscle or neurovascular structures. Mechanism will also have a direct impact on likely infection risk. When examining a wound, it is important to recall normal anatomy and function of the injured area and the underlying structures, to guide the examination and anticipate potential complications. The

involvement of deeper structures may affect normal function and such complications may indicate specialist referral.

Using the same systematic approach of inspection, palpation and movement to assess a wound ensures that the examination is thorough.

Inspection

Note the type of wound: abrasion, laceration, tissue avulsion, puncture, bite or a combination. A wound may be the only injury, as in the case of a single bite wound or laceration; or there may be multiple wounds of varying severity, location and depth, as in the case of a trauma or assault.

Note the shape, size and depth of the wound and whether underlying structures are visible at the deepest points of the wound bed. Inspect the colour and condition of the surrounding tissue. Dusky or mottled surrounding tissue may indicate poor circulatory perfusion. Wounds may be contaminated with debris or foreign bodies, which will need to be removed. The depth of the wound can often be concealed beneath a thrombus, the normal physiological response to injury. This will require evacuation for further examination.

Where wounds involve a limb, inspect the unaffected limb as a comparison, noting oedema and skin colour.

Palpation

Palpate the wound and surrounding tissue. Perfusion to surrounding tissues can be assessed by palpating surrounding tissue for colour, temperature and capillary refill time. Assess for changes or loss of sensation distal to the wound as an indication of nerve damage. It is not uncommon to find mild sensation differences due to the physiological response to injury and anxiety. However, there are several techniques that can be used to obtain objective information about sensory changes, including the two-point discrimination technique and assessing the discrimination between sharp and dull sensation. These are conducted distal to the wound. Test the sensation against the same area on the corresponding opposite side, i.e. the other arm, hand or foot. Where possible assess an unaffected area first to reduce the patient's anxiety and to provide an understanding of what is required.

Palpate arterial pulses distal to the wound. Deep lacerations may sever larger, vital vessels which could compromise perfusion. Where the injury involves a limb, compare quality of pulses between both limbs.

Where appropriate, palpate the underlying bony structures, noting crepitus or bony tenderness, which may indicate a fracture. Clear any debris and evacuate any thrombus to assess wound depth. If a wound appears to track, use a non-rigid sterile probe such as a wound swab. If the wound is large enough, the examiner's finger can be used to gently follow the course of any tracking and determine its depth and probability of damage to underlying structures. Note any palpable foreign body beneath the skin surface.

Movement

Move the underlying and adjacent areas and structures surrounding the wound, where appropriate, to establish any actual or potential loss of function. Assess through full range of motion, noting any loss in power. Deep hand lacerations involving tendons, for example, may affect subsequent function of the hand and/or digits. Where a wound affects a limb, compare motor function to the non-affected limb (Box 18.5).

Moving the joints adjacent to the wound will ascertain whether the wound is under tension, such as wounds over joint surfaces. This will affect choice of closure or dressing management.

Haemostasis

Thorough wound examination is dependent on establishing haemostasis to allow a detailed view of the wound. Haemostasis may have been achieved spontaneously through the normal physiological responses to injury, or in the pre-hospital setting through first-aid measures. Haemostasis may be difficult to achieve in patients with coagulopathies or those on medications affecting normal coagulation. Often, examining a wound will disrupt this process and bleeding will recommence. Haemostasis should be achieved by applying direct pressure and by elevating the wound. Local infiltration of the surrounding tissues with a local anaesthetic containing adrenaline can aid local vasoconstriction and haemostasis, after neurovascular assessment is complete.

In instances where haemostasis cannot be achieved and examination attempts result in gross haemorrhage, wound assessment is very difficult and indicates the involvement of larger vessels. Haemostasis is then the priority and referral may be indicated.

For limb injuries that continue to bleed, short-term tourniquet techniques can be used with caution, to establish a bloodless field for examination and wound care. Care must be taken to ensure that the tourniquet remains in place for the shortest period possible. A commonly used technique is the use of a sphygmomanometer cuff applied to the limb above the wound and inflated to 10 mmHg above systolic pressure or until bleeding ceases. Care must be taken to release the sphygmomanometer cuff slowly while maintaining pressure at the wound, to inhibit re-bleeding on re-perfusion of the wound.

Wound healing

The complex process of wound healing can be divided into four distinct, yet overlapping, phases:

1. Initial haemostasis
2. The inflammatory phase
3. The proliferative phase
4. The remodelling phase.

Within these four broad phases is a complex and coordinated series of events.[55] Table 18.1 outlines the overlapping phases and an approximate timeline of the phases of wound healing, excluding complications such as those listed above.

Wounds require a number of factors for healing to occur: adequate perfusion and temperature of the injured tissue, control of contamination and infection and good general health and nutrition of the injured patient.

Speed of wound healing varies depending upon the location of the wound. The face and scalp have a greater vascular supply and return than the foot, for example. This results in higher baseline skin temperature, better oxygen and nutrient delivery to the skin and therefore more rapid healing.

Infection results when there is an imbalance between the microbial load at the wound site and the host's immune response. Infection stalls and protracts wound healing and can result in greater scarring.

General health factors of the patient can inhibit healing. Conditions such as diabetes, obesity, haematological, vascular and renal disease, disease processes causing immunocompromise, advanced age and many drug therapies, such as corticosteroids, can inhibit the healing process.

Other factors such as poor nutrition, smoking, excessive alcohol use or other drug use can also inhibit the healing process. A lower socioeconomic background may limit the

---

BOX 18.5 Wound inspection

Inspect
- Type of wound
- Wound location
- Wound size
- Wound depth
- Wound contaminants—debris, foreign bodies
- Underlying visible structures
- Surrounding tissue integrity, colour

Palpate
- Surrounding tissue sensation
- Surrounding tissue perfusion—temperature, capillary refill time
- Pulses distal to the wound
- Underlying bony injury—crepitus, bony tenderness
- Wound tracking beneath skin surface

Move
If appropriate:
- Underlying and adjacent structures
- Assess for skin under high tension
- Assess range of motion
- Assess motor power

TABLE 18.1 Phases of wound healing[55]

PHASE	ACTIVITY
Haemostasis (immediate)	Local vasoconstriction
	Clotting to achieve haemostasis
Inflammatory phase (up to 3 days)	Release of vasoactive substances by damaged cells
	Local vasodilation and increased vascular permeability
	Migration of leucocytes and macrophages
	Bacterial balance restored
	Preparation of wound for healing
Proliferative/ reconstruction phase (3 days to 3 weeks)	Reconstruction of tissue
	Granulation tissue—new capillaries, fibroblasts, inflammatory cells, endothelial cells, connective tissue proteins, collagen deposition
	Epithelialisation—epithelial cells migrate across the granular tissue
	Contraction of wound size— myofibroblasts
Maturation phase (3 weeks to 1 year)	Scar development
	Matrix breakdown and reformation
	Continued collagen formation

patient's ability to appropriately care for their wound, or occupational commitments may restrict adherence to wound care advice, such as rest, elevation and keeping the wound dry. If any of these factors are suboptimal, the wound-healing process will be delayed or protracted.

Scarring

Scarring is an inevitable result of wound healing. Hypertrophic and keloid scarring can be unsightly and, depending upon the location of the wound, can cause problems with tissue and/or joint mobility as well as causing significant emotional distress to the patient. Methods such as compression, silicon based dressings, intralesional corticosteroid injection, dye laser and X-ray are used to flatten and improve the appearance of scars.[56]

There are several topical silicon-based products that have been developed with the objective of reducing or preventing such scarring, although the evidence to date is unequivocal.[57]

Managing wounds in the acute care setting

The decision to manage or refer a patient with an acute wound is based around a thorough, focused examination including investigations where appropriate. Wounds that fit into the criteria below may require referral to a specialist surgical team for evaluation. The referral will vary depending on local policy, geographical location and local expertise.

- *Is there evidence of injury to underlying structures?*
  Is there an underlying fracture? Is there neurovascular compromise? Is there motor function compromise?

- *Is the wound in a cosmetically sensitive area?*
  Does the wound involve the vermilion border of the lip, eyelid, nose or ear? Is there tissue avulsion of a cosmetically sensitive area, inhibiting primary closure?

- *Will the wound affect occupational function?*
  Will the patient's job be specifically affected by the injury; for example, a professional musician with a hand or digit injury?

- *Is closure of the wound technically challenging?*

- *Is the wound extensive?*
  Does the wound require significant debridement or further exploration to retrieve foreign bodies? Are the wound edges jagged or under excessive tension, making alignment difficult?

- *Is the patient cooperative?*
  Is the patient a young child, particularly anxious, or an elderly patient with dementia? Does the patient have an intellectual disability, where treatment may cause fear, refusal of or non-compliance with treatment?

Investigations in wound care

In the acute care setting, certain investigations may be useful to further assess the severity of an injury, prepare a patient for surgical wound repair and, in some instances, ensure the safe use of antibiotic prophylaxis.

Bedside investigations

A baseline bedside blood sugar level is indicated in patients where diabetes is confirmed or suspected to anticipate likelihood of satisfactory healing and to determine whether antibiotic prophylaxis may be indicated. Wound swabs are not indicated in the acute wound.

Pathology investigations

Blood pathology may be indicated to establish preoperative baseline values if surgical consultation for wound repair under general anaesthetic is required. Pathology may also be indicated if significant blood loss from the wound is suspected or confirmed, or where antibiotic prophylaxis is indicated and the patient has significant co-morbidities such as renal disease.

Radiological investigations

X-rays can be used to identify radio-opaque foreign bodies and underlying fractures. Ultrasound is useful to identify organic or non-radio-opaque foreign bodies, but is less accessible in the acute setting. Identification of foreign material via ultrasound images is generally reserved for cases where there is a confirmed or convincing story of non-radio-opaque or organic foreign material within the wound; it is not routinely used in the acute management of a wound.

Even if material is identified, be it by X-ray or ultrasound, size and location, it may still result in the foreign material not being removed in the initial stage. Removal of foreign bodies is discussed later in the chapter.

WHEN TO REFER A PATIENT FOR SPECIALIST OPINION

- Wounds involving underlying structures—ligaments, tendon, bone, amputations
- Wounds that result in neurovascular compromise
- Grossly contaminated wounds requiring debridement, washout
- Extensive wounds, where closure in the acute care setting is inappropriate
- Extensive wounds that may require skin grafting
- Concern about cosmetic outcome of wound closure
- Technically difficult wounds—eyelid lacerations, complex auricular cartilage injuries
- Patients who may be non-compliant with management in the acute care setting.

Anaesthesia of wounds

Given the high concentration of cutaneous nerve fibres, any trauma to the skin can cause significant pain. Examining and preparing a wound for closure or dressing can exacerbate pain and result in increased anxiety for the patient. Providing relief in the form of local anaesthesia and analgesia is essential to maximise wound preparation and compliance to treatment. Ensure that neurovascular assessment is complete before administering local anaesthetics.

Local anaesthetics work by temporarily inhibiting the influx of sodium through sodium-specific channels of the nerve cells. The result is a decrease of depolarisation and repolarisation of nerve cells and, subsequently, inhibition of both afferent and efferent conduction of impulses. Anaesthesia for wound care can be provided in a number of forms (Table 18.2).

Local infiltration of anaesthesia, commonly lignocaine, relies on the anaesthetic being injected intradermally and subcutaneously. It is the most common method of local anaesthesia administration. It can, however, distort the wound edges and may not be suitable if precise opposition of the wound edges is required. For wounds where haemostasis has not been achieved, lignocaine with adrenaline can be used to provide local vasodilation and anaesthesia, aiding in haemostasis and examination. Due to its vasoconstrictive quality, it should not be used on arterial endpoints such as digit tips or ears.

Local infiltration of anaesthetic is painful. The pain is caused by a combination of the solution temperature, its acidity and the infiltration pressure distorting the surrounding soft tissues. Techniques used to reduce pain include warming the anaesthetic solution to body temperature, using a slow injection rate, buffering the anaesthetic solution to neutralise its pH and using a small-bore needle to infiltrate the wound.

The solution can be warmed by holding the anaesthetic in a closed hand for several minutes. This can be done by the patient where appropriate, as equipment is set up. Of the most commonly used anaesthetics in the acute care setting, lignocaine has a pH of 6.5 and bupivacaine 4.0–6.5. The acidity of the anaesthetic can be buffered by adding 1 mL of sodium bicarbonate 8.4% (1 mmol/mL) to every 9 mL of lignocaine 1%. Buffering anaesthetic may decrease the time to onset of anaesthesia, but can maintain anaesthesia for longer.[58,60,61] A 27-gauge needle minimises pain on infiltration; where not available, it is suggested to use the smallest gauge available.

Topical application relies on dermal absorption of local anaesthetic. These preparations come in combinations of adrenaline, lignocaine and amethocaine (ALA); tetracaine, adrenaline and cocaine (TAC); or lignocaine, adrenaline and tetracaine (LAT). The combination gives both anaesthesia and local vasoconstriction. Adrenaline also serves to prolong the action of the anaesthetic and inhibit its systemic absorption. Again, due to its vasoconstrictive quality, it should not be used on arterial endpoints such as digit tips or ears. It is frequently used successfully on children with wounds to alleviate any anxiety surrounding the use of needles. Note that EMLA,

TABLE 18.2 Local anaesthetics commonly used in the acute care setting[56,57]

DRUG	DOSE	DURATION	ADVANTAGES/USES	DISADVANTAGES/EXCLUSIONS
Lignocaine 1%	3–5 mg/kg	0.5–2 hours	All locations	
Lignocaine with 1% adrenaline 1:100,000	5–7 mg/kg	2–5 hours	Areas likely to bleed Areas already bleeding Easier to see effect and where you are going	Regional blocks Wounds at end arterial points
Bupivacaine	2 mg/kg	2–12 hours	Longer-acting, useful for dental analgesia and situations where long duration is beneficial	Longer onset
Topical anaesthesia				
Lignocaine/adrenaline	Max: 0.1 mg/kg	20–30 minutes	Topical—no infiltration required	Wounds at end points
Amethocaine preparation	0.5–1 mL/cm of wound		Areas likely to bleed	Wounds larger than 5 cm Short duration

a topical dermal anaesthetic preparation of lignocaine and prilocaine, is not for use on open wounds.[59]

Anaesthesia can also be obtained through regional nerve blocks. Nerve fibres proximal to the wound are flooded with anaesthetic, blocking nerve conduction. This method is particularly useful for digit injuries and facial injuries, particularly the lip and intraoral injuries. It provides anaesthesia to larger areas without distorting the wound edges.

Local anaesthetics are relatively safe to use, but systemic responses can occur due to sensitivity or allergy, or if the recommended maximum dose is exceeded.

Wound cleansing/preparation

Studies have shown that potable, distilled, cooled boiled or high-quality tap water can be used to irrigate minor acute wounds, demonstrating infection rates to be similar regardless of the solution used.[62–64] Custom and patient expectation is still persuasive in the use of Normal saline over tap water for irrigation in clinical practice.

It is a relatively common practice to clean wound edges and surrounding tissues with cleansing solutions such as chlorhexidine or povidone–iodine, to inhibit migration of bacteria into the wound. While most sources recommend the use of Normal saline or potable tap water for wound irrigation, there is some evidence that the use of povidone–iodine diluted to 1% for grossly contaminated wounds in the initial wound-preparation process decreases the incidence of infection (Table 18.3). When used within the wound, however, these solutions can impair healing and immune response and should not be routinely used to cleanse wounds during ongoing wound care.[63,67]

There are conflicting recommendations on the ideal pressure of irrigation and the tools required to provide these pressures. Studies suggest that the ideal pressure for wound irrigation without causing tissue trauma is between 8 psi and 13 psi. Recommendations to achieve this pressure include using a 10 mL syringe and a 22-gauge needle; a 35 mL syringe and a 16/18-gauge needle; and a 20 mL syringe and 21-gauge needle.[63,64,68,69]

Regardless of the size of syringe and needle used, it is well recognised that copious irrigation of wounds forms the mainstay of wound cleansing and infection reduction.

Wound closure

Primary wound healing or healing by primary intention occurs when wound edges can be approximated and closed with suture material, topical adhesive or wound-closure strip dressings. There are several different types of tissue adhesives available, with no particular product proven to be superior in effect.[70] Healing begins within hours. Wounds closed by primary closure have a better cosmetic appearance and generally have fewer problems with abnormal scarring, presuming that the healing process is not complicated by infection or wound breakdown. Ideally, simple, non-contaminated wounds should be closed as soon as possible after injury. However, the maximum allowable time between injury and primary wound closure is yet to be clearly defined.[71,75,76] Various studies recommend that scalp and face wounds can be closed up to 24 hours after the injury with good outcome, while wounds of the body have a better healing outcome if closed within 12–18 hours of the injury.[67,72]

Secondary wound healing or healing by secondary intention involves no formal wound closure, allowing healing to occur by cellular regeneration from the base and edges of the wound. This form of wound management is used where there is overlying tissue loss which inhibits closure by primary intention. Closure by secondary intention has an increased risk of infection due to the lack of epidermis to provide a barrier to the external environment. After cleansing, wounds are dressed to optimise cellular regeneration and healing from the wound bed and

TABLE 18.3 Wound-cleansing solutions[31,66]				
SOLUTION	PROPERTIES	MECHANISM OF ACTION	USES	DISADVANTAGES
Normal saline	Isotonic, non-toxic	Simple washing action	In wound for irrigation	No antiseptic action
Chlorhexidine 0.1 w/v aqueous	Bacteriostatic	Antibacterial and washing action	Cleanse skin surrounding wound	Not near eyes (causes keratitis), perforated ear drum or meninges
Chlorhexidine 0.1% w/v + cetrimide 1% w/v	Bacteriostatic	Antibacterial and soap action, removes sebum, 'wetting' the skin	Cleanse skin surrounding wound	Not near mucous membranes, eyes (causes keratitis), perforated ear drum or meninges
Hydrogen peroxide (H_2O_2) 3%	Bacteriocidal to anaerobes	Forms superoxide radicals	Severely contaminated wounds with anaerobic-type pathogens	Obstruction of wound surface capillaries and subsequent necrosis
Povidone–iodine 10% w/v	Bacteriocidal, fungicidal, viricidal, sporacidal	Releases free iodine	On surrounding skin, or in severely contaminated wounds (dilute 1% w/v)	Use on/in large wounds, may cause acidosis due to iodine absorption

edges and require ongoing dressing changes and observation. It may take several weeks to even months for a wound to heal by secondary intention, and may be of considerable cost to the patient, both financially and socially.

Superficial wounds such as minor abrasions can be left to heal by secondary intention, with short-term use of simple dressings and/or soft white paraffin or antibiotic ointment in some instances.

Tertiary or delayed primary wound healing is reserved for heavily contaminated wounds. Wounds managed by delayed primary closure are not closed for 2–3 days to allow for passage of foreign material and exudate.[12,71] Frequent dressing changes are required to manage infection and promote debridement. Only when infection is resolved and the wound is free of debris is a decision made to close the wound. If there is an extensive delay to closure, the wound may no longer be suitable to close by primary intention. The wound is then left to heal by secondary intention or referred to a surgeon to be closed via skin grafting.

Wounds that expose vital structures, large wounds over joints or at cosmetically significant sites are not suitable for secondary intention healing. These require early referral to a surgeon for consideration of closure technique and possible skin grafting.

Dressings

Dressings have a number of purposes:

- to apply pressure to control bleeding
- to provide a barrier between the wound and surrounding tissue and the external environment
- to reduce pain
- to eliminate dead space
- to remove non-viable tissue
- to control exudate
- to optimise conditions for wound healing, by providing a moist wound environment and optimal wound bed temperature.

The goal of a wound dressing is to create the optimal environment for cellular regeneration and migration and assist in wound healing. Some specialised dressings are impregnated with antimicrobial substances which assist in the control of microbial load in infected wounds.

For acute wounds, the first objective is to achieve haemostasis, be it through direct digital pressure or a firm compression bandage. Where possible, it is best to use a simple dressing moistened with potable tap water or Normal saline, as bleeding is likely to recur on removal of a dry dressing that has adhered to the wound.

When a decision is made to apply a wound dressing, product choice is reliant on a number of factors. Consideration should be given to the nature of the wound and the goal of treatment, whether to promote moisture, control exudate or manage contamination. A rule of thumb is to keep dressings as simple as possible, avoid excessive wound dressing changes and minimise changing the type of products used at each dressing change. Studies have shown that in instances of non-infected wounds, less-frequent dressing changes supports healing through maintaining wound-bed temperature. Enzymatic and cellular function is at its optimum when the wound bed is at body temperature.[73] On each dressing change, the wound-bed temperature decreases due to exposure. The longer it is left exposed, the greater the temperature decrease. This is further exacerbated by using cool cleaning solutions. It can take several hours before the wound can return to body temperature for cellular regeneration and healing to recommence.

Dressing choice may also be affected by the circumstances of the patient. Issues to consider include whether the patient will be discharged or admitted to hospital, whether the patient will be able to care for the wound themselves with education and advice, and whether suitable wound care follow-up can be arranged. Consideration should also be given to the ongoing financial costs of dressings. In some instances, patients may need to purchase the dressing materials themselves, which may become a financial burden if dressings are expensive and required for extended periods. Local availability of products will also affect choice. Table 18.4 summarises the dressing types most frequently used in the acute care setting, and their purpose.

Prophylactic antibiotics

Intact and healthy skin is a poor medium for bacterial growth. It is when the skin is breached, or if it is overly moist and occlusive, that conditions support the growth of bacteria.

Thorough wound irrigation and cleansing techniques are the mainstay of antimicrobial treatment. Controversy still surrounds the use of prophylactic antibiotics for wounds in general. Antibiotic prophylaxis should be reserved for high-risk wounds only. High-risk wounds include bite and deep wounds to the hands, feet or face; over joints; grossly contaminated wounds; and wounds involving underlying structures. Contaminated wounds, where there is a delay in treatment, may also be considered high risk. There is debate over the exact time frame considered as 'delayed', but many sources suggest 8 hours.[75,76] Patients with co-morbidities affecting the immune system or wound healing, such as diabetes, and the elderly, are at greater risk of infection due to their inability to mount an adequate physiological response to infection. For these patients, infection may be the result of both normal skin commensals such as *Staphylococcus* and *Streptococcus* species, as well as opportunistic Gram-negative bacteria, such as *Pseudomonas* species. Antibiotic prophylaxis should be considered the exception rather than the rule in managing the acute wound.

There is growing concern regarding increasing resistance to antibiotic therapy. This has been attributed to inappropriate antibiotic selection, inappropriate use of antibiotics and over-prescribing. In Australia the National Prescribing Service (NPS) has published therapeutic guidelines to enhance the appropriate use and choice of therapy and, importantly, when they are not needed.[76] The risk of other complications to the patient such as adverse side effects and allergy should also not be overlooked. Antibiotic prophylaxis should be tailored to the individual circumstances of each patient.[75,77]

If prophylaxis is indicated, antibiotic choice is based on:

- knowledge of suspected pathogens involved
- local hospital or other health-setting policy
- national drug prescribing guidelines
- local availability

TABLE 18.4 Wound dressings commonly used in the acute care setting[66,72]

PRODUCT	CHARACTERISTICS/PURPOSE	EXAMPLES
Gauze	Provides absorption of exudate Supports debridement if applied and kept moist Maintains wound moisture if applied moistened Filter dressing in sinus tract	Numerous products available
Non-adherent dressings (woven or non-woven)	May be impregnated with saline, petroleum or antimicrobials Minimal absorbency	Adaptic Exu-dry Sofsorb Telfa Vaseline gauze Xeroform
Transparent films	Semipermeable membrane permits gaseous exchange between wound bed and environment For dry, non-infected wounds or wounds with minimal drainage Minimally absorbent—exudate at wound collects beneath dressing Protective barrier to bacteria	Acu-derm Biocclusive Blisterfilm Opsite Polyskin Tegaderm Transeal
Hydrocolloid	Occlusive dressing—no gaseous exchange between wound bed and external environment Occlusion—exudate collects at wound to promote moist wound environment Used for superficial and partial-thickness wounds—light to moderate drainage Not used in infected wounds Supports debridement and prevents secondary infections	Comfeel DuoDerm Intact Intrasite Restore Tegasorb Ultec
Polyurethane foams	Absorptive dressing—moderate to heavy amounts of exudate can be absorbed Can be used on infected wounds Used for partial- or full-thickness wounds with minimal to heavy drainage	Allevyn Epilock Hydrasorb Lyofoam Mitraflex Synthaderm
Absorption dressings	Large volumes of exudate can be absorbed Maintains moist wound surface Supports debridement Can be placed into wounds to obliterate dead space Used for partial- or full-thickness wounds Used for infected wounds	AlgoDERM Bard Absorption Debrisan DuoDerm Paste Hydragan Kaltostat Sorbsan
Hydrogel	Adds moisture to the wound bed Debridement because of moisturising effects—used to hydrate necrosis for debridement Available as a sheet or gel—mostly requires a secondary dressing Limited absorption of exudate (gel sheets) Used for partial- or full-thickness wounds, deep wounds with minimal drainage Used for necrotic wounds	Vigilon Elasto Gel Intrasite Gel Geliperm

- patient factors such as allergy or background medical conditions
- ease of antibiotic dosage regimen and maximisation of compliance.

The most likely contaminants of any wound are normal skin commensals such as Gram-positive *Staphylococcus* and *Streptococcus* species. Generally, penicillins are considered first-line treatment for antibiotic prophylaxis; or, if penicillin allergy exists, first-generation cephalosporins.[76] Bite wounds are also likely to be contaminated by a mixture of normal skin commensals and the oral flora of the causative animal (see the section on bite wounds later in the chapter).

Patient education regarding antibiotic use, including appropriate dosing, time intervals and completion of course, is vital to ensure effective results and limit the development of antibiotic resistance.

Delayed prescribing is an attempt to allow normal resolution of an infection before antibiotics are started by providing a prescription and advising the patient to wait for 24–48 hours while observing the wound, and only filling the prescription if antibiotics are indicated. Early signs of infection will generally begin to establish themselves within this timeframe. This 'wait and see' approach gives the patient some control over their health, prevents unnecessary antibiotic use and may prevent multiple trips to a healthcare facility for further advice. The approach is, however, reliant on thorough patient education and cooperation.

PRACTICE TIP
WOUNDS AT HIGHER RISK OF INFECTION

Wounds
- Grossly contaminated wounds
- Puncture wounds involving the hand, foot or face
- Cat and human bite wounds, some dog bite wounds
- Contaminated wounds with delay > 8 hours to irrigation treatment
- Wounds involving bone, joints, tendons and ligaments
- Open fractures
- Full-thickness intraoral wounds

Health of host
- Diabetes
- Obesity
- Immunocompromise/autoimmune/haematological disorders, malignancy
- Vascular disease
- Renal disease
- Elderly
- Malnutrition
- Medications—steroids, chemotherapy

Social factors
- Smoker
- Excessive alcohol/illicit drug use

Topical antibiotic ointment
The use of an antibiotic ointment such as chloramphenicol, particularly on sutured facial wounds as prophylaxis against infection, has been common recent practice.[78,79] However, more-recent reviews of this practice have found that the use of antibiotic ointment resulted in no clinically significant reduction in infection, although studies were limited to once-only application.[80–82] It is also believed that this practice may minimise scarring. The mechanism of scar reduction is unclear, but it is thought that chloramphenicol is a collagenase.[78,83] It can be argued that it is the massaging action of the application that reduces the scar, or the fact that the wound is kept moist. When using chloramphenicol ointment topically on wounds, consideration should be given to the potential for allergy or systemic side effects, such as pernicious anaemia, due to the active antimicrobial ingredient. Larger wounds may require a larger quantity of ointment, which may increase the risk of systemic side effects. Non-medicated soft white paraffin is a suitable alternative. More studies are required to further investigate the practice; clinicians should refer to local guidelines.

Tetanus immunisation
Tetanus is a systemic bacterial infection caused by *Clostridium tetani*. The bacterium can be found in the gastrointestinal tract of various animals, and as spores found in soil and dust. It is a hardy bacterium, and is resistant to many antiseptics and heat.

If a wound is contaminated by the *C. tetani* spore, the bacteria replicate anaerobically, incubating over a period of 2 days to 2 weeks. Once infection is established, the bacteria produce a toxin which acts on the central nervous system causing generalised muscle spasms and rigidity, resulting in trismus, fractures and muscle rupture. If left untreated, it can cause spasm of the ventilatory muscles, seizures, hypertension, cardiac dysrhythmia or arrest, and can be fatal.[84,85]

In Australia, as in many industrialised counties, the vast majority of deaths from tetanus occur in people over 70 years of age, with previous vaccination being a significant number of years prior to the injury; or in those from migrant populations who have had no previous vaccination at all.[83] Widespread immunisation programs beginning in childhood have been effective in limiting cases of tetanus. Boosters in adulthood are generally given on presentation to a medical facility to patients with a tetanus-prone wound, and are often given prophylactically prior to overseas travel.

Wounds that are considered prone to tetanus infection include:

- wounds contaminated by dirt or soil
- bite wounds
- deep, penetrating wounds
- wounds containing foreign materials
- crush injuries and open fractures.

Care should be taken to establish the immunisation history of any patient presenting with a wound and, where appropriate, a tetanus vaccination should be administered. For patients who have not received a primary course of three vaccinations, a tetanus immunoglobulin must also be administered with the initial vaccination, usually in the opposite arm. The Australian Tetanus Vaccination Guidelines are summarised in

Table 18.5 and provide a quick reference to ascertaining the tetanus vaccination requirements for a patient presenting with a wound.

Categories of wound

Abrasions

An abrasion is a wound caused by friction between the skin and a rough or hard surface, causing layers of the epidermis to be removed. There is superficial damage to the skin, involving the epidermis. A more-traumatic abrasion that removes deeper layers of skin is called an avulsion (see below).

Deep abrasions that remove the full thickness of epidermis can be painful, due to the exposure of superficial nerve endings. Management of abrasions includes wound irrigation and debridement, which may require either local anaesthesia or an inhaled anxiolytic. If debris such as gravel is left in the wound it may be visible through the epidermis after the wound has healed, as a tattoo. Care should be taken, particularly in cosmetically significant areas, to remove debris to avoid tattooing.

Abrasions should be kept moist to aid healing. This can be achieved with soft white paraffin or, in some instances, chloramphenicol ointment to retain moisture, and a non-adhesive dressing. Abrasions heal by secondary intention.

While different in mechanism, abrasions result in the same physiological effects as superficial or partial-thickness burns, including pain, fluid loss and loss of protective properties. It is suggested that widespread and deeper abrasions should be managed in the same way as superficial burns.

Avulsions

An avulsion refers to 'tearing away'. An avulsion of tissue results in the loss of both epidermis and dermis. In these instances, approximation of wound edges is not possible. Avulsion is also used to describe the 'tearing away' of a nail from the nail bed, as in the case of a nail avulsion (see earlier in the chapter). Degloving injuries are the result of a circumferential avulsion of skin over a larger surface, such as a digit, hand, foot or limb.

Management includes copious wound irrigation and debridement, which will require either local anaesthesia or possibly inhaled anxiolytics to perform. Avulsions can be successfully healed by secondary intention using dressings. Severe degloving injuries that involve larger areas of tissue loss will require referral to a surgeon for management under general anaesthesia and consideration for skin grafting.

Contusions and haematomas

A contusion occurs as a result of blunt trauma to the skin, causing rupture of blood vessels and subsequent diffuse bleeding into the local tissues. A contusion can be superficial, involving the skin, or can involve deeper structures such as muscle and bone. A 'corked muscle' is a muscle contusion resulting from a direct blunt trauma, normally to a limb, crushing the muscle

---

TABLE 18.5 Australian tetanus vaccination guidelines[106]

HISTORY OF TETANUS VACCINATION	TIME SINCE LAST DOSE	TYPE OF WOUND	DTPa, DTPa COMBINATION, dT OR dTpa AS APPROPRIATE	TETANUS IMMUNOGLOBULIN (TIG)*
≥ 3 doses	< 5 years	Clean minor wounds	No	No
		All other wounds†	No	No‡
	5–10 years	Clean minor wounds	No	No
		All other wounds†	Yes	No‡
	> 10 years	Clean minor wounds	Yes	No
		All other wounds	Yes	No‡
< 3 doses or uncertain§		Clean minor wounds	Yes	No
		All other wounds†	Yes	Yes

DTPa: infant/child formulation diphtheria–tetanus–acellular pertussis vaccine

dTpa: adult/adolescent formulation diphtheria–tetanus–acellular pertussis vaccine

dT: adult formulation diphtheria–tetanus vaccine

* The recommended dose for TIG is 250 IU, given by IM injection, as soon as practicable after the injury. If more than 24 hours have elapsed, 500 IU should be given. Because of its viscosity, TIG should be given to adults using a 21-gauge needle. For children, it can be given slowly using a 23-gauge needle.

† All wounds, other than clean minor wounds, should be considered 'tetanus-prone'.

‡ Individuals with a humoral immune deficiency (including HIV-infected persons who have immunodeficiency) should be given TIG if they have received a tetanus-prone injury, regardless of the time since their last dose of tetanus-containing vaccine.

§ Persons who have no documented history of a primary vaccination course (3 doses) with a tetanus toxoid-containing vaccine should receive all missing doses and must receive TIG.

against the underlying bone. Minor contusions cause minimal discomfort and pose no risk.

A more significant blunt trauma can result in a *haematoma*, a discrete interstitial collection of blood. Where it occurs beneath the surface of the skin it presents initially as a firm swelling. It progresses to a boggy swelling as the collection breaks down. The combination of the collection of blood and the swelling resulting from the local inflammatory process results in an increase in local pressure beneath the skin. This pressure can pose a risk to overlying skin integrity and is detected by local nerve endings causing the sensation of pain. Extravasated blood is an irritant to soft tissues and this also contributes to the pain sensation.

Initial treatment is compression, elevation where appropriate and ice to promote vasoconstriction and decreased flow from the ruptured vessels, maximising the environment for clot formation. If a larger vessel has ruptured, the clotting process alone may be unable to stem the blood flow. In this instance, the ruptured vessel may need to be sutured closed. Smaller vessels may be closed with sutures in the acute care setting, while injury to larger vessels may require urgent referral.

In most instances the haematoma will eventually be reabsorbed. Larger haematomas or those slow to resolve may need to be drained or evacuated to promote healing. Infection is a common complication of a haematoma, as the stagnant blood collection provides an excellent environment for bacteria colonisation.

Patients on anticoagulant therapies or with coagulopathies are at increased risk of developing haematomas from a relatively minor injury and risk significant loss of intravascular blood volume.

Lacerations

A laceration is a wound where the skin is torn or cut, following trauma (Fig 18.16). The skin is separated without tissue loss. Management includes wound irrigation and debridement, which may require local anaesthesia. Superficial lacerations involving the epidermis and dermis can be closed with topical adhesive or wound-closure strip dressings. Lacerations under tension, over moving joints or where the edges are not easily opposed may require closure with sutures. Deeper lacerations

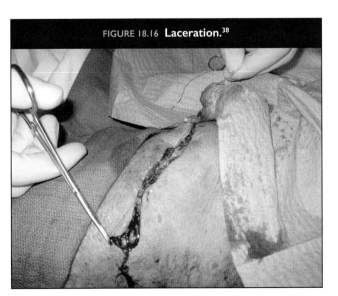

FIGURE 18.16 **Laceration.**[38]

may require closure in layers, using absorbable buried sutures at the wound base to oppose muscle facia. This inhibits the creation of dead space which is an ideal environment for bacteria colonisation. After closure, a non-adherent dressing should be applied for 48 hours until epithelial bridging has taken place, providing provisional coverage of the wound.[86]

Puncture wounds

A puncture wound is caused by penetration of the skin by a sharp object, creating a small hole. They are common on the feet after treading on objects and can be deceptive in their appearance. Minor puncture wounds rarely result in excessive bleeding. Deep wounds can appear relatively minor, yet can damage deeper structures. Objects causing puncture wounds can deposit foreign matter and infective organisms into the wound itself, leading to an increased risk of infection. Puncture wounds rapidly close, so cleansing to the wound base is difficult.

A high index of suspicion for retained foreign body should be held for puncture wounds, particularly if sustained on glass or other materials which may have broken off in the wound. Foreign bodies are discussed below.

Wound cleansing is often limited to the skin surface. Puncture wounds should not be closed, to allow the passage of debris and exudate. Dressings should provide wound coverage and manage any potential exudate.

Prophylactic antibiotics are only indicated in puncture wounds considered at high risk of infection. Factors to consider include the site and depth of the wound, involvement of underlying structures, risk of wound contamination by the inflicting implement and general health of the patient. Antibiotics are indicated, in particular, for significant plantar puncture wounds, which are commonly the result of a highly contaminated source.

Foreign bodies

Any wound caused by a foreign object can potentially leave foreign material at the wound site. The presence of foreign material instigates a local inflammatory process.

Certain foreign matter is radio-opaque, including glass > 2 mm long, metal, teeth, pencil graphite, certain plastics, gravel and sand, and may be visible on plain-film X-rays. Other, non-radio-opaque objects, such as wood, will often require ultrasound examination to detect. Organic material may also produce toxins, further intensifying the inflammatory response.

Any object, even those that are large, may be more difficult to locate and remove than it appears and may require specialist equipment such as image intensification. However, small, innocuous material that causes no discomfort or loss of function to the patient can in some instances be left in situ. Attempted removal can often cause more trauma to the local tissue, increase the size of the wound and the risk of scarring or infection or result in cosmetically poor outcomes, frequently without successful retrieval of the foreign material. The decision to leave or remove the foreign body should be based on the individual circumstances in each case.

Where an inert foreign body is left in place, a physiological response may occur at the site, where the foreign body is 'walled off' or encased, forming a foreign-body granuloma. Beneath the skin this can be felt as a firm, discreet swelling. Foreign-body granulomas have little clinical significance.

Impaled objects should be stabilised until safe removal can be assured, or referred to a surgeon.

Wounds sustained in fresh, salt or brackish water

Consideration should be given to wounds sustained in or around water. These often result from punctures or lacerations from foreign matter beneath the water's surface; for example, coral cuts, lacerations from boat motor propeller blades and embedded fish hooks. The most common water-borne organisms causing soft-tissue infection include *Aeromonas* species in fresh or brackish water, *Vibrio* species in salt water or brackish water and *Mycobacterium marinum* in fish tanks.[87] Ciprofloxacin or doxycycline are the recommended antibiotic treatments.[88]

Bite wounds

A bite wound can be caused by animals or humans. The resulting wound can be a combination of abrasion, laceration or puncture, and may involve underlying muscle, tendons, ligaments, bone, vasculature or organs. Not all animal bites are severe enough to prompt a patient to seek medical attention, and the significant risk to public health and safety is potentially underestimated. Animal bites comprise around 2% of emergency presentations each year.[89]

The severity of an injury must be considered in the context of the inflicting animal, the site of the injury and the general health of the patient. Bite wounds considered at high risk of infection include:

- all cat bite wounds
- complicated dog and human bite wounds
- all bite wounds involving the hand, foot, face and those over a joint
- puncture or crush wounds potentially penetrating underlying structures such as tendons, ligaments, bones or joints
- wounds resulting in vascular or lymphatic compromise

- wounds where there has a been a delay of more than 8 hours to cleansing, debridement and treatment
- co-morbidities, resulting in immunocompromise.[75,90]

Bite wounds require particular attention due to the high risk of contamination by a combination of the oral flora of the causative animal and the normal skin flora at the bite site (Fig 18.17). All bite wounds should be considered multimicrobial contaminated wounds. Gram-negative organisms such as *Pasteurella* and, less commonly, *Capnocytophaga* are particular to dog and cat bites. *Haemophilus* spp., *Eikenella corrodens* and other anaerobes are prevalent in human bites.[89,91]

Copious wound irrigation and debridement for any bite wound is vital to reduce the incidence of infection. Wounds are routinely managed by delayed primary closure. An exception to this is facial bite wounds, extensive lacerations and disfiguring wounds which require referral to a surgeon for washout and closure by primary intention.[92]

If prophylactic antibiotics are indicated, antibiotic selection should be based on the normal bacterial flora at the wound site, the likely oral flora of the offending animal and the patient's individual circumstances.[89] Amoxicillin and clavulanic acid combinations such as Augmentin in non-penicillin-allergic patients are considered first-line presumptive therapy. Refer to local guidelines to inform the decision for prophylactic antibiotics.[76]

Consider surgical referral for patients with cosmetically significant bites such as wounds of the face, extensive or disfiguring bite wounds or bites that involve underlying structures or fractures, particularly of the hand. These may require surgical washout. All bite wounds are considered tetanus-prone wounds and tetanus prophylaxis should be considered.

Dog bites

Dog bites are the most common bite injury, accounting for 80–90% of presentations.[89,91] Dog bites can result in abrasions, lacerations and/or avulsion of tissue. Due to the significant

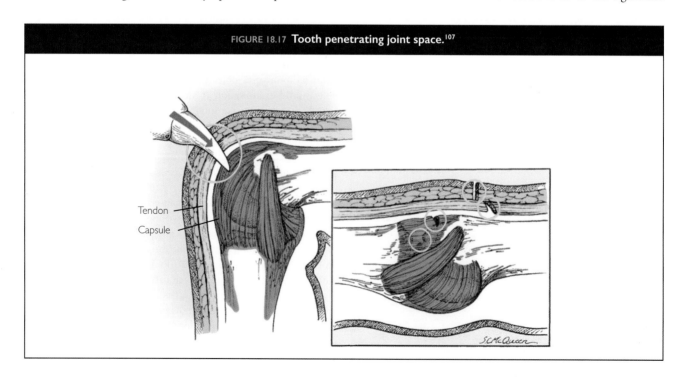

FIGURE 18.17 **Tooth penetrating joint space.**[107]

Tendon
Capsule

pressure exerted by the canine jaw, fractures are common. Studies indicate the infection rate of dog bite wounds is between 4% and 25%.[91,93]

Cat bites

Cat bite wounds most commonly result in puncture wounds, due to the shape of feline teeth. Bites commonly occur on the arm and hands. The infection rate of cat bites is greater than that of dog bites due to the penetrating nature of the bite. Cat bites press foreign debris and bacteria deep into the tissues, which is difficult to clear with wound cleansing as puncture wounds close over soon after injury. This traps foreign material in the tissues, increasing infection risk. Cat bites are therefore commonly treated prophylactically with antibiotics.[91]

Human bites

Human bite wounds are often the result of physical fighting and assault. These bite injuries commonly occur on the hand, face and head, including the ear. Mechanical falls can cause accidentally self-inflicted bite wounds to the lip and oral mucosa.

Human bite wounds often become infected due to the large load of normal oral flora contaminating the wound site. Human saliva can contain up to 190 different species of organisms.[94] Human bite wounds are associated with a 50% infection rate.[90] This is significantly reduced with the use of antibiotics.

There is a theoretical risk of blood-borne virus transmission from person to person following a human bite injury. Human bites have been shown to transmit hepatitis B, hepatitis C, herpes simplex virus (HSV), syphilis, tuberculosis, actinomycosis and tetanus.[94] An attack by an unknown person would raise concern regarding risk. If the patient's immunisation status against hepatitis B is unknown, it is generally recommended that the patient be administered hepatitis B immunoglobulin together with the first vaccination of an accelerated course of hepatitis B immunisation.[90] There is no active or passive vaccination for hepatitis C. Infection with HIV is negligible through a human bite. Many cases of bite injuries from known HIV/AIDS patients have been documented with no viral transmission; therefore the potential for salivary transmission of HIV is remote—blood-to-blood contact is necessary.[95–97]

Cosmetically significant wounds

Wounds to the face

Wounds to the face can be the cause of significant anxiety due to the potential for scarring or disfigurement.[98] This is particularly so in parents of young children with facial lacerations. Wounds are frequently caused by a blow to the face. Falls are common in the elderly, while punch injuries and assaults are common in younger adults. A blow to the face often results in underlying facial bone fractures. Examination should include assessment of underlying facial bones for crepitus or tenderness, and facial sensory and motor function to exclude damage to the branches of the facial and trigeminal nerves.

Facial skin is highly vascular, so simple, non-contaminated lacerations generally heal and are rarely complicated by infection. Skin develops along lines of tension (Fig 18.18). Lacerations following the direction of these lines generally have a better cosmetic outcome. Lacerations perpendicular to these lines often result in the scar widening, as the edges are under constant tension.

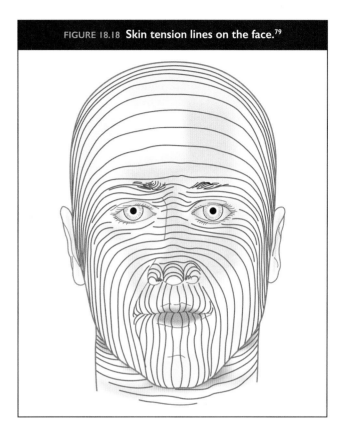

FIGURE 18.18 Skin tension lines on the face.[79]

Simple, non-contaminated facial wounds can be managed in the acute care setting. Wounds involving underlying fractures or those resulting in motor sensory deficit will require referral. Depending on the skills of the clinician, technically challenging wounds where cosmetic outcome is a concern may also be referred for surgical opinion. Wounds of the face are difficult to dress, and are frequently left uncovered and topical chloramphenicol ointment applied.

Oral mucosa and lip wounds

Lip and oral lacerations often occur as a result of a blow to the mouth, often the result of a fall or a blow to the face. Lacerations are often caused by the teeth, but can also be from the surface of the causative factor, such as a jewellery ring or the fingernail of an assailant. Oral wounds tend to bleed profusely at the time of injury, often resolving relatively quickly. Minor injuries are often seen in the acute care setting, as the patient equates the blood loss with significant injury.

When examining wounds sustained by a blow to the mouth, it is important to assess for broken or missing teeth, bite malocclusion or trismus (inability to fully open the mouth). Patients with crown fractures and misplaced teeth should be referred to a dentist for repair. Care of dental injuries is discussed later in this chapter and in more depth in Chapter 32. Patients with trismus or bite malocclusion may have a mandibular fracture and will require radiological investigation and referral. Consideration should be given to the location and possible involvement of the parotid and submandibular ducts and glands. Involvement of these structures will require referral.

Buccal mucosa and lips heal rapidly due to the nature of mucosal regeneration. Minor wounds not involving muscle or other buccal structures which have ceased bleeding do not require closure. For deeper wounds where a significant gaping or defect exists or the oral musculature is involved, layered closure using absorbable suture material may be required after careful, thorough wound preparation. Where a deep intraoral injury also involves a tooth fracture, explore the wound carefully to ensure the tooth fragment is not embedded in the wound.

In full-thickness 'through-and-through' lacerations there is a communication between the internal oral surface and the exterior skin surface. The external surface and intraoral musculature should be closed after careful wound preparation.

Minor tongue lacerations will heal with no cosmetic or functional deficit. Large tongue lacerations may need to be referred for closure, to avoid deformity.[99]

Lacerations to the surface of the lip may require closure to prevent cosmetic defect (Fig 18.19). Lacerations involving the vermilion border require precise approximation of edges. These lacerations are often closed using regional anaesthetic blocks such as mental nerve blocks, inferior alveolar nerve blocks or infraorbital nerve blocks, so that the wound edges are not distorted by local infiltration.

Meticulous oral hygiene is essential to avoid infection and promote healing. Normal saline mouth washes six times a day, particularly after meals, is advised. The patient should also be advised to avoid hot food and drinks and eat a soft diet.

There is no clear indication for antibiotic prophylaxis use in intraoral wounds. General practice reserves antibiotic prophylaxis for deep intraoral lacerations and through-and-through lacerations. Penicillin is the first-line choice.[79,99]

Dental injuries

Injuries to the mouth can result in injury to the teeth: tooth fractures, tooth avulsion or luxation. Tooth luxation refers to injury where the tooth remains in the socket but is displaced. The tooth can be twisted within the tooth socket space, pushed into the gum (intrusion) or incompletely pulled away from the gum line (extrusion). See Chapter 32 for more in-depth detail of dental injuries.

Where teeth are fractured and dental pulp is exposed (Fig 18.20), the injury can be very painful and may require local anaesthesia to manage. The fractured tooth and exposed pulp should be flushed with Normal saline and, if available, the pulp covered with a calcium hydroxide mix such as Dycal. Once set, the surface should be covered with glass ionomer

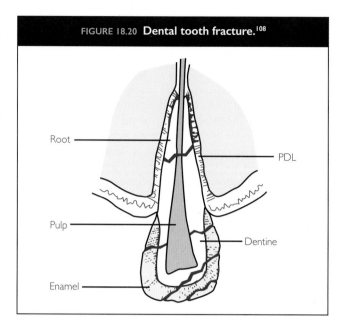

FIGURE 18.20 **Dental tooth fracture.**[108]

Root — PDL

Pulp — Dentine

Enamel

cement (GIC). Sealing the pulp will provide some pain relief, as the exposed dental nerves are sealed. This can also potentially save the tooth, reducing future dental costs for the patient.

Where the tooth is avulsed, best treatment is immediate re-implantation in the field, as soon as possible after the injury.[100] If the tooth is not immediately re-implanted, it is best transported in milk as this preserves the cells of the periodontal ligament (PDL) over the surface of the tooth root, as it is of similar pH to the PDL cells.[101] However, viability reduces after 3 hours. Where milk is not available, Normal saline is the next most appropriate solution to transport tooth survival. Re-implantation is generally unsuccessful where the tooth remains avulsed and is left to dry out.

To prepare a tooth for re-implantation, the tooth should be run under clean tap water or Normal saline, being careful not to remove or touch the root surface. The socket should be prepared by gentle irrigation with Normal saline and the lost tooth can be placed back into the tooth socket space. Ensure it is facing the correct way round. Re-implantation of deciduous or 'baby teeth' is not recommended. The avulsed tooth should then be secured in place by a splint. This can be achieved by using glass ionomer cement if available, but items such as

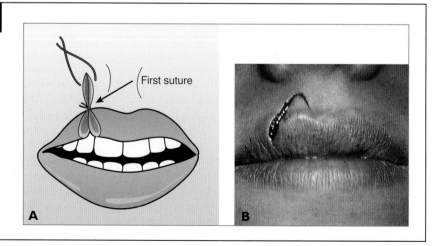

FIGURE 18.19 **Lip laceration.**

A, Position for first suture. **B**, Lacerated lip alignment.[38]

First suture

A   B

Blu-tac or aluminium foil can be fashioned as a splint. Patients who have a mouth guard or a dental retainer can also use these as a splint.

Luxations of teeth are at risk of neurovascular compromise if the nerves or vasculature are stressed or compressed. Therefore the tooth should be manipulated to the normal position under local anaesthetic block, and splinted.[102]

Dental injuries that are managed soon after the injury will increase the likelihood of a better outcome. Management in the acute care setting is only a temporary measure until definitive management by a dentist can be arranged. Patients should be advised to take a soft or preferably liquid diet, with no hot food or liquids, until dental review.

The use of antibiotic prophylaxis in the treatment of fractured and avulsed teeth is controversial. Some texts do not recommend the routine use of antibiotics, while other literature reviews recommend the use of antibiotics that cover mouth flora to decrease the inflammatory resorption of the root.[103–105] Where antibiotics are recommended, they are reserved for tooth fractures where pulp is exposed, and where the tooth socket or tooth is soiled or contaminated. Consideration should also be given to the patient's general health. Remember tetanus prophylaxis as indicated.

Wounds of the external ear

The pinna or auricle is the external, visible ear. The skin is highly vascular overlying avascular cartilage, which provides shape to the ear. Wounds to the ear are cosmetically important.

Lacerations of the external ear frequently involve laceration of the underlying cartilage. Due to lack of vascular supply, the cartilage is slower to heal. The goal of repairing auricular lacerations is to cover exposed cartilage. Some literature recommends avoiding using sutures to close auricular cartilage as this causes an increased risk of infection and subsequent delay in healing. Often the closure of the overlying skin laceration will approximate the cartilage edges without the need to suture the cartilage. Where cartilage deformity is significant it can cause distortion of the wound edges, making it difficult to close the overlying tissue.

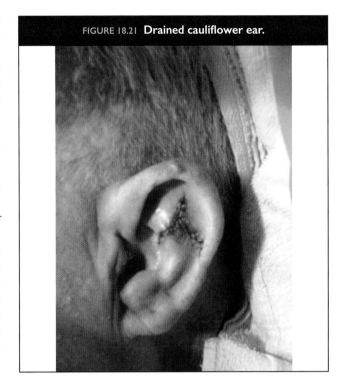

FIGURE 18.21 **Drained cauliflower ear.**

Management should include thorough irrigation and removal of debris. Debridement should be done with caution, as even a small loss of tissue may result in wound mal-union and cartilage exposure. Haematomas of the auricle should be drained, and a compressive bandage and ice applied to inhibit reformation (Fig 18.21). Auricular haematomas can result in deterioration of the underlying cartilage and a cosmetic defect known as a 'cauliflower ear'. This is often seen in players of full-contact sport. A compression bandage should be applied to all significant auricular injuries to prevent haematoma development. If injury to the external auditory canal or inner ear is suspected, referral is indicated. Antibiotic prophylaxis is reserved for contaminated wounds, and patients at high risk of infection.

SUMMARY

Minor injuries comprise a significant proportion of patients requiring pre-hospital and ED care. Timely and appropriate pre-hospital care can, where available, help to alleviate patient anxiety, their experience of pain, and most importantly can result in an overall reduction in severity of the injury and requirements of definitive in hospital treatment.

As with all physical assessment, minor injuries should be assessed using a systematic approach. The chapter has addressed the most commonly seen upper and lower limb injuries, their assessment and management. It has also covered wound examination, management of general and complex and special areas wounds and adjuncts to care including dressing choice, appropriate use of antibiotics and scar management.

CASE STUDY

Mrs Chan, a right-handed 54-year-old woman, presents to the ED after a trip and fall. She is normally well with no previous medical history. The triage nurse notes a painful right wrist and a laceration to her forehead. Although a little shaken, she looks and feels well, her vital signs are within normal limits and she reports there was no loss of consciousness. You begin to arrange some fast-tracking measures for her.

You decide to initiate some X-rays for Mrs Chan. On examination, she has a swollen wrist and is tender over her distal radius, ulna and scaphoid. On return from X-ray you manage her facial wound. It is a simple, superficial wound but requires closure with skin sutures to obtain a good cosmetic result. Mrs Chan recently immigrated to Australia and is unsure of her tetanus status. She does not recall ever having had a tetanus vaccine. You classify her wound as a clean, minor wound.

You must decide whether to provide antibiotic cover, as Mrs Chan is very concerned about the risk of a wound infection. She has no existing medical conditions and no drug allergies. Her X-ray examination does not demonstrate a fracture.

Questions

1. In what ways might you attempt to assess and relieve Mrs Chan's pain? Discuss both pharmacological and non-pharmacological measures.

2. Describe how you would systematically exclude other injuries to the right limb. What X-rays would you request? What are the issues with diagnosing scaphoid fractures on a plain X-ray?

3. What would be your choice of cleansing solution for the facial wound? How would you irrigate the wound adequately? Would you use a sterile procedure, as it is a facial wound?

4. What type of prophylaxis against tetanus would you give Mrs Chan now, and what additional injections should she be advised to have, and when, in the future?

5. What is the rationale behind your decision regarding antibiotics? Briefly discuss the explanation you give to your patient.

6. In view of Mrs Chan's scaphoid tenderness, how would manage her injury? Discuss this comparing the availability of further imaging resources where you presently work and what you would consider to be the gold standard.

Answers to Case Study Questions can be found on evolve
http://evolve.emergencytrauma.curtis

REFERENCES

1. McGinty J. Delivering a healthy WA—Fast-track for emergency patients helps cut waiting times. Ministerial Media Statements 2005. Online. www.mediastatements.wa.gov.au/ArchivedStatements/Pages/GallopLaborGovernmentSearch. aspx?ItemId=125074&minister=McGinty&admin=Gallop; accessed 10 Jan 2011.

2. Hullick C. John Hunter Hospital emergency department redesign, 2007. Online. www.hnehealth.nsw.gov.au/__data/assets/pdf_file/0010/38638/C7_JHH_ED_Redesign.pdf; accessed 15 Jan 2010.

3. O'Brien D, Williams A, Blondell K et al. Impact of streaming 'fast track' emergency department patients. Aust Health Rev 2006;30(4):525–32.

4. Fry M, Jones K. The clinical initiative nurse: Extending the role of the emergency nurse, who benefits? Australian Emergency Nursing Journal 2005;8(1–2):9–12.

5. Wallis M, Hooper J, Kerr D et al. Effectiveness of an advanced practice emergency nurse role in a minor injuries unit. Aust J Adv Nurs 2007;27(1):21–9.

6. Fry M, Rogers FT. The emergency transitional nurse practitioner role: implementation study and preliminary evaluation. Australas Emerg Nurs J 2009;12:32–7.

7. Wilson A, Shifaza F. An evaluation of the effectiveness and acceptability of nurse practitioners in an adult emergency department. Int J Nurs Pract 2008;14(2):149–56.

8. Derkson R, Coupe V, van Tulder M et al. Cost effectiveness of the SEN concept: Specialised Emergency Nurses (SEN) treating foot/ankle injuries. BMC Musculoskeletal Dis 2007;8:99.

9. Nash K, Zachariah B, Nitschmann J et al. Evaluation of the fast track unit of a university emergency department. J Emerg Nurs 2007;33(1):14–20.

10. Tachackra S, Deboo P. Comparing performance of ENPs and SHOs. Emerg Nurse 2001;9(7):36–9.

11. Sakr M, Angus J, Perrin J et al. Care of minor injuries by emergency nurse practitioners or junior doctors: a randomised controlled trial. Lancet 1999;354(9187):1321–6.

12. Primary surgery Vol. 2—Trauma: wounds. 54.1 Preventing infection—the wound toilet; 2008. Online. www.primary-surgery.org/ps/vol2/html/sect0026.html; accessed 08 Aug 2014.

13. Stone S, Carter W. Wound preparation—irrigation. In: Tintinalli J, Kelen G, Stapczynski J, eds. Emergency medicine: a comprehensive study guide. 6th edn. New York: McGraw-Hill; 2004.

14. American Academy of Orthopedic Surgeons. Emergency care and transportation of the sick and injured. 9th edn. Jones and Bartlett; 2006.

15. Bleakley C, McDonough S, MacAuley D. The use of ice in the treatment of acute soft-tissue injury: a systematic review of randomized controlled trials. Am J Sports Med 2004;32(1):251–61.

16. McCallum T. Pain management in Australian emergency departments: a critical appraisal of evidence based practice. Aust Emerg Nurs J 2004;6(2):9–13.

17. Moses K, Banks JC, Nara PB et al. Atlas of clinical gross anatomy. St Louis: Mosby; 2005.

18. England SP, Sundberg S. Management of common pediatric fractures. Pediatr Clin North Am 1996;43(5):991–1012.

19. Estephan A. Fracture, clavicle. Online. http://emedicine.medscape.com/article/824564-overview; accessed 08 Aug 2014.

20. Pujalte GG, Housner JA. Management of clavicle fractures. Curr Sports Med Rep 2008;7(5):275–80.

21. Kim W, McKee MD. Management of acute clavicle fractures. Orthop Clin North Am 2008;39(4):491–505.

22. Andersen K, Jensen PO, Lauritzen J et al. The treatment of clavicular fractures: Figure of eight bandage versus a simple sling. Acta Orthop Scand 1987;58:71–4.

23. Resch H. Fractures of the humeral head. Unfallchirurg 2003;106(8):602–17. Online. www.ncbi.nlm.nih.gov/pubmed/12955231; accessed 14 Jan 2014.

24. Appelboam A, Reuben AD, Benger JR et al. Elbow extension test to rule out elbow fracture: multicentre, prospective validation and observational study of diagnostic accuracy in adults and children. Br Med J 2008;337:a2428.

25. Skaggs DL, Mirzayan RJ. The posterior fat pad sign in association with occult fracture of the elbow in children. Bone Joint Surg Am 1999:81(10):1429–33.

26. McRae R, Esser M. Practical fracture treatment. 5th edn. Edinburgh: Elsevier; 2008.

27. Major NM, Crawford ST. Elbow effusions in trauma in adults and children: is there an occult fracture? Am J Roentgenol 2002;178(2):413–18.

28. Krul M, van der Wouden JC, van Suijlekom-Smit LWA et al. Manipulative interventions for reducing pulled elbow in young children. Cochrane Database Syst Rev 2009;(4). Online. www.cochrane.org/reviews/en/ab007759.html; accessed 08 Aug 2014.

29. Nguyen TV, Center JR, Sambrook PN et al. Risk factors for proximal humerus, forearm, and wrist fractures in elderly men and women: the Dubbo osteoporosis epidemiology study. Am J Epidemiol 2001;153(6):587–95.

30. Rennie L, Court-Brown CM, Mok JY et al. The epidemiology of fractures in children. Injury 2007;38(8):913–22.

31. Cameron P, Jelinek G, Kelly A et al. Textbook of adult emergency medicine. 2nd edn. Edinburgh: Churchill Livingstone; 2002.

32. Kendall JM, Allen PE, McCabe SE. A tide of change in the management of an old fracture? J Accid Emerg Med 1995;12(3):187–8.

33. Davidson JS, Brown DJ, Barnes SN et al. Simple treatment for torus fractures of the distal radius. J Bone Joint Surg Br 2001; 83(8):1173–5.

34. Salter RB, Harris WR. Injuries involving the epiphyseal plate. J Bone Joint Surg Am 1963:45(3):587–622.

35. Wardrope J, English B. Musculo-skeletal problems in emergency medicine. Oxford: Oxford University Press; 1998.

36. Scaphoid fracture. Online. www.scaphoidfracture.net.au; accessed 17 Jan 2014.

37. Salter RB, Harris WR. Injuries involving the epiphyseal plate. J Bone Joint Surg Am 1963:45(3):587–622.

38. Lammers RL. Methods of wound closure. In: Roberts JR, Hedges JR, eds. Clinical procedures in emergency medicine. 5th edn. Philadelphia: Saunders; 2010. pp. 592–633.

39. Costello J. Prophylactic antibiotics for subungual hematoma. BestBETs: Best evidence topics; 2004. Royal Preston Hospital. Online. www.bestbets.org/bets/bet.php?id=618; accessed 20 Jan 2010.

40. Stiell IG, Greenberg GH, Wells GA et al. Derivation of a decision rule for the use of radiography in acute knee injuries. Ann Emerg Med 1995;26(4):405–13.

41. Maffulli N, Binfield PM, King JB et al. Acute haemarthrosis of the knee in athletes: a prospective study of 106 cases. J Bone Joint Surg Br 1993;75(6):945–9.

42. Stiell IG, Greenberg GH, McKnight RD et al. A study to develop clinical decision rules for the use of radiography in acute ankle injuries. Ann Emerg Med 1992;21(4):384–90.

43. Bachmann LM, Kolb E, Koller MT et al. Accuracy of Ottawa ankle rules to exclude fractures of the ankle and mid-foot: systematic review. Br Med J 2003;326(7386):417.

44. Dowling S, Spooner CH, Liang Y et al. Accuracy of Ottawa ankle rules to exclude fractures of the ankle and midfoot in children: a meta-analysis. Acad Emerg Med 2009;16(4):277–87.

45. Dasan S. Split skin graft for pretibial lacerations. BestBETs: Best evidence topics. Mayday University Hospital, Surrey; 2005. Online. www.bestbets.org/bets/bet.php?id=197; accessed 08 Aug 2014.

46. Rubin A. Ankle ligament sprains. In: Sallis RE, Massimino F, eds. Essentials of sports medicine. American College of Sports Medicine. St Louis: Mosby Year-Book; 1997. pp. 450–2.

47. Kannus P, Renstrom P. Treatment for acute tears of the lateral ligaments of the ankle. Operation, cast, or early controlled mobilization. J Bone Joint Surg Am 1991;73(2):305–12.

48. Linde F, Hvass I, Jurgensen U et al. Compression bandage in the treatment of ankle sprains. A comparative prospective study. Scand J Rehabil Med 1984;16(4):177–9.

49. Watts BL, Armstrong B. A randomised controlled trial to determine the effectiveness of double Tubigrip in grade 1 and 2 (mild to moderate) ankle sprains. Emerg Med J 2001;18(1):46–50.

50. Lamb SE, Marsh JL, Hutton JL et al. Mechanical supports for acute, severe ankle sprain: a pragmatic, multicentre, randomised controlled trial. Collaborative Ankle Support Trial (CAST group). Lancet 2009;373(9663):575–81.

51. Simmonds FA. The diagnosis of the ruptured Achilles tendon. Practitioner 1957;179(1069):56–8.

52. Scott BW, Al Chalabi A. How the Simmonds-Thompson test works. J Bone Joint Surg Br 1992;74(2):314–15.

53. Mandell GL, Bennett JE, Dolin R. Mandell. Douglas and Bennett's principles and practice of infections diseases. 7th edn. Philadelphia: Churchill Livingstone; 2010.

54. Brannon H. Dermatology—epidermis. Online. About.com; 2009. http://dermatology.about.com/cs/skinanatomy/g/epidermis.htm; accessed 08 Aug 2014.

55. Doughty DB, Sparks-Defriese B. Wound healing physiology. In: Bryant RA, Nix DP, eds. Acute and chronic wounds. 3rd edn. St Louis: Mosby; 2007. pp. 56–81.

56. Anon. Local anaesthetics. Therapeutic guidelines: analgesic version 13. West Melbourne: Therapeutic Guidelines; 2007.

57. Murtagh JE. Managing painful pediatric procedures. Aust Prescr 2006;29:94–6.

58. Hoy EA Closure of complicated wounds, Medscape http://emedicine.medscape.com/article/1129806-overview#aw2aab6b2b1aa accessed 11 March 2015.

59. McGee DL. Local and topical anaesthesia. In: Roberts JR, Jerris R, eds. Clinical procedures in emergency medicine. 5th edn. Philadelphia: Saunders; 2009. pp. 481–99.

60. O'Brien L, Jones DJ. Silicone gel sheeting for preventing and treating hypertrophic and keloid scars. Cochrane Wounds Group, 2013.

61. Beam JW. Evidence-based medicine: acute wound management: cleansing, debridement and dressing. Athletic Ther Today 2008; 13(1):2–6.

62. Joanna Briggs Institute. Best practice: solutions, techniques and pressures in wound: cleansing. Joanna Briggs Institute 2006;10(2):1–4.

63. Joanna Briggs Institute JBI Solutions, techniques and pressure in wound cleansing. Best Practice 10(2):2006. http://connect.jbiconnectplus.org/ViewSourceFile.aspx?0=4341 accessed 11 March 2015.

64. Fernandez R, Griffiths R. Water for wound cleansing. Cochrane Database Syst Rev 2012;(1):CD003861. Pub 3.

65. Thompson S. Tap water is an adequate cleansant for minor wounds. BestBETs: Best evidence topics; 2003. Manchester Royal Infirmary. Online. www.bestbets.org/bets/bet.php?id=24; accessed 08 Aug 2014.

66. Wilson R. Wound management. In: Curtis K, Ramsden C, Friendship J, eds. Emergency and trauma nursing. Marrickville: Mosby; 2007.

67. Brancato JC. Minor wound preparation and irrigation. UpToDate, Inc; 2009. Online. www.uptodate.com/patients/content/topic.do?topicKey=~pT88X0sWkzg.kA; accessed 16 Jan 2011.

68. Daniels JH. Wound cleansing and irrigation. In: Proehl JA, editor. Emergency nursing procedures. 3rd edn. Philadelphia: Saunders; 2004.

69. Stevens RJ, Gardner ER, Lee SJ. A simple, effective and cheap device for the safe irrigation of open traumatic wounds. Emerg Med J 2009;26(5):354–6.

70. Reynolds T, Cole E. Techniques for acute wound closure. Nurs Stand 2006;20(21):55–64.

71. MacLellan DG. Chronic wound management. Aust Prescr 2000;23:6–9.

72. Lewis SM, Heitkemper MM, Dirksoen SR. Medical–surgical nursing: assessment and management of clinical problems. 5th edn. St Louis: Mosby; 2000.

73. Turnidge J. NPS Prescribing Practice Review 36: judicious antibiotic use in general practice; 2007. Online. www.nps.org.au/health_professionals/publications/prescribing_practice_review/current/judicious_antibiotic_use_in_general_practice; accessed 08 Aug 2014.

74. Anon. Post-traumatic wound infections. eTG complete [Internet]. Melbourne: Therapeutic Guidelines Limited; 2013 Novar. http://etg.hcn.com.au/desktop/index.htm?acc=36422; accessed 14 Jan 2014.

75. Farion KJ, Russell KF, Osmond MH et al. Tissue adhesives for traumatic lacerations in children and adults Primary closure versus delayed closure for non bite traumatic wounds within 24 hours post injury. Cochrane Database Syst Rev 2013;(10):CD008574.

76. Turnidge J. NPS News 50: back to the future: a world without effective antibiotics. Adelaide: Australian Government Department of Health and Ageing; 2007.

77. Eliya-Masamba MC, Banda GW. Primary closure versus delayed closure for non bite traumatic wounds within 24 hours post injury. Cochrane Database Syst Rev 2013; (10):CD008574.

78. University Hospital of South Manchester. Patient Information leaflet on the use of chloramphenicol 1% eye ointment topically on facial skin wounds; 2008. Online. www.uhsm.nhs.uk/patients/Pharmacy%20Documents/Patient%20info%20leaflet%20use%20of%20Chloramphenicol%20ointment.pdf; accessed 16 Jan 2011.

79. Simon B, Hern HG Jr. Wound management principles. In: Marx JA, ed. Rosen's emergency medicine. 7th edn. Philadelphia: Mosby; 2009.

80. Heal CF, Buettner PG, Cruickshank R et al. Does single application of topical chloramphenicol to high risk sutured wounds reduce incidence of wound infection after minor surgery? Prospective randomised placebo controlled double blind trial. Br Med J 2009;338:a2812.

81. Ford S. Chloramphenicol not effective against wound infection. Nursing times.net; 2009. Online. www.nursingtimes.net/whats-new-in-nursing/chloramphenicol-not-effective-against-wound-infection/1977746.article; accessed 08 Aug 2014.

82. Chan M, Fong P, Stern C. Evidence based medicine review: chloramphenicol wound infection prophylaxis. California Pharmacist: Fall 2009;LVI(4):56–8.

83. Anon. Talk: Chloramphenicol/wound healing. Hunter Drug Information Service; 2009. Online. www.asid.net.au/hicsigwiki/index.php?title=Talk:Chloramphenicol; accessed 01 Mar 2010.

84. Anon. Table 3.21.1. Guide to tetanus prophylaxis in wound management. Australian Immunisation Handbook. 10th edn. Australian Government; 2013.

85. Bruggemann H, Baumer S, Fricke WF et al. The genome sequence of Clostridium tetani, the causative agent of tetanus disease. Proc Natl Acad Sci USA 2003;100(3):1316–21.

86. Romo T, Pearson JM. Wound healing: skin. Emedicine.com; 2010. Online. http://emedicine.medscape.com/article/884594-overview; accessed 03 Mar 2010.

87. Baddour LM. Soft tissue infections following water exposure. UpToDate; 2008. Online. www.uptodate.com/patients/content/topic.do?topicKey=~yS844hB0.I0.Uky; accessed 07 July 2014.

88. Anon. Therapeutic Guidelines. Skin and soft tissue infections: Water-related infections. In: eTG complete [Internet]. Melbourne: Therapeutic Guidelines Limited; 2013 Nov. http://etg.hcn.com.au/desktop/index.htm?acc=36422; accessed 24 Dec 2013.

89. Dendle C, Looke D. Review article: animal bites: an update for management with a focus on infections. Emerg Med Australas 2008;20(6):458–67.

90. Hiller KM, Li J. Antibiotics—a review of ED use. Emedicine; 2009. Online. http://emedicine.medscape.com/article/810704-overview; accessed 23 Mar 2010.

91. Broom J, Woods ML. Management of bite injuries. Aust Prescr 2006; 29(1):6–8.

92. Baddour LM. Overview of puncture wounds. UpToDate; 2009. Online. http://utdol.com/online/content/topic.do?topicKey=skin_inf/5904&selectedTitle=1%7E52&source=search_result; accessed 01 Feb 2010.

93. Maurice S. Antibiotics are indicated following dog bites. BestBETs: Best evidence topics; 2001. Manchester Royal Infirmary. Online. www.bestbets.org/bets/bet.php?id=17; accessed 29 June 2015.

94. Revis DR. Human bite infections. Emedicine; 2009. Online. http://emedicine.medscape.com/article/218901-overview; accessed 23 Mar 2010.

95. Richman KM, Rickman LS. The potential for transmission of human immunodeficiency virus through human bites. J Acquir Immune Defic Syndr 1993;6(4):402–6.

96. Hui AY, Hung LC, Tse PC et al. Transmission of hepatitis B by human bite—confirmation by detection of virus in saliva and full genome sequencing. J Clin Virol 2005;33(3):254–6.

97. Tsoukas CM, Hadjis T, Shuster J et al. Lack of transmission of HIV through human bites and scratches. J Acquir Immune Defic Syndr 1988;1(5):505–7.

98. Tebble NJ, Thomas DW, Price P. Anxiety and self-consciousness in patients with minor facial lacerations. J Adv Nurs 2004;47(4):417–26.

99. Amsterdam JT. Oral medicine. In: Marx JA, ed. Rosen's emergency medicine. 7th edn. Philadelphia: Mosby; 2009.

100. Day P, Duggal M. Interventions for treating traumatised permanent front teeth: avulsed (knocked out) and replanted. Cochrane Database Syst Rev 2010;(1):CD006542.

101. Doshi D. Avulsed tooth brought in milk for replantation. BestBETs: Best evidence topics; 2009. Blackburn Royal Infirmary. Online. http://www.bestbets.org/bets/bet.php?id=187; 02 Mar 2010.

102. Skapetis T. Lecture notes: dental trauma. Clinical Director of Education, Westmead Centre for Oral Health, Westmead, NSW; 2009.

103. Andreasen JO, Jensen SS, Sae-Lim V. The role of antibiotics in preventing healing complications after traumatic dental injuries: a literature review. Endodontic Topics 2008;14(1):80–92.

104. Peng LF, Kazzi AA, Peng WP et al. Dental, avulsed tooth: treatment & medication. eMedicine; 2009. Online. http://emedicine.medscape.com/article/763291-treatment; 08 Aug 2014.

105. Benko K. Emergency dental procedures. In: Roberts JR, Jerris R, eds. Clinical procedures in emergency medicine. 5th edn. Philadelphia: Saunders; 2009. pp. 1217–34.

106. Department of Health. The Australian Immunisation Handbook 10th edn. Australian Government, January 2014. Table 4.19.1. p. 404. www.health.gov.au/internet/immunise/publishing.nsf/Content/Handbook10-home; accessed 16 March 2015.

107. Canale ST, Beaty JH. Campbell's operative orthopaedics. 11th edn. St Louis: Mosby; 2007.

108. Kliegman RM, Behrman RE, Jenson HS et al. Nelson textbook of pediatrics. 18th edn. Philadelphia: Saunders; 2007.

CHAPTER 19
PAIN MANAGEMENT
BILL LORD AND CLAIR RAMSDEN

Essentials

- Pain relief is an important component of the patient care process and is a basic human right.
- Unrelieved acute pain may be associated with morbidities, including the development of persistent pain due to changes in peripheral nerves, the spinal cord, pain pathways in the central nervous systems and sympathetic nerves.
- Pain is a highly personal experience, and the perception and expression of pain is influenced by factors that include prior pain experience, culture, gender, coping strategies, expectations of care and the social environment in which the pain occurs. There are no standards of pain expression, and interpersonal comparisons should not be used to set 'norms' for pain-related behaviour.
- Regular assessment of pain should be undertaken to inform pain-management decisions and to document the efficacy of care.
- Pain severity should be measured using validated tools. Wherever possible, the patient's self-report should be used to evaluate pain severity.
- Assessment of the presence and severity of pain in patients with communication difficulties or cognitive impairment should involve alternative tools which include assessment of pain-related behaviours.
- The type of pain and severity should inform the choice of analgesic interventions.
- Opioids should be given intravenously and titrated to achieve the desired effect; there are large interpatient variations in doses required to achieve pain relief and standard doses for adult patients may be ineffective in some cases.
- Intranasal administration of lipid-soluble opioids such as fentanyl produces effective analgesia and may be indicated where intravenous access is not possible.
- Adverse effects, such as respiratory depression, are associated with opioid use, but the risk can be reduced through careful titration and observation of sedation, as sedation is an early and more reliable sign of respiratory depression than a decrease in respiratory rate.
- Non-pharmacological interventions play an important role in the alleviation of pain.
- Although there are contraindications to specific analgesics, there are no contraindications to pain relief.

INTRODUCTION

Pain is a multidimensional phenomenon that results from a complex interaction of physiological and neurochemical effects, with psychosocial and environmental factors such as culture, context, previous pain experience, personality, coping styles and expectations of cure influencing the individual's perception and expression of pain. Although pain is considered an inevitable consequence of tissue injury, and its management is influenced by beliefs that pain in itself is not harmful, evidence shows that unrelieved pain is associated with significant morbidity. Unrelieved pain may increase the risk of delirium in older patients with hip fracture,[1] and may produce significant disability associated with 'emotional, behavioural and social disruption'.[2] Pain has been shown to inhibit immune function,[3] and can have detrimental effects on respiratory, cardiovascular, gastrointestinal and other body systems. Apart from the humane and moral considerations, it is imperative to relieve pain as the early relief of pain can have a significant effect on the overall health of the individual. Adverse effects of inadequately managed severe acute pain are listed in Box 19.1.

Pain is a common complaint that motivates people to seek emergency care, with evidence showing that over 60% of patients report pain on arrival at an emergency department (ED).[5] Patients expect their pain to be relieved in the ED, with a significant number expecting complete analgesia.[6] There is, however, evidence that these expectations are not always met, with low rates of analgesia for some painful conditions and evidence that some patients experience long delays between arrival at an ED and analgesic interventions.[7,8] Despite targeted strategies to improve the effectiveness of analgesia in cases of severe pain, recent research has failed to identify significant change.[9]

Disparities in the relief of pain in the ED setting have been associated with ethnicity[10] and age.[11] The very young and the elderly have been found to be at risk of inadequate analgesia, with these findings attributed to safety concerns associated with opioid administration as well as difficulties in assessing pain due to communication difficulties related to age or disease such as dementia. However, extremes of age should not result in disparities in the relief of pain. Patient gender has been found to influence pain management practice in the ED,[12] with the gender of the health provider also influencing practice.[13] Gender disparities have been demonstrated in the pre-hospital setting, with females treated by paramedics less likely to receive morphine, despite having more severe pain than males.[14] Race also appears to influence the odds of receiving analgesia in the pre-hospital setting.[15] Although pain management has been identified as a clinical priority in the pre-hospital setting, there is evidence of inadequate analgesia among patients treated by paramedics,[16] with children less likely to receive paramedic-initiated analgesia for painful injuries.[17]

Efforts to reduce disparities in care and to improve the healthcare professional's response to pain require a better understanding of factors that have contributed to inadequate management. Although multiple factors can contribute to ineffective pain management, barriers which have been documented include:

- lack of educational emphasis on pain management practices in nursing and medical school curricula and postgraduate training programs
- inadequate or non-existent clinical quality management programs that evaluate pain management
- a paucity of rigorous studies of populations with special needs that improve pain management in the ED, particularly in geriatric and paediatric patients
- clinicians' attitudes towards opioid analgesics that result in inappropriate diagnosis of drug-seeking behaviour and inappropriate concern about addiction, even in patients who have obvious acutely painful conditions and request pain relief
- inappropriate concerns about the safety of opioids compared with non-steroidal anti-inflammatory drugs (NSAIDs) that result in their under-use (opiophobia)
- unappreciated cultural and sex differences in pain reporting by patients and interpretation of pain reporting by providers
- bias and disbelief of pain reporting according to racial and ethnic stereotyping.[18]

Despite existence of these barriers, safe, effective and early control of pain is an appropriate and achievable goal for emergency care. Healthcare professionals can achieve these goals by ensuring that a comprehensive pain assessment is performed in the early stage of care, by using a reliable pain scale to measure pain severity, and by taking a lead role in the management of the patient's pain. This requires

---

BOX 19.1 Adverse effects of undertreated severe acute pain[4]

Cardiovascular
Tachycardia, hypertension, increased peripheral vascular resistance, increased myocardial oxygen consumption, myocardial ischaemia, altered regional blood flow, deep-vein thrombosis, pulmonary embolism

Respiratory
Reduced lung volumes, atelectasis, decreased cough, sputum retention, infection, hypoxaemia

Gastrointestinal
Decreased gastric and bowel motility, increased risk of bacterial transgression of bowel wall

Genitourinary
Urinary retention

Neuroendocrine
- Increased catabolic hormones—glucagon, growth metabolic hormone, vasopressin, aldosterone, renin and angiotensin
- Reduced anabolic hormones—insulin, testosterone
- This catabolic state leads to hyperglycaemia, increased protein breakdown, negative nitrogen balance; leading to impaired wound healing and muscle wasting

Musculoskeletal
Muscle spasm, immobility (increasing risk of deep-vein thrombosis), muscle wasting leading to prolonged recovery of function

Psychological
Anxiety, fear, helplessness, sleep deprivation, leading to increased pain

Central nervous
Chronic (persistent) pain due to central sensitisation

a sound knowledge of pain and its management, a more active role in the assessment and management of pain, and the development of evidence-based treatment plans to ensure safe and effective pain management. Clinical practice guidelines are available for the assessment and management of pain, and these should inform treatment plans.[19,20]

Definition of pain

The most widely used definition of pain is one recommended by the International Association for the Study of Pain (IASP): 'an unpleasant sensory and emotional experience associated with actual or potential tissue damage, or described in terms of such damage'.[21] This definition highlights the emotional interpretation and response to pain that is shaped by gender and cultural, environmental and social factors, as well as prior pain experience. This definition also acknowledges the fact that patients can experience very real pain without evidence of obvious pathology, such as phantom limb pain associated with amputation and some chronic pain syndromes.

It is important to remember that pain is a symptom that cannot be objectively verified in the same way that other clinical findings can. Attempts to judge the patient's pain should be resisted, as this often leads to a devaluing of the patient's experience. Instead, healthcare professionals need to actively seek and accept the patient's self-report of their pain. This is reinforced by a useful definition of pain promoted by Margo McCaffery: 'Pain is whatever the experiencing person says it is, existing whenever he says it does'.[22]

Pain can be defined as *acute* if it is of recent onset and probable limited duration. It usually has an identifiable temporal and causal relationship to injury or disease. In contrast, *chronic*—also known as persistent—pain may not have a clearly identifiable cause, has no obvious biological value, lasts longer than the time taken for injuries to heal (considered to be a duration of greater than 3 months) and may not respond to standard analgesic interventions.

Anatomy and physiology of pain

Several theories of pain exist, but none are complete. One of the first published theories to describe the physiology of pain was developed by the 17th century French philosopher René Descartes, who proposed a specific pain pathway between pain receptors in the skin and the brain. However, Descartes' purely mechanistic explanation of a stimulus–response model failed to acknowledge the interrelationships between the physical stimulus and the interpretation of the stimulus that is shaped by the individual's characteristics and experience of pain. This theory also assumes that the perception of pain arises from injury, and ignores the possibility that pain can have no obvious physical basis. Descartes' theory influenced the study and treatment of pain for the next three centuries, and it was the mid-1900s before research into pain began to more correctly describe the complexity of the somatosensory system and multifactorial influences on individual pain perception and expression.

A major breakthrough in the understanding of pain occurred in 1965, when Melzack and Wall described their 'gate theory'.[23] This theory suggested that sensory input from peripheral nerves is transmitted to the dorsal horn of the spinal cord, where it is modulated and then transmitted to the brain for perception. 'Gates' occur at afferent synapses in the spinal cord and brain that are responsible for pain signal transmission. When sensory stimulation associated with pain reaches the spinal cord the gates open and uninhibited signals from the periphery ascend via the spinothalamic tract to the brain, where pain is perceived. The pain can be moderated or inhibited if the gates are closed. Other sensory stimuli, such as gently rubbing the injured area, can help to close the gate by stimulating inhibitory neurons, which can reduce the pain an individual is experiencing. This concept forms the basis of transcutaneous electrical nerve stimulation (TENS), which is a therapeutic intervention that can reduce pain through sensory stimulation of the affected area.

Subsequent growth in understanding pain processing recognised that pain had several dimensions other than the obvious sensory dimension. Later work by Melzack proposed that the perception of pain involves:

- a sensory–discriminative system that enables the recognition of the location, intensity and duration of pain

- a motivational–affective component associated with reflexes and strategies designed to avoid or escape from the cause of the pain

- a cognitive–evaluative component that involves the comparison of contextual information about the current pain experience with past experiences in order to evaluate the pain, its significance and consequences, which, when combined with sensory and affective information, helps to inform response strategies.[24]

The ability to perceive and react to threats to our wellbeing is an important protective homeostatic process. In order to detect potential tissue-damaging stimuli, the body needs sensitive somatosensory nerve fibres to relay action potentials to multiple peripheral and central centres. Pain is experienced through pathways in the central, peripheral and autonomic nervous systems. The peripheral sensory organs are known as *nociceptors.* These are widely dispersed throughout the body, and can be identified in skin, periosteum, joints, muscle and viscera.

Two main types of nociceptor—A-delta fibres and C-fibres—give rise to the varied perceptions of pain. The A-delta fibres are myelinated fibres that are stimulated by heat and noxious mechanical injury. Action potentials travel rapidly (2 to 20 m/s) along these fibres towards the dorsal horn of the spinal cord, where they synapse with second-order neurons to finally convey signals to the brain. Stimulation of A-delta fibres gives rise to pain that is experienced as the initial sharp pain that follows injury. The throbbing, slowly building and sometimes burning pain that follows this initial injury is transmitted along C-fibres. These fibres are unmyelinated and conduct action potentials more slowly (< 2 m/s). C-fibres are activated by heat and by noxious chemical and mechanical stimuli. A C-fibre subclass—the C-fibre polymodal receptor—responds to heat, cold, pressure and chemical stimuli. These pain pathways are illustrated in Figure 19.1.

Tissue can be damaged by direct mechanical trauma (pressure, extremes of temperature or chemical), or by ischaemia and inflammation. Tissue injury causes the release of

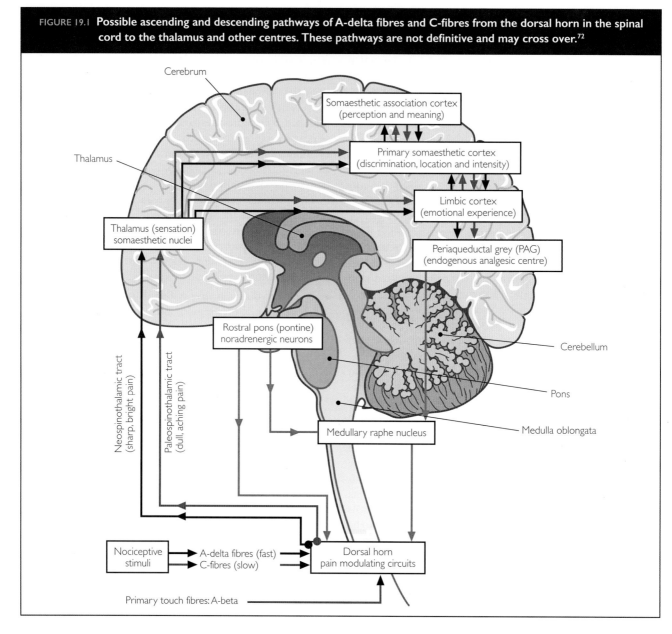

FIGURE 19.1 **Possible ascending and descending pathways of A-delta fibres and C-fibres from the dorsal horn in the spinal cord to the thalamus and other centres. These pathways are not definitive and may cross over.**[72]

chemical mediators such as bradykinins, substance P, histamine and arachidonic acid derivatives such as leukotrienes and prostaglandins. Several of these mediators are implicated in the stimulation and sensitisation of nociceptors.

Once a nociceptor is stimulated beyond its threshold, a signal is transmitted along the sensory nerve axon to the cell body in the dorsal root ganglion, and then on to a secondary neuron in the dorsal horn of the spinal cord. Nociceptive information can be processed within the spinal cord, as in the case of spinal reflexes, where the nociceptor neuron synapses with an interneuron within the cord. This then synapses with an anterior horn efferent nerve to produce an action such as skeletal muscle contraction to withdraw a hand from a hot surface.

Conscious awareness of pain requires the transmission of the nociceptive signal via the spinothalamic tracts and the dorsal columns. Neurons then transfer information from the thalamus to the sensory cortex of the brain. While this may appear to be a simple connection of neurons, the perception of pain relies on complex interconnections between other areas of the brain, such as the hypothalamus, brainstem nuclei and basal ganglia. Connections to the frontal lobe enable conscious interpretation of the experience and influence our emotional response to pain.[25]

The afferent input from nociceptors is moderated or inhibited by neurons that descend from the cerebral cortex via the periaqueductal grey (PAG) matter to the dorsal horns of the spinal cord. These can facilitate or inhibit the second-order neurons, modifying the sensory input and consequently the perception of pain.

Neurotransmitters associated with nociceptive transmission in the spinal cord and brain include substance P, glutamate, monoamines and opioid peptides. Inhibition of pain is a function of endogenous opioid peptides such as the dynorphins, endorphins and encephalins, which inhibit nociceptor transmission and pain perception by binding with specific opioid receptors. Exogenous opioids, such as morphine, also bind to these receptors, which are located in the spinal cord (substantia gelatinosa and primary afferent fibres) and brain (rostroventral medulla and midbrain periaqueductal grey). Receptors have been classified as mu (μ), kappa (κ) and delta (δ). The μ_1 subtype is responsible for the analgesic and euphoric effect of opioids, while activation of the μ_2 subtype produces side effects of opioid administration that include gastrointestinal slowing, constipation, sedation and respiratory depression. At this time there is no μ_1-specific analgesic available.

Pathophysiology

Pain is an important signal that tissue damage is occurring. Without the ability to perceive injury our life would be threatened, as organ ischaemia and inflammation would go undetected until major systemic derangement occurred. However, some pain does not have any obvious pathological basis, and this serves as the basis for the classification of pain. A useful clinical approach involves the classification of pain as *nociceptive* (with subcategories somatic and visceral), and *neuropathic* (with subcategories centrally generated pain or peripherally generated pain). A comparison of the clinical features associated with these major types of pain is outlined in Table 19.1.

Nociceptive pain

Somatic pain occurs following injury to the skin, bone, joints and skeletal muscle. An example of somatic pain is that arising from a laceration to the hand caused by a sharp knife. Pain from cutaneous sites is initially sharp and well localised,
although deeper structures such as muscle and joints may be more poorly localised. The initial pain may be followed by a duller, throbbing pain.

Visceral pain arises from stimulation of A-delta fibre and C-fibre nociceptors located near the surface of the organ. Ischaemia, stretching and pressure activate nociceptors, and pain from these structures is usually described as dull, cramp-like, diffuse and poorly localised. There may be associated autonomic stimulation as these afferent nerve fibres are located with sympathetic and sympathetic nerves innervating the same organs. Visceral pain can be referred to other areas of the body, possibly as a result of the fact that afferent fibres from the skin and viscera converge at the same secondary neurons within the spinal cord. This can produce pain that is perceived to be, for example, in the patient's left arm, if afferent signals from an ischaemic myocardium converge at the same level in the cord as cutaneous innervation from the arm. The classic descriptions of visceral pain can be gained from careful questioning, and this information helps to differentiate musculoskeletal and visceral pathologies. However, it should be remembered that patients could have pain arising from several anatomical sites concurrently (Fig 19.2).

When nociceptors are repeatedly stimulated their threshold for activation decreases, while the size of the response increases. This is known as *hyperalgesia*: an increased response to a painful stimulus. An associated term, *allodynia*, refers to pain produced by a stimulus that would not normally cause pain, and can be observed as the hypersensitive response to lightly stroking sunburnt skin.

TABLE 19.1　Classification of pain by inferred pathology[22]

TWO MAJOR TYPES OF PAIN			
I. Nociceptive pain		II. Neuropathic pain	
A. Somatic pain	B. Visceral pain	A. Centrally generated pain	B. Peripherally generated pain
Nociceptive pain: normal processing of stimuli that damages normal tissues or has the potential to do so if prolonged; usually responsive to non-opioids and/or opioids. Somatic pain: arises from bone, joint, muscle, skin or connective tissue. It is usually aching and is well localised. Visceral pain: arises from visceral organs, such as the gastrointestinal tract and pancreas. This may be subdivided: • Tumour involvement of the organ capsule that causes aching and fairly well-localised pain. • Obstruction of hollow viscus, which causes intermittent cramping and poorly localised pain.		**Neuropathic pain:** abnormal processing of sensory input by the peripheral or central nervous systems; treatment usually involves adjuvant analgesics. Centrally generated pain Deafferentation pain. Injury to either the peripheral or the central nervous system. Examples: phantom pain may reflect injury to the peripheral nervous system; burning pain below the level of a spinal cord lesion reflects injury to the central nervous system. Sympathetically maintained pain. Associated with dysregulation of the autonomic nervous system. Examples: may include some of the pain associated with reflex sympathetic dystrophy/causalgia (complex regional pain syndrome, type I, type II). Peripherally generated pain Painful polyneuropathies. Pain is felt along the distribution of many peripheral nerves. Examples: diabetic neuropathy, alcohol-nutritional neuropathy and those associated with Guillain-Barré syndrome. Painful mononeuropathies. Usually associated with a known peripheral nerve injury, and pain is felt at least partly along the distribution of the damaged nerve. Examples: nerve root compression, nerve entrapment, trigeminal neuralgia.	

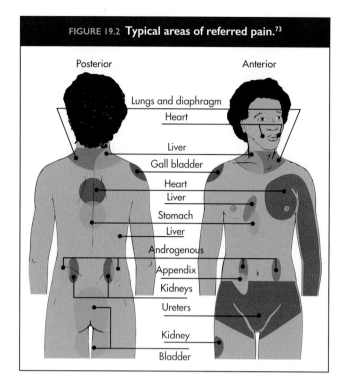

FIGURE 19.2 **Typical areas of referred pain.**[73]

Posterior   Anterior

Lungs and diaphragm
Heart
Liver
Gall bladder
Heart
Liver
Stomach
Liver
Androgenous
Appendix
Kidneys
Ureters
Kidney
Bladder

Neuropathic pain

Neuropathic pain—which may be acute or chronic—results from injuries or diseases that directly affect the nervous system. Acute neuropathic pain may result from lesions or entrapment of nerves; for example, an entrapped median nerve at the wrist causes burning pain or unpleasant tingling. Sensory neurons in the parasympathetic pathway generate impulses that fire spasmodically at the site of the injury or may be stimulated by movement, causing sharp or burning pain. Neuropathic pain syndromes are complex and difficult to treat.

Hyperalgesia is an exaggerated neuronal response that intensifies the sensory perception of pain intensity, especially in neuropathic pain. It can also be a feature of both somatic and visceral tissue injury and inflammation, occurring not only at the site of injury but also in the surrounding uninjured area (e.g. pharyngitis where swallowing can initiate severe pain).[26]

Chronic neuropathic pain is also referred to as *central pain*. Central pain is chronic pain that occurs as a result of a lesion or dysfunction in the central nervous system (CNS) rather than from receptor stimulation in the periphery. Diseases such as multiple sclerosis, stroke or traumatic spinal cord injury can produce central pain, and this may be associated with tactile allodynia (peripheral sensitisation). Central pain is usually diffuse and may extend over large areas, such as the whole right or left side or lower half of the body. Many symptoms and effects of central pain are congruent with acute neuropathic pain, and one of the main distinguishing features is the delay in the appearance of central pain after the causative event.[26]

Patient assessment

Approach to initial evaluation

To effectively manage pain, clinicians must recognise that pain has both physical and non-physical components. Specific components are the physical stimulus and the patient's cognitive and emotional interpretation of that stimulus. Interpretation of pain is influenced by a diverse range of factors that include the context in which the pain occurs, knowledge of the possible consequences of the injury or disease and trust and fear about interactions with healthcare professionals and health systems. Handling the subjectivity of pain can prove to be challenging, but a knowledgeable, calm, empathetic healthcare professional can do much to minimise the patient's fears and facilitate early pain management.

Pain may be the patient's chief complaint, or be one of several symptoms associated with disease or injury. Pain can be an important marker of serious pathology such as myocardial ischaemia, and a careful assessment of the quality of this symptom can inform clinical judgements regarding the likely cause of the pain and the most appropriate emergency interventions required. However, severe pain associated with significant soft tissue or musculoskeletal injury has the potential to distract the clinician from other clinical management priorities, and, as such, it is important to develop a systematic approach to patient assessment which ensures that, while pain is effectively managed, other priorities, such as airway patency and the patient's ventilation and perfusion status, are assessed and managed before lower-order priorities are addressed.

A comprehensive assessment is essential. A health history should be obtained to identify prior complaints and chronic pain conditions as well as risk factors that may be associated with the current episode. The assessment of pain includes the measurement of pain severity, and the evaluation of the clinical data to develop a management plan. As the existence of pain cannot be proved or disproved by an independent observer, it is accepted that the patient's self-report is the most reliable indicator of the existence and intensity of pain.

Physical examination

A focused assessment should be conducted to collect data about the patient's pain. The following mnemonic can assist assessment of pain, particularly when the cause of pain is not immediately obvious.

P **Provocation.** What activities were associated with the onset of pain? Did the pain occur during exercise, or did it occur at rest (unprovoked)? What makes the pain worse? Does deep inspiration, movement or palpation of the affected area change the intensity of the pain? When undertaking this assessment, it is important to avoid prompting the patient by asking leading questions and making inferences about the patient's pain.

Q **Quality.** How does the patient describe the pain? Is it dull, sharp, crushing, burning, shooting or cramping? Some of these descriptors are frequently associated with specific pathologies, and are therefore useful in identifying possible causes of the pain.

R **Region, radiation and relief.** Ask the patient to describe the region or site of the pain. Patterns of radiation should be elicited using open, non-leading questioning techniques. For example, instead of asking, 'Does the pain radiate to your back?', ask 'Can you tell me about where the pain is located, and whether it can be felt in other areas of your body?' Factors that relieve the pain should be explored. Does a particular body posture, such as lying supine with knees flexed, or sitting forward, help to relieve the pain? Patients should be questioned about prescription or over-the-counter (OTC) medications that they may have taken in an attempt to relieve their pain.

S Severity and associated symptoms. Patients should be asked to rate their pain severity using a validated pain scale. Paediatric scales should be used to assess pain in children who cannot understand the instructions used to score pain in adults. Triage decisions in the ED will need to consider the patient's reported level of pain. The Australasian Triage Scale requires assessment and treatment of severe pain from any cause within 10 minutes (triage code/category 2). Patients reporting moderately severe pain from any cause that will require analgesia should be assessed and treated within 30 minutes (triage code/category 3).[27] Associated symptoms, such as nausea and paraesthesia, should be sought.

T Time of onset and duration. Time of onset is important as this helps to differentiate acute and chronic pain. This information is also important if the patient is to receive thrombolytics for the management of cardiac pain, as the drug must be given within a narrow window of effectiveness (see Ch 22). Information should be sought about whether the pain is constant, or whether there have been periods of remission. Patients may have self-administered analgesics, or received analgesia from paramedics or other healthcare professionals prior to presenting at a healthcare facility. In these cases the drug, dose, time of last administration, analgesic effect and adverse events are important to note as this information informs the continuum of care.

It should be understood that patients might have difficulty describing key components of their pain. Language barriers, cultural differences, cognitive impairment and other physiological or psychosocial factors may make the assessment more difficult, and require an assessment strategy that addresses these limitations. A general recommendation where self-report is unavailable or unreliable is to seek evidence of pain-related behaviours, evidence of potential causes of pain, and to use estimates of pain by others such as carers and relatives who can describe changes in a patient's behaviour that may be associated with pain. Pain scales designed for the assessment of acute pain in cognitively impaired adults are available, and these may have utility in emergency health settings.[28] Physiological indicators such as vital signs have been shown to be an unreliable indicator of pain severity, and their use for this purpose is discouraged, unless a self-report is unavailable.[29,30]

Pain scales

Pain rating scales provide important information regarding the severity and nature of the patient's pain. Measurement of pain helps the clinician to:

- determine pain intensity, quality and duration
- aid in the diagnosis
- help determine the choice of therapy
- evaluate the relative effectiveness of the therapy.[31]

Evidence demonstrates that formal pain measurement reveals unrecognised or under-treated pain, with the consequence

that improved recognition of pain can lead to improved pain management practice.[32] Simple pain scales include the adjective rating scale (ARS), numeric rating scale (NRS) and visual analogue scale (VAS). The ARS involves the use of descriptions of pain severity, such as 'none', 'slight', 'moderate', 'severe' or 'agonising', with the patient asked to select the term that best describes their pain. By contrast, the NRS requires the patient to rate their pain between 0 and 10, with 0 representing no pain, and 10 representing the worst pain imaginable. The VAS involves the patient moving a slide on a mechanical scale to a point between two ends of a device that is marked 'no pain' at one end and 'worst pain imaginable' (or similar descriptors) at the other. The result is then read against a 100-point scale on the side that is not visible to the patient. Alternatively, the patient marks a point on a 100 mm line and the result is read as a pain score between 0 and 100. The NRS and VAS have been validated in the emergency health setting, and the resulting scores have good levels of correlation between each scale.

Pain is a dynamic process, which mandates frequent re-assessment. When using a pain-rating scale, it is important to use the same scale consistently with the patient. Using a simple scale is helpful for the patient and clinicians, as it minimises any confusion or misinterpretation that may occur. Several studies have shown that there is a poor correlation between the patient's pain rating and ratings estimated by the healthcare professional, with the latter tending to underestimate the patient's pain.[33] This underestimation may be a result of an individual's values, experience and biases influencing clinical

> **PRACTICE TIPS**
> ## AIMS FOR EFFECTIVE PAIN CONTROL
>
> - No single universally superior method of pain management exists. Pharmacological as well as non-pharmacological interventions should be considered to successfully manage pain.
> - The goal of pain management is to recognise relief of pain as a clinical priority and to relieve or prevent pain whenever possible. Pain relief may be more effective if initiated soon after onset of pain.
> - The underlying cause of pain and the severity of the pain are important considerations in selecting analgesia.
> - A calm, quiet patient—or one who is able to sleep despite reporting pain—does not preclude the presence of pain.
> - A patient's refusal to accept pain medication may be related to fear of addiction, sedation, loss of control, beliefs about pain or method of administration.
> - A patient's request for specific pain medication does not automatically mean he or she is a drug-seeker.
> - A patient's tolerance for pain is not directly proportional to the amount of analgesia required to relieve pain.
> - The endpoint of treatment relies on the patient's assessment of relief rather than achievement of a pre-determined reduction in pain score.
> - All pain is real. Pain is what a patient says it is.

judgements. As these attributes can lead to a devaluing of the patient's pain experience, it is important to recognise the detrimental effect that these attributes can have on the care of patients in pain. Clinicians must also remember that, while there is evidence for a minimally clinically significant change in pain score, the actual score reported by a patient is unique to that person, and interpersonal comparisons are unhelpful.

Assessing pain in children

Assessment tools and strategies for the paediatric patient vary from those used for adults. The ability of a child to accurately self-report pain depends on the stage of their cognitive and emotional development. While children aged eight years or more can generally use a visual analogue scale, those aged between three and eight may require different approaches to assessment of pain due to difficulties in communicating and interpreting instructions regarding the use of pain scales. Parents can contribute to assessing a child's pain by helping to distinguish usual behaviour from the child's current reactions.

Observing a child for pain-related facial expressions and body position augments assessment. This is particularly helpful in pre-verbal infants. Pain severity scales suitable for infants and children are described in Table 19.2.

TABLE 19.2 Pain rating scales for children		
DESCRIPTION	INSTRUCTIONS	RECOMMENDED AGE/COMMENTS
FACES pain rating scale, developed by Wong and Baker[34]		
Consists of six cartoon faces ranging from smiling face for 'no pain' to tearful face for 'worst pain'	*Original instructions:* Explain to child that each face is for a person who feels happy because there is no pain (hurt) or sad because there is some or a lot of pain. FACE 0 is very happy because there is no hurt. FACE 1 hurts just a little bit. FACE 2 hurts a little more. FACE 3 hurts even more. FACE 4 hurts a whole lot, but FACE 5 hurts as much as you can imagine, although you don't have to be crying to feel this bad. Ask child to choose face that best describes own pain. Record the number under chosen face on pain assessment record.	For children as young as 3 years. Using original instructions without affect words, such as *happy* or *sad*, or brief words resulted in same pain rating, probably reflecting child's rating of pain intensity. For coding purposes, numbers 0, 2, 4, 6, 8, 10 can be substituted for 0–5 system to accommodate 0–10 system.
	Brief word instructions: Point to each face using the words to describe the pain intensity. Ask child to choose face that best describes own pain and record the appropriate number.	The FACES provides three scales in one: facial expressions, numbers and words. Use of brief word instructions is recommended.

0 No hurt	1 or 2 Hurts a little bit	2 or 4 Hurts a little more	3 or 6 Hurts even more	4 or 8 Hurts a whole lot	5 or 10 Hurts worst

FLACC scale*, developed by Merkel et al[35]

The scale consists of descriptors of behaviours that are associated with pain.	The scale was first validated in the postoperative setting, but has subsequently been validated to score pain in infants and children with pain from injury and with procedural pain. The clinician should observe the patient for at least 1 minute with the legs and body uncovered and select the most appropriate score for each of the categories of behaviour listed. It may be necessary to reposition the patient to observe for pain-related behaviour on movement. The numbers for each category are summed to provide a score from 0–10. This scale should be used in conjunction with a self-report if the child is able to do this.	The authors validated this scale in children aged 2 months to 7 years. Further research has validated this scale in older children (up to 16 years) and in neonates. The scale is particularly useful in assessing pain in pre-verbal children or in those with cognitive impairment or communication difficulties.

TABLE 19.2 Pain rating scales for children—cont'd		
DESCRIPTION	**INSTRUCTIONS**	**RECOMMENDED AGE/COMMENTS**
Face	0	1	2
	No particular expression or smile	Occasional grimace or frown; withdrawn, disinterested	Frequent to constant frown, clenched jaw, quivering chin
Legs	0	1	2
	Normal position or relaxed	Uneasy, restless, tense	Kicking or legs drawn up
Activity	0	1	2
	Lying quietly, normal position, moves easily	Squirming, shifting back and forth, tense	Arched, rigid or jerking
Cry	0	1	2
	No cry (awake or asleep)	Moans or whimpers, occasional complaint	Crying steadily, screams or sobs; frequent complaints
Consolable	0	1	2
	Content, relaxed	Reassured by occasional touching, hugging or being talked to; distractible	Difficult to console or comfort

Each of the five categories is scored from 0–2, resulting in a final score of 0–10.

Management

Pain is a major human health problem throughout the world. Although relief from pain is considered a basic human right,[36] pain management practices in many healthcare settings have been shown to be deficient, leading to the use of the term 'oligoanalgesia' to describe low levels of analgesic use resulting in unrelieved pain.[37] Patients at particular risk for oligoanalgesia include children and the elderly, and those who are more seriously injured.[38,39] Managing pain is a multifaceted, multidimensional process. Co-existing medical conditions, age, social, cultural and psychological needs, beliefs and experiences, as well as individual variations to pain perception and response to therapy, all influence the process. The endpoint in the management of pain is not a predetermined reduction in pain severity score, as this endpoint varies between individuals. Rather, the aim is to achieve a reduction in pain that corresponds with the patient's assessment of satisfactory relief. This requires an assessment of the risk of dose-dependent adverse effects associated with commonly used analgesics.

There are many barriers to effective pain relief, including fear of addiction among both patients and healthcare professionals. This fear affects decisions regarding the administration of analgesics, but also affects the patient's acceptance of analgesia, particularly when opioids are recommended. This problem arises from a misunderstanding of the action of common analgesics, as well as terminology relating to addiction (see Table 19.3). The actual incidence of addiction in patients receiving opioids for pain management is often overestimated. A recent systematic review of the literature found a low risk of drug dependence in patients where opioids were used to treat pain.[44]

Addiction is defined as a chronic disease that is characterised by 'impaired control over drug use, compulsive use, continued use despite harm, and craving'.[45] It is important to note that patients taking analgesics for pain relief are using drugs for therapeutic reasons. This needs to be contrasted with the use of analgesics, particularly opioids, to satisfy a compulsive desire for the drug's non-analgesic effects such as euphoria. A useful analogy is to consider the therapeutic use of insulin in a patient with insulin-dependent diabetes mellitus. The patient depends on the regular injection of this drug. However, this is a physical dependence, rather than addiction. Physical dependence can occur in patients taking analgesics over time for chronic pain conditions. Withdrawal symptoms can occur by abruptly stopping drug administration, rapid dose reduction or administration of an antagonist that rapidly reverses the analgesic effect.

Tolerance is characterised by decreasing effects of a drug at a constant dose of the drug or, conversely, the need for a higher dose of a drug to maintain an effect. Tolerance to opioids is a natural physiological response that should be anticipated with long-term therapy. This response is typically seen in patients suffering chronic pain, particularly those with pain due to cancer, where very large doses of opioids may be required to achieve adequate analgesia. This finding is a reminder that opioids such as morphine have no ceiling effect—the dose of the drug can be continually increased to achieve analgesia while monitoring for potentially serious adverse effects. The assessment of tolerance is particularly important in managing acute pain in patients with opioid tolerance, whether due to addiction associated with illicit drug use or through long-term use for chronic pain. Patients taking an opioid antagonist such as naltrexone, which is used to manage addiction to alcohol or opioids, may represent a management challenge when they experience acute pain due to injury or disease as their pain may be unresponsive to opioids, requiring consideration of

TABLE 19.3 Definition of essential terms[73]

TERM	DEFINITION
Pharmacokinetics	The movement of drugs throughout the body.[40] The action following the administration of a drug such as an analgesic: its absorption, distribution, metabolism by the cells and elimination from the body, mainly by the kidneys and liver.
Bioavailability	The amount of drug absorbed through the gastrointestinal tract into the bloodstream that determines the subsequent plasma level available from each dose for analgesic effect.[40] Many factors can interfere with drug absorption and bioavailability, such as slower gastric emptying and peristalsis, or a decrease or increase in blood circulating volume and tissue perfusion.
Half-life	The length of time for the concentration of the drug in the bloodstream to be reduced by half.
Pain threshold	The least-intense stimulus that will cause pain or an intensity of stimulation below which pain is not perceived.
Pain tolerance	The level of pain accepted before intervention is requested or required.[41]
Drug tolerance	A decreased response to a drug dose requiring an increase in the dose to provide the original effect experienced.[42]
Physical dependence	Characterised by a tolerance to the drug causing a reduction in effectiveness of analgesia and an increase in dose requirements to relieve the existing pain. Withdrawal symptoms of agitation, anxiety, irritability, nausea and vomiting are likely if the drug is discontinued abruptly.[43]
Psychological dependence	Characterised by craving that influences mood and actions to acquire the drug. This dependence interferes with both the physical and the psychological health of the person concerned.
Minimum effective	The lowest concentration of drug in the blood required to provide a therapeutic effect such as minimum effective concentration (MEC) analgesia.
Titration	The dose adjustment to achieve and maintain the analgesic level within the therapeutic window.

non-opioid alternatives such as ketamine.[46–47] Patients on long-term opioid therapy may also experience opioid-induced hyperalgesia, which is seen as a heightened response to a stimulus that is not normally painful.

Clinicians may occasionally be faced with a patient who appears to be seeking drugs for non-therapeutic purposes. While this scenario has been found to be uncommon in one ED setting,[48] drug-seeking behaviour should be suspected when a patient: seeks injectable rather than oral opioids, or steadily increasing doses; seeks repeated supply of opioids; insists on a specific medication and refuses alternatives; requests supplies of opioid in more than one form (e.g. oral and injectable); requests opioids by name; gives a vague or evasive history or has atypical pain or non-anatomical distribution; has a lack of accompanying signs (e.g. no haematuria in renal colic); denies having a regular general practitioner and cannot provide names of previous doctors; attends multiple practitioners (history of 'doctor shopping'); is non-compliant with suggested treatment; in addition to requesting opioids requests other drugs that have known abuse potential (e.g. flunitrazepam and oxycodone (common brands are Hypnodorm and Oxycontin)). Research has identified that patient requests for parenteral medication and pain severity reports of greater than 10 out of 10 pain were most predictive evidence of drug-seeking.[49] However, none of these clues in isolation is completely reliable, and there is a risk that patients may be labelled as 'drug-seekers' when they are actually seeking drugs to relieve a genuine complaint of pain. Use clinical professional judgement; a complete history and thorough examination are of particular importance in such situations.

Choice of intervention

Selection of interventions for the relief of pain is influenced by a host of factors other than fears of addiction. Research has shown that tradition, intuition, stereotypes and ethnicity influence interventions selected for pain management. Burke and Jerrett[50] studied student nurses' perceptions of the best interventions for people of various ages who were in acute pain. Age was identified as a factor that influenced both the number and the type of interventions selected. In this study, student nurses selected more interventions for adolescents and adults, and fewer interventions for infants, toddlers, children and the elderly.

In a study of analgesic administration in the ED, Neighbor and colleagues[38] found that patients with trauma were less likely to receive opioids if they were young or elderly, intubated or had a lower Revised Trauma Score (RTS). Inadequate analgesia has also been documented in the pre-hospital setting.[51,53]

Alterations in levels of consciousness or cognitive disabilities related to age or illness can complicate the pain assessment and management process. Behavioural cues can be used to judge pain severity in the absence of a self-report. Patients with a decreased level of consciousness can experience severe pain and signs of agitation may be associated with nociception. As such it is important to attend to these patients' needs once other resuscitation priorities have been established and managed. In cases of altered levels of consciousness due to trauma, the motor component of the Glasgow Coma Scale (GCS) can be used to guide treatment decisions, as a motor score ≥ 3 indicates an intact reaction to painful stimuli. As such, analgesia should be considered in patients suffering trauma which is likely to be painful and where the motor component of the GCS is ≥ 3.[54]

An injury that may result in deterioration of neurological, pulmonary or haemodynamic status is not, in itself, an absolute contraindication for systemic analgesia. While there are contraindications associated with specific analgesics, there is no contraindication to analgesia. However, judicious choice of analgesic agent and careful titration of analgesia is mandatory to prevent complications.

There is strong evidence that early analgesic administration does not affect the diagnosis in cases of acute abdominal pain. Therefore, analgesia should not be withheld until a diagnosis is made in a patient presenting with abdominal pain.[19] Paramedics and nurses have important responsibilities for the provision of early and effective analgesia in patients experiencing pain. This role requires authority to administer a range of analgesics using appropriate clinical judgement that is supported by knowledge of contemporary pain management practices and by evidence-based clinical practice guidelines. Such guidelines should include protocols for nurse-initiated analgesia in the ED, as evidence has shown considerable patient benefits in establishing these programs.[55,56]

Pain management interventions include invasive techniques such as medication and non-invasive techniques such as distraction, cooling burns and splinting fractures. When selecting a technique for a specific patient, the healthcare professional should recognise that each patient is unique and that no single universally superior pain control method exists for all patients. The pathology responsible for the pain will influence the choice of analgesic. For example, in patients with renal colic, NSAIDs have been found to provide effective analgesia with a lower incidence of vomiting than opioids.[19] Patients should be evaluated individually and interventions tailored to each patient and their situation. The following sections discuss specific aspects of pain management.

Pharmacological pain management

Drugs that act as analgesics are divided into two groups: *non-opioids* and *opioids*. The term opioid includes natural and synthetic compounds that bind to opioid receptors in the nervous system. In 1986 the World Health Organization (WHO) released guidelines for the management of cancer pain, which included a three-step 'analgesic ladder' that advocated the addition of different analgesics to a patient's treatment regimen as pain severity increased.[57] Although this was designed to provide pain relief in patients with chronic pain due to cancer, this strategy can also be applied to the treatment of acute pain.

Non-opioids

Paracetamol and non-steroidal inflammatory drugs (NSAIDs) comprise this group of analgesics. Although the exact mechanism of action of paracetamol is unknown, it is believed to produce analgesia by blocking pain impulses through its prostaglandin inhibitory effect on the CNS. Paracetamol has few adverse effects, but, unlike aspirin, has no significant anti-inflammatory effects. Paracetamol is preferred for patients allergic to aspirin or those with platelet or gastrointestinal problems. The usual recommended daily dose of paracetamol should not exceed 4000 mg for adults.[58] Paracetamol has a low therapeutic index, and acute liver failure may occur in overdose due to the hepatocellular necrosis caused by an active metabolite. This metabolite is normally conjugated with glutathione in the liver to form a harmless compound that is excreted by the renal system. However, overdose of paracetamol may deplete glutathione stores leading to the accumulation of the toxic metabolite and consequent liver damage. This drug should be used with caution in patients with malnutrition or liver disease, who may have low levels of glutathione.

NSAIDs have an anti-inflammatory effect on the peripheral tissues. These drugs act by inhibiting prostaglandin synthesis by blocking cyclo-oxygenase (COX) production. Two forms (COX-1 and COX-2) exist. Many NSAIDs are non-selective. Examples of drugs in this category include aspirin, diclofenac, ibuprofen, indomethacin, ketoprofen, ketorolac, naproxen, piroxicam, sulindac and tiaprofenic acid. Selective (COX-2) inhibitors are less likely to cause the gastrointestinal adverse effects associated with COX-1 agents. Drugs in this class include celecoxib, meloxicam and parecoxib.

NSAIDs are insufficient for the management of severe pain, but can be a useful adjunct when used with opioids. These drugs have significant side effects, which are more common with long-term use. These include peptic ulceration and effects on renal and platelet function. Aspirin can precipitate bronchospasm in susceptible individuals with a history of asthma.

Paracetamol and NSAIDs are useful for the treatment of mild to moderate pain. However, as the common route of administration is oral, these drugs may not be appropriate in an emergency setting where a stress response may affect gastric motility and drug absorption. Readers are advised to consult a specialist pharmacology reference (e.g. MIMS) for advice regarding indications, dose, contraindications, adverse effects and preparation of these analgesics. Table 19.4 provides a summary of common non-opioid analgesics.

Opioids

All classes of analgesics can be used to manage acute pain, but opioids are considered the best agents for moderate to severe pain control. The effective use of opioids involves titration of the dose against pain relief while observing the patient for unwanted effects. Both exogenous and endogenous opioids bind to opioid receptors in the brain and spinal cord. These receptors are classified as mu (μ), delta (δ) and kappa (κ), and activation of these different receptors are responsible for the range of effects associated with opioid administration (Table 19.5).

The mu agonists (morphine-like) are the largest group and used most often. Examples of drugs in this category include morphine, codeine, fentanyl, hydromorphone, methadone, oxycodone and dextropropoxyphene. The mechanism of action of opioids is complex and not yet fully understood. In the spine, opioids inhibit the release of substance P from dorsal horn neurons. While opioids are considered to act on receptors in the CNS, there is evidence that there is also action of opioids at peripheral sites following tissue injury.

Although little difference is believed to exist among mu agonists and their ability to relieve pain, *morphine* is often

TABLE 19.4 Selected non-opioid analgesics and NSAIDs[73]

ANALGESIC	USUAL ADULT ORAL DOSAGE (mg/day)	DOSES/DAY	CLINICAL CONSIDERATIONS
Aspirin	2400–3600	4–6	Available in effervescent tablet, capsule, enteric coated, sustained release tablet, suppository
			Possibility of gastric irritation and bleeding
Paracetamol	2000–4000 (max. 4000)	4–6	Available in tablet, capsule, mixture, suppository
			Adverse effects rare in normal therapeutic doses
			Overdose can cause serious damage to liver and kidneys
Ibuprofen	1200–1600 (max. 2400)	3–4	Available in tablet and liquid
			Possibility of gastric irritation
Indomethacin	50–200 (max. 200)	2–4	Available in capsule, suppository
			Higher risk for GI effects
Celecoxib	100 (max. 400)	1–2	Does not affect platelet aggregation
			Long-term effects not established yet
Diclofenac	75–150 (max. 200)	2–3	Available in tablet and suppository
			Less effect on platelet aggregation
Naproxen	250–500 (max. 1000)	2	Available in tablet, controlled-release tablet and suppository
			Caution with patients on sodium-restricted diets

GI: gastrointestinal; NSAIDs: non-steroidal anti-inflammatory drugs

TABLE 19.5 Opioid receptor classification: current proposed terminology[4]

PROPOSED NOMENCLATURE	PREVIOUS NOMENCLATURE	EFFECTS
μ, mu, OP_3	β-endorphins, or MOP1 enkephalins, endomorphin-1, endomorphin-2	Analgesia, respiratory depression, euphoria, bradycardia, pruritus, miosis, nausea and vomiting, inhibition of gut motility, physical dependence
δ, delta, OP_1	Enkephalins, or DOP1 β-endorphins	Analgesia
κ, kappa, OP_2	Dynorphin A, or KOP1 dynorphin B, or KOP1 dynorphin B, α-neoendorphin	Analgesia, sedation, psychotomimetic effects, dysphoria, diuresis
NOP, OP_4, ORL-1	Nociceptin, orphanine FQ	Not opioid-like

the mu agonist of choice and is the standard against which other opioid analgesics are compared. In an emergency setting morphine should be given intravenously, with adults receiving 2.5–5 mg increments every 5 minutes until pain is relieved. While intramuscular administration is generally discouraged due to variations in absorption in the injured patient, this route of administration should be considered in haemodynamically stable patients where intravenous access is unavailable. If the intramuscular route is chosen, the initial dose of morphine should be based on the patient's weight: 0.1 mg/kg. However, the patient's weight may be poorly correlated with the dose required to achieve clinically significant pain relief, with up to a

10-fold variation in dose required to achieve analgesia between patients of similar age, irrespective of weight.

Immune-mediated reactions to morphine are rare, and the majority of reactions to morphine are classified as side effects rather than an allergy. When patients report an allergy they may be referring to an undesirable effect such as nausea, and it may be possible to pre-empt nausea by administering an antiemetic in cases where the patient reports previous episodes of nausea associated with morphine administration. Routine prophylactic use of antiemetics in conjunction with opioid administration is not recommended. Apart from nausea, some more common adverse effects of mu agonists include sedation, euphoria, dysphoria, pruritus, constipation and urinary retention. More serious adverse effects include hypotension and respiratory depression. Monitoring of the patient's respiratory status, perfusion and oxygenation is vital while administering opioids. However, respiratory rate is a poor indicator of respiratory depression. Instead, the level of sedation is a better early indicator of respiratory depression.[19] Common indicators of respiratory depression are listed in Box 19.2. The aim of opioid administration is to achieve satisfactory relief of pain while keeping the sedation score less than 2. It is important to note that respiratory depression in the setting of opioid administration usually results from decreased responsiveness to carbon dioxide within the medullary respiratory centre. Pulse oximetry will not reveal hypercapnia that may be associated with respiratory depression. It is therefore vital that a sedation score is regularly sought in patients receiving opioid therapy.

Tolerance to sedation and respiratory depression occur in patients receiving opioids over a period of several days. If clinically significant respiratory depression occurs following the administration of opioids, the patient's ventilations should be assisted. Decisions to reverse the opioid effect using an opioid antagonist such as naloxone should be made cautiously, as this will return the patient to their pre-opioid pain level and may induce withdrawal syndrome in the opioid dependent patient.

Fentanyl is a short-acting pure opioid agonist that binds to mu-receptors in the brain, spinal cord and other tissues. When administered intravenously, a dose of 100 µg is equivalent to 10 mg of intravenous morphine. Unlike morphine, fentanyl rarely causes significant histamine release. As such there is less potential for histamine-mediated hypotension following fentanyl administration. Fentanyl is showing great success in managing severe pain in the pre-hospital setting, and several

emergency medical services in Australia allow paramedic administration of fentanyl via the intranasal route using an atomising device attached to a 1 mL syringe. The efficacy of fentanyl delivered via the intranasal and intravenous routes has been shown to be similar.[59] However, the efficacy of this form of administration depends on delivery technique, as the drug must be atomised and dispersed across a large area of nasal mucosa to be effective. Research has shown that intranasal administration of this drug to children in pain is safe and effective.[60] This is a particularly effective route of administration in children who may have needle phobias. This study recommended the implementation of nurse-initiated administration of intranasal fentanyl in the ED.

Fentanyl is rapidly absorbed across mucous membranes as it is many times more lipid-soluble than morphine. However, bioavailability via the intranasal route is approximately 70% and a larger morphine-equivalent dose is required when administering the drug via this route. The initial intranasal dose for an adult is 200 µg. If the patient is aged more than 60 years or weighs less than 60 kg, half this dose (100 µg) should be used. The initial dose for children is 2 µg/kg. If the calculated dose volume exceeds 1 mL a more concentrated preparation must be used to reduce the total volume to be administered via the intranasal route. Onset of action is rapid, with duration of action approximately 30 minutes. Fentanyl has been associated with chest-wall rigidity in a small number of cases, which may make ventilation difficult.[54] A lozenge form for oral transmucosal administration is available and is approved for the treatment of breakthrough pain in palliative-care patients with cancer. While not currently approved for the treatment of acute or postoperative pain, this form of fentanyl has been shown to be effective in treating soldiers injured in combat.[61]

Oxycodone is a semisynthetic thebaine (opium alkaloid) derivative. This drug is a mu receptor agonist which also has affinity for delta and kappa opioid receptors in the brain and spinal cord. The drug is available in oral form for the treatment of moderate to severe pain, particularly chronic pain. The use of oxycodone has increased significantly in recent years, with much of this increase attributed to illicit drug use. It is often sought by individuals with opioid dependence who inject the drug, and its use as a substitute for drugs such as heroin (diamorphine) has led to the drug being known as 'hillbilly heroin' in the USA.

Other opioids have significant disadvantages in the emergency setting. *Codeine* is a weak opioid prodrug that is metabolised to morphine to provide an analgesic effect. However, up to 10% of the Caucasian population may lack the enzyme responsible for this conversion process (CYP2D6), rendering the drug ineffective in these individuals. The drug is available in combination with paracetamol or aspirin for oral administration for mild to moderate pain.

Pethidine is a synthetic opioid which was believed to be better than morphine in relieving the pain of renal colic. Research has subsequently shown that it is no more effective than morphine, while producing significant adverse effects due to the accumulation of the active metabolite, norpethidine.[19] This can produce CNS stimulation leading to muscle tremors, myoclonus and seizures. The use of this drug is no longer recommended.[19]

BOX 19.2 Commonly used indicators of respiratory depression[4]

Sedation score
1. Wide awake
2. Easy to rouse*
3. Constantly drowsy, easy to rouse but unable to stay awake (e.g. falls asleep during conversation); early respiratory depression
4. Severe; somnolent, difficult to rouse; severe respiratory depression.

Respiratory rate
- Fewer than 8 breaths/minute is often considered to be a sign of respiratory depression, but this is generally an unreliable indicator.
- Respiratory depression can co-exist with a normal respiratory rate.

Oxygen saturation
May also be unreliable, especially if the patient is receiving supplemental oxygen.

Some centres also add '1S', which indicates asleep but easy to rouse.

Tramadol is a weak opioid that acts on mu receptors, but also acts as a serotonin and noradrenaline re-uptake inhibitor. The active metabolite is mono-*O*-desmethyltramadol. However, this metabolism depends on the CYP2D6 isoenzyme of cytochrome P450, and patients who are lacking this enzyme may have a reduced analgesic effect (see discussion of codeine, above). The full analgesic action of this drug has not been completely explained. Although it causes less respiratory depression than an equivalent dose of morphine, nausea and vomiting occur at similar rates to other opioids. The interactions of tramadol with other drugs are similar to those of other opioids. However, particular attention should be given to interactions with drugs that increase serotonin by any mechanism, as this can lead to a serotonin syndrome.

Information comparing common opioids is shown in Table 19.6.

Inhalational analgesics

Nitrous oxide (N_2O) is an analgesic and is commonly used to induce anaesthesia. It is a mild analgesic and sedative when given with oxygen in a 50:50 mix. This analgesic is used in labour, during painful procedures such as changing burns dressings and in dental surgery. This is a safe analgesic with few side effects. However, if used over prolonged periods (6–8 hours), nitrous

TABLE 19.6 Opioid comparative information[57]			
When changing opioid, start at 50% of the approximate equianalgesic dose; then titrate according to response.			
DRUG	APPROXIMATE DOSE EQUIVALENT TO 10 mg IM/SC MORPHINE[a]	APPROXIMATE DURATION OF ACTION (HOURS)[b]	COMMENTS
Agonists			
codeine[c] (analgesic only)	200 mg oral	3–4	mild-to-moderate pain; not recommended
dextropropoxyphene	unknown		mild-to-moderate pain; not recommended; prescribing restrictions apply
fentanyl	100–150 mcg SC	1–2 (IM)	moderate-to-severe pain; preferred in renal impairment
hydromorphone[d]	1.5–2 mg SC/IM; 6–7.5 mg oral	2–4; 24 (controlled release)	moderate-to-severe pain
methadone (analgesic only)	complex; discuss conversion with a pain or palliative care specialist	8–24 (chronic dosing)	severe chronic pain
morphine[d]	30 mg oral	2–3; 12–24 (controlled release)	moderate-to-severe pain
oxycodone	15–20 mg oral	3–4; 12–24 (controlled release)	moderate-to-severe pain; preferred in renal impairment (adjust dose)
pethidine[d]	75–100 mg IM	2–3	not recommended
tapentadol[e]	75–100 mg oral	12 (controlled release)	moderate-to-severe chronic pain
tramadol[d]	100–120 mg IM/IV; 150 mg oral	3–6; 12–24 (controlled release)	moderate-to-severe pain
Partial agonists			
buprenorphine (analgesic only)	0.4 mg IM; 0.8 mg sublingual	6–8	not first line for analgesia

[a] dose equivalents are a guide only and may be greater than the maximum dose, see relevant monograph

[b] duration of action depends on dose and route of administration

[c] inactive; must be metabolised to morphine

[d] has an active metabolite; see monograph

[e] dose equivalence based on limited data; use caution

oxide can destroy the enzyme methionine synthetase (MS) and deplete vitamin B_{12} stores. Low levels of MS can affect DNA synthesis, resulting in rare but serious bone-marrow and neurological complications.[19] Patients and staff may experience adverse effects after long-term exposure to this gas if effective scavenging systems are not used. Its use in the community-based emergency health setting is becoming uncommon due to the bulk of the gas cylinder and administering apparatus, and safety concerns when the gas is used in confined spaces, including ambulances.

Methoxyflurane is classed as a volatile anaesthetic agent belonging to the fluorinated hydrocarbon group. It is a clear fluid with a distinctive odour that must be vaporised to be administered by inhalation. Unlike other volatile anaesthetics, at low concentrations this agent produces analgesia, which has been found to be effective in relieving acute pain in settings which include the ED.[62] This agent is currently used by several emergency medical services in Australia. The initial dose is 3 mL given via a disposable inhaler. The agent must be self-administered by the patient to avoid sedation. Duration of action is approximately 30 minutes, after which the initial dose may be repeated once. Patients should not be given more than 6 mL of methoxyflurane in 24 hours, and no more than 15 mL in a week. Contraindications include renal failure or impairment, as this agent has been shown to be nephrotoxic with long-term use or when high concentrations are given. Administration of this agent should be done in a well-ventilated environment.

N-methyl-D-aspartate receptor antagonists

Neurotransmitters such as glutamate, glycine and aspartate are involved in central nociceptive modulation, where they bind to *N*-methyl-D-aspartate (NMDA) receptors located in the postsynaptic interneurons and ascending neurons in the spinal cord. The action of these neurotransmitters appears to be linked to hyperalgesia and allodynia. Drugs such as ketamine and dextromethorphan block or antagonise these receptors and act as analgesics.

Ketamine has anaesthetic properties without reducing reflexes or muscle tone. At subanaesthetic doses it produces conscious sedation where the patient appears responsive but experiences analgesia while maintaining airway reflexes. The use of ketamine is becoming more widespread in managing severe pain in the pre-hospital and ED settings, and has been shown to be a safe and effective analgesic agent.[63] Analgesia is usually obtained with an intravenous dose of 0.3 mg/kg.[54] Ketamine stimulates sympathetic activity to increase cardiac output and blood pressure, reducing the risk of hypotension associated with some opioids. However, this may lead to increases in intraocular and intracranial pressure, so its use may be contraindicated in eye injuries and closed head trauma. At analgesic doses ketamine does not depress respiration in the way opioids can. While this drug has been successfully used in procedural sedation in children, its wider use as an analgesic has been constrained by a significant incidence of agitation, vivid dreams and hallucinations in older patients upon emergence from the dissociative state, and it is these properties that have seen an increase in the illegal use of this drug. These effects can, however, be managed by administering a short-acting benzodiazepine such as midazolam.[54]

Given its analgesic and anaesthetic properties, ketamine is particularly useful in disaster, transport and industrial accidents where patient extrication involves the manipulation of fractured limbs, or in cases of entrapment where amputation may be required and where the adverse effects of opioids complicate treatment. It should also be considered when managing severe acute pain in opioid-tolerant patients or in patients with poor response to opioids.

Adjuvants

Adjuvants are medications that are used in combination with opioid or NSAID analgesics to enhance pain relief or to treat symptoms that exacerbate pain. These drugs have analgesic properties but these properties are not their primary function. They are primarily used to treat chronic headaches, back pain and neuropathic pain. Examples of drugs in this group include:

- tricyclic antidepressants and selective serotonin reuptake inhibitors (SSRIs)
- corticosteroids—dexamethasone
- psychotropics—benzodiazepines and phenothiazines
- anticonvulsants—carbamazepine, gabapentin, sodium valproate
- alpha$_2$ agonists—dexmedetomidine, clonidine.

The type of pain determines the drug chosen; for example, patients with chronic continuous neuropathic pain have been shown to benefit from treatment with tricyclic antidepressants, which increase levels of noradrenaline and serotonin by inhibiting their uptake at adrenergic and serotonergic neurons.[19] This action may partly explain the action of tramadol in managing neuropathic pain. The route of administration for drugs in this group varies, but almost all adjuvants are available orally. Although not classified as analgesics, the drugs metoclopramide and prochlorperazine have been shown to be effective in reducing migraine pain.[64] These dopamine antagonists are commonly available in emergency health settings for the treatment of nausea and vomiting, and are also a useful adjunct or first-line agent for the relief of migraine in adults.

Non-pharmacological pain management

Distraction, hypnosis, imagery and relaxation are psychological interventions that may help to relieve pain. Physical adjuvant strategies include massage, application of heat and cold, transcutaneous electrical nerve stimulation (TENS) and acupuncture. These approaches are discussed briefly here.

Distraction

Distraction may facilitate pain management by assisting the patient to focus on a stimulus other than the pain. This technique may be of particular benefit in managing pain in young children. It may minimise, but does not entirely alleviate, pain. For distraction to be effective, the object of that distraction must be of interest to the patient. This can include pleasant images or music.[65] Multiple modes of distraction have been used to reduce pain in children with burns.[66]

Hypnosis, imagery and relaxation

Although hypnosis has been found to be useful in reducing pain during some medical procedures and in labour,[19] it is rarely used in emergency health settings because few clinicians have the knowledge, skills or time necessary to induce a trancelike state. However, the nurse or paramedic functioning in the capacity of patient advocate can assist the patient in pursuing this method of pain management by referring the patient to available community resources for continued pain management.

Using one's imagination to control pain is a form of distraction that produces relaxation. The imagination is used to develop images that promote pleasant sensations and diminish pain perception. For example, a patient may have decreased pain when imagining lying on the beach listening to the sound of waves washing over sand. By assisting in creating this imaginary setting, the nurse or paramedic can assist the patient with pain management. Effectiveness of imaging depends on familiarity of the image and its pleasantness for the patient and also depends on the environment, with noisy industrial settings or accidents in the middle of busy roads posing special challenges.

Relaxation techniques promote a state free from anxiety. When the patient is relaxed, skeletal muscle tension is minimal. Deep breathing is one way to promote relaxation. The nurse or paramedic can instruct the patient to inhale deeply through the nose and exhale slowly through the mouth. Repeating this sequence several times while concentrating on muscle relaxation may be an effective adjunct to pain management in the ED.

Cutaneous stimulation

This method refers to cutaneous techniques which stimulate the skin for the purpose of pain relief (e.g. vibration, superficial heat and cold, ice application, massage, methanol application to the skin, TENS and acupuncture). These techniques have been shown to be effective in some limited acute pain settings. For example, while acupuncture may help to relieve pain associated with childbirth, no evidence of analgesia has been associated with the use of TENS in the same clinical context.[19] Acupressure and TENS have been trialled in the paramedic practice setting.[67,68] However, the evidence for efficacy remains scant. Effects of cutaneous stimulation vary; nursing skill and preparation are required before this method is used as a pain management intervention. Emergency nurses and paramedics require appropriate initial and continuing education to use these techniques.

Anaesthesia

Local

Local anaesthesia refers to techniques that reduce or prevent pain without affecting consciousness. Drugs that provide local anaesthesia are often used for minor surgical procedures. These drugs block sodium channels and prevent the influx of sodium through membrane channels involved in depolarisation of the cell. This stops the propagation of action potentials along neurons, including nociceptor afferents. Although the intended site of action is the nerve cells responsible for the transmission of signals that are perceived as pain, all excitable tissue can be affected by sodium-channel blockade, including muscle cells and motor neurons. This action may produce paresis or paralysis. Autonomic neurons are also affected.

Lignocaine is a short-acting local anaesthetic, with a rapid onset and half-life of approximately 90 minutes. Longer-acting local anaesthetics include bupivacaine, ropivacaine and levobupivacaine. EMLA—a eutectic mixture of lignocaine and prilocaine—is useful as a topical preparation in reducing pain in procedures such as venous ulcer debridement. It is also used in procedural pain relief in children, particularly for venepuncture. However, EMLA needs to be applied at least 60 minutes prior to the procedure to be effective. A similar product with the same properties is AnGel, used topically to reduce pain.

Local anaesthetics may be injected into the epidural space to block transmission of afferent signals along thoracic, lumbar or sacral nerves.

Classification of local anaesthetics

Two groups of local anaesthetics can be described, based on their duration of action. The *amides* include lignocaine, bupivacaine, levobupivacaine and ropivacaine. These are slowly metabolised by the liver and have a long duration of action. In contrast, the *esters* are metabolised more quickly. Examples include procaine, cocaine, benzocaine, amethocaine, oxybuprocaine and proxymetacaine. The ester compounds are metabolised to *p*-aminobenzoic acid metabolites, which may be associated with allergic reactions in some patients.[69] The properties of common local anaesthetics are listed in Table 19.7.

Route of administration

Local anaesthetics can be given via several routes. *Topical* application produces anaesthesia when applied to mucous membranes, conjunctiva and damaged skin. Apart from EMLA and AnGel, local anaesthetics do not penetrate unbroken skin. A range of formulations is available for topical administration.

Infiltration involves subdermal and subcutaneous injections to produce an anaesthetic field around the injury or area to be repaired. Nerve blocks involve the injection of a drug such as lignocaine next to a peripheral nerve that may be some distance from the injury or pain-producing lesion. A femoral nerve block provides good analgesia distal to the injection, and is used to treat pain arising from injuries such as a fractured femur. However, ultrasound may be required to facilitate needle placement, and a related technique that does not require technology to guide needle placement and that has been shown to be effective in the prehospital setting is the fascia iliaca compartment block.[70]

Epidural anaesthesia involves injection of a local anaesthetic into the epidural space in the spinal canal where the drug remains localised. This procedure is used to relieve pain associated with labour and surgical procedures such as caesarean section and thoracic and abdominal surgery.

Subarachnoid (intrathecal) anaesthesia involves drug administration into the cerebrospinal fluid (CSF) within the subarachnoid space at a point below the third lumbar vertebra to avoid potential penetration of the spinal cord.

Local anaesthetics, opioids and combinations of both can be administered via the epidural route to provide analgesia while maintaining motor function. Opioids bind to opioid receptors in the substantia gelatinosa of the spinal cord to provide local analgesia without systemic effects. When administered by the epidural route, opioids diffuse into the CSF before reaching the cord. Local anaesthetics act on spinal roots and nerves as

TABLE 19.7 Properties of commonly used local anaesthetics[68]

NAME	TYPE/METABOLISM	USES	TOXICITY/NOTES
Short-acting (30–60 minutes)			
Procaine	Ester/plasma	Infiltration, nerve block, spinal	Least toxic LA; low lipid solubility; slow onset; potency 0.5 × lignocaine
Benzocaine	Ester/plasma	Topical: drops, gel, lozenges, paint, suppositories	Relatively non-toxic; very low potency; only active topically
Intermediate duration (1–3 hours)			
Lignocaine	Amide/liver	Infiltration, nerve block, spinal epidural, IV, topical	Prototype LA, potency = 1; more cardiotoxic than prilocaine; rapid onset
Prilocaine	Amide/liver	Infiltration, nerve blocks, caudal, epidural, IV	Lower systemic toxicity than lignocaine; equipotent with lignocaine; products of liver metabolism may cause methaemoglobinaemia
Lignocaine/prilocaine cream (EMLA®)	Amides/liver	Topical (venepuncture, cannulation, minor skin surgery)	Local irritation; risk in infants < 6 months old (methaemoglobinaemia); toxic if swallowed by small children
Mepivacaine	Amide/liver	Infiltration, nerve blocks, caudal, epidural	Less toxic than lignocaine; equipotent with lignocaine; avoid use in pregnancy
Articaine	Amide/liver	Dental	Combined with adrenaline 1:100,000 provides 1–3 hours of regional anaesthesia; no significant advantages over lignocaine
Long duration (3–10 hours)			
Bupivacaine, levobupivacaine, ropivacaine	Amides/liver	Infiltration, caudal, epidural, nerve blocks	More cardiotoxic than lignocaine; potency 4 × lignocaine; slow onset; adrenaline not needed; less motor blockade
Amethocaine (tetracaine)	Ester/plasma	Topical anaesthesia	Potency 5 × lignocaine; slow onset; high systemic toxicity; useful for analgesia for venous cannulation

IV: intravenous; LA: local anaesthetic

well as the spinal cord.[71] As the intrathecal technique provides direct access to the CNS, it is associated with an increased risk of infection and other adverse effects arising from medullary and sympathetic depression.

Intravenous regional anaesthesia of the forearm (Bier block) is used to provide analgesia in procedures such as wound debridement, foreign body removal and reduction of fractures and dislocations. After placing an intravenous cannula in the dorsum of the hand on the affected limb, the limb is exsanguinated by elevation and brachial artery compression, or by winding an Esmarch bandage proximally along the forearm. A blood-pressure cuff is placed over the upper arm and inflated to 100 mmHg above systolic blood pressure, and the arm is lowered. A local anaesthetic such as prilocaine is injected intravenously slowly via the cannula in the hand, with analgesia achieved within 5–10 minutes. The blood-pressure cuff should remain inflated for at least 20 minutes, but no longer than 60 minutes.[73] Continuous monitoring for evidence of systemic toxicity should be undertaken by nursing staff, particularly following release of the tourniquet. Chapter 17, p. 358, contains further information on administering regional anaesthesia.

Benefits of local anaesthetics

Local anaesthetics prevent or significantly reduce pain and discomfort associated with injury and medical procedures such as suturing, without affecting the patient's level of consciousness. For example, injecting a local anaesthetic such as lignocaine next to the digital nerve can effectively relieve pain associated with a crush injury to a digit. This technique—known as a nerve block—avoids the potential complications associated with administering a centrally-acting opioid, while providing an excellent level of analgesia. Although the use of digital and femoral nerve blocks has had limited use by nurses and paramedics, the wider use of these procedures offers a broader range of pain-control options, and their use could be extended with additional training.

Disadvantages and limitations of local anaesthetics

The interference with sodium-ion transport across cell membranes that results in anaesthesia when this transport is inhibited in afferent nociceptors can also influence the propagation of action potentials in other parts of the body, including the CNS and heart. This can lead to cardiac dysrhythmias and CNS stimulation if local anaesthetics such as lignocaine are injected intravenously, or if significant systemic absorption occurs following topical administration or infiltration in highly vascular areas. The addition of adrenaline can produce local vasoconstriction and restrict systemic absorption from the injection site. However, adrenaline may cause ischaemia in poorly perfused tissue and as such it must not be used on the digits, penis, ears or nose because of its vasoconstrictive effects.

Nursing implications for procedures involving local anaesthetics

Local anaesthetics are usually considered to be safe when administered in small doses prior to surgical procedures such as wound debridement. However, the patient's blood pressure, pulse rate and respiratory rate should be monitored during treatment with injectable agents because systemic toxicity may occur when the dose is too high or the drug is accidentally injected intravenously. Systemic toxicity can result in CNS stimulation and dysrhythmias such as ventricular fibrillation, heart block and asystole. Resuscitation equipment should be readily available and staff trained in resuscitation procedures.

In explaining the procedure, the nurse informs the patient that pain will be blocked but touch and pressure should remain intact during topical and infiltration administration. Pain management is facilitated if the patient is assisted into a comfortable position before initiating the procedure. As with all drug administration, contraindications to use should be assessed, such as known allergy or hypersensitivity to the drug. Local anaesthetics containing adrenaline should not be used in poorly perfused areas such as those previously described.

The maximum safe dose of a local anaesthetic should be calculated to avoid systemic side effects. Doses may need to be modified in children, pregnant patients, the elderly or patients with liver disease. Solutions containing adrenaline should be used with caution in hypertensive patients or those taking tricyclic and monoamine oxidase inhibitor antidepressants.

Other types and uses of anaesthesia

Procedural sedation refers to a technique of administering sedatives or dissociative agents with or without analgesics to induce a state that allows the patient to tolerate unpleasant procedures while maintaining cardiorespiratory function. This technique produces a reduced level of consciousness while maintaining airway reflexes. The continuum of sedation ranges from a state where the patient is able to respond purposefully to stimuli, to deep sedation where patients cannot be easily roused. Sedation that produces a drug-induced depression of consciousness to the point where patients do not respond to any stimuli is classified as *general anaesthesia*. This stage of sedation requires airway control and cardiorespiratory support, and requires considerable expertise in managing the patient and any complications that may arise. Procedural sedation requires that personnel providing procedural sedation and analgesia have an understanding of the drugs administered, have the ability to adequately monitor the patient's response to medications given and have the skills necessary to manage all potential complications. Chapter 17 contains information on how to test respiratory function (p. 334).

Informed consent should be obtained before initiation of analgesia. Patients should be given information regarding the nature of the procedure, risks and benefits and any potential complications. Contraindications for procedural sedation are clinical instability and refusal by a competent patient.

Although there are risks with procedural sedation, these can be minimised if the appropriate agent, dosage and route of administration are considered. Monitoring is mandatory, and should include level of consciousness, heart rate, blood pressure, ECG and respiratory rate and effort. Additionally, pulse oximetry and capnography to measure end-tidal carbon dioxide ($EtCO_2$) should be considered (see Ch 17, p. 323 for an

---

PRACTICE TIPS

ACTIONS FOR EFFECTIVE PAIN CONTROL

- Establish an effective, supportive relationship with the patient.
- Believe, collaborate with and respect the patient's response to pain and its management.
- Use a validated pain scale to measure pain severity; the scale used must be appropriate for age.
- Use an appropriate behavioural pain scale to assess pre-verbal children and patients with cognitive impairment, including patients with dementia.
- Tailor the treatment to suit the individual to accommodate inter-personal differences in response to analgesics.
- Ensure patient safety at all times. Monitoring the patient facilitates assessment of treatment effectiveness and minimises potential adverse occurrences. An opioid antagonist must be available for the management of serious adverse effects such as respiratory depression.
- Monitor the patient's response and effectiveness of treatment.
- Sedation is an early indicator of respiratory depression associated with opioid administration. Sedation should be routinely monitored in this setting.
- Consider other interventions when pain fails to respond to treatment; opioid-tolerant patients may require higher doses or non-opioid therapy such as ketamine to relieve severe pain.
- Inform the patient what they are likely to experience while in the ED to minimise fear of the unknown.
- Communicate effectively with the patient and healthcare professionals responsible for ongoing care regarding the treatment plan and its effectiveness.
- Maintain a calm, empathetic manner.
- Educate the patient about the occurrence, onset and duration of pain; methods of pain relief; and preventive measures.
- Research the multidimensional nature of pain, its assessment and subsequent management. Use this research in practice.
- Maintain current knowledge and competencies.

explanation on administering these). Pulse oximetry may not be as sensitive as $EtCO_2$ in identifying respiratory depression. As patients with respiratory depression will usually have an $EtCO_2$ of >50 mmHg, this finding may allow more-rapid identification of hypoventilation than pulse oximetry alone.

Opioids are the drug of choice, with the titrated IV route preferred. This is considered the safest approach to rapid analgesia. Opioids may be used alone or in combination with other analgesics and sedatives. A combination of fentanyl and midazolam has been found to be safe and effective when used in the ED. Propofol and ketamine are also recommended for procedural sedation. Before administering a drug it is important to determine the patient's history of drug use. Patients who have developed drug tolerance may require higher dosages; the elderly and the very young may require lower doses.

If respiratory depression occurs from induction with an opioid, it can be reversed with naloxone. For adults, naloxone can be slowly administered 0.4–2 mg IV, repeated every 2 minutes until the respiratory depression is reversed.

Patient assessment, patient monitoring and documentation are important before, during and after the procedure. Emergency nurses and doctors should be cognisant of their institution's policies on procedural sedation and accept responsibility for ensuring safe standards of practice.

SUMMARY

Pain is a common complaint in many healthcare settings. Paramedics, nurses and other healthcare professionals have an important role in assessing, evaluating, and managing a patient's pain. This requires a knowledge of contemporary principles of pain management practice, which includes the actions and indications of pharmacological agents used to manage pain. In addition, an understanding of non-pharmacological interventions is essential. However, the effectiveness of any care plan depends on the quality of the clinical decision-making process and awareness of the effect of bias on decisions. These include assumptions about pain-related behaviours based on gender, race and age. Being aware of these influences will help to ensure that equitable and effective analgesia is provided to relieve pain and improve the patient's quality of life.

CASE STUDY 1

A 40-year-old cyclist has collided with a car that turned into the path of the rider from a side street in a residential area. On examination the patient is conscious, orientated and is complaining of severe pain over the right lateral chest wall. The patient tells you that he was wearing a helmet and denies any loss of consciousness. He estimates that he was travelling at 20 km/h when he hit the side of the car. The patient's blood pressure is 110/80 mmHg, pulse is 120 beats/minute and skin is pale and sweaty. He is complaining of exacerbation of pain on inspiration (10/10 severity) but denies any other pain. Auscultation of the chest reveals decreased air entry in right lung fields but no adventitious sounds. However, the patient refuses to take a deep breath due to the pain. Examination of the chest wall reveals bruising over several ribs over the right anterior axillary line. This area is exquisitely painful on palpation. There is no obvious deformity, flail segment or paradoxical chest wall movement. A comprehensive 'nose to toes' examination does not reveal any other abnormalities other than abrasions over all extremities consistent with contact with the road surface. Further observations reveal a saturation of 90% on air by pulse oximetry. The patient's respiratory rate is 20 breaths/minute but his tidal volume appears low.

Questions

1. Propose causes for the observed decrease in oxygen saturation.

2. Are there any contraindications to analgesia in this case?

3. If you decide to use a pharmacological intervention to manage the patient's pain, what agent/s will you elect to use? Summarise the risks and benefits associated with each agent.

4. What is the end-point in analgesic administration in this case?

Answers to Case Study Questions can be found on evolve
http://evolve.emergencytrauma.curtis

CASE STUDY 2

A 32-year-old man is complaining of a sudden onset of severe abdominal pain. On examination the patient appears distressed and is restless. He occasionally paces the room before returning to a sitting position where he sits with knees drawn up. The patient describes the pain as 'agonising' and constant, starting abruptly approximately 20 minutes previously while he was at home. He tells you the pain is in his right flank and that the pain radiates to the umbilical region and groin. The pain is associated with nausea. On palpation the abdomen is soft with tenderness reported over all quadrants. The patient denies any constipation or other gastrointestinal tract symptoms. He denies any gross haematuria or recent trauma that may be associated with the pain. Vital signs show a pulse of 80 beats/minute, blood pressure of 130/85 mmHg, respiratory rate of 16 breaths/minute, and temperature of 37.2°C. The patient states that he is hepatitis C positive, and denies any current medications or drug use.

Questions

1. Are there any contraindications to analgesia in this case?

2. You note an absence of signs of sympathetic activity despite a report of severe pain. Describe the utility of vital signs in verifying pain in patients where a self-report is available.

3. Your colleague considers delaying analgesia until further diagnostic tests can be undertaken to rule out the possibility of drug-seeking behaviour. Discuss the clinical and ethical implications of this course of action.

4. If you decide to use a pharmacological intervention to manage the patient's pain, what agent/s will you elect to use? Summarise the risks and benefits associated with each agent.

 Answers to Case Study Questions can be found on evolve
http://evolve.emergencytrauma.curtis

REFERENCES

1. Morrison RS, Magaziner J, Gilbert M et al. Relationship between pain and opioid analgesics on the development of delirium following hip fracture. J Gerontol A Biol Sci Med Sci 2003;58(1):76–81.

2. Craig KD. Emotions and psychobiology. In: McMahon SB, Koltzenburg M, eds. Wall and Melzack's textbook of pain. 5th edn. Philadelphia: Churchill Livingstone; 2006. pp. 231–9.

3. Liebeskind JC. Pain can kill. Pain 1991;44(1):3–4.

4. Macintyre PE, Schug SA. Acute pain management: a practical guide. 3rd edn. Philadelphia: Saunders; 2007.

5. Cordell WH, Keene KK, Giles BK et al. The high prevalence of pain in emergency medical care. Am J Emerg Med 2002;20(3):165–9.

6. Fosnocht DE, Heaps ND, Swanson ER. Patient expectations for pain relief in the ED. Am J Emerg Med 2004;22(4):286–8.

7. Forero R, Mohsin M, McCarthy S et al. Prevalence of morphine use and time to initial analgesia in an Australian emergency department. Emerg Med Australas 2008;20(2):136–43.

8. Yeoh MJ, Huckson S. Audit of pain management in Australian emergency departments. Emerg Med Australas 2008;20(s1):A26–36.

9. Doherty S, Knott J, Bennetts S et al. National project seeking to improve pain management in the emergency department setting: Findings from the NHMRC-NICS National Pain Management Initiative. Emerg Med Australas 2013;25(2):120–6.

10. Anderson KO, Green CR, Payne R. Racial and ethnic disparities in pain: causes and consequences of unequal care. J Pain 2009;10(12):1187–204.

11. Jones JS, Johnson K, McNinch M. Age as a risk factor for inadequate emergency department analgesia. Am J Emerg Med 1996;14(2):157–60.

12. Raftery KA, Smith-Coggins R, Chen AH. Gender-associated differences in emergency department pain management. Ann Emerg Med 1995;26(4):414–21.

13. Safdar B, Heins A, Homel P et al. Impact of physician and patient gender on pain management in the emergency department: a multicenter study. Pain Med 2009;10(2):364–72.

14. Lord B, Cui J, Kelly AM. The impact of patient sex on paramedic pain management in the prehospital setting. Am J Emerg Med 2009;27(5):525–9.

15. Young MF, Hern HG, Alter HJ et al. Racial differences in receiving morphine among prehospital patients with blunt trauma. J Emerg Med 2013;45(1):46–52.

16. White LJ, Cooper JD, Chambers RM et al. Prehospital use of analgesia for suspected extremity fractures. Prehosp Emerg Care 2000;4(3):205–8.

17. Hennes H, Kim MK, Pirrallo RG. Prehospital pain management: a comparison of providers' perceptions and practices. Prehosp Emerg Care 2005;9(1):32–9.

18. Rupp T, Delaney KA. Inadequate analgesia in emergency medicine. Ann Emerg Med 2004;43(4):494–503.

19. Macintyre PE, Schug SA, Scott DA et al. APM-SE working group of the Australian and New Zealand College of Anaesthetists and Faculty of Pain Medicine. Acute pain management: scientific evidence. 3rd edn. Melbourne: Australian and New Zealand College of Anaesthetists and Faculty of Pain Medicine; 2010.

20. Institute for Clinical Systems Improvement. Health care guideline: assessment and management of acute pain. 6th edn. Bloomington: ICSI; 2008.

21. International Association for the Study of Pain (IASP). Part III: Pain terms, a current list with definitions and notes on usage. In: Merskey H, Bogduk N, eds. Classification of chronic pain. 2nd edn. Seattle: IASP Task Force on Taxonomy, IASP Press; 1994. pp. 209–14.

22. McCaffery M, Pasero C. Pain: clinical manual. 2nd edn. St Louis: Mosby; 1999.

23. Melzack R, Wall PD. Pain mechanisms: a new theory. Science 1965;150(699):971–9.

24. Melzack R, Katz J. Pain assessment in adult patients. In: McMahon SB, Koltzenburg M, eds. Wall and Melzack's textbook of pain. 5th edn. Philadelphia: Churchill Livingstone; 2006. pp. 291–304.

25. Liu M, Ferrante FM. Overview of pain mechanisms and neuroanatomy. In: Rosenberg AD, Grande C, Bernstein RL, eds. Pain management and regional anesthesia in trauma. London: WB Saunders; 2000.

26. Devor M. Response of nerves to injury in relation to neuropathic pain. In: McMahon SB, Koltzenburg M, eds. Wall and Melzack's Textbook of pain. 5th edn. Philadelphia: Churchill Livingstone; 2006. pp. 905–27.

27. Australasian College for Emergency Medicine. Guidelines for implementation of the Australasian Triage Scale in emergency departments 2013. Online. www.acem.org.au/Standards-Publications/Policies-Guidelines.aspx; accessed 18 Aug 2014.

28. Lord B. Paramedic assessment of pain in the cognitively impaired adult patient. BMC Emerg Med 2009;9(20). doi:10.1186/1471-227X-9-20.

29. Lord B, Woollard M. The reliability of vital signs in estimating pain severity among adult patients treated by paramedics. Emerg Med J 2010; http://emj.bmj.com/content/early/2010/10/06/emj.2009.079384.abstract; accessed 12 March 2015.

30. Marco CA, Plewa MC, Buderer N et al. Self-reported pain scores in the emergency department: lack of association with vital signs. Acad Emerg Med 2006;13(9):974–9.

31. Melzack R, Katz J. Pain assessment in adult patients. In: McMahon SB, Koltzenburg M, eds. Wall and Melzack's textbook of pain. 5th edn. Edinburgh: Churchill Livingstone; 2006.

32. Lee JS. Pain measurement: understanding existing tools and their application in the emergency department. Emerg Med (Fremantle) 2001;13(3):279–87.

33. Solomon P. Congruence between health professionals' and patients' pain ratings: a review of the literature. Scand J Caring Sci 2001;15(2):174–80.

34. Hockenberry MJ, Wilson D, eds. Wong's essentials of pediatric nursing. 8th edn. St Louis: Mosby; 2009.

35. Merkel SI, Voepel-Lewis T, Shayevitz JR, Malviya S. The FLACC: a behavioral scale for scoring postoperative pain in young children. Pediatr Nurs 1997;23(3):293–7.

36. Cousins MJ, Lynch ME. The Declaration Montreal: access to pain management is a fundamental human right. Pain 2011;152(12):2673–4.

37. Todd KH, Sloan EP, Chen C et al. Survey of pain etiology, management practices and patient satisfaction in two urban emergency departments. Can J Emerg Med 2002;4(4):252–6.

38. Neighbor ML, Honner S, Kohn MA. Factors affecting emergency department opioid administration to severely injured patients. Acad Emerg Med 2004;11(12):1290–6.

39. Silka PA, Roth MM, Geiderman JM. Patterns of analgesic use in trauma patients in the ED. Am J Emerg Med 2002;20(4):298–302.

40. Galbraith A, Bullock S, Manias E. Fundamentals of pharmacology: a text for nurses and allied health professionals. 4th edn. Sydney: Prentice Hall; 2004.

41. Bowsher D. Mechanisms of pain in man. London: TCI Publications; 1987.

42. Savage SR, Joranson DE, Covington EC et al. Definitions related to the medical use of opioids: Evolution towards universal agreement. J Pain Symptom Manag 2003;26(1):655–67.

43. Adriaensen HA. Opioid drugs in chronic non malignant pain. Acta Anaesth 1993;39(suppl 2):67–70.

44. Minozzi S, Amato L, Davoli M. Development of dependence following treatment with opioid analgesics for pain relief: a systematic review. Addiction 2013;108(4):688–98.

45. Heit HA. Addiction, physical dependence, and tolerance: precise definitions to help clinicians evaluate and treat chronic pain patients. J Pain Palliat Care Pharmacother 2003;17(1):15–29.

46. Vickers AP, Jolly A. Naltrexone and problems in pain management. Br Med J 2006;332(7534):132–3.

47. Huxtable CA, Roberts LJ, Somogyi AA, Macintyre PE. Acute pain management in opioid-tolerant patients: a growing challenge. Anaesth Intensi Care 2011;39(5):804–23.

48. McNabb C, Foot C, Ting J et al. Profiling patients suspected of drug seeking in an adult emergency department. Emerg Med Australas 2006;18(2):131–7.

49. Grover CA, Close RJH, Wiele ED et al. Quantifying Drug-seeking Behavior: A Case Control Study. J Emerg Med 2012;42(1):15–21.

50. Burke SO, Jerrett M. Pain management across age groups. West J Nurs Res 1989;11(2):164–78.

51. McEachin CC, McDermott JT, Swor R. Few emergency medical services patients with lower-extremity fracture receive prehospital analgesia. Prehosp Emerg Care 2002;6(4):406–10.

52. Vassiliadis J, Hitos K, Hill CT. Factors influencing prehospital and emergency department analgesia administration to patients with femoral neck fractures. Emerg Med (Fremantle) 2002;14(3):261–6.

53. Wisborg T, Flaatten H. Pain management in the pre-hospital/emergency medical service environment: on-site and transport. In: Rosenberg AD, Grande CM, Bernstein RL, eds. Pain management and regional anesthesia in trauma. London: WB Saunders; 1999. pp. 109–18.

54. Coman M, Kelly AM. Safety of a nurse-managed, titrated intravenous analgesia policy on the management of severe pain in the emergency department. Emerg Med 1999;11:128–31.

55. Fry M, Holdgate A. Nurse-initiated intravenous morphine in the emergency department: efficacy, rate of adverse events and impact on time to analgesia. Emerg Med (Fremantle) 2002;14(3):249–54.

56. World Health Organization. Cancer pain relief. Geneva: WHO; 1986.

57. Australian Medicines Handbook 2014 [online]. Adelaide: Australian Medicines Handbook Pty Ltd; www.amh.net.au; accessed 27 May 2015.

58. Rickard C, O'Meara P, McGrail M et al. A randomized controlled trial of intranasal fentanyl vs intravenous morphine for analgesia in the prehospital setting. Am J Emerg Med 2007;25(8):911–17.

59. Borland ML, Jacobs I, Geelhoed G. Intranasal fentanyl reduces acute pain in children in the emergency department: a safety and efficacy study. Emerg Med (Fremantle) 2002;14(3):275–80.

60. Kotwal RS, O'Connor KC, Johnson TR et al. A novel pain management strategy for combat casualty care. Ann Emerg Med 2004;44(2):121–7.

61. Grindlay J, Babl FE. Review—efficacy and safety of methoxyflurane analgesia in the emergency department and prehospital setting. Emerg Med Australas 2009;21(1):4–11.

62. Jennings PA, Cameron P, Bernard S. Ketamine as an analgesic in the pre-hospital setting: a systematic review. Acta Anaesthesiologica Scandinavica 2011;55(6):638–43.

63. Holdgate A, Kelly AM. Emergency care evidence in practice series: management of acute migraine. Melbourne: Emergency Care Community of Practice, National Institute of Clinical Studies; 2006.

64. Evans D. The effectiveness of music as an intervention for hospital patients: a systematic review. J Adv Nurs 2002;37(1):8–18.

65. Miller K, Rodger S, Bucolo S et al. Multi-modal distraction. Using technology to combat pain in young children with burn injuries. Burns 2010;36(5):647–58.

66. Simpson PM, Fouche PF, Thomas RE, Bendall JC. Transcutaneous electrical nerve stimulation for relieving acute pain in the prehospital setting: a systematic review and meta-analysis of randomized-controlled trials. Eur J Emerg Med 2014;21(1):10–17.

67. Lang T, Hager H, Funovits V et al. Prehospital analgesia with acupressure at the Baihui and Hegu points in patients with radial fractures: a prospective, randomized, double-blind trial. Am J Emerg Med 2007;25(8):887–93.

68. Bryant B, Knights K, Salerno E. Pharmacology for health professionals. 4th edn. Sydney: Mosby; 2014.

69. Lopez S, Gros T, Bernard N et al. Fascia iliaca compartment block for femoral bone fractures in prehospital care. Reg Anesth Pain Med 2003;28(3):203–7.

70. McQuay HJ, Moore RA. Local anaesthetics and epidurals. In: Wall PD, Melzack PR, eds. Textbook of pain. 4th edn. Edinburgh: Churchill Livingstone; 1999.

71. Fatovich DM, Brown AFT. Pain relief in emergency medicine. In: Cameron P, Jelinek G, Kelly AM et al. eds. Textbook of adult emergency medicine. 2nd edn. Edinburgh: Churchill Livingstone; 2000;626–34.

72. Brown D, Edwards H, eds. Lewis's Medical-surgical nursing. 2nd edn. Sydney: Elsevier; 2008.

73. Brown D, Edwards H, eds. Lewis's Medical-surgical nursing. 4th edn. Sydney: Elsevier; 2014.

CHAPTER 20
PHYSIOLOGY AND PATHOPHYSIOLOGY FOR EMERGENCY CARE

LEIGH KINSMAN, ADRIAN VERRINDER AND ALEX TZANNES

Essentials

- Physiological responses form the bases for signs and symptoms observed in emergency patients.
- The sympathetic nervous system is activated and the parasympathetic nervous system is slowed in most stressful situations.
- A physiological 'cascade' effect contributes to the death of cells in the vicinity of, or adjacent to, damaged or underperfused cells.
- Shock is the process resulting from inadequate cellular perfusion.
- The 'triad of death' (acidosis, hypothermia and coagulopathy) is linked to death following blood loss.
- Criteria used to determine level of trauma or illness include physiological responses.
- The early assessment and identification of abnormal physiology and shock are central to the work of emergency clinicians. Early sets of vital signs can provide an indication of the existence of shock and provide clinical cues that guide interventions.

INTRODUCTION

Physiology in emergency care forms the basis of the many signs and symptoms displayed in patients who use emergency health services. Many research articles and textbooks have been published on the physiological phenomena of the stress response, or 'general adaptation syndrome' (GAS), first introduced and popularised by Hans Selye.[1] Selye's research identified three very distinct phases within the GAS: *alarm*, *resistance* and *exhaustion* phases, triggered after the body's exposure to injury or illness, resulting in the disruption of homeostasis. This chapter examines these physiological principles that apply to patients seen in the pre-hospital and hospital emergency department (ED) setting and forms the basis for all applicable chapters within this textbook.

Fright, fight and flight

Sympathetic nervous system

Physiologically, emergencies are generally accompanied by the activation of the sympathetic nervous system (SNS). The resulting secretions of noradrenaline from sympathetic nerve endings, adrenaline from the adrenal medulla and cortisol from the adrenal cortex have a profound effect on the functioning of all organ systems. In evolutionary terms, the sympathetic nervous system prepares the body for physical activity: to fight or to run.

In most physiologically stressful situations, the sympathetic nervous system is activated and the parasympathetic nervous system slows. The majority of noradrenaline in a stress response is secreted from the sympathetic nerve endings. The adrenal medulla secretes adrenaline:noradrenaline in approximately 4:1 ratio. The noradrenaline and adrenaline then flood into the bloodstream to bind to any available receptors. The effect at a cellular level differs according to the subtype of adrenergic receptor activated by these hormones in various end organs. In the cardiovascular system, alpha-adrenergic receptors respond by causing a constriction of the arterioles of non-essential vascular beds—as in the gut, skin, kidneys and liver—while beta-adrenergic receptors respond by relaxing muscle arterioles and increasing the heart rate and contractile force of myocardium. The background vascular tone of muscle arterioles is simultaneously reduced by centres in the medulla oblongata. The resultant effect is to raise blood pressure, increase cardiac output and divert blood away from the temporarily non-essential organs to skeletal muscle.

In the liver, muscle and adipose tissue, adrenergic receptor stimulation leads to an increase in available levels of glucose and free fatty acids, as an immediate source of energy. In the lungs, beta-2 receptors lead to dilation of bronchial smooth muscle.

In extreme situations, excess adrenaline and noradrenaline can cause evacuation of the contents of the upper and lower digestive tract while the activity of the rest of the intestines is dramatically slowed, as blood is diverted from non-essential vascular beds to working muscle. The circulating adrenaline and noradrenaline also bring about increased alertness, anxiety and, at high levels, cognitive impairment, and sometimes nausea associated with slowing gastric motility.

Sympathetic activation also increases the secretion of adrenocorticotrophic hormone (ACTH) from the anterior pituitary gland, which increases the secretion of steroids from the adrenal cortex. This has the effect of inhibiting inflammation, retaining water and sodium and breaking down proteins and fats for their energy content.

The sympathetic nerves flow out of the spinal cord between the first thoracic and second lumbar vertebrae, synapse in the paravertebral ganglia and extend postsynaptic fibres back up to the head and down to the organs of the thorax and abdomen, the arms and the legs. The sympathetic nervous system is also directly wired to the adrenal medulla, which, when stimulated, secretes adrenaline and some noradrenaline directly into the bloodstream. These bind to receptors on cell membranes in addition to the noradrenaline that is secreted by the sympathetic nervous system.

Parasympathetic nervous system

The sympathetic nervous system is countered by the aptly named parasympathetic nervous system. Nearly every organ system has a dual supply of sympathetic and parasympathetic nerves which have largely opposite effects on the organs in question. A major exception is the vast majority of blood vessels which have, primarily, only sympathetic innervation.

The outflow of parasympathetic nerves from the central nervous system is mainly contained in the cranial nerves which service the head and most of the thorax and abdomen (via the vagus nerve). There is a small outflow in the sacral nerves at the base of the spine which service the bladder, genitals and the distal end of the digestive tract.

The sympathetic nerve endings generally secrete noradrenaline onto their target cells, while the parasympathetic nerve endings secrete acetylcholine.

The target organs have specific adrenergic and cholinergic receptors in their cell membranes to which the noradrenaline and acetylcholine specifically bind. This brings about changes in the target cells' activity by activating 'second messengers' in the cells and/or by opening ion channels in the cell membranes.

An example of this is the heart. It has both a sympathetic and a parasympathetic nerve supply. Both the sympathetic and the parasympathetic nerves are continuously secreting small amounts of noradrenaline and acetylcholine onto heart muscle. In cardiac pacemaker cells—for example, the sinoatrial node—an electrical potential difference is maintained across the cell membrane. This is due to the opposing effects of potassium and sodium ion concentrations in the intracellular compared with the extracellular fluid. A membrane protein 'pump' maintains the potential difference, termed polarisation. The resting electrical potential of the inside of the cell membrane compared to the outside is about −70 mV, comparable to other excitable cells. Highly regulated protein 'channels' allow specific ions to flow back down their concentration and/or electrical gradients leading to depolarisation. If a cell depolarises enough and reaches 'threshold', an 'action potential' is propagated by the pacemaker and conducting cells and that initiates contraction of the myocardium. The *rate* of discharge is affected by both the degree of baseline electrical polarisation across the cell membrane and the amount of channel leakage leading the cell to reach its threshold for action potential propagation. The sympathetic nerves thus increase the heart rate by speeding up the depolarisation of the pacemaker cells slightly (a few extra sodium channels are opened) and the parasympathetic nerves slow it down by hyperpolarising the cells slightly (a few extra potassium channels are opened). The resulting heart rate is essentially a net result of opposing sympathetic and parasympathetic activity. The administration of atropine, a potent blocker of parasympathetic transmission, would thus be expected to lead to an increase in heart rate.

The gastrointestinal tract also has a dual innervation, but in this instance the parasympathetic nervous system increases peristaltic activity and other aspects of digestion in the gut from the stomach to the colon while noradrenaline secreted by the sympathetic nervous system slows it down. Although the transmitters bind to very similar receptors on the gut cell membranes as on cardiac cells, they are linked to different second messengers and ion channels, and consequently mediate different cellular responses.

The sympathetic nerve terminals may also directly inhibit the output of parasympathetic nerve terminals, through pre-synaptic inhibition. Put simply, the parasympathetic nervous system plays the major role in our vegetative being—digesting food, for example, while the sympathetic nervous system mediates 'fight or flight'.

Capillaries and nutritive blood flow

During activation of the sympathetic nervous system the blood flow to non-essential organs is dramatically reduced. Normally organs are adequately supplied with oxygen, glucose, amino acids and fats and produce byproducts of cellular metabolism, such as carbon dioxide, lactate and other acids. Tissue perfusion through these capillary beds is tightly regulated at both a central and a local level. The sympathetic nervous system generally ensures an adequate flow of blood to organs by controlling the diameter of the feeding arterioles. In the perfused tissues, most of the time, the majority of the capillaries are actually closed off by pre-capillary sphincters that only open when waste products accumulate in the surrounding tissue. Under increased demand, metabolic byproducts accumulate, leading to dilation of these sphincters and hence increased local blood supply.

Oxygen, carbon dioxide, fats and urea are fat-soluble and can diffuse easily through capillary endothelium down their respective concentration gradients. Water-soluble components have to be filtered through 4-nm clefts in the capillary wall. This allows the flow of water and small molecules (glucose, amino acids, ions, etc), but not proteins, through the capillary walls. The proteins and other large molecules remaining in plasma are an important determinant of fluid equilibrium between the blood and extravascular tissue. By raising 'oncotic pressure' (a form of colloid osmotic pressure exerted by proteins, notably albumin, in the blood that pulls water into the circulatory system) they cause a tendency for fluid to move across the capillary wall into the vascular space. Opposing this is the *capillary hydrostatic pressure*, equal to the difference between capillary blood pressure and tissue pressure. At the arterial end of the capillary beds the hydrostatic pressure is greater than the colloid osmotic pressure and there is net flow of water and solute into the extravascular tissue. At the venous end of the capillary beds the hydrostatic pressure has fallen beneath the colloid osmotic pressure, and now there is a net flow of water and its dissolved components back into the capillaries. Hundreds of litres of fluid are shifted across capillary walls each day, but the process is usually finely balanced. A slight excess, roughly 500 mL per day, flows out into extravascular tissue and is collected and recirculated by the lymphatic system, ultimately draining via the cisterna chyli into the left supraclavicular vein.

If capillary hydrostatic pressure is elevated past a certain point, fluid will filter out through the 4-nm clefts in the capillary walls, accumulate in the extravascular tissues and cause swelling. The disturbance in this balance of oncotic and hydrostatic pressures is known as oedema. Capillary venous pressure might be elevated, as in the case of congestive cardiac failure or venous obstruction from thrombosis. Alternatively, the capillary hydrostatic pressure can be lower than normal; for example, by hepatic failure, malnutrition, protein-losing renal

diseases, or blockage, for example, by malignant infiltration. Then the protein in the blood can draw liquid out of the tissues and bolster blood volume. The section below on hypovolaemic shock is a case in point.

Another means of transporting blood molecules into the tissues is *vesicular transport*. This is used for transporting large molecules, especially proteins, out of capillaries and into the extracellular space. Proteins such as insulin or any of the anterior pituitary hormones are too large to get out of the 4-nm clefts in the capillary walls. Instead they bind to the surface of the endothelial cells lining the capillaries and are then surrounded by endothelial cell membrane, which forms a tiny vesicle around the protein. The vesicle then travels through the endothelial cell to the outer membrane and the contents are discharged into the tissue surrounding the capillary (the extravascular space). These transport mechanisms are protein-specific and highly regulated.

Physiological responses to tissue hypoperfusion

Tissue hypoperfusion may result from a systemic shock state, such as hypovolaemia, or may result from activation of the sympathetic nervous system in susceptible organs. Mechanisms exist to mitigate against this low flow state, with the dual problems of reduced oxygen and nutrient delivery, and reduced waste product removal. Commonly the blood flow is reduced to 25% of the normal blood flow, potentially reducing the supply of vital nutrients and reducing the removal of toxic wastes. The supply of water, soluble nutrients and those requiring vesicular transport will be reduced in proportion to the reduction in blood flow. The fat-soluble components fare a little better.

As we saw earlier, accumulation of CO_2 and various acids leads to relaxation of precapillary sphincters, allowing access to the perfusing blood. Flow is sluggish, but there *is* flow. Second, the acidic waste products cause haemoglobin to dissociate from most of the oxygen it is carrying, and consequently the perfusing blood can deliver up to four times as much oxygen to the tissue as it normally would. Similarly, hypoxic and acidic haemoglobin can take up and remove proportionately more carbon dioxide than in normal conditions. So even at a quarter of the normal flow, oxygen supply would remain adequate and carbon dioxide removal would keep pace. For details, see the sections below on oxygen and carbon dioxide transport.

The reduction in the supply of glucose and amino acids is countered by the effects of the stress hormone *cortisol* (from the adrenal cortex), which promotes the breakdown of cellular glycogen to glucose and also promotes the breakdown of some cellular protein to amino acids, both of which can be used to generate adenosine triphosphate (ATP) through glycolysis and through the Krebs cycle. This can supply some of the metabolic needs of cells in under-perfused tissues, but prolonged under-perfusion leads to cell starvation, cell death and ultimately multiple-organ failure.

Cell energetics

The internal environment of cells is quite different from the tissue fluid that surrounds them. The two media are separated and controlled by the cell membrane. This is comprised of a hydrophobic 'lipid bilayer' and a wide array of metabolically active proteins. An important example is the sodium–potassium exchange pump introduced earlier, which requires energy to move these ions up their respective concentration gradients. Forty per cent of the energy we extract from our diet is expended in maintaining the difference between the intracellular and extracellular environments.

Just about all cellular machinery use energy stored in the form of adenosine triphosphate (ATP). The whole process of carbohydrate metabolism is directed towards the extraction of energy from sugars and the manufacture of ATP, in which the extracted energy is temporarily stored then used for virtually all cellular processes. Primary among these is the operation of the ion pumps that actively pump sodium ions out of cells and potassium ions into cells, both up a concentration gradient. Not only does this generate an ion imbalance across the cell membrane (low sodium inside, high sodium outside), but it also creates a negative electrical potential of nearly a tenth of a volt between the inside and the outside of the cell. The rest of the energy is used in the manufacture of all the other molecular structures inside the cell. Many proteins are biological catalysts, or enzymes, which foster the conversion of ATP into adenosine diphosphate (ADP). The reconversion of ADP into ATP requires energy input. This is achieved by other enzymes that work in a series of steps to break down some form of metabolic fuel, such as simple carbohydrates (sugars), fatty acids, proteins or ketone bodies. Thus ATP can be thought of as the 'universal energy currency' of the body.

There are generally two processes inside cells which harvest the energy contained in the chemical bonds of sugars. The first is *glycolysis* which breaks glucose molecules in half and supplies a net gain of 2 ATP molecules for each glucose molecule used. It is rapid and, importantly, does not require oxygen to be supplied to the cell. The byproduct is pyruvate. In turn, pyruvate can be converted to the waste product lactic acid which diffuses out of the cells. In the presence of oxygen, the pyruvate can be processed through the *Krebs cycle* to carbon dioxide and water and the generation of over 30 high-energy molecules of ATP. The Krebs cycle takes place inside mitochondria—the powerhouses of the cell (Fig 20.1).[2]

In the presence of oxygen, pyruvate—a 3-carbon-atom compound—is converted to an acetyl group, a 2-carbon-atom compound, which binds to coenzyme A in the mitochondria for further processing by the Krebs cycle. The acetylcoenzyme A is processed by a series of enzymes attached sequentially to the inner membrane of the mitochondria. Essentially, the acetyl groups are de-constructed by these enzymes: the hydrogens are stripped off the carbon atoms, leaving CO_2 as a waste product. The protons and the electrons are removed from the carbons down a series of hydrogen carriers and an electron transport chain by the immense attraction between the protons and the strongly electronegative atomic oxygen at the end of the chain. Some of the energy of this attraction is captured and used to add a terminal phosphate group to ADP, generating an ATP supply. The oxygen ultimately combines with the hydrogen to form water molecules as a waste product. The resulting ATP is used as the energy currency of the cell.

Cell deterioration

This latter process, so-called oxidative phosphorylation, is dependent on the supply of oxygen to the cells. Generally,

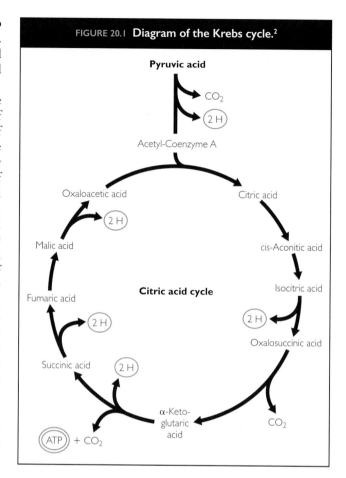

FIGURE 20.1 **Diagram of the Krebs cycle.**[2]

between 36 and 38 ATP molecules are formed for every glucose molecule that is metabolised through the Krebs cycle, compared with only two ATP molecules generated by glycolysis.

Under-perfused tissues are on the verge of oxygen starvation and frequently glycolysis alone cannot generate enough ATP to maintain cellular processes. This underperfusion may result from a global abnormality, such as asphyxia or haemorrhagic shock, or from local disruption of blood supply, such as during a stroke or myocardial infarct. The first thing that happens is that the energy dependent sodium–potassium exchange pump slows. Then the cell membranes start to lose their voltage and the membrane potential is gradually lost. This depolarisation can lead to catastrophic consequences for the cells in question *and* for the cells in the vicinity of the dying cells. A small number of dying cells can, literally, kill thousands of adjacent cells by inadvertently initiating a massive amplification of the initial disturbance. This amplification is called a 'cascade' effect. The important cascade effects on a cellular level may be electrical or chemical.

Electrical and chemical cascades

Electrical anomalies occur in excitable cells such as nerve cells and cardiac muscle. As the sodium-potassium-ATPase pumps fail and the cell starts to depolarise, the cell may experience electrical 'death shudders' in the form of abnormally triggered action potentials that stimulate other cells in the vicinity to follow suit. If confined to a small area of myocardium, this abnormal pacemaker is termed an ectopic focus. Spread of the action potential through the heart's conducting system and myocardium would give a mistimed but coordinated contraction called an ectopic beat. Under more critical conditions a greater amount of myocardial tissue may have a reduced threshold for action potential propagation. Abnormal electrical activity might spread in an uncoordinated fashion causing sustained ventricular fibrillation rather than effective rhythmic contractions.

Pathological depolarisation may precipitate calcium entry into the cell by the uncontrolled opening of voltage-regulated calcium channels in the plasma membrane, the endoplasmic reticulum and the mitochondria. The influx of calcium has a deleterious cascade effect on a number of cellular functions. These include maintaining the integrity of the mitochondrial membrane, cellular metabolism, neurotransmitter release in the nervous system and control of muscle cell contraction and relaxation

Loss of cell contents

The process of cellular death in an uncontrolled, widespread manner is termed necrosis. This is distinct from the orderly removal of individual senescent cells, termed apoptosis. One of the hallmarks of cellular necrosis is release of intracellular contents, such as potassium, intracellular enzymes and lactate. Clinically, the release of contents from a significant mass of dying cells may be detected by the presence of metabolic acidosis (a low arterial blood pH in the presence of a low bicarbonate level) and hyperkalaemia.

In addition, some of the cellular contents may appear in the blood. Depending on the type of tissue involved, specific intracellular contents might have diagnostic utility. For example, creatine kinase is part of the contractile apparatus of muscle cells and may be detectable in the blood after a crush injury to a limb. Various components of the enzyme troponin are specific to cardiac muscle. Their presence in blood is diagnostic of cardiac cellular necrosis, for example in the event of coronary arterial occlusion. When cardiac muscle cells are deprived of oxygen and depolarise and die, they release their contents, including troponin which can be detected by routine blood tests. Dead cells cannot maintain the integrity of their cell membranes and ultimately all the contents will spill out into the extracellular fluid.

All cells contain lysosomes, packets of digestive enzymes normally used for recycling proteins. Pancreatic cells, in particular, contain a variety of powerful digestive enzymes that can damage the protein and lipid components of surrounding tissue in an amplifying cascade of necrosis that characterises severe pancreatitis. One of these proteins is lipase, which when detectable in large quantities confirms the diagnosis.

The release of potassium from dying cells will also affect the electrical activity of neighbouring cells. This is due to the fact that membrane potential is primarily due to the ratio of the intracellular and extracellular potassium concentrations. If cells lose potassium into the extracellular space, the remaining cells will have a reduced ratio of potassium inside and outside the cell membrane, and consequently will have a lower (less-negative) membrane potential. This may tip adjacent cells into cell death, causing the release of even more potassium and hence initiating a potassium cascade.

Nerve cells may become ischaemic during a stroke, or due to systemic hypoxia. Normal cellular function rapidly ceases.

Within minutes, ongoing ischaemia cause the neurons to release excess glutamate (an excitatory amino acid neurotransmitter) as their electrical potential fails. This binds to and opens NMDA (*N*-methyl-D-aspartate) receptor-mediated calcium-ion channels in neighbouring cells, initiating a calcium cascade (see above), which causes the release of even more glutamate. This release results in a synergistic calcium and glutamate cascade,which propagates through nervous tissue, damaging cells in addition to those areas deprived of oxygen during the initial insult.

Cell protection: the blood–brain barrier

Specific tissues in the body depend on a tightly regulated environment to maintain optimal function. The most important example of this is the central nervous system (CNS), where we have seen that the orderly function of neurons is highly sensitive to changes in the extracellular milieu. The evolution of these intrinsically excitable cells was associated with the co-evolution of a protective barrier that tightly regulates the passage of molecules into the vicinity of the neurons.

The physical form of the blood–brain barrier comprises non-nerve cells (glial cells), called *astrocytes*, found throughout the nervous system. These cells interpose themselves between the perfusing capillaries and the neurons by wrapping their cytoplasmic processes around both capillary and nerve cells and acting as a cellular intermediary between the two. The CNS capillaries are relatively impermeable and have far fewer clefts between their endothelial cells than in other parts of the body. Most of the transport is by carrier-mediated facilitated diffusion through the endothelial cells themselves rather than through the clefts; thus the barrier can be highly selective in terms of the number of carriers that are manufactured by the cells forming the blood–brain barrier.

Water-soluble nutrients (glucose, amino acids, etc.) have specific carriers to supply the brain cells. In addition, some substances surplus to requirements are actively pumped out of the brain back into the capillaries. Conversely, the blood–brain barrier presents little impediment to fat-soluble substances, so oxygen, carbon dioxide, urea, etc. will diffuse in or out down their concentration gradients. Drugs that are highly lipid soluble are therefore more able to penetrate the blood–brain barrier and gain access to the CNS.

When damaged, the blood–brain barrier can lose its integrity, exposing the neurons to a less highly regulated extracellular environment. Normally excluded toxins may accumulate; in addition, lipid insoluble drugs may now have an effect on the CNS.

The blood–brain barrier is not uniform. The blood vessels in the hypothalamus are more permeable than most of the other regions of the nervous system, allowing the cells of the hypothalamus to sample the vascular components of blood and respond to any homeostatic imbalances that might be occurring. See the sections below on the control of plasma electrolytes, water and acid–base balance.

Homeostasis

Homeostasis may be defined as the body's maintenance of a relatively constant internal environment in the face of an ever-changing external environment. The factors that are being

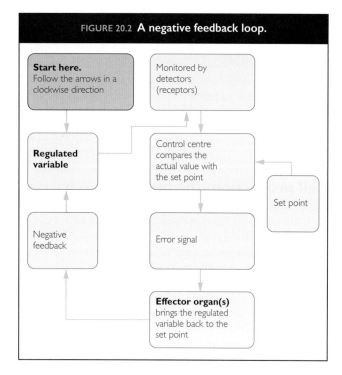

FIGURE 20.2 **A negative feedback loop.**

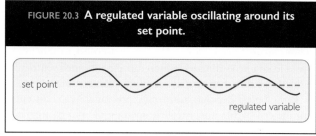

FIGURE 20.3 **A regulated variable oscillating around its set point.**

kept relatively constant are called *regulated variables*. Examples include the concentration of virtually all blood chemicals, core temperature, partial pressure of carbon dioxide, vertical posture, withdrawal reflexes, blood pressure, blood glucose, energy usage, metabolic rate—even weight.

In general, these variables are regulated by negative feedback loops (Fig 20.2). In order for any variable to be kept relatively constant there has to be a feedback loop which corrects (or negates) any deviation of that variable from the set point. This is the healthy range for every variable. In principle, every feedback loop must contain the following elements:

- set point—the level at which the regulated variable should be maintained, as determined by a process that is connected to the control centre, i.e. the control centre has to have some knowledge of what the set point should be
- receptors—sensitive cells or tissues that measure or monitor the regulated variable; this together with the neural or hormonal signalling mechanism is the *afferent* component.
- control centre—compares the regulated variable with the set point and initiates the 'error signal'
- error signal—a signal (electrical or chemical) initiated by the control centre in proportion to the difference between the regulated variable and the set point. The error signal brings about a response from the effector organ(s). This is the *efferent* component.
- effector organ(s)—the organ(s) that respond to the error signal and shift the regulated variable up or down towards the set point.

As a consequence, regulated variables are always oscillating around a set point, as shown in Figure 20.3.

If the regulated variable rises above the set point, this is monitored by receptors and the control centre compares this high value with the set point. The control centre sends an error

signal to the effector organs to bring the regulated variable back down towards the set point. The regulated variable then, generally, overshoots the set point; the lower value is detected by receptors and the control centre sends an error signal that causes the regulated variable to trend upwards, back to and over the set point—and so on.

A simple example is the control of core temperature when moving from a cool temperature to a slightly warmer one. The thermoreceptors in the hypothalamus constantly monitor the temperature of the blood. As it starts to warm, the control centre senses the difference between the temperature of the blood and the set point, and generates an error signal through the vascular portion of the sympathetic nervous system that controls the dilation and constriction of the small arterioles in the skin vascular beds. Dilation of these vessels allows the blood's heat to radiate into the environment. If too much heat is lost, constriction of the same vessels helps conserve heat. At more extreme changes of temperature, other mechanisms such as sweating and shivering are recruited to assist cooling and warming.

If any part of a feedback loop is damaged or missing, a loss of homeostasis may result. Feedback loops can become pathological when, rather than taking the regulated variable back to the set point, it moves it *further* from the set point. Instead of *negating* the difference between the regulated variable and the set point, a pathological feedback loop will increase and amplify the difference. This is called *positive feedback* and is a central principle in the pathophysiology of emergency care.

An example will help to make the point. Consider a panic attack. A patient becomes aware of their own heart beating (normally this cannot be felt). The anxiety caused by these palpitations increases the release of adrenaline, which causes the heart to beat faster and with increased force, which causes more anxiety, more adrenaline release and yet more rapid and forceful palpitations: even though the patient is not in danger, the 'fight or flight' feedback mechanism has entered a vicious cycle.

Examples of some relevant regulated variables, receptors, control centres, error signals, effector organs and outcomes are shown in Table 20.1.

Oxygen transport

The atmosphere at sea level has a pressure of 760 mmHg. Twenty-one per cent of this is oxygen, which has a proportionate, or *partial pressure*, of $0.21 \times 760 = 160$ mmHg. If this atmosphere is in contact with a body of fluid, the partial pressure of that particular gas dissolved in the fluid will equilibrate. The partial pressure can be thought of as the 'driving force' that causes the gas to dissolve in the fluid. The amount of gas in the fluid depends on other factors as well, in particular, the solubility.

TABLE 20.1 Receptor pathways for homeostasis

REGULATED VARIABLE	RECEPTOR	CONTROL CENTRE	SET POINT	ERROR SIGNAL	EFFECTOR ORGAN(S)	RESULT
Arterial partial pressure of carbon dioxide, $PaCO_2$	Central chemoreceptors— neurons in the medulla that are sensitive to CO_2 and hydrogen ions	Respiratory neurons in the pons and medulla	40 mmHg, determined by automatic neurons associated with the respiratory centres	Modulation of the medullary respiratory neurons that project down the spine	Intercostal and diaphragm muscles	Modulation of the rate and depth of respiration and maintenance of $PaCO_2$ at the set point
Plasma osmolarity	Hypothalamic osmoreceptors— neurons that shrink or swell depending on the particle content of the hypothalamic interstitial fluid. This changes their firing patterns depending on their degree of hydration	Paraventricular hypothalamic neurons whose axons project to the posterior pituitary	Approx. 300 Osm. Determined by automatic neurons associated with the hypothalamic control centre	Modulation of the secretion of ADH	Primarily the cells of the collecting ducts in the kidney	ADH binds to V-2 receptors in the kidney collecting-duct cell membranes, initiating an intracellular second messenger cAMP which promotes the manufacture and installation of aquaporins (water channels) in the apical and basolateral cell membranes. This increases their permeability to water and, providing the kidney medulla is of a higher osmolarity than the collecting ducts, water is reabsorbed and a more concentrated urine is produced.
Core temperature	Hypothalamic temperature receptors which change their discharge patterns depending on the temperature of the perfusing blood	Hypothalamic neurons whose axons connect to the vascular component of the sympathetic nervous system	37°C, determined by automatic neurons associated with the hypothalamic control centre	Modulation of discharge down the sympathetic nerves which control flow in the cutaneous circulation	The arterioles in the dermis of the skin	An increase in core temperature results in cutaneous vasodilation; a decrease in core temperature results in cutaneous vasoconstriction
Sodium and potassium— short route	Low plasma sodium or high plasma potassium stimulate the glomerulosa cells of the adrenal gland	Glomerulosa cells of the adrenal gland	Na^+ approx. 140 mmol/L; K^+ approx 4–5 mmol/L. Determined by the glomerulosa cells of the adrenal gland	Aldosterone secretion	Tubular cells of the distal convoluted tubule of the kidney	Aldosterone binds to nuclear receptors and stimulates the transcription of more Na^+-K^+-ATPase pumps. These retrieve more Na^+ from the filtrate and allow K^+ loss
Sodium and potassium— long route	A drop in blood pressure or volume or a lowering of plasma sodium stimulates the cells of the JGA in the kidney	Cells of the JGA	Na^+ approx. 140 mmol/L; K^+ approx. 4–5 mmol/L. Determined by cells of the JGA	Renin secretion → angiotensin I formation → angiotensin II formation → stimulates aldosterone secretion from glomerulosa cells of adrenal gland	Tubular cells of the distal convoluted tubule of the kidney	Aldosterone binds to nuclear receptors and stimulates the transcription of more Na^+-K^+-ATPase pumps. These retrieve more Na^+ from the filtrate and allow K^+ loss

Continued

TABLE 20.1 Receptor pathways for homeostasis—cont'd

REGULATED VARIABLE	RECEPTOR	CONTROL CENTRE	SET POINT	ERROR SIGNAL	EFFECTOR ORGAN(S)	RESULT
Calcium (Ca^{2+})	Low calcium detected by cells of the parathyroid gland	Cells of the parathyroid gland	Approx 5 mEq. Determined by cells of the parathyroid gland	Secretion of parathyroid hormone	(i) Bone, releases some Ca^{2+} from bone (ii) Gut, enhances Ca^{2+} absorption from the gut (iii) Kidney tubule cells, enhance Ca^{2+} reabsorption from kidney filtrate	Raises plasma calcium levels
	High plasma calcium stimulates interstitial cells in the thyroid gland	Interstitial cells of the thyroid gland	Approx. 5 mM. Determined by interstitial cells of the thyroid	Secretion of calcitonin	Opposes reabsorption of Ca^{2+} from bone	Lowers plasma calcium levels
Hydrogen ions and bicarbonate ions	The respiratory system controls hydrogen ions and bicarbonate ions (see above). The tubule cells of the kidney are sensitive to hydrogen ions	Kidney tubule cells	pH approx 7.4; 40 nM. Bicarbonate approx. 24 mmol/L. Determined by the kidney tubule cells	Activation of proton pumps when plasma is too acidic, inhibition if the plasma is too alkaline	Protons are pumped from the plasma into the tubular fluid and bicarbonate is retrieved. In alkalosis this is inhibited so acid accumulates and bicarbonate is lost	Plasma pH and bicarbonate concentrations are maintained within homeostatic limits
Mean arterial pressure (MAP)	Stretch receptors called baroreceptors in the carotid bifurcation and the aortic arch	Medulla cardiac and vasomotor centres	Approx. 100 mmHg (13.25 kPa). Determined by neurons associated with the cardiac and vasomotor centres in the medulla	Activation of sympathetic nerves to heart and blood vessels	Increases heart rate, stroke volume and constriction of arterioles in response to a drop in MAP	MAP is kept within homeostatic limits

ADH: antidiuretic hormone; cAMP: cyclic adenosine monophosphate; JGA: juxtaglomerular apparatus; K⁺: potassium ions; Na⁺: sodium ions.

Unlike carbon dioxide, oxygen is not very soluble in water or plasma. At 37°C, only 1.5% of the oxygen carried by 100 mL of blood is dissolved in plasma. The only reason that blood can carry a significant amount of oxygen is the presence of approximately 15 g of haemoglobin per 100 mL of blood. The haemoglobin is contained in the red blood cells. Haemoglobin is a globular protein with four subunits, each of which has a central iron atom capable of binding reversibly with one oxygen molecule, with an S-shaped affinity curve (Fig 20.4).

Under experimental conditions it is possible to vary the partial pressure of oxygen in blood, and measure the resulting

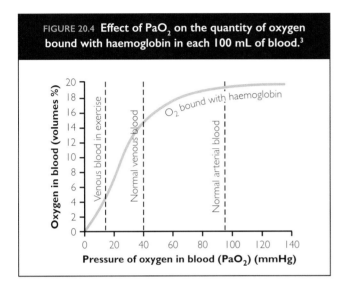

FIGURE 20.4 **Effect of PaO_2 on the quantity of oxygen bound with haemoglobin in each 100 mL of blood.**[3]

amount of bound *oxyhaemoglobin* as a percentage of total haemoglobin. This is termed the oxygen *saturation*. A gradient exists between alveolar air, across the alveolar wall, into the blood. At sea level, breathing room air, the typical partial pressure of oxygen in the arterial blood (PaO_2) in a healthy person is about 100 mmHg (Fig 20.5).

The oxygen–haemoglobin dissociation curve turns out to be S-shaped rather than linear. The shape of this curve (with a flat top) is primarily due to the fact that when all the haemoglobin molecules are carrying four oxygen molecules, no more oxygen can be carried by blood except if dissolved in the plasma. This dissolved amount is very small (0.3 mL O_2/100 mL plasma at 100 mmHg PaO_2). Each gram of haemoglobin can combine with a maximum of about 1.34 mL of oxygen, so an individual with 15 g of haemoglobin per 100 mL of blood can carry about 20 mL of oxygen per 100 mL of blood.[3] It can be seen that the vast majority of oxygen carried by the blood is bound to haemoglobin, thus even if the oxygen saturation approaches 100% a reduction in haemoglobin will lead to a reduction in the amount of oxygen delivered to tissues.

Symptoms of cardiac ischaemia may result from severe anaemia. No amount of supplemental oxygen will compensate for the reduced oxygen carriage in such a patient.

As foreshadowed above, another trick that haemoglobin has up its molecular sleeve is that its affinity for oxygen changes depending on the environment in which it is operating. Most of the time it flows from the lungs saturated with oxygen and is then pumped through working vascular beds, the tissue of which has relatively low metabolic rates. On average, each

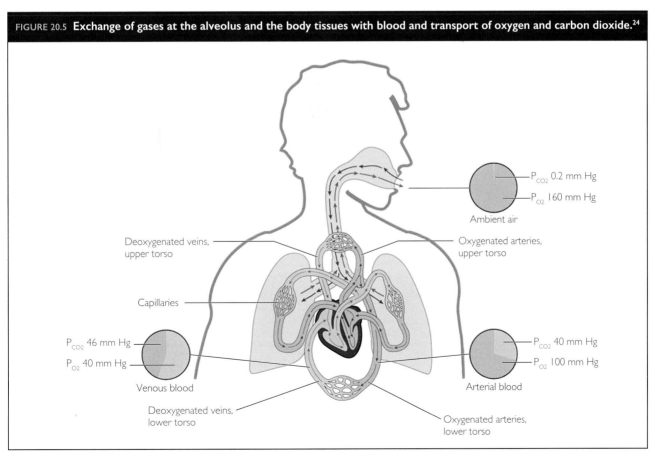

FIGURE 20.5 **Exchange of gases at the alveolus and the body tissues with blood and transport of oxygen and carbon dioxide.**[24]

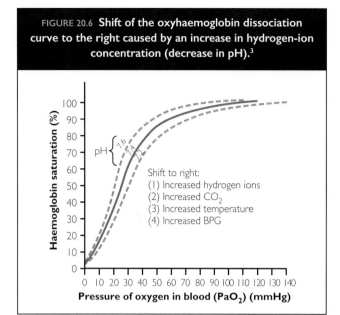

FIGURE 20.6 **Shift of the oxyhaemoglobin dissociation curve to the right caused by an increase in hydrogen-ion concentration (decrease in pH).**[3]

BPG: 2,3-bisphosphoglycertae.

haemoglobin molecule delivers only one oxygen molecule to the tissue and goes back to the heart and lungs still three-quarters saturated.

But in hardworking tissue like exercising muscle, the tissue is hot and acidic. This environment twists the haemoglobin molecule a touch and reduces the affinity between oxygen and haemoglobin so that more than one oxygen molecule is liberated from each haemoglobin molecule (see Fig 20.6). In extremely hot acidic working muscle, all the oxygen is stripped off the haemoglobin. In this way the oxygen supply to tissue can be increased four-fold without an increase in blood supply.

Carbon dioxide transport

Carbon dioxide does not bind to haemoglobin at the same sites as oxygen. It is carried as carbamino (N–COO⁻) compounds on all the blood protein molecules, including haemoglobin, but this only accounts for 18% of carbon dioxide carriage. Five per cent of carbon dioxide is carried dissolved in the plasma. Approximately 77% of carbon dioxide is carried as bicarbonate ions that result from the chemical reaction between carbon dioxide and water. Carbon dioxide easily diffuses into red cells and is hydrated by the enzyme carbonic anhydrase, producing

carbonic acid which ionises into bicarbonate ions and hydrogen ions:

$$CO_2 + H_2O \leftrightarrow H_2CO_3 \leftrightarrow HCO_3^- + H^+ \qquad (1)$$

The bicarbonate ions so produced diffuse out of the red cells and are replaced by chloride ions. In lung capillaries the opposite of this happens: bicarbonate ions are converted back into carbon dioxide and carbon dioxide flows down a concentration gradient out of the blood and into the alveoli of the lungs. As a result of this increased solubility and chemical buffering capacity in plasma and red blood cells, the carriage of CO_2 is more or less linearly proportional to its partial pressure. In arterial blood there is a partial pressure ($PaCO_2$) of about 40 mmHg (5.3 kPa), which represents around 400 mL of carbon dioxide per 100 mL of blood.

Capnography

Arterial $PaCO_2$ can be estimated by infrared assay of end-expiratory air samples. This air, essentially alveolar air, in normal haemodynamic and pulmonary states has a PCO_2 approximately 1–5 mmHg (0.14–0.68 kPa) below that of arterial blood. End-expiratory, or end-tidal, CO_2 ($EtCO_2$) reflects a combination of the arterial CO_2 level and the amount of pulmonary perfusion. Regions of the lung ventilated but not perfused are known as 'dead space', and this increases as a result of decreased pulmonary perfusion. These areas do not contribute to gas exchange between the blood and the atmosphere and thus decrease the efficiency of the lung as a functional unit. An increase in dead space results in an increased gradient between arterial CO_2 and end-expiratory CO_2. As the gradient between $EtCO_2$ and $PaCO_2$ may be significant in ill or injured patients, it is good practice to obtain a measure of arterial PCO_2 and correlate this with the $EtCO_2$.

Capnography is the real-time graphical representation of sampled CO_2 in air inspired and expired by the patient. It has become a standard monitoring tool for intubated patients in the pre-hospital setting and ED for several reasons. First, the presence of expired CO_2 confirmed by the monitor waveform (see Fig 20.7) indicates that the endotracheal tube is in the trachea and not the oesophagus.[4] Second, in brain injured patients, for example, controlling ventilation to maintain arterial PCO_2 in normal ranges has been associated with improved outcomes. Lastly the level of expired CO_2 during steady ventilation is a reflection of pulmonary perfusion and hence a useful indicator of cardiac output.[5] During cardiac arrest, for example, the $EtCO_2$ can reflect the adequacy of

FIGURE 20.7

Normal findings on a capnogram.[5]
A→B indicates the baseline;
B→C, expiratory upstroke;
C→D, alveolar plateau; D, partial pressure of end-tidal carbon dioxide;
D→E, expiratory downstroke.

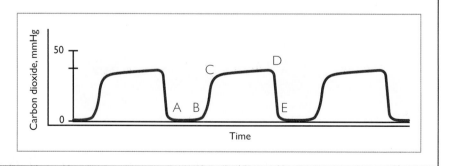

CPR. See Chapter 17, p. 323, for information on capnography and EtCO$_2$ monitoring.

Oxygen/carbon dioxide homeostasis

Due to the crucial role of CO$_2$ in the maintenance of acid–base balance via carbonic anhydrase, the respiratory system controls PaCO$_2$ very tightly (see Fig 20.8 and Table 20.1).

When the PaCO$_2$ gets above 40 mmHg (5.3 kPa), there is a reflex increase in the rate and depth of respiration, so more carbon dioxide diffuses from the blood into the alveoli and is 'blown off'.

When the PaCO$_2$ drops below 40 mmHg (5.3 kPa), there is a reflex decrease in the rate and depth of respiration, so more carbon dioxide is retained.

The respiratory muscles, the diaphragm and the intercostals, are the effector organs. They are driven by motor neurons in the spinal cord which are in turn driven by descending motor neurons that originate in the medulla oblongata. In the medulla and pons are respiratory centres; they consist of pacemaker cells which determine the rate of respiration, and amplifier circuits which determine the depth of respiration. These respiratory centres are influenced by central chemoreceptors that are sensitive to PaCO$_2$ and hydrogen-ion concentration ([H$^+$]) and by peripheral chemoreceptors situated in the aortic arch and carotid bodies that are sensitive to arterial PaCO$_2$, [H$^+$] and also PaO$_2$, but only if oxygen drops to dangerously low levels. This hypoxic sensitivity and the associated respiratory drive are, essentially, emergency devices.

Hyperventilation (may be voluntary or caused by anxiety or fever) blows off carbon dioxide. PaCO$_2$ may by reduced to as low as 20 mmHg (2.6 kPa; normally 40 mmHg, 5.3 kPa), thus reducing the respiratory drive. Hyperventilation cannot, however, increase the amount of oxygen carried in arterial blood if all the haemoglobin is already fully saturated and has no further carrying capacity. Consider the effects of hyperventilation on the equation:

$$CO_2 + H_2O \leftrightarrow H_2CO_3 \leftrightarrow HCO_3^- + H^+ \qquad (1)$$

As carbon dioxide is 'blown off', the equation will be *pulled* from right to left reducing the concentration of HCO$_3^-$ and H$^+$ (i.e. the pH will increase—respiratory alkalosis).

Consider the effects of breath-holding or hypoventilation on the same equation: carbon dioxide will accumulate and *push* the equation from left to right thus *increasing* the concentration of HCO$_3^-$ and H$^+$ (i.e. the pH will decrease—respiratory acidosis). Therefore, in the ordinary daily moment-to-moment control of the blood gases oxygen and carbon dioxide, the regulated variable is, largely, carbon dioxide. If the arterial PaCO$_2$ is kept at around 40 mmHg (5.3 kPa) then the blood, ordinarily, will be close to fully saturated with oxygen.

If the respiratory system is compromised, for example, by brain injury, and respiration is reduced, the brain becomes relatively insensitive to the rising carbon dioxide levels and at a certain point the peripheral chemoreceptors, which alone monitor oxygen content of arterial blood, kick in and provide a significant drive to respiration. As noted above, this is an emergency mechanism that may lead to intermittent (Cheyne-Stokes) breathing patterns. The oxygen-sensitive peripheral chemoreceptors do not provide a significant amount of drive to the respiratory centres until the arterial blood is approaching the PaO$_2$ of venous blood (PaO$_2$ 40–50 mmHg, 5.3–6.6 kPa), by which time cyanosis may well be evident.

In chronic respiratory acidosis (lasting more than an hour or so), the kidney tubule cells progressively increase their expulsion of hydrogen ions into the urine and retain bicarbonate ions in

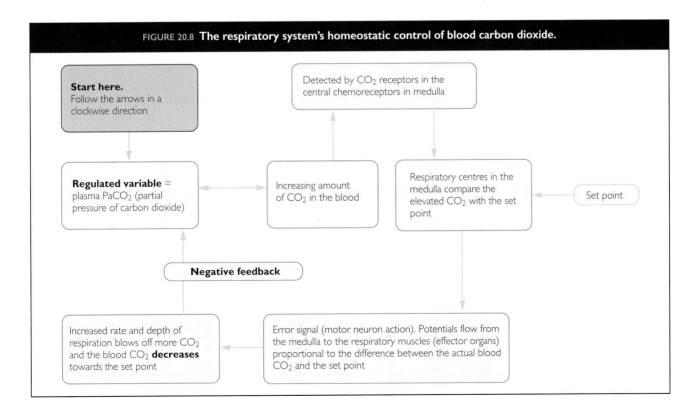

FIGURE 20.8 **The respiratory system's homeostatic control of blood carbon dioxide.**

the plasma in an attempt to maintain normal pH levels in the blood. A more comprehensive discussion of the measurement of acid–base balance and interpretation of arterial and venous blood gases is provided in Chapter 17 (pp. 329–32) and Chapter 21: Respiratory Emergencies.

Oxygen therapy

The provision of oxygen at a greater concentration than room air (i.e. above 21%) is a commonly performed procedure in emergency situations. Very high concentrations of oxygen are also toxic. Particularly in premature infants, breathing 100% oxygen can damage lung tissue due to the activity of oxygen-free radicals (atomic oxygen) that occur in the gas. The unpaired electrons of atomic oxygen damage structural and functional proteins in the lung. However, in the first 24 hours it is important to titrate oxygen delivery according to oxygen saturation measurements, but oxygen should not be withheld for fear of toxicity in adults.[6]

The most common delivery devices used in emergency environments are nasal cannulae, masks or masks with reservoir bags. The approximate percentage oxygen delivery for each device is presented in Table 20.2.[6]

Temperature control

In normal health, core body temperature is a regulated variable. The normal body temperature (recorded via a tympanic thermometer) is in the range of 35.4–37.8°C, and has a slight diurnal variation.[7] The detectors and control centre are temperature-sensitive receptors in the skin, and specialised neurons in the hypothalamus. In other species, and in human infants, metabolically active 'brown' adipose tissue plays a role in temperature homeostasis. In adults the principal effector organs are the blood vessels and sweat glands in the skin. In temperate climates, the skin serves as an adjustable radiator for heat loss and heat retention and, depending on the requirement to either eliminate or retain heat, blood is redistributed either to or from the peripheral skin circulation. A change in temperature below the 'set point' of the body's thermostat is detected by skin and hypothalamic receptors, and results in vasoconstriction of the skin arterioles, reducing the rate of heat loss. Conversely, if the body core starts to heat up vasodilation results, increasing skin blood flow and dissipating excess heat into the environment. In low-melanin persons this can be seen as a change in skin colour—pale in cold and pink in warm environments.

TABLE 20.2 Variable-performance oxygen delivery systems[6]

APPARATUS	OXYGEN FLOW (L/MIN)	OXYGEN CONCENTRATION (%)
Nasal catheters	1–4	24–40
Semi-rigid mask	6–15	35–60
Semi-rigid mask with double O_2 supply	15–30	Up to 80
Semi-rigid mask with reservoir bag	12–15	60–90

In response to more extreme changes in temperature, other mechanisms are used to warm or cool the body. As ambient temperature approaches body temperature, radiant heat loss becomes less effective and is augmented by sweating and evaporative cooling. The sweat glands are also under the control of the sympathetic nervous system. When water evaporates it has to draw heat from the skin to change it from a liquid to a gas. This can provide a cooling effect, even if the ambient temperature is above body temperature. However, the effectiveness is reduced in the presence of humid heat, and excessive sweating also reduces plasma volume, serum sodium and potassium and urinary output (see Ch 28, which discusses environmental emergencies). Individuals acclimatise to heat over several days to weeks, with an increase in sweat production and a reduction in sweat sodium losses.

When the body is exposed to extreme cold, the drop in core temperature detected in the hypothalamus results in shivering—involuntary contractions of skeletal muscles that produce some waste heat. At the same time the contraction of the arrector pili muscles at the base of each hair follicle (goose-bumps) is an ancient reflex harking back to our evolutionary heritage when humans were a lot hairier. The generalised erection of body hair improves the skin's insulating properties.

Fluid and electrolyte balance

The amount of fluid, water and the concentration of electrolytes are all under the control of homeostatic mechanisms. Ultimately the kidney is the main effector organ. Life processes depend on water and electrolytes being kept within strict limits.

Water

An increase in osmotic pressure (i.e. particle concentration in the blood) is caused, for example, by a loss of water when sweating is detected by osmoreceptors in the hypothalamus. Essentially the osmoreceptors are neurons that swell or shrink depending on the solute concentration of the perfusing fluid and change their electrical discharge rates as a result. The information is processed by the nearby control centre, also in the hypothalamus. The nerves that emerge from the control centre descend to the posterior pituitary and secrete the peptide antidiuretic hormone (ADH), also known as vasopressin. The ADH is secreted into the bloodstream and ultimately binds to V-2 receptors mainly on the collecting ducts deep in the medulla of the kidney. The ADH-receptor complex initiates the manufacture of the second messenger cyclic adenosine monophosphate (cAMP) in the cytoplasm of cells, which in turn brings about the incorporation of aquaporins—water pores—in the apical and basolateral membranes of the collecting duct tubules. This increases the permeability of the membranes, allowing water to be drawn back into the relatively hyperosmotic (dry) kidney medulla and subsequently back into systemic circulation. A concentrated urine is produced; it has up to four times the osmotic concentration of blood. The hypothalamus also governs the subjective feeling of thirst, leading to increased oral water intake.

Excess water has the opposite effect: in the presence of hypo-osmolar plasma ADH secretion is inhibited and excess water is allowed to pass through the collecting ducts producing a dilute urine (see Table 20.1).

The osmoreceptors in the hypothalamus are not the only receptors involved in the ADH reflex. Baroreceptors in the aortic arch and at the bifurcation of the carotid arteries detect pressure. If the pressure is lowered due to blood loss or dehydration, the reduced pressure also results in increased ADH release from the posterior pituitary and retention of water. This accounts for about 10–15% of the response.

Importantly, both ADH and the baroreceptor reflex cause vasoconstriction of both the resistance vessels (arterioles) and the capacitance vessels (venules). Sensibly, when faced with loss of blood volume the vasculature contracts, both keeping the pressure up on the arterial side and reducing the capacitance on the venous side. This accommodates the reduced circulating volume and preserves venous return of blood to the heart.

As noted earlier, the constriction of the arterioles generally reduces the capillary blood hydrostatic pressure, and so tissue fluid is drawn into the circulation in capillaries where the osmotic pressure of the blood exceeds the capillary hydrostatic pressure. This bolsters blood volume.

The antidiuretic effect of ADH and the baroreceptors is opposed to some extent by atrial natriuretic peptide (ANP). ANP is secreted by the atria of the heart in response to stretch, and therefore helps regulate intravascular volume. The secretion of ANP is inhibited when blood volumes are reduced and venous return to the heart reduced. When venous return increases, ANP secretion follows suit. ANP antagonises the effects of ADH by inhibiting its release, both from the posterior pituitary and at its site of action in the collecting duct of the kidney. ANP, as the term 'natriuretic' suggests (from the Latin word for sodium, 'natrium'), also antagonises the effects of aldosterone and reduces renin production (see next section) and promotes sodium, and hence water, loss from the kidney by reducing reabsorption in the distal convoluted tubule. Finally, it has vasodilatory properties and effects on fat metabolism.

In the face of congestive cardiac failure, the filling pressures of the heart increase abnormally, and myocardium can become hypertrophic in response. In addition to its beneficial modulation of blood volume in this situation, ANP is thought to have a protective effect on cardiac muscle by directly limiting this 'remodelling'.

Electrolytes

Sodium and potassium

The levels of sodium and potassium in the blood are ultimately controlled by action of the steroid hormone aldosterone, mainly on the distal convoluted tubules of the kidney. Essentially, aldosterone binds to nuclear receptors in the nuclei of tubular cells and promotes the transcription of genes for specific proteins that increase the number of sodium channels in the cell membranes and also increase the number of sodium-potassium-ATPase pumps in the basolateral membrane that pump sodium back in to the kidney capillaries and allow potassium to be lost in the urine. The relative abundance of aldosterone will determine how much sodium is being retained and potassium is lost, and vice versa.

There are two feedback loops that control the secretion of aldosterone from the adrenal cortex. First, the cells of the adrenal cortex itself sense reductions in plasma sodium levels

and secrete aldosterone as a response. Second, some sensitive tissue (the juxtaglomerular apparatus, JGA), lodged between the glomeruli and the distal convoluted tubules of the kidney, senses the loss of sodium and releases the enzyme renin as a result. Renin, when released into the plasma, converts angiotensinogen into angiotensin I; this is converted in turn by angiotensin-converting enzyme (ACE) into angiotensin II, which causes the release of aldosterone from the adrenal cortex. In addition, angiotensin II causes vasoconstriction of arterioles and venules.

Calcium

Ninety-nine per cent of the body's calcium is in the form of calcium phosphate in bone. Calcium in plasma exists in an ionised, or free, form and an electrically neutral form bound to albumin and other plasma proteins. Only the ionised form is biologically active, and is important for many cellular functions, including nerve transmission, blood coagulation and muscle contraction. A reduction in plasma albumin or acidosis tends to favour an increase in the ionised, active form. Conversely, alkalosis tends to decrease ionised calcium. A clinical example is respiratory alkalosis caused by hyperventilation. The profound reduction in ionised calcium causes paraesthesia and tetany of skeletal muscles, which is reversible once normal ventilation is restored.

The total concentration of calcium in plasma is controlled by two hormones—parathyroid hormone (PTH) and calcitonin—secreted, respectively, by the parathyroid gland and the interstitial cells of the thyroid gland. When plasma calcium starts to drop this is detected by the cells of the parathyroid gland and increased amounts of PTH are released. PTH has three actions:

1. It stimulates the synthesis of calcitriol, which increases the number of calcium pumps in the gut epithelium, thereby increasing the absorption of calcium from the gut.

2. It binds to PTH receptors in the kidney tubules and via a second messenger increases the number of calcium pumps in the tubules, thereby increasing the reabsorption of calcium from the kidney tubules back into the blood.

3. It recruits calcium from bone by stimulating the recruitment of osteoclasts.

As the plasma calcium concentration rises, the release of PTH is progressively inhibited and the release of calcitonin is progressively stimulated.

Calcitonin opposes the effects of PTH. There is some evidence that, paradoxically, pulsatile release of PTH and some PTH fragments have the effect of increasing calcium deposition in bone rather than decreasing it.[8]

Magnesium

The control of plasma magnesium concentration is primarily under the control of the tubular cells of the proximal convoluted tubules of the kidney and the loops of Henle. These tubes convey the glomerular filtrate through the kidney, and the cells of these tubes are sensitive to plasma and tubular levels of magnesium and reabsorb magnesium as required. This may vary from almost total reabsorption during time on a low-magnesium diet to low reabsorption on a high-magnesium diet.

Acid–base regulation

All biological enzyme systems are dependent on a very tight control of acid–base balance for optimal function. pH is a mathematical expression of the degree of acidosis or alkalosis in a solution:

$$pH = -\log_{10}[H]$$

Hence for each decrease in pH by 1, there is an increase in hydrogen ion concentration by a factor of 10. The physiological range of plasma pH is 7.35 to 7.45. Two interrelated systems, the respiratory system and the renal system, are responsible for maintaining this critical acid–base balance, by contributing hydrogen ions or bicarbonate ions to the various *buffers* present in body fluid. A buffer is a system of molecules that exists in equilibrium in a solution, and which, by gaining or losing a bicarbonate or a hydrogen ion in response to an alkali or acid load, tends to resist changes in pH. An important example was outlined above in the case of carbon dioxide and bicarbonate, catalysed by carbonic anhydrase. By increasing or decreasing ventilation, the respiratory system has the capacity to blow off or retain carbon dioxide and hence can control pH over a course of minutes to hours.

The kidney, by altering the acidity of urine, has an even more profound influence on body pH maintenance, albeit exerted over a longer time frame of hours to days. The renal tubule has several mechanisms to control H^+ excretion and HCO_3^- reabsorption, in response to pH, sodium and potassium concentration and hormonal influences. Essentially, carbon dioxide is distributed evenly through the kidney but inside tubular cells the enzyme carbonic anhydrase catalyses a chemical reaction between carbon dioxide and water. This results in the production of bicarbonate ions and hydrogen ions (as in Equation 1). The hydrogen ions are pumped by an ATP-powered proton pump into the tubular fluid where they are mostly buffered by phosphate and ammonium ions. The bicarbonate is retrieved back into the peritubular capillaries and then into the systemic circulation. The buffered and unbuffered hydrogen ions are voided in the urine.

Extended accounts of the mechanisms of gas carriage, temperature control and water and electrolyte homeostatic mechanisms can be found in the relevant chapters of the Guyton and Hall text.[3]

Shock

Shock refers to an insufficient circulatory state leading to inadequately perfused body tissues. The lack of oxygen and nutrients and the non-removal of waste products impair normal metabolism. The cells cannot generate enough ATP for their metabolic requirements and are consequently prone to cell death. When cells die, as outlined in the cell deterioration section earlier in the chapter, their membranes allow the cell contents to leak into the extracellular space and generate an even more toxic environment for the adjacent cells—resulting in even more cell death. This is yet another example of a positive (vicious-cycle) feedback mechanism (see Fig 20.9).

A review of the normal functioning of the cardiovascular system will demonstrate the major reasons for inadequate perfusion. In order to function adequately, the cardiovascular system requires the following components:

- an adequate blood volume with sufficient oxygen-saturated haemoglobin that is circulating through the arteries, arterioles, capillaries, venules and veins
- an adequate pump (i.e. the heart) to provide circulatory force
- sufficient vascular tone (i.e. degree of arteriolar constriction) to resist blood flow and maintain adequate arterial pressure, yet allow adequate tissue perfusion
- sufficient vascular tone in the venules to supply a capacitance that is related to the blood volume, and in the venous system to ensure blood return to the heart
- Finally, the major vessels must be free of any kind of functional obstruction, such as pulmonary emboli or pericardial tamponade.

Variations in any of these factors may give rise to inadequate perfusion of the tissues. The process of shock is an example of the positive (or vicious-circle) feedback system causing further physiological derangement if left uninterrupted (see Fig 20.9).

PRACTICE TIP

Timely interventions such as oxygen therapy early in the shock process can impede the positive feedback mechanism that leads to cellular death and organ failure. These interventions are generally directed by treatment protocols established to respond to vital signs.

Stages and causes of shock

Varying any of the critical elements in the cardiovascular system beyond homeostatic limits will give rise to inadequate tissue perfusion. These are summarised in Table 20.3. It can be helpful for the clinician to approach a patient in shock using the following classification, as defining the type of shock can yield clues to the specific diagnosis and suggest a course of treatment:

- *hypovolaemic*—resulting from a loss of intravascular volume
- *cardiogenic*—resulting from pump failure, due to a problem with myocardial contractility, heart rate or rhythm or valvular apparatus
- *obstructive*—resulting from any impedance to flow in the major vessels.
- *distributive*—resulting from a loss of vasomotor tone (i.e. resistance) in the arterioles and the venules. Distributive shock results from a drop of pressure due to the drop in arteriole resistance and a reduction in venous return due to the loss of tone in the post-capillary venules. Distributive shock may be further categorised as:
  - *septic shock:* caused by infection; either toxins from the pathogenic organism or an adverse effect of the host's immune response (an excess of the periphery's own antibacterial gas (nitric oxide, a potent vasodilator))

FIGURE 20.9 Different types of positive feedback that can lead to the progression of shock.[3]

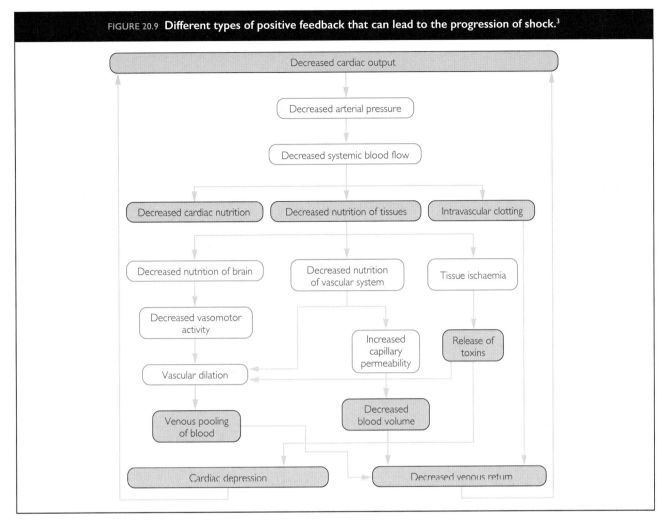

- *neurogenic shock:* where the descending sympathetic control of vascular tone is disrupted, e.g. in spinal cord injury, again relaxing the arterioles and venules
- *anaphylactic shock:* a hypersensitivity to a substance leading to an overproduction of vasodilator mediators resulting in a gross relaxation of blood vessels.

Compensatory responses

Neural control of blood pressure and flow
Although the cardiovascular system is primarily concerned with perfusing tissue, thereby providing an adequate supply of oxygen and nutrients and removing waste products, by and large the regulated variable in the cardiovascular system is systemic pressure (Table 20.1). Blood pressure is maintained by an adequate pump discharging into a vascular resistance that both maintains systemic pressure and allows enough blood through to the downstream tissues to keep those tissues alive. Equally, having perfused the tissues the blood must return through the venules and the veins back to the heart to ensure a continuity of flow.

The arterial pressure is monitored by baroreceptors in the aortic arch and the carotid bifurcation. This pressure information is continually fed, beat by beat, up the vagus and glossopharyngeal nerves to the control centres in the medulla oblongata. If the systemic pressure drops, two centres in the medulla oblongata respond through connections to the autonomic nervous system to increase the heart rate and stroke volume (i.e. increase the cardiac output) and mildly constrict the systemic arterioles and the venules below the heart to increase the pressure and direct flow towards the head. Unless affected by some form of autonomic dysfunction, this happens every time an individual stands up from a lying position. In addition to the sympathetic nervous system providing continuing tonic constriction of the vasculature, some tonic constriction is provided by circulating and local hormones.

Endocrine and paracrine control of blood pressure and flow
Adrenaline and noradrenaline from the adrenal medulla and sympathetic nerve terminals constrict the skin, gut ('splanchnic') and kidney circulation through alpha-receptors. The second messenger system involves the inositol triphosphate–calcium–calmodulin pathway. Adrenaline also binds to beta-receptors in muscle blood vessels and activates the cyclic-GMP (guanosine monophosphate) pathway that leads to smooth muscle relaxation and dilation of the muscle blood vessels. Additionally, adrenaline also binds to beta-receptors in the heart and increases both the force of contraction and the heart rate.

As noted above, hormones involved in fluid and electrolyte balance, ADH and angiotensin II, also provide some of the

TABLE 20.3 Classification and precipitating factors of shock[9]

LOW BLOOD FLOW	MALDISTRIBUTION OF BLOOD FLOW
Cardiogenic shock	**Neurogenic shock**
Systolic dysfunction: inability of the heart to pump blood forward (e.g. myocardial infarction, cardiomyopathy)	Haemodynamic consequence of injury and/or disease to the spinal cord at or above T5
Diastolic dysfunction: inability of the heart to fill during diastole (e.g. cardiac tamponade)	Spinal anaesthesia
Dysrhythmias (e.g. bradycardia, tachycardia)	Vasomotor centre depression (e.g. severe pain, drugs, hypoglycaemia, injury)
Structural factors: valvular abnormality (e.g. stenosis or regurgitation), papillary muscle dysfunction, acute ventricular septal defect	**Septic shock**
Hypovolaemic shock	Infection (e.g. urinary tract, respiratory tract, invasive procedure, indwelling lines and catheters)
Absolute hypovolaemia	At-risk patients: older adults, patients with chronic diseases (e.g. diabetes mellitus, chronic renal failure, congestive heart failure), patients receiving immunosuppressive therapy or who are malnourished or debilitated
Loss of whole blood (e.g. haemorrhage from trauma, surgery, GI bleeding)	Gram-negative bacteria most common; also Gram-positive bacteria, viruses, fungi and parasites
Loss of plasma (e.g. burn injuries)	**Anaphylactic shock**
Loss of other body fluids (e.g. vomiting, diarrhoea, excessive diuresis, diaphoresis, diabetes insipidus, diabetes mellitus)	Contrast media, blood/blood products, drugs, insect bites, anaesthetic agents, food/food additives, vaccines, environmental agents, latex
Relative hypovolaemia	
Pooling of blood or fluids (e.g. ascites, peritonitis, bowel obstruction)	
Internal bleeding (e.g. fracture of long bones, ruptured spleen, haemothorax, severe pancreatitis)	
Massive vasodilation (e.g. sepsis)	

GI: gastrointestinal

background vasoconstriction. Angiotensin II binds to AT_1 receptors and, again, via the inositol triphosphate–calcium–calmodulin pathway cause the constriction of vascular smooth muscle. This latter effect provides the rationale for using ACE inhibitors and angiotensin II receptor antagonists as drugs to lower blood pressure.

Also contributing at the tissue level are local pressure and flow mediators, notably nitric oxide (a vasodilator) and endothelin (a vasoconstrictor). A number of other local mediators produced by damaged or inflamed tissue affect local vascular tone and the permeability of the capillaries in those vascular beds. Vascular compensation for various types of shock depends on the origin of the problem.

Systemic response to a drop in blood pressure

The body's responses to a drop in arterial pressure are summarised in Figure 20.10.[8] The drop in pressure is detected by the baroreceptors which cause a reflex increase in heart rate and stroke volume and a generalised vasoconstriction if this is possible. This assists with venous return to the heart and should assist with cardiac output. The sympathetic nervous system also restricts renal blood flow and triggers the release of renin which leads to the production of angiotensin II, causing further vasoconstriction and the release of aldosterone. Aldosterone increases renal sodium reabsorption, which in turn causes

more water to be reabsorbed in the kidney tubules. If the drop in pressure is not too severe, these homeostatic mechanisms will maintain blood pressure and reasonably adequate tissue perfusion.

Hypovolaemic shock

Hypovolaemic shock is the loss of circulating volume (see Fig 20.11).[8] The resulting drop in pressure generally results in a baroreceptor reflex which initiates a massive vasoconstriction that holds up the systemic pressure but may drastically restrict the perfusion of most organs. In extreme shock blood flow to the peripheries and the splanchnic circulation is sacrificed and diverted to 'vital organs' (brain, heart and lungs). Arteriolar constriction results in a drop in capillary hydrostatic pressure. Unopposed oncotic pressure from plasma proteins in the capillary blood draw tissue fluid out of the interstitial space, bolstering the plasma volume by up to 30% over the ensuing 24 hours. The massive constriction on the venous side ensures that no blood pools in the capacitance vessels. Often the systemic pressure remains within normal limits, even though tissue perfusion, particularly of the skin, gut and kidney, may be reduced.

A clue to the presence of vasoconstriction is the rise in diastolic pressure and hence a reduction in pulse pressure. Peripheral pulses may be reduced in amplitude or entirely absent.

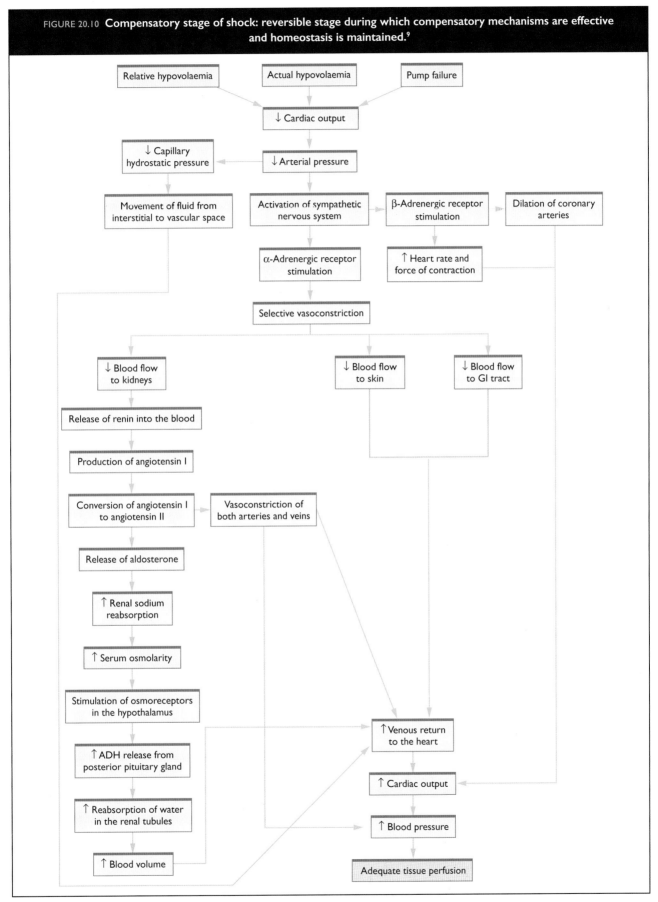

FIGURE 20.10 Compensatory stage of shock: reversible stage during which compensatory mechanisms are effective and homeostasis is maintained.[9]

ADH: antidiuretic hormone; GI: gastrointestinal.

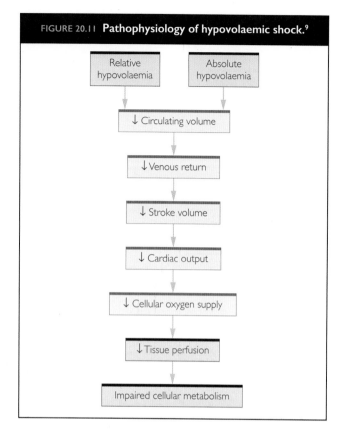

FIGURE 20.11 **Pathophysiology of hypovolaemic shock.**[9]

TABLE 20.4 Signs for each class/stage of hypovolaemic shock

	HEART RATE	BLOOD PRESSURE	PERIPHERY
Class II	↑	unchanged	Cool, pale
Class III	↑	↓	Cool, pale
Class IV	↓	↓	Cool, cyanosed

Traditionally, hypovolaemic shock has been classified into four stages according to typical signs expected with increasing degrees of volume loss. Much variation exists between individuals, however, and this classification is often misleading (Table 20.4).

Clinical manifestations are produced according to the degree to which tissue perfusion is compromised and the response of the body's compensatory mechanisms. Physiological responses can be related to the level of fluid loss.[10] Tachypnoea is often present, particularly after haemorrhage; this is a respiratory compensation associated with the reduction of circulating haemoglobin, and may also reflect a 'thoracic pump' mechanism to augment venous return. Acute haemorrhage represents one end of a spectrum of hypovolaemia, where fluid is lost from the intravascular space. Circumstances such as diabetic ketoacidosis, diarrhoea or heat stress may also lead to a reduction in interstitial, intracellular and intravascular volume. This is identified by clinical manifestations of shock plus evidence of dehydration such as dry tongue, reduced skin turgor and excessive thirst.

General fluid resuscitation is discussed in Chapter 15. Trauma-induced coagulopathy, the triad of death and principles of management of traumatic hypovolaemic shock are discussed in Chapter 44 and burns in Chapter 52.

Trauma induced coagulopathy and the triad of death
Shock by definition involves the under-perfusion of tissues and thus there is a reduced supply of oxygen. This severely limits cellular oxidative processes. This has three effects:

1. ATP can only be produced by anaerobic glycolysis, resulting in lactic acidosis.

2. The heat produced as a by-product of the use of ATP is dramatically reduced.

3. Tissue damage and associated inflammatory response.

This accounts for the frequently-observed acidosis and hypothermia. The microcirculation plays a crucial contributory role. Haemorrhage and resuscitation induce cellular changes that are characteristic of ischaemia–reperfusion injury—for example, production of reactive oxygen species, activation of inflammation and apoptotic cell death. In severe shock, a large range of inflammatory mediators, cytokines and oxidants are almost instantaneously produced and released in large quantities (Fig 20.12).[11]

Coagulopathy, known as trauma induced coagulopathy, usually accompanies severe haemorrhage in trauma patients and commences within minutes of injury.[12] It is characterised by systemic anticoagulation and fibrinolysis.[13] As many as 25% of severely injured trauma patients have an established coagulopathy when they arrive in the emergency department.[14] It is driven by severe shock in the presence of some degree of physical tissue trauma,[15] and the protein C feedback system has a central role.[16] Within a normal coagulation cascade, protein C is intended to deactivate clotting factors once they have performed their 'duty' of clotting and ceasing bleeding. However in the major trauma patient, it appears that protein C is present in elevated levels, and continues to deactivate clotting factors, even though clots haven't formed or more clotting is required. Early control of bleeding and haemostatic resuscitation, incorporating correction of coagulopathy and minimal volume replacement, are likely to improve outcomes at least in part by facilitating recovery in the microcirculation (discussed further in Ch 44).

Hypothermia is known to be an indicator and result of severe injury (rather than an independent predictor of mortality), which has its own impacts on coagulopathy and the shock process by impacting on both platelet function and the oxyhaemoglobin dissociation curve. Hypothermia causes sequestration and inhibited release of platelets, thereby diminishing clotting capacity,[17] while shifting the oxyhaemoglobin curve to the left and impairing oxygen availability to cells.[18] Along with hypoperfusion and coagulopathy, hypothermia feeds back into the vicious circle: the 'triad of death' (also see Ch 28).

There is some evidence of benefit where therapeutic hypothermia is used for the management of isolated traumatic brain injury and this is covered in Chapter 45.[19]

FIGURE 20.12 **Microcirculatory changes in haemorrhagic shock and resuscitation.**[11]

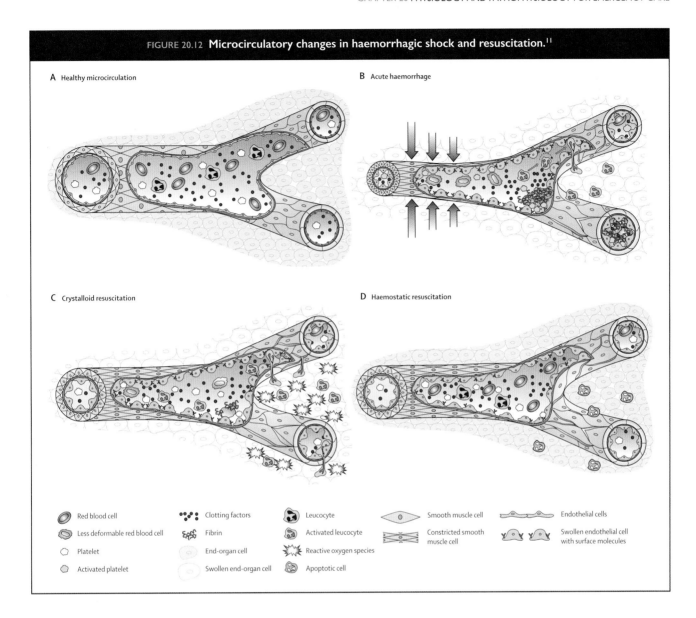

A Healthy microcirculation

B Acute haemorrhage

C Crystalloid resuscitation

D Haemostatic resuscitation

Red blood cell	Clotting factors	Leucocyte	Smooth muscle cell	Endothelial cells
Less deformable red blood cell	Fibrin	Activated leucocyte	Constricted smooth muscle cell	Swollen endothelial cell with surface molecules
Platelet	End-organ cell	Reactive oxygen species		
Activated platelet	Swollen end-organ cell	Apoptotic cell		

Distributive shock

Distributive shock is due to a loss of vascular tone in the systemic arterioles and venules. The three types of distributive shock—septic, anaphylactic and neurogenic—are all associated with hypotension but differentiated by the cause. With septic and anaphylactic shock, the drop in pressure detected by the baroreceptors is compensated for initially by an increase in force and rate of the heart, but no increase in peripheral resistance as the vasomotor centre and the sympathetic supply to blood vessels and the autonomic nervous system are overridden by peripheral mediators (Fig 20.13). In contrast to hypovolaemic shock, anaphylactic and septic shock are often characterised by a bounding pulse and warm, pink skin.

Sepsis and septic shock

Sepsis is a systemic response to a severe, usually bacterial, infection, characterised by varying degrees of cardiovascular and other organ system dysfunction. The source of the infection may be anywhere in the body, but tends to occur with organisms that produce endotoxins or that incite a dis-

proportionate and destructive immune response. The various inflammatory mediators, including nitric oxide, interleukins, cytokines and prostaglandin, are responsible for many of the features of the 'systemic inflammatory response syndrome', such as tachycardia, fever and leukocytosis, which are the hallmarks of sepsis. The hypotension is the result of a relaxation of the arterioles and venules due partly to bacterial endotoxins and partly to the nitric oxide gas released by macrophages in an attempt to kill off the pathogens. Nitric oxide is a potent vasodilator.

Septic shock is identified by the presence of hypotension with evidence of infection. The evidence of infection can be fever and an elevated white blood cell count and an identifiable source of infection, such as a wound or chest infection. The high metabolic demands of sepsis result in a high cardiac output, and often the key clinical manifestation is a bounding pulse in the presence of hypotension. Later, circulating cardiac depressants may add to the worsening haemodynamic state.[20]

Treatment of septic shock requires a combination of fluid resuscitation to fill the expanded vascular space, vasopressor

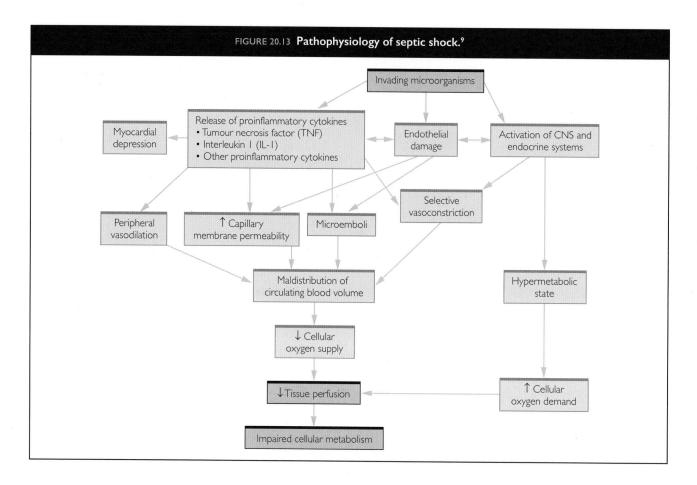

FIGURE 20.13 **Pathophysiology of septic shock.**[9]

drugs (such as noradrenaline) to constrict the vasculature and identification and eradication of the infective process. Management of sepsis is discussed in Chapter 27.

Most common causes of sepsis:

1. pneumonia (*n* = 138/324, 42.6%)
2. urinary tract infection (*n* = 98/324, 30.2%)

Common interventions within 6 hours of presentation to ED:

3. intra-arterial catheter (*n* = 144/324, 44.4%)
4. central venous catheter (*n* = 120/324, 37.0%)
5. vasopressor infusion (*n* = 104/324, 32.1%)
6. mechanical ventilation (*n* = 60/324, 18.5%)

Admission to ICU rate: 52.4% (*n* = 170/324)

7. In-hospital mortality rate: 23.1% (*n* = 75/324)

Anaphylactic shock

Anaphylaxis results from an exaggerated antibody–antigen reaction after exposure to an antigen to which the patient is allergic. Prior exposure to the antigen is a prerequisite, and 'primes' mast cells with antibodies. Subsequent exposure to the same antigen causes degranulation of mast cells and a massive release of histamine and other vasodilatory substances. Vascular smooth muscle relaxes, resulting in a drop in the total peripheral resistance and a consequent drop in blood pressure. The smooth muscle on the venous side of the circulation also relaxes, causing blood to pool and reducing venous return to the heart with a consequent reduction in cardiac output. The antigen–antibody reaction also causes bronchoconstriction in the lungs, and increased vascular permeability in the laryngeal mucosa, resulting in oedema. Death can be rapid, particularly when a compromised circulation is combined with the dual threats of upper airway obstruction and bronchospasm. At times, the diagnosis of anaphylaxis may be obvious, for example urticaria, wheeze and collapse following a bee sting in a patient with a known hypersensitivity. At other times the manifestations may be subtle or confounded by other causes of hypotension; for example, a severely injured trauma patient who becomes difficult to ventilate and then arrests following induction of general anaesthetic.

Neurogenic shock

Neurogenic shock is produced by a lesion of the spinal cord that disrupts the sympathetic nervous system. Spinal shock is a separate phenomenon describing a complete but usually transient disruption of all spinal cord activity below the level of an acute injury.

Parasympathetic nerves are largely unaffected as these are located in cranial nerves. A complete collapse of the sympathetic nervous system allows all the peripheral vessels to relax, dramatically increasing vascular capacity.[3] If the spinal cord lesion is above the lower cervical segments then the sympathetic supply to the heart is also disrupted, leading to a paradoxical bradycardia in the face of hypotension. Common examples of lesions or interventions that may block impulses from spinal nerves include spinal trauma, spinal anaesthetic and epidural infusion.

Treatment of neurogenic shock comprises support of blood pressure and/or heart rate. If fluid resuscitation alone is ineffective, vasopressor and chronotropic drugs may be required. If possible, the underlying cause needs to be addressed, for example shock due to spinal or epidural interventions requires reduction or removal of the anaesthetic or infusion. Neurogenic shock as a result of trauma is discussed in Chapter 49.

Cardiogenic shock

Cardiogenic shock is the reduction of cardiac output and a consequent reduction in blood pressure. This precipitates a baroreceptor response to increase the heart rate and stroke volume and initiate a fight or flight response that, through peripheral vasoconstriction, limits flow to the skin, gut and kidneys favouring flow to the brain, heart and lungs. The reduction in kidney blood flow precipitates water retention by way of ADH and the renin–angiotensin–aldosterone system, further increasing the load on the heart. This is another example of a damaged feedback loop making matters worse rather than returning the system to its set point. It explains the use of diuretics in heart failure.

The clinical manifestations of cardiogenic shock relate to the inadequate cardiac output and evidence of cardiac damage or failure. Hypotension, significant peripheral shutdown, tachycardia, oliguria and extreme lethargy reflect the low cardiac output. The classic presentation of the patient with cardiogenic shock is a person with chest pain or cardiac failure who develops hypotension. The treatments of cardiogenic shock are provided in greater detail in Chapter 22. In principle, the treatment involves minimising cardiac damage due to acute myocardial infarction, maximising oxygen delivery and minimising oxygen consumption. Cardiogenic shock is associated with a high mortality rate. Irreversible cardiogenic shock is reached when other organs fail due to inadequate perfusion.

Obstructive shock

Obstructive shock occurs when, despite a relatively healthy cardiovascular system and operating baroreceptor reflexes, tissue perfusion is compromised by an obstruction in a major vessel; for example, an embolus in a major artery, lung or major vein. The reduction in flow again initiates baroreceptor reflexes that restrict blood flow to non-essential organs.

Clinical manifestations of obstructive shock vary according to the site of the obstruction. There may be signs of reduced blood flow and hypoxaemia, such as a cold periphery and cyanosis, combined with typical signs of shock, including tachycardia, hypotension and oliguria. Identification and management of the cause, such as a pulmonary embolus, tension pneumothorax, cardiac tamponade or aortic aneurysm, are covered in detail in Chapters 21 and 47.

Unique population groups

Paediatric, elderly and pregnant patients may respond differently to hypovolaemia and other causes of shock. Normal physiological responses and indicators of shock may be compromised; these are summarised in Table 20.5.[22]

Complications of shock

The positive (or vicious-circle) feedback processes associated with shock result in worsening tissue perfusion and oxygen deficit. When the mean systemic pressure drops below 50 mmHg (6.6 kPa), the baroreceptors fail and the cardiovascular system is essentially out of control because a vital part of the feedback loop is missing. If tissues continue to be grossly under-perfused, multiple-organ failure will result followed by death. Typical complications include adult respiratory distress syndrome (ARDS), DIC and acute kidney injury. These are reviewed in Chapters 21, 25 and 29. Figure 20.14 shows the progression of shock, systemic inflammatory response and multiple-organ dysfunction syndrome. Minimisation of the severity and duration of the dysfunctional

---

TABLE 20.5 Shock in the paediatric, elderly or pregnant patient[25]

PATIENT	DESCRIPTION
Paediatric	Increases cardiac output by increasing heart rate; fixed stroke volume; sustains arterial pressure despite significant volume loss; loses 25% of circulating volume before signs of shock occur; hypotension and lethargy are ominous signs. Early clinical manifestations are tachycardia, tachypnoea, pallor, cool mottled skin and delayed capillary refill; volume replaced with 20 mL/kg bolus of crystalloid
Elderly	Shock progression often rapid; normal physiological changes of ageing reduce compensatory mechanisms; predisposed to hypothermia; pre-existing disease states contribute co-morbidities
Pregnant	Hypervolaemia of pregnancy means patient can remain normotensive with up to a 1500 mL blood loss; compression of inferior vena cava by gravid uterus reduces circulating volume by 30%; place patient on left side, manually displace uterus to the left or elevate right hip with towel; risk for aspiration resulting from decreased gastric motility and decreased gastric emptying; treat suspected hypovolaemia to prevent placental vasoconstriction associated with catecholamine release; potential for fetal distress exists despite maternal stability

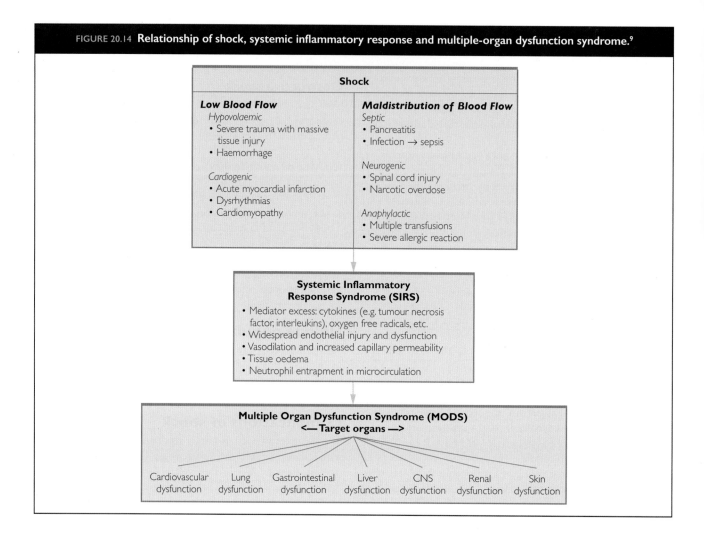

FIGURE 20.14 **Relationship of shock, systemic inflammatory response and multiple-organ dysfunction syndrome.**[9]

microcirculatory response in the first minutes and hours after injury might prevent complications.[11] Early control of bleeding and haemostatic resuscitation, incorporating correction of coagulopathy and minimal volume replacement, are likely to improve outcomes at least in part by facilitating recovery in the microcirculation.[23]

SUMMARY

Physiology is the study of feedback loops, while pathology is the study of failing feedback loops. As a consequence, an understanding of pathology requires an appreciation of the underlying physiology. Failure of any links in the physiological chain will affect the whole mechanism. The feedback loops explored in this chapter include gas carriage, temperature control, fluid and electrolyte balance, and the control of tissue perfusion.

Health is adversely affected when negative feedback mechanisms that usually keep the regulated variables close to the set point actually do the reverse—shifting the regulated variables away from the set point and initiating mechanisms that move the regulated variables even further away from the set point; so-called positive feedback. Ideally, clinical interventions are aimed at restoring the damaged physiological link(s) so that the regulated variables return to their set points.

CASE STUDY

Dale is a 24-year-old man who has crashed his car head-on into a power pole. He was the only occupant. The accident occurred in a 60 km/h zone, but witnesses report that the car was speeding. The car is quite old and has no airbags; the front of the car is caved in against the pole but the windscreen is intact. When the paramedics arrive, Dale is sitting on the footpath beside the vehicle. He is noted to be conscious and alert, and there is no obvious external trauma or bleeding. He is complaining of pain in his lower abdomen and is pale and sweaty; his skin is cool to touch. Dale's vital signs are: heart rate 126 beats/minute, blood pressure 85/50 mmHg, respiratory rate 28 breaths/minute, oxygen saturation 96% and Glasgow Coma Scale score 15.

Spinal Motion Restriction practices are applied, oxygen applied via a mask at 8 L/minute, intravenous access obtained and intravenous analgesia administered. Dale is prepared for transfer to the local hospital and intravenous fluids are commenced en route. The paramedics transfer Dale to the nearest trauma centre where his vital signs are: heart rate 128 beats/minute, blood pressure 90/60 mmHg, respiratory rate 26 breaths/minute, oxygen saturation 99% and Glasgow Coma Scale score 15. He is receiving oxygen via mask at 8 L/minute, and continues to complain of lower abdominal pain. The following blood tests are ordered: full blood count, urea and electrolytes, blood glucose and blood cross-matching. A trauma radiology series is also requested, including plain chest, cervical spine and pelvis X-rays. Prior to X-rays being taken an abdominal ultrasound is performed and a significant amount of intraperitoneal blood is detected.

Questions

1. Explain the physiological basis for the vital-sign findings—the patient has no significant medical history and is not taking any medications that may cause vital sign changes.

2. What determines the affinity between oxygen and haemoglobin, and how does hypothermia impact this affinity?

3. In the presence of hypotension, what changes will occur to heart rate and peripheral perfusion in the following types of shock?
   a. hypovolaemic
   b. septic
   c. neurogenic
   d. anaphylactic
   e. cardiogenic.

4. What mechanism initiates a systemic response to a reduction in blood pressure? Briefly outline the main stages of the body's response to a reduction in blood pressure and describe potential masking agents.

 Answers to Case Study Questions can be found on evolve
http://evolve.emergencytrauma.curtis

ACKNOWLEDGEMENTS

We wish to extend our thanks to the following for their appraisal of this chapter: Susan Furness RN MICA NAPA ACAP, Paramedic Lecturer, FHS La Trobe University, Bendigo; Associate Professor Simon Cooper PhD RN, School of Nursing and Midwifery, Monash University, Australia.

REFERENCES

1. Selye H. The stress of life. New York: McGraw-Hill; 1956.

2. Porth CM, Curtis RL. Cell and tissue characteristics. In: Porth CM, ed. Pathophysiology concepts and altered states. 4th edn. Philadelphia: JB Lippincott; 1994:16.

3. Guyton AC, Hall JE. Textbook of medical physiology. 12th edn. Philadelphia: Elsevier; 2011.

4. Urden L, Stacy K, Lough M. Thelan's Critical care nursing: diagnosis and management. 6th edn. St Louis: Mosby; 2009.

5. Frakes M. Measuring end-tidal carbon dioxide: clinical applications and usefulness. Crit Care Nurse 2001;21(5):23.

6. Cameron P, Jelinek G, Kelly A-M et al. Textbook of adult emergency medicine. 4th edn. Sydney: Elsevier; 2014.

7. Sund-Levander M, Forsberg C, Wahren LK. Normal rectal, tympanic and axillary body temperature in adult men and women: a systematic literature review. Scand J Caring Sci 2002;16(2):122–8.

8. Rang HP, Dale MM, Ritter JM et al. Rang and Dale's pharmacology. 6th edn. Edinburgh: Churchill Livingstone; 2007.

9. Lewis SM, Collier IC, Heitkemper MM. Medical–surgical nursing: assessment and management of clinical problems. 9th edn. St Louis: Mosby; 2013.

10. Porth CM, Matfin G. Pathophysiology: concepts of altered health states. 8th edn. Philadelphia: Lippincott Williams & Wilkins; 2009. p. 627.

11. Gruen RL, Brohi K, Schreiber M et al. Haemorrhage control in severely injured patients. The Lancet 2012;380(9847):1099–108.

12. Floccard B, Rugeri L, Faure A et al. Early coagulopathy in trauma patients: an on-scene and hospital admission study. Injury 2012;43:26–32.

13. Brohi K, Cohen MJ, Ganter MT et al. Acute coagulopathy of trauma: hypoperfusion induces systemic anticoagulation and hyperfibrinolysis. J Trauma Injury Infect Crit Care 2008;64:1211–17.

14. Brohi K, Singh J, Heron M, Coats T. Acute traumatic coagulopathy. J Trauma Injury Infect Crit Care 2003;54:1127–30.

15. Frith D, Goslings JC, Gaarder C et al. Definition and drivers of acute traumatic coagulopathy: clinical and experimental investigations. J Thromb Haemost 2010;8:1919–25.

16. Brohi K, Cohen MJ, Ganter MT et al. Acute traumatic coagulopathy: initiated by hypoperfusion: modulated through the protein C pathway? Ann Surg 2007;245:812–18.

17. Boffard KD, ed. Manual of definitive surgical trauma care. 3rd edn. CRC Press: USA; 2011.

18. Bacher A. Effects of body temperature on blood gases. In: M Pinsky, L Brochard, G Hedenstierna, M Antonelli, eds. Applied physiology in intensive care medicine 1. 2013. Springer-Verlag: Heidelberg.

19. Rhodes J. Therapeutic hypothermia in traumatic brain injury. Critical Care 2012;16(suppl 2):A11.

20. Jozwiak M, Persichini R, Monnet X, Tebou J-L. Management of myocardial dysfunction in severe sepsis. Seminars in Respiratory Critical Care 2011;32(2):206–14.

21. Peake SL, Bailey M, Bellomo R et al. Australasian resuscitation of sepsis evaluation (ARISE): a multi-centre, prospective, inception cohort study. Resuscitation 2009;80:811–18.

22. Holleran R. Shock emergencies. In: Howard P, Steinmann R, eds. Sheehy's emergency nursing. 6th edn. St Louis: Mosby; 2009.

23. Duchesne JC, McSwain NE, Cotton BA et al. Damage control resuscitation: the new face of damage control. J Trauma 2010;69:976–90.

24. Boundless.com Gas Exchange across the Alveoli. Boundless Biology. 3 Jul. 2014. www.boundless.com/biology/textbooks/boundless-biology-textbook/the-respiratory-system-39/gas-exchange-across-respiratory-surfaces-220/gas-exchange-across-the-alveoli-836-12081/; accessed 3 April 2015.

25. Newberry L, ed. Sheehy's emergency nursing. 5th edn. St Louis: Mosby; 2003:514.

CHAPTER 21
RESPIRATORY EMERGENCIES
STEPHEN ASHA, JEFF KENNEALLY AND ALISTER HODGE

Essentials

- Respiratory compromise is a common reason for seeking assistance from healthcare providers, with common clinical presentations including chronic obstructive pulmonary disease, asthma, pneumonia, pulmonary oedema and pulmonary emboli.

- A comprehensive respiratory assessment should include a patient history and physical assessment incorporating inspection, percussion, palpation and auscultation.

- Pre-hospital decisions must be based on comparatively little information with an emphasis on identifying key assessment findings that prompt initial management options.

- Physical assessment can be further informed by appropriate use of investigations such as pulse oximetry, capnography, arterial or venous blood gases, radiography, peak flows and spirometry.

- The level of respiratory support required will vary. Non-invasive ventilation or invasive mechanical ventilation may be required to support gas exchange in some patients.

- Accurate respiratory assessment should inform investigations and plan of care, as well as resource and environment allocation to maintain patient safety.

INTRODUCTION

Respiratory complaints account for a significant proportion of emergency presentations. Symptoms experienced by the patient may range from mild to immediately life-threatening. It is essential that the emergency care provider has the ability to identify early signs of respiratory compromise or the patient at immediate risk. Subsequent to assessment, the clinician must be able to implement appropriate interventions to maintain patient safety, provide adequate respiratory support and prevent further deterioration. This chapter will discuss the physiological changes that occur in respiratory failure and will present a methodical approach for assessing respiratory function, explore respiratory support strategies and detail five common adult respiratory emergencies.

Respiratory failure

As many as one in ten Australians have some form of lung disease. This translates to as many as 14% of all deaths in Australia being from lung disease. This definition includes chronic obstructive pulmonary disease (COPD), asthma, bronchiectasis, lung cancer, influenza and pneumonia.[1] Respiratory compromise is a common clinical presentation seen by healthcare providers; the causes are extensive (Table 21.1).[2] Common presentations, including asthma, COPD, pneumonia, pulmonary oedema and pulmonary emboli, will be specifically covered in this chapter, although it is acknowledged there are many other clinical presentations which healthcare providers may encounter in their practice.

Regardless of the cause of respiratory failure, it is important to understand how physiological changes associated with respiratory failure contribute to alterations in gas exchange and increased work of breathing. Respiratory failure occurs when either function of gas exchange—the exchange of oxygen and of carbon dioxide between the lungs and the atmosphere—fails. Respiratory failure is said to occur when the partial pressure of arterial oxygen (PaO_2) falls below 60 mmHg (hypoxaemia) or the partial pressure of arterial carbon dioxide ($PaCO_2$) rises above 50 mmHg (hypercapnia).[3] This definition may be accurate yet not sufficient for pre-hospital responders where access to the tools required may be incomplete or entirely absent. The differentiation between respiratory distress and failure may have to rely more generally on physical signs that the patient has been overwhelmed by hypoxaemia or hypercapnia. Arguably a critical finding will be a failure of respiration to maintain sufficient gas levels to allow for maintenance of normal consciousness.

Respiratory failure may be acute or chronic in nature, and can occur in patients with a normal respiratory system as well as in those with existing chronic pulmonary disease. Acute respiratory failure is characterised by life-threatening derangements in PaO_2, $PaCO_2$ and acid–base balance. Those with chronic respiratory failure may have alterations in their arterial blood gas values but these are usually not life-threatening. Chronic patients may have very different 'normal for them' vital signs and presentations that will have to be appreciated when establishing any baseline with which to make comparisons.

Respiratory failure is an important complication that may be associated with both respiratory and non-respiratory causes. Patients with pre-existing lung disease and those who smoke are at particular risk. A number of clinical conditions may also increase the chance of patients developing respiratory failure, including cardiac failure, renal failure and hepatic disease.[4] The mortality rate associated with respiratory failure is somewhat dependent on the underlying cause. Although the mortality rates for most causes of respiratory failure are poorly described, it is estimated that the mortality rate for patients with COPD is approximately 4.4% of Australians aged 55 and over, while that for asthma is 0.3% of all deaths.[5] Despite being difficult to determine, estimates suggest COPD is a leading cause of death in Australia after heart disease, stroke and cancer.[7] It is a major burden on pre-hospital and emergency medical providers. In contrast 378 asthma deaths in Australia were reported in 2011.[8] This is internationally high though numerically small, yet it is still estimated that up to 10% of the Australian population have current asthma making it also a burden for emergency responders.[7]

Mechanisms of gas exchange

For gas exchange to occur effectively there must be good matching between alveolar ventilation and pulmonary capillary blood flow. During normal respiration the lungs are in balance and every litre of alveolar ventilation is matched (approximately) by a litre of pulmonary capillary blood flow. Changes in this balance are expressed as a ratio, called the ventilation–perfusion ratio (V/Q). A high V/Q is indicative of greater than normal ventilation and lower than normal perfusion, or both. A low V/Q is indicative of lower than normal ventilation and greater than normal perfusion, or both (Fig 21.1).[4] Alterations in V/Q matching can contribute to both hypercapnia and hypoxaemia.

Hypercapnia, the increase in $PaCO_2$, occurs because of a decrease in tidal volume and/or respiratory rate (minute

TABLE 21.1 Causes of respiratory compromise[4]	
CATEGORY	DISEASE
Chest wall disorders	Chest wall restriction such as severe kyphosis or scoliosis
	Flail chest
Pleural abnormalities	Pneumothorax
	Haemothorax
	Pleural effusion
	Empyema
Restrictive lung disorders	Aspiration
	Atelectasis
	Bronchiectasis
	Bronchiolitis
	Pulmonary fibrosis
	Pulmonary oedema
	Acute respiratory distress syndrome
Obstructive pulmonary disease	Asthma
	Chronic obstructive pulmonary disease
Respiratory tract infections	Pneumonia
	Tuberculosis
	Abscess formation and cavitation
	Acute bronchitis
Pulmonary vascular disease	Pulmonary embolism
	Pulmonary artery hypertension

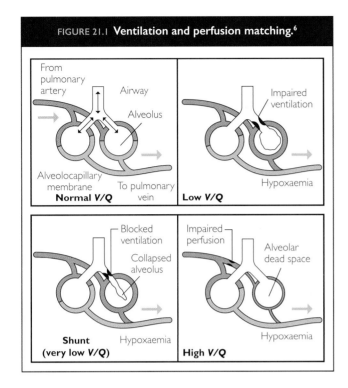

FIGURE 21.1 Ventilation and perfusion matching.[6]

TABLE 21.2 Causes of hypoxia[4]

MECHANISM	COMMON CLINICAL CAUSES
Decrease in FiO_2	High altitude
	Low oxygen concentration of gas mixture
	Suffocation
Hypoventilation of the alveoli	Lack of neurological stimulation of the respiratory centre
	Defects in chest wall mechanics
	Large airway obstruction
	Fatigue/exhaustions in conditions causing prolonged increased work of breathing
Ventilation–perfusion mismatch	Asthma
	Chronic obstructive pulmonary disease
	Pneumonia
	Atelectasis
	Pulmonary embolism
	Acute respiratory distress syndrome
Alveolocapillary diffusion abnormality	Oedema
	Fibrosis
	Emphysema
Reduced oxygen carrying capacity of blood	Anaemia
	Methaemoglobinaemia
	Carbon monoxide poisoning
Inability of cells to utilise oxygen	Carbon monoxide and cyanide poisoning
Decreased pulmonary capillary perfusion (shunting of de-oxygenated venous blood to the systemic arterial circulation)	Intracardiac defects (e.g. atrial and ventricular septal defects)
	Intrapulmonary arteriovenous malformations

ventilation), which decreases alveolar ventilation and CO_2 removal and can contribute to alterations in acid–base balance.[9] Hypercapnia can be determined through arterial blood gas analysis or capnography, but is difficult to determine through physical assessment because the rate and depth of breathing may appear normal in many patients. For pre-hospital responders where blood gas analysis is not available and capnography typically restricted to intensive care paramedics, physical assessment tools and guides are critical to follow.

Hypoxaemia occurs when oxygenation in the arterial blood is decreased. Hypoxia (reduced cellular oxygenation) may occur without alterations in pulmonary function and may be attributed to systemic abnormalities such as cardiac failure. Mechanisms that contribute to hypoxaemia include decreased alveolar oxygenation; decreased diffusion of oxygen from the alveoli into the pulmonary capillary; and decreased pulmonary capillary perfusion.[9] Clinical causes associated with these mechanisms are detailed in Table 21.2.[4]

Respiratory assessment

Primary survey

As with any emergency presentation, patient assessment of a respiratory complaint begins with a primary survey of airway, breathing, circulation, disability, exposure and a set of vital signs. The purpose of the primary survey is to identify life-threatening conditions and manage them immediately.[10] A comprehensive description of a primary survey is detailed in Chapters 14 and 44. Gross signs of respiratory compromise that may be identified during the primary survey and require immediate intervention include evidence of airway obstruction evidenced by audible inspiratory noise called stridor; increased respiratory effort and marked accessory muscle use; tachypnoea; decreased speech tolerance; pallor or cyanosis; hypoxia despite oxygen therapy; paradoxical chest wall movement; decreased

air entry; and altered level of consciousness.[11] With very limited access to past history and without more complex assessment tools these findings will be critical for paramedics in respiratory assessment.

At the completion of the primary survey and before proceeding further, clinicians must first reflect on their assessment findings and consider the following questions:

• Are immediate interventions required?

• Does the patient's condition warrant escalation, re-triage to higher category or transfer to an area of higher acuity within the department?

- Will pre-hospital responders require other resources, including people and devices to help extricate and move the patient and intensive care support to assist with advanced airway and ventilation management?

If the answer is 'yes' to any question, it may be necessary to immediately commence treatment or summon further assistance before a history and comprehensive physical examination are carried out.[12] If no immediate interventions are required, continue on with the respiratory assessment.

Clinical history

The aim of respiratory assessment is to identify the adequacy of gas exchange, tissue oxygenation and the excretion of carbon dioxide.[13] During a comprehensive respiratory assessment it is vital to review the patient's clinical history (Table 21.3) as this will guide the remainder of the examination and aid interpretation of clinical findings.[14]

Detailed patient history is a relative luxury for the pre-hospital responder. What has happened in the past to the patient will come from the patient, family and, less commonly, general practitioner or nursing notes. Doctor information may come from a co-attendance, hospital discharge or handover letters or available telephone number. Nursing notes may come from district nursing notes left with the patient. Other past history findings will include medications, hospital patient information books, including old electrocardiographs and medical devices in the vicinity of the patient, such as nebulisers, CPAP therapy devices and oxygen cylinders. The other element of patient history is the description of current events, including defining why help has been requested at this time, duration of the current illness episode and what therapies may have been employed already. The pattern of previous similar episodes will be critical in predicting likely course of events on this occasion.

The medical history will generally provide most of the information vital to determining the aetiology of the patient's respiratory distress. The first step is to determine what the current symptoms are (such as chest pain, breathlessness, cough) and the duration. However, as many respiratory and cardiac conditions share similar symptoms, it is vital to question the patient for disease specific symptoms (for example, haemoptysis and risk factors for pulmonary embolism; fever and cough for pneumonia; nocturnal dyspnoea, peripheral oedema and a history of cardiac disease for congestive cardiac failure).

The past medical history is the next important aspect of history-taking. In a patient with a known chronic respiratory illness, the cause of their current respiratory symptoms will most commonly be due to an exacerbation of this chronic respiratory disease or a complication related to it. Likewise, a past history of cardiac failure should heighten suspicion for a cardiac cause of the patient's respiration distress.

Physical assessment

Physical assessment includes inspection, palpation, percussion and auscultation. Using a systematic format during physical assessment has merit: it helps the clinician avoid missing subtle signs while practising in the chaotic emergency environment. A head-to-toe format is used here to detail inspection, palpation, percussion and auscultation; however, another method may be

used to identify relevant elements from each domain while assessing a body section before moving to the next. Although a comprehensive respiratory physical assessment is detailed, clinical judgement should be used to identify the relevant aspects of respiratory assessment in relation to the particular patient presentation—e.g. seeking evidence of inhalation injury in a patient with possible airway burns. Once signs of respiratory compromise are located, escalation of care and implementation of appropriate interventions should take priority. It can be relatively easy to assess the patient in respiratory distress as most of the findings can be visibly observed. This is unlike pain, for example, where examination requires questioning and more subjective determinations.

> ### PRACTICE TIP
>
> The aim of respiratory assessment is to determine respiratory status, identify deterioration in patients at risk, and guide and evaluate the effectiveness of treatment.

Inspection

Inspection involves critical, purposeful direct observation utilising vision, hearing and smell. The aim of inspection is to identify abnormalities, paying attention to both subtle and obvious changes.[13] Inspection begins with a general inspection, then inspection of the head, neck and thorax.

General inspection

Note skin and mucous membrane colour as an indication of haemoglobin oxygen saturation.[15] Is the patient pink, pale, mottled or cyanotic? Peripheral cyanosis is noted in the extremities; central cyanosis is a late sign and is noted in the oral mucous membranes as a bluish colour. Cyanosis may become visible when arterial saturation drops below 85%;[13] however, it may not be visible during severe anaemia as there is insufficient haemoglobin present.[4,12] Peripheral cyanosis secondary to vasoconstriction, decreased cardiac output or vascular occlusion can occur in the presence of normal systemic oxygen saturation.[12] A mottled appearance to the skin can indicate poor tissue perfusion as may occur with sepsis and septic shock.

During general inspection, the patient's level of consciousness should be assessed. A baseline Glasgow Coma Scale (GCS) score is critical to note deterioration or improvement. Changes in GCS are very significant in respiratory distress. Confusion or drowsiness with GCS 14 or even presentations with lesser GCS scores indicate severe distress or even respiratory failure.[16,17] More common though is a subtler change in consciousness, including patient behaviour. An increase in agitation or anxiety or an altered consciousness level may be an indication of cerebral hypoxia or inadequate ventilation and resultant hypercapnia.[13]

Observe the patient's speech pattern, noting if they are speaking in sentences, phrases or words, or unable to talk. The degree of respiratory distress is reflected in a decreasing tolerance for speech.[15]

Identify the posture and activity of the patient and how much exercise the patient can tolerate prior to experiencing dyspnoea. Patients experiencing respiratory distress may sit forward in a position known as 'tripoding', with their hands on

TABLE 21.3 Clinical history of a patient with respiratory compromise[12,14,18,136]	
AREA OF FOCUS	RATIONALE
Presenting complaint	A statement as to why the patient has attended the ED, e.g. 'increased shortness of breath'. This provides a starting point to guide specific areas of questioning relevant to the problem.
Allergies	Identifies whether an allergic reaction is a factor in the current presentation, and avoidance of future exposure to known drug allergies during the hospital stay.
Medications	Identify what medications the patient is currently taking. Take notice of drug classes that may inform interpretation of physical assessment findings; e.g. beta-blocker drugs will inhibit sympathetic compensatory mechanisms such as increased heart rate.
	Medications may also give an indication of medical conditions that the patient forgets/doesn't understand, or may allude to severity of disease process and potential for future deterioration.
Past medical/surgical history	Identify conditions the patient has been diagnosed with and treated for in the past. Identify chronic illnesses such as chronic obstructive pulmonary disease, asthma, cystic fibrosis, heart failure, hypertension and cancer.
	Enquire if the patient is on a specific management plan and whether they adhere to it.
	Past surgical procedures and historical risk features that may be relevant to the current presentation should be identified; e.g. previous admission to ICU/HDU, previous deterioration requiring intubation or invasive interventions.[147]
Last menstrual period/ last meal	Possible pregnancy should be identified prior to radiation exposure, e.g. chest X-ray, computed tomography pulmonary angiogram (CTPA).
	Identify last meal if surgery and elective intubation are a possibility.
Familial history	Identify family history of pulmonary and cardiac disease.
Social history	Explore tobacco use (number of pack-years); inhaled drugs, e.g. marijuana.
	Identify recent overseas travel and exposure to environmental hazards such as chemicals, allergens, extreme heat/cold, animals within the home or work site.
Events leading to presentation and associated signs and symptoms	Identify the sequence of events that led to the patient coming to hospital, and any associated symptoms. The sequence of events, mechanism of injury and associated symptoms provide clues to the underlying pathophysiology of the complaint, and may indicate particular investigations and interventions.
Dyspnoea	Questions regarding dyspnoea include: Does it occur with exercise? Does it relate to position, e.g. worse when lying down/better when sitting up, or time of day?
Chest pain	Identify the presence of any pain/pressure/tightness in the chest, or radiation of pain to jaw/shoulder/arm. If the patient has had a complaint of chest pain, further questioning aims to help differentiate cardiac ischaemia, pleuritic or musculoskeletal origin.
	A useful mnemonic to assess chest pain is PQRST: P—precipitating and palliating factors; Q—quality; R—region and radiation; S—severity, pain scale 1–10; T—time of onset and duration.
Sputum	Questions regarding sputum include changes in amount and colour. Yellow, green and brown sputum typically represent bacterial infection.[10] Clear or white may notify the absence of bacteria. Mucoid, viscid or blood-streaked may be a sign of viral infection. Frothy white or pink-tinged sputum can be a clinical symptom of pulmonary oedema.[10]
Cough	Coughs have various precipitants, such as inflammation to the respiratory mucosa, smoking, allergies, asthma and certain medications. Relevant questions involve identifying onset, precipitant factors, timing, frequency and whether or not it is productive.[16]

HDU: high-dependency unit; ICU: intensive care unit

their knees or a table. This helps to elevate the clavicles, giving a slightly greater ability to expand the chest on inspiration.[14] Alternatively the patient who is slumped and unable to support themselves suggests a state of respiratory failure.

Identify evidence of vasodilation as an indication of hypercapnia. High levels of CO_2 result in dilation of vasculature,[4] and may be apparent in surface capillaries. Hypercapnia may also produce a flapping tremor noticeable in the hands.[4,12]

Look for evidence of clubbing of fingertips. Clubbing is an abnormal enlargement, thinning and change in the angle of the fingernail bases, or less commonly those of the toes, and is associated with chronic hypoxia.[4,12,13]

Head

Respiratory distress evidence on the head and face include pursed-lip breathing, nasal flaring, mouth breathing versus via the nose, cyanosis of mucous membranes, decreased speech tolerance and alterations to level of consciousness.[13,18,19] Pursed lip breathing in particular is a technique often performed spontaneously but can be taught to patients to use as an adjunct. It involves providing resistance to expiration prolonging time for gas exchange and combatting airway collapse and is particularly useful in COPD.[20,21]

Listen for sounds of upper airway obstruction, evidenced by a snoring, stridor or gurgling noise on inspiration.[22] Stridor is a high-pitched crowing-type noise, occurring only on inspiration (or louder during inspiration). Stridor is caused by upper airway, laryngeal or tracheal obstruction and indicates an airway emergency.[23]

Inspect for foreign bodies in the oropharynx.[24] Where the patient is conscious this may include looking for signs of choking, such as clutching the throat, sudden onset of coughing, wheezing from partly obstructed airways or unequal lung sounds. The unconscious patient may require visualisation under laryngoscopy and require aggressive methods including suctioning, forceps and chest compressions to dislodge. In hospital methods may require further intervention including removal of the item under bronchoscopy. Clinical history will often fail to recognise the problem, but remains nonetheless particularly important in diagnosis.[25,26] Signs of vomitus may be evident on the mouth, clothing or near the patient, suggestive of foreign body or aspiration occurrence. If inhalation burns are suspected, search for relevant evidence, including facial and nasal hair singeing, soot particles in mouth or nose, carbonaceous sputum, intra oral oedema or stridor, or hoarse voice.[27] Inspect for signs of trauma, deformity or bruising that may affect the airway.[22]

Neck

Inspect for signs of trauma, bruising or swelling around the neck.[24] Identify if the trachea is midline or deviated to the left or right.[13] A deviated trachea can indicate mediastinal shift, which may occur with tension pneumothorax, haemothorax or pleural effusion, which pushes the trachea away from the affected side.[13] The trachea can also be pulled towards the affected side with atelectasis, fibrosis, tumours or phrenic nerve palsy.[14] Neck vein distension may be observed as jugular venous pressure rises. This may be associated with ventricular dysfunction and may be useful in assessing patients with cardiac disease and breathing difficulty.[28]

Chest

The chest should be fully exposed to facilitate examination. Pre-hospital examination of the chest can be very different to the in-hospital examination. Great care must be taken when exposing any patient where public view is possible. This may still be the case even if only other family members or friends are present or where particular observances are encountered, such as religious. Physical exposure of patients can also increase the risk of environmental hazard if the temperature is cold or there is wind. Pre-hospital responders may have to consider moving a patient to a more protected location to allow a thorough chest examination. Similarly, the presence of an appropriate witness or adult may be sought where the patient is a child, female or has religious observances that could be problematic.

Observe for symmetrical movement of the chest wall during breathing. Asymmetry may indicate bronchial obstruction, pneumothorax, fibrosis or collapse of lobes.[13] Paradoxical movement is seen when some or the entire chest wall moves inwards during inspiration and outwards on expiration.[12] This may be seen in the presence of a flail segment of ribs, or severe respiratory distress in a young child.[12,13,29] Pardoxical breathing can also be seen where there is spinal cord injury and altered nervous control of the normal respiratory muscles.[30]

Observe for accessory muscle use. During breathing at rest, the diaphragm contracts and the intercostal muscles contract, pulling the ribs upwards and outwards.[4,15] This causes an increase in intrathoracic volume and negative pressure, causing net movement of air into the lungs.[4,15] A patient who is in respiratory distress will use additional muscles to aid the respiratory effort.[15] These include abdominal muscles that aid the diaphragm to increase vertical diameter, and the sternocleidomastoid, scalenes and trapezii, which all contract to increase the anteroposterior (AP) and transverse diameters of the thorax.[4,12,15]

The respiratory rate and rhythm should be carefully assessed. A normal rate is between 10 and 18 breaths/minute, with an inspiratory : expiratory ratio of 1:2.[15] Alterations to rate, rhythm or this ratio may indicate underlying conditions. Hypoventilation (rate <10) can suggest a number of conditions, including opioid overdose causing depression of respiratory centre, or increased intracranial pressure.[13] Tachypnoea is a respiratory rate >18 and is often the first sign of respiratory distress.[13] Kussmaul respirations—breaths that are rapid, deep and caused by stimulation of the respiratory centre secondary to metabolic acidosis—may be observed if there is an attempt to increase removal of CO_2.[13] Prolongation of the expiratory phase of respiration may be noted in some respiratory disease, including COPD and asthma.

Examine the chest wall for signs of trauma, bruising, deformity and scars from previous injury or surgery.[14] The shape of the thorax should also be inspected. The chest wall should be symmetrical, with the transverse diameter larger than the AP diameter. Barrel-shaped chests (where transverse and AP diameter are equal) are commonly associated with chronic obstructive respiratory disorders such as emphysema.[4,12] Other irregular anatomical features affecting the thorax and function include: pectus excavatum, where the sternum is depressed inwards; pectus carinatum, where the sternum and costal cartilages project outwards; kyphosis, a forward curvature of the spine; and scoliosis, a lateral curvature of the spine.[4,12]

Intercostal muscle recession may be commonly seen in children who have underdeveloped intercostal muscles, or thin or elderly patients.[14,18] Intercostal recession occurs during inspiration where the intercostal muscles are sucked backwards between the ribs by intrathoracic negative pressure.[14]

COMPONENTS OF INSPECTION DURING RESPIRATORY ASSESSMENT

General

Level of consciousness:

- Agitation/anxiety
- Speech
  - sentences/phrases/words/unable to speak
  - quality (hoarseness)

Skin colour:

- Pallor/cyanosis
- Exercise tolerance/body position

Head and neck:

- Nasal flaring
- Pursed-lip breathing
- Mouth vs nose breathing
- Evidence of trauma: deformity, bruising, wounds, swelling, burns
- Tracheal position
- Tracheal tug

Thorax:

- Symmetry of chest wall movement
- Accessory muscle use, recession
- Rate, rhythm, pattern of breathing
- Evidence of trauma, wounds, deformity, flail, bruising, scars
- Anteroposterior vs transverse diameter of chest
- Alignment of spine: presence of kyphosis, scoliosis

Extremities:

- Clubbing
- Oedema
- Peripheral cyanosis

Palpation

Palpate structures in the neck and thorax to locate abnormalities.

Neck

Palpate the position of the trachea. The trachea should be midline above the suprasternal notch.[12,14] Deviation from centre suggests a mediastinal shift.[12] Palpate for subcutaneous emphysema.[24]

Chest

Palpate the thorax systematically, comparing left with right.[12] Commence above each clavicle and progress down the anterior wall, followed by palpation of each axilla and posterior chest wall.[12] Identify areas of bony or soft tissue tenderness, crepitus, depressions, bulges, pulsations, paradoxical movement and subcutaneous emphysema.[12] Subcutaneous emphysema is a condition caused by a disruption to the alveoli, allowing air into the subcutaneous tissue.[14] The cause may be mechanical trauma, barotrauma from a high peak inspiratory pressure (PIP) or use of positive end-expiratory pressure (PEEP). Palpation

of subcutaneous emphysema is likened to the sensation of rice paper under the skin.[14]

Respiratory excursion (expansion) is checked by standing behind the patient, placing the palmar surface of the hands on the patient's back with thumbs next to one another along the spinal processes at the approximate level of the 10th rib.[12] The thumbs should separate symmetrically on inspiration. An absence of symmetry indicates a problem with respiratory excursion on one or both sides of the chest.[12]

The final stage of palpation is to identify tactile fremitus. This is the palpable vibration of the chest wall during speech. Assessment of tactile fremitus is completed by placing the ulnar aspect of one hand on the chest wall and requesting the patient to say 'ninety-nine'.[12] Vibration is better transmitted through solid- than air-filled structures. A decrease in vibration transmission to the hand may be felt when air is present between lung and chest wall, such as with a pneumothorax; or when there is an increase of air per unit of lung tissue, e.g. with emphysema.[14] An increase in vibration may be present with lung consolidation.[12]

Auscultation

Auscultation of the chest involves listening and interpreting the sounds transmitted through the thorax with a stethoscope.[12] A structured approach should be taken: auscultating the anterior, posterior and lateral aspects of the chest, comparing the left and right sides and listening throughout inspiration and expiration.[14]

Breath sounds in the normal chest are created by airflow in the airways.[12] These are described as vesicular (normal) or bronchial (abnormal).[14]

- Vesicular sounds are heard in normal lung parenchyma where air flows through smaller bronchioles; the inspiratory phase is longer than the expiratory phase and the sound is soft and low-pitched.[12,14]

- Bronchial breath sounds are heard over areas of lung where the alveoli are filled with fluid (most commonly caused by pneumonia). The sounds of air flow through bronchi are efficiently transmitted through the abnormal fluid to the chest wall. The sound is high-pitched, harsh and loud.[12,14]

Adventitious noises are abnormal sounds created by fluid or sputum accumulation, obstruction, bronchoconstriction, inflammation or pleural lining pathology.[12,14] Common adventitious noises are crackles, wheezes, rhonchi and pleural rubs.[12,14]

- Crackles are caused by the opening of collapsed alveoli, or from fluid in the smaller airways.[12] The sound is a soft, high-pitched, brief clicking or popping sound, heard more commonly during inspiration.[12,14] They are often described as fine or coarse. Coarse crackles occur with fluid accumulations, as may occur if the patient had pneumonia.[10] Crackles also occur with congestive cardiac failure, atelectasis of lung tissue and sometimes in an acute exacerbation of asthma. These sounds can pose a particular difficulty for paramedics during examination where history may be partly unclear and there is no access to detailed medical records or more complex assessment methods, including X-ray. A focus on past and current history may offer further clues in assessment. Management options selected may have to be mindful of an uncertain diagnosis where the different possible options may conflict with each other.

- Wheezes are caused by air movement through narrowed or partially obstructed airways due to bronchoconstriction, increased sputum, mucosal oedema or foreign bodies.[12] Wheezes have a continuous musical sound.[12,14] The degree of airway narrowing may be indicated by the pitch of the wheeze, higher pitches being associated with greater obstruction.[12]
- Rhonchi are a different type of continuous sound typified by a low-pitched rumbling noise.[14] They are caused by secretions in the larger airways and may be cleared sometimes by coughing.[14]
- A pleural rub, or friction rub, is more commonly heard on inspiration and is a grating or crackling sound.[12] It is caused by the rubbing together of inflamed parietal and visceral pleura.[14]

Whispered pectoriloquy refers to being able to hear clear, loud sounds through the stethoscope when the patient whispers.[14] Normally the whispered voice is heard only faintly and indirectly while auscultating.[14] An increase in sound transmission indicates the presence of consolidation or fluid, such as in pneumonia, pulmonary oedema or haemothorax.[14]

Absent air sounds over lung tissue indicate absence of air movement. This may be due to consolidation or obstruction. The absence of sound, or a quiet chest in a patient displaying increased respiratory effort, is an emergent sign requiring immediate escalation and intervention.[23]

As with exposing the chest to allow examination to occur, auscultation may also pose some difficulties for pre-hospital responders. Exposure to the environment or breaching privacy can be problematic. The emergency presentation is often sudden and allows the patient little or no time to prepare. The clothing they are wearing is not intended to allow chest auscultation and often many items of clothing have to be removed to allow access to the posterior and anterior chest. The temptation to leave out auscultation, perform only part assessment or listen over clothing should be avoided as the pre-hospital assessment is already compromised for detail.

Percussion

During percussion, one hand is placed flat to the chest wall with fingers separated. The other hand is used as a hammer, swinging from the wrist, the fingers striking the middle-finger distal inter-phalangeal joint (DIPJ) of the hand on the chest.[12] Percussion should be performed systematically starting from above the clavicles, comparing left and right of the chest, at 3–4 cm intervals.[12] The quality of the sound heard indicates the nature of the structures beneath the hand.[12,14] A dense structure such as consolidated tissue or liquid will give a dull sound, whereas air-filled structures will give a louder, hollow sound called tympany.[12,14]

Pre-hospital considerations for respiratory complaints

Respiratory complaints comprise a significant proportion of emergency medical service (EMS) responses. The assessment and management priorities remain the same for a respiratory complaint (primary survey approach), whether or not the patient is in the pre-hospital or emergency department (ED) environment. Utilisation of the appropriate protocol and related interventions must be dictated by the patient's clinical history and physical assessment. Severe airway and respiratory compromise must be identified early and used to determine the need for a priority call notification and/or additional support for interventions that may fall outside the scope of practice of the attending EMS provider. Respiratory difficulty may be the primary complaint or it may be an element of another problem such as associated with chest pains, trauma, infection or metabolic disorder. Managing the respiratory problems may be assisted by managing the associated problem instead of or concurrently with.

Diagnostics and monitoring

Pulse oximetry

Pulse oximetry non-invasively monitors the saturation of haemoglobin in tissue capillaries by transmitting a beam of light through tissue to a receiver.[13] The amount of saturated haemoglobin alters the wavelengths of the transmitted light, which is then translated by the receiver into a percentage of haemoglobin saturation.[13] The oxygen saturation as measured by pulse oximetry (SpO_2) has a normal range of 95–99% at sea level when breathing room air.[14] The displayed value is an average of multiple readings over a 3–10 second window, reducing the effect of waveform variation caused by patient movement.[14]

Limitations of SpO_2 monitoring should be taken into consideration when using this technology:

- Nail polish should be removed from the digit used.[13]
- Poor peripheral perfusion due to shock or peripheral vasoconstriction will contribute to an inaccurate reading.[13]
- SpO_2 in an anaemic patient is an unreliable indication of oxygen transport to tissues. SpO_2 is only an indication of available haemoglobin saturation, rather than oxygen-carrying capability.[13,14] For example, a patient with haemoglobin of 60 g/L and SpO_2 of 99% will still have reduced capacity for oxygen transport to the tissues.
- During carbon monoxide (CO) poisoning, CO binds preferentially to haemoglobin. Pulse oximetry cannot differentiate between carboxyhaemoglobin and oxyhaemoglobin, and consequently in such cases pulse oximetry will not accurately indicate oxygen saturation of available haemoglobin.[13,14,31,32]
- Movement can affect the ability of emitted light to travel between the diode and receiver, affecting the accuracy of the results.[13]

The SpO_2 value only reflects a part of the ventilation equation. Carbon dioxide is also important and any oxygen reading must be maintained in an overall patient context. Asthma in particular can incur significant rise in CO_2 capable of taking the patient into altered consciousness and respiratory failure,[33] despite being able to maintain normally tolerable pulse oximetry levels. Relying on pulse oximetry alone as a guide to severity of illness can be deceiving. Similarly, patients with COPD may have lower oxygen and higher carbon dioxide values than other patients as a normal finding for them. In such instances the value of trend monitoring can be more important than any one finding alone.

Pulse oximetry is only an indication of saturation of available haemoglobin. Values should be interpreted in conjunction with clinical conditions such as low haemoglobin, poor peripheral perfusion and clinical history, such as exposure to carbon monoxide.

Capnography

End-tidal carbon dioxide ($EtCO_2$) monitoring, known as capnography, quantifies the amount of CO_2 at the end of expiration. It can be used to monitor a patient's level of arterial CO_2 when alveolar carbon dioxide ($PACO_2$) closely approximates the carbon dioxide dissolved in the arterial blood ($PaCO_2$).[14] The $EtCO_2$ is usually 2–5 mmHg lower than the patient's $PaCO_2$.[14] Normal values for $PaCO_2$ range between 35 and 45 mmHg.[14] See Chapter 17, p. 323, for an explanation on applying capnography and end-tidal monitoring.

$EtCO_2$ monitoring is indicated immediately post-intubation as a gold-standard initial confirmation of endotracheal tube placement in the trachea. Thereafter, $EtCO_2$ monitoring can be used to gauge adequacy of mechanical ventilation and guide adjustment of minute volume.[23,34–36] Correlation between $EtCO_2$ and $PaCO_2$ should be confirmed by arterial blood gas measurement at the commencement of invasive ventilation.[23] Conflict exists over the strength of this approximation ranging between reasonable[37] to inability to produce such correlation between values.[38] For pre-hospital responders the use of $EtCO_2$ can be important given the absence of more invasive blood gas assessment[39] extending beyond use as a confirmatory tool for endotracheal intubation placement.

Occasionally clinical problems may necessitate knowledge of the $EtCO_2$ for reasons other than to maintain normal levels, monitor trends or endotracheal tube placement. Patients with diabetic ketoacidosis develop a progressive metabolic acidosis and $EtCO_2$ may be useful in assessment and ongoing maintenance of any compensatory respiratory alkalosis.[40] Similarly, it may be useful in monitoring $EtCO_2$ values in patients being intentionally hyperventilated to create a therapeutic respiratory alkalosis following tricyclic acid medication overdose.[41]

Arterial blood gases

The arterial blood gas (ABG) is an investigation that provides information regarding respiratory function in areas of acid–base balance, oxygenation, ventilation, tissue perfusion and compensation.[4,14] This information can be used to guide the respiratory management plan and interventions. Chapter 17 contains information on ABGs (p. 323) and blood glucose level sampling (p. 329).

ARTERIAL BLOOD GAS (ABG)

The normal ranges for components of an ABG are as follows:[42]

pH	7.35–7.45	$PaCO_2$	35–45 mmHg
PaO_2	80–100 mmHg	HCO_3^-	22–26 mmol/L
SaO_2	95–99%		

pH is a measurement of hydrogen-ion concentration within the blood, and indicates acidity or alkalinity. A pH of < 7.35 indicates acidosis; a pH of > 7.45 indicates alkalosis.[14]

An ABG measures two factors that alter pH: $PaCO_2$ and bicarbonate (HCO_3^-).[42,44]

- $PaCO_2$ is the respiratory component of the blood gas, and measures CO_2 dissolved in the blood.[14] High levels of $PaCO_2$ will contribute to acidosis; low levels to alkalosis. CO_2 is a byproduct of cellular metabolism and diffuses across the alveolar–capillary membrane for removal during alveolar ventilation.[45] Any changes to the steps of gas transport and ventilation will affect $PaCO_2$ levels.[4]

- HCO_3^- is a buffer produced by the kidneys, and the metabolic component of the blood gas.[42] If the body produces more acid than the kidneys can buffer (HCO_3^- < 22 mmol/L), acidosis will result; if too much HCO_3^- is produced (HCO_3^- > 26 mmol/L), alkalosis will result.[42]

PaO_2 assesses the amount of oxygen dissolved in the blood.[42] After oxygen dissolves, it binds to haemoglobin to form oxyhaemoglobin.[4] The SaO_2 refers to the percentage of haemoglobin binding sites that have been attached to oxygen in arterial blood.[14] In line with increasing common practice and availability, pulse oximetry this become a frequent substitute to invasive oxygen monitoring provided its limitations are recognised.[44]

Six-step process to ABG analysis[42]

1. Analyse the pH
   - Determine if the pH is normal (7.35–7.45), acidotic (< 7.35) or alkalotic (> 7.45).
   - If the pH is within normal limits, establish if it is on the acidotic side of normal (7.35–7.39) or on the alkalotic side of normal (7.41–7.45).

2. Analyse the $PaCO_2$ changes (respiratory component of blood gas).
   - A low $PaCO_2$ of < 35 mmHg can be caused by hyperventilation and will result in respiratory alkalosis by removal of high amounts of CO_2.
   - Conversely, hypoventilation causes less CO_2 removal and causes the $PaCO_2$ to increase, resulting in respiratory acidosis (> 45 mmHg).

3. Analyse the HCO_3^- (metabolic component).
   - A value of < 22 mmol/L indicates acidosis; a value of > 26 mmol/L indicates alkalosis.

4. Match either $PaCO_2$ or HCO_3^- with the pH.
   - If $PaCO_2$ is high (acidosis) and pH low (acidosis), there is respiratory acidosis.
   - If $PaCO_2$ is low (alkalosis) and pH high (alkalosis), there is respiratory alkalosis.
   - If HCO_3^- is low (acidosis) and pH is low (acidosis), there is metabolic acidosis.
   - If HCO_3^- is high (alkalosis) and pH is high (alkalosis), there is metabolic alkalosis.

5. Determine if $PaCO_2$ or HCO_3^- move in the opposite direction to the pH.
   - If this occurs, compensation is present. Compensation aims to return the pH to normal parameters and can happen via respiratory (CO_2) or metabolic

(HCO_3^-) compensation. The respiratory system can begin compensation immediately; however, metabolic compensation can take many hours.

- If there is no change in the $PaCO_2$ or HCO_3^-, then compensation is not occurring.
- If compensation is occurring (as seen by a change in the $PaCO_2$ or HCO_3^-), but the pH has not returned to within normal limits, this is termed a partial compensation. Full compensation is reflected by a pH within normal limits.

6. Analyse the PaO_2 and SaO_2 for hypoxaemia. This must be interpreted in the context of the inspired oxygen concentration. For example, the normal range for PaO_2 is usually between 80 and 100 mmHg when breathing room air, but a patient who has a PaO_2 in this range when receiving high flow supplemental oxygen is most likely to have serious pulmonary pathology impairing gas exchange.

Examples of ABG results

1. pH 7.20
   $PaCO_2$ 50 mmHg
   HCO_3^- 25 mmol/L
   PaO_2 70 mmHg
   SaO_2 90%
   The pH is acidotic, and this corresponds with a high $PaCO_2$ which is also acidotic. The HCO_3^- is normal so does not reflect an attempt at compensation. The PaO_2 is low and suggests hypoxaemia. Therefore, this ABG reflects a patient with an uncompensated respiratory acidosis with hypoxaemia.

2. pH 7.50
   $PaCO_2$ 30 mmHg
   HCO_3^- 24 mmol/L
   PaO_2 80 mmHg
   SaO_2 95%
   The pH is alkalotic, and this corresponds with a low $PaCO_2$ that also reflects alkalosis. The HCO_3^- is normal and therefore there are no attempts at compensation. The PaO_2 and SaO_2 are normal. Therefore, this ABG reflects a patient with an uncompensated respiratory alkalosis.

3. pH 7.20
   $PaCO_2$ 38 mmHg
   HCO_3^- 19 mmol/L
   PaO_2 85 mmHg
   SaO_2 96%
   The pH is acidotic which corresponds with a low HCO_3^- (acidosis). The $PaCO_2$ is within the normal range, suggesting no attempts at compensation; the PaO_2 and SaO_2 are also normal. This ABG reflects a patient with an uncompensated metabolic acidosis and normal arterial oxygenation.

4. pH 7.50
   $PaCO_2$ 38 mmHg
   HCO_3^- 29 mmol/L
   PaO_2 85 mmHg
   SaO_2 96%

The pH is alkalotic which corresponds with a high HCO_3^- (alkalosis). The $PaCO_2$, PaO_2 and SaO_2 are normal. This ABG reflects a patient with an uncompensated metabolic alkalosis and normal arterial oxygenation.

5. pH 7.34
   $PaCO_2$ 50 mmHg
   HCO_3^- 30 mmol/L
   PaO_2 85 mmHg
   SaO_2 96%
   The pH is acidotic which corresponds with a high $PaCO_2$ (acidosis). The HCO_3^- is high (alkalosis). The acidotic pH and acidotic $PaCO_2$ suggest a respiratory acidosis. Because the HCO_3^- is alkalotic (opposite to the pH), this suggests an attempt at compensation. As the pH has not returned to normal limits, the compensation is not complete. This ABG reflects a patient with a partially compensated respiratory acidosis with normal PaO_2 and SaO_2 levels, suggesting adequate arterial oxygenation.

6. pH 7.44
   $PaCO_2$ 50 mmHg
   HCO_3^- 31 mmol/L
   PaO_2 70 mmHg
   SaO_2 92%
   The pH is normal and on the alkalotic side of normal, which corresponds with the HCO_3^- (alkalosis). The $PaCO_2$ is acidotic which is opposite to the pH, indicating that compensation is occurring; because the pH is in normal limits, there is full compensation. The PaO_2 and SaO_2 are low. Therefore, this is a fully compensated metabolic alkalosis with hypoxaemia.

Venous or arterial blood gas? When is a venous blood gas enough?

Arterial puncture for the purpose of obtaining ABGs brings additional risk to the patient and is often a painful investigation; it is also another potential exposure to a sharp for the healthcare professional.[45,46] Due to these considerations—and like any investigation—there should be a clear clinical necessity to obtain an arterial sample. The sample should provide clinical information that will influence diagnosis, management and interventions or referral that cannot be gained from a method that exposes the patient to less risk and pain. Much information that has been traditionally acquired from an ABG can be inferred from a venous blood gas (VBG).

PRACTICE TIP

VENOUS BLOOD GAS (VBG)

Normal VBG values are as follows:

pH	7.35–7.38
$PvCO_2$	44–48 mmHg
PvO_2	40 mmHg
HCO_3^-	21–22 mmol/L

The VBG cannot replace an ABG in all circumstances. While a VBG does give reliable correlations to arterial pH and

HCO_3^- values, and can be used to evaluate acid–base balance, oxygenation is much more difficult to reliably assess on a VBG. Measurement of pH on a VBG will be –0.04 less than for an arterial sample.[45] For example, if a VBG pH is 7.33, the arterial sample is likely to be 7.37. Likewise, a venous HCO_3^- value is on average 0.52 mmol/L less than that of an arterial sample.[46] However, in acute illness there is a non-linear relationship between venous and arterial oxygen content. This means that PvO_2 cannot reliably be used as an indicator of PaO_2 in acutely or critically ill patients.

A study comparing VBG and ABG values for PCO_2 in acute respiratory illness or respiratory compromise found fair agreement between samples, with venous PCO_2 ($PvCO_2$) on average 5.8 mmHg higher than in arterial samples.[48] $PvCO_2$ was recommended as a screening test for hypercarbia; however, there was not sufficient agreement between samples to replace an ABG for evaluation of respiratory function.[48] A meta-analysis considering this question also found insufficient correlation to allow for VBG to be used as a reliable substitute for ABG.[44]

If frequent ABG sampling is necessary, for example, with an unstable invasively ventilated patient, consider whether the insertion of an arterial line may be more appropriate to minimise trauma associated with frequent arterial puncture.

> **PRACTICE TIP**
>
> The risks and benefits of measuring ABGs should be considered in relation to information that may be more easily obtained through VBGs or non-invasive means such as $EtCO_2$ monitoring and pulse oximetry.

Peak flow and spirometry

Two methods of assessing airflow limitations and obstruction have been commonly available in the ED environment: peak flow and spirometry.

Peak flow testing may also be used in the community, and paramedics should seek information about peak flow if the patient routinely records this information as part of their management plan. The peak flow test measures 'peak expiratory flow', which is the maximum flow achievable from a forced expiration starting at full inspiration.[49] It only reflects resistance through the larger conducting airways and the reading is reached within the first tenth of a second on expiration.[49] Peak flow is most commonly used for home monitoring of asthma.[49]

More-sensitive information can be gained from *spirometry*. Spirometry measures two main values: forced vital capacity (FVC), which is the maximum volume of air expired from the point of maximal inspiration,[14] and forced expiratory volume (FEV_1), which is the volume of air exhaled during the first second of the exercise.[50] The ratio of these two measurements is then calculated (FEV_1:FVC).[51] A value of < 80% of the predicted norm is indicative of an airflow limitation.[51] The predicted norm is calculated based on sex, height, age and race, and graphs depicting normal values across a range of parameters are commonly available.[4,51] In obstructive diseases such as COPD or exacerbation of asthma, airflow is reduced. This will be reflected with a decrease in FEV_1, and greater time taken to expire the full breath.[51]

> **BOX 21.1 A guide to systematic chest X-ray interpretation[53]**
>
> **Chest X-ray review:**
>
> A. Appearance—chest view (AP, lateral, PA), airway, additional apparatus (ETT/tracheostomy, ECG leads, NGT), lung fields captured
>
> B. Bones—fractures
>
> C. Cardiac shadow—cardiac and costophrenic angles, aortic arch and width of mediastinum
>
> D. Diaphragm—shape, breadth, depth (8th ribs viewed) in lung field
>
> E. Exposure—are the posterior spinous processes visible?
>
> F. Fine lines (normal lung markings out to edge of lung field); fat lines (congested fluid volume); fuzzy lines (infection)
>
> G. Gastric bubble
>
> H. Hylus markings
>
> I. Identification (MRN, name), position of patient
>
> *AP: anteroposterior; PA: posterior–anterior; ECG: electrocardiogram; ETT: endotracheal tube; MRN: Medical Records Number; NGT: nasogastric tube*

To gain a spirometry reading, position the patient as either sitting or standing, instruct them to take as deep a breath as possible, and immediately place the tube between their teeth. The patient should make a firm seal around the tube with their lips, then exhale as hard and as long as possible. The test should be repeated a minimum of three times. An average (mean) of the three readings is then recorded.[50] After therapy is instituted, a second reading should be taken to gauge efficacy of treatment.

> **PRACTICE TIP**
>
> Spirometry is a more sensitive method than peak flow monitoring for assessing respiratory limitation.

Chest X-ray

The chest X-ray is an extremely common and informative diagnostic tool for pulmonary and thoracic assessment within the ED. The image is used to assess lung fields, disease processes, the presence of trauma sequelae such as fractures, haemo- or pneumothorax, as well as the position of invasive lines and tubes. For a guide to systematic chest X-ray interpretation, see Box 21.1.[53]

Support of respiratory function

Oxygen therapy

The administration of supplemental oxygen therapy has long been considered one of the most fundamental components of emergency medical and trauma management. Even colloquially referred to as 'the good gas', it was long thought to be unable to do any harm. In recent years the entire role of oxygen administration has come into question. Already widely criticised in use when managing exacerbations of COPD, particularly pre-hospital,[55,56] the oxygen therapy debate has widened to consider that it may in fact be able to do harm to a wider patient cohort. There is a growing body of evidence that routine oxygen administration for acute coronary syndrome patients can be associated with increased infarct size and mortality,[57–59] and that oxygen may constrict coronary vessels and, in fact, worsen ischaemia.[60–62] Similarly, high concentration oxygen-induced vasoconstriction has been shown to cause reduction in cerebral blood flow and worsen outcomes in some acute neurological emergencies, including stroke severity and one-year survival.[58,63] Increasingly, pre-hospital and emergency practitioners are being guided by true hypoxia and pulse oximetry to guide oxygen administration rather than indiscriminately applied therapy. There is no evidence that patients who are normoxaemic with or without the complaint of breath shortage benefit from oxygen therapy.[60] Patients with no history of COPD should have a normal target saturation range of 94–98% in most cases with critical illnesses other than COPD maintained over 90%.[60]

Oxygen therapy devices are categorised as low-flow or high-flow devices that provide either a fixed or a variable concentration of oxygen. *Low-flow devices*, such as standard nasal cannula, deliver flows of gas usually between 1–3 L/min, and no more than about 6–8 L/min as rates higher than this are poorly tolerated due to discomfort caused by drying of the nasal

mucosa. This rate of flow is well below the normal inspiratory flow demand of 30 L/min, and consequently the remainder of airflow is obtained from room air. The entrainment of room air that occurs with low-flow devices means that the fraction of inspired oxygen (FiO_2) varies from breath to breath and is dependent on the patient's minute ventilation. In contrast, *high-flow devices* are able to accommodate a patient's inspiratory demand and maintain a fixed FiO_2 irrespective of the patient's respiratory rate and tidal volume. A choice regarding appropriate oxygen therapy and delivery device should be dictated by the patient's support requirements, whether in the pre-hospital or the emergency setting. The most commonly used oxygen therapy devices are described in Table 21.4.[54] See Chapter 17 (pp. 314–322) for an explanation of inserting a range of airway management devices.

In addition to commonly used oxygen therapy devices, the use of humidified high-flow nasal cannulae (HHFNCs) has become an additional way of delivering oxygen to spontaneously breathing patients who may have high oxygen requirements. It is also being increasingly used in patients with blunt chest trauma. With HHFNCs the aim is to exceed the patient's inspiratory flow demands so that dilution of delivered oxygen does not occur. With the delivery of high flows directly into the nares, a

TABLE 21.4 Common oxygen therapy devices[64]		
DEVICE	TYPE	DESCRIPTION AND DELIVERY RATES
Nasal cannula	Low flow	Delivers flow rates of 6 L/min or less
		Delivers FiO_2 of 0.24 (at 1 L/min) to 0.40 (at 5–6 L/min)*
Simple mask	Low flow	Design acts as an oxygen reservoir. Holes in the mask allow entrainment of room air
		CO_2 accumulates in the mask, so oxygen flow rates of at least 5 L/min are required to flush CO_2 out of the mask
		Delivers FiO_2 of 0.3–0.6 at flow rates of 5–10 L/min*
Partial-rebreathing mask	Low flow	Simple facemask with the addition of a 300–600 mL reservoir bag
		Oxygen flow should be set so that the bag remains inflated on inspiration (usually 8–15 L is sufficient)
		Delivers FiO_2 of 0.3–0.6 at flow rates of 5–10 L/min*
Non-rebreathing mask	Low flow	Design similar to partial-rebreathing mask, but with a one-way valve between the mask and the reservoir bag. During exhalation the reservoir fills with 100% oxygen. Mask port valves close on inspiration, preventing entrainment of room air
		Oxygen flow rate should be set so that the bag remains inflated on inspiration
		Delivers FiO_2 of 0.6–0.8 at flow rates of 10–15 L/min
Air-entrainment mask (e.g. Venturi mask or Multi-vent mask)	High flow	Consists of a facemask, jet nozzle and entrainment ports.
		Oxygen is delivered through the jet nozzle which increases velocity. Entrainment of ambient air occurs because of viscous shearing forces between the gas travelling through the nozzle and the ambient air
		FiO_2 is dependent on the size of the nozzle and the entrainment ports, and can vary from 0.24 to 0.70
		Flow to the mask must exceed the patient's peak inspiratory flow in order to deliver a fixed FiO_2

*Assuming a constant tidal volume, inspiratory–expiratory ratio, inspiratory time and respiratory rate

flushing effect occurs in the pharynx.[64,67] The anatomical dead space of the upper airway is flushed by the high incoming gas flows. This creates a reservoir of fresh oxygen available for each and every breath, minimising rebreathing of carbon dioxide (CO_2).[64,67] When using HHFNCs the mean airway pressure may increase,[65] although this may be influenced by a number of factors, including the flow rate, structure of the upper airway, cannula size and whether the patient breathes through the nose or the mouth.[64,67] An increasing body of evidence is being added regarding the effectiveness of HHFNCs as an oxygen-delivery method in adults. It does appear that they are effective in improving oxygenation in patients with respiratory failure,[65–69] and are reasonably well tolerated by patients. HHFNCs may also contribute to a decrease in work of breathing and provide a minimal level of end-expiratory pressure.

The administration of oxygen is required when hypoxia is present and should be provided in the amount required to overcome hypoxia. Some patients with chronic respiratory disease will exhibit both hypoxia and hypercarbia. The notion of a hypoxic drive theory which proposed that oxygen administration to this group of patients could result in apnoea, cardiorespiratory arrest and death because administration of oxygen removed the patient's stimulus to breathe has long been associated with acute COPD exacerbation management. It has almost as long been questioned and challenged.[70] There is no evidence to suggest that patients with hypoxia and hypercarbia should not receive oxygen therapy sufficient to address the hypoxia, and failure to do so may result in further clinical deterioration.[71,72] When oxygen is administered, elevations in $PaCO_2$ may be observed in some patients. This increase in $PaCO_2$ appears to be related to changes in ventilation–perfusion matching in the lung and to the Haldane effect, which causes an increase in $PaCO_2$ as more oxygen attaches to the haemoglobin molecule, and is not the consequence of changes in the patient's respiratory drive, respiratory rate or tidal volume.[71] In short, when oxygen is administered $PaCO_2$ will increase, but not because the patient stops breathing. The clear message for patients who exhibit both hypercarbia and hypoxia is that sufficient oxygen needs to be administered to ensure an adequate PaO_2 for the patient, being mindful that excessive amounts of oxygen will needlessly worsen V/Q matching and gas exchange. The critical determinant is what constitutes hypoxia in the patient with COPD. While a normal SpO_2 target may be 94% or greater the desired target range in a patient with COPD may in fact be as low as 88–92% with supplemental oxygen only required below that.[75–77] There is good evidence that pre-hospital responders administer greater oxygen therapy concentrations than are required without providing sufficient ongoing patient assessment.[73,74]

PRACTICE TIP

Patients, including those with COPD, require sufficient supplemental oxygen to reverse hypoxia. Oxygen should be titrated to individual patient requirements. Hypoxia in the COPD patient may be defined differently to other clinical problems with intentionally lower targets used to guide management.

Non-invasive ventilation

In the absence of an endotracheal tube, non-invasive ventilation (NIV), delivered through the application of positive pressure, can be used as a respiratory support strategy. Compared with invasive mechanical ventilation, the use of NIV has benefits that include improved survival, fewer complications, increased comfort and decreased cost.[75,80] Though the efficacy of NIV is well established in hospitals, only relatively recently has pre-hospital application gained similar support. Prospective and retrospective studies of pre-hospital CPAP looking typically at APO, and less commonly COPD, asthma and pneumonia, have all been able to demonstrate clinical patient vital sign improvement, decreased intubation rates and in some cases decreased mortality.[79,81–87]

Appropriately applied NIV is usually adequate to support the work of breathing required for adequate ventilation. While reduced ventilator effort is particularly important in the patient with respiratory failure, NIV may also alter cardiac load and therefore contribute to a decrease in cardiac oxygen demands and adrenergic stimulation. With application of NIV a decrease in respiratory work occurs which improves the balance between oxygen delivery and demand, and results in increased mixed venous PO_2 and PaO_2.[79] Improvements in oxygenation may also be attributed to the increase in mean airway pressure.

In the setting of acute respiratory failure the goal of NIV is to rest the respiratory muscles and increase alveolar ventilation. Importantly, alveolar collapse is reduced leading to substantially reduced work of breathing in re-opening them. Through these processes, gas exchange is enhanced. In the ED, NIV is most commonly used as a respiratory support strategy for patients presenting with respiratory failure because of cardiogenic pulmonary oedema, acute exacerbation of COPD, asthma, hypoxaemic respiratory failure and community-acquired pneumonia.[79,89–92] Current research supports the effectiveness of NIV for exacerbations of COPD and acute cardiogenic pulmonary oedema. Evidence supporting the use of NIV in asthma and hypoxaemic respiratory failure is not as abundant and may be conflicting.[95–97,100]

For NIV to be effective as a respiratory support strategy, there must be careful consideration of patient suitability and selection of appropriate equipment, such as the ventilator and the patient interface.

Patient selection

Success rates with NIV are dependent on its use in appropriate patient populations. NIV is being used increasingly to treat patients with respiratory failure who otherwise meet criteria for intubation and intensive care unit admission, but where underlying poor health prognosis makes this undesirable.[98,99] This can include the elderly and those with chronic or even palliative illnesses. Knowledge of factors that are indicative of success or failure can assist with determining for which patients NIV might be suitable. Patient selection is detailed in Box 21.2.[79,94,100] It must be remembered that non-invasive ventilation is only capable of supporting spontaneous ventilation and not substituting for absent or inadequate respiratory effort. Any patient in whom consciousness has been impaired is suggestive that spontaneous respiration may no longer be sufficient for NIV to assist.[101] An important general consideration is that NIV is not suitable for patients with advanced respiratory failure as evidenced by significant CO_2 retention and acidaemia.[100] Additional contraindications for NIV are listed in Box 21.3.

Equipment selection

There are many different ventilators through which NIV can be delivered, including those designed specifically for NIV; critical care ventilators designed for invasive mechanical ventilation; and portable positive-pressure ventilators designed for use in the home. The choice of ventilator will be dependent on availability and suitability for patient need.[94]

For pre-hospital responders any NIV device must be lightweight and compact, easy to use and not excessively expensive. A critical determinant is the need to be sparing in oxygen consumption given the limited capacity for gas storage. There are few such devices and these have only become available since about 2005.

In the ED, bilevel pressure-limited ventilators are the most common although critical care ventilators can also be used, some of which may have a specific NIV setting. Bilevel pressure-limited ventilators deliver pressure-assist or pressure-support ventilation. Bilevel ventilators deliver a pre-set inspiratory positive airway pressure (often referred to as IPAP) and positive end-expiratory pressure (often referred to as PEEP or EPAP). Support of ventilation is provided by the difference between these two set pressure levels. Most ventilators provide

a maximum pressure of 20–35 cmH_2O and have the capacity to deliver supplemental oxygen. What makes these ventilators particularly useful for NIV (where it may be difficult to achieve a leakproof seal with the mask) is the ability to increase inspiratory flow and provide leak compensation. Some bilevel pressure-limited ventilators have limited capability to delivery an FiO_2 above 0.50, and therefore may not be suitable for patients with hypoxaemic respiratory failure.

Bilevel pressure-limited ventilators differ from critical-care ventilators in that they usually have a single ventilator tube. This design may contribute to rebreathing and increased $PaCO_2$.[102] Rebreathing can be minimised by using masks with in-mask exhalation ports or non-rebreathing valves.[100] Ensuring the EPAP is greater than 4 cmH_2O provides higher flow during exhalation, which assists with removal of CO_2 from the mask and tubing.[102]

There are a variety of interfaces available and in an acute care setting it is useful to have a selection at hand so that the most appropriate mask can be rapidly applied. The oronasal mask is the most common mask used in the ED setting, although its use has been associated with leaks.[103] The advantages and disadvantages of patient interfaces used in NIV are listed in Table 21.5. The most common challenge with the patient interface is leak minimisation. Using a mask that is too large will often contribute to an increase in leaks.[104] As a general guide the smallest mask should be selected. When assessing best fit of nasal masks, the landmarks that should come closest to the interface are the nasal bridge, the skin on the side of the nares and just above the upper lip. For oronasal masks the landmarks should be just outside the sides of the mouth, the area just below the lower lip and the nasal bridge.[93] More recently, full-face masks have been developed that provide better patient comfort and tolerance and often fewer problems with air-leaks.

Initiation and management of NIV

The most important step in initiating NIV is patient education and emotional support from the nurse or paramedic. It is often useful to allow the patient, if they are able, to hold the mask in place in the initial stages of commencing NIV. To enhance patient comfort it is best to begin with lower pressure levels; inspiratory pressures of 8–12 cmH_2O and expiratory pressures of 4–5 cmH_2O may provide a useful starting point. Upward titration of these levels (by 1–2 cmH_2O with each adjustment) can occur as the patient begins to tolerate NIV.[105] NIV can be used with continuous positive airway pressure (CPAP), where only an expiratory pressure is applied, or with bilevel ventilation, which has both an inspiratory pressure and an expiratory pressure.[106]

Patient tolerance and comfort are key to successful use of NIV. Patient tolerance is identified through a decrease in the respiratory rate, and a reduction in inspiratory muscle activity and compliance with NIV itself. If these clinical signs are not evident, then steps should be made to improve tolerance. This may include refitting the mask, adjusting the ventilator settings and, most importantly, providing ongoing patient support. Ongoing patient monitoring should include heart rate, respiratory rate and pulse oximetry. After the patient has had an opportunity to adjust to NIV, an ABG may be taken to assess gas exchange. An improvement in PaO_2, $PaCO_2$ and pH should be evident. If the patient has chronic hypercapnia,

TABLE 21.5 Advantages and disadvantages of patient interfaces used in non-invasive ventilation[94,105]

INTERFACE	ADVANTAGES	DISADVANTAGES
Nasal mask	Easy to fit	Mouth leaks
	Less feeling of claustrophobia	Eye irritation
	Low risk of aspiration	Facial skin irritation
	Allows patient to cough and clear secretions	Nasal bridge ulceration
	Maintains ability to speak and eat	Oral dryness
	Minimal dead space	Nasal congestion
		Increased resistance through nasal passage
Facemask (oronasal mask)	Reduces air leakage through the mouth	Increased risk of aspiration
	Less airway resistance	Increased risk of asphyxia
		Increased dead space
		Claustrophobia
		Difficult to secure and fit
		Facial skin irritation
		Nasal bridge ulceration
		Patient must remove mask to eat, drink, expectorate
Total facemask	Reduced risk of pressure sores	Increased risk of aspiration
	Less claustrophobic	Increased risk of asphyxia
		Increased dead space

an improvement in $PaCO_2$ may occur over a longer period of time.[93]

Common problems encountered with NIV include mask-related problems, air-pressure and air-flow-related problems, air leaking and asynchrony. Suggested remedies are provided in Table 21.6. Occasionally patients may become restless during therapy. Some pre-hospital guidelines allow for mild sedation to facilitate providing respiratory support. Where this occurs great caution must be taken to ensure that consciousness and respiratory effort are not compromised. Sedation may also be used in hospital with the intention of allowing for application of therapy while maintaining the patient sufficiently awake,[108] however, the safety and efficacy of this practice remains in question with association with failure of NIV and increased mortality.[109]

Adjuncts to NIV include humidification of the gas. Excessive drying of the mucosa may occur during NIV and may contribute to patient discomfort and non-compliance. Humidification of inspired gases is generally recommended, except for patients with acute cardiogenic pulmonary oedema. Humidification should be achieved through the use of a passover-type heated humidifier, as heated bubble humidifiers and heat–moisture exchangers (HME) can increase airway resistance and the work of breathing.[94,110]

The initial stages of NIV may require considerable nursing time and expertise. Consequently, appropriate patient allocation should occur with, whenever possible, the nurse or paramedic providing care to the one patient only.[111]

When to initiate therapy in pre-hospital practice can require careful consideration. The usual intention of pre-hospital care is to safely convey a patient from place found to higher medical care. This movement itself can compromise patient presentation and create difficulties if attempting to provide concurrent care. Preferred posturing of the patient can be challenging as can the logistics of concurrent movement of equipment and ongoing therapies. It is sometimes more advantageous to settle patients with initial therapies, including NIV, then plan careful extrication and movement rather than a more hurried extraction. Movement of patients with NIV, oxygen cylinders and ongoing vital sign monitoring typically requires suitable equipment and sufficient personnel for the safety of all concerned. The patient with respiratory distress in particular can deteriorate with even mild exertion or if left briefly without sufficient respiratory support. Conveying patients to medical care is a balance between critical at-scene management and in transit therapies. The further balance of providing other concurrent therapies including sublingual, nebulised or intravenous medications must similarly be addressed during patient movement.

PRACTICE TIP

Nursing management and patient support is critical to the success of non-invasive ventilation. Pre-hospital movements of patients require careful planning, appropriate equipment and sufficient personnel for safety and effectiveness.

TABLE 21.6 Complications of non-invasive ventilation and possible solutions[94]

COMPLICATIONS	SOLUTION
Mask-related problems	
Discomfort	Decrease strap tension
Nasal redness, ulceration	Check mask fit
Poor fit	Try new mask
Air-pressure- and air-flow-related problems	
Sinus and ear pain	Lower mask pressure
Nasal dryness	Humidification
Nasal congestion	Decongestants, nasal steroids
Gastrointestinal insufflations	Lower pressures
Air leaks	
Under mask	Re-seat mask, tighten straps
Through mouth	Use chin strap to close mouth
Into eyes	Tighten straps, use new mask
Asynchrony	
Failure to trigger	New ventilator
Failure to cycle	Shorten inspiratory time
Failure to ventilate	Use leak-compensating ventilator

Invasive mechanical ventilation

The objectives of mechanical ventilation are to reduce respiratory distress and reverse acute respiratory failure. Patients who require respiratory support, but for whom NIV may not be appropriate, will require endotracheal intubation and mechanical ventilation (see Ch 15 for information about intubation and airway management, and Ch 17, p. 314, for techniques on applying airway management devices). Once intubated, a decision must be made regarding the most appropriate ventilation strategy for the patient:

- With full ventilator support the ventilator maintains effective alveolar ventilation irrespective of patient effort.
- Partial ventilator support is provided when the patient is capable of participating in work of breathing and contributes to maintaining alveolar ventilation.

In the ED the degree of respiratory distress may mean that full ventilator support is required. However, it is important that patient assessment occurs to avoid inappropriate use of full ventilator support, which may contribute to muscle wasting and atrophy.

Principles of mechanical ventilation

There are numerous mechanical ventilators in use across Australia and worldwide. Many EDs and EMS providers use critical-care ventilators which are commonly seen in the

intensive care setting, while others may use ventilators that have less versatility.[112] It is critical to appreciate the capabilities and limitations of the ventilator being used, as key features, such as spontaneous breathing and pressure support, may not be possible with the simpler devices.

Understanding the principles of mechanical ventilation enables healthcare providers to effectively and safely use a wide variety of devices. The four variables that are controlled during inspiration are pressure, flow, volume and time. The primary variable that the ventilator adjusts during inspiration is referred to as the control variable. When volume is controlled, the inspiratory pressure varies. Conversely, when pressure is controlled, volume and flow are variable. Because ventilators are microprocessor-controlled, the ventilator can change, breath by breath, which variable is controlled on inspiration.

There are four phases to the delivery of a single breath: the change from expiration to inspiration (commonly referred to as triggering); the inspiratory phase; the change from inspiration to expiration (commonly referred to as cycling); and exhalation. Table 21.7 provides a description of each phase of the respiratory cycle, and Table 21.8 provides a description of common breath-delivery strategies used in the ED.

Consideration also needs to be given to setting delivery parameters on the ventilator. The respiratory rate, tidal volume (or inspiratory pressure), FiO_2, positive end-expiratory pressure and inspiratory:expiratory ratio all need to be set. A general guide to setting ventilation parameters is provided in Table 21.9; however, clinicians are reminded that these settings will need to be modified with consideration for the patient's clinical condition, age and respiratory function. Healthcare practitioners who commonly work with ventilated patients and who make clinical decisions about ventilation strategies are encouraged to read more widely in this area.[114]

Management of the ventilated patient

While the ED is not designed to provide ongoing care to critically ill patients who require invasive mechanical ventilation, resource allocation at times prevents timely admission to the intensive care unit. For this reason it is imperative that a nurse working in the ED has a sound foundational knowledge of mechanical ventilation.[115,223] Patients who are receiving mechanical ventilation in the pre-hospital setting or ED are likely to have received sedation, analgesia and neuromuscular blockade. The effect of these drugs means that ventilated patients will require frequent and diligent fundamental care, including, but not limited to, mouth care, eye care, pressure-area care, positioning and psychological support (see Ch 14).[116] Specific issues that relate to the care of the ventilated patient include patient assessment, troubleshooting ventilation and transportation of the intubated and ventilated patient.

> **PRACTICE TIP**
>
> The importance of fundamental care for the mechanically ventilated patient, such as mouth care, eye care, pressure-area care and psychological support, should not be underestimated.

	TABLE 21.7 Phases of the respiratory cycle	
PHASE	DESCRIPTION
Beginning of inspiration— triggering	*Time-triggered* when the ventilator delivers a breath after a set time.
	Pressure-triggered when patient effort is sufficient to decrease circuit pressure to the pre-set pressure sensitivity level.
	Flow-triggered when the patient effort is sufficient to drop the flow in the circuit to the pre-set flow trigger level.
Inspiration	Inspiration occurs from the beginning of inspiratory flow until the beginning of expiratory flow.
	Pressure, flow, volume or time can be limited during inspiration. The variable is limited but this does not end inspiration.
	Pressure limiting allows pressure to rise but not to exceed the specified pressure. Pressure-limited breaths may be used where lung compliance is poor.
	Volume limiting establishes the maximum volume to be delivered. If patient lung compliance is poor, volume-limited breaths may be terminated before all volume has been delivered (to avoid generation of excessive airway pressures).
	Flow limiting is not in the interests of the patient, as this limits the flow of gas that can be received. Some older ventilators can limit flow (such as when a specified flow rate is set). More-modern ventilators allow patients to access increased flow to accommodate any increase in demand.
Beginning of expiration— cycling	Pressure, flow, volume or time can be the variable which cycles the breath out of inspiration, but only one can function for each individual breath.
	Volume and time cycling are not influenced by changes in lung compliance and may result in increased airway pressures.
	Pressure cycling is greatly influenced by lung compliance, and the volume delivered is dependent on the flow delivered, the length of inspiration, lung characteristics and the set pressure.
	Flow cycling functions on a pressure-supported breath in that the exhalation valve opens when a predetermined flow rate is reached.
Exhalation	Exhalation is passive. The baseline pressure can be altered and is usually positive.
	Positive end-expiratory pressure (PEEP) is usually applied as this helps to prevent early airway closure and alveolar collapse at end of expiration. The increase in functional residual capacity assists in improving oxygenation.

Patient assessment

The use of positive pressure ventilation has a direct effect on the pulmonary system, but also affects the cardiovascular, renal and other organ systems. Ongoing assessment of heart rate, temperature, blood pressure and physical examination of the chest are required in any patient receiving mechanical ventilation. Table 21.10 provides a summary of the physiological effects of positive pressure ventilation and related nursing assessment and management. Comprehensive information about assessment of the mechanically ventilated patient is discussed elsewhere.[117]

Assessment of respiratory support equipment

Assessment of equipment, including the ventilator, is a fundamental aspect of caring for the mechanically ventilated patient.[117] A self-inflating manual resuscitation bag with appropriate-sized face mask should be readily available and able to be quickly attached to supplemental oxygen. High-flow suction with a Yankauer sucker and endotracheal suction catheters need to be checked for availability and functioning. Checks should be made to ensure that the ventilator is connected to an uninterrupted power supply and that appropriate ventilator alarm limits have been set. Specific assessment of the endotracheal tube and humidification equipment should also be made.

Assessment of the endotracheal tube

Following intubation, the position of the endotracheal tube (ETT) should be assessed by chest radiograph. The tip of the ETT should be positioned approximately 5 cm above the carina. If the carina is not visible, the tip of the ETT should be positioned at the level of T3 or T4. Once confirmed, the nurse or paramedic should check markers on the ETT to determine the level at which the tube is inserted. This is measured as the distance from the tip of the ETT to the teeth, using the 1 cm gradated markings on the tube.

Pre-hospital assessment of endotracheal tube placement is more difficult but just as critical. Radiograph assessment is not available, but use of ultrasonography has been shown to be reliable.[118] End tidal carbon dioxide confirmation is 'gold standard' and should be available wherever intubation occurs.

TABLE 21.8 **Breath-delivery strategies in mechanical ventilation**		
BREATH-DELIVERY STRATEGY	**CLINICAL APPLICATION**	**NURSING IMPLICATIONS**
Continuous mandatory ventilation (CMV): can be pressure- or volume-controlled. Breaths are time-triggered.	Only appropriate if the patient cannot make the effort to breathe. This mode should not be used unless the patient is sedated and paralysed.	Patients on CMV may not be able to breathe spontaneously. If spontaneous drive is intact, distress may occur.
Assist-control (A/C) ventilation: can be pressure- or volume-controlled. Breaths are patient- or time-triggered. A minimum rate is set and the patient can trigger additional breaths if required.	A minimum breath rate is set and these mandatory breaths, plus any additional breaths, are delivered at the set volume or pressure (whichever is the control variable).	High rates in A/C ventilation may lead to hyperventilation and respiratory alkalosis.
Synchronised intermittent mandatory ventilation (SIMV): delivers a set rate and allows the patient to breathe spontaneously.	Mandatory breaths are time-triggered and deliver the set pressure or volume. Assisted breaths may be initiated by the patient and deliver the set pressure or volume. Patient effort and the level of pressure support determine the volume of spontaneous breaths.	Volume-control SIMV may result in increased airway pressures. If these exceed the pressure-alarm limits, pre-set volume may not be delivered. Pressure-control SIMV results in variable tidal volume. High tidal volume can contribute to volutrauma and hypocapnia. Low tidal volumes may contribute to hypercapnia and respiratory acidosis.
Pressure-support ventilation: a pre-set positive pressure is used to augment the patient's inspiratory effort. The patient controls the rate, inspiratory flow and tidal volume.	Pressure-support ventilation requires a stable respiratory drive and sufficient respiratory muscle strength to overcome airway and equipment resistance. May be used in conjunction with SIMV.	Patients must have an intact respiratory drive and sufficient respiratory muscle strength to generate a tidal volume sufficient for CO_2 clearance. With low rates or tidal volumes, hypoventilation may occur.
Continuous positive airway pressure (CPAP): on most ventilators, CPAP refers to spontaneous breathing with positive end-expiratory pressure.	As with pressure-support ventilation, CPAP requires a stable respiratory drive and sufficient respiratory muscle strength to achieve an acceptable tidal volume.	Hypoventilation may occur with low respiratory rates and low tidal volumes (or both). Patients will need to overcome circuit resistance and this increases work of breathing.

Secondary assessment tools, including chest and epigastric auscultation and pulse oximetry, should be considered as adjuncts only.

The ETT must be adequately secured to prevent accidental extubation or tube migration. Methods for securing the ETT vary and there is no evidence to suggest the best way to do so. Whatever method is used to secure the tube, careful consideration must be given to the potential for this to produce pressure areas or cause skin damage. Almost invariably patients will be moved in the pre-hospital setting. This makes securing the endotracheal tube a critical factor along with appropriate continuous supervision. Even minor patient head movements or inattentive pulling on equipment can cause tube displacement and continued vigilance is required. Each patient movement must be carefully coordinated by the airway supervisor. Following each movement correct tube placement should be reconfirmed. This should be finally affirmed on transfer of patient to destination facility with agreed confirmation provided by the airway attendant taking over responsibility. Patient tolerance of the ETT (and of ventilation itself) may vary, and often sedation is required to achieve patient comfort and tolerance of the tube and ventilator.

The high-volume, low-pressure cuff on the ETT is designed to prevent oropharyngeal secretions from entering the airway.

Cuff pressures should be kept below 25 cmH$_2$O to avoid mucosal damage.[119] The ETT cuff should be inflated using a minimal occlusion technique that adjusts cuff inflation volume so that during inspiration a leak around the ETT cuff cannot be heard. Enough air should be removed from the cuff to first identify the leak, and then volume slowly added until the leak just disappears. Cuff pressure should be assessed once per shift. Best practice for cuff measurement involves the use of a manometer attached to the ETT cuff balloon, to achieve cuff pressures of not more than 25 cmH$_2$O—the aim being to maintain the pressure below tracheal mucosal perfusion pressure (34 cmH$_2$O).[120]

Humidification equipment

During mechanical ventilation the upper airway is bypassed, and consequently inspired gases should be warmed and humidified.[121,122] This can be achieved using either a heat–moisture exchanger (Fig 21.2) or a heated humidifier (Fig 21.3). As the duration of mechanical ventilation increases, humidification becomes particularly important to prevent retention of secretions and maximise mucociliary function. Humidification systems have limitations to consider in use. They can contribute to dead space and increase airway resistance when used, adversely affecting patients by increasing the

	TABLE 21.9 Setting the ventilator[196,197]	
VENTILATOR PARAMETER	SETTING	RATIONALE
Tidal volume	6–10 mL/kg	The injured lung has reduced inspiratory capacity and is more susceptible to further damage as a result of increased volumes and pressures to the lung during mechanical ventilation. For patients with acute respiratory distress syndrome or similar bilateral alveolar processes, the lower end of this range (e.g. 6 mL/kg) should be used.
Respiratory rate	Hypoxic respiratory failure, 20–30 breaths/minute	In hypoxic respiratory failure, respiratory rates < 20 breaths/minute are usually poorly tolerated because of existing rapid shallow breathing.
	Hypercapnic respiratory failure, 8–15 breaths/minute	Ventilator respiratory rates should be closely set to the patient's requirements. Clinicians should be mindful of the contribution of respiratory rate to the overall minute ventilation and CO_2 removal.
	Asthma, 12–14 breaths/minute	High respiratory rates should be avoided as these contribute to the development of intrinsic PEEP. With a tidal volume of 8–9 mL/kg, respiratory rates below 12 breaths/minute have not demonstrated significant impact on gas trapping. Lower rates may be indicated when hyperinflation is marked or when small reductions in hyperinflation have significant clinical impact.
Inspiratory pressure	< 30 cmH_2O	Lung inflation beyond total lung capacity increases the chance of barotraumas (extra-alveolar air). At total lung capacity the transpulmonary pressure is 25 cmH_2O and the alveolar pressures are 35 cmH_2O. Consensus regarding the safety of pressures < 30 cmH_2O is lacking.
Inspiratory ratio	1:2 to 1:3	Longer inspiratory times will bring the I:E closer to 1:1 and may improve alveolar recruitment. However, this can be associated with adverse haemodynamic effects and is generally poorly tolerated by the patient (in the absence of sedation and paralysis).
Flow rate	40–90 L/min	Higher flow rates may be required for some patients and may improve comfort, decrease work of breathing and help slow the respiratory rate. Higher flow rates will increase the peak airway pressure, although most of this is dissipated along the length of the endotracheal tube. Flow waveforms can be selected on some ventilators. Selection of decelerating flow waveforms in volume ventilation will extend the inspiratory time.
Positive end-expiratory pressure (PEEP)	5–20 cmH_2O	There is general agreement that a PEEP > 5 cmH_2O should be used in patients with injured lungs, and in this group of patients a starting point of 10 cmH_2O should be considered. However, there is little consensus about target endpoints for PEEP. Adjustments to PEEP should be made during evaluation of ventilator graphics and evidence of lung recruitment.
Trigger sensitivity	Pressure trigger: 0.5–2.0 cmH_2O Flow trigger: 1–3 L/min	Triggering that is too sensitive to the patient's inspiratory effort will result in excessive breaths being delivered, or self-cycling of the ventilator. Insensitive triggering will result in increased work of breathing and patient anxiety or discomfort.
FiO_2	0.21–1.0	The FiO_2 should be adjusted to achieved the desired PaO_2 and SaO_2. Prolonged high levels of oxygen should be avoided if possible. Manipulation of PEEP increases mean alveolar pressure, and may also improve the PaO_2 and SaO_2.

I:E: inspiratory:expiratory ratio; FiO_2: fraction of inspired oxygen; PaO_2: arterial partial pressure of oxygen; SaO_2: arterial oxygen saturation

work of breathing, particularly where low tidal volumes are being used for lung protection.[121,122]

Troubleshooting and problem-solving mechanical ventilation

Ventilators, like other complex equipment, can contribute to and help identify problems. Alarm systems on ventilators are designed to identify when there might be a problem with the ventilator or the patient. The two most common alarms

are the high pressure and low pressure alarms. Reasons why these alarms might be triggered, and suggested management strategies, are given in Table 21.11.

Ventilators can also be the source of problems for the patient. The delivery of gas under positive pressure and imposition of mandatory breaths may be uncomfortable for some patients. Patient–ventilator dyssynchrony results when the delivery of ventilator breaths is no longer in synchrony with the patient's spontaneous respiratory effort, and may result

	TABLE 21.10 Physiological effect of positive pressure ventilation	
SYSTEM	**PHYSIOLOGICAL EFFECT**	**ASSESSMENT**
Cardiovascular	Increased pressure reduces venous return to the right heart, reducing right ventricular preload. Increased intrathoracic pressures and PEEP also reduce venous return to the left heart and reduce cardiac output.	Close monitoring of blood pressure, especially when ventilation is commenced or when inspiratory pressures are changed.
	Increased pulmonary vascular resistance, making the right ventricle work harder.	Closely monitor patients with known or suspected right ventricular compromise.
	Increased intrathoracic pressure may decrease coronary perfusion.	Monitor patients for signs of myocardial ischaemia.
Neurological	The decrease in cardiac output may result in a decrease in cerebral perfusion pressure (CPP). CPP may also be reduced because of an increase in CVP.	Patients at greatest risk are those with increased intracranial pressure and who may develop cerebral oedema.
Renal	Decreased cardiac output can lead to a decrease in renal blood flow and glomerular filtration rates.	Monitor urine output.
	Redistribution of blood flow within the kidneys so that flow to the outer cortex decreases and flow to the inner cortex and outer medullary tissue increases.	Monitor urine output and creatinine levels.
Liver and gastrointestinal	Decreased cardiac output, downward movement of the diaphragm against the liver, a decrease in portal blood flow and/or increase in splanchnic resistance may contribute to liver ischaemia.	Monitor liver function through blood chemistry.
	Increases in splanchnic resistance may contribute to gastric mucosal ischaemia.	Assess for clinically important gastric bleeding. Treat with histamine-2 receptor antagonists or proton pump inhibitors.
	Gastric distension may occur from swallowing air that leaks around the ETT cuff.	Assess gastric distension and insert a nasogastric tube as required.
Pulmonary	Barotrauma (subcutaneous emphysema, pneumothorax, pneumomediastinum, etc) can occur secondary to increased positive pressure.	Monitor peak airway pressure.
	Volutrauma occurs with overdistension of the alveoli.	Monitor tidal volumes. Tidal volumes of 4–10 mL/kg ideal bodyweight can be used for adults, and of 5–10 mL/kg ideal bodyweight for children. The lower range of tidal volume should be used when lung pathology is present.
	Hospital-acquired infections, such as ventilator associated pneumonia, may occur secondary to aspiration of subglottic secretions.	Respiratory assessment including chest X-ray is important. Prevention measures include mouth care, head-of-bed elevation 45°, suctioning subglottic secretions.

CVP: central venous pressure; ETT: endotracheal tube; PEEP: positive end-expiratory pressure

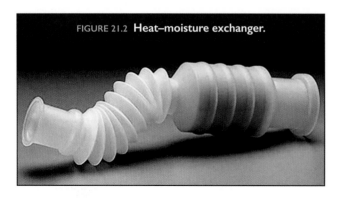

FIGURE 21.2 **Heat–moisture exchanger.**

in signs of respiratory distress or increased patient anxiety. Patient–ventilator dyssynchrony can result from patient- or ventilator-related problems.

Patient-related problems

There are many different patient-related problems that may contribute to the development of patient–ventilator dyssynchrony. One of the most common problems is the retention of secretions which increase work of breathing, and this is usually easily rectified by suctioning the endotracheal tube. Bronchospasm, normally managed with common bronchodilators, can result in increased work of breathing and the

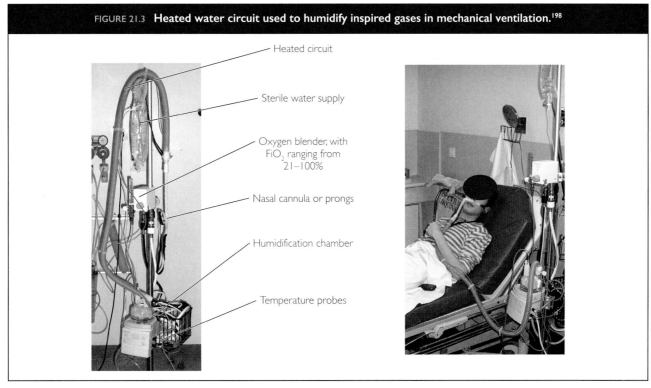

FIGURE 21.3 Heated water circuit used to humidify inspired gases in mechanical ventilation.[198]

- Heated circuit
- Sterile water supply
- Oxygen blender, with FiO_2 ranging from 21–100%
- Nasal cannula or prongs
- Humidification chamber
- Temperature probes

Shows the device of HFNC. Air and oxygen are mixed through a blender to achieve the desired Fio_2 and flow. The gas mixture is admitted to the humidification chamber where it is heated and humidified. It is then delivered to the patient via a heated circuit to avoid heat loss and condensation and finally via wide bore nasal prongs or cannula.

generation of high-peak inspiratory airway pressures and/or difficulty in delivering the set tidal volume.

General anxiety associated with endotracheal tube placement and the imposition of mechanical ventilation is usually well managed with low levels of sedation. It is important to determine the cause of patient–ventilator dyssynchrony in order to implement appropriate strategies to alleviate the problem. Increasing sedation is only appropriate when all other physical and mechanical problems have been investigated and corrected. For a more detailed discussion of patient-related problems, readers are encouraged to access publications that specifically focus on this topic.[124,125,197]

Ventilator-related problems

Ventilator-related problems include leaks, inadequate ventilator support, trigger sensitivity and inadequate flow. Leaks can occur within the ventilator circuitry, especially at the junctions where connections exist, or around the ETT cuff. Less commonly, the presence of a pleural drainage system can contribute to system leak. Before connecting the patient to a ventilator, a leak check should be performed to assess the system.[123]

Inadequate ventilator support may occur when the prescribed minute ventilation cannot be delivered. This can occur as a result of circuit leaks, or may be attributed to failure to deliver the prescribed tidal volume because peak inspiratory pressures have been reached.

Trigger sensitivity can be set too low or too high. When the trigger sensitivity is too low, autotriggering will result. Setting the trigger sensitivity too high means that, despite patient respiratory effort, the ventilator will not deliver a spontaneous or assisted breath. This can lead to a considerable increase in

work of breathing, patient discomfort and patient–ventilator dyssynchrony.

Inadequate flow can be identified by patient–ventilator dyssynchrony, increased respiratory effort and high negative pressures generated on inspiration. Increasing the flow rate or shortening the inspiratory time can rectify this. If a volume-control ventilation strategy is used, consideration should be given to changing to a pressure-control strategy.

Transporting the patient on mechanical ventilation

Patients who require mechanical ventilation in the ED are also likely to need to be transferred to the intensive care unit (ICU) or to other departments in the hospital for diagnostic tests or therapeutic procedures. When planning to transport a mechanically ventilated patient, it is important that time is taken to stabilise haemodynamics, oxygenation and ventilation. The team transporting the patient will be dependent on local policies, but should take into consideration the severity of illness and the degree of support required. Transport equipment should be lightweight, small, portable and rugged.[120]

Many hospitals have a common ventilator for use in the ICU and the ED. This simplifies transport somewhat, as the patient can remain on the one ventilator from initiation of mechanical ventilation to discontinuation. Additionally, the ventilator used for transport will not be limited in its capabilities. When selecting a ventilator for transport, the power source is an important consideration. Pneumatically powered and operated ventilators are preferable for transport, but consume gas to function and therefore may quickly deplete

TABLE 21.11 Ventilator alarms—causes and solutions

CAUSE	SOLUTION
Low-pressure alarm: should be set 5–10 cmH$_2$O below peak inspiratory pressure	
Patient disconnection	Reconnect patient to the ventilator
Circuit leaks	Check all connections are secure
	Assess ventilator tubing for cracks or holes
	Check exhalation valves are correctly seated
Cuff leak	Use minimum occlusion technique for inflating the ETT cuff
	Check pilot balloon
	Check position of ETT as migration into the upper airway (above the vocal cords) can cause leaking
Chest tube leaks	Assess degree of leak. Consider readjusting the low pressure alarm
High-pressure alarm: should be set about 10 cmH$_2$O above peak inspiratory pressure	
Coughing	Usually self-limiting and does not require treatment. Secretions loosened during coughing may need to be cleared by suctioning
Increased secretions	Suction as required
Patient is biting on the endotracheal tube (ETT)	Consider sedation or use of a bite block
ETT is kinked	Check ETT through visual inspection, and check on X-ray
ETT migration	Check position of ETT on X-ray
ETT cuff herniation	Attempt to pass a suction catheter. If unable to do so, deflate the ETT cuff and reposition the tube before reinflating
Heat–moisture exchanger (HME) blocked	Check and replace HME if indicated
Inspiratory circuit kinked	Assess ventilator tubing
Accumulation of water in the circuit	Drain circuit
Increased airway resistance	Auscultate the chest. Consider bronchodilators
Decreased compliance	Re-evaluate the ventilation strategy

the gas supply. If the ventilator is an electronically controlled device, consideration should be given to battery longevity.

In addition to the ventilator, a cardiac monitor, pulse oximeter, wave-form capnography, bag-valve-mask ventilation device and supply of pharmacology agents and intravenous fluids should be available. During transportation, airway management is of utmost concern and should be a responsibility dedicated to one member of the healthcare team. The person responsible for airway management should be skilled in emergency intubation. Transport of patients receiving mechanical ventilation therapy by pre-hospital responders varies considerably between primary and secondary transport and jurisdictions. Mechanical ventilation is usually restricted in primary roles to intensive care paramedics. Devices used often either lack complexity or have only a few of their capabilities used. Most commonly the purpose of ventilation for pre-hospital responders is to care for paralysed and intubated patients. The

key is to provide the patient with suitable respiratory rate and tidal volume sufficient to maintain suitable oxygen saturation and end tidal capnography. To this might be included PEEP as indicated in support of positive pressure ventilation.

Ventilators may also be used in secondary hospital transfers and patient retrievals. These transport teams may vary in discipline, including mixtures of paramedics, nurses and doctors. The complexity of ventilator used may vary depending on purpose.

The most common ventilator setting used is synchronised intermittent mandatory ventilation (SIMV). The value of this setting is that a predetermined baseline of ventilation will be provided, yet spontaneous breathing by the patient can be detected and allowed for by the device. Where this spontaneous breathing proves ineffective and problematic the patient may be paralysed to allow for better operator control. Paralysing patients, common in initial patient management by intensive care paramedics, reduces, but does not negate, the value of SIMV. As these patients are intubated the intrinsic autoPEEP formed by the glottis closing is lost. Typically a small amount of PEEP, usually 5 cmH$_2$O, is added to compensate for this. Another variable to be considered by paramedics is the fraction of inspired oxygen. Given the usual emergency nature of most calls the fraction is usually high and typically 1.0.

The device chosen will be restricted by the same problems that confront all pre-hospital equipment. It must be lightweight and compact. Even in a larger ambulance space is a premium with great competition to place the device near to the patient for immediate use. In sedans, helicopters and fixed wing aircraft size and weight becomes even more of an issue. Before embarking on any patient response a suitable oxygen supply must be ascertained. Typically this will include at least one and probably two 1500 mL cylinders with regulator attached. Similarly, battery life will have to be assured. Ideally, battery life will be long and beyond the anticipated duration of transfer. Spare batteries should be present and, where possible, the ventilator should be able to run on external power while in the vehicle.

Transferring intubated patients incurs some risk. The endotracheal tube can become dislodged with relatively small amounts of movement shifting from the trachea to the oropharynx or even oesophagus without being noticed. All movements should be coordinated by a team leader with secure hold of the endotracheal tube. The patient's head and body should be moved as one each time. It is frequently easier to disconnect the endotracheal tube briefly during movement to reduce any pressure that may be placed on it by hoses. If it is not disconnected the length of hose available must be inspected first to ensure that there is sufficient to accommodate the move. At the completion of each move the tube placement should be reconfirmed with capnography and chest auscultation. Monitoring devices must be kept close to the patient at all times during transfer, including pulse oximetry and end tidal capnography. The most appropriately qualified paramedic must remain constantly nearby to the patient's airway to maintain constant scrutiny of the endotracheal tube and ongoing ventilation. Concurrent management of the main presenting problems will usually continue whether primary response or secondary retrieval.

Acute pulmonary oedema

Acute pulmonary oedema (APO) is a pathophysiological state typified by fluid in the alveolar space, resulting in gas-exchange problems and decreased lung compliance.[125] APO is most commonly cardiogenic in origin as a result of heart failure.[4]

Assessment

On presentation most patients are normotensive or hypertensive; the presence of hypotension indicates a concurrent cardiogenic shock.[125] Patients demonstrating a thready pulse, pale or cyanosed skin and delayed capillary refill may be systemically hypo-perfused despite an adequate systolic blood pressure that is maintained by severe vasoconstriction.[126] Patients are commonly diaphoretic due to sympathetic activation.[126]

Left ventricular failure results in a decreased ventricular ejection fraction and a decrease in cardiac output.[127] Problems

with ventricular emptying result in increased left-side heart-filling pressures and a back-up of pressure into the pulmonary vasculature.[4] The increase in pressure within the pulmonary capillaries manifests as increased hydrostatic pressure (the mechanical force exerted by a fluid against the walls of a vessel). When the hydrostatic pressure exceeds the oncotic pressure (the osmotic pull of a fluid into a compartment), the fluid will begin to move out of the capillary into the interstitial space between the vessel and the alveolus.[4,128] At first, the fluid in the interstitium is removed via lymphatic drainage; however, when the movement out of the capillary exceeds the ability of the lymphatic system to remove it, the fluid then starts to move into the alveolar space.[4,128] When the alveolus is filled with fluid, it is no longer able to participate in gas exchange.[4] Alterations in gas exchange are reflected in reduced SpO$_2$, indicating hypoxaemia,[127] and increased PaCO$_2$. Hypoxaemia and hypercarbia, in conjunction, may be reflected in the patient being agitated, anxious, restless or have a decreased consciousness level.[125,127] The fluid within the alveolus and interstitium results in reduced pulmonary compliance and reduced functional residual capacity, and is reflected in clinical findings of dyspnoea and diffuse moist crackles on auscultation. Progression to peri-bronchial oedema may cause wheezing or rhonchi. Pulmonary oedema may cause the patient to have a productive cough producing white- or pink-tinged frothy sputum. The chest may be dull to percussion, especially over the bases. The patient strives to remain in an upright position,[125] and there is marked accessory muscle use with tachypnoea.[127] The left and right sides of the heart do not function in isolation from each other, so that failure of the left side of the heart will lead to deterioration in function of the right side, manifesting as lower limb oedema and raised jugular venous pressure.[125]

Non-cardiogenic pulmonary oedema is an uncommon phenomenon thought to be due to changes in pulmonary vascular permeability allowing excess fluid into the interstitial space, or problems with lymphatic drainage.[4] It can be precipitated by intra-cerebral events such as subarachnoid haemorrhage.

Diagnostics and monitoring

Consider including the following blood tests: full blood count to identify anaemia; electrolytes, urea and creatinine to identify electrolyte disturbances and renal function; consider troponin for evidence of myocardial injury.[127] An upright chest X-ray will aid differentiation of pulmonary oedema from other causes of dyspnoea. An early ECG is essential for recognition of dysrhythmia and for identification of acute coronary syndrome. Pulse oximetry allows a non-invasive indication of oxygenation.[127]

Pre-hospital recognition of the patient in acute pulmonary oedema must be made on rudimentary clinical examination findings. A past history of cardiac disease and previous episodes of pulmonary oedema can be helpful. Clinical findings of breathing difficulty when supine may be noted or be more prevalent at night. These presenting signs and symptoms may not be specific to acute pulmonary oedema.[130] Jugular venous distension may be observed. Audible crackles on chest auscultation may be heard, but these may be difficult to differentiate from infective crackles or overshadowed by other sounds such as wheezing.

Treatment

- *Oxygen therapy*—all patients presenting with APO should be given supplemental oxygen to match their needs.[125,130] This should be guided by pulse oximetry, and patients with oxygen saturations of 95% or more on room air do not need supplementation.
- *Nitrates*—nitrates initially cause venous dilation and reduction in preload.[125,127] At higher doses, nitrates precipitate arterial dilation leading to a concurrent decrease in afterload and resultant drop in systolic blood pressure.[125,130] Coronary artery dilation results in greater myocardial blood flow and oxygen delivery.[125,130] Overall, nitrates achieve decreased demand on the myocardium while increasing oxygen delivery.[125,130]
- *Ventilation support*—patients who have a severe decrease in consciousness level, agonal breaths or respiratory arrest require intubation and mechanical ventilation.[125,130] For patients not fitting the above exclusion criteria, NIV has allowed many to avoid intubation and its associated risks. The application of CPAP works by aiding the redistribution of intra-alveolar fluid and splinting the alveoli open, resulting in an increased area for gas exchange, increased lung compliance and a decrease in the work of breathing.[125,129] A Cochrane Review of recent studies in APO management using NIV, both CPAP and BiPAP, has recommended CPAP as the first choice in NIV strategy, as evidence supporting use of bilevel NIV for APO remains inconclusive.[129] CPAP is increasingly becoming the mainstay of pre-hospital management of acute episodes of APO with all other therapies taking on the role of adjunct therapies.[79–87]
- *Frusemide*—this is thought to decrease preload by initially causing venous dilation, and then increasing diuresis and a further reduction in preload.[125] Diuretics are recommended in patients with evidence of significant fluid overload;[130,131] however, caution is advised to avoid unnecessary diuresis in patients that are normovolaemic.[132] Loop diuretics have the potential to reduce glomular filtration rate and produce electrolyte disturbances; hence, although diuretics may aid in symptom relief, their impact on mortality has not been well studied.[131]
- *Opioids* are no longer a mainstay of treatment for acute pulmonary oedema. Morphine is primarily used to relieve chest pain resistant to nitrates.[125] Morphine also acts upon the sympathetic response and has anxiolytic properties. Resultant decreased heart rate, blood pressure, contractility and vasodilation cause a decrease in myocardial oxygen demand and workload.[125] Negative aspects of morphine that must be taken into consideration include respiratory and central nervous system depression; therefore the administration of morphine to patients with decreased conscious levels, hypotension or respiratory depression is not recommended.[125,126]

Disposition

In the majority of patients who respond to standard therapy, consider admission to a coronary care unit if there are ongoing cardiac issues such as pain and/or dysrhythmias, and close monitoring is still required. In other cases, such as elderly patients who have had a brief decompensation of chronic heart failure, admission to a non-monitored medical bed may be appropriate.[126]

Asthma
Assessment

Asthma is a common respiratory presentation characterised by bronchial hyper-responsiveness and inflammation that cause episodic reversible bronchospasm and increased mucous production and oedema.[4] This leads to widespread but variable airway obstruction that is often reversible, either spontaneously or with treatment.[133] Inflammation resulting in hyper-reactivity of the airways is the hallmark pathological feature of asthma.[4,133]

Allergen- or irritant-induced mast cell degranulation releases a large number of inflammatory mediators such as histamine, and chemotactic factors that cause bronchial infiltration by white cells.[4] These inflammatory mediators produce bronchial smooth muscle spasm, increased permeability, oedema formation, vascular congestion, mucous production and impaired mucociliary function.[4] The resultant airway obstruction causes resistance to air flow, increased physiological dead space, hyperventilation, air trapping and impaired gas exchange. This manifests as dyspnoea, wheeze, a feeling of chest tightness, cough, prolonged expiration,[133] hypoxaemia and hypercapnia and respiratory muscle fatigue.[4] Patients with long-term asthma have the potential to develop lung function impairment that becomes irreversible. This is not fully understood, but is thought to be different to COPD and independent of a smoking history.[134]

High-risk features in a clinical history include a previous serious episode of asthma requiring ventilatory support, or having taken a course of steroids within the last six months.[136] Physical assessment findings that highlight a potentially life-threatening episode include an inability to talk normally, a quiet or silent chest on auscultation, agitation or decreased level of consciousness (Table 21.12).[136] While peak expiratory flow rate (PEFR) or a FEV_1 < 80% of that expected is recognised also as an indication of severity, it is an impractical tool for use in the ED in patients who are markedly short of breath and in distress, and are simply unable to complete this test. Severity of asthma is defined by the ability for it to be controlled, particularly the medications required to do so, and is divided into untreated, difficult to treat and treatment-resistant severe asthma.[137] Severe asthma is also considered in terms of non-medication features of presentation including symptom frequency, the ability to become life-threatening and the severity of symptoms.[138] Severe asthma should have alternative diagnoses excluded, trigger factors removed and the patient should be compliant with medication. Where this has all occurred yet the asthma remains poorly controlled or there are more than two severe exacerbations per year or there is dependency on corticosteroids to avoid exacerbations, this is also considered severe asthma.[139]

Diagnostics and monitoring

In the pre-hospital setting, protocol-driven therapy is primarily in response to physical assessment findings. The level of assessment for pre-hospital responders is largely based on clinical observations. Audible wheeze and prolonged expiratory phase

	MILD/MODERATE:	SEVERE:	LIFE-THREATENING:
TABLE 21.12 Initial assessment of acute asthma in adults[141]			
Speech	Can finish a sentence in one breath	Can only speak a few words in one breath	Can't speak
Posture	Can walk	Unable to lie flat due to dyspnoea	Collapsed or exhausted
Breathing	Respiratory distress is not severe	Paradoxical chest wall movement: inward movement on inspiration and outward movement on expiration (chest sucks in when person breathes in) Use of accessory muscles of neck or intercostal muscles or 'tracheal tug' during inspiration Subcostal recession	Severe respiratory distress Poor respiratory effort (indicates respiratory exhaustion and impending respiratory arrest)
Consciousness	Alert	Alert	Drowsy or unconscious
Skin colour	Normal	Normal	Cyanosis
Respiratory rate	<25 breaths/min	≥25 breaths/min	≥25 breaths/min Bradypnoea (indicates respiratory exhaustion and impending respiratory arrest)
Heart rate	<110 beats/min	≥110 beats/min	≥110 beats/min Bradycardia (indicates impending cardio-respiratory arrest)
Chest auscultation	Wheeze or Normal lung sounds	Wheeze and reduced breath sounds	Markedly reduced breath sounds with few wheezes Silent chest
Oxygen saturation	>94%	90–94%	<90% Cyanosis
Blood gas analysis	Not indicated	Not indicated	PaO_2 <60 mmHg $PaCO_2$ >50 mmHg $PaCO_2$ within normal range despite increased work of breathing may indicate the patient is tiring and may need respiratory support pH <7.35

are important clues. Past history will be useful in diagnosis, as will perusal of current medications being taken. Of particular interest will be previous hospital and intensive care admissions as some form of guide to underlying severity and possible course of acute illness. Pulse oximetry is an adjunct to severity though is often not a great clue until the episode is severe. By this point other clinical findings such as consciousness, ability to speak freely and involvement of accessory respiratory muscles will provide more guide.

In the emergency setting, further investigations should be considered. In asthma of mild and moderate severity, investigations should be limited to spirometry or peak flow to compare lung volumes or flow rates with the predicted norm.[136] A chest X-ray is indicated if physical examination suggests possible pneumonia or pneumothorax.[136] In severe asthma, a chest X-ray is necessary. ABGs are not considered routine, but may be useful to gain a full respiratory picture in the following cases: SpO_2 < 92%; if the patient is not responding to treatment; if the patient is tiring; and if intubation is being considered.[133,136] In severe asthma, an ABG may initially show a respiratory alkalosis with hypoxaemia as the patient raises their respiratory rate to maintain oxygenation; as deterioration occurs, a respiratory acidosis will develop as airway obstruction worsens and the patient tires.[136]

Treatment

The management of asthma is determined by episode severity. Presentations of asthma are assessed against objective criteria into three classes of severity—mild, moderate and severe—as articulated by the National Asthma Council of Australia.[140] The mainstay of asthma management surrounds the administration of beta-2 agonists such as salbutamol for bronchodilation, a possible addition of ipratropium bromide and systemic corticosteroids.[136,141] Ipratropium bromide may relieve cholinergic bronchomotor tone and lessen mucosal oedema and secretions, resulting in bronchodilation, and can be delivered via metered-dose inhaler or nebulised.[142] Ipratropium is generally only recommended for severe exacerbations of asthma. Salbutamol can be delivered via metered-dose inhaler with a spacer, or nebulised. Both methods of delivery are equally efficacious, but for most situations delivery by metered-dose inhaler with a spacer has advantages over the nebuliser: it is faster to deliver the dose; it is cheaper; it can be taken home with the patient for continued treatment without the need to hire/buy expensive and cumbersome equipment as required for home nebulisation; it is safer for infection control as respiratory viruses can be transmitted by the nebulised aerosol to nearby patients or staff. However, in severe exacerbations of asthma the nebuliser is generally used as it is more practical for the delivery of continuous aerosolised salbutamol. Finally, salbutamol can be administered as an intravenous infusion in extreme cases, although it is unclear if this offers a benefit over continuous nebulised salbutamol. Corticosteroids can be given orally or intravenously and act upon the inflammatory cascade.[133,144] Other therapies include magnesium sulphate[145] and adrenaline. All offer some bronchial smooth muscle benefit but evidence is limited as to whether there is any advantage over nebulised or aerosol therapy. The most likely role is where the patient remains unresponsive or deteriorates following initial therapies.[144] Aminophylline is no longer considered a favoured drug but there may be some limited occasional role.[144]

Oxygen therapy to maintain an $SaO_2 > 95\%$ and ventilatory support are dictated by clinical need.[136] High concentration oxygen therapy has been shown to increase transcutaneous partial pressure of carbon dioxide during severe asthma exacerbation. Instead it should be titrated to provide the minimal oxygen therapy to maintain adequate pulse oximetry.[146] As with other respiratory presentations, there is growing evidence of a role for NIV in the management of acute, severe asthma with decreased drug therapy requirement and shortened hospital stays as observed benefits.[147] Heliox is a blend of helium and oxygen, and is thought to provide advantages in acute asthma due to better gas-flow dynamics.[136] A recent Cochrane Review concluded that the evidence did not support routine use of heliox in patients with acute asthma; however, it was stated that treatment with heliox may improve pulmonary function in the most severe acute asthma patients, in conjunction with other evidence-based treatments.[143,148] Management of adults with acute asthma can be seen in Table 21.13.

Disposition
Moderate and severe cases of asthma will require admission to hospital; severe cases responding poorly to therapy will require ICU admission. Mild cases of asthma, and moderate exacerbation responding promptly to therapy, typified by absence of physical exhaustion or decreased speech tolerance, pulse rate less than 100, normal oxygen saturation, variable wheeze intensity and $FEV_1 > 75\%$ of predicted,[135] can usually be discharged home after treatment in the ED and at least 1 hour of observation, and the formulation of a treatment plan.[136]

Chronic obstructive pulmonary disease

Chronic obstructive pulmonary disease (COPD) has been defined by the Global Initiative for Chronic Obstructive Disease (GOLD), a multinational collaboration sponsored by the World Health Organization, as pulmonary disease characterised by airflow limitation that is not fully reversible.[148] The airflow limitation is usually progressive and associated with an abnormal inflammatory response of the lungs to noxious particles or gas.[149]

Assessment

The continued division of patients with COPD into chronic obstructive bronchitis 'blue bloaters' and emphysema 'pink puffers' is outdated, as many patients do not fit within these stereotypes. However, most patients with COPD have a varying prominence of the two main pathologies of COPD: emphysema and chronic obstructive bronchitis.[150] Obstruction to airflow and decrease in FEV_1 is primarily caused by inflammation which is evident from the trachea down to the smallest peripheral airways that become progressively more scarred and narrow. Obstruction to airflow is further impeded by an increased number and size of mucous-secreting goblet cells that create mucous plugs.[150] Ability to clear bacteria and mucous is impeded by damage to the epithelium which impairs mucocilliary function. Lung parenchyma is damaged over time, most commonly in a pattern of centrilobular emphysema.[150] This is typified by a destruction of alveoli, loss of lung elasticity and collapse of small airways that require the support of surrounding connective tissues for patency during expiration. The decrease in lung elasticity and parenchymal destruction further contributes to airflow obstruction,[151] and causes problems with gas exchange.[150] Gas-exchange abnormalities produce hypoxaemia and hypercapnia.[151] Pulmonary hypertension may develop late in the progression of the disease, and this is attributed to hypoxic vasoconstriction of small pulmonary arteries.[148]

In patients where chronic obstructive bronchitis is the predominant pathology, cough is more prominent due to increased mucous production.[150] When coughing is vigorous, it results in expectoration of sputum. The presence of severe bronchopulmonary secretions is evidenced on auscultation by scattered crackles and wheeze, especially at the lung bases.[150] The primary symptom of airflow obstruction/limitation is chronic and progressive dyspnoea.[150] Gas exchange abnormality is often present with carbon dioxide retention, and hypoxaemia contributes to cyanotic appearance, and when hypoxaemia is severe may lead to decrease in consciousness level. If emphysema is a minor component, the anterior posterior diameter of the chest will be normal.[150]

When emphysema characteristics predominate, the patient is commonly thin, alert and orientated, dyspnoeic, tachypnoeic and using accessory muscles to ventilate.[150] They often assume a 'tripod' position, hunched forward to aid chest expansion, and create positive end expiratory pressure (PEEP) through pursed-lip breathing during exhalation. The additional PEEP provides increased intraluminal bronchial pressure and internal

TABLE 21.13 Initial management of adults with acute asthma[141]			
	MILD/MODERATE	SEVERE	LIFE-THREATENING
Immediately	Give 12 puffs salbutamol via MDI and spacer (100 mcg/puff)	Give 12 puffs salbutamol via MDI and spacer (100 mcg/puff) Use intermittent nebulised salbutamol (5 mg) if patient cannot breathe through spacer Drive nebuliser with air unless oxygen needed Provide oxygen if oxygen saturation less than 95% (titrate to target oxygen saturation of 92–95%)	Give continuous nebulised salbutamol (commence with 2 × 5 mg nebules. Keep the nebuliser chamber approximately half full by 'topping-up' with nebuliser solution) Start oxygen (if oxygen saturation less than 95%) and titrate to target oxygen saturation of 92–95% Ventilatory assistance if required (non-invasive ventilation; intubation/ventilation)
Re-assess response to treatment			
Over 1 hour	Repeat dose every 20 mins in the first hour (or sooner if needed)	Repeat dose every 20 mins in the first hour (or sooner if needed)	Continuous nebulisation until dyspnoea improves. Then change to intermittent bronchodilator therapy via MDI plus spacer or intermittent nebuliser
	If poor response, add ipratropium bromide 8 puffs via MDI and spacer (21 mcg/puff) Repeat every 4–6 hours as needed	Give ipratropium bromide 8 puffs via MDI and spacer (21 mcg/puff) or 500 mcg nebule via nebuliser added to nebulised salbutamol every 20 minutes for the first hour	Give ipratropium bromide 8 puffs via MDI and spacer (21 mcg/puff) or 500 mcg nebule via nebuliser added to nebulised salbutamol every 20 minutes for the first hour
	Give steroids. Oral prednisolone 37.5–50 mg then continue 5–10 days OR If oral route not possible hydrocortisone 100 mg IV every 6 hours		
Re-assess response to treatment			
Consider add-on treatments for persisting severe or life-threatening asthma		IV magnesium sulphate 2 g (20 mmol) infused over 20 minutes IV salbutamol Loading dose 5 mcg/kg/min over 1 hour, then 1–2 mcg/kg/min Non-invasive positive pressure ventilation Consider if starting to tire or signs of respiratory failure If no improvement, intubate and start mechanical ventilation	

MDI: metered dose inhaler

support for bronchial walls that have decreased support due to destruction of surrounding connective tissues.[150] Parenchymal destruction and loss of elasticity results in gross overinflation of the lungs, increased antero-posterior thorax diameter and a low diaphragm. Percussion of the chest demonstrates hyper-resonance, while decreased breath sounds are heard during auscultation. The patient experiences dypsnoea due to extensive lung parenchyma destruction; however, near-normal ABG values are maintained, while increased mucous production contributes to clinical features of productive cough.[148]

Diagnostics and monitoring

Pulse oximetry is used to evaluate the oxygenation status[152] and spirometry can be used to confirm degree of obstruction.[152] An ECG should be taken to identify concurrent dysrhythmias, ischaemic changes and right-side heart hypertrophy.[149] A chest

X-ray helps to rule out alternative diagnoses that can mimic an exacerbation and to identify the presence of co-existing diseases requiring specific interventions, e.g. pneumonia, pneumothorax or pleural effusion.[152] An ABG is not universally indicated; however, in a severe exacerbation, one may provide information regarding acute versus chronic gas-exchange problems and monitor improvement or deterioration against interventions.[152]

Other tests that may be useful, but will have little effect on initial management in the acute setting, include full blood count to identify polycythaemia and raised white cells, and assessing serum electrolyte levels for abnormalities.[152]

Management

- Oxygen therapy—this remains the cornerstone of acute treatment of COPD. However, there is growing evidence regarding more controlled and targeted administration.[60,140] For the hypoxic patient it is critical that sufficient oxygen is administered to correct oxygen deficits. This oxygen therapy should be titrated to the minimum delivery to maintain tolerable pulse oximetry between 88% and 92%.[60] This has been shown to significantly reduce the risk of respiratory failure and mortality when compared with high-flow oxygen therapy and is particularly applicable to pre-hospital responders in acute emergencies.[56] Uncontrolled oxygen administration can lead to hypercapnia.[153] In non-emergency situations supplemental oxygen therapy to assist with normal daily life and activity is considered differently and plays an important role in maintaining activity and quality of life.[154] For most patients, this targeted oxygen therapy will not produce clinically significant CO_2 retention.[152]

- Ventilation—the use of NIV, both CPAP and BiPAP, has provided consistent positive results in acute respiratory failure.[149] NIV improves respiratory acidosis, decreases the work of breathing, decreases respiratory rate and dyspnoea and also, importantly, decreases rates of intubation.[140] For some patients, the use of invasive ventilation may be more appropriate. If volume ventilation is used, it is recommended that the tidal volume not exceed 7–9 mL/kg. An inspiratory to expiratory (I:E) ratio of 1:3 should also be used to avoid the development of cumulative air-trapping.[152] This phenomenon (also known as breath stacking) is due to the collapse of small airways during expiration which traps air in the distal lung airspaces. If the expiratory time is too short to allow this gas to escape, more air becomes trapped with each breath leading to progressive hyperinflation of the lungs. The increased intrathoracic pressure can impair venous return to the heart and, in extreme cases, cardiac arrest. If air-trapping is such that haemodynamic compromise results, then fluid resuscitation may be indicated to maintain adequate preload and cardiac output.[152] However, measures to reverse the air trapping need to be addressed. This may include reducing ventilator PEEP to zero, reducing the respiratory rate and increasing the expiratory phase of the respiratory cycle. In extreme situations external manual thoracic compression in time with expiration can be attempted, although the effectiveness of

this technique has not been well studied. Air trapping may develop more readily in the patient with COPD because of changes in pulmonary flow resistance, expiratory flow limitation and decreased respiratory system compliance.[155]

- Bronchodilators—these are used because of a possibility of a small reversible component of the airway obstruction.[152] Beta-2 agonists, such as salbutamol, and an anticholinergic agent, such as ipratroprium bromide, are the most commonly used agents.[152] Variation in responsiveness to bronchodilators appears to be inversely related to the severity of the COPD and not all patients will benefit from bronchodilator therapy.[156] Bronchodilator therapy is an appropriate starting point for therapy; however, alternative therapy options such as NIV should be considered where necessary.

- Glucocorticosteroids are recommended as an addition to other therapies in an acute exacerbation.[148]

- Antibiotics may be indicated if specific symptoms exist of increased sputum production and increased purulence of sputum, and for patients who require mechanical ventilation for the exacerbation.[148]

- Exertion should be kept to an absolute minimum during acute exacerbations. This is particularly so for pre-hospital responders where movement of the patient will be imposed. Transfer should involve the use of lifting devices, wheelchairs and mobile stretchers. Patient sliding or standing self-transfers or standing, ambulation or positioning the patient in any way other than their own preference are all capable of worsening breathing difficulty and causing patient deterioration.

Disposition

A decision regarding admission is based upon the severity of exacerbation, how well the patient responds to therapy and how easily correctable the precipitating factor is.[152] For discharge home, the emergency care provider must ensure appropriate social support, including a check that home conditions are suitable and that follow-up care, such as community nursing or a respiratory chronic care program, has been organised.

Pneumonia

Pneumonia is an infection of the lower respiratory tract caused by bacteria, viruses and other organisms. Many individuals in the community are susceptible to the development of pneumonia, particularly the elderly. Other factors that increase the risk of pneumonia include immune system compromise, alcoholism, smoking, malnutrition and immobilisation.[4] Table 21.14 lists conditions that may predispose the patient to pneumonia. Community-acquired pneumonia is likely to be the most common type of pneumonia seen in the ED. Causative organisms include *Streptococcus pneumoniae* which can be identified in approximately 14% of presentations, *Mycoplasm pneumoniae* (9%) and viral pathogens such as influenza (15%).[158]

In the context of community-acquired pneumonia, airborne pathogens released through coughing and sneezing can be inhaled and enter the respiratory system. Airborne pathogens can also be released from aerosolised water. An example of this is when cooling towers are implicated in an outbreak of *Legionella* infection.

TABLE 21.14 Precipitating conditions of pneumonia[158]	
CONDITION	AETIOLOGIES
Depressed epiglottal and cough reflexes	Unconsciousness, neurological disease, endotracheal or tracheal tubes, anaesthesia, ageing
Decreased ciliary activity	Smoke inhalation, smoking history, oxygen toxicity, hypoventilation, intubation, viral infections, ageing, COPD
Increased secretions	COPD, viral infections, bronchiectasis, general anaesthesia, endotracheal intubation, smoking
Atelectasis	Trauma, foreign-body obstruction, tumour, splinting, shallow ventilations, general anaesthesia
Decreased lymphatic flow	Heart failure, tumour
Fluid in alveoli	Heart failure, aspiration, trauma
Abnormal phagocytosis and humoral activity	Neutropenia, immunocompetent disorders, patients receiving chemotherapy
Impaired alveolar macrophages	Hypoxaemia, metabolic acidosis, cigarette smoking history, hypoxia, alcohol use, viral infections, ageing

COPD: chronic obstructive pulmonary disease

The first line of defence is the protective mechanisms of coughing and mucociliary clearance. If organisms are able to bypass these, alveolar macrophages are the next line of defence—but this will only be effective if the virulence and load of the bacteria or virus is low. If this defence is not effective, then the immune system will be activated. Release of inflammatory mediators and immune complexes damage bronchial mucous membranes and alveolocapillary membranes, causing the terminal bronchioles to fill with debris and exudates and results in patients experiencing dyspnoea, pleuritic chest pain, cough with expectoration of purulent sputum, crackles or wheezing and bronchial breath sound on auscultation. Changes in ventilation–perfusion matching contribute to hypoxia. CO_2 levels may remain normal, as it diffuses more easily than oxygen. Pre-existing respiratory compromise may further compromise and complicate the patient's clinical presentation. It is important to remember that the elderly and those with weaker immune systems may have fewer and less-severe symptoms, or non-specific symptoms such as acute confusion/delirium or deterioration of baseline function.

Diagnostics and monitoring

Pulse oximetry is used to evaluate the oxygenation status.[148,152] A chest X-ray will demonstrate one or more areas of airspace opacification, and helps to rule out alternative diagnoses. Patients with a pleural effusion greater than 5 cm on an upright posterior–anterior chest X-ray may be considered for a diagnostic thoracocentesis with fluid sent for cell count, pH, culture and Gram stain.[152,160]

A full blood count may demonstrate an elevated white count; however, this information rarely alters diagnostic or management decisions. Creatinine and electrolytes are useful in the elderly to determine renal function, which may alter dosing of drugs that are eliminated by the kidneys. Sputum cultures, which take 24–48 hours for results, rarely change the choice of antibiotics already made, and are not routinely required. They may be useful in patients at risk of unusual pathogens, such as those with pre-existing chronic lung disease (e.g. bronchiectasis, cystic fibrosis) and immunocompromised patients. Blood cultures are not routinely required although may be considered for higher-risk patients admitted with community-acquired pneumonia.[159] For young patients who are otherwise healthy and have an uncomplicated case of pneumonia, testing can be limited to a chest X-ray and pulse oximetry.

Management

The vast majority of patients with community-acquired pneumonia can be treated successfully with narrow-spectrum beta-lactam treatment, such as penicillin combined with doxycycline or a macrolide.[158] Pneumonia of a viral origin may be treated with antivirals. Patients who are severely affected may require supportive therapy, such as NIV or invasive ventilation.

The majority of patients presenting with pneumonia are able to be managed outside the hospital environment, with approximately 20% of pneumonia patients being admitted.[161]

PRACTICE TIP

'RED FLAGS' INDICATING SEVERE COMMUNITY-ACQUIRED PNEUMONIA REQUIRING HOSPITAL ADMISSION[165]

Clinical

Respiratory rate greater than 30 breaths/min
Systolic blood pressure less than 90 mmHg
PR > 125 beats/min
Oxygen saturation less than 92%
Acute onset confusion

Investigations

Arterial (or venous) pH less than 7.35
Partial pressure of oxygen (PaO_2) less than 60 mmHg
Multilobar involvement on chest X-ray

An assessment of pneumonia severity is essential to inform decisions regarding the need for admission. Refer to the Practice Tip below (red flags indicating severe CAP requiring hospital admission) for 'red flags' in clinical features and investigations that should prompt hospital admission.

Australian studies have developed two severity scoring systems—CORB and SMART-COP—to aid disposition and management decisions of community-acquired pneumonia in adults. These scales are based on predictors of likely requirement of intensive respiratory or vasopressor support, and direct attention to clinical features that predict clinical deterioration, and are therefore now the preferred tools for assessing pneumonia severity.[164] Patients considered for treatment outside the hospital environment should not display high-risk features and should score mild severity or mild–moderate severity on one of the scoring systems.[161]

Pulmonary emboli

Pulmonary emboli cause occlusion of the pulmonary vascular bed. Thrombi, tissue fragments, lipids, foreign bodies and air bubbles can all cause emboli, although the vast majority of emboli occur as a result of deep vein thrombosis.[4] Risk factors for the development of pulmonary emboli are therefore linked to deep vein thrombosis formation and also include hypercoagulability, venous stasis and injuries to the endothelial lining of blood vessels.

Pathophysiology

The impact of the embolism is dependent on the size of the emboli and how much blood flow is obstructed. Emboli can cause massive occlusion, such as to the pulmonary artery, and can contribute to infarction of lung tissue. Some patients may develop multiple emboli and experience recurrent pulmonary emboli.

Occlusion of the pulmonary circulation results in ventilation–perfusion mismatch. Hypoxic vasoconstriction, decreased surfactant, atelectasis and the development of pulmonary oedema all contribute to the alterations in ventilation–perfusion matching.

Approximately 90% of patients with non-infarcting PE experience dyspnoea. This is most likely the clinical manifestation caused by ventilation–perfusion mismatch where alveoli are ventilated but not perfused. This same V/Q mismatch is also the likely primary cause of hypoxaemia in a patient with PE, although not all patients experiencing a PE will actually be hypoxaemic.[166]

If the PE is large enough to result in occlusion of an artery leading to tissue necrosis, the patient can experience a sharp, pleuritic, focal chest pain. In later days after infarction, the infarcted section of lung tissue will become consolidated on chest X-ray and develop a pleural effusion due to the accompanying inflammatory process.[166]

When a PE obstructs >50% of vasculature, it can result in increased right ventricular pressure, and in the most severe cases arterial hypotension can eventuate. This is associated with a four-fold increase in risk of death.[166]

Diagnostics and monitoring

Diagnosis of pulmonary emboli (PE) starts with an estimation of probability. Patient history is important, and questioning should focus on risk factors for pulmonary emboli and deep vein thrombosis. The most commonly used tool to aid decision making is the 'Wells criteria/scoring for PE' (Table 21.15).[167]

A second very useful clinical decision aid that works in concert with the Wells scoring system is the pulmonary embolism rule out criteria (PERC) rule. In patients who are considered unlikely to have a pulmonary embolism, the PERC rule can be applied to rule out a PE based on clinical criteria alone, avoiding the problems associated with the frequent false positive D-dimer test. The PERC rule consists of eight items, all of which must be answered 'No' to rule out a PE. The items are age ≥50, pulse rate ≥100, oxygen saturation <95%, previous history of DVT or PE, recent trauma or surgery, haemoptysis, drug therapy containing oestrogens and unilateral leg swelling.[168,169]

The chest X-ray rarely shows diagnostic features for PE, but is useful for detecting alternative causes for the patient's symptoms, such as pneumothorax, pneumonia and cardiac failure. Arterial blood gases may be taken and may show hypoxaemia and hypocarbia. In patients considered unlikely to have a PE on Wells risk criteria but who cannot have PE ruled out using the PERC rule should have a D-dimer test. If positive, further testing is required to make the diagnosis. Ventilation–perfusion lung scan is a useful modality in young patients with no pre-existing lung disease and a clear CXR, and may be the preferred test in this population due to the lower radiation exposure. For other patients, spiral computed tomography (CT) is more useful in making the diagnosis of pulmonary emboli, and has the added benefit of identifying alternative diagnoses such as pneumonia and aortic dissection. Echocardiography may be used for rapid and accurate risk-stratification of patients with pulmonary embolism.[162]

Management

Prevention is the best strategy for managing pulmonary emboli. If pulmonary emboli are diagnosed, anticoagulant therapy

---

TABLE 21.15 Wells criteria and scoring for pulmonary embolism

PRESENT	SCORE
Clinical signs and symptoms of DVT	+3
PE is No. 1 diagnosis or equally likely diagnosis	+3
Heart rate >100	+1.5
Immobilisation at least 3 days, or surgery in the previous 4 weeks	+1.5
PREVIOUS	
Objectively diagnosed PE or EVT?	+1.5
Haemoptysis?	+1
Malignancy with treatment within 6 months, or palliative?	+1

Pre-test clinical probability of a PE:

Wells Score > 4: PE likely, consider diagnostic imaging

Wells Score ≤ 4: PE unlikely, consider D-dimer to rule out PE

(heparin, warfarin, or both) will usually be prescribed. Patients are increasingly being treated with new oral anticoagulants (e.g. dabigatran, rivaroxiban, apixaban) which have the benefit of rapid onset of action and no need for blood testing to monitor the level of anti-coagulation. If the pulmonary emboli are life-threatening, pulmonary angiography may be used to locate and extract the emboli or inject thrombolytic agents to dissolve the clot. If thrombolysis is contraindicated, surgical embolectomy may be required.[169] There is limited evidence on the efficacy of using vena caval filters to trap emboli from deep veins.[170]

Disposition

Haemodynamically unstable patients, or those with significant hypoxia, should be admitted to ICU. The majority of patients diagnosed with a pulmonary embolism can be admitted to a ward; however, early discharge home with low-molecular-weight heparin can be considered with small pulmonary emboli.[171]

Respiratory outpatient care programs

Various models of outpatient respiratory care programs have been developed in different locations. The aim of these programs may incorporate some or all of the following areas: to facilitate early discharge from hospital with follow-up care in the home; development of action plans to guide management of future exacerbations, thereby reducing admission rate; provide pulmonary rehabilitation services, and specialist review services within the home or hospital for acute exacerbations.[172] Successful respiratory care programs have been instrumental in decreasing hospital presentation and admission rates for chronic respiratory patients, and decreasing hospital length of stay for some patients by continuing therapy post-discharge in the home.[172]

If a patient is involved with a respiratory outpatient program, early contact should be made with the program to enable input towards management, and determine what supports are available in the home environment. Early liaison with the respiratory outpatient program may present other options for management than admission to an acute hospital bed.

Inhalation injuries

Three factors to consider when evaluating a patient with an inhalation injury are exposure to asphyxiants (carbon monoxide, cyanide), thermal or heat injury of the airways (see Ch 28) and inhalation of pulmonary irritants (smoke particles and other gases produced by a fire). Exposure to asphyxiants is the most frequent cause of early mortality, with carbon monoxide (CO) the most frequent asphyxiant from a fire.

Carbon monoxide

Carbon monoxide is extremely common, being produced by the incomplete combustion of carbon-containing fuels, including petrol, coal, wood and gas. It is produced in domestic heating, motor vehicles, industry and cigarette smoking. It is also produced naturally within the body as a byproduct of haemoglobin breakdown. It has no colour, no smell and cannot be detected by human senses. It diffuses into the lungs in a similar way to oxygen, but has an affinity for attaching to haemoglobin over 200 times greater forming carboxyhaemoglobin. Carbon

monoxide also binds to key proteins within the mitochondria of cells that use oxygen for the production of cellular energy (ATP). Cellular respiration is impaired by the failure to deliver expected quantities of oxygen attached to haemoglobin, and the inability of cells to use the oxygen that is delivered. Oxygen that diffuses into the blood remains highly reactive and is more available to form unwanted radical substances. The resultant cellular changes and dysfunction include inflammation, capillary changes and oedema. These are most notable in the brain where susceptible oxygen-demanding tissue can be found including white matter, cerebral cortex and basal ganglia.[174-176]

Significant exposure, such as from a suicide attempt or exposure to smoke from house or building fire, will typically raise suspicions of carbon monoxide exposure. In other instances, such as a malfunctioning gas heater, it may be completely unrecognised or overlooked. There may be clues that help, such as other people or animals being unwell or being winter time with obvious heater usage increase. Patients who may also appear to improve and then have a return of symptoms in certain locations can assist with identifying the cause.[174]

Exhaust fumes containing carbon monoxide was once a well-recognised method of committing suicide; however, changes to vehicle emission laws have produced a steady reduction in available gas and resultant fatalities.[177]

Carboxyhaemogloblin (COHb) levels greater than 10% may indicate smoke inhalation; however, smokers or individuals exposed to automobile exhaust fumes can have baseline COHb levels of 10–15%. Fetal haemoglobin binds even more quickly with CO, so the fetus is at greater risk for injury from smoke inhalation.

The signs and symptoms of acute CO poisoning can be related to the concentration at the time of exposure. Acute exposure to CO usually causes central nervous system and cardiovascular toxicity. Tissues in these regions have high blood flow and oxygen demand. Table 21.16 summarises the signs and symptoms and Table 21.17 summarises the clinical features of CO poisoning.

TABLE 21.16 Signs and symptoms related to carboxyhaemoglobin (COHb) level at time of exposure to CO[186]

COHb LEVEL (%)	SIGNS AND SYMPTOMS
0	None
10	Frontal headache
20	Throbbing headache, shortness of breath on exertion
30	Impaired judgement, nausea, fatigue, visual disturbances, dizziness
40	Confusion, loss of consciousness
50	Seizures, coma
60	Hypotension, respiratory failure
70	Death

TABLE 21.17 Clinical features of carbon monoxide poisoning[186]

SYSTEM	SYMPTOMS	PATHOLOGY	DIAGNOSTIC
Central nervous system	Early—confusion, coma, seizures	Brain oedema, encephalopathy	EEG
	Late—psychoses, dementia, parkinsonism, ataxia, peripheral neuropathy, gait disturbance	Cerebral atrophy, basal ganglia lesions	CT scan
Cardiac	Dysrhythmias, hypotension angina, tachycardia	Myocardial ischaemia	ECG, CK, CK–MB, troponin
Pulmonary	Shortness of breath	Pulmonary oedema	Chest X-ray
Ophthalmological	Visual disturbances	Flame-shaped retinal haemorrhages, cerebral lesions, retrobulbar neuritis, papillo-oedema	Fundoscopy
Renal	Acute failure	Myoglobinuria	Renal function tests, serum myoglobin, urine myoglobin
Muscular	Ischaemia	Compartment syndrome, rhabdomyolysis	
Auditory and vestibular	Hearing loss, nystagmus, tinnitus		

CK: creatine kinase; CK–MB: creatine kinase–MB enzyme (primarily produced by the heart muscle); CT: computed tomography; ECG: electrocardiogram

Diagnosis of CO poisoning

The presenting signs and symptoms of carbon monoxide poisoning are often vague and non-specific. They can be easily confused with or dismissed as other problems. Even severe illness can be mistaken for another diagnosis, including stroke and seizure.[178] The most common initial complaints are fatigue, nausea, headache and dizziness.

Neurological signs include confusion and anxiety. Ataxia and vision impairment can develop. Reduced consciousness with decreasing GCS score and convulsions occur at higher levels of exposure. Even after recovery some of these complaints can persist for several weeks with reports of symptoms persisting beyond 1 year.[174,176] The onset of Parkinsonism following exposure has been described.[179,180] Even in patients who present with only mild acute exposure to carbon monoxide, symptoms of headache and dizziness can continue for more than 4 weeks.[181]

Early cardiovascular signs of tachycardia and hypertension are frequently noted.[179,182] Myoglobin has an even stronger affinity for carbon monoxide. This increases the likelihood of cardiovascular problems.[178,183,184] Angina, hypotension and myocardial infarction can be caused by significant carbon monoxide exposure. Acute pulmonary oedema can occur.[32,174,179,182]

Cardiovascular complications can be loosely divided into two different groups. The first is the younger comparatively healthy patient with significant signs of cardiac failure following exposure to large concentrations of carbon monoxide. The second is the person with existing coronary artery disease exacerbated by lesser concentrations.[32,182] Cardiovascular signs and symptoms commonly suggest higher exposure levels in acute incidents.[185] Death from carbon monoxide that occurs very quickly is likely to be due to lethal dysrhythmia following myocardial ischaemia.[183]

Carboxyhaemoblobin is a redder colour than oxyhaemoglobin and this has led to the belief that redness in skin colour can be useful in diagnosis. This is not, however, of any use in assessment as the redness only becomes apparent when concentrations become near lethal.[187]

The diagnosis of carbon monoxide poisoning is based on a history of exposure to the gas, the presence of symptoms of exposure and a finding of elevated carboxyhaemoglobin level in the blood. Venous and arterial blood will have the same reading.[187] Patient presentations may be varied where there were other gases also exposed, such as cyanides that can be found in house fires. The diagnosis of CO poisoning should be considered whenever multiple members of the same family or from the same workplace present with non-specific symptoms, especially headache within 24 hours of each other.

Carboxyhaemoglobin levels in non-smokers are normally close to zero of total haemoglobin. Light smokers may have 1% and heavy smokers as much as 15% as a normal finding. After 3% high-risk groups, including the elderly, those with cardiovascular disease and children, will begin to show effects.[183,188] Children may recover more quickly and this is most likely to be due to increased minute ventilation.[174,176] Pregnant women have increased risk with the fetus having even greater affinity than adults.[174,185,189] In non-smokers 10% will usually produce symptoms; by the time 25% produce symptoms severe poisoning will have occurred, and loss of consciousness and fatality will have occurred by 40%.[189]

Evaluation of blood levels of carboxyhaemoglobin is an accurate way to determine levels. Devices that can measure exhaled levels of carbon monoxide are also accurate.[173,189]

However, the correlation between levels found in the blood and presentation is unreliable. This is because as soon as exposure ceases, carbon monoxide begins to disassociate from haemoglobin and is exhaled. This process is faster if the patient is given oxygen, for example, while being transported by ambulance to hospital. By the time a blood sample is taken in hospital the carboxyhaemoglobin level may have decreased substantially. Severe presentations can therefore have comparatively low measured levels of carbon monoxide and clinical improvements in presentation do not always correlate with clearance.[31]

Pulse oximeters are unable to differentiate between oxyhaemoglobin and carboxyhaemoglobin. This makes them useless for determining severity of exposure and unreliable at providing oxygenation information.[174,187] There is commercially available carbon monoxide pulse oximetry (SpCO) but while they are potentially useful their reliability remains in question.[31,187,191,192] However, where these are used and readings are obtained their use as a guide to exposure should be supported by clinical examination and detailed history.

Management

Pre-hospital management of the patient exposed to carbon monoxide is comparatively simple and straightforward. The first key is to remove the patient from further exposure. Increasing the partial pressure of oxygen available will displace carbon monoxide bound to haemoglobin. High-concentration oxygen therapy should be utilised with either a non-re-breathing mask or bag-valve-mask with high-flow oxygen therapy attached.[31,174,176,189]

Hyperbaric oxygen therapy involving high concentrations of oxygen delivered under greater than atmospheric air pressure is supported but controversial. Numerous studies have demonstrated a variety of patient improvements in both short- and long-term evaluations.[176,193] That said, a Cochrane review was less definitive in regard to any advantage of such therapy.[194,195] Hyperbaric oxygen administration has been shown to reduce the half-life of carboxyhaemoglobin from 320 minutes to 80 minutes with 100% oxygen therapy then reduced again to only 22 minutes with hyperbaric therapy. The benefit of this therapy, though, must be provided within 6 hours of exposure. Overall, patient benefit and improvement is not as reliable and predictable.[174]

Cardiac monitoring for dysrhythmias and 12-lead ECG should be performed.[176,184] Intravenous cannulation and blood testing for full blood count, electrolyte imbalance, urea and creatinine, COHb, blood sugar level and cardiac enzymes should be performed. Measurement of an elevated COHb concentration confirms the diagnosis; ABG analysis may demonstrate an acidosis, with an elevated lactate level. Where lactate levels are measured above 10 mmol/L, concomitant cyanide poisoning should be considered. Blood gas machines calculate the oxygen saturation from measured partial pressure and give a falsely elevated result in CO poisoning.

Other acute presenting problems associated with exposure, including cardiac chest pain, dysrhythmias, acute pulmonary oedema, hypotension, dehydration, external and airway burn injuries, pain and bronchospasm, may have to be managed concurrently depending on the nature of the exposure and examination findings.

An additional consideration with CO poisoning in the setting of fires and smoke in enclosed spaces is the potential for exposure to cyanide. Cyanide can be produced during the combustion of wool, silk, plastics, paper products, rubber and polyurethane (see Ch 30).[172]

CASE STUDY

A 72-year-old woman presents to triage with increased shortness of breath. Her accompanying husband reports recent chest infection, and worsening shortness of breath over the past 2 days. Physical examination reveals that the patient is leaning forward with hands on knees, she is speaking in short phrases, and is tachypnoeic with a respiratory rate of 38 breaths/minute. She is using pursed-lip breathing, is pale and her nails reveal clubbing and are dusky coloured. On palpation, the radial pulse is rapid and thready. The patient has a Glasgow Coma Scale (GCS) score of 15, and is becoming increasingly agitated.

Questions

1. Within which area of the ED could this patient be adequately managed?
   A. Waiting room
   B. Subacute
   C. Acute
   D. Resuscitation bay

2. Which physical assessment findings would indicate acute deterioration?
   A. Recent chest infection with increased shortness of breath
   B. Tripoding, short phrases, peripheral cyanosis, tachypnoea, pursed-lip breathing
   C. Clubbing of fingernails
   D. Being elderly

3. The patient is moved into a resuscitation bay for prompt assessment and management. The first priority of the resuscitation nurse is to complete:
   A. Introduction
   B. Primary survey of ABCD
   C. Intravenous access
   D. Humidified oxygen

4. A decision is made to commence non-invasive ventilation. The initial settings utilised are IPAP 10 cmH$_2$O, EPAP 6 cmH$_2$O, FiO$_2$ 0.50. Half an hour

later the patient is reviewed and the nurse finds the following information:

- Observations: respiratory rate 34 breaths/minute, blood pressure 110/65 mmHg, heart rate 120 beats/minute, GCS 15.
- ABG: pH 7.30, $PaCO_2$ 55 mmHg, HCO_3^- 29 mmol/L, PaO_2 70 mmHg

Interpret the blood gas results:

A. Partially compensated respiratory acidosis with hypoxaemia

B. Uncompensated respiratory acidosis with hypoxaemia

C. Uncompensated metabolic acidosis with hypoxaemia

D. Partially compensated respiratory alkalosis with hypoxaemia

5. To decrease the $PaCO_2$ and correct the pH, the ventilation strategy should increase which of the following?

A. FiO_2

B. Minute volume

C. Respiratory rate

D. Positive end-expiratory pressure

6. Using non-invasive ventilation, what strategies can you use to alter the minute volume?

A. Increase the respiratory rate

B. Increase the pressure support, and therefore the IPAP value

C. Increase the EPAP

D. Minute volume cannot be altered in non-invasive ventilation

7. One of the doctors makes a significant change to the ventilator settings, to EPAP 10 cmH_2O, IPAP 20 cmH_2O. The next set of observations post ventilation reflect a deterioration in haemodynamic status: blood pressure 90/45 mmHg, heart rate 125 beats/min. What is a probable cause for this sudden change in the scenario?

A. Dehydration

B. High settings of positive-pressure ventilation contributing to obstructive shock by raising intrathoracic pressure

C. Hypoxia resulting in a haemodynamic decompensation

D. Acute myocardial infarction

 Answers to Case Study Questions can be found on evolve
http://evolve.emergencytrauma.curtis

ACKNOWLEDGEMENT

The contributors would like to acknowledge and thank Diane Inglis for her assistance on this chapter.

REFERENCES

1. The Australian Lung Foundation. http://lungfoundation.com.au/general-information/statistics as at 25 September 2014.
2. Calverley PMA, Gorini M. Chronic respiratory failure. In: Nicolino A, Goldstein RS, eds. Ventilatory support for chronic respiratory failure. New York: Informa Healthcare; 2008:12.
3. Kaynar AM, Sharma S. Respiratory failure. 2009. Online. http://emedicine.medscape.com/article/167981-followup; accessed 25 Jan 2010.
4. Brashers V. Alterations of pulmonary function. In: McCance KL, Huether SE, eds. Pathophysiology: the biological basis for disease in adults and children. 4th edn. St. Louis: Mosby; 2010.
5. Poulos LM, Cooper SJ, Ampon R et al. Mortality from asthma and COPD in Australia. Australian Institute of Health and Welfare, Cat. No. ACM 30. Canberra: AIHW, 2014.
6. McCance KL, Huether SE. Understanding pathophysiology. 5th edn. St Louis: Mosby; 2011.
7. Australian Institute of Health and Welfare 2012. Australia's health 2012. Australia's health series no.13. Cat. no. AUS 156. Canberra: AIHW.
8. Australian Bureau of Statistics. Causes of death, Australia; 2011.
9. Laghi F, Tobin MJ. Indications for mechanical ventilation. In: Tobin MJ, ed. Principle and practice of mechanical ventilation. 2nd edn. New York: McGraw-Hill; 2006:129–62.
10. Gumm K. Emergency department trauma management. In: Curtis K, Ramsden C, Friendship J, eds. Emergency and trauma nursing. Sydney: Mosby; 2006.
11. Pandit R. I can't breathe. In: Jacques T, Fisher M, Hillman K et al. eds. Detecting deterioration, evaluation, treatment, escalation and communicating in teams. 2nd edn. Sydney: NSW: Clinical Excellence Commission. Online.

12. Simpson H. Respiratory assessment. Br J Nurs 2006;15(9):484–8.

13. Moore T. Respiratory assessment in adults. Nurs Stand 2007;21(49):48–56.

14. Rempher K, Morton P. Patient assessment: respiratory system. In: Morton P, Fontaine D, Hudak C et al, eds. Critical care nursing: a holistic approach. 8th edn. Philadelphia: Lippincott Williams & Wilkins; 2005.

15. Higginson R, Jones B. Respiratory assessment in critically ill patients: airway and breathing. Br J Nurs 2009;18(8):456–61.

16. Campbell ML, Templin T, Walch J. A respiratory distress observation scale for patient's unable to self report dyspnea. Journal of Palliative Medicine 2010;13(3):285–90.

17. Barbas CSV, Lopes GC, Vieira DF et al. Respiratory evaluation of patients requiring ventilator support due to acute respiratory failure. Open Journal of Nursing 2012;2:336–40.

18. Bradley R. Improving respiratory assessment skills. JNP 2007:3(4):276–7.

19. Hunter J, Rawlings-Anderson K. Respiratory assessment. Nurs Stand 2008;22(41):41–3.

20. Martin AD, Davenport PW. Extrinsic threshold PEEP reduces post exercise dyspnea in COPD patients: a placebo controlled, double-blind cross-over study. Cardiopulm. Phys Ther J 2011;22(3):5–10.

21. Visser FJ, Ramlal S, Dekhuijzen PNR, Heijdra YF. Pursed lips breathing improves inspiratory capacity in chronic obstructive pulmonary disease. Respiration 2011;81:372–8.

22. Macken L, Manning R. Facial trauma. In: Cameron P, Jelinek G, Kelly A-M et al, eds. Textbook of adult emergency medicine. 4th edn. Sydney: Churchill Livingstone; 2014.

23. Mohamad N, Sjam'un A, Ismail F et al. Acute stridor diagnostic challenges in different age groups presented to the emergency department. Emergency Med 2012;2:7.

24. Gaudry P, Finckh A, Alford J. Securing the airway, ventilation and procedural sedation. In: Fulde GW, ed. Emergency medicine: the principles of practice. 5th edn. Sydney: Elsevier; 2009.

25. Orji FT, Akpeh JO. Tracheobronchial foreign body aspiration in children: how reliable are clinical and radiological signs in the diagnosis? Clinical Otolaryngology 2010;35(6):479–85.

26. Boyd M, Chaterjee A, Chiles C, Chin R. Tracheobronchial foreign body aspiration in adults. Southern Medical Journal. 2009; 102(2):171–4.

27. Alfred Health. Victorian Burns Units website: www.vicburns.org.au/about.html; accessed 27 March 2015.

28. Meyer P, Ekundayo OJ, Adamopolous C et al. A propensity matched study of elevated jugular venous pressure and outcomes in chronic heart failure. Am J Cardiol 2009;103(6):839–44.

29. Aylott M. Observing the sick child: Part 2a. Respiratory assessment. Paediatric Nursing 2006;18(9):38–44.

30. Castriotta RJ, Murthy JN. Hypoventilation after spinal cord injury. Semin Respir Crit Care Med 2009;30:330–8.

31. Hampson NB, Piantdosi CA, Thom SR, Weaver LK. Practice recommendations in the diagnosis, management and prevention of carbon monoxide poisoning. Am J Respiratory Crit Care Med 2012;186(11):1095–101.

32. Kalay N, Ozdogru I, Cetinkaya Y et al. Cardiovascular effects of carbon monoxide poisoning. Am J Cardiol. 2007;99(3):322–4.

33. Nagurka R, Bechmann S, Gluckman W et al. Utility of initial pre-hospital end tidal carbon dioxide measurements to predict poor outcomes in adult asthmatic patients. Pre-hospital Emergency Care. Posted online 8 January 2014. doi:10.3109/10903127.2013.851306

34. Bernard S. Advanced airway management. In: Cameron P, Jelinek G, Kelly A-M et al, eds. Textbook of adult emergency medicine. 4th edn. Sydney: Churchill Livingstone; 2014.

35. Minkler MA, Mistovich JJ, Krost WS et al. Beyond the basics: capnography. EMS Mag 2008:37(1):74–8.

36. Ramirez R, Pickar T, Cappon J. Capnography: a better way? J Respir Care Pract 2009;22(1):30–3.

37. Cinar O, Acar YA, Arzimam I et al. Can mainstream end tidal carbon dioxide measurement accurately predict the arterial carbon dioxide level of patients with acute dyspnea in ED. The Am J Emerg Med 2012;30(2):358–61.

38. Pekdemir M, Cinar O, Yilmaz S et al. Disparity between mainstream and sidestream end tidal carbon dioxide values and arterial carbon dioxide levels. Respiratory Care 2013;58(7):1152–6.

39. Manifold CA, Davids N, Villers LC, Wampler DA. Capnography for the non intubated patient in the emergency setting. J Emerg Med 2013;45(4):626–32.

40. Soleimenpour H, Taghizadieh A, Niafar M et al. Predictive value of capnography for suspected diabetic ketoacidosis in the emergency department. West J Emerg Med 2013;14(6):590–4.

41. Bradbury SM, Thanacoody HKR, Watt BE et al. Management of the cardiovascular complications of tricyclic antidepressant poisoning. Toxicological Reviews 2005;24(3):195–204.

42. Thorborg PAJ. Blood gas analysis. In: Papadakos PJ, Lachmann B, eds. Mechanical ventilation: clinical applications and pathophysiology. Philadelphia: Saunders; 2008.

43. Woodruff DW. Take these 6 easy steps to ABG analysis. Nursing Made Incredibly Easy 2006;4(1):4–7.

44. Byrne AL, Bennett M, Chatterji R et al. Peripheral venous and arterial blood gas analysis in adults: are they comparable? A systematic review and meta-analysis. Respirology 2012;19(2):168–75.

45. Woodrow P. Arterial blood gas analysis. Nurs Stand 2004;18(21):45–52.

46. Kelly AM, McAlpine R, Kyle E. Venous pH can safely replace arterial pH in the initial evaluation of patients in the emergency department. Emerg Med J 2001;18(5):340–2.

47. Middleton P, Kelly AM, Brown J et al. Agreement between arterial and central venous values for pH, bicarbonate, base excess, and lactate. Emerg Med J 2006;23(8):622–4.

48. Sherman SC, Schindlbeck M. When is venous blood gas analysis enough? Emerg Med 2006;38(12):44–8.

49. Kelly A-M, Kyle E, McAlpine R. Venous pCO_2 and pH can be used to screen for significant hypercarbia in emergency patients with acute respiratory disease. J Emerg Med 2002;22(1):15–19.

50. Booker R. Good use of spirometry in general practice. Pract Nurs 2009;20(10):490–5.

51. Macintyre NR. Spirometry for the diagnosis and management of chronic obstructive pulmonary disease. Respir Care 2009; 54(8):1050–7.

52. Booker R. Interpretation and evaluation of pulmonary function tests. Nurs Stand 2009;23(39):46–56.

53. Johns D, Pierce R. Spirometry: The measurement and interpretation of ventilatory function in clinical practice. The Thoracic Society of Australia and New Zealand; 2008. Available: www.nationalasthma.org.au/images/stories/manage/pdf/spirometer_handbook_naca.pdf; 22 Jan 2010.

54. Kent B, Dowd B. Assessment, monitoring and diagnostics. In: Elliot D, Aitkin L, Chaboyer W, eds. ACCCN's critical care nursing. Sydney: Mosby; 2nd edn, 2011.

55. Wijesinghe M, Perrin K, Healy B et al. Pre-hospital oxygen therapy in acute exacerbations of chronic obstructive pulmonary disease. Internal Medicine Journal 2011;41(8):618–22.

56. Austin MA, Wills KE, Blizzard L et al. Effect of high flow oxygen on mortality in chronic obstructive pulmonary disease patients in pre-hospital setting: randomised controlled trial. BMJ 2010;341:c5462.

57. Wijesinghe M, Perrin K, Ranchord A et al. Routine use of oxygen in the treatment of myocardial infarction: a systematic review. Heart. 2009;95:198–202.

58. Iscoe S, Beasley R, Fisher JA. Supplementary oxygen for nonhypoxemic patients: O_2 much of a good thing? Critical Care 2011;15:305.

59. Meier P, Ebrahim S, Otto CM, Casas JP. Oxygen therapy in acute myocardial infarction—good or bad? (editorial) Cochrane Database of Systematic Reviews 2013;8:ED000065.

60. Kane B, Decalmer S, O'Driscoll BR. Emergency oxygen therapy: from guideline to implementation. Breathe. 2013;9(4):246–53.

61. Kones R. Oxygen therapy for acute myocardial infarction—then and now. A century of uncertainty. Am J Med 2011;124(11):1000–05.

62. Burls A, Cabello JB, Emparanza JI et al. Oxygen therapy for acute myocardial infarction: a systematic review and meta-analysis. Emerg Med J 2011;28:917–23.

63. Cornet AD, Kooter AJ, Peters MJL, Smulders YM. Supplemental oxygen therapy in medical emergencies: more harm than benefit? Arch Intern Med 2013;172(3):289–90.

64. Saposnick A, Hess D. Oxygen therapy: Administration and management. In: Hess DR, MacIntyre NR, Mishoe SC et al, eds. Respiratory care: principles and practice. Philadelphia: WB Saunders; 2002.

65. Dysart K, Miller TL, Wolfson MR et al. Research in high flow therapy: mechanisms of action. Respir Med 2009;103(10):1400–5.

66. El-Khatib MF. High flow nasal cannula oxygen therapy during hypoxemic respiratory failure. Respiratory Care 2012;57(10):1696–8.

67. Parke R, McGuiness S, Eccleston M. A preliminary randomized controlled trial to assess effectiveness of nasal high flow oxygen in intensive care patients. Respiratory Care 2011;56(3):265–70.

68. Sztrymf B, Messika J, Mayot T et al. Impact of high flow nasal cannula oxygen therapy on intensive care unit patients with acute respiratory failure: a prospective observational study. J Crit Care 2012;27(3):324e9–13.

69. Maggiore SM, Idone FA, Fest RV et al. Nasal high flow versus venturi mask oxygen therapy after extubation. Effects on oxygenation, comfort and clinical outcome. Amer J Resp and Crit Care Med. 2014;(190(3):282–8.

70. Kernick J, Magarey J. What is the evidence for the use of high flow nasal cannula oxygen in adult patients admitted to critical care units? A systematic review. Aust Crit Care 2010;23(2):53–70.

71. Hoyt JW. Debunking myths of chronic obstructive lung disease. Crit Care Med 1997;25(9):1450–1.

72. Cornet AD, Kooter AJ, Peters MJL, Smulders YM. Supplemental oxygen therapy in medical emergencies: more harm than benefit. Arch Intern Med 2012;172(3):289–90.

73. Beasley R, Patel M, Perrin K, O'Driscoll BR. High concentration oxygen therapy in COPD. The Lancet, 2011;378(9795):969–70.

74. Johnstone J, Malpas L, Johnstone F, Malpas M. Emergency oxygen use and monitoring in the pre-hospital and acute hospital setting—the significance of a common problem. ERJ 2012;40(56):4297.

75. Cornet AD, Kooter AJ et al. The potential harm of oxygen therapy in medical emergencies. Critical Care 2013;17:313.

76. Cameron L, Pilcher J, Weatherall M et al. The risk of serious adverse outcomes associated with hyoxaemia and hyperoxaemia in acute exacerbations of COPD. Postgrad Med J 2012;88:684–9.

77. Pilcher J, Perrin K, Beasley R. The effect of high concentration oxygen therapy on $PaCO_2$ in acute and chronic respiratory disorders. Translational Respiratory Medicine 2013;1:8.

78. Pilcher J, Cameron L, Braithwaite I et al. Comparative audit of oxygen use in the pre-hospital setting in acute COPD exacerbation over 5 years. Emerg Med J. http://emj.bmj.com/content/early/2013/11/15/emermed-2013-203094.short; accessed 29 Sept 2014.

79. Ducros L, Logeart D, Vicaut E et al. CPAP for acute cardiogenic pulmonary oedema from out of hospital to cardiac intensive care unit: a randomized multicenter study. Intensive Care Med 2011;37(9):1501–09.

80. Mariani J, Macchia A, Belziti C et al. Non invasive ventilation in acute cardiogenic pulmonary edema: a meta analysis of randomized controlled trials. J Cardiac Failure 2011;17(10):850–9.

81. Bledsoe BE, Anderson E, Hodnick R et al. Low fractional oxygen concentration continuous positive airway pressure is effective in the pre-hospital setting. Pre-Hospital Emergency Care 2012;16(2)217–21.

82. Dib JE, Matin SA, Luckert A. Pre-hospital use of continuous positive airway pressure for acute severe congestive heart failure. The Journal of Emergency Medicine 2012;42(5):553–8.

83. Roessler MS, Schmid DS, Michels P et al. Early out of hospital non invasive ventilation is superior to standard medical treatment in patients with acute respiratory failure: a pilot study. Emergency Medical Journal 2012;29:409–14.

84. Simpson PM, Bendall JC. Pre-hospital non invasive ventilation for acute cardiogenic pulmonary oedema: an evidence based review. Emerg Med J 2011;28:609–12.

85. Warner GS. Evaluation of the effect of pre-hospital application of continuous positive airway pressure therapy in acute respiratory distress. Pre-hospital and disaster medicine. 2010;25(1)87–91.

86. Williams TA, Finn J, Perkins GA, Jacobs IG. Pre-hospital continuous positive airway pressure for acute respiratory failure: a systematic review and meta analysis. Pre-Hospital Emergency Care 2013; 17(2)261–73.

87. Williams B, Boyle M, Robertson N, Giddings C. When pressure is positive: a literature review of the pre-hospital use of continuous positive airway pressure. Pre-Hospital and Disaster Medicine 2013;28(1):52-60

88. Marini JJ, Hotchkiss JR, Bach JR. Noninvasive ventilation in the acute care setting. In: Bach JR, ed. Noninvasive mechanical ventilation. Philadelphia: Hanley & Belfus; 2002.

89. Chandra D, Stamm JA, Taylor B et al. Outcomes of noninvasive ventilation for acute exacerbations of chronic obstructive pulmonary disease in the United States, 1998–2009. American Journal of Respiratory and Critical Care Medicine 2012;185(2):152–9.

90. Elliot MW. Non invasive ventilation in acute exacerbations of chronic obstructive pulmonary disease: a new gold standard? App Physiol Int Care Med 2 2012;335–8.

91. Okpala PC, Alexander JL, Ewing H, Tulp OL. The use of non invasive positive pressure ventilator (NIPPV) and conventional medical care to treat respiratory failure arising from acute exacerbation of COPD: A systematic review. J App Med Sci 2013;2(2):31–41.

92. Schnell D, Timsit JF, Darmon M et al. Non invasive mechanical ventilation in acute respiratory failure: trends in use and outcomes. Int Care Med 2014. Online: DOI 10.1007/s00134-014-3222-y.

93. Marini JJ, Hotchkiss JR, Bach JR. Noninvasive ventilation in the acute care setting. In: Bach JR, ed. Noninvasive mechanical ventilation. Philadelphia: Hanley & Belfus; 2002.

94. Hill NS. Non-invasive ventilation. In: MacIntyre NR, Branson RD, eds. Mechanical ventilation. 2nd edn. St Louis: Saunders; 2009.

95. Lim WJ, Mohammed Akram R et al. Non invasive positive pressure ventilation for treatment of respiratory failure due to severe acute exacerbations of asthma. Cochrane database of systematic reviews 2012(12):CD004360

96. Murase K, Tomii K, Chin K et al. The use of non invasive ventilation for life threatening asthma attacks: changes in the need for intubation. Respirology 2010;15(4):714–20.

97. Yasui H, Fujisawa T, Karayama M et al. Usefulness of non invasive positive pressure ventilation (NPPV) for acute exacerbation of asthma. American Thoracic Society International conference abstracts in AJRCCM. B48. Non invasive ventilation. 1 May 2012, A3141.

98. Azoulay E, Demoule A, Jaber S et al. Palliative noninvasive ventilation in patients with acute respiratory failure. Intensive Care Medicine. 2011;37(8):1250–7.

99. Naval S, Grassi M, Fanfulla F et al. Non-invasive ventilation in elderly patients with acute hypercapnic respiratory failure: a randomised controlled trial. Age Ageing 2011;40(4):444–50.

100. Gramlich T. Basic concept of noninvasive positive pressure ventilation. In: Pilbeam SP, Cairo JM, eds. Mechanical ventilation: physiological and clinical applications 4th edn. St Louis: Mosby; 2006.

101. Shirakabe A, Hata N, Yokayama S et al. Predicting the success of noninvasive positive pressure ventilation in emergency room for patients with acute heart failure. Journal of Cardiology 2011;57(1):107–14.

102. Pertab D. Principles of non-invasive ventilation: a critical review of practice issues. Br J Nurs 2009;18(16):1004–8.

103. Ferguson GT, Gilmartin M. CO_2 rebreathing during BiPAP ventilatory assistance. Am J Respir Crit Care Med 1995;151(4):1126–35.

104. Kwok H, McCormack J, Cece R et al. Controlled trial of oronasal versus nasal mask ventilation in the treatment of acute respiratory failure. Crit Care Med 2003;31(2):468–73.

105. Saatci E, Miller DM, Stell IM et al. Dynamic dead space in face masks used with noninvasive ventilators: a lung model study. Eur Respir J 2004;23(1):129–35.

106. Hostetler MA. Use of noninvasive positive-pressure ventilation in the emergency department. Emerg Med Clin North Am 2008;26(4):929–39, viii.

107. Wilbeck J, Fischer M. Noninvasive ventilation in emergency care. Adv Emerg Nurs J 2009;31(2):161–9.

108. Hilbert G, Clouzeau B, Nam Bui H, Vargas F. Sedation during non invasive ventilation. Minerva Anestsiologica. 2012;78(7):842–6.

109. Arroliga AC, Frutos-Vivar F, Anzueto A et al. The use of sedatives and analgesics in patients receiving non invasive positive pressure mechanical ventilation. 2012. American Thoracic Society international conference abstracts. D94 non invasive ventilation and weaning by the bay. 1164/ajrccm-conference.2012.185.1_MeetingAbstracts.A6490.

110. Massie CA, Hart RW, Peralez K et al. Effects of humidification on nasal symptoms and compliance in sleep apnea patients using continuous positive airway pressure. Chest 1999;116(2):403–8.

111. Holland AE, Denehy L, Buchan CA et al. Efficacy of a heated passover humidifier during noninvasive ventilation: a bench study. Respir Care 2007;52(1):38–44.

112. Rose L, Gerdtz MF. Mechanical ventilation in Australian emergency departments: survey of workforce profile, nursing role responsibility, and education. Aust Emerg Nurs J 2009;12(2):38–43.

113. Rose L, Gerdtz M. Invasive ventilation in the emergency department Part 1: What nurses need to know. Aust Emerg Nurs J 2007;10:21–5.

114. Papadakos PJ, Lachmann B, eds. Mechanical ventilation: clinical applications and pathophysiology. Philadelphia: Saunders; 2008.

115. Tobin MJ, ed. Principles and practice of mechanical ventilation. 2nd edn. New York: McGraw-Hill; 2006.

116. Rose L, Gerdtz MF. Invasive ventilation in the emergency department part 2: implications for patient safety. Aust Emerg Nurs J 2007;10:26–9.

117. Coyer FM, Wheeler MK, Wetzig SM et al. Nursing care of the mechanically ventilated patient: what does the evidence say? Part two. Intensive Crit Care Nurs 2007;23(2):71–80.

118. Couchman BA, Wetzig SM, Coyer FM et al. Nursing care of the mechanically ventilated patient: what does the evidence say? Part one. Intensive Crit Care Nurs 2007;23(1):4–14.

119. Chou HC, Chong KM, Sim SS et al. Real time tracheal ultrasonography for confirmation of endotracheal tube placement during cardiopulmonary resuscitation. Resuscitation 2013;84(12):1708–12.

120. Branson RD. The patient–ventilator interface: ventilator circuit, airway care and suctioning. In: MacIntyre NR, Branson R, eds. Mechanical ventilation 2nd edn. St Louis: Saunders; 2009.

121. Stauffer JL. Complications of translaryngeal intubation. In: Tobin MJ, ed. Principles and practice of mechanical ventilation. 2nd edn. Philadelphia: Saunders; 2006.

122. Restropo RD, Walsh BK. Humidification during invasive and noninvasive mechanical ventilation. Respiratory Care. 2012;57(5):782–8.

123. Ashry HAS, Modrykamien AM. Humidification during mechanical ventilation in the adult patient. Biomed research international vol. 2014, Article ID 715434.

124. Pilbeam SP. Problem solving and troubleshooting. In: Pilbeam SP, Cairo JM, eds. Mechanical ventilation: physiological and clinical applications. 4th edn. St Louis: Mosby; 2006.

125. MacIntyre NR, Branson RD, eds. Mechanical ventilation. Philadelphia: Saunders; 2008.

126. O'Brien J, Hunter C. Heart Failure. In: Marx J, Hockberger R, Walls R, eds. Rosen's emergency medicine. Concepts and clinical practice. 8th edn. Philadelphia. Elsevier Saunders 2014:1075–90.

127. Lightfoot D. Assessment and management of acute pulmonary oedema. In: Cameron P, Jelinek G, Kelly A-M et al, eds. Textbook of adult emergency medicine. 4th edn. Sydney: Churchill Livingstone; 2014.

128. Brown AFT. Acute pulmonary oedema. In: Fulde GWO, ed. Emergency medicine: the principles of practice. 5th edn. Sydney: Elsevier; 2009.

129. O'Brien J, Falk J. Heart failure. In: Marx J, Hockberger R, Walls R et al, eds. Rosen's emergency medicine: concepts and clinical practice. 7th edn. Philadelphia: Mosby/Elsevier; 2009.

130. McMurray JJV (Chairperson) The Task Force for the Diagnosis and Treatment of Acute and Chronic Heart Failure 2012 of the European Society of Cardiology. Developed in collaboration with the Heart Failure Association (HFA) of the ESC. ESC guidelines for the diagnosis and treatment of acute and chronic heart failure 2012. European Heart Journal. 2012;33:1787–847.

131. Vital FM, Saconato H, Ladeira MT et al. Non-invasive positive pressure ventilation (CPAP or bilevel NPPV) for cardiogenic pulmonary edema. Cochrane Database Syst Rev 2008(3):CD005351.

132. Jessup M, Abraham WT, Casey DE et al. 2009 focused updated: ACCF/AHA guidelines for the diagnosis and management of heart failure in adults. Circulation 2009;119(14):1977–2016.

133. Colucci W. Treatment of acute decompensated heart failure in acute coronary syndromes. UptoDate; updated 27 Oct 2010. Online. www.uptodate.com/patients/content/topic.do?topicKey=~FJHFJRp3PWozlbY; 5 Dec 2010.

134. Nowak R, Tokarski G. Asthma. In: Marx J, Hockberger R, Walls R et al, eds. Rosen's emergency medicine: concepts and clinical practice. 7th edn. Philadelphia: Mosby/Elsevier; 2009.

135. Lange P. Persistent airway obstruction in asthma. Amer J Resp and Crit Care Med. 2013;187(1):1–2.

136. Kelly A-M. Asthma. In: Cameron P, Jelinek G, Kelly A-M et al. eds. Textbook of adult emergency medicine. 4th edn. Sydney: Churchill Livingstone; 2014.

137. Bousquet J, Mantzouranis E, Cruz AA et al. Uniform definition of asthma severity, control and exacerbations: document presented for the World Health Organization consultation on severe asthma. J Allergy and Clin Imm 2010;126(5):926–38.

138. Jarjour NN, Erzurum SC, Bleecker ER et al. Lessons learned from the national heart, lung and blood institute severe asthma research program. Amer J Resp and Crit Care Med 2012;185(4).

139. Bel EH, Sousa A, Fleming L et al. Diagnosis and definition of severe refractory asthma: an international consensus statement from the innovative medicine initiative (IMI). Thorax 2010 http://thorax.bmj.com/content/early/2010/11/23/thx.2010.153643.full; accessed 29 Sept 2014.

140. National Asthma Council Australia. Asthma management handbook 2006. South Melbourne: National Asthma Council; 2006.

141. National Asthma Council Australia. Australian asthma handbook, quick reference guide, version 1.1. Melbourne, 2015. www.asthmahandbook.org.au; accessed 18 March 2015.

142. Hore C, Roberts J. Respiratory emergencies: the acutely breathless patient. In: Fulde GW, ed. Emergency medicine: the principles of practice. 5th edn. Sydney: Elsevier; 2009.

143. Plotnick LH, Ducharme FM. Combined inhaled anticholinergics and beta2-agonists for initial treatment of acute asthma in children. Cochrane Database Syst Rev 2000;(3):CD000060.

144. Sellers WFS. Inhaled and intravenous treatment in acute severe and life threatening asthma. British Journal of Anaesthesia 2013;110(2):183–90.

145. Song WJ, Chang YS. Magnesium sulphate for acute asthma in adults: a systematic literature review. Asia Pacific Allergy 2012;2(1):76–85.

146. Perrin K, Wijesinghe M, Healy B et al. Randomised controlled trial of high concentration versus titrated oxygen therapy in severe exacerbations of asthma. Thorax 2011;66:937–41.

147. Gupta D, Nath A, Agarwal R, Behera D. A prospective randomised controlled trial on the efficacy of non invasive ventilation in severe acute asthma. Respiratory Care 2010;55(5):536–43.

148. Rodrigo G, Pollack C, Rodrigo C et al. Heliox for non-intubated acute asthma patients. Cochrane Database Syst Rev 2006;(4):CD002884.

149. Rodrigo G, Pollack C, Rodrigo C et al. Heliox for non-intubated acute asthma patients [updated 18 Aug 2009]. The Cochrane Library. 2010:(1).

150. Swadron S, Gruber G. Chronic obstructive pulmonary disease. In: Marx J, Hockberger R, Walls R, eds. In: Marx: Rosen's Emergency Medicine. Concepts and Clinical Practice. 8th edn. Philadelphia. Elsevier Saunders. 2014:956–65.

151. Rabe KF, Hurd S, Anzueto A et al. Global strategy for the diagnosis, management, and prevention of chronic obstructive pulmonary disease. Am J Respir Crit Care Med 2007;176:532–55.

152. Swadron SP, Mandavia DP. Chronic obstructive pulmonary disease. In: Marx J, Hockberger R, Walls R et al, eds. Rosen's emergency medicine: concepts and clinical practice. 7th edn. Philadelphia: Mosby/Elsevier; 2009.

153. Abdo WF, Heunks LMA. Oxygen induced hypercapnia in COPD: myths and facts. Critical Care. 2012;16:323

154. Stoller JK, Panos RJ, Krachman S et al. The long term oxygen treatment trial research group. Oxygen therapy for patients with COPD: Current evidence and the long term oxygen treatment trial. Chest 2010;138(1)179–87.

155. Duffy M. Chronic obstructive airways disease. In: Cameron P, Jelinek G, Kelly A-M et al, eds. Textbook of adult emergency medicine. 2nd edn. Sydney: Churchill Livingstone; 2004:286–90.

156. Hanania NA, Celli BR, Donohye JF, Martin UJ. Bronchodilator reversibility in COPD. Chest. 2011;140(4):1055–63.

157. Khirani S, Polese G, Appendini L et al. Mechanical ventilation in chronic obstructive pulmonary disease. In: Tobin MJ, ed. Principles and practice of mechanical ventilation. 2nd edn. New York: McGraw-Hill; 2006.

158. Urden LD, Stacy KM, Lough ME. Thelan's Critical care nursing: diagnosis and management. 5th edn. St Louis: Mosby; 2006.

159. Charles PG, Whitby M, Fuller AJ et al. The etiology of community-acquired pneumonia in Australia: why penicillin plus doxycycline or a macrolide is the most appropriate therapy. Clin Infect Dis 2008;46(10):1513–21.

160. Moran G, Talan D. Pneumonia. In: Marx J, Hockberger R, Walls R, eds. In: Marx: Rosen's Emergency Medicine. Concepts and Clinical Practice. 8th edn. Philadelphia. Elsevier Saunders. 2014:978–87.

161. Nazarian DJ, Eddy OL, Lukens TW et al. Clinical policy: critical issues in the management of adult patients presenting to the emergency department with community-acquired pneumonia. Ann Emerg Med 2009;54(5):704–31.

162. Wilkes G. Community-acquired pneumonia. In: Cameron P, Jelinek G, Kelly A-M et al, eds. Textbook of adult emergency medicine. 2nd edn. Sydney: Churchill Livingstone; 2004:275–85.

163. Mookadam F, Jiamsripong P, Goel R et al. Critical appraisal on the utility of echocardiography in the management of acute pulmonary embolism. Cardiol Rev 2010;18(1):29–37.

164. eTG (2014) Assessing pneumonia severity. http://etg.hcn.com.au/desktop/index.htm?acc=36422; accessed 15 Jan 2014.

165. eTG. (2014) Box 2.5 'Red Flags' indicating severe community-acquired pneumonia requiring hospital admission. http://etg.hcn.com.au/desktop/index.htm?acc=36422; accessed 15 Jan 2014.

166. Kline J. Pulmonary embolism and deep vein thrombosis. In: Marx J, Hockberger R, Walls R, eds. In: Marx: Rosen's Emergency Medicine. Concepts and Clinical Practice. 8th edn. Philadelphia. Elsevier Saunders. 2014:1157–69.

167. Wolf S, McCubbin T, Feldhaus K et al. Prospective validation of Wells criteria in the evaluation of patients with suspected pulmonary embolism. Annals of Emergency Medicine 2004;44(5):503–10.

168. Kline JA, Courtney DM, Kabrhel C et al. Prospective multicenter evaluation of the pulmonary embolism rule-out criteria. J Thromb Haemost 2008;6(5):772–80.

169. Singh B, Parsaik AK, Agarwal D et al. Diagnostic accuracy of pulmonary embolism rule out criteria: A systematic review and meta-analysis. Annals of Emergency Medicine 2012 June;59(6):517–20.

170. Todoran TM, Sobieszczyk P. Catheter-based therapies for massive pulmonary embolism. Prog Cardiovasc Dis 2010;52(5):429–37.

171. Young T, Tang H, Hughes R. Vena caval filters for the prevention of pulmonary embolism. Cochrane Database Syst Rev 2010:(2).

172. Cameron P, Jelinek G, Kelly A-M et al, eds. Textbook of adult emergency medicine. 4th edn. Sydney: Churchill Livingstone; 2014.

173. McKenzie D, Dunford M, Wilcox N. Respiratory coordinated care program. Improved management of patients with respiratory infection, acute respiratory failure and chronic and complex respiratory disease: a GMCT proposal for a new model of care. North Sydney: NSW Health; 2007.

174. Harper A, Croft-Baker J. Carbon monoxide poisoning: undetected by both patients and their doctors. Age and Ageing 2004;33:105–09.

175. Prockchop LD, Chichkova RI. Carbon monoxide intoxication: an updated review. Journal of the Neurological Sciences 2007; 262(1-2):122–30.

176. Weaver LK. Carbon monoxide poisoning. The New England Journal of Medicine 2009;360:1217–25.

177. Studdert DM, Gurrin LC, Jatkar U, Pirkis J. Relationship between vehicle emissions laws and incidence of suicide by motor vehicle exhaust gas in Australia, 2001–06: an ecological analysis. PLoS Med. 2010;7(1):e1000210.

178. Mehta SR, Niyogi M, Kasthuri AS et al. Carbon monoxide poisoning. The Journal of the Association of Physicians of India. 2001; 49:622–25.

179. Choi IS. Parkinsonism after carbon monoxide poisoning. European Neurology. 2002;48(1):30–3.

180. Young SH, Yong J, Hyun SK, Joo HI, Jin-Soo K. The brain lesion responsible for Parkinsonism after carbon monoxide poisoning. Archives of Neurology. 2000;57(8):1214–18.

181. Annane D, Shevret S, Jars-Guincestre M et al. Prognostic factors in unintentional mild carbon monoxide poisoning. Intensive Care Medicine 2001;27(11):1776–81.

182. Jang W, Park JH. Transient left ventricular systolic dysfunction associated with carbon monoxide toxicity. J Cardiovascular Ultrasound 2010;18(1):12–15.

183. Lippi G, Rastelli G, Meschi T et al. Pathophysiology, clinics, diagnosis and treatment of heart involvement in carbon monoxide poisoning. Clinical Biochemistry 2012;45(16–17):1278–85.

184. Henry CR, Satran D, Lindgren B et al. Myocardial injury and long term mortality following moderate to severe carbon monoxide poisoning. JAMA 2006;295(4):398–402.

185. Aubard Y. Carbon monoxide poisoning in pregnancy. BJOG: An International Journal of Obstetrics and Gynaecology 2000;107(7):833–8.

186. Cruise DC. Carbon monoxide. In: Cameron P, Jelinek G, Kelly A et al, eds. Textbook of adult emergency medicine. 4th edn. Edinburgh: Churchill Livingstone; 2014.

187. Hampson NB. Non invasive pulse CO-oximetry expedites evaluation and management of patients with carbon monoxide poisoning. Am J Emerg Med 2012;30(9):2021–24.

188. Teksam O, Gumus P, Bayrakci B et al. Acute cardiac effects of carbon monoxide poisoning in children. European Journal of Emergency Medicine 2010;17(4):192–6.

189. Smollin C, Olson K. Carbon monoxide poisoning (acute). Clinical Evidence (Online) 2010;2010:2103.

190. Dunn KH, Devaux I, Stock A, Naeher LP. Application of end exhaled breath monitoring to assess carbon monoxide exposures at wildland firefighters at prescribed burns. Inhalational Toxicology 2009;21(1):55–61.

191. Piatkowski A, Ulrich D, Grieb G, Pallua N. A new tool for the early diagnosis of carbon monoxide intoxication. Inhalation toxicology 2009;21(13):1144–7.

192. Roth D, Hubmann N, Havel C et al. Victim of carbon monoxide poisoning identified by carbon monoxide oximetry. J Emerg Med 2011;40(6):640–2.

193. Hawkins M, Harrison J, Charters P. Severe carbon monoxide poisoning: outcome after hyperbaric oxygen therapy. British Journal of Anaesthesia 2000;84(5):584–6.

194. Juurlink DN, Buckley NA, Stanbrook MB et al. Hyperbaric oxygen for carbon monoxide poisoning. Cochrane Database Syst Rev 2005;1:CD002041.

195. Buckley NA, Juurlink DN, Isbister G et al. Hyperbaric oxygen for carbon monoxide poisoning. Cochrane Database of Systematic Reviews 2011;4:CD002041.

196. Holets S, Hubmayr RD. Setting the ventilator. In: Tobin M, ed. Principles and practice of mechanical ventilation. 2nd edn. New York: McGraw-Hill; 2006:163–82.

197. Huang Y-CT, Singh J. Basic modes of mechanical ventilation. In: Papadakos PJ, Lachmann B, eds. Mechanical ventilation: clinical applications and pathophysiology. Philadelphia: Saunders; 2008.

198. Sztrymf B, Messika J, Mayot T et al. Impact of high-flow nasal cannula oxygen therapy on intensive care unit patients with acute respiratory failure: A prospective observational study. Journal of Critical Care 2012;27(3):324e9–324e13.

CHAPTER 22
CARDIOVASCULAR EMERGENCIES
SUZANNE DAVIES AND CLAIR RAMSDEN

Essentials

- A comprehensive history is of paramount importance in the assessment of the cardiac patient.
- It is necessary to understand the anatomy, physiology and blood flow through the heart.
- Significant changes that occur on the electrocardiogram will determine treatment interventions.
- Identification of cardiac risk is vital to assess management of the cardiac patient.
- Appropriate management of patients with acute coronary syndromes is essential.

INTRODUCTION

The 2008 Australian National Health Survey reported that an estimated 3.4 million people had a cardiovascular disease (CVD) in 2007–08.[1] Despite a significant and consistent decrease in the death rate from CVD since the late 1960s, it was still Australia's biggest killer in 2009—recorded as the underlying cause of 46,100 deaths. This is more than any other single disease group, and is a characteristic of developed, and increasingly developing, countries.[2] It is estimated that more than 50,000 Australians suffered an acute myocardial infarction in 2009, costing the Australian community over a quarter of a million dollars per event. More than 3,000,000 Australians are affected by cardiovascular disease and some are more likely to suffer than others: Aboriginal and Torres Strait Islander people are 2.6 times more likely to die from heart, stroke and vascular disease than other Australians.[3] A recent Australian economic evaluation estimated that the total cost to Australians arising from the morbidity and mortality associated with Acute Coronary Syndromes exceeds $17 billion dollars per year.[4] Complications of acute coronary syndrome represent a major burden of disease in Australia.[5]

This chapter discusses the essential steps in assessing emergencies of the heart and the great vessels, outlines serious cardiovascular conditions and describes their subsequent paramedic and nursing management.

Anatomy and physiology

The normal human heart is cone-shaped and located within the thoracic cavity with one-third to the right of the sternum and the remaining two-thirds to the left. The average human heart is about the size of the clenched fist of the individual. Unusually, the top of the heart is referred to as the *base*; this is comprised of the left atrium and a small part of the right atrium. The pointed lower section is the *apex*, which lies at the 5th left intercostal space at the midclavicular line.[6–8]

The heart is a four-chambered, fibromuscular, hollow organ. The function of the heart is to pump blood around the body, and two highly specific pumps (a left and a right), each with its own set of valves, allow this to happen.[6–8]

Blood flow through the heart

Deoxygenated blood is returned to the right side of the heart from the body via the superior and inferior venae cavae. Blood enters the right atrium then flows through the tricuspid valve and into the right ventricle. From here it is forced through the pulmonary valve during systole and into the pulmonary circulation where it becomes oxygenated in the lungs. This is the *pulmonary circuit*.[6–8]

Oxygenated blood is returned to the left side of the heart from the lungs via the pulmonary veins. Blood enters the left atrium then flows through the mitral valve and into the left ventricle. From here it is forced through the aortic valve during systole and into the circulation, which supplies blood to the body. This is the *systemic circuit* (Fig 22.1).[6–8]

Chambers of the heart

The human heart has four chambers—right and left atria, and right and left ventricles. The heart also contains two atrioventricular valves, the tricuspid and mitral valves, and two semilunar or cardiac valves, the pulmonary (or pulmonic) and aortic valves.[6,8]

The annuli fibrosi is a fibrous skeleton within the heart that consists of rings of fibrous connective tissue. This tissue surrounds the cardiac valves and provides an internal supporting structure for the heart. The atria and the ventricles are divided by the fibrous skeleton which also serves as an electrical insulator.[6,8]

The atria are relatively thin-walled, as they are not under a great amount of pressure. The two atria are separated by a fibromuscular septum. The heart is filled passively: 70% occurring during diastole; and atrial contraction (atrial kick) contributing approximately 30% to complete ventricular filling.[6,7] The right ventricle is smaller than the left and has thinner walls as it pumps blood into the low-pressure pulmonary circulation. The left ventricular wall is 2–3 times thicker than the right ventricular wall as it pumps blood into the high-pressure systemic circulation.[6,8] The left ventricle must generate great force to eject blood into the aorta, and it is for this reason

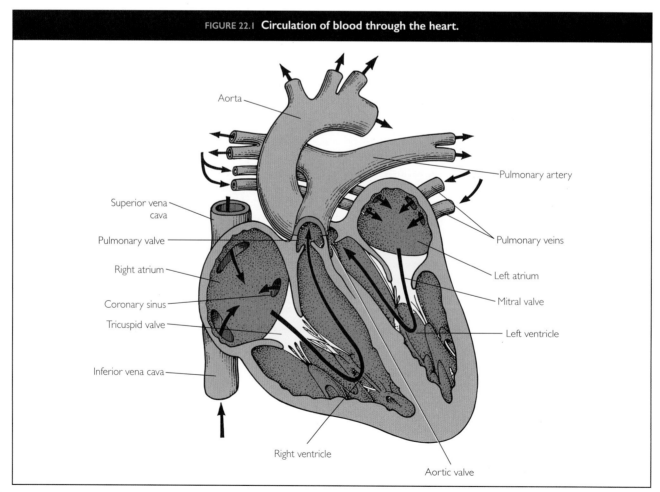

FIGURE 22.1 **Circulation of blood through the heart.**

Arrows indicate direction of flow.[9]

that the left ventricle is considered to be the major pump of the heart. The approximate thicknesses of the chamber walls are as follows: right atrium 2 mm; right ventricle 3–5 mm; left atrium 3 mm; left ventricle 13–15 mm.[6,8]

Valves of the heart

The *atrioventricular valves* are the tricuspid valve and the mitral valve (Fig 22.2). The tricuspid valve is situated between the right atrium and the right ventricle and consists of three cusps or leaflets. The mitral (bicuspid) valve is situated between the left atrium and the left ventricle and consists of two cusps or leaflets. Both valve leaflets are composed of fibrous tissue covered by endothelium.[6,8] The valve leaflets attach to the fibrous skeleton of the heart and are anchored by fibrous cords called chordae tendineae. These cords attach the ends of the valve to papillary muscle and the ventricular wall. The opening and closing of the valves is passive and depends on pressure gradients. The structure of the valves and the attachment of the leaflets to the ventricle walls allow only one directional blood flow (Fig 22.2).[6,8]

The *semilunar valves* are the pulmonary valve and the aortic valve. Both semilunar valves consist of three cusps, all of about equal size, which are attached to the fibrous skeleton. The leaflets of the semilunar valves are comprised of fibrous connective tissue covered by endothelium. These valves separate the ventricles from their outflow arteries.[6,8] The *aortic valve* is the strongest of all the heart's valves as it is exposed to the greatest pressures during the cardiac cycle. The leaflets of the aortic valve are attached to the annuli fibrosi that forms part of the sinus of Valsalva; the coronary arteries open near the upper part of this sinus. The three cusps of the aortic valve are named from the coronary arteries that lie behind each semilunar cusp: the right coronary aortic cusp, the left coronary artery aortic cusp and the non-coronary aortic cusp (Fig 22.3).[6–8]

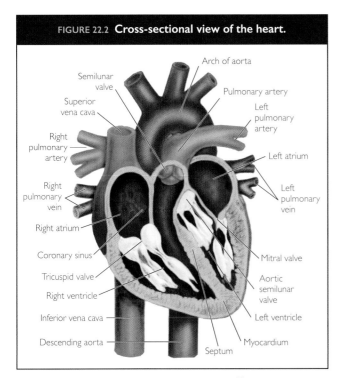

FIGURE 22.2 **Cross-sectional view of the heart.**

Note the position of the four cardiac valves.[10]

Layers of the heart

The *pericardium*, or parietal pericardium, is the outermost layer of the heart; it holds the heart in a fixed position and provides a physical barrier against infection.

The *epicardium*, or visceral pericardium, completely encloses the external surface of the heart. Together the pericardium and the epicardium form a sac around the heart. This sac normally contains a small amount of pericardial fluid. This clear serous fluid (approximately 10–30 mL) lubricates the moving surface of the heart.[6–8]

The *myocardium* is the thick middle muscular layer that forms the bulk of the heart and is the muscle that is damaged during a myocardial infarction.

The *endocardium* is the innermost layer and is composed of a layer of endothelial cells. The endocardium is continuous with the internal lining of adjoining blood vessels—the tunica intima.

The coronary circulation

The coronary circulation consists of the blood vessels that supply oxygenated blood to the heart muscle (*coronary arteries*) and those that return deoxygenated blood to the circulation (*coronary veins*). Coronary arteries originate at the base of the aorta in the region of the sinus of Valsalva. They extend over the epicardial surface of the heart and branch many times. Two coronary arteries originate at the aorta: the left coronary artery (LCA) and the right coronary artery (RCA). Coronary arteries are supplied with blood during diastole. As the heart relaxes and the aortic valve closes, blood flows down the coronary arteries and the myocardium is perfused. During this passive, diastolic phase, ventricular filling also occurs.[8,11]

The left main coronary artery is a short vessel that divides into the left anterior descending branch (LAD) and the circumflex branch (Cx). In most people the right coronary artery (RCA) supplies the right atrium and right ventricle. It also supplies the sinoatrial (SA) node and the atrioventricular (AV) node. The LAD supplies the anterior surface of the left ventricle and the interventricular septum. The Cx supplies the lateral aspect and part of the posterior aspect of the left ventricle.[5,8] (See Fig 22.4 and Box 22.1.) There is considerable variation in the normal anatomy of the coronary circulation. In approximately 90% of people, the RCA is the origin of the posterior descending artery (PDA); in the remaining cases, the PDA arises from the left circumflex artery. The RCA also supplies the SA nodal artery in 60% of cases, the left circumflex artery in the remaining 40%.

The conduction system

The specialised conductive system that controls and propagates cardiac contraction is the *conduction pathway*. This consists of three main areas of impulse generation: the sinoatrial (SA) node, the atrioventricular (AV) node and the His/Purkinje system.[6,8,11]

The *SA node* is referred to as the pacemaker of the heart, as it has the highest degree of automaticity or highest intrinsic rate: 60–100 times per minute. The SA node initiates each cardiac cycle. It is located on the posterior surface of the right atrium near the superior vena cava. Its anatomical position ensures that the atria are depolarised before the ventricles. Cells within the SA node initiate a wave of electrical depolarisation and the

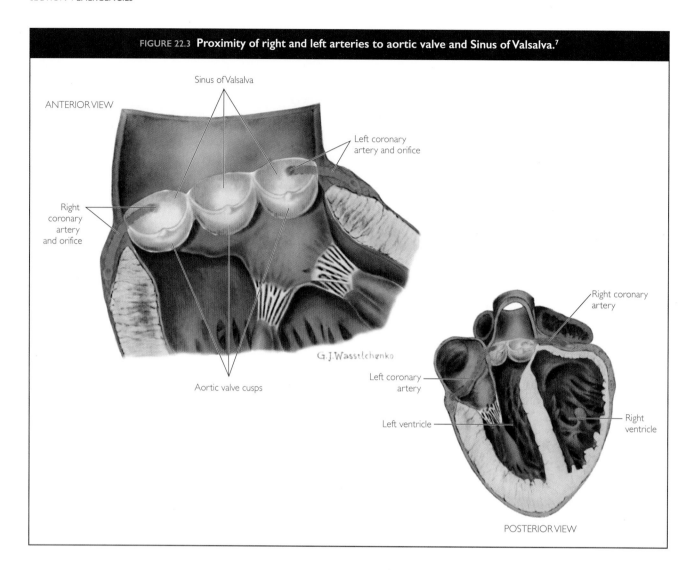

FIGURE 22.3 Proximity of right and left arteries to aortic valve and Sinus of Valsalva.[7]

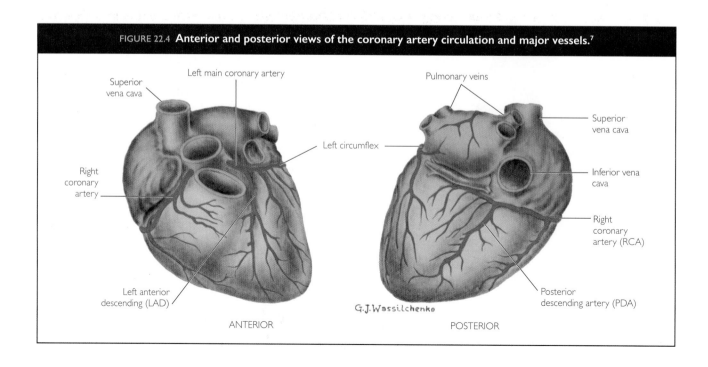

FIGURE 22.4 Anterior and posterior views of the coronary artery circulation and major vessels.[7]

BOX 22.1 Coronary arteries in myocardial infarction[12]

Right coronary artery

Supplies the following:

- right atrium
- right ventricle
- inferior/diaphragmatic surface of left ventricle
- sinoatrial node (55%)
- atrioventricular node (90%)
- bundle of His

Blockage causes the following:

- infarction of posterior or inferior wall of left ventricle
- right ventricle infarction
- in inferior myocardial infarction (leads II, III, aV$_F$), anticipate second-degree heart block or Mobitz type I block (Wenckebach)

Left coronary artery

Left circumflex branch

Supplies the following:

- left atrium
- lateral wall of left ventricle
- sinoatrial node (45%)
- atrioventricular node (10%)
- posterior/inferior division of left bundle

Blockage causes the following:

- lateral wall infarction
- posterior wall infarction (near base)
- in lateral wall myocardial infarction, electrocardiogram changes seen in leads I, AV$_L$, and V$_5$ and V$_6$

Left anterior descending branch

Supplies the following:

- anterior wall of left ventricle
- interventricular septum
- bundle of His
- right bundle
- posterior/inferior division of left bundle
- apex of left ventricle

Blockage causes the following:

- infarction of anterior wall of left ventricle
- effect on papillary muscle (which attaches to mitral valve)
- in anterior myocardial infarction (leads V$_2$, V$_3$, V$_4$), anticipate second-degree heart block, Mobitz type II block or third-degree block

---

cardiac impulse spreads from the SA node to the AV node by myocardial cell-to-cell conduction.[6,11]

The *AV node* also possesses pacemaker cells that depolarise at an intrinsic rate that is less than that of the SA node—about 40–60 times per minute. The AV node is located on the right, posterior side of the interatrial septum. Non-conductive tissue separates the atria and the ventricles, and as the depolarisation arrives at the AV node from the SA node there is a slight delay. This delay allows optimal time for ventricular filling to occur and ensures that the ventricles do not respond to excessively rapid atrial rates.[6,11]

The *bundle of His* conducts the electrical depolarisation from the AV node to the ventricles. The impulse is conducted rapidly through the bundle of His into the upper part of the interventricular septum. The intrinsic rate of the His/Purkinje system is approximately 15–40 times per minute.[6,8,11] Approximately 10–12 mm away from the AV node, the bundle of His divides into the right and left bundle branches. The right bundle branch consists of one fascicle, which continues down the right side of the interventricular septum and radiates towards the right ventricular apex.[6,8,11] The left bundle branch consists of two sets of fibres, referred to as the anterior and posterior fascicles. The anterior fascicle courses over the left ventricular wall to the papillary muscle. The left posterior fascicle travels inferiorly and posteriorly across the left ventricular outflow tract. Where one of the left bundle branches is blocked or damaged and hence non-conducting, it is referred to as a hemiblock or fascicular block.[6-8,11]

Basic electrocardiogram interpretation

The electrocardiogram (ECG) records the electrical change in the heart. The 12-lead ECG is an important diagnostic tool used in critical care areas within both pre-hospital and hospital settings. The ECG identifies electrical activity of the heart's depolarisation during the cardiac cycle.

- The direction of electrical activity in atrial depolarisation is downwards and towards the left; this creates the P wave on the ECG.[7,10,14]

- In ventricular depolarisation the overall direction of electrical activity is again downwards and to the left, due to the thicker muscle mass of the left ventricle compared with the thinner right ventricle. This produces the QRS complex on the ECG.

- The T wave on the ECG represents ventricular repolarisation. An electrical impulse travelling towards an ECG lead will create a positive or upwards deflection on the ECG. An electrical impulse travelling away from a lead will create a negative or downwards deflection, and an impulse travelling perpendicular to a lead will create a biphasic (both positive and negative) deflection.[7,14]

The 12-lead ECG consists of six limb leads (standard leads) and six chest or praecordial leads. Twelve 'views' of the heart are obtained from an ECG. The limb leads (Fig 22.5) should be positioned on each wrist and ankle; however, modification may be required. The six chest leads are positioned in specific places on the chest wall around the praecordium as shown in Figure 22.6.[8,13,14]

Ischaemia and infarction

The changes that occur on the ECG are a result of changes in the electrical flow of the current and can identify myocardial ischaemia, indicated by ST-segment depression, T-wave inversion, or a combination of both. Myocardial injury or infarction causes ST-segment elevation. Myocardial necrosis is identified by the formation of a pathological Q wave.[7,8,14] The ECG can aid in the identification of the coronary arteries involved in the ischaemia or infarction, as discussed in Box 22.1.

In myocardial infarction (MI), ST segment elevation can occur within minutes of total occlusion of a coronary artery, and can remain elevated for up to 24 hours. Within a few hours, T-wave inversion occurs; the subsequent formation of Q waves develops at around 24 hours (Fig 22.7). Q waves need to be 25% of the height of the QRS to be significant indicators of transmural damage. In general, Q-wave MIs are associated with larger amounts of myocardial cell damage and therefore a higher cardiac enzyme result (see Figs 22.8 to 22.11).[6,8,14,15]

Despite the usually specific placement of the chest leads, they may be positioned in different places on the chest wall to aid diagnosis and assess the extent of myocardial damage of the right ventricle or posterior wall of the left ventricle.[6,14,15] For example, when a right ventricular infarction is suspected the right ventricle can be assessed by swapping the position of leads V_3 to V_6 to a mirror-image position on the right side of the chest; should right-ventricular damage be present these

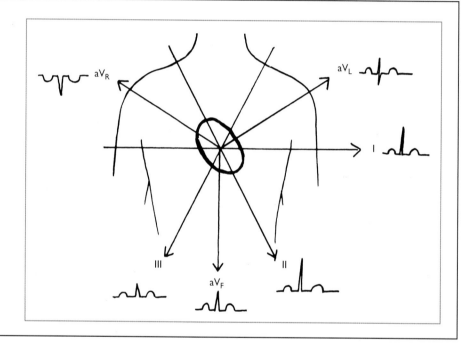

FIGURE 22.5

Six limb lead (leads I, II, III, aV$_R$, aV$_L$ and aV$_F$) normally appear as shown.

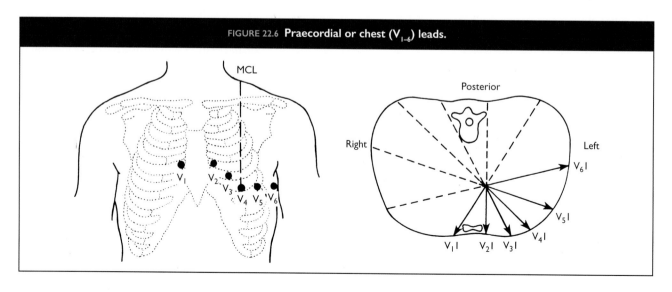

FIGURE 22.6 **Praecordial or chest (V$_{1-6}$) leads.**

FIGURE 22.7 **Electrocardiogram changes.**

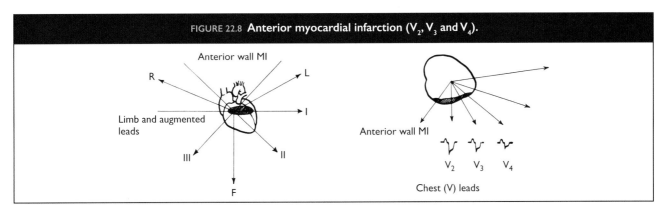

Normal

Ischaemia
Decreased blood supply
T wave inversion
May indicate ischaemia
without myocardial infarction

Injury
Acute or recent;
the more elevated
the ST segment,
the more recent
the injury

Infarct
Significant Q wave
greater than 1 mm
wide and half the
height + depth of
the entire complex
indicates myocardial
necrosis

FIGURE 22.8 **Anterior myocardial infarction (V$_2$, V$_3$ and V$_4$).**

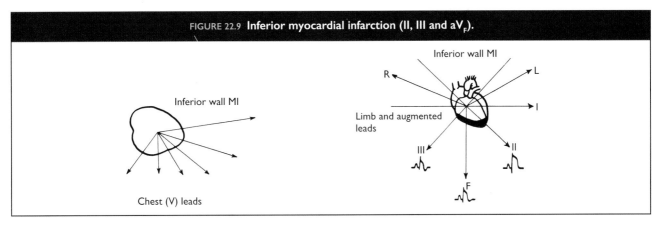

FIGURE 22.9 **Inferior myocardial infarction (II, III and aV$_F$).**

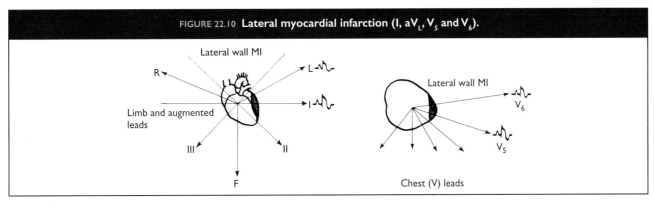

FIGURE 22.10 **Lateral myocardial infarction (I, aV$_L$, V$_5$ and V$_6$).**

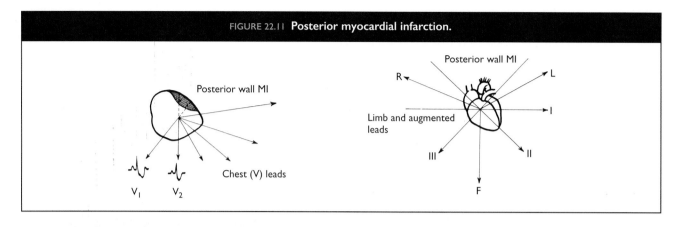

FIGURE 22.11 **Posterior myocardial infarction.**

BOX 22.2 **Lead placement for right ventricular and posterior leads**

Right ventricular leads

V_{3R} = Between V_1 and V_{4R}

V_{4R} = Fifth intercostal space right midclavicular line

V_{5R} = Fifth intercostal space right anterior axillary line

V_{6R} = Fifth intercostal space right midaxillary line

Posterior leads

V_7 = Fifth intercostal space posterior axillary line

V_8 = Fifth intercostal space between V_7 and V_9

V_9 = Fifth intercostal space next to vertebral column

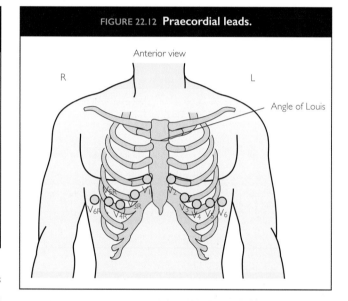

FIGURE 22.12 **Praecordial leads.**

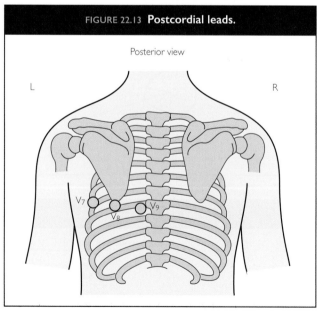

FIGURE 22.13 **Postcordial leads.**

---

leads will show an injury pattern on the ECG. These leads should be clearly labelled on the ECG as V_{3R}, V_{4R}, V_{5R} and V_{6R} (Box 22.2).[14,15]

When an infarction of the posterior wall of the left ventricular is suspected, it can be assessed by continuing the leads from V_6 around the back of the patient to V_7, V_8 and V_9 by replacing V_1 to V_6 with V_4 to V_9 (see Figs 22.12 and 22.13). Obtaining a posterior lead ECG can be a challenge as patient positioning is difficult and artefact is often a problem; however, valuable clinical information may be obtained. Both techniques should always be considered in any inferior, right ventricular infarction and posterior infarction.[6,8,14,15]

Cardiac axis

Cardiac axis refers to the mean (overall) direction of a wave of ventricular depolarisation. The mean vector (electrical activity) travels downwards and towards the left due to the increased muscle mass of the left ventricle towards lead II. The mean vector can be plotted on a graph known as the hexaxial reference system. Lead I is the zero reference point. The normal range of cardiac axis is −30° to +110°. An axis lying > −30° is referred to as a left-axis deviation and an axis > +110° is referred to as a right-axis deviation. Axis deviation can be caused by hypertrophy of the ventricle, bundle branch blocks, Wolff-Parkinson-White syndrome, fascicular blocks or MI.[7,8,14]

Accurate assessment of cardiac axis can be achieved by examining all six limb leads. The hexaxial reference system shows that the flow of depolarisation towards a lead results

in a positive deflection, away from a lead results in a negative deflection and at 90° to a lead results in an equiphasic (equal amounts of positive and negative deflection) QRS complex.[7,8,13,16] The steps to follow are:

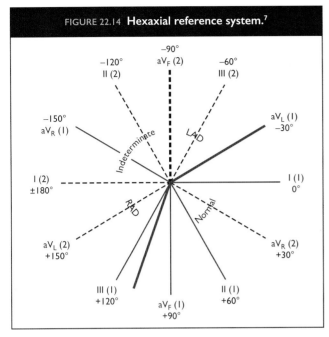

FIGURE 22.14 **Hexaxial reference system.**[7]

LAD: left-axis deviation; RAD: right-axis deviation.

1. Choose the lead that has the smallest or most equiphasic QRS complex. The axis lies approximately 90° to the right or left of this lead.
2. Using the hexaxial reference system, find the lead that is perpendicular (at a right-angle) to the lead chosen in step 1.
3. If the deflection of the lead in which you are now looking is positive, then the axis is in this direction. If the deflection of the lead is negative, then it is the opposite pole that is the direction of the axis.[7,8,13,16]

Refer to Figures 22.14 and 22.15.

Acute chest pain

The 2011 Addendum to the National Heart Foundation of Australia/Cardiac Society of Australia and New Zealand Guidelines for the Management of Acute Coronary Syndromes (ACS) 2006 recommends urgent assessment of patients with prolonged or recurrent chest discomfort. Patients should be assessed by a doctor within 10 minutes of arrival to the emergency department (ED) (Australasian Triage Scale category—see Ch 13). In the absence of trauma, the primary focus of an initial assessment is the exclusion of potentially

FIGURE 22.15

Patterns of axis deviation and associated conditions.[12]

LBBB: left bundle branch block; LPH: left posterior hemiblock; LVH: left ventricular hypertrophy; RBBB: right bundle branch block; RVH: right ventricular hypertrophy; WPW: Wolff-Parkinson-White syndrome.

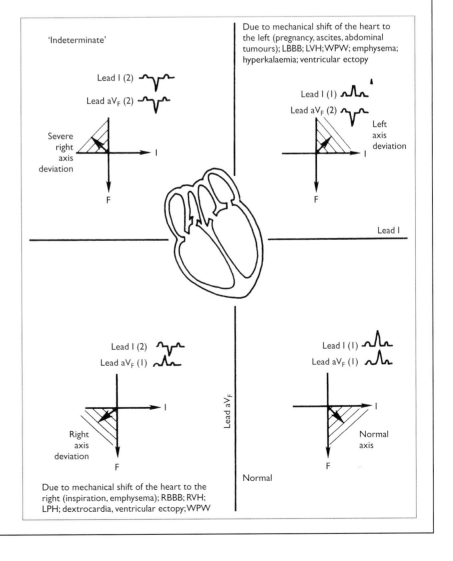

fatal conditions; pulmonary embolism, aortic dissection, spontaneous pneumothorax and acute coronary syndromes (ACS). Of these ACS is by far the most common, and this section will deal with the identification and treatment of ACS.

For chest pain patients managed in the out-of-hospital setting, the principles remain the same. Each patient should be assessed immediately and appropriately, and transported to the nearest appropriate facility.[5] Paramedics should approach the assessment and treatment of the chest pain patient in a step-wise manner, including continual monitoring and re-assessment of vital signs. A 12-lead ECG should be obtained as soon as practicable, and either transmitted to the receiving hospital or the results communicated to the receiving hospital according to local or state protocol. Aspirin, analgesia and nitrates are considered front-line therapy; however, the routine administration of high-flow oxygen to normoxic patients is now not widely recommended. The National Heart Foundation of Australia/Cardiac Society of Australia and New Zealand Guidelines recommend that oxygen therapy should be initiated if the patient is breathless, hypoxaemic (oxygen saturations of < 93%) or signs of heart failure or shock are present. Non-invasive monitoring of oxygen saturation may be used to decide on the need for oxygen administration.[5,18]

Patient assessment by either a nurse or a paramedic should include the following:

- Obtain and examine a rhythm strip and a 12-lead ECG as soon as possible. This is for the early and accurate identification of patients with an ST-segment elevation infarction (STEMI) and enables timely emergency reperfusion if not contraindicated. In the in-hospital setting, blood is taken for initial cardiac biomarker (enzyme) assessment.

- Measure heart rate, blood pressure, respiratory rate, oxygen saturation, work of breathing and central and peripheral perfusion. Assess neurological status. Auscultate the chest, noting abnormal heart and valve sounds and adventitious lung sounds.

- Ascertain the patient's past medical and social history (especially previous cardiac events/interventions and high-risk lifestyle choices), their present symptoms and the nature of their chest pain (or discomfort). Various mnemonics exist to aid in the assessment of pain including: PQRST (**P**rovokes/palliates, **Q**uality, **R**adiates, **S**everity,

Time) or DOLOR (**D**escription, **O**nset, **L**ocation, **O**ther signs/symptoms, **R**elieving factors). It is critical to remember that many patients suffering an infarct or an ACS may not report chest pain, instead presenting with 'atypical' symptoms, including gastrointestinal pain, back pain, shoulder pain or simply a vague feeling of being 'unwell' or fatigued: refer to Table 22.1 for chest pain assessment.[17] Women may describe symptoms that are different to males. Women are perceived as being a lower risk of ACS than men, thus making diagnosis more difficult. Diagnosis of ACS in women may be under-recognised or undertreated. Chest pain or discomfort is still a common sign in women, but it is important to know that other signs women may experience include shortness of breath, nausea and vomiting and back or jaw pain.[19]

- Be aware of the differential diagnoses to consider in patients who present with a complaint of chest pain (Table 22.2). However, remember to retain a high index of suspicion of an ACS, as it is not possible to accurately and safely exclude an ACS in the pre-hospital setting. Table 22.3 highlights aetiological factors related to differential diagnosis of chest pain.[4,8,14,15]

- Record current medication usage, including prescription, over-the-counter, recreational and herbal remedies. Remember to assess compliance with current medication regimen.

- Identify and record other symptoms including dyspnoea, nausea, vomiting, diaphoresis and neck vein distension, even if these symptoms may be considered 'atypical' of an ACS.

PRACTICE TIP

The aim of a cardiac assessment is to determine cardiac status, identify deterioration in patients at risk and guide and evaluate the effectiveness of treatment. Ongoing assessment is required regularly.

Acute coronary syndromes

ACS represents a spectrum of disease that includes unstable angina pectoris (UAP), non-ST-segment elevation MI (NSTEMI) and ST-segment elevation MI (STEMI). The terminology used to describe ACS is evolving and 'non-ST-segment elevation acute coronary syndrome' (NSTEACS) is now used to refer collectively to unstable angina and NSTEMI. This reflects a more contemporary approach to clinical management, given its broad spectrum of risk—moving away from defining a diagnosis at presentation and focusing on early risk stratification to guide timely management.

At presentation, the initial working diagnosis should focus on risk stratification to direct treatment strategies, as the establishment of a definitive diagnosis often takes some time, particularly to assess myocardial necrosis in elevated biochemical cardiac markers.[5]

ACSs without an ECG showing evidence of ST-segment elevation are collectively referred to as NSTEACSs, since both NSTEMI and UAP share the same pathogenesis.[8] This grouping

---

BOX 22.3 Cardiac risk factors: patient characteristics and high-risk behaviours[12]

Ageing	New onset of fatigue within the past month (particularly in women)
Cocaine or stimulant use	
Diabetes	Obesity
Emotional stress	Previous myocardial infarction, angina, cardiac surgery or peripheral vascular disease
Hyperlipidaemia	
Hypertension	
Immediate family history	Smoking
Lack of exercise	

		TABLE 22.1 CHEST PAIN mnemonic for chest pain assessment[17]	
LETTER	TRIGGER WORDS	ASSESSMENT
C	Commenced when?	When did the pain start?
		Was onset associated with anything specific? Exertion? Activity? Emotional upset?
H	History/risk factors	Do you have a history of heart disease?
		Is there a primary relative (parent/sibling) with early onset and/or early death related to heart disease?
		Do you have other risk factors, e.g. diabetes, smoking, hypertension or obesity?
E	Extra symptoms?	What else are you feeling with the pain? Are you nervous? Sweating? Is your heart racing? Are you short of breath? Do you feel nauseated? Dizzy? Weak?
S	Stays/radiates	Does the pain stay in one place?
		Does it radiate or go anywhere else in the body? Where?
T	Timing	How long does the pain last? How long has this episode lasted? How many minutes?
		Is the pain continuous or does it come and go? When did it become continuous?
P	Place	Where is your pain? Check for point tenderness with palpation.
A	Alleviates	What makes the pain better? Rest? Changing position? Deep breathing?
	Aggravates	What makes the pain worse? Exercise? Deep breathing? Changing position?
I	Intensity	How intense is the pain? Rate the pain from 0 to 10.
N	Nature	Describe the pain. (Listen for descriptors such as sharp, stabbing, crushing, dull, burning, elephant sitting on my chest.) Do not suggest descriptors.

is beneficial because urgent reperfusion is not indicated as in STEMI, and risk stratification is very often complex.[5,14,15]

Unstable angina is defined as myocardial ischaemia without ECG or biochemical evidence of necrosis, while NSTEMI involves sub-endocardial or intramural (partial thickness) myocardial wall damage. STEMI involves full-thickness myocardial wall damage or necrosis. It is considered more appropriate to describe a myocardial infarct as the presence or absence of significant ST elevation, and this classification reflects the differences in pathophysiology between STEMI and NSTEMI.[5,8,14,15]

Atherosclerosis affects the coronary arteries. It is a progressive disease that is characterised by the accumulation of lipids (lipid oxidation) and the proliferation of smooth muscle within the intimal lining of these arteries, known as plaques. Atherosclerosis is described in three stages: (1) birth of plaque, (2) plaque progression and (3) plaque rupture.[11] Previous suggestions that atherosclerosis was simply a 'plumbing problem' have recently been debunked, with evidence now suggesting that inflammatory processes are the key factor in the development of atherosclerotic plaques that are more vulnerable to rupture.[7,8,11] These plaques protrude into the lumen of the artery and impede or obstruct blood flow, which may result in myocardial ischaemia, particularly when myocardial oxygen demand increases as in exertion or stress. Atherosclerotic plaques are subject to continuing structural weakening from turbulent blood flow, calcification and internal inflammatory-driven changes. This may cause them to rupture, exposing highly thrombogenic plaque contents to the circulation. Platelets in the blood accumulate around the rupture site, resulting in the formation of a platelet plug. The formation of this platelet plug activates the coagulation system, resulting in the formation of a thrombus superimposed on the plaque, totally or subtotally occluding the arterial lumen (Fig 22.16).[7,8,11,14,15]

Neither signs and symptoms nor cardiac markers alone are sufficient to diagnose acute MI or ischaemia in the first 4–6 hours in the pre-hospital or hospital setting. The 12-lead ECG in the pre-hospital and ED setting is crucial to the initial triage of patients, offering strong, positive, predictive value for patients experiencing possible ACS.[8,13–15,18] A pre-hospital 12-lead is also vital in triaging STEMI patients to appropriate coronary catherisation laboratories, or for the pre-hospital administration of fibrinolytic therapy.[11] It is also important to note that despite the predictive nature of 12-lead ECGs, the most common reason for inappropriate discharge of patients who are subsequently diagnosed with an ACS is a normal or non-specific 12-lead ECG; therefore highlighting the complexities in cardiovascular management.[15]

PRACTICE TIP

The 12-lead ECG in the pre-hospital and ED setting is crucial to the initial triage of patients, offering strong positive predictive value for patients experiencing possible ACS. It is imperative that the ECG is reviewed by a senior doctor for diagnosis and treatment early.

TABLE 22.2 Differential diagnosis of chest pain[12]

CAUSE	ONSET OF PAIN	CHARACTERISTICS OF PAIN	LOCATION OF PAIN	HISTORY	PAIN WORSENED BY	PAIN RELIEVED BY	OTHER
Acute myocardial infarction	Sudden onset; lasts more than 30 minutes to 1 hour	Pressure, burning, aching, tightness, choking	Across chest; may radiate to jaws and neck and down arms and back	Age 40–70 years; may or may not have history of angina	Movement, anxiety	Nothing; not movement, stillness, position, or breath holding; only relieved by medication (morphine sulfate)	Shortness of breath, diaphoresis, weakness, anxiety
Angina	Sudden onset; lasts only a few minutes	Ache, squeezing, choking, heaviness, burning	Substernal; may radiate to jaw and neck and down arms and back	May have history of angina; precipitating circumstances; pain characteristic; response to glyceryl trinitrate	Lying down, eating, effort, cold weather, smoking, stress, anger, worry, hunger	Rest, glyceryl trinitrate	Unstable angina occurs even at rest
Dissecting aortic aneurysm	Sudden onset	Excruciating, tearing	Centre of chest; radiates into back; may radiate to abdomen	Nothing specific, except that pain is usually worse at onset		Nothing	Blood pressure difference between right and left arms, murmur of aortic regurgitation
Pericarditis	Sudden onset or may be variable	Sharp, knifelike	Retrosternal; may radiate up neck and down left arm	Short history of upper respiratory infection or fever	Deep breathing, trunk movement, maybe swallowing	Sitting up, leaning forward	Friction rub, paradoxic pulse over 10 mmHg
Pneumothorax	Sudden onset	Tearing, pleuritic	Lateral side of chest	None	Breathing	Nothing	Dyspnoea, increased pulse, decreased breath sounds, deviated trachea
Pulmonary embolus	Sudden onset	Crushing (but not always)	Lateral side of chest	Sometimes phlebitis Deep vein thrombosis Recent surgery	Breathing	Not breathing	Cyanosis, dyspnoea, profound anxiety, hypoxaemia, cough with haemoptysis

TABLE 22.2 Differential diagnosis of chest pain[12]—cont'd

CAUSE	ONSET OF PAIN	CHARACTERISTICS OF PAIN	LOCATION OF PAIN	HISTORY	PAIN WORSENED BY	PAIN RELIEVED BY	OTHER
Hiatus hernia	Sudden onset	Sharp, severe	Lower chest; upper abdomen	May have none	Heavy meal, bending, lying down	Bland diet, walking, antacids, semi-Fowler position	
Gastrointestinal disturbance or cholecystitis	Sudden onset	Gripping, burning	Lower substernal area, upper abdomen	May have none	Eating, lying down	Antacids	
Degenerative disk (cervical or thoracic spine) disease	Sudden onset	Sharp, severe	Substernal; may radiate to neck, jaw, arms and shoulders	May have none	Movement of the neck or spine, lifting, straining	Rest, decreased movement	Pain usually on outer aspect of arm, thumb or index finger
Degenerative or inflammatory lesions of shoulder, ribs, scalenus anterior	Sudden onset	Sharp, severe	Substernal; radiates to shoulder	May have none	Movement of arm or shoulder	Elevation of arm, support to shoulder; postural exercises	
Hyperventilation	Sudden onset	Vague	Vague	Hyperventilation, anxiety, stress, emotional upset	Increased respiratory rate	Slowing of respiratory rate	Be sure hyperventilation is from non-medical cause

TABLE 22.3 Aetiological factors to be considered in the differential diagnosis of chest pain[12]

AETIOLOGICAL FACTORS	P—PRECIPITATING/PALLIATING	Q—QUALITY	R—RADIATING/REGION	S—SEVERITY/SYMPTOMS	T—TIME/TEMPORAL
Ischaemia/angina	Precipitating factors: effort-related activity, large meals, emotional stress Palliation: ceases with activity abatement, relief with glyceryl trinitrate, relief with rest	Tightness, burning, deep, constrictive	Retrosternal, area affected the size of the palm of the hand Pain may radiate to left shoulder, left hand (e.g. especially the fourth and fifth fingers), epigastrium trachea, larynx Never involves region above the level of the eye	Associated symptoms: profuse diaphoresis, weakness, shortness of breath, nausea, vomiting	Gradual onset of pain builds up to maximum pain intensity; usually anginal pain lasts 1–5 minutes
Myocardial infarction	Precipitating factors: effort-related activity, large meals, emotional stress	Severe chest pain	Chest pain; may have radiation of pain to back, jaw or left arm	Associated symptoms: palpitations, dyspnoea, diaphoresis, nausea, vomiting, dizziness, weakness, sense of impending doom	Usually pain has lasted 30 minutes or more
Acute pericarditis	Precipitating factors: may occur after AMI; also may be related to viral, collagen or vascular disorders	Chest pain may be due to severe and crushing type of pain	Anterior chest pain with radiation to the neck, arms or shoulders; pain may be intensified by deep inspiration	Associated symptoms: fever (i.e. between 38.3°C and 38.9°C); pericardial friction rub; electrocardiogram; ST-segment elevation in all leads except V_I and aV_R	May be hours to days
Dissecting aortic aneurysm	Sudden onset	Severe, ripping, tearing type of pain	Anterior and posterior chest Often radiates from anterior chest to intrascapular region or to abdomen Pain may move with progression of aortic dissection	Associated symptoms: dyspnoea, tachypnoea, CHF (i.e. because of aortic regurgitation caused by dissection); also, CVA, syncope, paraplegia and pulse loss associated with dissecting aneurysm	Sudden onset
Oesophageal disorders (oesophageal reflux, oesophageal spasm)	Precipitating factors: often triggered by exercise or by food (large meal, spicy foods, acidic foods, cold foods) or ethanol intake	Burning or pressure-like pain May be severe	May radiate to neck, ear, jaw or lower abdomen	Associated symptoms: dysphagia, aspiration	Minutes to days
Cocaine-induced	Precipitating factors: cocaine use Palliation: relieved with glyceryl trinitrate	Severe pain	Substernal location, with radiation to both arms	Associated symptoms: tachycardia, palpitations, diaphoresis, nausea, dizziness, syncope, dyspnoea	Occurs 1–6 hours after cocaine use

TABLE 22.3 Aetiological factors to be considered in the differential diagnosis of chest pain[12]—cont'd

AETIOLOGICAL FACTORS	P—PRECIPITATING/PALLIATING	Q—QUALITY	R—RADIATING/REGION	S—SEVERITY/SYMPTOMS	T—TIME/TEMPORAL
Postoperative coronary artery bypass graft (CABG) after harvest of internal mammary artery (IMA)	Precipitating factors: use of IMA for graft of CABG patient	Mild to severe chest pain, burning, prickling and dull type of sensations	Anterior chest; may radiate over entire chest wall and particularly over the site of the graft; may radiate to neck or axilla	Associated symptoms: numbness, tenderness on palpation of the sternum, hyperaesthesia along the incisional line, delayed healing of the sternum	Persistent type of pain Shooting-type pain may last for several seconds and occur several times per day
Mitral valve prolapse	Palliation: relief in recumbent position, no relief with glyceryl trinitrate	Dull and aching; although also may be sharp	Non-retrosternal chest pain	Associated symptoms: systolic murmur, unexplained dyspnoea, weakness, midsystolic (apical) click	Onset may be sudden or recurrent May last for a few seconds, or be persistent for days
5-Fluorouracil (5-FU) therapy	Precipitating factors: following infusion of 5-FU Palliation: relief with glyceryl trinitrate	Mild to severe pain	Central chest pain; radiates to left shoulder and left arm	Associated symptoms: nausea, vomiting, tachycardia, hypertension	Occurs several days after intravenous bolus or infusion of 5-FU No chest pain between treatment
Spontaneous pneumothorax	COPD, chronic asthma	Sharp or stabbing; described as moderate to severe	Usually pain of entire lung region (hemithorax); may radiate to back and neck	Associated symptoms: decreased or absent breath sounds; pneumothorax per chest radiograph	Continuous pain until treated
Tachydysrhythmias	Precipitating factors: anxiety, digitalis toxicity, exercise, organic heart disease Palliation: terminated by antidysrhythmics, direct current shock, vagal manoeuvres	Sharp, stabbing type of chest pain May have palpitations, 'skipped beats'	Praecordial chest pain	Associated symptoms: weakness, fatigue, lethargy, palpitations, dizziness, vertigo	Paroxysmal in onset Lasts briefly to hours
Anxiety disorders	May have history of depression or anxiety	Pain may be vague, diffuse; may be further described as disabling	Anterior chest and abdomen	Associated symptoms: dyspnoea, fatigue, anorexia	Variable; often continuous for hours to days
Monosodium glutamate	Occurs with ingestion of food high in monosodium glutamate	Burning type of chest pain	Retrosternal chest pain	Associated symptoms: facial pain, nausea, vomiting	Occurs shortly after meals up to several hours after meal
Musculoskeletal	Precipitating factors: pain with inspiration or with musculoskeletal movement	Generalised aching stiffness with point tenderness, swelling	Tenderness of the anterior chest wall	Persistent chest pain without relief with rest	

AMI: acute myocardial infarction; CHF: congestive heart failure; COPD: chronic obstructive pulmonary disease; CVA: cerebrovascular accident

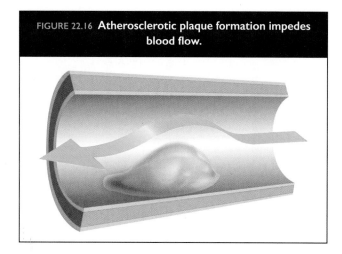

FIGURE 22.16 **Atherosclerotic plaque formation impedes blood flow.**

Unstable angina

Unstable angina is commonly associated with atherosclerotic changes in the coronary arteries and the rupture of an atherosclerotic plaque. In conjunction with the rupture of the plaque comes the release of vasoconstrictor substances, which may induce clotting and therefore precipitate the formation of a thrombus.[7,8,11] This thrombus is usually sub-occlusive and intermittently obstructs the blood flow within the coronary artery. Platelet aggregation, vasoconstriction and intermittent thrombosis can impede blood flow without producing detectable myocardial damage.[7,8,11]

Unstable coronary syndromes are a group of disorders that may present in many different ways. Most patients will present with prolonged angina-type pain at rest and lasting over 20 minutes. If there has been no elevation in cardiac markers, the patient is said to have UAP. Both UAP and NSTEMI are collectively referred to as non ST-elevation acute coronary syndrome (NSTEACS). These patients will be at differing levels of risk. All patients should be risk-stratified for progression to myocardial infarction or death.[16]

Any patient presenting with chest discomfort or other symptoms suggestive of cardiac ischaemia should undergo risk stratification using a risk stratification tool or model. The Thrombolysis in Myocardial Infarction (TIMI) or Global Registry of Acute Coronary Events (GRACE) tools can be useful to assist in the assessment of the patient and indicate risk of death from ACS.[5,18]

Table 22.4 compares the characteristics of the three types of angina: stable angina, unstable angina and Prinzmetal angina.

Non-ST-segment elevation Acute Coronary Syndrome (NSTEACS)

There has been considerable advancement in the understanding of NSTEACS aetiology over the past decade. NSTEACS occurs when there is an incomplete thrombosis, as in unstable angina or when early lysis of the thrombus occurs. In 80% of patients this thrombogenesis occurs at a vulnerable 'soft' plaque site, which is defined by a large lipid pool and weakened fibrosis cap. This causes minimal necrosis of myocardial tissue in the region supplied by the coronary artery[6,8] and a rise in blood troponin levels with no ST-segment elevation on the 12-lead ECG. NSTEACS can be defined as ST-segment depression, T-wave inversion or a combination of both, and represent up

to 25% of all acute MIs.[5,18] Approximately a quarter of patients presenting with UAP or NSTEACS are at significant risk for progression to a STEMI, with NSTEACSs carrying similar 1-year mortality rates as STEMIs.[5,18]

Early coronary angiography and revascularisation is recommended in patients with high-risk features in NSTEACS. One valuable and validated risk-assessment tool is the TIMI risk score, which identifies early risk in NSTEACS (see Box 22.4). This risk stratification may be a contributing factor in the decision to transfer patients for early revascularisation where funding may be constrained. Appropriate patients should be transferred within 48 hours if symptoms do not increase and thus indicate the need for earlier angiography.[5]

In the pre-hospital setting, patients suffering an NSTEACS should be continuously monitored, and administered appropriate analgesia, glyceryl trinitrate, aspirin and oxygen titrated to normoxia. They should be transported to the nearest, most appropriate hospital, recognising that NSTEACS have the potential to evolve into STEMIs. This approach should also apply to patients suffering UAP. Currently, no pre-hospital risk-stratification tool is available to paramedics for in-field assessment of NSTEACs.

Figure 22.17 shows the common sites and areas of pain experienced by a patient with angina or MI.[6,8,14,15]

Myocardial infarction

Chest pain that is indicative of an acute myocardial infarction (AMI) is usually central, crushing, retrosternal pain which occurs at rest, lasts longer than 30 minutes and is unrelieved by glyceryl trinitrate (GTN). The pain can radiate to the neck, jaw or back and can be associated with nausea and vomiting.[4,7,8,11]

Chest pain can manifest from a variety of musculoskeletal and gastrointestinal pathologies as a result of a shared neurological pathway with abdominal and thoracic organs. Patients experiencing MI can also present with atypical symptoms such as toothache, fatigue or sensations of discomfort.[4,7,14,15]

Total occlusion of a coronary artery may result from thrombus formation, spasm or haemorrhage. Myocardial cell necrosis starts approximately 20 minutes after coronary arterial occlusion and proceeds from the subendocardium (inside) to the epicardium (outside). The surrounding myocardium becomes hypoxic and zones of ischaemia and necrosis form in the heart muscle around the site of occlusion.[6,8,11] The areas of myocardial necrosis and cell death are called *zones of infarction*. This infarcted tissue is surrounded by the *zone of injury*, which comprises severely ischaemic yet still potentially viable tissue. The outermost zone is the *zone of ischaemia* which contains viable myocardial cells dependent on the rapid restoration of blood flow and revascularisation of the coronary artery.[6,8,11] The hypoxic myocardial tissue can become irritable and result in various dysrhythmias, and damage to the myocardium can predispose the patient to pump failure.[6,11]

Haemodynamic changes occur with AMI because of the decreased pumping function of the heart which results in a reduced cardiac output and decreased coronary artery perfusion pressures. The reduced cardiac output will eventually result in a lowered blood pressure which in turn activates a sympathetic response producing vasoconstriction. The sympathetic response redistributes blood flow to the heart and brain. Blood vessels in

	TABLE 22.4 Comparison of characteristics of angina[12]		
CHARACTERISTIC	STABLE ANGINA	UNSTABLE ANGINA	PRINZMETAL ANGINA
Location of pain	Substernal; may radiate to the jaw, neck and down arms or back	Substernal; may radiate to the jaw, neck and down arms or back	Substernal; may radiate to the jaw, neck and down arms and back
Duration of pain	1–15 minutes	Occurs progressively more frequently with episodes lasting as along as 30 minutes	Occurs repeatedly at about the same time of day. Episodes tend to cluster between midnight and 8 am
Pain characteristics	Commonly referred to as an aching, squeezing, choking, heaving or burning discomfort	Same as stable angina, but more intense	Distinctly painful
Severity of pain	Generally severity is the same as previous episodes	The severity, duration or frequency of events increases over time	Extremely severe
Other symptoms	None for most patients	Diaphoresis, weakness, S3 or S4 heart sound, pulsus alternans, transient pulmonary crackles	Diaphoresis, weakness, S3 or S4 heart sound, pulsus alternans, transient pulmonary crackles
Pain worsened by	Exercise, activity, eating, cold weather, reclining	Exercise, activity, eating, cold weather, reclining	Occurs at rest
Pain relieved by	Rest, glyceryl trinitrate, isosorbide	Rest, glyceryl trinitrate and isosorbide may provide only partial relief	Glyceryl trinitrate may be helpful
Electrocardiogram findings	Transient ST segment depression that disappears with pain relief	Patients often have ST segment depression or T wave inversion but the electrocardiogram may be normal	Episodic ST segment elevation with pain. ST segment returns to baseline when the pain subsides. Patients are prone to develop ventricular dysrhythmias
Additional characteristics	Most common in middle-aged and elderly males and postmenopausal females	Most common in middle-aged and elderly males and postmenopausal females; often referred to as preinfarction angina	Generally occurs in younger patients; thought to result from coronary artery spasm

BOX 22.4 TIMI risk score for NSTEACS[20]

Score one point for each of the following:

- Age over 65 years
- Three or more coronary risk factors (hypertension, hyper-cholesterolaemia, diabetes, family history, smoking)
- Aspirin use within the last 7 days
- Known coronary disease (> 50% stenosis at angiography)
- More than two anginal events in previous 24 hours
- Raised troponin (or other cardiac biomarker)
- ST deviation (depression or transient elevation)

Risk of major coronary event in 14 days:

- 0–2 points = low risk (5–8%)
- 3–4 points = medium risk (13–20%)
- 5–7 points = high risk (26–41%)

the skin, lungs, kidneys and gastrointestinal tract also constrict in response to sympathetic activation.[6,8,11]

In the renal circulation, hormonal compensation takes place when blood flow decreases. Renin and angiotensin are produced as a result of reduced blood flow, and subsequent production of aldosterone occurs. The increase in levels of aldosterone brings about the retention of sodium and water which increases the circulating volume that the already damaged and failing heart has to pump.[4,7,8,14,15,21]

Changes which occur on the 12-lead ECG that are indicative of AMI or STEMI are ST-segment elevation in two or more anatomically contiguous leads on the ECG, > 1 mm in the limb leads and > 2 mm in the chest leads, or a new left bundle branch block (LBBB). ST-segment elevation occurs in the leads which 'look at' that area of myocardium (see Box 22.1 and Fig 22.18).

Paramedical and nursing management of AMI should focus on a prompt and comprehensive assessment of the

FIGURE 22.17

Common sites for anginal pain.

A, Upper part of chest. **B**, Beneath sternum, radiating to neck and jaw. **C**, Beneath sternum, radiating down left arm. **D**, Epigastric. **E**, Epigastric, radiating to neck, jaw and arms. **F**, Neck and jaw. **G**, Left shoulder. **H**, Intrascapular.[12]

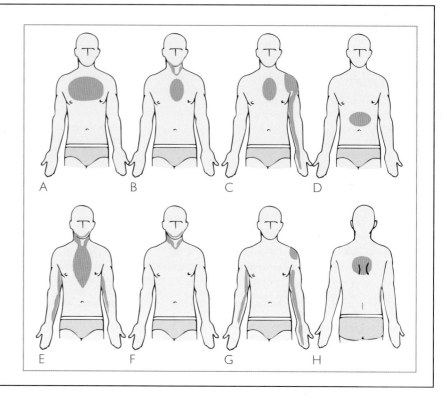

A   B   C   D

E   F   G   H

FIGURE 22.18 Zone of ischaemia, zone of injury and zone of infarction, shown through ECG waveforms and reciprocal waveforms corresponding to each zone.[12]

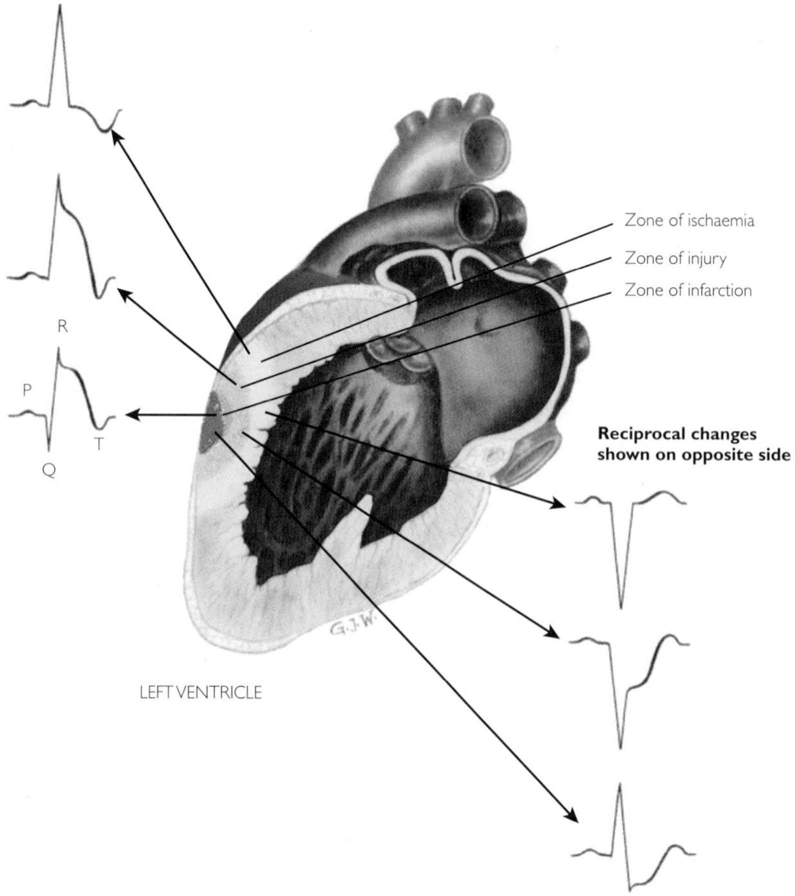

Zone of ischaemia
Zone of injury
Zone of infarction

R

P

Q   T

Reciprocal changes shown on opposite side

LEFT VENTRICLE

G.J.W

patient. A 12-lead ECG should be obtained as soon as possible, assuring that lead placement is precise. Given the evidence supporting the improved patient outcomes associated with early reperfusion, many Australian (and international) pre-hospital providers routinely obtain and transmit 12-lead ECGs for chest pain patients.[5,21–23,26] A 12-lead ECG performed by paramedical staff can facilitate pre-hospital diagnosis, and transmission of the ECG to a hospital to confirm a STEMI pattern allows for prompt triage to an appropriate Percutaneous Coronary Intervention (PCI) facility by activation of the catheterisation laboratory, the nearest hospital for thrombolysis or the paramedics may be advised to administer lysis at the scene, in accordance with local clinical practice guidelines.[5,8,24]

PRACTICE TIP

Chest pain that is indicative of an acute myocardial infarction (AMI) is usually central, crushing, retrosternal pain which occurs at rest, lasts longer than 30 minutes and is unrelieved by glyceryl-trinitrate (GTN). Management should include appropriate analgesia, oxygen, ongoing assessment of vital signs and continuous ECG monitoring to ensure prompt treatment and management of potential dysrhythmias.

At all times clinicians should be calm and reassuring, as increased anxiety may also increase endogenous catecholamine levels and place extra demands on myocardial delivery.[14,15,21]

Prompt treatment to restore and maintain blood flow to the myocardium reduces the mortality and morbidity associated with AMI. Time to reperfusion is critical, as the longer myocardium is without blood flow, the greater the chance of permanent damage—'minutes mean myocardium'. Current guidelines recommend that fibrinolytic therapy should be delivered within 30 minutes of the patient presenting to the ED ('door to needle time') and intervention with percutaneous coronary intervention (PCI) should occur within 60 minutes of arrival at hospital ('door to balloon time').[4,21,22] These guidelines also apply to the pre-hospital context, with evidence supporting pre-hospital fibrinolytic administration, particularly in systems with strong education, training and professional development programs.[5] Current Australian registry data suggests significant improvements are still required in door-to-needle and door-to-balloon times, both within the hospital and in the pre-hospital context.[21]

Management should include appropriate analgesia, ongoing assessment of vital signs and continuous ECG monitoring to ensure prompt treatment and management of potential dysrhythmias.[14,15] The NHFA ACS guideline recommends that patients should be advised to take aspirin while still at home or that pre-hospital clinicians should administer an initial dose of 150–300 mg while in transit to the hospital (Table 22.5).[14,15,21–23,25,26,28]

Cardiac markers

As myocardial cells die because of infarction, intracellular cardiac proteins are released into the bloodstream. The presence of these proteins, generally troponin or creatine kinase-MB, in the circulation is the most common method used to confirm

a diagnosis of MI, to estimate the amount of irreversible myocardial cell damage and to stratify the risk of further episodes of ACS. Troponins are an intracellular contractile protein found in all muscle types.[6–8] Some troponins, namely Troponin-T and Troponin-I, are unique to myocardial cells, and it is these that are used to diagnose MI. Cardiac troponins are currently considered the gold-standard biomarkers for AMI diagnosis.[15] Pre-hospital cardiac point-of-care biomarker assays have been shown to be effective tools in confirming MIs; however, given the potential for high false-negative rates, it is uncertain whether pre-hospital cardiac marker assays can reduce time delays to percutaneous cardiac intervention (see later in the chapter).[30,31]

Serial measurements of cardiac biomarkers are required to show diagnostic changes in blood concentrations, and the time in which a cardiac biomarker peaks then returns to baseline provides essential information to identify and manage patients with cardiac chest pain. Each cardiac biomarker has a specific pattern of elevation and return to baseline. Table 22.6 shows each biomarker's specific pattern.[6–8]

Cardiogenic shock

Cardiogenic shock results from the inability of the heart to pump blood forwards, and can occur with right or left ventricular dysfunction or when the heart rate and rhythm are compromised, causing impairment of myocardial contraction.[6,11]

The most common cause of cardiogenic shock is acute MI. Development of cardiogenic shock is directly related to the extent of myocardial cell necrosis from an MI, producing inadequate contractility of the heart muscle (pump failure). Cardiogenic shock is generally associated with the infarction of a critical mass of myocardium and a loss of up to 40% of the left ventricle (Box 22.5).[7,8,11]

Cardiogenic shock is defined as a reduced systemic blood flow, affecting renal and cerebral blood flow, or the inability of the heart to deliver sufficient blood flow to the tissues to meet resting metabolic demands. Cardiogenic shock results from failure of the myocardium to pump adequately. It progresses in four stages: initial, compensatory, progressive and refractory.[3,4,8]

Pathophysiology of cardiogenic shock

In MI some cardiac muscle fibres are not functioning and others are too weak to contract; consequently the overall pumping ability of the affected ventricle is depressed and cardiac output (CO) is reduced (Fig 22.19).[6,11]

The reduced CO from a damaged left ventricle results in inadequate perfusion of the tissues due to a reduction in blood flow. The failing ability of the left ventricle to sustain an adequate stroke volume causes blood flow within the chambers of the heart to slow down. There will therefore be a backflow of blood to the lungs, where gaseous exchange will be impaired as a result of an increase of fluid in the lung tissues or interstitial space (pulmonary oedema). This results in hypoxaemia of arterial blood and the complications of hypoxia and acidosis. This is the *initial stage* of shock.[6,8,11]

In the first stage of shock there is a fall in CO and blood pressure because of the inability of the myocardium to expel an adequate stroke volume (SV). As a consequence of the hypotension, compensatory mechanisms follow. These

TABLE 22.5 'MONA' medications for the patient with myocardial infarction

MEDICATION	DOSE	COMMENTS
Morphine sulfate	2–4 mg IV push given slowly over 1 to 5 minutes. Repeat every 5–30 minutes; titrate to effect. No maximum dose	The drug of choice for ischaemic chest pain. Also reduces preload and decreases myocardial oxygen demand
		Hold for significant hypotension
Oxygen	4 L/min via nasal cannula or Hudson mask for patients with a PaO_2 less than 93% on room air.	Recent evidence suggests that high-flow oxygen may be harmful for the chest pain patient with normal oxygen saturations. Avoid hyper-oxygenation.
Glyceryl trinitrate (**N**itroglycerine)	*Sublingual tablets:* 0.3–0.4 mg; repeat as needed every 5 minutes for up to 3 doses	Establish IV access before giving GTN to a patient who has never previously received it
	Sublingual spray: spray for 0.5–1 second (provides 0.4 mg per dose). Repeat as needed every 5 minutes for up to 3 doses. Do not shake the container before spraying because this affects the dose delivered	Monitor BP before and after GTN administration
		Limit SBP changes to a 10% decrease in the patient with MI who is normotensive, or a 30% decrease if hypertensive. Hold further doses for an SBP ≤ 90 mmHg
	Intravenous: give patient bolus of 12.5–25 μg followed by an infusion of 10–20 μg/min. Titrate to pain relief	Maximum IV dose is 200 μg/min. Drug concentration should not exceed 400 μg/mL
		Side effects include hypotension, tachycardia, ischaemia and headache
		Avoid giving GTN to patients with right ventricular infarction, hypotension, severe bradycardia or severe tachycardia
		GTN is contraindicated in patients who have taken sildenafil citrate or vardenafil within previous 24 hours
		May interfere with the anticoagulant effect of heparin; monitor activated partial thromboplastin time and prothrombin time (international normalised ratio)
Aspirin	160–325 mg orally. Chew for faster absorption	Administer as soon as possible after chest pain starts
		The antiplatelet activity of aspirin decreases mortality after acute MI
		Do not give to patients hypersensitive to salicylates
		Patients on daily aspirin therapy can receive an additional tablet safely at chest pain onset

BP: blood pressure; GTN: glyceryl trinitrate; IV: intravenous; MI, myocardial infarction; SBP: systolic blood pressure

TABLE 22.6 Cardiac markers for acute myocardial infarction

CARDIAC MARKER	INITIAL ELEVATION AFTER ACUTE MYOCARDIAL INFARCTION (H)	MEAN PEAK TIME (H)	TIME TO RETURN TO BASELINE
Myoglobin	1–4	6–7	18–24 hours
Troponin-I (cTn I) (cardiac-specific)	3–12	10–24	3–7 days
Troponin-T (cTn T) (cardiac-specific)	3–12	12–48	10–14 days
Creatine kinase-MB (CK-MB)	4–12	10–24	48–72 hours
CK-MB subforms: MB1 and MB2	1–6	18	Unknown
Lactate dehydrogenase (LDH)	8–12	24–48	10–14 days

Note: an LDH-1/LDH-2 ratio > 0.76 is significantly associated with acute myocardial infarction

---

BOX 22.5 Aetiological factors in cardiogenic shock[7]

Primary ventricular ischaemia:
- acute myocardial infarction
- cardiopulmonary arrest
- open heart surgery

Structural problems:
- septal rupture
- papillary muscle rupture
- free wall rupture
- ventricular aneurysm
- cardiomyopathies
- congestive
- hypertrophic
- restrictive
- intracardiac tumour
- pulmonary embolus
- atrial thrombus
- valvular dysfunction
- acute myocarditis
- cardiac tamponade
- myocardial contusion

Dysrhythmias:
- bradydysrhythmias
- tachydysrhythmias

---

homeostatic mechanisms are intricately interrelated and include neural, hormonal and chemical changes. This is the *compensatory stage* of shock (Box 22.6).[6,8,11]

As CO falls, arterial blood pressure decreases and this activates neural compensation by the baroreceptor reflex. Within seconds, baroreceptors in the aorta and carotid artery junctions detect the decrease in blood pressure and inform the vasomotor centre (VMC) in the medulla oblongata of the brainstem, resulting in peripheral arterial vasoconstriction. This sympathetic response redistributes blood flow to the heart and brain. Blood vessels in the skin, lungs, kidneys and gastrointestinal tract constrict in response to sympathetic activation. If the vasoconstriction is sufficiently great, the blood pressure may be kept at or close to normal levels at the expense of producing localised tissue hypoxia. Strong sympathetic stimulation also affects the heart by temporarily strengthening the functional muscle, increasing pumping ability and heart rate.[6,8,11] Because of a reduced blood flow to the skin and reduced perfusion of the tissues, a pallor and cold and clammy skin is often evident. Adrenaline, produced by sympathetic response, stimulates sweat glands, causing clamminess. Lactic acid is produced by anaerobic metabolism in poorly perfused tissue.[6–8,11]

In the renal circulation, hormonal compensation takes place when blood flow to the kidneys is decreased. The juxtaglomerular junction in the renal nephron produces renin. Renin released into the bloodstream activates the chemical

---

FIGURE 22.19

The pathophysiology of cardiogenic shock.[12]

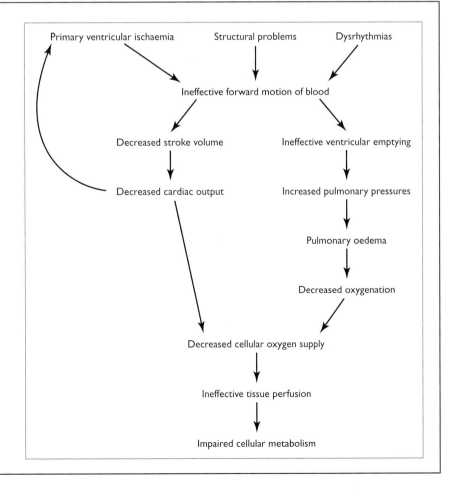

BOX 22.6 **Clinical manifestations of cardiogenic shock**[7]

- Systolic blood pressure < 90 mmHg
- Heart rate >100 beats/minute
- Weak, thready pulse
- Diminished heart sounds
- Change in sensorium
- Cool, pale, moist skin
- Urine output < 30 mL/h
- Chest pain
- Dysrhythmias
- Tachypnoea
- Crackles
- Decreased cardiac output
- Cardiac index < 2.2 L/min/m^2
- Increased pulmonary artery occlusion pressure
- Increased right atrial pressure
- Increased systemic vascular resistance

angiotensinogen to produce angiotensin I. This circulates in the blood to the lungs, where it is converted to angiotensin II. This powerful vasoconstrictor aids in the maintenance of blood pressure. Angiotensin II also stimulates the adrenal gland to produce the hormone aldosterone. This stimulates the re-absorption of sodium ions and when blood levels increase, the pituitary gland in the brain releases antidiuretic hormone (ADH) which further reduces urine production to increase circulatory volume.[6–8,11]

Chemical compensation comes from a reduction in pulmonary circulation, which causes a ventilation/perfusion imbalance, impaired gas exchange and hypoxaemia. Hypoxaemia increases the rate and depth of ventilation, which results in the exhalation of large amounts of carbon dioxide and a respiratory alkalosis. As a result of decreased arterial oxygen and carbon dioxide tension and alkalosis, the patient's level of consciousness is affected.[6–8,11]

The third, *progressive stage* of shock leads to multi-organ failure. Compensatory mechanisms eventually fail to maintain perfusion of the vital organs, which reduces arterial blood pressure, which in turn reduces coronary artery perfusion, resulting in myocardial hypoperfusion. An imbalance between myocardial oxygen supply and demand further depresses CO and cardiac function. In the kidneys, if the blood flow or pressure is reduced to a critical point, arteriolar blood bypasses the nephron and flows back into the venuole. The nephron dies as a result of hypoxia and acute tubular necrosis (ATN) develops.[6,8,11]

Prolonged vasoconstriction leads to gastrointestinal dysfunction caused by splanchnic vasoconstriction. Endotoxin is released from the bodies of the dead intestinal bacteria; it causes vascular dilation and increases cellular metabolism. Cell deterioration occurs and, as the pancreas becomes ischaemic, myocardial depressing factor (MDF) is released. MDF circulates in the blood and further depresses myocardial contractility.[6,8,11]

The *refractory* or irreversible stage of shock is when it is so profound, and cell destruction so severe, that death is inevitable as a result of the hypoxia in the liver, kidneys, heart or brain. Neurological insults diminish the sympathetic response. Specifically, the VMC fails to continue the sympathetic compensatory outflow. As a result, the heart rate slows, blood pressure falls and intractable circulatory failure develops. This refractory stage of shock ultimately leads to total body failure and death.[6,8,11]

Management of cardiogenic shock

In patients with cardiogenic shock secondary to AMI, therapy and management should focus on establishing immediate reperfusion through either thrombolysis or emergency angioplasty. Treatment of cardiogenic shock should be early and aggressive to ensure optimal patient outcomes. Either pharmacological or mechanical agents may be utilised to improve cardiac output and subsequent tissue perfusion.[6,8,11]

Inotropic agents commonly used in the treatment of cardiogenic shock are dobutamine, dopamine, adrenaline and noradrenaline. A positive inotrope is a drug given by intravenous infusion to increase myocardial contractility. Many are also chronotropes and therefore increase the heart rate. This effect is desirable, as cardiac output is determined by heart rate multiplied by stroke volume (the amount of blood ejected every contraction).[6,8,11] Dobutamine increases cardiac contractility and is chronotropic, yet to some degree causes peripheral vasodilation which decreases the afterload of the heart. The other inotropic agents mentioned can exacerbate an already failing heart, as they increase myocardial oxygen demands and bring about peripheral vasoconstriction thereby increasing afterload.[6–8,11]

The inadequate contractile force of the myocardium is the major clinical complication of acute heart failure. The reduction in contractility is a result of a decreased oxygen supply to the failing heart muscle and an increase in cardiac workload.

Mechanical therapy includes the use of intra-aortic balloon pump (IABP) counterpulsation. A helium-filled balloon approximately 10 cm long is inserted (usually in a cardiac catheter laboratory or in an operating theatre) into the aorta via the femoral artery, just below the aortic arch. The purpose of IABP therapy is to restore the balance between myocardial oxygen supply and demand, by reducing the workload of the heart, thereby reducing demand; at the same time improving myocardial oxygen supply.[6–8,11,32] The balloon is activated with every beat of the heart by an ECG trigger or arterial pressure waveform. During diastole, when the ventricles fill and the coronary arteries are perfused the balloon inflates and creates a greater than normal pressure in the aortic arch which assists in pushing blood back down the coronary arteries to improve myocardial perfusion and oxygen delivery. Just prior to systole the balloon deflates, thereby reducing the pressure in the aorta immediately before contraction and reducing the workload of the left ventricle as afterload is markedly decreased. This improves cardiac output and equalises myocardial oxygen supply and demand. One application of intra-aortic balloon counterpulsation in Australia is in the setting of cardiogenic shock. IAB therapy can be used pre-coronary bypass surgery and has shown to reduce mortality by 30% and for patients that are considered high-risk undergoing PCI.[6–8,11,32]

Percutaneous coronary intervention

Percutaneous coronary intervention (PCI) includes primary, rescue and elective PCI. A patient's access to primary angioplasty is dependent upon the availability of cardiac interventional services at the local or nearby hospitals. Primary PCI should be performed within 60 minutes of presentation to hospital. Time to PCI is the time from hospital presentation to balloon inflation, and is not calculated from the time of arrival at the PCI facility of the cardiac catheter laboratory, although the argument has been made that this should be calculated from the time the patient first presents to pre-hospital clinicians. Timely PCI has benefits over fibrinolytic therapy, as thrombolysis does not have any effect on coronary artery stenosis; however, both will reperfuse the hypoxic myocardium.[6,8,21]

The choice of reperfusion therapy is usually between PCI and fibrinolysis. PCI is the most effective treatment when provided promptly by an appropriately qualified cardiologist at an appropriate facility. Cardiologists performing PCI should have expertise in both management of an AMI and coronary angioplasty. On-site surgical backup is not a requirement for primary PCI, and therefore the establishment of more centres providing these facilities is possible throughout rural Australia.[5,24]

The procedure is performed in a cardiac catheterisation laboratory. A catheter 'sheath' is inserted into the femoral artery or radial artery and a balloon-tipped catheter is inserted through the sheath and is guided through the arterial circulation, down the aorta and into the relevant coronary artery. The balloon is then positioned within the atherosclerotic lesion of the coronary artery and is intermittently inflated to expand the diameter of the vessel and push the atherosclerotic lesion back into the wall of the vessel.[6,8] A stent is a tubular metal scaffold which is then expanded into the atherosclerotic lesion of the vessel by the angioplasty balloon. Stents can be either bare metal or drug eluting, and are inserted to maintain the patency of the occluded vessel after balloon angioplasty; this prevents closure of the coronary artery and enables adequate blood flow by ensuring the artery remains open (Fig 22.20).[6,8,21]

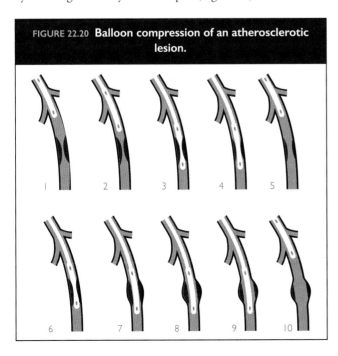

FIGURE 22.20 Balloon compression of an atherosclerotic lesion.

It is essential that pre-hospital clinicians and ambulance dispatch centres know which hospitals have PCI facilities, appropriate cardiac intervention staff and the 24-hour availability of these services. Maintaining a seamless patient-care continuum from pre-hospital to hospital is critical in order to minimise delays in patients receiving PCI. Reduction in door-to-balloon times for STEMI patients has been reported with the implementation of pre-hospital 12-lead ECG acquisition and transmission to local cardiac interventional centres.[5,14,24]

Pharmacological management

Fibrinolytic therapy

Fibrinolytic agents are administered to dissolve a thrombus occluding a coronary artery in an attempt to restore vital blood flow to the myocardium and cease the process of infarction. Fibrinolytic agents bring about lysis by targeting elements of the clotting process to degrade the fibrin clot.[3-5] The fibrinolytic agents differ in their action; Table 22.7 compares agents currently used in Australian hospitals. Indications for fibrinolytic therapy include: acute chest pain less than 12 hours in duration with accompanying ST-segment elevation evident on the 12-lead ECG or a new left bundle branch block. Absolute contraindications include haemorrhagic stroke, internal bleeding or suspected aortic dissection. Fibrinolytic agents may be used cautiously in hypertension, trauma and recent surgery.[6-8,21,22,23,25]

The major complication of fibrinolytic therapy is bleeding and haemorrhage. Clinical management should focus on hypotension, tachycardia, monitoring for reperfusion dysrhythmias and allergic reactions (see Table 22.7).[6-8,22,23,25]

The administration of pre-hospital fibrinolysis minimises delays in patients receiving reperfusion therapy, and evidence to date has shown it to be safe and effective.[5,22,33] One meta-analysis of studies comparing pre-hospital and in-hospital thrombolysis reported that pre-hospital thrombolysis reduced time for fibrinolysis to be administered and improved patient mortality.[20] In another study, investigators found that patients treated with pre-hospital recombinant tissue plasminogen activator (rt-PA) demonstrated an improved 5-year mortality rate compared to those receiving primary angiography.[33] Pre-hospital fibrinolysis has the same associated risks as in-hospital fibrinolytic therapy, and therefore should be administered with the same, if not increased, caution.

Anticoagulation

Anticoagulants include injections of low-molecular-weight heparins (LMWH) and the more traditional infusion of unfractionated heparin. Anticoagulants do not dissolve already-formed blood clots as do fibrinolytic agents, but they do inhibit any further formation of thrombin.[6,8] Anticoagulants are indicated for patients with ST-segment depression on an ECG and unstable angina and for all patients with AMI. Anticoagulants are used with fibrinolytic agents to prevent clot formation and subsequent re-occlusion of the affected vessel.[6-8,21]

The advantages of low-molecular-weight heparins include the dosage and the administration via subcutaneous injection and a reduction in the need to monitor the activated partial thromboplastin time (APTT); however, a disadvantage of

	TABLE 22.7 Comparison of fibrinolytic agents[12]		
AGENT	ACTION	DOSE	COMMENTS
Streptokinase	Exogenous plasminogen activator; not clot-specific	*IV:* 1.5 million units IV over 1 hr *Intracoronary:* 10,000 to 30,000 units; followed by maintenance infusion of 2000 to 4000 units/min until thrombolysis occurs (e.g. 150,000 to 500,000 units total)	Half-life in plasma is 18 minutes; has a prolonged effect on coagulation because of depletion of fibrinogen, which persists for 18–24 hours; antibodies to the drug may be present in persons who have been exposed to Streptococcus infection resulting in allergic reactions (e.g. rash, fever or chills); patients should not be re-treated with streptokinase for a period of 2 weeks to 1 year after initial administration because of secondary resistance to development of antibodies
Alteplase	Proteolytic enzyme; direct activator of plasminogen; high degree of clot specificity	*IV:* 15 mg IV bolus over 1–2 minutes; then 50 mg over 30 minutes; then 35 mg over 60 minutes	Half-life in plasma is 5–7 minutes; may cause sudden hypotension; inline IV filters can remove as much as 47% of the drug
Reteplase	Activates the conversion of plasminogen to plasmin; high degree of clot specificity	*IV:* 10 units over 2 minutes; then repeat 10 units in 30 minutes after initiation of first bolus	Give normal saline fluid before and after administration of reteplase Reconstitute just before administration and use within 4 hours after reconstituting
Tenecteplase	Activates clot-bound plasminogen to plasmin	*IV:* 30–50 mg bolus over 5 seconds Dosing based on patient weight: < 60 kg = 30 mg TNKase ≥ 60 to < 70 kg = 35 mg TNKase ≥ 70 to < 80 kg = 40 mg TNKase ≥ 80 to < 90 kg = 45 mg TNKase ≥ 90 mg = 50 mg TNKase	More fibrin specificity and less incidence of bleeding than alteplase

IV: intravenous; TNKase: tenecteplase

LMWH is its longer half-life, and this could delay access to cardiac angiography.

Antiplatelet agents

Platelet aggregation is essential in the early stages of thrombus formation. Antiplatelet aggregating agents have a primary role in the prevention of MI and ischaemic cerebrovascular accident. They are also effective in reducing the re-occlusion of arteries following stent insertion.[6,22,23]

Early treatment should be initiated in patients (unless contraindicated) from low- to high-risk NSTEACS. Aspirin is recommended in all low- to high-risk patients. Clopidogrel should be given, preferably before coronary intervention, but avoided in those who may require emergency coronary bypass surgery. Glycoprotein IIb/IIIa inhibitors are particularly recommended in high-risk patients and should be commenced as soon as features of high risk are identified.[5,29]

- *Aspirin*—activated platelets synthesise and release a powerful and potent vasoconstrictor thromboxane A$_2$. Aspirin inhibits and thereby blocks thromboxane A$_2$ synthesis in platelets. In doing this it reduces the aggregating properties of the platelet and, because the

inhibition is irreversible, the effect lasts for the 7- to 10-day life span of the platelet.[11,26,28]

- *Clopidogrel*—adherent platelets are activated and release substances. These substances released from activated platelets recruit additional platelets from the circulation to the site of injury and mediate the process of aggregation. Clopidogrel irreversibly inhibits the binding of adenosine diphosphate to its receptor on the platelet, thereby preventing the transformation of the glycoprotein inhibitor (GP IIb/IIIa) receptor into its active form.[26,27]

- *Prasugrel*—a drug similar to clopidogrel works by irreversibly inhibiting the activation of the GP IIb/IIIa complex. It has a more rapid onset of action and stronger inhibitory effect than clopidogrel and studies suggested that STEMI and diabetic patients may derive a greater benefit from more platelet inhibition with prasugrel, yet elderly (age >75 years) patients weighing <60 kg and those with a history of stroke have a potential unfavourable bleeding risk.[7,8]

- *Ticagrelor*—is a new class of antiplatelet agent, it is reversible, has a shorter half-life and requires twice daily dosing. It acts in a dose-dependent manner with

TABLE 22.8 Overview of glycoprotein IIb/IIIa inhibitors[12]		
GLYCOPROTEIN IIB/IIIA INHIBITOR	DOSAGE	POTENTIAL SIDE EFFECTS
Abciximab	0.25 mg/kg over 10–60 minutes 0.125 mg/kg/min for 12 hours	Potential for increased bleeding, hypotension, bradycardia, nausea and vomiting, diarrhoea
Eptifibatide	180 µg/kg over 1 to 2 minutes 2 µg/kg/min for up to 72 hours	Potential for increased bleeding, hypotension
Tirofiban	0.4 µg/kg/min for 30 minutes 0.1 µg/kg/min for 12–24 hours	Potential for increased bleeding, nausea, bradycardia

its antiplatelet effect having a rapid onset and offset. In the acute ACS setting where surgery may be required and cessation of antiplatelet therapy, ticagrelor would be ideally suited.[7,8] For high risk groups of patients undergoing PCI, such as diabetes and stent thrombosis, prasugrel and ticagrelor should be considered as an alternative to clopidogrel. However, careful assessment of the bleeding risks should be undertaken prior to using these agents.[5]

- *Glycoprotein inhibitors (GP IIb/IIIa)*—the GP IIb/IIIa complex is the most abundant receptor on the platelet surface. Platelet activation converts GP IIb/IIIa into a competent receptor, enabling it to bind to fibrinogen and von Willebrand factor (vWF). It is this process of platelet aggregation that serves as a target for antiplatelet therapy with GP IIb/IIIa antagonists. Glycoprotein inhibitors act by inhibiting the platelet GP IIb/IIIa receptor. They inhibit fibrinogen and vWF from binding to the IIb/IIIa receptor. Although they block the final common pathway of platelet aggregation, GP IIb/IIIa antagonists do not prevent platelet adhesion, secretion of platelet products or thrombin activation (Table 22.8).[26,27,30]

Beta-blocker therapy

Beta-blockers are effective in controlling hypertension and angina pain, and are considered essential post AMI as secondary prophylaxis (Table 22.9). Beta-blockers block the beta-adrenoreceptors in the heart, bronchi and vascular smooth muscle. They are divided into two subtypes:

- beta-1 receptors: found in heart muscle (cardio-selective)
- beta-2 receptors: found in bronchial and vascular smooth muscle (non-cardioselective).[11]

Beta-blockers were designed to counteract the cardiac effects of adrenergic stimulation (fight or flight response). This stimulation increases myocardial oxygen demand by increasing heart rate, blood pressure and force of contraction. The bradycardic and negative inotropic effects of beta-blockers are relevant to the therapeutic effect in angina, as these changes reduce myocardial oxygen demand.[8,31,32]

In the post-infarct phase, beta-blockers reduce mortality by 30–45%. The mechanisms of action are not fully understood, but may be related to a lower incidence of ventricular fibrillation (VF) and limitation of infarct size. Beta-blockers

TABLE 22.9 Beta-blocker therapy for the patient with myocardial infarction[12]	
MEDICATION	DOSE
Esmolol	0.5 mg/kg bolus over 1 minute followed by a continuous infusion at 0.5 mg/kg/min. Maximum dose is 0.3 mg/kg/min. Titrate to effect. The half-life is short (2–9 minutes)
Metoprolol	5 mg slow intravenous (IV) push. Repeat as needed at 5-minute intervals to a total of 15 mg. Give 25–50 mg orally within 15 minutes of the last IV dose (unless contraindicated). Oral dose is 50 mg bid for 24 hours; then increase to 100 mg bid
Propranolol	0.1 mg/kg slow IV push, divided into three equal doses, at 2- to 3-minute intervals. Do not infuse faster than 1 mg/min. Repeat after 2 minutes if necessary
Atenolol	5 mg IV over 5 minutes, wait 10 minutes, and then give second 5 mg dose over 5 minutes. In 10 minutes (if tolerated well) start 50 mg orally and then 50 mg orally bid. Oral dose is 100 mg daily
Labetalol	10 mg IV push over 1–2 minutes. May repeat or double labetalol dose every 10 minutes to a maximum of 150 mg. Another option is to give the initial dose as a bolus and then start a labetalol infusion at 2–8 mg/min

have been shown to reduce the incidence of recurrent MIs (Table 22.9).[31-33]

Angiotensin-converting enzyme inhibitors

Angiotensin-converting enzyme (ACE) inhibitors are well supported by evidence for use in patients post AMI or with heart failure. ACE inhibitors act on the renin–angiotensin–aldosterone system by inhibiting the conversion of angiotensin I to angiotensin II, a powerful vasoconstrictor.[8,15] In patients post MI, ACE inhibitors reduce mortality, improve left ventricular (LV) function, have a beneficial effect on the LV remodelling and delay the progression of heart failure. They are used in patients with signs and symptoms of heart failure or in patients with significant LV dysfunction, anterior wall infarctions and patients with LV ejection fraction less than 40%.[8,15,34,35]

Dysrhythmias

Cardiac dysrhythmias require continuous ECG monitoring to obtain a real-time electrical interpretation of the patient's cardiac rhythm. Chapter 17, p. 336, contains information on administering cardiac monitoring. In order for this monitoring to be of any therapeutic benefit to the patient in the ED, the emergency nurse must have knowledge of rhythm interpretation, presenting symptoms and potential complications associated with cardiac dysrhythmias.[5,8]

Heart rate affects ventricular filling and coronary artery perfusion. Heart rate and stroke volume determine cardiac output and subsequent blood pressure; therefore, when a patient presents with symptoms including dizziness, syncope, chest pain, breathlessness and palpitations the rapid assessment of the underlying cardiac rhythm is essential to avoid serious complications associated with a low cardiac output (Box 22.7).[8,11]

Dysrhythmias can occur throughout the cardiac conduction pathway (as discussed earlier in the chapter) and can originate in the SA node, the atria, the AV node or junction and the ventricles. A dysrhythmia is a rhythm that is not a sinus rhythm (SR) and can be the result of a heart rate outside 60–100 beats/minute (bpm), failure of the SA node to initiate an impulse, a delay or blockage in the conduction pathway, activation of aberrant conduction pathways and other foci initiating impulses causing ectopy (Table 22.10).[5,8,15,36]

Sinus rhythm

This is the normal rhythm of the heart originating from the SA node, the natural cardiac pacemaker. The rate is between 60 and 100 beats/minute, the rhythm is regular, P waves are present and precede every QRS complex, all intervals are within normal limits and the conduction is through the typical pathway. Figure 22.21 illustrates the conduction in sinus rhythm. Table 22.11 lists the ECG criteria for l sinus rhythm.[8,11,15]

Sinus bradycardia

Sinus bradycardia occurs when the SA node takes longer to depolarise than normal as a result of increased vagal (parasympathetic) stimulation. This produces a heart rate slower than 60 beats/minute, but fulfills all the other criteria for normal sinus rhythm.[5,8] Diastole is of a longer duration in sinus bradycardia, which means ventricular filling and coronary artery perfusion may not be reduced, but the heart rate may be insufficient to meet the demands of the body. Sinus bradycardia may then lead to a reduction in cardiac output that may not be tolerated well in patients with underlying coronary heart disease (CHD).[8,11,14,15] Primary causes include stimulation

BOX 22.7 Systematic evaluation of cardiac rhythms
Rate Bradycardia: < 60 beats/minute Normal rate: 60 to 100 beats/minute Tachycardia: > 100 beats/minute **Rhythm** Is the rhythm regular or irregular? **P waves** Are P waves present? Does one P wave appear before each QRS? Is P wave deflection normal? **QRS complex** Normal is 0.06–0.12 second. Are the QRS complexes normal shape and configuration? Does QRS complex follow every P wave? **PR Interval** Normal is 0.12–0.2 second. Is the interval prolonged? Shortened?

TABLE 22.10 Cardiac rhythms by point of origin[12]	
ORIGIN	RHYTHM
Sinus node	Normal sinus rhythm
	Sinus tachycardia
	Sinus bradycardia
	Sinus dysrhythmia
Atria	Premature atrial complexes
	Atrial flutter
	Atrial fibrillation
	Wandering atrial pacemaker
	Multifocal atrial tachycardia
Atrioventricular junction	Supraventricular tachycardia
	Premature junctional complexes
	Junctional escape rhythm
	Accelerated junctional rhythm
	Junctional tachycardia
Atrioventricular blocks	First-degree atrioventricular block
	Second-degree atrioventricular block, type I
	Second-degree atrioventricular block, type II
	Third-degree atrioventricular block
Ventricles	Premature ventricular complexes
	Ventricular tachycardia
	Ventricular fibrillation
	Idioventricular rhythm
	Accelerated idioventricular rhythm
Other	Pulseless electrical activity
	Asystole

FIGURE 22.21

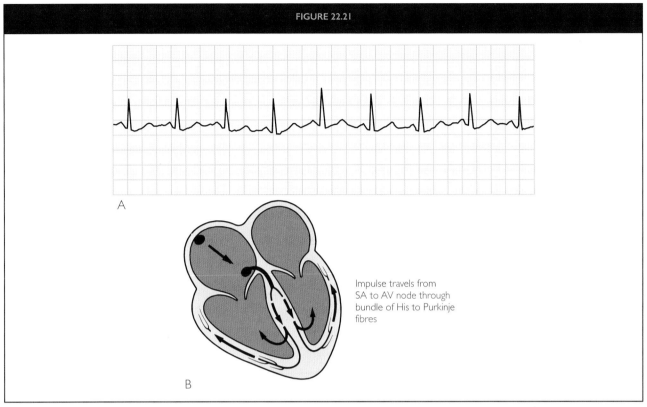

A, Normal sinus rhythm. B, Conduction pathway for normal sinus rhythm.[12] *SA, sinoatrial; AV, atrioventricular.*

TABLE 22.11	Normal sinus rhythm[12]
Rate	60 to 100 beats/minute
Rhythm	Regular
P waves	Present
QRS complex	Present; normal duration 0.04–0.11 second
P/QRS relationship	P wave precedes each QRS complex
PR interval	Normal 0.12–0.20 second

of the vagus nerve, for example, carotid sinus massage, vagal attacks, vomiting or straining to pass a stool. Sinus bradycardia occurs in a healthy athletic heart, during sleep, anoxia, MI, raised intracranial pressure, hypothermia and hypothyroidism and post direct current (DC) cardioversion, and can also be produced by some drugs, including beta-blockers and digitalis (Fig 22.22 and Table 22.12).[5,8,14,15]

Therapeutic interventions

- Observe for signs of decreased cardiac output, low blood pressure, low urine output and pallor.
- Cease all medications which may affect the heart rate and/or blood pressure until consultation with the patient's doctor or cardiologist.
- Severe symptoms can be treated with intravenous atropine or temporary transvenous or external cardiac pacing.[8,15,36]

Sinus tachycardia

Sinus tachycardia occurs when the SA node depolarises more quickly than normal. This produces a heart rate faster than 100 beats/minute and again fulfils all the other criteria for normal sinus rhythm.[5,8] Diastole is of a shorter duration in sinus tachycardia, which means ventricular filling and coronary artery perfusion are reduced. Sinus tachycardia may lead to a reduction in cardiac output which may not be tolerated well in patients with underlying CHD.[5,8,14,15]

Primary causes include stimulation of the sympathetic nervous system through, for example, pain, anxiety, stress, hyperthyroidism or a physiological response to hypotension and hypovolaemia. Sinus tachycardia can also occur during exercise and be associated with caffeine and nicotine use (Fig 22.23 and Table 22.13).[5,8,15]

Therapeutic interventions

- Sinus tachycardia is a symptom. Treat the underlying cause.
- Observe for signs of decreased cardiac output, low blood pressure, low urine output and pallor.
- In MI or stimulant overdose, a beta-blocker may be considered to reduce rate and therefore myocardial oxygen demand.[8,15,36]

Sinus dysrhythmia

Sinus dysrhythmia occurs when there is a cyclic variation in a sinus rhythm, usually because of changes in stimulation of the vagus nerve; this usually coincides with respiration and a change in intrathoracic pressure. The SA node speeds up a little at the end of inspiration and slows down at the end of expiration. It is

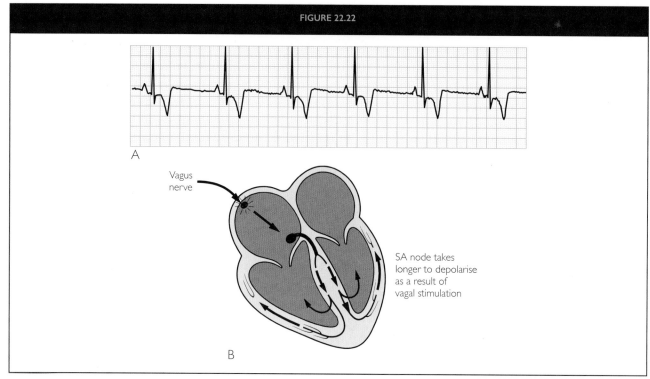

FIGURE 22.22

A, Sinus bradycardia. **B**, Conduction pathway for sinus bradycardia.[12]

TABLE 22.12 Sinus bradycardia[12]	
Rate	Fewer than 60 beats/minute (age-dependent)
Rhythm	Regular
P waves	Present
QRS complexes	Present; normal duration
P/QRS relationship	P wave precedes each QRS complex
PR interval	Normal

found more in young healthy adults and paediatric individuals, and if not related to respiration may indicate SA node disease or inferior MI (Table 22.14 and Fig 22.24).[8,15,36]

Premature atrial complexes

Premature atrial complexes (PACs) are stimulated from irritable atrial cells and may precede atrial fibrillation. The pathway is abnormal as it does not originate from the SA node and results in an abnormal, premature P wave followed by a normal QRS complex. Causes of atrial irritation include fatigue, alcohol, nicotine, electrolyte imbalance, digitalis toxicity, hypoxia and ischaemia (Fig 22.25 and Table 22.15).[8,15,36]

Atrial fibrillation

Atrial fibrillation (AF) is the most commonly recognised form of tachycardia and is frequently found in the elderly. It occurs when multiple atrial foci fire chaotically, causing the atria to quiver or fibrillate but with no effective atrial contraction. Fibrillatory waves are seen on the ECG and the atrial rate is around 400–600 beats/minute.[5,8] The ventricular rate is determined by the AV node and is irregular and can also be rapid. Conduction is then via the normal pathway with a normal QRS complex.[5,8] Cardiac output may be affected due to the loss of atrial kick. The ventricles lose approximately 25% of their filling because of the absence of atrial contraction. The primary causes of AF include CHD, ischaemia/hypoxia, hypertensive heart disease, mitral valve disease, congestive heart failure and pulmonary embolus (Fig 22.26 and Table 22.16).[8,15,36]

Therapeutic interventions

- Evaluate ventricular response by comparison of ECG and apex beat.
- Attempt rate control for haemodynamically stable patients with beta-blockers or digitalis.
- Severely symptomatic patients will require emergency synchronised DC cardioversion.
- If the AF lasts longer than 48 hours, an intra-cardiac thrombus may have developed. Anticoagulation is indicated prior to cardioversion to prevent thromboembolism unless excluded by a trans-oesophageal echocardiogram (TOE).
- Anticoagulation with unfractionated heparin or low-molecular-weight heparin should begin. Anticoagulation with vitamin K antagonists such as warfarin has been shown to be superior treatment to aspirin and clopidogrel in general patients with atrial fibrillation.[37]
- Chemical cardioversion can be achieved with several drugs, including amiodarone.[5,8,15,36]

Atrial flutter

A re-entry circuit within the right atria is thought to be responsible for atrial flutter. The atrial focus depolarises at a

FIGURE 22.23

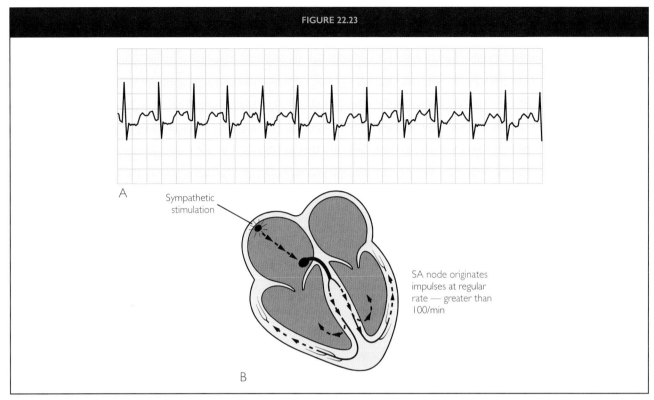

A, Sinus tachycardia. **B**, Conduction pathway for sinus tachycardia.[12] *SA, sinoatrial.*

TABLE 22.13 Sinus tachycardia[12]	
Rate	100 to 180 beats/minute (age-dependent)
Rhythm	Regular
P waves	Present, may merge with T waves
QRS complexes	Present; normal duration (width)
P/QRS relationship	P wave precedes each QRS complex
PR interval	Normal

rapid rate of around 300 beats/minute but most impulses are blocked by the AV node, usually to a regular, slower rate.[5,8] The AV node will allow every second, third or fourth flutter wave to reach the ventricles; consequently there may be four flutter waves to every ventricular beat (4:1) or three or two flutter waves to every ventricular beat (2:1). Atrial flutter may be regular or irregular and although the atria do not contract well and thrombus formation may occur, it is less common than in atrial fibrillation.[5,8,15] Primary causes of atrial flutter include CHD, right heart enlargement, chronic pulmonary disease, heart failure and thyrotoxicosis (Fig 22.27 and Table 22.17).[8,15,36]

Therapeutic interventions

• Control rapid atrial response rates with beta-blockers, digitalis, calcium channel blockers and amiodarone.

• If the patient is symptomatic, consider synchronised DC cardioversion.

• Treat any underlying condition.

Paroxysmal supraventricular tachycardia

Supraventricular tachycardia (SVT) is the term used for the narrow complex tachycardia that originates when the atria or the AV junction act as the heart's pacemaker.[5,8] The term *paroxysmal supraventricular tachycardia* (PSVT) is used when the dysrhythmia begins and ends abruptly. The rate may be as high as 280 beats/minute, the P wave is not clear or absent and the QRS complex is normal.[5,8,15,36] In some circumstances there may be two accessory pathways within the AV node and an electrical circuit or loop may be formed which can continuously stimulate the ventricles to depolarise; thus called a re-entrant tachycardia. With such a rapid tachycardia cardiac output may be compromised.

Primary causes of SVT include alcohol, nicotine, caffeine and stress, and it can occur in a normal heart, but may be associated with hypoxia, ischaemia, electrolyte imbalance and MI (Fig 22.28 and Table 22.18).[8,15,36]

Therapeutic interventions

• Record rhythm and a 12-lead ECG to aid correct diagnosis.

• AV nodal re-entry tachycardias are usually self-limiting or can be easily terminated with vagal manoeuvres such as coughing, the Valsalva manoeuvre or carotid sinus massage.

• Intravenous adenosine may be used. It depresses conduction through the AV node. This action can interrupt re-entry circuits involving the AV node and

FIGURE 22.24

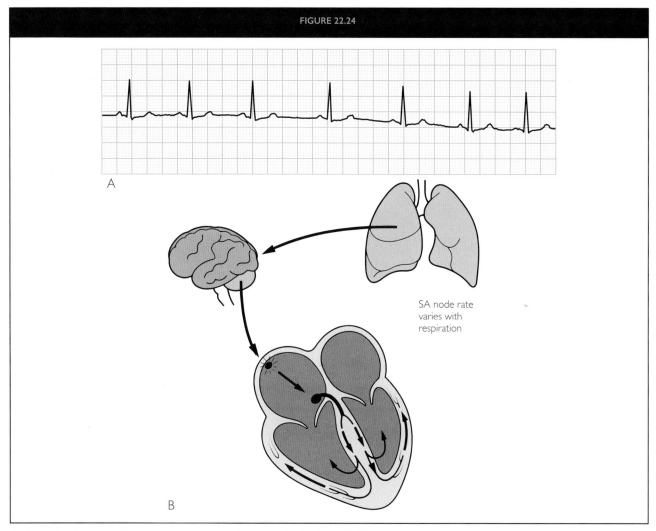

SA node rate varies with respiration

A

B

A, Sinus dysrhythmia. **B**, Conduction pathway for sinus dysrhythmia.[12] *SA, sinoatrial.*

TABLE 22.14	Sinus dysrhythmia[12]
Rate	60–100 beats/minute; may increase with inspiration and decrease with expiration
Rhythm	Slightly irregular; may be obvious on a rhythm strip but undetectable by palpation
P waves	Present
QRS complexes	Present; normal duration
P/QRS relationship	P wave precedes each QRS complex
PR interval	Normal

restore normal sinus rhythm in patients with paroxysmal SVT. As adenosine causes short-lived AV node blockade (10–20 seconds), cardiac monitoring and resuscitation equipment need to be immediately available.[36]

- Haemodynamically unstable patients may require synchronised DC cardioversion.

- Permanent prevention of recurrent SVT can be achieved by radiofrequency catheter ablation of the accessory pathway.

First-degree atrioventricular block

A first-degree AV block exists when the impulse is delayed in the AV node longer than normal, resulting in a prolonged PR interval. There is a P wave for every QRS. This is frequently an asymptomatic dysrhythmia but may precede a more severe heart block (Fig 22.29 and Table 22.19).[8,15,36]

Therapeutic interventions

Treatment is unnecessary unless associated with other symptoms.

Second-degree atrioventricular block, type I

Second-degree AV block, type I is also known as Mobitz type I or Wenckebach. It exists when the delay in conduction through the AV node progressively worsens over each consecutive beat. The PR interval gradually lengthens with each beat until it results in a non-conducted P wave and a resultant dropped QRS complex; then the cycle begins again. It is as if the P wave is 'walking back' from its QRS complex (Table 22.20 and Fig 22.30).[8,15,36]

FIGURE 22.25

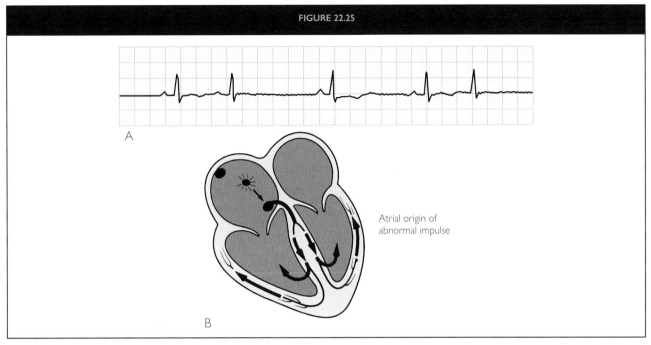

A, Premature atrial complexes (PAC). **B**, Conduction pathway for PAC.[12]

TABLE 22.15 Premature atrial complexes[12]	
Rate	60–100 beats/minute
Rhythm	Irregular because of early beats
P waves	Present, but (because they do not originate in the sinoatrial node) premature P waves have a different configuration
QRS complexes	Present; normal duration; noncompensatory pause
P/QRS relationship	A P wave precedes each QRS complex. If an ectopic P wave appears early in the cardiac cycle, a QRS complex may not follow (non-conducted premature atrial complex)
PR interval	Normal or prolonged

Therapeutic interventions
- Treatment is not usually necessary.
- Observe for symptomatic bradycardia and progression to second-degree type II or third-degree blocks.
- Discontinue digitalis and obtain serum digoxin levels.[8,15,36]

Second-degree atrioventricular block, type II
Second-degree AV block, type II is also known as Mobitz type II and exists when there is an intermittent block of the atrial impulse by the AV node to the ventricles.[5,12] The block may occur in a pattern of 2:1 or 3:1, etc. The PR interval is normal when there is a P wave with each QRS complex, but not every P wave will precede a QRS complex. Progression

to complete heart block is not uncommon with this rhythm (Fig 22.31 and Table 22.21).[15,36]

Therapeutic interventions
- Ensure close cardiac monitoring.
- Provide supplemental oxygen and do regular recording of vital signs.
- Consider intravenous atropine, isoprenaline infusion or temporary cardiac pacing.[8,15,36]

Third-degree heart block (complete heart block)
Third-degree heart block is also known as complete AV disassociation and exists when there is no conduction of the atrial impulse through the AV node to the ventricles. In response to the complete block by the AV node, a junctional or ventricular pacemaker will take over ventricular depolarisation.[8,15] The atria and the ventricles are working completely independently of each other. The atrial rate is around 60 beats/minute as it is initiated by the SA node, and the ventricular rate can be between 20–40 beats/minute depending on the site of the ventricular pacemaker. If the impulse originates within the ventricle, the QRS complex will be wide.[8,15,36]

Cardiac output falls because of loss of atrial filling and a potential bradycardia. If the heart block occurs gradually, as with fibrosis associated with the ageing process, compensatory mechanisms will help maintain homeostasis. However, when cardiac output is compromised or the heart block occurs suddenly (as in MI), rapid treatment may be necessary (Fig 22.32 and Table 22.22).[8,15,36]

The primary causes of heart blocks include CHD, degenerative disease, infarction of the conduction pathway as in anterior MI, inferior MI and reversible ischaemia of the AV node, aortic valve disease (degenerative), drugs (digoxin, beta-blockers, other anti-dysrhythmics, carbamazepine), acute rheumatic fever, atrial septal defect, dilated cardiomyopathy and connective tissue disorders.[8,15,36]

FIGURE 22.26

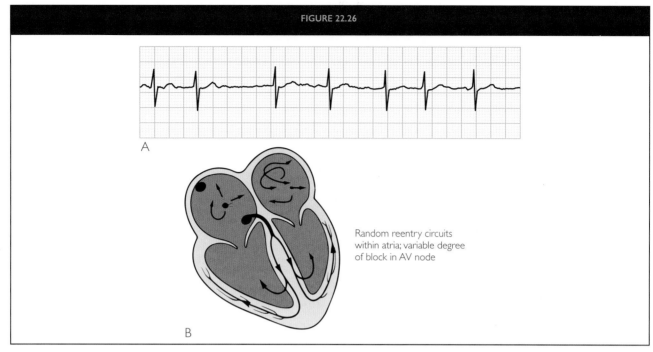

A, Atrial fibrillation. **B**, Conduction pathway for atrial fibrillation.[12] *AV: atrioventricular.*

Random reentry circuits within atria; variable degree of block in AV node

TABLE 22.16 Atrial fibrillation[12]

Rate	Atrial rate 400 beats/minute or more; ventricular rate varies
Rhythm	The ventricular rhythm is always irregular
P waves	No identifiable P waves
QRS complexes	Present, normal duration
P/QRS relationship	None identified; irregular ventricular response
PR interval	Not applicable

Therapeutic interventions

- Closely observe ventricular rate. If the patient becomes symptomatic (syncope, chest pain, altered level of consciousness) cardiac failure will soon follow.
- Perform cardiac pacing either permanent, temporary trans-venous or temporary transcutaneous (external).
- Be prepared to provide basic and advanced life support as necessary.[8,15,36]

Premature ventricular complexes

Premature ventricular complexes (PVCs) are referred to by a number of names, including premature ventricular ectopic beats (VEBs) and extrasystoles. They are stimulated from irritable ventricular cells and indicate an irritable ventricle. The abnormal impulse is initiated from an ectopic focus within the ventricle.[8,15] Factors that can cause PVCs include electrolyte imbalance, digitalis toxicity, hypoxia, ischaemia and acidosis. Causes of ventricular irritation include fatigue, alcohol and nicotine. When a single focus of the ventricle initiates an impulse, the complex will have the same configuration and is therefore said to be unifocal.[8,15] When multiple foci are involved in initiating ventricular impulses, the complexes present in a variety of configurations and are said to be multifocal.[8,15]

> **PRACTICE TIP**
>
> Bigeminy is a repetitive pattern of PVCs which occurs every other beat; and in trigeminy, PVC occurs every third beat.

A pair of PVCs is known as a couplet and three consecutive PVCs are known as a triplet. Three or more PVCs constitute a run of non-sustained ventricular tachycardia (Fig 22.33 and Table 22.23).[8,15,36]

Ventricular tachycardia

Ventricular tachycardia (VT) is a rhythm usually associated in patients with underlying heart disease, and all rhythms that originate within the ventricle are considered to be the most dangerous and potentially life-threatening.[8,15,18] The impulse originates in the ventricle and has a broad QRS complex on the ECG. Because of the rapid rate of VT and the loss of atrial function, haemodynamic compromise can occur rapidly. Any wide-complex tachycardia should be considered VT until proven otherwise. The following criteria support VT diagnosis: > 0.12 second QRS; > 100 beats/minute; > 3 consecutive beats; usually regular, dissociated P waves. In VT associated with a pulse rate of approximately 130 beats/minute the patient may become dizzy, and loss of consciousness can occur with rates of approximately 200 beats/minute.[8,15] However, any VT, despite the rate, may not produce a palpable pulse and is therefore considered to be a cardiac arrest situation.[15,18]

Monomorphic VT is usually associated with LV dysfunction and coronary heart disease. Polymorphic VT (torsades

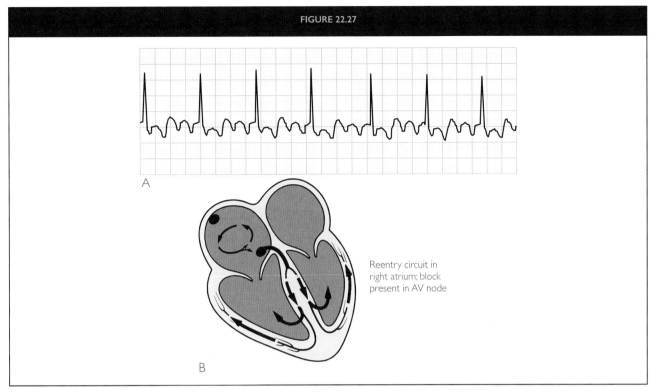

FIGURE 22.27

Reentry circuit in right atrium; block present in AV node

A, Atrial flutter. **B**, Conduction pathway for atrial flutter.[12] *AV: atrioventricular.*

TABLE 22.17	Atrial flutter[12]
Rate	Atrial rate of 230 to 350 beats/minute; ventricular rate varies from normal to rapid
Rhythm	Regular if there is a fixed conduction ratio (a constant number of F waves to QRS complexes); irregular if there is a variable conduction ratio
P waves	A saw-toothed pattern of flutter waves (F waves)
QRS complexes	Present; normal duration
P/QRS relationship	Because of the rapid atrial rate, there will be two or more flutter waves for every QRS; the rhythm may be regular or irregular
PR interval	Not applicable

de pointes) can be induced by medications that prolong the Q–T interval, such as amiodarone, or by toxicity due to drugs including tricyclic antidepressants (Table 22.24 and Fig 22.34).[8,15,36]

Therapeutic interventions

- Monomorphic VT in conscious but unstable patients is treated with synchronised DC cardioversion.
- Pulseless VT is treated as ventricular fibrillation and requires immediate DC cardioversion.

- Stable VT is treated with antidysrhythmic drugs such as amiodarone or lignocaine.

PRACTICE TIP

Polymorphic VT treatments include stopping all medications that prolong the QT interval, correction of electrolytes and intravenous magnesium sulfate and *possibly* lignocaine.[8,15,18,26]

Ventricular fibrillation (VF)

Ventricular fibrillation exists when there is a rapid firing of ventricular ectopic sites at the same time, causing a fibrillatory waveform that originates in the ventricles.[8,15] This rhythm produces no effective ventricular contraction and therefore no cardiac output. Without immediate intervention it becomes a fatal dysrhythmia—death occurs within 4–6 minutes if the rhythm persists without advanced life-support techniques (Fig 22.35 and Table 22.25).[8,15,18,36]

Therapeutic interventions

- Immediate initiation of basic and advanced life support.
- Early defibrillation, administer 100% oxygen and minimise interruptions to cardiac compressions.

Asystole

Asystole is the complete absence of any ventricular activity. Atrial impulses may or may not be present. This rhythm usually implies that the patient has been in cardiopulmonary arrest for a prolonged time, and mortality is high.[8,15,36] P waves can be seen on the ECG with the absence of the QRS complex. This can be referred to as P-wave asystole or ventricular standstill;

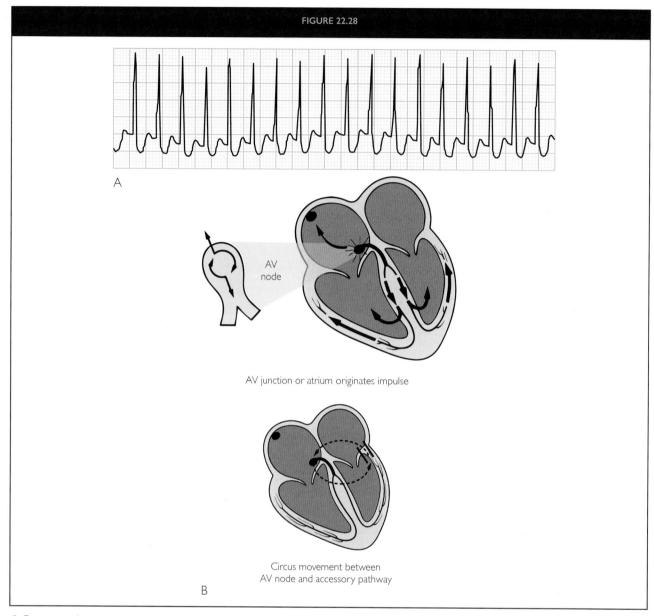

FIGURE 22.28

A

AV node

AV junction or atrium originates impulse

Circus movement between
AV node and accessory pathway

B

A, Paroxysmal supraventricular tachycardia. **B,** Conduction pathway for paroxysmal supraventricular tachycardia.[12] *AV: atrioventricular.*

TABLE 22.18 Paroxysmal supraventricular tachycardia[12]	
Rate	100 to 280 beats/minute
Rhythm	Regular; sudden start and stop
P wave	May occur before the QRS; often distorted or buried within the QRS complex
QRS complexes	Present; duration is usually normal though the QRS may be wide
P/QRS relationship	A P wave for each QRS or none seen (buried in QRS complex)
PR interval	Short or none

the outcome remains the same. The aim is to treat or correct the cause of asystole if known (Fig 22.36 and Table 22.26).

Therapeutic interventions

- Immediately initiate basic and advanced life support.
- Administer 100% oxygen and intravenous adrenaline.
- Confirm asystole in another ECG lead.
- Consider sodium bicarbonate administration in prolonged resuscitation attempts.
- Consider termination of resuscitation efforts after excluding all potentially reversible causes.[7,15,18,36]

For management of dysrhythmias refer to your local policies, procedures and guidelines as availability of drugs and therapeutic equipment will govern choice of agent and clinician preference.

Refer to Chapter 15 for more information regarding resuscitation.

FIGURE 22.29

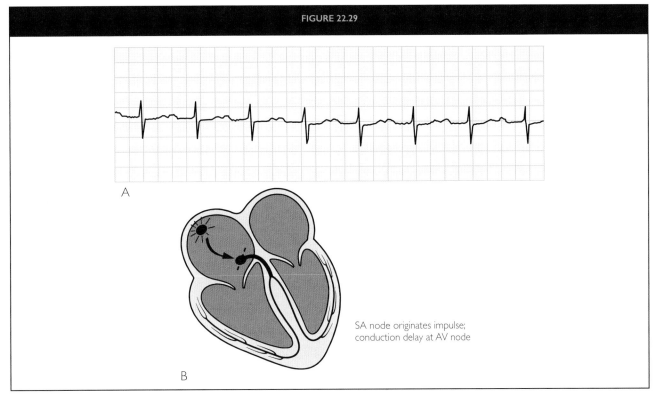

A, First-degree AV block. **B**, Conduction pathway for first-degree AV block.[12] *SA: sinoatrial; AV: atrioventricular.*

TABLE 22.19	First-degree atrioventricular block[12]
Rate	Usually 60 to 100 beats/minute
Rhythm	Regular
P waves	Present
QRS complexes	Present; normal duration
P/QRS relationship	A P wave precedes each QRS complex
PR interval	Prolonged (> 0.20 second) but consistent

Pulseless electrical activity (PEA)

Pulseless electrical activity (PEA) is defined as organised electrical activity, with no detectable cardiac output. Patients who exhibit PEA generally have a poor prognosis, unless the underlying reversible cause is identified and treated rapidly. Hypovolaemia, as a result of either a disease process or trauma, is the most common cause of PEA.

Therapeutic interventions

- Immediately initiate basic and advanced life support.
- Administer 100% oxygen and intravenous adrenaline 1mg IV/IO.
- Consider termination of resuscitation efforts after excluding all potentially reversible causes.[7,15,18,36]

For management of dysrhythmias refer to your local policies, procedures and guidelines as availability of drugs and thera-peutic equipment will govern choice of agent and clinician preference.

Refer to Chapter 15 for more information regarding resuscitation.

Pacemakers

The most common methods used to enable cardiac pacing include the transvenous or transcutaneous approach; however, cardiac pacing can be achieved by the insertion of epicardial pacing wires post cardiothoracic surgery, and transthoracic where a myocardial pacing electrode is inserted via a cardiac needle into the right ventricle.[6,8]

Temporary transcutaneous pacing

Transcutaneous or external cardiac pacing can be utilised for the emergency treatment of an unstable patient with an abnormally slow heart rate, as it is non-invasive, relatively straightforward to undertake and most defibrillators have a cardiac pacing function. (See Ch 17, p. 337, for information on applying cardiac pacing.) After appropriate analgesia and sedation, one electrode is placed anteriorly on the chest over the cardiac apex at the V_3 position and a second electrode is placed posteriorly and level with the inferior aspect of the left scapula, avoiding as best as possible medication patches, implanted devices and injured areas.[6,8] Positioning over bone may increase the amount of energy required. The pacemaker generates an electrical impulse that causes depolarisation of myocardial tissue. The rate and energy level can be adjusted to maintain adequate capture and optimise patient comfort.[6,8]

Temporary transvenous pacing

This is a common procedure in coronary care units and is performed when the patient is haemodynamically

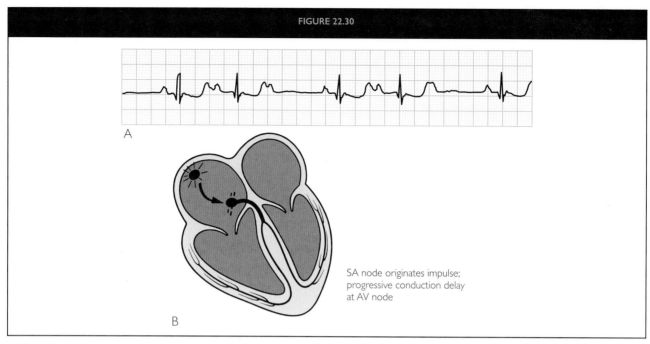

A, Second-degree AV block, type I. **B**, Conduction pathway for second-degree AV block, type I.[12] *SA: sinoatrial; AV: atrioventricular.*

TABLE 22.20	Second-degree atrioventricular block, type I[12]
Rate	Normal
Rhythm	Atrial beats are regular; ventricular beats are irregular
P waves	One P wave precedes each QRS complex until the QRS is dropped. This pattern recurs at regular intervals
QRS complexes	Cyclic missed conduction; when the QRS complex is present, it is of normal duration
P/QRS relationship	A QRS complex follows each P wave and then is dropped (absent) at patterned intervals
PR interval	Lengthens with each cycle until a QRS complex is dropped, and then the pattern repeats

compromised. The method involves the insertion of a pacing electrode into the right ventricle via the subclavian or external jugular venous route, under fluoroscopy or with a flotation-pacing catheter under guidance by the ECG. The electrodes are connected to a pulse generator where the output can be selected in milliamps along with the rate.[6,8] Either type of pacemaker can be at a fixed-rate mode or demand mode. Fixed rate is rarely used as it can have potential complications by delivering an impulse on the T wave and precipitating VF. Demand mode senses the patient's own QRS complexes and only generates an impulse when the heart does not produce its own intrinsic QRS complex.[6,8]

Temporary cardiac pacing is indicated in symptomatic sinus bradycardia, sick sinus syndrome, heart blocks, usually second degree type II and complete heart block, and ventricular standstill or P-wave asystole when P waves are present in the absence of any QRS complexes.[8,14]

External cardioverter defibrillators

Defibrillation delivers an electrical counter-shock that interrupts the chaotic heart rhythm by depolarising a critical mass of myocardium, thus stopping the heart. This then allows the heart's pacemaker to regain its normal electrical activity.

There are two types of external defibrillator available: monophasic and biphasic.

- The monophasic defibrillator delivers a single pulse of electricity that travels in one direction between the paddles or pads applied to the chest.
- The biphasic defibrillator discharges the electrical current then reverses itself and travels in two directions.

Unlike monophasic units, biphasic units are able to compensate for differences in thoracic impedance, which is the resistance to current flow created by an individual's chest size and tissue density. It automatically measures the impedance and adjusts the waveform for each shock, thus increasing the likelihood that the first shock will work.

Biphasic waveforms of defibrillation at lower energy levels have been shown to be as effective as monophasic waveforms for successfully terminating VF.[18,38,39] Biphasic shock defibrillators have become increasingly available and are replacing monophasic defibrillators.[36–38]

Defibrillation is improved by good electrode contact and correct positioning. Self-adhesive pads are the preferred mode of delivery as they allow minimal interruptions to cardiac compressions and are a safer method of defibrillation than manual paddles.[41] The self-adhesive pads can be used

FIGURE 22.31

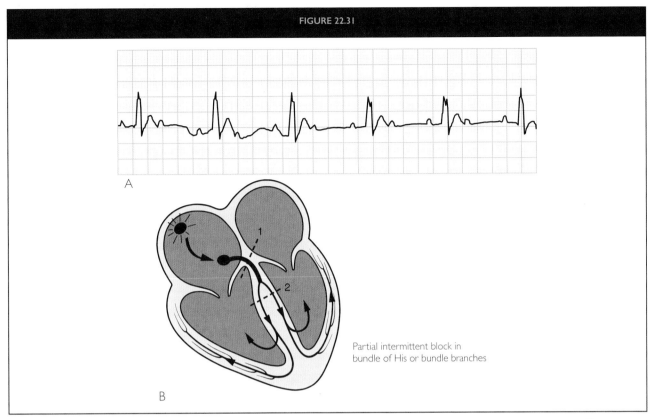

Partial intermittent block in
bundle of His or bundle branches

A, Second-degree AV block, type II, with 2:1 conduction. B, Conduction pathway for second-degree AV block, type II.[12]

TABLE 22.21	Second-degree atrioventricular block, type II[12]
Rate	Atrial rate of 60 to 100 beats/minute; ventricular rate is often slow
Rhythm	Atrial rhythm is regular; ventricular rhythm is regular with a consistent conduction pattern but is irregular if conduction pattern is variable
P waves	One or more for every QRS complex
QRS complexes	When present, normal or prolonged duration
P/QRS relationship	One or more P waves for each QRS complex
PR interval	Normal or delayed for the P wave that conducts the QRS complex

with all defibrillators in both manual and automatic external defibrillator (AED) modes.[15,38–40,43]

Internal cardioverter defibrillators

Sudden cardiac deaths from ventricular tachycardias or dysrhythmias post MI are now effectively treated with an implantable cardioverter defibrillator (ICD). ICDs are implanted in patients with increased risk of sudden death from recognised heart disease, low ejection fractions post MI, heart-failure patients and patients with cardiomyopathies.[44,45] The ICD is inserted in the same way as a permanent pacemaker—the generator is implanted under the skin and subcutaneous tissue and the wires are directly inserted into the atria, ventricles or both. The ICD has many functions, including dysrhythmia detection and acting as a pacemaker if heart rate drops below the device's set parameters. It can anti-tachycardia (overdrive) pace—the ability to pace the heart at a rate that is faster than the intrinsic rhythm—until capture occurs, then reduce the pacing rate which in turn slows down the heart rate.[44,45] This is particularly effective as the common dysrhythmia in patients requiring ICD therapy is VT. The ICD has the ability to perform synchronised cardioversion in order to bring the heart back into a normal rhythm, and also defibrillate.[44,45]

Heart failure

Chronic heart failure (CHF) occurs in 1.5–2% of Australians and increases markedly with age. It affects approximately 1% of the population aged between 50 and 59 years, 10% in those 65 years and older and 50% in people aged 85 years or older. CHF is the most common reason for hospital admission and GP consultation in people aged 70 years and older.[42,45] Heart failure has several definitions and can be described as a systolic or diastolic dysfunction of the ventricles or both. CHF is a complex syndrome in which typical symptoms of dyspnoea and fatigue can occur at rest. There is an underlying structural abnormality or dysfunction impairing the filling or emptying ability of the ventricles.[8,15,41] It is due to poor contraction or relaxation of the heart muscle and is characterised by haemodynamic, renal, neural and hormonal

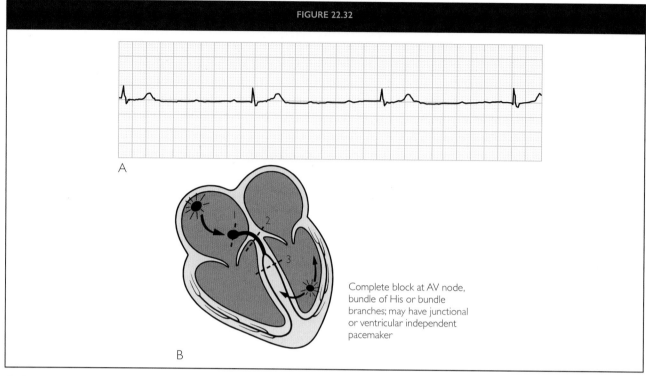

FIGURE 22.32

Complete block at AV node, bundle of His or bundle branches; may have junctional or ventricular independent pacemaker

A, Third-degree heart block. **B,** Conduction pathway for third-degree heart block.[12] *AV, atrioventricular.*

TABLE 22.22	Third-degree heart block[12]
Rate	Atrial rate of 60 to 100 beats/minute; ventricular rate usually less than 60 beats/minute
Rhythm	Regular
P waves	Occurring regularly
QRS complexes	Slow; narrow if the QRS is a junctional escape beat, wide (≥ 0.12 second) if it is a ventricular escape beat
P/QRS relationship	The P wave and QRS complex are completely independent of each other
PR interval	Inconsistent

responses. Presenting signs and symptoms include exertional dyspnoea, orthopnoea, dry and irritating cough, fatigue or weakness, dizzy spells or palpitations, which may indicate a dysrhythmia. Symptoms related to fluid retention may indicate a more advanced CHF.[8,15,42] Common causes of CHF are ischaemic heart disease, hypertension, dilated cardiomyopathy and diabetes (Table 22.27).[46,47]

Systolic dysfunction of the left ventricle is the most common cause of heart disease in Western societies and although both systolic and diastolic CHF coexist, distinguishing between the two is relevant to therapeutic management.[8,47,48]

Recommended management of chronic heart failure focuses on:

- Lifestyle modifications to improve diet and exercise
- ACE inhibitors in all patients to achieve the highest tolerated dose
- beta-blockers: recommended unless not tolerated or contraindicated
- diuretics used to maintain volume in patients with fluid overload
- angiotensin II receptor antagonists: used when patients are unable to tolerate ACE inhibitors.[8,42,47]

Patients with CHF experience symptoms that severely affect their everyday life, including shortness of breath, reduced exercise tolerance and lethargy. The NHFA consumer resource focuses on patients learning how to manage their CHF to reduce symptoms and hospitalisation by adhering to self-management strategies. These strategies include restricting fluid intake, adhering to a complex medication regimen, maintaining a low-sodium diet and engaging in physical activity.[32,33,42]

Some CHF patients may have asynchronous contraction of the left ventricle, especially if the duration of the QRS on the ECG is prolonged. Evidence suggests benefits from the use of biventricular pacing in heart failure, as this resynchronises cardiac contraction, improves ventricular performance and reduces frequency of hospitalisation.[42] Implantable cardioverter defibrillators (ICDs) have a role in the prophylaxis of dysrhythmia management in patients with significant LV dysfunction from ischaemic heart disease and therefore CHF. Prophylactic implantation of ICDs may be considered in patients with a low ejection fraction (<35%), however, funding is a significant constraint to patients receiving therapy.[8,15,42,46–48]

For further information from the Australian Heart Foundation on heart failure visit the website (www.heartfoundation.com.au).

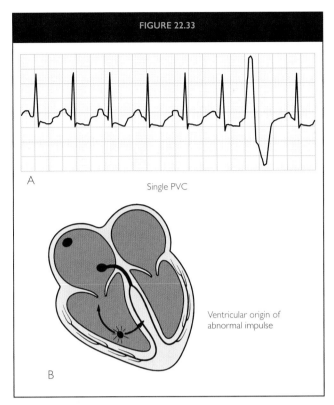

FIGURE 22.33

A

Single PVC

B

Ventricular origin of
abnormal impulse

A, Premature ventricular complexes (PVCs). **B**, Conduction
pathway for PVC.[12]

TABLE 22.23 Premature ventricular complexes (PVCs)[12]

Rate	Varies with underlying rhythm
Rhythm	Irregular because of early beats
P waves	Present with each sinus beat; P waves do not precede premature ventricular complexes (PVCs)
QRS complexes	Sinus-initiated QRS complexes are normal; the QRS complexes of PVCs are wide (> 0.12 second) and bizarre and usually have a T wave of opposite polarity. Look for a full compensatory pause
P/QRS relationship	A P wave precedes each QRS complex in the normal sinus beats; no P wave precedes PVCs
PR interval	Normal in sinus beats; none in PVCs

Acute pericarditis

Acute pericarditis is inflammation of the pericardium, a
sac containing serous fluid that surrounds the myocardium
and maintains lubrication. Pericarditis occurs more often in
adult males than in females and can be caused by infection,
MI, malignancy or medications, or it can be idiopathic.
When caused by a viral infection, it is also referred to as viral
pericarditis (Table 22.28).[15,49,52]

Chest pain, fever and a pericardial friction rub are among
the common signs and symptoms. Chest pain usually occurs
suddenly and is typically a persistent, sharp, stabbing pain
aggravated by deep inspiration and coughing. Relief is felt
when sitting upright and leaning forward. A pericardial rub is
produced by the movement of the inflamed pericardial layers
moving against one another and is best heard with the patient
sitting upright, forward and on expiration.[15] A complication
of pericarditis is cardiac tamponade which happens when
a pericardial effusion occurs at a rapid rate. The rapid
accumulation of fluid within the pericardial sac compresses
the heart, preventing the ventricles from filling adequately. The
ECG is a useful tool in diagnosing pericarditis; typical changes
include ST-segment elevation in all leads except aV_R and V_1,
though this is not to be misinterpreted as AMI when ST-
segment elevation occurs in two or three leads with reciprocal
changes in opposite leads.[49,50]

Treatments should include pain relief with analgesia, non-
steroidal anti-inflammatory medications, treatment of the
underlying cause and cardiac monitoring for observation of
complications.[15,49,50]

Aortic aneurysm

The two atherosclerotic diseases of the aorta are discussed here:
aortic aneurysm and aortic dissection.

Aortic aneurysm is the localised weakness of the arterial
wall that results in a bulge or alteration in shape of the artery
and therefore an alteration in blood flow. The weakness of the
arterial wall may predispose the vessel to thrombus formation,
embolisation or rupture.[14,15] Optimal cardiovascular risk
management should focus on statin therapy, antihypertensives,
antiplatelets and smoking cessations as most cases of aortic
aneurysm involve patients with a history of atherosclerosis
and its associated risk factors such as systemic hypertension
and hypercholesterolaemia.[51] The incidence of aneurysm
is higher in men than in women and can occur anywhere
along the aorta, but occurs more frequently in the abdominal
region than the thoracic region.[52-54] There are three types of
aneurysm:

- a *fusiform aneurysm*, where the aneurysmal area radiates
  around the whole diameter of the vessel
- a *sacculated aneurysm*, which involves only one side of
  the vessel, usually the ascending aorta
- a *pseudoaneurysm*, which involves a dissection of the
  intimal layer of the vessel creating a false channel or
  lumen.

Aortic aneurysms are often discovered incidentally during
routine examination. Symptoms include chest, back, groin or
flank pain usually depending on the location of the aneurysm.[52]

Aortic dissection

The most common initial presenting complaint in over 90%
of acute aortic dissections is severe pain often described as
'tearing', 'sharp' or 'ripping'. Dissection can occlude nearby
vessels that branch off from the aorta, including the coronary
arteries, carotid, spinal, mesenteric and renal arteries. A chest
X-ray is the most common diagnostic test to identify aortic
aneurysm—by a widened mediastinum. Reduced or absent
carotid or femoral pulses usually indicate aortic dissection, and

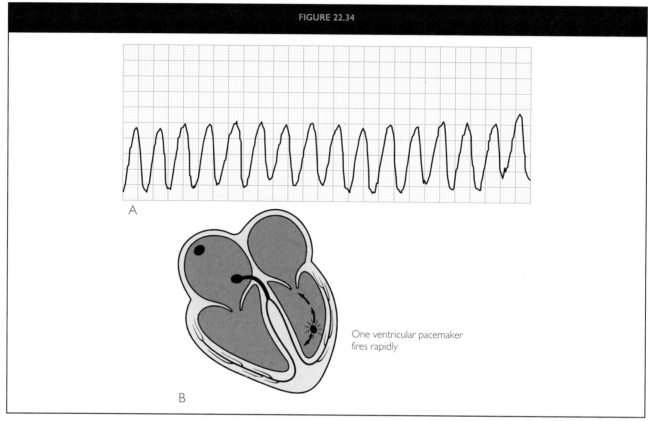

FIGURE 22.34

One ventricular pacemaker
fires rapidly

A, Ventricular tachycardia (VT). **B,** Conduction pathway for VT.[12]

TABLE 22.24 Ventricular tachycardia[12]	
Rate	100 to 250 beats/minute
Rhythm	Regular
P waves	Not seen
QRS complexes	Wide, regular, monomorphic
P/QRS relationship	None

acute MI or ischaemia may involve occlusion of the coronary arteries.[14,15,52,54] Pericardial involvement will be indicated by a pericardial rub, diminished heart sounds and cardiac tamponade and its complications can result in sudden death. Neurological deficits may include an altered level of consciousness and syncope.[14,15,52–54]

Immediate medical management should focus on the control of hypertension and analgesia. Observation and ongoing treatment should focus on maintaining blood pressure and intervention in the case of shock. Beta-blockade is useful in reducing blood pressure, and vasodilators are additional agents but can increase the force of ventricular contraction. Antihypertensive therapy should be carefully titrated and if blood pressure cannot be controlled, preparation for surgery should be considered to prevent aortic rupture or cardiac tamponade.[14,15,52–53]

Hypertensive emergencies

Raised blood pressure is a risk factor for heart disease. Blood pressure is a result of both cardiac output and peripheral vascular resistance; in hypertension either one or both of these components are elevated. Complications from uncontrolled hypertension include increased risk of stroke, heart disease and heart failure, renal disease and death.[14,15]

Malignant hypertension is defined as a sudden blood pressure increase. Immediate intervention is required. A hypertensive emergency develops rapidly over hours and involves a significant elevation in blood pressure that requires treatment within an hour to prevent end-organ damage. Hypertensive urgency develops over days and requires treatment within 24 hours of presentation.[14,15,52,55]

Hypertensive crisis is manifested by a diastolic blood pressure above 120 mmHg and central nervous system compromise, altered level of consciousness and headache, cardiovascular compromise, chest pain, angina, MI and heart failure, renal compromise, haematuria, oliguria and renal failure. Common causes of hypertensive crisis include noncompliance with medications, illegal drug usage, renal disease, pre-eclampsia and eclampsia.[57]

Intravenous medications should be administered to reduce the blood pressure by 30% within 30 minutes. Several medications are available, including vasodilators such as GTN and sodium nitroprusside (SNP). GTN dilates both arteries and veins and has its greatest effect on the venous system. SNP dilates both veins and arteries equally and reduces

FIGURE 22.35

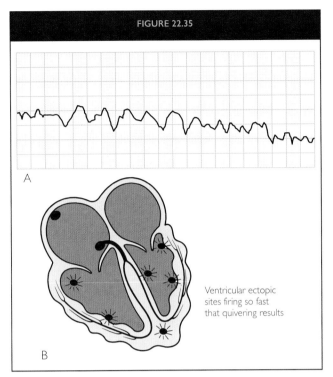

A, Ventricular fibrillation (VF). **B**, Conduction for VF.[12]

TABLE 22.25 Ventricular fibrillation[12]	
Rate	Rapid, disorganised
Rhythm	Irregular amplitude and wavelength (polymorphic)
P waves	Not seen
QRS complexes	None
P/QRS relationship	None
PR interval	None

pre and afterload with a minimal effect on cardiac output. Beta-blockers and ACE inhibitors are also effective. Nursing management for the hypertensive patient should focus on the reduction of blood pressure without the introduction of adverse complications as a result of drug therapy. Observation of CNS and cardiovascular systems will allow early interventions if either is compromised.[14,15,55,56]

FIGURE 22.36

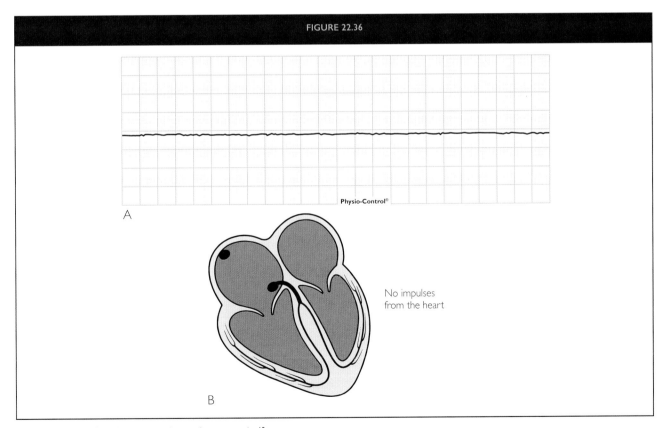

A, Asystole. **B**, Conduction pathway for asystole.[12]

TABLE 22.26 Asystole[12]	
Rate	None
Rhythm	None
P waves	May or may not appear
P/QRS relationship	None
PR interval	None

TABLE 22.27 Causes of heart failure by type[12]	
TYPE	CAUSE
Left ventricular failure	Systemic hypertension, aortic stenosis, aortic regurgitation, mitral regurgitation, cardiomyopathy, bacterial endocarditis, myocardial infarction
Right ventricular failure	Mitral stenosis, pulmonary hypertension, bacterial endocarditis on the right side of the heart, right ventricular infarction
Biventricular failure	Left ventricular failure, cardiomyopathy, myocarditis, dysrhythmias, anaemia, thyrotoxicosis

TABLE 22.28 Causes of pericarditis	
CATEGORY	DISCUSSION
Idiopathic	May follow a viral or febrile illness but the cause is often never established
Viral	Echovirus, coxsackievirus, adenovirus, varicella, Epstein-Barr, cytomegalovirus, hepatitis B, human immunodeficiency virus
Bacterial	*Staphylococcus, Streptococcus, Haemophilus, Salmonella, Legionella, Mycobacterium tuberculosis*
Fungal	*Candida, Aspergillus, Histoplasma capsulatum, Coccidioides immitis*
Parasitic	*Entamoeba histolytica, Toxoplasma gondii, Echinococcus*
Neoplasms	Lung, breast, lymphoma, leukaemia, melanoma, radiation therapy
Drugs	Procainamide, hydralazine, dantrolene, fibrinolytic agents
Connective tissue disease	Systemic lupus erythematosus, rheumatoid arthritis, scleroderma
Others	Uraemia, haemodialysis, myocardial infarction, chest trauma, aortic dissection, pancreatitis, irritable bowel syndrome

SUMMARY

Cardiovascular emergencies are commonplace in any ED. In the evolving arena of cardiovascular medicine, research and treatment interventions, the paramedic and the ED nurse are constantly challenged to remain up to date as new evidence is published.

Sound knowledge of anatomy and physiology and the pathophysiology of cardiovascular disease will enable the paramedic and ED nurse to critically assess and predict potential complications in patients presenting with a wide variety of cardiovascular complaints.

CASE STUDY

Mr Smith is a 65-year-old man who has called for an ambulance after having a 2-hour history of central chest pain. He has no known history of cardiac disease. He is a smoker and is overweight. He has been unwell for the past few days with indigestion-type symptoms.

Mr Smith is transported to the emergency department (ED) at his local hospital. He is triaged and has a 12-lead ECG taken (Fig 22.CS1). His vital signs are recorded; blood pressure is 122/88 mmHg, pulse regular 83 beats/minute and respiratory rate 24 breaths/minute.

Questions

1. Describe the initial assessment and treatment by the ambulance personnel on arrival at Mr Smith's home.
2. What other management options could be considered by the paramedics?
3. Describe the ongoing assessment of Mr Smith by the ED nurse, after arrival at the ED.
4. What other treatment and investigations could be performed by the ED nurse?
5. Describe the changes shown on the ECG (Fig 22.CS1).
6. Discuss the treatment options available for Mr Smith.

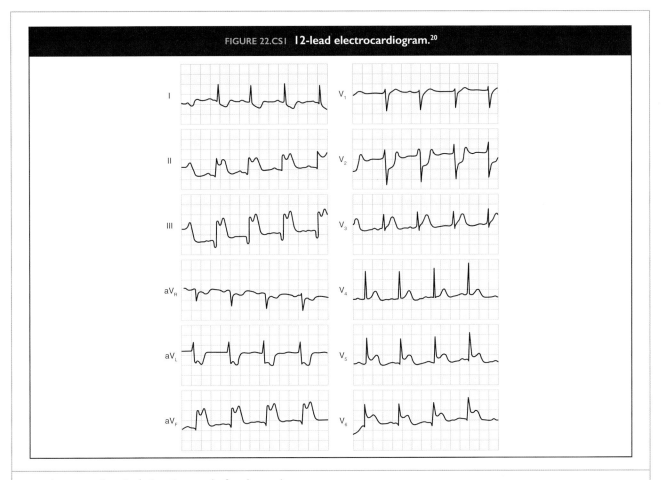

FIGURE 22.CS1 12-lead electrocardiogram.[20]

Answers to Case Study Questions can be found on evolve
http://evolve.emergencytrauma.curtis

REFERENCES

1. Australian Bureau of Statistics. National Health Survey 2007–2008. Online. http://www.abs.gov.au.
2. Australian Institute of Health and Welfare 2012. Australian Institute of Health. Cat. no. AUS 156. Canberra: AIHW.
3. Heart Foundation of Australia. Heart, stroke and vascular diseases. Australian Facts 2004. Online. www.aihw.gov.au/WorkArea/DownloadAsset.aspx?id=6442454948; accessed 3 June 2015.
4. Access Economics. The economic costs of heart attack and chest pain (acute coronary syndromes). 2009. Access Economics. Online. www.bakeridi.edu.au/Assets/Files/FullReport%20-%20the%20economic%20costs%20of%20heart%20attack%20and%20chest%20pain%20(emilable.pdf; accessed 27 March 2015.
5. Addendum to the National Heart Foundation of Australia/Cardiac Society of Australia and New Zealand. Guidelines for the management of acute coronary syndromes 2006. Heart, Lung and Circulation 2011; 20:487–502.
6. Woods SL, Sivarajan Froelicher ES, Halpenny JC et al. Cardiac nursing. 6th edn. Philadelphia: Lippincott; 2010.
7. Urden LD, Stacy KM, Lough ME. Thelan's critical care nursing: diagnosis and management. 6th edn. St Louis: Mosby; 2010.
8. Hatchett R, Thompson D, eds. Cardiac nursing: a comprehensive guide. 2nd edn. Edinburgh: Churchill Livingstone; 2008.
9. Atkinson LJ, Fortunato NM. Berry & Kohn's operating room technique. 8th edn. St Louis: Mosby; 1996.
10. Thompson JM, McFarland GK, Hirsch JE et al. Mosby's clinical nursing. 5th edn. St Louis: Mosby; 2002.
11. Tortora G, Grabowski S. Principles of anatomy and physiology. 8th edn. New York: Harper Collins College Publishers; 1996.
12. Newberry L, ed. Sheehy's emergency nursing principles and practice. 6th edn. St Louis: Mosby; 2005.
13. Drew BJ, Califf RM, Funk M et al. AHA Scientific Statement: practice standards for electrocardiographic monitoring in hospital settings: an American Heart Association Scientific Statement from the Councils on Cardiovascular Nursing, Clinical Cardiology, and Cardiovascular Disease in the Young: Endorsed by the International Society of Computerized Electrocardiology and the American Association of Critical Care Nurses. J Cardiovasc Nurs 2005;20(2):76–106.
14. Barnason S. Cardiovascular emergencies. In: Newberry L, ed. Sheehy's emergency nursing: principles and practice. 5th edn. St Louis: Mosby; 2003.
15. Gloe DS, Ballard NM. In: Newberry L, ed. Sheehy's manual of emergency care. 6th edn. St Louis: Mosby; 2005.
16. Meek S, Morris F. ABC of clinical electrocardiography. Introduction. I—leads, rate, rhythm and cardiac axis. Br Med J 2002;324(7334):415–18.
17. Newberry L, Barret G, Ballard N. A new mnemonic for chest pain assessment. J Emerg Nurs 2005;31:84–5.

18. Bossaert L, O'Connor RE, Arntz H-R et al on behalf of the Acute Coronary Syndrome Chapter Collaborators. Part 9: Acute coronary syndromes. 2010 International Consensus on Cardiopulmonary Resuscitation and Emergency Cardiovascular Care Science with Treatment Recommendations. Resuscitation 2010;81S:e175–e212.

19. Australian Institute of Health and Welfare (AIHW). Women and heart disease. Cardiovascular profile of women in Australia (June 2010).

20. Jowett N, Thompson D. Comprehensive coronary care. 4th edn. Edinburgh: Elsevier/Bailliere Tindall; 2007.

21. National Heart Foundation of Australia. Guidelines on reperfusion therapy for AMI. Adapted from management of unstable angina guidelines 2000. Online. http://circ.ahajournals.org/content/102/10/1193.full; accessed 3 June 2015.

22. GISSI. Effectiveness of intravenous thrombolytic therapy in acute myocardial infarction. Lancet 1986;ii:397–401.

23. ISIS-2. Second International study of Infarct Survival. Lancet 1988;ii:349–60.

24. Theologou T, Field ML. Pre operative IABP in high risk patients undergoing CABG. HSR Proceedings in Intensive Care and Cardiovascular Anaesthesia 2011, Vol. 3.

25. An international randomized trial comparing four thrombolytic strategies for acute myocardial infarction. The GUSTO investigators. N Engl J Med 1993;329:673–82.

26. Awtry EH, Loscalzo J. Aspirin. Circulation 2000;101(10):1206–18.

27. CAPRIE Steering Committee. A randomised, blinded trial of clopidogrel versus aspirin in patients at risk of ischaemic events (CAPRIE). Lancet 1996;348(9038):1329–39.

28. Fuster V, Dyken ML, Vokonas PS et al. Aspirin as a therapeutic agent in cardiovascular diseases: special writing group. Circulation 1993;87(2):659–75.

29. American College of Cardiology, American Heart Association. ACC/AHA guidelines for the evaluation and management of chronic heart failure in the adult. Online. http://circ.ahajournals.org/cgi/content/full/112/12/e154; accessed 28 Dec 2010.

30. Kong DF, Califf RM, Miller DP et al. Clinical outcomes of therapeutic agents that block the platelet glycoprotein IIb/IIIa integrin in ischaemic heart disease. Circulation 1998;98(25):2829–35.

31. CIBIS-II Investigators and Committees. The cardiac insufficiency bisoprolol study II (CIBIS-II): a randomised trial. Lancet 1999;353(9146):9–13.

32. Merit-HF Study Group. Effect of metoprolol CR/XL in chronic heart failure: metoprolol CR/XL randomised intervention trial in congestive heart failure (Merit-HF). Lancet 1999;353(9169):2001–7.

33. Gottlieb SS, Mc Carter RJ, Vogel RA. Effects of beta-blockade on mortality among high-risk and low-risk patients after myocardial infarction. N Engl J Med 1998;339:489–97.

34. Pfeffer MA, McMurray JJ, Velazquez EJ et al. Valsartan, captopril, or both in myocardial infarction complicated by heart failure, left ventricular dysfunction or both. N Engl J Med 2003;349:1893–906.

35. Kleinert S. HOPE for cardiovascular disease prevention with ACE-inhibitor ramipril. Heart outcomes prevention evaluation. Lancet 1999;354(9181):841.

36. Holmes DR, Curzen N. Handbook of cardiovascular emergencies. rev. edn. Manchester: Science Press; 2005.

37. American College of Cardiology/American Heart Association/European Society of Cardiology. Guidelines for the management of patients with atrial fibrillation 2006. A report of the ACC/AHA Task Force on Practical Guidelines and the ESC Committee for Practice Guidelines. J Am Coll Cardiol 2006;48(4):149–246.

38. Jones JL, Tovar OH. Electrophysiology of ventricular fibrillation and defibrillation. Crit Care Med 2000;28(11 suppl):N219–21.

39. Nussbaum G, Hartwick S. Biphasic defibrillators: headed your way? RN 2002;65(9):28ac2–6.

40. Tang W, Weil M, Sun S. Low-energy biphasic waveform defibrillation reduces the severity of post resuscitation myocardial dysfunction. Crit Care Med 2000;28(11):222.

41. Electrical Therapy for Adult Advanced Life Support. Guideline 11.4. Australian Resuscitation Council. December 2010.

42. Guidelines for the prevention, detection and management of chronic heart failure in Australia. Updated July 2011. National Heart Foundation of Australia and the Cardiac Society of Australia and New Zealand.

43. Vincent R. Resuscitation. Heart 2003;89:673–80.

44. Gura MT. Implantable cardioverter defibrillator therapy. J Cardiovasc Nurs 2005;20(4):276–87.

45. Angerstein RL, Thompson B, Rasmussen MJ. Preventing sudden cardiac death in post-myocardial infarction patients with left ventricular dysfunction. J Cardiovasc Nurs 2005;20(6):397–404.

46. National Heart Foundation of Australia and The Cardiac Society of Australia and New Zealand. Guidelines for the prevention, detection and management of chronic heart failure in Australia. Updated July 2011. Online. www.heartfoundation.com.au; 2011.

47. Eisenberg MJ, Gioia L. Angiotensin II receptor blockers in congestive heart failure. Cardiol Rev 2006;14(1):26–34.

48. Turer AT, Rao SV. Device therapy in the management of congestive heart failure. Cardiol Rev 2005;13(3):130–8.

49. Carter T, Brooks CA. Pericarditis. Inflammation or infarction? J Cardiovasc Nurs 2005;20(4):239–44.

50. Spodick DH. Acute pericarditis. Current concepts and practice. JAMA 2003;289(9):1150–3.

51. Rodriguez MA, Kumar SK, De Caro M. Hypertensive crisis. Cardiology in Review 2010;18(2):102–7.

52. Klein DG. Thoracic aortic aneurysms. J Cardiovasc Nurs 2005;20(4):245–50.

53. Finklemeier BA, Marolda D. Aortic dissection. J Cardiovasc Nurs 2001;15(4):15–24.

54. Latimer W, Harlamert E. Diagnosing an aortic dissection. Physicians Assistant 2003;27(4):45–7.

55. National Heart Foundation of Australia. Guide to management of Hypertension. Online. www.heartfoundation.org.au/SiteCollectionDocuments/HypertensionGuidelines2008to2010Update.pdf; accessed 27 March 2015.

56. Rosenow DJ, Russell E. Current concepts in the management of hypertensive crisis: emergencies and urgencies. Holistic Nurse Pract 2001;15(4):12–21.

57. Behan MW, Chew DP, Aylward PE. The role of antiplatelet therapy in the secondary prevention of coronary artery disease. Curr Opin Cardiol 2010 Jul;25(4):321–8.

CHAPTER 23

NEUROLOGICAL EMERGENCIES
JULIE CONSIDINE

Essentials

- Altered conscious state is a known predictor of poor patient outcomes and high mortality adverse events such as cardiac arrest and unplanned intensive care unit admissions.
- Adequate oxygenation and blood pressure are key priorities in the management of a patient with altered conscious state.
- Transient ischaemic attack (TIA) and stroke are a continuum: TIA is a major risk factor for stroke.
- Stroke is a medical emergency: early diagnosis and access to specialist services are pivotal to improved outcomes for stroke survivors.
- Physiological monitoring and maintenance of normal physiological parameters (oxygenation, blood glucose, temperature) are fundamental to optimal stroke management.
- Seizure management should be aimed at rapid seizure control, identifying precipitating factors and prevention of complications.
- Routine laboratory investigations and imaging are not warranted for patients with an uncomplicated first-time seizure and who make a complete recovery, and there is no evidence to currently support routine lumbar puncture in patients with seizure who are alert, afebrile and not immunocompromised.
- Head computed tomography is indicated in patients following seizure if the patient has focal neurological signs, does not recover fully or has a history of head trauma.
- Persistent or severe postictal confusion should not be presumed to be a consequence of the seizure and should be fully investigated.
- Severity of headache is an unreliable indicator of underlying pathology.
- Neuroimaging is recommended for patients with new headache and abnormal neurological assessment findings; new, sudden-onset severe headache; HIV-positive patients with new headache; and patients older than 50 years with new headache.

INTRODUCTION

Neurological emergencies relate to either illness or injury and can present as a minor discomfort or a severe life-threatening emergency requiring urgent medical and/or surgical intervention. Altered conscious state is a known predictor of adverse outcomes and is a recurrent antecedent to cardiac arrest.[1–3] As many as 42% of hospitalised patients have an altered conscious state prior to cardiac arrest,[3] and 18% of patients with physiological abnormalities preceding cardiac arrest had a neurological problem (decreased consciousness, seizures or agitation).[4] It is imperative that paramedics and emergency nurses pay attention to subtle changes in conscious state and recognise behavioural disturbance, anxiety, restlessness and agitation as signs of clinical deterioration rather than dismissing these signs as disruptive behaviours or psychosomatic symptoms. The focus of this chapter is to provide a review of neuroanatomy and physiology, a guide to structured assessment of a patient with a neurological problem and an overview of the management of common neurological conditions. Chapter 45 discusses trauma as it relates to brain injuries.

Anatomy and physiology of the nervous system

Meninges

The three membranes which cover the brain and spinal cord are the meninges (Fig 23.1).[5,6] The outer layer is called the dura mater and is composed of fibrous connective tissue that supports and separates brain structures.[5,6] The arachnoid mater is a delicate layer of connective tissue membrane and the pia mater is the innermost layer of transparent fibrous membrane.[5,6] Two important folds in the dura mater that separate areas of the brain are the *falx cerebri* and the *tentorium cerebelli*.[5,6] The falx cerebri creates a longitudinal fissure that separates the two cerebral hemispheres and the tentorium cerebelli separates the hemispheres from and covers the cerebellum.[5,6] In between the meninges are spaces. The *epidural space* is the space between dura and skull and contains fat, connective tissue and blood vessels. The *subdural space* is the space between dura and arachnoid mater that contains serous fluid, and the *subarachnoid space* is the space between arachnoid and pia mater and contains circulating *cerebrospinal fluid*.[5,6]

Brain

The adult brain is one of the largest organs of the body, weighing approximately 1300 g or 2% of total bodyweight.[5,7] Structurally the brain is divided into three parts: the cerebrum, cerebellum and brainstem (Fig 23.2).[5,7] The *cerebrum* accounts for about 80% of the total weight of the brain. The cerebrum is divided into the left and right cerebral hemispheres (Fig 23.3).[5]

Each hemisphere is made up of grey matter (nerve cell bodies and dendrites) and white matter (myelinated nerve fibres),[5,6] and the hemispheres are connected by a bundle of fibres called the corpus callosum. The corpus callosum relays information between the two hemispheres.[5,7] Each cerebral hemisphere has four lobes that are responsible for specific aspects of cerebral function (Table 23.1).

The *cerebellum* is a butterfly-shaped structure located below the cerebrum.[5] The cerebellum controls subconscious skeletal muscle contractions required for coordination, posture and balance.[5]

The *brainstem* contains vital centres and is composed of the medulla oblongata, the pons and the midbrain. The *medulla* is continuous with the upper spinal cord and forms part of the inferior brainstem. The medulla contains ascending and descending tracts that relay motor and sensory impulses between the brain and spinal cord.[5] Many tracts cross (or decussate) as they pass through the medulla,[5] which is why the right side of the brain controls the left side of the body and vice versa. Vital reflex centres are located in the medulla.[5] The cardiac centre controls heart rate and force of contraction, the medullary rhythmicity area controls respiratory pattern and the vasomotor area controls blood-vessel diameter.[5] The medulla also contains non-vital reflex centres such as those required for swallowing, vomiting, coughing and sneezing.[5] The *pons* lies directly above the medulla and relays impulses within the brain and between the brain and spinal cord.[5] The pons contains the pneumotaxic area and the apneustic area, both of which control respiration along with the medullary rhythmicity area.[5] The *midbrain* relays motor impulses from cerebral cortex to pons and spinal cord, and relays sensory impulses from spinal cord to thalamus.[5]

The thalamus and hypothalamus are situated on top of the brainstem. The *thalamus* surrounds the third ventricle and is an interpretation centre for sensory impulses (e.g. pain,

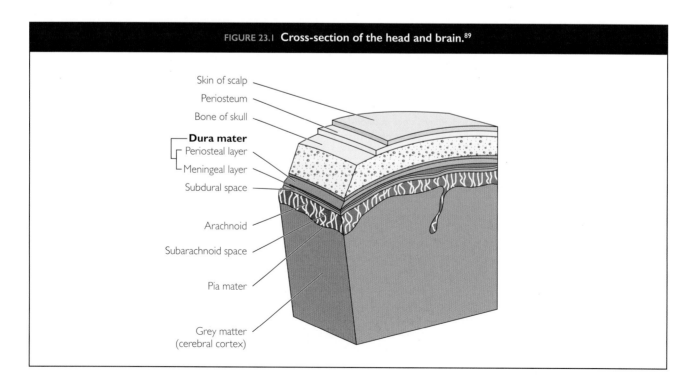

FIGURE 23.1 **Cross-section of the head and brain.**[89]

Skin of scalp
Periosteum
Bone of skull
Dura mater
  Periosteal layer
  Meningeal layer
Subdural space
Arachnoid
Subarachnoid space
Pia mater
Grey matter (cerebral cortex)

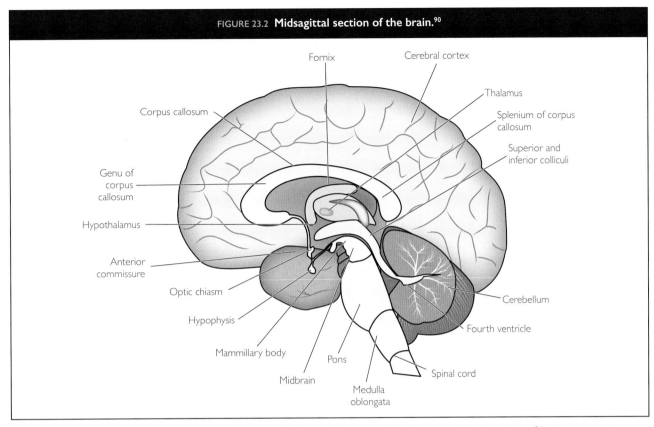

FIGURE 23.2 **Midsagittal section of the brain.**[90]

Fornix
Cerebral cortex
Corpus callosum
Thalamus
Splenium of corpus callosum
Superior and inferior colliculi
Genu of corpus callosum
Hypothalamus
Anterior commissure
Optic chiasm
Cerebellum
Hypophysis
Fourth ventricle
Mammillary body
Pons
Spinal cord
Midbrain
Medulla oblongata

Note the relationships among the cerebral cortex, cerebellum, thalamus and brainstem and the location of various commissures.

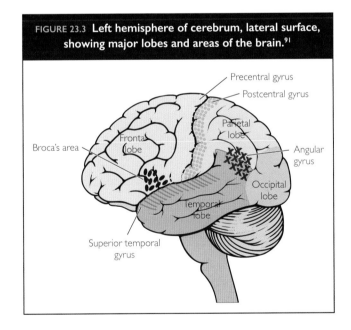

FIGURE 23.3 **Left hemisphere of cerebrum, lateral surface, showing major lobes and areas of the brain.**[91]

Precentral gyrus
Postcentral gyrus
Parietal lobe
Broca's area
Frontal lobe
Angular gyrus
Occipital lobe
Temporal lobe
Superior temporal gyrus

temperature, touch and pressure).[5] The *hypothalamus* is located inferior to the thalamus[5] and controls vital functions (e.g. water balance, blood pressure, sleep, appetite and body temperature) and regulates the autonomic nervous system. The hypothalamus stimulates smooth muscle, controls heart rate and strength of contraction, controls gland secretions, receives and interprets sensory impulses from the viscera and is the main connection between the nervous system and the endocrine system.

Spinal cord

The spinal cord is located in the vertebral canal (cavity formed by the vertebral foramina) and is covered by the meninges.[5,6] The spinal cord is continuous with the brainstem, beginning as a continuation of the medulla oblongata and terminating at the level of the second lumbar vertebra.[5] The spinal cord is composed of H-shaped grey matter (nerve cell bodies) surrounded by white matter (nerve tracts and fibres). The spinal cord contains bundles of fibres called tracts: ascending tracts conduct impulses up the spinal cord (sensory) and descending tracts conduct impulses down the spinal cord (motor).[5] These features are illustrated in Figure 23.4. The *filum terminale* is a section of non-nervous fibrous tissue that extends inferiorly from below the lumbar enlargement to the coccyx, and the *cauda equina* is the tail-like collection of roots of spinal nerves at the inferior end of the spinal canal.[5]

Spinal nerves

There are 31 pairs of spinal nerves which are named and numbered according to the spinal cord region from which they emerge.[5] Each spinal nerve has two connections to the spinal cord: the *posterior or dorsal root* receives sensory input from sensory receptors and the *anterior or ventral root* contains a combination of efferent (motor) fibres.[5] Close to the spinal cord, spinal nerves divide into branches called *rami* and the anterior rami form networks with adjacent nerves called *plexuses*.[5] The *cervical plexus* supplies the skin and muscles of the head, neck and upper shoulders and innervates the diaphragm. The phrenic nerves also arise from the cervical plexus.[5] The *brachial plexus* innervates the upper extremities

PART	LOCATION	FUNCTION
TABLE 23.1 Location and function of the parts of the cerebrum[91]		
CORTICAL AREAS		
Motor		
Primary	Precentral gyrus	Controls initiation of movement on opposite side of body
Supplementary	Anterior to precentral gyrus	Facilitates proximal muscle activity, including activity for stance and gait, and spontaneous movement and coordination
Sensory		
Somatic	Postcentral gyrus	Registers body sensations (e.g. temperature, touch, pressure, pain) from opposite side of body
Visual	Occipital lobe	Registers visual images
Auditory	Superior temporal gyrus	Registers auditory inputs
Association areas	Parietal lobe	Integrates somatic and special sensory inputs
	Posterior temporal lobe	Integrates visual and auditory inputs for language comprehension
	Anterior temporal lobe	Integrates past experiences
	Anterior frontal lobe	Controls higher-order processes (e.g. judgement, insight, reasoning, problem solving, planning)
OTHER AREAS		
Language		
Comprehension	Wernicke's area	Integrates auditory language (understanding of spoken words)
Expression	Broca's area	Regulates verbal expression
Basal ganglia	Near lateral ventricles of both cerebral hemispheres	Controls and facilitates learned and automatic movements
Thalamus	Below basal ganglia	Relays sensory and motor inputs to cortex and other parts of cerebrum
Hypothalamus	Below thalamus	Regulates endocrine and autonomic functions (e.g. feeding, sleeping, emotional and sexual responses)
Limbic system	Lateral to hypothalamus	Influences affective (emotional) behaviour and basic drives, such as feeding and sexual behaviour

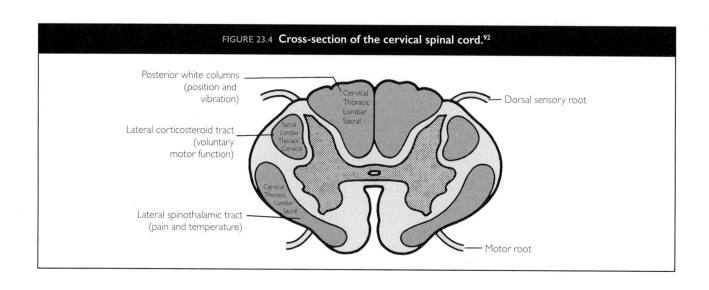

FIGURE 23.4 **Cross-section of the cervical spinal cord.[92]**

and shoulder region; the radial, median and ulnar nerves arise from the brachial plexus.[5] The *lumbar plexus* innervates the anterolateral abdominal wall and parts of the lower extremities, and is the origin of the femoral nerve. The sciatic nerve arises from the *sacral plexus*, which innervates the buttocks, perineum and lower extremities.[5]

The spinal nerves originating from T2 to T11 do not form plexuses and are known as the *intercostal nerves*.[5] Nerve

T2 supplies the intercostal muscles of the second intercostal space, the skin of the axilla and the posteromedial aspect of the arm; nerves T3 to T6 supply intercostal muscles and the skin of the anterior and lateral chest; and nerves T7 to T11 supply intercostal muscles, abdominal muscles and overlying skin. The areas of skin that are innervated by specific spinal-cord segments are called *dermatomes* (Fig 23.5).

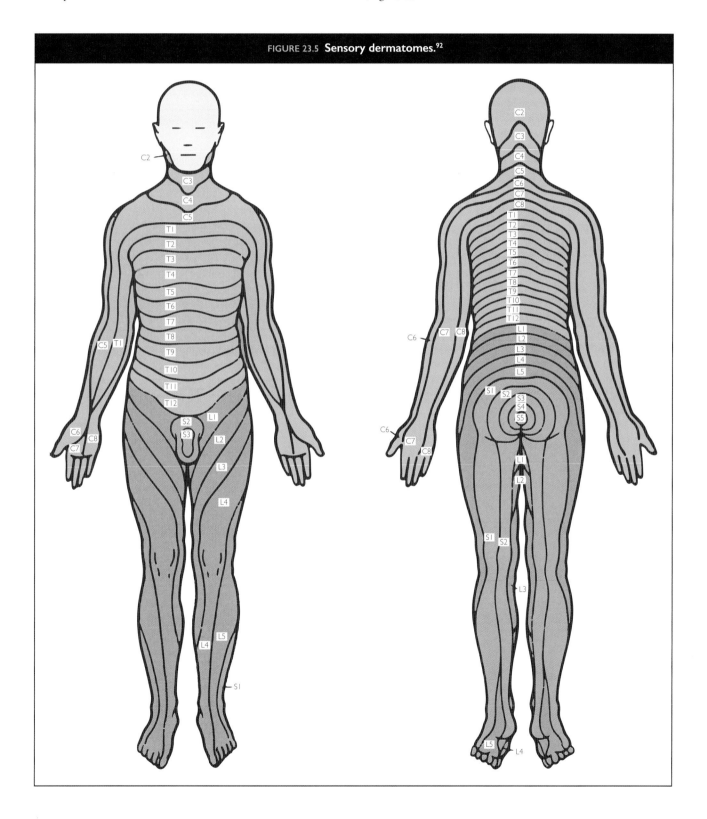

FIGURE 23.5 **Sensory dermatomes.**[92]

Cranial nerves

There are 12 pairs of cranial nerves, each with a name and numbered using Roman numerals.[5] The numbers indicate the order in which the nerves arise from the brain (front to back), and the name indicates the function of each nerve pair. Cranial nerve functions are not consciously controlled; therefore, assessment of cranial nerves provides an accurate picture of brainstem activity and neurological function.[7] Table 23.2 outlines the functions of each cranial nerve, discussed further in Chapter 45.

Cerebrospinal fluid

Cerebrospinal fluid (CSF) is produced in the cerebral ventricles by the choroid plexus and circulates through the cerebral ventricles and subarachnoid space.[5] CSF is a clear, colourless fluid containing oxygen, glucose, proteins, urea and salts.[5] Normally, the central nervous system contains 80–150 mL of CSF, and 20 mL of CSF is produced per hour.[5] CSF has protective and circulatory functions. It is a shock-absorbing medium for the brain and spinal cord and prevents the brain and spinal cord crashing against bony structures. CSF also delivers nutrients filtered from the blood to the brain and spinal cord, and removes wastes produced by the brain and spinal-cord cells.[5] CSF also compensates for changes in intracranial pressure and volume.[5] The blood–CSF (or blood–brain) barrier is the interface between the peripheral circulation and the central nervous system and is made up of specialised endothelial cells.[8] The blood–brain barrier serves as protective mechanism that prevents passage of certain substances from blood to CSF and then to the brain,[5] but also enables the maintenance of central nervous system homeostasis.[8] The blood–brain barrier has controlled reversible openings that are essential for normal cerebral physiological function.[8] Disruption to the blood–brain barrier from conditions such as stroke, head injury and cerebral inflammatory diseases often causes increased permeability, resulting in injurious substances causing further damage to the underlying brain.[8]

Cerebral blood flow

The brain requires a continuous oxygen and glucose supply—although the brain comprises only 2% of total bodyweight, it uses 20% of the body's oxygen and 25% of the body's glucose.[5] Adequate cerebral perfusion is required to ensure a continuous oxygen and glucose supply.[5] The arterial circle or circle of Willis is formed by the posterior cerebral, posterior communicating, internal carotid, anterior cerebral and anterior communicating arteries (Fig 23.6). This circular structure allows compensation if blood flow from one of the major contributing arteries is reduced, and provides collateral circulation to the brain.[6,7] The internal carotid arteries supply the anterior brain and vertebral arteries supply the posterior brain.[7] Venous blood drains from the brain through sinuses in the dura mater into the internal jugular veins.[7]

Intracranial pressure

Intracranial pressure (ICP) is the pressure within the cranial cavity; normal ICP ranges from 5 to 15 mmHg.[9] The cranial cavity contains brain tissue (80%), blood (10%) and CSF (10%),[6] and increased ICP occurs when the volume of any of these components increases.[9] Small alterations in brain tissue, blood or CSF volume do not cause increased ICP because a small increase in volume of one component is compensated for by a decrease in the volume of the other components (Monro-Kellie hypothesis).[10] CSF is the most easily displaced, and CSF volume is reduced via reabsorption.[11] If ICP remains elevated following CSF displacement, cerebral blood volume is reduced via vasoconstriction and compression of small intracranial veins.[9] Cerebral vessel diameter is a key determinant of cerebral blood volume. In normal circumstances, cerebral blood vessel diameter is regulated by the autonomic nervous system and fluctuations in the arterial partial pressure of carbon dioxide

	TABLE 23.2 Cranial nerves and their functions	
NUMBER	NAME	FUNCTION
I	Olfactory	Smell
II	Optic	Vision
III	Oculomotor	Elevate upper lid, pupillary constriction, most extraocular movements
IV	Trochlear	Downward, inward movement of the eye
V	Trigeminal	Chewing, clenching the jaw, lateral jaw movement, corneal reflexes, face sensation
VI	Abducens	Lateral eye deviation
VII	Facial	Facial motor, taste, lacrimation and salivation
VIII	Acoustic	Equilibrium, hearing
IX	Glossopharyngeal	Swallowing, gag reflex, taste on posterior tongue
X	Vagus	Swallowing, gag reflex, abdominal viscera, phonation
XI	Spinal accessory	Head and shoulder movement
XII	Hypoglossal	Tongue movement

FIGURE 23.6

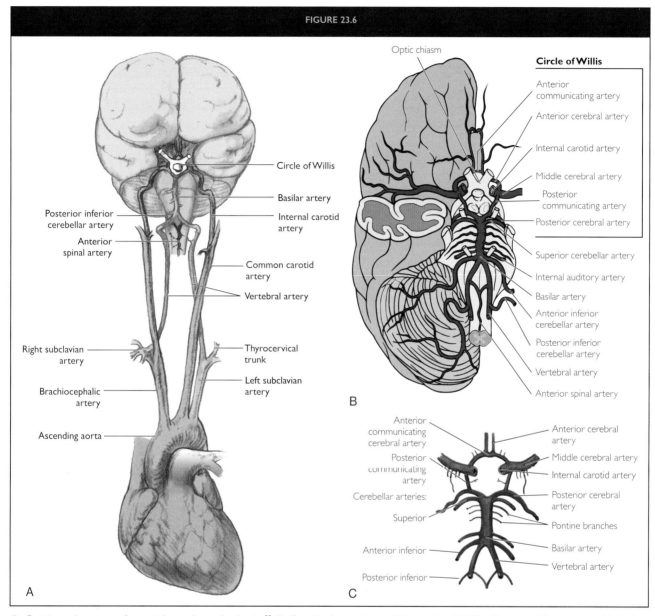

A, Origin and course of arterial supply to the brain.[93] **B**, Cerebral arteries and the circle of Willis. The tip of the temporal lobe has been removed to show the course of the middle cerebral artery.[93] **C**, Arteries at the base of the brain. The arteries that compose the circle of Willis are the two anterior cerebral arteries joined to each other by the anterior communicating cerebral artery and to the posterior cerebral arteries by the posterior communicating arteries.[93]

and oxygen (PaCO$_2$ and PaO$_2$). Increased PaCO$_2$ results in generalised vasodilation (including vasodilation of cerebral blood vessels) and increased ICP.[10]

Cerebral perfusion pressure (CPP) is the pressure required to perfuse the brain. CPP is the difference between mean arterial blood pressure (MAP) and ICP; i.e. CPP = MAP – ICP.[10] Normal CCP ranges from 60 to 100 mmHg.[9,10]

Understanding the relationship between ICP, blood pressure and cerebral perfusion is important for the management of increased ICP and preservation of cerebral perfusion. A patient with normal ICP who is hypotensive will have inadequate cerebral perfusion. Similarly, a patient with increased ICP from a head injury or stroke and normal blood pressure will also have reduced cerebral perfusion. Cerebral

perfusion will be especially compromised in the patient with increased intracranial pressure and concurrent hypotension. When ICP approaches or exceeds MAP, cellular hypoxia and death occur (Fig 23.7).[9,10]

Divisions of the nervous system

The major functions of the neurological system are to sense, interpret and respond to changes within the body and the outside environment.[5] The major divisions of the nervous system are the central and peripheral nervous systems. The *central nervous system* (CNS) is responsible for organising and coordinating all body system responses, including consciousness and cognition, while the *peripheral nervous system* (PNS) acts as the information pathway.[12]

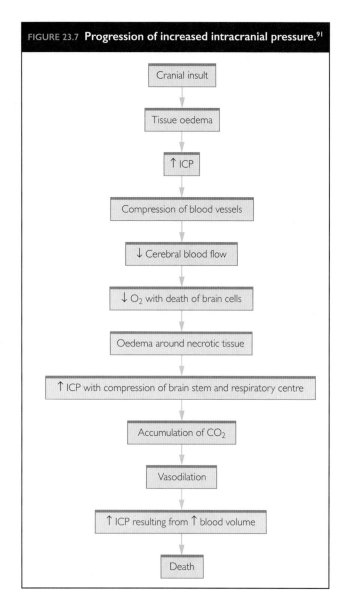

FIGURE 23.7 **Progression of increased intracranial pressure.**[91]

Cranial insult → Tissue oedema → ↑ ICP → Compression of blood vessels → ↓ Cerebral blood flow → ↓ O₂ with death of brain cells → Oedema around necrotic tissue → ↑ ICP with compression of brain stem and respiratory centre → Accumulation of CO₂ → Vasodilation → ↑ ICP resulting from ↑ blood volume → Death

Central nervous system

The CNS consists of the brain and the spinal cord.[5,6] Sensations are relayed from peripheral receptors to the CNS, then interpreted. The CNS is also responsible for the nerve impulses that stimulate the contraction of muscles and the excretion of glands.[5]

Peripheral nervous system

The PNS is the processor that connects the brain with receptors, muscles and glands. It is divided into the *afferent (sensory)* system, which relays information from sensory receptors to the CNS, and the *efferent (motor)* system, which relays information from the CNS to muscles and glands.[5] The efferent nervous system is further divided into the *somatic nervous system*, which relays information from CNS to skeletal muscles, and the *autonomic nervous system* (ANS), which relays information from CNS to smooth muscle, cardiac muscles and glands.[5] The ANS is divided into the sympathetic nervous system and the parasympathetic nervous system.[5] These systems are discussed further in Chapter 20.

Autonomic nervous system

The ANS controls smooth muscle, cardiac muscle and gland function.[5] ANS activity is regulated by the centres in the cerebral cortex, hypothalamus and brainstem, and functions without conscious control or awareness.[5] The ANS is divided into the sympathetic and parasympathetic nervous systems.[5] Table 23.3 compares sympathetic and parasympathetic functions.

Sympathetic division

The sympathetic nervous system is responsible for the 'fight or flight' response and activates energy stores when required.[5,6] Sympathetic division domination occurs during fear, embarrassment, exercise, rage and emergency situations. It causes dilation of the pupils, increased heart rate and force of contraction, increased blood pressure, bronchodilation, decreased perfusion of gastrointestinal and genitourinary organs and increased glucose production and release.[5]

Parasympathetic division

The parasympathetic nervous system conserves and restores energy, resulting in effects that oppose sympathetic nervous system effects.[5,6] Parasympathetic stimulation results in decreased heart rate, bronchoconstriction and constriction of the pupils, and activities such as salivation, lacrimation, urination, defecation and digestion.[5]

Neurons

Neurons are the structural and functional units of the nervous system. Neurons consist of three parts: a *cell body*, *dendrites* (or processes) that convey messages to the cell body and an *axon* (or nerve fibre) which carries impulses away from the cell body and towards another neuron, muscle fibre or gland cell (Fig 23.8).[5] Propagation of impulses is known as the *action potential*. The junction between two neurons or a neuron and muscle or gland cell is called a *synapse*.[5,6] The synapse is the point at which impulses are transmitted between the axon of one neuron and the dendrite of another.

- **Nerve impulse transmission**—synapses may be electrical or chemical.[5] Electrical synapses are faster than chemical synapses and can synchronise large groups of neurons or muscle fibres.[5] As a result, electrical synapses are commonly found in visceral smooth muscle and cardiac muscle.[5]
- **Electrical transmission**—at electrical synapses, impulses are conducted directly between adjacent cells through gap junctions.[5] At gap junctions, ions flow from one cell to the next through tunnel-like structures called *connexons*, resulting in the transfer of action potential.[5]
- **Chemical transmission**—transmission of impulses between two neurons, a neuron and a muscle cell or a neuron and a glandular cell is controlled by *neurotransmitters* (Fig 23.9).[5] Examples of neurotransmitters include acetylcholine, dopamine, noradrenaline, adrenaline and serotonin.[5,6] Neurotransmitters are partially responsible for pleasure, sexual desire, sadness, appetite, memory, anxiety and humour.

TABLE 23.3 Effect of sympathetic and parasympathetic nervous systems[94,95]

VISCERAL EFFECTOR	EFFECT OF SYMPATHETIC NERVOUS SYSTEM*	EFFECT OF PARASYMPATHETIC NERVOUS SYSTEM†
Heart	Increase in rate and strength of heartbeat (beta-receptors)	Decrease in rate and strength of heartbeat
SMOOTH MUSCLE OF BLOOD VESSELS		
Skin blood vessels	Constriction (alpha-receptors)	No effect
Skeletal muscle blood vessels	Dilation (beta-receptors)	No effect
Coronary blood vessels	Dilation (beta-receptors), constriction (alpha-receptors)	Dilation
Abdominal blood vessels	Constriction (alpha-receptors)	No effect
Blood vessels of external genitals	Ejaculation (contraction of smooth muscle in male ducts [e.g. epididymis, ductus deferens])	Dilation of blood vessels causing erection in male
SMOOTH MUSCLE OF HOLLOW ORGANS AND SPHINCTERS		
Bronchi	Dilation (beta-receptors)	Constriction
Digestive tract, except sphincters	Decrease in peristalsis (beta-receptors)	Increase in peristalsis
Sphincters of digestive tract	Contraction (alpha-receptors)	Relaxation
Urinary bladder	Relaxation (beta-receptors)	Contraction
Urinary sphincters	Contraction (alpha-receptors)	Relaxation
EYE		
Iris	Contraction of radial muscle, dilation of pupil	Contraction of circular muscle, constriction of pupil
Ciliary	Relaxation, accommodation for far vision	Contraction, accommodation for near vision
Hairs (pilomotor muscles)	Contraction producing 'goose bumps' or piloerection (alpha-receptors)	No effect
GLANDS		
Sweat	Increase in sweat (neurotransmitter, acetylcholine)	No effect
Digestive (e.g. salivary, gastric)	Decrease in secretion of saliva; not known for others	Increase in secretion of saliva and gastric hydrochloric acid
Pancreas, including islets	Decrease in secretion	Increase in secretion of pancreatic juice and insulin
Liver	Increase in glycogenolysis (beta-receptors), increase in blood glucose level	No effect
Adrenal medulla‡	Increase in adrenaline secretion	No effect

*Neurotransmitter is noradrenaline unless otherwise stated.

†Neurotransmitter is acetylcholine unless otherwise stated.

‡Sympathetic preganglionic axons terminate in contact with secreting cells of the adrenal medulla. Thus, the adrenal medulla functions as a 'giant sympathetic postganglionic neuron'.

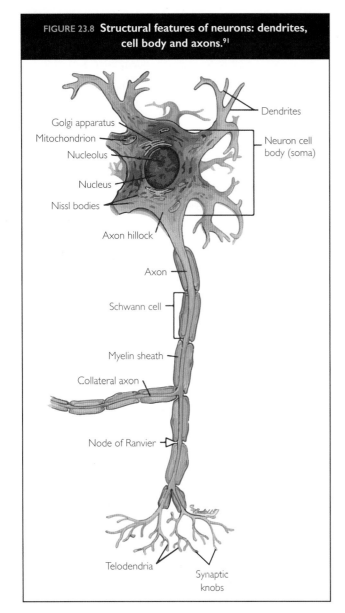

FIGURE 23.8 Structural features of neurons: dendrites, cell body and axons.[91]

Golgi apparatus
Mitochondrion
Nucleolus
Nucleus
Nissl bodies
Dendrites
Neuron cell body (soma)
Axon hillock
Axon
Schwann cell
Myelin sheath
Collateral axon
Node of Ranvier
Telodendria
Synaptic knobs

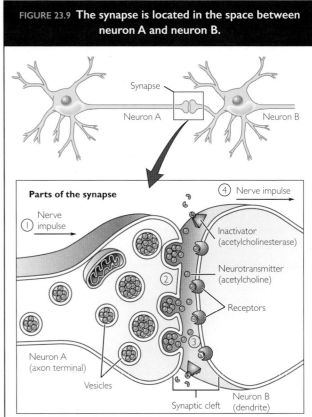

FIGURE 23.9 The synapse is located in the space between neuron A and neuron B.

Synapse
Neuron A
Neuron B

Parts of the synapse
Nerve impulse (1)
Nerve impulse (4)
Inactivator (acetylcholinesterase)
Neurotransmitter (acetylcholine)
Receptors
Neuron A (axon terminal)
Vesicles
Synaptic cleft
Neuron B (dendrite)

Parts of the synapse include the neurotransmitters, inactivators and receptors. The neurotransmitters are located in the vesicles of neuron A. The inactivators are located on the membrane of neuron B. The receptors are located on the membrane of neuron B.[91]

- Consider the need for cervical spine immobilisation if altered conscious state is potentially the cause of, or results in, injury.
- Associated symptoms—headache, seizures, nausea, vomiting, fevers, motor or sensory impairment, changes to speech, vision, memory, alterations to bladder and/or bowel function.
- Past medical history—similar episodes, past and concurrent medical and surgical history (particularly history of chronic neurological disorders or existing neurological deficits, headaches, seizure disorders, stroke/TIA (transient ischaemic attack), mental illness, results of previous investigations, allergies, medications.
- Social and employment history—patterns of drug and alcohol use, environmental factors, stressors.
- Specific considerations for extremes of age—developmental delay, intellectual disability, cognitive impairment, dementia, delerium (see Chs 36 and 39).

Even when there is a history of illness that may easily explain an altered conscious state, all sudden deterioration should be treated as an acute event and thoroughly investigated.

Physical assessment

As discussed earlier in this chapter, the brain is highly dependent on a continuous supply of oxygen and glucose.[7]

Assessment of the patient with altered consciousness

A focused history and thorough physiological assessment are fundamental to early identification and treatment of life-threatening neurological emergencies and are addressed in the following section.

History

Obtaining an accurate history in a patient with an altered level of consciousness can be difficult, therefore family members, police, local medical officers and carers are valuable sources of information.[13] Causes of an altered level of consciousness are listed in Box 23.1. The following information should be elicited:

- History of presenting problem—time and acuity of onset, history of trauma including falls, consistency or fluctuation in symptoms, possibility of drug or alcohol use, environmental exposures (e.g. carbon monoxide exposure).

BOX 23.1 Causes of alteration in conscious state[96]

Structural insults

Supratentorial

Haematoma
- epidural
- subdural

Cerebral tumour

Cerebral aneurysm

Haemorrhagic stroke

Infratentorial

Cerebellar arteriovenous malformation

Pontine haemorrhage

Brainstem tumour

Metabolic insults

Loss of substrate

Hypoxia

Hypoglycaemia

Global ischaemia

Shock
- hypovolaemia
- cardiogenic

Focal ischaemia
- transient ischaemic attack/stroke
- vasculitis

Derangement of normal physiology

Hypo- or hypernatraemia

Hyperglycaemia/hyperosmolarity

Hypercalcaemia

Hypermagnesaemia

Addisonian crisis

Seizures
- status epilepticus
- postictal

Post-concussive

Hypo- or hyperthyroidism

Cofactor deficiency

Metastatic malignancy

Psychiatric illness

Toxins

Drugs
- alcohol
- illicit
- prescription

Endotoxins
- subarachnoid blood
- liver failure
- renal failure

Sepsis
- systemic

Focal
- meningitis
- encephalitis

Environmental
- hypothermia/heat exhaustion
- altitude illness/decompression
- envenomations

Assessment priorities therefore include the identification and treatment (or exclusion and prevention) of hypoxia, hypotension and hypoglycaemia as causes of altered level of consciousness. The initial and ongoing assessment of patients with a neurological emergency is primarily aimed at identifying increasing ICP or evaluating the response to treatment for increased ICP. Frequent monitoring of vital signs (respiratory rate and pattern, heart rate and rhythm, blood pressure and oxygen saturation) provide important indicators of cerebral oxygenation and cerebral perfusion. Temperature should be measured to detect hypothermia, which may be a cause of altered level of consciousness (see Ch 28). Conversely, an elevated temperature may suggest an infective cause for an altered level of consciousness.

As the brain is extremely sensitive to oxygen deprivation, a decreased level of consciousness is an early and reliable indicator of increased ICP.[10] Conscious state changes can be subtle (restlessness, agitation, anxiety) or obvious (confusion, drowsiness and unconsciousness).[10] The Glasgow Coma Scale (GCS) assesses state of consciousness in adults, and in children the Paediatric Glasgow Coma Scale is used. The AVPU scale (Alert, responds to Voice, responds to Pain and Unresponsive) is useful as a rapid assessment tool but should not replace formal assessment of GCS. Both of these scores assess eye opening, verbal response and motor response. The use of these scales in the emergency department (ED) is discussed in depth in Chapter 14.

Assessment of pupil size, equality and reactivity provides information regarding the presence and level of brainstem dysfunction.[9] Pressure on the oculomotor nerve (cranial nerve III) causes pupil dilation; however, this is a late sign of increasing ICP. Patients with an altered conscious state should have a blood glucose test to exclude hypoglycaemia (see Ch 17, p. 332, for blood glucose sampling techniques).[13] Hypoglycaemia is easily treated, quickly reversed and can present in many ways: agitation, confusion, restlessness, hemiplegia, slurred speech, fitting and unconsciousness. Hyperglycaemia may cause alterations in level of consciousness (see Chapter 2). Assessment of other symptoms such as pain, vomiting, fever, photophobia, urinary retention and under-sedation in the intubated patient should also be conducted, as they may further exacerbate increased ICP. Assessment of the unconscious patient is summarised in Box 23.2.

Herniation

If untreated, increased ICP will result in herniation of brain tissue—lateral (transtentorial), downward (central transtentorial) or medial (cingulate).[7,9,10]

- During *lateral herniation,* pressure on the oculomotor nerve results in sluggish, then fixed and dilated, pupils.[9]
- If herniation occurs laterally, pupillary changes will occur first in the ipsilateral pupil and then in the contralateral pupil.[9]
- During *central herniation*, pupils will be bilaterally small but reactive to light and then progress to bilateral fixed and dilated pupils.[9]
- If increased ICP continues, ischaemia of the vasomotor centre in the brainstem results in increased systemic blood pressure[10] in an attempt to improve cerebral perfusion.[7]

BOX 23.2 Assessment of the unconscious patient[78]

PRIMARY SURVEY ASSESSMENT

Airway	Conscious state—capacity to protect airway
Cervical spine	Possible need for cervical spine immobilisation if neurological deficit cause or result of associated injury
Breathing	Respiratory rate
	Oxygen saturation—possible hypoxia
	Respiratory effort/pattern
Circulation	Heart rate
	Blood pressure—possible hypo/hypertension
	Skin status
	12-lead ECG—possible cardiac dysrhythmia, cardio-embolic event
Disability	AVPU
	GCS
	Assessment of pupils
	BSL—possible hypo/hyperglycaemia
Other	Temperature—possible sepsis

FOCUSED SYMPTOM ASSESSMENT USING THE NOPQRST MNEMONIC

Normal health status	Patient's usual health status: • allergies? • medications? Complimentary therapies? Drugs? Alcohol? • past medical and surgical history • past history of neurological disorders (seizure disorders, TIA/stroke, migraines/headaches) Patient's usual level of neurological function: • pre-existing hemiparesis/paralysis/neuropathy/cognitive impairment Social history • who does patient live with? • occupation if working
Onset	When did symptoms start? Was the onset gradual or sudden?
Palliating/ provoking factors	Known risk factors for: • headache, migraine • TIA/stroke/intracerebral haemorrhage • seizure disorders • dementia/delirium History of prescription medication/social or illicit drugs/alcohol use
Quality and quantity	Can the patient describe their symptoms? Are there other associated symptoms? • fevers: possible CNS infection/sepsis • rash: possible sepsis, allergy • headache: possible migraine/headache syndromes/intracerebral haemorrhage • tongue trauma/incontinence/soft-tissue injuries: possible seizure • paralysis: unilateral = possible stroke; ascending = Guillain-Barré syndrome • signs of head trauma: haematoma, soft-tissue injuries, Battle's sign, periorbital ecchymosis, rhinorrhoea, otorrhoea Do symptoms interrupt activities of daily living—sleeping, eating, bathing, walking?
Region/radiation	Headache? Do neurological symptoms affect other areas of the body—limbs, breathing?
Severity	How severe are the symptoms (pain/neurological deficits)? • 0 to 10 rating scale • qualitative measures: mild, moderate, severe
Timing	How long does the symptom last? How often do symptoms occur? Are symptoms related to a particular time of day or a particular activity?

AVPU: Alert, Voice, Pain, Unresponsive; BSL: blood sugar level; CNS: central nervous system; GCS: Glasgow Coma Scale; ECG: electrocardiogram; TIA: transient ischaemic attack

- *Cushing's reflex* is a triad of the following signs: hypertension, widening pulse pressure and bradycardia;[10] and is a **late indicator** of increased ICP indicating significant brainstem ischaemia.[10]
- *Cheyne-Stokes respiration* (deep, rapid breathing with periods of apnoea) and abnormal posturing will also be seen if brain herniation occurs.[10]

The structural changes that occur during herniation are shown in Figure 23.10.

Investigations

Investigations for the patient with neurological emergency may include routine blood tests such as urea and electrolytes, full blood examination and coagulation profile. Specific tests that may be indicated, depending on history and nature of presentation, may include drug levels, serum lactate, septic work-up and venom detection kits.[13] Routine drug screens are of limited clinical value.[13] A 12-lead electrocardiogram (ECG) should be performed to identify potential sources of cardiogenic emboli, cardiac dysrhythmias, specific rhythm changes related to hypokalaemia (J wave) and hypothermia (U wave) and myocardial ischaemia or infarction as potential sources of shock.[13]

Lumbar puncture

Lumbar puncture (LP) examines the CSF, most commonly for CNS infections (meningitis, encephalitis), subarachnoid haemorrhage, measuring ICP, radiological imaging and cytological examination.[13] Contraindications to LP include local infection at LP site, bleeding disorders, risk of CNS herniation.[14] There is ongoing debate regarding obtaining head computed tomography (CT) before LP because of the concern of the lumbar puncture causing herniation. Current recommendations suggest that adult patients with signs of increased intracranial pressure (for example, papilloedema,

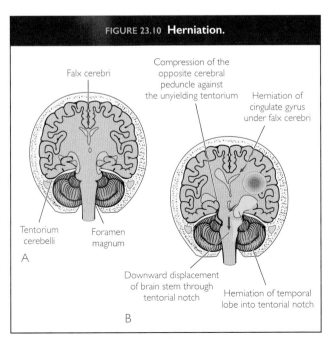

FIGURE 23.10 Herniation.

Falx cerebri

Compression of the opposite cerebral peduncle against the unyielding tentorium

Herniation of cingulate gyrus under falx cerebri

Tentorium cerebelli

Foramen magnum

A

Downward displacement of brain stem through tentorial notch

Herniation of temporal lobe into tentorial notch

B

A, Normal relationship of intracranial structures. **B**, Shift of intracranial structures.[91]

altered mental status, focal neurological deficits, signs of meningeal irritation) should have neuroimaging CT prior to lumbar puncture. In the absence of signs of increased ICP, lumbar puncture can be performed without neuroimaging.[15] Intracranial imaging is most often performed using CT brain scan and, depending on the nature of the presentation, a contrast-enhanced CT scan or MRI (magnetic resonance imaging) may also be performed.[13] All children should have some form of local anaesthetic for lumbar puncture. Topical anaesthetic cream (AnGEL) should be used (except where specimens are required urgently) and subcutaneous lignocaine should be used in addition to topical anaesthetic. Oral sucrose should be used for infants <3 months and sedation, including nitrous oxide, should be considered for those older than 6 months with normal conscious state.[16]

As an LP is a stressful procedure, reassurance and explanation is vital. In children, the most important determinant of a successful lumbar puncture is a strong, calm, experienced assistant to hold the patient.[16] Patient position is critical. The patient should be positioned lying on their side with their back parallel to the edge of the bed. The patient's knees are flexed up to the chest with the chin touching the knees so that the back is arched. Alternatively, the patient may sit up leaning over a bed table. Ask the patient to slouch rather than bend from their hips.[14] Avoid over-flexing the neck, especially in infants, as this may cause respiratory compromise.[16]

LP is a sterile procedure. Following preparation and draping of the site, vertebrae L3 and L4 are located and local anaesthetic is injected into the skin. The use of pencil-point (also known as blunt, atraumatic or non-cutting) needles reduces the risk of headache in adults.[17] Following the procedure, brief pressure and a dressing should be applied, such as a Band-aid or occlusive dressing (e.g. Tegaderm).

Post lumbar puncture care

It is important to monitor for and be aware of potential complications related to LP. Neurological and routine observations should be performed hourly post procedure and any change reported immediately to medical staff. Monitor all sedated or seriously ill patients with continuous pulse oximetry.

The most common LP-related complication is headache (sometimes called postdural puncture headache, PDPH) and this affects as many as 32% of patients.[18] Onset of PDPH is usually 24–48 hours after LP, but can occur up to 12 days post procedure.[18] Headache is rarely present immediately following LP, so any headache present immediately post procedure should be investigated to exclude increased ICP or displacement of intracranial structures.[18] PDPHs are typically dull or throbbing, often start in frontal or occipital regions but can become generalised, may radiate to neck and shoulders and may be associated with lower back pain, nausea, vomiting, vertigo and tinnitus.[27] PDPH is exacerbated by sitting upright, head movement or activities that increase intracerebral pressure (coughing, sneezing).[18]

The cause of PDPH is CSF leakage through a dural hole from the subarachnoid to the epidural spaces, producing a low-CSF-pressure headache. This causes traction on the pain-sensitive structures in the brain and vasodilation of the cerebral vessels when the patient is upright. The headache will continue until the hole heals and CSF pressure is restored; this headache typically lasts a few days and rarely more than 1 week. The risk of PDPH is related to age, sex, needle size and shape and LP technique.[18,19] Factors that increase risk of PDPH are younger patient age, female gender, low body mass index, history of chronic headaches or previous PDPH.[19,20] Factors that do *not* increase risk of PDPH include patient position during LP, number of LP attempts, experience of clinician performing LP, volume of CSF removed and bed rest following LP.[18,20] There is evidence to support use of small-gauge (22 gauge) needles, particularly of the pencil-point design, as they are associated with a lower risk of headache than traditional cutting-point needle-tip needles.[20]

Most PDPHs (approximately 85%) will resolve without any specific treatment[18] and management, if required, is focused on symptom control. The patient should be encouraged to lie in a position of comfort (will commonly be supine position due to postural influence on symptoms). Supportive treatments such as rehydration, simple analgesics, opioids and antiemetics may be helpful for mild headache.[18,20] Specific treatment is indicated if PDPH lasts longer than 72 hours to prevent risk of complications such as subdural haematoma and seizures.[18] The most common treatment is 'blood patch' which involves injecting 20–30 mL of the patient's blood into the epidural space so that the clot seals the dural perforation and prevents further CSF leak.[18,20] After the blood patch procedure, the patient should lie still for 1–2 hours in a supine position.[18] Blood patch is contraindicated in patients with fever, local infection at the LP site and bleeding disorders.[18] Oral or intravenous caffeine has been promoted as a treatment option in the past; however, headaches often reoccur after caffeine treatment and the evidence to support the effectiveness of caffeine is scant. In theory, caffeine acts as a cerebral vasoconstrictor and blocks adenosine receptors; however, there is also a risk that caffeine can cause side effects such as tachydysrhythmias and CNS toxicity.[18] As a last resort, surgical closure of the dural gap may be considered when other treatments have failed.[18] PDPH is the commonest complication of LP; however, other serious but uncommon complications can include cerebral herniation, spinal haematoma, iatrogenic spinal cord tumour and induced meningitis.[14,21]

Patient management

Management priorities for the pre-hospital and ED care of patient with an altered level of consciousness are preservation of airway, breathing and circulation, and optimisation of cerebral oxygenation and perfusion by ensuring adequate oxygenation and systemic blood pressure. Endotracheal intubation may be indicated for patients with a decreased level of consciousness if the patient is unable to maintain or protect his or her airway (see Ch 17, p. 318, for intubation procedures). A GCS score ≤8 is often used to indicate the need for endotracheal intubation, particularly in poisoned patients (see Ch 31).[22] Supplemental oxygen or assisted ventilation may be warranted if hypoxia, hypercapnia or hypoventilation is present. Hypotension should be treated by fluid resuscitation and/or inotropes. In the setting of increased ICP, hypercapnia and acidosis should be avoided and current recommendations are that $PaCO_2$ be maintained on the lower edge of normal (30–35 mmHg)[13] and evaluated by frequent arterial blood gas analysis.

The 'coma cocktail'—glucose, thiamine and naloxone—previously recommended for all unconscious patients, has come under scrutiny.[23] The routine use of these agents is no longer advocated,[13] although some agents may be useful, depending on the history and nature of the presentation. Although there is currently no evidence that 50% glucose will cause harm to an already hyperglycaemic patient,[13] the routine use of 50% glucose is questionable, given that bedside blood glucose measurement is a quick and simple test (see Ch 17, p. 332, for blood glucose sampling procedure). Administration of naloxone may be warranted if there is a history suggestive of opiate use and clinical signs such as pinpoint pupils and hypoventilation, and in this context naloxone may be both therapeutic and diagnostic.[13] Naloxone should be used with caution, as the reversal of opiate effects may result in danger to staff from an aggressive or unpredictable patient and from needlestick injury; or, in the case of a multi-medication overdose, reversal of opiate effects may allow drugs with seizure or dysrhythmic properties to dominate.[13] Thiamine administration is recommended in patients in whom alcohol abuse or hepatic encephalopathy is suspected (see Ch 41).[13,23] There is no evidence to support recommendations that thiamine should be administered prior to glucose administration and that correction of hypoglycaemia should occur prior to thiamine administration.[13,23]

Osmotic diuretics such as mannitol may be considered to decrease intravascular volume;[23] however, mannitol administration may also exacerbate haemodynamic instability resulting in a further decrease in cerebral perfusion and secondary insult.[13] The management of head injuries is discussed in Chapter 45. Depending on the pathology, other medications may be considered: for example, steroids, anticonvulsants or antibiotics.[12]

> **PRACTICE TIP**
>
> **MANAGEMENT PRIORITIES IN THE PATIENT WITH ALTERED CONSCIOUS STATE**
>
> - Airway—position, endotracheal intubation
> - Breathing—treat/prevent hypoxaemia, prevent hyperoxia
> - Circulation—ensure adequate blood pressure to increase cerebral perfusion pressure
> - Disability—treat/prevent hypo/hyperglycaemia

Transient ischaemic attacks

Transient ischaemic attack (TIA) was historically defined as 'rapidly developed clinical signs of focal or global disturbance of cerebral function lasting fewer than 24 hours, with no apparent non-vascular cause'.[24,25] However, the arbitrary duration of 24 hours for TIA is now recognised to be unhelpful, because up to 50% of TIAs (including even brief TIAs lasting minutes) are associated with infarction on diffusion-weighted MRI, so, therefore, those patients have suffered an acute ischaemic stroke.[26,27]

Stroke and TIA are now considered a continuum based on degree of tissue damage.[26] Early identification and management of TIA by paramedics and emergency nurses is important because progression of TIA to stroke often results in significant mortality and morbidity.[26,28] The risk of stroke following TIA is significant.[29–31] TIA symptoms occur in 15% to 30% of patients with ischaemic stroke, and some of those patients have TIA symptoms on the same day.[31] The risk of stroke following TIA is highest within the first 24 hours,[28] and meta-analysis of the risk of stroke early after a TIA found that the cumulative risk of stroke at 7 days was 5.2%.[28,30] An accurate history is important in the diagnosis of TIA.[28] Persistent neurological symptoms should be treated as suspected stroke rather than TIA,[24,28] and may influence pre-hospital decision making about transport to a stroke centre. Abrupt onset of maximal symptoms is predictive of a final diagnosis of TIA but there was no statistically significant difference between duration of symptoms in patients with TIA and TIA mimics (commonly epileptic seizures and migraines).[32] Key aspects of the history that are useful to help identify TIA from other conditions are as follows.[32]

- Age and other demographics: is there a high probability of a cerebrovascular event from hypertension, ischaemic heart disease, diabetes, smoking, haematological disease?
- Nature of the symptoms: positive symptoms indicate an 'excess' of central nervous system activity and may include visual, somatosensory or motor disturbances. Negative symptoms indicate a loss or reduction of central nervous system function, such as loss of vision, hearing, sensation or limb power.
- Onset and progression
- Duration: TIAs nearly always last less than 1 hour
- Precipitating factors
- Associated symptoms: tongue trauma and muscle pains are commonly associated with seizures. Vomiting is common after migraine and occasionally follows syncope, but is extremely rare in TIA or seizures. Nausea, sweating, pallor and a need to urinate or defecate commonly precede or follow syncope.

Assessment

All patients with actual or suspected TIA should have a thorough clinical assessment, baseline blood tests, ECG and brain imaging.[24] It is essential that emergency nurses and paramedics obtain a thorough history in order to establish the risk of stroke. ABCD2 is a well-validated risk-stratification tool that identifies the following five factors as risks for early stroke after TIA:[26]

1. Age over 60 years.
2. Diabetes mellitus.
3. Symptom duration greater than 10 minutes.
4. TIA with motor or speech symptoms.
5. Hypertension (systolic blood pressure > 140/90 mmHg).[33,34]

ABCD, later to become ABCD2, is the most common risk assessment tool for stroke following TIA.[35] Independent validations of the ABCD system showed good predictive value, with the exception of some studies.[35] ABCD2 has a total score of 7, and a score greater than 4 indicates high risk of stroke.[36] Details of the ABCD2 risk-stratification tool and scoring system are shown in Box 23.3. ABCD2 should also be used by paramedics and triage personnel to inform triage decisions for patients presenting with TIA.[37]

Vital-sign monitoring in both pre-hospital and ED

BOX 23.3 ABCD2 risk-stratification tool for stroke following transient ischaemic attack (TIA)

Age	> 60 years	1 point
Blood pressure	> 140/90 mmHg	1 point
Clinical features	Unilateral weakness	2 points
	Speech impairment without weakness	1 point
Duration	> 60 minutes	2 points
Diabetes	History of diabetes	1 point

Interpretation of scores
Johnston et al[34]—risk of stroke in 2 days following TIA
6–7: high risk of stroke (8.1%)
4–5: moderate risk (4.1%)
0–3: low risk (1.0%)

Bray et al[36]
< 4: low risk
> 4: high risk

---

environments should aim to ensure adequate ventilation, oxygenation and cerebral perfusion, and frequent neurological observations should be performed to identify neurological deterioration or symptom progression. Blood glucose level should be measured to exclude hypoglycaemia as a cause for symptoms and to identify diabetes as a potential risk factor (see Ch 17, p. 332, for blood glucose sampling procedure).[38] As many as 44% of patients with TIA have ECG abnormalities,[39] so an ECG should be performed to identify sources of cardiogenic emboli, such as atrial fibrillation or recent acute myocardial infarction (AMI) and signs of pre-existing cardiac disease.[29,38] Brain imaging options include CT scan, MRI, ultrasonography (Doppler) and angiography;[24,38] however, the majority of patients will have a CT scan in the ED to exclude haemorrhage or other pathology. Current recommendations are that patients classified as high risk (ABCD2 score > 4) should have an urgent CT brain scan (urgent defined as soon as possible, but definitely within 24 hours).[24] Cardiac imaging such as transthoracic or transoesophageal echocardiogram may also be warranted.[29]

Management

Management of TIA aims to identify and treat the cause and prevent progression to stroke.[40] Both the EXPRESS[41] and SOS-TIA[42] studies have shown that urgent specialist management reduces the risk of early stroke following TIA. Initial TIA management by emergency nurses and paramedics should focus on restoring/maintaining ventilation, oxygenation and cerebral perfusion, and establishing the risk of stroke. The major treatment modalities for TIA are risk-factor modification, antiplatelet therapy and carotid endarterectomy.[29] Hypertension, diabetes, hyperlipidaemia, smoking and lack of exercise are all well-known risk factors for vascular disease, so patients with TIA should be referred to appropriate services for risk-factor reduction.[38]

Hypertension is a common feature in ED patients with TIA. To maintain cerebral perfusion, aggressive blood-pressure reduction should generally be avoided.[38] If it is suspected that hypertension is causing neurological features, long-term oral antihypertensive therapy should be commenced; however, urgent blood-pressure reduction in the ED is not indicated and may be harmful.[38]

Antiplatelet therapy is the most common treatment for TIA.[38] Aspirin is beneficial and prevents subsequent vascular events by approximately 13%.[43,44] Newer antiplatelet agents such as clopidogrel, ticlodipine and aspirin-dipyridamole are also reasonable first-line options.[38] Carotid endarterectomy is beneficial for patients with TIA and greater than 50–70% carotid stenosis.[38] Angioplasty and carotid artery stenting may also be promising treatment alternatives for TIA.[38] Comparisons of aspirin and warfarin have shown no difference in TIA and stroke recurrence,[44] and therefore anticoagulation is not recommended as routine management of TIA. Anticoagulation is not superior to antiplatelet therapy for non-cardioembolic stroke or TIA and carries higher haemorrhage risk.[45]

Disposition and follow-up of patients with TIA will be dependent on institutional resources and patient risk factors. High-risk patients may warrant admission, whereas other patients may be discharged with antiplatelet therapy and neurology or primary-care follow-up. Irrespective of the source, early follow-up is important in patients who have suffered a TIA. The EXPRESS showed that the risk of recurrent stroke at 90 days in patients with TIA or minor stroke was 10.3% in those patients whose follow-up occurred after a median of 3 days, compared with 2.1% in those assessed in a median of 1 day.[41]

> **PRACTICE TIP**
>
> **TIA**
>
> Any patient with prolonged symptoms of TIA (greater than I hour) should be treated as if they are having a stroke.

Vertebrobasilar attacks

Vertebrobasilar insufficiency is used to describe TIA syndromes of the posterior circulation.[46] Vertigo is the most common symptom of vertebrobasilar ischaemia; however, other symptoms include dysarthria, dysphagia, diplopia, hemianopia, hemiparesis and sensory deficits.[5,46] Motor deficits are typically unilateral with similar degrees of weakness in the arm, leg and face.[36] Sensory deficits can be either contralateral or crossed (e.g. contralateral deficits involving the body suggest medial medullary infarct, and ipsilateral deficits involving the face suggest lateral medullary infarct).[46] Vertebrobasilar attacks may be a cause of collapse, syncopal episode or sudden loss of consciousness.[46,47] Vertebrobasilar (basilar artery) occlusion from a thrombosis or embolism can result in 'locked in' syndrome.[47] Patients with 'locked in' syndrome are paralysed and unable to speak, while having intact consciousness and understanding.[46,48]

Investigations of symptoms include Doppler/ultrasound, CT or MRI angiography. Management is dependent on cause and symptoms.[46]

Stroke

Stroke is an acute neurological injury that is caused by interruption to the blood flow to an area of the brain.[29,49] Stroke is Australia's second biggest killer after coronary heart disease and a leading cause of disability.[50] In 2012, about 50,000 Australians suffered new and recurrent strokes, 30% of stroke survivors were aged under 65, and the total financial costs of stroke in Australia were estimated to be $5 billion.[50]

Strokes can be classified according to cause as ischaemic or haemorrhagic.[29]

Ischaemic stroke

Approximately 80% of strokes are ischaemic, resulting from three major pathophysiological processes: thrombi, emboli and hypoperfusion.[49] The most common cause of stroke is thrombosis, or blood-vessel narrowing secondary to clot formation.[18] Atherosclerosis is the most common cause of thrombotic stroke; however, other causes include vasculitis, polycythaemia and infectious diseases. Embolic stroke occurs when a normal cerebral blood vessel is occluded by fragments from a clot arising from outside the brain, commonly the heart and major vessels.[49] Cardiogenic emboli may result from atrial fibrillation, AMI, valve disease resulting in vegetations and atrial or ventricular septal defects.[49] Less-common causes of embolic stroke are fat emboli, emboli arising from intravenous drug use or septic emboli.[49] Hypoperfusion is an uncommon cause of ischaemic stroke and occurs most often as a consequence of cardiac failure (AMI, cardiac dysrhythmias).[49] Hypoperfusion causes more diffuse injury than thrombotic or embolic strokes.[49]

Cerebral injury from ischaemic stroke is directly related to lack of blood supply. As neurons are highly dependent on a continuous supply of oxygen and glucose, when blood flow is interrupted they die within a few minutes.[49] Even with complete occlusion of a cerebral blood vessel, collateral blood flow and local tissue pressure gradients preserve some perfusion to the ischaemic area.[49] Cell death occurs at the centre of the ischaemic area and this is surrounded by an area of potentially reversible injury (the penumbra).[49] The viability of cells in the penumbra is dependent on the severity and duration of the occlusion and the timing of re-perfusion.[49]

Haemorrhagic stroke

Approximately 20% of strokes are haemorrhagic and the common cause of haemorrhagic stroke is hypertension.[49] Other causes include haemorrhage from ruptured aneurysms, vascular malformations, tumours and head trauma.[9] Cerebral injury occurs as a result of increased intracranial pressure, local compression and decreased perfusion.[49]

Subarachnoid haemorrhage

When a spontaneous subarachnoid haemorrhage (SAH) occurs, blood leaks into the subarachnoid space from a cerebral vessel,[49] in 85% of occurrences from a cerebral aneurysm rupture.[51] The incidence of subarachnoid haemorrhage is around nine cases per 100 000 person-years.[52] Aneurysmal SAH occurs most commonly in the 40- to 60-year age group. A sudden onset of severe headache is a key feature of SAH.[53] In a recent study, 99% of patients with confirmed SAH reported 'the worst headache of their life' and 82% of patients described a 'thunderclap' headache that instantly peaks.[53] Vomiting was present in 66% of patients and 76% of patients complained of neck stiffness.[53] The Ottawa SAH decision rule shows that age 40 years or older, neck pain or stiffness, witnessed loss of consciousness or onset during exertion had 98.5% sensitivity and 27.5% specificity for subarachnoid haemorrhage. Adding 'thunderclap headache' (instantly peaking pain) and 'limited neck flexion on examination' resulted in 100% sensitivity and 15.3% specificity.[53]

Patients are classified into clinical grades according to their conscious state and neurological deficit (Table 23.4). Survival rates have increased by 17% over the past 3 decades and is around 65%.[52] Approximately 12% of patients who have a subarachnoid haemorrhage die immediately; however, most patients who survive the initial weeks are functionally independent.[52]

Risk factors

Non-modifiable risk factors for stroke include age (stroke rate doubles for every 10 years after age 55), male gender and positive family history.[29] Hypertension is the single-most important risk factor that is amenable to change, and effective antihypertensive therapy has been shown to reduce the incidence of stroke. Risk of stroke is increased by risk factors for atherosclerosis (smoking, hyperlipidaemia, diabetes).[9] Atrial fibrillation is the most significant cardiac risk factor; however, other cardiac risk factors include endocarditis, cardiac valve prostheses, recent AMI and mitral stenosis.[29] Carotid stenosis or a carotid bruit in asymptomatic patients is also a risk factor for stroke.[29]

TABLE 23.4 Clinical grading schemes for patients with SAH[96,98]

GRADING SCHEME OF HUNT AND HESS

Grade	Symptoms
1	No symptoms or minimal headache, slight nuchal rigidity
2	Moderate to severe headache, no neurological deficit other than cranial nerve palsy
3	Drowsy, confused, mild focal deficit
4	Stupor, moderate to severe hemiparesis, vegetative posturing
5	Deep coma, decerebration, moribund

GRADING SCHEME OF WORLD FEDERATION OF NEUROLOGICAL SURGEONS

GCS	Motor deficit
15	No
13–14	No
13–14	Yes
7–12	Yes or no
3–6	Yes or no

GCS: Glasgow Coma Scale

Signs and symptoms of stroke

The signs and symptoms of stroke are variable and clinical differentiation between an ischaemic and haemorrhagic stroke is unreliable.[29] As discussed earlier in this chapter, cerebral blood supply is divided into the anterior and posterior circulations. The signs and symptoms of ischaemic stroke depend on the brain area affected.

The anterior circulation supplies the optic nerve, retina and fronto-parietal and temporal lobes.[29] Signs and symptoms associated with anterior circulation disruption include visual disturbance, motor and sensory facial deficits, dysphasia, difficulty writing and calculating numbers, unilateral neglect (usually left-sided) and difficulties dressing.[29] Less-common features are those associated with disruption to the supply from the anterior cerebral artery. These include sensory and motor changes commonly affecting the leg rather than the arm, subtle personality changes, conjugate gaze and urinary dysfunction.[29]

The posterior circulation supplies the cerebellum, brainstem, thalamus and temporal and occipital lobes.[29] Signs and symptoms associated with posterior circulation disruption include visual disturbance, motor and sensory deficits that may be unilateral or bilateral, cerebellar signs (ataxia, vertigo, nystagmus) and cranial nerve palsies resulting in dysarthria, vertigo and diplopia.[29]

Brainstem strokes are characterised by ipsilateral cranial nerve or cerebellar signs.[29] Altered level of consciousness occurs when there is reticular-activating-system ischaemia.[29] Signs and symptoms associated with haemorrhagic stroke may include history of prolonged hypertension, sudden onset of symptoms, headache, vomiting, collapse and history of anticoagulant medications.[29]

Assessment

Stroke is a medical emergency and the triage of stroke patients should reflect the fact that early diagnosis, treatment and referral to specialist services is pivotal to improving patient outcomes and preventing complications.[24] Current guidelines recommend that ED clinicians use a validated stroke screening tool (such as ROSIER: Recognition of Stroke in the Emergency Room or NIHSS: National Institute of Health Stroke Scale).[24] An important part of acute stroke management and decreasing stroke-related mortality is preventing complications within the first 24–48 hours.[37] Early assessment and management of acute stroke should focus on optimal triage decisions, physiological surveillance, fluid management, risk management and prevention of complications, and early referral to specialists.[37]

Paramedics play a key role in prioritising transfer to hospital and early notification to EDs to facilitate efficient stroke management.[24] Triage decisions are a key determinant of care for patients with actual or potential acute stroke. The National Stroke Foundation 'FAST' test is useful for identifying patients with actual or potential stroke in both pre-hospital and ED environments.[54] 'FAST' stands for:[54]

- Face: has the patient's mouth drooped?
- Arms: can they lift both arms?
- Speech: is their speech slurred? Do they understand you?
- Time: time is critical in patients with any of the above signs.

As thrombolysis is a time-critical intervention in acute stroke, facilitation of rapid assessment and identification of patients who may be eligible for thrombolysis or transfer for thrombolysis should be a major priority for pre-hospital and ED triage personnel.[37]

Although current stroke guidelines do not make clear recommendations about triage category allocation in actual or suspected stroke,[24] the American Heart Association/American Stroke Association guidelines[55] recommend that 'patients with suspected acute stroke should be triaged with the same priority as patients with acute myocardial infarction or serious trauma, regardless of the severity of the deficits'.[55] In addition, the American Heart Association/American Stroke Association guidelines recommend a 'door to doctor' time of less than 10 minutes.[55] In Australia, these recommendations equate to Category 2 of the Australasian Triage Scale,[56] and this is reflected in local ED guidelines for emergency nursing management of acute stroke.[37] It is important to understand organisational systems such as 'Code Stroke' and stroke team activation where available.

History is an important factor in the diagnosis and management of stroke (see the case study at the end of this chapter). Accurate information regarding onset of symptoms is vital to assist in deciding the treatment options available for patients. For example, current National Stroke Foundation Guidelines recommend that thrombolytics may be beneficial in selected patients with acute ischaemic stroke if administered up to 4.5 hours after symptom onset.[24] Issues related to thrombolysis administration in acute stroke are discussed later in this chapter.

Investigations

All patients with actual or suspected stroke should have a thorough examination, baseline blood tests, ECG and brain imaging.[24,55] Frequent neurological observations should be performed to identify neurological deterioration or progression of symptoms.

ECG changes are not uncommon in patients with acute stroke.[39,57,58] Common ECG changes include prolonged QT, T-wave abnormalities, prominent U waves and abnormal ST-segments.[58,59] Atrial fibrillation is also a common dysrhythmia in patients with acute stroke; however, atrial fibrillation can occur as the cause of stroke or secondary to cerebral infarction.[58] An ECG should be performed to identify sources of cardiogenic emboli, such as atrial fibrillation or recent AMI, and signs of pre-existing cardiac disease.[29]

Computed tomography

Non-contrast CT is the most common investigation for completed stroke.[37]

Both the National Stroke Foundation[24] and The European Stroke Organisation[73] recommend 'urgent brain CT' for acute stroke, and the National Stroke Foundation defines urgent as 'immediately where facilities are available but within 24 hours. Patients who are candidates for thrombolysis should undergo brain imaging immediately'.[24]

The American Heart Association/American Stroke Association guidelines recommend that CT initiation should occur within 25 minutes of arrival in the ED and be interpreted within 45 minutes of ED arrival.[55]

CT is most often performed to exclude intracerebral haemorrhage prior to anticoagulation or thrombolytic therapy.[29] Many CT scans will be normal in the first few hours following ischaemic stroke, and changes at 24 hours after symptom onset will be evident in approximately 50% of patients.[37] MRI is superior to CT in terms of identifying early signs of infarction and 90% of MRIs will show changes within 24 hours.[29] There is some evidence to suggest that MRI is equivalent to CT in diagnosing intracerebral haemorrage, and this may result in patients going directly to MRI in facilities where it is available.[29]

Management

The management priorities for a patient with stroke are dependent on the nature and site of the stroke, the underlying cause and assessment of treatment risks and benefits.[29]

Restoration of airway, breathing and circulation is the first priority for all patients, including patients with stroke.[37] For patients with stroke, adequate ventilation, oxygenation and cerebral perfusion are essential. Airway support by endotracheal intubation may be indicated in patients with decreased conscious state (see Ch 17, p. 318, for intubation procedures). Impaired swallowing is associated with increased mortality following stroke,[24] so patients with stroke should remain nil by mouth until ability to swallow safely has been formally assessed.[37]

Assessment of oxygen saturation is important, as one early study showed that patients with acute stroke had a lower oxygen saturation than matched controls,[60] and hypoxia increases cerebral injury following stroke.[61] Supplemental oxygen is indicated in patients who are hypoxaemic (peripheral oxygen saturation less than 95%).[24] The use of supplemental oxygen in non-hypoxic patients is controversial, as no survival benefit has been shown for this patient group and some researchers suggest that hyperoxia may also increase cerebral injury.[61]

Hypotension should be treated aggressively with intravenous fluids and, if indicated, inotropes or vasopressors in order to maintain cerebral perfusion and minimise infarct size. Hypertension is often associated with stroke and is a physiological response to preserve cerebral perfusion pressure in the setting of cerebral ischaemia and increased intracranial pressure.[29] Aggressive blood-pressure reduction is not recommended as this may further compromise cerebral perfusion.[29,61] In the case of severe hypertension (systolic blood pressure greater than 220 mmHg), some guidelines recommend cautious and controlled blood-pressure reduction using drugs such as glyceryl trinitrate or sodium nitroprusside that can be readily titrated;[29] however, there is currently no high-level evidence to support this approach in patients with stroke.[29] The use of oral or sublingual agents is not recommended as this may result in rapid and uncontrolled blood-pressure reduction.[29] Other causes for hypertension, such as pain, vomiting or urinary retention, should be considered and, if present, treated appropriately.[29]

There are a number of pathways and guidelines for management of acute stroke,[24,55,62] and implementation of local guidelines focused on emergency care of acute stroke have been shown to improve specific elements of stroke care: the principles of these guidelines may also be applied in the pre-hospital context.[63] The emergency care of the patient with acute stroke is summarised in Box 23.4. The management of cerebral oedema and increased ICP is discussed in detail in Chapter 45.

Specialist referrals and interventions

Early referral to specialists (stroke units, specialist stroke nurses and doctors, and allied health personnel) is an important part of ED stroke management.[37] In some organisations there are pager-activated team responses to stroke; in other organisations,

the process of involving specialist stroke personnel will be less structured. There is high-level evidence that standardised stroke care in an organised stroke unit improves patient outcomes;[62] however, emergency nurses and paramedics have the skills and knowledge to provide the same standard of care in their respective environments.

Three important interventions for patients with stroke are management of fever, glucose levels and swallowing. The recent landmark Quality in Acute Stroke Care (QASC) study was a single-blind cluster randomised controlled trial involving Acute Stroke Units in New South Wales, Australia.[64] Patients in intervention stroke units received care according to treatment protocols to manage fever, hyperglycaemia and swallowing dysfunction. The results showed that, irrespective of stroke severity, patients in the intervention group were 16% less likely to be dead or dependent at 90 days ($p = 0.002$).[64] This study is

---

BOX 23.4 Emergency care of the patient with stroke[37]

Triage

- Stroke is a medical emergency: patients with **suspected or actual** stroke should be triaged to Australasian Triage Scale Category 2
- Use the FAST criteria to identify stroke:
  - **F**acial weakness (can patient smile?)
  - **A**rm weakness (can patient raise both arms?)
  - **S**peech difficulty (can patient speak clearly and understand what you say?)
  - **T**ime to act (should be seen < 10 mins)
- Use ABCD2 risk-stratification (see Box 23.3) to identify patients with TIA at high risk of stroke
- Patients with a high risk of stroke or prolonged TIA symptoms (> 60 mins) should be triaged as stroke

Initial assessment

Airway:
- conscious state
- nil by mouth

Breathing:
- respiratory rate
- respiratory effort
- SpO$_2$—supplemental oxygen if SpO$_2$ < 92%
- chest auscultation

Circulation:
- heart rate
- blood pressure
- 12-lead electrocardiogram/cardiac monitoring
- IV cannula—consider IV fluids if clinical signs of dehydration or maintenance fluids if nil by mouth

Disability:
- neurological observations (GCS and pupils)
- blood sugar level

Other:
- temperature

Ongoing care

Vital signs (RR, HR, BP, SpO$_2$, temperature):
- hourly for 4 hours; then 2-hourly if normal
- report abnormalities; continue hourly vital signs if abnormal

Neurological observations:
- half-hourly for first 2 hours; then hourly for following 2 hours; then 4-hourly for 24 hours
- any deterioration in GCS—neurological observations half-hourly and notify treating team

Blood sugar levels:
- 4-hourly (even if no history of diabetes)—report abnormalities

Fluid management:
- maintenance IV fluids if nil by mouth
- treat dehydration if clinical signs
- aim to maintain normovolaemia and not overload
- maintain fluid balance chart

Venous thromboembolism prophylaxis:
- as per organisational/ED policy

Pressure area assessment and prophylaxis:
- as per organisational/ED policy

Nil by mouth:
- until swallowing assessment completed

Limb care:
- prevent shoulder subluxation (support affected arm with pillow, do not pull on shoulder, consider collar and cuff sling)

Continence care:
- avoid use of indwelling catheters as initial management of incontinence

Head CT:
- check head CT prior to leaving ED[79] (or earlier if clinically indicated)

Aspirin:
- 300 mg orally or by nasogastric tube if no haemorrhage
- consider clopidogrel if allergic to aspirin

Allied health referrals:
- speech pathology
- physiotherapy
- dietitian

BP: blood pressure; CT: computed tomography; ED: emergency department; GCS: Glasgow Coma Scale; HR: heart rate; IV: intravenous; RR: respiratory rate; SpO$_2$: peripheral oxygen saturation; TIA: transient ischaemic attack

important as it highlights the impact of evidence-based nursing care on patient outcomes (death and dependency).[64]

Hyperthermia in the early phase of acute stroke increases mortality and infarct size. A meta-analysis of hyperthermia and stroke outcomes showed that patients who were febrile following stroke had a 19% increase in mortality.[65] Hyperthermia (temperature greater than 37.5°C) occurs in 20–50% of patients in the first few days of acute stroke.[64] Current guidelines recommend antipyretic therapy (paracetamol and/or physical cooling) when fever occurs; however, a clear definition of fever is not provided.[24] The QASC study recommended temperature monitoring every 4 hours and treatment of temperatures ≥ 37.5°C with intravenous, rectal or oral paracetamol.[64]

Up to 50% of patients become hyperglycaemic following acute stroke,[64] and hyperglycaemia can occur in diabetic and non-diabetic patients.[24] Blood glucose level over 8 mmol/L is predictive of mortality following stroke, even when adjusted for age, stroke severity and stroke type.[66] Hyperglycaemia following stroke is also associated with increased infarct size and decreased functional outcomes.[24,61,62] Current guidelines recommend early blood glucose monitoring (see Ch 17, p. 332, for technique); however, aggressive maintenance of euglycaemia early in acute stroke is not recommended.[24] The QASC study protocol was to monitor blood glucose every 6 hours for the first 3 days and commence insulin if the blood glucose is between 8 mmol/L and 11 mmol/L and patient is diabetic, or between 8 mmol/L and 16 mmol/L and patient is not diabetic.[64]

Dysphagia affects as many as 47% of patients following acute stroke and is associated with increased death, disability, pulmonary complications and prolonged length of stay.[62] Patients should be screened for dysphagia by a trained assessor using a validated tool before receiving food, drinks or oral medications: assessment of gag is an unreliable indicator of swallowing.[24] Swallow screening should ideally be performed as soon as possible, and definitely within 24 hours of admission.[24] The personnel performing dysphagia screening and swallow assessment will vary: in some organisations, speech pathologists are part of the stroke team, while in others nurses perform initial dysphagia screening. If the patient is delayed in the ED, then early referral to allied health or the stroke unit to facilitate dysphagia screening is a key emergency nursing responsibility.[37] Dehydration and malnutrition are also associated with an increase in poor outcomes following acute stroke.[24] All patients with acute stroke should be screened for malnutrition and at-risk patients (including those with dysphagia) should have dietitian assessment within 48 hours.[24]

Up to 51% of deaths in the first 30 days after ischaemic stroke are due to complications of immobility and over 62% of these complications occur in the first week.[24] Early mobilisation (< 48 hours) decreases complications, improves functional outcomes and decreases depression and anxiety for patients with acute stroke,[55,67] so patients experiencing delays to inpatient care should have an ED referral to physiotherapy.[37]

Urinary and/or faecal incontinence can occur due to stroke-related impairments such as weakness, cognitive impairment and decreased mobility.[24] Incontinence is associated with stroke-related complications such as depression,[24] can precipitate other adverse events such as falls or can result in prolonged recovery.[37] Thorough assessment of continence may not occur in the ED,

but it is important that use of indwelling catheters as initial management of incontinence should be avoided.[24]

Ischaemic stroke management

Numerous trials have shown that aspirin administration within 48 hours of onset of symptoms in acute stroke reduces the rates of early death and recurrent stroke.[29,68] Current recommendations are that intracerebral haemorrhage be excluded by CT prior to aspirin administration.[24]

For patients with acute ischaemic stroke, there is no evidence that anticoagulation decreases morbidity, mortality or early recurrent stroke, and routine use of low-molecular-weight heparin is not recommended.[24,83] However, exclusion of intracerebral haemorrhage by CT scan and a neurological consultation should occur prior to commencement of heparin in patients with stroke secondary to cardiogenic emboli.[69] The use of thrombolytic agents in the management of acute ischaemic stroke may be appropriate for selected patients.[24]

Current National Stroke Foundation guidelines (2010)[24] state that thrombolysis (rt-PA) should be given 'as early as possible in carefully selected patients' and that therapy should 'commence in the first few hours but may be used up to 4.5 hours after stroke onset'. Clinicians should consult their organisational guidelines for the indications, contraindications and relative contraindications for thrombolysis in acute ischaemic stroke.

A recent Cochrane review of thrombolytic doses, agents and routes of administration for ischaemic stroke reviewed 20 unconfounded randomised and quasi-randomised trials involving 2527 patients.[70] They found that higher doses of thrombolytic agents may lead to higher bleeding rates; however, there currently is not enough evidence to make conclusions about the optimum dose, agent or route of administration.[70] Wardlaw et al[70] state that 'at present, intravenous rt-PA at 0.9 mg/kg appears to represent best practice and other drugs, doses or routes of administration should only be used in randomised controlled trials'.

Seizures occur in approximately 5% of patients with acute ischaemic stroke and anticonvulsant agents (e.g. phenytoin) are indicated in these patients.[24] There are no clear guidelines or randomised trials regarding when to initiate anticonvulsant therapy in patients with acute stroke, and the optimal timing and type of antiepileptic treatment for patients with post-stroke seizures has not been established.[71] Therefore, a decision regarding anticonvulsant therapy will be based on individual patient status.[71]

Haemorrhagic stroke management

The management of intracerebral haemorrhage is dependent on the location, cause, neurological deficit and patient's clinical condition.[29] Cerebral oedema and increased ICP tend to occur more acutely in haemorrhagic strokes; however, ischaemic strokes can also have haemorrhagic complications that can occur spontaneously or as a result of anticoagulant or thrombolytic treatments.[29] Neurosurgical referral should occur early for patients with potential for surgical intervention.[29] Management of SAH is directed at maintaining oxygenation, reducing hypertension and increased ICP,[49] and surgical aneurysm clipping.[51] Re-bleeding and vasospasm are major complications of SAH.[49] Re-bleeding is most likely to occur in the first

24 hours, and blood-pressure control (mean arterial pressure of 110 mmHg) decreases the risk of re-bleeding and is associated with decreased mortality.[49] Cerebral ischaemia secondary to vasospasm can occur up to 3 weeks following aneurysm rupture. Oral nimodipine has been shown to decrease both the incidence and the severity of vasospasm in patients with SAH, and to improve patient outcome.[49] Other management strategies include anticonvulsant therapy if seizures occur, management of pain by administering analgesia, dimming lights and removing stimuli. Vomiting should be treated with antiemetics.[49] Surgical clipping of the neck of the aneurysm remains the definitive treatment of choice for ruptured cerebral aneurysm, as it prevents re-bleeding and removes the clot. It is essential that emergency nurses and paramedics monitor the patient's blood pressure and GCS frequently, and facilitate transfer to definitive care as soon as possible.

Seizures

A *seizure* is an 'episode of abnormal neurological function caused by abnormal discharge of brain neurons'.[72] A *convulsion* is an 'episode of excessive and abnormal motor activity'.[72] These definitions are important, as seizures can occur with or without convulsion.[72] A seizure can be an acute event or can be the result of a past neurological insult (e.g. stroke, head injury or hypoxic brain injury). A first-time seizure is a major event for patients and their families. Not only are there short-term health concerns, but concerns regarding long-term occupational, social and quality-of-life implications are also valid.[72]

The focus for seizure activity is a group of neuronal cells which have highly permeable plasma membranes and are therefore in a hypersensitive state.[9] Hyperexcited neurons fire impulses that increase in frequency and amplitude until impulses spread to adjacent normal neurons.[9] Excitation of the subcortical areas of the basal ganglia, thalamus and brainstem areas results in the *tonic phase* of seizure (muscle contraction with excessive tone), autonomic signs and symptoms, apnoea and loss of consciousness.[9] Hyperexcitation is interrupted by inhibitory neurons in the cortex, anterior thalamus and basal ganglia, resulting in the *clonic phase* of seizure (alternating muscular contraction and relaxation). During a seizure, energy demands are increased by 250%, there is a 60% increase in cerebral oxygen consumption and cerebral blood flow also increases by 250% in an attempt to keep up with cerebral oxygen and glucose demands.[9] Tonic–clonic seizures may be preceded by an aura or partial seizure that occurs immediately prior to a generalised tonic–clonic seizure.[9] The patient may also experience prodromal symptoms in the hours or days preceding a seizure.[9]

The International Classification of Epileptic Seizures classifies epileptic seizures as either partial or generalised, as discussed below.[72]

Partial seizures

Partial (or focal) epileptic seizures are classified as simple partial, complex partial or secondary generalised seizures, according to whether or not there is loss of consciousness.[72] Conscious state is not affected during a simple partial seizure; however, there is impaired consciousness in complex partial seizures and loss of consciousness in secondary generalised seizures.[9,72]

Simple partial seizures can have the following local effects without impairment of conscious state:[9]

- Focal motor signs that are usually clonic movements, and can occur with or without 'Jacksonian march' (Jacksonian marching is the spread of seizure activity in an organised manner to adjacent areas).[9]
- Somatic sensory symptoms can include altered sensation such as numbness, tingling, 'pins and needles' or visual, olfactory, auditory dysfunction.
- Autonomic signs and symptoms that are particularly characteristic of temporal lobe seizures and may include lip-smacking, chewing, facial grimacing, patting or picking at clothing.
- Psychic symptoms such as feelings of familiarity in an unfamiliar setting (déjà vu) or unfamiliarity in a familiar setting (jamais vu).[7]

During a complex partial seizure, consciousness is impaired and ability to respond to external stimuli is reduced.[9] Complex partial seizures may occur as a simple partial seizure followed by impaired conscious state, or conscious state may be impaired from the onset of seizure activity.[9] If impaired conscious state is delayed, symptoms as described above may occur. A secondary generalised seizure is thus a progression of a simple partial seizure that results in loss of consciousness.[9] During a simple partial seizure, the patient is conscious if the seizure is confined to one cerebral hemisphere. However, if seizure activity spreads to the other cerebral hemisphere and deeper brain structures, the patient will become unconscious.[9]

Generalised seizures

Generalised epileptic seizures are further classified as:

- generalised tonic–clonic seizures (formerly referred to as grand mal seizures)
- non-convulsive seizures that include absence seizures (formerly referred to as petit mal seizures), myoclonic, tonic and atonic seizures.[72]

The American College of Emergency Physicians further classifies seizures as provoked (seizures from electrolyte abnormalities, CNS infections, drug or alcohol withdrawal) and unprovoked (seizures from epilepsy).[73] Tonic–clonic seizures are usually characterised by sudden loss of consciousness, falling to the ground, stiffening and extension of arms and legs and forceful closure of the jaw (often resulting in tongue-biting).[7,9] A shrill cry may occur as air is forcibly exhaled through closed vocal cords and urinary and/or faecal incontinence may occur.[7,9] During the tonic phase the patient is apnoeic, may become cyanosed and the pupils are dilated and unresponsive to light.[7,9] The tonic phase is usually short, lasting less than 1 minute. During the clonic phase, there is alternating muscular contraction and relaxation.[7,9] Hyperventilation, eye-rolling, excessive salivation, profuse sweating and tachycardia also occur during the clonic phase.[7,9] The clonic movements usually decrease over 30 seconds.

During the postictal period following a tonic–clonic seizure, the patient may have a decreased conscious state and limp muscle tone. As conscious state improves, the patient may be confused, irritable and may complain of headache, fatigue and muscle aches.[7,9] Usually there is no recollection of the seizure.[7,9]

Absence seizures occur in children aged older than 4 years and prior to the onset of puberty.[10] Absence seizures are characterised by abrupt cessation of activity with momentary loss of consciousness.[7,9] A vacant stare or eye-rolling may occur and the lips may droop or twitch; however, the child will be responsive to verbal stimuli.[9] The duration of absence seizures is usually 5–10 seconds, after which the child usually resumes their previous activity.[9]

Status epilepticus

Status epilepticus is defined as 5 minutes or more of (i) continuous clinical and/or electrographic seizure activity or (ii) recurrent seizure activity without recovery (returning to baseline) between seizures.[74] Status epilepticus is easily recognised when it involves convulsive seizures, but it can also be non-convulsive involving partial seizures or absence seizures; the latter presents significant diagnostic difficulties.[74]

One of the major pathophysiological issues with status epilepticus is that compensatory mechanisms which usually occur during seizures begin to fail as the duration of seizure activity increases.[72] Prolonged seizure activity causes direct neuronal damage, and secondary neuronal injury occurs from hypoxia, hypoglycaemia, hyperpyrexia and acidosis.[72] There is also evidence to suggest that excitatory neurotransmitters such as glutamate and aspartate contribute to brain damage from prolonged status epilepticus.[72] The likelihood of permanent brain injury increases with the duration of status epilepticus: the mortality rate increases from 2.7% for seizures lasting less than 1 hour to 32% for seizures lasting longer than 1 hour.[72]

Assessment

Assessment of the patient with seizure can be difficult, as many patients arrive in the ED after the seizure has resolved. History is an extremely important diagnostic factor in these patients.[72] Factors that should be considered include head trauma, drug and alcohol use and underlying or associated illnesses.[72] It is estimated that alcohol is a factor in 50% of ED presentations related to seizures and most alcohol-related seizures are due to withdrawal.[72] Acute drug and/or alcohol toxicity and alcohol withdrawal can also precipitate seizures, and seizures in the setting of acute drug overdose are associated with significant mortality and morbidity.[72] Pregnancy status should be ascertained in women of childbearing age because pregnancy will influence patient disposition and anticonvulsant drug therapy choices. In advanced pregnancy or the early postpartum period, eclampsia should be considered (see Ch 35).

The signs and symptoms of seizures can vary, and seizures can affect motor, sensory and autonomic activity, level of consciousness, emotions, memory, cognition and behaviour. Tongue-biting, broken teeth and distal limb injuries commonly occur with generalised seizures.[72] If an altered conscious state is present, it should not be automatically attributed to a postictal state: thorough assessment and investigation is warranted.[72] When assessing the associated conditions and treatable causes of seizure, cause of seizures may be considered using the following categories:[9,72]

- acute symptomatic seizures that occur as a result of neurological insult during an acute illness or injury (e.g. hypoxia, hypoglycaemia, head injury, CNS infections, metabolic and electrolyte derangement, drug overdose, drug withdrawal, cerebral tumours or stroke)
- remote symptomatic seizures that occur in patients without a history of neurological insult
- progressive encephalopathy seizures that occur in association with a progressive neurological disease
- febrile seizures that occur almost exclusively in children
- idiopathic seizures (that are usually classified as epilepsy).

Routine laboratory investigations and imaging are not warranted for patients with an uncomplicated first-time seizure and who make a complete recovery.[72,75] However, glucose abnormalities and hyponatraemia are the most common laboratory abnormalities in patients with seizure disorder,[75] so blood glucose level is useful during initial patient assessment. Serum sodium may be indicated, depending on patient history and examination results.[75] There is no evidence to currently support routine lumbar puncture (LP) in patients with seizure who are alert, afebrile and not immunocompromised.[75] However, LP is indicated in patients with suspected CNS infection or subarachnoid haemorrhage or immunocomprised patients even if they are afebrile.[75] There is debate regarding the indication for head CT scan in patients with first-time seizure[75] and local and logistic factors will often be a major influence on imaging decisions.[72] Between 3% and 40% in patients with first-time seizure will have abnormalities on noncontrast CT scan; however, the risk of finding an abnormality is increased if the patient has a focal neurological finding, focal seizure onset or a history of malignancy or HIV.[75] Current recommendations suggest that CT should be performed in the ED for patients with first-time seizure if possible. However, outpatient neuroimaging is a safe alternative, provided there is reliable follow-up. Outpatient EEG may also be considered.[72] Head CT is indicated in patients: (1) with focal neurological signs; (2) who do not recover fully; and (3) with a history of head trauma.[72]

Management

Key aims in general seizure management are highlighted in Box 23.5. Pharmacological agents that may be used in the treatment of status epilepticus include benzodiazepines and phenytoin. There are a number of benzodiazepines that may be used in this context (diazepam, midazolam, clonazepam);

BOX 23.5 Aims of seizure management

- Airway protection and prevention of aspiration (lateral position, suction)
- Restoration and preservation of oxygenation (supplemental oxygen)
- Injury prevention (removing objects, use of pillows, bedrails)
- Cessation of seizure activity (intravenous access, drug therapy)
- Identify and treat precipitating factors
- Identify and treat complications
- Provide seizure prevention/management plan to optimise seizure control and quality of life

however, currently there is no evidence to suggest that one agent is superior to the others. All benzodiazepines can cause respiratory depression and hypotension.[72] The IV route is preferred but intramuscular or rectal administration are other options. Rectal administration of diazepam is highly effective in children, but the onset of action of rectal diazepam in adults can be slow and unpredictable.[72]

Phenytoin is a commonly used anticonvulsant drug. The dose is 15–20 mg/kg and should be given slowly, at a rate of no more than 50 mg/min.[72] Rapid phenytoin administration can cause hypotension and bradydysrhythmias.[72] The common practice of administering 1 g in adults is inadequate for many patients and a weight-related dose should be given.[72] The clinical effects of phenytoin are not apparent until 40% of the dose has been given; therefore phenytoin should be commenced early and given in conjunction with benzodiazepines.[72]

Other treatment issues for the patient suffering from status epilepticus are the management of secondary problems such as hypoxia, hypotension, hypoglycaemia, hyperpyrexia and cerebral oedema.[72]

PRACTICE TIP

PRIORITIES FOR THE MANAGEMENT OF A PATIENT HAVING A SEIZURE

- Maintain safety and prevent injury.
- Record the duration of the seizure.
- Once seizure activity stops: ensure airway patency, provide supplemental oxygen if hypoxaemic, assess vital signs and GCS, check blood glucose level, reassure the patient.

Headache

Headaches are a common health problem. Although most headaches are innocuous,[76] it is essential that emergency nurses and paramedics can rapidly identify life-threatening causes of headache. The management priorities for patients presenting with headache are pain relief and accurate diagnosis.

Headache, like many other painful symptoms, is not a disease state, but is the symptom of a pathological process.[76] The pathological processes that can result in headache are:

- tension of neck and head muscles
- traction on intracranial structures
- vasodilation of cerebral blood vessels
- inflammation.[76]

It is thought that headache pain is transmitted from the blood vessels of the pia mater and dura mater via the trigeminal nerve.[15] Response to analgesia is an unreliable indicator of the seriousness or aetiology of headache.[15]

Headache may be classified as primary and secondary headache syndromes.[77] Primary headache syndromes include migraine headache, tension headache and cluster headaches (Table 23.5). Secondary headache syndromes may be considered in terms of extracranial or intracranial causes.[77]

Intracranial causes may include cerebrovascular conditions such as haemorrhage or temporal arteritis, CNS infections and CNS tumours.

Extracranial causes of headache may include non-CNS infections such as systemic infection, herpes zoster or sinusitis, ophthalmic pathology, such as glaucoma, iritis and optic neuritis, referred pain from dental or optic conditions, and other conditions such as nitrate administration, hypercapnia that results in vasodilation, carbon monoxide poisoning and hypertension.

Causes of headache types are presented in Table 23.6.

TABLE 23.5 Comparison of tension-type, migraine and cluster headaches[91]

PATTERN	TENSION-TYPE HEADACHE	MIGRAINE HEADACHE	CLUSTER HEADACHE
Site	Bilateral, band-like pressure at base of skull, in face or in both	Unilateral (in 60%), may switch sides, commonly anterior	Unilateral, radiating up or down from one eye
Quality	Constant, squeezing tightness	Throbbing, synchronous with pulse	Severe, bone-crushing
Frequency	Cycles for several years	Periodic; cycles of several months to years	May have months or years between attacks; attacks occur in clusters: one to three times a day over a period of 4–8 weeks
Duration	Intermittent for months or years	Continuous for hours or days	30–90 minutes
Time and mode of onset	Not related to time	May be preceded by prodromal stage; onset after awakening; gets better with sleep	Nocturnal; commonly wakens patient from sleep
Associated symptoms	Palpable neck and shoulder muscles, stiff neck, tenderness	Nausea or vomiting, oedema, irritability, sweating, photophobia, phonophobia, prodrome of sensory, motor or psychic phenomena; family history (in 65%)	Vasomotor symptoms such as facial flushing or pallor, unilateral lacrimation, ptosis and rhinitis

TABLE 23.6 Classic clinical complexes and cause of headache[96]

SIGNS AND SYMPTOMS	CAUSE
Preceded by an aura	Migraine
Throbbing unilateral headache, nausea	
Family history	
Sudden onset	Subarachnoid haemorrhage
Severe occipital headache; 'like a blow'	
Worst headache ever	
Throbbing/constant frontal headache	Sinusitis
Worse with cough, leaning forward	
Recent URTI	
Pain on percussion of sinuses	
Paroxysmal, fleeting pain	Neuralgia
Distribution of a nerve	
Trigger manoeuvres cause pain	
Hyperalgesia of nerve distribution	
Unilateral with superimposed stabbing	Temporal arteritis
Claudication on chewing	
Associated malaise, myalgia	
Tender artery with reduced pulsation	
Persistent, deep-seated headache	Tumour: primary or secondary
Increasing duration and intensity	
Worse in morning	
Aching in character	
Acute, generalised headache	Meningitis
Fever, nausea and vomiting	
Altered level of consciousness	
Neck stiffness ± rash	
Unilateral, aching, related to eye	Glaucoma
Nausea and vomiting	
Raised intraocular pressure	
Aching, facial region	Dental cause
Worse at night	
Tooth sensitive to heat, pressure	

Assessment and management

Baseline vital signs and neurological observations score should be recorded (see Ch 14). When headache is a key feature, history is of paramount importance.[76] The NOPQRST mnemonic (see Box 23.2) provides a useful guide for focused symptom assessment.[78] Specific aspects of past medical history that are important to note are hypertension and a history of neurological problems or seizure disorders. Specific considerations may include gender: migraine headaches are more common in women and may be influenced by hormonal factors.[77] In pregnant women, pre-eclampsia should be excluded as a cause of headache (see Ch 35).

The investigations that may be warranted in patients with headache include LP, CT scan or MRI.[77] In patients with acute headache, LP may be indicated. Because of concerns regarding causing herniation as a consequence of lumbar puncture, adult patients with headache and signs of increased ICP should have a head CT prior to LP.[79] In the absence of signs of increased ICP, LP can be performed without neuroimaging.[79] Approximately 14% of ED patients with headache have imaging performed and, of those, 5.5% had a diagnosis of intracranial pathology.[79] Neuroimaging is recommended for:

- patients with new headache and abnormal neurological assessment findings
- patients with new sudden-onset severe headache
- HIV-positive patients with new headache
- patients older than 50 years presenting with new headache.[79]

The aim of neuroimaging in these patients is to identify a treatable lesion (for example, tumours, vascular malformations, aneurysms, subarachnoid haemorrhage, cerebral venous sinus thrombosis, subdural and epidural haematomas, infections, stroke, hydrocephalus, and others).[15] Sudden onset of new headache is a major risk factor for intracerebral haemorrhage, and patients with advanced HIV disease are at risk of CNS pathology including infections and space-occupying lesions.[79] Pregnant women are at increased risk of stroke that may involve headache as a symptom, and risk of subarachnoid haemorrhage is thought to be increased during pregnancy, delivery and the puerperium.[79,80]

For the majority of patients with migraine, investigations are not indicated. Investigations for suspected meningitis are discussed later in this chapter. CT scan or MRI may be indicated to exclude space-occupying lesion.

Migraine

Migraine is a recurring headache disorder with gradual onset and lasting 4–72 hours, characterised by throbbing pain, a triggering event and manifestations associated with neurological and autonomous nervous system dysfunction which increases with physical activity.[76,77,81] Migraines are often accompanied by nausea, photophobia and phonophobia.[76,77] Many patients who suffer from migraine headaches are able to manage their symptoms without hospital care, so when patients present to the ED it is often because self-medication has failed[76] or symptoms are unusually prolonged or severe. Migraine headaches are more common in women and may be influenced by hormonal factors such as menstruation, use of oral contraceptives, pregnancy and menopause.[77]

The pathophysiology of migraine is unclear; however, it is thought interaction between the brain and cranial circulation in susceptible patients may contribute to migraine.[76] The phenomenon of aura is thought to be the result of 'cortical spreading depression', whereby there is a brief wave of depolarisation that moves across the cerebral cortex.[76] This state of excitability is followed by prolonged nerve-cell depression.[76,77]

Some patients describe a preceding aura of symptoms such as visual disturbance, diplopia, hemiparaesthesia, hemiparesis or speech difficulties[76] that develop gradually and usually last less than 60 minutes.[77] Migraine headache usually follows within 1 hour.[76] If migraine aura is associated with neurological deficits (such as weakness, visual disturbance, sensory disturbance, speech impairments), symptoms should resolve prior to discharge from the ED. Emergency nurses and paramedics should have a high index of suspicion of significant pathology in patients with 'migraine' that is notably different from their usual migraine headache.[77]

There are a number of pharmacological agents that can be used in the treatment of migraine, but current evidence suggests that phenothiazines and selective serotonin receptor agonists (triptans) are the most effective agents.[76] Aspirin and metoclopramide are also recommended in recent National Institute of Clinical Studies evidence-based guidelines.[82]

Temporal arteritis

Temporal arteritis is a form of systemic vasculitis[83] that commonly occurs in older patients (over 50 years of age)[77] and is more common in women.[77] Headache is the most common symptom of temporal arteritis and occurs in 60–90% of patients.[77] The headache is usually severe and is often located in the temporal region.[77,83,84] The cardinal feature of headache in temporal arteritis is that it is new and often occurs in older patients with no history of headaches.[83] Other classic signs and symptoms include jaw or tongue claudication, visual disturbance (usually diplopia or loss of vision), fever and polymyalgia rheumatica (pain and stiffness in shoulders, neck and hips that is worse in the mornings and improves throughout the day).[77,83,85]

The signs and symptoms of temporal arteritis are due to local arterial inflammation causing endovascular damage, vessel stenosis and occlusion, resulting in tissue ischaemia or necrosis.[83] The most devastating complication of temporal arteritis is irreversible blindness, usually due to ischaemic optic neuritis.[85] Blindness is rarely the first symptom of temporal arteritis, so there is always an opportunity to prevent permanent loss of vision.[83] Early identification, referral for temporal artery biopsy and treatment are therefore extremely important.[85] Diagnostic criteria for temporal arteritis are:

- age > 50 years
- new onset of localised headache
- temporal artery tenderness or decreased pulse
- elevated erythrocyte sedimentation rate (ESR)
- abnormal temporal artery biopsy findings.[77]

The aim of treatment of temporal arteritis is to prevent vision loss[83] using corticosteroid therapy (usually prednisolone).[77]

Cluster headaches

Cluster headaches are rare and usually self-limiting.[77] Unlike migraine headaches, cluster headaches are more common in men.[77] Cluster headaches are thought to be related to trigeminal nerve dysfunction and are characterised by severe unilateral, orbital, supraorbital or temporal pain that lasts from 15 minutes to several hours.[77] Cluster headaches are usually associated with at least one of the following symptoms that occur on the ipsilateral side: conjunctival injection,

lacrimation, nasal congestion, rhinorrhoea, facial swelling, miosis or ptosis.[77]

Oxygen has been shown to be effective in the relief of cluster headaches, as has sumatriptan and dihydroergotamine.[77] Given the short duration of cluster headaches, oral agents are unlikely to be effective but non-steroidal anti-inflammatory agents may be useful in decreasing the frequency and severity of future cluster headaches.[77]

Inflammatory brain conditions

A comparison of inflammatory brain conditions is presented in Table 23.7.

Meningitis

Meningitis is an infection of the pia mater, arachnoid mater and subarachnoid space.[5] It is a neurological emergency and an infectious disease emergency. Meningitis is typically classified as bacterial (purulent) meningitis or viral (lymphocytic or aseptic) meningitis.[5]

Bacterial meningitis

The most common bacterial agents causing meningitis are *Streptococcus pneumoniae*, *Haemophilus influenzae* and *Neisseria meningitidis*.[5] The incidence of *H. influenzae* in children has decreased in recent years as a result of the *H. influenzae* vaccine.[5] Other pathogens include *Staphylococcus aureus*, *Listeria monocytogenes* and *Escherichia coli*.[86]

Bacterial meningitis is associated with significant mortality and morbidity. The mortality rate is estimated to be 25% in adults,[5,9] and as many as 61% of infants who survive Gram-negative bacterial meningitis have significant developmental and neurological issues.[5] Risk factors for meningitis include head trauma with basilar skull fractures, otitis media, sinusitis or mastoiditis, neurosurgery, systemic sepsis and immuno-compromise.[5]

Common symptoms of bacterial meningitis include those associated with systemic infection, such as fevers, chills, tachycardia, petechial rash and generalised back, abdominal or limb pain.[5,9] Signs that result from meningeal irritation include severe headache, neck stiffness, photophobia, Kernig's sign (resistance to leg extension when lying with hip flexed at a right-angle), and Brudzinski's sign (neck flexion causes hip and knee flexion).[5,9] Kernig's and Brudzinski's signs are related to painful stretching of inflamed meninges from the lumbar region to the head.[5] Neurological signs may include altered conscious state, seizures, focal neurological deficits, nausea and vomiting.[5] Hydrocephalus and cranial nerve damage (particularly XIII cranial nerve resulting in deafness) can occur as a complication of bacterial meningitis.[5] Other signs and symptoms may be specific to the causative agent (e.g. petechial rash, a non-blanching rash with small purple or red dots on the skin surface or mucous membranes, is associated with meningococcal meningitis).[5]

Diagnosis of bacterial meningitis is made by history, physical examination and lumbar puncture.[5] Lumbar puncture findings are usually cloudy, purulent CSF that is under increased pressure.[5] CSF analysis shows increased polymorphonuclear white blood cells, increased protein content and decreased glucose.[5] Bacteria can also be seen on smear and culture.[5] Adult patients with headache and signs of increased intracranial pressure should have neuroimaging prior to lumbar puncture.[79]

TABLE 23.7 Comparison of cerebral inflammatory conditions[91]

	MENINGITIS	ENCEPHALITIS	BRAIN ABSCESS
Causative organisms	Bacteria (*Streptococcus pneumoniae*, *Neisseria meningitidis*, group B *Streptococcus*, viruses, fungi)	Bacteria, fungi, parasites, herpes simplex virus (HSV), other viruses (e.g. Murray Valley encephalitis)	Streptococci, staphylococci through bloodstream
CSF			
Pressure (normal: 60–150 mmH$_2$O)	Increased	Normal to slight increase	Increased
WBC count (normal: 0–8 × 10^6/L)	*Bacterial*: > 1000 × 10^6/L (mainly PMN) *Viral*: 25–500/mL (mainly lymphocytes)	< 5 × 10^6/L, PMN (early), lymphocytes (later)	0.25–3 × 10^6/L (PMN)
Protein (normal, 0.15–0.45 g/L)	*Bacterial*: > 5 g/L *Viral*: 0.5–5 g/L	Slight increase	Normal
Glucose (normal, 2.8–4.4 mmol/L)	*Bacterial*: decreased *Viral*: normal or low	Normal	Low or absent
Appearance of CSF	*Bacterial*: turbid, cloudy *Viral*: clear or cloudy	Clear	Clear
Diagnostic studies	Gram stain, smear, culture, PCR*	EEG, MRI, PET, PCR, IgM antibodies to virus in serum or CSF	CT scan, EEG, head X-ray
Treatment	Antibiotics, supportive care, prevention of ICP	Supportive care, prevention of ↑ ICP, aciclovir for HSV	Antibiotics, incision and drainage Supportive care

CSF: cerebrospinal fluid; CT: computed tomography; EEG: electroencephalogram; ICP: intracranial pressure; MRI: magnetic resonance imaging; PCR: polymerase chain reaction; PET: positron emission tomography; PMN: polymorphonuclear cells; WBC: white blood cell

*PCR is used to detect viral RNA or DNA.

Early antibiotic administration (which may include pre-hospital administration) is important in preventing death or serious disability in patients with bacterial meningitis. Agents that may be considered are third-generation cephalosporins and benzylpenicillin. There is also some evidence to support the use of corticosteroids in conjunction with antibiotic therapy.[5] Clinicians should have a low threshold for considering this potentially devastating illness. Supportive management includes preservation and monitoring of airway, breathing and circulation, and conscious state, analgesia, hydration and seizure management.[87] Depending on the causative agent (e.g. meningococcal meningitis), close contacts may be offered prophylactic antibiotic therapy.[5]

Viral meningitis

Viruses are the leading cause of meningitis.[87] Although viral meningitis most commonly affects children and young adults, older adults can also be affected.[9,87] In many instances the causative agent is not identified;[5,87] however, common viral agents include enterovirus, mumps virus, coxsackievirus, Epstein-Barr virus and herpes simplex virus 2 (HSV 2), varicella zoster virus and HIV.[5,9,87]

The clinical signs of viral meningitis are similar to those of bacterial meningitis, but are generally less severe[5] as the infection is limited to the meninges.[9] CSF analysis shows increased lymphocytes and moderate increase in protein and normal glucose content.[5] Acute viral meningitis is self-limiting and treatment is largely symptomatic, as described above.[5] Antiviral agents may be used in specific circumstances, for example aciclovir may be given for meningitis caused by HSV 2.[5]

Guillain-Barré syndrome

Guillain-Barré syndrome is an acquired inflammatory condition that causes demyelination of peripheral nerves.[9] The syndrome can affect both children and adults and has a 4–6% mortality rate.[9] *Campylobacter jejuni* is the causative organism in 60% of cases.[9]

Guillain-Barré syndrome may be preceded by a mild infectious episode (typically respiratory, gastrointestinal or viral illness), surgical procedures or viral immunisations.[9] Signs and symptoms of Guillain-Barré syndrome include bilateral ascending paralysis, sensory symptoms such as paraesthesia, pain and numbness, and decreased or absent deep tendon reflexes.[9] However, presenting symptoms of Guillain-Barré syndrome are variable and misdiagnosis is common.[88]

Early diagnosis of Guillain-Barré syndrome is important: respiratory failure and complications secondary to ventilation are the major causes of morbidity and mortality.[88] Respiratory muscle weakness requiring ventilator support occurs in 10–30% of patients.[9] It is therefore important to thoroughly assess the respiratory function in patients with actual or suspected Guillain-Barré syndrome (see Ch 17, p. 334, for techniques on testing respiratory function).[88] Cranial nerve weakness may result in facial weakness and difficulties swallowing, chewing and coughing.[9] Autonomic dysfunction causes heart rate and blood pressure changes and profuse or decreased sweating.[9] Inappropriate secretion of antidiuretic hormone and hypernatraemia is common, particularly in ventilated patients.[9] Diagnostic studies may include CSF studies, nerve conduction studies and electromyography (EMG). CSF findings in patients with Guillain-Barré syndrome include elevated protein levels.[9,88]

Emergency management of Guillain-Barré syndrome is aimed at preservation of oxygenation and circulation, and ongoing management involves supportive care for respiratory failure and management of autonomic dysfunction.[9,88] Aggressive rehabilitation is warranted to return functional status.[9]

SUMMARY

Preservation or restoration of airway, breathing and circulation are key priorities in the initial assessment and management of the patient with a neurological emergency. Neurological emergencies can have significant consequences for patients. Life-threatening conditions obviously carry a risk of mortality, but even non life-threatening neurological conditions can have major effects on quality of life. Many neurological emergencies can have subtle or non-specific symptoms, making accurate symptom assessment and history important elements of patient assessment. Frequent monitoring of vital signs and level of consciousness and the correct and consistent application of assessment tools such as the GCS are vital to the early identification of deterioration. Paramedics and emergency nurses have a professional responsibility to ensure that their knowledge of assessment and management of neurological emergencies is current, based on the best available evidence and is regularly reviewed.

CASE STUDY

Joan is a 68-year-old woman who collapsed while out shopping with her husband. She suddenly grabbed his arm and said she felt dizzy, before becoming weak at the knees and slumping to the floor. Her husband says he helped her to the floor so she did not fall, but she was 'out to it' for a couple of minutes. When she woke, she was confused: she recognised her husband but did not know where she was, what day it was or what had happened. As she tried to stand up, she fell to the floor again as a result of a left hemiparesis. Her husband also states that her speech is slightly slurred.

Questions

1. What questions will you ask in this scenario to determine historical and clinical indicators of urgency and relevance?

2. Describe each aspect of your physical assessment and explain each step.

3. What investigations will you perform and why?

4. What ongoing monitoring will you provide?

Answers to Case Study Questions can be found on evolve
http://evolve.emergencytrauma.curtis

REFERENCES

1. Berben SAA, Meijs THJM, van Dongen RTM et al. Pain prevalence and pain relief in trauma patients in the Accident & Emergency department. Acute Pain 2008;10:105.

2. Considine J, Botti M. Who, when and where? Identification of patients at risk of an in-hospital adverse event: implications for nursing practice. International Journal of Nursing Practice 2004;10:21–31.

3. Schein RM, Hazday N, Pena M et al. Clinical antecedents to in-hospital cardiopulmonary arrest. Chest 1990;98:1388–92.

4. Goldhill DR, McNarry AF. Physiological abnormalities in early warning scores are related to mortality in adult inpatients. British Journal of Anaesthesia 2004;92:822–4.

5. Tortora GJ, Derrickson BH. Principles of anatomy and physiology. Hoboken, NJ: John Wiley & Sons; 2012.

6. Sugerman RA. Structure and function of the neurological system. In: McCance K, Huether S, Brashers V, Rote N, eds. Pathophysiology: The biological basis for disease in adults and children, 7th edn. St Louis: Mosby; 2013:477–83.

7. Brown A, King D. Neurologic emergencies. In: Kunz Howard P, Steinmann RA, eds. Sheehy's emergency nursing: principles and practice. 6th edn. St. Louis: Mosby Elsevier; 2010:457–66.

8. Lawther BK, Kumar S, Krovvidi H. Blood–brain barrier. Continuing Education in Anaesthesia, Critical Care & Pain 2011;11:128–32.

9. Boss BJ, Heuther SE. Disorders of the central and peripheral nervous systems and neuromuscular junction. In: McCance K, Huether S, Brashers V, Rote N, eds. Pathophysiology: The biological basis for disease in adults and children. 7th edn. St Louis: Mosby; 2013:581–632.

10. Book D. Disorders of brain function. In: Porth CM, Matfin G, eds. Pathophysiology: Concepts of altered health states. 8th edn. Philadelphia: Lippincott Williams & Wilkins; 2009:1299–337.

11. McCance K, Huether S, Brashers V, Rote N, eds. Pathophysiology. The biological basis for disease in adults and children. 7th edn. St Louis: Mosby; 2013.

12. Barker E. Neuroanatomy and physiology of the nervous system. In: Barker E, ed. Neuroscience Nursing: a spectrum of care. 3rd edn. St Louis: Mosby; 2007:3–52.

13. Hew R. Altered conscious state. In: Cameron P, Jelinek G, Kelly A et al. eds. Adult Textbook of Emergency Medicine. 3rd edn. Sydney: Churchill Livingstone; 2009:386–91.

14. Wright BLC, Lai JTF, Sinclair AJ. Cerebrospinal fluid and lumbar puncture: A practical review. Journal of Neurology 2012;259:1530–45.

15. Edlow JA, Panagos PD, Godwin SA et al. Clinical policy: Critical issues in the evaluation and management of adult patients presenting to the emergency department with acute headache. Annals of Emergency Medicine 2008;52:407–36.

16. Clinical Practice Guideline: Lumbar Puncture Royal Childrens' Hospital, nd. www.rch.org.au/clinicalguide/cpg.cfm?doc_id=5251; accessed 4 April 2013.

17. Arendt K, Demaerschalk BM, Wingerchuk DM, Camann W. Atraumatic lumbar puncture needles: after all these years, are we still missing the point? The Neurologist 2009;15:17–20.

18. Ahmed SV, Jayawarna C, Jude E. Post lumbar puncture headache: Diagnosis and management. Postgraduate Medical Journal 2006; 82:713–16.

19. Amorim JA, Gomes De Barros MV, Valença MM. Post-dural (post-lumbar) puncture headache: Risk factors and clinical features. Cephalalgia 2012;32:916–23.

20. Frank RL. Lumbar puncture and post-dural puncture headaches: implications for the emergency physician. Journal of Emergency Medicine 2008;35:149–57.

21. Majed B, Zephir H, Pichonnier-Cassagne V et al. Lumbar punctures: Use and diagnostic efficiency in emergency medical departments. International Journal of Emergency Medicine 2009;2:227–35.

22. Kelly CA, Upex A, Batemen DN. Comparison of conscious level assessment in the poisoned patient using the alert/verbal/painful/unresponsive scale and the Glasgow Coma Scale. Annals of Emergency Medicine 2004;22:108–13.

23. Huff JS. Altered mental status and coma. In: Tintinalli J, Stapczynski JS, Cline DM et al, eds. Emergency medicine: a comprehensive study guide. 7th edn. New York: McGraw Hill; 2011.

24. National Stroke Foundation. Clinical guidelines for stroke management Melbourne. www.strokefoundation.com.au/clinical-guidelines: National Stroke Foundation; accessed 25 Feb 2011.

25. Easton JD, Saver JL, Albers GW et al. Definition and evaluation of transient ischemic attack: A scientific statement for healthcare professionals from the American Heart Association/American Stroke Association Stroke Council; Council on Cardiovascular Surgery and Anesthesia; Council on Cardiovascular Radiology and Intervention; Council on Cardiovascular Nursing; and the Interdisciplinary Council on Peripheral Vascular Disease: The American Academy of Neurology affirms the value of this statement as an educational tool for neurologists. Stroke 2009;40:2276–93.

26. Nadarajan V, Perry RJ, Johnson J, Werring DJ. Transient ischaemic attacks: Mimics and chameleons. Practical Neurology 2014;14:23–31.

27. Morgenstern LB, Sánchez BN. Tissue is the issue in transient ischemic attack and stroke. Annals of Neurology 2014;75:171–2.

28. Chandratheva A, Mehta Z, Geraghty O et al. Population-based study of risk and predictors of stroke in the first few hours after a TIA. Neurology 2009;72:1941–7.

29. Aplin P. Stroke and transient ischaemic attacks. In: Cameron P, Jelinek G, Kelly A et al. eds. Adult textbook of emergency medicine. 3rd edn. Sydney: Churchill Livingstone; 2009:372–86.

30. Giles MF, Rothwell PM. Risk of stroke early after transient ischaemic attack: a systematic review and meta-analysis. The Lancet Neurology 2007;6:1063–72.

31. Rothwell PM, Warlow CP. Timing of TIAs preceding stroke: Time window for prevention is very short. Neurology 2005;64:817–20.

32. Amort M, Fluri F, Schäfer J et al. Transient ischemic attack versus transient ischemic attack mimics: frequency, clinical characteristics and outcome. Cerebrovascular Diseases 2011;32:57–64.

33. Rothwell PM, Giles MF, Flossmann E et al. A simple score (ABCD) to identify individuals at high early risk of stroke after transient ischaemia attack. Lancet 2005;366:28–36.

34. Johnston SC, Rothwell PM, Nguyen-Huynh MN et al. Validation and refinement of scores to predict very early stroke risk after transient ischaemic attack. Lancet 2007;369:283–92.

35. Giles MF, Rothwell PM. Systematic review and pooled analysis of published and unpublished validations of the ABCD and ABCD2 transient ischemic attack risk scores. Stroke 2010;41:667–73.

36. Bray JE, Coughlan K, Bladin C. Can the ABCD Score be dichotomised to identify high-risk patients with transient ischaemic attack in the emergency department? Emergency Medicine Journal 2007;24:92–5.

37. McGillivray B, Considine J. Implementation of evidence into practice: development of a tool to improve emergency nursing care of acute stroke. Australasian Emergency Nursing Journal 2009;12:110–19.

38. Nanda A, Singh N. Transient ischemic attack treatment and management. eMedicine 2014: http://emedicine.medscape.com/article/1910519-treatment; accessed 2 May 2014.

39. Christensen H, Christensen AF, Boysen G. Abnormalities on ECG and telemetry predict stroke outcome at 3 months. Journal of Neurological Sciences 2005;234:99–103.

40. Perry JJ, Sharma M, Sivilotti MLA et al. A prospective cohort study of patients with transient ischemic attack to identify high-risk clinical characteristics. Stroke 2014;45:92–100.

41. Rothwell PM, Giles MF, Chandratheva A et al. Effect of urgent treatment of transient ischaemic attack and minor stroke on early recurrent stroke (EXPRESS study): a prospective population-based sequential comparison. The Lancet 2007;370:1432–42.

42. Lavallée PC, Meseguer E, Abboud H et al. A transient ischaemic attack clinic with round-the-clock access (SOS-TIA): feasibility and effects. The Lancet Neurology 2007;6:953–60.

43. The Dutch TIA Trial Study Group. A comparison of two doses of aspirin (30 mg vs 283 mg a day) in patients after a transient ischemic attack or minor ischemic stroke. New England Journal of Medicine 1991;325:1261–6.

44. UK-TIA Study Group. United Kingdom transient ischaemic attack (UK-TIA) aspirin trial: interim results. British Medical Journal 1988;296:316–20.

45. De Schryver E, Algra A, Kappelle L et al. Vitamin K antagonists versus antiplatelet therapy after transient ischaemic attack or minor ischaemic stroke of presumed arterial origin. Issue 9. Art. No.: CD001342. DOI: 10.1002/14651858.CD001342.pub3. Cochrane Database of Systematic Reviews 2012: accessed 2 May 2014.

46. Lang E, Afilalo M. Vertebrobasilar Atherothrombotic Disease eMedicine 2012: http://emedicine.medscape.com/article/794678-overview; accessed 2 May 2014.

47. Savitz SI, Caplan LR. Current concepts: Vertebrobasilar disease. New England Journal of Medicine 2005;352:2618–26.

48. Smith E, Delargy M. Locked-in syndrome. British Medical Journal 2005;330:406–9.

49. Go S, Worman DJ. Stroke, transient ischemic attack and cervical artery dissecton. In: Tintinalli J, Stapczynski JS, Cline DM et al, eds. Emergency Medicine: A Comprehensive Study Guide. 7th edn. New York: McGraw Hill; 2011.

50. National Stroke Foundation. Top 10 facts about stroke. 2013: https://strokefoundation.com.au/health-professionals/tools-and-resources/facts-and-figures-about-stroke/; accessed 2 May 2014.

51. Rosengarten P. Subarachnoid haemorrhage. In: Cameron P, Jelinek G, Kelly A et al, eds. Adult textbook of emergency medicine. 3rd edn. Sydney: Churchill Livingstone; 2009:381–6.

52. Rinkel GJE, Algra A. Long-term outcomes of patients with aneurysmal subarachnoid haemorrhage. The Lancet Neurology 2011; 10:349–56.

53. Perry JJ, Stiell IG, Sivilotti ML et al. Clinical decision rules to rule out subarachnoid hemorrhage for acute headache. JAMA 2013;310:1248–55.

54. National Stroke Foundation. Signs of stroke FAST. 2014: Online. http://strokefoundation.com.au/what-is-a-stroke/signs-of-stroke/; accessed 2 May 2014.

55. Jauch EC, Saver JL, Adams HP et al. Guidelines for the early management of patients with acute ischemic stroke: A guideline for healthcare professionals from the American Heart Association/American Stroke Association. Stroke 2013;44:870–947.

56. Gerdtz M, Considine J, Sands N et al. Emergency triage education kit. Canberra: Australian Government Department of Health and Ageing; 2007.

57. van Bree MD, Roos YB, van der Bilt IA et al. Prevalence and characterization of ECG abnormalities after intracerebral hemorrhage. Neurocritical care 2010;12:50–5.

58. Popescu D, Laza C, Mergeani A et al. Lead electrocardiogram changes after supratentorial intracerebral hemorrhage. Mædica 2012;7:290.

59. Khechinashvili G, Asplund K. Electrocardiographic changes in patients with acute stroke: a systematic review. Cerebrovascular diseases 2002;14:67–76.

60. Elizabeth J, Singarayar J, Ellul J et al. Arterial oxygen saturation and posture in acute stroke. Age Ageing 1993;22:269–72.

61. Bhalla A, Wolfe CDA, Rudd AG. Management of acute physiological parameters after stroke. QJM: An International Journal of Medicine 2001;94:167–72.

62. Stroke Unit Trialists' Collaboration. Organised inpatient (stroke unit) care for stroke. Cochrane Database of Systematic Reviews Issue 4 Art No: CD000197 DOI: 101002/14651858CD000197pub2 2007.

63. Considine J, McGillivray B. An evidence-based practice approach to improving nursing care of acute stroke in an Australian Emergency Department. Journal of Clinical Nursing 2010;19:138–44.

64. Middleton S, McElduff P, Ward J et al. Implementation of evidence-based treatment protocols to manage fever, hyperglycaemia, and swallowing dysfunction in acute stroke (QASC): a cluster randomised controlled trial. The Lancet 2011;378:1699–706.

65. Hajat C, Hajat S, Sharma P. Effects of poststroke pyrexia on stroke outcome: a meta-analysis of studies in patients. Stroke 2000;31:410–14.

66. Weir CJ, Murray GD, Dyker AG, Lees KR. Is hyperglycaemia an independent predictor of poor outcome after acute stroke? Results of a long-term follow-up study. British Medical Journal 1997;314:1303–6.

67. Cumming TB, Tyedin K, Churilov L et al. The effect of physical activity on cognitive function after stroke: A systematic review. International Psychogeriatrics 2012;24:557–67.

68. Coull BM, Williams LS, Goldstein LB et al. Anticoagulants and antiplatelet agents in acute ischemic stroke. Report of the Joint Stroke Guideline Development Committee of the American Academy of Neurology and the American Stroke Association. Stroke 2002;33:1934–42.

69. Albers GW, Caplan LR, Easton JD et al. Transient ischaemic attack—proposal for a new definition. New England Journal of Medicine 2002;347:1713–16.

70. Wardlaw JM, Koumellis P, Liu M. Thrombolysis (different doses, routes of administration and agents) for acute ischaemic stroke. The Cochrane database of systematic reviews 2013;5.

71. Balami JS, Chen R-L, Grunwald IQ, Buchan AM. Neurological complications of acute ischaemic stroke. The Lancet Neurology 2011;10:357–71.

72. Wilkes G. Seizures. In: Cameron P, Jelinek G, Kelly A et al. eds. Adult textbook of emergency medicine. 3rd edn. Sydney: Churchill Livingstone; 2009:392–7.

73. Huff JS, Melnick ER, Tomaszewski CA et al. Clinical policy: Critical issues in the evaluation and management of adult patients presenting to the emergency department with seizures. Annals of Emergency Medicine 2014;63:437–47.

74. Brophy GM, Bell R, Claassen J et al. Guidelines for the evaluation and management of status epilepticus. Neurocritical care 2012;17:3–23.

75. Jagoda A, Gupta K. The emergency department evaluation of the adult patient who presents with a first-time seizure. Emergency medicine clinics of North America 2011;29:41–9.

76. Kelly A-M. Headache. In: Cameron P, Jelinek G, Kelly A et al. eds. Adult textbook of emergency medicine. 3rd edn. Sydney: Churchill Livingstone; 2009:368–72.

77. Denny CJ, Schull M. Headache and facial pain. In: Tintinalli J, Stapczynski JS, Cline DM et al, eds. Emergency Medicine. 7th edn. New York: McGraw Hill; 2011.

78. Morton P, Tucker T. Patient assessment: cardiovascular system. In: Morton PG, Fontaine DK, Hudak CM, Gallo BM, eds. Critical care nursing: a holistic approach. 8th edn. Philadelphia: Lippincott Williams & Wilkins; 2005:211–91.

79. Edlow JA, Panagos PD, Godwin SA et al. Clinical policy: critical issues in the evaluation and management of adult patients presenting to the emergency department with acute headache. Annals of Emergency Medicine 2008;52:407–36.

80. Digre KB. Headaches during pregnancy. Clinical Obstetrics and Gynecology 2013;56:317–29.

81. Beddoes L. Chronic neurological problems. In: Brown D, Edwards H, eds. Lewis's medical-surgical nursing. Sydney: Elsevier; 2005:1549–81.

82. Holdgate A, Kelly AM. Emergency care evidence in practice series: management of acute migraine. Emergency care community of practice. National Institute of Clinical Studies; 2006. www.nhmrc.gov.au/_files_nhmrc/file/nics/material_resources/Management%20of%20acute%20migraine%20colour.pdf; accessed 1 Jan 2010.

83. Hellman DB. Temporal arteritis. A cough, toothache and tongue infarction. JAMA 2002;287:2996–3000.

84. Smetana GW, Shmerling RH. Does this patient have temporal arteritis? JAMA 2002;287:92–101.

85. Widico CR, Newman DH. Does this patient have temporal arteritis? Annals of Emergency Medicine 2005;45:85–6.

86. Meyer CN, Sammuelsson JS, Galle M, Bansborg JM. Adult bacterial meningitis: aetiology, penicillin susceptibility, risk factors, prognostic factors and guidelines for empirical antibiotic treatment. Clinical Microbiology and Infection 2004;10:709–17.

87. Nowak DA, Boehmer R, Fuchs HH. A retrospective clinical laboratory and outcome analysis in 43 cases of acute aseptic meningitis. European Journal of Neurology 2003;10:271–80.

88. McGillicuddy DC, Walker O, Shapiro NI, Edlow JA. Guillian Barre syndrome in the Emergency Department. Annals of Emergency Medicine 2006;47:390–3.

89. Adapted from MedicineNet, Inc., eMedicine health. Hematoma. Online. www.emedicinehealth.com/hematoma/page3_em.htm; accessed 6 July 2015.

90. Koeppen B, Stanton B. Berne and Levy, Physiology, 6th edn. St. Louis: Mosby; 2010.

91. Lewis SM, Collier IC, Heitkemper MM. Medical-surgical nursing: assessment and management of clinical problems. 8th edn. St Louis: Mosby; 2011.

92. Rund DA, Barkin RM, Rosen P. Essentials of emergency medicine. 2nd edn. St Louis: Mosby; 1996.

93. Davis JH, Drucker WR. Clinical Surgery. vol 1. St Louis: Mosby; 1987.

94. Brown D, Edwards H. Lewis' Medical–Surgical Nursing. Sydney: Mosby; 2005.

95. Thibodeau GA, Patton KT. Anatomy and Physiology. 5th edn. St Louis: Mosby; 2003.

96. Cameron P, Jelinek G, Kelly A et al. Adult textbook of emergency medicine. 3rd edn. Sydney: Churchill Livingstone; 2009.

97. Hunt WE, Hess RM. Surgical risk as related to time of intervention in the repair of intracranial aneurysms. Journal of Neurosurgery 1968;28:14–20.

98. Sawin P, Loftus C. Diagnosis of spontaneous subarachnoid hemorrhage. American family physician 1997;55:145–56.

CHAPTER 24
GASTROINTESTINAL EMERGENCIES

WAYNE VARNDELL

Essentials

- Abdominal pain is a symptom of disease, not a diagnosis.
- Management of acute abdominal pathology involves a combination of prudent history taking and physical examination, and is aided by diagnostic studies.
- Examination always begins with a primary survey. The airway, breathing and circulatory status must be addressed to include airway patency, breathing pattern including rate, pulse, blood pressure/capillary refill time and postural changes. The brain must be adequately perfused and the level of consciousness will provide a useful indicator.
- Fluid resuscitation must be considered immediately if derangements in circulation are evident.
- Complete assessment must include accurate fluid balance. Output must be maintained.
- Peritonism or abdominal rigidity is an abdominal emergency.
- Early consultation and referral is essential for all gastrointestinal bleeding, especially when there is haemodynamic instability.
- Hypotension is a late sign in the dehydrated or shocked child. Do not delay fluids in children who are dry, pale, lethargic, tachycardic or show signs of peripheral shut-down.
- Be certain to consider pathology outside the abdomen.
- Repeat examination and assessments, including vital signs. The trend and changes are key to a deteriorating patient.

INTRODUCTION

Diseases of the digestive system account for more hospital separations in Australia than any other principal diagnosis.[1] Although conditions of a gastrointestinal nature are a common reason for calls to ambulance services and visits to the ED, they must be approached in a serious manner. The complexity of gastrointestinal (GI) conditions can make the assessment, diagnosis and management difficult, as the nature of presentations may constitute acute illness, chronic illness or a combination of both. GI emergencies vary from minor problems to the more serious, including life-threatening conditions. Vigilance in assessment, observation and management aims to ensure that underlying abdominal pathophysiology is identified and treated promptly and appropriately.

A patient's condition may be variable. Changes in a condition may be related to clinical improvement, patient deterioration or a response to intervention. It is important to assess and elicit an understanding about the direction of clinical change. Pre-hospital assessment of patients with gastrointestinal emergencies includes a systematic history of the pain and identification of any high-risk symptoms/patients as detailed herein, coupled with examination as part of an

ABC approach to formulate ideas about the nature and cause of the pain and associated symptoms. In the pre-hospital setting, it can be difficult to differentiate between the many GI and non-GI causes of abdominal complaints. The chief aims of pre-hospital management consists of pain relief, early initiation of therapies such as fluid resuscitation to stabilise the patient and prompt transportation of patients with life-threatening injuries/symptoms to hospital. Where critically ill patients require prompt transportation to hospital, an alert message should be sent to the receiving ED detailing the mechanism/medical complaint, injuries/information about the complaint, symptoms and treatment initiated.[2] Early communication of the patient's status enables the ED to prepare for the patient's arrival. On arrival to ED, patients are rapidly assessed by the triage nurse to establish the patient's level of clinical urgency. Triage of the patient is a dynamic process and provides a snapshot view of the progression of illness. Within an ED, the patient's triage assessment is categorised according to clinical acuity and is placed into one of the five Australasian Triage Scale categories (Category 1 being of the highest priority). Ongoing re-assessment, professional communication and clinical hand-over at every stage of patient care is vital to the management of the patient.

Classic indications of dysfunction in the GI system include heartburn, nausea, vomiting, constipation, diarrhoea, belching, bloating, chest pain, abdominal pain, back pain and bleeding.[3] This chapter focuses on those conditions seen most often in the emergency department (ED). A brief review of anatomy and physiology is followed by discussion relating to patient assessment, physical examination and the relevant screening (e.g. urinalysis, blood sugar level) and diagnostic investigations (e.g. haematology, biochemistry) most often carried out. Treatment provided is based upon the history, assessment, investigation and findings. Pain relief is humane, and the most often prescribed initial treatment. Specific GI conditions will be covered and include: gastroenteritis, gastrointestinal bleeding, bowel obstruction, diverticulitis, gastro-oesophageal reflux disease (GORD), appendicitis, cholecystitis, pancreatitis and liver failure. Trauma of the GI system is discussed in Chapter 48.

Anatomy and physiology

Normal GI function requires ingestion of nutrients and fluids and is followed by elimination of waste products formed from metabolic activities. Major organs and structures of the GI system are the mouth, oesophagus, stomach, large and small intestines, liver, pancreas, gallbladder and peritoneum (Fig 24.1).

Mouth

The beginning of the digestive process starts normally in the mouth. The bite, movement of the tongue and pushing against the walls of the mouth begin the physical breakdown of food. Food is chewed and mixed with saliva, which begins one of many chemical interactions within the GI system. Saliva lubricates the tissues of the mouth and creates a semi-solid of the food being eaten. Salivary amylase, the enzyme of saliva, begins carbohydrate metabolism.

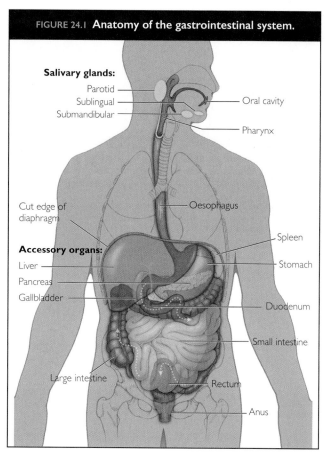

FIGURE 24.1 Anatomy of the gastrointestinal system.

Salivary glands:
Parotid
Sublingual
Submandibular
Oral cavity
Pharynx
Cut edge of diaphragm
Oesophagus
Spleen
Stomach
Accessory organs:
Liver
Pancreas
Gallbladder
Duodenum
Small intestine
Large intestine
Rectum
Anus

http://www.medicalartlibrary.com/gastrointestinal-system.html

Pathology of the mouth includes trauma and dental and gum disease. Infection may occur in any part of the mouth, including the salivary glands or ducts; parotid, submandibular and sublingual. Further information on oral and dental emergencies can be found in Chapter 32 and on faciomaxillary trauma in Chapter 46.

Oesophagus

The major function of the oesophagus is movement of food. The oesophagus, a straight, collapsible tube approximately 25 cm long and up to 3 cm in diameter, extends from the pharynx to the stomach. Distinct oesophageal layers are the mucous membrane, submucosa and muscular layer. Secretions from mucous glands scattered throughout the submucosa keep the inner lining moist and lubricated. Striated muscle in the upper oesophagus is gradually replaced by smooth muscle in the lower oesophagus and GI tract. The upper oesophageal sphincter is at the proximal end of the oesophagus, with the lower oesophageal sphincter (also called the cardiac sphincter) at the distal junction of the oesophagus and stomach. The lower oesophageal sphincter prevents regurgitation from the stomach into the oesophagus.

Stomach

Stomach functions include food storage, combining food with gastric juices, limited absorption and moving food into the small intestine. The stomach is a J-shaped organ located below the diaphragm between the oesophagus and the small intestine. Recognised regions of the stomach are the pylorus,

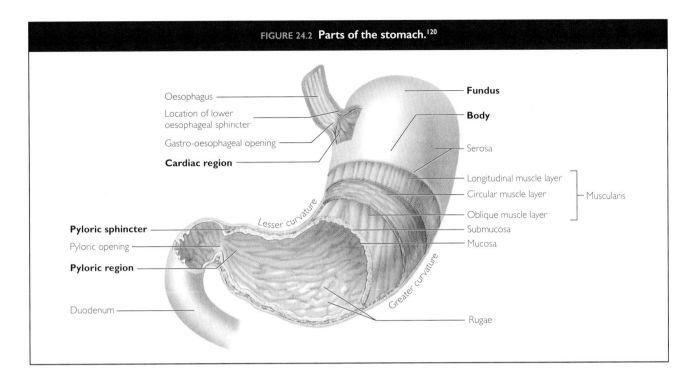

FIGURE 24.2 **Parts of the stomach.**[120]

fundus, body and antrum (Fig 24.2). The pyloric sphincter controls food movement from stomach to duodenum. Distinct layers of the stomach wall are outer serosa, muscular layer, submucosa and mucosa. The mucosal layer contains multiple wrinkles called rugae that straighten as the stomach fills to accommodate more volume. Completely relaxed, the stomach holds up to 1.5 L.[4] Gastric juices containing pepsin, hydrochloric acid, mucous and intrinsic factor are secreted by glands in the submucosa. These agents begin food breakdown. Acids in the stomach maintain the pH of gastric juices at 1.0. Absorption of some substances, including alcohol, actually begins in the stomach.[5]

Intestines

The small intestine is a tubular organ extending from the pyloric sphincter to the proximal large intestine. Secretions from the pancreas and liver complete digestion of nutrients in *chyme*—the semi-liquid mixture of food and gastric secretions. The small intestine absorbs nutrients and other products of digestion and transports residue to the large intestine. Segments of the small intestine are the duodenum, jejunum and ileum.[4] The duodenum attaches to the stomach at the pyloric sphincter in the retroperitoneal space, and represents the only fixed portion of the small intestine. The duodenum is approximately 25 cm long and 5 cm in diameter. The jejunum and ileum are mobile and lie free in the peritoneal cavity.

Segments of the large intestine are the caecum, colon, rectum and anal canal. The large intestine is approximately 1.5 m long, beginning in the lower right side of the abdomen where the ileum joins the caecum. The colon is divided into ascending colon, transverse colon, descending colon and sigmoid colon (Fig 24.3A, B and C). Primary functions of the large intestine are absorption of water and electrolytes, formation of faeces and storage of faeces. Approximately 1500 mL of chyme pass through the ileocaecal valve each day.[4]

Liver

The liver (Fig 24.4), located in the right upper quadrant of the abdomen, is divided into right and left lobes. Functional units of the liver called *lobules* contain sinusoids and Kupffer cells. Each lobule is supplied by a hepatic artery, sublobular vein, bile duct and lymph channel (Fig 24.5). The liver is extremely vascular; approximately 1450 mL of blood flows through the liver each minute, accounting for 29% of resting cardiac output.[4] Sinusoids in lobules act as a reservoir for overflow of blood and fluids from the right ventricle. A thick capsule of connective tissue, known as Glisson's capsule, covers the liver. The liver is involved in hundreds of metabolic functions, including metabolism of nutrients, gluconeogenesis and drug metabolism.

Table 24.1 summarises functions related to nutrition and waste removal. Production of bile is a major function of the liver: 600–1200 mL of bile is secreted each day. Bile is essential for digestion, absorption and excretion of bilirubin and excess cholesterol. Bilirubin is an end-product of haemoglobin destruction. Figure 24.6 illustrates processes involved in bilirubin conjugation.

Pancreas

The pancreas is approximately 20 cm long, lobulated, contains endocrine and exocrine cells and lies deep in the abdomen behind the stomach.[4] The organ is divided into the head, body and a thin, narrow tail that extends towards the spleen (Fig 24.7). Cells in the islets of Langerhans secrete insulin and regulate glucose levels. The exocrine cells form 98% of the pancreatic tissue and consist of clusters of acini cells. These are responsible for secretion of enzymes required for the digestion of fats, carbohydrates, proteins and nucleic acids.[6] Pancreatic enzymes enter the intestines through the pancreatic duct at the same juncture as the bile duct from the liver and gallbladder. The pancreatic and bile ducts join at a short, dilated tube

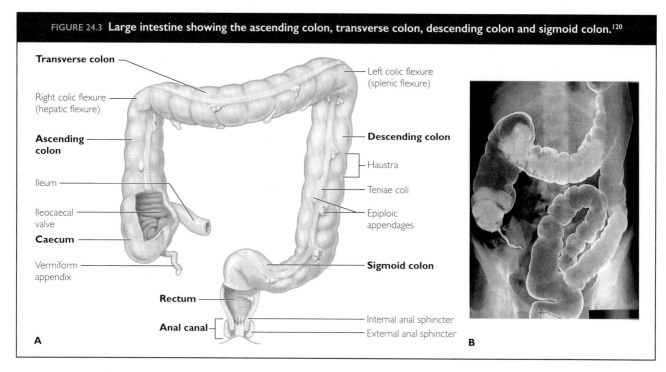

FIGURE 24.3 **Large intestine showing the ascending colon, transverse colon, descending colon and sigmoid colon.**[120]

Transverse colon

Left colic flexure (splenic flexure)

Right colic flexure (hepatic flexure)

Descending colon

Ascending colon

Haustra

Ileum

Teniae coli

Ileocaecal valve

Epiploic appendages

Caecum

Vermiform appendix

Sigmoid colon

Rectum

Internal anal sphincter

Anal canal

External anal sphincter

A

B

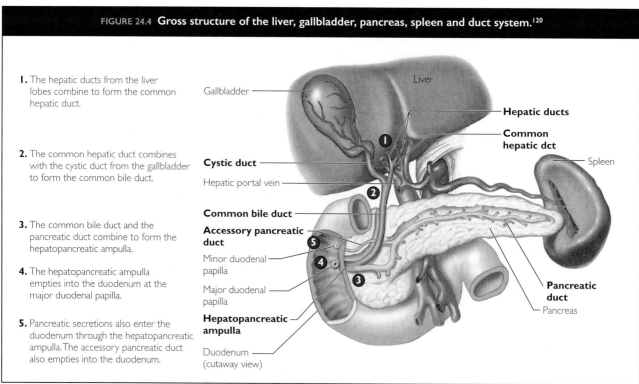

FIGURE 24.4 **Gross structure of the liver, gallbladder, pancreas, spleen and duct system.**[120]

1. The hepatic ducts from the liver lobes combine to form the common hepatic duct.

Liver

Gallbladder

Hepatic ducts

Common hepatic dct

2. The common hepatic duct combines with the cystic duct from the gallbladder to form the common bile duct.

Spleen

Cystic duct

Hepatic portal vein

3. The common bile duct and the pancreatic duct combine to form the hepatopancreatic ampulla.

Common bile duct

Accessory pancreatic duct

Minor duodenal papilla

4. The hepatopancreatic ampulla empties into the duodenum at the major duodenal papilla.

Major duodenal papilla

Pancreatic duct

Pancreas

5. Pancreatic secretions also enter the duodenum through the hepatopancreatic ampulla. The accessory pancreatic duct also empties into the duodenum.

Hepatopancreatic ampulla

Duodenum (cutaway view)

called the ampulla of Vater. A band of smooth muscles, called the sphincter of Oddi, surrounds this area and controls exit of pancreatic enzymes and bile. In a normally functioning pancreas, the enzymes are prevented from being activated until they reach the intestines.[6]

Gallbladder

The gallbladder is a pear-shaped sac located in a depression on the inferior surface of the liver. The organ's main functions are collection, concentration and storage of bile. Maximum volume is 30–60 mL; however, input from the liver can reach 450 mL over 12 hours. Concentration of bile in the gallbladder can be 5–20 times that of bile in the liver.[4] Bile is predominantly (80%) water, with the remaining volume comprised of bile acids (10%), phospholipid (4% to 5%) and cholesterol (1%).[7]

Peritoneum

The peritoneum is a serous membrane covering the liver, spleen, stomach and intestines which acts as a semipermeable membrane; it contains pain receptors and provides proliferative

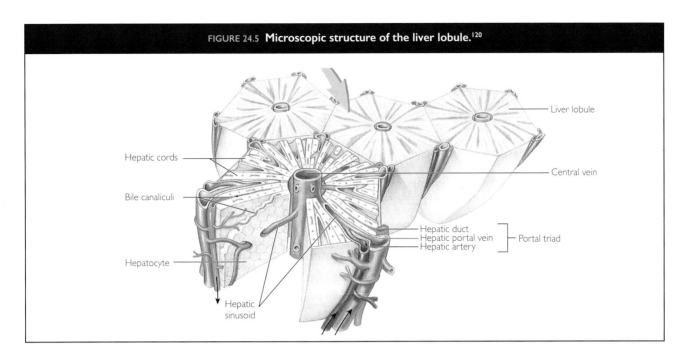

FIGURE 24.5 **Microscopic structure of the liver lobule.**[120]

TABLE 24.1 **Major functions of the liver**[121]

FUNCTION	DESCRIPTION
METABOLIC FUNCTIONS	
Carbohydrate metabolism	Glycogenesis (conversion of glucose to glycogen), glycogenolysis (process of breaking down glycogen to glucose), gluconeogenesis (formation of glucose from amino acids and fatty acids)
Protein metabolism	Synthesis of non-essential amino acids, synthesis of plasma proteins (except gamma-globulin), synthesis of clotting factors, urea formation from NH_3 (NH_3 formed from deamination of amino acids and by action of bacteria on proteins in colon)
Fat metabolism	Synthesis of lipoproteins, breakdown of triglycerides into fatty acids and glycerol, formation of ketone bodies, synthesis of fatty acids from amino acids and glucose, synthesis and breakdown of cholesterol
Detoxification	Inactivation of drugs and harmful substances and excretion of their breakdown products
Steroid metabolism	Conjugation and excretion of gonadal and adrenal steroids
BILE SYNTHESIS	
Bile production	Formation of bile, containing bile salts, bile pigments (mainly bilirubin) and cholesterol
Bile excretion	Bile excretion by liver about 1 L/day
Storage	Glucose in form of glycogen; vitamins, including fat-soluble (A, D, E, K) and water-soluble (B_1, B_2, cobalamin and folic acid); fatty acids; minerals (iron and copper); amino acids in form of albumin and beta-globulins
MONONUCLEAR PHAGOCYTE SYSTEM	
Kupffer cells	Breakdown of old red blood cells, white blood cells, bacteria and other particles, breakdown of haemoglobin from old red blood cells to bilirubin and biliverdin

cellular protection. Technically, all abdominal organs are behind the peritoneum and therefore are retroperitoneal; however, the liver, spleen, stomach and intestines are suspended into the peritoneum and considered intraperitoneal organs.[7] Omenta are folds of peritoneum that surround the stomach and adjacent organs. The greater omentum drapes the transverse colon and loops of small intestine. It is extremely mobile and spreads easily into areas of injury to seal off potential sources of infection.

The lesser omentum covers parts of the stomach and proximal intestines but is not as movable as the greater omentum.

The peritoneum is permeable to fluid, electrolytes, urea and toxins. Somatic afferent nerves sensitise the peritoneum to all types of stimuli. In acute abdominal conditions, the peritoneum can localise an irritable focus by producing sharp pain and tenderness, voluntary or involuntary abdominal muscle rigidity and rebound tenderness.[7]

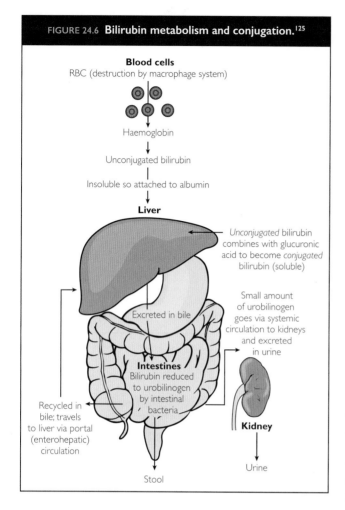

FIGURE 24.6 Bilirubin metabolism and conjugation.[125]

Blood cells
RBC (destruction by macrophage system)

Haemoglobin

Unconjugated bilirubin

Insoluble so attached to albumin

Liver

Unconjugated bilirubin combines with glucuronic acid to become *conjugated* bilirubin (soluble)

Excreted in bile

Small amount of urobilinogen goes via systemic circulation to kidneys and excreted in urine

Intestines
Bilirubin reduced to urobilinogen by intestinal bacteria

Recycled in bile; travels to liver via portal (enterohepatic) circulation

Kidney

Urine

Stool

General assessment

Assessment of a patient with a GI emergency should initially focus on airway (e.g. vomiting, obstruction), breathing pattern (rate, work of breathing) and circulation, including vital signs.[8] A completed primary assessment then allows a systematic and focused assessment. The patient's general appearance will provide an important first impression (pale, grey, jaundiced, flushed, sweaty). A patient who is still and responding to questioning is initially easier to assess than one who is extremely agitated and distressed due to pain. An air of control and calm needs to be obtained, as a distressed patient coupled with a distressed clinician makes for difficult work.[9]

The initial assessment will provide a cue to recognition of an underlying GI-related disorder, such as severe dehydration, intense pain, shock and metabolic and biochemical disturbances. The respiratory system may be activated to assist with maintaining normal blood pH (see Ch 21). Abdominal pain may also affect breathing and lead to shallow respirations. Heart rate is often elevated as a result of a number of causative factors. Pain alone may increase heart rate; however, underlying pathology, such as fever, sepsis or shock, will also increase the heart rate and it is important to remain objective about physiological observations. Care must be taken not to assume that pain is the only factor to raise the heart rate. Blood pressure (BP) must be obtained to detect life-threatening hypotension which may be associated with severe fluid shifts and poor perfusion. Temperature may be elevated when infection is an underlying causative factor. Consideration must be given to the very young, older or immunosuppressed patient who may have a serious infection and not be able to mount a significant fever in response to infection.[10,11] Observe skin colour, diaphoresis, rashes, scars, wounds, abdominal-wall abnormalities and characteristics of any pain.

Patient history

Obtaining a complete focused patient history is the cornerstone of accurate symptom evaluation, appropriate test ordering and diagnosis. The history should be as complete as possible and include description of the patient's pain and associated symptoms. In addition, patient past medical, surgical and social history should be elicited to aid in directing decisions regarding further work-up. High-yield historical questions have been posited within the literature,[10,12,13] a summary of which is provided in Table 24.2.

> **PRACTICE TIP**
>
> Not all abdominal symptoms are caused by GI disease. Take a broad and detailed history.

Pain

The nature and quality of abdominal pain are key clues as to the potential cause and diagnosis; it is therefore important to undertake a detailed assessment. While the assessment of pain using the mnemonic PQRST (see Ch 19) may provide for a systematic approach to assessing pain in general, it does not allow for a smooth patient interview regarding abdominal pain. An alternative pain assessment mnemonic SOCRATES may better suit the evaluation of abdominal pain and the patient interview (Table 24.3).[149] As part of assessing abdominal pain, the clinician must consider individual and cultural variations in expressions of pain. Each person reacts differently to pain. Older patients may not exhibit the same level of pain as younger patients;[10] men may hide pain because expression of pain is not considered masculine in many cultures. Conversely, dramatic expression of pain may be expected in some cultures. It is important to remember that pain is a symptom, not a diagnosis.[14] Interventions should focus on identification and treatment of the source of pain.

Location

Potential causes based on location of pain are listed in Table 24.4; Table 24.5 reviews pain descriptions associated with certain conditions. The location of pain may assist in localising the area of pathology; however, this may be misleading, especially if the pain is referred. Further, decreased perception of pain in advancing age, patients with diabetes, delirium/confusion or widespread abdominal pain may be unable to localise pain.[10,15] Obtain details about the presenting problem and drill to specifics as much as possible. Often the only symptom is abdominal pain, which may or may not be related to the GI tract. Abdominal pain may be visceral, somatic or referred.

- *Visceral pain*, caused by stretching of hollow viscus, is described as cramping or a sensation of gas. Pain

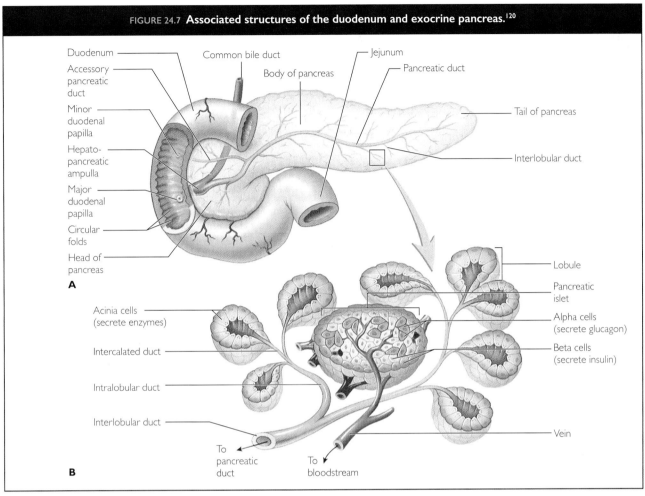

FIGURE 24.7 Associated structures of the duodenum and exocrine pancreas.[120]

A, The head of the pancreas lies within the duodenum curvature, with the pancreatic duct emptying into the duodenum. B, Histology of the pancreas showing both the acini and the pancreatic duct system.

intensifies then decreases, and is usually centred on the umbilicus or below the midline.[16] Diffuse pain makes localisation of pain difficult, due to intraperitoneal organs being bilaterally innervated resulting in stimuli being perceived by both sides of the spinal cord. For example, stimuli from visceral fibres in the appendix enter the spinal cord at about T10, resulting in midline periumbilical pain. Other symptoms such as diaphoresis, nausea, vomiting, hypotension, tachycardia and abdominal-wall spasms may be present.[16] Conditions associated with visceral pain are appendicitis, acute pancreatitis, cholecystitis and intestinal obstruction.

- *Somatic pain* is produced by bacterial or chemical irritation of nerve fibres.[17] Pain is sharp and usually localised to one area. A patient lies with legs flexed and knees pulled to the chest to prevent stimulation of the peritoneum and subsequent increase in pain. Associated findings include involuntary guarding and rebound tenderness.
- *Referred pain* occurs at a distance from the original source of the pain, and is thought to be caused by development of nerve tracts during fetal growth and development.[18] Biliary pain can be referred to the subscapular area, whereas a peptic ulcer and pancreatic disease can cause back pain

(see Chs 19 and 26). Referred pain to the shoulder tip (Kehr's sign) can be an important sign of diaphragmatic irritation, due to blood or fluid accumulation from intra-abdominal pathology. This may be present following abdominal surgery, injury, trauma or a spontaneous perforation.

PRACTICE TIPS

- 'Abdominal pain' is a symptom, not a diagnosis.
- Abdominal pain with vomiting, no flatus or bowel movements and a midline abdominal scar suggests small bowel obstruction unless otherwise excluded.
- Constipation, gastroenteritis, irritable bowel syndrome and non-specific abdominal pain are diagnoses of exclusion.

Physical examination

A systematic approach is recommended for clinical assessment of the abdomen: a sequence of inspection, auscultation, percussion and palpation. Patient position should be noted because patients assume positions of comfort.[9]

TABLE 24.2 High-yield historical questions[12]
How old are you?
Advanced age is associated with increased hospitalisation, surgical intervention and mortality.
Which came first, pain or vomiting?
Pain worse before vomiting suggests surgical disease.
How long have you had the pain?
Pain lasting less than 48 hours is more likely to be caused by surgical disease.
Have you ever had abdominal surgery?
Previous abdominal surgery increases the risk of adhesions or obstruction.
Is the pain constant or intermittent?
Constant pain is more likely to be caused by surgical disease.
Have you ever had this before?
No previous episode is more likely to be caused by surgical disease.
Do you have a history of cancer, diverticulosis, pancreatitis, kidney failure, gallstones or inflammatory bowel disease?
All are suggestive of more serious pathology.
Are you immunocompromised (e.g. receiving chemotherapy, on immunosuppressant therapy)?
Consider occult infection of drug-related pancreatitis.
How much alcohol do you drink per day?
Consider pancreatitis, hepatitis or cirrhosis.
Are you pregnant?
Test for pregnancy; consider ectopic pregnancy.
Are you taking any antibiotics or steroids?
May potentially mask infection.
Did the pain start centrally and migrate to the right lower quadrant?
High specificity for appendicitis.
Do you have a history of vascular or heart disease, hypertension or atrial fibrillation?
Consider mesenteric ischaemia or abdominal aneurysm.

TABLE 24.3 SOCRATES pain assessment mnemonic
Site: Where is the pain? Where is the maximal site of pain?
Onset: When did the pain start, and was it sudden or gradual?
Character: What is the pain like?
Radiation: Does the pain radiate anywhere?
Associations: Are there any other signs or symptoms associated with the pain?
Tempo: Does the pain follow any pattern?
Exacerbating or relieving factors: Does anything change the pain?
Severity: How bad is the pain?

noisy environment. Auscultate bowel sounds in all four quadrants, determining frequency, quality and pitch.
- Normal bowel sounds are irregular, high-pitched gurgling sounds occurring 5–35 times per minute.
- Decreased or absent bowel sounds suggest peritonitis or paralytic ileus, whereas hyperactive bowel sounds associated with nausea, vomiting and diarrhoea suggest gastroenteritis.
- Frequent, high-pitched bowel sounds occur with bowel obstruction.
- Vascular sounds such as venous hums or bruits are abnormal findings (see Ch 21).

- *Percussion* is performed in all four quadrants. Dull sounds occur over solid organs or tumours, whereas tympanic sounds occur over air masses. Tympany is the normal sound heard when percussing the abdomen. Like performing auscultation, environmental noise can reduce the effectiveness and specificity of this assessment and thus the value of the findings.
- *Palpation* is important. Feeling the abdomen provides rapid and useful clinical information to underlying pathology. Initially, palpate away from areas of pain, noting areas of tenderness, guarding, rigidity or masses. Gently palpate towards the painful area last. Tenderness, guarding, rigidity and peritonism are all important clinical pointers to a patient suffering an acute abdominal event. Care is to be taken, as a soft and non-tender abdomen is not necessarily without pathology; it may be intermittent or transient and the patient as a whole must be considered with other clinical findings and history.
- *Specific abdominal signs* have been described within the literature as being associated with specific diagnosis (Table 24.6). Sensitivity and specificity varies between patient populations and pathologies. However, the sensitivity and specificity of all abdominal signs or assessment techniques is not known.

Another common finding with most GI emergencies is nausea and vomiting. Specific treatment varies with the suspected

- *Inspection* is often the first approach. Observe the patient's face (a central perspective) for facial expression, signs of discomfort, diaphoresis and skin colour, e.g. flushed, pale. Look at the abdomen for colour, e.g. pale, jaundice, mottled; the abdominal wall for pulsations, movement, masses, symmetry or surgical scars.
- *Auscultation* should be done before palpation/percussion to prevent the creation of false bowel sounds by palpation. Auscultation can be difficult to perform in a

TABLE 24.4 Potential sources of abdominal pain, by location		
LOCATION	POTENTIAL CAUSE	
Right upper quadrant	Cholecystitis	Pancreatic abscess
	Hepatic abscess	Duodenal ulcer perforation
	Hepatitis	Right lung pneumonia
	Hepatomegaly	Right renal pain
Left upper quadrant	Pancreatitis	Left renal pain
	Splenic rupture	Pericarditis
	Myocardial infarction	Left lung pneumonia
	Gastritis	
Right lower quadrant	Appendicitis	Ovarian cyst
	Cholecystitis	Pelvic inflammatory disease
	Perforated ulcer	Endometriosis
	Intestinal obstruction	Right ureteral calculi
	Meckel's diverticulum	Incarcerated hernia
	Abdominal aortic aneurysm, dissection or rupture	Gastric ulcer perforation
	Ruptured ectopic pregnancy	Colon perforation
	Twisted right ovary	Urinary tract infection
Left lower quadrant	Appendicitis	Left ureteral calculi
	Intestinal obstruction	Left renal pain
	Diverticulum of the sigmoid colon	Urinary tract infection
	Ruptured ectopic pregnancy	Incarcerated hernia
	Twisted left ovary	Perforated descending colon
	Ovarian cyst	Regional enteritis
	Endometriosis	

TABLE 24.5 Description of pain associated with certain clinical conditions	
PAIN DESCRIPTION	ASSOCIATED CLINICAL CONDITIONS
Severe, sharp pain	Infarction or rupture
Severe pain controlled by medication	Pancreatitis, peritonitis, small bowel obstruction, renal colic, biliary colic
Dull pain	Inflammation, low-grade infection
Intermittent pain	Gastroenteritis, small-bowel obstruction

PRACTICE TIP

Patients unable to tolerate fluid without vomiting are not suitable for discharge.

Gain an understanding about the patient's dietary and fluid input (anorexia, increased thirst) as well as output in terms of urination (anuria, oliguria, polyuria, dysuria) and bowel motion activity (constipation/diarrhoea, consistency, colour). Past medical history provides essential clinical information; however, maintain a view that this presentation may differ from that of previous presentations (see Ch 14). Obtain a social history. Information may be gleaned from the patient, family members, friends, other healthcare professionals or old medical records.[6] Historical assessment should include questions related to respiratory, cardiovascular, gynaecological and genitourinary (GU) symptoms as they may also cause abdominal pain, nausea and vomiting. When appropriate, a complete assessment should also gain understanding about sexual contacts or sexual history, drug and alcohol use and any recent overseas travel. Information related to food and fluid intake and tolerance should also be noted.

Findings such as fever and chills are usually found with infective processes. Intractable vomiting or faeces in emesis suggest bowel obstruction. Blood in emesis occurs with

underlying cause. Care must be taken to understand the causes of vomiting. Vomiting may be related to a condition of the GI system that directly initiates vomiting, for example a toxin or virus. Alternatively, the vomiting may be secondary to a mechanical condition such as a bowel obstruction or a sign of raised intracranial pressure. If vomiting is present, observe or enquire if it contains blood or bile. Gain an understanding into the frequency; several times versus many or intractable. Table 24.7 lists various drugs that may be used for nausea and vomiting.

TABLE 24.6 Specific signs in patients with abdominal pain

SIGN	DESCRIPTION	ASSOCIATION
Cough test	Post-tussive abdominal pain.	Peritonitis (sensitivity 50–85%; specificity 38–79%)[128–133]
Cullen's sign	Periumbilical ecchymosis	Retroperitoneal haemorrhage, 37% increase in mortality rate[134]
Grey-Turner's sign	Flank ecchymosis	Retroperitoneal haemorrhage, 37% increase in mortality rate[134]
Heel-drop sign	Pain at RLQ on dropping heels to floor from standing on tiptoes, or from forcefully banging the patient's right heel with clinician's hand	Appendicitis (sensitivity 74–93%)[135,136]
Kehr's sign	Severe pain radiating to left shoulder tip, especially when the patient is supine.[137]	Intraperitoneal bleeding
McBurney's sign	Tenderness located 2/3 distance from anterior iliac spine to umbilicus on right side.[138]	Appendicitis (sensitivity 50–94%; specificity 75–86%)[95,129,139]
Murphy's sign	Exquisite pain is elicited by applying gentle pressure below the right sub-costal arch below the liver margin during deep inspiration.[9]	Acute cholecystitis (sensitivity 48–97%; specificity 48–98%)[140–143]
Obturator's sign	The right hip and knee is flexed and then right hip is internally rotated.	Appendicitis (sensitivity 8%; specificity 94%)[144]
Psoas sign	With the patient lying down on the left side, the right hip is then hyperextended. Painful hip extension is the positive response.[145]	Appendicitis (sensitivity 13–42%; specificity 79–97%)[144,146,147]
Rovsing's sign	Pain at RLQ when palpating LLQ	Appendicitis (sensitivity 7–68%; specificity 58–96%)[92,95,130,146,148]

TABLE 24.7 Drug therapy in nausea and vomiting[150]

CLASSIFICATION	DRUG
Antiemetic and antipsychotic	Chlorpromazine
	Haloperidol
	Perphenazine
	Prochlorperazine
	Trifluoperazine
Antihistamine	Dimenhydrinate
	Diphenhydramine
	Promethazine
Prokinetic	Domperidone
	Metoclopramide
Serotonin antagonist	Dolasetron
	Ondansetron
	Tropisetron
Antimuscarinic	Hyoscine
Other	Dexamethasone

gastritis, upper GI bleeding or mucosal tearing. Diarrhoea occurs with gastroenteritis; black, tarry stools suggest upper GI bleeding; and clay-coloured stools are found with biliary tract obstruction. Fatty, foul-smelling, frothy stools occur with pancreatitis. Table 24.8 presents the factors that increase the probability of non-benign diarrhoea and Table 24.9 describes causes of infectious diarrhoea.

Investigations

Abdominal complaints can represent a spectrum of conditions from benign and self-limited disease to surgical emergencies. Despite an in-depth history and physical exam, many patients may not present 'classically', therefore further diagnostic testing may, in the context of the patient's history, risk factors and physical examination, aid in determining the diagnosis.

Bedside

- *Urinalysis*: Urinalysis is an important screening test for all patients presenting with any type of abdominal pain. Women of childbearing age (even if uncertain about pregnancy status) should have a screening urine pregnancy test, in the setting of abdominal pain.[19] Pregnant women should undergo routine urine screening for the presence of protein, glucose or infection. The purpose for urine testing is to test pH (identifying acid–base disturbances), the presence of glucose (glucosuria, hyperglycaemic states), protein (proteinuria, renal damage), ketones (ketonuria, metabolic anomaly), blood (haematuria, renal damage,

TABLE 24.8 Factors increasing probability of non-benign diarrhoea[125]

FACTOR	SPECIFIC PATHOGEN(S)/OTHER CONSIDERATIONS
Presentation to a healthcare facility	Degree of illness overall greater in patients presenting for evaluation; increased probability of 'not norovirus' aetiology to 50%
Travel history	Especially foreign travel and to endemic areas of dysenteric disease
Recent hospitalisation	*Clostridium difficile* from antibiotic exposure
Day-care attendance	Rotavirus, *Shigella*, *Giardia*
Nursing-home residence	*C. difficile*, medication side effects, tube feedings, ischaemic colitis, faecal impaction and overflow diarrhoea
Wilderness exposure	*Giardia* or *Cryptosporidium*
Antibiotic therapy	*C. difficile*, antibiotic side effects
Raw shellfish, farm animals and show livestock, pet reptiles or amphibians, petting zoos	*Salmonella* spp, *Escherichia coli* O157:H7 and non-O157 Shiga-toxin-producing *E. coli*, *Vibrio* spp.
Epidemic of multiple patients with a short time of onset	Norovirus; less commonly, *Campylobacter jejuni*, *Salmonella* spp, *Cryptosporidium*
Acute vomiting and diarrhoea after suspected contaminated food	*Bacillus cereus*, *Clostridium botulinum*, *Staphylococcus aureus*
Epidemic of severe gastroenteritis traced to eggs, poultry, meat or dairy products	*C. jejuni*, *Salmonella* spp
Oral-anal sexual practices (anilingus)	*Giardia lamblia*, *Entamoeba hystolytica*
Abdominal pain	
Nausea, vomiting	
Bloody stool	
Fever	
Rectal pain	
Tenesmus	Severe bacterial infections: *Salmonella*, *Campylobacter*, *Shigella*, EPEC, *Yersinia* or *Vibrio* spp
Also consider surgical abdomen, GI bleeding	
Inflammatory bowel disease	
Diarrhoea > 7–14 days' duration	Protozoa and microsporidia, *C. difficile*, *Campylobacter*, Shiga-toxin-producing *E. coli*
Haemolytic uraemic syndrome	*E. coli* O157:H7 or other species
Stool WBC count	Not reliable for diagnosis of bacterial aetiology
Colonic ulcerations	Inflammatory bowel disease
Proctitis	Bacterial aetiology highly probable
Pseudomembranes	Toxic megacolon, *C. difficile*
Chronic disease (e.g. cirrhosis, DM)	Complicated course expected with any form of diarrhoeal illness
Organ transplantation	Abnormally severe illness from rotavirus and adenovirus
Increased frequency of cytomegalovirus	
Severe illness from dysenteric diarrhoea	
Spore-forming protozoa and microsporidia	
HIV infection, other immunodeficiency disorders	Severe illness from common bacteria/spore-forming protozoa and microsporidia
Increased frequency of cytomegalovirus and *Mycobacterium avium* complex	

DM: diabetes mellitus; EPEC: enteropathogenic E. coli; HIV: human immunodeficiency virus; WBC, white blood cell

TABLE 24.9 Pathogen-specific syndromes

CAUSATIVE AGENT	INCUBATION PERIOD	DURATION OF ILLNESS	PREDOMINANT SYMPTOMS	FOODS COMMONLY IMPLICATED
Bacteria				
Campylobacter jejuni	3–5 days	2–5 days, occ. > 10 days	Sudden onset of diarrhoea, abdominal pain, nausea, vomiting	Raw or undercooked poultry, raw milk, meat, untreated water
Escherichia coli enteropathogenic, enterotoxigenic, enteroinvasive, enterohaemorrhagic	12–72 hours (enterotoxigenic); longer in others	3–14 days	Severe colicky abdominal pain, watery to profuse diarrhoea, sometimes bloody. May cause haemolytic uraemic syndrome	Many raw foods, unpasteurised milk, contaminated water, minced beef
Salmonella serovars	6–72 hours	3–5 days	Abdominal pain, diarrhoea, chills, fever, malaise	Meat, chicken, eggs and egg products
Shigella spp.	12–96 hours	4–7 days	Malaise, fever, vomiting, diarrhoea commonly with blood and/or mucus	Any contaminated food or water
Yersinia enterocolitica	3–7 days	1–21 days	Acute diarrhoea sometimes bloody, fever, vomiting	Raw meat and poultry, milk and milk products
Vibrio cholerae	Few hours to 5 days	3–4 days	Asymptomatic to profuse dehydrating diarrhoea	Raw seafood, contaminated water
Vibrio parahaemolyticus	12–24 hours	1–7 days	Abdominal pain, moderate diarrhoea/vomiting of moderate severity	Raw and cooked fish, shellfish, other seafoods
Viruses				
Small round structured viruses (SRSVs) such as astrovirus, adenovirus, calicivirus	24–48 hours	12–48 hours	Severe vomiting, diarrhoea	Oysters, clams, other food contaminated by human Norwalk virus, excreta
Rotaviruses	24–72 hours	3–7 days	Malaise, headache, fever, vomiting, diarrhoea	Contaminated water
Parasites				
Cryptosporidium	1–12 days	4–21 days	Profuse watery diarrhoea	Contaminated water and food
Giardia lamblia	1–3 weeks	1–2 weeks to months	Loose pale greasy stools, abdominal pain	Contaminated water, food contaminated by infected food-handlers
Entamoeba histolytica	2–4 weeks	Weeks–months	Colic, mucus or bloody diarrhoea	Contaminated water and food
Toxin-producing bacteria				
Bacillus cereus (toxin in food)	1–6 hours	< 24 hours	Nausea, vomiting, diarrhoea, cramps	Cereals, rice, meat products, soups, vegetables
Clostridium perfringens (toxin in gut)	8–20 hours	24 hours	Sudden-onset colic, diarrhoea	Meats, poultry, stews, gravies (often reheated)
Staphylococcus aureus (toxin in food)	30 mins–8 hours	24 hours	Acute vomiting, purging, may lead to collapse	Cold foods (much-handled during preparation), milk products, salted meats

Victorian Government Department of Health Services. The blue book: guidelines for the control of infectious diseases; 2005.[151] Reproduced with kind permission of the Victorian Government.

coagulopathy), bilirubin (liver and gallbladder states), specific gravity (indication of urine osmolarity), nitrates and leucocytes (markers of infection). The test is simple, quick, inexpensive and may uncover remarkable underlying causes or associated conditions related to the presentation. The test should not be limited to patients with abdominal pain but extended to most patients who pass urine, and more so the unwell patient. Conditions such as diabetes or its complications, urinary tract infections, bleeding disorders, metabolic disturbances, dehydration, renal pathology and pregnancy are some of the important findings that can be revealed upon urinalysis.

> ## PRACTICE TIP
>
> There are many other abdominal causes of pyuria and microhaematuria such as appendicitis, pyelonephritis and renal abscess or tumour.

- *ECG*: Patients experiencing acute coronary artery events may present with a variety of atypical symptoms, some of which manifest as abdominal conditions: epigastric pain, nausea, vomiting and indigestion.[20] Further, atypical acute coronary events may present more frequently in patients aged over 75 years, in women, and in patients with diabetes, chronic renal failure or dementia.[21,22] It is therefore important that an ECG be performed in cases where Acute Coronary Syndrome (ACS) is suspected.
- *Capillary blood sugar*: Patients with diabetic ketoacidosis may present with symptoms and signs imitating the acute abdomen: abdominal pain (especially in children due to gastric distension or stretching of the liver capsule), vomiting, polyuria, polydipsia and diarrhoea.[23]

Laboratory tests

Diagnosing patients who present in the ED with acute abdominal pain is challenging. In addition to history-taking and physical examination, laboratory tests may be required to exclude diagnoses that can mimic acute abdominal pain. Appropriate laboratory test ordering will vary depending upon the clinical presentation;[24] however, the clinical value of most laboratory tests ordered in differentiating surgical from non-surgical abdominal pain is limited. Commonly ordered laboratory tests in the evolution of acute abdominal pain are: full blood count, C-reactive protein, amylase, lipase and liver function tests.

Inflammatory markers, such as white cell count (WCC) and C-reactive protein (CRP), are commonly part of the main battery of tests ordered in ED in the evaluation and differentiation of abdominal pain.[12,25] More recently, procalcitonin (PCT), the pro-hormone form of calcitonin secreted by the extra-thyroid immune cells, has also been promoted as a biomarker in the assessment and diagnosis of abdominal pain.[26,27] The role of WCC, CRP and PCT in differentiating abdominal pain, as exemplified in diagnosing appendicitis, is not perfect and in some instances misleading.[25,26,28–31] Earlier studies[32,33] examining raised WCC found that 10–60% of patients with surgically proven appendicitis had WCCs within the normal range.

More recent studies examining the diagnostic value of WCC, CRP and PCT further demonstrated wide-ranging sensitivity and specificity.[26,34–36] In terms of accuracy, CRP has shown the greatest accuracy followed by WCC and procalcitonin in diagnosing appendicitis.[36] Inflammatory biomarkers have been studied as an aid to differentiating between minor illness and more serious disease. Most of the studies have shown a moderate relationship between raised inflammatory biomarkers and the target condition, but conclude that if used in isolation are insufficient to rule in or out the condition safely.[37]

Serum lipase is the principal biomarker used for diagnosing acute pancreatitis, and has largely replaced amylase in terms of diagnostic value.[38] While both lipase and amylase are produced by the acinar cells of the pancreas, amylase is also produced by the salivary glands, small intestine mucosa, ovaries, placenta, liver and fallopian tubes, thus limiting its sensitivity and specificity in diagnosing pancreatitis.[39] In the setting of acute pancreatitis, both lipase and amylase become elevated at about the same time (4–8 hours), but lipase may rise to a greater extent and remain elevated much longer (7–10 days versus 12–72 hours respectively). The degrees to which serum lipase levels elevate are not proportional to the severity of the disease. Further, in some instances, both serum lipase and amylase levels may be normal in patients with recurrent pancreatitis or alcoholism.[40] These limitations notwithstanding, lipase is the most useful test in patients suspected of pancreatitis.

Liver function tests consist of total bilirubin, conjugated bilirubin, alkaline phosphatase, alanine aminotransferase, aspartate aminotransferase, gamma-glutamyl transpeptidase, serum albumin and serum globulin. The term 'liver function test' is a misnomer as few of the tests actually assess liver function; the majority are based upon some property of the damaged hepatocyte (serum aminotransferases), biliary tract disorder (serum alkaline phosphatase, GGT) or synthetic function (serum albumin and prothrombin time/international normalised ratio). While abnormal liver-enzyme levels may signal liver damage or alternation in bile flow, abnormal results are frequently detected in patients who are asymptomatic.[41] Therefore, the decision to obtain LFTs should be determined in conjunction with information gathered from the history, identification of risk factors and physical examination of the patient.[42] Similarly, interpreting LFT results should be done with reference to this information as well as the pattern of LFT abnormality.[43] LFT abnormalities can often be grouped into one of three patterns: hepatocellular, cholestatic or isolated hyperbilirubinaemia.

Patients presenting with a hepatocellular process (e.g. alcoholic liver disease, hepatotoxicity) generally have a disproportionate elevation in serum aminotransferases compared with alkaline phosphatase (AP), while those with a cholestatic process (e.g. biliary flow obstruction) have the opposite findings. In the setting of cholestasis, whether extrahepatic or intrahepatic biliary obstruction, alkaline phosphatase is typically elevated to at least four times the upper limit of normal.[44] Differentiating between extra- and intrahepatic cholestasis is achieved through right upper quadrant ultrasonography. The presence of biliary dilation on ultrasonography suggests extrahepatic cholestasis (e.g. gallstones, strictures or malignancy). The absence of dilation suggests intrahepatic cholestasis (e.g. primary biliary cirrhosis or viral hepatitis). Lesser degrees of alkaline phosphatase elevation are non-specific and may suggest several other types of liver disease. High serum GGT may also assist in confirming hepatobiliary disease; however, elevated levels can be attributed to a wide variety of other clinical conditions such as pancreatic disease, MI, renal failure, COPD, diabetes, alcoholism and in patients taking phenytoin and barbiturates.[43]

> **PRACTICE TIP**
>
> Normal vital signs, laboratory results, history and physical exam findings are not reassuring in the older patient presenting with abdominal pain. Take the worst-first approach.

Rectal and pelvic examination

The inclusion of digital rectal examination (DRE) in all patients with abdominal pain has a longstanding history as a mainstay component in a complete physical exam,[45–47] despite being unsupported by the literature.[48–50] Studies examining clinicians' use of DRE in the management of acute, undifferentiated abdominal pain in the ED concluded that it contributes no additional information that could not be obtained from history taking and abdominal examination, and further, it has minimal predictive value.[49,51–53]

Pelvic examination is a key part of the evaluation of a women presenting with abdominal pain or vaginal bleeding to the ED. Examining the pelvic organs may yield further information regarding the possible gynaecological or obstetric causes of abdominal pain in women. Pelvic examination begins with inspecting the external genitalia for discharge, erythaemia, ulceration, atrophy, masses and old scars. This is then followed by speculum examination of the cervix and bimanual palpation of the pelvic organs.[9] Consideration of testicular pathology in men presenting with lower abdominal pain is also important (see Chapter 25).

Imaging

Plain X-rays

Abdominal radiography is often requested in ED, but contributes little to patient treatment while exposing patients to significant doses of unnecessary radiation.[54] Current indications for abdominal X-ray are few: suspected bowel obstruction, oesophageal foreign body (chest X-ray to be performed first) and suspected sharp/poisonous foreign body.[54–57] With the exception of these indications, abdominal radiography sensitivity and specificity is poor (23% and 38% respectively) in patients presenting with non-traumatic acute abdominal pain.[58,59] For patients requiring investigation beyond clinical history, physical examination and lab results, the clinician should be encouraged to request more definitive imaging such as ultrasound and CT.

Ultrasound

Ultrasound is a rapid non-invasive examination that does not involve exposing the patient to ionising radiation. Most solid intra-abdominal organs (e.g. liver, spleen, gallbladder, pancreas and kidneys) can be imaged using ultrasound. Focused bedside ultrasound examination has significantly impacted

upon the detection and management of abdominal aortic aneurysm (>3 cm), ectopic pregnancy and in the presence of free-fluid, haemoperitoneum bleeding.[60] Ultrasound sensitivity and specificity is largely operator-dependent; however, patient characteristics such as obesity, bowel gas and surgical emphysema can also reduce image quality. Within the context of the emergency care setting, bedside ultrasound is an appropriate first-line approach to assessing, monitoring and triaging abdominal pain;[61,62] however, further diagnostic modalities may be required, such as computer tomography.

Computer tomography

Computer tomography (CT) imaging has been demonstrated to have a positive effect on the accuracy and certainty in the clinical diagnosis of patients with abdominal pain,[62–65] and direct decisions regarding patient management.[66] However, while CT imaging has been associated with improving timely diagnosis and treatment of patients presenting with abdominal pain, it is costly[67,68] and is a growing source of exposure to radiation in adults.[69,70] The frequency of CT imaging and subsequent exposure to radiation in some instances could be reduced by initially screening abdominal pain patients using ultrasound.[62]

Specific gastrointestinal emergencies

Infection, structural abnormalities or pathological processes may cause GI emergencies. Heredity and lifestyle also play a role. For example, excessive alcohol consumption can lead to GI bleeding, cirrhosis or oesophageal varices. Regardless of aetiology, non-traumatic GI emergencies are a common occurrence in any ED—ranging from minor inconvenience to life-threatening problems. Diseases of the digestive system account for the highest proportion of hospital admissions in Australia.[71]

Gastrointestinal bleeding

Gastrointestinal bleeding is a relatively frequent problem encountered in the ED.[72] The initial triage assessment must gain an understanding of clinical risk based on several factors. Patients at increased risk include age > 60 years, hypotension, tachycardia, the presence of comorbidities and evidence of blood in the vomit or stool. Bleeding can originate anywhere in the GI tract and can occur at any age.[73,74] The age group most often affected is individuals 50–80 years of age. Factors associated with high morbidity rates are haemodynamic instability, repeated haematemesis, haematochezia and a co-existent organ-system disease.[75] Bleeding is functionally categorised by location—upper or lower GI bleeding. Figure 24.8 highlights various sites and causes of GI bleeding. Upper GI bleeding is more common in males,[74] whereas lower GI bleeding is seen more often in females.[73] Patients may have bright-red blood from mouth or rectum or black, tarry stools indicating bleeding from within the GI tract.

Bleeding stops spontaneously in 80% of hospitalised patients.[72] In the initial stages of presentation to the ED, patients suspected of GI bleeding should be initially nil by mouth (NBM) and if the bleeding is significant a nasogastric tube should be passed.[76] This will rest the gut, reduce additional pressure in the stomach and reduce the likelihood of vomiting. If a patient is NBM, consideration must be made

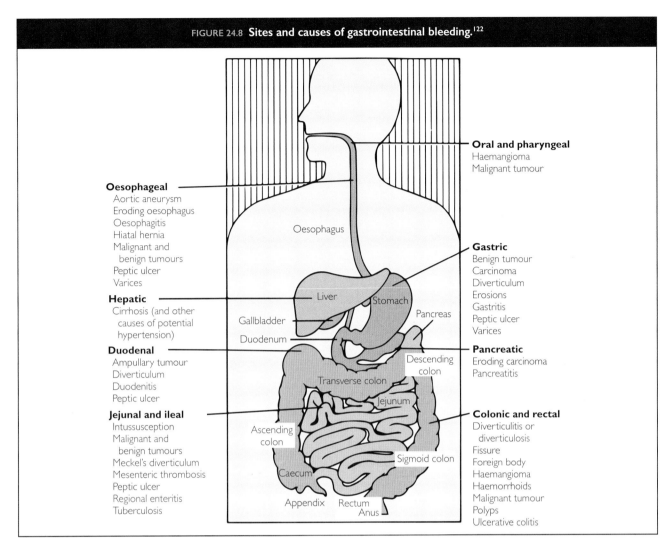

FIGURE 24.8 **Sites and causes of gastrointestinal bleeding.**[122]

to the underlying fluid balance status with supplementation of intravenous (IV) fluids.

Upper gastrointestinal bleeding

Upper GI bleeding refers to blood loss between the upper oesophagus and duodenum at the ligament of Treitz. Bleeding is categorised as variceal or non-variceal. The risk for death is greater with variceal bleeding because of the occurrence of haemorrhage in these patients.[77] Gastro-oesophageal varices are enlarged venous channels and are dilated by portal hypertension. As portal hypertension increases, varices continue to enlarge and eventually rupture, causing massive haemorrhage. Cirrhosis, mainly from alcohol and chronic viral hepatitis, is the most important cause of portal hypertension in the Western world, while schistosomiasis is the leading cause in developing countries.[78] Figure 24.9 highlights systemic manifestations of cirrhosis. Bleeding from varices requires immediate intervention and close observation following initial control of bleeding. More than 40% of patients with variceal bleeds will re-bleed within 48–72 hours.[79] Non-variceal bleeding is due to erosion or ulceration of the oesophageal or gastroduodenal mucosa which extends into an underlying blood vessel.

Peptic ulcer disease is an infectious process caused by *Helicobacter pylori*, and is the most common cause of upper GI bleeding in adults and children.[79] Peptic ulcers account for half of major upper GI bleeding, with a mortality rate of 4%. Improvements in the prevention and management of ulcers are seeing a decline in bleeding complications from ulcers in certain parts of the world. This is perhaps due to control of *H. pylori*, safer use of non-steroidal anti-inflammatory drugs (NSAIDs) and prophylaxis with proton pump inhibitors.[74]

Other causes of upper GI bleeding include: drug-induced erosions (e.g. aspirin); retching and vomiting which cause lacerations in the gastro-oesophageal mucosa (Mallory-Weiss syndrome); vascular anomalies; and gastritis.

Clinical signs and symptoms are variable, and may be life-threatening. They include pallor, dizziness, lethargy, abdominal pain, nausea, vomiting blood or dark 'coffee grounds' (haematemesis) and passing of dark or bright blood in the stool (malaena or haematochezia). Fluid volume status is important to assess, and signs of hypovolaemia such as tachycardia, postural hypotension, dizziness, confusion or syncope may also occur.

Assessment and management
Assessment and management begins with control of the ABCs, and a full assessment of the vital signs including heart rate, blood pressure, baseline mental status or Glasgow Coma Scale

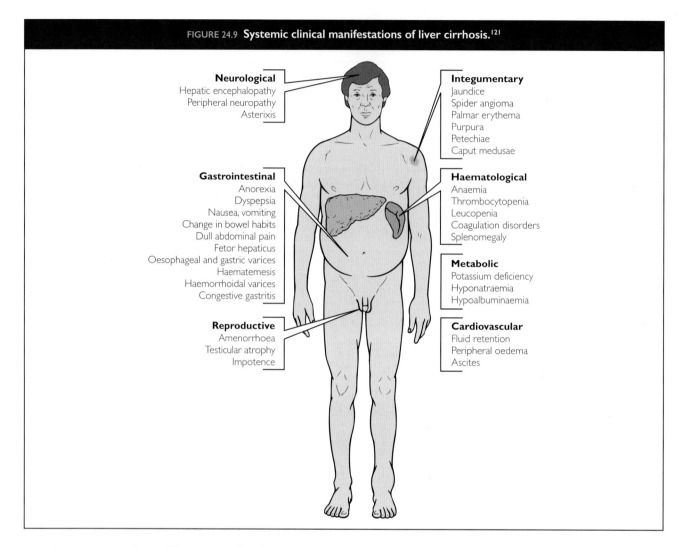

FIGURE 24.9 **Systemic clinical manifestations of liver cirrhosis.**[121]

Neurological
Hepatic encephalopathy
Peripheral neuropathy
Asterixis

Integumentary
Jaundice
Spider angioma
Palmar erythema
Purpura
Petechiae
Caput medusae

Gastrointestinal
Anorexia
Dyspepsia
Nausea, vomiting
Change in bowel habits
Dull abdominal pain
Fetor hepaticus
Oesophageal and gastric varices
Haematemesis
Haemorrhoidal varices
Congestive gastritis

Haematological
Anaemia
Thrombocytopenia
Leucopenia
Coagulation disorders
Splenomegaly

Metabolic
Potassium deficiency
Hyponatraemia
Hypoalbuminaemia

Reproductive
Amenorrhoea
Testicular atrophy
Impotence

Cardiovascular
Fluid retention
Peripheral oedema
Ascites

score (GCS) and capillary refill time (see Ch 14). A thorough approach to observation is vital to understanding trends and responses to treatment. Administer high-flow oxygen via non-rebreather mask for patients with evidence of decreased oxygen saturation. Fluid replacement begins with crystalloid or colloid solutions, followed by blood (packed red blood cells [PRBCs] or whole blood) replacement if the patient's condition does not improve.

Using a cardiac monitor and continuous measurement of heart rate, blood pressure and pulse oximetry is recommended for patients with actual or potential significant blood loss. Be aware that patients with considerable blood loss have lost a large amount of red blood cells and thus oxygen-carrying ability, so are at risk of hypovolaemia and ischaemic conditions such as myocardial infarction. The older patient with poor compensatory mechanisms is further predisposed to ischaemic conditions and can deteriorate rapidly.

A nasogastric tube is recommended for patients with upper GI bleeding. Aspiration of blood or suspicious-coloured dark material confirms a source of bleeding. However, a non-bloodstained return may signify that bleeding is occurring outside the stomach, e.g. the duodenum. Concerns that passage of a nasogastric tube may provoke bleeding are unwarranted.[74]

Monitoring of fluid balance is essential and may involve passing a urinary catheter to monitor output or if oliguria is present. A complete abdominal assessment should involve a rectal examination and testing for faecal occult blood.

Baseline laboratory studies include full blood count (FBC), 'group type and hold' or cross-match (for a minimum of 2 units) depending upon clinical picture, electrolytes, urea, creatinine and serum glucose. Normal creatinine with increased urea suggests bleeding with breakdown of blood in the gut, dehydration or diuretic therapy. Liver function and coagulation studies are also recommended to rule out coagulopathies or liver disease. An upright chest X-ray can provide valuable information if perforation is suspected; however, this is not feasible if significant haemodynamic compromise is present. An electrocardiogram (ECG) should be obtained to assess for dysrhythmias or ischaemic changes related to blood loss.

Treatment modalities include endoscopy to identify the source of bleeding and control if needed, medications and surgical interventions. Medical therapy for non-variceal bleeding includes administration of proton pump inhibitors, antacids and H$_2$ antagonists (Table 24.10). If, on endoscopy, a bleeding ulcer is detected, it is often managed by an adrenaline injection or cautery into the base of the lesion and a proton pump inhibitor.[74] Gastro-oesophageal variceal bleeding is treated with balloon tamponade (e.g. Sengstaken-Blakemore tube) or one of the variants to control bleeding. Peptic ulcer disease is treated endoscopically with thermal coagulation or injection therapy,

TABLE 24.10 Drug therapy in gastrointestinal (GI) bleeding[123]

DRUG	SOURCE OF GI BLEEDING	MECHANISM OF ACTION
Antacids	Duodenal ulcer, gastric ulcer, acute gastritis (corrosive, erosive and haemorrhagic)	Neutralises acid and maintains gastric pH above 5.5; elevated pH inhibits activation of pepsinogen
H_2-receptor antagonists Cimetidine Famotidine Nizatidine Ranitidine	Duodenal ulcer, gastric ulcer, oesophagitis, acute gastritis (especially haemorrhagic)	Inhibits action of histamine at H_2 receptors on parietal cells and decreases HCl secretion
Proton pump inhibitors Omeprazole Esomeprazole Lansoprazole Pantoprazole		Inhibits activity of proton pump and binds to hydrogen–potassium ATP at secretory surface of gastric parietal cell, blocking gastric acid production
Vasopressin	Oesophageal varices	Causes vasoconstriction and increases smooth muscle activity of the GI tract; reduces pressure in the portal circulation and arrests bleeding
Octreotide	Upper gastrointestinal bleeding, oesophageal varices	Somatostatin analogue that decreases splanchnic blood flow; decreases HCl secretion via decrease in release of gastrin

ATP: adenosine triphosphate; HCl: hydrochloric acid.

whereas gastro-oesophageal varices are treated endoscopically with injection sclerotherapy or variceal band ligation. Endoscopic procedures may be done on a limited basis in EDs across the country. Surgical intervention may be necessary for variceal or non-variceal bleeding.

Complications related to upper GI bleeding include aspiration, pneumonia, respiratory failure and hypovolaemic shock. Maintain NBM patients with attention to mouth care.

Lower GI bleeding

Lower GI bleeding is bleeding that occurs below the ligament of Treitz. Common causes are haemorrhoids, diverticulitis (diverticular disease), angiodysplasia, colonic polyps, colon cancer or colitis. Diverticulitis and angiodysplasia are common causes of lower GI bleeding in the older patient, whereas haemorrhoids, anal fissures and inflammatory bowel disease occur most often in younger patients. Diverticulitis refers to pouch-like herniations on the colon (Fig 24.10). What initially appears to be lower bleeding may in fact often be upper GI bleeding. Consideration should always be given to conditions of the upper GI tract when assessing patients with GI bleeding.

Haemorrhoids are the most common aetiology of lower GI bleeding.[73] Figure 24.11 depicts internal and external haemorrhoidal veins, where haemorrhoids often erupt. Internal haemorrhoids are rarely associated with pain, whereas external haemorrhoids can cause significant discomfort.

Assessment and management

Eighty-five per cent of patients with lower GI bleeding experience acute bleeds that are self-limiting and do not cause significant changes in haemodynamic status. Most patients with mild lower GI bleeding who are haemodynamically

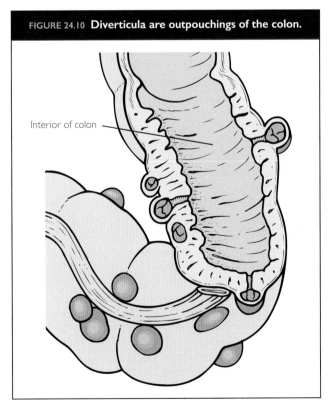

FIGURE 24.10 Diverticula are outpouchings of the colon.

Interior of colon

When they become inflamed, the condition is diverticulitis. The inflammatory process can spread to the surrounding area in the intestine.[121]

FIGURE 24.11 Anatomical structures of the rectum and anus with internal and external haemorrhoids.[123]

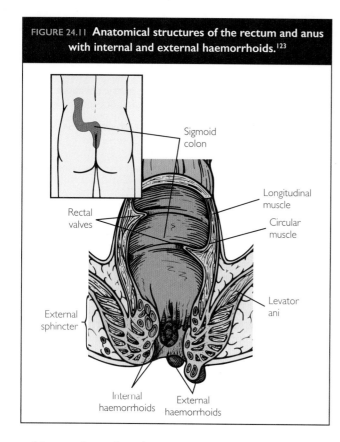

Sigmoid colon

Longitudinal muscle

Circular muscle

Rectal valves

Levator ani

External sphincter

Internal haemorrhoids

External haemorrhoids

BOX 24.1 Factors affecting lower oesophageal sphincter pressure[123]

INCREASE PRESSURE	
Bethanechol	Metoclopramide
DECREASE PRESSURE	
Alcohol	Tea, coffee (caffeine)
Anticholinergics	Beta-adrenergic blockers
Chocolate (theobromine)	Calcium channel blockers
Fatty foods	Diazepam
Nicotine	Morphine sulfate
Peppermint, spearmint	Nitrates
Progesterone	Theophylline

stable may be evaluated on an outpatient basis. Treatment includes identifying the source of bleeding with anoscopy, flexible sigmoidoscopy or barium enema. Patients with severe symptomatic lower GI bleeding require hospital admission for resuscitation, diagnosis and treatment. Colonoscopy may be performed to determine the source of bleeding after the patient is stabilised.[73]

The cardinal sign of lower GI bleeding is haematochezia. Patients may have bright blood or maroon stools, or there may be occult blood in the stool. Cramp-like abdominal pain may be present. Explosive diarrhoea with foul odour is frequently present. Painless bleeding also occurs. Pallor, diaphoresis and decreased capillary refill are present with significant bleeding. Postural changes in pulse or BP occur in many patients. Pedal oedema can occur with chronic bleeding because of protein depletion. The first priority is management of the ABCs and full assessment of the vital signs. Patients with signs or symptoms of hypovolaemia require immediate intervention, high-flow oxygen, ECG, BP and oxygen saturation monitoring, large-bore IV access and fluid resuscitation. Vigilant monitoring of fluid balance status is essential.

Baseline laboratory studies include FBC, platelet count and coagulation studies. Administration of PRBCs may be necessary in cases of significant blood loss. Determining the source of bleeding is a priority. Colonoscopy, bleeding scans or angiography may be performed, with surgical intervention required in some cases.

Gastro-oesophageal reflux disease

Transient gastro-oesophageal reflux is a normal physiological event that occurs at various intervals without causing disease or symptoms. Rosen suggests that it occurs daily in 7% of patients

and at least monthly in 15%.[80] Regardless, those who experience an increased frequency of reflux will experience some type of symptoms. Reflux disease is common in Australia. Between 15% and 20% of adults experience heartburn and indigestion each week, and it is estimated that the prevalence of general-practitioner-diagnosed GORD in Australia is approximately 10% of patients attending GPs.[81] Conditions associated with GORD are decreased lower oesophageal sphincter (LOS) pressure, decreased oesophageal motility and increased gastric emptying time. Box 24.1 lists specific causes for each situation. It is of interest that acid secretion does not increase in patients with GORD.

Assessment and management

Chest pain or heartburn is the most common symptom associated with this condition. Patients experience a variance of pain or discomfort ranging from mild to quite severe. Relaxation of the LOS during pregnancy increases the occurrence of heartburn during pregnancy; at least 25% of pregnant women experience daily heartburn. Chest pain as the only symptom of GORD is reported in 10% of patients with the disease.[82] A key aspect of pain associated with GORD is that it radiates, usually to the neck, jaws, shoulders, arms and abdomen. Similarities to the clinical presentation of ischaemic heart disease require thoughtful consideration. It is often difficult to distinguish between these very different conditions in the ED. The healthcare professional should pay close attention to the appearance of the patient, the history, clinical assessment and changes in vital signs and clinical condition. Characteristics unique to GORD include worsening of symptoms with stooping, lying or leaning forward. Other symptoms associated with GORD are summarised in Box 24.2.

Consider the classic presentation for ischaemic heart disease, and note the similarities and differences in presentation of patients who present with epigastric discomfort or chest pain of a GI origin. This is an important consideration, as both may have very similar presentations and symptoms, although one is immediately life-threatening while the other is not. Therefore, management of GORD in the emergency

---

BOX 24.2 Clinical symptoms of GORD

TYPICAL	ATYPICAL
Chest pain	Non-cardiac chest pain
Heartburn	Asthma
Dysphagia	Persistent cough
Odynophagia	Hiccups
Regurgitation	Hoarseness
Water brash	Frequent throat clearing
Belching	Nocturnal choking
Early satiety	Sleep apnoea
Nausea	Recurrent pneumonia
Anorexia	Recurrent ENT infections
Weight loss	Loss of dental enamel
	Halitosis

ENT: ear–nose–throat; GORD: gastro-oesophageal reflux disease

---

sense begins with elimination of other conditions that are more lethal (e.g. myocardial infarction).[82,83] Vital signs must be obtained, with the regularity of observations dependent on the clinical picture. Patient assessment and studies such as ECG, chest radiograph and pathology investigations are primarily used to rule out other conditions. Additional imaging studies include endoscopy and barium studies. Specific treatment in the ED includes symptomatic relief through use of antacids, H_2 blockers and other medications.[82,83] Antacids are given with viscous lignocaine to increase effectiveness. Table 24.11 highlights specific medications and their actions.

Achalasia (cardiospasm)

In achalasia, peristalsis of the lower two-thirds (smooth muscle) of the oesophagus is absent. Pressure in the LOS is increased, along with incomplete relaxation of the sphincter. Obstruction of the oesophagus at or near the diaphragm occurs. Food and fluid accumulate in the lower oesophagus.[80] The result of the condition is dilation of the lower oesophagus (Fig 24.12). The altered peristalsis is a result of impairment of the neurons that innervate the lower oesophagus. There is a selective loss of inhibitory neurons, resulting in unopposed excitation of the LOS. Achalasia affects all ages and both genders. The course of the disease is chronic. It is linked to increased incidence of carcinoma, possibly secondary to food stasis.

Assessment and management

Dysphagia (difficulty in swallowing) is the most common symptom and occurs with both liquids and solids.[84] Patients may report a globus sensation (a lump in the throat). Substernal chest pain (similar to the pain of angina) occurs during or immediately after a meal. Halitosis (foul-smelling breath) and the inability to eructate (belch) are other symptoms. Another common symptom is regurgitation of sour-tasting food and liquids, especially when the patient is in the horizontal position. Patients with achalasia may also report symptoms of GORD (e.g. heartburn).[82] Weight loss is typical.

Diagnosis is usually by radiological studies, manometric studies of the lower oesophagus and endoscopy. The exact

---

TABLE 24.11 Drug therapy for GORD[123]

MECHANISM OF ACTION	EXAMPLES
Increase LOS pressure	
Cholinergic	Bethanechol chloride
Dopamine antagonist	Metoclopramide
	Cisapride
Serotonin antagonist	
Neutralise acid	
Antacids	Alka-Seltzer: $NaHCO_3$ and/or $KHCO_3$
	Andrews Antacid: $CaCO_3$, $MgCO_3$
	Equate: $Al(OH)_3$ and $Mg(OH)_2$
	Gaviscon: $Al(OH)_3$
	Maalox (liquid): $Al(OH)_3$ and $Mg(OH)_2$
	Maalox (tablet): $CaCO_3$
	Milk of magnesia: $Mg(OH)_2$
	Pepto Bismol: $C_7H_5BiO_4$
	Pepto-Bismol Children's: $CaCO_3$
	Rolaids: $CaCO_3$ and $Mg(OH)_2$
	Tums: $CaCO_3$
	Mylanta: contains $Al(OH)_3$
	Eno
	Gelusil (tablet, syrup)
	Alusil MPS (tablet)
Antisecretory	
Histamine H_2-receptor antagonists	Ranitidine
	Cimetidine
	Famotidine
	Nizatidine
Proton pump inhibitors	Esomeprazole
	Omeprazole
	Lansoprazole
	Pantoprazole
	Rabeprazole
Cytoprotective	
Alginic acid antacid	Gaviscon: contains alginic acid and $NaHCO_3$
Antacids	Gelusil, Mylanta
Acid-protective	Sucralfate

LOS: lower oesophageal sphincter; $Al(OH)_3$: aluminium hydroxide; $C_7H_5BiO_4$: bismuth subsalicylate; $CaCO_3$: calcium carbonate; $KHCO_3$: potassium bicarbonate; $MgCO_3$: magnesium carbonate; $Mg(OH)_2$: magnesium hydroxide; $NaHCO_3$: sodium bicarbonate

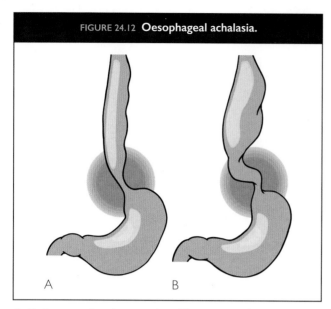

FIGURE 24.12 **Oesophageal achalasia.**

A, Early stage, showing tapering of lower oesophagus.
B, Advanced stage, showing dilated, tortuous oesophagus.[123]

cause of achalasia is not known, so treatment is focused on symptoms. Treatment consists of dilation surgery and the use of drugs. Drug therapy is used to manage early achalasia when there is no significant dilation. Drug therapy is used as a short-term measure and is considered as an alternative only in patients unfit to undergo surgery. Drugs used in management of achalasia include anticholinergics, calcium channel blockers (e.g. nifedipine) and long-acting nitrates, which act by relaxing the smooth muscle.[83]

Appendicitis

Obstruction of the appendiceal opening decreases blood supply and leads to bacterial invasion. Untreated, inflammation progresses so that the appendix becomes non-viable and gangrenous; at worst it may eventually lead to a rupture into the peritoneal space.[85] Appendicitis affects both sexes and all ages, is most common in the 10- to 30-year age range and rarely occurs in infants less than 2 years old. Appendicitis is the most common problem requiring surgery in children. Approximately 6% of the population develops appendicitis in their lifetime. One in 2200 pregnant women develops appendicitis, making it the most common surgical procedure during pregnancy.[80] Surgical removal of the appendix was first documented in 1735.[80]

Assessment and management
Patients may have abdominal pain or abdominal cramping, nausea, vomiting, tachycardia, malaise and anorexia. Chills and fever also occur. Abdominal pain may be initially diffuse and periumbilical and may later become intense and localised to the lower right quadrant. Classic pain associated with appendicitis is located in the right iliac fossa (inside the iliac crest at McBurney's point). Older patients are often afebrile and do not exhibit this classic pain. Pressure on the lower left abdomen intensifies pain in the right lower quadrant (Rovsing's sign).[86] Pain may not always occur in this classic location because of normal variations in the location of the appendix. The position of comfort for most patients is supine with hips

and knees flexed. Women may exhibit tenderness when the cervix is moved.[80,83]

If the appendix ruptures, peritoneal signs increase and involuntary guarding develops. Increased fever and rebound tenderness occur. Diagnosis is made by assessment of clinical signs and symptoms in tandem with physical examination. Diagnostic data may demonstrate an elevation of white blood cell (WBC) count with increased neutrophils, though this is not invariable.[84] Ultrasound may occasionally demonstrate an enlarged appendix or collection of periappendicial fluid, with 88–100% sensitivity and a specificity approaching 100%.[76] Urinalysis should be performed to rule out GU problems and pregnancy in women of childbearing age. CT has been used effectively in certain patients, but its broad use as a diagnostic tool for appendicitis has not been established.

Definitive therapy for appendicitis is surgical intervention, with laparoscopic surgery as the preferred method. Obtain IV access, administer prophylactic broad-spectrum antibiotic if clinically indicated, intravenous analgesia and instruct the patient to be NBM. Complications such as perforation, peritonitis and abscess formation can occur when treatment is delayed.

Cholecystitis

Inflammation of the gallbladder (cholecystitis) causes distension as the cystic duct becomes obstructed. Bacterial invasion, usually by *Escherichia coli*, *Streptococcus* or *Salmonella*, also causes cholecystitis. The most common cause of biliary colic and cholecystitis is cholelithiasis (gallstones). Gallstones arise from the precipitation of cholesterol and calcium salts in saturated bile.[87] It is estimated that between 2% and 12% of patients suffering cholecystitis do not have gallstones.[80] Gallbladder disease is a significant condition affecting Australians: over 70,000 people are hospitalised each year for illness relating to the gallbladder and biliary tree.[15] Cholecystitis usually affects obese, fair-skinned women of increasing age and parity. The female population is affected 3:1 with respect to males.[87]

Assessment and management
Symptoms include sudden-onset abdominal pain—usually after ingestion of fried or fatty foods.[84] Pain may radiate from the epigastrium to the right upper quadrant or may be referred to the right supraclavicular area. Patients usually describe pain as colicky or intermittent in nature, waxing and waning in intensity. The symptoms are experienced when the gallbladder is contracting against an obstruction.[88] Eventual accumulation of fluid and bacterial proliferation may result. Local and rebound tenderness may also be present. Marked tenderness and inspiratory limitation on deep palpation under the right subcostal margin (Murphy's sign) may also be present. Low-grade fever (38°C), tachycardia, nausea, vomiting and flatulence are common findings.[80] If the common bile duct is obstructed, the patient may appear slightly jaundiced, with a history of pale stools. Untreated and progressive worsening of the condition may lead to deterioration, with a clinical picture of bacteraemia and sepsis. Table 24.12 highlights clinical signs associated with obstructed bile flow.

Diagnostic tests include urinalysis, FBC, serum electrolytes, urea, creatinine, serum glucose and serum bilirubin levels; however, results may be non-specific. Elevated amylase suggests

TABLE 24.12 Clinical manifestations caused by obstructed bile flow[123]

CLINICAL MANIFESTATION	AETIOLOGY
Obstructive jaundice	No bile flow into duodenum
Dark amber urine, which foams when shaken	Soluble bilirubin in urine
No urobilinogen in urine	No bilirubin reaching small intestine to be converted to urobilinogen
Clay-coloured stools	As above
Pruritus	Deposition of bile salts in skin tissues
Intolerance for fatty foods (nausea, sensation of fullness, anorexia)	No bile in small intestine for fat digestion
Bleeding tendencies	Lack of or decreased absorption of vitamin K, resulting in decreased production of prothrombin
Steatorrhoea	No bile salts in duodenum, preventing fat emulsion and digestion

BOX 24.3 Drug-induced pancreatitis[125]

DEFINITE

Azathioprine	Tetracycline
Cisplatin	Thiazides
Frusemide	Sulfonamides
Colapase	

PROBABLE

Paracetamol	Mefenamic acid
Cimetidine	Opiates
Oestrogens	Sodium valproate
Indomethacin	

POSSIBLE

Bumetanide	Isoniazid
Carbamazepine	Isotretinoin
Chlorthalidone	Methyldopa
Clonidine	Metronidazole
Colchicine	Nitrofurantoin
Corticosteroids	Pentamidine
Cyclosporin	Piroxicam
Cytarabine	Procainamide
Enalapril	Rifampicin
Ergotamine	Salicylates
Ethacrynic acid	Sulindac

pancreatitis rather than cholecystitis.[79] Leucocytosis may be mild to pronounced. Ultrasound is sensitive, specific and extremely useful in the emergency setting for detection of a thickened gallbladder wall and gallstones. An ECG should be obtained to exclude the presentation with cardiac involvement. A cardiac cause should be considered especially in patients with significant risk factors such as age, smoking, hyperlipidaemia, hypertension or previous cardiac pathology. Additional differentials include renal calculi, pancreatitis, gastritis and ulcer disease.[80]

Treatment of cholecystitis includes administration of IV crystalloid solution and medications for nausea and vomiting. A nasogastric tube may be necessary for gastric decompression. Monitor vital signs and intake and output. Broad-spectrum antibiotics are indicated if microbial infection is suspected. Narcotic analgesics are recommended for pain control. Definitive treatment for cholecystitis is surgery with traditional laparotomy or laparoscopic cholecystectomy.[87]

Acute pancreatitis

Acute pancreatitis results from inflammation of the pancreas.[89] Causes of acute pancreatitis are variable, and include: bile or duodenal reflux, bacterial infection, pancreatic enzyme activation with autolysis and ductal hypertension. Some 70–80% of pancreatitis cases are due to biliary disease with probable obstruction of the common bile duct resulting in ductal hypertension and pancreatic enzyme activation.[80] Alcohol abuse causes toxic metabolites that injure the pancreas, leading to inflammation. Other causes include chronic hypercalcaemia, surgery, abdominal trauma, infections (mumps, cytomegalovirus infection), drugs, toxins

(organophosphate insecticides) or endoscopic retrograde cholangiopancreatography.[90] More than 85 drugs have been identified as causative agents for pancreatitis (Table 24.3).[125]

There exist both similarities and distinct differences between acute and chronic pancreatitis. Acute pancreatitis, with a mortality rate of <5%, may occur as isolated or recurring attacks where the gland is normal before the attack, returning to normal after the episode. In severe pancreatitis, there is pronounced inflammation, tissue necrosis and hemorrhaging of the gland, which gives rise to a systemic inflammatory response; the mortality rate is 10 to 50%.[91] After 5 to 7 days, necrotic pancreatic tissue can become infected by enteric bacteria. In contrast, chronic pancreatitis results in permanent structural changes to the pancreas which impair the endocrine and exocrine functions of the gland.[6,90]

Regardless of mechanism, pancreatitis is characterised by acinar cell damage that leads to necrosis, oedema and inflammation. Acute pancreatitis affects 1.5 people per 100,000 population, but varies with the population.[92] Pancreatitis is the second most frequent pancreatic emergency seen in the ED, a frequency exceeded only by diabetes mellitus.[6,90] (See also Ch 26.)

Assessment and management

A clinical hallmark in 95% of patients with pancreatitis is abdominal pain originating in the epigastric region and radiating to the back. Abdominal tenderness, rebound and guarding are usually present. Nausea, vomiting and abdominal distension may be present. Patients may be febrile with tachycardia, tachypnoea and hypotension. Decreased gastric motility causes hypoactive or absent bowel sounds. The presence of Cullen's or Turner's sign resulting from acute pancreatitis is associated with a mortality estimate of nearly 40%.

Certain laboratory values can aid in diagnosis of acute pancreatitis (Table 24.13). An elevated serum lipase level, and to some lesser degree raised amylase levels, is pathognomonic for pancreatitis. Serum lipase is considered a more sensitive marker as it is only produced by the pancreas and persists after the onset of the attack. Lipase concentrations rise within 4–8 hours of the attack, peak at 24 hours and return to normal after 8–14 days.[6,90] Leucocytosis, decreased haematocrit, hyperglycaemia and glucosuria may also be present.[89] Continuing decreases in haematocrit suggest haemorrhagic pancreatitis. Persistent hypocalcaemia is associated with poor prognosis.[76] Serum amylase may be normal in patients with pancreatitis related to alcohol abuse or elevated triglycerides, or if testing is delayed. Amylase is a small molecule rapidly cleared by the kidneys, therefore abnormally high levels in acute pancreatitis may be short-lived. Conversely, in patients with renal disease, a higher threshold of the upper normal values should be considered.

Radiographic studies are useful. A chest X-ray may reveal pleural effusions or pulmonary infiltrates, and the ileus may be detected on abdominal X-ray. Abdominal ultrasound can allow visualisation of dilated pancreatic ducts, ascites or the presence of gallstones as an underlying cause. An abdominal CT scan may also contribute to the diagnosis of acute pancreatitis by identification of pancreatic oedema or fluid around the pancreas.[76,90]

Management includes maintaining strict NBM status. Obtain IV access for fluid and electrolyte replacement with balanced salt solution to ensure renal perfusion. Antiemetics are administered for nausea and vomiting, and to minimise further fluid loss. Pain control is a high priority for the patient with pancreatitis. Table 24.14 highlights drugs used for management of acute and chronic pancreatitis.

Nasogastric suction helps alleviate nausea, vomiting and abdominal distension. Ongoing monitoring of respiratory, cardiovascular and renal functions and fluid balance is recom-

mended.[84] Prophylactic administration of antibiotics should be considered.

Acute pancreatitis is a serious condition with significant

TABLE 24.14 Drug therapy in acute and chronic pancreatitis[6,123]

DRUG	MECHANISM OF ACTION
Acute pancreatitis	
Morphine, fentanyl	Relief of pain
Glyceryl trinitrate or papaverine	Relaxation of smooth muscles and relief of pain
Antispasmodics (e.g. propantheline bromide)	Decrease of vagal stimulation, motility, pancreatic outflow (inhibition of volume and concentration of bicarbonate and enzymatic secretion); contraindicated in paralytic ileus
Carbonic anhydrase inhibitor (acetazolamide)	Reduction in volume and bicarbonate concentration of pancreatic secretion
Antacids	Neutralisation of gastric HCl secretion and subsequent decrease in secretin, which stimulates production and secretion of pancreatic secretions
Proton pump inhibitors	Decrease in HCl secretion (HCl stimulates pancreatic activity)
Insulin	Treatment of hyperglycaemia
Chronic pancreatitis	
Pancreatin, pancrelipase	Replacement therapy for pancreatic enzymes
Insulin	Treatment for diabetes mellitus if it occurs or for hyperglycaemia

HCl: hydrochloric acid.

TABLE 24.13 Diagnostic studies for acute pancreatitis[6,123]

LABORATORY TEST	ABNORMAL FINDING	AETIOLOGY
Primary tests		
Serum amylase	Increased	Pancreatic cell injury
Serum lipase	Elevated	Pancreatic cell injury
Urinary amylase	Elevated	Pancreatic cell injury
Secondary tests		
Blood glucose	Hyperglycaemia	Impairment of carbohydrate metabolism resulting from beta-cell damage and release of glucagons
Serum calcium	Hypocalcaemia	Saponification of calcium by fatty acids in areas of fat necrosis
Serum triglycerides	Hyperlipidaemia	Release of free fatty acids by lipase

mortality. Severe and life-threatening complications with acute pancreatitis are pleural effusion, fluid loss, abscess formation, jaundice, acute renal failure and adult respiratory distress syndrome. Respiratory complications can occur in 30–50% of patients.[80] Significant hypovolaemia can lead to hypovolaemic shock and ischaemia of lungs, heart and kidneys. Electrolyte imbalances such as hyperglycaemia and hypocalcaemia also occur. Septic complications include formation of pancreatic abscesses.[89]

Diverticulitis

Diverticula are small pouches that develop in the large intestines secondary to ageing (see Fig 24.10). Diverticular disease accounts for over 42,000 hospitalisations per year in Australia; it affects more women than men.[71] Weakened areas that predispose the colon to herniation of inferior tissue layers in combination with a low-fibre diet lead to this primarily painless disorder.[85] Fewer than 10% of patients with diverticulosis experience pain. However, pain is the most-reported complaint when diverticula become inflamed and diverticulitis develops. Inflammation develops when faecal material is trapped in the pouches, causing trauma to the intestinal lining, which ultimately leads to inflammation. Persistent pain associated with diverticulitis is localised in the left lower quadrant.[76] Fever, chills, nausea and vomiting are seen when infection is present; other symptoms include cramping and constipation. The older, those on corticosteroids and patients who are immunosuppressed may have an unremarkable clinical examination. Complications of diverticulitis include intestinal obstruction, haemorrhage, perforation, abscess, stricture and fistula.[83,86]

Assessment and management

Diagnostic evaluation includes FBC and urinalysis. Results of the FBC show a left shift resulting from infection. The presence of WBCs and RBCs in urine is also a common finding. Supine and upright abdominal X-rays are obtained to rule out perforation or obstruction.[93] Abdominal CT is the preferred diagnostic modality because it is more effective in identification of processes outside the colon's lumen (i.e. diverticulitis).[94] Barium enema, endoscopy and ultrasonography may also be used.

Treatment of patients with diverticulitis includes rehydration with a saline solution, resting the bowel by making the patient NBM and inserting a gastric tube if persistent vomiting is present.[85] Anticholinergics are used to reduce colonic spasms, with opiates reserved for more-aggressive pain management. Oral or parenteral antibiotics may be given depending on clinical presentation. Emergency surgery is required when there is evidence of peritonitis.[95]

Ulcerative colitis

Ulcerative colitis is characterised by inflammation and ulceration of the colon and rectum. It may occur at any age, but peaks between the ages of 15 and 25 years. There is a second, smaller, peak of onset between 60 and 80 years of age. Ulcerative colitis affects both genders equally.[86]

The inflammation of ulcerative colitis is diffuse and involves the mucosa and submucosa, with alternating periods of exacerbation and remission. The disease usually begins in the rectum and sigmoid colon and extends up the colon in a continuous pattern. The ulcerations also destroy the mucosal epithelium, causing bleeding and diarrhoea.[85] Losses of fluid and electrolytes occur because of the decreased mucosal surface area for absorption. Breakdown of cells results in protein loss through the stools. Areas of inflamed mucosa form pseudopolyps that have the appearance of tongue-like projections into the bowel lumen.[94] Granulation tissue develops and the mucosal musculature becomes thickened, shortening the colon. Although the precipitating factors involved in ulcerative colitis are poorly understood, it is clear that, once initiated, the inflammatory response is involved.

Assessment and management

Ulcerative colitis may appear as an acute fulminating crisis or, more commonly, as a chronic disorder with mild to severe acute exacerbations that occur at unpredictable intervals over many years.[85] The major symptoms of ulcerative colitis are bloody diarrhoea and abdominal pain. Pain may vary from the mild lower abdominal cramping associated with diarrhoea to severe, constant abdominal pain that may be associated with perforations. In severe cases, diarrhoea is bloody, contains mucus and occurs 10–20 times per day. In addition, fever, weight loss, tachycardia and dehydration are present.[86]

Diagnostic studies include full blood count (FBC), serum electrolyte levels and serum protein level. The FBC typically shows iron-deficiency anaemia from blood loss. An elevated WCC may indicate toxic megacolon or perforation. A decrease in serum electrolyte levels, such as sodium, potassium, chloride, bicarbonate and magnesium, are due to fluid and electrolyte losses from diarrhoea and vomiting.[76] Hypoalbuminaemia is present in severe cases and is due to protein loss from the bowel. The stool should be examined for blood and pus; a sample should be cultured to rule out an infectious cause of inflammation. Drug therapy is an extremely important aspect of treatment (see Table 24.15).

Crohn's disease

Crohn's disease is a chronic, non-specific inflammatory bowel disorder of unknown origin that can affect any part of the GI tract from the mouth to anus. Crohn's disease may occur at any age but occurs most often between the ages of 15 and 30 years. When it occurs in older adults, the morbidity and mortality rates are higher because of other chronic problems that may be present. Both genders are affected, with higher incidences in women. The incidence of Crohn's disease is slightly lower than that of ulcerative colitis.[86]

Crohn's disease is characterised by inflammation of segments of the GI tract. It can affect any part of the GI tract but is most often seen in the terminal ileum, jejunum and colon. Involvement of the oesophagus, stomach and duodenum is rare. The inflammation involves all the layers of the bowel wall; the radiographic appearance in some patients with Crohn's disease is a section of normal bowel interspersed with segments of affected bowel (skip lesions).[80] Typically, ulcerations are deep and longitudinal, and penetrate between islands of inflamed oedematous mucosa, causing a classic cobblestone appearance. Thickening of the bowel wall occurs, as well as narrowing of the lumen with stricture development. The area of inflammation can extend through all the layers of the bowel wall. Abscesses or fistula tracts that communicate with other loops of bowel, skin, bladder, rectum or vagina may develop.[83]

The manifestation of the disease depends largely on the anatomical site of involvement, extent of the disease process and presence or absence of complications. The onset of Crohn's disease is usually insidious, with non-specific complaints such as diarrhoea, fatigue, abdominal pain, weight loss and fever.

Assessment and management
Crohn's disease is a chronic disorder with unpredictable periods of recurrence and remission. Attacks are intermittent and subside spontaneously, usually recurring over a period of several weeks to months, with diarrhoea and abdominal pain which can be quite debilitating.[94] During a period of pain and inflammation, it is important to rest the GI tract and initially, in the acute phase, this may mean a short period of fasting or fluids only. During recovery, particular attention needs to be focused on a diet which is light and non-irritating.

Diagnosis of Crohn's disease can be made by means of a thorough history and physical assessment to establish clinical signs and symptoms. Barium studies will show characteristic inflammatory studies. Laboratory studies may determine electrolyte disturbance and presence of anaemia. Treat symptoms while in the ED, arrange for appropriate follow-up, discharge information and resource access to modify lifestyle or dietary approach, should this be necessary. Drug therapy for Crohn's disease is presented in Table 24.15.

Bowel obstruction

Bowel obstruction occurs in either sex, at any age, and from a variety of causes.[6] The most common cause is adhesions from previous abdominal surgery, followed by incarcerated inguinal hernia.[5] Other causes include foreign bodies, volvulus, intussusception, strictures, tumours, congenital adhesive bands, faecal impaction, gallstones and haematomas (Fig 24.13).

Bowel obstructions are classified as mechanical or non-mechanical.

- Mechanical obstruction results from a disorder outside the intestines or blockage inside the lumen of the intestines (Fig 24.14A and B). Intussusception, telescoping of the bowel within itself by peristalsis, is an example of a mechanical obstruction (Fig 24.15). Figure 24.16 is a radiographic illustration of a small bowel obstruction.

TABLE 24.15 Drug therapy in inflammatory bowel disease[125]

CATEGORY	ACTION	EXAMPLES
Antimicrobials	Prevent or treat secondary infection	Metronidazole
5-aminosalicylic acid (5-ASA)	Decrease GI inflammation*	Systemic Sulfasalazine Mesalazine Olsalazine Rectal suppository Sulfasalazine
Corticosteroids	Decrease inflammation	Systemic: corticosteroids (cortisone, prednisolone, budesonide) Enemas: prednisone Rectal suppository: prednisone
Anticholinergics	Decrease GI motility and secretions and relieve smooth-muscle spasms†	Propantheline bromide
Sedatives	Reduce anxiety and restlessness	Diazepam
Antidiarrhoeals	Decrease GI motility†	Diphenoxylate
Immunosuppressants	Suppress immune response	Azathioprine, cyclosporin
Immunomodulators	Inhibit the cytokine tumour necrosis factor-alpha (TNF-α) Block lymphocyte adhesion to blood vessel walls and subsequent migration into tissues	Infliximab
Haematinics and vitamins	Correct iron-deficiency anaemia and promote healing	Oral ferrous sulfate, ferrous gluconate; iron polymaltose injection Vitamin B$_{12}$, zinc

GI, gastrointestinal

Mechanism of action unknown, possibly antimicrobial, as well as antiinflammatory.

†Used with caution during severe disease because of potential to produce toxic megacolon.

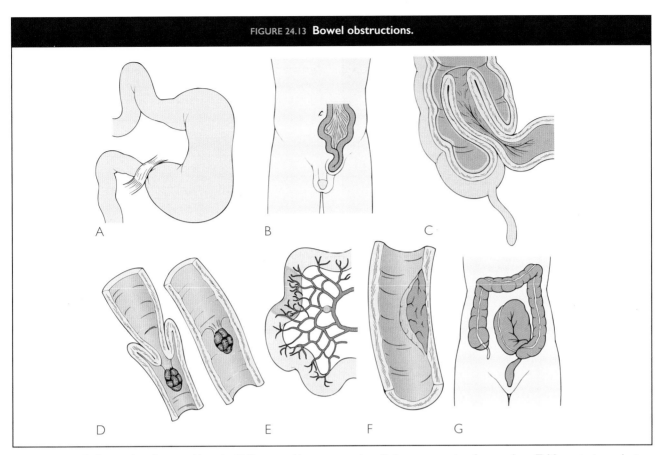

FIGURE 24.13 Bowel obstructions.

A, Adhesions. **B**, Strangulated inguinal hernia. **C**, Ileocaecal intussusception. **D**, Intussusception from polyps. **E**, Mesenteric occlusion. **F**, Neoplasm. **G**, Volvulus of the sigmoid colon.[123]

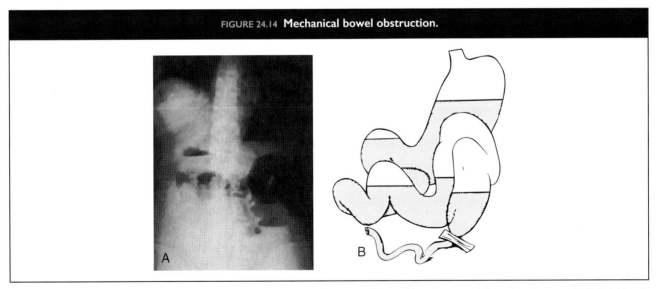

FIGURE 24.14 Mechanical bowel obstruction.

A, Localised air-fluid levels seen on upright film of abdomen. **B**, Diagram shows dilated proximal bowel and stomach air-fluid levels and adhesive band causing obstruction.[124]

- Non-mechanical obstruction results when muscle activity of the intestine decreases and movement of contents slows (i.e. paralytic ileus) (Fig 24.17).

When obstruction occurs, bowel contents accumulate above the obstruction. This leads to rapid increase in anaerobic and aerobic bacteria, which causes an increase in methane and hydrogen production.[95] McQuaid indicates that 'the more proximal the obstruction, the greater the discomfort' and the shorter the time between symptom onset and presentation.[79] Peristalsis increases so more secretions are released, which worsens distension, causes bowel oedema and increases capillary permeability. Plasma leaks into the peritoneal cavity with fluid

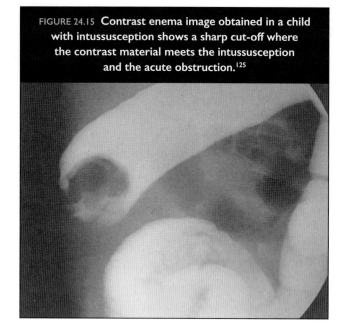

FIGURE 24.15 **Contrast enema image obtained in a child with intussusception shows a sharp cut-off where the contrast material meets the intussusception and the acute obstruction.**[125]

trapped in the intestinal lumen, so absorption of fluid and electrolytes decreases.

Assessment and management

Clinical signs vary with the location of the obstruction. Table 24.16 compares clinical manifestations of obstructions in the large and small intestines. Symptoms include colic, cramping and intermittent and wavelike abdominal pain. At times pain may be severe, and analgesia should be titrated accordingly. Abdominal distension may also be present. Patients may have diffuse abdominal tenderness, rigidity and constipation. Hyperactive bowel sounds or absent bowel sounds may be noted. The patient may also be febrile, tachycardic and hypotensive with nausea and vomiting. Emesis (secondary to reverse peristalsis) usually has an odour of faeces from proliferation of bacteria.[79]

Laboratory studies include FBC, urea, serum glucose, electrolytes, creatinine, amylase and arterial blood gas measurements. A WBC count greater than 20×10^9/L suggests bowel gangrene, whereas elevations greater than 40×10^9/L occur with mesenteric vascular occlusion.[5] An ECG should be obtained to confirm no cardiac involvement or an acute cardiac event presenting like a GI presentation. Abdominal X-rays show dilated, fluid-filled loops of bowel with visible air-fluid levels.[96] Table 24.17 highlights radiographic differences with specific obstructions.

Management includes IV access for fluid and electrolyte replacement using crystalloid solution to maintain haemodynamic values and renal perfusion.[85] Fluid balance monitoring is important along with an understanding of the balances of intake and output and patient response to therapy, which should be monitored. Early identification of reduced renal blood flow or hypovolaemia by recognising oliguria is vital to prevent an unwell patient deteriorating further. Bowel sounds should be evaluated frequently to identify changes. A nasogastric tube is inserted to decompress the stomach and reduce vomiting.[72] Evaluate pain for worsening of the condition.

Prophylactic administration of antibiotics is recommended. Surgical intervention may be required for some patients.

Life-threatening complications of bowel obstruction include peritonitis, bowel strangulation or perforation, renal insufficiency, aspiration, hypovolaemia, intestinal ischaemia or infarction, and death. Untreated obstruction that progresses to shock has a 70% mortality rate.[5]

> **PRACTICE TIP**
>
> Mesenteric ischaemia can present covertly in the older patient; have a higher degree of suspicion.

Constipation

Constipation is a decrease in the frequency of bowel movements from what is 'normal' for the individual. Hard, difficult-to-pass stools, a decrease in stool volume and retention of faeces in the rectum is the usual clinical pattern.[85] Normal bowel elimination may vary from 3 times a day to once every 3 days. Because of this it is important for the clinician to ascertain the patient's normal pattern. It is important to remember that changes in bowel habits may also indicate bowel obstruction produced by a tumour. Constipation itself can become quite a severe bowel obstruction.

Constipation may frequently be due to insufficient dietary fibre, inadequate fluid intake, medications and lack of exercise. Constipation may also be due to environmental constraints, ignoring the urge to defecate, chronic laxative abuse and multiple organic causes (Table 24.18). Conditions that affect nerve function may also have an impact on bowel motility function.

Changes in diet, mealtime or daily routines are some of the few environmental factors that may cause constipation. Depression and stress can also result in constipation. For many patients it is not possible to identify the underlying cause.[86] Some patients believe that they are constipated if they do not have a daily bowel movement. This can result in chronic laxative use and subsequent cathartic colon syndrome. In this condition, the colon becomes dilated and atonic. The clinical presentation of constipation may vary from a chronic discomfort to an acute event mimicking acute abdomen. Haemorrhoids are the most common complication of chronic constipation.

Assessment and management

In the presence of constipation or faecal impaction secondary to constipation, especially in the older patient, colonic perforation may occur. Perforation of the colon, which is life-threatening, causes abdominal pain, nausea, vomiting, fever and an elevated WBC count. An abdominal X-ray shows the presence of free air, which is diagnostic of perforation.[93]

A thorough history and physical assessment should be performed so that the underlying cause of constipation can be identified and treatment started (see Table 24.19). Laxatives should always be used cautiously because with chronic overuse they may become a cause of constipation. See Table 24.20 for cathartic agents.

Patient and family education should emphasise the need for a high-fibre diet, ensuring adequate water intake and a regular exercise regimen (Box 24.4).

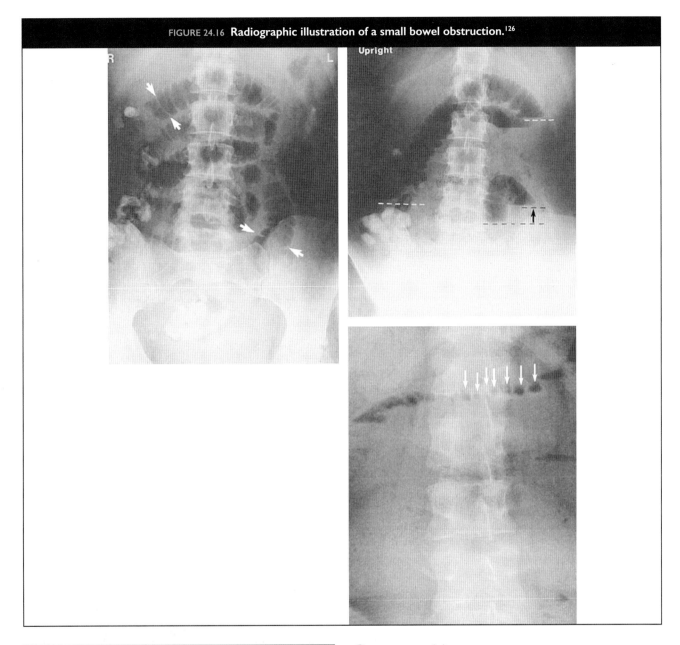

FIGURE 24.16 **Radiographic illustration of a small bowel obstruction.**[126]

Gastroenteritis

Gastroenteritis is inflammation of the stomach and intestinal lining caused by viral, protozoal, bacterial or parasitic agents (see Table 24.9). Bacterial infection accounts for 20% of acute diarrhoea disease.[14] Gastroenteritis may be caused by an imbalance of the normal flora (*E. coli*) resulting from the ingestion of contaminated food. Patients have nausea, vomiting, diarrhoea and abdominal cramps. Hyperactive bowel sounds, fever and headaches may also be present. Anal excoriation occurs with frequent episodes of diarrhoea. Diarrhoea accounts for 5 million to 10 million deaths annually in Asia, Africa and Latin America.[14]

Assessment and management

Laboratory data include FBC, electrolytes measurement, stool for ova and parasites, and stool culture.[80] Obtain IV access for replacement of fluid and electrolytes. Administer anti-emetics and analgesics as needed. Antibiotics are determined by patient history and presenting symptoms (see Box 24.5). Successful

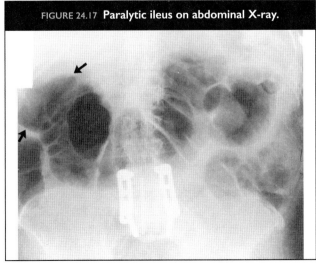

FIGURE 24.17 **Paralytic ileus on abdominal X-ray.**

Note dilated loops of bowel.[127]

TABLE 24.16 Clinical manifestations of small and large intestinal obstructions[123,125]

CLINICAL MANIFESTATION	SMALL INTESTINE	LARGE INTESTINE
Onset	Rapid	Gradual
Vomiting	Frequent and copious	Rare
Pain	Colicky, cramp-like, intermittent	Low-grade, cramping abdominal pain
Bowel movement	Faeces for a short time	Absolute constipation
Abdominal distension	Minimally increased	Greatly increased

TABLE 24.17 Radiographic and clinical evidence of specific bowel obstructions[123]

TYPE	RADIOGRAPHIC FINDINGS	CLINICAL SIGNS AND SYMPTOMS
Bowel obstructions (general)	Air-fluid levels may appear as 'string of beads' and thus serve as important diagnostic clue to mechanical obstructions. More than two air-fluid levels reflect mechanical obstruction, adynamic ileus, or both. Fluid-filled loops form a proximal impediment and are indicative of bowel obstruction	Pain, distension, vomiting, obstipation and constipation
	Routine films or contrast studies show air-fluid levels, distortion, abscess formation, narrow lumens, mucosal destruction, distension and deformities at site of torsion	
Strangulation obstruction	'Coffee bean' sign appears on radiograph (dilated bowel loop bent on itself, assuming shape of coffee bean)	Abdominal tenderness, hyperactive bowel sounds, leucocytosis, rebound tenderness, fever
	Gas- and fluid-filled loops may have unchanging locations on multiple projection films	
	Pseudotumour (closed-loop obstruction filled with water that looks like tumour) may be present	
Gallstones	Air in gallbladder tree, distension of small bowel and visualisation of stone	
Hernia		Extra-abdominal or intra-abdominal hernia may be present: in men, most commonly inguinal; in women, right-sided femoral hernias
Volvulus		Torsion of mesenteric axis creating digestive disturbances
Intussusception	'Coiled spring' appearance seen on contrast radiograph	

treatment is based on identifying the causative agent and resting the intestinal tract.

Oral hydration with clear liquids is possible in most patients. Suggested fluids should be dilute and gentle to the mucosa of the gastrointestinal tract and include various teas, ginger ale, broth and electrolyte replacement drinks or electrolyte ice blocks. Fluid replacement in children is critical to prevent dehydration. Electrolyte replacement substances such as ice blocks are an ideal first place to start. Oral rehydration is the preferred route to begin rehydration. Parenteral rehydration is reserved for patients unable to tolerate oral substances and demonstrating clinical signs of dehydration (dry mucous membranes, tachycardia, hypotension, lethargy and weakness). Rice, apple sauce, bananas and toast can be started as soon as diarrhoea subsides. Feeding should begin as soon as possible in children and adults, but only following an ability to tolerate fluids.

Liver failure and cirrhosis

When damage to the liver parenchyma is so severe that metabolic functions are no longer possible, liver failure occurs. Irrespective of the cause of liver insult, the syndrome of acute liver failure (ALF) develops.[78] The clinical features are characterised by jaundice, ascites, coagulopathy, hepatic encephalopathy, haemodynamic changes, electrolyte disturbance and renal failure (hepatorenal syndrome [HRS]).[97–99] ALF is associated with multiple organ failure and a poor prognosis. Alcohol is the leading cause of liver failure; however, other aetiologies include

---

TABLE 24.18 Causes of constipation[123]

COLONIC DISORDERS	SYSTEMIC DISORDERS
Luminal or extraluminal obstructing lesions	*Metabolic/endocrine*
Inflammatory strictures	Diabetes mellitus
Volvulus	Hypothyroidism
Intussusception	Pregnancy
Irritable bowel syndrome	Hypercalcaemia/hyperparathyroidism
Diverticular disease	Phaeochromocytoma
Rectocoele	*Collagen vascular disease*
Drug induced	Systemic sclerosis (scleroderma)
Antacids (calcium and aluminium)	Amyloidosis
Antidepressants	*Neurological disorders*
Anticholinergics	Hirschsprung's megacolon
Antipsychotics	Neurofibromatosis
Antihypertensives	Autonomic neuropathy (secondary to diabetes mellitus)
Barium sulfate	Multiple sclerosis
Iron supplements	Parkinson's disease
Bismuth	Spinal cord lesions or injury
Calcium supplements	Stroke
Laxative abuse	

TABLE 24.19 Nursing assessment in constipation[123]

SUBJECTIVE DATA	OBJECTIVE DATA
Important health information	*General*
Past health history—colorectal disease, neurological dysfunction, bowel obstruction, environmental changes, cancer, irritable bowel syndrome	Lethargy
	Integumentary
Medications—use of aluminium and calcium antacids, anticholinergics, antidepressants, antihistamines, antipsychotics, diuretics, narcotics, iron, laxatives, enemas	Anorectal fissures, haemorrhoids, abscesses
Functional health patterns	*Gastrointestinal*
Health perception/health management—chronic laxative or enema abuse; rigid beliefs regarding bowel function; malaise	Abdominal distension; hypoactive or absent bowel sounds; palpable abdominal mass; faecal impaction; small, hard, dry stool; stool with blood
Nutritional/metabolic—changes in diet or mealtime; inadequate fibre and fluid intake; anorexia, nausea	*Possible findings*
Elimination—change in usual elimination patterns; hard, difficult-to-pass stool, decrease in frequency and amount of stools; flatus, abdominal distension; tenesmus, rectal pressure; faecal incontinence (if impacted)	Positive faecal occult blood test (but should not do if patient is constipated); abdominal X-ray demonstrating stool in lower colon
Activity/exercise—change in daily activity routines; immobility; sedentary lifestyle	
Cognitive/perceptual—dizziness, headache, anorectal pain; abdominal pain on defecation	
Coping/stress tolerance—acute or chronic stress	

---

chronic hepatitis B or C, biliary obstruction, haemochromatosis, chemical toxins, fatty liver disease and cirrhosis.[98]

Cirrhosis is often a 'silent' disease, with patients remaining asymptomatic until decompensation occurs.[98] Cirrhosis refers to a progressive, diffuse, fibrosing nodular condition that disrupts the entire normal architecture of the liver. The sequela of cirrhosis is liver failure. Risk factors for cirrhosis include alcohol as the major precipitant; others include hepatitis B or C, cystic fibrosis, biliary obstruction, haemochromatosis and autoimmune causes[97] (see Ch 41).

TABLE 24.20 Drug therapy in cathartic agents[123]

CATEGORY	MECHANISMS OF ACTION	EXAMPLE	ONSET OF ACTION	COMMENTS
Bulk-forming	Absorbs water; increases bulk, thereby stimulating peristalsis	Metamucil, Konsyl, Citrucel	Usually within 24 hours	Contraindicated in patients with abdominal pain, nausea and vomiting and in patients suspected of having appendicitis, biliary tract obstruction or acute hepatitis; must be taken with fluids
Stool softeners and lubricants	Lubricate intestinal tract and soften faeces, making hard stools easier to pass; do not affect peristalsis	Mineral oil, dioctyl sodium, sulfosuccinate, Colace, Doxidan	Softeners up to 72 hours, lubricants up to 8 hours	Can block absorption of fat-soluble vitamins such as vitamin K, which may increase risk of bleeding in patients on anticoagulants
Saline and osmotic solutions	Cause retention of fluid in intestinal lumen caused by osmotic effect	Magnesium salts: magnesium citrate, milk of magnesia; Sodium phosphates: Fleet enema, Phospho-Soda; Lactulose; Polyethylene glycol saline solutions	15 minutes to 3 hours	Magnesium-containing products may cause hypermagnesaemia in patients with renal insufficiency
Stimulants	Increase peristalsis by irritating colon wall and stimulating enteric nerves	Anthraquinone drugs: cascara sagrada, senna	Usually within 12 hours	Cause melanosis coli (brown or black pigmentation of colon); are most widely abused laxatives; should not be used in patients with impaction or obstipation

BOX 24.4 **Patient and family teaching guide in constipation (Adult)**[123]

The following are teaching guidelines for the patient and family:

Eat dietary fibre
Eat 20–30 g of fibre per day. Gradually increase the amount of fibre eaten over 1–2 weeks. Fibre softens hard stools and adds bulk to stool, promoting evacuation.

Foods high in fibre: raw vegetables and fruits, beans, breakfast cereals (All Bran, oatmeal)

Fibre supplements: Metamucil, Mucilax

Drink fluids
Drink plenty of clear fluids but not excessively and no more than 1 extra litre a day.

Exercise regularly
Walk, swim or ride a bike at least three times per week. Contract and relax abdominal muscles when standing or by doing sit-ups to strengthen muscles and prevent straining. Exercise stimulates bowel motility and moves stool through the intestine.

Establish a regular time to defecate
First thing in the morning or after the first meal of the day is a good time because people often have the urge to defecate at this time.

Do not delay defecation
Respond to the urge to have a bowel movement as soon as possible. Delaying defecation results in hard stools and a decreased 'urge' to defecate. Water is absorbed from stool by the intestine over time. The intestine becomes less sensitive to the presence of stool in the rectum.

Record your bowel elimination pattern
Develop a habit of recording on your calendar when you have a bowel movement. Regular monitoring of bowel movement will assist in early identification of a problem.

Avoid laxatives and enemas
Do not overuse laxatives and enemas because they can actually cause constipation. The normal motility of the bowel is interrupted and bowel movements slow or stop.

BOX 24.5 Antibiotic treatment regimens for gastroenteritis[151,152]

Giardia lamblia

Tinidazole 2 g orally as a single dose. Children: 50 mg/kg/day up to adult dose

OR

Metronidazole 400 mg orally, 8-hourly for 7 days

Amoebiasis

Metronidazole 600 mg orally, 6-hourly for 6–10 days. Children: 45 mg/kg/day up to adult dose in three divided doses

PLUS

Diloxanide furonate 500 mg orally 8-hourly for 10 days. Children: 20 mg/kg/day up to adult dose in three divided doses (to prevent relapse)

Shigellosis

Norfloxacin 400 mg orally, 12-hourly for 7–10 days (not in children)

OR

Ampicillin 1 g orally, 6-hourly for 7–10 days. Children: 100 mg/kg/day up to adult dose in four divided doses

OR

Co-trimoxazole (sulfamethoxazole and trimethoprim in ratio 1:5) 80 mg/400 mg orally, 12-hourly for 7–10 days. Children: 8/40 mg/kg/day up to adult dose in two divided doses

Campylobacter

Erythromycin 500 mg orally, 6-hourly for 7–10 days. Children: 40 mg/kg/day up to adult dose in four divided doses

Traveller's diarrhoea

Norfloxacin 800 mg orally as a single dose or 400 mg orally 12-hourly for 3 days (not in children)

OR

Co-trimoxazole (trimethoprim and sulfamethoxazole in ratio 1:5) 320/1600 mg orally, as a single dose or 160/800 mg orally, 12-hourly for 3 days. Children: 8/40 mg/kg/day up to a maximum of 160/800 mg/day in two divided doses orally for 3 days

Clostridium difficile

Metronidazole 400 mg orally 8-hourly for 7–10 days. Children: 30 mg/kg/day up to adult dose in three divided doses

If unresponsive or severe disease: vancomycin 125 mg orally 6-hourly for 1–2 weeks. Children: 5 mg/kg up to adult dose.

The clinical features of cirrhosis include jaundice, organomegaly, ascites and encephalopathy. The following summarises important considerations in the presentation and physical appearance of cirrhosis and liver failure.[99,100]

- Stigmata of chronic liver disease include spider naevi, palmar erythema, gynaecomastia, caput medusa.
- Oesophageal varices develop as a consequence of portal hypertension, and bleeding may initially present with small or significant haematemesis, malaena or rectal bleeding.

- Hepatorenal syndrome is a functional disorder whereby renal failure develops (elevated serum creatinine) in the context of liver failure, ascites and structurally normal kidneys.
- Ascites is the pathological accumulation of fluid in the peritoneal cavity. Approximately 85% of patients with ascites have cirrhosis.
- Sepsis may occur due to the immunosuppressive nature of cirrhosis. The clinician should have a low threshold for severe infection in unwell patients who have cirrhosis. The classic febrile state may not always be seen in immunocompromised patients. Consider also other markers of sepsis and shock such as tachycardia, hypotension and poor peripheral perfusion. Particular attention should be given to the possible development of spontaneous bacterial peritonitis (SBP), especially in patients with ascites. Empirical antibiotic therapy is recommended.
- Encephalopathy may be mild and be manifested only as low-grade confusion or sleep disturbances. Conversely, the encephalopathy may be severe and be associated with a marked reduction in level of consciousness. Note that hepatic encephalopathy is a diagnosis of exclusion, and other possible causes to an altered mental state must be excluded.
- Jugular venous distension, a sign of right-side heart failure, suggests hepatic congestion.
- Abdominal examination should focus on the size and consistency of the liver and spleen, and the presence of ascites.

Assessment and management

Investigations into liver function can be assisted by laboratory evaluation, radiographic studies and biopsy. Utilising pathology is useful; however, the standard liver function assays do not reflect the function of the liver correctly. When interpreting the biochemistry along with the clinical picture, an impression of certain liver diseases may evolve.[97]

When liver disease is suspected, FBC with platelets; prothrombin time; enzymes aspartate transaminase (AST) and alanine transaminase (ALT); alkaline phosphatase; gamma glutamyl transferase; bilirubin; and albumin are useful.[101] Rather than a single measurement of a value, repeated testing over a period of time is warranted and may prove useful in assisting diagnosis. Imaging such as ultrasonography is a valuable first-line modality, as it provides information regarding the gross appearance of the liver and associated anatomy. It is relatively inexpensive, does not pose a radiation risk and does not require potentially toxic contrast. CT and MRI have limitations in detecting early changes with cirrhosis. They can accurately demonstrate nodularity, atrophy or hypertrophic changes, as well as ascites and varices in advanced disease. CT and MRI are valuable in follow-up studies.[78]

The goals of treatment include resuscitation and stabilisation initially. Airway protection is vital and aspiration is a risk in any vomiting patient. Early pharmacology (vasoactive drugs, e.g octreotide, to reduce portal pressures) and endoscopy improves outcomes for variceal haemorrhage. Sepsis is frequently a feature in liver failure, therefore septic screening and use of antibiotics are recommended. Renal function needs to be closely monitored. Removal of hepatotoxic agents and liver insults is important to reduce the impact and effect of cirrhosis and liver failure. Eliminating alcohol, drugs and medications which are known to be toxic to the liver are vital to ensure what function is left is operating at maximum ability.[98,101]

> ### PRACTICE TIP
>
> Patients with alcoholism may have a combination of pancreatitis, hepatitis and gastritis.

Bariatric surgery

Bariatric surgical procedures have increased exponentially in an effort to combat obesity. Presently there are two main forms of surgical therapy undertaken to promote weight loss and reduce patient morbidity and mortality; these are laparoscopic adjustable gastric banding and laparoscopic gastric bypass. Gastric bypass refers to any surgical procedure that first divides the stomach to leave a small pouch, which is then connected through rearranging the small intestine. In relation to Roux-en-Y gastric bypass surgery, this is commonly achieved laparoscopically. Similarly, in gastric banding an adjustable band is placed laparoscopically just below the gastro-oesophageal junction at a 45° angle towards the left shoulder, leaving a 50–80 mL size gastric pouch. Although the benefits and relative low mortality of bariatric surgery are clear,[102] postoperative abdominal pain is one of the most common and vexing problems increasingly presenting to ED. Clinical presentations are highly variable and evaluation may be complicated by the fact that obese patients feel abdominal symptoms more intensely compared to lean patients.[103] Therefore, a broad evaluation directed by history and clinical presentation is required. As a result, emergency clinicians have required increasing knowledge and expertise in managing patients presenting post bariatric surgery with abdominal pain to the ED. It is imperative that ED clinicians remain vigilant in the evaluation and management of patients presenting following bariatric surgery, and seek surgical consultation as soon as possible. The assessment and management of both gastric banding and bypass surgery are discussed jointly below.

Assessment and management

Common emergencies occurring early (<30 days) post gastric bypass surgery include: anastomotic leakage leading to peritonitis (1–6%);[104] acute distension of the bypassed division of the stomach, typically developing in less than 7 days post surgery, patients will present with nausea, dry-retching, left upper quadrant bloating and hiccups[105] and bleeding. Hepatobiliary complications in the form of gallstones occurs most frequently (32%) postoperatively, due to rapid weight loss and resultant bile stasis with biliary sludge formation.[106] In open gastric bypass, incisional hernias occur much more frequently (15–20%)[107] compared to using a laparoscopic approach (6%.)[108] Late gastric bypass surgical emergencies include: stomal stenosis, small bowel obstruction may occur in the early or late post-operative period and has been described in up to 5% of Roux-en-Y gastric bypass. Aetiologies of small bowel obstruction post gastric bypass surgery include: adhesion,

internal hernia and intussusception.[104] A further potential complication post-bariatric surgery, whether by bypass or by banding, is pulmonary embolism secondary to deep vein thrombosis. Pulmonary embolism is the second-most common cause of death after bariatric surgery with an incidence of 2% and a mortality of 20–30%.[102] Nutritional complications are more common with gastric bypass surgery than gastric banding, frequently resulting in iron-deficiency anaemia (20–49%) and B_{12} deficiencies (26–70%).[109] Similar complications have also been observed following laparoscopic gastric banding.

Laparoscopic adjustable gastric banding has gained popularity for treatment of morbid obesity worldwide, but has been associated with various complications. Pouch enlargement can occur in up to 12% of patients following gastric banding.[110] Pouch enlargement can frequently (77%) be resolved by deflating the band and conservative management (low calorie diet, re-enforcement of portion size control).[110] Band slippage can occur in up to 22% of patients, potentially leading to gastric perforation, necrosis, upper gastrointestinal bleeding and aspiration pneumonia.[111] Patients normally present complaining of dysphagia, vomiting, regurgitation and food intolerance,[112,113] and require surgical correction. Band erosion, whereby the band erodes through the stomach wall and into the gastric lumen, is uncommon (<1%).[111] However, despite its low incidence, ED clinicians should have a high index of suspicion as most patients present asymptomatically. When symptomatic, patients will complain of loss of restriction, vague epigastric pain, gastrointestinal bleeding, intra-abdominal abscesses or port site infection. Management involves the removal of the gastric band, which is made increasing difficult by the extensive inflammatory response around the proximal stomach and left lobe of the liver. Port-site infections, breakages and tubing malfunction can also occur. Port-site infections that manifest early following surgery often present with the cardinal signs of erythaema, swelling and pain. Early infections with cellulitis alone can normally be managed with oral antibiotics, yet if the response is inadequate, then intravenous antibiotic administration should be trialled. Should this fail, and the infection is limited to the port, then the port should be removed and the tubing knotted and left inside the abdomen. Once the infection is resolved, a new port can be reconnected to the tubing. Late onset post-site infections are caused by delayed band erosion with ascending infection which manifests several months after surgery.[111,114] Late onset port-site infections are normally unresponsive to antibiotic therapy. Left untreated, late port-site infections can develop into life-threatening intra-abdominal sepsis. Early gastroscopy and removal of the band is required. Damage to the port resulting in breakage typically presents as a slow leak, loss of injected fluid volume on aspiration. It is essential to only access ports with non-coring Huber needles to maintain port septum integrity. Any adjustment required of the gastric band must by undertaken using fluoroscopy. Similarly, assessing for tube leakage can be undertaken by injecting dilute nonionic iodinated contrast into the port under fluoroscopy.[111,113]

Analgesia

Pain relief is a humane practice. The historical practices of withholding the administration of narcotic or other similar analgesia until a confirmed diagnosis is made or surgical consult obtained continues despite the overwhelming evidence that it does not lead to diagnostic error.[115,116] Evidence supports the early administration of analgesia to patients with abdominal pain, including children (see Chs 19 and 36) and adults, finding that it enhances patient examination and facilitates diagnosis.[115] Education programs have also been researched and established throughout Australian EDs to facilitate early narcotic and non-narcotic analgesia.[117]

For patients with severe (≥7/10) pain, pain management options include IV morphine sulphate[118] or IV fentanyl[119] depending on patient age and haemodynamic stability. For patients with less severe pain, pain management includes paracetamol with the addition of oxycodone (immediate release) for those in moderate pain.[117]

SUMMARY

GI emergencies can be minor or life-threatening. Most GI emergencies present with similar clinical manifestations, so triage history and physical assessment play an important role in the management of these patients. Ability to differentiate conditions that require immediate attention is a requisite skill for the emergency healthcare professional (Fig 24.18A–D).

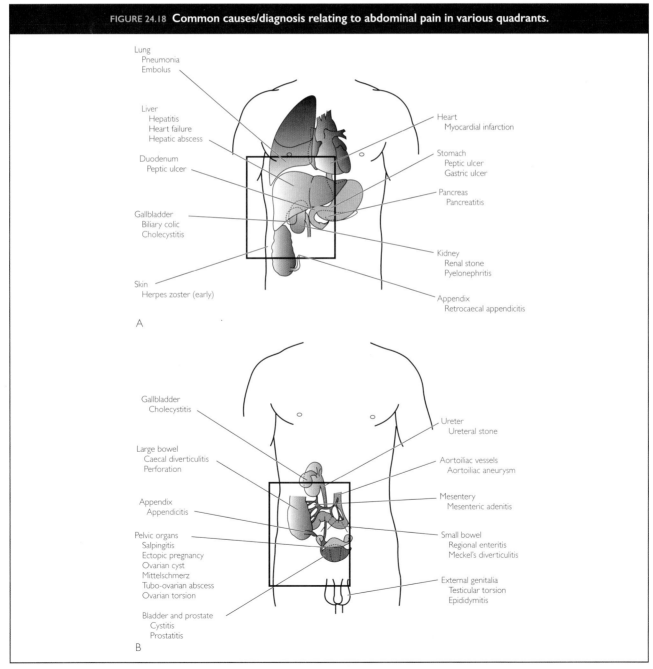

FIGURE 24.18 **Common causes/diagnosis relating to abdominal pain in various quadrants.**

Continued

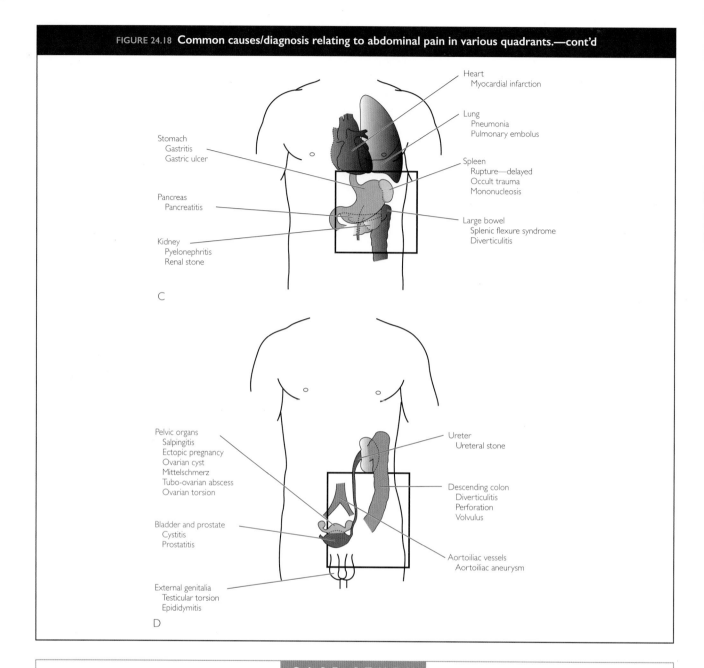

FIGURE 24.18 **Common causes/diagnosis relating to abdominal pain in various quadrants.—cont'd**

C

Heart
 Myocardial infarction

Lung
 Pneumonia
 Pulmonary embolus

Stomach
 Gastritis
 Gastric ulcer

Spleen
 Rupture—delayed
 Occult trauma
 Mononucleosis

Pancreas
 Pancreatitis

Large bowel
 Splenic flexure syndrome
 Diverticulitis

Kidney
 Pyelonephritis
 Renal stone

D

Pelvic organs
 Salpingitis
 Ectopic pregnancy
 Ovarian cyst
 Mittelschmerz
 Tubo-ovarian abscess
 Ovarian torsion

Ureter
 Ureteral stone

Descending colon
 Diverticulitis
 Perforation
 Volvulus

Bladder and prostate
 Cystitis
 Prostatitis

Aortoiliac vessels
 Aortoiliac aneurysm

External genitalia
 Testicular torsion
 Epididymitis

CASE STUDY

A 24-year-old man complains of increasing abdominal pain, with nausea and shortness-of-breath when sitting or lying down for the past four hours. In the course of your assessment you obtain information about the onset of his symptoms and past medical history. The previous evening following work, the patient had played rugby from 1830 hrs. During the match the patient was substituted off the field after being shoulder-charged in the abdomen and then vomiting. After the match ended, the patient went home, had a small dinner and took paracetamol (1 gram) for 'stomach pain'. On exploring the patient's past medical history, the patient describes no significant medical history, denies smoking or recreational drug use. The patient works at the weekend as a bartender, and attends university

during the week where he is studying for a law degree. His observations are:

• blood pressure 134/65 mmHg
• heart rate 122 beats/minute and regular
• temperature 36.8°C
• oxygen saturation 98% on room air
• respiratory rate 28 breaths/minute, breaths are short and staggered
• Glasgow Coma Scale score 15.

On asking the patient to describe the location and nature of the abdominal pain, he states that the pain is primarily over the upper left quadrant, increasingly intense when sitting or lying down, with pain radiating to the left shoulder tip when lying down. The patient rates the pain as 6/10 when standing and 10/10 on sitting or lying down. On examination the patient finds it difficult to lie still as he finds it painful to straighten his body. On visual examination of the abdomen, there is no bruising or signs of injury. On light palpation, the patient is tender in the epigastric region and left upper quadrant. Deep palpation over the left upper quadrant elicits guarding. No tenderness noted elsewhere on palpating the abdomen; bowel sounds are normal.

Questions

1. Your immediate intervention on presentation following triage is to:
   A. Obtain a family history
   B. Provide pain relief
   C. Conduct a primary survey
   D. Obtain a blood sample to measure serum lactate.

2. The next clinical intervention is likely to be:
   A. Intravenous cannulation and blood sampling
   B. Arterial line insertion to monitor blood pressure
   C. Abdominal or girth measurement
   D. Urinalysis.

3. The best type of analgesia for this patient would be:
   A. Oral medication
   B. Nil at present; he needs to be assessed by a surgeon in case he has a surgical emergency requiring theatre
   C. Start with a non-steroidal anti-inflammatory drug and titrate response
   D. Intravenous narcotic analgesia.

4. Pain radiating to the left shoulder tip suggests which specific abdominal sign?
   A. Murphy's sign
   B. Kehr's sign
   C. Cullen's sign
   D. Grey-Turner's sign.

5. The best type of bedside diagnostic test for this patient would be:
   A. Urinalysis
   B. FAST scan
   C. Abdominal X-ray
   D. Blood sugar level.

6. Ancillary tests are conducted to assist the diagnosis. The most useful initial blood tests for this patient would be:
   A. Full blood count; urea electrolytes and creatinine; amylase and lipase
   B. Full blood count; blood group and cross-match
   C. Lipase, troponin, full blood count
   D. Coagulation profile, liver and renal function tests, lipase and amylase.

7. Radiology will assist in diagnosis, and the inclusion or exclusion of other conditions. A useful initial investigation would be:
   A. Abdominal ultrasound
   B. Abdominal CT
   C. Abdominal magnetic resonance imaging
   D. Chest X-ray.

8. Blood tests reveal:
   - White blood cell count 13,000/mm^3
   - Haemoglobin 149 g/L
   - Packed cell volume 29%
   - Serum amylase 445 U/L
   - Serum lipase 65 U/L
   - Urea 5.4 mmol/L
   - Creatinine 7.9 µm/L
   - Sodium 141 mmol/L
   - Potassium 3.9 mmol/L
   - Chloride 104 mmol/L
   - Gamma GT (gamma-glutamyl transpeptidase) 41 U/L
   - ALT (alanine amino transferase) 31 U/L
   - AST (aspartate amino transferase) 21 U/L

   What are your findings?
   A. Pancreatitis
   B. Cholecystis
   C. Splenic rupture
   D. Myocardial infarction

9. If treated appropriately, most patients with acute pancreatitis will recover well. There are several complications associated with the disease of pancreatitis, and they include:
   A. Liver failure
   B. Coagulopathies and deep venous thrombosis
   C. Pulmonary complications and effusions
   D. Renal calculi.

Answers to Case Study Questions can be found on evolve
http://evolve.emergencytrauma.curtis

REFERENCES

1. Principal diagnosis of admitted patients. 2010. www.aihw.gov.au/publications/hse/ahs95-6/ahs95-6-c05a.pdf; accessed January 2011.

2. Bost N, Crilly J, Patterson E, Chaboyer W. Clinical handover of patients arriving by ambulance to a hospital emergency department: a qualitative study. International Emergency Nursing 2012;20(3):133–41.

3. Makrauer F, Greenberger N. Acute abdominal pain: basic principles and current challenges. In: Greenberger N, Blumberg R, eds. Current diagnosis and treatment: gastroenterology, hepatology and endoscopy. 2nd edn. New York: McGraw-Hill; 2011.

4. Gordon C, Craft J. The structure and function of the digestive system. In: Craft J, Gordon C, Tiziani A, eds. Understanding pathophysiology. Sydney: Mosby; 2011.

5. Tortora G, Grabowski S. Principles of anatomy and physiology. 13th edn. New York: John Wiley; 2011.

6. Sargent S. Pathophysiology, diagnosis and management of acute pancreatitis. British Journal of Nursing 2006;15(18):999–1005.

7. Porth C, Grossman S. Porth's Pathophysiology: Concepts of Altered Health States. 9th edn. Sydney: Lippincott Williams & Wilkins; 2013.

8. Rossoll L. Abdominal emergencies. Emergency nursing core curriculum. 6th edn. Philadelphia, PA: Saunders; 2007.

9. Thomas J, Monaghan T, eds. Oxford Handbook of Clinical Examination and Practical Skills. Oxford: Oxford Medical Publications; 2006.

10. Laurell H, Hansson L, Gunnarsson U. Acute abdominal pain among elderly patients. Gerontology 2006;52(6):339–44.

11. Yim V, Graham C, Rainer T. A comparison of emergency department utilization by elderly and younger adult patients presenting to three hospitals in Hong Kong. International Journal of Emergency Medicine 2009;2:19–24.

12. Colucciello S, Lukens T, Morgan D. Assessing abdominal pain in adults: a rational, cost-effective, and evidence-based strategy. Emergency Medicine Practice 1999;1(1):1–20.

13. Lewis L, Banet G, Blanda M et al. Etiology and clinical course of abdominal pain in senior patients: a prospective, multicentre study. The Journals of Gerontology, Series A, Biological Sciences and Medical Sciences 2005;60(8):1071–6.

14. Makrauer F, Greenberger N. Acute abdominal pain: basic principles and current challenges. In: Greenberger N, Blumberg R, Burakoff R, eds. Current diagnosis and treatment: gastroenterology, hepatology and endoscopy 2011.

15. Zwakhalen S, Hamers J, Abu-Saad H, Berger M. Pain in elderly people with severe dementia: a systematic review of behavioural pain assessment tools. BMC Geriatrics 2006;6(3).

16. Handbook AM. Australian Medicines Handbook Online. 2013; www.amh.net.au/online/; accessed March 2014.

17. Burridge N, Deidum D, eds. Australian Injectable Drugs Handbook. 5th ed: Society of Hospital Pharmacists of Australia; 2011.

18. Cerner Corporation. Kansas City, MO 2009.

19. O'Brien M. Acute abdominal pain. In: Tintinalli J, Stapczynski J, Ma O et al, eds. Tintinalli's emergency medicine, 7th edn. Sydney: McGraw-Hill; 2010.

20. Hamm CW, Bassand J-P, Agewall S et al. ESC Guidelines for the management of acute coronary syndromes in patients presenting without persistent ST-segment elevation: The Task Force for the management of acute coronary syndromes (ACS) in patients presenting without persistent ST-segment elevation of the European Society of Cardiology (ESC). European Heart Journal 2011;32(23):2999–3054.

21. Canto J, Fincher C, Kiefe C et al. Atypical presentations among Medicare beneficiaries with unstable angina pectoris. American Journal of Cardiology 2002;30:248–53.

22. Culic V, Eterovic D, Miric D, Silic N. Symptom presentation of acute myocardial infarction: influence of sex, age, and risk factors. American Heart Journal 2002;144:1012–17.

23. Umpierrez G, Freire A. Abdominal pain in patients with hyperglycemic crises. Journal of Critical Care 2002;17(1):63–7.

24. Australasia College of Emergency Medicine and the Royal College of Pathologists of Australia. Guideline on pathology testing in the emergency department. 2013.

25. Panagiotopoulou I, Parashar D, Lin R et al. The diagnostic value of white cell count, C-reactive protein and bilirubin in acute appendicitis and its complications. Annals of the Royal College of Surgeons of England 2013;95(3):215–21.

26. Wu J, Chen H, Lee S et al. Diagnostic role of procalcitonin in patients with suspected acute appendicitis. World Journal of Surgery 2012;36(8):1744–9.

27. Bezmarevic M, Mirkovic D, Soldatovic I et al. Correlation between procalcitonin and intra-abdominal pressure and their role in prediction of the severity of acute pancreatitis. Pancreatology 2012;12(4):337–43.

28. Schellekens D, Hulsewé K, van Acker B et al. Evaluation of the diagnostic accuracy of plasma markers for early diagnosis in patients suspected for acute appendicitis. Academic Emergency Medicine 2013;20(7):703–10.

29. Al-gaithy Z. Clinical value of total white blood cells and neutrophil counts in patients with suspected appendicitis: retrospective study. World Journal of Emergency Surgery 2012;7(1):32–9.

30. Meyer Z, Schreinemakers J, van der Laan L. The value of C-reactive protein and lactate in the acute abdomen in the emergency department. World Journal of Emergency Surgery 2012;7:22–8.

31. Albu E, Miller B, Choi Y et al. Diagnostic value of C-reactive protein in acute appendicitis. Diseases of the Colon and Rectum 1994;37(1):49–51.

32. Lyons D, Waldron R, Ryan T, O'Malley E. An evaluation of the clinical value of the leucocyte count and sequential counts in suspected acute appendicitis. British Journal of Clinical Practice 1987;41(6):794–6.

33. Lau W, Ho Y, Chu K, Yeung C. Leucocyte count and neutrophil percentage in appendicectomy for suspected appendicitis. The Australian and New Zealand Journal of Surgery 1989;59(5):395–8.

34. Sand M, Trullen X, Bechara F et al. A prospective bicentre study investigating the diagnostic value of procalcitonin in patients with acute appendicitis. European Surgical Research 2009;43(3):291–7.

35. Anielski R, Kuśnierz-Cabala B, Szafraniec K. An evaluation of the utility of additional tests in the preoperative diagnostics of acute appendicitis. Langenbecks Archives of Surgery 2010;395(8):1061–8.

36. Yu C, Juan L, Wu M et al. Systematic review and meta-analysis of the diagnostic accuracy of procalcitonin, C-reactive protein and white blood cell count for suspected acute appendicitis. British Journal of Surgeons 2013;100(3):322.

37. van Ravesteijn H, van Dijk I, Darmon D et al. The reassuring value of diagnostic tests: a systematic review. Patient Education and Counseling 2012;86(1):3–8.

38. Yang R, Shao Z, Chen Y et al. Lipase and pancreatic amylase activities in diagnosis of acute pancreatitis in patients with hyperamylasemia. Hipatoniliary and Pancreatic Disease International 2005;4(4):600–3.

39. Prinzen L, Keulemans J, Bekers O. The diagnostic benefits of lipase values in acute pancreatitis. Nederlands Tijdschrift voor Geneeskunde 2013;157(35):A6432.

40. Sutton P, Humes D, Purcell G et al. The role of routine assays of serum amylase and lipase for the diagnosis of acute abdominal pain. Annals of the Royal College of Surgeons of England 2009;91(5):381–4.

41. Pratt D, Kaplan M. Evaluation of abnormal liver-enzyme results in asymptomatic patients. The New England Journal of Medicine 2000;342:1266.

42. Limdi JK, Hyde GM. Evaluation of abnormal liver function tests. Postgraduate Medical Journal 2003;79(932):307–12.

43. Gopal D, Rosen H. Abnormal findings on liver function tests: Interpreting results to narrow the diagnosis and establish a prognosis. Postgraduate Medicine 2000;107(2):24.

44. Davern T, Scharschmidt B. Biochemical liver tests. In: Feldman M, Friedman L, Sleisenger M, eds. Sleisenger & Fordtran's Gastrointestinal and Liver Disease: Pathophysiology, Diagnosis and Management. 8th edn. Philadelphia: Saunders; 2006.

45. Zhang B, Nakama H, Fattah A, Kamijo N. Lower specificity of occult test on stool collected by digital rectal examination. Hepatogastroenterology 2002;49(43):165–7.

46. Bini E, Reinhold J, Weinshel E et al. Prospective evaluation of the use and outcome of admission stool guaiac testing: the digital rectal examination on admission to the medical service (DREAMS) study. Journal of Clinical Gastroenterology 2006;40(9):821–7.

47. Orkin B, Sinuykin S, Lloyd P. The digital rectal examination scoring system (DRESS). Disease of the Colon and Rectum 2010;53(12):1656–60.

48. Kessler C, Bauer S. Utility of the digital rectal examination in the emergency department: a review. Journal of Emergency Medicine 2012;43(6):1169–204.

49. Quaas J, Lanigan M, Newman D et al. Utility of the digital rectal examination in the evaluation of undifferentiated abdominal pain. American Journal of Emergency Medicine 2009;27(9):1125–9.

50. Manimaran N, Galland R. Significance of routine digital rectal examination in adults presenting with abdominal pain. Annals of the Royal College of Surgeons of England 2004;86(4):292–5.

51. Dixon J, Elton R, Rainey J, Macleod D. Rectal examination in patients with pain in the right lower quadrant of the abdomen. British Medical Journal 1991;302(6773):386–9.

52. Bonello J, Abrams J. The significance of a 'positive' rectal examination in acute appendicitis. Disease of the Colon and Rectum 1979;22(2):97–101.

53. Werner J, Zock M, Khalil P et al. Evidence for the Digital Rectal Examination in the Emergency Assessment of Acute Abdominal Pain—Abstract. Zentralbl Chirurgie 2011;December.

54. Smith J, Hall E. The use of plain abdominal X-rays in the emergency department. Emergency Medicine Journal 2009;26:160–3.

55. Maglinte D, Reyes B, Harmon B et al. Reliability and role of plain film radiography and CT in the diagnosis of small-bowel obstruction. American Journal of Roentgenology 1996;225(1):159–64.

56. Ahn S, Mayo-Smith W, Murphy B et al. Acute Nontraumatic Abdominal Pain in Adult Patients: Abdominal Radiography Compared with CT Evaluation. Radiography 2002;225(1):159–64.

57. Suri S, Gupta S, Sudhakar P et al. Comparative evaluation of plain films, ultrasound and CT in the diagnosis of intestinal obstruction. Acta Radiologica 1999;40(4):442–8.

58. Sharma S, Mohan A, Kadhiravan T. HIV-TB co-infection: epidemiology, diagnosis and management. Journal of Medical Research 2005;121(4):550–67.

59. MacKersie A, Lane M, Gerhardt R et al. Nontraumatic acute abdominal pain: unenhanced helical CT compared to with three-view acute abdominal series. Radiography 2005;237(1):114–22.

60. Poletti P, Kinkel K, Vermeulen B. Blunt abdominal trauma: should US be used to detect both free fluid and organ injuries? Journal of Trauma 2003;227(1):95–103.

61. van Randen A, Lameris W, Wouter van Es H et al. A comparison of the accuracy of ultrasound and computer tomography in common diagnoses causing acute abdominal pain. European Radiology 2011;21(7):1535–45.

62. Laméris W, van Randen A, van Es HW et al. Imaging strategies for detection of urgent conditions in patients with acute abdominal pain: diagnostic accuracy study. BMJ 2009;338.

63. Allemann F, Cassina P, Rothlin M, Largiader F. Ultrasound scans done by surgeons for patients with acute abdominal pain: a prospective study. European Journal of Surgery 1999;165(10):966–70.

64. Sala E, Watson C, Beadsmoore C et al. A randomized, controlled trial of routine early abdominal computed tomography in patients presenting with non-specific acute abdominal pain. Clinical Radiology 2007;62(10):961–9.

65. Ng C, Watson C, Palmer C et al. Evaluation of early abdominopelvic computer tomography in patients with acute abdominal pain of unknown cause: prospective randomised study. British Journal of Medicine 2002;325(7377):1387.

66. Esses D, Birndaum A, Bijur P et al. Ability of CT to alter decision making in elderly patients with acute abdominal pain. American Journal of Emergency Medicine 2004;22(4):270–2.

67. Broder J, Warshauer D. Increased utilization of computer tomography in the adult emergency department, 2000–2005. Emergency Radiology 2006;13(1):25–30.

68. Mitka M. Costly surge in diagnostic imaging spurs debate. Journal of American Medical Association 2005;293(6):663–7.

69. Brenner D, Hall E. Computer tomography—an increasing source of radiation exposure. New England Journal of Medicine 2007;357(22):2277–84.

70. Griffey R, Sodickson A. Cumulative radiation exposure and cancer risk estimates in emergency department patients undergoing repeat or multiple CT. American Journal of Roentgenology 2009;192(4):887–92.

71. National hospital morbidity database (2009–2010). Australian Institute of Health and Welfare; accessed 26 December 2013.

72. Goralnick W, Meguerdichian D. Gastrointestinal bleeding. In: Marx J, Hockberger R, Walls R, eds. Rosen's emergency medicine—concepts and clinical practice: expert consult premium edition. 8th edn. Philadelphia, PA: Saunders; 2013.

73. Lo B. Lower gastrointestinal bleeding. In: Tintinalli J, Stapczynski J, Ma O et al, eds. Tintinalli's Emergency Medicine, 7th edn. Sydney: McGraw-Hill; 2010.

74. Overton D. Upper gastrointestinal bleeding. In: Tintinalli J, Stapczynski J, Ma O et al, eds. Tintinalli's Emergency Medicine, 7th edn. Sydney: McGraw-Hill; 2010.

75. Seeley R, Vanputte C, Regan J, Russo A, eds. Anatomy and Physiology. 10th edn. New York: McGraw-Hill; 2013.

76. Tintinalli J, Stapczynski J, Ma O et al. eds. Tintinalli's emergency medicine: a comprehensive study guide. 7th edn. Sydney: McGraw-Hill; 2010.

77. Roline C, Reardon R. Disorders of the small intestine. In: Marx J, Hockberger R, Walls R, eds. Rosen's emergency medicine—concepts and clinical practice: expert consult premium edition. 8th edn. Philadelphia, PA: Saunders; 2013.

78. Feldman M, Friedman L, Brandt L, eds. Sleisenger and Fordtran's gastrointestinal and liver disease pathphysiology/diagnosis/management. 9th edn. Philadelphia, PA: Saunders; 2010.

79. McQuaid K. Gastrointestinal disorders. In: McPhee S, Papadakis M, eds. Current medical diagnosis and treatment. New York: McGraw-Hill; 2010.

80. Marx J, Hockberger R, Walls R, eds. Rosen's emergency medicine—concepts and clinical practice. 8th edn. St. Louis: Mosby; 2013.

81. Knox S, Harrison C, Britt H, Henderson J. Estimating prevalence of common chronic morbidities in Australia. Medical Journal of Australia 2008;189(2):66–70.

82. Gastroenterological Society of Australia. Gastro-oesophageal reflux disease in adults. GESA; 2011.

83. Society of Gastroenterology Nurses and Associates. Gastroenterology nursing: a core curriculum. SGNA; 2008.

84. Wyatt J, Illingworth R, Graham C, Hogg K, eds. Oxford handbook of emergency medicine. New York: Oxford University Press; 2012.

85. Peterson M. Disorders of the large intestine. In: Marx J, Hockberger R, Walls R, eds. Rosen's emergency medicine—concepts and clinical practice: expert consult premium edition. 8th edn. Philadelphia, PA: Saunders; 2013.

86. Lewis S, Dirksen M, Heitkemper M, Bucher L. Medical–surgical nursing: assessment and management of clinical problems. 9th edn. St. Louis: Mosby; 2013.

87. Elwood D. Cholecystitis. The Surgical Clinics of North America 2008;88(6):1241–52.

88. Craft J, Gordon C, Tiziani A. Understanding Pathophysiology. Sydney: Mosby; 2011.

89. Hernphill R, Saten S. Disorders of the pancreas. In: Marx J, Hockberger R, Walls R, eds. Rosen's emergency medicine—concepts and clinical practice: expert consult premium edition. 8th edn. Philadelphia, PA: Saunders; 2013.

90. Amerine E. Get optimum outcomes for acute pancreatitis patients. Nurse Practitioner 2007;32(6):44–8.

91. Freedman S. Pancreatitis. In: Porter R, Kaplan J, eds. The Merck manual of diagnosis and therapy. 19th edn. Whitehouse Station, NJ: Merck Sharp & Dohme Corp.; 2011.

92. Andersson R, Hugander A, Ghazi S et al. Diagnostic value of disease history, clinical presentation, and inflammatory parameters of appendicitis. World Journal of Surgery 1999;23(2):133–40.

93. Otto C, ed. ABC of emergency medicine. London: Blackwell Publishing Ltd; 2013.

94. Cameron P, Jelinek G, Kelly A-M et al. eds. Textbook of adult emergency medicine. 3rd edn. Edinburgh: Churchill Livingstone 2009.

95. Andersson R, Sward A, Tingstedt B, Akerberg D. Treatment of acute pancreatitis: focus on medical care. Drugs 2009;69(5):505–14.

96. Raby N, De Lacey G, Berman L, eds. Accident and emergency radiology. 2nd edn. London: Saunders Ltd.; 2005.

97. Larson A. Diagnosis and management of acute liver failure. Current Opinon in Gastroenterology 2010;26(3):214–21.

98. Friedman S, Runyon B, Travis A. Clinical manifestations and diagnosis of alcoholic fatty liver disease and alcoholic cirrhosis. 2013; http://www.uptodate.com/contents/clinical-manifestations-and-diagnosis-of-alcoholic-fatty-liver-disease-and-alcoholic-cirrhosis. Accessed September, 2013.

99. Heidelbaugh J, Bruderly M. Cirrhosis and chronic liver failure: part 1—diagnosis and evaluation. American Family Physician 2006;74(5):756–62.

100. Macnaughtan J, Thomas H. Liver failure at the front door. Clinical Medicine 2010;10(1):73–8.

101. Friedman S, Chopra S, Travis A. Approach to the patient with abnormal liver biochemical and function tests 2013; www.uptodate.com/contents/approach-to-the-patient-with-abnormal-liver-biochemical-and-function-tests; accessed 27 March 2015.

102. Flum D, Dellinger E. Assessing the impact of bariatric surgery on survival. Journal of American College of Surgeons 2004;199:551.

103. Foster A, Richards W, McDowell J et al. Gastrointestinal symptoms are more intense in morbidly obese patients. Surgical endoscopy 2003;17(11):1766–8.

104. Carucci L, Turner M. Radiologic evaluation following Roux-en-Y gastric bypass surgery for morbid obesity. European Journal of Radiology 2005;53:353–65.

105. Gorecki P, Wise L, Brolin R, Champion J. Complications of combined gastric restrictive and malabsorptive procedures: part 1. Current Surgery 2003;60(138–44):138.

106. Sugerman HJ, Brewer WH, Shiffman ML et al. A multicenter, placebo-controlled, randomized, double-blind, prospective trial of prophylactic ursodiol for the prevention of gallstone formation following gastric-bypass-induced rapid weight loss. American Journal of Surgery 1995;169(1):91–7.

107. Byrne T. Complications of surgery for obesity. Surgical Clinics of North America 2001;81:1181–93.

108. Comeau E, Gagner M, Inabnet W et al. Symptomatic internal hernias after laparoscopic bariatric surgery. Surgical Endoscopy 2005;19:34–9.

109. Podnos Y, Jimenez J, Wilson S et al. Complications after laparoscopic gastric bypass: a review of 3464 cases. Archives of Surgery 2003;138:957–61.

110. Moser F, Gorodner M, Galvani C et al. Pouch enlargement and band slippage: two different entities. Surgical Endoscopy 2006;20(7):1021–9.

111. Eid I, Birch D, Sharma A et al. Complications associated with adjustable gastric banding for morbid obesity: a surgeon's guide. Canadian Journal of Surgery 2011;54(1):61–6.

112. Suter M. Laparoscopic band repositioning for pouch dilatation/slippage after gastric banding: disappointing results. Obesity Surgery 2001;11:507–12.

113. Tran D, Rhoden D, Cacchione R et al. Techniques for repair of gastric prolapse after laparoscopic gastric banding. Journal of Laparoendoscopic and Advanced Surgical Techniques, Part A 2004;14(2):117–20.

114. Msika S. Surgery for morbid obesity: 2. Complications. Results of a technological evaluation by the ANAES. Journal de chirurgie (Paris) 2003;140(1):4–21.

115. National Institute of Clinical Studies. Pain medication for acute abdominal pain. Canberra: National Health and Medical Research Council; 2008.

116. Manterola C, Vial M, Moraga J, Astudillo P. Analgesia in patients with acute abdominal pain. Cochrane Database System Review 2011;19(1):1–33.

117. National Health and Medical Research Council. Emergency Care Acute Pain Management Manual. Canberra: NHMRC; 2011.

118. MIMSOnline. Fentanyl for injection. 2014; www.mimsonline.com.au.acs.hcn.com.au/Search/FullPI.aspx?ModuleName=ProductInfo&searchKeyword=Fentanyl&PreviousPage=~/Search/QuickSearch.aspx&SearchType=&ID=3690001_2; accessed March 2014.

119. Considine J, Kropman M, Kelly E, Winter C. Effect of Emergency Department fast track on Emergency Department length of stay: a case-control study. Emergency Medicine Journal 2008;25:815–19.

120. Seeley R, Stephens T, Tate P, eds. Anatomy and physiology. 2003.

121. Lewis S, Heitkemper M, Dirksen S, eds. Medical-surgical nursing: assessment and management of clinical problems. 5th edn. St. Louis: Mosby; 2000.

122. Society of Gastroenterology Nurses and Associates. Gastroenterology nursing: a core curriculum. St. Louis: Mosby; 1993.

123. Lewis S, Collier I, Heitkemper M, eds. Medical-surgical nursing: assessment and management of clinical problems. 7th ed. St. Louis: Mosby; 2007.

124. Liechty R, Soper R. Fundamentals of surgery. 6th edn. St. Louis: Mosby; 1989.

125. Marx J, Hockberger R, Walls R et al, eds. Rosen's emergency medicine: concepts and clinical practice, volume 1. 7th edn. St. Louis: Mosby; 2010.

126. Mettler F, Guibertereau M, Voss C, Urbina C. Primary care radiology. Philadelphia: WB Saunders; 2000.

127. Dettenmeier P. Radiographic assessment for nurses. St. Louis: Mosby; 1995.

128. Bennett D, Tanmbeur L, Campbell W. Use of cough test to diagnose peritonitis. British Medical Journal 1994;308(6940):1336.

129. Golledge J, Toms A, Franklin I et al. Assessment of peritonism in appendicitis. Annals of the Royal College of Surgeons of England 1996;78(1):11–14.

130. Jahn H, Mathiesen F, Neckelmann K et al. Comparison of clinical judgment and diagnostic ultrasonography in the diagnosis of acute appendicitis: experience with a score-aided diagnosis. European Journal of Surgery 1997;163(6):433–43.

131. Fenyö G, Lindberg G, Blind P et al. Diagnostic decision support in suspected acute appendicitis: validation of a simplified scoring system. European Journal of Surgery 1997;163(11):831–8.

132. Mahadevan M, Graff L. Prospective randomized study of analgesic use for ED patients with right lower quadrant abndominal pain. American Journal of Emergency Medicine 2000;18(7):753–6.

133. Hallan S, Asberg A, Edna T. Estimating the probability of acute appendicitis using clinical criteria of a structured record sheet: the physician against the computer. European Journal of Surgery 1997;163(6):427–32.

134. Mookadam F, Cikes M. Cullen's and Turner's signs. New England Journal of Medicine 2005;353(13):1386.

135. Markle G. Heel-drop jarring test for appendicitis. Archives of Surgery 1985;120(2):243.

136. Markle G. A simple test for intraperitoneal inflammation. American Journal of Surgery 1975;125:721–2.

137. Donoghue v Stevenson. AC 562 at 580, 1932.

138. White M, Counselman F. Troubleshooting acute abdominal pain. Emergency Medicine 2002;34(1):16–27.

139. Lane R, Grabham J. A useful sign for the diagnosis of peritoneal irritation in the right iliac fossa. Annals of the Royal College of Surgeons of England 1997;79:128–9.

140. Fernandes J, Lopez P, Montes J, Cara M. Validity of tests performed to diagnose acute abominal pain in patients admitted at an emergency department. Revista Española de Enfermedades Digestivas 2009;101(9):610–18.

141. Singer A, McCracken G, Henry M et al. Correlation among clinical, laboratory, and hepatobiliary scanning fingings in patients with suspected acute cholecystitis. Annuals of Emergency Medicine 1996;28(3):267–72.

142. Adedeji O, McAdam W. Murphy's sign, acute cholecystitis and elderly people. Journal of the Royal College of Surgeons of Edinburgh 1996;41(2):88–9.

143. Mills LD, Mills T, Foster B. Association of clinical and laboratory variables with ultrasound findings in right upper quadrant abdominal pain. Southern Medical Journal 2005;98(2):155–61.

144. Berry J, Malt R. Appendicitis near its centenary. Annals of Surgery 1984;200(5):567–75.

145. Wagner J, McKinney M, Carpenter J. Does this patient have appendicitis? Journal of American Medical Association 1996; 276(19):1589–94.

146. Izbicki J, Knoefel W, Wilker D et al. Accurate diagnosis of acute appendicitis: a retrospective and prospective analysis of 686 patients. The European Journal of Surgery 1992;158(4):227–31.

147. John H, Neff U, Keleman M. Appendicitis diagnosis today: clinical and ultrasound deductions. World Journal of Surgery 1993; 17(2):243–9.

148. Alshehri M, Ibrahim A, Abuaisha N et al. Value of rebound tenderness in acute appendicitis. East African Medical Journal 1995;72(8):504–6.

149. Clayton H, Reschak G, Gaynor S, Creamer J. A novel program to assess and manage pain. MedSurg Nursing 2000;9(6):317–22.

150. Brown D, Edwards H, eds. Lewis's medical-surgical nursing: assessment and management of clinical problems. Sydney: Elsevier; 2005.

151. Victorian Government Department of Health Services. The blue book: guidelines for the control of infectious diseases. 2005; http://docs.health.vic.gov.au/docs/doc/FE2665DB66894C46CA2578B0001BE87E/$FILE/bluebook.pdf; accessed 3 June 2015.

152. Therapeutic Guidelines. Antibiotics: gastrointestinal tract infections. 2011.

CHAPTER 25
RENAL AND GENITOURINARY EMERGENCIES

ANN BONNER

Essentials

- Urinalysis is an important, simple, quick and non-invasive assessment.
- Early and aggressive treatment of hypotension or hypovolaemia will prevent the development of acute kidney injury.
- Acute kidney injury can result from nephrotoxic agents such as contrast media.
- Chronic kidney disease should be considered likely in people with diabetes or hypertension regardless of whether or not it is diagnosed.
- Arteriovenous fistulae should be regularly assessed for patency and should never be cannulated.
- Peritonitis is the most common complication associated with peritoneal dialysis.
- Urinary tract infections and pyelonephritis can be the cause of septicaemia, particularly in older people.
- The pain associated with renal calculi requires regular assessment and administration of appropriate analgesia.
- Scrotal pain needs urgent assessment and referral to preserve testicular function.

INTRODUCTION

Genitourinary (GU) problems are a common complaint in the community and the emergency department (ED). Urinary tract infections (UTIs) are the second most-common bacterial disease, and up to 20% of women will experience at least one UTI in their lifetime. UTIs are mostly managed by general practitioners.[1] Nephrolithiasis (renal calculi) affects over 1,000,000 Australians and it is likely that the hot, dry climate causes more stone formation than in many other countries in the world. Acute kidney injury (AKI) is a common complication of any trauma. Hypovolaemia results in severe hypotension and this precipitates the development of acute tubular necrosis and subsequent AKI. The global incidence of chronic kidney disease (CKD) is rapidly rising in developed and developing nations. CKD is classified into five stages, with those in stage 5 classified as being in end-stage kidney disease (ESKD). It is estimated that one in three adults are at risk of developing CKD, and 10% of the Australian and New Zealand population does have CKD. Dialysis is the leading cause of hospitalisation and accounts for 13% of separations from all public and private hospitals in Australia.[2] Indigenous populations from both countries (Aboriginals, Torres Strait Islanders, Maori and Pacific Islanders) are over-represented in the number of people with all stages of CKD.

Patients with compromised renal function often require the assistance of paramedics and will arrive at the ED with life-threatening fluid and electrolyte imbalances.

Specific GU emergencies discussed in this chapter are acute kidney injury, rhabdomyolysis, chronic kidney disease, UTIs, acute urinary retention, urinary calculi, testicular torsion, epididymitis and priapism. Refer to Chapter 34 for discussion of sexually transmitted infections (STIs) in women and to Chapter 48 for discussion of genitourinary trauma.

Anatomy and physiology

The genitourinary tract consists of the kidneys, ureters, urinary bladder, urethra and external genitalia. Urine is produced by the kidneys as a way to regulate fluid volume and electrolyte balance. The kidneys also have a major role in acid–base balance, regulation of blood pressure, excretion of toxins (such as urea, creatinine and drugs), production of erythropoietin and synthesis of vitamin D.[3] Ureters transport urine to the bladder for temporary storage. The urine is drained from the bladder to the outside by the urethra. Figure 25.1 shows structures of the GU system. External structures of the male GU system have reproductive functions.

Kidneys

The kidneys are located on the posterior abdominal wall behind the peritoneum on either side of the vertebral column. The kidney is shown in cross-section in Figure 25.2. On the medial aspect of each kidney is the *hilum*, where the renal artery and nerve enter and the renal vein and ureter exit. The hilum opens into the *renal pelvis*, an enlargement of the urinary channel. Renal calyces, shaped like the cup of a flower, open into the renal pelvis. Each kidney contains 20 minor calyces that open into 2–3 major calyces. The kidney has an outer *cortex* and an inner layer or *medulla*. Cone- or triangular-shaped structures called *medullary pyramids* located in the renal medulla open into a minor calyx. The cortex surrounds the medulla and extends between pyramids in columns to the renal pelvis. Blood flow to the kidney is supplied by the *renal artery*, which branches off the abdominal aorta and enters the kidney through the renal sinus. Blood leaves the kidney through the *renal vein*, which empties into the abdominal inferior vena cava.

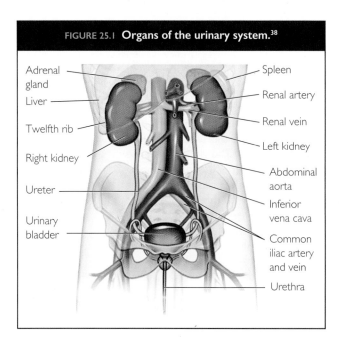

FIGURE 25.1 **Organs of the urinary system.**[38]

Adrenal gland
Liver
Twelfth rib
Right kidney
Ureter
Urinary bladder

Spleen
Renal artery
Renal vein
Left kidney
Abdominal aorta
Inferior vena cava
Common iliac artery and vein
Urethra

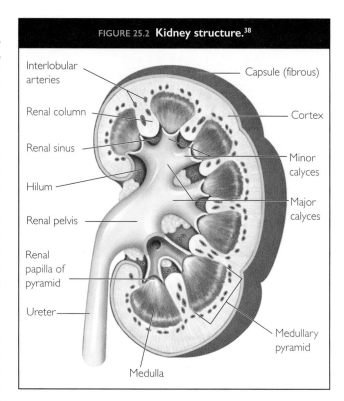

FIGURE 25.2 **Kidney structure.**[38]

Interlobular arteries
Renal column
Renal sinus
Hilum
Renal pelvis
Renal papilla of pyramid
Ureter

Capsule (fibrous)
Cortex
Minor calyces
Major calyces
Medullary pyramid
Medulla

Nephron

The *nephron*, the functional unit of the kidney, is composed of the renal corpuscle, proximal convoluted tubule, loop of Henle, distal convoluted tubule and collecting ducts (Fig 25.3). Each kidney contains an estimated 1,000,000 nephrons that are individually capable of producing urine. These nephrons cannot be reproduced once destroyed. The renal corpuscle contains the *glomerulus*, a web of tightly convoluted capillaries, and *Bowman's capsule*, which surrounds and supports these structures. Blood flows through the afferent arteriole into the glomerulus and out the efferent arteriole. Each minute approximately 1–1.5 L of blood (25% of cardiac output) is passed through the 2,000,000 glomeruli, where ultrafiltration takes place.[3]

Specialised cells called *juxtaglomerular cells* are located at the entrance to the glomerulus of the afferent arteriole in 15% of nephrons. Juxtaglomerular cells form a cuff and combine with the *macula densa*, a portion of the distal convoluted tubule that lies adjacent to the renal corpuscle between afferent and efferent arterioles.[3] The juxtaglomerular cells and the macula densa form the *juxtaglomerular apparatus*, which senses changes in pressure and sodium concentration and plays a role in the renin–angiotensin–aldosterone (RAA) system. Juxtaglomerular nephrons have a greater capacity to concentrate urine because they have longer loops of Henle, which extend into the medulla.

Filtration of plasma in the renal corpuscle is the first step in urine production and helps the kidneys rid the body of wastes and retain water and essential solutes.[3] Pressure, generated as blood, courses through the tight web of capillaries in the glomerulus. Along with oncotic pressure within the blood, it is greater than pressure created by Bowman's capsules, so plasma or filtrate and small solutes cross the semipermeable epithelial capillary lining. Injury to the glomerulus, such as

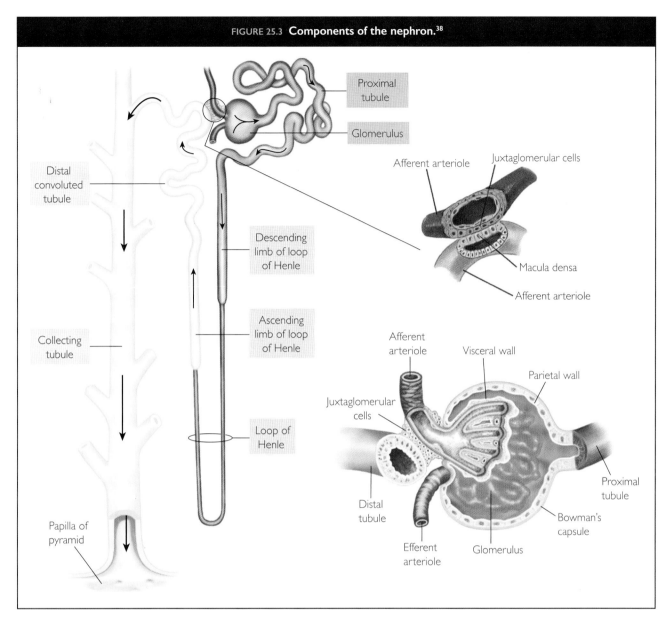

FIGURE 25.3 **Components of the nephron.**[38]

ischaemia or inflammation, increases permeability of the capillary membrane and allows larger molecules (red blood cells [RBCs], epithelial casts, protein or white blood cells [WBCs]) to cross. Decreased oncotic pressure, often the result of decreased serum albumin levels or decreased pressure within

the glomerulus produced by systemic hypotension, decreases glomerular filtration rate (GFR) and eventually urine output. GFR in the average adult is 125 mL/min or 180 L/day.[3] The functions of the segments of the nephron are summarised in Table 25.1.

TABLE 25.1 **Functions of nephron segments**[40]

COMPONENT	FUNCTION
Glomerulus	Selective filtration
Proximal tubule	Reabsorption of 80% of electrolytes and water, glucose, amino acids, HCO_3^-. Secretion of H^+ and creatinine
Loop of Henle	Reabsorption of Na^+ and Cl^- in ascending limb and water in descending loop. Concentration of filtrate
Distal tubule	Secretion of K^+, H^+, ammonia. Reabsorption of water (regulated by ADH) and HCO_3^-. Regulation of Ca^{2+} and PO_4^{2-} by parathyroid hormone. Regulation of Na^+ and K^+ by aldosterone
Collecting duct	Reabsorption of water (ADH required)

ADH: antidiuretic hormone; Ca^{2+}: calcium; Cl^-: chloride; H^+: hydrogen; HCO_3^-: bicarbonate; K^+: potassium; Na^+: sodium; PO_4^{3-}: phosphate

Tubules, loops of Henle and collecting ducts excrete waste products (e.g. urea, nitrogen, creatinine, drug metabolites), reabsorb water and solutes (potassium, sodium, chloride, hydrogen, glucose, amino acids) from filtrate and secrete excess solutes the body doesn't need into filtrate.[3] Osmosis, diffusion and active transport occur between the nephron and surrounding capillaries. Hormonal control regulates reabsorption and secretion in the nephron. Tubular cells have the capacity to regenerate following ischaemia (e.g. acute tubular necrosis).

Renin–angiotensin–aldosterone mechanism

The RAA system (Fig 25.4) and antidiuretic hormone (ADH) are feedback loop systems within the body that maintain homeostasis. Serum osmolarity increases and causes stimulation of the hypothalamus, which releases ADH. Nephron permeability increases, so additional water is absorbed, serum osmolarity returns to normal and ADH release stops.[3] Pressure changes in the glomerulus are overcome by vasodilation and constriction of the afferent arteriole by a process called *autoregulation*. This autoregulation keeps pressure in the glomerulus within a wide range of systolic blood pressures. When the range is exceeded, autoregulation fails and epithelial damage occurs, with eventual scarring and sclerosis followed by decreased permeability, GFR and urine output. Inadequate nephron perfusion stimulates the reabsorption of sodium and water by the nephron under the influence of the RAA mechanism.[3] Perfusion to the nephron increases and the cycle is altered.

Without a functioning kidney and adequate urine production, homeostasis is severely impaired. Fluid, electrolyte and acid–base imbalance, accumulation of urea and creatinine, decreased excretion of drug metabolites and inadequate reabsorption of amino acids and glucose occur. The kidneys also help convert vitamin D into the active form (1,25-vitamin D_3)

to ensure calcium absorption from intestines, and they secrete erythropoietin for stimulation of RBC production in bone marrow. Consequently, altered renal function causes severe electrolyte disturbances and decreases bone mineralisation and the oxygen-carrying capacity of the blood. A detailed discussion of the RAA mechanism and homeostasis can be found in Chapter 20.

Reproductive organs

External genitalia are also part of the GU system.[4] Female genitalia consist of the *vestibule*, the space into which the urethra and vagina open, and surrounding *labia minora* and *majora* (Fig 25.5). Anatomical position and the short length of the female urethra are responsible for the high frequency of UTIs in females.

Male external genitalia include *penis, scrotum* and *scrotal contents* (Fig 25.6). Scrotal contents include the *testes,* tubules that carry developing sperm cells and secrete testosterone, and the *epididymis* which lies along the posterior testes and is the final maturation area for sperm. The *prostate* is glandular and muscle tissue which surrounds the urethra at the base of the bladder. Enlargement of the prostate can cause outlet obstruction and urinary retention. The penis consists of three columns of erectile tissue that become engorged with blood, producing erection (Fig 25.7). Two columns of *corpora cavernosa* form the dorsum and sides of the penis and the *corpus spongiosum* forms the base and glans.[4] Clinical manifestations of GU disease frequently involve external genitalia.

Patient assessment

History

General health assessment of the GU system should determine history of hypertension, diabetes, previous infections, prostatitis, urethritis, bladder or urethral damage during

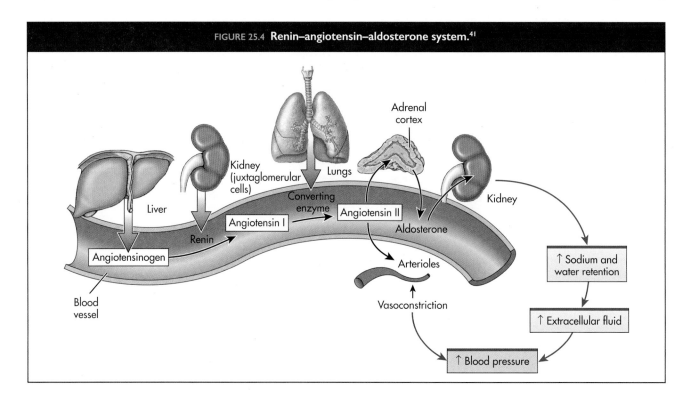

FIGURE 25.4 **Renin–angiotensin–aldosterone system.**[41]

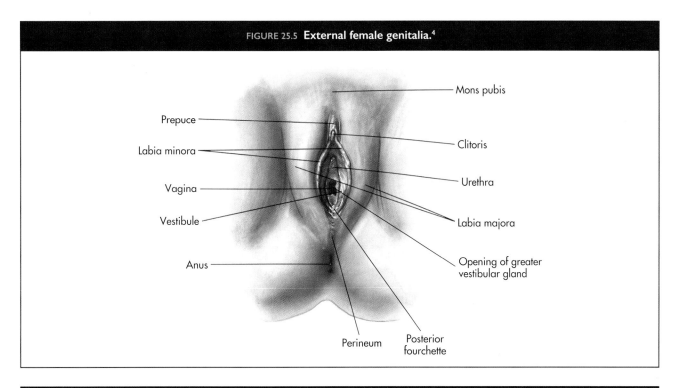

FIGURE 25.5 **External female genitalia.**[4]

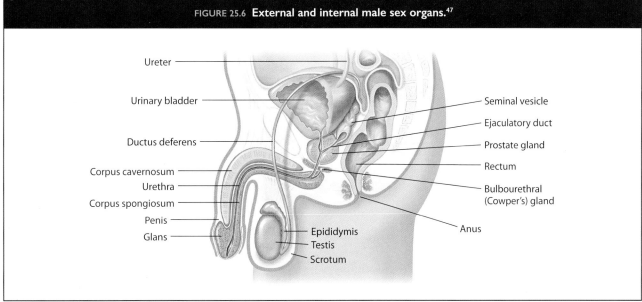

FIGURE 25.6 **External and internal male sex organs.**[47]

childbirth, history of renal calculi and recurrent urinary tract infections.[5] A detailed drug list, including prescription, over-the-counter (OTC) and illegal drugs, should be obtained. Recent medical and surgical history can also be important, such as urethral instrumentation (catheterisation) or other urological procedures (e.g. transurethral resection of prostate [TURP], uterine prolapse repair [Colpopexy]). Identification of any history of exposure to chemicals or toxins, including recent intravenous contrast media (e.g. for computed tomography or angiography) or those encountered in the workplace, may identify contact with substances that could cause nephrotoxicity (Table 25.2). Sexual history should include discussion of risk factors that can cause GU symptoms (e.g. use of contraceptive jellies or creams, multiple partners, abnormal

penile or vaginal discharges, unsafe sexual practices, history of STDs). GU complaints often arise from changes in urinary patterns; for example frequency, dysuria, urgency, dribbling, nocturia or incontinence. In a patient currently receiving kidney replacement therapy (i.e. haemodialysis, peritoneal dialysis or functioning kidney transplant), additional renal-specific history should be obtained.

Physical assessment

Inspection

Inspection of the patient with renal or urological dysfunction may reveal characteristic changes.[6]

- *Skin*—pallor, yellow-grey, excoriations, changes in turgor, bruising (particularly thorax, abdomen and flank have the

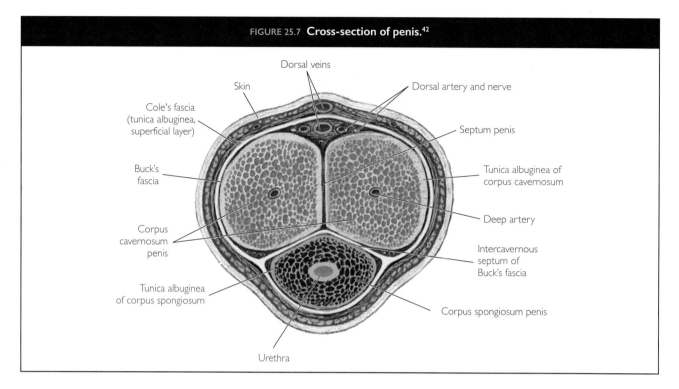

FIGURE 25.7 **Cross-section of penis.**[42]

TABLE 25.2 Potentially nephrotoxic agents[40]		
ANTIBIOTICS	OTHER DRUGS	OTHER AGENTS
Amphotericin B	Captopril	Gold
Cephalosporins	Cimetidine	Heavy metals
Gentamicin	Cisplatin	
Neomycin	Cocaine	
Polymyxin B	Cyclosporin	
Streptomycin	Ethylene glycol	
Sulfonamides	Heroin	
Tobramycin	Lithium	
Vancomycin	Methotrexate	
	Nitrosoureas (e.g. carmustine)	
	Non-steroidal antiinflammatory drugs (e.g. ibuprofen, indomethacin)	
	Phenacetin	
	Quinine	
	Rifampicin	
	Salicylates (large quantities)	

potential for injury to the renal and genitourinary system), texture (e.g. rough, dry skin).

- *Mouth*—stomatitis, ammonia breath odour.
- *Face and extremities*—generalised oedema, peripheral oedema, bladder distension, masses, enlarged kidneys, presence, site and type of vascular access for dialysis.
- *Abdomen*—skin changes described earlier, as well as striae, abdominal contour for midline mass in lower abdomen (may indicate urinary retention) or unilateral mass (occasionally seen in adult, indicating enlargement of one or both kidneys from large tumour or polycystic kidney), presence of peritoneal dialysis catheter exit-site and whether the site is inflamed, leaking or encrusted.
- *Genitourinary*—presence of blood at the urinary meatus is a strong indication of trauma to the urethra; visualisation of genitalia may reveal injuries.
- *Weight*—current and ideal weight, weight gain secondary to oedema; weight loss and muscle wasting in renal failure.
- *General state of health*—fatigue, lethargy and diminished alertness.

Palpation

As the kidneys are posterior organs protected by the abdominal organs, the ribs and the heavy back muscles, it is rare to palpate a normal-sized left kidney. Occasionally the lower pole of the right kidney is palpable. A landmark useful in locating the kidneys is the costovertebral angle (CVA) formed by the rib cage and the vertebral column.[5,6]

To palpate the right kidney, the examiner's left hand is placed behind and supports the patient's right side between the rib cage and the iliac crest (Fig 25.8). The right flank is elevated with the left hand, and the right hand is used to palpate deeply for the right kidney. The lower pole of the right kidney may be felt as a smooth, rounded mass that descends on inspiration. If the kidney is palpable, its size, contour and tenderness should be noted. Kidney enlargement is suggestive of neoplasm or other serious renal pathological conditions. The urinary bladder is normally not palpable unless it is distended with urine. If the bladder is full, it may be felt as a smooth, round, firm organ and is sensitive to palpation.

Percussion

Percussion is used to determine tenderness in the flank area. This technique is performed by striking the fist of one hand

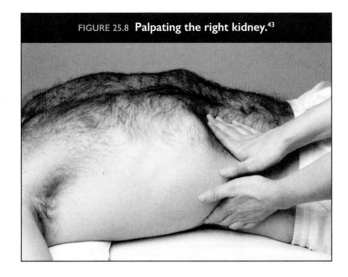

FIGURE 25.8 **Palpating the right kidney.**[43]

against the dorsal surface of the other hand (kidney punch), which is placed flat along the posterior CVA margin.[6] Normally a firm blow in the flank area should not elicit pain. If CVA tenderness and pain are present, it may indicate a kidney infection or polycystic kidney disease.

Auscultation

The diaphragm of the stethoscope may be used to auscultate over both CVAs and in the upper abdominal quadrants. With this technique, the abdominal aorta and renal arteries are auscultated for a bruit (an abnormal murmur), which indicates impaired blood flow to the kidneys.[6] Arteriovenous fistula and grafts should also be auscultated with a stethoscope to determine the presence of a bruit which indicates the vascular access is patent. See Chapter 17, p. 339, for further information and vascular access techniques. Bladder ultrasound, if available, can be used to verify urine volume.

Table 25.3 presents clinical manifestations of disorders of the urinary system and Table 25.4 presents common assessment abnormalities.

Urinalysis

In evaluating disorders of the urinary tract, one of the first studies done is a urinalysis (Table 25.5). This test may provide information about possible abnormalities, indicate what further studies need to be done and supply information on the progression of a diagnosed disorder. For a routine urinalysis, a specimen may be collected at any time of the day. The specimen should be examined within 1 hour of urinating.[5] If it is not, bacteria multiply rapidly, RBCs haemolyse, casts (moulds of renal tubules) disintegrate and the urine becomes alkaline as a result of urea-splitting bacteria. If it is not possible to send the specimen to the laboratory immediately, it should be refrigerated. The results of a urinalysis usually include a description of the appearance, specific gravity (mass and density), pH, glucose, ketones and protein in the urine and a microscopic examination of urine sediment for WBCs, RBCs, crystals and casts (Table 25.5). It is preferable to avoid an invasive procedure such as urinary catheterisation to collect a urine specimen for routine urinalysis.

If the urinalysis indicates a likelihood of infection, a reliable method to collect a mid-stream urine is required. In patients with severe cognitive impairments[7] or non-toilet-trained children,[8] insertion of a urethral catheter (e.g. in/out catheter) will enable a non-contaminated urine specimen to be collected.

Haematuria

Haematuria, the presence of blood in the urine, may be the primary complaint or may accompany other symptoms,[6] and is a sign of a serious underlying problem. Macroscopic haematuria is the hallmark of GU trauma and is also commonly associated with urological cancer, benign prostatic hypertrophy, renal disease, infection or renal calculi.[9] A detailed medication and diet history may uncover other causes for discolouration of urine. Box 25.1 highlights possible causes of red or dark-red urine. Microscopic haematuria is found during urinalysis. Early-stream haematuria suggests

---

TABLE 25.3 Signs and symptoms of urinary system disorders[40]

GENERAL SIGNS AND SYMPTOMS	OEDEMA	PAIN	PATTERNS OF URINATION	URINE OUTPUT	URINE COMPOSITION
Fatigue	Facial (periorbital)	Dysuria	Frequency	Anuria	Concentrated
Headaches	Ankle	Flank or costovertebral angle	Urgency	Oliguria	Dilute
Blurred vision	Ascites		Hesitancy of stream	Polyuria	Haematuria
Elevated blood pressure	Anasarca	Groin	Change in stream		Pyuria
Anorexia	Sacral	Suprapubic	Retention		Colour (red, brown, yellowish green)
Nausea and vomiting			Dysuria		
Chills			Nocturia		
Itching			Incontinence		
Excessive thirst			Stress incontinence		
Change in body weight			Dribbling		
Cognitive changes					

TABLE 25.4 Common assessment abnormalities of the urinary system[40]

FINDING	DESCRIPTION	POSSIBLE AETIOLOGY AND SIGNIFICANCE
Anuria	Technically no urination (24-hour urine output <100 mL)	Acute kidney injury, end-stage kidney disease, bilateral ureteral obstruction
Burning on urination	Stinging pain in urethral area	Urethral irritation, urinary tract infection
Dysuria	Painful or difficult urination	Sign of urinary tract infection, interstitial cystitis, and wide variety of pathological conditions
Enuresis	Involuntary nocturnal urination	Symptomatic of lower urinary tract disorder
Frequency	Increased incidence of urination	Acutely inflamed bladder, retention with overflow, excess fluid intake, intake of bladder irritants
Haematuria	Blood in the urine	Cancer of genitourinary tract, blood dyscrasias, kidney disease, urinary tract infection, stones in kidney or ureter, medications (anticoagulants)
Hesitancy	Delay or difficulty in initiating urination	Partial urethral obstruction, benign prostatic hyperplasia
Incontinence	Inability to voluntarily control discharge of urine	Neurogenic bladder, bladder infection, injury to external sphincter
Nocturia	Frequency of urination at night	Kidney disease with impaired concentrating ability, bladder obstruction, heart failure, diabetes mellitus, finding after renal transplant, excessive evening and night time fluid intake
Oliguria	Diminished amount of urine in a given time (24-hour urine output of 100–400 mL)	Severe dehydration, shock, transfusion reaction, kidney disease, end-stage kidney disease
Pain	Suprapubic pain (related to bladder), urethral pain (irritation of bladder neck), flank (CVA) pain	Infection, urinary retention, foreign body in urinary tract, urethritis, pyelonephritis, renal colic or stones
Pneumaturia	Passage of urine containing gas	Fistula connections between bowel and bladder, gas-forming urinary tract infections
Polyuria	Large volume of urine in a given time	Diabetes mellitus, diabetes insipidus, chronic kidney disease, diuretics, excess fluid intake, obstructive sleep apnoea
Retention	Inability to urinate even though bladder contains excessive amount of urine	Finding after pelvic surgery, childbirth, catheter removal, anaesthesia; urethral stricture or obstruction; neurogenic bladder
Stress incontinence	Involuntary urination with increased pressure (sneezing or coughing)	Weakness of sphincter control, lack of oestrogen, urinary retention

CVA, costovertebral angle.

bleeding from the urethra, haematuria throughout the stream indicates upper GU tract bleeding and bleeding at the end of the void suggests bladder neck or urethral bleeding. The majority of patients with haematuria will need to be admitted for further investigation.

Presence of gross blood at the urethral meatus strongly suggests urethral injury, generally associated with pelvic fractures (see Chapter 50 for further details). An indwelling urinary catheter (IDC) should not be inserted without first doing a retrograde urethrogram to ensure urethral integrity, or consultating with senior medical/urology clinicians.[9] If required, a suprapubic catheter will be inserted in the ED. In non-traumatic situations, patients with haematuria will need an IDC inserted. Where possible, determine from the patient the colour of the urine and the presence of clots.

PRACTICE TIP

Thick bloody urine with clots frequently requires a 22 F three-way IDC which enables the bladder to be continually washed and irrigated to prevent clot retention.

Pain

Pain should be assessed using the PQRST mnemonic—**P**rovocation, **Q**uality, **R**egion or radiation, **S**everity and **T**iming (see Ch 19 for further details).

The most severe pain associated with the GU system is renal colic caused by calculi (nephrolithiasis). Increased pressure and dilation of the kidney and urinary collecting system cause sudden, unbearable pain. The patient usually presents

		TABLE 25.5 Urinalysis findings[40]	
TEST	NORMAL	ABNORMAL FINDING	POSSIBLE AETIOLOGY AND SIGNIFICANCE
Colour	Amber yellow	Dark, smoky colour	Haematuria
		Yellow-brown to olive green	Excessive bilirubin
		Orange-red or orange-brown	Phenazopyridine
		Cloudiness of freshly voided urine	Infection
		Colourless urine	Excessive fluid intake, kidney disease or diabetes insipidus
Odour	Aromatic	Ammonia-like odour	Urine allowed to stand
		Unpleasant odour	Urinary tract infection
Protein	Random protein (dipstick): 0–trace	Persistent proteinuria	Characteristic of acute and chronic kidney disease, especially involving glomeruli. Heart failure
	24-hour protein (quantitative): <150 mg/day		In absence of disease: high-protein diet, strenuous exercise, dehydration, fever, emotional stress, contamination by vaginal secretions
Glucose	None	Glycosuria	Diabetes mellitus, low renal threshold for glucose reabsorption (if blood glucose level is normal). Pituitary disorders
Ketones	None	Present	Altered carbohydrate and fat metabolism in diabetes mellitus and starvation; dehydration, vomiting, severe diarrhoea
Bilirubin	None	Present	Liver disorders May appear before jaundice is visible (see Ch 40)
Specific gravity	1.003–1.030 Maximum concentrating ability of kidney in morning urine (1.025–1.030)	Low	Dilute urine, excessive diuresis, diabetes insipidus
		High	Dehydration, albuminuria, glycosuria
		Fixed at about 1.010	Renal inability to concentrate urine; end-stage kidney disease
Osmolality	300–1300 mOsm/kg (300–1300 mmol/kg)	<300 mOsm/kg >1300 mOsm/kg	Tubular dysfunction. Kidney lost ability to concentrate or dilute urine (not part of routine urinalysis)
pH	4.0–8.0 (average, 6.0)	>8.0	Urinary tract infection. Urine allowed to stand at room temperature (bacteria decompose urea to ammonia)
		<4.0	Respiratory or metabolic acidosis
RBCs	0–4/hpf	>4/hpf	Calculi, cystitis, neoplasm, glomerulonephritis, tuberculosis, kidney biopsy, trauma
WBCs	0–5/hpf	>5/hpf	Urinary tract infection or inflammation
Casts	None Occasional hyaline	Present	Moulds of the renal tubules that may contain protein, WBCs, RBCs or bacteria. Non-cellular casts (hyaline in appearance) occasionally found in normal urine
Culture for organisms	No organisms in bladder <10⁴ organisms/mL result of normal urethral flora	Bacteria counts >10⁵/mL	Urinary tract infection; most common organisms are *Escherichia coli*, enterococci, *Klebsiella*, *Proteus* and streptococci

hpf, high-powered field.

with restlessness and pallor, and complains of flank pain that often radiates to the abdomen and groin, often termed *loin-to-groin pain*.[6,11] If the stone lodges in the bladder, urinary frequency and urgency develop. Pain can cause tachypnoea and tachycardia with elevated blood pressure, although patients with these symptoms should not have other causes lightly

---

BOX 25.1 Non-haematuria causes of abnormal colour changes in urine[48,49]

Food	Drugs	Pathological conditions
Beetroot (red)	Adriamycin (red)	Chyluria (white milky)
Rhubarb (red)	Aminosalicylic acid (red)	Jaundice (yellow to brown)
Blackberries (red)	Ibuprofen (red)	Myoglobinuria (red/brown/rust)
Food colouring (rhodamine B) (red)	Methyldopa (red)	Porphyrins (red to black)
Senna (yellow to brown, red)	Metronidazole (dark yellow)	Uric acid crystalluria (pink)
	Nitrofurantoin (brown)	
	Phenytoin (Dilantin) (red)	
	Rifampicin (red)	

---

excluded. Relief of renal colic requires substantial amounts of analgesia, as discussed later in the chapter.

Oliguria

Oliguria, defined as urine output less than 400 mL in 24 hours, or anuria, less than 100 mL in 24 hours, may be the presenting symptom.[5] Dehydration or obstruction are the usual causes of oliguria; anuria is more likely to be due to acute kidney injury or end-stage kidney disease. However, blood chemistries should be evaluated for elevated urea and creatinine (azotaemia), which indicates renal failure from prolonged obstruction, leading to hydronephrosis or other causes. If the patient has a urinary catheter in place, patency should be assessed. A physical examination can identify acute urinary retention by palpating the bladder as a firm mass above the symphysis pubis, with an urge to void on palpation (more detail later in this chapter).

Specific conditions

Acute kidney injury

Acute kidney injury (AKI) is the rapid and sudden deterioration of renal function resulting in the retention of metabolic wastes (azotaemia) and impaired fluid and electrolyte balance.[11] It usually develops over hours or days and usually follows severe, prolonged hypotension or hypovolaemia or exposure to a nephrotoxic agent. AKI is usually accompanied by a reduction in urine output and an increase in serum creatinine.[12] Unlike chronic kidney disease, AKI is potentially reversible if the precipitating factors can be removed or corrected before permanent kidney damage has occurred. Despite advances in renal replacement therapies, AKI continues to have a mortality rate of approximately 50%.[12]

The acronym RIFLE (**R**isk, **I**njury, **F**ailure, **L**oss and **E**nd-stage kidney disease) is used to classify the severity (R, I, F) and the outcome (L, E) (Table 25.6).[13] The causes of AKI are commonly categorised as *prerenal* (55–60%), *intrarenal* (35–40%) and *postrenal* (< 5%).[13]

Prerenal

Prerenal causes are more commonly seen in the ED, as this form of AKI results from any external factors which cause a sudden and severe reduction in blood flow to the kidneys and subsequent reduction in glomerular perfusion and filtration rate.[14] Hypovolaemia, decreased cardiac output, decreased peripheral vascular resistance and vascular obstruction can all decrease the effective circulating volume of the blood. Oliguria occurs as the kidneys respond to the decreased blood flow by activating the RAA mechanism. This compensation by the kidneys results in sodium and water conservation. Decreased renal perfusion also decreases clearance of wastes (azotaemia). As decreased perfusion continues, the kidneys lose their ability to engage in compensatory mechanisms, and intrarenal damage to renal tissue occurs. The result is low urine output due to the kidneys' inability to excrete water, a rise in serum urea and creatinine proportional to each other (ratio of > 10:1), and the inability of the kidneys to conserve sodium. Prolonged hypotension and/or hypovolaemia will result in acute tubular necrosis (ATN). Causes of AKI, specific pathophysiology, general treatment and diagnostic markers are listed in Box 25.2. Table 25.7 highlights clinical manifestations of AKI.

Intrarenal

Acute tubular necrosis is a type of intrarenal AKI usually resulting from prolonged ischaemia, nephrotoxins (e.g. amino-glycoside antibiotics, contrast media), haemoglobin released from haemolysed red blood cells (RBCs), myoglobin released from necrotic muscle cells or toxins released from severe sepsis.[13] Those at greatest risk of developing ATN include the elderly, patients who have diabetes or those with a history of CKD. Paramedics and ED nurses should be alert to the potential for AKI in these types of patients particularly if there has been recent exposure to contrast media or other nephrotoxins. Ischaemic and nephrotoxic ATN are responsible for 90% of intrarenal AKI cases.[13] Primary renal diseases, such as acute glomerulonephritis and systemic lupus erythematosus, may also cause AKI.

ATN typically develops following prolonged ischaemia when perfusion to the kidney is considerably reduced, and in some patients ATN can eventuate after only a few hours of hypovolaemia or hypotension.[14] The renal protective mechanisms of autoregulation of renal blood vessels and activation of the RAA system are able to increase renal perfusion during the early stages of AKI. If, however, the blood flow is reduced for longer than 1 hour, these protective mechanisms begin to weaken, triggering a variety of factors which result in the development of ATN.

TABLE 25.6 RIFLE criteria for staging acute kidney injury[40]		
STAGE	GFR CRITERIA	URINE OUTPUT CRITERIA
Risk	Serum creatinine increased × 1.5 or GFR decreased by 25%	Urine output <0.5 mL/kg/hr for 6 hr
Injury	Serum creatinine increased × 2 or GFR decreased by 50%	Urine output <0.5 mL/kg/hr for 12 hr
Failure	Serum creatinine increased × 3 or GFR decreased by 75% or Serum creatinine >4 mg/dL with acute rise ≥0.5 mg/dL	Urine output <0.3 mL/kg/hr for 24 hr (oliguria) or Anuria for 12 hr
Loss	Persistent acute kidney failure; complete loss of kidney function >4 wk	—
End-stage kidney disease	Complete loss of kidney function >3 months	—

GFR, Glomerular filtration rate; AKI: acute kidney injury
*All serum creatinine references are based on changes from baseline.

BOX 25.2 Common causes of acute kidney injury[40]

Prerenal
Hypovolaemia

- Dehydration
- Haemorrhage
- GI losses (diarrhoea, vomiting)
- Excessive diuresis
- Hypoalbuminaemia
- Burns

Decreased cardiac output

- Cardiac dysrhythmias
- Cardiogenic shock
- Heart failure
- Myocardial infarction

Decreased peripheral vascular resistance

- Anaphylaxis
- Neurological injury
- Septic shock

Decreased renovascular blood flow

- Bilateral renal vein thrombosis
- Embolism
- Hepatorenal syndrome
- Renal artery thrombosis

Intrarenal
Nephrotoxic injury

- Drugs: aminoglycosides (gentamicin), amphotericin B
- Contrast media
- Haemolytic blood transfusion reaction
- Severe crush injury
- Chemical exposure: ethylene glycol, lead, arsenic, carbon tetrachloride

Interstitial nephritis

- Allergies: antibiotics (sulfonamides, rifampicin), non-steroidal antiinflammatory drugs, ACE inhibitors
- Infections: bacterial (acute pyelonephritis), viral (CMV), fungal (candidiasis)

Other causes

- Prolonged prerenal ischaemia
- Acute glomerulonephritis
- Thrombotic disorders
- Toxaemia of pregnancy
- Malignant hypertension
- Systemic lupus erythematosus

Postrenal
Benign prostatic hyperplasia

Bladder cancer

Calculi formation

Neuromuscular disorders

Prostate cancer

Spinal cord disease

Strictures

Trauma (back, pelvis, perineum)

ACE: angiotensin-converting enzyme; CMV: cytomegalovirus; GI: gastrointestinal

Postrenal

Postrenal AKI results from an obstruction of urine outflow from the kidneys. The obstruction can occur in the kidneys (e.g. renal cell carcinoma), ureter (e.g. renal calculi), bladder (e.g. cancer) or urethra (e.g. prostatic hypertrophy). Prostatic hypertrophy is the most common underlying problem.[14]

TABLE 25.7 Manifestations of acute kidney injury[39]

BODY SYSTEM	CLINICAL MANIFESTATIONS
Urinary	↓ Urinary output
	Proteinuria
	Casts
	↓ Specific gravity
	↓ Osmolality
	Urinary sodium
Cardiovascular	Volume overload
	Congestive heart failure
	Hypotension (early)
	Hypertension (after development of fluid overload)
	Pericarditis
	Pericardial effusion
	Dysrhythmias
Respiratory	Pulmonary oedema
	Kussmaul respirations
	Pleural effusions
Gastrointestinal	Nausea and vomiting
	Anorexia
	Stomatitis
	Bleeding
	Diarrhoea
	Constipation
Haematological	Anaemia (development within 48 hours)
	Susceptibility to infection
	Leucocytosis
	Defect in platelet functioning
Neurological	Lethargy
	Seizures
	Asterixis
	Memory impairment
Metabolic	Urea
	Creatinine
	↓ Sodium
	Potassium
	↓ pH
	↓ Bicarbonate
	↓ Calcium
	Phosphate

Urinary tract obstruction causes an increase in pressure proximal to the obstruction which often leads to dilation of the proximal collecting system (i.e. hydroureter and hydronephrosis). The elevated pressure in the collecting system is transmitted back into the tubular network and eventually stops glomerular filtration. Postrenal AKI is a urological emergency that requires immediate relief of the obstruction and decompression of the urinary system, otherwise permanent renal damage can occur.

Management of acute kidney injury

AKI is potentially reversible if the basement membrane of the glomerulus is not destroyed and the tubular epithelium regenerates. Prerenal and postrenal AKI resolve relatively easily when they are identified early and treatment is commenced quickly.[15] Intrarenal failure and ATN have a prolonged course of recovery because actual parenchymal damage has occurred. Clinically, AKI usually progresses through four phases: initiating, oliguric, diuretic and recovery.[12,15] In some situations, the patient does not recover from AKI and chronic kidney disease results.

The primary goals of treatment are to eliminate the cause, manage the signs and symptoms and prevent complications while the kidneys recover.[15]

> **PRACTICE TIP**
>
> The first step is to determine if there is adequate intra-vascular volume and cardiac output to ensure adequate perfusion of the kidneys; an important responsibility of paramedics. Urine output may be increased or decreased. This is assessed by the administration of volume expanders (e.g. Gelofusin) or bolus amounts of crystalloids along with diuretics (e.g. frusemide). This is assisted by monitoring jugular vein distension and vital signs (including mean arterial pressure [MAP]) or by invasive lines such as central venous pressure catheters.

If AKI is already established, forcing fluids and diuretics will not be effective and may, in fact, result in life-threatening fluid overload and pulmonary oedema. It is essential that paramedics accurately document and communicate fluids given, and the ED nurse commences and maintains an accurate fluid-balance chart, including fluids given pre-hospital.

Hyperkalaemia, hyponatraemia, hypocalcaemia, hyperphosphataemia and volume overload are the most common fluid and electrolyte imbalances resulting from loss of the kidney's ability to excrete potassium and phosphorus, conserve sodium and eliminate excess volume.[15] Other symptoms may include short-term weight gain or loss, nausea and vomiting, haematemesis, dysrhythmias, dyspnoea, stupor or coma. Compromise of airway, breathing, circulation and neurological function requires prompt intervention. Fever may be associated with infectious or inflammatory events. Thus, regular reassessment of vital signs is essential.

Hyperkalaemia is a medical emergency.[16] An electrocardiogram (ECG) may reveal tall peaked T waves, widened QRS and a prolonged P–R interval secondary to hyperkalaemia. The various therapies used to treat elevated potassium levels are listed in Box 25.3. Both intravenous (IV) insulin and sodium bicarbonate shift potassium into the cells within 15–30 minutes, but it will eventually shift back out. IV calcium gluconate works within minutes by raising the action potential threshold at which dysrhythmias will occur, but duration is short, as evidenced by return of ECG changes. Nebulised salbutamol can be used as adjuvant therapy, although this is more commonly used in children. Only sodium (or calcium) polystyrene sulfonate (e.g. Resonium) and dialysis actually remove potassium from the body. Sodium (or calcium) polystyrene sulfonate's onset of action is 60 minutes when given rectally and 120 minutes for oral administration.

After initial stabilisation, history and diagnostic testing focus on identifying the cause of AKI. Tests include serial blood chemistries, urinalysis with sodium and potassium concentrations, chest radiograph, renal ultrasounds and

---

BOX 25.3 Treatment alternatives for elevated potassium levels[40]

Regular insulin IV
- Potassium moves into cells when insulin is given.
- IV glucose is given concurrently to prevent hypoglycaemia.
- When effects of insulin diminish, potassium shifts back out of cells.

Sodium bicarbonate
- Therapy can correct acidosis and cause a shift of potassium into cells.

Calcium gluconate IV
- Generally used in advanced cardiac toxicity (with evidence of hyperkalaemia ECG changes).
- Calcium raises the threshold for excitation, resulting in dysrhythmias.

Haemodialysis
- Most effective therapy to remove potassium.
- Works within a short time.

Sodium polystyrene sulfonate
- Cation-exchange resin is administered by mouth or retention enema.
- When resin is in the bowel, potassium is exchanged for sodium.
- Therapy removes 1 mmol of potassium per gram of drug.
- It is mixed in water with sorbitol (or lactulose) to produce osmotic diarrhoea, allowing for evacuation of potassium-rich stool from body.

Salbutamol
- Shifts potassium into the cells
- Administer via nebuliser

Dietary restriction
- Potassium intake is limited to 40 mmol/day.
- Primarily used to prevent recurrent elevation; not used for acute elevation.

IV: intravenous

Doppler studies or computed tomography (CT) scan. Imaging procedures are usually done without contrast media because of toxic effects of the media on renal tubules. Acetylcysteine can also be used to prevent the nephrotoxic effects of contrast media in people at high risk of developing AKI, although this is controversial. If a patient requires the use of contrast media during imaging, adequate pre and post procedure hydration and close follow-up are more effective in avoiding AKI.[17]

Indications for emergency dialysis include stupor or coma (caused by rising nitrogen waste products in blood and metabolic changes), volume overload and pulmonary oedema, dangerous hyperkalaemia and metabolic acidosis.[18] Emergency haemodialysis requires vascular access (usually a temporary femoral or subclavian dual-lumen catheter) and an artificial kidney (dialyser) to act as a semipermeable membrane. The dialysate is used on one side of the semipermeable membrane and blood is on the other; then the processes of diffusion and osmosis occur. A blood pump is required to move blood through the dialyser (Fig 25.9). The ED nurse should be prepared to transfer the patient to the intensive care or dialysis unit, be familiar with transport equipment and have documented preceding events and communicated with the patient and their family.

Monitoring fluid volume status is the most important nursing and paramedic intervention of all patients at risk for the development of AKI or during the course of AKI.[14,15] Accurate measurements of blood pressure, pulse, body weight, urine output and jugular or central venous pressure, as well as assessment of lung fields, skin turgor, mucous membranes and presence of oedema, are all vital in determining the patient's fluid volume status. Monitoring the use, as well as careful administration, of potentially nephrotoxic agents is also an important nursing responsibility.

Rhabdomyolysis

Skeletal muscle destruction with subsequent release of myoglobin into the circulatory system causes rhabdomyolysis, which can lead to AKI.[19] There are a number of different causes of rhabdomyolysis, including crush injuries, compartment syndrome, excessive physical exertion (e.g. long-distance running), muscle ischaemia (e.g. immobile or comatose person), drug or toxin ingestion, envenomation, infection, burns, temperature extremes or metabolic disturbances. Drugs, toxins and venoms are the largest causes of rhabdomyolysis. Crush injuries may be caused by entrapment, such as prolonged compression of the abdomen or a limb during a motor vehicle crash. Police cadets and military recruits are at risk of developing rhabdomyolysis due to excessive physical exertion. See Chapter 50 for a detailed discussion of compartment syndrome and crush injuries.

When there is breakdown of muscle tissue and ensuing cell deterioration and death, there is a rapid release of myoglobin and potassium into the plasma circulation. Fluid shifts from the intravascular space into the interstitial space can cause the patient to become profoundly hypovolaemic. Dehydration results from hypovolaemia and causes hypoperfusion of the kidneys, thereby decreasing the GFR. The electrolyte abnormalities that can occur with rhabdomyolysis include hyperkalaemia (which can be rapidly increasing), hypocalcaemia, hyperphosphataemia and hyperuricaemia.[19] There is a massive increase in serum creatinine phosphokinase (CK)

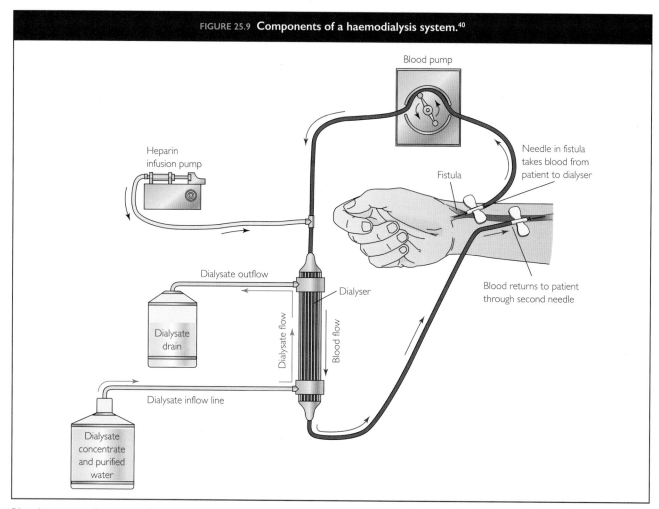

FIGURE 25.9 Components of a haemodialysis system.[40]

Blood is removed via a needle inserted in a fistula or via catheter lumen. It is propelled to the dialyser by a blood pump. Heparin is infused either as a bolus pre-dialysis or through a heparin pump continuously to prevent clotting. Dialysate is pumped in and flows in the opposite direction to the blood. The dialysed blood is returned to the patient through a second needle or catheter lumen. Old dialysate and ultrafiltrate are drained and discarded.

levels; anywhere from 10,000 to 200,000 U/L.[19] The urine may have a characteristic reddish brown colour ('tea-coloured'). Myoglobin reacts with the haemoglobin reagent on urine dipsticks causing a positive result; however, no RBCs are seen during microscopic examination. Proteinuria is also noted on urinalysis. Presenting signs and symptoms include complaints of muscle aches or acute muscle pain. General malaise, fever and muscle tenderness may occur.

Treatment of rhabdomyolysis consists of early and aggressive fluid-volume replacement, monitoring and maintenance of electrolyte balance.[14,19] Increasing the urine output helps flush myoglobin through the kidneys. Sodium bicarbonate may be added to IV fluids to alkalinise the urine which decreases the precipitation of myoglobin. If sodium bicarbonate is used, urine pH and serum bicarbonate, calcium and potassium levels should be monitored, and if the urine pH does not rise after 4–6 hours of treatment or if symptomatic hypocalcaemia develops, alkalinisation should be discontinued and hydration continued with normal saline.[19] If the patient progresses to acute kidney injury (AKI), management is the same as previously described. For further discussion on the management of rhabdomyolysis, refer to Chapter 50.

Chronic kidney disease

One in three Australians is at risk of developing chronic kidney disease (CKD) due to the increasing number of people with risk factors such as hypertension, obesity, smoking or diabetes. CKD is characterised by a progressive and irreversible destruction of renal function that occurs over varying periods of time, ranging from a few months to decades.[20] There are five stages of CKD, and the prognosis and course of CKD are highly variable, depending on the aetiology, patient's condition and age and adequacy of medical follow-up. The vast majority of individuals with CKD stages 2–3 live normal, active lives, whereas others may rapidly progress to stage 5 (ESKD). The Indigenous populations of both Australia and New Zealand are over-represented in the number of people with CKD. The major causes of CKD stage 5 in Australia are diabetes mellitus (31%), glomerulonephritis (25%) and hypertension (16%).[2] Regardless of the stage of CKD, it is also possible to develop AKI, particularly due to the administration of nephrotoxic agents such as contract media or antibiotics. Consequences of CKD are hypertension, elevated urea and creatinine levels, and anaemia.[12] In ESKD, oedema, electrolyte imbalances, metabolic acidosis and multisystem effects of uraemia develop (see Fig 25.10). When an individual

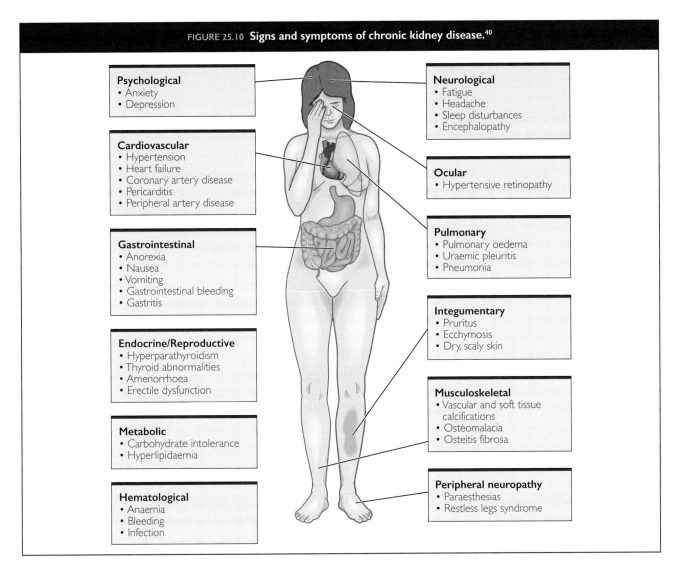

FIGURE 25.10 **Signs and symptoms of chronic kidney disease.**[40]

Psychological
• Anxiety
• Depression

Cardiovascular
• Hypertension
• Heart failure
• Coronary artery disease
• Pericarditis
• Peripheral artery disease

Gastrointestinal
• Anorexia
• Nausea
• Vomiting
• Gastrointestinal bleeding
• Gastritis

Endocrine/Reproductive
• Hyperparathyroidism
• Thyroid abnormalities
• Amenorrhoea
• Erectile dysfunction

Metabolic
• Carbohydrate intolerance
• Hyperlipidaemia

Hematological
• Anaemia
• Bleeding
• Infection

Neurological
• Fatigue
• Headache
• Sleep disturbances
• Encephalopathy

Ocular
• Hypertensive retinopathy

Pulmonary
• Pulmonary oedema
• Uraemic pleuritis
• Pneumonia

Integumentary
• Pruritus
• Ecchymosis
• Dry, scaly skin

Musculoskeletal
• Vascular and soft tissue calcifications
• Osteomalacia
• Osteitis fibrosa

Peripheral neuropathy
• Paraesthesias
• Restless legs syndrome

has severely impaired kidney function (Stage 4 and 5 CKD), extra care should be taken with the rapid administration of intravenous fluids; in some patients greater than 1000 mL in 8 hours can cause substantial fluid overload and/or pulmonary oedema can quickly result.

Dialysis complications
Kidney replacement therapy (KRT) is needed for people with CKD stage 5 (ESKD) in order to sustain life.[13] KRT may be provided by haemodialysis, peritoneal dialysis or a kidney transplant. There are increasing numbers of satellite haemo-dialysis units which are often isolated from the main hospital or located in separate community facilities. These units are only staffed by nurses who in an emergency may call the paramedic team. In addition, there are increasing numbers of patients who are performing haemodialysis at home—with or without a dialysis partner (e.g. spouse) in the home. Typically, a patient with ESKD who is being managed with haemodialysis will receive a minimum of 4 hours of treatment on three occasions each week, although home haemodialysis patients may dialyse overnight.

Regardless of the reason for presentation to an ED, all patients with an arteriovenous (AV) fistula require special precautions to prevent infection and clotting of the vascular access. There are three main types of vascular access: AV native fistula, AV grafts and central lines. An AV fistula is a surgical connection of an existing artery (e.g. radial) with an existing vein (e.g. cephalic) in any extremity, but particularly the wrist, forearm and upper arm.[13,21] See Chapter 17, p. 339, for further information on types of vascular access and techniques. Alternatively, an AV fistula can be created with the use of material (e.g. Gortex) to form the AV connection (Fig 25.11).

PRACTICE TIP

Regardless of the type of vascular access, it is crucial that ED staff and paramedics are aware of the presence of an AV fistula in a patient and that the access should be assessed (and preserved) at all times. For patients performing haemodialysis at home, emergency discontinuation involves stopping the blood pump, clamping all lines and leaving cannula in situ (flush with normal saline). If time permits and trained assistance is available (e.g. spouse) then blood in the circuit can be returned. If time does not permit disconnect and discard blood-filled circuit.

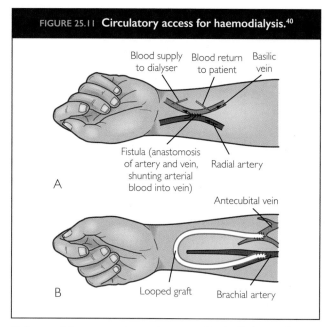

FIGURE 25.11 **Circulatory access for haemodialysis.**[40]

Blood supply to dialyser
Blood return to patient
Basilic vein
Fistula (anastomosis of artery and vein, shunting arterial blood into vein)
Radial artery
Antecubital vein
A
Looped graft
Brachial artery
B

A, Internal (permanent) arteriovenous fistula. **B**, Internal (permanent) arteriovenous graft.

Assessment of patency should be routinely and regularly undertaken and involves two steps: first, palpation over the anastomosis site to determine the presence of a thrill; and second, auscultation with a stethoscope to determine the presence of a bruit. The bruit and thrill are created by arterial blood rushing into the vein. A limb with a fistula should never have a blood pressure cuff applied, insertion of IV lines or venepuncture. An AV fistula will clot during episodes of hypotension or constriction of blood vessels (e.g. application of tourniquet, circumferential bandaging or blood-pressure cuffs).

Clotted vascular access frequently brings patients with ESKD to the ED and should be dealt with urgently in order to restore circulation through the fistula, with the patient being referred to the vascular surgeon or renal team. AV fistula and catheter insertion sites also become infected and may progress to septicaemia. Local symptoms include redness, drainage or oedema. Blood cultures and a full blood count (FBC) should be obtained to rule out systemic infection.

Peritoneal dialysis involves instilling 2–3 L of dialysate fluid containing varying amounts of glucose, sodium, magnesium, calcium, chloride, lactate and water into the abdomen.[12] The peritoneal membrane acts as a semipermeable pathway for exchange of solutes and water between the vascular peritoneal space and dialysate by osmosis and diffusion (Fig 25.12). Access to the peritoneal cavity is achieved through a plastic catheter held in place by a Dacron cuff (Fig 25.13). Although there are several different techniques for peritoneal dialysis, the most common are continuous ambulatory peritoneal dialysis (CAPD) and automated peritoneal dialysis (APD). CAPD requires the individual to manually change the dialysate in the peritoneal cavity four or five times each day. APD is normally performed overnight where a machine exchanges the dialysate.

Regardless of the type of peritoneal dialysis, peritonitis and exit site infections are the most common complications and often bring the patient to the ED with complaints of abdominal pain, nausea and vomiting, fever and cloudy dialysate fluid.[13]

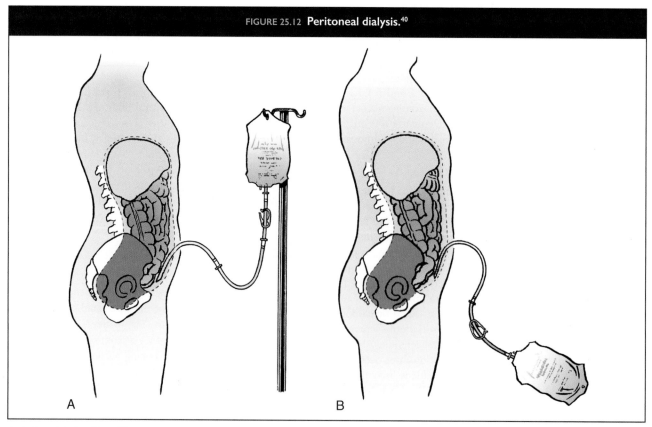

FIGURE 25.12 **Peritoneal dialysis.**[40]

A
B

A, Inflow. **B**, Outflow (drains to gravity).

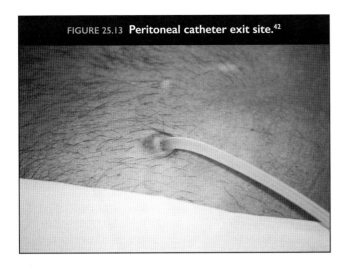

FIGURE 25.13 **Peritoneal catheter exit site.**[42]

PRACTICE TIP

Patients with ESKD receiving peritoneal dialysis have been instructed by the renal unit to bring the most recent bag exchange (i.e. effluent) to the ED (providing it has been stored in the refrigerator); paramedics should ensure the patient is accompanied by the bag.

Peritonitis is a potentially life-threatening complication, so the patient needs to be assessed urgently, a sample of effluent sent to the microbiology department and the patient commenced on antibiotics which are often added to the dialysate (IP) or may be given IV.[13] If this is unsuccessful, the catheter is removed and haemodialysis initiated until the peritonitis clears. Unless scarring impairs permeability of the peritoneal membrane, the catheter can be surgically replaced and peritoneal dialysis reinitiated.

Kidney transplantation is also an option for most patients with ESKD. The donor kidney is placed in the iliac fossa and native kidneys are not removed. Immunosuppression (e.g. prednisone, mycophenolate and cyclosporin) is required to avoid rejection.[13] Kidney transplant recipients commonly present to the ED with cardiovascular events or infections, particularly severe pyelonephritis.

Urinary tract infections

Urinary tract infections are a frequent presenting problem to the ED, particularly for older adults[22] and young children.[23] It is the source of infection in 30% of patients presenting to Australian and New Zealand EDs.[24] Symptoms include pyuria, haematuria, chills and fever, leucocytosis, nausea, vomiting and signs of bladder irritability, such as frequency, dysuria and urgency. With renal involvement, dull flank pain and costovertebral angle tenderness are associated with pyelonephritis. Older adults may not experience these symptoms and often experience non-localised abdominal discomfort.[22] In addition they are at risk of confusion or cognitive impairment and rapid progression to sepsis. UTI occurs in about 5–10% of children and should be considered in all febrile infants.[23] A minority of UTIs can be due to vesicoureteric reflux (VUR) and referral to a paediatrician may be required.

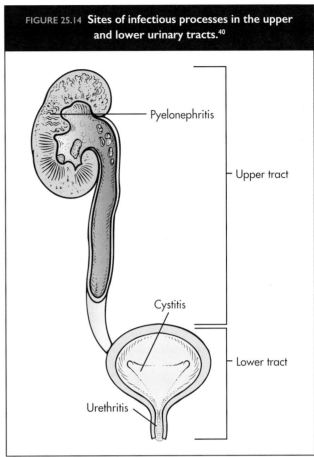

FIGURE 25.14 **Sites of infectious processes in the upper and lower urinary tracts.**[40]

Figure 25.14 illustrates infectious processes of the urinary system. Diagnosis is made by history, presenting signs, urinalysis, urine culture and sensitivity and FBC with differential. A KUB (kidneys–ureters–bladder) radiograph may show a hazy outline of the kidney secondary to oedema, although it is not always warranted.[25] Blood urea nitrogen (BUN), creatinine and electrolyte values are obtained to rule out alteration in renal function.

Approximately 80% of uncomplicated infections are caused by Gram-negative bacilli such as *Escherichia coli, Klebsiella pneumoniae, Enterobacter, Proteus* and *Serratia*.[25] Table 25.8 compares common GU tract infections that present to the ED. Persistent microscopic or gross haematuria, symptoms of obstruction or presence of urea-splitting bacteria associated with staghorn renal calculi require work-up with renal ultrasound, cystogram or intravenous pyelogram. Infection with *Chlamydia trachomatis* or *Neisseria gonorrhoea* should be considered with urethral infection and pyuria that has a negative culture.

In uncomplicated UTIs, commonly used antimicrobial therapy includes trimethoprim-sulfamethoxazole (TMP-SMX) and cephalexin.[25] Older patients, particularly from nursing homes, often have an infection that is resistant to TMP-SMX so ciprofloxacin, nitrofurantoin or cephalexin are used.[22,25] Antimicrobial therapy is adjusted once culture and susceptibility are known. Collaborative interventions involve antibiotics, adequate fluid intake and urinary alkaliniser[21] (Box 25.4). Intravenous rehydration may be needed in severe cases. Hot packs can relieve the discomfort associated with a

TABLE 25.8 Common genitourinary infections

TYPE	DESCRIPTION	ADDITIONAL SIGNS AND SYMPTOMS	INTERVENTIONS	COMPLICATIONS AND COMMENTS
Pyelonephritis	Involves renal parenchyma and pelvis Usually unilateral Kidneys enlarged by oedema More prevalent in women and diabetics Most commonly caused by ascending *Escherichia coli* infection from lower GU tract		Antibiotics specific to C & S Antipyretics and antiemetics Adequate hydration Monitor intake and output Bed rest	Complications uncommon but may include septicaemia Follow-up urine C & S to ensure effective antibiotic therapy Recurrence may require continuous antibiotic prophylactic suppression
Urethritis	More common in women; *E. coli* most common organism Associated behavioural factors include sexual intercourse, diaphragm and/or spermicide use, not voiding within 10–15 minutes after intercourse		Short-term antibiotics May need continuous antibiotic, prophylactic suppression or postcoital antibiotic	Associated behaviours UTIs Direction of wiping after defecation Tampon use Bubble bath Douche Tight clothing Carbonated beverages, coffee, alcohol Resisting urge to void Decreasing oral fluids Synthetic underwear
Epididymitis	Bacterial infection in older men Usually preceded by STI or urethritis in young men	P—lifting, sexual excitement, trauma Q—dull ache, sharp R—scrotum, lower abdomen S—increased with sex, decreased with elevation and support T—gradual onset Scrotum red, swollen and warm	Antibiotics Posttreatment culture Bed rest Scrotal support Avoid heavy lifting and straining	Teach safe sex and condom use, complete antibiotic regimen
Prostatitis	Expressed prostate secretions have more WBCs than urine	May have bladder outlet obstruction Low back pain Tender, boggy, hot prostate on manual exam	Antibiotics, urinalysis C & S and expressed prostate fluid C & S	
Non-specific urethritis	Causative agents: *E. coli, Staphylococcus, Klebsiella, Pseudomonas*	White discharge Urethral itching Perineal, suprapubic or testicular pain	Antibiotics as result of discharge C & S	

C & S: culture and sensitivity; GU: genitourinary; STI: sexually transmitted infection; UTIs: urinary tract infections; WBCs: white blood cells

---

BOX 25.4 Collaborative care in urinary tract infection[40]

Diagnostic studies
- History and physical examination
- Urinalysis
- Urine for culture and sensitivity (if indicated)
- Imaging studies of urinary tract (e.g. IVP, cystoscopy) (if indicated)
- Collaborative therapy

Uncomplicated UTI:
- Antibiotic, 1- to 3-day treatment regimen: trimethoprim-sulfamethoxazole, nitrofurantoin
- Adequate fluid intake
- Urinary alkaliniser
- Counselling about risk of recurrence and reduction of risk factors

Recurrent, uncomplicated UTI:
- Repeat urinalysis and consideration of need for urine culture and sensitivity testing
- Antibiotic, 3- to 5-day treatment regimen: trimethoprim-sulfamethoxazole, nitrofurantoin
- Sensitivity-guided antibiotic (ampicillin, amoxycillin, first-generation cephalosporin, fluoroquinolone)
- Consider 3- to 6-month trial of suppressive antibiotics
- Adequate fluid intake
- Urinary alkaliniser
- Counselling about risk of recurrence and reduction of risk factors
- Imaging study of urinary tract in selected cases

IVP: intravenous pyelogram; UTI: urinary tract infection

BOX 25.5 Risk factors for urinary tract calculi[40]

Metabolic
Abnormalities that result in increased urine levels of calcium, oxaluric acid, uric acid or citric acid
Climate
Hot climates that cause increased fluid loss, low urine volume and increased solute concentration in urine
Diet
Large intake of dietary proteins that increases uric acid excretion
Excessive amounts of tea or fruit juices that elevate urinary oxalate level
Large intake of calcium and oxalate
Low fluid intake that increases urinary concentration
Genetic factors
Family history of stone formation, cystinuria, gout or renal acidosis
Lifestyle
Sedentary occupation, immobility

UTI. Education about the risk of recurrence and reduction of risk factors is important (Box 25.5). Contrary to public opinion, there is insufficient robust evidence to support the use of cranberry juice or tablets as an effective treatment for UTIs.[26]

Acute pyelonephritis

Acute pyelonephritis is an infection of the upper urinary tract, commonly caused by ascending organisms, that may result in permanent renal damage.[27] Acute pyelonephritis occurs more frequently in women who present with costovertebral angle pain and tenderness, often accompanied by fever greater than 38°C.[27] Urinalysis and urine culture confirm the diagnosis of acute pyelonephritis, with *E. coli* responsible for more than 80% of cases. Blood cultures do not need to be routinely collected because they are not always positive and do not significantly alter therapy in adult patients.[27]

Acute pyelonephritis can usually be managed with oral antimicrobial therapy such as trimethoprim-sulfamethoxazole or ciprofloxacin. Severe systemic symptoms of infection (high fever, haemodynamic instability and nausea or vomiting) warrant IV therapy and hospitalisation (see also septic shock in Ch 27). An aminoglycoside, such as gentamicin, remains appropriate first-line therapy, although ceftriaxone, cefotaxime, piperacillin, ticarcillin, imipenem or meropenem can be used.[25,27] In older children, acute pyelonephritis can be treated with trimethoprim-sulfamethoxazole or cephalexin. Infants are usually hospitalised and receive IV therapy with ceftriaxone.[23,28]

Urinary calculi

Calculi formation (urolithiasis) is more common in Australia due to the hotter and drier climate, affecting approximately 4–8% of the population.[29] A primary risk factor for calculi is hypercalciuria; however, there is also an association with UTI, gout, excessive ingestion of certain foods, family history, dehydration and pregnancy (Box 25.5). Although different substances can form stones, the most commonly occurring are calcium oxalate (60%), calcium phosphate (10%), infective (struvite) (25%) or metabolic (cystine and urate) (5%).[30] Calculi are asymptomatic until movement causes intermittent backache, urge to void, dysuria, renal colic and haematuria. The pain caused by either a partial or a complete obstruction to the flow of urine in the renal pelvis is referred to as *renal colic*.

Renal colic typically presents with flank pain that radiates to the groin and is often described as a constant, gnawing ache in the costovertebral region (the point on the back corresponding to the 12th rib and lateral border of sacrospinal muscle). The symptoms of renal colic can be so severe that patients find it impossible to be still, and writhe in agony. The pain can cause a sympathetic response of nausea, vomiting, pallor and cool, clammy skin.[10] Bacteraemia and proteinuria may also be present. Diagnostic studies include FBC, BUN, creatinine, electrolytes, uric acid, urinalysis with culture and sensitivity (C and S), KUB and IVP. Non-contrast helical CT scans are now considered to be the primary diagnostic study of choice when investigating an episode of acute renal colic.[30,31] Figure 25.15 shows a calculus on a CT scan. Ninety per cent of stones exit spontaneously; however, if unpassed, they may be removed by laparoscopy, lithotripsy or surgically.[30]

Initial management includes insertion of an IV cannula, the commencement of IV fluids and administration of analgesia. Once in the ED, nursing interventions include

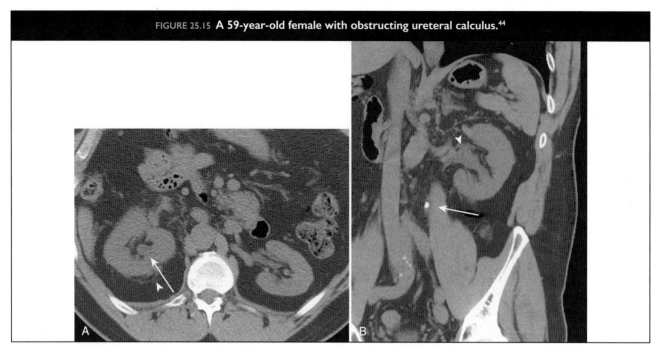

FIGURE 25.15 **A 59-year-old female with obstructing ureteral calculus.**[44]

A, Axial unenhanced computed tomography (CT) image demonstrates mild, diffuse enlargement of the right kidney with hydro-nephrosis (arrow) and mild perinephric stranding (arrowhead). **B,** Coronal unenhanced CT image demonstrates hydronephrosis (arrowhead) and the ureteral stone (arrow).

ongoing analgesia, urinalysis, fluid balance monitoring and increased fluids. Current Australian recommendations are that all urine should be strained for 48 hours following an episode of ureteric colic and any calculi submitted for chemical analysis. Pain assessment and management is critical in these patients because of the severity of their pain. Depending on the severity of the pain, either opioids (morphine sulfate via IV injection) or non-steroidal anti-inflammatory drugs (NSAIDs; ketorolac, naproxen) administered orally or rectally can be used; a combination of these is usually most effective.[30] Current evidence suggests that patients receiving NSAIDs achieve greater reduction in pain scores and are less likely to require further analgesia in the short term. Opioids, particularly pethidine, are associated with a higher rate of vomiting than NSAIDs, although NSAIDs are contraindicated in patients at risk for gastrointestinal bleeding or CKD.[30] Current Australian recommendations are for a single bolus of NSAID rather than an opioid; if opioids are to be used because of either contraindications to NSAIDS or ability to more easily titrate doses, pethidine should not be given.[32] Intavenous paracetamol (1 g) can also be used as first-line analgesia in patients with renal colic.

Tamsolusin, an oral alpha-blocker (adrenergic alpha$_1$-receptor antagonist) more commonly used in the non-surgical treatment of benign prostatic hypertrophy, has been shown to be effective in increasing the expulsion rate of renal calculi and reducing analgesic requirements. It can be used for a short period (2–4 weeks) and requires follow-up with a urologist.[30]

Complications of renal calculi include ischaemia at obstructive site, altered elimination and UTI. Approximately 10% of presentations will result in an admission, often due to need for frequent analgesia, large-diameter stones, solitary kidney, ileus, bladder stones and infection.[30] If the patient is discharged,

information should be provided to them about returning to the ED in case of increasing pain, excessive vomiting or fever and chills. Urological follow-up will be required. A high fluid intake (approximately 3 L per day) is recommended to produce a urine output of at least 2 L per day. High urine output prevents supersaturation of minerals (i.e. dilutes the concentration) and flushes them out before the minerals have a chance to precipitate and form a stone. Increasing the fluid intake is especially important for the patient who is active in sports, lives in a dry climate, performs physical exercise, has a family history of stone formation or works in an occupation that requires outdoor work or a great deal of physical activity that can lead to dehydration. Water is the preferred fluid, and consumption of colas, coffee and tea should be limited, because high intake of these beverages tends to increase rather than diminish the risk of recurring urinary calculi.[30]

Dietary intervention may be important in the management of urinary calculi. In the past, calcium restriction was routinely implemented for the patient with kidney stones. However, more-recent research suggests that a high dietary calcium intake, which was previously thought to contribute to kidney stones, may actually lower the risk by reducing the urinary excretion of oxalate, a common factor in many stones.[30] Initial nutritional management should include limiting oxalate-rich foods and thereby reducing oxalate excretion.

Acute urinary retention

Acute urinary retention (AUR) is the sudden, painful inability to urinate spontaneously and is one of the most common GU emergencies.[33] It is characterised by lower abdominal pain, complete or partial urinary retention, overflow incontinence, bladder distension and irritative voiding. Elderly men are at the highest risk because of prostatic enlargement.[33] History will reveal progressive lower urinary tract symptoms (LUTS), such as decreased urinary stream, hesitancy, nocturia and dribbling (often secondary to an enlarged prostate); rarely AUR can occur following a transurethral resection of the prostate. Medications may also cause AUR, such as anticholinergics, antihistamines, decongestants, hypnotics, NSAIDs and narcotics. A neurological examination should be performed to rule out spinal cord injury or disease that can interfere with the micturition reflex. Assessment includes bladder palpation/ultrasonography and digital rectal examination of the prostate.

AUR requires prompt recognition and rapid and complete bladder decompression through indwelling urethral or suprapubic 2-way catheters,[33] with the catheter left in place to allow the bladder to decompress, even if the volume is greater than 500 mL. A Coudé catheter can be used in preference to a Foley's catheter in men with suspected prostatic hypertrophy as the cause of the AUR. This catheter is more rigid than other straight catheters and has a tapered, curved tip. If a catheter cannot be inserted without force, a suprapubic catheter or assistance from a urologist may be necessary. If AUR is due to haematuria (i.e. clots), then a three-way catheter should be used so that continuous bladder irrigation can be established. The insertion technique is the same as a two-way catheter.[34] Figure 25.16 shows different urinary catheters.

> **PRACTICE TIP**
>
> In the acute setting use aseptic technique when catheterising.[34] A Coudé catheter is inserted with tip pointing upwards.[34] There is no evidence to support the clamping of urinary catheters as a strategy to avoid post-obstructive diuresis, hypotension and haematuria from rapid bladder decompression.[33] Bladder irrigation for acute obstruction using a 60 mL syringe (either sterile water or Normal saline) is recommended, but vigorous flushing/aspiration should be avoided due to damaging bladder mucosa.[34]

If sufficient oral hydration cannot be maintained during the diuresis phase or if marked polyuria (>200 mL/h) occurs, then IV fluid replacement is required.[33] If the residual volume is minimal (<100 mL), further diagnostic evaluation is aimed at identifying the cause.

Patients with uncomplicated AUR are not admitted, but hospitalisation is indicated when there is renal failure or urosepsis, or for patients unable to manage a urinary catheter at home.[33] Simple discharge instructions should be provided on the management of the catheter and drainage bags. Referral to the urologist and community nurse is also required.

Testicular torsion

Testicular torsion causes vascular compromise of the testes within 6–12 hours and can lead to infarction with resultant atrophy and loss of spermatogenesis. Most cases occur in adolescent males, 50% during sleep, and are associated with congenital abnormality of the tunica vaginalis, the canal from which the testes descend.[35] Recognition by paramedics and triage nurses can help in the immediate management of patients through referral pathways that will improve the long-term prognosis.[36]

Clinical manifestations include upwardly retracted testes with redness and oedema to the site of the torsion, abdominal pain and nausea and vomiting.[36] Figure 25.17 compares normal testicular structures with testicular torsion. It can be difficult to differentiate between testicular torsion and epididymitis.[36] Scrotal examination is urgently required in case there is torsion. Prehn's sign may be helpful in differentiating testicular torsion from epididymitis.

> **PRACTICE TIP**
>
> To assess for Prehn's sign, the scrotum is gently elevated to the level of the symphysis. In testicular torsion, pain increases; however, in epididymitis, a decrease in pain is noted.[36] Colour Doppler ultrasound can be used to confirm the diagnosis and to determine blood flow to the testis.

Analgesia should be administered as necessary and urological or paediatric consultation is urgently sought, as surgery

FIGURE 25.16 **Different urinary catheters.**[45]

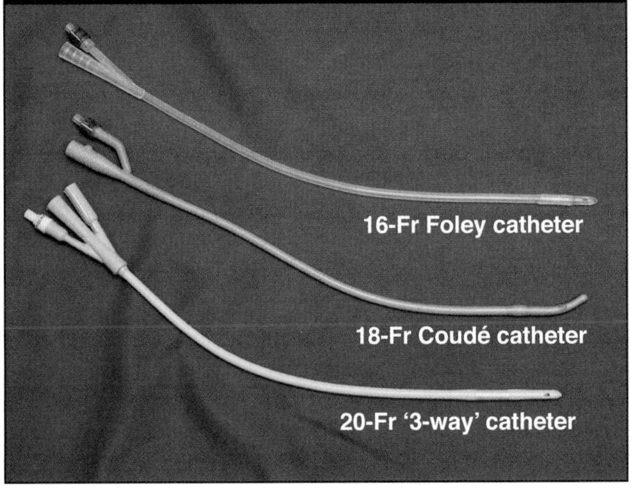

16-Fr Foley catheter

18-Fr Coudé catheter

20-Fr '3-way' catheter

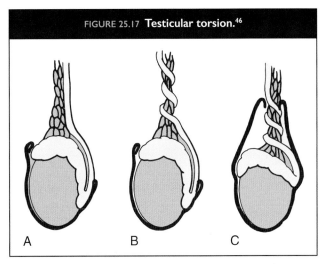

FIGURE 25.17 **Testicular torsion.**[46]

A   B   C

A, Normal tunica vaginalis insertion. **B**, Extravaginal torsion. **C**, Intravaginal torsion with abnormally high vaginalis insertion.

must be performed within 6 hours or orchidectomy may be necessary.[35] Manual detorsion may also be performed under local anaesthesia. Good communication skills are required as patients are often embarrassed young males.

Epididymitis

Epididymitis results from inflammation of the epididymis secondary to an infection (sexually or non-sexually transmitted). It is most common in sexually active males between 18 and 50 years of age and is the fifth most common urinary emergency.[36] The causative organism is most often *Chlamydia trachomatis* or *Neisseria gonorrhoeae*. Extreme physical strain or exertion can also cause epididymitis. Orchitis can also be a consequence; this is termed epididymo-orchitis.

Signs and symptoms of epididymitis include severe scrotal pain, which can radiate into the abdomen, tenderness along the spermatic cord, oedema, fever, pyuria and, possibly, urethral discharge. A positive Prehn's sign may also be observed. On laboratory assessment of the FBC, an elevated WBC count will be present, and urinalysis will reveal bacteria.

Treatment of epididymitis includes administration of antibiotics (e.g. fluoroquinolones or doxycycline), antipyretics and analgesics. Supportive care includes scrotal support and elevation, ice packs to the affected area and sitz baths to assist in pain relief.[36] Sexual activity and physical strain should be avoided.

Priapism

Priapism is persistent, painful erection not associated with sexual desire.[37] Engorgement is limited to the corpora cavernosa; the corpus spongiosum and glans are not involved.[37] Obstruction of venous drainage causes build-up of viscous deoxygenated blood, interstitial oedema and eventual fibrosis. Pain severity increases with duration, and with urinary obstruction and bladder distension, pain can last as long as 24 hours. Aetiologies include diabetes mellitus, spinal cord injury, multiple sclerosis, psychotropic drugs, prolonged sexual activity and marijuana or cocaine use. In addition, many common medications such as anticoagulants, corticosteroids and prazosin can result in priapism. Priapism from use of papaverine for impotence is occurring more frequently. Prolonged priapism is a medical emergency.[37]

Acute detumescence is accomplished surgically with a large-bore needle after a regional nerve block is administered (Ch 17 contains information on administering a regional nerve block, see p. 358). Surgical stenting may be necessary by tissue removal to relieve obstruction or by anastomosis of veins between glans and cavernosa. Fifty per cent of cases require a urinary catheter for bladder obstruction and distension. Development of fibrosis and scarring in cavernous spaces related to the duration of priapism and decompression can cause impotence. Paramedics and triage nurses need to be aware that men will often be embarrassed when calling for paramedic assistance or when presenting to the ED.

SUMMARY

Genitourinary emergencies require careful evaluation of renal function to identify any kidney involvement, particularly AKI. The GU system functions to maintain homeostasis, so disruption of renal function interrupts almost all organ systems. In addition, emerging strains of resistant bacteria are challenging healthcare professions in prevention and management. The role of the emergency nurse and paramedic are important and crucial in the detection and prevention of GU diseases.

CASE STUDY

Mrs Barbara Dunlop, a 71-year-old woman with type 2 diabetes (treated with metformin, frusemide and perindopril), complains of arthritis pain to her GP, who prescribes Nurofen. Five days later, Mrs Dunlop is visited by her daughter, who finds her complaining of nausea and feeling too weak to stand. An ambulance is called, and on arrival the paramedic notes the following assessment:

- pulse 102 beats/minute
- respiratory rate 32 breaths/minute
- blood pressure 140/85 mmHg
- Mrs Dunlop is conscious but confused as to time.

Her daughter confirms that her mother was well the previous evening (approximately 16 hours ago). An intravenous cannula (IVC) is inserted and 1000 mL Normal saline at 100 mL/h is commenced. Mrs Dunlop is transported to the emergency department (ED) of the local hospital. On arrival her temperature is 36.3°C; other vital signs are similar to earlier. She is transferred to a bed where an ECG reveals peaked T waves and QRS duration of 0.12 seconds. Urgent biochemistry reveals the following:

- sodium 138 mmol/L
- potassium 6.8 mmol/L
- urea 11.8 mmol/L
- creatinine 168 μmol/L
- bicarbonate 12 mmol/L
- blood glucose level 18.7 mmol/L

Questions

1. What questions will you ask in this scenario to determine historical and clinical indicators of urgency and relevance?

2. What ongoing nursing assessment and monitoring will you provide? Why?

3. Mrs Dunlop has most likely developed which of the following:
   - intrarenal acute kidney injury (AKI)
   - chronic kidney disease (CKD)
   - acute on chronic kidney disease
   - prerenal AKI

4. Which of the following medication combinations is the likely cause of her hyperkalaemia? Why?
   - Metformin and frusemide
   - Perinodopril and Nurofen
   - Nurofen and metformin
   - Triple whammy (Nurofen, perindopril and frusemide)

5. The most important treatment for a patient with a serum potassium level of 7.6 mmol/L would be:
   - intravenous neutral insulin
   - oral resonium
   - haemodialysis
   - intravenous bicarbonate

 Answers to Case Study Questions can be found on evolve
http://evolve.emergencytrauma.curtis

USEFUL WEBSITES

Caring for Australasians with Renal Impairment, www.cari.org.au/index.php

Kidney Health Australia, www.kidney.org.au

Lions Australian Prostate Cancer Web Site, www.prostatehealth.org.au

New Zealand Kidney Foundation, www.kidneys.co.nz/

Urological Society of Australia and New Zealand, www.usanz.org.au

REFERENCES

1. McGuire T. Urinary tract infection: urinary symptoms are a common presentation in community pharmacy. How can pharmacists play an effective role in UTI management? Pharmacy News 2012;Sept:39–44.

2. Australian Institute of Health and Welfare. Projections of the incidence of treated end stage kidney disease in Australia 2010–2020. Cat no PHE 150. Australian Institute of Health and Welfare; 2011.

3. Skelly D. The structure and function of the urinary system. In: Craft J, Gordon C, Tiziani A, eds. Understanding pathophysiology. 2nd edn. Sydney: Elsevier; 2014.

4. Thibodeau G, Patton K. Anatomy and physiology. 8th edn. Sydney: Elsevier; 2012.

5. Bonner A. Nursing assessment: urinary system. In: Brown D, Edwards H, Seaton L, Buckley T eds. Lewis's medical–surgical nursing: assessment and management of clinical problems. 4th edn. Sydney: Elsevier; 2014.

6. Forbes H, Watt E. Jarvis's physical examination and health assessment, Australian and New Zealand edition. Sydney: Elsevier; 2011.

7. Agata E. Challenges in assessing nursing home residents with advanced dementia for suspected urinary tract infections. J Am Geri Soc 2013; 61(1):62–6.

8. Freedman A. Urethral catheterization in children—whom does it hurt? J Urol 2013;189(4):e262–3.

9. Swallow D. Guidelines for the management of haematuria. In Dawson C, Nethercliffe J, eds. ABC of urology. 3rd edn. Oxford: Wiley & Sons; 2012;5–8.

10. Manjunath A, Skinner R, Probert J. Assessment and management of renal colic. BMJ 2013;346:f985.

11. Wang HE, Muntner P, Chertow G et al. Acute kidney injury and mortality in hospitalized patients. Am J Neph 2012;35(4):349–55.

12. Bonner A. Nursing management: acute renal failure and chronic kidney disease. In: Brown D, Edwards H, Seaton L, Buckley T eds. Lewis's medical–surgical nursing: assessment and management of clinical problems. 4th edn. Sydney: Elsevier; 2014.

13. Singbartl K, Kellum J. AKI in the ICU: definition, epidemiology, risk stratification, and outcomes. Kid Int 2012;81(9):819–25.

14. Yaklin K. Acute kidney injury: an overview of pathophysiology and treatments. Nephrol Nurs J 2011;38(1):13–18,30.

15. Kellum J, Lameire N et al. Clinical practice guidelines for acute kidney injury: KDIGO. Kid Int 2012;(Suppl 1):1. www.kdigo.org/clinical_practice_guidelines/pdf/KDIGO%20AKI%20Guideline.pdf; accessed 27 March 2015.

16. Pepin J, Shields C. Advances in diagnosis and management of hypokalemic and hyperkalemic emergencies. Emerg Med Pract 2012;14:1–17.

17. Marenzi G, Cabiati A, Milazzo V, Rubino M. Contrast-induced nephropathy. Int & Emerg Med 2012;7(3,3):S181–3.

18. Ostermann M, Dickie H, Barrett N. Renal replacement therapy in critically ill patients with acute kidney injury: when to start. Nephrol Dial Transplant 2012;27(6):2242–8.

19. El-Abdellati E, Eyselbergs M, Sirimsi H et al. An observational study on rhabdomyolysis in the intensive care unit. Exploring its risk factors and main complication: acute kidney injury. Annals Int Care 2013;3(1):8.

20. Kidney Health Australia. Chronic kidney disease management in general practice. 2nd edn. Melbourne: Kidney Health Australia; 2012.

21. Asano M, Thumma J, Oguchi K et al. Vascular access care and treatment practices associated with outcomes of arteriovenous fistula: International comparisons from the dialysis outcomes and practice patterns study. Nephron Clin Pract 2013;124:23–30.

22. Rowe T. Diagnosis and management of urinary tract infection in older adults. Infect Dis Clin North Am 2014; 28(1):75–89.

23. Williams GJ, Hodson EH, Isaacs D, Craig JC. Diagnosis and management of urinary tract infection in children. J Paed Child Hlth 2012;48(4):296–301.

24. Peake SL, Bailey M, Bellomo R et al. Australian resuscitation of sepsis evaluation (ARISE): a multi-centre, prospective, inception cohort study. Resus 2009;80:811–18.

25. Nicolle LE. Urinary tract infection. Crit Care Clin 2013;29(3):699–717.

26. Jepson R. Cranberries for the prevention of urinary tract infections. Nephrol 2013;18(5):388–9.

27. Abraham G, Reddy YNV, Gautam G. Diagnosis of acute pyelonephritis with recent trends in management. Nephrol Dialysis Transplant 2012;27(9):3391–4.

28. Gea E, Avellanet M, Estrada J, Medina M. Management of urinary tract infection in a paediatric emergency department. Int J Clin Pharm 2013;35(5):965.

29. Kidney Health Australia. What are kidney stones? www.kidney.org.au/ForPatients/Management/KidneyStones/tabid/838/Default.aspx; accessed 27 March 2015.

30. Miller J, Stoller ML. Renal colic and obstructing kidney stones: Diagnosis and management. In Wessells H, ed. Urological emergencies: a practical approach. 2nd edn. New York: Springer; 2013:221–38.

31. Dalziel PJ, Noble VE. Bedside ultrasound and the assessment of renal colic: A review. Emerg Med J 2013;30(1):3–8.

32. Thomas M. Caring for Australians with renal impairment (CARI) guideline. Clinical diagnosis of kidney stones. Nephrol 2007;12:S1–3.

33. Shih C, Yang CC. Urgent and emergent management of acute urinary retention. In Wessells H, ed. Urological emergencies: a practical approach. 2nd edn. New York: Springer; 2013:251–60.

34. European Association of Urology Nurses. Evidence-based guidelines for best practice in urological health care, catheterisation indwelling catheters in adults—urethral and suprapubic. 2012. www.nursing.nl/PageFiles/11870/001_1391694991387.pdf; accessed 27 March 2015.

35. Kern A. Testicular torsion and trauma. In Parsons JK, Eifler JB, Han M, eds. Handbook of urology. Oxford: Wiley Blackwell; 2014:75–84.

36. Srinath H. Acute scrotal pain. Fam Phys 2013;42(11):790–2.

37. Sundi D, Bivalacqua TJ. Priapism. In Parsons JK, Eifler JB, Han M, eds. Handbook of urology. Oxford: Wiley Blackwell; 2014:88–95.

38. McCance KL, Huether SE. Pathophysiology: the biologic basis for disease in adults and children. 6th edn. St Louis: Mosby; 2010.

39. Brown D, Edwards H, eds. Lewis's medical–surgical nursing. 3rd edn. Sydney: Elsevier; 2008.

40. Brown D, Edwards H, eds. Lewis's medical–surgical nursing. 4th edn. Sydney: Elsevier; 2014.

41. Herlihy B, Maebius N. The human body in health and illness. 2nd edn. Philadelphia: Saunders, 2003.

42. Thompson JM, McFarland GK, Hirsch JE et al. Mosby's clinical nursing. 5th edn. St Louis: Mosby; 2001.

43. Brundage DJ. Renal disorders. St Louis: Mosby, 1992.

44. Soto JA, Lucey BC. Emergency radiology: the requisites. Philadelphia: Elsevier; 2009.

45. Roberts JR. Roberts and Hedges' Clinical Procedures in Emergency Medicine, 6th edn, Ch 55. Saunders, Elsevier; 2015:1113-1154.e2

46. Price SA, Wilson LM. Pathophysiology: clinical concepts of disease processes. 5th edn. St Louis: Mosby; 1997.

47. Thibodeau GA, Patton KT. The human body in health and disease. 3rd edn. St Louis: Mosby, 2002.

48. Fogazzi GB, Verdesca S, Garigali G. Urinalysis core curriculum 2008. Am J Kidney Dis 2008;51(6):1052–67.

49. Patel JV, Chambers CV, Gomella LG. Hematuria: etiology and evaluation for the primary care physician. Can J Urol 2008;15(suppl 1):54–62.

CHAPTER 26
ENDOCRINE EMERGENCIES
THOMAS BUCKLEY AND MARGARET MURPHY

Essentials

- One of the key roles of the endocrine system is to maintain an optimal internal environment throughout the life span.
- Endocrine emergencies are rare and therefore constitute only a fraction of ED workload. The most frequent endocrine emergencies are related to diabetes.
- Diabetes is the fastest growing chronic condition in Australia.
- Clinicians should be aware of potential red flags for endocrine emergencies and not delay initiation of treatment while awaiting investigation results.
- It is also imperative that involvement of the endocrine team occur in a timely manner once endocrine involvement is suspected.
- Clinical assessment should follow the ABCDEFG algorithim and interventions initiated if any of these parameters are compromised using Rapid Response Systems.

INTRODUCTION

The endocrine system is comprised of glands capable of synthesising and releasing chemical messengers known as hormones. One of the key roles of the endocrine system is to maintain an optimal internal environment throughout the life span, and, in the context of acute or critical illness, to initiate adaptive responses when emergency demands occur. Endocrine emergencies constitute only a fraction of emergency department (ED) workload, and, as such, healthcare professionals working in pre-hospital and emergency care may have limited experience in early detection and management of such emergencies. The most frequent endocrine emergencies are related to diabetes. With early detection and early interventions, diabetic emergencies may be successfully managed. In this chapter diabetic ketoacidosis is discussed, as well as other, less common endocrine emergencies, with emphasis on early assessment and initial management strategies.

Anatomy and physiology

The endocrine system consists of the hypothalamus, pituitary, pineal gland, thyroid, parathyroid, adrenals, pancreas, testes (in males) and ovaries (in females) (Fig 26.1). Hormone molecules are transported via blood to their target tissues, where each hormone exerts its characteristic regulatory function at a cellular and molecular level.[1] An overview of the major endocrine glands, hormones produced and functions is presented in Table 26.1.

Most hormones are proteins and are synthesised and produced in endocrine glands throughout the body. Hormone release occurs in response to altered cellular environment and are regulated by one or more of the following mechanisms:

- chemical factors
- endocrine factors
- neural control.[3]

The most important regulatory mechanism is the *negative feedback system* where the endocrine system is controlled through negative feedback loops. An example of negative feedback is where thyroid-stimulating hormone (TSH) released from the anterior pituitary stimulates the synthesis and secretion of thyroid hormones. TSH secretion is regulated by thyrotropin-releasing hormone primarily in the hypothalamus and is inhibited by the thyroid-secreted hormones thyroxine (T_4) and, to a lesser extent, triiodothyronine (T_3).

Negative feedback systems maintain a delicate balance to ensure that hormone levels remain within physiological levels. Pathological conditions occur when there is a lack of negative-feedback inhibition resulting in excessive hormonal levels. Alerted renal and liver function, and external factors, such as pain, fear and stress, all influence hormone release. Neural stimulation, for example sympathetic activation during stress, results in increased levels of hormones such as adrenaline and

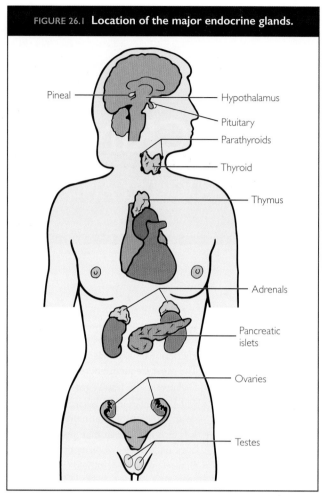

FIGURE 26.1 Location of the major endocrine glands.

Pineal — Hypothalamus — Pituitary — Parathyroids — Thyroid — Thymus — Adrenals — Pancreatic islets — Ovaries — Testes

The parathyroid glands actually lie on the posterior surface of the thyroid gland.

HORMONES	TARGET TISSUE	FUNCTIONS
TABLE 26.1 Primary endocrine glands and hormones[2]		
Anterior pituitary (adenohypophysis)		
Growth hormone (GH)	All body cells	Promotes protein anabolism (growth, tissue repair) and lipid mobilisation and catabolism
Thyroid-stimulating hormone (TSH)	Thyroid gland	Stimulates synthesis and release of thyroid hormones, growth and function of thyroid gland
Adrenocorticotrophic hormone (ACTH)	Adrenal cortex	Fosters growth of adrenal cortex; stimulates secretion of corticosteroids
Gonadotrophic hormones	Reproductive organs	Stimulate sex-hormone secretion, reproductive organ growth, reproductive processes
Follicle-stimulating hormone (FSH)		
Luteinising hormone (LH)		
Melanocyte-stimulating hormone (MSH)	Melanocytes in skin	Increases melanin production in melanocytes to make skin darker in colour
Prolactin	Ovary and mammary glands in females	Stimulates milk production in lactating women; increases response of follicles to LH and FSH; has unclear function in men

TABLE 26.1 Primary endocrine glands and hormones²—cont'd

HORMONES	TARGET TISSUE	FUNCTIONS
Posterior pituitary (neurohypophysis)		
Oxytocin	Uterus; mammary glands	Stimulates milk secretion, uterine contractility
Antidiuretic hormone (ADH) or vasopressin	Renal tubules, vascular smooth muscle	Promotes reabsorption of water, vasoconstriction
Thyroid		
Thyroxine (T_4)	All body tissues	Precursor to T_3
Triiodothyronine (T_3)	All body tissues	Regulates metabolic rate of all cells and processes of cell growth and tissue differentiation
Calcitonin	Bone tissue	Regulates calcium and phosphorus blood levels; decreases serum calcium levels
Parathyroids		
Parathyroid hormone (PTH)	Bone, intestine, kidneys	Regulates calcium and phosphorus blood levels; promotes bone demineralisation and increases intestinal absorption of calcium; increases serum calcium levels
Adrenal medulla		
Adrenaline	Sympathetic effectors	Response to stress; enhances and prolongs effects of sympathetic nervous system
Noradrenaline	Sympathetic effectors	Response to stress; enhances and prolongs effects of sympathetic nervous system
Adrenal cortex		
Corticosteroids (e.g. cortisol, hydrocortisone)	All body tissues	Promotes metabolism, response to stress
Androgens (e.g. testosterone, androsterone) and oestrogen	Reproductive organs	Promotes masculinisation in men, growth and sexual activity in women
Mineralocorticoids (e.g. aldosterone)	Kidney	Regulates sodium and potassium balance and thus water balance
Pancreas		
Islets of Langerhans		
Insulin (from beta cells)	General	Promotes movement of glucose out of blood and into cells
Glucagon (from alpha cells)	General	Promotes movement of glucose from glycogen (glycogenolysis) and into blood
Somatostatin	Pancreas	Inhibits insulin and glucagon secretion
Pancreatic polypeptide	General	Influences regulation of pancreatic exocrine function and metabolism of absorbed nutrients
Gonads		
Women: ovaries Oestrogen	Reproductive system, breasts	Stimulates development of secondary sex characteristics, preparation of uterus for fertilisation and fetal development; stimulates bone growth
Progesterone	Reproductive system	Maintains lining of uterus necessary for successful pregnancy
Men: testes Testosterone	Reproductive system	Stimulates development of secondary sex characteristics, spermatogenesis

glucagon resulting in increasing heart rate, blood pressure and serum blood sugar levels. When the stress reduces, adrenaline and glucagon levels decrease and symptoms subside. Intrinsic rhythms (e.g. circadian rhythms) vary from hours to weeks and provide another method of hormone control.[3,4]

Once secreted into the circulatory system, hormones may be either water soluble or lipid soluble or circulate in a free or active form. Water-soluble hormones usually have a short half-life (e.g. insulin with a half-life of 3–5 minutes), whereas lipid-soluble hormones (e.g. cortisol or thyroxine) have a considerably longer half-life. Some hormones, such as cortisol, also have small amounts of unbound, circulating, free cortisol in addition to the bound form.[1,3]

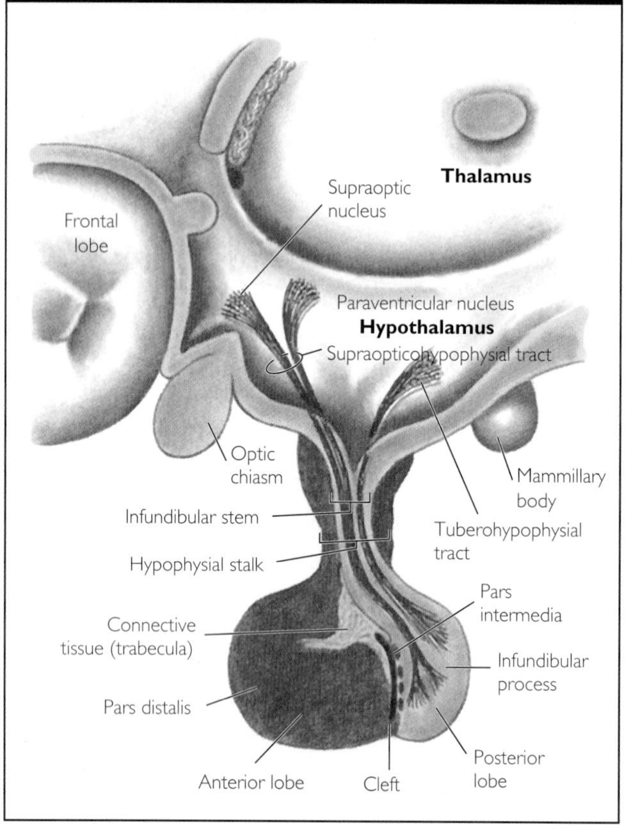

Hypothalamus

The hypothalamus creates part of the walls and floor of the third ventricle of the brain and has been described as an automatic nervous centre (Fig 26.2). Although the hypothalamus is small in size, centres in the anterior and posterior hypothalamus are responsible for performing numerous vital functions, most of which relate either directly or indirectly to the regulation of visceral activities (Table 26.2). The hypothalamus is responsible for limbic (emotional) regulation, as well as instinctual functions.[1,3]

The hypothalamus lies close to the pituitary and is linked to the brain by nerves and blood vessels. It produces neurosecretory chemicals that regulate anterior pituitary action through the stimulation or suppression of various hormones. These hormones are responsible for the regulation of other endocrine glands via the negative feedback loop. As the hypothalamus is one of the most vital structures of the body, dysfunction can have a serious effect on the autonomic, somatic or psychic functions of the body.[1,3]

Pituitary

The pituitary is located on the inferior aspect of the brain in the region of the diencephalon, and lies within the sella turcica of the middle cranial fossa (Fig 26.2). Pituitary secretions are controlled by the hypothalamus, as well as negative feedback from target glands. It is rounded and pea-shaped, measuring approximately 1 cm in diameter and is attached to the hypothalamus by the infundibular stalk.[1] The pituitary gland is structurally and functionally divided into the anterior and posterior regions. The anterior region contains secretory cells, and secretes trophic hormones—the term *trophic* meaning 'food'. The anterior pituitary hormones do not target food;

FIGURE 26.2 Anatomy of the hypothalamus and pituitary.[5]

TABLE 26.2 Control centres of the hypothalamus

POSTERIOR HYPOTHALAMUS		ANTERIOR HYPOTHALAMUS	
Control centre	Effect	Control centre	Effect
Posterior hypothalamus	Increased blood pressure; pupillary dilation; shivering	Paraventricular nucleus	Oxytocin release; water conservation
Dorsomedial nucleus	Gastrointestinal stimulation	Medical preoptic area	Bladder contraction; decreased heart rate; decreased blood pressure
Perifornical nucleus	Hunger; increased blood pressure; rage	Supraoptic nucleus	Vasopressin release
Ventromedial nucleus	Satiety; neuroendocrine control	Posterior preoptic and anterior hypothalamic area	Temperature regulation; panting, sweating, thyroid-stimulating hormone
Mammillary body	Feeding reflexes		
Arcuate nucleus and periventricular zone	Neuroendocrine control		
Lateral hypothalamic area	Thirst, hunger		

rather they result in hypertrophy of their targets when levels are high, and result in atrophy of target organs when levels are low. Hormones that are secreted by the anterior pituitary include growth hormone, adrenocorticotrophic hormone (ACTH), thyroid-stimulating hormone (TSH), prolactin, follicle-stimulating hormone and luteinising hormone.[1]

The posterior pituitary consists of neural cells that serve as a supporting structure for nerve fibres and nerve endings, and secretes two hormones into the circulation: antidiuretic hormone (ADH) and oxytocin. Both ADH and oxytocin are produced by the hypothalamus and stored in the pituitary's posterior lobe until required.[1,6]

Thyroid

The thyroid is the largest of the endocrine glands. It is butterfly shaped and positioned just below the larynx, partially surrounding the trachea (Fig 26.3). It consists of two lobes that lie on either side of the trachea which are connected anteriorly by a broad isthmus.[1,3] The initiating hormone is thyrotropin-releasing hormone (TRH) which is synthesised and stored in the hypothalamus and released into the hypothalamic–pituitary portal system, circulates to the pituitary and stimulates the release of TSH. TSH stimulates the thyroid gland to produce thyroid hormone, a process that requires iodide. Ninety per cent of thyroid hormone is in the form of thyroxine (T_4), and the remainder triiodothyronine (T_3). These hormones are essential for proper growth and development, neurological function and the determination of basal metabolic rate (BMR).[1] Generally, thyroid hormones exert a number of permissive effects on many organs but abnormally high or low levels can exert pronounced effects.

Adrenals

The adrenal glands (also called the suprarenal glands) are paired organs located in the retroperitoneal area above the upper pole of each kidney and embedded against the muscles of the back in a protective layer of fat. The adrenal glands are generally pyramidal in appearance, measuring approximately 50 mm long, 30 mm wide and 10 mm deep.[4] Like the pituitary,

the adrenal glands have dual origin. Each gland consists of an outer cortical layer and an inner medullary layer. They are functionally two different endocrine tissues, located in the same organ, and each secretes different hormones that are regulated by different control systems.

The bulk of the gland is made up by the *adrenal cortex*, which is divided into three zones. These are the outer zona glomerulosa, intermediate zona fasciculata and inner zona reticularis. The adrenal cortex secretes more than 50 steroid hormones, classified as glucocorticoids, mineralocorticoids and androgens.[1,3] Cortisol, the most abundant glucocorticoid, is necessary for the maintenance of life and protection from stress. Cortisol has a half-life of approximately 90 minutes and increases blood glucose levels through the promotion of hepatic gluconeogenesis by facilitating conversion of amino acids to glucose and inhibiting protein synthesis.[7] Pathophysiologically, high levels of aldosterone have been associated with hypertension, atherosclerosis and heart failure.[8] Aldosterone is a potent mineralocorticoid that maintains extracellular fluid volume, regulated primarily by the renin–angiotensin–aldosterone system to alter serum sodium levels.

The *adrenal medulla* is composed of tightly packed clusters of cells, innervated by sympathetic neurons that are arranged around blood vessels. Impulses are initiated from the hypothalamus via the spinal cord when the sympathetic division of the autonomic nervous system (ANS) is stimulated. The cells of the medulla secrete the catecholamines adrenaline and noradrenaline in a ratio of approximately 4 : 1. Approximately 30% of adrenaline is secreted from the adrenal medulla; the remainder comes from nerve terminals. Adrenaline is up to 10 times more potent than noradrenaline, although the latter has a longer duration of action.[1,3] Once released, catecholamines remain in the plasma for a very short duration, just several seconds, but result in increased cardiac output and heart rate, dilated coronary blood vessels, increased mental alertness, increased respiratory rate and elevated metabolic rate. Activation of the adrenal medulla together with sympathetic division of the ANS prepares the body for greater physical performance, the 'fight or flight' response.

Excessive stimulation of the adrenal medulla can result in depletion of the body's energy reserves and a high level of corticosteroid secretion from the adrenal cortex. This can significantly impair the immune system. The major functions of catecholamines are summarised in Table 26.3.

Pancreas

The pancreas is situated behind the stomach and anterior to the first and second lumbar vertebrae, in the retroperitoneal space. The body of the pancreas extends horizontally across the abdominal wall with the head in the curve of the abdomen and the tail touching the spleen. It is a soft, lobular gland (Fig 26.4). The pancreas has both endocrine and exocrine functions. Acini are exocrine cells that release amylase, lipase and other enzymes that aid digestion. The endocrine portion of the pancreas consists of scattered clusters of cells called the pancreatic islets, or islets of Langerhans. The islets account for less than 2% of the gland and consist of three types of hormone-secreting cells that produce hormones responsible for serum glucose regulation. Alpha cells produce and secrete glucagon, beta cells

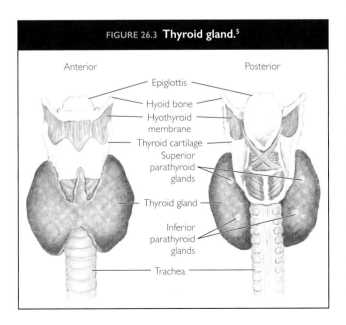

FIGURE 26.3 **Thyroid gland.**[5]

Anterior   Posterior

Epiglottis
Hyoid bone
Hyothyroid membrane
Thyroid cartilage
Superior parathyroid glands
Thyroid gland
Inferior parathyroid glands
Trachea

TABLE 26.3 Catecholamine functions

CLASS AND FUNCTION	ALPHA-ADRENERGIC	BETA-ADRENERGIC	DOPAMINERGIC
Agonist	Noradrenaline	Adrenaline	Dopamine
Antagonist	Phentolamine	Propranolol	Haloperidol
Actions			
Cardiac		Inotropic and chronotropic	Inotropic
Smooth muscle	Contracts	Relaxes	Mixed
Metabolic		Lipolysis	
		Glycogenolysis	
		Gluconeogenesis	
Molecular	Decreases cAMP	Increases cAMP	Increases cAMP

cAMP: cyclic adenosine monophosphate; this is a second messenger and regulates the effects of adrenaline and glucagon

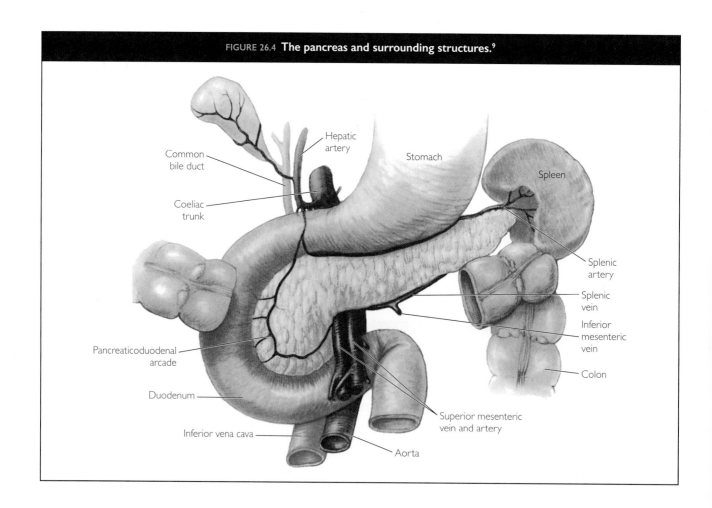

FIGURE 26.4 **The pancreas and surrounding structures.**[9]

produce and secrete insulin and delta cells secrete somatostatin, which inhibits glucagon and insulin release.

Insulin, synthesised from the precursor proinsulin, is stimulated by increased serum glucose levels, the amino acids arginine and lysine, serum free-fatty acids and parasympathetic stimulation. Conversely, insulin secretion reduces in response to low serum glucose, high levels of insulin through the beta-cell negative feedback system and sympathetic stimulation. The primary role of insulin is to facilitate glucose uptake into cells; it is an anabolic hormone, promoting synthesis of proteins, lipids and nucleic acids resulting in increased metabolism (Table 26.4).

TABLE 26.4 Action of insulin[10]			
	LIVER	ADIPOSE TISSUE	MUSCLE
Anticatabolic effects	↓ glycogenolysis	↓ lipolysis	↓ protein catabolism
	↓ gluconeogenesis		↓ amino acid output
	↓ ketogenesis		↓ amino acid oxidation
Anabolic effects	↑ glycogen synthesis	↑ glycerol synthesis	↑ amino acid uptake
	↑ fatty acid synthesis	↑ fatty acid synthesis	↑ protein synthesis
			↑ glycogen synthesis

Glucagon acts primarily in the liver, stimulating glycogenolysis and gluconeogenesis in response to hypoglycaemia, resulting in increased blood glucose.

Diabetes

Diabetes is a chronic disease caused by relative or absolute insulin insufficiency. Diabetes is the fastest growing chronic condition in Australia. In Australia, 280 people develop diabetes every day. Over 100,000 Australians have developed diabetes in the past year. Almost 1.1 million Australians currently have diagnosed diabetes.[11] This includes:

- 120,000 people with type 1 diabetes
- 956,000 people with type 2 diabetes
- 23,600 women with gestational diabetes.[11]

Type 1 diabetes is characterised by destruction of insulin-producing beta cells caused by an autoimmune abnormality. Onset is usually rapid, although latent autoimmune diabetes (LADA) is a more slowly progressive autoimmune diabetes in adults. The exact cause of type 1 diabetes remains unknown and incidence has a strong family link. Type 2 diabetes is the most common form of diabetes in Australia, affecting 85–90% of all people with diabetes.[11,12] Traditionally, type 2 diabetes has been associated with later adulthood, although incidence is increasing in children. Type 2 diabetes may range from predominant insulin resistance to a predominant insulin secretory defect, with or without insulin resistance.[13] Gestational diabetes refers to glucose intolerance with onset during pregnancy. Between 3% and 8% of pregnant women develop gestational diabetes around the 24th to 28th week of pregnancy. Women who develop gestational diabetes are at higher risk of developing type 2 diabetes.[11,12]

Other specific and less-common types of type 2 diabetes include:[3,13]

- genetic defects of beta cell function (e.g. MODY1–MODY6 sulfonylurea receptor [KCNJ11] genes)
- genetic defects in insulin action (e.g. type A insulin resistance and leprechaunism)
- diseases of the exocrine pancreas (e.g. pancreatitis, cystic fibrosis, haemochromatosis); endocrinopathies (e.g. Cushing syndrome)

- drug-induced or chemical-induced diabetes (e.g. glucocorticoids)
- infections (e.g. congenital rubella, cytomegalovirus)
- uncommon but specific forms of immune-mediated diabetes (e.g. 'stiff-man' syndrome and anti-insulin-receptor antibodies)
- other genetic syndromes sometimes associated with diabetes (e.g. Down syndrome, Wolfram syndrome, Turner's syndrome and myotonic dystrophy).

Diabetic ketoacidosis

Diabetic ketoacidosis (DKA) is an acute, life-threatening condition characterised by hyperglycaemia, the presence of ketones in urine or blood and acidosis (arterial pH < 7.3 or HCO_3^- <16). It has long been assumed that DKA is pathognomic of type 1 diabetes with most presentations occurring in individuals with type 1 disease. However, it is now recognised that it can also occur in type 2 diabetes, especially in African-American and ethnic minority populations.[3,11–13] Among patients who develop DKA, mortality rates are between 5% and 15%. Seventy per cent of diabetes-related deaths in children are attributed to DKA. It occurs in 20–30% of all new-onset presentations of diabetes; therefore, acute presentation often results in a diagnosis of diabetes.[11,13]

Hyperglycaemia is a result of severe insulin deficiency, either absolute or relative, which impairs peripheral glucose uptake and promotes fat breakdown. Relative glucagon excess promotes hepatic gluconeogenesis. Overall, metabolism in DKA shifts from the normal fed state characterised by carbohydrate metabolism to a fasting state characterised by fat metabolism (Fig 26.5). Secondary consequences of the primary metabolic derangements include ketosis, caused by a switch to fat metabolism, leading to free fatty acid oxidation in the liver. As a result the ketone bodies acetoacetic acid and 3-hydroxybutyric acid are formed. The dissociation of the ketone bodies (weak acids) results in acidosis due to depletion of extracellular and cellular buffers. As a consequence of hyperglycaemic state, renal threshold is surpassed and glucose is secreted in the urine, known as osmotic diuresis. This hyperglycaemia-induced osmotic diuresis depletes sodium, potassium, phosphates and water as well as ketones and glucose, resulting in absolute dehydration and electrolyte depletion.

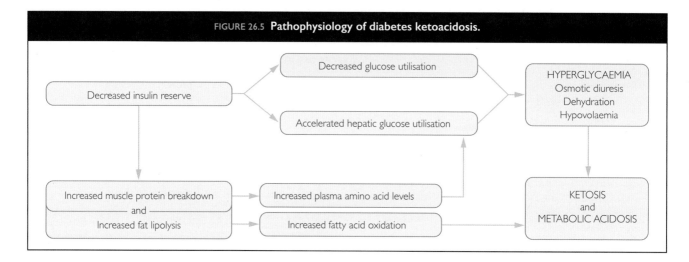

FIGURE 26.5 **Pathophysiology of diabetes ketoacidosis.**

DIABETIC KETOACIDOSIS (DKA)

- DKA is a serious medical problem in patients with diabetes.
- Reducing the occurrence and severity of DKA depends on early detection of elevated serum blood ketones.
- All people with diabetes should test for ketones during acute illness, stress, when blood glucose levels are consistently elevated, during pregnancy or when there are symptoms suggestive of ketoacidosis, e.g. nausea, vomiting, abdominal pain, excessive thirst, polyuria.
- Insulin binds to plastic containers and tubing. Thus when administering insulin via tubing the correct procedure should be followed. This involves priming the line with the insulin/saline solution. Leave for a minimum of 1 minute and then flush the solution from the tubing (4 mL), replacing it with fresh solution prior to commencing the infusion.
- Insulin infusion should be maintained until there is biochemical evidence that ketoacidosis has resolved. The most common mistake is to reduce the rate of insulin as the blood glucose falls before the acidosis is reversed.
- It takes up to 24 hours to reverse ketoacidosis. This is evidenced by normal pH, HCO_3^- and blood ketones < 0.5 mmol.
- Never cease insulin completely. The patient will be commenced on subcutaneous insulin and then the infusion ceased when ketoacidosis is ceased, plasma glucose levels are stable and patient is tolerating oral fluids/diet.

Clinical features

Diabetic ketoacidosis tends to occur in leaner, young, type 1 diabetes patients and although symptoms may be present for several days, the presentation of DKA is usually rapid and predictable. DKA may be precipitated by factors that result in increased circulating levels of stress hormones, such as adrenaline, growth hormone and cortisol, and the resulting increase in insulin resistance reduces the effectiveness of any residual insulin production or injected insulin. Examples of precipitating causes may include infection, myocardial infarction, cerebrovascular causes, influenza, surgical emergencies, cocaine use or stress.[14,15] These conditions often present with their own complex set of signs and symptoms, and therefore the possibility of DKA needs to always be considered in any diabetic patient presenting with the potential triggers listed above. Additionally, errors of insulin administration or patient manipulation with insulin treatment may be the precipitant of an acute DKA episode.

After prolonged insulin deficiency, hyperglycaemia leads to thirst, polyuria, dehydration, electrolyte depletion and metabolic acidosis. Patients with DKA often complain of non-specific symptoms such as malaise and fatigue. Nausea, vomiting and abdominal pain are common and although it is not fully understood why these symptoms occur, it is thought to be the result of delayed gastric emptying, ileus, subacute pancreatitis, oesophagitis with ulceration or bowel ischaemia.[15,16]

Physical signs include evidence of dehydration such as tachycardia; hypotension may be the result of volume depletion, sepsis or both. Additionally, skin examination may reveal diminished skin turgor, and dry mucous membranes due to dehydration. The most frequent cardiac rhythm is sinus tachycardia; however, dysrhythmias can occur secondary to electrolyte disturbances. The patient may also be tachypnoeic with Kussmaul respirations and a fruity odour to their breath as a result of exhaled acetone.[13,15,16] The clinical features of DKA are summarised in Table 26.5.

Assessment and diagnosis

The first priority is to establish the severity of the presenting problem and hence the need for immediate intervention. The initial clinical examination follows the ABCD mnemonic to assess the potential or actual threat to Airway, Breathing, Circulation and Disability. Interventions may need to be initiated if these parameters are compromised. A focused secondary assessment then follows, usually directed by the presenting signs and symptoms.

In determining the severity of the patient's illness and the need for intervention, it is important to determine the history of the presenting illness. Most patients presenting with DKA have a known history of diabetes, making differential diagnosis

TABLE 26.5 Clinical manifestations of diabetic ketoacidosis

SYSTEM	CLINICAL MANIFESTATIONS
Neurological	Lethargy, malaise and fatigue, possible confusion and coma in extreme cases
Respiratory	Kussmaul respirations, fruity acetone breath
Cardiovascular	Tachycardia, hypotension, dysrhythmias
Integumentary	Flushed skin, dry mucous membranes, poor skin turgor, fever if infection
Renal	Thirst, polyuria, ketonuria, glucosuria
Gastrointestinal	Nausea, vomiting, abdominal cramps or pain

fairly uncomplicated. However, as patients may also have signs and symptoms related to the precipitant factor, or trigger, of the DKA, laboratory tests will be needed to confirm DKA. The signs and symptoms may develop rapidly, but there is usually a history of being unwell for days, predominantly with gastrointestinal symptoms, such as vomiting, excessive thirst or urination and abdominal pain. In more advanced stages the patient may be confused or obtunded. The patient's breathing pattern may be described as rapid, referred to as Kussmaul's respirations with a distinctive 'sweet-smelling' odour. Dehydration, occasionally associated with hypotension, tachycardia and delayed capillary refill, may also be present. However, there may also be excessive

urinary output in a hypoperfused patient with significant weight loss (up to 5 kg/week).

Bedside testing of capillary blood glucose and beta-hydroxybutyrate levels using point-of-care testing, in patients with the above presentation, will confirm the diagnosis of diabetic ketoacidosis (see Ch 17, p. 332, for information on blood glucose testing techniques). A diligent search for the precipitant is also essential. These causes may include infection, cessation of insulin, trauma or acute myocardial infarction (may be painless), to name a few. Other bedside testing that may assist this process include urinalysis, electrocardiogram and vital signs monitoring.

Laboratory investigations

Laboratory tests should be obtained as early as possible. Diagnosis of DKA is confirmed in the presence of four clinical features:

1. Hyperglycaemia with serum glucose higher than 13.8 mmol/L
2. Ketones in urine or blood
3. Metabolic acidosis with pH < 7.3
4. Dehydration.[15]

Other possible laboratory findings are summarised in Table 26.6.[15,16,17]

Patient management

While DKA generally requires specialist treatment, early assessment and initial treatments should commence as soon as possible in the pre-hospital setting. Once initial treatments have been commenced, most patients with DKA can be nursed in high-dependency units or even general medical wards. Only patients with severe DKA or critical illness

TABLE 26.6 Laboratory findings in diabetic ketoacidosis (DKA)

LABORATORY ASSESSMENT	POSSIBLE FINDING	CLINICAL RELEVANCE
Sodium	For each 5.5 mmol/L increase in glucose from normal, serum sodium is lowered by 1.6 mmol/L	Increased sodium results from extravascular water movement to intervascular space due to the osmotic effect of hyperglycaemia
Potassium	Initial serum potassium levels may be normal or slightly elevated	Potassium levels can rapidly decrease after commencement of insulin as potassium moves into the cells
Beta-hydroxybutyrate	Levels greater than 0.5 mmol/L are considered abnormal, and levels of 3 mmol/L correlate with need for DKA treatment	Beta-hydroxybutyrate, the more common ketone body, is not detected by Ketostix. Serum or capillary beta-hydroxybutyrate can be used to follow response to treatment.
Osmolality	Blood levels may be increased due to intravascular dehydration	DKA patients who are comatosed typically have values > 330 mOsm/kg. If the osmolality is less than this in a patient who is comatose, other causes of obtundation should be investigated
Amylase	Hyperamylasaemia	Hyperamylasaemia may be seen even in absence of pancreatitis. It is not understood why this occurs, but it occurs in up to 75% of patients with DKA
White cell count	Elevated white cell count > 15 × 10⁹/L	Elevated white cell count may suggest underlying infection
Urea and creatinine	Elevated	Serum levels may be elevated due to dehydration

that precipitated the event usually require admission to the intensive care unit.

While most institutions have DKA management protocols to guide overall management, the generally agreed principles of DKA management are to correct fluid depletion, decrease the blood glucose level, correct the electrolyte imbalance and treat the precipitating causes.[13,15,16] To ensure efficacy and safety of treatments, patients with DKA will require close monitoring of clinical and metabolic status to monitor response to treatments and recognise changes to the patient's condition. For example, onset of headaches or decreased level of consciousness may indicate the development of cerebral oedema and the need for more-focused assessment and interventions in such patients.

Fluid depletion

Intravascular fluid depletion in adults with DKA can be significant. In the absence of heart failure, the fluid of choice in the resuscitation phase is sodium chloride 0.9%. If the patient is hypotensive (systolic blood pressure below 90 mmHg) 500 mL sodium chloride 0.9% is given intravenously over 10–15 minutes while requesting senior medical review.[13] This rehydration therapy can be commenced by pre-hospital responders when treating adult patients. When the systolic blood pressure is above 90 mmHg fluid replacement for most people of average weight is 1000 mL within the first hour.[16] Fluids should then be reduced to 1000 mL over 2 hours for 2 consecutive hours and after that, titrated to maintain adequate blood pressure, pulse, urinary output and mental status. Correcting intravascular dehydration will reduce plasma osmolarity and blood glucose levels. Care needs to be taken in cases of younger patients with DKA as rapid fluid infusion may result in cerebral oedema, which has a high mortality rate. For this reason many pre-hospital guidelines do not advocate this therapy. As a guide, the aim should be to reduce serum osmolarity not more than 3 mOsm/L/h or decrease sodium concentration by less than 1 mmol/hr to avoid potential cerebral oedema due to large fluid shifts. Additionally, if serum sodium rises above 155 mmol/L, switching to 0.45% sodium chloride may need to be considered, although the optimal time to use 0.45% sodium chloride remains uncertain.[16]

Many DKA protocols will recommend commencing glucose (5% dextrose) at 80–120 mL/h to prevent hypoglycaemia when blood glucose levels approach 15 mmol/L.[14,18] The glucose rate is adjusted to achieve a target blood glucose level (BGL) of 10–15 mmol/L. Occasionally 10% glucose may be needed. Normal saline will be continued if hydration status requires.

Blood glucose level

Intravenous insulin will lower blood glucose concentration through increased glucose utilisation in peripheral tissues and a decrease in hepatic glucose production. Insulin will decrease ketone release, thereby correcting metabolic acidosis. Initial commencement of insulin infusion at a rate of approximately 5 units/hour (or 0.1 units/kg/h) is generally recommended to encourage a steady fall in blood glucose levels. However, infusions may need to be increased if initial rates do not reduce blood glucose levels after 1–2 hours. It is imperative that insulin therapy is continued until ketonaemia is resolved.

Blood glucose levels should be monitored at least hourly, with the aim to prevent blood sugar levels falling below 10 mmol/L, and 5% dextrose should be added to the fluid replacement regimen once blood sugar levels approach 12–14 mmol/L.[14,18] It is recommended that a mechanical pump or syringe driver is used to deliver the infusion. All intravenous tubing must be flushed with the prepared insulin solution prior to patient administration to ensure tubing is coated with insulin solution as insulin adheres to the tubing. If intravenous infusion is not possible, then intramuscular-route infusion may be considered and can be successful in delivering 8–10 units of insulin hourly.[13]

The transition from intravenous insulin to subcutaneous injections can be initiated once glucose level is < 11 mmol/L, serum bicarbonate level > 18 mmol/L, venous pH > 7.30 and the patient has been eating and drinking for at least 24 hours.[14,16] Transition to subcutaneous insulin can be challenging, and involvement of the diabetes team is recommended. Normal diet should be resumed prior to ceasing the infusion. The subcutaneous insulin or anti hyperglycaemic therapy is given with the next meal. An overlap time between the intravenous and subcutaneous insulin will be allowed depending on the type of insulin. Cease infusion 2 hours after giving regular insulin (i.e Actrapid, Humulin R, Mixtard 30/70, Mixtard 50/50, Humulin 30/70) or 1 hour after oral anti-hyperglycaemic therapy or rapid-acting insulin (i.e. Novarapid, Humalog, Apidra, Nova Mix 30, Humalog Mix 25, Humalog Mix 50).

Electrolyte imbalance

Total body depletion of potassium can occur in DKA, despite initial normal or slightly elevated serum levels (Table 26.6). To prevent acute hypokalaemia after fluid and insulin therapy, potassium replacement should be considered once the patient's serum levels are known and adequate renal output established. The aim is to maintain serum potassium levels at between 4 and 5 mmol/L. Most DKA protocols will advocate commencing potassium replacement at a rate of 20 mmol/h if potassium levels are < 3.5 mmol/L, adjusted in the succeeding hours to a replacement rate of 10 mmol/h to maintain a serum potassium level of 3.5–5.5 mmol/L.[13]

Cease potassium infusion when the serum potassium is greater than 5.5 mmol/L.

While there are many slight variations on how to replace potassium, initial and 2-hourly monitoring of serum potassium and, if possible, continuous electrocardiogram are recommended during the resuscitation and treatment phases of DKA management. An example guide to potassium replacement is presented in Box 26.1.

BOX 26.1 Potassium replacement guideline

- Serum potassium < 3 mmol/L, consider potassium 40 mmol/hour
- Serum potassium 3 to 4 mmol/L, consider potassium 30 mmol/hour
- Serum potassium 4 to 5 mmol/L, consider potassium 10 mmol/hour
- Serum potassium > 5 mmol/L, cease potassium infusion

Bicarbonate replacement in patients with initial metabolic acidosis remains controversial, with no clear benefit in clinical trials. However, in patients with severe acidosis (i.e. pH < 7), infusion of sodium bicarbonate may be considered after consultation with an endocrinologist when pH is < 7.0 and the HCO_3^- is <5.[16,18] It is important to note that infusion of sodium bicarbonate is likely to lower serum potassium levels significantly. Sodium bicarbonate may be administered at a rate of 1–2 mmol/kg or 70–100 mL (8.4%) over 20–30 minutes.[13]

Although serum phosphate depletion is frequently observed in patients with DKA, replacement is not routinely recommended with no clear benefit and a potential increased risk of hypocalcaemia and hypomagnesaemia.[18] Serum phosphate level is often normal at presentation and may decrease with insulin therapy. Phosphate replacement may be considered necessary in patients with cardiac dysfunction, anaemia or respiratory depression if their serum phosphate level is less than 1.0 mg/dL. Replacement in such circumstances may consists of 20–30 mEq/L potassium phosphate in intra-venous fluids.[18] In less urgent circumstances, if phosphate replacement is considered necessary, oral supplementation may be safer.[16]

Pre-hospital responders may be confronted by patients in a poor conscious state presenting with hyperventilation to produce compensatory respiratory alkalosis. Some intensive care paramedic guidelines may allow for drug-facilitated intubation to assist with airway protection and ventilation maintenance. See Chapter 17, p. 318, for intubation techniques. In such instances the preservation of the compensatory alkalosis is imperative with end-tidal carbon dioxide values determined before any therapy is provided.

Investigations and consider precipitating causes

Identification of the precipitating cause is important both to prevent further occurrence and if appropriate to treat confounding illness. This will involve the following investigations:

- Baseline arterial blood gases (hypoxia, lactic acidosis) (see Ch 17, p. 329, for techniques)
- Electrolytes (Ca, Mg, PO_4, urea, creatinine)
- Liver function tests, amylase, lipase
- ECG and troponins
- Septic screen (blood cultures, CRP, chest X-ray, MSU)
- Pregnancy test in females of child-bearing age
- Serum cortisol, if adrenal insufficiency is considered
- Alcohol and drug screen if drug use is suspected because acidosis will not resolve.

Assessment by a diabetes educator as early as possible after presentation is also highly recommended, as it is estimated that ongoing diabetes education and follow-up care may prevent unnecessary hospital admissions in about 50% of presentations. Co-existing illness such as pelvic or rectal abscess, pneumonia and silent myocardial infarction should be excluded prior to discharge.[15] Special concern exists in the pregnant woman presenting with DKA. Fetal mortality rate may be as high as 30% and up to 60% with ketoacidosis coma. Fetal death mainly occurs in women with overt diabetes, but may occur in gestational diabetes.[15]

Hyperglycaemic, hyperosmolar syndrome

Hyperglycaemic, hyperosmolar syndrome (HHS) is characterised by hyperglycaemia and high plasma osmolality without significant ketoacidosis (Fig 26.6). In the HHS state, blood sugar levels rise slowly and patients become progressively unwell. In most cases, sufficient insulin exists to prevent ketone formation and therefore metabolic acidosis is normally not present, except in extreme cases. In contrast to DKA, patients with HHS present with an increase in serum bicarbonate levels, usually exceeding 18 mmol/L, and serum sodium levels frequently 140 mmol/L or higher. Serum osmolality levels will also be significantly elevated, in the region of 350 mOsm/kg, and serum blood glucose levels will usually be < 50–60 mmol/L.

The HHS state occurs in type 2 diabetes and usually has gradual onset occurring over several weeks, not days. Patients presenting with HHS usually have an underlying medical condition exacerbating often-undiagnosed type 2 diabetes. Traditionally, patients presenting with HHS are usually middle-aged or elderly, but awareness of increased reports of type 2 diabetes in younger adults and children make presentations in these groups possible.

Differentiation between HHS and DKA may be difficult initially (Table 26.7). However, the treatment approach initially is similar to DKA, with a few modifications:

- If serum sodium is greater than 155 mmol/L, it is recommended to use 0.45% sodium chloride as initial fluid replacement.[13,14]
- As with DKA, insulin replacement is usually required initially but blood sugar levels tend to fall rapidly with hydration; after recovery, not all patients will require insulin treatment.

For many presenting with HHS, this may be their first diagnosis with type 2 diabetes and therefore the diabetes team should be alerted early and involved in the patient's ongoing and future care.

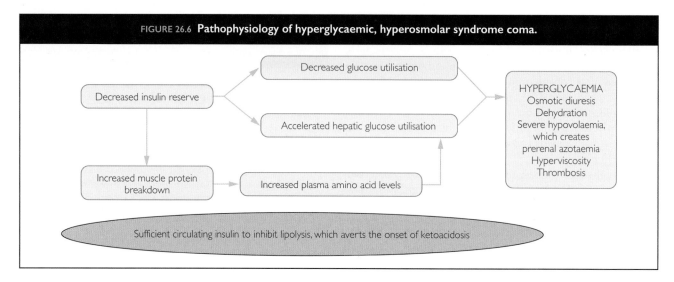

FIGURE 26.6 **Pathophysiology of hyperglycaemic, hyperosmolar syndrome coma.**

TABLE 26.7 Comparison of hyperosmolar, hyperglycaemic syndrome (HHS) and diabetic ketoacidosis (DKA)[19]

CLINICAL PICTURE	HHS	DKA
General	More dehydrated, not acidotic	More acidotic and less dehydrated
	Frequently comatose	Rarely comatose
	No hyperventilation	Hyperventilation
Age frequency	Usually elderly	Younger patients
Type of diabetes mellitus	Type 2 or non-insulin-dependent	Type 1 or insulin-dependent
Previous history of diabetes mellitus	In only 50%	Almost always
Prodromes	Several days duration	Less than 1 day
Neurological symptoms and signs	Very common	Rare
Underlying renal or cardiovascular disease	About 85%	About 15%
Laboratory findings		
Blood glucose	More than 800 mg/dL	Usually less than 800 mg/dL
Plasma ketones	Less than large in undiluted specimen	Positive in several dilutions
Serum sodium	Normal, elevated, low	Usually low
Serum potassium	Normal or elevated	Elevated, normal or low
Serum bicarbonate	More than 16 mEq	Less than 10 mEq
Anion gap	0–12 mEq	More than 12 mEq
Blood pH	Normal	Less than 7.35
Serum osmolality	More than 350 mOsm/L	Less than 330 mOsm/L
Serum urea	Higher than DKA	Not as high as in HHNS
Free fatty acids	Less than 1000 mEq/L	More than 1500 mEq/L
Complications		
Thrombosis	Frequent	Very rare
Mortality	20–50%	1–10%
Diabetes treatment after recovery	Diet alone or oral agents (sometimes)	Always insulin

HHNS: hyperosmolar, hyperglycaemic non-ketotic state

HYPERGLYCAEMIC, HYPEROSMOLAR SYNDROME (HHS)

- Traditionally, the majority of patients with HHS are elderly and have an underlying medical condition.
- The choice of fluid used in the HHS state should consider age, serum sodium, degree of dehydration and patient's co-morbidities.
- Incorrect resuscitation may cause an increase in plasma sodium levels and a further increase in plasma osmolality, which has been associated with pontine myelinolysis.
- Serious complications related to treatment for HHS are rare, but may include cerebral oedema and adult respiratory distress syndrome.

Hypoglycaemia

Hypoglycaemia most commonly occurs in type 1 diabetes, although it may also occur in type 2 diabetics.[13,16] Most episodes of hypoglycaemia are related to insulin treatment, although sulfonylurea drugs may also cause hypoglycaemic episodes.[20] Sulfonylurea medications act by binding to a high-affinity receptor on the surface of the pancreatic islet beta cells, potentiating normal glucose-stimulated insulin release in the presence of a pancreas with functioning beta cells.[13] An inevitable consequence of tight glycaemic control, most hypoglycaemic episodes are managed by the patients themselves, a family member or ambulance services.

Hypoglycaemia should be considered in any unresponsive patient until proven otherwise, and insulin overdose considered in patients who present with hypoglycaemia that requires continuing doses of intravenous glucose to maintain blood glucose above 5 mmol/L. A lack of dietary intake, increased physical stress, liver disease, changes in insulin or oral medication regimens, pregnancy, pancreatitis, pituitary insufficiency, Addison's disease, alcohol ingestion and drugs such as non-steroidal anti-inflammatory drugs, phenytoin, thyroid hormones and propanolol can all contribute to hypoglycaemia.[13,15] It is also worth noting that beta-blockers can mask the adrenergic warning symptoms, making symptoms sudden and unexpected in patients on such therapy.[13]

Definitions of hypoglycaemia

The normal blood glucose level (BGL) is 4.0–8.0 mmol/L. When the blood glucose level is < 2.5 mmol/L this is defined as severe hypoglycaemia.[16] A blood glucose level of < 3.5 mmol/L is considered moderate hypoglycaemia.[13]

Additionally, hypoglycaemic symptoms may occur when a very high blood glucose level falls too rapidly (e.g. a blood glucose level of 16.7 mmol/L falling quickly to 10 mmol/L). This is especially true for patients with chronically elevated blood sugar levels.[21] Symptoms tend to be grouped as either:

- autonomic (i.e. sweating, warm sensation, anxiety, nausea, palpations and possibly hunger) or
- neurological (i.e. tiredness, visual disturbance, drowsiness, altered behaviour, confusion and, if untreated, seizures or coma).

Autonomic-related symptoms frequently occur with blood sugar levels around 3.5 mmol/L, whereas neurological symptoms tend to be present with blood sugar levels closer to 2.5 mmol/L. A combination of sweating and reduced activity, along with depleted energy reserves, predisposes hypoglycaemic patients to hypothermia. Close attention to rewarming and protecting the patient from further heat loss is required during initial management.

Treatment

Mild to moderate hypoglycaemia

If the patient is conscious and cooperative, a readily available and fast-acting glucose-containing food or drink (60–130 mL fruit juice, 75–150 mL lemonade, jelly beans, honey, 15 g of glucose in adults) may be considered, followed by a lower-glycaemic-load carbohydrate meal (sandwich, dried fruit).[13]

Severe hypoglycaemia

In episodes of severe hypoglycaemia, the person is likely to be unconscious or confused, requiring assistance. Treatment recommendations for hypoglycaemia in adults are glucose 50% given intravenously (into the antecubital vein if possible), 0.5–2 mg intramuscular (IM) glucagon or subcutaneous (SC) glucagon 1 mg (treatment of choice for non-healthcare professionals), depending on availability and clinical setting.[13] The IM route has a quicker release rate and rectifies the blood sugar levels more quickly, while the SC route is slower and more sustained. Response would be expected within 5–6 minutes of injection (either glucose or glucagon). However, prolonged hypoglycaemia associated with a seizure may take several hours for recovery of full consciousness and cognition. In the pre-hospital setting, use of glucose 50% is not advocated and glucose 10% by intravenous infusion (see below) or glucagon are preferred treatment choices.

Following successful reversal of hypoglycaemia, blood glucose should be monitored every 1–2 hours initially, and then revert to the patient's usual testing regimen. Consultation with the diabetic specialist team is advisable to determine the cause of the hypoglycaemia; consider medication dose changes and commence education to prevent further episodes. Most patients are usually discharged home if the cause of the hypoglycaemic event can be identified unless they are on oral antihyperglycaemic medications that have a longer half-life.

HYPOGLYCAEMIA

Blood glucose level is < 2 mmol/L or severe symptoms of hypoglycaemia:

- Administer 50% glucose 25–50 mL intravenously or Glucagon 0.5–2 mg intramuscularly.
- Pre-hospital responders can administer 10% glucose 150 mL intravenously for adults or 3 mL/kg intravenously for children. This can be followed by a further 100 mL or 2 mL/kg respectively if response is inadequate or alternatively Glucagon 0.5–2 mg intramuscularly.
- Consider hypothermia as a possible complication with the intent to maintain normothermia and protect from further heat loss.

Continued

- If on insulin infusion:
  - cease insulin
  - bolus 100 mL 5% glucose
  - administer 50% glucose 25 mL (if asymptomatic) or 50% glucose 50 mL (if symptomatic) intravenously
  - if the pump is the patient's own insulin administration device, ask a carer or relative for assistance if uncertain how to operate it. Recovery can still occur even if it is left operating.
- In all cases repeat BGL measurement every 15 minutes
- Resume insulin at half the rate when BGL > 4.0 mmol/L if on insulin infusion

Blood glucose level is > 2 mmol/L or minor symptoms of hypoglycaemia:
- Administer 200 mL soft drink or fruit juice or 6 jelly beans
- Where access to sugar-containing products is difficult, pre-hospital responders can use 15 g oral glucose paste as an alternative
- Repeat BSL every 15 minutes
- Give complex carbohydrate meal
- If on insulin infusion:
  - cease insulin
  - bolus 100 mL 5% glucose
  - Resume insulin at half the rate when BGL is >4.0 mmol/L

BGL: blood glucose level; BSL: blood sugar level test

Alcoholic ketocidosis

Alcoholic acidosis usually occurs in patients with chronic alcoholism in the setting of prolonged fasting, protracted vomiting and large alcohol ingestion.[22] The patient usually presents with severe hypoglycaemia but will have concurrent accumulation of ketoacids and lactic acid. Insulin deficiency, depleted glycogen stores and volume depletion provide an appropriate milieu for the development of alcoholic keto-acidosis. Hypoglycaemia occurs, as gluconeogenesis is inhibited by ethanol and glycogenolysis is exhausted by a significant fasting state. If insulin levels are decreased, metabolism of glucose is altered leading to the utilisation of fat and muscle tissue for energy. This results in ketosis which, together with profound dehydration, continues the cycle of ketosis and acidosis.[22,23]

Management
The focus of treatment in the ED is rehydration with Normal saline and correction of hypoglycaemia with 5% dextrose. This treatment modality is usually sufficient to reverse the acidosis. Adjunctive therapy includes parental thiamine administration. Thiamine is often given before glucose administration to prevent precipitating Wernicke's encephalopathy, a neurological syndrome associated with ataxia, ophthalmoplegia and mental status changes.[17] Vital signs and neurological assessment are imperative to the nursing care of these patients, together with accurate monitoring of fluid, hydration and electrolyte status. Monitor also for signs of alcohol withdrawal.

Adrenal insufficiency

Adrenal insufficiency is a condition that occurs when glucocorticoid production is inadequate to meet metabolic requirements (Fig 26.7).[19] It may be caused by structural or functional lesions of the adrenal cortex (*primary adrenal insufficiency*) or anterior pituitary gland/hypothalamus (*secondary adrenal insufficiency*).

The presenting signs and symptoms can vary from non-specific clinical features, such as tiredness, nausea, anorexia, lethargy, mild hypotension, fever and abdominal pain, through to potentially life-threatening cardiovascular collapse. Historical indicators of the potential for adrenal insufficiency to occur include history of long-term glucocorticoid treatment and/or known adrenal failure.[16]

Precipitating factors and aetiology

The aetiology of adrenal insufficiency is also diverse. It may result from abrupt withdrawal of glucocorticoid therapy or the onset of an acute illness or stressor, such as infection or trauma in steroid-dependent patients. Causes that are specific to the adrenal gland include autoimmune disorders, adrenal haemorrhage or infiltrates (carcinoma, sarcoidosis), bilateral adrenalectomy or drugs (ketoconazole). Pituitary and hypothalamic causes of adrenal insufficiency may be due to tumours, apoplexy or granulomatous disease.[14]

Clinical management

As with all emergency presentations, the clinical assessment follows the ABCD mnemonic and interventions are initiated if a threat to any of these parameters is established. Fluid resuscitation with intravenous Normal saline 0.9% is usually required, titrated to the clinical response. Hydrocortisone infusion is commenced immediately at 4 mg/h and maintained for 24 hours.[13,14]

Following the primary survey, the healthcare should continue with a focused assessment to identify any precipitating event. Broad-spectrum antibiotic therapy may be indicated if infection is expected. Having stabilised the patient, blood is sampled for random cortisol and adrenocorticotrophic hormone (ACTH) levels. This test is time-sensitive and needs to reach the laboratory within 30 minutes. The blood sample must be placed on ice for transport. Diagnosis is confirmed by performing a short ACTH stimulation (Synacthen) test. Hydrocortisone therapy will be slowly reduced over the following 24–48 hours. The maintenance dose of gluco-corticoid is usually hydrocortisone 10 mg twice per day.[14]

Discharge advice

A patient with adrenal insufficiency should be educated on the following key features of self-care on discharge. Patient education on glucocorticoid therapy is very important following an acute crisis. This education will include instructions to increase glucocorticoid dose at times of intercurrent illness. Wearing a 'medical alert' bracelet or necklace is advocated. Instructions on the use of an emergency injection pack (hydrocortisone), particularly when away from medical care, may also be included as part of the discharge advice. Above all, the early recognition of signs and symptoms suggestive of an adrenal crisis (nausea, vomiting, dehydration, feeling faint) are emphasised.

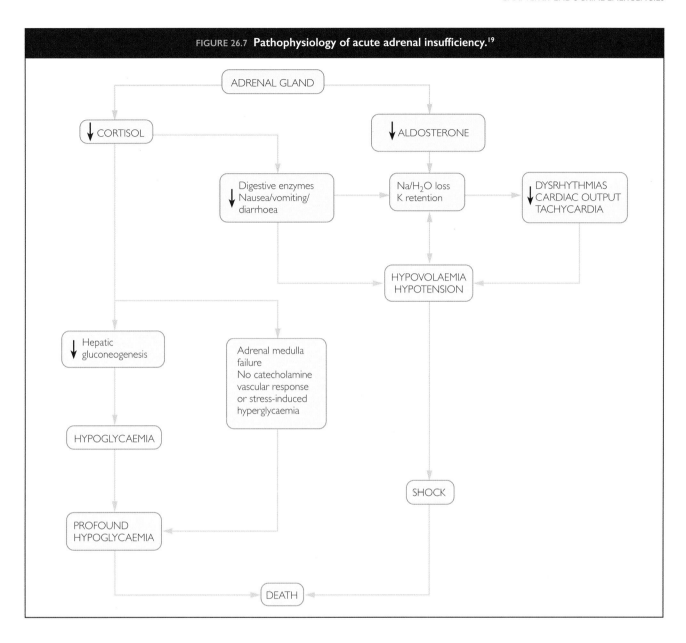

FIGURE 26.7 **Pathophysiology of acute adrenal insufficiency.**[19]

Acute pituitary apoplexy

This rare disorder is caused by infarction or haemorrhage of the pituitary gland associated with trauma, hypertension, anticoagulation, cardiac surgery and a large number of other conditions. Acute pituitary apoplexy in uncommon, affecting both males and females equally with an incidence of 0.6–9.1%.[14]

Clinical features

The clinical signs and symptoms are similar to those seen in raised intracranial pressure and include headache, vomiting, photophobia and altered level of consciousness. Neuro-ophthalmic signs, such as visual field defects and loss of vision, may also be present.[16]

Treatment

As with all emergency presentations, the clinical assessment follows the ABCD mnemonic and the initiation of interventions to support these systems. Hydrocortisone therapy is started immediately by administering hydrocortisone 4 mg/h

intravenously.[13,14] Blood levels are taken prior to commencing steroid therapy. They include the following:

- cortisol
- prolactin
- follicle-stimulating hormone, luteinising hormone, oestradiol (women), testosterone (men)
- thyroid-stimulating hormone
- adrenocorticotrophic hormone.

Diagnosis is confirmed by urgent magnetic resonance imaging or computed tomography. A critical referral is then made for a neurosurgical consult, with operative management associated with improved outcomes especially in visual acuity.[14]

Thyroid storm

Thyroid emergencies are very rare but can be life-threatening.[24] Abnormality, either hyperactivity or hypoactivity, can result in multisystem symptoms. Thyroid storm (hyperactivity or thyrotoxicosis) commonly occurs as a complication of Graves' disease, primarily in women aged between 30 and 40 years. The hypothalamic–pituitary–thyroid counterregulatory system is responsible for normal thyroid function.

Precipitating factors and aetiology

Thyroid crisis occurs when any part of the circuit malfunctions. It is unusual for untreated hyperthyroidism to present as thyroid storm, as there are usually precipitating events. Hyperthyroidism can be divided into three categories: *true* (i.e. excessive thyroid hormones), *drug-induced* or *thyroid injury*. True hyperthyroidism is characterised by an overactive thyroid gland and excessive production of thyroid hormones. In Graves' disease, thyroid-stimulating immunoglobulins increase thyroid activity. Tumours and thyroid nodules also increase thyroid activity. A type of thyroid toxicosis occurs with an increased amount of circulating hormones without concurrent overactivity from the thyroid, as in thyroiditis or ingestion of thyroid hormones. Drugs such as iodine and iodine-containing agents such as amiodarone and lithium may potentially induce hyperthyroidism. Other thyroid-specific precipitation factors in thyroid storm may include thyroid injury such as palpation, infarction or an adenoma.[3,14,16]

Clinical features

Thyroid storm, an endocrine emergency first described in 1926, remains a diagnostic and therapeutic challenge.[24] Thyroid storm occurs with rapid elevation in thyroid hormone levels and is a clinical diagnosis. General precipitating factors include: infection, non-thyroidal trauma or surgery, psychosis, parturition, myocardial infarction or other medical problems.[14] A concise medical history is imperative to the treatment of these patients, as it is unusual for untreated hyperthyroidism to present as thyroid storm. Assessment should include history of recent illnesses and medications. Red flags to observe for include recent weight loss despite increased appetite and increased caloric intake; abdominal pain is also a common complaint. The patient may be restless with a reduced attention span and prone to changing discussion topics frequently. Tremors and manic behaviours are also common. In the late stages, an alteration in mental status occurs, which can progress to coma. In extreme cases hyperthermia can occur with temperatures reaching 40.5–41°C, as well as tachycardia with heart rates of 200–300 beats/minute, which increase the risk of cardiac failure and arrest.[24] Rales secondary to cardiac failure may be heard. The skin can progress from warm and diaphoretic to hot and dry as dehydration worsens. Increased gastric motility can cause nausea, vomiting and diarrhoea. Hepatic tenderness, jaundice and thinning of the hair may also occur. Goitre, an enlarged thyroid gland, develops as the condition progresses. Eyes become protuberant, periorbital oedema develops and the patient has a staring gaze with heavy eyelids. The clinical manifestations of thyroid storm are summarised in Table 26.8.

Treatment

Treatment should be initiated promptly targeting all steps of thyroid hormone function, release and action.[25] Thyroid hormone levels can help differentiate the causative factor; however, the hormone levels are frequently not readily available, making differentiation between thyroid storm and thyrotoxicosis difficult. If thyroid storm is suspected, therapy needs to be aggressive and rapid so that hormone levels

TABLE 26.8 Clinical manifestations of thyroid storm

SYSTEM	CLINICAL MANIFESTATIONS
Neurological	Nervousness, restlessness, tremors, confusion
Pulmonary	Tachycardia, dysrhythmias, hypertension
Respiratory	Shortness of breath, dyspnoea, rales, congestive heart failure
Gastrointestinal	Hyperactive bowel, abdominal pain, decreased appetite, weight loss, diarrhoea, jaundice
Ocular	Exophthalmos, lid lag, staring gaze
Integumentary	Hyperthermia, flushed, diaphoresis, poor turgor

are reduced and haemodynamic integrity is preserved. The treatment principles are to decrease the production and release of thyroid hormones, inhibit the peripheral effects of thyroid hormones using beta-blockers and identify and deal with the underlying precipitating factors.

Propanolol can be given intravenously to reduce the heart rate. Younger patients and those in an acute crisis often require larger than normal doses. The propanolol acts to block the conversion of the T_4 to T_3. In cases where beta-blockers are contraindicated (e.g. in diabetes, pregnancy and asthma), digitalis may be used.[14,16]

Propylthiouracil, which inhibits thyroid hormone synthesis, and methimazole may be used to further block hormone synthesis. This can be given orally or through a gastric tube. Onset of action occurs within an hour; however, full potential is not reached for 3–6 weeks.[3,14] Iodine may be given 1 hour after antithyroid medications to slow the release of stored thyroid hormones from the thyroid gland. Iodine can be given orally or by intravenous infusion. Patients with Graves' disease and thyroid crisis metabolise and use cortisol faster than normal. Glucocorticosteroids, such as dexamethasone or hydrocortisone, have been found to increase survival rates, as they prevent adrenal compromise and inhibit T_4 and T_3 conversion.[25,26]

Approaches to supportive therapy may include fluid resuscitation if required and reduction in core body temperature.

PRACTICE TIPS
THYROID STORM

- Thyroid storm is very rare.
- In a patient with existing thyrotoxicosis, thyroid storm may be caused by intercurrent illness or by direct injury to the thyroid.
- Treatment includes the rapid inhibition of thyroid hormone synthesis with propylthiouracil, inhibition of the effects of excess thyroid hormone using beta-blockers and correction of the underlying cause.

Myxoedema coma

Myxoedema coma is a rare but potentially serious complication of untreated hypothyroidism.

Precipitating factors and aetiology

The incidence of myxoedema coma is greater in men than in women. Precipitating causes include hypothermia, infection, myocardial infarction or congestive heart failure, cerebral vascular accidents, drug-induced respiratory depression (e.g. sedatives, anaesthetics or tranquillisers), trauma or gastro-instestinal blood loss.[14,16] The disease usually progresses insidiously over months to years, with coma developing when the patient is subjected to stress. It is known to also affect elderly women who have long-standing hypothyroidism and those with undiagnosed hypothyroidism. The latter tends to occur in the winter months. Survival rates are increased when prompt hormone replacement with intense supportive care is received. Mortality rates, however, approach 50%.[27]

Clinical features

A hypoactive thyroid results in reduced metabolic rate and activity. Pronounced fatigue, decreased activity tolerance, episodes of shortness of breath and weight gain may be displayed. Tongue swelling or macroglossia are common complaints. Patients may display elements of confusion and be slow to answer questions (Table 26.9). This alteration in mental status can result in coma. Psychiatric symptoms such as hallucinations, paranoia, depression, combativeness and decreased concern for personal appearance may also present, and are often referred to as 'myxoedema madness'.

Angio-oedema can result in airway occlusion in an unconscious or semiconscious patient. Weak respiratory effort with decreased respiratory drive results in alveolar hypoventilation and can predispose patients to infections. Alveolar hypoventilation also results in hypercarbia, which can cause alteration in mental status. Obesity-related sleep apnoea could further compromise the respiratory system (Table 26.9).

Cardiac changes include bradycardia, decreased stroke volume and decreased cardiac output. Widespread ST and T-wave changes may be evident, with prolonged QT intervals.

TABLE 26.9 Clinical manifestations of myxoedema coma

SYSTEM	CLINICAL MANIFESTATIONS
Neurological	Confusion, lethargy, coma
Pulmonary	Decreased stroke volume, decreased cardiac output, bradycardia, peripheral vasoconstriction, inverted T waves, prolonged QT interval
Respiratory	Macroglossia, obesity-related sleep apnoea, pneumonia, hypoventilation, hypercarbia
Gastrointestinal	Hypoglycaemia, constipation
Renal	Decreased renal blood flow, decreased sodium reabsorption, hyponatraemia

Body temperature will be low and the skin pale and cool due to peripheral vasoconstriction. In myxoedema coma, the glomerular filtration rate and renal blood flow decreases. Generalised non-pitting oedema as a result of increased insulin sensitivity and decreased oral intake and constipation may also occur. Biochemical abnormalities may include hyponatraemia, increased creatine phosphokinase and lactate dehydrogenase, hypoglycaemia and normocytic or macrocytic anaemia.[16] Thyroid-stimulating hormones may be modestly low in primary hypothyroidism or low in secondary hypothyroidism, but free thyroxine levels are usually low.[16]

Treatment

Even with prompt treatment, mortality can be as high as 30% in myxoedema coma. Care is primarily focused on hormone replacement after initial ABC assessment and stabilisation. Hormone replacement may take the form of intravenous T_4 (levothyroxine). Large doses are used to saturate empty sites and replenish the circulating levels. T_4 avoids adverse cardiac effects that might occur with a sudden increase in T_3. Some doctors may recommend a combination of both T_3 and T_4. As myxoedema coma is a rare condition, a lack of clinical trials to suggest best methods is lacking, and management is likely to be guided by an endocrinology specialist. Electrocardiogram monitoring during careful titration of thyroid replacement is recommended.[14]

> **PRACTICE TIPS**
> ## MYXOEDEMA COMA
> - This condition carries a high mortality rate.
> - The aim of treatment is prompt recognition, immediate thyroid replacement therapy, treatment of precipitating cause and supportive therapy (ventilation).

Cushing's syndrome

Cushing's syndrome is a rare endocrine disorder involving the hypothalamic–pituitary–adrenal glands, which results in excessive cortisol levels.[28,29] Cortisol, a steroid hormone produced by the adrenal gland and normally produced in response to stress, can trigger physiological changes resulting in a wide range of health problems including hypertension, hyperglycaemia, muscle wastage and osteoporosis. Causes of Cushing's syndrome include:

- iatrogenic factors—prolonged administration of a glucocorticoid such as prednisone to treat conditions such as asthma or rheumatoid arthritis
- ectopic factors—production of cortisol by adrenal adenoma or carcinoma (e.g. lung cancer can produce ACTH which when added to the normal pituitary production of ACTH leads to excessive cortisol secretion)
- problems in the hypothalamic–pituitary–adrenal axis resulting in excessive cortisol secretion from the adrenal glands due to overstimulation of the adrenal glands by ACTH.[29]

Features that best discriminate Cushing's syndrome from other common conditions

- *Skin*—Easy bruising, facial plethora, purple striae
- *Musculoskeletal system*—Proximal muscle weakness and/or myopathy; early osteoporosis with or without vertebral fractures or osteonecrosis of femoral or humeral head

Other features

- *Skin and hair*—Thin skin, poor wound healing, hirsutism or scalp thinning
- *Body habitus*—Weight gain and central obesity; dorsocervical fat pad ('buffalo hump'), supraclavicular fat pads, facial fullness ('moon face')
- *Reproductive system*—Menstrual irregularity, infertility
- *Psychiatric effects*—Depression, psychosis, irritability, insomnia, fatigue
- *Metabolic effects*—Diabetes
- *Cardiovascular effects*—Congestive cardiac failure, hypertension, thrombosis (including deep vein thrombosis and myocardial infarction)
- *Immune system*—Immunosuppression causing recurrent and atypical infection, including tuberculosis.[29]

Assessment and investigations

The diagnosis of Cushing's syndrome is generally based on laboratory investigations. Serum ACTH levels determine the aetiology of the excessive cortisol secretion.

- An elevated ACTH indicates ACTH-dependent disease, with further pituitary investigations required to identify the source.
- Normal ACTH levels identify the need for abdominal computed tomography scanning to investigate the possibility of an adrenal tumour.

Other laboratory tests indicated include:

- serum glucose to establish if hyperglycaemia is present
- full blood count and white blood cell count may reveal elevated levels of both, but a decrease in lymphocytes
- electrolytes, particularly serum potassium which may be decreased
- 24-hour urine collection may also be commenced to measure cortisol levels.[28,29]

Treatment

Treatment modalities are centred on removing the precipitating cause. Endogenous Cushing's syndrome requires surgical removal of the tumour causing the oversecretion of cortisol. Patients will require glucocortisol replacement therapy for a period of time post surgery due to adrenal insufficiency. Pharmacological blockade of cortisol production may be the treatment of choice in some patient populations, using metyrapone or mitotane. If the cause is iatrogenic due to long-term glucocorticoid therapy, the prescribed dose of steroids is gradually reduced.

Metyrapone

- Action—reversibly inhibits the biosynthesis of cortisol, corticosterone and aldosterone in the adrenal cortex.
- Indications:
  - to establish the diagnosis of adrenocortical hyperfunction in Cushing's syndrome
  - following pituitary surgery.
- Contraindications—adrenocortical insufficiency.
- Adverse reactions—nausea, vomiting, dizziness, light-headedness, abdominal pain.
- Dosage—500–1000 mg orally 3 times a day. [13]

Mitotane

Mitotane is not registered for use in Australia but is available via the Special Access Scheme. Dosage is 500 mg orally initially, increasing up to 4–6 g daily.[13]

PRACTICE TIP

- Consider the diagnosis of Cushing's syndrome in patients who have discriminating signs (such as early osteoporosis, myopathy, or easy bruising) or multiple features, especially if becoming progressively more severe (such as refractory diabetes and hypertension associated with end organ complications).
- Delayed diagnosis can cause life-threatening illness and irreversible organ damage and may compromise the management options of any underlying tumour.
- If endogenous Cushing's syndrome is suspected, refer to an endocrinologist; possible screening tests include urinary free cortisol, salivary cortisol and an overnight dexamethasone test.[29]

SUMMARY

Endocrine emergencies are rare, and diabetic ketoacidosis is the most frequently encountered. Most institutions and health services have established protocols which should be utilised when available. Clinicians should be aware of potential red flags for endocrine emergencies and not delay initiation of treatment while awaiting investigation results. It is also imperative that involvement of the endocrine team occur in a timely manner once endocrine involvement is suspected.

Mrs Riley, a 40-year-old woman, presents to the emergency department (ED) by ambulance following a 000 call by her husband. She was found by her husband to be drowsy and disorientated following a collapse.

The following handover was given by the paramedic:

- 40-year-old female found by her husband with a decreased level of consciousness.

- Patient has been recently treated for a tooth abscess by her dentist for which she was taking flucloxacillin 500 mg 6-hourly. Yesterday she complained of abdominal pain and persistent vomiting and has been unable to tolerate even clear fluids for the past 48 hours.

Her observations by the paramedics on arrival were:

- blood pressure 90/30 mmHg
- pulse rate 145 beats/minute
- temperature 38.6°C
- respiratory rate 45 breaths/minute
- oxygen saturation 93%
- Glasgow Coma Scale (GCS) score 13–14
- BGL on glucometer was HHH.

The treatment initiated was oxygen therapy and the establishment of an intravenous line. 1 L NaCl 0.9% was commenced. Haemodynamic monitoring was initiated by the paramedics. En route the patient's condition deteriorated and on arrival in ED her Glasgow Coma Scale score was 7 and she was tolerating an oral adjunct (Guedel's airway).

She has no known allergies. She was previously healthy with no known medical conditions except hypertension.

In ED the patient was allocated a triage category 1 and directed to the resuscitation area. The first priority was to establish the severity of Mrs Riley's symptoms and hence the need for medical intervention. This determination was made within seconds of the primary assessment. It was established that there was an actual threat to her airway, breathing, circulation and disability; interventions were required immediately. This included the establishment of a definitive airway via endotracheal intubation, and ventilatory support to achieve adequate oxygenation and ventilation. Mrs Riley was sedated and paralysed using rapid sequence induction (thiopentone and suxamethonium) to facilitate the intubation process. Circulatory support was established by infusing 3 L Normal saline 0.9% via a large-bore cannula to correct the hypotension. A blood glucose level was recorded as 'HI' using point-of-care testing. Following the establishment of hyperglycaemia in this acutely ill patient, the next bedside test was serum ketone monitoring. The result was a serum ketone level of 4.1 mmol/L.

Ketosis and hyperglycaemia are distinct metabolic problems. When these abnormal states occur together, diabetic ketoacidosis (DKA) may result. In determining the severity of Mrs Riley's illness (DKA), it was necessary to consider a combination of clinical assessment findings, historical factors, diagnostic and laboratory testing and the outcome of interventions. A secondary assessment outlying these findings is given in Table 26.CS1.

TABLE 26.CS1 Focused clinical assessment

	CLINICAL FINDING	FINDING/INTERVENTION
E	Exposure	Potential site of infection
	Expose patient to identify all injuries:	Commenced on antibiotic therapy
	recent tooth extraction	Septic screening, including chest X-ray
F	Fluids	Circulatory support was established
	The circulatory system was assessed and the following vital signs established:	Fluid resuscitation: 3 L NaCl 0.9% were infused in the first 2 hours followed by 1 L NaCl 0.9% over the next hour
	• blood pressure 110/70 mmHg	Indwelling catheter was inserted, which initially drained 650 mL dilute urine.
	• heart rate 112 beats/minute	
	• respiratory rate—ventilated	Hourly urinary measures were commenced to ensure a urinary output of 0.5 mL/kg/h
	• GCS 3 (sedated and paralysed)	
	• pupils (equal and reacting to light)	ECG recorded—Sinus tachycardia with no acute changes
	• SpO₂ 99%	Haemodynamic monitoring was commenced via arterial line and continuous cardiac monitoring
	• Temperature 37.9°C	

Continued

	TABLE 26.CS1 Focused clinical assessment—cont'd	
	CLINICAL FINDING	**FINDING/INTERVENTION**
G	Glucose	Formal blood sugar 28.4 mmol/L
		Serum ketones 4.1 mmol/L
		Commenced on insulin infusion therapy
		(50 units Actrapid in 50 mL NaCl infusing at 5 units/h)
H	History	Hypertension
		Not a known diabetic (gestational diabetes only)
		Referred by GP and seen in ED 2 days prior with:
		• an impacted infected left tooth
		• persistent vomiting with 3 kg loss in 1 week
		• Blood pressure 115/50 mmHg
H	Head-to-toe assessment	
	Head/neck	Left upper molar extraction
		CT head/facial bones: NAD
	Respiratory	Clear
		Ventilated: SIMV
		ABG: severe acidosis
		pH: 6.7
		$PaCO_2$ 28.4 mmHg
		HCO_3^- 4.9 mmol/L
		BE −27.1 mmol/L
		Lactate: 0.9 mmol/L
	Cardiovascular	Cool peripheries
		Dual heart sounds
		CK < 20 μmol/L (normal limits are: male 60–120 μmol/L, female 40–90 μmol/L)
		Troponin negative
	Abdomen	Soft and non-tender
		Bowel sounds present
		Beta-hCG negative
		LFTs normal
		Amylase and lipase normal
	Renal	Very good urinary output
		Potassium 4.2 mmol/K (potassium replacement commenced at 10 mmol/h)
		Sodium 139 mmol/L; corrected sodium 153 mmol/L
		Anion gap 23 mmol/L
I	Inspect the back	Nil abnormality found

ABG: arterial blood gas; BE: base excess; CK: creatine kinase; CT: computed tomography; GCS: Glasgow Coma Scale; hCG: human chorionic gonadotrophin; HCO_3^-: bicarbonate level; LFT: liver function test; $PaCO_2$: arterial pressure of carbon dioxide; SIMV: synchronised intermittent mandatory ventilation; SpO_2: peripheral oxygen saturation

With respect to the circulation and metabolic derangements that Mrs Riley suffered, the management goals were to:

- replace salt and fluid losses
- restrain lipolysis and inhibit glucose production with insulin
- identify and correct precipitant
- re-establish normal physiology.

The greatest dangers to Mrs Riley are acidosis and electrolyte disturbances, especially hypokalaemia, not hyperglycaemia. The first priority was rapid fluid resuscitation to improve tissue perfusion and the tissue's response to insulin. Fluids also decrease the blood sugar level by 30%. Correcting Mrs Riley's hypotension would also decrease the secretion of counterregulatory hormones and improve acidosis. As there was clear clinical evidence of ketoacidosis, the next priority was the commencement of an insulin infusion. The initial infusion rate was 5 units/h. The blood glucose level progressively decreased from 28.4 mmol/L by 4.5–5.5 mmol/L over the next few hours. When Mrs Riley's blood glucose level dropped to 14 mmol/L, a 5% dextrose infusion was commenced at 80 mL/h. This allowed the blood glucose level to be maintained until the acidosis was reversed by the insulin therapy. The next most-critical management step was the recognition of the need to replace potassium. Potassium replacement was commenced at 10 mmol/h, and close monitoring was initiated in anticipation of a further fall in serum potassium due to the commencement of insulin therapy and the correction of the acidosis. Identification of the precipitating factor was the next vital step. This was identified as the infected and impacted left tooth. She was commenced on ceftriaxone, metronidazole and gentamycin. Mrs Riley was then transferred to the intensive care unit 4 hours after presenting to the ED.

During her ICU stay, she was further resuscitated and stabilised. Her acidosis and hyperglycaemia were corrected slowly. She was successfully extubated 3 days later. The maxillofacial and endocrine teams were consulted on her care. Mrs Riley was discharged home on insulin 9 days later.

Questions

1. What are the main characteristics of DKA?
2. What are the key physical signs seen in patients presenting with DKA?
3. What is the first priority in managing the patient in the above case?
4. What are the overarching key principles of managing this patient presenting with DKA?
5. What are the most common errors when managing a patient with DKA?

 Answers to Case Study Questions can be found on evolve
http://evolve.emergencytrauma.curtis

REFERENCES

1. Guyton AC, Hall JE. Textbook of medical physiology. 12th edn. Philadelphia: Saunders; 2011.
2. Brown D, Edwards H, eds. Lewis's Medical–surgical nursing. 3rd edn. Sydney: Elsevier; 2012:1337.
3. Jones RE, Huether SE. Alterations of hormonal regulation. In: McCance KL, Huether SE, Parkinson CF, eds. Pathophysiology: the biological basis for disease in adults and children. 6th edn. St. Louis: Mosby; 2010.
4. Newberry L, Sheehy SB, Emergency Nurses Association. Sheehy's emergency nursing: principles and practice. 6th edn. St. Louis: Mosby; 2010.
5. Thompson JM, McFarlance GK, Hirsch JE et al. Mosby's clinical nursing. 5th edn. St Louis: Mosby; 2001.
6. Goodman HM. Basic medical endocrinology. 4th edn. Philadelphia: Saunders; 2009.
7. Herlihy B. The human body in health and illness. 4rd edn. St. Louis: Saunders; 2011.
8. Sech, LA, Colussi G, Di Fabio A, Catena C. Cardiovascular and renal damage in primary aldosteronism: outcomes after treatment. American Journal of Hypertension 2010;23(12):1253–60.
9. Davis JH et al. Surgery: a problem-solving approach. Vol 2. 2nd edn. St Louis: Mosby; 1995.
10. Magkos F, Wang X, Mittendorfer B. Metabolic actions of insulin in men and women. Nutrition 2010;26(7–8):686–93.
11. Australia Diabetes Association. Understanding diabetes. Online. www.diabetesaustralia.com.au/Understanding-Diabetes/Diabetes-in-Australia; accessed 30 March 2015.
12. Australian Institute of Health and Welfare. Diabetes prevalence in Australia: an assessment of national data sources; 2009. Online. www.aihw.gov.au/publications/index.cfm/title/10639; accessed 30 March 2015.
13. Therapeutic guidelines. Therapeutic guidelines: endocrinology. 5th edn. North Melbourne: Therapeutic Guidelines; 2014.
14. Savage MW, Mah PM, Weetman AP et al. Endocrine emergencies. Postgrad Med J 2004;80(947):506–15.
15. Westerberg DP. Diabetic ketoacidosis: evaluation and treatment. American Family Physician 2013;87(5):337–46.

16. Kearney T, Dang C. Diabetic and endocrine emergencies. Postgrad Med J 2007;83(976):79–86.

17. Cameron P. Textbook of adult emergency medicine. 3rd edn. Edinburgh: Churchill Livingstone; 2009.

18. Pollock, F, Funk DC. Acute diabetes management: adult patients with hyperglycemic crises and hypoglycemia. AACN Advanced Critical Care 2013;24(3):314–24.

19. Kozak G, ed. Clinical diabetes mellitus. Philadelphia: WB Saunders; 1982.

20. Seaquist ER, Anderson J, Childs B et al. Hypoglycemia and diabetes: a report of a workgroup of the American Diabetes Association and the Endocrine Society. Diabetes Care 2013;36(5):1384–95.

21. Boyle PJ, Schwartz NS, Shah SD et al. Plasma glucose concentrations at the onset of hypoglycemic symptoms in patients with poorly controlled diabetes and in nondiabetics. N Engl J Med 1988;318(23):1487–92.

22. Marinella MA. Alcoholic ketoacidosis presenting with extreme hypoglycemia. Am J Emerg Med 1997;15(3):280–1.

23. Yanagawa Y, Sakamoto T, Okada Y. Six cases of sudden cardiac arrest in alcoholic ketoacidosis. Internal Medicine 2008;47(2):113–17.

24. Chiha M, Samarasinghe S, Kabaker AS. Thyroid storm: an updated review. J Int Care Med 2015;30(3):131–40.

25. Tietgens ST, Leinung MC. Thyroid storm. Med Clin North Am 1995;79(1):169–84.

26. Sercombe CT, Kletti CA. Adrenal and pituitary disorders. In: Wolfson AB, Harwood-Nuss A, eds. Harwood-Nuss' Clinical practice of emergency medicine. 4th edn. Philadelphia: Lippincott Williams & Wilkins; 2005:863–8.

27. Beynon J, Akhtar S, Kearney, T et al. Predictors of outcome in myxoedema coma. Critical Care 2008;12(1):111.

28. Holcomb S. Confronting Cushing's syndrome. Nursing 2005;35(9):1–6.

29. Prague JK, May S, Whitelaw BC. Cushing's syndrome. British Medical Journal 2013;346: f945.

CHAPTER 27
HEALTHCARE-ASSOCIATED INFECTIONS AND COMMUNICABLE DISEASES

RAMON Z SHABAN AND TERRI REBMANN

Essentials

The following *Standard Precautions* apply when providing emergency healthcare.[1]

Hand hygiene

- Hand hygiene must be performed before and after every episode of patient contact. This includes before touching a patient, before a procedure, after a procedure or body-fluid-exposure risk, after touching a patient and after touching a patient's surroundings.
- Hand hygiene must also be performed after removal of gloves.
- Alcohol-based hand rubs containing at least 70% v/v ethanol or equivalent should be used for all routine hand hygiene practices in the healthcare environment. If hands are visibly soiled, hand hygiene should be performed using soap and water.

Personal protective equipment (PPE)

- Aprons or gowns should be appropriate to the task being undertaken. They should be worn for a single procedure or episode of patient care and removed in the area where the episode of care takes place.
- A surgical mask and goggles must be worn during procedures that generate aerosols, splashes or sprays of blood, body fluids, secretions or excretions into the face and eyes.
- Gloves must be worn as a single-use item for each invasive procedure, contact with sterile sites and non-intact skin or mucous membranes; and for any activity that has been assessed as carrying a risk of exposure to blood, body fluids, secretions and excretions.
- Gloves must be changed between patients and after every episode of individual patient care.
- Sterile gloves must be used for aseptic procedures and contact with sterile sites.

Handling and disposal of sharps

- Sharps must not be passed directly from hand to hand and handling should be kept to a minimum.
- Needles must not be recapped, bent, broken or disassembled after use.
- The person who has used the sharp must be responsible for its immediate safe disposal.
- Used sharps must be discarded into an approved sharps container at the point-of-use. Do not fill above the mark that indicates the bin is three-quarters full.

Routine environmental cleaning

- Clean frequently touched surfaces with detergent solution at least daily, and when visibly soiled and after every known contamination.
- Clean general surfaces and fittings when visibly soiled and immediately after spillage.

- Clean touched surfaces of shared clinical equipment between patient uses with detergent solution.
- Use surface barriers to protect clinical surfaces (including equipment) that are touched frequently with gloved hands during the delivery of patient care, are likely to become contaminated with blood or body substances, or are difficult to clean (e.g. computer keyboards).
- Spills of blood or other potentially infectious materials should be promptly cleaned as follows: wear utility gloves and other PPE appropriate to the task; confine and contain spill, clean visible matter with disposable absorbent material and discard the used cleaning materials in the appropriate waste container; and clean the spill area with a cloth or paper towels using detergent solution.
- Use of chemical disinfectants should be based on assessment of risk of transmission of infectious agents from that spill.

In addition, three specific levels of *transmission-based precautions* apply in particular circumstances.

Contact precautions

- In addition to standard precautions, implement contact precautions in the presence of known or suspected infectious agents that are spread by direct or indirect contact with the patient or the patient's environment.
- When working with patients who require contact precautions, perform hand hygiene, put on gloves and gown upon entry to the patient care area, ensure that clothing and skin do not contact potentially contaminated environmental surfaces and remove gown and gloves and perform hand hygiene before leaving the patient care area.
- To facilitate the mechanical removal of spores, meticulously wash hands with soap and water and pat dry with single-use towels.
- Use of alcohol-based hand rubs alone may not be sufficient to reduce transmission of *Clostridium difficile*.
- Use patient-dedicated equipment or single-use non-critical patient-care equipment (e.g. blood pressure cuffs).
- If common use of equipment for multiple patients is unavoidable, clean the equipment and allow it to dry before use on another patient.

Droplet precautions

- In addition to standard precautions, implement droplet precautions for patients known or suspected to be infected with agents transmitted by respiratory droplets (i.e. large-particle droplets > 5 μm in size) that are generated by a patient when coughing, sneezing or talking, or during suctioning.
- When entering the patient-care environment, put on a surgical mask.
- Place patients who require droplet precautions in a single-patient room when available.

Airborne precautions

- In addition to standard precautions, implement airborne precautions for patients known or suspected to be infected with infectious agents transmitted person-to-person by the airborne route (i.e. airborne droplet nuclei or particles < 5 μm in size).
- Wear a correctly fitted P2 (N95) respirator when entering the patient-care area when an airborne-transmissible infectious agent is known or suspected.
- Patients on airborne precautions should be placed in negative-pressure rooms or in a room from which the air does not circulate to other areas. Exceptions to this should be justified by risk assessment.
- Implement transmission-based precautions for all patients colonised or infected with a multi-resistant organism, including:
  - Put on gloves and gowns before entering the patient-care area.
  - Use patient-dedicated or single-use non-critical patient-care equipment (e.g. blood-pressure cuff, stethoscope).
  - Use a single-patient room or, if unavailable, cohort patients with the same strain of multi-resistant organism in designated patient-care areas; and ensure consistent cleaning and disinfection of surfaces in close proximity to the patient and those likely to be touched by the patient and healthcare workers.

INTRODUCTION

Communicable diseases are those where the causative agent passes or is carried from one person to another directly or indirectly. Generally speaking, healthcare-associated infections are acquired in healthcare facilities ('hospital-acquired' infections) or are infections that occur as a result of healthcare interventions ('iatrogenic' infections) and which may manifest after people leave the healthcare facility.[1,2] A variety of like and related definitions exist that are determined by, among other things, the setting or context in which they occur.[3] Community-acquired infections are those that are acquired and detected within 48 hours of hospital admission in patients without previous contact with healthcare service.[3] A hospital-acquired infection (HAI) is a localised or systemic condition that results from adverse reaction to the presence of an infectious agent(s) or its toxin(s) and was present 48 hours or more after hospital admission and not incubating at hospital admission time.[3,4] In clinical and epidemiological terms, healthcare-associated infections (HCAIs) are those where an infection is detected within 48 hours of hospital admission in patients who had previous contact with healthcare service within 1 year.[3]

It is estimated that there are more than 200,000 cases of HCAI in Australian acute healthcare facilities each year, making them the most common complication affecting patients in clinical settings.[1] The average excess hospital length of stay due to a surgical site infection in Australia is estimated to be between 3.5 and 23 hospital bed days, depending on the type of infection.[5] The average annual total national number of bed days due to surgical site infections in Australian is estimated to be 206,527 bed days.[5,6] Antimicrobial resistance is a leading worldwide threat to the wellbeing of patients, and the safety and quality of healthcare globally.[7] With effective antimicrobial stewardship for optimal use of antimicrobials and containment of antimicrobial resistance, $300 million of the Australian national healthcare budget could be redirected to more effective use every year.[7,8] Fundamentally, HCAIs, cross-contamination and the spread of infection and communicable disease are risks in all healthcare settings.[9]

The human, financial and societal costs of HCAIs are significant. Approximately 1 in 10 hospitalised patients will acquire an infection after admission, resulting in substantial economic cost. The financial and health systems costs of HCAIs are typically reflected in increasing length of stay, rates of re-admission, increasing access block and bed block and additional diagnostic and therapeutic interventions. The human cost, by way of unnecessary pain and suffering for patients and their families and prolonged hospital stays, is difficult to quantify, but it is significant.[1] HCAIs lead to substantial morbidity, and, in some cases, death.

HCAIs are, however, largely preventable adverse events rather than unpredictable complications. It is possible to significantly reduce the rate of HCAIs through effective infection control.[1] Effective infection prevention and control is thus a prerequisite for high-quality healthcare for patients and a safe working environment for those who work in healthcare settings. Successful approaches for preventing and reducing harm arising from HCAIs involve applying a risk-management framework to manage 'human' and 'system' factors associated with the transmission of infectious agents. Understanding the modes of transmission of infectious organisms and knowing how and when to apply the basic principles of infection control is critical to the success of an infection-control program. This responsibility applies to everybody working and visiting a healthcare facility, including administrators, staff, patients and carers.[1]

Although the risk of infection and transmission of communicable diseases exists in all healthcare settings, some contexts present particular challenges.[10] The context of emergency nursing and paramedic practice are two such settings. The demand for emergency healthcare nationally and internationally is high.[11] Emergency nurses and paramedics provide clinical care to patients where there is a serious, unexpected or potentially dangerous situation requiring immediate action. The demands placed upon these healthcare professionals to render life-saving care to the sick and injured are complex, time-pressured and challenging. Patients often present with complex, severe injuries and infections requiring rapid and aggressive intervention. The presentation of acute or chronic infections presents emergency nurses and paramedics with many challenges.

The ability to recognise infections and to determine their relative severity is critical to the practice of emergency nursing and paramedic practice. Severe or life-threatening infections, such as meningococcal septicaemia and sepsis[12] require rapid identification[13] and intervention to ameliorate the high levels of morbidity and mortality. If the care and interventions that emergency nurses and paramedics employ are to be effective and efficient, the strategies for infection prevention and control must be both high-quality and safe. With increasing rates of presentations, increasing complexity of illness and disease, and a well-documented workforce shortage of skilled staff, healthcare professionals are expected to do more with less.[1,7] One of the consequences of this is that emergency nurses and paramedics are taking on new roles, extending their scope of practice, and consequently are more accountable for their clinical practice than ever before.[14] The rapid changes in the healthcare environment continue to precipitate challenges for healthcare professions regarding the sufficiency of professional practice standards,

education and training, and clinical policy and procedures that ensure quality, safety and accountability in healthcare. As healthcare provided in primary and emergency care settings becomes more complex, so too do the complexities and risks of infection.

Overview of infection and communicable disease

Infections and outbreaks

From time to time, new infections emerge to which individuals and populations around the world have little or no immunity. Infectious diseases account for approximately 25% of the 57 million deaths worldwide. Globally they are the leading cause of death for people under the age of 50 years.[15] The World Health Organization estimates that new diseases are occurring at a rate of at least one per year. Occasionally, these outbreaks become pandemic. Historically, humankind has faced significant threats from infectious disease. The global 'Spanish flu' pandemic of 1918 caused an estimated 40–50 million deaths around the world. Influenza pandemics in 1957 and 1968 caused widespread morbidity and more than a million deaths worldwide, causing significant economic and social disruption.[16]

Australia has sustained relatively few outbreaks of infectious disease compared with the rest of the world. Although the demographic consequences have been minimal, the human and social impact on individuals and communities has been significant. The smallpox epidemics of 1881–82 and 1913–17 in Sydney, and the plague epidemic of 1900, led to the emergence of formal policies of isolation, quarantine, fumigation, cleansing and vaccination.[17] There have been a few notable cases that captured public attention and were responsible for widespread fear, panic and hysteria; they are listed in Table 27.1.

Many of the infectious diseases that threatened public health and safety in the past continue to do so today. However, not all encounters with infectious agents lead to infection. For an infection to occur, a number of scientific conditions must be met. Understanding the science of infection and disease, including the modes of transmission of infectious organisms and knowing how and when to apply the basic principles of infection control, is critical to the success of an infection-control program.

Microorganisms are responsible for infectious disease. They are ubiquitous, and a necessary element of the environment. Not all of them, however, result in infection; not all are pathogenic all of the time. For microorganisms to cause infection, a number of criteria must be satisfied.

- There must be an agent that has the ability to cause disease.
- It must gain entry to the body of a susceptible host in sufficient numbers to overcome the body's defence mechanism.[18]
- The body must succumb to the infection, and for the spread to be sustained, it must leave the organism and spread to another.

This is referred to as the 'chain of infection', and is illustrated in Figure 27.1.

TABLE 27.1 Notable infectious disease outbreaks in Australia[49]

YEAR	DISEASE
1789–1790	Smallpox
1828	Smallpox
1857	Smallpox, influenza
1866/67	Measles
1875/76	Scarlet fever
1881/82	Smallpox
1894	Plague
1900/09	Plague
1913/17	Smallpox
1918/19	Spanish Influenza
1921	Plague
1937–1955	Polio
1940	Rubella
1957/58	Asian Influenza
1968/69	Hong Kong Influenza
1977/78	Russian Influenza
1997/98	Cryptosporidiosis
1997	Hepatitis A
2000	Psittacosis
2009	Dengue fever (Queensland)
2009	H1N1 influenza
2014	Ebola

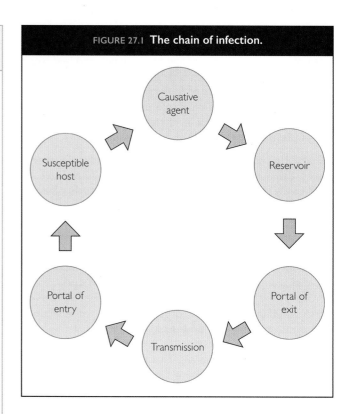

FIGURE 27.1 **The chain of infection.**

For infection to occur, therefore, there must be a source of infection, a susceptible host and a means of transmission, and the *chain of infection* must be satisfied.

The chain of infection

The chain of infection consists of six process points, each of which must occur concurrently for the spread of infection to be sustained.

1. Causative agent

First, there must be a causative agent. It may be caused by a variety of agents, such as a bacterium, virus, fungus or parasite. The property of an infectious agent that determines the extent to which overt disease is produced, or the power of an organism to produce disease, is called *pathogenicity*. Some agents are highly pathogenic and almost always produce disease, whereas others multiply without invasion and rarely cause disease.[19]

2. Reservoir

The causative agent that causes infection, such as bacteria, viruses, fungi, parasites and prions, can be involved in either colonisation or infection, depending on the susceptibility of the host.

- With *colonisation*, there is a sustained presence of replicating infectious agents on or in the body, without the production of an immune response or disease.
- With *infection,* invasion of infectious agents into the body results in an immune response, with or without symptomatic disease.[1]

Most microorganisms that cause disease in humans can only survive for limited periods outside the human body unless they are provided with an environment that will satisfy their requirements. Another animal or a non-living environment, such as soil or water, may provide an alternative environment or *reservoir* which will support the organism.

3. Susceptible host

To cause disease, the infectious agent must gain entry to a susceptible host. A susceptible host is one who lacks effective resistance to a pathogenic agent. Characteristics that influence susceptibility include age, sex, medical history, underlying pathology, lifestyle, nutrition, immunisation, medications and specific insult to the body, such as trauma.[19,20] The nature of the host response elicited by the pathogen often determines the pathology of a particular infection. The outcome of an infection depends on the balance between an effective host response that eliminates a pathogen, and an excessive inflammatory response that is associated with an inability to eliminate a pathogen and with resultant tissue damage that leads to disease.

In healthcare settings, the most common susceptible hosts are patients and healthcare workers. Patients may be exposed to infectious agents from themselves (endogenous infection) or from other people, instruments and equipment, or the environment (exogenous infection). The level of risk relates to the healthcare setting (specifically, the presence or absence of infectious agents), the type of healthcare procedures performed and the susceptibility of the patient. Healthcare workers may be exposed to infectious agents from infected or colonised patients, instruments and equipment, or the environment. The level of risk relates to the type of clinical contact healthcare workers have with potentially infected or colonised patient groups, instruments or environments, and the health status of the healthcare worker (e.g. immunised or immunocompromised).[1]

Vaccination renders hosts non-susceptible to infection. Vaccination is the process whereby a person is deliberately exposed to an agent which is antigenic, but not pathogenic, to provide immunity to that specific antigen. Since the introduction of vaccination, the burden of many bacterial and viral diseases has been reduced. Healthcare workers have the potential to come into contact with a number of vaccine-preventable diseases. Vaccination against or proof of immunity to diphtheria, tetanus, pertussis, hepatitis B, varicella, measles, mumps, rubella, influenza and tuberculosis are recommended for healthcare workers throughout Australasia.[1]

4. Portal of entry

The major portals of entry are via the skin following trauma and via the mucous membranes that line the wall of the respiratory, gastrointestinal and genitourinary tracts. Pathogens may have a preferred portal of entry that gives access to an environment suitable for the establishment of growth. For example, *Bordetella pertussis*, which causes whooping cough, a disease of the respiratory system, enters via the mouth or nose.[21]

5. Transmission

There are five ways in which the causative agent may be transmitted: contact, inhalation, inoculation, ingestion and transplacenta, although in healthcare settings the main modes of transmission of infectious agents are contact (including bloodborne), droplet and airborne.[1]

The *contact route* consists of two subcategories: direct and indirect contact. The primary difference between the two is whether or not an environmental source is involved in disease transmission.

- With *direct contact* there is no environmental source involved in disease transmission; the susceptible person comes into direct contact with an infected individual's contaminated bodily fluids.
- *Indirect contact* spread involves an intermediary contaminated environmental source between the infected person and the susceptible person.

In most situations, contact spread occurs when a healthcare worker's hands become contaminated with infectious particles and proper hand hygiene is not performed. Diseases such as scabies and methicillin-resistant *Staphyloccocus aureus* (MRSA) are spread by contact transmission.[1]

The *droplet route* involves respiratory droplets. Respiratory droplets are large, heavy drops that are released from the respiratory tract via the nose or mouth when people sneeze, cough, talk or even breathe. These droplets contain millions of bacteria and viruses. Respiratory droplets are believed to travel ~1 m from the infected person. If a healthcare worker is within

approximately 1 m of the patient when these droplets are released, they could inhale the infectious particles. The person's respiratory tract (the mucous membranes of the nose, mouth or pharynx) then becomes the portal of entry for the germs to enter the body. Once the agent enters the body, it can replicate and cause an infection. Direct contact with an infected person's respiratory secretions can also transmit infection. Infections such as tuberculosis are spread via inhalation.[1]

The *airborne route* of transmission occurs when airborne droplet nuclei, small particles < 5 μm in size, are expelled when infected individuals sneeze, cough, talk or breathe. Because of their small size, these particles can attach themselves to dust particles and be carried by air currents for long distances. Eventually, these particles will settle to the ground, but they can remain suspended in the air for hours unless they are removed by ventilation or filtration systems. As long as droplet nuclei are airborne, they remain a risk to nearby susceptible people who can inhale the particles and become infected. The respiratory tract (the mucous membranes of the nose, mouth or pharynx) again becomes the portal of entry for the germs to enter the body. Once the agent enters the body, it can replicate and cause an infection.[1]

Other modes of transmission also occur. *Trans-placental infections* are those that are transmitted vertically between mother and her embryo or fetus. Such infections are transmitted from the mother, who acts as the reservoir of infection. These infections include syphilis, rubella and viral hepatitis. Some infections are transmitted by *ingestion*, a form of contact, such as hepatitis A; and others via *inoculation*, such as hepatitis B and C. The modes of transmission vary by type of organism. In some cases the same organism may be transmitted by more than one route, such as influenza which can be transmitted by contact and droplet routes.[1]

6. Portal of exit

The agent may be transmitted in a variety of mediums, including blood, saliva, faeces, vomitus, discharge (wounds), urine and semen or in other body tissues and/or fluids. The portal of exit is disease- and organism-specific. Some organisms present in one portal cannot be transmitted successfully in another. For example, hepatitis A exits the body via faeces, and hepatitis B and C by blood, and not vice versa.

PRACTICE TIP

Interrupting the cycle of infection is fundamental to infection control and prevention.

When infection strikes: the immune response

The ability of the human body to resist infection depends on two major human defence mechanisms:[22] the *innate or non-specific* immune response and the *specific* immune response. These are outlined below.

Innate or non-specific immune response

The *innate or non-specific immunity* is the body's first line of defence. It relies on natural, mechanical and local barriers, does not discriminate one agent from another and acts in a similar way each time the same agent enters (or attempts to enter) the body. The function of the innate or non-specific immune response is to prevent the entry of pathogens into the tissues of the body, or to destroy them immediately if they do manage to enter. The skin and mucous membranes, certain cells, inflammation, various antimicrobial proteins and fever contribute to the body's non-specific response to a pathogen.[18]

The *skin* and *mucous membranes* are the body's first line of defence against invasion by microorganisms.[18] Intact skin and epithelial surfaces do not provide a friendly environment for microorganisms. The skin is dry, and mucosa have an established microflora and secretions with antimicrobial properties.[23] The skin consists of two distinct layers, the *epidermis* and the *dermis*. The epidermis is the tough outer layer and represents a formidable barrier to most organisms. The dermis contains sebaceous and sweat glands whose secretions inhibit the growth of some microorganisms. However, the bacteria that form the normal flora of the skin are tolerant and able to survive in the conditions created by the secretions.[18]

The human body's *cellular defence* system is activated when microorganisms or foreign substances enter the tissues. Phagocytes and natural killer cells perform a most important role in this system.

- *Phagocytes* ingest and break down foreign particles and dead tissue, and remove cellular debris from the tissues; macrophages and neutrophils are the two major types of phagocytes. Macrophages, the largest of the phagocytic cells, are located in most tissues and organs of the body. Neutrophils, the most abundant of the white blood cells, are active in the bloodstream but also migrate into tissues in the early stages of infection and inflammation.
- *Natural killer cells* are large granular lymphocytes, which are able to destroy cancer cells and virus-infected cells. They do not recognise specific cells, but attack a variety of targets.

Inflammation is the body's response to any injury or infection. The function of the acute inflammatory response is to prepare the injured area for the repair process by clearing the injured site of cellular debris and foreign material or pathogens. Once the injury has occurred, there is activation or release of a variety of chemicals, which cause dilation of the arterioles in the damaged area, increase the permeability of local capillaries and create an influx of phagocytic cells. This process creates the four main signs of acute inflammation: redness, heat, swelling and pain. *Chronic inflammation* occurs when the body is unable to clear the organisms or foreign particles from the damaged area.

Various *antimicrobial proteins*, the most important of which are the complement proteins, interferon and acute-phase proteins, also act non-specifically against foreign cells in the body. The complement system's major function is to enhance phagocytosis, produce inflammation and directly lyse foreign cells.

The hypothalamus (the body's thermostat) normally controls the body's temperature at around 37°C. *Fever*, a higher-than-normal body temperature, is the systemic response to invading microorganisms. Chemical substances called pyrogens that originate from within the body (endogenous) or outside the body (exogenous) produce fever. High fevers above 40°C may damage nerve cells and produce convulsions. However, a mild or moderate fever may be of benefit to the body, as temperatures above 37°C slow the rate of cell division of bacteria.

Specific immune response

Acquired or specific immunity is the body's second line of defence and is activated when microorgaisms evade the non-specific defence mechanism. The specific and non-specific response systems overlap and interact with each other to protect the body.[18]

When a microbe evades the non-specific defences, the body reacts by producing an antigen-specific response. The specific immune response is tightly regulated and has unique properties: specificity for antigens, the ability to turn off the response once an exposure is cleared, and memory with augmentation, such that repeated exposure results in a more rapid and enhanced response.[23]

The specific or acquired immune system consists of a variety of cells, especially lymphocytes and macrophages, and various organs. There are two major populations of lymphocytes: the B lymphocytes (B cells) and the T lymphocytes (T cells). The B cells are mainly responsible for humoral immunity (immunity provided by antibodies), and the T cells provide cell-mediated immunity.[18]

Antibodies produced and secreted by plasma cells (derived from B cells) circulate in the blood and other body fluids. They bind to the invading microorganism and are most effective against bacteria and viruses before they enter host cells. An initial encounter with an antigen prompts a primary immune response, followed by a lag time during which there is activation and proliferation of B cells specific for the antigen. Specific serum antibody level will peak within several weeks and decline in weeks to months. If the body is exposed to the same microorganism a second time, then a secondary immune response occurs that is faster, stronger and longer-lasting. The response is prompt because of the priming of the immune system during the initial exposure when large numbers of memory B lymphocytes were produced.[18] This previously described process of antibody production is classified as *naturally-acquired active immunity*.

Immunity may also be acquired in other ways: *artificially-acquired active immunity* following vaccination; *artificially-acquired passive immunity* resulting from the transfer of pre-made antibodies from an immune person to a non-immune person; and *naturally-acquired passive immunity* when maternal antibodies pass across the placenta. Passive immunity provides only short-term protection against disease.

T cells (cellular immunity) deal with intracellular pathogens by directly lysing the cells, or by releasing chemicals that enhance the inflammatory response and/or activate other defence cells to destroy the target cells. They are required for the proper functioning of both humoral and cell-mediated immunity. T-cell deficiency increases the susceptibility to viruses, intracellular bacteria and other intracellular parasites.[18]

Breaking the chain—preventing infection

Principles of infection prevention and control

The control and prevention of HCAIs and communicable diseases are high on the political and public agenda. The unacceptable burden of HCAIs in economic and human terms is significant, with increasing patient length of hospital stay, re-admission, suffering, morbidity and mortality. Ultimately, everyone pays the price for such infections.

The Australian Commission on Safety and Quality in Health Care (ACSQHC) recognises the community concerns requiring urgent national consideration, and the role that infection prevention and control has on reducing HAIs. The Commission's Healthcare Associated Infection Program[9] enables a national approach to reducing HAIs by identifying and addressing systemic problems and gaps and ensuring that comprehensive actions are undertaken in a nationally coordinated way by leaders and decision-makers in both the public and the private health sectors.[24]

Infection prevention programs

The control and prevention of HCAIs is a core function of all healthcare workers, including emergency nurses and paramedics. Infection prevention and control programs are formal structures and processes that together prevent, reduce and control transmission of HCAI and the spread of infectious disease and enable the provision of safe and high-quality healthcare. Effective infection prevention guidelines and strategies for the control and prevention of HAIs are required for all health contexts and settings, from large hospitals to emergency home and practice settings. Specific settings require tailored programs and elements, but infection prevention principles remain the same across all healthcare settings. The success of infection prevention and control strategies relies on six key elements,[1] as shown in Figure 27.2.

The Australian Guidelines for the Prevention and Control of Infection in Healthcare (2010) is the authoritative text for infection prevention and control across the range of healthcare establishments in Australia and New Zealand.[1] The recommendations for each setting should be implemented in concert with state or territory legislative requirements that affect work practices at the local level. When using these guidelines, it is important to note that statutory requirements of the jurisdiction take precedence when difference exists. A range of resources and support materials are available for health professionals and agencies.[53]

Infection control management plans

Work practices at the local level occur through the design, development and implementation of an infection-control management plan (ICMP), a formal and systematic clinical governance process that enables institutions to meet their infection prevention and control obligations within the broader corporate mission and goal.[1] They are designed to ensure that institutions and their people demonstrate accountability for quality in areas of infection prevention and control. Infection control management plans should risk-manage and reduce the incidence of preventable HAIs within organisational frameworks and systems that ensure quality and safety in healthcare.

ICMPs should embrace, build and extend the organisational strategic plan, where they define the scope of an infection-prevention program within the boundaries of areas such as client demographics, epidemiology of infection and restricted resources. The plan allows organisations to prioritise infection-prevention activity in accordance with principles of risk management and to develop appropriate professional and program performance measures; thereby demonstrating professional and public accountability of the infection-prevention program in terms of cost-effectiveness and/or cost–benefit. Key elements of an infection-control program are outlined below (Fig 27.3).

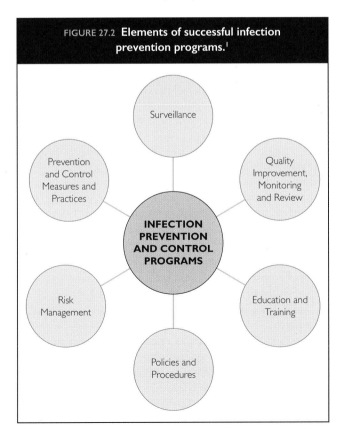

FIGURE 27.2 **Elements of successful infection prevention programs.**[1]

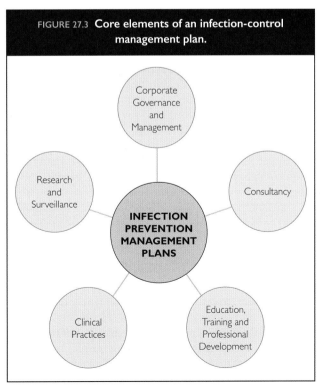

FIGURE 27.3 **Core elements of an infection-control management plan.**

An ICMP must incorporate all practice contexts, including the emergency care setting. The plan provides a strategic evidence base to guide work practices. The intentions documented in the strategic plan or activities outlined in the operational plan should form the basis of the infection control committee's (ICC) agenda, thereby assisting the ICC to steer activity.

Good infection-control outcomes rely on clinicians and service providers complying with infection-control principles/ standards and reporting various risk factors and/or situations that may lead to a risk of infection transmission. As such, leadership is required to obtain stakeholder buy-in at every level of the organisation. Key stakeholder input is required when setting policies/guidelines, targets and performance measures, as in most instances the performance being measured is that of the stakeholders. This fact needs to be clear for clinicians or service providers to be held accountable for their actions and outcomes.

In 2013, the Australian Commission on Safety and Quality in Health Care released National Safety and Quality Health Service (NSQHS) Standards to improve the quality of health service provision in Australia. The Standards provide a nationally consistent statement of the level of care consumers should be able to expect from health service organisations. There are 10 NSQHS Standards focusing on areas that are essential to drive the implementation and use of safety and quality systems, of which Standard 3 is *Preventing and Controlling Healthcare Associated Infections*. The aim of Standard 3 is to prevent patients acquiring preventable healthcare-associated infections and to effectively manage infections when they occur using evidence-based strategies.[5]

For this to be successful, a variety of measures are required as outlined in Box 27.1.[5] There must be formal governance and management systems for healthcare-associated infections that operate systemically within quality assurance systems. Healthcare agencies and professionals must develop and enact strategies for the prevention and control of healthcare-associated infections. Patients that present with or acquire an infection or colonisation during an episode or following episodes of care must be identified promptly and receive timely management and treatment, and they must be informed about their treatment and care. The healthcare environment must be clean and hygienic in accordance with best evidence and practice standards, in particular instrument and equipment reprocessing. Finally, safe and appropriate antimicrobial prescribing is a strategic goal of the clinical governance system.[5] The Commission has the published tools and resources to assist emergency nurses, paramedics and other health professionals with the implementation of Standard 3.[2]

Basic measures—standard and transmission-based precautions

Central to the success of the implementation of NSQHS Standard 3 *Preventing and Controlling Healthcare Associated Infections* is the implementation of systematic infection control practices. The emergency nurse and paramedic must adopt work practices that adhere to the two-tiered system of *Standard* and *Transmission-based* precautions.

> **BOX 27.1 Standard 3 Criteria—Preventing and Controlling Healthcare Associated Infections Standard[2]**
>
> **Governance and systems for infection prevention, control and surveillance**
> Effective governance and management systems for healthcare-associated infections are implemented and maintained.
>
> **Infection prevention and control strategies**
> Strategies for the prevention and control of healthcare-associated infections are developed and implemented.
>
> **Managing patients with infections or colonisations**
> Patients presenting with, or acquiring, an infection or colonisation during their care are identified promptly and receive the necessary management and treatment.
>
> **Antimicrobial stewardship**
> Safe and appropriate antimicrobial prescribing is a strategic goal of the clinical governance system.
>
> **Cleaning, disinfection and sterilisation**
> Healthcare facilities and the associated environment are clean and hygienic. Reprocessing of equipment and instrumentation meets current best practice guidelines.
>
> **Communicating with patients and carers**
> Information on healthcare-associated infections is provided to patients, carers, consumers and service providers.

PRACTICE TIP

Standard and Additional Precautions are used to break the Cycle of Infection, and apply to everyone including patients and visitors.

Standard Precautions

Standard precautions are practices and procedures that are employed during the care of all patients to achieve a basic level of infection prevention and control. They are work practices that ensure that a basic level of infection control is applied to everyone, regardless of their perceived or confirmed infectious status. Implementing standard precautions as a first-line approach to infection control in the healthcare environment minimises the risk of transmission of infectious agents from person to person, even in high-risk situations.[1] The core elements of standard precautions include the following.

- Aseptic technique, including appropriate use of skin disinfectants.
- Personal hygiene practices, particularly hand-washing and hand hygiene, and cough etiquette.
- Use of personal protective equipment (PPE).
- Appropriate handling and disposal of sharps and clinical waste.
- Appropriate reprocessing of re-usable equipment and instruments, including appropriate use of disinfectants.
- Environmental controls, including design and maintenance of premises, cleaning and spills management.
- Appropriate provision of support services, such as laundry and food services.

In the clinical environment, transmission of an infectious agent to a susceptible host occurs by direct and indirect contact. Inappropriate hand hygiene is the most significant reason for HAI. In the absence of a true emergency, personnel should always perform hand hygiene in accordance with the Five Moments for Hand Hygiene (Fig 27.4). Hand hygiene must be performed before and after every episode of patient contact. This includes before touching a patient, before a procedure, after a procedure or body-fluid-exposure risk, after touching a patient and after touching a patient's surroundings. Hand hygiene must also be performed after removal of gloves. Alcohol-based hand rubs containing at least 70% v/v ethanol or equivalent should be used for all routine hand hygiene practices in the healthcare environment. Alcohol-based products may be used as an adjunct to traditional hand-washing. However, visible soil must be removed by hand-washing before using antiseptic products formulated for use without water.[1]

Transmission-based precautions
Transmission-based precautions are required in extra work-practice situations where standard precautions alone may be insufficient to prevent infection (e.g. for patients known or suspected to be infected or colonised with infectious agents that may not be contained with standard precautions alone; Table 27.2).[1]

These precautions are tailored around specific infections or organisms, and may involve measures to prevent contact, airborne or droplet transmission (such as source isolation). Transmission-based precautions are also used in the event of an outbreak (e.g. gastroenteritis), to assist in containing the outbreak and preventing further infection, and must be tailored to the particular infectious agent involved and its mode of transmission.[1] This may involve a combination of the practices included in Box 27.2.

Transmission of infectious agents can occur in a number of ways:

- Indirect or direct *contact transmission*, when healthcare workers' hands or clothing become contaminated, patient-care devices are shared between patients, infectious patients have contact with other patients or environmental surfaces are not regularly decontaminated.

- *Droplet transmission*, when healthcare workers' hands become contaminated with respiratory droplets and are transferred to susceptible mucosal surfaces such as the eyes, when infectious respiratory droplets are expelled by coughing, sneezing or talking, and are either inhaled or come into contact with another's mucosa (eyes, nose or mouth), either directly into or via contaminated hands.

- *Airborne transmission*, when attending healthcare workers or others inhale small particles that contain infectious agents.[1]

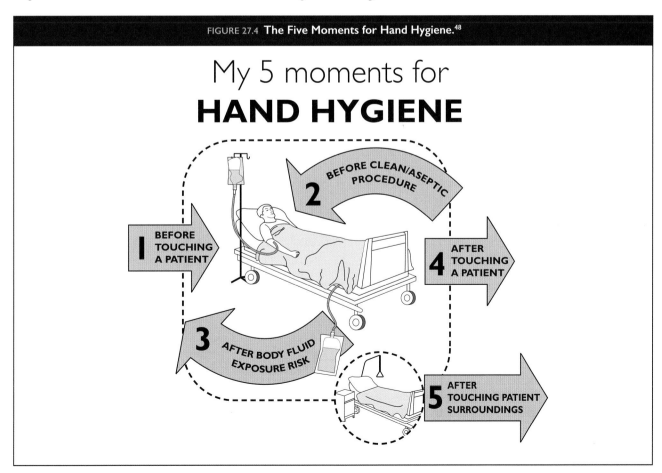

FIGURE 27.4 **The Five Moments for Hand Hygiene.**[48]

My 5 moments for
HAND HYGIENE

1 **BEFORE TOUCHING A PATIENT**

2 **BEFORE CLEAN/ASEPTIC PROCEDURE**

3 **AFTER BODY FLUID EXPOSURE RISK**

4 **AFTER TOUCHING A PATIENT**

5 **AFTER TOUCHING PATIENT SURROUNDINGS**

TABLE 27.2 Infections warranting transmission-based precautions before laboratory confirmation of infection[1]

INFECTION	TYPE	TRANSMISSION
Chickenpox and shingles (varicella zoster)	Viral	Airborne
Creutzfeldt–Jakob disease	Prion	Contact (CNS instruments)
Gastroenteritis	Bacterial	Contact (faecal–oral)
Gastroenteritis	Viral	Airborne
Hepatitis A	Viral	Contact (faecal–oral)
Influenza (during outbreaks)	Viral	Droplet
Measles	Viral	Airborne
Meningococcal infection	Bacterial	Droplet
Norovirus	Viral	Droplet (aerosolised vomitus)
Parvovirus B19	Viral	Droplet
Respiratory syncytial virus	Viral	Droplet (oral, fomites)
Rotavirus	Viral	Contact (faecal–oral)
Rubella	Viral	Droplet
Severe acute respiratory syndrome (SARS)	Viral	Droplet
Staphylococcal infection	Bacterial	Droplet
Tuberculosis	Bacterial	Airborne
Viral haemorrhagic fevers	Viral	Contact
Whooping cough (pertussis)	Bacterial	Droplet

CNS: central nervous system

BOX 27.2 Transmission-based precautions[1]

- Allocating a single room to an infected patient (isolation).
- Placing patients colonised or infected with the same infectious agent in a room together (cohorting).
- Personal protective equipment that is specific to the task being performed.
- Using disinfectants effective against the specific infectious agent.
- Providing a dedicated toilet.
- Use of specific air-handling techniques.
- Restricting movement of both patients and healthcare workers.

PRACTICE TIP

Transmission-based precautions can have adverse effects on patients and their families, including anxiety, mood disturbances and social isolation. Explain to patients and their families how and why these precautions are needed.

For diseases that have multiple routes of transmission, more than one transmission-based precaution category is applied. Whether used singly or in combination, transmission-based precautions are always applied *in addition* to standard precautions, as outlined in Table 27.3.

Transmission-based precautions remain in effect for limited periods of time until signs and symptoms of the infection have resolved or according to recommendations from infection-control practitioners specific to the infectious agent.[1] In Australia, a national system of surveillance operates to track the control and prevention of the organism for which transmission-based precautions are used, referred to as 'notifiable diseases'. The National Notifiable Diseases Surveillance System (NNDSS) was established in 1990 under the auspices of the Communicable Diseases Network Australia. It coordinates national surveillance of more than 50 communicable diseases or disease groups. Under this scheme, notifications are made to the state or territory health authority under the provisions of the public health legislation in their jurisdiction. Computerised, de-identified unit records of notifications are supplied to the Australian Government Department of Health and Ageing on a daily basis, for collation, analysis and publication on the internet and in the quarterly journal *Communicable Diseases Intelligence*.[1]

TABLE 27.3 Application of standard and transmission-based precautions[1]

	TYPE OF PRECAUTION			
	STANDARD	CONTACT	DROPLET	AIRBORNE
EXAMPLES OF INFECTIOUS AGENTS	Standard practices for all patients	Scabies, MRSA, VRE	Influenza, norovirus, pertussis	Pulmonary TB, varicella, measles
HAND HYGIENE	✓	✓	✓	✓
SINGLE ROOM/ COHORT TRANSPORT	✗	✓	✓	✓ Negative pressure
GLOVES	⊙	✓	✓	✓
GOWN	⊙	✓	✓	✓
MASK	⊙	✓ Surgical mask if in sputum	✓ Surgical mask	✓ P2 (N95) respirator
EYE PROTECTION	⊙	⊙	⊙	✓
EQUIPMENT HANDLING	⊙	Single use or reprocess	Single use or reprocess	Single use or reprocess
VISITORS	✗	⊙	Restrict number, and precautions as for staff	Restrict number, and precautions as for staff

MRSA: methicillin-resistant Staphylococcus aureus; *TB: tuberculosis; VRE: vancomycin-resistant* Enterococcus

⊙ *As required—gloves to be worn whenever potential exposure to body fluids; gown if contamination with blood, body fluids, secretions or excretions likely; face and/or eye protection if splash likely (including during aerosol-generating procedures).*

Specific challenges for infection prevention in emergency care

There are a variety of other special challenges in infection prevention and communicable diseases for emergency nurses and paramedics.

Infections in older populations

Elderly individuals are at an increased risk of morbidity and mortality from infection due to normal physiological changes, such as decreased mobility, impaired sight and hearing and declining response to immunisations and medications. In addition, cognitive impairment and/or altered mental status changes put the elderly at risk from infection and make diagnosis more difficult. The frail elderly and those who live in institutionalised settings, such as long-term care or nursing homes and assisted living, tend to have limited mobility and co-morbidities that put them at increased risk for infection.[10]

Emergency department (ED) and emergency medical services personnel can expect to see infections frequently among older individuals and populations. Infection is the primary reason for hospital admissions among elderly individuals who reside in long-term care facilities such as nursing homes.[1] Infection may be difficult to diagnose in the elderly because most older individuals have a pulse/temperature dissociation that masks the signs of infection.[10] Diagnosis of infection may also be difficult because other normal signs of infection may be absent among the elderly. Often, a change in behaviour or cognitive functioning, loss of appetite or tachypnoea is the only symptom that indicates an infection is present in older individuals.[1]

Infections in children and young populations

Children are at increased risk from infection for a variety of reasons. First, very young children are dependent upon adult caregivers to ensure that proper hygiene needs are met. Secondly, children's immune systems are not as advanced as adults, putting them at risk from infections that are generally not an issue in adults. In addition, young children tend to put objects into their mouth, which increases the risk of faecal–oral and contact transmission of infectious agents. Children also have a higher respiratory rate than adults and a disproportionate ratio of body surface area to weight, which puts them at risk from inhaling aerosolised infectious agents. Lastly, children are more at risk from vaccine-preventable diseases because they often have not yet developed full immunity to these agents. Similar to adults, children are at risk from HAIs, multi-resistant organisms (MROs) and respiratory illnesses. Newborns and children with immunodeficiencies are at an increased risk from infection, especially during an infectious-disease outbreak.

EDs need to be prepared to address the risks to children and young people in relation to infection prevention, including the need for special medical equipment/supplies that are specific to children. Examples of such equipment include different doses of medications (based on the child's weight), smaller endotracheal tubes, needles, intravenous kits, linen and other equipment.[1]

Bioterrorism

Bioterrorism has emerged as a key public health issue in the 21st century that presents unique challenges for emergency nurses and paramedics. Surprisingly, such challenges are not new. For many years numerous published papers, protocols and guidelines have focused on the serious public health threat posed by the deliberate release of agents such as influenza, anthrax and smallpox.[25] As a phenomenon, bioterrorism comprises acts that are politically or religiously motivated and employ or threaten the use of biological agents/toxins to create deliberate harm or fear.[25] The threat of biological weapons and bioterrorism has been dramatically heightened since anthrax-tainted letters followed the terrorist attacks in the USA in September 2001.[26] In 2001 in the USA, two mailed letters containing anthrax spores resulted in 22 cases of anthrax and five deaths. These incidents led to considerable emergency anxiety, confusion and mistrust, and demand for chemoprophylaxis and increased overall demand on health service delivery. Similar events occurred in Australia in 2001, which received international attention, although no mortality or morbidity occurred.

Of all the infectious agents that pose challenges to humanity, few constitute significant threats in terms of their use in bioterrorism. Risk assessments are based on the severity and consequence of clinical disease, mode of transmission, potential for major public health impact and possible effects on public panic and social disruption. The most devastating potential bioterrorism threats are from smallpox, anthrax, botulism, plague and viral haemorrhagic fevers, such as Ebola, Marburg and Lassa fever.[27] Smallpox and anthrax are considered the greatest bioterrorism risk in Australia, although naturally-occurring smallpox was last seen globally in 1977.[25] Other important biological threats such as plague and viral haemorrhagic fevers are not endemic in Australia.[27]

Responding to bioterrorism, whether real or threatened, requires public-health preparedness at an individual, emergency and societal level. Healthcare workers, particularly emergency-based individuals, lack adequate training, resources and opportunities for clinical education in bioterrorism preparedness.[25,26] An outbreak of avian influenza or another infectious disease spread via bioterrorism would have widespread social and economic impact on communities. Infections of pandemic magnitude have the potential to be catastrophic. Even with close collaboration between healthcare providers and the public health system, difficulties in early detection and diagnosis would compound the problems of containing the spread of disease and dealing with mass care, mass prophylaxis and mass fatality management.[28] Achieving the best health outcome in outbreaks depends on having a plan that will facilitate the rapid identification and treatment of affected and potentially exposed people, appropriate containment and robust communication mechanisms between clinical services, public health services and emergency services.[25] Adequate training and preparedness of clinicians in recognition and management of infection is vital for those working in emergency contexts. Swift and decisive responses and effective communication and collaboration between law enforcement officials, clinicians and public health officials are essential to contain outbreaks.[28,29]

Emergency nurses and paramedics should, in all instances, seek specialist assistance from local and state public health officials such as Australian Emergency Management, the Department of Health and the Communicable Diseases Network Australia. National emergency response and disaster management is coordinated by the Office of the Minister for Justice. Emergency nurses and paramedics must understand the specific nature of the various commonwealth, state and local health threats and participate in preparing and testing comprehensive plans to manage the health threat within their facility.[25]

Wounds, sepsis, antibiotics and multi-drug resistance

Wounds, particularly chronic ones, present emergency nurses and paramedics with challenges. Wounds are often chronic and complex in nature, and emergency nurses and paramedics often manage them in resource-poor environments that may compound the complexity of wound care. Wound care is made more complex with multiple resistant organisms such as MRSA. The emergence and re-emergence of rapid-spread MROs is an ongoing international health priority.

When *Staphylococcus aureus* or another organism overcomes the body's defence mechanisms, as described earlier in the chapter, infection occurs. Local signs of infection include oedema, erythema and purulent exudate. If the infection becomes vascular, patients may deteriorate into septic shock, a form of distributive shock. In this event, fluid shift in the peripheral vasculature occurs, where extravascular spaces result in pooling of fluid, hypotension and poor tissue perfusion as described in Chapter 15. In septic shock, patients present with systemic vasodilation, bounding pulse, tachycardia, bradycardia, hypoxia, altered mental state, alterations in core temperature and, in the late stages, a fall in blood pressure and oliguria. At the cellular level, there are alterations in microvascularity, vasodilation, poor perfusion, capillary endothelial leak and anaerobic respiration within the cell leading to the production of lactic acid.[30] Septic shock ultimately results in a cellular hypoxia, anaerobic metabolism and respiration and irreversible cell injury. Treating the infection is critical for resuscitation to be successful.

Treating and preventing infection, or sepsis, is a major challenge in emergency trauma and care. In instances of septic shock, patients require aggressive resuscitation and rapid, broad-spectrum antibiotic therapy until such time as microbiological culture and sensitivities, and antibiograms, can be performed. Box 27.3 summarises important principles of treatment for septic shock.

Historically, *Staphylococcus aureus* has been a major cause of sepsis, septic shock and HIA. It is the leading cause of healthcare-associated pneumonia and surgical-site infections, and the second leading cause of healthcare-associated bloodstream infections. It is responsible for infections such as osteomyelitis, septic arthritis, skin infections, endocarditis and meningitis.[31] MRSA continues to challenge the safety and quality of modern healthcare, and in some settings MRSA can constitute as many as 20% of all hospital-acquired infections. Endemic in most hospitals and epidemic in others, approximately 30% of all *S. aureus* infections present with some form of drug resistance.[32] First reported in 1961, MRSA is internationally endemic and one of the most challenging bacterial pathogens affecting clients in hospitals, including the ED. More recently, community-acquired MRSA (CA-MRSA) presents particular challenges. It occurs in otherwise healthy individuals with no

---

BOX 27.3 Principles of treatment for septicaemia and septic shock

- Oxygen therapy (high-flow)
- Fluid resuscitation
- Urinalysis to ensure output of > 0.05 mL/kg/h
- Blood and wound cultures
- Broad-spectrum antibiotic therapy pending microbiological culture/sensitivity and antibiograms
- Blood gas and haemodynamic monitoring, especially for lactic acidosis (see Ch 17, pp. 332 and 345, for procedural techniques)
- Other interventions including glycaemic regulation, vasopressors (such as dopamine, adrenaline, noradrenaline and vasopressin), inotropic support (such as dobutamine), bicarbonate therapy (consideration for advanced acidosis), steroids[51,52]

---

risk factors for MRSA (such as recent hospitalisation, surgical procedure or antibiotic administration). The prevalence of CA-MRSA in EDs is increasing, especially in children and young people patient settings.

PRACTICE TIP

Patients are often confused about what 'colonisation' and 'infection' mean in terms of multidrug resistant organisms. Explain these clearly to patients within an appropriate risk framework.

The main route of MRSA transfer is from one client to another. Individuals transmit infection by failing to decontaminate their hands effectively before and after contact with individuals colonised or infected with MRSA. Attempts to eliminate endemic MRSA in hospitals have proven difficult, costly and largely unsuccessful. In some settings, identification of known carriers, prospective surveillance of clients and hospital workers and use of nasal mupirocin have helped control drug-resistant *S. aureus* infection rates.[32,33] Reported costs of a healthcare-acquired infection vary because of the wide range of study populations, sites of infection and methods used.[32]

Sometimes sepsis is due to MROs, making treatment even more challenging. Another MRO that is resulting in increased morbidity is *Clostridium difficile*. *C. difficile* infections are on the rise in hospitals around the world, including Australia. Emergency room staff are likely to encounter a patient with *C. difficile* infection; when this occurs, contact precautions should be utilised to prevent healthcare-associated spread.[7]

Fundamentally, good hand hygiene is central to controlling and preventing the spread of infection.[1] Frequent and thorough hand hygiene and decontamination practices must be employed by emergency nurses and paramedics. Australian research suggests that nurses rely on facilities provided by the client for hand hygiene, and in the main nurses 'make do' when facilities, tools, inclination or time are inadequate.[34] Alcohol hand gels and rubs for use at 'point of care' are particularly useful in emergency care settings. Emergency nurses and

paramedics require an understanding of microbiology, and how and why microorganisms develop resistance to antibiotics. This prepares them for preventing the spread of MROs, and equips them with the knowledge they need to teach clients and their families about infection control and antibiotic management.[7] Continued investment in comprehensive infection control programs that focus on sound hand hygiene practices, surveillance and rational and justified use of antibiotics are essential for emergency nursing and paramedic practice.

SARS, influenza and other respiratory infections

Respiratory viruses present considerable challenge when it comes to infection prevention and control. SARS (severe acute respiratory syndrome) emerged in the human population in 2002 in the Guangdong province of China, and avian influenza H5N1 re-emerged in Vietnam in 2003. SARS, caused by a coronavirus, is thought to have originated from contact with semi-domesticated animals, such as the palm civet or the dog raccoon. Avian influenza, caused by a subtype of influenza A strain virus, occurs in the wild bird population and has spread to domestic poultry and humans in Asia, the Middle East, Africa and Europe. The SARS virus was introduced to Hong Kong and then spread to 26 other countries around the world (including Australia), with an overall case-fatality rate of approximately 11%. Avian influenza H5N1 does not yet demonstrate the ability for direct, sustained human-to-human transmission. It is thought that the droplet and contact routes may predominantly transmit both viruses, although during the SARS outbreak the airborne and possibly the faecal–oral routes may also have transmitted outbreaks of coronavirus. Healthcare workers in contact with SARS or avian H5N1 influenza cases are advised to use standard precautions plus adhere to strict contact, droplet and airborne precautions.[35] Both diseases are notifiable by law, and must be notified in Australia to the medical officer of health and in New Zealand to the local health authority.

Influenza is a contagious and acute viral infection that attacks the respiratory system. Influenza has evolved over hundreds of years, surviving the passing of time and the rising and falling of populations, to remain a significant global challenge. Over many years, multiple strains of influenza have been encountered globally. The 'Spanish flu' of 1918–19 was estimated to have killed 40–50 million people worldwide, including 11,500 in Australia—in an age before mass commercial air travel.[16] Outbreaks of avian influenza in bird flocks have affected many countries in Asia, the Middle East, Europe and Africa;[36,37] there are as many as 15 different groups of avian influenza virus present in wild bird populations. The virus is largely asymptomatic in host populations. Humans appear to be accidental hosts of this infection, which is spread through bird faeces and contaminated water or dust. The pathogenicity of avian influenza changes as the virus mutates and spreads between host populations, and can result in severe disease. Those strains with the highest mortality rates are referred to as 'highly pathogenic avian influenza' (HPAI) and are thought to have evolved from the 2003 strain (H5N1) found in Asia that spread to most parts of the world through migratory birds and the poultry trade. Strict quarantine and infection-control measures successfully halted the spread of earlier infection; however, the current strain has moved across continents worldwide.[36]

Although H5N1 can cause severe and sometimes fatal infections in humans, the actual number of human cases around the world has been small relative to the levels of infection in host bird populations. Human cases have been in people who had close contact with infected poultry, usually from their own farms.[37] There is evidence that supports effective human-to-human spread of H5N1 infection.[37] An outbreak of H5N1, if significant, could have devastating economic and social impacts on Australia. Outbreaks of HPAI have occurred in Australia and around the world, and while outbreaks are quickly eradicated or are self-limiting there is evidence and growing concern of contact between farmed poultry and wild waterfowl.[16]

Infection prevention for influenza is best aimed at reducing emergency risk and household transmission.[38] Personal hygiene, such as hand hygiene and cough etiquette, is an important infection-control measure in deterring household infection transmission, particularly for respiratory infections such as influenza.

EDs and emergency medical services are at the forefront of Australia's health disaster response, providing immediate patient care and system-wide patient facilitation. The H1N1 influenza outbreak in 2009 demonstrated the diversity of roles of EDs in disease containment and management, but also provided an opportunity to describe the extended clinical impact of pandemic disease. Public awareness of H1N1 influenza 2009 led to a large number of patients presenting to both EDs and primary health services (including general practitioners) with flu-like illness. This impact occurred at a time when Australian and New Zealand emergency health services were confronting continual problems of overcrowding associated with access block and growing demand. EDs and ambulance services have responded to this demand, and have adopted standard and transmission-based precautions to manage these patients, protect staff members and protect non-affected patients and visitors from potential cross-contamination. The response by EDs to the recent H1N1 influenza outbreak occurred during a period of evolving knowledge about the disease. Initial reports from Mexico raised serious concerns regarding the severity and mortality rate. Although the severity was subsequently shown to be less serious, the response by EDs and ambulance services was, and always will be, based on the information available at the time. Such events highlight the importance of pandemic planning by emergency health services.[39]

Recent research indicates that Australian and New Zealand hospitals have experienced significant increases in demand for service during the peak period of seasonal respiratory infections, in some states as high as a 10-fold increase, resulting in increased access block, ED overcrowding and ambulance ramping, all known to be associated with increased morbidity and mortality.[11,39] Other research indicates that many hospitals in Australia and around the world were unable to order sufficient supplies to care for H1N1 patients, including transport media for laboratory testing, masks, N95 respirators, disinfectant wipes, oseltamivir (e.g. Tamiflu) and other products needed for infection prevention.[40] While research demonstrates that prophylactic administration reduces time to first alleviation of symptoms, there are side-effects associated with its use

and the evidence supporting clinically significant effects on complications from infection is limited. Moreover, the value and utility of stockpiling, particular in economic terms, relative to potential benefits, has been questioned.[41]

> **PRACTICE TIP**
>
> Teach patients to look for the signs and symptoms of infection.

Tuberculosis

Tuberculosis (TB) is one of the oldest diseases known to affect humans. Bacteria belonging to the *Mycobacterium tuberculosis* complex cause tuberculosis. The complex includes *M. tuberculosis*, *M. bovis*, *M. africanum*, *M. microti* and *M. canettii*.[42] In humans, the most frequent and important agent of disease is *M. tuberculosis*. The aetiological agent can be identified only by culture of the organisms. *M. tuberculosis* is a rod-shaped, non-spore-forming, aerobic bacterium which is often neutral on Gram staining. However, once stained, the colour is not removed by acid alcohol, and therefore has the classification of acid-fast bacilli (AFB). *M. tuberculosis* grows very slowly compared with other bacteria.[21] Australia has one of the lowest rates of TB in the world. However, specific populations within Australia, such as Indigenous peoples and people born overseas, have rates many times those of non-Indigenous Australian-born persons.[42]

The incubation period from infection to demonstrable primary lesion or significant tuberculin reaction is about 4–12 weeks.[20] The degree of communicability depends on the number of bacilli in the droplets, the virulence of the bacilli, adequacy of ventilation, exposure of bacilli to sun or ultraviolet light and opportunities for aerosolisation. Theoretically, as long as viable tubercle bacilli are discharged in the sputum, a person may be infectious.[20] Effective antimicrobial chemotherapy usually eliminates communicability within a few weeks.[43]

The disease usually affects the lungs, but it may affect any organ or tissue in the body. The sites of infection as a result of extrapulmonary TB include meninges, pleura, pericardium, kidneys, bones and joints, larynx, skin, intestines, peritoneum and eyes.[21] Extrapulmonary TB occurs more frequently among people infected with HIV. Pulmonary tuberculosis can be categorised as primary or secondary.

Primary pulmonary tuberculosis occurs when there is an initial infection with tubercle bacilli. The lesion formed in the lung at this time may not be detectable on chest X-ray, and in the majority of cases it will heal spontaneously.[42] In general, persons infected with tuberculosis have approximately a 10% risk for developing active TB during their lifetime. The risk is greatest during the first two years after infection.[20] In children and in immunocompromised people, primary tuberculosis may progress rapidly to clinical illness.

Secondary pulmonary tuberculosis results from endogenous reactivation of latent infection, and is usually localised to the apical and posterior segments of the upper lobes.[42]

Diagnosis of TB is usually made by clinical signs and symptoms, including chest X-ray findings and results of tuberculin skin testing (see below). Confirmation of infection is demonstrated by the presence of AFB in sputum or tissue.[21] Primary TB is usually asymptomatic in immunocompetent people, and lesions in the lungs may not be detectable on chest X-ray. In symptomatic cases and/or secondary pulmonary TB, the signs and symptoms of disease may be non-specific and often insidious. Commonly there is fever and night sweats, weight loss, anorexia, general malaise and weakness. As the disease progresses a cough develops, accompanied by the production of purulent sputum. The sputum often becomes blood-streaked because of erosion of a blood vessel. Chest X-ray may reveal infection, usually localised to the apical and posterior segments of the upper lobes. Eventually, because of extensive disease, there may be dyspnoea and adult respiratory distress syndrome (ARDS).[21]

Directly observed treatments are recommended for TB infection. Australia has implemented this strategy with some modifications because of the low incidence of TB in the country. The treatment of TB may be protracted, particularly in cases of multi-drug resistance, where treatment may continue for many months. Drugs used to treat TB are classified into first-line and second-line agents. First-line agents are the most effective and are a necessity for any short-course therapeutic regimen. Contact tracing is an essential component of TB control. The TB prevention and control services or health department must always carry out contact tracing. The estimated risk of transmission of TB should guide the priority and rapidity of the contact management. The case should be categorised according to the likely degree of infectiousness (sputum smear result, and presence of symptoms), and the contacts according to risk of disease acquisition (i.e. the amount of time and type of contact they have had with the index case).

PRACTICE TIP

Managing active TB requires specialist care and additional precautions.

Patients diagnosed with pulmonary TB, or those where there exists a high index of suspicion, require transmission-based precautions for airborne transmission. The patient should be placed in a single, negative-pressure room with the door closed. People (healthcare workers and visitors) should wear a particulate filter mask when in the room. The patient should wear a surgical mask during transport. Receiving departments must be notified of the additional precautions required for patient management.[1] Diagnosis of TB is notifiable by law, and must be notified to the TB prevention and control service and health department, for follow up contact tracing.[1]

The benefit of BCG (Bacille Calmette-Guérin) vaccine in adolescents and adults is not certain. BCG is recommended for the following: Aboriginal neonates living in regions of high incidence (Australia); neonates with one or both parents who identify as being Pacific people (New Zealand); neonates born to patients with leprosy or TB; children under the age of 5 years who will be travelling to live in countries of high TB prevalence for longer than 3 months; and children and adolescents aged less than 16 years (unable to be treated with antibiotics) who continue to be exposed to an individual with active pulmonary TB.[44]

Human immunodeficiency virus and acquired immune deficiency syndrome

Human immunodeficiency virus (HIV) is a retrovirus. Once inside the body, HIV replicates within white cells called CD4 cells. CD4 cells normally help coordinate the body's immune response; as the infection progresses, these cells are destroyed and the CD4 count gradually falls, reducing the ability of the immune system to ward off infections. As a result, HIV-infected people become susceptible to illnesses caused by the collapse of the body's immune system. Acquired immune deficiency syndrome (AIDS) is a severe, life-threatening consequence of HIV infection. This syndrome represents the late clinical stage of infection with HIV and is most often the result of progressive damage to the immune and other organ systems.

Within several weeks to months after infection with HIV, many individuals develop an acute, self-limited mononucleosis-like illness lasting for 1–2 weeks. Infected individuals may then be free of clinical signs or symptoms for months to years. Onset of clinical illness is usually insidious, with non-specific symptoms such as lymphadenopathy, anorexia, chronic diarrhoea, weight loss, fever and fatigue. Many opportunistic infections are considered AIDS-related illnesses, including several cancers, pulmonary and extrapulmonary tuberculosis, recurrent pneumonia, wasting syndrome, neurological disease (HIV dementia or sensory neuropathy) and invasive cervical cancer.[20]

HIV is transmitted by direct contact with blood or infected body fluids, through mucous membranes, non-intact skin or through percutaneous injury. The three significant routes of transmission for HIV are infected blood or blood products, infected sexual fluids and from infected mother to baby during pregnancy and delivery.[9] Antibodies to HIV usually develop within 2–8 weeks, typically within 12 weeks. However, most people do not feel unwell or develop symptoms of disease for years. All persons in the acute or chronic stage of infection who are HIV-antibody-positive are potentially infectious. The period of infectivity is believed to begin shortly after primary infection and to continue throughout life.[44] Epidemiological evidence suggests that infectivity increases with increasing immune deficiency, clinical symptoms and presence of other sexually transmitted infections.[20]

The most commonly used screening test for HIV, enzyme-linked immunoassay, is highly sensitive and specific. When this test is reactive, an additional test such as the Western blot or indirect immunofluorescence assay (IFA) should be obtained. Most individuals infected with HIV develop detectable antibodies within 1–3 months.

Susceptibility to HIV infection is universal. The risk of transmission of disease is dependent on the type of exposure and the concentration of HIV in the bloodstream of the source at the time of exposure. The risk of HIV transmission varies according to the type of exposure: 0.1% per act of unprotected sexual intercourse, 30% from mother to baby during pregnancy and delivery, and close to 100% if transfused with HIV-infected blood. The risk to healthcare workers of acquiring HIV from an occupational exposure is very small, with the average risk for HIV infection estimated to be 0.3% after percutaneous exposure (needlestick injury) and 0.09% following mucous membrane exposure.[44]

Patients with HIV are rarely treated in the ED, as it is a highly specialised field with the patient treated for the most part as an outpatient. However, the ED is often the first point of contact for these patients when they have an acute exacerbation of symptoms secondary to their disease, in the presence or absence of a diagnosis.

Hepatitis

Hepatitis is injury and inflammation of the liver. Viruses are a major cause of hepatitis, but other microorganisms or non-infectious causes may also be responsible.[45,46] The non-viral causes include drugs and chemicals such as carbon tetrachloride, ethylene glycol, rifampicin, methotrexate, monoamine oxide (MAO) inhibitors, chlorpromazine and paracetamol.[1,47] Inflammation of the liver caused by the hepatitis viruses may produce a variety of features. The common signs and symptoms of viral hepatitis include jaundice, fatigue, abdominal pain, arthralgia, anorexia, nausea and vomiting. During the acute phase, marked increases in the liver enzymes serum alanine aminotransferase (ALT) and serum aspartate aminotransferase (AST) can be detected. Liver failure or liver cancer may occur in more-severe manifestations of the disease.[46] Definitive diagnosis of the causative virus can only be made on laboratory testing. Table 27.4 outlines the characteristics of all viral hepatitis. Those most commonly encountered in Australia and New Zealand are hepatitis A, B and C.

Gastrointestinal diseases

Many microorganisms are capable of producing symptoms of diarrhoeal disease. Gastrointestinal disease causes fluid loss and dehydration in people, regardless of the cause. Outbreaks of infectious diseases can occur sporadically and there are organisms that cause infections seasonally. Infections in healthcare may arise from staff, clients, visitors, air, food, water, sterile products, the environment and vermin. Most pathogens will enter the gastrointestinal tract via the faecal–oral route, from contaminated hands, food or fluids.[46] Diarrhoea may be caused by many viral, bacterial and parasitic pathogens, including (but not limited to) adenovirus, rotavirus, norovirus, *Campylobacter* spp, *Clostridium difficile*, *Salmonella* spp, *Yersinia*, *Cryptosporidium* and *Giardia lamblia*.

Norovirus (formerly known as Norwalk-like viruses) is a common cause of non-bacterial gastroenteritis. Outbreaks have been reported in the ED, hospitals and aged-care facilities. Norovirus commonly occurs in winter months, and is a syndrome of acute nausea, vomiting and explosive diarrhoea. Symptoms usually last between 24 and 48 hours, with an incubation period of the same; viral shedding continues for approximately 24 hours after the symptoms cease. The Norwalk-like viruses are small, structured ribonucleic acid (RNA) viruses classified as caliciviruses. This virus is transmitted via the faecal–oral route. Vomiting causes widespread aerosol dissemination of viral particles, resulting in environmental contamination and subsequent spread.

TABLE 27.4 Characteristics of viral hepatitis[50]

	HEPATITIS				
	A	B	C	D	E
VIRUS	Picornavirus	Hepadnavirus	Flavivirus	RNA virus—classified with plant virus satellites	RNA virus
TRANSMISSION	Faecal–oral (person–person or epidemics)	Blood/body fluid. Perinatal vertical transmission	Parenteral. Possible other routes, e.g. sexual, perinatal	Parenteral (as for HBV) HDV requires HBV (enveloped with HBsAg)	Faecal–oral. Central and South America, Asia and Africa
INCUBATION PERIOD	15–45 days	40–180 days	20–120 days	30–180 days	40 days
HEPATITIS SEVERITY	Mild to moderate. Increases with age	Moderate to severe 1% fulminant hepatic failure	Mild	Severe	Mild to moderate
MORTALITY	Overall: < 0.2%. > 40 years: 1%	0.2–2%	< 1%	2–20%	0.2–1%; up to 20% in pregnancy
CHRONICITY	No	Yes; 2–7% in adults, > 90% in newborns	Yes; up to 80%	Yes; 1–3% of co-infections; 70–80% of superinfection (with HBV)	No
VACCINATION	Yes	Yes	No	Indirectly via HBV immunisation	No

HBsAg: hepatitis B surface antigen; HBV: hepatitis B virus; HDV: hepatitis D virus; RNA: ribonucleic acid

Other vaccine-preventable communicable diseases, such as respiratory infections, measles, pertussis and varicella, require particular management practices and precautions, including contract tracing given their high communicability and the risk they present to particular populations that are immuno-compromised, such as the neutropenic patients.[1,47] The general principles of infection prevention and control apply when providing care for clients in the emergency setting. Standard precautions expect strict hand hygiene after contact with clients who have signs and symptoms of gastrointestinal disease. Healthcare providers should encourage clients to practise good hand hygiene and toilet hygiene. Healthcare providers themselves should not attend work when symptomatic of gastrointestinal disease of unknown or infectious origin.

SUMMARY

In this chapter we have explored some contemporary challenges of healthcare-associated infection and communicable diseases and their control and prevention in emergency nursing and paramedic practice in the Australasian emergency care context. Recognition of the potential for disease transmission in emergency care is essential. Contacts between staff and patients are frequent and varied, allowing many opportunities for the transmission of infectious agents. All patients should be deemed a potential source of infection and standard precautions adopted to minimise the risk for disease transmission. The emergency nurse or paramedic should be aware of the modes of disease transmission and adopt the appropriate additional precautions when the airborne, droplet or contact routes transmit the infectious agent responsible for causing disease. Infection prevention and control is critical to providing high-quality, safe and timely emergency care. The practice environment of the emergency nurse and paramedic presents unique challenges requiring specialist knowledge and evidence.

CASE STUDY 1

You and your road partner are ambulance paramedics. You have been dispatched to a road traffic crash on a major highway 20 minutes from the station. It is reported to be a head on-collision between a passenger car and motorcyclist, with five patients, two of whom died instantly at the scene. On arrival, the mangled wreckage is off the side of the road in a shallow, muddy creek bed. There is mud and water everywhere. Of the three surviving patients, one patient (A) is trapped and unconscious, and the other two patients (B) and (C) self-extricated. Patient A has open head, chest and lower limb trauma. Patient B has a closed head injury and superficial grazes, and Patient C has an open fracture of the femur that has been contaminated by the mud from the creek. Both patients B and C are reported as consuming beer at the local hotel prior to the accident. The three surviving patients are transported to hospital, and all are admitted to the intensive care unit. Patient A develops a consolidated pneumonia two days post admission.

Questions

1. What are the particular infection risks for each of the patients in this situation?

2. What prophylactic measures would be considered appropriate for each patient with respect to particular infectious diseases?

3. Would the pneumonia infection be classified as healthcare-associated? What factors would need to be considered for this assessment to be made?

 Answers to Case Study Questions can be found on evolve
http://evolve.emergencytrauma.curtis

CASE STUDY 2

You are the triage nurse when Mrs V is brought in by ambulance to the emergency department (ED). She is hypoxic, cyanotic and has a productive, purulent and unrelenting cough. She returned from an overseas holiday to Africa where she spent 3 months on a safari tour. She is stabilised in the ED and an urgent microscopy of her sputum reveals acid-fast bacillus and active pulmonary tuberculosis.

Questions

1. What are the implications of this scenario with respect to infection prevention and control?

2. What are the risks of the spread of infection to the paramedics and hospital staff, and what follow-up is required?

3. How should this incident be managed?

 Answers to Case Study Questions can be found on evolve
http://evolve.emergencytrauma.curtis

REFERENCES

1. National Health and Medical Research Council. Australian guidelines for the prevention and control of infection in healthcare. In: Australian Commission on Safety and Quality in Healthcare. Canberra: Australian Government; 2010.

2. Australian Commission on Safety and Quality in Health Care. Standard 3—Preventing and controlling healthcare associated infections—safety and quality improvement guide. Sydney: Australian Commission on Safety and Quality in Health Care; 2012.

3. Cardoso T, Almeida M, Friedman ND et al. Classification of healthcare-associated infection: a systematic review 10 years after the first proposal. BMC Medicine 2014;12:40.

4. Pop-Vicas AE, D'Agata EM. The rising influx of multidrug-resistant Gram negative bacilli into a tertiary care hospital. Clinical Infectious Disease 2005;40:1792–8.

5. Australian Commission on Safety and Quality in Healthcare. Preventing and controlling healthcare associated infections—Standard 3 Factsheet. 2012. www.safetyandquality.gov.au/wp-content/uploads/2012/01/NSQHS-Standards-Fact-Sheet-Standard-3.pdf; accessed 19 December 2013.

6. Graves N, Halton K, Robertus L. Costs of healthcare associated infection. In: Cruickshank M, Ferguson J, eds. Reducing harm to patients from healthcare associated Infection: the role of surveillance. Sydney: Australian Commission on Safety and Quality in Health; 2008:307–55.

7. Shaban RZ, Cruickshank M, Christiansen K, Antimicrobial Resistance Standing Committee. National surveillance and report of antimicrobial resistance and antibiotic usage for human health in Australia. Sydney: Antimicrobial Resistance Standing Committee; 2013: www.safetyandquality.gov.au/publications/national-surveillance-and-reporting-of-antimicrobial-resistance-and-antibiotic-usage-for-human-health-in-australia/.

8. Australian Commission on Safety and Quality in Health Care. Windows into safety and quality in health care 2009. Sydney: Australian Commission on Safety and Quality in Health Care; 2009.

9. Australian Commission on Safety and Quality in Health Care. Reducing harm to patients from healthcare associated infections: an Australian infection prevention and control model for acute hospitals. Canberra: Commonwealth of Australia; 2009.

10. Johnson A, Roush RE, Howe JL et al. Bioterrorism and Emergency Preparedness in Aging (BTEPA). Gerontology and Geriatrics Education. 2008;26(4):23.

11. Lowthian JA, Curtis AJ, Jolley DJ et al. Demand at the emergency department front door: 10-year trends in presentations. Medical Journal of Australia 2012;196(2):128–32.

12. Patocka C, Turner J, Xue X, Segal E. Evaluation of an emergency department triage screening tool for suspected severe sepsis and septic shock. Journal for Healthcare Quality 2014;36(1):52.

13. Clinical Excellence Commission. Sepsis Kills. www.cec.health.nsw.gov.au/programs/sepsis; accessed 20 March 2014.

14. Shaban RZ. Paramedic knowledge of infection control principles and standards in an Australian emergency medical system (EMS). Australian Infection Control 2006;11(1):7.

15. World Health Organization. Primary health care: now more than ever. Geneva, Switzerland: WHO; 2008.

16. Parliament of Australia. Australia's capacity to respond to an infectious disease outbreak. In: Services DoP, ed. Canberra: Australian Government; 2004.

17. Hess I, Curson P, Plant A. Bug breakfast in the bulletin: Outbreaks: The past, present and future. New South Wales Public Health Bulletin. 2005;16(6):2.

18. Lee G. The body's defence systems. In: Lee G, Bishop P, eds. Microbiology and infection control for health professionals. 5th edn. Sydney: Pearson Education Australia; 2012.

19. Bishop P. Epidemiology: how diseases are spread. In: Lee G, Bishop P, eds. Microbiology and infection control for health professionals. 4th ed. Sydney: Pearson Education Australia; 2010:152–75.

20. Newberry L. Sheehy's emergency nursing: principles and practice. 5th edn. St Louis: Mosby; 2003.

21. Lee G. Respiratory tract infections. In: Lee G, Bishop P, eds. Microbiology and infection control for health professionals. 5th edn. Sydney: Pearson Education Australia; 2012:397–423.

22. Doolan K. Infectious and communicable diseases. In: Curtis K, Ramsden C, Friendship J, eds. Emergency nursing and care. Sydney: Elsevier; 2008:420–34.

23. Borysiewicz LK. The host's response to infection. In: Warrell DA, Cox TM, Firth JD, eds. Oxford textbook of medicine. 4th edn. Oxford: Oxford University Press; 2003.

24. Australian Commission on Safety and Quality in Healthcare. Healthcare Associated Infection Program. 2014; www.safetyandquality.gov.au/our-work/healthcare-associated-infection/; accessed 2 January 2014.

25. McCall BJ, Looke D. The infection control practitioner and bioterrorism: threats, planning, preparedness. Australian Infection Control 2003;8(2):5.

26. Shadel BN, Rebmann T, Clements B et al. Infection control practitioners' perceptions and educational needs regarding bioterrorism: Results from a national needs assessment survey. American Journal of Infection Control 2003;31(3):129–34.

27. Department of Health and Ageing. Overview of biological agents that could be used in a terrorist act. Canberra: Australian Government; 2006.

28. Flowers LK, Mothershead JL, Blackwell TH. Bioterrorism preparedness II: the community and emergency medical services systems. Emergency Medicine Clinics of North America 2002;20(2):19.

29. Bratberg J, Deady K. Development and application of a bioterrorism emergency management plan. Prehospital and Disaster Medicine 2012;20(S3):158–9.

30. Banasik JL. Shock. In: Copstead LC, Banasik JL, eds. Pathophysiology. St Louis, Missouri: WB Saunders; 2014.

31. Lee G. Cardiovascular and multisystem infections. In: Lee G, Bishop P, eds. Microbiology and infection control for health professionals. 5th ed. Sydney: Pearson Education Australia; 2012.

32. Rubin RJ, Harrington CA, Poon A et al. The economic impact of *Staphylococcus aureus* infection in New York City hospitals. Emerging Infectious Diseases 1999;5(1):18.

33. Casewell MW. New threats to the control of methicillin-resistant *Staphylococcus aureus*. Journal of Hospital Infection 1995;30, Supplement(0):465–71.

34. Praxis KB. Research and issues in community nursing: hand washing in the community setting. ACCNS Journal of Community Nurses 2002;7(2):3.

35. Fauci AS. Emerging and re-emerging infectious diseases: the perpetual challenge. In: Robert H, ed. New York: Milbank Memorial Fund; 2005.

36. World Health Organization. Epidemic and pandemic alert and response: avian influenza. Geneva: WHO; 2006.

37. Department of Health and Ageing. Avian influenza. In: Department of Health and Ageing, ed. Canberra: Australian Government; 2008.

38. Weber JT, Hughes JM. Beyond Semmelweis: Moving Infection Control into the Community. Annals of Internal Medicine 2004; 140(5):397–8.

39. Fitzgerald GJ, Shaban RZ, Arbon P et al. Emergency department impact and patient profile of H1N1 influenza 09 outbreak in Australia: a national study. Paper presented at: H1N1 Influenza 09. Canberra: Urgent Research Forum 2009; Canberra.

40. Rebmann T, Wagner W. Infection preventionists' experience during the first months of the 2009 novel H1N1 influenza A pandemic. American Journal of Infection Control 2009;37(10):e5–16.

41. Jefferson T, Jones M, Doshi P et al. Oseltamivir for influenza in adults and children: systematic review of clinical study reports and summary of regulatory comments. British Medical Journal 2014;348.

42. Communicable Diseases Network Australia. National strategic plan for TB control in Australia beyond 2000. Canberra: Commonwealth Department of Health and Ageing; 2002.

43. Tally N, Martin C. Clinical gastroenterology: a practical problem based approach. Sydney: MacLennan & Petty; 1996.

44. Department of Health and Ageing. Infection control guidelines for the prevention of transmission of infectious diseases in the health care setting. Canberra: Biotext; 2004.

45. Wasley A, Miller JT, Finelli L, (CDC) CfDCaP. Surveillance for acute viral hepatitis—United States 2005. MMWR Surveillance Summary. 2007;56(3):24.

46. Lee G, Bishop P. Gastrointestinal tract infections. In: Lee G, ed. Microbiology and infection control for health professionals. 5th edn. Sydney: Pearson Education Australia; 2012.

47. Lee G, Bishop P. Microbiology and Infection Control for Heath Professionals. Sydney: Pearson; 2012.

48. World Health Organization. WHO guidelines on hand hygiene in health care. Geneva, Switzerland: WHO; 2009.

49. Curson P. Epidemics and pandemics in Australia. Sydney: University of Sydney; 2010.

50. The Merck manual of diagnosis and therapy. 18th edn. Whitehouse Station NJ: Merck, Sharp and Dohme; 2006.

51. Dellinger RP, Levy MM, Carlet J et al. Surviving Sepsis Campaign: International guidelines for management of severe sepsis and septic shock: 2008. Critical Care Medicine 2008;36(1):31.

52. Hicks P, Cooper DJ, Australian and New Zealand Intensive Care Society (ANZICS). The surviving sepsis campaign: international guidelines for management of severe sepsis and septic shock: 2009. Critical Care and Resuscitation 2009;10(1):1.

53. Australian Commission on Safety and Quality in Health Care. www.safetyandquality.gov.au/our-work/healthcare-associated-infection/national-infection-control-guidelines/; accessed 1 April 2015.

CHAPTER 28
ENVIRONMENTAL EMERGENCIES AND PANDEMICS

JANE MATEER, LYNETTE CUSACK AND JAMIE RANSE

Essentials

- The severity of heat stress depends on the degree of heat, amount of humidity and length of exposure.
- Heat rash and heat oedema are compensated forms of heat stress that do not involve a rise in optimal core temperature.
- The lack of neurological sequelae is a significant difference between heat exhaustion and heat stroke.
- The focus of treatment in heat stroke is two-fold: rapid cooling of core temperature and life support.
- Supplemental oxygen is essential for altitude sickness, although peripheral shutdown may confound the use of oximetry as an indicator for oxygen administration.
- As gas exchange between the air and the human body is dependent upon a pressure gradient involving atmospheric pressure at sea level, a reduced partial pressure at altitude will inhibit oxygen transfer, thus making hypoxia at altitude a significant problem.
- Hypoxaemia is at the maximum point during sleep, thus the sleeping altitude is the critical point to consider.
- Pandemics—good hygiene, use of personal protective equipment, avoiding practices that generate aerosol droplets and separating those individuals who are infected from those who are not are essential infection control practices.

INTRODUCTION

Interaction with the natural environment through a range of human activities is historically responsible for exposing people to the potential for injury or illness and unpredictable emergency situations. Now climate change is expected to influence an increase in the frequency and intensity of environmental (natural) disasters, including cyclones, heatwaves, droughts, storms, bushfires and floods.[1] In addition to the challenge of widespread disaster events, those working in primary healthcare, pre-hospital emergency medical services and emergency departments (EDs) should be aware of, and able to respond to, environmental emergencies. The focus of this chapter is on environmental emergencies resulting from a range of human-induced and natural events, including exposure to extreme weather conditions, changes in atmospheric pressure, drowning, pandemics and mass gatherings.

Temperature-related emergencies

Anatomy and physiology

The temperature around us is the ambient temperature, which is a product of environmental temperature and humidity (the amount of moisture dissolved in the air). Increases in humidity will increase the ambient temperature, even when the environmental temperature remains constant. Optimal functioning of the human body and normal cellular function occur within a carefully regulated temperature window between 36°C and 37.3°C, which is maintained by autonomic and endocrine feedback loops (Ch 20). Metabolism of fuel supplies a range of biochemical functions, with endogenous heat being one by-product. The sum of all biochemical reactions is the basal metabolic rate (BMR), which, if unchecked by cooling processes, would increase body temperature by 1.1°C per hour.[2] Hyperthermia is less well tolerated than hypothermia.[4]

Factors influencing temperature gain and loss include the heat transfer properties of water and air (convection, evaporation, conduction, radiation). Water is able to conduct heat at a rate greater than air, so is an ideal medium for both cooling and heating.[5] However, as indicated in Table 28.1, the higher the wind speed the greater the heat loss, though this effect is reduced in humid environments above 32°C.[6] Conversely, no wind will inhibit the body's ability to reduce heat, especially in humid conditions. Wet clothing can have a significant influence on the development of cold injury. The severity of heat or cold injury is related to the degree of temperature and length of exposure.

The significant effect of body temperature on metabolism and, thus, oxygenation is outlined in Table 28.2. For example, for every 1°C rise in temperature, there is a correlating rise in oxygen consumption; and with each drop of 1°C in temperature below 36°C, there is a corresponding drop in both BMR and oxygen demand. Hyperthermia will produce a right shift on the oxygen–haemoglobin (O_2–Hb) dissociation curve, while hypothermia will produce a left shift (see Ch 20). These responses are increased in non-acclimatised individuals. Acclimatisation is a process by which physiological adaptations occur in response to repeated exposures to heat or cold stress. Children and the elderly are at most risk of developing heat-related illness. Children have a greater body surface area by ratio to body mass and lose heat more easily (Ch 36). Further, very young children have a reduced ability to shiver

TABLE 28.1 Body temperature and metabolism

IF BODY TEMPERATURE RISES TO _°C	METABOLISM INCREASES BY _%
38	13
39	26
40	39
41	52
42	Insufficient oxygen to meet cellular needs

TABLE 28.2 Wind chill effect

WIND (km/h)	TEMPERATURE (°C)					
Calm	15	10	5	0	−5	−10
8	14	8	2	−4	−10	−17
16	11	6	1	−6	−12	−20
24	9	3	0	−7	−14	−22
32	6	0	−1	−8	−15	−23
40	2	−2	−4	−9	−16	−24

in response to cold and therefore to increase body temperature in the presence of cold environmental temperature. Children are more reliant on others to ensure an adequate fluid intake to prevent dehydration and associated heat stress. Those over the age of 50 may have impaired thermoregulation, a reduced sweating response and comorbidities associated with usage of medications which inhibit thermoregulatory control, which increases the risk of developing hyperthermia. For example, beta blockers inhibit the body's ability to shunt hypothermic blood away from the core.[7]

Heat-related emergencies

By definition, hyperthermia is a core temperature above 38°C[2,4,9] and the term 'thermal maximum' measures the magnitude and duration of heat that cells can encounter before damage occurs.[7] In humans, this point is 42°C, beyond which the greater the increase in temperature the more rapidly damage occurs, including progressive denaturing of a number of vital cellular proteins, failure of energy-producing functions and loss of cell membrane function. Hyperthermia produces a shift to the right in the curve representing affinity of Hb for O_2, which essentially means Hb is less inclined to bind to O_2, leading to more O_2 offloaded to hot tissue, increasing cellular level oxygenation and meeting increased metabolic demand. However, while more oxygen is delivered to tissues, it takes a higher partial pressure in the lungs to bind O_2 to Hb and therefore ongoing supply is ultimately dependent on good respiratory function. At an organ system level, heat-influenced changes may manifest as rhabdomyolysis (Ch 50), acute pulmonary oedema (APO) (Ch 21), disseminated intravascular coagulopathy (DIC) (Ch 29), acute respiratory distress syndrome (ARDS), cardiovascular dysfunction, electrolyte disturbance, acute kidney injury, liver failure and permanent neurological damage.

Heat illness will affect anyone whose body is pushed past its ability to maintain thermal control and compensate for excessive heat production, either internally or externally. There is a risk of heat illness while exercising in ambient temperatures above 23°C. Because of our ability to lose heat we can develop our capacity to maintain high levels of exercise without overheating, although good physical condition does not preclude heat illness. Dehydration and intravascular volume depletion aggravate the risk in all age groups and fitness levels. Box 28.1 outlines the risk factors for heat-related illness. With heat waves historically attributed to significant morbidity and mortality, rising baseline temperatures, especially at night, and longer periods of high daytime heat due to climate change are likely to worsen the incidence of heat-related emergencies. Where heat oedema and heat cramps are mild heat-related conditions, heat emergencies include heat exhaustion and heat stroke. Differential diagnoses are listed in Box 28.2.

Prevention of heat-related illness is essential, particularly as it exacerbates the risk of cardiac arrest in individuals with preexisting comorbidities. Education to the community, both pre hospital and prior to ED discharge, should stress the critical importance of adaptive behaviour to reduce ambient heat by choosing a cool environment, reduce activity to keep BMR low and maintain hydration. Reliance on air conditioning has reduced effective behaviours for staying cool on hot days, leaving many without options during power failures. Websites such as Environmental Health (see Useful websites, p. 705) provide useful community tools, such as the 'staying healthy in the heat' brochure. Problems occur when people

exercise (relative to age and condition) during periods of high heat, the elderly or ill go outside when temperatures are over 40°C, when they do not need to, houses are not closed up to reduce radiant heat and hydration and electrolyte balance are not maintained (using appropriate fluids). Importantly, many people do not understand that heat illness occurs more rapidly after the first instance during any period of heat stress, and rest for at least 12 hours afterwards is essential. For those who are required to work during periods of high heat, heat–work–rest and water consumption tables, which incorporate thermal heat indexes, should be used. Included in OH&S regulations, examples include the tables used by the Australian military and Workplace Health and Safety in each state.

Heat illness is generally associated with thermal regulation and therefore sunburn is not a heat-related illness. More information can be found in Chapter 52 (Burns).

Heat rash and oedema
Heat rash is a fine, red, papular rash occurring on the torso, neck and in skin folds. The rash occurs when sweat ducts are obstructed and become inflamed, inhibiting sweat excretion. The rash usually occurs in warm weather, but has also been reported in cold weather as a result of excess clothing.[10]

Heat oedema is characterised by swelling of feet, ankles and fingers and usually occurs in non-acclimatised individuals who exercise after prolonged periods of standing or sitting. The cause is believed to be cutaneous vasodilation and orthostatic pooling of interstitial fluid in gravity-dependent extremities following exposure to a hot environment.[6] It is self-limiting and resolves in hours to days. Treatment includes rest and elevation. While it is important to rule out other causes of peripheral oedema, especially in the elderly, overly vigorous diagnostic evaluation is unnecessary.[6,11]

Heat cramps
Anatomy and physiology
Heat cramps are painful, involuntary muscle cramps (brief and intermittent), usually in the lower extremities, that develop suddenly after periods of exercise in a hot or humid environment in individuals who have sweated profusely. Heat cramps are presumed to be a result of hyponatraemia caused by replacing lost fluid with hypotonic solutions.[4,6,11] The greater the

intake of water without added electrolytes, the greater the risk of hyponatraemia. In muscles relying on calcium for relaxation, the reduction in sodium is believed to produce cramps. In this manner they differ from the cramps experienced by athletes during exercise, which can be relieved with rest and massage.[4,11]

Patient assessment and clinical interventions

Signs and symptoms may include weakness, nausea and tachycardia. As a form of compensated heat stress, the core temperature remains in the normal range as thermoregulation is not affected. Treatment includes removal from heat, rest and electrolyte replacement with oral or parenteral fluids.

PRACTICE TIP

Discharge instructions are essential and should *stress* the importance of rest and hydration as discussed earlier, including no further activity for at least 12 hours.

Heat exhaustion

Anatomy and physiology

Heat exhaustion occurs during periods of constant exercise in relatively high environmental heat, when there is a failure to maintain fluid intake equal to losses through perspiration and respiration. It is not uncommon to lose a litre or more of fluid per hour during periods of extreme heat stress.[7] Cardiac output declines in response to a reduction in circulating fluid volume and poor venous return induced by vasodilation secondary to thermoregulatory demands. The subsequent response of the body to reduced cardiac output is peripheral vasoconstriction, thus preventing the usual mechanisms of heat loss through transfer to occur. Unable to cool itself, the body may heat up to a core temperature of 40°C.[4,7] In essence, heat exhaustion primarily involves significant volume depletion in the presence of an elevated temperature, following exposure to heat stress. The dehydration associated with heat exhaustion occurs in one of two forms. The first is *water depletion*, where the primary problem is a loss of water with subsequent reduced circulating volume. The second is *salt depletion*, with subsequent hyponatraemia and a milder degree of water depletion and associated hypovolaemia.

Patient assessment

Signs and symptoms include diaphoresis, pallor, hypotension, tachycardia, reduced urine output, nausea and vomiting, frontal headache, thirst, myalgia and syncope. Heat cramps may exist in the patient with salt depletion. The patient with heat exhaustion may be mildly confused, but does not demonstrate other mental-state changes or neurological sequelae. Because of the relatively ill-defined range of signs and symptoms, heat exhaustion is a diagnosis of exclusion.[6]

Clinical interventions

Treatment is primarily focused on active cooling and fluid and electrolyte replacement. Cooling involves removing the patient from the source of heat, rest and removal of clothing. The application of moist cloths will improve heat lost by evaporation. Where the core temperature is around 40°C, ice packs may be used in the armpit, groin and behind the neck to enable rapid cooling. Fluid therapy is titrated to haemodynamic

response and electrolyte replacement is based on serum electrolyte levels. Fluid and electrolyte replacement may be done orally if tolerated by the patient. All oral replacement is by commercially prepared oral rehydration solution (ORS). Where oral rehydration is not possible, intravenous therapy is used. If the patient is haemodynamically compromised and requires bolus fluid administration, the primary choice is 0.9% saline solution (Normal saline). It is not uncommon for a fit young adult who has been exercising in the heat to receive up to 5 or 6 L of fluid replacement.

Core temperature should be monitored hourly (preferably continuously by central thermometer) to ensure it is decreasing. Active cooling should be ceased once core temperature reaches 38°C,[12] as shivering may occur and core temperature rise again. Admission should be considered for any patient who does not improve significantly within 3–4 hours of emergency treatment. Heat exhaustion is believed by some to be on the continuum to heat stroke, and therefore should be identified and treated early.[11]

Heat stroke

Anatomy and physiology

Heat stroke is an uncommon but life-threatening form of heat-related illness. While difficult to define, heat stroke is always associated with altered mental status due to heat-induced encephalopathy in combination with a core temperature greater than 40.5°C.[4,6,13] As heat stroke is an interplay between the effects of heat and a range of inflammatory and coagulopathic responses, it has been argued that it should also be classified as a systemic inflammatory response syndrome (SIRS).[13] However, unlike sepsis, the most familiar SIRS, heat stroke is commonly associated with rhabdomyolysis and guidelines for initial fluid resuscitation are less defined.[2,7,12,13]

Thermoregulatory failure will occur universally at ambient temperatures above 42°C, and has a variable presentation at temperatures between 40°C and 42°C.[4,7,11,13] While a lack of sweating is classically considered a key sign, sweating may initially persist despite the presence of thermoregulatory failure, so dry skin and no sweating are not sensitive indicators. Mortality in heat stroke is dependent on the duration and intensity of hyperthermia. The more rapidly the condition is treated, the lower the incidence of both mortality and morbidity.

Heat stroke may be classified in two ways: *non-exertional* and *exertional*. Non-exertional heat stroke—also known as classic heat stroke—occurs as a result of prolonged exposure to sustained, high ambient temperatures and humidity. While anyone can be affected, the most susceptible are the elderly, children, the incapacitated, the chronically ill and those with mental health or substance-use disorders or suffering disordered perception. This is in part due to the inability of these populations to initiate behavioural changes which will improve heat transfer, as well as the side effects of some medications. They have a diminished capacity to thermoregulate, adapt to hot climates and increase cardiac output. Paralysed and intoxicated patients are often unable to initiate autonomic responses to improve heat transfer. The elderly are more likely to suffer cardiac disease, which may limit their ability to increase cardiac output in response to heat stress, particularly in the presence of rate-controlling medication. In children, the younger the child, the greater their inability to thermoregulate and the more responsive they are to ambient temperature. Non-exertional heat stroke has been the cause of death in children locked in cars on warm to hot days. A car acts like an oven, with the temperature inside rising rapidly in the first 10–20 minutes.

Exertional heat stroke is, by definition, the consequence of exercise or work. This type of heat stroke usually occurs in the presence of high surrounding ambient temperatures, where heat production exceeds the internal heat elimination mechanisms. It is most commonly seen in athletes and soldiers. Individuals with one or more risk factors (Box 28.1) are at much greater risk for hyperthermia when exacerbating environmental conditions are present.[14] Heatwaves are environmental events, with significant potential to contribute to both non-exertional and exertional heat stroke and to exacerbate the risk of other adverse health events

Patient assessment

Signs and symptoms of heat stroke are varied and the final outcome is multiple organ failure. In 80% of cases, the onset of heat stroke is usually sudden.[11] However, heat stroke may be preceded by a period of several hours, during which heat illness progresses from an initial appearance of heat exhaustion. In the initial stages of heat stroke, central nervous system (CNS) dysfunction is observed. These are the first signs of thermoregulatory failure. Changes in mental state include anxiety, confusion, hallucinations, ataxia (cerebellar dysfunction), combativeness and unconsciousness. Seizures occur most commonly during cooling. Direct thermal damage to cerebral tissue combined with decreased cerebral blood flow often produces cerebral oedema, further exacerbating CNS dysfunction. The cerebellum is particularly sensitive to thermal injury and thus the range of neurological sequelae is broad.

> **PRACTICE TIP**
>
> The degree of neurological injury is directly related to the duration and height of maximum body temperature.[4]

Initially, peripheral vascular beds dilate in an attempt to improve heat transfer, in turn producing a functional hypovolaemia, hypotension and tachycardia. Eventually excessive sweating and inability to maintain adequate fluid intake in correlation with losses produces significant volume depletion.[9,11,14] Sympathetic compensation reduces renal blood flow and subsequently urine output. Hepatic damage is indicated by an elevated serum aspartate aminotransferase (AST) and alanine aminotransferase (ALT) and is so common that its absence should raise doubts as to the diagnosis of heat stroke.[4,11] Coagulopathies are common. While platelets may suffer heat damage, DIC is believed to occur secondary to a SIRS response.[4,13] Additional complications include rhabdomyolysis, multiple organ failure, hypoglycaemia, acid–base imbalance and ARDS. It is important to take into account pre-hospital care, as a patient may present with a normal temperature and ALT and still have demonstrated all the characteristics of heat stroke during initial care.[11]

Clinical interventions

Early definitive airway intervention is important, as aspiration and seizures are common. Administer supplemental oxygen by the method most appropriate for the patient's level of consciousness and available resources. The use of non-depolarising agents to facilitate intubation and ventilation offers the advantage of improving heat loss through muscle paralysis.

Fluid replacement is essential and correction of hypovolaemia with cool, crystalloid isotonic fluids will reduce temperature and support cardiac output. The volume delivered is titrated to response. As the body cools and thermoregulatory control is regained, the true extent of fluid deficit will be easier to assess and treat. The use of isotonic fluid is important to avoid cerebral and pulmonary oedema. This most commonly involves Normal saline or Hartmann's solution. However, if hepatic damage is suspected, lactated products should be avoided because of problems with metabolism. In this situation, Normal saline use in the pre-hospital setting is warranted.

Continuous monitoring should include haemodynamics, urine output, core body temperature, blood glucose level and oxygenation. (Refer to Ch 17 for techniques relating to the different types of monitoring.) It is important to observe for myoglobin in the urine, as rhabdomyolysis may occur secondary to heat damage of peripheral tissues. Regular assessment of serum liver enzymes and coagulation studies are useful in identifying complications. Corticosteroid therapy may be used to treat cerebral oedema.

Active cooling

Every minute the patient remains overheated, they are at increased risk of potential sequelae and mortality. Rapid cooling without producing over-cooling has demonstrated the best longterm outcomes.[12] Cooling should occur simultaneously with primary survey intervention and may include removing the source of heat, undressing the patient, immersion in cold water or ice pack application. Whilst the practice may complicate the provision of other life-supporting measures, cold water immersion is recognised as the most effective strategy for rapid cooling.[5,12] Nine minutes in a cool bath to a rectal temperature of 38.6°C is recommended.[5] However, where it is not achievable, ice packs should be applied over and under the patient. Use of a fan is also effective, preferably in conjunction with ice, as water conducts heat at a far greater rate than air and the application of moving air over moisture further increases heat transfer. If necessary, ice-water peritoneal lavage may be used to initiate rapid cooling. Cooling should never produce shivering in the patient, as this will increase core temperature and oxygen consumption. Pharmacological agents such as chlorpromazine, benzodiazepine and paralysing agents may be considered to prevent shivering during the cooling process.[6,9,11]

> **PRACTICE TIP**
>
> Aspirin and paracetamol have not proved effective in reducing hyperthermia secondary to heat stroke.[6]

Cold-related emergencies

In general, cold-related emergencies occur with prolonged exposure to cold ambient temperatures or immersion in cold water, and severity depends on the extent and speed of the cold encountered. Compared to heat injuries, the body is better able to cope with cold exposure,[4] which is aggravated by the use of alcohol or pre-existing conditions, such as diabetes, renal and cardiac disease. Cold injuries are classified as *localised* or *systemic*. Although uncommon, it is possible for localised and systemic cold injuries to occur concurrently. Localised injuries are almost uniquely peripheral, partly because human homeostasis places a priority on maintaining core temperature at the expense of peripheries.[11] In humans adapted to cold, a reflex develops when a cold-induced vasodilation occurs at regular intervals to provide peripheral protection against the hypoxic effects of vasoconstriction.[15] Thus, most cold injuries occur in poorly prepared, unadapted individuals who fail to protect their peripheries with adequate clothing. Localised injuries can be categorised as *freezing* or *non-freezing* in nature. Frostbite is the primary localised freezing injury, while non-freezing injuries include chilblains, immersion and trench foot.

Immersion and trench foot
Anatomy and physiology
Immersion and trench foot are the result of prolonged or constant exposure of a foot to both water and cold. The term 'trench foot' was coined in World War I—the era of trench warfare—when feet remained in the same boots, in subzero temperatures, deep in stagnant water for days. It is seen today among people who wear wet boots for long periods in temperate or cold, damp conditions. Immersion foot is a more severe form of trench foot and has been identified among sailors and downed pilots, who may spend days in life rafts with their feet submersed in cold water. Soft-tissue injury occurs with prolonged cooling of the foot and is accelerated by wet conditions.[6] Primary injury is to peripheral nerves and vascular fields.

Patient assessment and clinical interventions
Progression of the injury occurs over days and on initial assessment the foot will be cold, damp, pale, numb or anaesthetic, pulseless and oedematous. The warming process produces vasodilation, erythema, intense burning and tingling, with perfusion returning to the foot over several days. In severe cases anaesthesia may persist for many weeks after re-warming and may be permanent. Severe cases may also complicate with lymphangitis, cellulitis or liquefaction gangrene, requiring surgical intervention.

Treatment is focused on drying and warming the foot. Re-warming should occur gradually and is best achieved by exposing the area to warm air or soaking in warm water (37–39°C). Injury is reversible with timely treatment, a factor dependent on early presentation to care. Hospitalisation is only required in the presence of complications, which usually occur as the result of a delay in commencing treatment. Prevention is based on good-fitting boots, allowing feet exposure to air for at least 8 hours a day (during sleep if possible), changing into dry socks and allowing footwear to dry. If trench or immersion foot is identified in the field, the focus should be on drying, warming and elevating the feet immediately.

Chilblains
Chilblains, also known as *pernio*, are an acute mild inflammatory response to cold, damp, non-freezing ambient temperatures seen in people chronically exposed to cold environments. Less than 24 hours after acute exposure, cold-induced vasospasm and vasculitis produce areas of localised itching, erythema and mild oedema.[11,15] Most commonly, the face, ears, hands, pretibial regions and feet are affected because they are exposed or poorly protected from the cold. Women, children and those with peripheral vascular disease are most susceptible.

Chilblain management is focused on prevention and warming the affected part. Ideal warming is gradual and should avoid direct heat sources, as direct heat may exacerbate vasospasm and oedema. Some patients may develop tender blue nodules after warming. Elevation of the affected area decreases oedema, which improves circulation. Topical corticosteroids have been shown to have some effect.[6,15]

Frostbite
Anatomy and physiology
Frost nip is the transient tingling and numbness after cold exposure, which resolves with warming and leaves no permanent damage. The lack of damage distinguishes frost nip from frostbite. Frostbite occurs with exposure to below freezing temperatures. The risk is increased if the affected body part is covered with damp clothing. Cycles of warming and freezing are particularly damaging. As the temperature drops below 10°C, cutaneous sensation is lost. Simultaneously vasoconstriction reduces perfusion, blood viscosity increases and endothelial damage leads to interstitial leakage.

When skin temperature drops below freezing, ice crystals form initially in extracellular spaces.[11] Crystal formation is increased if cold ambient temperatures occur in the presence of wind and moisture. Extracellular crystals prevent water movement in and out of cells, eventually resulting in cell dehydration and damage.[4] Intracellular crystal development enlarges and compresses cells, leading to membrane rupture. Cell rupture interrupts enzymatic activity and alters intracellular metabolic processes. After thawing, in addition to the architectural damage produced by crystal formation, sludging and microvascular collapse secondary to thrombosis occur. Reduced vascular flow is exacerbated by hyperviscosity and endothelial damage. Anaerobic metabolism eventually produces ischaemia and necrosis. Damage to the microvasculature ultimately determines the degree of permanent injury.[4,16] The extent of frostbite is dependent on the degree and length of cold exposure, and estimation of the extent of injury may not be possible until several days after exposure. Table 28.3 summarises frostbite according to severity.

Patient assessment
All patients with frostbite will have some degree of sensory deficit. Areas at greatest risk are extremities: nose, digits, ears and penis. The most common symptoms include tingling, numbness or a burning sensation. Complete anaesthesia is the result of ischaemic nerve damage and should be considered an indicator of severe injury. Skin may appear white and waxy and frozen skin feels cold and stiff. After thawing the patient may feel a hot, stinging sensation or, more commonly, a dull continuous ache. Mottling and blisters may develop within hours to days of the injury (Fig 28.1), progressing to gangrene if ischaemia is not resolved. Commonly, a dry black eschar will form over several weeks (Fig 28.2). Oedema of the area is expected and in severe cases can persist for months.

TABLE 28.3 Frostbite classifications according to severity

CLASSIFICATION	DESCRIPTION	SYMPTOMS
Superficial		
First degree	Partial skin freezing	Transient stinging, burning
	Erythema, oedema, no blisters or necrosis	Some throbbing pain ± hyperhidrosis
Second degree	Full-thickness skin freezing	Numbness ± vasomotor disturbance
	Erythema, significant oedema, vesicles	
	Blisters which desquamate to form a black eschar	
Deep		
Third degree	Full-thickness skin and subcutaneous freezing	Anaesthesia
	Haemorrhagic or violaceous blisters	Tissue 'feels like a block of wood'
	Skin necrosis, blue-grey discolouration	After re-warming—pain, burning, aching
Fourth degree	Full-thickness skin, subcutaneous, muscle, tendon and bone freezing	Anaesthesia
	Almost no oedema	Tissue 'feels like a block of wood'
	Initially mottled, deeply red or cyanotic	After re-warming—pain, burning, aching
	Eventually dry, black and mummified	Possible joint discomfort

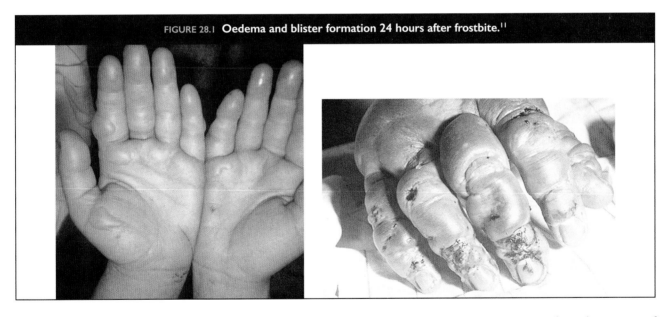

FIGURE 28.1 Oedema and blister formation 24 hours after frostbite.[11]

Clinical interventions

In the pre-hospital environment, the focus of treatment is hypothermia, removal of constricting jewellery or material from the affected part and ideally, gentle handling, moderate elevation and deferment of re-warming, if it is not possible to guarantee the part will not re-freeze.[4,16,17]

If rewarming can be achieved without subsequent re-freezing, use the processes outlined below. Air dry and do not rub the affected area, which is very fragile, and if an extremity has been thawed, immobilise, protect with soft, thick dressings and elevate. This will continue in the ED. During the treatment phase warm the room (or vehicle) in which the patient is kept. Preventing the onset of (or managing existing) hypothermia

through core temperature monitoring, the judicious use of warm blankets, head coverings and warmed fluids is essential, as hypothermia is life-threatening and further aggravates frostbite. Rapid re-warming of the part under controlled conditions is the ideal for maintaining tissue viability. Thaw in a warm bath (40–42°C) for up to 30 minutes until the part is pliable and erythematous.[4,16,17] Alternatively, the application of warm wet dressings (at a similar temperature) and elevation provides gentle re-warming and improves vascular flow. This method is useful for areas such as the ears and face, although the dressings must be kept warm (changed as required). Avoid heavy dressings, blankets and clothes over the injured area, as it is fragile. Ensure hydration to reduce the effect of

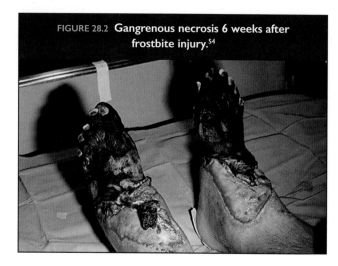

FIGURE 28.2 **Gangrenous necrosis 6 weeks after frostbite injury.**[54]

TABLE 28.4 Hypothermia aetiologies[18]	
ENVIRONMENTAL	Cold, wet, windy ambient conditions
	Cold-water immersion
	Exhaustion
TRAUMA	Multitrauma (entrapment, resuscitation, head injury)
	Minor trauma and immobility (e.g. #NOF)
	Major burns
DRUGS	Ethanol
	Sedatives (e.g. benzodiazepines) in overdose
	Phenothiazines (impaired shivering)
NEUROLOGICAL	CVA
	Paraplegia
	Parkinson's disease
ENDOCRINE	Hypoglycaemia
	Hypothyroidism
	Hypoadrenalism
SYSTEMIC ILLNESS	Sepsis
	Malnutrition

CVA: cerebrovascular accident; #NOF: fractured neck of femur

intravascular sludging on microvascular flow. All intravenous or oral fluids should be warmed prior to administration.

Wound management includes not debriding haemorrhagic blisters, tetanus prophylaxis, avoidance of vasoconstrictors, prohibition of weight bearing on the affected part and fasciotomy for compartment syndrome. Antibiotics are only used for identified infections. Dress the thawed wound with dry, non-restrictive dressings and elevate the part. As the severity of injury usually takes a couple of weeks to months to determine, amputation is not considered during the early phase of treatment, although a surgical opinion is essential early. Eschars are allowed to develop as part of the demarcation process. Over time, viable tissue will reveal itself and wounds will be managed surgically.[9,17]

As the process of thawing frozen tissue is extremely painful, administration of analgesia is recommended. Intravenous narcotics are often required initially and non-steroidal anti-inflammatory drugs (NSAIDs) are used for ongoing analgesia. Complications include secondary infections, tetanus, gangrene and ongoing paraesthesia.

Hypothermia

Anatomy and physiology

Hypothermia is defined as a core temperature below 35°C, with moderate hypothermia occurring below 32.2°C and severe hypothermia below 26°C.[5,18] Primary hypothermia is essentially caused by exposure to the environment, secondary hypothermia as a result of medical illness (for example, any condition leading to a decreased BMR, including hypoglycaemia and CNS conditions interfering with thermoregulation or disrupting muscle movement—limiting the shiver response) and therapeutic hypothermia is used in the post resuscitation period for specific cases. Controlled hypothermia can play a positive role in the management of a patient post VF arrest, where the effects of hypothermia are used to protect the patient from the detrimental effects of reduced cerebral perfusion. However, research has demonstrated inconsistent outcomes in the use of hypothermia to treat brain injury and in trauma in general, the consequences of hypothermia, particularly for the development of coagulopathy, lead to well-demonstrated poor outcomes (see Chs 23, 44, 45).

Primary hypothermia resulting from accidental exposure can be classified as *immersion-induced* or *non-immersion-induced*. Immersion hypothermia generally develops more rapidly because water conducts heat much faster than air. The lower below 21°C the temperature of the water, the more profound and rapid the hypothermia is likely to be.[6] Non-immersion hypothermia occurs in damp, windy environments. Common aetiologies of hypothermia are listed in Table 28.4. Behavioural patterns, including drug and alcohol use and social situations such as homelessness, may alter a person's ability to prevent the onset of hypothermia. The aged are more prone to hypothermia as a result of taking medications that alter body defences and decreases in the following: body fat, energy releases, basal metabolic rate, shivering response and sensory perception.[6,11] Importantly, the process of resuscitation can cause hypothermia due to continuous exposure, poor circulation and cold fluids. It is essential to monitor temperature, keep the patient covered, re-warm the cold patient and administer warmed intravenous fluids.

Patient assessment

The physiological effects of hypothermia produce symptoms and signs as indicated at the following core body temperatures:

- 35°C—cold, pale skin, poor muscle coordination, tachypnoea, piloerection and shivering, all designed to raise core temperature by retaining and generating heat.
- 35°C to 32°C—decreased respiratory rate and carbon dioxide (CO_2) production.[18] This will be seen initially affecting the CNS as lethargy, weakness, slurred speech,

impaired reasoning, poor coordination and ataxia. Shivering may cease.

- 32°C to 30°C—muscle rigidity, poor reflexes, dilated pupils, hypotension, bradycardia, coma.
- 30°C to 28°C—flaccid muscles, fixed dilated pupils, dysrhythmias, cardiac arrest.[11]
- A core temperature below 25.6°C is generally considered fatal.

The slowing of metabolic processes reduces cerebral oxygen requirements and is believed to provide some protection against hypoxic damage. A slowing of respiratory effort produces CO_2 retention, hypoxia and eventually acidosis. Oxygen delivery to the tissues is inhibited by a leftward shift on the oxygen–haemoglobin dissociation curve, which represents an increased affinity of Hb for O_2. Consequently, Hb picks up O_2 more easily in the lungs, but is reluctant to offload it, leading to hypoxia at the tissue level. This is further aggravated by hypoperfusion due to peripheral shutdown.

Cough and gag reflexes are depressed, increasing the risk of aspiration. While much has been said about the accuracy of arterial blood gases (ABGs) in hypothermic patients and the need to correct them prior to interpretation, it is recommended that ABGs be interpreted in their uncorrected form.[4,6] (See Ch 17, p. 329, for arterial blood gas sampling techniques.)

Hypothermia produces bradycardia in proportion to the reduction in temperature, leading to reduced cardiac output and hypotension. Stroke volume is not affected. Concurrent hypovolaemia produced by dehydration will aggravate haemodynamic compromise. The cardiac conduction system is suppressed by hypothermia, with myocardial necrosis a well-known complication.[4] Due to AV node and action potential (AP) disruption, prolonged QT and QRS occur on the electrocardiogram (ECG), as often do characteristic Osborne (J) waves (Fig 28.3). An Osborne wave is a sharp, positive deflection at the end of the QRS complex, most prominent in leads II and V_3–V_6.[4,11,19] Dysrhythmias, particularly VF, are a potential hazard once core temperature falls below 30°C, with the risk rising as core temperature declines. This is largely due to myocardial irritability, which is aggravated by rough handling and it is possible to potentiate dysrhythmias by turning the patient. Thus gentle handling to avoid cardiac arrest is essential. The typical sequence for the progression of dysrhythmias is sinus bradycardia, atrial fibrillation with a slow ventricular response, ventricular fibrillation (VF) and eventually asystole.[4,6,19] The temperature of 28°C is commonly considered the most likely point at which the patient will develop VF. Unfortunately, hypothermia increases transthoracic impedance and reduces the effectiveness of defibrillation below 30°C. As a rule, it is necessary to warm the patient before defibrillation can be effective. Antidysrhythmics have generally been shown to have little effect,[4] and may worsen AV and AP disturbance.

Haemoconcentration, increased blood viscosity and reduced peripheral circulation have a tendency to produce thromboemboli, with subsequent complications. Platelet function and the coagulation cascade are inhibited by cold, leading to a tendency to bleed (Ch 20). As coagulation tests are performed at 37°C, cold-induced coagulopathies evident by clinical bleeding may not be confirmed in laboratory testing.[4,6,18]

The ability of the kidneys to concentrate urine is reduced in hypothermia, leading to a 'cold diuresis'. This results in volume losses, dehydration and a subsequent drop in urinary output. A failure of the kidney to concentrate urine makes the use of specific gravity and output poor indicators of haemodynamic status. In addition, the hypothermic patient who is immobile is at risk of rhabdomyolysis, myoglobinuria and renal failure.

Endocrine function is generally well preserved at low temperatures, with normal hormonal levels maintained. However, persistent shivering eventually uses glycogen stores, resulting in hypoglycaemia. In a percentage of patients,

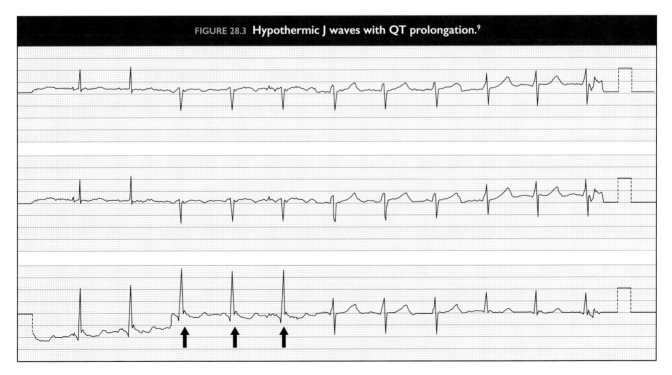

FIGURE 28.3 Hypothermic J waves with QT prolongation.[9]

hyperglycaemia occurs secondary to reduced insulin release and decreased glucose use. A slowing in circulation reduces hepatic clearance, thus medication half-lives are extended and toxicity risks are increased. Below 30°C there will be inadequate circulation and no hepatic clearance.

> ### PRACTICE TIP
>
> The use of intravenous medications should be limited to those patients whose core temperature is greater than 30°C.

Clinical interventions

Treatment of hypothermia is focused on re-warming and life support. If there is any detectable movement, pulse or cardiac rhythm capable of sustaining life, CPR should not be commenced in the field, due to the risk of precipitating VF.[5] However, where cardiac arrest has already occurred, CPR is appropriate and prolonged CPR in combination with rapid rewarming of patients in VF has resulted in neurologically intact survival.[5] Re-warming procedures are active or passive, based on external warming or internal warming. The choice of warming technique is dependent upon the severity of hypothermia and the need to warm the patient in order to maximise the effectiveness of resuscitation. Table 28.5 outlines the options for re-warming.

The patient with mild hypothermia (32–35°C) requires simple external re-warming techniques to prevent further heat loss and to re-warm as rapidly as possible. Passive re-warming raises the temperature 1–2°C per hour.[17,18] Place the patient in a warm room, remove wet clothing and provide dry clothes and warm blankets. Warming blankets such as a Bair Hugger and radiant heat lamps are all useful for more rapid and aggressive warming. All intravenous fluids should be warmed and ideally include a percentage of glucose unless bolus fluid is required. Use hot, sweet drinks if the patient can tolerate fluids. Sugar is important as this produces heat through metabolism. Some patients may require additional warming via the use of warmed, humidified oxygen. Re-warming will produce vasodilation, which in turn may precipitate hypotension as volume redistributes into warmed peripheries. As the patient re-warms and renal flow improves, urinary output will become a more predictive tool for haemodynamic status.

In the hypothermic patient with a core temperature below 32°C it is necessary to use both active external and internal (core) re-warming techniques. The American Heart Association has established 30°C as the temperature for initiation of aggressive internal re-warming procedures.[14] Active internal rewarming can include simple procedures such as heated inhalations via an endotracheal tube or warmed intravenous fluid; to more advanced procedures such as administration of warmed fluid via peritoneal lavage, gastrointestinal irrigation, bladder irrigation or around the pleura via an ICC. Because of the technical challenges posed by some of these procedures and negative impacts on organ function, such as lung expansion, bladder irrigation using a three-way system and peritoneal lavage are simpler to facilitate. In critical cases, extracorporeal re-warming via cardiopulmonary bypass and haemodialysis may be used.

Re-warming shock

Re-warming shock is a condition in which core temperature continues to drop after re-warming is initiated. The improvement in blood flow with re-warming shunts cold, acidotic, potassium-rich peripheral blood to the central circulation,

TABLE 28.5 Options for re-warming patients

TEMPERATURE	WARMING OPTIONS	INTERVENTIONS
Less than 35°C but greater than 32°C	Passive external warming	Remove cold, wet clothing and dry the patient
		Warm the room
		Cover with warm blankets
	Active external warming	Infrared radiant lamp (over bare skin)
		Heating blankets (e.g. Bair Hugger)
		Heating pads
Less than 32°C	Active core/internal warming	Warmed IV fluids at 39°C
		Warmed humidified oxygen at 42°C
		Gastric or bladder lavage with Normal saline 20 mL/kg cycled 15 minutes at 42°C
		Peritoneal lavage with K+-free dialysate 20 mL/kg cycled every 15 minutes at 42°C
	Extracorporeal	Haemodialysis
		Cardiopulmonary bypass

IV: intravenous; K+: potassium ion

increasing ventricular irritability and leading to VF. This is compounded by peripheral vasodilation, which can precipitate hypotension and cardiovascular collapse. To this end, VF can occur on both the decline and the increase in temperature. This necessitates treating the patient very carefully and continuing warming methods until normal core temperature is reached. Active internal (core) warming may cease once the patient reaches 32°C, at which point re-warming continues via external methods. Active re-warming should discontinue when core temperature reaches 35°C, in order to prevent the onset of hyperthermia. Successful re-warming depends on the patient's age, general condition before the hypothermic event and length of exposure.[14,18]

> ### PRACTICE TIP
>
> It is important to remember that a patient cannot be declared deceased until they are warm and dead.

There is one exception to the rule given in the Practice Tip. Body temperature decreases 2°C in the first hour after death and 1.5°C for every hour thereafter. A persistently declining temperature despite aggressive efforts to warm internally and externally, or a temperature that will not rise above 33°C despite aggressive actions, is the only time when patient can be declared deceased and still cold.[6,11]

Drowning

Historically, drowning is defined as death within 24 hours from asphyxia associated with submersion in a fluid, with near-drowning as any degree of recovery with survival beyond 24 hours from the point of submersion.[4,6] In 2002 ILCOR (International Liaison Committee On Resuscitation) established a simpler definition which does not discriminate between the two, and defines 'drowning' as a process of respiratory impairment resulting from immersion in a liquid regardless of the survival outcome.[20,21] Drowning is the third leading cause of death by injury in Australia and New Zealand and one of the highest causes of death in childhood.[22,23] In 2012–13[22] in Australia, 344 people died from unintentional drowning, an increase on the previous 2 years; however, it was an overall reduction since 2002. Of these 31 were aged under 4 years and, more significantly, a sharp increase was seen in the 114 who were aged over 55 years. The number of beach-drowning deaths has increased by 35%. Despite improvements in public health promotion and laws mandating safety measures such as pool fencing reducing drowning deaths in some age groups, the risk of drowning has increased in other areas due to drug and alcohol consumption, underlying medical conditions and visitor status. The last is important, as the majority of drownings at beaches in particular is by people not familiar with the area, tourists and new arrivals in Australia, who are at particular risk due to lack of knowledge about the risks found at beaches.[22]

Submersion events may be precipitated by trauma, risk-taking behaviour, hypothermia, syncope or seizures or disaster events such as flooding, and thus assessment for additional injury, intoxication or illness should be part of drowning management.

Anatomy and physiology

Initial immersion will elicit the diving reflex (parasympathetic stimulation), also known as the cold–shock response, producing peripheral vasoconstriction and lowering the heart and respiratory rates. Once thought to provide some protection against cerebral insult, it is now believed that the sympathetic stimulation associated with submersion of the head blunts the diving reflex in adults, although the diving reflex eventually predominates.[6,21,24] Moreover, only 15% of fully clothed adults demonstrate a significant diving reflex response to submersion.[14] However, submersion in cold water may provide protection due to rapid CNS cooling prior to the development of significant dysrhythmias.[14] Between the first 20 seconds and 5 minutes of immersion, a point is reached at which time the individual will breathe. This usually results in water entering the airway, producing laryngeal spasm and subsequent apnoea. Hypoxia, acidosis, convulsions and cardiac arrest follow.

There is a theoretical distinction between 'wet' and 'dry' drowning, separating those who aspirate and those in whom no obvious aspiration of fluid occurs and asphyxiation is secondary to laryngeal spasm obstruction.[14,21,25] Inhalation of fluid is usually broken up into occurrence in fresh or in salty water, although despite differences in the effects each solution will have on the lungs, the type of water has no bearing on prognosis. Inhalation of salt water is believed to diffuse fluid from the pulmonary capillary network into the alveoli, resulting in pulmonary oedema, hypovolaemia and electrolyte disturbance. By contrast, fresh water exerts an osmotic force on the lungs that pushes water into the capillary network, potentially resulting in haemodilution and hypervolaemia. In reality, the amount of aspirated water is usually no greater than 3–4 mL/kg and the volumes are usually inadequate to have any significant effect on cardiovascular status.[14,25]

Patient assessment

Early basic life support is critical to increasing survival without neurological sequelae due to hypoxia. This should be complemented by rapid and aggressive management by paramedics with urgent transfer to an ED. Without detracting from patient resuscitation, it is important to obtain a patient history. This should always include submersion time, medium, risk of water contaminants, temperature, level of consciousness (LOC) at the scene, first aid rendered and any other events that led to the incident.[12]

It is possible for patients to present as relatively asymptomatic, although most will demonstrate respiratory distress ranging from shortness of breath to apnoea, pallor and a degree of cyanosis. Hypotension is common secondary to bradycardia or other dysrhythmias. Profound bradycardia in combination with vasoconstriction may present as a pulseless patient, from hypoxia, hypothermia or head injury. Peripheral vasoconstriction will produce pale, often mottled extremities, pupils will be dilated and the patient will be extremely cold. The conscious patient may be vomiting and mildly confused. Evaluate the confusion as secondary to hypoxia early. Assess for signs of aspiration and other injury, particularly of the head and spine. Table 28.6 describes the association of presenting mental status post near-drowning with neurological outcome.

TABLE 28.6 Conn/Modell classification of mental status following near-drowning[18]

GRADE	DESCRIPTION OF MENTAL STATUS	EQUIVALENT GCS SCORE	EXPECTED LIKELIHOOD OF GOOD OUTCOME (NEUROLOGICALLY INTACT) (%)
A	Awake/alert	14–15	100
B	Blunted	8–13	100
C	Comatose	6–7	> 90
C1	Decerebrate	5	> 90
C2	Decorticate	4	> 90
C3/4	Flaccid coma or arrest	3	< 20

GCS: Glasgow Coma Scale

Clinical interventions

Early airway establishment with cervical spine control, if indicated, is critical. High-flow oxygen therapy administration for the conscious patient or intubation and ventilation for patients with a reduced GCS or persistent low arterial oxygen pressure (PaO_2) should occur.[6,14,20,21] See Chapter 17 for various airway management techniques, including intubation (p. 318). Positive end-expiratory pressure (PEEP) is often used to improve the relationship of ventilation to perfusion and therefore gas exchange. Continuous cardiac, temperature and peripheral oxygen saturation (SpO_2) monitoring should be commenced, although SpO_2 monitoring may be impaired in the patient with hypothermia. Chapter 17 contains information on cardiac monitoring techniques (p. 336).

A chest X-ray should be performed and is useful for evaluating the risk of aspiration or the presence of other trauma.[6,20] ABGs are useful for determining acid–base balance and gas exchange. An ECG should be performed, especially in the absence of a palpable pulse, as hypothermia is a significant cause of pulseless electrical activity (PEA). CPR is required in the pulseless patient and should continue until a palpable pulse is produced and the patient is warm. Fluid resuscitation is often required, although it should be administered judiciously, titrated to urine output, and the use of crystalloid fluids is recommended.[14] Inotropes may be required to support cardiac output and blood pressure. Gastric decompression will be required to remove gastric water and reduce the risk of aspiration. Concurrent hypothermia is not uncommon and should be treated aggressively.[26]

There is a high incidence of injury associated with immersion, so a full secondary survey is essential (Ch 44). Check glucose levels in all patients, particularly children and the hypothermic. Laboratory studies should include creatinine phosphokinase (CK) because of the reported risk of rhabdomyolysis; and urine drug screen where the cause of submersion is questioned.[11] Depending on the events surrounding the submersion incident, total haemoglobin (Hb), free Hb, myoglobin and electrolyte levels may be useful investigations (Table 28.7).[14,20]

Primary complications are pulmonary, cerebral and cardiovascular, including pulmonary oedema, pneumonitis, ARDS, encephalopathy and cardiopulmonary arrest. Later complications are related to poor circulation and include cerebral oedema, DIC and renal failure.

Atmospheric-pressure-related emergencies

Anatomy and physiology

Atmospheric pressure is pressure of atmospheric gas and water, at any given altitude or depth. *Barometric pressure* is pressure (weight of air) exerted by the atmosphere against an object or human. At sea level, the human body is at zero on the atmospheric pressure scale and 760 mmHg barometric pressure. Atmospheric pressure drops with the rise to higher altitude, as air becomes less dense and drier. Conversely, with descent to depth, pressure rises because total pressure is a combination of both water and air. With every metre of descent, water exerts approximately 70 mmHg of pressure on the diver which equates to exerting 1 atmosphere of pressure (700 mmHg) for every 10 m of descent.[27,28] The pressure changes on the diver are far greater and more significant with smaller distance changes than with altitude. For example, where a mountain climber needs to ascend to 5486 m (18,000 ft) to reduce atmospheric pressure by 50%, a diver needs to descend only 10 m (33 ft) to increase total pressure by 50%. Further, atmospheric pressure will vary with weather patterns and seasonal fluctuations.

Understanding the effects of pressure on the body requires an appreciation of several laws of physics and a few concepts. The human body and the environment are made of substances that are solid, liquid or gas. These substances are affected to varying degrees by pressure and temperature.

- Depending on its consistency, a *solid* experiences almost no change in the presence of either pressure or temperature.
- A *liquid*, while unaffected by pressure, will expand or contract with temperature. Pascal's law states that a pressure applied to a liquid will be transmitted equally throughout the liquid.
- *Gas* volumes experience the greatest changes in the presence of both pressure and temperature. As the majority of the human body is water, only the air-filled cavities demonstrate the effects of changes in pressure.[11,27,28] Chapter 16 includes a discussion on the effect of gas laws on aeromedical retrieval. Atmospheric

TABLE 28.7 Emergency management of submersion injuries[54]

AETIOLOGY	ASSESSMENT FINDINGS	INTERVENTIONS
Inability to swim or exhaustion while swimming	**Pulmonary**	**Initial**
	Ineffective breathing	Manage and maintain ABCs
Entrapment or entanglement with objects in water	Dyspnoea	Assume cervical spine injury in all drowning victims and stabilise and/or immobilise cervical spine
Loss of ability to move secondary to trauma, stroke, hypothermia, acute MI	Respiratory distress	
	Respiratory arrest	Provide 100% oxygen via non-rebreather mask or BVM
Poor judgement due to alcohol or drugs	Crackles	
	Cough with pink frothy sputum	Anticipate need for intubation if gag reflex is absent
Seizure while in water	Cyanosis	
	Cardiac	Establish IV access with two large-bore catheters for fluid resuscitation and infuse warmed fluids if appropriate
	Tachycardia	
	Bradycardia	Assess for other injuries
	Dysrhythmia	Remove wet clothing and cover patient with warm blankets
	Hypotension	
	Cardiac arrest	Obtain temperature and begin re-warming if needed
	Other	
	Panic	Obtain cervical spine and chest X-rays
	Exhaustion	Insert gastric tube
	Coma	**Ongoing monitoring**
	Co-existing illness (e.g. acute MI) or injury (e.g. cervical spine injury)	Monitor ABCs, vital signs, level of consciousness
	Core temperature slightly elevated or below normal depending on water temperature and length of submersion	Monitor oxygen saturation, cardiac rhythm
		Monitor temperature and maintain normothermia
		Monitor for signs of acute respiratory failure

ABCs: airway, breathing, circulation; BVM: bag–valve–mask; IV: intravenous; MI: myocardial infarction

pressure changes are greatest near sea level. A change of 1 atmosphere in water (10 m) will halve a gas volume on descent and double a gas volume on ascent.

> **PRACTICE TIP**
>
> The greatest changes in pressure and therefore the greatest risk for pressure-related trauma (barotrauma), occur during the last 10 m of ascent from depth. This is one of the most significant laws in respect of diving-related illness.

For example, if a diver with a residual volume of 1200 mL at the surface holds their breath and descends 10 m, they will end up with a residual volume of 600 mL. However, divers continually breathe compressed air, allowing their lungs to operate at normal volumes and thus maintaining normal lung capacity at all times. This works as long as they continually

breathe in and out during the dive. On ascent a failure to exhale will result in a doubling of lung volume with every 10 m rise. If they start with a total lung capacity of 5000 mL at 30 m depth and rise without exhaling, they will have a total volume of 10,000 mL at 10 m and 20,000 mL at the surface. This will produce significant barotrauma and has been responsible for diver mortality.

The rate of change in the pressure–volume relationship described by Boyle (Ch 16) relies on a constant temperature. However, temperature variations occur at both depth and altitude. For example, for every 300 m rise in altitude, temperature drops 2°C.[29] The effect of temperature on both the pressure and the volume of a gas is described by Charles's Law, which states that a change in temperature will result in a directly proportional change in volume and therefore gas pressure. Thus, as temperature rises, gas volume and subsequently pressure go up. The opposite is true with a drop in temperature. Equally, increasing a gas volume will result in an increase in temperature.

Every gas, based on its volume and consistency, will exert a pressure on the environment it is in. The pressure it exerts is known as a *partial pressure*. Thus, as described by Dalton, the total pressure exerted by a mixture of gases is equal to the sum of the partial pressures of each gas in the mix. For example, atmospheric total pressure is 760 mmHg and is made up of approximately 21% oxygen (158 mmHg), 0.3% carbon dioxide (0.4 mmHg), 78% nitrogen (596 mmHg) and 0.7% water (5.7 mmHg). During an ascent to higher altitude, atmospheric pressure drops and thus the partial pressure of each gas in the mix drops. This means that while oxygen remains at 21%, at higher altitudes it has a lower partial pressure than at sea level.

Henry's Law refers to the dissolution of a gas in a liquid. At a given temperature, there is a directly proportional relationship between the partial pressure of a gas and how much of the gas will dissolve in a liquid. At higher pressures, more gas will dissolve in a liquid. This explains the accumulation of nitrogen in tissues and blood, increasing with depth and length of a dive. Ascent to a lower atmospheric pressure will result in the gas dissolving out of the liquid. With a controlled, carefully timed ascent, this allows for dissolved gas to be exhaled via the lungs. However, if the ascent is rapid, nitrogen will dissolve out, forming bubbles and potentially blocking the microcirculation.

Moderate (intermediate) altitude is defined as between 1528 m and 2438 m (5000–8000 ft).[29] At these heights, exercise tolerance drops and minute ventilation rises. A number of the world's population lives at high altitude (above 2438 m). Those populations living at high altitude are largely not at risk of altitude-related emergencies as they have adapted to the environment in which they live. Physiological adaptations (*acclimatisation*) to altitude include a relatively rapid increase in minute volume (MV) [hyperventilation] resulting in a decrease in $PaCO_2$ and a subsequent increase in PaO_2.[30] Over days to months changes occur with reduction in total body water, bicarbonate concentration, haematocrit and haemoglobin. Cardiovascular compensation for maintaining near normal oxygen delivery to the tissues includes initial tachycardia, elevated blood pressure and peripheral vasoconstriction; eventually returning to near-sea-level resting heart rate and blood pressure.[30] Extremely high altitudes occur above 5800 m (18,000 ft), and acclimatisation above this is not possible because of progressive physiological deterioration associated with chronic, profound hypoxia.

Rapid ascent has been enhanced by the advent of air and car travel and improved mountaineering equipment. Most significant altitude illness occurs above 3000 m (10,000 ft), with pathophysiological effects being noted once arterial oxygen saturation drops below 90%,[31] causing hypoxia, hypoxaemia and subsequent pathophysiological changes such as oedema. The shape of the oxygen–haemoglobin dissociation curve prevents significant desaturation until approximately 3658 m (12,000 ft), when desaturation occurs rapidly with small increases in altitude. The development of hypoxia is influenced by altitude, the rate of ascent, duration at altitude, individual tolerance and physical fitness, exercise at altitude, environmental temperatures and the use of medications or toxic substances.[30,32,33] Prevention of altitude illness focuses on controlling the rate of ascent, with the altitude at which

someone is able to sleep (*sleeping altitude*) the most important indicator of safe altitude. Altitude illness syndromes are a result of oedema formation initiated by the pathophysiological changes secondary to decreased PaO_2.

Altitude emergencies
Acute mountain sickness
A relatively benign, self-limiting illness, acute mountain sickness (AMS) usually develops over several hours after ascent to critical altitude. *Critical altitude* is the point at which an individual can no longer maintain normal gas exchange, leading to hypoxia. In most people this occurs around 2438 m (8000 ft). A lack of fitness, underlying respiratory disease and anaemia will predispose to AMS. The primary signs and symptoms of AMS as defined by the Lake Louise consensus criteria are a headache and at least one of the following: anorexia, nausea, vomiting, fatigue, dizziness and insomnia in the setting of moderate to high altitude.[30,31,32]

PRACTICE TIP

Treatment for all cases of AMS is to cease ascent and reduce altitude if symptoms persist or increase or there are pulmonary or cerebral signs. A 500–1000 m of descent is usually adequate to reverse symptoms.[30,33]

For mild cases, rest and increased fluid intake is usually adequate, allowing time for acclimatisation; with symptomatic relief of headache (aspirin, paracetamol) and nausea (antiemetics) useful. For moderate or severe cases, acetazolamide—which aids the normal process of ventilatory acclimatisation by stimulating breathing, particularly during sleep when hypoxaemia is maximal—is indicated and multiple trials support this.[30,31,33,34] It helps to maintain cerebral blood flow despite hypocapnia and opposes fluid retention associated with AMS. The recommended dose is 125 mg twice daily.[33] Supplemental oxygen may be beneficial and immediate descent for severe or persistent moderate cases is required. Dexamethasone may have a benefit in severe cases as it improves oxygen saturation and provides symptomatic relief.[30,31,33] Untreated and ignored AMS could potentially lead to high-altitude cerebral oedema (HACE) or high-altitude pulmonary oedema (HAPE).

High-altitude cerebral oedema
HACE is a life-threatening condition developing over several days of exposure to critical altitude (usually above 3657 m [12,000 ft]) or with rapid ascent. As HACE is considered to be the end stage of AMS, clinically, the prevention and treatment for both is on a continuum.[33,35] Hypoxaemia leads to cerebral hypoxia, increasing blood–brain barrier permeability, increasing cerebral blood flow, producing cerebral oedema and increasing intracranial pressure. Primary signs and symptoms may initially appear as severe AMS. However, the headache will remain severe and be unrelieved by analgesia.[30,32,33] Ataxia will develop early, nausea and vomiting, altered mental state, seizures and unconsciousness may occur.[30,33,35] Treatment for all cases is immediate descent, oxygen, dexamethasone, rest, symptomatic treatment and, if available, hyperbaric therapy.

High-altitude pulmonary oedema

HAPE is a life-threatening condition developing over several days of exposure to critical altitude or with very rapid ascent. Hypoxaemia leads to fluid retention, increased pulmonary blood volume, pulmonary artery hypertension and peripheral vasoconstriction secondary to cerebral hypoxia.[36] The primary signs and symptoms are shortness of breath at rest, tachypnoea (worse at night), an initial dry cough which becomes moist, fatigue, rales and tachycardia.[30,33,36]

PRACTICE TIP

As with HACE, treatment for all cases of HAPE is to cease ascent and descend immediately, and give oxygen if available.

Mild cases usually respond to rest, while moderate cases require supplemental oxygen. Oxygen provides excellent results in alleviating HAPE, although it may be required for more than 36 hours, so while it is recommended oxygen is titrated to an SpO_2 of 90%, it is more critical in the field to conserve oxygen supplies for the duration of treatment.[30] Severe cases may require nifedipine, which lowers pulmonary artery pressure, assisting in progressive clearing of alveolar oedema, and hyperbaric oxygen. The decision to give nifedipine should take into account the risk of hypotension and concurrent HACE, where nifedipine may reduce cerebral perfusion.

Diving emergencies

Diving is pursued in a variety of environments, including caves, lakes, oceans and rivers, and is central to tourism in many parts of Australia and New Zealand, to commercial fishing interests and military endeavours. With an increase in the availability and affordability of diving equipment and training, the number of divers has increased. This, in turn, has increased the risk of diving-related accidents. Combined with human error, unexpected events and the tendency of some to push to the boundaries of safety, incidents occur. While the greatest risk is from changes in pressure (*dysbarism*), divers are at risk from injuries commonly associated with environmental exposure and aquatic activity (cold, underwater hazards, drowning and envenomation). The injuries discussed in this section include squeeze, barotrauma, nitrogen narcosis and decompression illness.

Squeeze

A 'squeeze' occurs when air is trapped on descent. The ears, sinuses, lungs, gastrointestinal tract, teeth and added air space, such as the facemask, are all potential areas for a squeeze. During descent, external pressure exceeds the pressure inside air-filled cavities in the body. To avoid a squeeze it is important that divers equalise their eustachian tubes and breathe slowly, and regularly. Symptoms and signs include pain in the affected cavity, oedema, capillary rupture and bleeding. Treatment is to ascend until the pain is alleviated. The diver may then attempt to descend again or ascend completely for further treatment. Therapy is symptomatic and includes decongestants and NSAID analgesia. Antibiotics may be required in the presence of tympanic membrane (TM) rupture.[27] Prevention includes not diving with an upper respiratory tract infection and not using decongestants to assist with eustachian tube equalising during descent.

Barotrauma

Barotrauma refers to injury produced as the result of volume increases in air-filled cavities expanding on ascent. Therefore, any gas-filled cavity susceptible to a squeeze is susceptible to barotrauma. Barotrauma is avoidable and occurs when air becomes trapped and cannot equalise with the surrounding environment.

Patient assessment and clinical interventions

Barosinusitis is pain in the ethmoid, frontal or maxillary sinuses due to air entrapment during ascent or descent. It may be associated with epistaxis and is essentially self-limiting. Decongestants and antihistamines have proven useful, and antibiotics are only required if evidence of infection exists.[6,11,27] *Barodentalgia* is the pain associated with air trapped in a poorly filled dental cavity. The condition will self-limit and only requires analgesia until pain subsides.

A failure to equalise the *middle ear* during ascent will produce the opposite of a squeeze. This usually only occurs when the diver has a pre-existing infection or inflammation of the middle ear or eustachian tubes. The initial symptom will be sudden acute pain, progressing to TM rupture if the diver continues to ascend and fails to equalise. If the TM ruptures, the ear is then exposed to cold water, producing a caloric response with subsequent nystagmus, vertigo, nausea and vomiting. Treatment is symptomatic.

Inner ear barotrauma involves injury to the cochleovestibular apparatus and, while less common than barotrauma of the middle ear, is associated with a greater level of morbidity. Initially there is a failure to equalise, with increasing middle-ear pressure. The pressure is transferred via the ossicles to the oval window where a pressure wave is created in the perilymph of the cochlea. This produces an outward distension of the round window. If there is a sudden equalising of pressure or a harsh Valsalva, the round window may rupture. Clinically the patient will present with severe nystagmus, positional vertigo, ataxia and vomiting. The patient may have associated hearing loss or tinnitus. History and examination are primary in the initial diagnosis. Treatment is symptomatic and referral to ENT is necessary.

Pulmonary barotrauma involves a number of conditions caused by expansion of gas on ascent, or occasionally volume reduction on descent. The traditional term 'pulmonary overpressurisation syndrome' (POPS) is now considered inadequate to describe the causes of pulmonary barotrauma. Volume increases can be prevented as long as the diver exhales continuously on ascent to the surface. The most common causes of pulmonary barotrauma are panic, running out of air and buoyancy problems. Respiratory illness predisposes barotrauma. The clinical conditions associated with pulmonary barotrauma include pneumothorax, pneumomediastinum and arterial gas embolism (AGE). Pulmonary signs may include interstitial emphysema, mild substernal chest pain and shortness of breath. A chest X-ray will reveal a pneumomediastinum or pneumopericardium.[6,11,27] Where either of these conditions are present, the patient should be assessed for neurological signs indicating AGE (discussed later). Interstitial emphysema without a pneumothorax will usually resolve without treatment. See Chapter 47 for assessment and management of a pneumothorax. Mechanical ventilation should be carefully considered, avoiding high pressures which may aggravate barotrauma.

Nitrogen narcosis

Nitrogen narcosis is the term describing the neurodepressant effect of high levels of nitrogen on the human body.[27,37] This effect varies in individuals, with some divers having a far greater tolerance to the effects of nitrogen. While nitrogen narcosis does not directly result in death, it can contribute significantly to death or diving injury by directly impairing a diver's judgement. In the words of Jacques Cousteau, nitrogen narcosis can be described as 'rapture of the deep', producing a euphoric state in which the diver becomes unaware of their condition and the need to surface.[27] Symptoms and signs begin to appear at depths of 30 m (100 ft) or deeper, and resolve with ascent. Initially the diver may feel euphoric and exhibit impaired judgement. Motor responses may slow and proprioception is lost. Below 60 m (200 ft) the diver is unable to work and unconsciousness occurs at approximately 90 m (300 ft). Prevention is primarily by limiting dive depth and frequency over a given period.

Decompression illness

Injury mechanism

Decompression illness (DCI) is the current term which describes injury resulting from gas release and bubble formation as a result of diving.[27,38] Previously, diving incidents were divided into *decompression sickness* (DCS), a result of nitrogen bubbles, and *arterial gas embolism* (AGE), a result of pulmonary barotrauma releasing air into the circulation. The current encompassing term considers that although their aetiology differs, DCS and AGE are hard to distinguish clinically and their pre recompression management is identical.

Arterial gas embolism

AGE is second only to drowning as cause of death among divers and has a mortality of 5% in divers who reach a compression chamber alive.[39] An AGE occurs during a rise to the surface. As the diver rises, gas expands, increasing lung volume. If the diver fails to breathe out on the ascent, air is unable to escape the lungs, pressure builds up and alveoli rupture. Air leaks into the circulatory system, migrating via the heart to the arterial system to produce an AGE. Clinical signs of AGE are related to vascular obstruction by emboli. AGE most commonly appears within seconds to 10 minutes of ascent and alveolar rupture. Rarely, AGE can occur when a patent foramen ovale ruptures during diving, as a result of a change in the normal cardiac gradient from left to right.

> **PRACTICE TIP**
>
> Symptoms of arterial gas embolism almost always begin within 10 minutes of surfacing and are primarily neurological in nature.

Cerebral emboli signs include vertigo, headache, visual changes, cranial nerve palsies, asymmetric multiplegia, confusion, seizures and loss of consciousness.[11,27,38] Coronary artery emboli may present as an acute myocardial infarction or dysrhythmia. Emboli may be widespread and cause shortness of breath or interruption to the vascular flow to the spinal cord, leading to spinal cord injury.

Decompression sickness

Known as 'the bends' and *Caisson's disease* (because DCS is also a problem for miners who spend time, or are trapped, deep underground in mines, surrounded by compressed gases, for long periods), the risk of developing DCS increases with the number of sequential and long, deep dives. When the nitrogen absorbed into the body's tissues during a dive as a result of pressure changes (Henry's Law) does not have time to diffuse from the tissue back into the bloodstream and be eliminated by the lungs, nitrogen forms bubbles in the tissue, blood or lymphatic system. Bubbles of nitrogen impair tissue perfusion and in the arterial system obstruct flow. Any organ in the body may be affected.

Symptoms of DCS usually begin within 6 hours of ascent and may be delayed up to 36 hours.[38] Onset within 10 minutes suggests AGE. However, some individuals (30%) will exhibit symptoms before or on surfacing.[11,38] Obstruction of lymphatic tissue produces oedema, cellular distension and membrane rupture. Ischaemia in the pulmonary vasculature leads to dyspnoea, pleuritic chest pain, pulmonary oedema, cough or haemoptysis (the 'chokes'). Neurological symptoms include headache, fatigue, dizziness, paraesthesia, unconsciousness and seizures. Joint pain is a classic sign and, because of its tendency to reduce joint movement, gave rise to the name 'the bends'.

> **PRACTICE TIP**
>
> Joint pain can occur at depths less than 10 m (33 ft), and any joint pain within 24–48 hours of a dive should be treated as DCS.

The upper extremities are more susceptible than the legs. If a blood-pressure cuff around the affected joint is inflated to 200 mmHg and the pain subsides, there is a very high chance that the problem is DCS.[11] Spinal cord involvement occurs in up to 60% of cases, probably due to venous infarction of the cord, obstruction of the epidural vertebral venous plexus, inflammation or bubble emboli.[27] For this reason, back pain occurring within 24 hours of a dive should be evaluated for DCI. Diagnosis is primarily based on history and clinical findings. It is possible for DCS to exist simultaneously with an AGE or barotraumas. A variety of rashes can be caused by cutaneous bubbles.

Patient assessment and clinical interventions

The diagnosis of DCI is made on history and examination, including a full dive history. Cold water, older age, fatigue, peripheral vascular disease, heavy work during or immediately after diving, multiple ascents, uncontrolled ascents and poor physical fitness aggravate the severity of DCI. Obesity lengthens the time during which the diver is at risk of DCI, as nitrogen is slowly absorbed and slowly released.[37] Moreover, children are increasingly learning to dive, with potential associated risks. The key issues are whether, in addition to the physical strength to undertake diving, they have the emotional and intellectual capacity to remain calm in a crisis, to understand and apply multiple rules and technological requirements associated with avoiding adverse gas pressure changes. This means they need to be able to recognise the dangers, equalise safely, descend and ascend using the right timings, provide buddy assistance if their adult supervisor gets into trouble and obey strict commands.

A full set of vital signs should be conducted and blood glucose levels measured in any patient with diabetes or an altered level of consciousness. (See Ch 17, p. 332, for techniques relating to testing blood glucose levels.) One hundred per cent oxygen therapy should be applied to aid oxygenation and increase excretion of nitrogen by increasing the concentration gradient of nitrogen across the respiratory membrane. If intubation is required, the cuff should be inflated with saline rather than air to avoid a change in volume on recompression. The patient should be left supine or in the left lateral position. Traditionally the Trendelenburg position was used to reduce cerebral bubble emboli; however, it has since been shown to cause cerebral oedema and is not advocated. A full blood count is useful, as intravascular fluid depletion is common and haemoconcentration may be affected. A chest X-ray is indicated if pulmonary barotrauma is suspected.

Intravenous crystalloids should be commenced and titrated in response in acute presentations. Importantly, note that fluid loading will affect microcirculation and may potentiate damage to vascular endothelium, in combination with the effect of bubbles. Glucose-containing fluids may exacerbate CNS injury. Hypothermia should be corrected.[27,38] For patients diagnosed unequivocally with cerebral AGE, a 48-hour lignocaine infusion may be of benefit to reduce the incidence of neuropsychiatric abnormalities.[27]

PRACTICE TIP

Definitive treatment for DCI is recompression and should be sought as soon as possible.[27,38]

Hyperbaric oxygen is beneficial as it reduces bubble size, aiding diffusion of nitrogen. It reduces obstruction and inflammation, and relieves ischaemia and hypoxia.[27] If air transport is the best option for timely patient transfer, every attempt should be made to avoid altitudes exceeding 30 m (100 ft). The higher the aircraft flies, the more the change in pressure will adversely affect the patient. Flying after diving can precipitate DCI. Even if there are no bubbles at the end of the dive, excess nitrogen will still be in the tissues waiting to be diffused and exhaled. Altitude can produce bubbles or enlarge existing asymptomatic ones. Current guidelines advise against flying for 12 hours after a single short dive, and 24 hours after multiple and decompression dives.[27] It is recommended that further diving not be done within 4 weeks of DCI symptom resolution. Twenty-four-hour assistance is available through the Divers Emergency Service 1800 088 200 (Australia), or 0800 4 DES 111 or 0800 4 337 111 (New Zealand).

Pandemics

During the previous three decades, the world has experienced a number of global respiratory threats. Influenza A (H5N1) or

'avian flu' was reported to be transmitted to humans in Hong Kong[40] and subsequently spread throughout many countries. Severe acute respiratory syndrome (SARS) emerged in China in 2002 and, like H5N1, spread throughout many countries resulting in a large number of deaths. More recently, influenza A (H1N1) or 'swine flu' was reported to be transmitted between humans in Mexico in 2009. During 2009, the WHO indexed H1N1 2009 influenza as being a global pandemic, which had resulted in over 10,580 deaths worldwide.[41]

Pandemic challenges

A number of lessons have been learnt from the above-mentioned pandemics of respiratory diseases, particularly in relation to the workforce. For example, staff may be isolated at their workplace for a period greater than a week, personal protective equipment, such as gloves, gowns and masks, need to be specifically ordered for individuals to ensure they fit appropriately, and staff may not be available to work as they have caring responsibilities within their family home.[42]

During pandemics, a goal for health authorities is to prevent the further spread of disease. This is challenging given the rate of international travel, mass gatherings and likely close contact of individuals at workplaces, shopping centres, schools and homes. Implementing processes that slow the spread of the disease is a significant challenge for many community medical services, emergency medical services and hospital care providers. In general, infection control practices, such as good hygiene, use of personal protective equipment, avoiding practices that generate aerosol droplets, such as nebulisers, and separating those individuals who are infected from those who are not, are essential in preventing the spread of disease.[43]

H1N1 2009 influenza: a pandemic example

In June 2009, the H1N1 2009 influenza reached its height in Australia. Emergency medical services and health facilities had a heightened awareness about the potential implications of the somewhat unknown epidemiology and transmission of this novel and infective variant of influenza.

Anecdotally, paramedics attending to patients with respiratory distress or influenza-like symptoms approached these patients with caution, as if they had H1N1 2009 influenza. This response involved paramedics wearing gowns, gloves and masks as part of their routine care. Communication was required between emergency medical services and hospital EDs to ensure that patients with influenza-like symptoms were appropriately placed and secluded on arrival to the ED.

On arrival in the ED environment, possible patients were diverted from the general ED patient population. They were placed in single isolation rooms or co-located with other patients who had influenza-like symptoms, or were diverted to co-located 'flu clinics' or influenza assessment clinics.[44,45] Influenza assessment clinics were a suitable model in diverting low-acuity patients with influenza-like symptoms. The majority of patients who presented to the ED and influenza assessment clinic during the pandemic were discharged home.[44] Approximately 13% of patients were admitted to hospital for ongoing management of their influenza-like illness, and of these 13% required an intensive care admission.[46] Those requiring intensive care admissions commonly had pre-existing comorbidities.

Mass gatherings

Mass gatherings present particular challenges in the prevention, harm minimisation and emergency response capacities. Mass gatherings are events in which crowds gather; they are variably defined, commonly based on spectator and participant numbers. These events are not well understood, and are surprisingly more hazardous than would be expected, with the potential for delayed health response because of the context, limited egress or other features of the environment and location,[47] and a higher incidence of injury and illness than in the general population, even though participants and spectators are 'well persons'.[48–50]

On any given day, events are conducted that attract crowds large and small, at varying types and styles of venues. The quality and quantity of planning and preparation for health and safety aspects of these events vary considerably. This may be due to many factors, such as the number of spectators, the nature of the event, the type of environment and the promoter's experience.

Several of the features of mass gatherings have been discussed in the literature, and are considered important influences on the demand for healthcare. These key characteristics include:

- the weather (temperature and humidity)
- the duration of the event
- whether the event is predominantly an outdoor or an indoor event
- whether the crowd is predominantly seated or mobile within the venue
- whether the event is bounded (fenced or contained) or unbounded
- the type of event
- the crowd mood
- availability of alcohol and drugs
- the crowd density
- the geography of the event (or terrain/locale)
- the average age of the crowd.[51]

While this is not an exhaustive or complete list of the characteristics of mass gatherings that need to be considered in the development of health plans, it is clear that we are developing sufficient evidence to underpin more evidence-based practice in the field of mass-gathering healthcare.

On-site medical care providers are interested in the 'patient presentation rate' of spectators and participants at mass gatherings, as this is a predictor of workload. Models exist that predict such workloads.[51,52] Similarly, the rate of 'patient transportations to hospital' is of interest to emergency medical services and EDs. Once again, these rates are somewhat predictable. The types of injury and illness that present will vary significantly depending on the nature of the event. It has been identified that between 0.5% and 1.5% of concert-goers will require some form of medical assistance, regardless of the character, locale, physical layout and size of the concert. Alcohol and drug use is common at most festivals and is the primary diagnosis in greater than 10% of patients.[53] Other common complaints include lacerations, fractures and sprains, burns, sunburn, heat stroke, seizures, asthma and exposure.

Planning for the provision of medical care for both spectators and participants is essential, for both humanitarian and legal reasons. In addition, the provision of on-site first aid or medical care will significantly reduce the demand on the EDs of local hospitals in the area of the event. Local health authorities should be notified of details of events and provided with emergency plans for a major incident. Inadequate planning can increase risks associated with insufficient or ineffective spectator management or service provision. The evidence lies in the large number of public events where multiple injuries, illness and deaths have occurred. There are a number of issues that must be considered from both a public and an emergency health perspective. A health response includes public health and health promotion as well as emergency management. Public health issues could include:

- safe and adequate water supply
- food safety
- sanitation requirements and waste management
- water and swimming pool safety
- pest/vector control
- infectious disease prevention and investigation
- standards for activities involving skin penetration, such as tattooing and body piercing
- building safety
- noise and other nuisance issues
- public health emergency management/planning.

Public events provide an excellent opportunity to promote health messages and to encourage event organisers and service providers, such as food vendors, to participate. Health promotion activities could include sunsmart, no smoking, nutrition, safe sex, alcohol and other drugs, hearing protection, nutrition and prevention of transmission of blood-borne viruses through activities such as tattooing and body piercing.[53]

Major-incident management is discussed in Chapter 12.

> **PRACTICE TIP**
>
> A health planning response for a mass gathering includes public health and health promotion as well as emergency management.

SUMMARY

It is important to understand, recognise and effectively manage the effect of environmental impacts on the human body, such as temperature, submersion and environmental pressure. Onset may be insidious and difficult to identify, thus warranting a high index of suspicion when assessing and managing patients who have potentially been exposed to environmental hazards. Treatment should be timely and often based on clinical assessment, without the necessary benefit of diagnostic confirmation. Where appropriate, timely first aid and transfer to a facility capable of implementing required treatment is essential for positive outcomes and reduced morbidity and mortality.

CASE STUDY

Approximately 30,000 people aged 15 years or older attended the Big Day Out music festival in Sydney in 2014. It commenced at 11 am and finished at midnight. The event consists of a number of popular overseas and local bands, performing in eight primary areas of entertainment, including large stages and disco environments. In planning for patient presentation and transportation rates to hospital there are a number of factors that must be considered in determining the mass-gathering profile and potential risks. In this situation the profile consisted of:

- being bounded or fenced within a defined area
- both mobile and seated participants
- available alcohol
- being held primarily outdoors
- held both during the day and at night.

During this event, voluntary members of St John Ambulance Australia provided the first aid assessment and response. These members consisted of a range of skilled personnel, including laypersons with first-aid qualifications and experience in providing advanced first aid, and first-responder services, which included nurses, paramedics and medical officers. Additionally, the government emergency medical services were available if required. Participants at the event can present with a range of health issues from sunburn; dehydration; heat stress; crushed toes, to alcohol poisoning, fractures and head injuries. A local hospital, approximately 5 km away, provided emergency admissions if medical treatment was required.

Extra planning for such an event is required between paramedics, first aid officers and event planners if the temperatures and humidity are going to be high. It is known that temperature has an effect on increasing presentation

TABLE 28.8 Pre-hospital presentations to St John Ambulance at the Big Day Out			
	FRIDAY	SATURDAY	TOTAL
Patient presentations	873	666	1539
Transported to hospital	16	15	31

rates at mass gatherings. Table 28.8 shows the numbers of people presenting and needing to be transported to hospital over the course of one festival.

Questions

1. Consider the different levels of clinical care available at this mass gathering (first aid and first-responder, emergency medical service, local emergency department (ED), tertiary referral centre). What types of injuries or illnesses would you expect at each level of clinical care?

2. What strategies could the event organisers employ to reduce patient presentation rates?

3. What role should the emergency medical services and the ED play in the planning of a medical response to this mass gathering?

4. Differentiate between heat exhaustion and heat stroke.

5. How does an increase in temperature cause an alteration in physiological function?

6. Outline the options for cooling hyperthermic patients in the community as well as the emergency department.

 Answers to Case Study Questions can be found on evolve
http://evolve.emergencytrauma.curtis

USEFUL WEBSITES

Climate Institute, www.climateinstitute.org.au/verve/_resources/heatwaves_fact_sheet_oct_3_07.pdf

Defining Heatwaves: The Centre for Australian Weather and Climate Research

http://www.cawcr.gov.au/publications/technicalreports/CTR_060.pdf

Environmental: Knowledge Hub, Australian Emergency Management

http://www.emknowledge.gov.au/category/?id=5

Environmental Health: www.health.vic.gov.au/environment/heatwaves.htm

Heat Events: Public Health, Department of Health, Government of Western Australia

http://www.public.health.wa.gov.au/3/1299/2/heat_events.pm

Heat Waves: Department of Health, Victoria, Australia http://www.health.vic.gov.au/environment/heatwaves.htm

Protecting human health and safety during severe and extreme heat events: A national framework

www.pwc.com.au/industry/government/assets/extreme-heat-events-nov11.pdf

State Health Sub Plan, Emergency New South Wales

www.emergency.nsw.gov.au/media/1355.pdf

REFERENCES

1. Hanna E, Harley D, Xu C, McMichael A. Overview of climate change impacts on human health in the Pacific region. Draft report to Commonwealth of Australia, Dept of climate change and energy efficiency. 1 Dec 2011.

2. Helman R. Heatstroke. Medscape 16 Oct 2012.

3. Hammond B, Zimmerman P, eds. Sheehy's manual of emergency care. 7th edn. St Louis: Elsevier; 2013.

4. Delaney K, Goldfrank L. Thermal extremes in the work environment. In Rom W, ed. Environmental and Occupational Medicine, 4th edn. Philadelphia: Wolters Kluwer: Lippincott Williams Wilkins, 2007.

5. Gagnon D, Lemire B, Casa D. Cold-water immersion and the treatment of hyperthermia: using 38.6°C as a safe rectal temperature cooling limit. J athletic training 2010;45(5):439–44.

6. Tintinalli J, Kelen GD, Stapczynski JS, eds. Emergency medicine: a comprehensive study guide. 7th edn. New York: McGraw-Hill; 2010.

7. Glazer J. Management of heatstroke and heat exhaustion. American family physician 2005;71(11): 2133–140.

8. NOAA's National Weather Service (NWS). NWS windchill chart. Online. Available: www.nws.noaa.gov/om/windchill/index.html. Accessed 12 Dec 2013.

9. Rogers I, Williams A. Heat related illness. In: Cameron P, Jelinek G, Kelly AM et al, editors. Textbook of adult emergency medicine. 3rd edn. Edinburgh: Churchill Livingstone; 2009:848–51.

10. Bucher L, Parkinson S. Emergency care situations. In: Brown D, Edwards H, editors. Lewis's Medical–surgical nursing: assessment and management of clinical problems, 2nd edn. Sydney: Elsevier; 2008.

11. Marx J, Walls R, Hockberger R, eds. Rosen's emergency medicine: concepts and clinical practice. 8th edn. St Louis: Saunders; 2013.

12. Smith J. Cooling methods used in the treatment of exertional heat illness. Br J Sports Med 2005;39:503–7.

13. Horseman M, Rather-Conally J et al. A case of severe heatstroke and review of the pathophysiology, clinical presentation and treatment. J Intensive Care Med 2013;28:334–40.

14. Bersten A, Soni N. Oh's Intensive care manual. 7th edn. Edinburgh: Butterworth–Heinemann; 2013.

15. Almahameed A, Pinto D. Pernio (Chillblains). Current treatment options in cardiovascular med 2008;10:128–35.

16. Zafren K. Frostbite: prevention and initial management. High alt med biol 2013;14(1): 9–12.

17. McIntosh S, Hamonko M, Freer L et al. Wilderness Medical Society practice guidelines for the prevention and treatment of frostbite. Wilderness environ med 2011;22(2):156–66.

18. Rogers I. Hypothermia. In: Cameron P, Jelinek G, Kelly AM et al, eds. Textbook of adult emergency medicine. 3rd edn. Edinburgh: Churchill Livingstone; 2009.

19. Wesley, K. Huszar's basic dysrhythmias and acute coronary syndromes: interpretation and management. 4th edn. St Louis: Mosby Elsevier; 2011.

20. Auerbach P. Wilderness Medicine. London: Elsevier. 2012.

21. Szpilman D, Joost M, Bierens M et al. Drowning. N Engl J Med 2013;22:2102–10.

22. Royal Lifesaving Society–Australia. National drowning report 2013. Online. www.royallifesaving.com.au/__data/assets/pdf_file/0003/9759/RLS_NationalDrowningReport_2013.pdf; accessed 12 Dec 2013.

23. New Zealand Injury Prevention Strategy. The strategy. Wellington: New Zealand Government. Online. www.nzips.govt.nz/ Accessed 12 Dec 2013.

24. Gagnon D, Pretorius T, McDonald G et al. Cardiovascular and ventilator responses to dorsal, facial and whole head water immersion in eupnea. Aviat Space Environ Med 2013;84(6):573–83.

25. Datta A, Tipton M. Respiratory responses to cold water immersion: neural pathways, interactions, and clinical consequences awake and asleep. J Appl physiol 2006;100:2057–64.

26. Giesbrecht G, Hayward J. Problems and complications with cold water rescue. Wilderness environ med 2006;17(1):26–30.

27. Smart DR. Dysbarism. In: Cameron P, Jelinek G, Kelly AM et al. ed. Textbook of adult emergency medicine. 3rd edn. Edinburgh: Churchill Livingstone; 2009.

28. Tetzlaff K, Thorsen E. Breathing at depth: physiologic and clinical aspects of diving while breathing compressed gas. Clin chest med 2005;26:355–80.

29. American meteorological society. The atmosphere aloft teacher's guide. Project Atmosphere, 2012. Online. Available at: http://www.ametsoc.org/amsedu/proj_atm/modules/AtmAloft.pdf Accessed 12 Dec 2013.

30. Davis P, Pattinson K, Mason N et al. High altitude illness. J R army med corps 2005;151:243–9.

31. Imray C, Wright A, Subudhi A, Roach R. Acute mountain sickness: pathophysiology, prevention and treatment. Progress in cardiovascular diseases 2010;52:467–84.

32. Rogers I, O'Brien D. Altitude illness. In: Cameron P, Jelinek G, Kelly AM et al. eds. Textbook of adult emergency medicine. 3rd edn. Edinburgh: Churchill Livingstone; 2009.

33. Luks A, McIntosh S, Grissom C et al. Wilderness Medical Society consensus guidelines for the prevention and treatment of acute altitude illness. Wilderness and Environmental Med 2010;21:146–55.

34. Low E, Avery A, Gupta V et al. Identifying the lowest effective dose of acetazolamide for the prophylaxis of acute mountain sickness: systematic review and meta-analysis. BMJ 18 Oct 2012.

35. Wilson M, Newman S, Imray C. The cerebral effects of ascent to high altitudes. Lancet 8 Feb 2009.

36. Hall D, Duncan K, Baillie J. High altitude pulmonary oedema. J R army med corps 2011;157(1):68–72.

37. Fowler B, Ackles K, Porlier G. Effects of inert gas narcosis on behaviour—a critical review. Undersea biomed res 1985;12(4): 369–402.

38. Schipke J, Gams E, Kallweit O. Decompression sickness following breath hold diving. Res sports med 2006;14(3):163–78.

39. McClelland A. Diving related deaths in New Zealand 2000–2006. Diving Hyperbaric med 2007;37(4)174–88.

40. Monto AS. The threat of an avian influenza pandemic. N Engl J Med 2005;352(4):323–5.

41. World Health Organization [WHO]. Pandemic (H1N1) 2009—update 79; 2009. Online. Available: www.who.int/csr/don/2009_12_18a/en/index.html; 29 Dec 2009.

42. Arbon P, Ranse J, Cusack L, Considine J et al. Australasian emergency nurses' willingness to attend work in a disaster: A survey. Australasian Emergency Nursing Journal 2013;16(2):52–7.

43. Collignon PJ, Carnie JA. Infection control and pandemic influenza. Med J Aust 2006;185(10 Suppl):S54–7.

44. Ranse J, Lenson S, Luther M et al. H1N1 2009 influenza (human swine influenza): a descriptive study of the response of an influenza assessment clinic collaborating with an emergency department in Australia. Australas Emerg Nurs J 2010;13:46–52.

45. Lum ME, McMillan AJ, Brook CW et al. Impact of pandemic (H1N1) 2009 influenza on critical care capacity in Victoria. Med J Aust 2009;191(9):502–6.

46. Department of Health and Ageing. Australian influenza surveillance summary report, No. 32, 2009, reporting period: 12 Dec 2009–18 Dec 2009. Online. Available: www.healthemergency.gov.au/internet/healthemergency/publishing.nsf/Content/ozflu2009.htm/$File/ozflu-no32-2009.pdf; accessed 29 Dec 2009.

47. Ranse J, Zeitz K. Chain of survival at mass gatherings: a case series of resuscitation events. Prehosp Disaster Med 2010;25(5):457–63.

48. Franaszek J. Medical care at mass gatherings. Ann Emerg Med 1986;15(5):600–1.

49. Zeitz K, Bolton S, Dippy R et al. Measuring emergency service workloads at mass gathering events. Aust J Emerg Manage 2007; 22(3):23–30.

50. Thompson JM, Savoia G, Powell G et al. Level of medical care required for mass gatherings: the XV Winter Olympic games in Calgary, Canada. Ann Emerg Med 1991;20(4):385–90.

51. Arbon P, Bridgewater FH, Smith C. Mass gathering medicine: a predictive model for patient presentation and transport rates. Prehosp Disaster Med 2001;16(3):150–8.

52. Zeitz KM, Zeitz CJ, Arbon P. Forecasting medical work at mass-gathering events: predictive model versus retrospective review. Prehosp Disaster Med 2005;20(3):164–8.

53. Emergency Management Australia. Safe and healthy mass gatherings: Manual 12; 2009. Australian Emergency Manual Series. Commonwealth of Australia. Australia: Better Printing Service. Online. Available: www.ag.gov.au/www/emaweb/rwpattach. nsf/VAP/(3273BD3F76A7A5DEDAE36942A54D7D90)~Manual12-SafeAndHealthyMassGatherings.pdf/$file/Manual12-SafeAndHealthyMassGatherings.pdf.

54. Lewis SM, Collier IC, Heitkemper MM. Medical–surgical nursing: assessment and management of clinical problems. 7th edn. St Louis: Mosby; 2007.

55. Rosen P, Barkin RM, Hockberger RS et al. Emergency medicine: concepts and clinical practice, vol. 1. 3rd edn. St Louis: Mosby; 1992.

CHAPTER 29
HAEMATOLOGICAL EMERGENCIES
RUTH DUNLEAVEY

Essentials

- An understanding of normal blood physiology and how to interpret a full blood count are important in the management of both patients with haematological diseases and patients admitted for other reasons. Recognising the signs and symptoms of anaemia and appreciating its possible causes are essential in implementing appropriate management strategies.

- Haematology patients may present with a number of life-threatening or highly debilitating syndromes, such as sickle cell crisis, hyperviscosity, cord compression, superior vena cava obstruction, hypercalcaemia and disseminated intravascular coagulation. Early recognition, prompt intervention and appropriate nursing management reduces morbidity and mortality.

- Early recognition and intervention of febrile neutropenic patients correlates highly with patient outcome.

- Administration of blood products, while commonplace in hospital, is hazardous. An understanding of the risks and of how to administer blood products safely is essential for nurses and emergency department staff.

INTRODUCTION

Haematological emergencies may involve problems with red or white blood cells, or platelets. They may result from the disease process, from the therapy used to treat it, or from a combination of the two. Diseases of the blood can be divided into two groups: malignant haematological conditions and non-malignant haematological conditions. This chapter looks in particular at malignant conditions, and examines how they may affect emergency health professionals.

The chapter begins with an outline of the composition of blood, the mechanism of normal haemopoiesis, and what happens when this is deranged, either because of the primary illness or by toxicities from treatment. A brief summary of the leukaemias, lymphomas and the haematological conditions most commonly encountered in the emergency department (ED) is also provided.

Many haematology patients have chronic conditions that are generally managed at home but sometimes require emergency treatment and hospitalisation. Others require aggressive therapy for their disease which renders them at risk of life-threatening toxicities. Still others may not be receiving aggressive, curative therapy and may even have palliative status. For all patients, however, recognition of the 'emergency' situations described below can be of great significance in extending the length or quality of life—or both.

Aspects of blood composition

Blood volume is composed of 55% plasma, 45% RBCs, and 1% WBCs and platelets.[1] The manufacture of blood cells (haematopoiesis) begins with the haematopoetic stem cell in the bone marrow, which has the capability of differentiating into any of the three main cell lineages: red blood cells (RBCs [erythrocytes]), white blood cells (WBCs [leucocytes]) or platelets (Fig 29.1).

A full blood count (FBC), also called a full blood examination (FBE), is a laboratory test that provides details of the respective levels of the cellular components of blood. Table 29.1 illustrates an abnormal FBC and also provides the normal ranges for each value. Normal ranges may vary slightly between different laboratories, but not hugely. Some normal ranges, such as haemoglobin (Hb), will be different for men and women and may also vary with age. The different blood cells measured in a FBC are described below, together with their role in a healthy individual.

Red blood cells (erythrocytes)

Adults have approximately 5 million RBCs per microlitre of blood; the number of RBCs is slightly higher in men. The primary role of RBCs is to transport oxygen and carbon dioxide and to assist in maintaining acid–base balance. Erythrocytes have no nucleus and cannot reproduce. They are soft, pliable cells that change shape easily, allowing them to pass through tiny capillaries. The cell membrane is very thin to facilitate the diffusion of gases.

Reticulocytes

Reticulocytes are erythrocyte precursors and mature within 24–48 hours of release into the circulation. The life span of an RBC is only 120 days, so new cells must be constantly produced. Production occurs in the bone marrow but is regulated by the kidneys. When oxygen levels drop, the kidneys release erythropoietin, which stimulates reticulocyte production by the bone marrow. An FBC that shows increased reticulocytes indicates increased bone marrow activity.

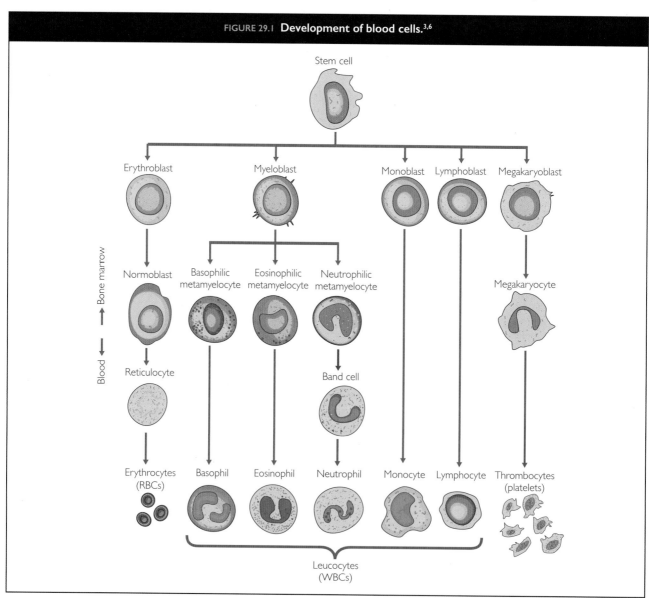

FIGURE 29.1 **Development of blood cells.**[3,6]

RBCs, red blood cells; WBCs, white blood cells.

TABLE 29.1 Example of an abnormal full blood count

ASPECT OF TEST	EXAMPLE VALUE	NORMAL RANGE	UNIT
WBCs	0.4	4.0–11.0	10^9/L
RBCs	3.0	3.8–5.8	10^{12}/L
Haemoglobin	85	115–165	g/L
Haematocrit	0.36	0.37–0.47	
MCV	90	76–96	fL
Platelets	35	150–400	10^9/L
Differential	0		
Neutrophils	0	2.0–7.5	10^9/L
Lymphocytes	0	1.5–4.0	10^9/L
Monocytes	0	0.2–1.0	10^9/L
Eosinophils	0	0.0–0.4	10^9/L
Basophils	0	0.0–0.1	10^9/L

MCV: mean cell volume; RBCs: red blood cells; WBCs: white blood cells

Haemoglobin

The outer stroma of the RBC contains the antigens A, B and Rhesus factor, whereas the inner stroma contains haemoglobin. Haemoglobin is a complex protein–iron compound composed of haem (the iron component) and globin (a simple protein), and is the primary vehicle for oxygen transport (see Ch 20). Haemoglobin concentration is reduced in anaemia and increased in polycythaemia.

Mean cell volume

Mean cell volume (MCV) provides an indication of the average size of the RBCs. If they are larger than normal, the MCV is elevated and the RBCs are described as macrocytic (this can occur with vitamin B_{12} or folic acid deficiency). A low MCV, indicating a small RBC size, occurs in iron-deficiency anaemia and thalassaemia.

Haematocrit or packed cell volume

This is the MCV multiplied by the red cell count. It provides an indication of the proportion of the blood that is occupied by the RBCs. A normal total red cell mass combined with an elevated haematocrit indicates dehydration.

White blood cells (leucocytes)

One of the body's main defences against infection is the leucocyte or WBC. There are six types of leucocytes in the blood: neutrophils, eosinophils, basophils, monocytes, lymphocytes and, occasionally, plasma cells (Table 29.2). A standard FBC will not always provide details of each subtype (the differential), which may need to be specifically requested on the blood form. Where the WBC count is very low, it may not be possible to obtain a differential electronically and a manual differential will be required.

Lymphocytes

Lymphocytes originate from stem cells in the bone marrow and thymus gland, and have the capacity to react to specific antigens and maintain an immunological 'memory'. There are two types of lymphocyte: B-lymphocytes and T-lymphocytes. B-lymphocytes are involved in antibody production. Natural killer (NK) cells are one type of T-lymphocyte.

Lymphocytes interact with various antigens at the lymph nodes. The lymph nodes can be seen as a sort of filter, 'sampling' lymphatic fluid for bacteria, viruses and foreign particles[2] (Fig 29.2). Lymph nodes can be enlarged for a variety of reasons, infection being one. Some malignant diseases, such as lymphoma and leukaemia, can be also associated with enlarged nodes. Significant enlargement of nodes may result in pressure on vital organs, possibly leading to a medical emergency (see sections on superior vena cava obstruction and cord compression, later in the chapter).

TABLE 29.2 Leucocytes: functions and characteristics[4,5]

NAME	% OF TOTAL WHITE BLOOD CELLS	FUNCTION	CIRCULATORY LIFE SPAN
Neutrophils	62	Attack and destroy bacteria and viruses through phagocytosis, especially during the early phase of inflammation	4–8 hours
Eosinophils	2.3	Phagocytosis (not as effective as neutrophils): attach to surface of parasites, then release substances that kill the organism; detoxify inflammatory substances that occur in allergic reactions	4–8 hours
Basophils	0.4	Limited phagocytosis: prevent coagulation and speed fat removal from blood after a fatty meal, release of bradykinin, heparin, histamine and serotonin	4–8 hours
Monocytes	5.3	Phagocytosis: consume bacteria, viruses, necrotic tissue and other foreign material	10–20 hours
Lymphocytes	30.0	Provide immunity against acquired infections: basis for antibody formation with a cellular and humoral immune response	2–3 hours

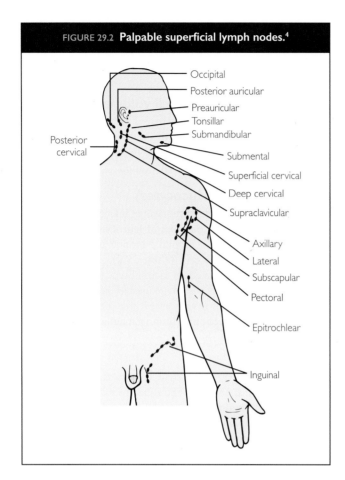

FIGURE 29.2 **Palpable superficial lymph nodes.**[4]

Occipital
Posterior auricular
Preauricular
Tonsillar
Submandibular
Posterior cervical
Submental
Superficial cervical
Deep cervical
Supraclavicular
Axillary
Lateral
Subscapular
Pectoral
Epitrochlear
Inguinal

Platelets or thrombocytes

The primary function of thrombocytes or platelets is to aid blood clotting by assisting haemostasis at the site of injury. These granular, disc-shaped fragments form when a parent cell breaks into thousands of cell pieces. The parent cell has no nucleus, so it cannot divide. Platelet life span is 9–12 days. Approximately one-third of the body's platelets are stored in the spleen as a reserve.

Clotting factors V, VIII and IX are found on the platelet surface. Platelets contribute to haemostasis by clumping at the site of injury to form a platelet plug and seal bleeding capillaries. Substances such as ethanol and aspirin interfere with platelet aggregation by impairing their ability to 'clump'.

Plasma

Plasma is a clear, yellow fluid containing blood cells, electrolytes, gases, amino acids, glucose, fats and non-protein nitrogens such as urea, creatine and uric acid. These and other substances may be dissolved in the plasma or may bind with various plasma proteins for transport. The proteins suspended in the plasma include antibodies, growth factors and hormones. Albumin, the primary plasma protein, maintains blood volume by providing colloid osmotic pressure, regulates pH and electrolyte balance and transports substances, including many drugs. Plasma also includes the proteins that bring about clotting (Table 29.3). Plasma without the clotting factors is known as serum.

Lymph

At the arterial end of the capillaries, water and some solutes leak out into the tissue spaces to form interstitial fluid. Most of this will return into the capillaries at the venous end. However, some will enter the lymphatic system. Tissue fluid which enters

FACTOR	SYNONYMS	DESCRIPTION/FUNCTION
I	Fibrinogen	Fibrin precursor
II	Prothrombin	Is converted to thrombin in the presence of thromboplastin and calcium
III	Tissue thromboplastin	Thrombin precursor
IV	Calcium	Essential for prothrombin activation and fibrin formation
V	Labile factor, proaccelerin	Accelerates conversion of prothrombin to thrombin
VII	Prothrombin conversion accelerator	Accelerates conversion of prothrombin to thrombin
VIII	Antihaemophilic factor (AHF) A	Associated with factors IX, XI and XII; essential for thromboplastin formation
IX	Christmas factor, AHF-B	Associated with factors VIII, XI and XII; essential for thromboplastin formation
X	Thrombokinase factor, Stuart-Prower factor	Triggers prothrombin conversion; requires vitamin K
XI	Plasma thromboplastin antecedent, AHF-C	Formation of thromboplastin in association with factors VIII, IX and XII
XII	Contact factor, Hageman factor	Activates factor XI in thromboplastin formation
XIII	Fibrin-stabilising factor	Strengthens fibrin clot

TABLE 29.3 **Coagulation factors**

BOX 29.1 Causes of splenomegaly[2]

Haematological
Lymphomas, leukaemias, haemolytic anaemias, haemoglobinopathies

Infectious
Acute—bacterial endocarditis, glandular fever
Chronic—tuberculosis
Parasitic—malaria and a range of parasitic infections

Other
Portal hypertension—liver cirrhosis, right-sided heart failure
Immunological—rheumatoid arthritis, systemic lupus erythematosus, sarcoidosis
Other—cysts, malignancies (rare), hyperthyroidism

---

lymphatic vessels is known as lymph. Lymphatic vessels are present in almost all tissues and organs of the body.

The spleen

The spleen is an organ which is involved in the physiology of blood at various different stages. The functions of the healthy spleen can be classified into four groups:

1. Erythropoietic: production of RBCs during fetal development.
2. Filtering: the spleen removes old and defective erythrocytes from the circulation.
3. Immunity: the spleen contains a rich supply of lymphocytes and monocytes. Splenectomy renders individuals at a very high risk of sepsis, and is discussed more fully below.
4. Storage of platelets: an increase in spleen size (splenomegaly) results in an increase in the splenic platelet pool to the point that it might account for up to 90% of total body platelets. This leads to peripheral thrombocytopenia.

The spleen may become enlarged in a number of haematological (and other) conditions, as described in Box 29.1.

Haematological emergency assessment

The haematological and oncological conditions described in the sections below may present as the primary reason for admission or may be secondary to other medical conditions requiring therapy. In either situation the first challenge for clinicians is assessment (see Table 29.4).

Sometimes assessment is relatively straightforward (for example, with known haematology patients presenting with expected disease or treatment related problems). However, more often than not, the haematological signs will be subtle and easy to miss.

Be on the alert for general systemic indications of a reduced blood count, such as new onset of fever, weakness, cough, rash, dyspnoea, increased/unusual bruising and spontaneous bleeding (e.g. epistaxis, bleeding gums, haematemesis, melaena, dark urine or haemoptysis). Identification of pre-existing haematological diseases, a family history of haematological diseases and surgical procedures, such as splenectomy, should all raise suspicions of a haematological illness.

History should also determine the extent of alcohol use. Alcohol is caustic to the gastrointestinal (GI) mucosa, with chronic abuse causing GI tears, haematemesis, compromised platelet function and liver damage (the liver is the site of production of clotting factors and so coagulation is compromised in alcoholic patients). Assessment of a patient suspected of having a haematological problem should include a medication history, detailing both prescription and over-the-counter medications. Long-term anti-coagulation therapy can lead to insidious occult blood loss and, consequently, anaemia. Some herbal medications may affect clotting including evening primrose, garlic and skull cap (thought to increase clotting time). Ginseng, cinnamon and parsley are claimed to decrease clotting time.

Patient medications and medication lists should be transported with the patient.

The patient who is anaemic

Anaemia is an abnormally low haemoglobin concentration in the blood. More specifically, it can be defined as haemoglobin concentration, written [Hb], below 130 g/L in a male or 115 g/L in a female. The diagnosis is normally made on the basis of a FBC.

Anaemia can be acute or chronic and may indicate either a reduction in red cell production or excessive red cell loss.

The anaemic patient is possibly:

- not producing enough haemoglobin (e.g. due to iron deficiency, vitamin B_{12} deficiency, folate deficiency)
- producing abnormal RBCs (e.g. sickle cell disease, thalassaemia)
- destroying RBCs too quickly (e.g. intra- or extravascular haemolysis)
- producing inadequate red cells (e.g. marrow disorders, such as leukaemia)

or

- bleeding.

There are a number of different anaemias, and in order to instigate the correct therapy it is important to establish the type (Table 29.5).

Frequently encountered in ED is anaemia as a result of blood loss—either acute (e.g. trauma-related haemorrhage) or chronic (slow haemorrhage from the GI or renal tracts, uterus or nasal mucosa). Iron deficiency is the most common cause of anaemia worldwide[6] and may be related to deficient iron intake and/or chronic blood loss. Deficiencies of folate and vitamin B_{12} (also required for haemoglobin manufacture) lead to anaemia.

The most common cause of anaemia in the elderly is chronic disease, followed by nutritional deficiencies.[6] Cancer patients are also known to experience chronic anaemia which has been shown to negatively affect their quality of life. This may be significantly improved when their anaemia is corrected.[7]

Signs and symptoms

Symptoms of anaemia vary from vague complaints of tiredness, lethargy and impaired performance to shortness of breath on exertion, dizziness, restlessness, confusion and collapse (Table 29.4). Co-morbid conditions such as ischaemic heart disease may be exacerbated. Physical findings may include pallor of the skin, mucous membranes and lips, fatigue, dyspnoea, palpitations, headache and tinnitus.[2]

TABLE 29.4 Common assessment abnormalities of the haematological system[6]

FINDING	DESCRIPTION	POSSIBLE AETIOLOGY AND SIGNIFICANCE
Skin		
Pallor of skin or nail beds	Paleness; decreased or absence of skin colouration	Low haemoglobin level (anaemia)
Flushing	Transient, episodic redness of skin (usually around face and neck)	Increase in haemoglobin (polycythaemia), congestion of capillaries
Jaundice	Yellow appearance of skin and mucous membranes	Accumulation of bile pigment caused by rapid or excessive haemolysis or liver damage
Cyanosis	Bluish discolouration of skin and mucous membranes	Reduced haemoglobin, excessive concentration of deoxyhaemoglobin in blood
Excoriation	Scratch or abrasion of skin	Scratching from intense pruritus
Pruritus	Unpleasant cutaneous sensation that provokes the desire to rub or scratch the skin	Hodgkin's disease, increased bilirubin
Leg ulcers	Prominent on the malleoli on the ankles	Sickle cell disease
Angioma	Benign tumour consisting of blood or lymph vessels	Most are congenital; some may disappear spontaneously
Telangiectasis	Small angioma with tendency to bleed; focal red lesions, coarse or fine red lines	Dilation of small vessels
Spider naevus	Form of telangiectasis characterised by a round red central portion and branching radiations resembling the profile of a spider; usually develop on face, neck or chest	Elevated oestrogen levels as in pregnancy or liver disease
Purpura	Any of a small group of conditions characterised by ecchymosis or other small haemorrhages in skin and mucous membranes	Decreased platelets or clotting factors resulting in haemorrhage into the skin; vascular abnormalities; break in blood vessel walls resulting from trauma
Petechiae	Pinpoint, non-raised, perfectly round area > 2 mm; purple, dark red or brown	Same as above
Ecchymosis (bruise)	Small haemorrhagic spot, larger than petechiae; non-elevated; round or irregular	Same as above
Haematoma	A localised collection of blood, usually clotted	Same as above
Eyes		
Jaundiced sclera	Yellow appearance of the sclera	Accumulation of bile pigment resulting from rapid or excessive haemolysis or liver disease
Conjunctival pallor	Paleness; decreased or absence of colouration in the conjunctiva	Low haemoglobin level (anaemia)
Mouth		
Gingival and mucous membrane changes	Pallor	Low haemoglobin level (anaemia)
	Gingival/mucosal ulceration, swelling or bleeding	Neutropenia; inability of impaired leucocytes to combat oral infections; thrombocytopenia
Smooth tongue	Tongue surface is smooth and shiny; mucosa is thin and red from decreased papillae	Pernicious anaemia, iron-deficiency anaemia
Lymph nodes		
Lymphadenopathy	Lymph nodes are enlarged (> 1 cm); may be tender to the touch	Infection, foreign infiltrations or systemic disease such as leukaemia, lymphoma, Hodgkin's disease or metastatic cancer

TABLE 29.4 Common assessment abnormalities of the haematological system[6]—cont'd

FINDING	DESCRIPTION	POSSIBLE AETIOLOGY AND SIGNIFICANCE
Heart and chest		
Tachycardia	Heart rate > 100 beats/minute	Compensatory mechanism in anaemia to increase cardiac output
Sternal tenderness	Abnormal sensitivity to touch or pressure on sternum	Leukaemia resulting from increased bone marrow cellularity, causing increase in pressure and bone erosion; multiple myeloma as a result of stretching of periosteum
Abdomen		
Hepatomegaly	Palpable liver	Leukaemia, cirrhosis or fibrosis secondary to iron overload from sickle cell disease or thalassaemia
Splenomegaly	Palpable spleen	Anaemia, thrombocytopenia, leukaemia, lymphomas, leucopenia, glandular fever, malaria, cirrhosis, trauma, portal hypertension
Nervous system		
Paraesthesias of feet and hands; ataxia	Numbness sensation and extreme sensitivity experienced in central and peripheral nerves; impaired muscle movement	Cyanocobalamin (vitamin B_{12}) deficiency
Weakness	Lacking physical strength or energy	Low haemoglobin level (anaemia)
Musculoskeletal system		
Bone pain	Pain in pelvis, ribs, spine, sternum	Multiple myeloma related to enlarged tumours that stretch periosteum; bone invasion by leukaemia cells; bone demineralisation resulting from various malignancies; sickle cell disease
Arthralgia	Joint pain	Sickle cell disease from haemarthrosis

Assessment and management

Assessment of the anaemic patient should include a dietary history which may indicate poor iron, folate or B_{12} intake or absorption (e.g. because of excessive alcohol consumption). A medication history will alert for other causes of anaemia and a family history of anaemia may suggest inherited causes.

History should also assess possible sources of bleeding. A menstrual history is particularly important in women as this can be the cause of significant blood loss. Where intestinal bleeding is suspected, stool testing for faecal occult blood may be indicated.

Anaemia causes cardiac output to increase in order to maintain adequate oxygenation of the tissues and thus may result in tachycardia. In patients with severe anaemia or pre-existing heart disease, hyperdynamic circulatory changes can lead to cardiac ischaemia and therefore cardiac monitoring and electrocardiogram (ECG) may be appropriate. Supplementary bloods for folate and iron studies are called for if deficiency is suspected.

Once the cause of anaemia has been established, corrective treatment can be instigated. This may be as simple as oral supplementation with iron, folate or B_{12}. Iron is usually given in the form of ferrous sulfate tablets. They must be continued for 4–6 months in order to replenish iron stores. Iron supplements can be constipating and may cause the stools to become

black. Rarely, parenteral iron (intramuscular or intravenous) will be necessary if the patient has malabsorbtion or cannot tolerate the iron tablets. Intravenous iron infusion is associated with a number of potential toxicities. Delayed hypotension, arthralgias, myalgias, malaise, abdominal pain, nausea and vomiting have all been reported following intravenous iron infusion, as well as life-threatening anaphylaxis during the infusion.

> **PRACTICE TIP**
>
> Consult your institutional pharmacist or policy manual before giving intravenous iron. Close monitoring will be required and the administration of a test dose before commencing the infusion.

Where anaemia is severe (< 70 g/L) treatment will include an RBC transfusion. If the source of bleeding or cause of anaemia is not obvious—particularly in older patients—admission may be required for investigation. Decisions to admit or discharge depend on red cell reserves, the patient's cardiorespiratory status and home circumstances.[8] If the cause of anaemia is an underlying disease process, the disease must be treated in conjunction with the anaemia.

TABLE 29.5 Types of anaemia

TYPE OF ANAEMIA	CAUSE/EXAMPLES	TREATMENT
Not producing enough RBCs		
Iron deficiency	Diet, blood loss, decreased absorption (e.g. after gastrectomy), increased requirements (e.g. pregnancy)	Iron supplements—oral or parenteral
Vitamin B_{12} deficiency	Dietary, intrinsic factor deficiency, intestinal malabsorbtion (e.g. Crohn's disease)	Oral or IM B_{12} supplements
Pernicious anaemia	Autoimmune chronic type of gastritis which leads to lack of intrinsic factor and thus poor B_{12} absorption	Correct cause; IM B_{12} supplements
Folate deficiency	Dietary, increased requirement (e.g. pregnancy), increased loss (e.g. dialysis), drugs (ethanol, trimethoprim, anticonvulsants, possibly contraceptive pill)	Correct cause; folate supplements
Aplastic anaemia	Pancytopenia of bone marrow	Stem cell transplant
Invasive marrow diseases	Bone metastases	Treat cause; supportive measures
Chronic renal failure		Erythropoeitin
Producing abnormal RBCs/destroying RBCs too quickly		
Hereditary cell defects	Thalassaemia or sickle cell syndromes	Transfuse, but with caution—chelation therapy may be required to prevent iron overload
Myelodysplastic syndromes	Dysplasia of bone marrow cells	Supportive care with transfusion, possibly chemotherapy or (rarely) stem cell transplant
Bleeding		
Anaemia due to blood loss	Chronic or acute haemorrhage	Address cause; transfuse

IM: intramuscular; RBCs: red blood cells

Sickle cell syndromes

Sickle cell disease (SCD) is not very common in Australasia although it is probably increasing in incidence because of increased migration. The Royal Children's Hospital in Victoria documented 535 sickle cell admissions in a 10.5 year period.[9]

SCD is a genetically determined condition prevalent in tropical Africa and parts of the Mediterranean, Middle East and India, occurring only rarely in Caucasian people. While most serious acute complications of SCD occur during childhood, chronic symptoms are ongoing and worsen with age. It is a condition requiring comprehensive, multidisciplinary, life-long management.[10] It is unfortunate that because of poor infrastructure, some adults with SCD become over-reliant on ED services (as opposed to ambulatory services) for their ongoing support.[11]

Sickle cell anaemia results from the production of abnormal haemoglobin—HbS. HbS differs from HbA (normal haemo-globin) in that when it becomes deoxygenated it elongates into a sickle shape. Re-oxygenation can reverse the process, but after repeated episodes the red cells become irreversibly sickled.[2] Obstruction of blood vessels may occur (vaso-occlusion), and infarction of the distal tissue. It may also result in premature destruction of the red calls (haemolysis), causing anaemia.[2]

There are different sickle cell syndromes dependent on the genotype of the individual. While sickle cell anaemia is the most serious form of the disease, some individuals with a less-strong genetic predisposition may suffer from milder forms. *Sickle cell trait* (heterozygous inheritance of HbS) has a protective effect against malaria, which is perhaps why the condition has remained in the gene pool for this length of time.[2]

Signs and symptoms

The sickle cell patient will experience periods of wellbeing interspersed with multifocal painful episodes that can occur spontaneously and in any part of the patient's body.[12] These periodic episodes of pain, anaemia or jaundice are called *sickle cell crises*. Crises may be precipitated by infection or dehydration and may occur quite often or only once every few years. In between crises, the affected person is usually quite well.

Sickle cell crises can be classified into:[12]

- haemolytic—resulting in anaemia
- aplastic—the predominant sign is marrow hypoplasia with increased reticulocytes and decreased haemoglobin

- vaso-occlusive—pain from areas of ischaemia
- sequestration—massive trapping of RBCs, e.g in liver and spleen
- sickle cell/endothelial cell interaction resulting in organ damage to lung, brain and kidneys
- mixed—two or more of the above.

Assessment and management

Identification of a sickle cell crisis can be difficult. Presenting signs and symptoms are extremely variable, but will classically include pain, particularly in the bones and joints. The duration of a crisis may range from minutes and hours to years. Different organs are affected in different ways and can result in the following common presentations:

- joint/bone pain; ischaemia can cause avascular necrosis and subsequent local infection
- chest pain or shortness of breath/hypoxia—from pulmonary vascular occlusion
- abdominal pain—from mesenteric occlusion
- decreased urinary output/acute renal failure—from medullary damage in the kidneys
- fever—secondary to tissue necrosis
- neurological impairment—transient ischaemic attack, stroke, decreased level of consciousness
- skin—chronic leg ulcers.

The majority of painful episodes are probably managed at home with analgesia, hydration and rest. However, during a crisis an individual may require hospitalisation. Management will include providing oxygen, IV hydration, warmth, analgesia and antibiotics if necessary. Often high doses of opiates are required for adequate pain control, and close monitoring is necessary to avoid potential respiratory problems.

PRACTICE TIP

It has been demonstrated that a proportion of SCD patients die from the complications of opioid analgesia.[13] Close monitoring of vital signs, respiratory function, fluid balance and neurological function is essential while the patient is receiving opiates.

Prophylaxis of sickle cell crises remains the mainstay of treatment (i.e. avoiding infection or other physiological stressors, such as excessive physical exertion). Other prophylactic measures include:

- pneumococcal, meningococcal and Hib vaccines
- penicillin prophylaxis
- folic acid supplements
- avoiding factors that might precipitate a crisis
- prompt treatment of infection
- blood and exchange transfusions when necessary
- prevention of iron overload.

The patient who is bleeding

Bleeding in the ED population will commonly be the result of gastro-intestinal or traumatic injury (see Chs 24 and 44). However, bleeding may also be caused by deficient/ dysfunctional platelets or by coagulopathies. These will be examined below, but first a review of normal haemostasis and the coagulation cascade.

Haemostasis refers to the processes that prevent blood loss after vascular damage (i.e. vascular spasm, platelet aggregation, coagulation and fibrinolysis). When injury occurs, the initial response is reflex vasoconstriction. Arterioles contract, reducing blood flow by decreasing vessel size and pressing endothelial surfaces together. Serotonin and histamine release also bring about vasoconstriction and decreased blood flow to the injured area. Vasoconstriction is followed by platelet aggregation at the injury site, which prevents bleeding by sealing capillaries. This temporary measure may last for 20–30 minutes, allowing time for clotting factors to work.

Clot formation requires activation of the coagulation cascade (Fig 29.3). The coagulation cascade is a complex network of 12 different clotting factors (see Table 29.3), and a defect of any clotting factor or an injury that overwhelms the entire system can cause its failure, leading to life-threatening haemorrhage. The coagulation cascade consists of two pathways: the intrinsic and the extrinsic. Physiologically the two pathways work together, resulting in the stimulation of factor X, which (in the presence of factor V) activates the conversion of prothrombin to thrombin. The end result of the coagulation cascade is formation of a clot—a protein mesh made of fibrin strands.

The process of haemostasis must also include clot resolution. The fibrinolytic system maintains the blood in a fluid state by removing clots that are no longer needed. Without this system, circulation to affected areas may be permanently lost because of obstructed blood vessels.

In the clinical situation, blood coagulation is measured by performing a coagulation screen. The different elements of this screen are described in Table 29.6.

Platelet problems

A reduced platelet count is referred to as thrombocytopenia. Among patients with known haematological disorders or patients who are receiving cytotoxic therapy (or both), thrombocytopenia is not unusual. People with haematological diseases can still lead an active life with platelet counts that are substantially lower than the normal value of $150–400 \times 10^9$/L. Indeed, some haematology patients function in the community with counts as low as 5×10^9/L. Among this population, thrombocytopenia per se is not an emergency situation; it only becomes one when complicated by bleeding. While there are some indications for using prophylactic platelet transfusions for patients with very low platelet counts, this can lead to transfusion-associated problems and will not necessarily provide any benefit.[14] However, in situations in which the thrombocytopenic patient is actively bleeding, platelets will be required. Some of the special transfusion requirements of the haematology patient are discussed at the end of this chapter.

Normal platelet production is controlled by negative feedback (i.e. it is regulated by the number of circulating platelets; see Ch 20). The body produces a number of substances to stimulate platelet production and release, including thrombopoietin, interleukin-3 (IL-3) and granulocyte–macrophage colony-stimulating factor (GM-CSF), which stimulates the megakaryocytes from which platelets are made.

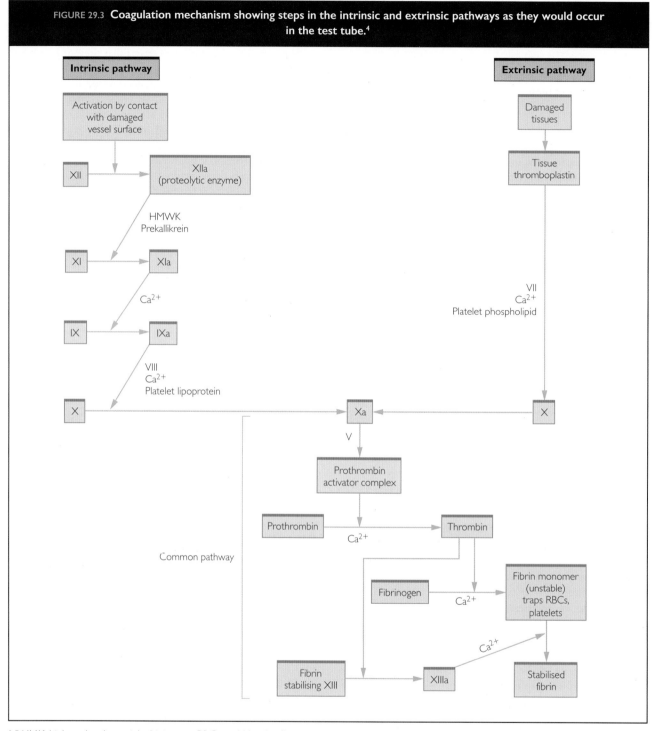

FIGURE 29.3 Coagulation mechanism showing steps in the intrinsic and extrinsic pathways as they would occur in the test tube.[4]

HWMK: high-molecular-weight kininogen; RBCs: red blood cells.

Platelet function can be disrupted by either a reduced number of platelets or faulty platelets. Platelet numbers can be reduced for a variety of reasons, some of which are discussed below.[15]

Decreased platelet production

This may be the result of disease or treatment. Each of the following factors can lead to decreased platelet production:

- aplastic anaemia—a disease of the bone marrow in which there are reduced/defective bone marrow stem cells and consequent pancytopenia

- bone marrow infiltration—due to metastatic carcinoma, leukaemia, lymphoma, myeloma, etc, in which infiltration of the bone marrow by malignant cells can cause a reduction in blood cell counts

- drugs (e.g. chemotherapy agents, alcohol)—different drugs affect platelets in different ways. Chemotherapy agents may have direct effects on the DNA, and alcohol has a direct toxic effect on the production, survival time and function of platelets.[16]

TABLE 29.6 Coagulation screen

PARAMETER	NORMAL VALUE	WHAT IS BEING MEASURED	REASONS FOR ELEVATED VALUE
Prothrombin time (PT)—the international normalised ratio (INR) is calculated from the PT to take into account other coagulation variables	11–15 s	The time required for a fibrin clot to form via the extrinsic pathway	Liver disease, clotting factor deficiencies or patient on oral anticoagulants (where therapeutic goal is typically to maintain the value at 1.5–2.5 times the control value)
Partial thromboplastin time (PTT) or activated partial thromboplastin time (APTT)—APTT is a slightly more sensitive test	60–70 s; 25–38 s	The time required for a fibrin clot to form via the intrinsic pathway	Unfractionated heparin therapy, liver disease and clotting factor deficiencies (e.g. haemophilia), DIC, high-dose warfarin
Fibrinogen	200–400 mg/dL	Also known as factor I	Inflammatory response, acute infection, liver disease, DIC, menstruation, pregnancy, hyperthyroidism
D-dimer	400–500 ng/mL	D-dimer is a fibrin degradation product, indicating breakdown of the fibrin clot by plasmin	Pulmonary embolism, deep vein thrombosis, DIC, recent surgery, myocardial infarction/sepsis

DIC: disseminated intravascular coagulation

Splenic sequestration

There are many different causes of splenomegaly (Box 29.1) and the degree of enlargement varies with the disease. A large spleen results in abdominal pain and, depending on the cause, a splenectomy may be indicated. After splenectomy, immunological deficiencies may develop (IgM levels are reduced), and patients have a lifelong risk of infection, especially from organisms such as *Pneumococcus*, which is reduced by immunisation.

> **PRACTICE TIP**
>
> People who have had a splenectomy should be vaccinated with pneumococcal, *Haemophilus influenzae* type B and meningococcal vaccines at the time of surgery and should receive appropriate booster and annual influenza vaccines thereafter.

Patients who have had a splenectomy can present with overwhelming sepsis from encapsulated bacteria (most commonly *Pneumococcus* and *Neisseria meningitidis*). Such patients can deteriorate extremely quickly and require immediate treatment with intravenous antibiotics in the same way as febrile neutropenic patients.

The Victorian Spleen Register, based at the Alfred Hospital in Melbourne, facilitates the provision of up-to-date information to patients and is also a resource for healthcare professionals.

Dilutional thrombocytopenia

Massive blood transfusion can result in a shortage of platelets (and other clotting factors). Whole blood that has been stored for more than 24 hours contains very few viable platelets because they only have a short half-life.

Decreased platelet survival

Decreased platelet survival (i.e. platelet destruction) may be immune- or non-immune-related. Blood loss and disseminated intravascular coagulation can cause platelet loss. Certain drugs can precipitate an immune thrombocytopenia (e.g. quinine). Another example of an immune-system-mediated thrombocytopenia is idiopathic thrombocytopenic purpura (ITP).

Idiopathic thrombocytopenic purpura

ITP is a self-limiting post-viral illness, most common among under-10-year-olds. The platelet count is often less than 20×10^9/L. The cause is not fully understood, but it is hypothesised that it develops because of antibody complexes forming as the result of an immune response following an infection. These complexes bind to platelets and destroy them.

Over 80% of patients recover without treatment, but in 5–10% of cases a chronic form of the disease develops.[15] ITP can also occur in adults—mostly in 15- to 50-year-olds; it is more common among women than men. It does not resolve spontaneously as often as in children, and tends to be characterised by relapses and remissions.[15]

Signs and symptoms

Patients present with petechiae, epistaxis and menorrhagia. In adults the onset is usually insidious, with no history of a recent viral infection. The disease sometimes arises in conjunction with other immune system disorders, such as systemic lupus erythematosus (SLE).

Thrombotic thrombocytopenic purpura

Thrombotic thrombocytopenic purpura (TTP) is an example of non-immune platelet destruction. It is a rare but serious disorder that most commonly affects young adults. It is associated with fever, haemolysis, transient neurological defects and renal failure. Microthrombi (platelets and fibrin) are deposited in arterioles and capillaries, causing thrombocytopenia and anaemia. The mortality rate associated with TTP approached 100% until the 1980s, but is now closer to 25% with early diagnosis and treatment with therapeutic plasma exchange (TPE).[17]

Pregnancy and the postpartum state account for 12–25% of cases of TTP[17] and the disorder is also often associated with cancer. Other causes include toxins (e.g. from *Escherichia coli*), spider and bee venoms (see Ch 31) or human immunodeficiency virus (HIV).

Signs and symptoms

Thrombotic thrombocytopenic purpura can present with very few clinical features and is therefore notoriously difficult to diagnose. Early signs include abdominal pain, nausea, vomiting, weakness, acute renal insufficiency and fever. Purpura are common, and some patients will present with haemorrhage (e.g. haematuria, epistaxis, menorrhagia or retinal haemorrhage).[18] Some symptoms are linked to platelet-clumping-induced ischaemia. The brain is a common target, with ischaemia present in 75% of TTP cases.[17] The clinical triad of thrombocytopenia, haemolytic anaemia and neurological abnormalities is suggestive of the condition.[19]

Management

The mainstay of treatment is to arrest any obvious bleeding and provide supportive therapy.[20] The role of plasma infusion exchange with fresh frozen plasma has significantly increased the survival rate in recent years. Prompt plasma exchange is associated with better recovery. A number of other therapies have been utilised to prolong remission, including steroids and treatment with various medications, but none has been definitively proven.[20] Platelet transfusion is contraindicated because it is associated with rapid deterioration.

Haemolytic uraemic syndrome (HUS) is a disorder similar to TTP that affects infants and young children, often following infections with *E. coli* or other enteric pathogens.

Other clotting cascade problems

There are also a number of places in the clotting cascade at which problems can occur and lead to a risk of bleeding. These are the result of clotting-factor abnormalities rather than platelet deficiency. Factor abnormalities may be either inherited or acquired. Haemophilia is a hereditary clotting factor disorder of factor VIII. Acquired factor abnormalities include vitamin K deficiency, liver disease or disseminated intravascular coagulation (DIC).

Hereditary clotting-factor abnormalities

Haemophilia

Haemophilia refers to a number of clotting disorders, including haemophilia A, haemophilia B and von Willebrand's disease. Haemophilia is an inherited, gender-linked disorder that occurs almost always in males. Females carry the disease and pass it on to their children. Currently there are approximately 2800 people in Australia with haemophilia[21] and approximately 300 in New Zealand.[22] Severity ranges from mild (6–60%) to severe (<1%). The primary defect in haemophilia is absence or dysfunction of a specific clotting factor.

Haemophilia A, or classic haemophilia, is due to a factor VIII disorder. In the majority of patients with haemophilia A, factor VIII is not missing—it may even be present in excess quantities; however, available factor VIII does not function adequately. Disease severity is directly related to the functional activity of factor VIII.

Haemophilia B, or Christmas disease, occurs less often than haemophilia A. It is caused by the absence or functional deficiency of factor IX.

Von Willebrand's disease is usually less severe than haemophilia A or B and occurs in both genders. The specific coagulation defect in this type of haemophilia is defective platelet adherence coupled with decreased levels of factor VIII. Von Willebrand's factor (vWF) is required for the stabilisation and transport of factor VIII.

Signs and symptoms

Haemophilia A and B have similar clinical presentations. Patients with von Willebrand's disease exhibit less severe symptoms, with a lower incidence of bleeding into joints and deeper tissues. Children usually manifest these diseases when they start crawling, although first-time presentations in adulthood have occurred and the bleeding may be severe. Bleeding tends to be spontaneous or following trauma, with even minor trauma sometimes causing major bruises or injury. Emergency conditions include haemarthroses—bleeding into a joint.

Haemarthroses usually begin in adolescence and involve primarily the knees, ankles and elbows. Patients almost always come to the ED because of severe joint pain rather than actual bleeding. Improperly managed haemarthrosis can lead to arthritis and ultimately joint destruction. Bleeding into tissue planes and tense haematomas in limbs can cause compartment syndromes. Bleeding into the neck or mouth may cause airway compromise. Central nervous system bleeding can be caused by minor head trauma, and patients will require hospital assessment and computed tomography (CT) scanning. If intracranial pathology is suspected, replacement therapy with appropriate clotting factors should be commenced prior to radiological investigation. Retroperitoneal bleeding should be considered if there is evidence of acute blood loss and the source cannot be found. Patients may also present with a complication of therapy, such as hepatitis or HIV as a result of exposure to viruses prior to the introduction of extensive screening of blood products.

Identification of the specific type of haemophilia is crucial, because haemophilia A and haemophilia B present the same clinical picture but require treatment with different clotting factors.

Management

Haemophilia is a disease that requires lifetime medical management, and the development of a comprehensive disease-management plan involves a complex interrelationship between the patient, family and healthcare team.[23] The goals of treatment are to prevent and treat bleeding. Replacement of deficient clotting factors is the primary means of support.

For mild haemophilia A and certain subtypes of von Willebrand's disease, desmopressin acetate (DDAVP), a synthetic analogue of vasopressin, may be used to stimulate an increase in factor VIII and vWF, which subsequently binds with factor VIII thus increasing its concentration. It can be

---

BOX 29.2 Interventions for acute haemophilia presentations[98,99]

1. Stop topical bleeding as quickly as possible by applying direct pressure, ice, packing the area with Gelfoam or fibrin foam and applying topical haemostatic agents such as thrombin.
2. Administer the specific coagulation factor to raise the patient's level of the deficient coagulation factor.
3. When joint bleeding occurs, in addition to administering replacement factors, it is important to rest the injured joint totally until bleeding has stopped to prevent crippling deformities from haemarthrosis. The joint may be packed in ice. Analgesics are given to reduce pain, keeping in mind that those agents which affect clotting such as aspirin should never be used.
4. Monitor closely for life- and limb-threatening complications that may develop as a result of bleeding: airway obstruction from haemorrhage into the neck, decreased level of consciousness from acute head injury indicating cerebral bleeding, compartment syndrome developing from limb injuries.
5. Monitor for signs of ongoing blood loss such as hypovolaemic shock: tachycardia, tachypnoea, altered level of consciousness, hypotension, pallor, diaphoresis, decreased capillary refill.

BOX 29.3 Potential causes of disseminated intravascular coagulation (DIC)

DIC can be brought about by shock of any type and the following triggers:

- infection—Gram-negative sepsis accounts for 30–50% of cases of DIC[100]
- malignancy (e.g. acute promyelocytic leukaemia)
- obstetric complications—amniotic fluid embolism, eclampsia, retained placenta, incomplete abortion
- hypersensitivity reactions
- major trauma
- widespread tissue damage (e.g. following burns)
- vascular abnormalities
- snake bites
- hypothermia
- liver disease
- heat stroke
- acute hypoxia
- recreational drugs.

---

administered intravenously and the beneficial effects are seen within 30 minutes and last for more than 12 hours.

Patients with moderate and severe haemophilia A will require factor VIII concentrate. Most haemophiliacs have personalised management plans and are able to manage minor incidents and administer factor VIII at home, but are aware that certain events—a large bleed, ongoing bleeding, severe pain, swelling of a muscle that restricts movement, head injury, swelling in the neck or mouth, haematuria, melaena and wounds in need of suturing—require medical attention. Acute interventions are related primarily to stopping the bleeding and are listed in Box 29.2. Some patients, particularly those with severe hereditary haemophilia and the elderly or, less commonly, patients with autoimmune disease, who are pregnant or who are taking certain medications (notably penicillin) develop antibodies to factor VIII, known as inhibitors.

Acquired clotting factor abnormalities

Disseminated intravascular coagulation

A number of clinical conditions may be associated with disseminated intravascular coagulation (DIC). It can be the presenting symptom of certain haematological disorders (e.g. acute promyelocytic leukaemia), or result from another precipitating factor (Box 29.3). DIC never occurs de novo, but is always secondary to another condition.

DIC is a paradoxical condition characterised by both bleeding and thrombosis. It results from the release of pro-inflammatory cytokines such as the interleukins and tumour necrosis factor (TNF) as a response to one of the triggers listed in Box 29.3. It is characterised by simultaneous activation of blood coagulation, consumption of clotting proteins, generation of thrombin, activation of platelets and secondary activation of the fibrinolytic system. Microclots form within the capillaries and deplete clotting factors in the circulating blood faster than the liver and bone marrow can replace them, resulting in haemorrhage. Intravascular clots obstruct the capillaries causing ischaemia in the tissues. The fibrinolytic system is activated to dissolve the clots and potent fibrin degradation products trigger further bleeding.

DIC may be associated with a fulminant haemorrhagic/thrombotic syndrome or run a less severe course. Some patients with cancer may develop a subacute form of DIC that produces abnormal laboratory values without the evidence of thrombosis or haemorrhage. The incidence of DIC among patients with metastatic cancer is 10–15%, and 15% among patients with acute leukaemia.[23]

Signs and symptoms

Signs and symptoms vary depending on the severity of DIC, and may include both bleeding and thrombotic events. Major bleeding is in fact seen only with a minority of patients[24]—more common is the occurrence of organ failure.[25]

Initial signs and symptoms are often subtle and may be overlooked until a catastrophic event occurs, such as cerebrovascular accident, myocardial infarction, massive haemorrhage or acute renal failure.[26] Microvascular thrombosis may manifest itself as peripheral cyanosis. Neurological signs may include severe headache or altered behaviour, mood or level of consciousness. Patients may also exhibit haemodynamic instability (tachycardia and hypotension) and a whole range of other potential symptoms, depending on the organs involved.[26]

Laboratory abnormalities are the most reliable way of diagnosing the disorder. Characteristically these will show:[26]

- prolonged PT, TT (thrombin time) and APTT
- low platelet count
- low fibrinogen level

- elevated D-dimer
- reduced fibrinogen
- reduced protein C
- reduced antithrombin.

Management

The key to reversing DIC is through addressing the causative factors. However, this may be difficult and may constitute a longer-term goal. In the short term, various more immediate measures can be implemented, including maintenance of organ perfusion, restoration of blood components and drug therapy. The patient requires immediate transfer to a tertiary care hospital environment. While in transit, monitor vital signs, maintain airway, assess and document extent of haemorrhage or thrombosis, and correct hypovolaemia as required.[27]

- *Maintaining organ perfusion*—DIC is made worse by hypotension, hypoxia and acidosis (otherwise known as the *triad of death*—see Chapter 20 for physiology and Chapter 44 for early management of trauma and massive transfusion protocols). Unfortunately, aggressive intravenous fluid therapy can exacerbate the problem by diluting clotting factors and naturally-occurring prothrombins which could help to reverse the cascade. Infusion of a vasopressor such as dopamine may be necessary.

- *Restoring blood components*—imbalances in RBCs and platelets can be corrected by transfusions, and clotting factors can be replaced by the infusion of fresh frozen plasma and cryoprecipitate where necessary. Platelet transfusion should be used cautiously as it may aggravate thrombosis.[26] Platelet or plasma transfusions are recommended only for those actively bleeding.[25]

- *Drug therapies*—low-molecular-weight heparin has traditionally been administered with the rationale that although it would not dissolve existing clots, it might prevent the formation of new ones. However, a beneficial effect of this practice on clinically relevant factors has never been demonstrated in a randomised, controlled trial.[26,28] The administration of recombinant human activated protein C (drotrecogin alfa) was thought to be beneficial in the management of DIC,[29] but this was not replicated in subsequent studies and the drug has been withdrawn from the market.[30] Some still believe it has a role in selected patient groups.[29]

The patient with leucocyte abnormalities

Some patients will present to ED with disorders of the white blood cells (leucocyte). These abnormalities will often be the result of malignant disease or of the therapy used to treat it.

Leukaemia

Leukaemia is a malignant disorder of blood and blood-forming organs characterised by excessive, abnormal growth of leucocyte precursors in the bone marrow. An uncontrolled increase in immature leucocytes decreases production and function of normal leucocytes (and other cell lineages).

In New Zealand leukaemia accounts for 2.8% of all new cancer registrations and 3.4% of all cancer deaths.[31] In Australia, over 2500 people a year are diagnosed with leukaemia.[32] It is the most common form of cancer among children, although more than 90% of the people diagnosed with leukaemia are adults. Different types of leukaemia peak at different ages, with acute myeloid leukaemia being most common in the over-60s and acute lymphoblastic leukaemia more common in children.[2] Factors affecting the development of leukaemia are not clear, but may include a person's genetic history and exposure to intense radiation and certain chemicals and viruses like the human T-cell leukaemia virus.

Leukaemia can affect either the granulocte (myeloid) or lymphocyte (lymphocytic) lines, and may be either acute or chronic. Chronic leukaemias affect the blood cells when they are comparatively well-differentiated. Acute leukaemia affects cells earlier in their maturation process, when they are closer to the undifferentiated stem cell (see Fig 29.1). There are four main leukaemias: acute myeloid leukaemia, chronic myeloid leukaemia, acute lymphoblastic leukaemia and chronic lymphoblastic leukaemia. Regardless of type, leukaemic cells have the capacity to invade the spleen, lymph nodes, liver and other vascular regions.

Presentation with leukaemia may be subtle or acute. Clinical manifestations include fatigue, fever and weight loss. The patient may also complain of bone pain. Elevated uric acid levels, lymph node enlargement, hepatomegaly and splenomegaly are usually present. Neurological findings include headache, vomiting, papillo-oedema and blurred vision. Some patients are simply diagnosed following routine blood tests, whereas others present with extremely elevated white blood counts in a critical condition. Treatment for acute leukaemia generally begins within 24 hours of diagnosis and can include chemotherapy, radiotherapy, bone marrow or stem cell transplantation, or a combination of these.

Lymphoma

In Australia, lymphoma is the leading form of haematological cancer, with almost 5000 people diagnosed per year.[32] In New Zealand non-Hodgkin's lymphoma is the sixth most commonly registered cancer, accounting for 3.7% of all new cancer registrations and 3.1% of all deaths from cancer.[31] Lymphomas are a heterogeneous group of disorders caused by malignant lymphocytes which usually accumulate in lymph nodes, leading to the characteristic clinical features of lymphadenopathy. They occasionally spill over into the blood or infiltrate organs outside the lymphoid tissue, and the normal structure of the lymph nodes is destroyed. The cause of lymphoma is not known; however, several key factors are thought to play a role in its development. These include infection with Epstein-Barr virus (EBV), genetic predisposition and exposure to occupational toxins such as herbicides, pesticides and benzene. Lymphomas are divided into Hodgkin's lymphoma (HL) and non-Hodgkin's lymphoma (NHL). A total of 85–90% of lymphomas are of the non-Hodgkin's variety[33] and do not generally carry as favourable a prognosis as HL. Five years after diagnosis, about 85% of people will have survived HL as opposed to 62% of people with NHL.[34]

Multiple myeloma

Multiple myeloma is a neoplastic proliferation of bone marrow plasma cells (a type of lymphocyte). These cells can be thought of as factories whose energy is devoted to producing a single immunoglobulin.[35] Myeloma involves overproduction of an abnormal immunoglobulin, known as a 'paraprotein', by the malignant plasma cell or lymphocyte. It is characterised by lytic bone lesions, plasma cell accumulation in the bone marrow and the presence of monoclonal protein in the serum and urine.[36] The cause of multiple myeloma is unknown, although exposure to radiation, organic chemicals (e.g. benzene), herbicides and insecticides may play a role, as may genetic factors and viral infection. Each year in Australia, approximately 1200 people are diagnosed with myeloma.[37] Overall it is a rare disease, accounting for 1.2% of all cancers diagnosed and 2% of cancer deaths.[38] Myeloma is uncommon in people under 40 years of age, with almost 80% of all new cases diagnosed in people over the age of 60. It occurs more frequently in men than in women, possibly because of greater occupational exposure to potential carcinogens.[39]

Disease-related emergencies of the leukaemias and lymphomas

Hyperviscosity syndromes

Derangement of the balance of cellular or non-cellular components of blood is a characteristic of the haematological malignancies. Excessive production of one protein or cell can lead to hyperviscosity of the blood which can cause leucostasis and inadequate organ perfusion—an emergency situation. Hyperviscosity may arise because of a massive increase in the cellular components of the blood, as in the case of acute leukaemia, or an increase in plasma proteins, as seen in multiple myeloma.

Hyperleucocytosis and leukaemia

Hyperleucocytosis (i.e. WBCs greater than 100×10^9/L) occurs as a presenting feature in a small proportion of new patients with acute leukaemia. Some 5–30% of adult patients with acute leukaemia and approximately 8% of children with acute lymphoblastic leukaemia will present in this way.[40,41] These patients have a 20–40% increased risk of death from severe pulmonary and neurological complications and have also been found to have a poorer response to chemotherapy than acute leukaemic patients who do not have hyperleucocytosis.[42]

Signs and symptoms

Hyperleucocytosis is a haematological emergency because it may result in leucostasis and consequently impaired organ perfusion. It is associated with the following symptoms:[43]

- neurological (headache, tinnitus, confusion, potential spontaneous cranial haemorrhage)
- anaemia (although patients should not be transfused until the hyperviscosity has been rectified)
- visual (retinal haemorrhage, blurred vision)
- renal failure

- respiratory failure
- severe metabolic abnormalities: hyperkalaemia, hyperphosphataemia, hyperuricaemia.

Management

Management of hyperviscosity requires immediate cytotoxic treatment and possibly apheresis. Apheresis is performed using a machine called a Cell Separator. The patient requires two large gauge cannulae or a double lumen central line. Blood is drawn off via one cannula or lumen and returned via the other. The anticoagulated blood is separated into different blood components by either centrifugation or membrane filtration. The undesired components are removed and the remaining 'depleted' blood reinfused, together with replacement fluid.[44] By reducing the number of circulating blasts, it is also hoped that further toxic sequelae resulting from commencing chemotherapy (e.g. tumour lysis syndrome) may be avoided.

Specific guidelines as to when apheresis should be performed are unclear. Some centres will perform apheresis when the leucocyte count is in excess of $200–400 \times 10^9$/L[41] and/or in the presence of metabolic abnormalities such as increasing serum lactate levels.[45] However, the role of apheresis in leucostasis has never been definitively proved in a randomised, controlled trial.[46] It has been argued that the procedure may not necessarily prevent death more efficiently than fluid therapy and the prompt initiation of chemotherapy.[42]

Hyperviscosity and multiple myeloma

Paraprotein proliferation may result in hyperviscosity of the plasma, especially in certain subtypes of myeloma such as Waldenström's macroglobulinaemia, which involves over-production of immunoglobulin M (IgM)—a very large protein. Hyperviscosity may be a presenting feature of the disease or may occur in its later stages.

Signs and symptoms

Signs and symptoms of hyperviscosity occur when plasma viscosity exceeds three times the normal value, and are similar to those of hyperleucocytosis. They include lassitude, confusion, blurred vision, dizziness, vertigo, diplopia and a bleeding tendency, especially oronasal bleeding. Patients may also present in renal failure due to congestion of the renal tubules.[47] Hyperviscosity occurs in less than 5% of myeloma patients but may be fatal if untreated and hence is classified as a haematological emergency.[48]

Management

Treatment is by therapeutic plasma exchange (TPE) in combination with chemotherapy. TPE (also used in the management of TTP, as described earlier in the chapter) involves the removal of a volume of diseased plasma and its replacement with healthy plasma or plasma substitute. The procedure uses the same apheresis machine that is used for hyperleucocytosis, but instead of removing white blood cells it removes plasma. Coagulation is checked pre- and post-procedure as replacement of clotting factors may be required.

Tumour Lysis Syndrome (TLS)

A small proportion of oncology patients will develop severe metabolic disturbances after commencing treatment for their disease—a condition known as tumour lysis syndrome (TLS).

The initiation of cytotoxic therapy—particularly in patients with a high tumour burden—brings about large-scale cellular death causing the release of potassium, phosphorus and nucleic acids into the blood stream. High-risk patients may go on to develop life-threatening hyperkalaemia, hyperphosphataemia, hypocalcaemia and hyperuricaemia. Identification of at-risk populations coupled with appropriate prophylactic treatment has reduced the incidence of this oncological emergency.[49] Futhermore, it is unlikely to be frequently encountered in the ED as it is generally a treatment-related issue, more commonly seen post-hospital admission, once therapy has commenced (ideally) on the ward.

Cord compression

Cord compression results from either an intradural or more commonly an extradural metastasis pressing onto the spinal cord. It is seen in up to 5% of cancer patients,[50] and is included here because it is an occasional complication of lymphoma, arising in approximately 3% of all systemic lymphomas.[50] It is also seen in myeloma and other metastatic cancers where there may be bone metastases.

In 85% of cases, cord damage arises from extension of a vertebral body metastasis into the epidural space, but other mechanisms of damage include vertebral collapse (e.g. secondary to lytic lesions in myeloma), direct spread of tumour through the intervertebral foramen (as is often found with lymphoma) and interruption of the vascular supply.[50]

Spinal cord compression is not immediately life-threatening in itself but can cause severe neurological morbidity.[51] Preservation of function is therefore the primary goal of therapy, and this is why it is classified as an emergency: intervention needs to be timely in order to avoid irreparable damage to the spinal cord.

Cord compression may be associated with metastatic disease or may be a presenting feature (e.g. with lymphoma). As a presenting feature it does not necessarily mean poor prognosis.[52] In the metastatic setting it is generally indicative of a poor prognosis, with a median survival rate of approximately 4 months from diagnosis.[53]

Signs and symptoms

Cord compression is not always easy to recognise—especially among children.[54] Symptoms are often put down to a number of other factors, especially in cases of advanced disease.

The most common presenting feature noted by 83–95% of patients before diagnosis is back pain.[55] This may sometimes be associated with root irritation creating a girdle or 'band' of pain that tends to be worse on coughing or straining. Increasing compression of the spinal cord is often—but not always—marked by improvement or resolution of the back pain.

Other neurological symptoms and signs can vary enormously according to the rapidity of development of the lesion and its location. Leg weakness indicates progressive spinal damage and may initially be described as a feeling of stiffness rather than weakness, with tingling and numbness starting in both feet and ascending the legs. Pain generally pre-dates the onset of weakness by some weeks. Whereas the onset of pain may be gradual, the onset of weakness is generally sudden.

Late neurological signs include urinary and bowel symptoms such as hesitancy, retention or constipation. Both urinary and bowel symptoms are suggestive of extensive cord damage, except if the lesion is at the level of the cauda equina.[56]

Assessment and management

Expedited radiological imaging is required for thorough assessment. Ideally this is with CT or magnetic resonance imaging (MRI), although for patients unable to tolerate these, plain X-rays can provide some information if there are gross changes to the spinal cord. Physical assessment should consist of regular neurovascular observations, and at paramedical or nursing hand-over time these should be conducted with the receiving clinician to maintain consistency. Any alterations or deterioration should immediately be communicated with the treating medical team. Treatment is generally with high-dose corticosteroids plus radiotherapy. Rarely, surgical approaches may be used. With some chemotherapy-sensitive tumours, such as Burkitt's lymphoma, chemotherapy and steroids are the treatment of choice.[51]

Prompt diagnosis and appropriate intervention in cases of cord compression can have significant impact on quality of life. Neurological status at the start of treatment is the most important factor influencing outcome: if treatment is started within 24–48 hours of onset of symptoms, neurological damage may be reversible. After palliative radiotherapy, about one-third of patients who were not mobile *but not paraplegic* before treatment will regain the ability to walk, but only 2–6% of patients *who were already paraplegic* will regain this ability.[57]

Superior vena cava syndrome

Superior vena cava syndrome (SVCS) refers to pressure on the superior vena cava that may arise from occlusion by extrinsic pressure, intraluminal thrombosis or direct invasion of the vessel wall. The result of this is reduced blood flow to the lungs and a backlog of blood in the venous circulation. Most commonly today SVCS results from a mediastinal malignancy (such as a lymphoma or lung cancer) or from the insertion of an intravascular device.[58] About 3% of patients with carcinoma of the bronchus and 8% of those with lymphoma will develop superior venal caval obstruction.[50]

In recent years it has been argued that SVCS is not, in fact, an oncological emergency because outcome is unrelated to duration of symptoms.[59] Nevertheless, it has been included here because traditionally it has been considered to be one, causing either death by airway obstruction from laryngeal and bronchial oedema or coma and death as a result of cerebral oedema.[60]

Signs and symptoms

The majority of patients present after having developed symptoms over days to weeks.[58] These include:

- neck swelling
- distended veins along chest
- shortness of breath
- hoarse voice
- swelling in one or both arms
- tracheal oedema and shortness of breath
- cerebral oedema with headache worse on stooping
- visual changes
- dizziness and syncope
- swelling of face, particularly periorbital oedema
- rapid breathing
- cyanosis.

Management

Initial management includes basic supportive measures such as elevating the head, providing oxygen and expedited transport to hospital. On arrival at hospital the mainstays of treatment include diuretics to reduce intravascular volume and at least a short course of parenteral steroids (dexamethasone, 4 mg every 6 hours) to decrease oedema and tumour burden. Both these therapies remain unproven.[58,60] CT or MRI scanning is used to identify the extent of tumour and is also useful for radiotherapy planning if this is the preferred treatment. Sometimes CT angiography is used to assess for thrombus formation.

PRACTICE TIP

Steroid therapy can be associated with sleep disturbance and it is therefore preferable to administer doses (where possible) earlier in the day. Avoid gastric irritation by administering with food or with some form of gastritis prophylaxis.

Further management is dependent on diagnosis and will require histology if this is the first presentation of disease. For potentially curable diseases such as lymphomas or germ cell tumours, chemotherapy and radiotherapy are often given. High-dose corticosteroids and surgical stenting of the superior vena cava are also treatment options.

Hypercalcaemia

Hypercalcaemia is defined as an increase in serum calcium > 1 mg/mL above the normal range.[61] The normal range for calcium varies between laboratories, but is generally between 2.2 and 2.5 mmol/L (8.5–10.2 mg/dL). As more than 50% of calcium binds to protein (principally albumin), albumin levels must also be considered when assessing calcium levels (Box 29.4).

Hypercalcaemia occurs in 20–30% of patients with cancer at some time during their disease, and its detection indicates a poor prognosis—approximately 50% of patients with hypercalcaemia will die within 30 days.[62] It is an oncological emergency because it can lead to serious renal toxicity and cardiac dysrhythmias which may be life-threatening. The condition is most commonly seen among patients with multiple myeloma: at diagnosis 25% of myeloma patients have serum calcium concentrations greater than 2.76 mmol/L (11.5 mg/dL) after correction for serum albumin;[47] it is also seen in patients with metastatic breast cancer, non-small-cell lung cancer and a number of other malignancies.[62]

Hypercalcaemia is caused by the inappropriate release of parathyroid hormone-related peptide (PTHrp) from tumour cells, resulting in a triad of processes: enhanced osteoclastic bone resorption, enhanced renal tubule reabsorption of calcium and enhanced intestinal absorption of calcium. These physiological changes bring about pathological bone fractures and other symptoms of hypercalcaemia.

Signs and symptoms

Signs and symptoms may be acute or gradual, but classically they include:

- polydipsia
- polyurea
- nausea and vomiting
- constipation
- loss of appetite
- depression
- apathy
- drowsiness
- somnolence
- confusion.

A rapid rise in calcium is more likely to produce marked neurological symptoms than a gradual one, and these may be exacerbated by sedatives or narcotics.[63] Hypercalcaemia causes renal tubular damage resulting in rising blood urea and creatinine levels. Patients are generally dehydrated as a result of their renal damage, worsened by decreased oral intake because of nausea, vomiting or both.[63] Elevated calcium levels also cause cardiac changes. An ECG reveals a shortened QT interval and the patient may develop dysrhythmias.[64]

Management

Prompt, effective therapy will minimise the severity of hypercalcaemia and reduce the possibility of renal failure.[47] Management involves:

- rehydration—200–500 mL/hr dependent on renal and cardiac status
- loop diuretics—but only when dehydration has been rectified
- medications—principally bisphosphonates such as pamidronate and zoledronic acid. The former has been used for longer, but takes 2 hours to administer as opposed to 15 minutes for zoledronic acid
- chemotherapy—the key to controlling hypercalcaemia is to control the malignant process, and therefore cytotoxic therapy must be commenced as soon as possible[63]
- dialysis—may be used in severe cases and with patients who are likely to respond to cancer therapy[63]
- calcitonin—reduces calcium levels by inhibiting bone resorption and increasing renal excretion, but resistance develops after repeated doses
- corticosteroids—sometimes helpful in haematological malignancies.

Treatment-related haematological emergencies

Cytotoxic chemotherapy

Oncologists and haematologists have embraced the trend towards shorter hospitalisations and increased ambulatory care. Many chemotherapy regimens that once required hospital

---

BOX 29.4 Corrected calcium (Ca) formula[61]

$$\text{albumin-corrected Ca (mmol/L)} = \text{total Ca (mmol/L)} + [0.02 \times (41.33 - \text{albumin (g/L)})]$$

The use of such formulae is, however, sometimes inaccurate and ionised calcium values are more reliable.

admission are now given to outpatients. The trend away from hospitalisation has been facilitated by a number of factors, such as:

- better drugs to control side effects of chemotherapy (e.g. better antiemetics)
- indwelling central lines such as portacaths and Hickman lines
- a change in philosophy which focuses more heavily on quality of life
- recognition that the hospital environment affords little protection against infections and is indeed the source of many
- availability of haematopoietic growth factors
- new treatment modalities such as peripheral blood stem cell transplantation which allow earlier discharge from hospital.

The result of this is that many more patients are managed at home and in haematology day-units. Unfortunately, when something untoward occurs out of hours, these units may be closed and the patients are inevitably directed to the ED.

Some patients will present to the ED with problems associated with their cytotoxic chemotherapy. This could be protracted nausea and vomiting, dehydration or diarrhoea. Such symptoms are managed with appropriate supportive care, as they would be with non-chemotherapy patients. Box 29.5 provides some information about management of patients who may present a cytotoxic risk to healthcare professionals.

Other oncology and haematology patients will present with more life-threatening treatment-associated problems. These are often sequelae of bone marrow suppression and are discussed in the following section.

Bone marrow suppression

The most common treatment-related complication among haematology patients today is bone marrow suppression as a result of cytotoxic chemotherapy regimens. While such regimens can also cause anaemia, this is rarely an acute problem and is generally monitored and managed in a routine manner in the ambulatory unit. Far more significant in the acute setting is the effect of chemotherapy on the WBC and platelet counts, which can drop to very low levels. Whereas neutropenia and thrombocytopenia per se are not considered to be emergencies, haemorrhage while thrombocytopenic or the acquisition of an infection during a neutropenic period (febrile neutropenia) are life-threatening situations. Management of the patient who is bleeding has already been discussed above. In the following section, management of the neutropenic patient with an infection is examined.

Febrile neutropenia

The normal WBC count is $4{-}10 \times 10^9$/L with neutrophils making up approximately 40–60% of this. There are several grades of neutropenia, the most profound of which is classified as Grade IV, meaning the neutrophil count is less than 0.5×10^9/L. The depth and duration of neutropenia is the principal factor determining whether a patient will acquire an infection, with most infections occurring when the neutrophil count falls below 0.1×10^9/L.[65,66] The risk of infection among haematology and oncology patients is further increased when there are other factors causing immunosuppression (Box 29.6).

It is not usually the aim of outpatient chemotherapy regimens to render the patient severely neutropenic, but it is a potential toxicity. This is especially the case in recent years during which doses of cytotoxics have been significantly increased to maximise efficacy. The neutrophil nadir can occur at any time from a few days to weeks post chemotherapy administration, depending on the agents used. Patients receiving chemotherapy are at greatest risk of becoming neutropenic following their first or second cycle.[67]

One of the most significant changes in haematology and oncology units over the last two decades has been in the management of the neutropenic patient. In the past neutropenia was treated with a great deal of mystique and units adopted complex practices to protect the patients from potential pathogens. These included measures such as protective isolation (isolating patients in positive-air-pressure rooms and restricting entrance into this protective environment to only a very few people); donning protective clothing when nursing patients with neutropenia (gown, mask, overshoes); restricting the diet of neutropenic patients so that they were exposed to minimal organisms, for example, omitting fresh fruit and salad.

Most of these measures were not evidence-based and today many centres have abandoned some or all of them. It is

---

BOX 29.5 Cytotoxic precautions

- Patients who are receiving infusional chemotherapy or have received chemotherapy within the last 48 hours may have cytotoxic residue in their blood, and therefore their body fluids should be treated as cytotoxic. This means avoiding handling body fluids (blood, urine, vomit, sputum) where possible. If contact is unavoidable, personal protective equipment should be used—cytotoxic gloves (purple), goggles and a cytotoxic gown (long-sleeved Tyvek gown).
- Note that it is only necessary to wear protective clothing if handling body fluids—otherwise, contact with the patient should be completely normal.
- Disposal of cytotoxic waste should be in the purple cytotoxic bin.

BOX 29.6 Risk factors for febrile neutropenia

- Disease process (especially with haematology patients)
- Mucosal integrity—mucositis is a potential toxicity from chemotherapy and increases the possibility of infection
- Presence of central venous catheters or other invasive devices
- Poor nutritional status
- Age and other immunocompromising factors
- Corticosteroid therapy (steroids and old age may mask the signs of infection, and so a patient may be septic without having a temperature)

instead recognised that the majority of infections developed by the neutropenic patient are caused by endogenous flora.[68] In hospitalised patients almost half of these infections are caused by organisms acquired during hospitalisation.[68] Manipulation of the environment to render it pathogen-free is no longer considered to be the solution to preventing infection in the neutropenic population. Strong evidence is, however, available in support of good hygiene.[69] Practitioners should be aware of and follow their institutional policies regarding care of the neutropenic patient, bearing in mind the particular importance of hand-washing.

Assessment and management

Most septic patients will present with a fever, although some will present with hypothermia, malaise or an isolated incidence of hypotension. An elevation in temperature during a neutropenic period is known as febrile neutropenia. This can be defined as a single temperature of > 38.3°C or ≥ 38°C over at least 1 hour and/or an absolute neutrophil count (ANC) of < 0.5 × 10^9 or of < 1.0 × 10^9 with predicted rapid decline to 0.5 × 10^9.[70]

Local policies may vary, but in general, management of oncology patients with febrile neutropenia requires a detailed history to be taken, determining the date of the last chemotherapy administration and the drugs used, an FBC to assess whether the patient is neutropenic and a set of blood cultures (see Box 29.7). In general, if the patient has an indwelling venous catheter and this is considered to be a likely source of infection, one set of cultures is taken from there and another from peripheral blood.[71] Sputum, urine and stool specimens should also be taken as soon as possible although it is sometimes impossible to obtain all of these before antibiotics commence.

National Cancer Institute data show that whereas in 1963 70% of cancer deaths were caused by infection, today the figure is less than 30%.[72] This improvement in mortality is because it is now recognised that antibiotic therapy needs to be implemented immediately for neutropenic septic patients. More than 70% of patients will respond to antibiotics if given within the first 24 hours, compared with only 22% if they are delayed to the third day following the development of symptoms.[73] For this reason, patients with febrile neutropenia should be treated with clinical urgency—generally as Australian Triage Scale category 2 (to be seen by a medical officer within 10 minutes; see Ch 13). However in spite of this, there is some evidence to suggest that these patients can wait for prolonged periods in the ED before treatment.[74]

Colony-stimulating factors such as granulocyte colony-stimulating factor (G-CSF) are sometimes added to accelerate neutrophil recovery, although this has not been found to necessarily improve survival for all patients with febrile neutropenia. It can, however, reduce the amount of time spent in hospital.[75]

PRACTICE TIP

Colony-stimulating factors administered to boost the neutrophil count are given as subcutaneous injections and are generally well tolerated. Toxicities include injection site reactions, arthralgias and myalgias, usually managed with paracetamol.

BOX 29.7 Practice tips for the febrile neutropenic patient

Assessment

If febrile neutropenia is suspected, outcome is significantly improved by expedited action. Remember that a neutropenic patient may not necessarily have a temperature but may still be septic; for example, paracetamol and corticosteroids can mask a temperature. Treat any abnormal signs with suspicion (e.g. confusion, decreased level of consciousness, hypotension, tachycardia, etc). Also:[77]

- note presence of indwelling venous catheter
- note symptoms or signs suggesting an infection focus
  - respiratory system
  - gastrointestinal tract
  - skin
  - perineal region/genitourinary discharges
  - oropharynx
  - central nervous system.

Investigations

- Blood testing—full blood count; electrolytes, urea and creatinine (EUC); coagulation; C-reactive protein (CRP)
- Blood cultures (minimum two sets), including cultures from indwelling venous catheter
- Urinalysis and culture
- Sputum microscopy and culture
- Stool microscopy and culture (if diarrhoea present)
- Skin lesions (aspirate/biopsy/swab)
- Chest X-ray
- It may be helpful to also take a cross-match at this time.

On some occasions there may be a delay in obtaining some samples (e.g. stool, sometimes chest X-ray). If delay is unavoidable and likely to be protracted, antibiotics should be commenced immediately.

Therapy

- Intravenous hydration and if necessary oxygen therapy should be commenced immediately.
- As soon as septic screen is completed, intravenous antibiotics should be given. It is important to start these as soon as possible—do not wait, for example, for the next scheduled dose time.
- Some institutions have programs treating neutropenic patients with oral antibiotics on an outpatient basis. These patients will have to meet certain criteria in order to establish that they are 'low risk' and institutional guidelines should be followed.

Sepsis

Unsuccessful management or late presentation of the febrile neutropenic patient will result in sepsis. The incidence of sepsis ranges from 50–300 cases per 100,000 population and it carries a short-term mortality of 20–25%, reaching to up to 50% when shock is present.[76] The phases of sepsis are defined in the 'septic syndrome' which can be seen as a continuum beginning with the systemic inflammatory response syndrome (SIRS) and culminating in septic shock[77] (Box 29.8). (See also Chs 20 and 27).

BOX 29.8 Sepsis definitions[77]

1. Systemic inflammatory response syndrome (SIRS) is the presence of two or more of the following:
   – temperature > 38°C or < 36°C
   – heart rate > 90 beats/minute
   – respiratory rate > 20 breaths/minute or a $PaCO_2$ < 32 mmHg
   – WBC count > 12.0×10^9/L or < 4.0×10^9/L or the presence of more than 0.10 immature neutrophils.
2. Sepsis in a patient with a documented infection.
3. Severe sepsis (the term 'sepsis syndrome' has been discarded) refers to sepsis complicated by organ dysfunction, as indicated by lactic acidosis, oliguria or an acute change in mental status.
4. Septic shock is defined as sepsis with hypotension, despite adequate fluid resuscitation, associated with hypoperfusion abnormalities that include, but are not limited to, lactic acidosis, oliguria or an acute alteration in mental status.

$PaCO_2$: arterial pressure of carbon dioxide; WBC: white blood cell

---

Just as the management of DIC is problematic because of a lack of high level evidence, so is the management of the septic patient. Both are critical conditions in which it is difficult to conduct multicentre randomised trials. A patient with sepsis is around five times more likely to die than a patient who has suffered a heart attack or stroke, and yet many still do not appreciate its seriousness.[79] Globally the incidence of sepsis continues to rise.[80]

A seminal study some years ago by Rivers et al[81] identified that the implementation of early goal-directed therapy resulted in better outcomes for septic patients. This means that potentially septic patients are monitored closely to ensure a number of important physiological endpoints (vital signs, urine output, etc) fall within specific ranges. If they do not then interventions are implemented *systematically* and *early*. Early sepsis intervention strategies are associated with increased survival rates with one life being saved for every seven treated. The Adult Sepsis Pathway is illustrated in Fig 29.4.

Optimal sepsis management involves timely *recognition*, *resuscitation* and *referral*.

- *Recognition* of the septic patient is facilitated by identifying risk factors such as:
  - increased respiratory rate
  - increased heart rate
  - decreased blood pressure
  - reduced urine output
  - alterations in temperature.
- *Resuscitation* involves provision of antibiotics within the first hour of recognition and administration of intravenous fluids.
- *Referral* of the patient to appropriate retrieval or in-patient teams is essential for optimal care.

Management

The 'Surviving Sepsis Campaign Guidelines for Management of Severe Sepsis and Septic Shock',[82] first formulated in 2008, were updated in 2013.[83] Some of the major recommendations for management of the severely septic or shock patient include:

- early resuscitation of the septic patient
- maintaining oxygen saturation at >95%
- monitoring respiratory rate, heart rate, blood pressure, oxygen saturation, temperature and fluid balance (see Ch 17 for techniques relating to these)
- administration of broad spectrum antibiotics within an hour of recognition of septic shock. Blood cultures should be sent before antibiotic therapy which should be commenced immediately without waiting for results
- fluid resuscitation with crystalloid—20 mL/kg stat followed by another 20 mL/kg if no response and no sign of pulmonary oedema. Aim to maintain MAP >65 mmHg and urine output >0.5 mL/kg/hr
- if no response to IV fluid, commencing vasopressors as per local policy
- imaging studies to promptly identify source of infection
- obtaining FBC, UEC, coagulation tests (coags), LFTs, glucose, cross-match and serial lactate levels
- avoidance of hydroxyethyl starch products
- avoiding use of intravenous hydrocortisone in adult septic shock patients
- haemoglobin target of 7–9 g/dL in the absence of tissue hypoperfusion, ischaemic coronary artery disease or acute haemorrhage
- monitoring patients' vital signs, level of consciousness and lactate levels regularly. Ongoing treatment will be dictated by the patient's response.

While acknowledging that the evidence base for some of these recommendations is limited, the level of consensus between committee members was high. Implementation of formal guidelines many provide a better-controlled environment for future clinical studies. Clearly identifying evidence-based guidelines is the key to optical clinical support for this patient group.

Blood-product administration in haematology patients

Within the ED, blood transfusion for trauma occurs frequently and is often massive. This may lead to problems such as coagulation imbalances, hypocalcaemia, hyper- and hypokalaemia and hypothermia (see Chs 20 and 44 for early management of trauma and massive transfusion protocols). For patients with haematological problems, an additional set of difficulties is presented. These are immunological considerations related to the frequency of these patients' exposure to blood products, rather than to the volumes infused.

Over the last decade there has been increased concern about the potential problems of blood product transfusion. It is now thought to contribute to organ dysfunction and transfusion-related acute lung injury in the acute setting. It seems to be particularly poorly tolerated in the critically ill, where sepsis, trauma, pneumonia or respiratory failure may stimulate an inflammatory response that is exacerbated by blood products.[85,86] Thus the decision to transfuse should not be undertaken lightly.[87] In order to reduce the risks of repeated transfusion, it has been found that it is safer to restrict blood transfusions to situations in which the haemoglobin level is < 70 g/L—even among ED patients.[88,89]

Frequent blood transfusion may be required for patients with haematological diseases, either as primary therapy or to support treatment-related toxicities. In the past it was necessary to use special leucocyte filters when administering blood products to certain groups of haematology patient. Today all blood products in Australasia are leucodepleted prior to arriving on the ward and so this is no longer necessary—standard blood-giving sets are adequate. Chronic blood transfusion has a number of other damaging sequelae including iron overload, a small risk of allo-immunisation (despite leucocyte depletion) and the very small risk of transmission of infection (despite modern screening

methods). These are discussed more fully below, and some nursing guidelines are outlined in Box 29.9.

Haemolytic blood-transfusion reactions

Major blood incompatibility is an infrequent but potentially lethal event occurring when the recipient has anti-A or anti-B antibodies that react with the transfused cells, resulting in a haemolytic transfusion reaction. The risk of an ABO-incompatible transfusion being administered is thought to be 1:100,000.[87,90] Most major transfusion incompatibilities are the result of human error.[91]

Management strategies for haemolytic blood transfusions rest with prevention. Each hospital adopts its own policies, generally based on the guidelines set out by the Australian and New Zealand Society of Blood Transfusion (ANZSBT).[92] Guidelines apply to all stages of the transfusion procedure from taking the cross-match sample to administering the final product.

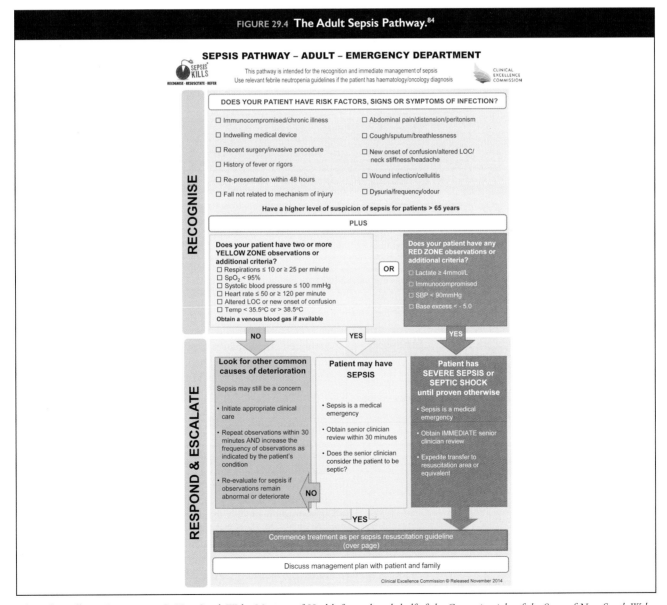

FIGURE 29.4 **The Adult Sepsis Pathway.**[84]

Clinical Excellence Commission, © New South Wales Ministry of Health for and on behalf of the Crown in right of the State of New South Wales, http://www.cec.health.nsw.gov.au/programs/sepsis/sepsis-tools?

Continued

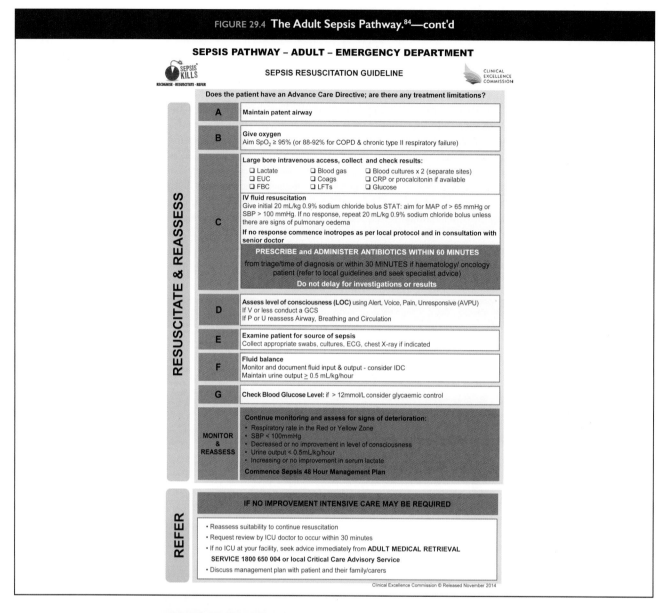

FIGURE 29.4 **The Adult Sepsis Pathway.**[84]—cont'd

SEPSIS PATHWAY – ADULT – EMERGENCY DEPARTMENT

SEPSIS RESUSCITATION GUIDELINE

Does the patient have an Advance Care Directive; are there any treatment limitations?

RESUSCITATE & REASSESS

A — Maintain patent airway

B — Give oxygen
Aim SpO₂ ≥ 95% (or 88-92% for COPD & chronic type II respiratory failure)

C — Large bore intravenous access, collect and check results:
- Lactate
- EUC
- FBC
- Blood gas
- Coags
- LFTs
- Blood cultures x 2 (separate sites)
- CRP or procalcitonin if available
- Glucose

IV fluid resuscitation
Give initial 20 mL/kg 0.9% sodium chloride bolus STAT: aim for MAP of > 65 mmHg or SBP > 100 mmHg. If no response, repeat 20 mL/kg 0.9% sodium chloride bolus unless there are signs of pulmonary oedema
If no response commence inotropes as per local protocol and in consultation with senior doctor

PRESCRIBE and ADMINISTER ANTIBIOTICS WITHIN 60 MINUTES
from triage/time of diagnosis or within 30 MINUTES if haematology/ oncology patient (refer to local guidelines and seek specialist advice)
Do not delay for investigations or results

D — Assess level of consciousness (LOC) using Alert, Voice, Pain, Unresponsive (AVPU)
If V or less conduct a GCS
If P or U reassess Airway, Breathing and Circulation

E — Examine patient for source of sepsis
Collect appropriate swabs, cultures, ECG, chest X-ray if indicated

F — Fluid balance
Monitor and document fluid input & output - consider IDC
Maintain urine output ≥ 0.5 mL/kg/hour

G — Check Blood Glucose Level: if > 12mmol/L consider glycaemic control

MONITOR & REASSESS — Continue monitoring and assess for signs of deterioration:
- Respiratory rate in the Red or Yellow Zone
- SBP < 100mmHg
- Decreased or no improvement in level of consciousness
- Urine output < 0.5mL/kg/hour
- Increasing or no improvement in serum lactate
Commence Sepsis 48 Hour Management Plan

REFER

IF NO IMPROVEMENT INTENSIVE CARE MAY BE REQUIRED

- Reassess suitability to continue resuscitation
- Request review by ICU doctor to occur within 30 minutes
- If no ICU at your facility, seek advice immediately from **ADULT MEDICAL RETRIEVAL SERVICE 1800 650 004 or local Critical Care Advisory Service**
- Discuss management plan with patient and their family/carers

Clinical Excellence Commission © Released November 2014

BOX 29.9 Blood-product transfusion[91,101]

- The standard blood-component-giving set should be primed with blood component or Normal saline—not dextrose.
- One giving set is used for 2–4 units of blood or up to 8 in the emergency setting, but should be changed every 8 hours.
- A RBC-giving set should never be subsequently used for platelets because the red cell debris in the filter would trap the platelets.
- Blood-giving sets should never be 'piggy-backed'.
- Medications should never be given through a blood-component-giving set.
- Platelets aggregate if static and therefore should be agitated until administered to the patient.

RBC: red blood cell

Cross-matching of blood aims to identify and prevent potential incompatibilities. The cross-matching procedure involves testing a specimen of the patient's blood to identify their ABO and Rhesus groups. Next, an antibody screen is performed to determine whether they have antibodies to any other red cell antigens. Approximately 3% of samples obtained for cross-match contain an unexpected antibody.[93] The final cross-match testing involves mixing the patient's serum with the donor blood red cells and inspecting to see if there is agglutination.

The sooner a transfusion reaction is detected, the more effective intervention is likely to be. Traditionally, transfusions have been monitored through the taking of 'blood obs'. Most centres have regional recommendations for the taking of observations during a transfusion, although there is some variation between centres.[91] The ANZSBT[92] recommendations state that the patient should be closely observed for signs of a transfusion reaction, particularly for the first 15 minutes following commencement of the unit of blood. In the event of a reaction, the steps that should be taken are outlined in Box 29.10.

BOX 29.10 Steps to be taken in the event of a blood-transfusion reaction[91]

The most common adverse transfusion outcome is a rise in the patient's temperature. This may be due to the transfusion or incidental and as a result of the patient's underlying illness. A temperature rise to >38°C or >1°C above baseline (if baseline >37°C) should prompt the interruption of the transfusion and a clinical assessment of the patient.

The following could be considered signs of a mild transfusion reaction:

- Isolated temperature rise <1.5°C above baseline without any signs of a serious reaction (including any of those listed below)
- Localised rash/pruritis.

If a mild transfusion reaction is suspected:

- **STOP the transfusion**
- maintain IV access
- monitor and record the patient's temperature, pulse, respirations and blood pressure
- repeat all clerical and identity checks of the patient and blood pack
- contact medical staff immediately for further management and investigation.

If the temperature rise is <1.5°C above baseline or the patient has only localised rash or pruritis, the patient observations are stable and the patient is otherwise well, an antipyretic or antihistamines may be administered at the discretion of the doctor and the transfusion then continued with caution and close observation. If signs or symptoms persist, develop or deteriorate subsequently, STOP the transfusion and manage as for a severe transfusion reaction (following).

Moderate to severe transfusion reactions

Any of the following could be considered signs of a moderate to severe transfusion reaction:

- Temperature ≥1.5°C above baseline
- Hypotension/shock OR hypertension
- Tachycardia
- Tachypnoea, wheeze, stridor
- Rigors or chills
- Nausea, vomiting or pain (local, chest, back).

If a moderate or severe transfusion reaction is suspected the following steps MUST be undertaken:

- **STOP the transfusion immediately and seek urgent medical advice;** Medical Emergency Team (MET) support may be required, depending on the specific clinical situation.
- Maintain venous access using a new administration set and 0.9% sodium chloride (normal saline), but do not discard the blood administration set and do not flush the original line.
- Repeat all clerical and identity checks of the patient and blood pack.
- Immediately report the reaction to the transfusion service provider, who will advise on returning the implicated product and administration set, and any further blood or urine samples required from the patient.
- Monitor and record the patient's temperature, pulse, respirations and blood pressure.
- Record the volume and colour of any urine passed (looking for evidence of haemoglobinuria).

PRACTICE TIP

The recommendations made by the ANZSBT[92] are that vital signs are taken at the beginning of each unit and at the end of the transfusion episode. The patient should be monitored closely for the first 15 minutes. The timing for taking vital signs after this is discretionary and should be guided by the clinical condition of the patient.

Non-haemolytic transfusion reactions

A non-haemolytic transfusion reaction can be defined as an increase in body temperature of at least 1°C within 4 hours of the onset of transfusion.[93] These reactions are not exclusive to blood transfusions and are also seen with platelets. They are mediated by proteins and cytokines released from the breakdown of leucocyte contaminants in stored blood products and can occur in up to 30% of transfusions among patient populations who require chronic transfusion support.[93] Non-haemolytic transfusion reactions are much less common since leucodepletion of blood products was introduced. Typically, reactions may be characterised by a rash or mild broncho-constriction. Rare but severe responses include subglottic oedema, severe bronchoconstriction and anaphylaxis with cardiovascular collapse.

Non-haemolytic reactions can be managed by pre-medication with steroid and antihistamine 'cover' prior to infusion. Patients who experience repeated reactions may also be given 'washed' blood.

Platelet allo-immunisation

Repeated exposure to leucocytes and other contaminants of transfusion can lead to the recipient developing antibodies to the platelet antigens on donor platelets. Such patients become refractory to platelet transfusions (i.e. the patient fails to achieve a therapeutic platelet increment post transfusion).[93] Leucodepletion of blood products and minimising transfusions reduces the risk of this occurring. Such patients may also require HLA-matched (human leucocyte antigen) platelets in order to avoid an immune reaction.

Transmission of infection via blood products

Cytomegalovirus (CMV) is a virus in the herpes family which may lie dormant in the tissues and leucocytes of infected people. Many healthy individuals have been exposed to it and carry CMV antibodies. Some people, however, have never had exposure and have no immunity to the virus. Primary exposure to the virus during a period of extreme immunosuppression such as a course of chemotherapy could result in CMV-associated gastroenteritis, retinitis, pneumonia or hepatitis. At-risk haematology patients who are CMV-negative should receive CMV-negative blood. Blood for transfusion is screened for HIV and hepatitis C; however, there is still debate as to whether the neurodegenerative disease Creutzfeldt-Jakob disease (CJD) is transmitted via blood components[92] and there are no screening tests for this yet.[87]

Graft-versus-host disease

Even leucodepleted, packed cells may still retain some donor lymphocytes which, on rare occasions, proliferate within the recipient's bloodstream, recognising the recipient as foreign and mounting an immune response. Graft-versus-host disease (GVHD) will typically become manifest 10–12 days after the transfusion; the symptoms include diarrhoea, skin rashes, abnormal liver function tests and ultimately bone marrow failure. GVHD is a particular problem for the immuno-suppressed, and for this reason at-risk populations such as bone marrow or peripheral blood stem cell transplant patients receive irradiated blood products. The irradiation renders inactive any viable lymphocytes in the transfusion.

Venous access

Many oncology and haematology patients are exposed to multiple venepunctures and their veins subsequently become scarred and difficult to cannulate. Intensive chemotherapy regimens for haematology patients today often require insertion of an indwelling venous catheter. The development of indwelling central venous catheters has revolutionised cancer treatment by facilitating intensive, long-term chemotherapy regimens, infusional chemotherapy and venous access in patients without the need for repeated cannulations. As a result, many oncology, and particularly haematology, patients who present to the ED will have a central venous device of some description.

Central venous access devices vary between institutions, but include untunnelled central venous catheters (single-, double- or triple-lumen), tunnelled central venous catheters (e.g. Hickman lines), peripherally inserted central catheter (PICC)

lines and surgically implanted devices (e.g. portacaths). The devices are similar in that they consist of a long venous catheter which is inserted under sterile conditions into the vena cava or top part of the right atrium. Catheters are designed to remain in situ for weeks to months. Policies developed for accessing lines should be put into place in the ED, taking into consideration the recommended practices outlined in Box 29.11.[94–97] See Chapter 17 for techniques on applying central venous catheters (p. 346).

BOX 29.11 Vascular access policies[95–97]

- Dressing the exit site of the line—tunnelled lines are ultimately left undressed. Non-tunnelled lines may be dressed with gauze or transparent polyurethane dressings; there are currently no clear data as to which is better.
- Infection-control practices in accessing the line—hand hygiene is required prior to using the line and the bung should be decontaminated using alcohol solution prior to use.[26]
- Flushing the line—there are now data to suggest that flushing with saline is as effective as flushing with low-dose heparin.
- 'Heparin locking'—some institutions 'lock' the line by injecting small volumes of high-dose heparin into it when de-accessing.
- Anticoagulation policies—some centres prescribe low-dose warfarin (1 mg/day) for patients with indwelling central venous catheters. This practice is probably safe among patients who are otherwise well, although most of the newer studies do not support it as a method of reducing thrombosis.

SUMMARY

Because of a general shift towards outpatient care, haematology patients are using emergency services more frequently. Some of the disease- and treatment-related complications of this population have been discussed here. ED clinicians will be faced with acute complications of chronic disorders as well as newly-presenting haematology patients. Management of the former calls for particular sensitivity as these patients are well versed in their disease and often have strong opinions as to its management. Management of the latter requires a good

understanding of the physiology of blood and of supportive care.

Particularly important areas for ED professionals include the management of neutropenic sepsis and the competent administration of blood products. Changes in haematological treatment strategies coupled with a growing awareness of quality-of-life issues is likely to further involve ED healthcare professionals in the management of haematology populations in the years to come.

CASE STUDY

Michael's partner called 000 for an ambulance when he came home to find Michael 'shaking all over' and 'in a terrible state'. Michael was 46 years old and had been diagnosed with non-Hodgkin's lymphoma 6 months previously. He

was receiving chemotherapy (CHOP-14) and had been given his fourth cycle in the haematology outpatients unit 5 days before. Until his lymphoma diagnosis, Michael had been quite well, apart from occasional asthma which was mild and controlled with a salbutamol inhaler without the need for any other medication. His chemotherapy to date had been uneventful except for some venous access problems—he was told that he had 'difficult veins'. For this reason a portacath had been inserted prior to his last chemotherapy cycle. The portacath was not currently accessed.

Paramedical staff arrived to find Michael in bed, experiencing a rigor. He was conscious, but slightly disorientated and confused (Glasgow Coma Scale score 14). His vital signs were:

- temperature 35.6°C
- pulse 120 beats/minute
- blood pressure 90/40 mmHg
- respiratory rate 30 breaths/minute
- oxygen saturation 92%

His partner, John, was present. He was anxious and a little verbally aggressive. He was insistent that the patient be taken immediately to the Haematology and Oncology Ambulatory Care Unit for assessment by his haematology team. He was confident that 'they will fix him up—they know him and have all his records'.

The paramedics assessed the patient and considered it likely that he was neutropenic and septic. They provided supplementary oxygen and attempted to insert a peripheral cannula in order to fluid-resuscitate. Not only were Michael's veins scarred and difficult to cannulate, but he was also peripherally shut-down. After three unsuccessful attempts, the paramedic team decided to expedite the patient to hospital (the closest hospital was 5 minutes away). They felt he was acutely unwell and needed to be transported straight to ED.

On arrival at the ED, the patient was given a triage category 2 and transferred to a resuscitation bay. Cardiac monitoring was commenced, O_2 therapy was applied and vital signs and a GCS were recorded. A full blood count, EUC, clotting screen, lactate, cross-match and blood cultures were taken. The results confirmed that Michael was indeed neutropenic (neutrophils $0.4 \times 10^9/L$) and also thrombocytopenic (platelets $34 \times 10^9/L$). Another three attempts were made to insert a peripheral cannula—one in his foot—but this was unsuccessful.

Michael's blood pressure had now fallen to 80/35 mmHg, his pulse was 130 beats/minute and his temperature 38.5°C. He remained conscious and responsive, but a little disorientated (GCS 14). Adequate venous access was urgently required for antibiotics, fluid replacement and possibly blood products. The nurse caring for Michael

contacted the ambulatory chemotherapy unit to see if someone could access his portacath and shortly after this a nurse arrived and was able to do this. This nurse also advised the ED staff that Michael had experienced a severe platelet transfusion reaction on a previous occasion and that pre-medication with hydrocortisone and antihistamine would be recommended if he required platelets.

Fluids were commenced immediately and antibiotics (as per institutional policy) were 'piggy-backed' on to the IV line. The haematology team had by this time attended and prescribed 5 units of irradiated platelets. These were given stat (half an hour after the prescribed pre-medication) and after the first litre of fluid had finished. By this time Michael's blood pressure was improving. No other intravenous products were 'piggy-backed' with the platelets.

The nurse who put up the platelets was concerned that she was unable to draw blood back from the portacath and so contacted the chemotherapy nurse. She was reassured, however, that this particular central venous access device was 'temperamental' and did not always 'draw back'. She documented this in the patient's notes.

A bed was found on the haematology ward and Michael was transferred there when haemodynamically stable. By this time he was afebrile and showed no signs of confusion. No obvious focus for the infection was ever found and the blood cultures came back negative. Michael was discharged home 5 days later when his blood counts recovered and his fever abated. His next cycle of chemotherapy was delayed and dose-reduced.

Questions

1. Where was the most appropriate place for the paramedics to take this patient? Could the paramedics have taken any additional steps to improve his care on transferring him to the hospital?

2. What signs raised the paramedic's suspicion that Michael may be (a) neutropenic and (b) septic?

3. Michael needed fluids, platelets and intravenous antibiotics. In what order should these be given and why?

4. Should the nurse have used the portacath in view of the fact that she could not draw blood back?

5. How would the nurse have recognised that Michael was having a platelet transfusion reaction, and what should she do?

6. Could this whole hospital admission have been prevented. If so, how?

USEFUL WEBSITES

Transfusion www.transfusion.com.au/

Haematological disorders

www.haemophilia.org.au

www.haemophilia.org.nz

www.lymphoma.org.au/

www.allg.org.au

www.leukaemia.org.nz

www.spleen.org.au

Sepsis www.cec.health.nsw.gov.au

REFERENCES

1. Widmaier EP, Raff H, Strang KT. Vander's human physiology, 12th edn. McGraw Hill, 2011.
2. Kitchen G. Immunology and haematology. Edinburgh: Mosby; 2012.
3. Patton KT & Thibodeau GA, Anatomy and physiology, 8th edn, St Louis: Mosby, 2013.
4. Lewis SM, Collier IC, Heitkemper MM. Medical–surgical nursing: assessment and management of clinical problems. 7th edn. St Louis: Mosby; 2007.
5. Newberry L, ed. Sheehy's emergency nursing. 5th edn. St Louis: Mosby; 2003.
6. Shelton BK, Rome SI, Lewis SL Nursing assessment: haematological system. In: Brown D, Edwards H, eds. Lewis's medical–surgical nursing. Sydney: Elsevier; 2008.
7. Lind M, Vernon C, Cruickshank D et al. The level of haemoglobin in anaemic cancer patients correlates positively with quality of life. Br J Cancer 2002;86(8):1243–9.
8. Maclaren H. Anaemia. In: Cameron P, Jelinek G, Kelly A-M et al, eds. Textbook of adult emergency medicine. Sydney: Elsevier; 2009.
9. Teoh Y, Greenway A, Savola H et al. Hospitalisations for sickle cell disease in Australian Paediatric Population. J Paediatr Child Health 2013;49(1);68–71.
10. Kanter J, Kruse-Jarres R. Management of sickle cell disease from childhood through adulthood. Blood Reviews 2013;27(6):279–87.
11. Blinder M, Vekeman F, Sasane M. ISPOR 18th Annual International Meeting Research Abstracts Age-related emergency department reliance (EDR) and health care resource utilization in patients with sickle cell disease (SCD). Value in Health. 2013;16(3):A198.
12. De D. Acute nursing care and management of patients with sickle cell. Br J Nurs 2008;17(13):819–23.
13. National Confidential Enquiry into Patient Outcome and Death. A sickle crisis? A report of the National Confidential Enquiry into Patient Outcome and Death. UK: NCEPOD; 2008.
14. Estcourt L, Stanworth S, Doree C et al. Prophylactic platelet transfusion for prevention of bleeding in patients with haematological disorders after chemotherapy and stem cell transplantation. Cochrane Database Syst Rev. 2012;5:CD004269.
15. Kitchen G. Immunology and haematology. Edinburgh: Mosby; 2007:113–15.
16. Rodak BF, Fritsma GA, Keohane EM. Haematology. Clinical principles and applications. Elsevier Saunders, 2012.
17. Veyradier A, Meyer D. Thrombotic thrombocytopenic purpura and its diagnosis. J Thromb Haemost 2005;3(11):2420–7.
18. Cox D, Coyer F. A case study of thrombotic thrombocytopenic purpura: a 'powerful poison'. Aust Crit Care 2004;17(2):54–64.
19. Patel A, Patel H, Patel A. Thrombotic thrombocytopenic purpura: the masquerader. South Med J 2009;102(5):504–9.
20. Elliott EJ, Ridley GF, Hodson EM et al. Interventions for haemolytic uraemic syndrome and thrombotic thrombocytopenic purpura. Cochrane Database Syst Rev CD003595; 2009.
21. Haemophilia Foundation Australia. Fast Facts. Online: www.haemophilia.org.au/bleedingdisorders/cid/27/parent/0/pid/1/t/bleedingdisorders/title/fast-facts; accessed 20 Nov 2013.
22. Haemophilia Foundation of New Zealand. Online. www.haemophilia.org.nz/page.php?onClickbd=bd&page_id=16; accessed 20 Nov 2013.
23. Levi M, Ten Cate H. Disseminated intravascular coagulation. N Engl J Med 1999;341(8):586–92.
24. Dhainaut JF, Shorr AF, Macias WL et al. Dynamic evolution of coagulopathy in the first day of severe sepsis: relationship with mortality and organ failure. Crit Care Med 2005;33(2):341–8.
25. Levi M. Disseminated intravascular coagulation. Crit Care Med 2007;35(9):2191–5.
26. Toh CH, Dennis M. Disseminated intravascular coagulation: old disease, new hope. Br Med J 2003;327(7421):974–7.
27. Horwitz L. Disseminated intravascular coagulation First Consult. Elsevier. Revised: 25 Oct 2012.
28. Levi M. Current understanding of disseminated intravascular coagulation. Br J Haematol 2004;124(5):567–76.
29. Bernard GR, Vincent JL, Laterre PF et al. Efficacy and safety of recombinant human activated protein C for severe sepsis. N Engl J Med. 2001;344(10):699–709.
30. Vincent JL The rise and fall of drotrecogin alfa (activated). Lancet Infectious Diseases 2012;12(9):649–51.
31. New Zealand Health Information Service. Online. www.health.govt.nz/publication/cancer-new-registrations-and-deaths-2010; accessed 19 Nov 2013.

32. Australian Institute of Health and Welfare. Online. www.aihw.gov.au/cancer/data/acim_books/leukaemia.xls; accessed 19 Nov 2013.

33. Australian Institute of Health and Welfare. Cancer survival and prevalence in Australia—cancers diagnosed from 1982–2004. Cancer Series no. 42. Canberra: AIHW; 2008.

34. Leukaemia Foundation. Fact sheet: lymphomas; 2008. Online. http://leukaemia.org.au/fileadmin/dl-docs/factsheets2/FactSheet_LF_Lymphomas.pdf; accessed 1 Dec 2009.

35. Hillman RS, Ault KA. Haematology in clinical practice. 3rd edn. New York: McGraw-Hill; 2002:284.

36. Hillman RS, Ault KA. Haematology in clinical practice. 3rd edn. New York: McGraw-Hill; 2002:215.

37. Australian Institute of Health and Welfare. ACIM (Australian Cancer Incidence and Mortality) books. AIHW: Canberra; 2007.

38. Leukaemia Foundation. Myeloma. Fast sheet: myeloma; 2008. Online. www.leukaemia.org.au/fileadmin/dl-docs/factsheets2/FactSheet_LF_Myeloma.pdf; accessed 1 Dec 2009.

39. Lope V, Perez-Gomez B, Aragones N et al. Occupation, exposure to chemicals, sensitizing agents and risk of multiple myeloma in Sweden. Cancer Epidemiol Biomarkers Prev 2008;17(11):3123–7.

40. Majhail NS, Lichtin AE. Acute leukemia with a very high leukocyte count: confronting a medical emergency. Cleve Clin J Med 2004;71(8):633–7.

41. Lowe EJ, Pui CH, Hancock ML et al. Early complications in children with acute lymphoblastic leukemia presenting with hyperleukocytosis. Pediatr Blood Cancer 2005;45(1):10–15.

42. Porcu P, Farag S, Marcucci G et al. Leukocytoreduction for acute leukaemia. Ther Apher 2002;6(1):15–23.

43. Haut C. Oncological emergencies in the pediatric intensive care unit. AACN Clin Issues 2005;16(2):232–45.

44. Zarkovic M, Kwaan HC. Correction of hyperviscosity by apheresis. Semin Thromb Hemost 2003;29(5):535–42.

45. Stemmler J, Wittmann GW, Hacker U et al. Leukapheresis in chronic myelomonocytic leukaemia with leukostasis syndrome: elevated serum lactate levels as an early sign of microcirculation failure. Leuk Lymphoma 2002;43(7):1427–30.

46. Ganzel C, Becker J, Mintz PD et al. Hyperleukocytosis, leukostasis and leukapheresis: Practice management. Blood Reviews 2012;26(3):117–22.

47. Hussein MA, Oken MM. Multiple myeloma, macroglobulinemia, and amyloidosis. In: Furie B, Cassileth PA, Atkins MB et al, eds. Clinical hematology and oncology: presentation diagnosis and treatment. Edinburgh: Churchill Livingstone; 2003:581–600.

48. Drew MJ. Therapeutic plasma exchange in hematologic diseases and dysproteinemias. In: McLeod BC, Price TH, Weinstein R, eds. Apheresis: principles and practice. 2nd edn. Bethesda, MD: AABB Press; 2003:345–73.

49. Will A, Tholouli E. The clinical management of tumour lysis syndrome in haematological malignancies. Brit J Haematol 2011;154:3–13.

50. Falk S, Fallon M. ABC of palliative care: emergencies. Br Med J 1997;315(7121):1525–8.

51. Matsubara H, Watanabe K, Sakai H et al. Rapid improvement of paraplegia caused by epidural involvements of Burkitt's lymphoma with chemotherapy. Spine (Phila Pa 1976) 2004;29(1):E4–6.

52. Chahal S, Lagera JE, Ryder J et al. Hematological neoplasms with first presentation as spinal cord compression syndromes: a 10-year retrospective series and review of the literature. Clin Neuropathol 2003;22(6):282–90.

53. Guo Y, Young B, Palmer JL et al. Prognostic factors for survival in metastatic spinal cord compression: a retrospective study in a rehabilitation setting. Am J Phys Med Rehabil 2003;82(9):665–8.

54. Grattan-Smith PJ, Ryan MM, Procopis PG. Persistent or severe back pain and stiffness are ominous symptoms requiring prompt attention. J Paediatr Child Health 2000;36(3):208–12.

55. Abrahm JL, Banffy MB, Harris MB. Spinal cord compression in patients with advanced metastatic cancer: all I care about is walking and living my life. JAMA 2008;299(8):937–46.

56. Frewin R, Henson A, Provan D. ABC of clinical haematology: haematological emergencies. Br Med J 1997;314(7090):1333–6.

57. Prasad D, Schiff D. Malignant spinal-cord compression. Lancet Oncol 2005;6(1):15–24.

58. Cheng S. Superior vena cava syndrome: a contemporary review of a historic disease. Cardiol Rev 2009;17(1):16–23.

59. Gauden SJ. Superior vena cava syndrome induced by bronchogenic carcinoma: is this an oncological emergency? Aust Radiol 1993;37:363–6.

60. Rowell NP, Gleeson FV. Steroids, radiotherapy, chemotherapy and stents for superior vena caval obstruction in carcinoma of the bronchus. EBM Reviews—Cochrane Database of Systematic Reviews Cochrane Lung Cancer Group Cochrane Database of Systematic Reviews 4, 2012.

61. Ariyan CE, Sosa JA. Assessment and management of patients with abnormal calcium. Crit Care Med 2004;32(4 Suppl):S146–54.

62. Shepard MM, Smith JW. Hypercalcemia. Am J Med Sci 2007;334(5):381–5.

63. Stewart AF. Hypercalcemia associated with cancer. N Engl J Med 2005;352(4):373–9.

64. Richman S. Hypercalcaemia. In: Furie B, Cassileth PA, Atkins MB et al, eds. Clinical hematology and oncology: presentation diagnosis, and treatment. Edinburgh: Churchill Livingstone;2003:191–5.

65. Bodey G. Infections in patients with cancer. In: Holland JF, Frei E, eds. Cancer medicine. Philadelphia: Lea and Febinger;1982:1339–72.

66. Bodey GP, Buckley M, Sathe YS et al. Quantitative relationships between circulating leukocytes and infection in patients with acute leukemia. Ann Intern Med 1966;64:328–40.

67. Lyman GH, Kuderer NM. The economics of the colony-stimulating factors in the prevention and treatment of febrile neutropenia. Crit Rev Oncol Hematol 2004;50(2):129–46.

68. Schimpff SC, Young VM, Greene WH et al. Origin of infection in acute nonlymphocytic leukemia: significance of hospital acquisition of potential pathogens. Ann Intern Med 1972;77:707–14.

69. Nirenberg A, Bush AP, Davis A et al. Neutropenia: state of the knowledge Part II. Oncol Nurs Forum 2006b;33(6):1202–8.

70. Infectious Disease Society of America. Guidelines for the use of antimicrobial agents in neutropenic patients with cancer. Clin Infect Dis 2002;34:730–51.

71. Cohen J, Brun-Buisson C, Torres A et al. Diagnosis of infection in sepsis: an evidence-based review. Crit Care Med 2004;32(11 Suppl): S466–94.

72. Katz JT, Baden LR. Febrile neutropenia. In: Furie B, Cassileth PA, Atkins MB et al, eds. Clinical practice of hematology and oncology. Edinburgh: Churchill Livingstone; 2003:1173–8.

73. Bodey GP, Jadeja L, Elting L. Pseudomonas bacteremia: retrospective analysis of 410 episodes. Arch Intern Med 1985;145:1621–9.

74. Nirenberg A, Mulhearn L, Lin S et al. Emergency department waiting times for patients with cancer with febrile neutropenia: a pilot study. Oncol Nurs Forum 2004;31(4):711–15.

75. Clark OA, Lyman G, Castro AA et al. Colony stimulating factors for chemotherapy induced febrile neutropenia. 2009 Cochrane Database of Systematic Reviews 4.

76. Annane D, Bellissant E, Cavaillon JM. Septic shock. Lancet 2005;365(9453):63–78.

77. ACCP/SCCM. American College of Chest Physicians/Society of Critical Care Medicine Consensus Conference: definitions for sepsis and organ failure and guidelines for the use of innovative therapies in sepsis. Crit Care Med 1992;20(6):864–74.

78. Marti Marti F, Cullen MH, Roila F (ESMO Working Group). Management of febrile neutropenia: ESMO clinical recommendations. Ann Oncol 2009;20(4):iv166–9.

79. Reinhart K, Daniels R, Kisson N et al. The burden of sepsis—a call to action in support of World Sepsis Day. J Crit Care 2013;28(4):526–8.

80. Hall MJ, Williams SN, DeFrances CJ et al. Inpatient care for septicemia or sepsis: a challenge for patients and hospitals. NCHS data brief. Hyattsville, MD: National Center for Health, Statistics; 2011:62.

81. Rivers E, Nguyen B, Havstad S et al. Early goal directed therapy in the treatment of severe sepsis and septic shock. The New England Journal of Medicine 2001;345(19):1368–77.

82. Dellinger RP, Levy MM, Carlet JM et al. Surviving sepsis campaign: international guidelines for management of severe sepsis and septic shock. Crit Care Med 2008;36(1):296–327.

83. Dellinger RP, Levy MM, Rhodes A et al. Surviving sepsis campaign: international guidelines for management of severe sepsis and septic shock: 2012. Crit. Care Med. Feb 2013;41(2):580–637.

84. Clinical Excellence Commission, © New South Wales Ministry of Health for and on behalf of the Crown in right of the State of New South Wales, http://www.cec.health.nsw.gov.au/programs/sepsis/sepsis-tools; accessed 5 June 2015.

85. Gong MN, Thompson BT, Williams P et al. Clinical predictors of and mortality in acute respiratory distress syndrome: potential role of red cell transfusion. Crit Care Med 2005;33(6):1191–8.

86. Jackson WL, Shorr AF. Blood transfusion and the development of acute respiratory distress syndrome: more evidence that blood transfusion in the intensive care unit may not be benign. Crit Care Med 2005;33(6):1420–1.

87. Davis K, Hui CH, Quested B. Transfusing safely: a 2006 guide for nurses. Aust Nurs J 2006;13(6):17–20.

88. Hill SR, Carless PA, Henry DA et al. Transfusion thresholds and other strategies for guiding allogeneic red blood cell transfusion. Cochrane Database Syst Rev 1 18 April 2005.

89. McIntyre L, Hebert PC, Wells G et al. Is a restrictive transfusion strategy safe for resuscitated and critically ill trauma patients? J Trauma 2004;57(3):563–8.

90. Stainsby D, Russell J, Cohen H et al. Reducing adverse events in blood transfusion. Br J Haematol 2005;131:8–12.

91. Australian and New Zealand Society of Blood Transfusion. Guidelines for the administration of blood components. Australia: ANZSBT; 2004. Online: www.anzsbt.org.au/publications/documents/AdminGiudelinesOct2004.pdf.

92. Angelbeck JH, Ortolano GA. Universal leukocyte reduction. J Infus Nurs 2005;28(4):273–81.

93. Wilkinson J, Wilkinson C. Administration of blood transfusions to adults in general hospital settings: a review of the literature. J Clin Nurs 2001;10(2):161–70.

94. ANZICS 2012 'Central Line Insertion and Maintenance Guideline' Australian and New Zealand Intensive Care Society Publication (see www.clabsi.com.au and www.anzics.com.au)

95. Gillies D, O'Riordan L, Carr D et al. Gauze and tape and transparent polyurethane dressings for central venous catheters. Cochrane Database Syst Rev 1 most recent update 29 Aug 2003.

96. Kuter DJ. Thrombotic complications of central venous catheters in cancer patients. Oncologist 2004;9:207–16.

97. Stevens LC, Haire WD, Tarantolo S et al. Normal saline versus heparin flush for maintaining central venous catheter patency during apheresis collection of peripheral blood stem cells (PBSC). Transfus Sci 1997;18:187–93.

98. Brack S. Nursing management of haematological problems. In: Lewis SM, Collier IC, Heitkemper MM, eds. Medical–surgical nursing: assessment and management of clinical problems. 7th edn. St Louis: Mosby;2007:709.

99. Maclaren H. Anaemia. In: Cameron P, Jelinek G, Kelly A et al, eds. Textbook of adult emergency medicine. 3rd edn. Edinburgh: Churchill Livingstone; 2009.

100. Dalainas I. Pathogenesis, diagnosis and management of disseminated intravascular coagulation: a literature review. Europ Rev Med Pharmacol Sci 2008;12(1):19–31.

101. van der Meer PF, Gulliksson H, AuBuchon JP et al. Interruption of agitation of platelet concentrates: effects on in vitro parameters. Vox Sang 2005;88:227.

CHAPTER 30
TOXICOLOGICAL EMERGENCIES
IOANA VLAD AND KANE GUTHRIE

Essentials

- A standardised approach to the management of all poisonings allows the appropriate use of interventions in a timely, sequential manner.
- The risk assessment is of prime importance in guiding subsequent management decisions.
- Acute poisoning is a dynamic presentation, and deterioration can usually be predicted and managed effectively.
- Attention to airway, breathing and circulation will ensure the survival of the vast majority of patients.
- Antidotal therapy is occasionally used in the resuscitation phase of acute poisoning, but more often is considered after immediate life-threats have been treated.

INTRODUCTION

Clinical toxicology is a rapidly expanding area of core knowledge for paramedics and nurses working in emergency care. While virtually any agent ingested at sufficient dose is potentially toxic, so too all agents have a threshold dose below which they are relatively harmless; hence the need to have a thorough understanding of common agents and their particular toxic kinetics.

Demographics and common presentations

poisonings may occur across the spectrum of the population. In 2009–10 poisonings accounted for approximately 6% of all admissions to Australian hospitals and approximately 2.1% of emergency department (ED) admissions. The most common substances involved were anti-epileptic, sedative-hypnotic and psychotropic drugs (39% of cases). Benzodiazepines were the most commonly involved (16%), followed by antidepressants (5%) and antipsychotics (5%). In 2007, New Zealand data showed that the incidence of self-harm was approximately 64 per 100,000. Of these, the most common form of self-harm was self-poisoning.[1-4] New Zealand Health Information Service data documented 2678 hospitalisations for deliberate self-poisonings in 2007. The highest percentage of deliberate self-poisonings were patients in the 15–19-year-old group (15%).[5-8]

Accidental overdose may occur as a result of lack of information regarding the substance, causing incorrect dosage or the ingestion of substances that are contraindicated. Confusion—such as in the early stages of dementia—may lead to a person taking larger doses than prescribed. Prescribed medications that have a therapeutic range pose risks, if not monitored carefully, of a rise above the therapeutic dose to a toxic level. Misuse of regular medication such as digitalis, lithium or warfarin may lead to a toxicological presentation.

Children generally fall under the accidental exposure category, either by incorrect dosage or because the inquisitive child gains access to a dangerous substance. However, within the adolescent age group deliberate overdose is becoming more common.[9] Approximately 50 Australian children present per week with toxicology-related presentations: 7 out of 10 of these are ingestion of medication; these data correspond with the New Zealand data relating to presentations of children under 5 years.[4,8,10]

The effective management of toxicology patients requires a systematic approach of resuscitation, followed by the formulation of a risk assessment that guides all further management decisions. An appropriate approach to assessment and management is outlined in Box 30.1.

Out-of-hospital management of the poisoned patient

Deliberate or accidental poisoning is a common cause of altered mental state or presentation to hospital. This should always be considered prior to departing the scene, particularly in the unconscious patient. If any empty packets or containers of chemical are found at the scene, they should be placed in a bag and brought to hospital with the patient.

Poisoned patients who require out-of-hospital resuscitation should be managed along the same lines as other critically unwell patients, with some specific differences:

- In cardiac arrest due to tachydysrhythmias after hydrocarbons abuse (e.g. glue sniffing), the pathophysiological mechanism is myocardial sensitisation to catecholamines, so adrenaline administration should be avoided. In hospital settings, beta-blockers are used in the treatment of these ventricular tachydysrhythmias.
- In patients poisoned with paraquat, decontamination takes priority over resuscitation. In these patients, oxygen

should be avoided, unless the oxygen saturation drops below 90%. If this occurs, oxygen administration is titrated to achieve saturation not higher than 91%.

- Glucagon has no role in the management of hypoglycaemia secondary to poisoning. Dextrose should always be used to treat hypoglycaemia in the poisoned patient.

Decontamination is the priority in ingested paraquat poisoning, when food or soil should be administered at the scene to decrease gastric absorption. Fuller's earth is traditionally recommended, but it is not readily available and has no advantage over activated charcoal.

If transporting a patient whose skin or clothes are contaminated, normal personal protective equipment (PPE—gown, gloves, and safety glasses) should be worn.

Triaging of the poisoned patient

The triage of the poisoned patient is a vital part in the assessment and management. The aim of triaging the poisoned patient is to risk stratify a given overdose to predict clinical deterioration and potential for complications. Triaging the poisoned patient is often a complex task due to the subjective nature of triage and the confounding factors that often go along with deliberate self-harm, including psychiatric backgrounds, behavioural components and suicidality of the patient, which can often make it difficult to take a history and confirm medication and doses taken. To effectively and competently triage a poisoned patient the triage nurse needs to possess excellent history-taking skills, have a high index of suspicion and use resources available to them. FACEMs, pharmacists and calling the Poisons Information Centre (Australia 13 11 26 or New Zealand 0800 POISON/0800 764 766) can all be of assistance.

High risk triage pitfalls to be aware of:

- cardiac medications (beta-blockers, calcium channel blockers)
- heavy metals (lithium, iron, potassium)
- oral hypoglycaemic agents, insulin
- organophosphates
- paraquat
- unusual chemicals
- sustained release preparation
- paediatric presentations.

Resuscitation

Poisoning is a leading cause of death in patients under the age of 40 years and is high in the differential diagnosis when cardiac arrest occurs in a young adult. Unlike cardiac arrest in the older population, resuscitation following acute poisoning may be associated with good neurological outcomes, even after prolonged periods (hours) of cardiopulmonary resuscitation (CPR). Thus, while poisoning is considered part of the differential diagnosis in a patient with cardiac arrest, resuscitation should continue until expert advice can be obtained. Attempts at decontamination of the skin or gastrointestinal decontamination almost never take priority over resuscitation and institution of supportive care measures (except for paraquat poisoning). Therefore, clinicians should wear appropriate PPE, including gown, gloves, goggles and appropriate mask, at all times. Depending on the toxic substance, higher levels of PPE may be needed, which ultimately may require staff specially

---

BOX 30.1   Risk assessment-based approach to poisoning[12]

Resuscitation
- Airway
- Breathing
- Circulation
- Control seizures
- Correct hypoglycaemia
- Correct hyperthermia
- Consider resuscitation antidotes

Risk assessment
- Agent
- Dose

Time since ingestion
- Clinical features and course
- Patient factors

Supportive care and monitoring

Investigations
- Screening—12-lead ECG, paracetamol
- Specific investigations
- Decontamination
- Enhanced elimination
- Antidotes
- Disposition

trained in hazardous material decontamination (see Ch 28). In these instances, topical decontamination becomes a priority.

Airway, breathing and circulation

Acute poisoning is a dynamic medical illness and patients may deteriorate within minutes or hours of presentation. Altered level of consciousness, loss of airway protective reflexes and hypotension are common threats to life in the poisoned patient. As in all life-threatening emergencies, attention to airway, breathing and circulation are paramount and ensures the survival of the vast majority of patients.

Clinical scores such as the Glasgow Coma Scale (GCS) or Alert-Verbal-Pain-Unresponsive (AVPU) system, although commonly used to describe a patient's mental status, have never been validated in poisonings. A patient's ability to guard their airway is not well correlated to the GCS and may change dramatically in a short period of time. An increased risk of aspiration has been noted with GCS scores of less than 12.[11]

Control of seizures

Toxic seizures are generalised, and can usually be controlled with intravenous benzodiazepines (e.g. diazepam, midazolam, lorazepam or clonazepam). Barbiturates are second-line therapy for refractory seizures in acute poisoning and pyridoxine is a third-line agent that may be indicated in intractable seizures secondary to isoniazid. Phenytoin is not indicated in the management of seizures related to acute poisoning.

The presence of focal or partial seizures indicates a focal neurological disorder that is either a complication of poisoning or the result of a non-toxicological cause, and further investigation is required.

Venlafaxine, tramadol and amphetamines are the most common causes of seizures in poisoned patients in Australasia.

Hypoglycaemia

Hypoglycaemia is an easily detectable and correctable cause of significant neurological injury. Bedside serum glucose estimation should be performed as soon as possible in all patients with altered mental status.

If the serum glucose is less than 4.0 mmol/L, 50 mL of 50% dextrose should be given intravenously (5 mL/kg of 10% dextrose in children) to urgently correct hypoglycaemia.

Insulin, sulfonylureas, beta-blockers, quinine, chloroquine, salicylates and valproic acid are the most common causes of hypoglycaemia in poisoned patients in Australasia.[12]

Hyperthermia

Hyperthermia is associated with a number of life-threatening acute poisonings and is associated with poor outcome. A temperature > 38.5°C during the resuscitation phase of management is an indication for continuous core temperature monitoring. A temperature > 39.5°C is an emergency that requires immediate management to prevent multiple organ failure and neurological injury. Neuromuscular paralysis with intubation and ventilation leads to a cessation of muscle-generated heat production and a rapid reduction of temperature.

Antidotes

Administration of antidotes is sometimes indicated during the resuscitation phase of management. Examples include intravenous sodium bicarbonate ($NaHCO_3$) in tricyclic antidepressant poisoning, naloxone in severe opioid intoxication, digoxin-specific antibody fragments in suspected digoxin intoxication and high-dose insulin euglycaemic therapy in severe calcium channel blocker poisoning.

Risk assessment

Risk assessment should occur as soon as possible in the management of the poisoned patient. Only resuscitation takes a greater priority. It is the pivotal step in predicting the likely clinical course and potential complications.[13] The five key components of the history and examination required to construct a risk assessment are listed in Box 30.2.

All subsequent management steps (supportive care and monitoring, investigations, decontamination, enhanced elimination, antidotes and disposition) are determined by the risk assessment. Patients with a normal mental status are generally able to give a good history from which an accurate risk assessment can be constructed. If altered mental status precludes obtaining a direct history, back-up strategies are employed to gather necessary information. These include:

- asking paramedics or family to search for agents
- counting tablets to determine quantity missing
- checking medical records for previous prescriptions
- questioning relatives about agents potentially available to the patient
- findings on clinical examination, such as the presence of track marks and transdermal patches.

Under these circumstances, the risk assessment is less accurate and may, at least initially, be based on a 'worst-case scenario'. This is commonly the case with small children where ingestion is rarely witnessed. As the clinical course progresses, the risk assessment and management plan are refined.

In unknown ingestions, the patient's clinical status is correlated with knowledge of the agents commonly prescribed in that geographical area. For example, central nervous system (CNS) and respiratory depression associated with miotic pupils would indicate opioid intoxication in a young adult male in urban Australia, but is more likely to indicate organophosphate intoxication in rural Australia.

The agent, dose and time since ingestion should correlate with the patient's current clinical status. If they do not, the risk assessment needs to be revised. Acute poisoning is a dynamic process and important decisions can often be made at particular time-points. For example, following deliberate self-poisoning with a tricyclic antidepressant, life-threatening events occur within 6 hours (and usually within the first 2 hours) of ingestion. Therefore, low-risk patients can be identified on clinical grounds at 6 hours post-ingestion. By contrast,

---

BOX 30.2 Steps for construction of a risk assessment

Takes into account:
1. Agent(s)
2. Dose(s)
3. Time since ingestion
4. Clinical features and progress
5. Patient factors (weight and co-morbidities)

following deliberate self-poisoning with sustained-release calcium channel blockers, patients may not exhibit clinical features of poisoning during the first few hours. Indeed, the risk assessment anticipates delayed severe cardiovascular effects.

In the majority of cases, risk assessment allows early recognition of medically trivial poisonings. This reassures attending staff, family and patient, and prevents unnecessary investigations, interventions and observation. Supportive care may be instituted and early psychosocial assessment and discharge planning may begin. This usually shortens hospital length of stay. Less commonly, but very importantly, risk assessment allows early identification of potentially serious poisoning and the implementation of a tailored proactive management plan. Balanced decisions about gastrointestinal decontamination can be made and appropriate investigations selected. If a specialised procedure or antidote might be required in the next few hours, early communication and disposition planning should begin.

Supportive care

Following resuscitation and risk assessment, supportive care and disposition planning can begin.

Poisoning morbidity and mortality usually results from the acute effects of the toxin on the cardiovascular, central nervous or respiratory systems. Support of these and other systems for the duration of the intoxication will ensure a good outcome in the vast majority of acute poisonings. Monitoring of the clinical status is essential to detect the progress of the intoxication and the timing of the institution, escalation and withdrawal of supportive care and other measures.

An initial period of close observation in the ED is usually appropriate. During this time the patient's clinical status is monitored closely to ensure that it correlates with the previous risk assessment. If early complications are expected (e.g. decreased level of consciousness requiring intubation in the following 2 hours), preparations can be made to secure the airway as soon as the intoxication declares itself, and before the patient is moved elsewhere. If unexpected deterioration occurs at any time, the clinician's priorities revert to resuscitation prior to revising the risk assessment. To ensure a comprehensive assessment is ongoing the patient should have:

- regular intervals of assessment of vital signs—the timeframe is determined by the severity of the presentation and the potential risks of the toxic substance
- cardiac monitoring until it is established that there is no further risk for cardiac complications (see Ch 17, p. 336, for cardiac monitoring techniques)
- neurological assessment
- haemodynamic monitoring including fluid input and urine output (see Ch 17, p. 345, for haemodynamic monitoring techniques)
- general physical assessment for signs such as diaphoresis, rashes or injuries caused through seizures or agitation
- psychological assessment to determine ongoing risks of self-harm or risks which may develop for psychotropic toxins.

If specific complications are anticipated, the chosen inpatient clinical area must be resourced to detect and manage them. The accuracy and skill of the initial management and risk assessment are wasted if the subsequent plan of management is not documented and communicated to the treating team.

Good practice includes the documentation of a comprehensive management plan that informs the team looking after the patient of:

- expected clinical course
- potential complications according to the individual risk assessment
- type of observation and monitoring required
- endpoints that must trigger notification of the treating doctor or further consultation
- management plans for agitation or delirium
- criteria for changing management
- risk of developing venous thromboembolism in certain groups, mainly due to coma and prophylaxis should be provided early in the clinical course
- patients at risk for coma/drowsiness should have regular pressure care attended to
- bladder care urinary retention is common (anticholinergic effects)
- psychosocial risk assessments with a contingency plan should the patient attempt to abscond prior to formal psychosocial assessment.

The emergency observation unit is appropriate for the ongoing management of most acute poisonings, where the general supportive measures outlined below can be provided.

Criteria for admission to the *emergency observation unit* following acute poisoning include:

- ongoing cardiac monitoring not required
- patient not displaying agitated behaviour
- clinical deterioration not anticipated.

Criteria for admission to the *intensive care unit* following acute poisoning include requirements for:

- airway control
- ventilation
- prolonged or invasive haemodynamic monitoring or support
- haemodialysis.

Investigations

Investigations in acute poisoning are employed either as screening tests or for specific purposes.

Screening tests

Screening refers to the performance of a medical evaluation and/or diagnostic test in asymptomatic persons in the hope that early diagnosis may lead to improved outcome. In the acutely poisoned patient, screening tests aim to identify occult toxic ingestions for which early specific treatment is indicated. The recommended screening tests for acute poisoning are the 12-lead electrocardiogram (ECG) and the serum paracetamol level.

The ECG is a readily available non-invasive tool that assists in the identification of potentially lethal cardiac conduction abnormalities, such as those seen in tricyclic antidepressant cardiotoxicity.

Paracetamol is a ubiquitous analgesic in the Western world. Deliberate self-poisoning with paracetamol is common, comprising up to 15% of adult poisoning presentations in Australia. Life-threatening paracetamol poisoning may be occult in the early stages and death can be prevented by timely administration of *N*-acetylcysteine. For this reason, it is advisable to

BOX 30.3 Indications for specific investigations

To:
- refine risk assessment or prognosis
- exclude or confirm an important differential diagnosis
- exclude or confirm an important specific poisoning
- exclude or confirm a complication that requires specific management
- establish an indication for antidote administration
- establish an indication for institution of enhanced elimination
- monitor response to therapy or define an endpoint for a therapeutic intervention.

TABLE 30.1 Gastrointestinal decontamination

POTENTIAL BENEFITS	POTENTIAL RISKS
Improved clinical outcome (morbidity and mortality)	Pulmonary aspiration
More benign clinical course requiring lower level of supportive care	Distraction of staff from resuscitation and supportive care priorities
Reduced need for other potentially hazardous interventions or expensive antidotes	Gastrointestinal complications – bowel obstruction – perforation
Reduced hospital length of stay	Diversion of departmental resources for performance of procedure

screen for paracetamol in all cases of known or suspected acute deliberate self-poisoning. The screening paracetamol level may be performed at presentation and does not need to be delayed until 4 hours after ingestion. A non-detectable paracetamol level greater than 1 hour after ingestion excludes significant paracetamol ingestion and further paracetamol level tests are not required.

If paracetamol poisoning is suspected after the initial risk assessment, then a screening paracetamol level check is not required. Instead, a timed paracetamol level should be performed as soon as possible after 4 hours post-ingestion.

Specific investigations

After appropriate risk assessment and the institution of supportive care, the patient may require no further investigation beyond the screening ECG and serum paracetamol measurement. Other investigations are ordered selectively as shown in Box 30.3.

Serum drug levels are indicated for only a few agents. These include lithium, salicylate, iron, theophylline, digoxin and CNS depressants such as sodium valproate, carbamazepine and barbiturates.

Qualitative urine screens for drugs of abuse (e.g. opioids, benzodiazepines, amphetamines, cocaine, barbiturates and cannabinoids) rarely alter the management of the acutely poisoned patient.[14] Patients with acute intoxication with one or more of these agents may be managed according to their clinical presentation. A positive result from a patient without corresponding symptoms of intoxication rarely alters acute medical management. Electrolyte levels are a common assessment and are useful for identifying other underlying pathology; beta human chorionic gonadotrophin (beta-hCG) is useful for establishing pregnancy status, and urinalysis for assessing underlying pathology or the potential of rhabdomyolysis causing myoglobinuria associated with some toxic substances. Other pathology investigations will depend on the presentation and may include renal and liver function tests, full blood count (FBC) and arterial/venous blood gases (see Ch 17, p. 329, for details on collecting arterial blood gases). Abdominal X-ray may be requested for evaluating radio-opaque substances such as iron, lithium, lead or arsenic (refer to Box 30.3).

Gastrointestinal decontamination

Historically, various methods have been employed in the reasonable expectation that by reducing the dose absorbed they will also reduce the subsequent severity and duration of clinical

toxicity. The Australian Poisons Information Centre and the New Zealand National Poisons Centre are available 24 hours a day and should be consulted for the most current treatment protocols for specific poisons.

Unfortunately, the tendency has been to overestimate the potential benefits while underestimating the potential hazards of gastrointestinal decontamination procedures. These procedures do not provide significant benefit when applied to unselected deliberately self-poisoned patients and are no longer considered routine. The decision to decontaminate is one of clinical judgement in which the potential benefits are weighed against the potential risks and the resources required to perform the procedure (see Table 30.1).

By employing this rationale, gastrointestinal decontamination is reserved for cases where the risk assessment predicts severe or life-threatening toxicity and where supportive care or antidote treatment alone is insufficient to ensure a satisfactory outcome. Before proceeding, there should be reasonable grounds to believe that a significant amount of agent remains unabsorbed and is amenable to removal by the selected procedure. This requires some knowledge of the absorption kinetics of the agent(s) involved. For most ingested agents, absorption is virtually complete within 1 hour.

Gastrointestinal decontamination is never performed to the detriment of basic resuscitation or supportive care. To avoid pulmonary aspiration, the procedure is not performed without first securing the airway in a patient with a depressed level of consciousness or where the risk assessment indicates a potential for imminent seizures or decline in level of consciousness.

Single-dose activated charcoal

Oral activated charcoal consists of fine porous particles suspended in water or sorbitol. It reversibly adsorbs most ingested toxins and prevents them from being further absorbed by the gastrointestinal tract. However, it does not improve clinical outcome when applied to unselected patients with self-poisoning and should not be regarded as routine.[15]

Oral activated charcoal is indicated where it is likely that toxin remains in the gastrointestinal tract (within the first hour for most agents), and where the potential benefits outweigh the potential risks (see Table 30.1).

TABLE 30.2 Agents poorly bound to activated charcoal

HYDROCARBONS AND ALCOHOLS	METALS	CORROSIVES
Ethanol	Lithium	Acids
Isopropyl alcohol	Iron	Alkalis
Ethylene glycol	Potassium	
Methanol	Lead	
	Arsenic	
	Mercury	

Activated charcoal is contraindicated if:

- risk assessment indicates good outcome with supportive care and antidote therapy alone
- risk assessment suggests potential for imminent onset of seizures or decreased level of consciousness
- there is decreased level of consciousness, delirium or poor patient compliance (unless airway protected by endotracheal intubation)
- the agent ingested is poorly adsorbed to charcoal (see Table 30.2).

The major risk is charcoal pulmonary aspiration due to loss of airway reflexes associated with impaired level of consciousness or seizures. There are no data to support the use of activated charcoal in sorbitol or another cathartic agent over activated charcoal in water.

Induced emesis

Emptying the stomach by inducing emesis has long been a tradition in clinical toxicology. However, the benefits of administration rarely, if ever, outweigh the risks of induced vomiting and its use is no longer advocated.

Gastric lavage

Gastric lavage involves the sequential administration and aspiration of small volumes of fluid from the stomach via an orogastric tube to empty the stomach of toxic substances. This previously widely favoured method of gastrointestinal decontamination has now been all but abandoned and few EDs remain experienced in its use.

The amount of toxin removed by gastric lavage is unreliable and negligible if performed after the first hour. There are few situations where the expected benefits of this procedure might be judged to exceed the risks involved and where administration of charcoal would not be expected to provide equal or greater efficacy of decontamination.

Whole-bowel irrigation

This aggressive and labour-intensive form of gastrointestinal decontamination attempts to cleanse the entire bowel by administering large volumes of osmotically-balanced poly-ethylene glycol–electrolyte solution (PEG-ELS). It is rarely performed because risk–benefit analysis reserves this intervention for life-threatening ingestions of sustained-release preparations or other agents, as outlined in Box 30.4.

Nursing care of whole-bowel irrigation

- Dedicated area
- 1:1 nursing care

BOX 30.4 Conditions in which whole-bowel irrigation may be potentially useful

- Iron overdose > 60 mg/kg
- Slow-release potassium chloride ingestion > 2.5 mmol/kg
- Life-threatening slow-release verapamil or diltiazem ingestions
- Symptomatic arsenic trioxide ingestion
- Lead ingestion
- Body packers

BOX 30.5 Techniques of enhanced elimination and amenable agents

Multiple-dose activated charcoal
- Carbamazepine
- Dapsone
- Phenobarbitone
- Theophylline
- Quinine
- Amanita phalloides mushroom

Haemodialysis and haemofiltration
- Lithium
- Metformin lactic acidosis
- Potassium
- Salicylate
- Theophylline
- Toxic alcohols
- Valproic acid

Urinary alkalinisation
- Phenobarbitone
- Salicylate
- MCPA (herbicide)

Charcoal haemoperfusion
- Theophylline

- Place nasogastric tube (NGT) and confirm placement
- Give activated charcoal 50 g or 1 g/kg in children via NGT if it is an agent that binds to activated charcoal
- Commence polyethylene glycol electrolyte solution (PEG-ELS) at a rate of 2 litres per hour
- Keep hydrated
- Position patient on a bedside commode if possible as they will develop diarrhoea
- Monitor until passing clear liquid stools (it may take several hours).

Enhanced elimination

Techniques of enhanced elimination (see Box 30.5) are employed to increase the rate of removal of an agent with the aim of reducing the severity and duration of clinical intoxication. These interventions are indicated if they reduce mortality, length of stay, complications or the need for other more invasive interventions. In practice, these techniques are useful only in the treatment of poisoning by a few agents that are characterised by:

- severe toxicity
- poor outcome despite good supportive care and antidote administration
- slow endogenous rates of elimination
- suitable pharmacokinetic properties.

Enhanced elimination is never carried out to the detriment of resuscitation and good supportive care, and once the decision is made to initiate a technique of enhanced elimination, it is essential to establish clinical or laboratory endpoints for therapy.

Multiple-dose activated charcoal

Repeated administration of oral activated charcoal progressively fills the gut lumen with charcoal. This enhances the elimination of agents that enter the enterohepatic circulation and those that are lipid-soluble with low protein binding and have a small volume of distribution (see Box 30.5).

Potential complications of administering multiple-dose activated charcoal include all those associated with single-dose activated charcoal, with the added risk of mechanical bowel obstruction.

Urinary alkalinisation

The production of an alkaline urine pH promotes the ionisation of highly acidic drugs and prevents their reabsorption across the renal tubular epithelium, thus promoting excretion in the urine. For this method to be effective the drug must be filtered at the glomerulus, have a small volume of distribution and be a weak acid (e.g. salicylate overdose).

Antidotes

Antidotes are drugs that correct the effects of poisoning. Contrary to popular belief, there is not an antidote for every poison. In fact, only a few exist and these are used for a limited number of poisonings, with many being used extremely rarely (e.g. chelating agents). Like all pharmaceuticals, antidotes have specific indications and contraindications, and optimal administration methods, monitoring requirements, appropriate therapeutic endpoints and adverse effect profiles.

An antidote is administered when the potential therapeutic benefit is judged to exceed the potential adverse effects, cost and resource requirements. While some antidotes, such as naloxone and benzodiazepines, are commonly used, many antidotes are rarely prescribed, expensive and not widely stocked. Planning for the stocking, storage, access, monitoring, training and protocol development are essential components of rational antidote use.[16] It is often appropriate for stocking to be coordinated on a regional basis in association with regional policies concerning the treatment of poisoned patients. It is frequently cheaper and safer to transport an antidote to a patient rather than vice versa. Commonly used antidotes are discussed with their specific target drugs in the following pages.

Disposition

A medical disposition is required for all patients who present with poisoning or potential exposure to a toxic substance. Those who have deliberately self-poisoned also require psychiatric and social review. Patients must be admitted to an environment capable of providing an adequate level of monitoring and supportive care and, if appropriate, where staff and resources are available to undertake decontamination, administration of antidotes or enhanced elimination techniques. Early risk assessment in the out-of-hospital setting, usually by poisons information centre staff, often allows non-intentional exposures to be observed outside of the hospital environment. For those who present to hospital, this can minimise the duration and intensity of monitoring. Frequently patients can be 'cleared' for medical discharge directly from the ED immediately following assessment or following a few hours of monitoring. At other times the risk assessment will indicate the need for ongoing observation, supportive care or the need for specific enhanced elimination techniques or antidote administration. Under these circumstances, the patient must be admitted to an environment capable of providing a level of care appropriate for the anticipated clinical course. In many hospitals in Australia, this is now the emergency observation unit rather than the general medical ward. Where ongoing airway control, ventilation or advanced haemodynamic support is required, then admission to an intensive care unit is appropriate.

PRACTICE TIPS

- Risk assessment, after resuscitation, is the most important step in the management of the poisoned patient as it determines subsequent management steps and patient disposition.
- Call the Poisons Information Centre (13 11 26 in Australia or 0800 POISON/0800 764 766 in New Zealand) when dealing with a time-critical toxicological emergency or for any toxicology advice.
- Meticulous supportive care and monitoring is sufficient to ensure a good outcome in most poisonings.
- Perform paracetamol levels and an electrocardiogram as screening tests in the poisoned patient.
- Gastrointestinal decontamination, enhanced elimination techniques and specific antidotes are rarely required, but in specific circumstances may be life-saving.
- Most episodes of acute poisoning are an exacerbation of an underlying psychosocial disorder, which may determine the patient's final disposition.
- Administration of sodium bicarbonate prior to intubation may prevent deterioration from progressive acidosis in sodium channel blocker toxicity (e.g. tricyclic antidepressants).
- Absence of oral or lip burns does not exclude significant gastro-oesophageal injury following corrosive ingestions.
- Consider cyanide toxicity in the collapsed patient with severe lactic acidosis, especially following a house fire.

Commonly ingested agents
Alcohol and toxic alcohols
Ethanol

Ethanol ingestion causes rapid, dose-related CNS depression, with a high degree of inter-individual variability. The dose may be estimated if the number of standard drinks consumed is known. A standard drink contains approximately 10 g ethanol, which is equivalent to a 375 mL can of mid-strength beer (3.5%), a 100 mL glass of wine or a 30 mL shot of spirits.

Co-ingestion of other CNS depressants (e.g. sedative–hypnotic agents, opioids, antidepressants) increases the risk of CNS and respiratory depression. Other acute clinical effects include disinhibition, nystagmus, vomiting, tachycardia, seizures (in the setting of ethanol intoxication or withdrawal) and hypoglycaemia, particularly in children.

Ethanol is rapidly absorbed following oral administration and is distributed readily across the total body water (volume of distribution 0.6 L/kg). Ethanol is oxidised by cytosolic and microsomal cytochrome P-450 (2E1 and 1A2) alcohol dehydrogenase to form acetaldehyde, which in turn is metabolised by aldehyde dehydrogenase to acetylcoenzyme A.

Investigations and management

Serum ethanol levels assist risk assessment in patients with CNS depression, but must not be assumed to be the sole contributor to CNS depression, and an appropriate evaluation for other causes such as co-ingestants or trauma is required.

- Serum ethanol concentration is approximately 10% higher than the 'whole blood ethanol level', which is used to define legal driving limits. Breath ethanol estimation is a useful tool in the ED, providing a convenient bedside estimation of blood ethanol concentration, but the accuracy is influenced by minute ventilation, body temperature and presence of vomit or blood in the mouth.

Management of ethanol intoxication is supportive with airway protection and adequate IV hydration. In alcoholic patients, this should include the administration of thiamine (200 mg TDS initially, that can then be changed to 100 mg OD orally) and the recognition that intoxication may be followed by alcohol withdrawal.

The major pitfalls are failure to regard an intoxicated patient as having a potential life-threat, and failure to detect co-ingestants or co-existent injuries or medical conditions.

Toxic alcohols

Toxic alcohols include ethylene glycol, methanol and isopropyl alcohol.

Ethylene glycol and methanol cause rapid-onset CNS effects similar to ethanol. Of note, both agents are metabolised by the alcohol dehydrogenase enzyme pathway to form acids, and the intentional ingestion of > 1 mL/kg ethylene glycol or 0.5 mL/kg methanol can result in potentially lethal metabolic acidosis.[17] Ethylene glycol also causes hypocalcaemia and acute renal failure, while methanol classically causes optic nerve injury and blindness. Small accidental ingestions of less than a mouthful are benign, as are dermal exposures, but deliberate self-poisonings are assumed to be potentially lethal.

Isopropyl alcohol causes significant CNS depression. As little as 1 mL/kg of a 70% solution causes symptoms of inebriation. Ingestion of more than 4 mL/kg causes coma and respiratory depression.

Investigations and management

The diagnosis of both ethylene glycol and methanol toxicity can be made by a combination of history, clinical examination and biochemistry. Very few centres in Australia can perform ethylene glycol or methanol level measurements; however, the measurement of serum osmolality (to calculate an osmolar gap), serum lactate, pH and bicarbonate are usually adequate to confirm the diagnosis. In the absence of ethanol, a raised osmolar gap (> 10 mmol/L), hyperlactaemia and development of high anion-gap metabolic acidosis is suggestive of ethylene glycol or methanol poisoning. The presence of calcium oxalate crystals in the urine is pathognomonic of ethylene glycol intoxication, and readily detectable with a Woods lamp. However, the absence of crystals does not exclude the diagnosis.

Significant ethylene glycol or methanol intoxication is initially treated with oral or intravenous (IV) ethanol. Ethanol competitively inhibits the formation of toxic metabolites (acids) by having a greater affinity for the enzyme alcohol dehydrogenase. Fomepizole is an alternative agent used to inhibit the action of alcohol dehydrogenase, but is not currently available in Australasia. Inhibition of toxic alcohol metabolism is, however, only a temporising measure and definitive treatment with haemodialysis must be arranged as soon as possible.

A common pitfall in management is not to recognise that co-ingestion of ethanol prior to presentation will delay metabolism of the toxic alcohols and may mask their presence. It should also be noted that 'methylated spirits' in Australia does not contain methanol, but does in New Zealand.

Isopropyl alcohol does not cause a metabolic acidosis, but will cause an osmolar gap, which can be measured to confirm diagnosis. Treatment is supportive, as for ethanol. Haemodialysis is effective at removing isopropyl alcohol, as it is with ethanol, but is rarely clinically indicated.

Analgesics

Aspirin (salicylates)

Salicylate toxicity occurs following irreversible inhibition of cyclo-oxygenase enzymes (COX-1 and COX-2) and resultant decreased prostaglandin synthesis. This manifests as hyperventilation and respiratory alkalosis secondary to respiratory centre stimulation, and progressive metabolic acidosis as a result of oxidative phosphorylation uncoupling.[18]

Acute salicylate toxicity causes mild symptoms with ingested acetylsalicylate (aspirin) doses of < 150 mg/kg, but is potentially lethal with doses > 500 mg/kg. Methylsalicylate, found in numerous topical products such as oil of wintergreen, is more potent, with 1 g equivalent to 1.5 g of acetylsalicylate. Due to delayed absorption, symptoms may not occur for many hours post-ingestion.

Initial clinical features include profuse vomiting, tinnitus and diaphoresis (salicylism). Complicated acid–base disturbances occur in salicylate toxicity. The first of these is respiratory alkalosis due to hyperventilation (typically with increased tidal volumes rather than respiratory rate). This is caused by direct stimulation by salicylate of the medullary respiratory centre. Following this, metabolic acidosis occurs by an inhibition of the Krebs cycle, causing an increase in lactic acid production. In addition, lipid metabolism and protein catabolism is increased, leading to increased production of ketone bodies and amino acids respectively. The worsening acidosis enhances salicylate movement into the brain, resulting in cerebral oedema with coma and seizures. Hypoglycaemia can also develop, further complicating management of the patient.

In contrast, chronic intoxication is more common in the

elderly and usually presents with non-specific clinical features such as dehydration, confusion, fever and acidosis. The diagnosis is frequently missed and, as a consequence, morbidity and mortality are greater in chronic intoxication.

Investigations and management

Specific investigations include venous or arterial blood gases and salicylate levels. (See Ch 17, p. 329, for details on collecting arterial blood gases.) Serial salicylate levels correlate poorly with actual toxicity, but are useful in determining treatment regimens and monitoring response to therapy.

Management consists of meticulous supportive care, decontamination and institution of enhanced elimination techniques.[17] Activated charcoal adsorbs salicylate very effectively and should be administered in patients with intact mental state even many hours post-ingestion, as salicylates may form pharmacobezoars, which result in ongoing delayed absorption.[18]

Salicylates are eliminated by hepatic metabolism in therapeutic doses, but this capacity is exceeded in overdose and enhanced renal elimination is the management of choice. All symptomatic patients should be commenced on a sodium bicarbonate infusion to induce alkaline urine (target urine pH 7.5) and enhance renal elimination of salicylate.[18]

Patients with confusion, acidaemia, renal failure or high salicylate levels should be referred for urgent haemodialysis. Deterioration in conscious state is an ominous sign in salicylate poisoning, and may require intubation while definitive therapy with haemodialysis is organised. Failure to maintain hyperventilation after intubation and ventilation of the patient with severe salicylate poisoning may lead to catastrophic deterioration from worsening acidosis.

Paracetamol

Paracetamol toxicity is a complicated subject that cannot adequately be covered in this chapter. Instead, the salient points are presented here and further reading is recommended.[12,19]

Paracetamol in acute overdose or with supratherapeutic administration has the potential to cause life-threatening hepatotoxicity. Hepatotoxicity is caused by the metabolism of paracetamol to *N*-acetyl-p-benzoquinone imine (NAPQI), which causes glutathione depletion and consequent hepatonecrosis. Other organ effects include nephrotoxicity, which may occur independently of hepatotoxicity, and coma, which is seen with massive ingestions.

Investigations and management

Specific investigations include paracetamol levels, hepatic transaminase levels, international normalised ratio (INR), FBC and renal function.

For acute ingestions the threshold for toxicity is now considered to be > 200 mg/kg in adults and children.[19] If the time of ingestion is known, a paracetamol level at 4–16 hours can be plotted on the paracetamol treatment nomogram for Australia and New Zealand published in 2008.[19] If the level is above the treatment line, for example, > 150 mg/L (1000 µmol/L) at 4 hours, treatment with *N*-acetylcysteine is indicated. If the level is below the treatment line, the patient may be medically cleared. If the time of ingestion is not known, the decision to treat can be based on either a worst-case scenario (i.e. earliest possible time of ingestion), or the presence of a raised paracetamol level or abnormal liver transaminases.

Treatment with *N*-acetylcysteine, which replaces glutathione, is 100% life-saving if given within 8 hours of an acute ingestion. Every effort should be made to commence it within this timeframe if toxic ingestion is suspected or confirmed. Outside this period, safe management is to commence *N*-acetylcysteine prior to investigation if the risk assessment infers a potentially toxic dose. While there is a significant risk of anaphylactoid reaction with the infusion (approx 15% of patients during the first or start of the second IV bag), this is easily managed by slowing or ceasing the infusion, treating with an antihistamine such as loratadine and recommencing therapy at a lower rate. The safety and efficacy of *N*-acetylcysteine mean that decontamination with oral activated charcoal is rarely justified.

Supratherapeutic administration of paracetamol is, in contrast to acute ingestions, a greater risk in children than adults. The decision to treat is based on abnormal hepatic transaminase levels (alanine aminotransferase [ALT] or aspartate aminotransferase [AST] > 50 IU/L) and/or raised paracetamol levels. These decisions should be made in consultation with a clinical toxicologist.

Anticonvulsants

Carbamazepine

Carbamazepine is structurally similar to the tricyclic antidepressant imipramine. It inhibits inactivated sodium channels, blocks noradrenaline re-uptake and is an antagonist at muscarinic and nicotinic receptors.

Intentional ingestion of carbamazepine causes CNS depression, anticholinergic symptoms and, in massive doses, dysrhythmias and haemodynamic instability. Clinical features are dose-dependent, but onset is dependent on the type of preparation ingested (immediate or controlled-release) and the patient may not become symptomatic for 8–12 hours.

Doses of 20–50 mg/kg predictably cause mild to moderate CNS effects, such as nystagmus, dysarthria, ataxia, sedation, delirium, mydriasis, ophthalmoplegia and myoclonus; and anticholinergic effects such as urinary retention, tachycardia and dry mouth. If > 50 mg/kg is ingested there is risk of coma requiring intubation, hypotension, dysrhythmias and the potential for sudden death.

Carbamazepine is slowly and erratically absorbed. Following large overdoses, ileus secondary to anticholinergic effects may result in ongoing absorption for several days.

Investigations and management

Carbamazepine levels are useful to confirm ingestion and to monitor intubated patients. There is little benefit in performing repeat levels on patients who are awake and who can be monitored clinically. The therapeutic range is 8–12 mg/L (34 to 51 µmol/L) and coma is expected at > 40 mg/L (170 µmol/L).

Management is based on good supportive care and airway protection as required. In massive ingestions, ventricular dysrhythmias are managed with sodium bicarbonate. Carbamazepine is well adsorbed by activated charcoal and elimination is enhanced by the use of repeat-dose activated charcoal. In life-threatening cases, haemodialysis may be required. Avoidable pitfalls include failure to detect urinary retention from anticholinergic effects, bowel obstruction from multiple dose activated charcoal in the context of an anticholinergic ileus and failure to appreciate the potential for delayed onset of toxicity.

Carbamazepine is teratogenic and overdose in the first trimester warrants referral for further antenatal assessment.

Sodium valproate

Valproate increases levels of gamma-aminobutyric acid (GABA), a central inhibitory neurotransmitter, and in large doses interferes with numerous mitochondrial metabolic pathways. It is usually well absorbed following oral administration but absorption may be slow and erratic following overdose. Peak levels may be delayed up to 18 hours.

Most valproate overdoses result in CNS depression and are managed successfully with supportive care. Large overdoses can cause multiple organ failure and death, which is preventable with early haemodialysis.

Clinically, patients develop CNS depression that correlates with rising serum levels. Miosis, tachycardia and mild hypotension may be seen. Ingested doses < 200 mg/kg are generally asymptomatic, with risk of coma developing at 400 mg/kg. With doses above this, patients are at risk of multi-organ toxicity with haemodynamic instability, cerebral oedema and bone marrow suppression. A dose of 1 g/kg is potentially fatal.

Investigations and management

Serial valproate levels can be used to confirm poisoning and guide therapy, particularly in the intubated patient. Levels of > 500 mg/L (3500 µmol/L) usually manifest as coma, and levels > 1000 mg/L (7000 µmol/L) are frequently associated with severe systemic toxicity. The valproate level on arrival can be normal even in a life-threatening overdose, so the level should be repeated if there is clinical deterioration. Hypernatraemia, hypocalcaemia, hypoglycaemia, elevated lactate and hyperammonaemia are all associated with significant valproate toxicity.

Mainstays of treatment are good supportive care and airway protection. Valproate is well adsorbed to activated charcoal and this should be administered in the patient with a protected airway who has taken > 400 mg/kg. Serum levels or evidence of systemic toxicity guide the use of haemodialysis, which can be life-saving in the severely poisoned patient.

Antidepressants

Tricyclic antidepressants

Tricyclic antidepressant (TCA) poisoning remains a major cause of morbidity and mortality, despite the decline in their use. Deliberate self-poisoning may lead to the rapid onset of CNS and cardiovascular toxicity. Prompt intubation, hyperventilation and sodium bicarbonate administration are life-saving.

TCAs are noradrenaline and serotonin re-uptake inhibitors, as well as GABA-A and muscarinic receptor blockers. However, their major toxic effect is through fast sodium channel blockade, which results in dysrhythmias, hypotension and seizures. TCAs are rapidly absorbed, highly protein-bound and have a large volume of distribution.

Ingestion of > 10 mg/kg is usually associated with major toxicity, which is manifest within 1–2 hours. Doses < 5 mg/kg cause minimal symptoms, and 5–10 mg/kg is associated with mild sedation and anticholinergic symptoms.

Investigations and management

The most useful investigation in TCA toxicity is the ECG. Sodium channel blockade causes prolongation of the P–R and QRS intervals and a prominent terminal 'R' wave in aV$_R$. A QRS width of > 110 ms is associated with an increased risk of seizures and one of > 160 ms with ventricular tachycardia.[20]

Severe toxicity is characterised by rapid deterioration in clinical status within 1–2 hours of ingestion. Patients may present alert and orientated only to rapidly develop coma, seizures, hypotension and cardiac dysrhythmias. This clinical situation is managed by endotracheal intubation, hyperventilation to a pH of 7.5–7.55 and the administration of 1 mEq/kg bolus of NaHCO$_3$ repeated every 3–5 minutes, as required. Adjunctive treatment measures include benzodiazepines for seizures and intravenous fluid boluses and vasopressors for hypotension.

Activated charcoal should only be administered once the airway has been secured. Intralipid rescue therapy can be considered in the event of refractory cardiac arrest.

Management of smaller ingestions is generally supportive, although anticholinergic symptoms may be problematic. Patients with a normal ECG and mental state at 6 hours may be removed from cardiac monitoring and referred for psychiatric assessment as appropriate.

Selective serotonin re-uptake inhibitors

Deliberate self-poisoning with the selective serotonin re-uptake inhibitor (SSRI) antidepressants is common and usually follows a benign course.

The SSRIs are rapidly absorbed following oral administration, are protein bound and have large volumes of distribution. They undergo hepatic metabolism to form less-active and water-soluble metabolites, and elimination half-lives are approximately 24 hours.

Clinically, most patients are asymptomatic or have mild symptoms, which resolve completely within 12 hours.

Ingestions may uncommonly be associated with seizures or the development of symptoms of serotonin toxicity, particularly with co-ingestion of other serotonergic agents. These agents include monoamine oxidase inhibitors (MAOIs), serotonin reuptake inhibitors (SSRIs and SNRIs—selective serotonin and noradrenaline re-uptake inhibitors), TCAs, lithium, tramadol, pethidine, sympathomimetic recreational drugs (such as amphetamines or ecstasy) and herbal preparations.

Serotonin syndrome manifests as agitation, tremor, tachycardia, mydriasis and hypertonia and clonus in the lower limbs. When severe it is associated with profound mental state changes, rigidity and hyperthermia that are life-threatening.[21] Two SSRI antidepressants, escitalopram and citalopram, apart from the risk of serotonin toxicity, can also cause QT prolongation and lower the threshold for seizures.

Investigations and management

A 12-lead ECG and serum paracetamol level are the only baseline investigations required following SSRI ingestion. Among the SSRIs, citalopram and escitalopram have the ability to cause dose-dependent Q–T interval prolongation. Following citalopram overdose of > 600 mg, all patients should have cardiac monitoring until 8 hours post-ingestion (see Ch 17, p. 336, for cardiac monitoring techniques). A normal ECG at this time allows cardiac monitoring to cease.[21] If the ingested dose is > 1000 mg, or the Q–T interval is > 450 ms, cardiac monitoring is continued and serial ECGs performed for at least 12 hours post-ingestion until resolution occurs. Cardiac dysrhythmias, such as wide complex bradycardia or torsades de pointes, may occur, but are rare and are managed with magnesium and overdrive pacing.

Patients with SSRI overdose other than citalopram who have a normal ECG do not require ongoing cardiac monitoring.

Seizures are usually short-lived and heralded by agitation and tachycardia, and are managed with benzodiazepines. Symptoms of serotonin toxicity are also well managed in almost all cases with benzodiazepines. Serotonin antagonists, such as cyproheptadine and olanzapine, can also be used in patients requiring large amounts of benzodiazepines. Life-threatening mental state changes, rigidity and hyperthermia require immediate intubation, paralysis and active cooling.[21]

Activated charcoal is rarely indicated as most ingestions are benign, and there is a risk of seizures in more significant ingestions. The exception to this may be early administration in large citalopram ingestions (< 4 hours post-ingestion).

Monoamine oxidase inhibitors

Toxicity with monoamine oxidase inhibitors (MAOIs) may be broadly classified into two groups:

- irreversible non-selective monoamine oxidase inhibitors such as phenelzine and tranylcypromine are associated with potentially lethal serotonin toxicity in overdose and cause significant adverse reactions, even with therapeutic dosing
- isolated overdose of the newer reversible and selective agents such as moclobemide are associated with a benign clinical course, but severe serotonin syndrome occurs when they are taken in combination with other serotonergic agents.[21]

MAOIs act by decreasing the metabolism of sympathomimetic amines, in particular dopamine, serotonin and noradrenaline. They are rapidly absorbed orally, and metabolised prior to elimination.

Clinical features of significant ingestions include agitation, hypertonia, altered mental state, seizures, hyperthermia and cardiovascular instability with severe hyper- or hypotension. When symptoms occur they are generally prolonged and may last for several days.

Investigations and management

There are no blood tests specific to these poisonings. Baseline investigations are the 12-lead ECG and paracetamol level. Ingested doses of > 3 g moclobemide have been associated with Q–T prolongation.

Management of severe toxicity is based around good supportive care and airway protection as required. Benzodiazepines, control of hyperthermia with paralysis if required and other anti-serotonergic agents such as cyproheptadine may be indicated. Hypertensive crises are best treated with titratable vasodilators (e.g. sodium nitroprusside, glyceryl trinitrate), as autonomic instability may result in profound hypotension and beta-blockers are contraindicated. Activated charcoal may be administered to intubated patients. Severely poisoned patients who require intubation and paralysis for hyperthermia may have prolonged ICU admissions.

Antipsychotics

Typical antipsychotic agents

Phenothiazines (e.g. chlorpromazine, pericyazine) and butyrophenones (e.g. haloperidol, droperidol) are therapeutic antagonists at central dopamine receptors. They are known as 'typical' antipsychotics because they were the initial agents used for psychotic disorders; however, they are rarely prescribed now for outpatient treatment. They have a number of adverse effects at alpha$_1$-adrenergic and cholinergic receptors, and in overdose they cause CNS depression, orthostatic hypotension and anticholinergic effects. Cardiotoxicity is secondary to sodium and potassium channel-blocking effects. Thioridazine, in particular, is associated with cardiac conduction abnormalities and high rates of ventricular dysrhythmias. Extrapyramidal effects (dystonic reactions, akathisia and tardive dyskinesia) may occur after small ingestions, especially in children, and these may be delayed over the next few days.

Investigations and management

The clinical features of intoxication occur within 2–4 hours of overdose. Sedation may occasionally require intubation for airway protection, and hypotension usually responds to volume resuscitation. Urinary retention is common, and anticholinergic delirium may complicate recovery from coma. Serial ECGs and cardiac monitoring are required if there are signs of toxicity (QRS widening and Q–T prolongation) and should be continued until these abnormalities resolve. See Chapter 17, p. 336, for details on cardiac monitoring techniques, including ECGs.

Atypical antipsychotics

This group includes quetiapine, olanzapine, clozapine, amisulpride, aripiprazole and ziprasidone. They are classified as atypical due to their decreased propensity to cause dystonia or extrapyramidal effects, and have become an extremely common cause of drug-induced coma requiring intubation. All these agents have anticholinergic effects and the potential for mild hypotension.[22]

Following overdose, patients typically present with early-onset dose-related sedation, significant tachycardia, mild Q–T prolongation and occasionally hypotension. Seizures are rare. Large ingestions of amisulpride and ziprasidone have been associated with Q–T prolongation, delayed broad-complex tachycardias and life-threatening cardiovascular collapse. Clozapine is associated with profuse salivation in overdose, and with agranulocytosis and cardiotoxicity with therapeutic use. Management of poisoning with these agents is for the most part supportive, although the management of broad-complex tachycardias with amisulpride includes magnesium, sodium bicarbonate and overdrive pacing.

Cardiac drugs

Beta-blockers

Overdose involving the vast majority of beta-blockers is relatively benign and results in minimal toxicity only. However, large ingestions of propranolol or sotalol may be life-threatening.[23]

Beta-blockers are competitive antagonists at beta$_1$ and beta$_2$ receptors, leading to bradycardia and hypotension in overdose. In addition, propranolol has sodium-channel blocking effects (QRS widening and ventricular dysrhythmias) and crosses the blood–brain barrier (reduced seizure threshold). Sotalol blocks cardiac potassium channels, disrupting cardiac repolarisation, and may lead to Q–T prolongation and, potentially, torsades de pointes.

The response to overdose is highly variable, but usually most significant in elderly patients with underlying heart or lung disease, or on regular treatment with calcium channel blockers or digoxin.

Investigations and management

Acute beta-blocker poisoning is a potentially life-threatening emergency that should be managed in an area equipped for cardiorespiratory monitoring and resuscitation. Bradycardia may be temporarily relieved with IV boluses of atropine 0.01–0.03 mg/kg, and in patients with concomitant significant hypotension, an infusion of adrenaline or isoprenaline should be considered.[24]

The threshold dose for severe toxicity from propranolol is approximately 1 g (15 mg/kg in children). Severe toxicity is characterised by rapid deterioration in clinical status within 1–2 hours of ingestion. Patients may present alert and orientated only to rapidly develop coma, seizures, hypotension and cardiac dysrhythmias. This clinical situation is similar to severe TCA toxicity and is also managed by endotracheal intubation, hyperventilation to a pH of 7.5–7.55 and the administration of 1 mEq/kg bolus of $NaHCO_3$ repeated every 3–5 minutes, as required. The endpoints of successful treatment are an improvement in QRS duration or return of spontaneous circulation, and the cessation of seizures.

Sotalol can cause Q–T prolongation in therapeutic dosing and in overdose. If torsades de pointes develop, treatment options include intravenous magnesium, overdrive pacing with isoprenaline or the insertion of a transvenous pacemaker.

Glucagon is no longer recommended for the treatment of beta-blocker poisoning as it offers no advantages over standard inotropic and chronotropic management. High-dose insulin euglycaemic therapy may have an emerging role in the management of severe and refractory beta-blocker toxicity.

Calcium channel blockers

Verapamil and diltiazem cause life-threatening cardiovascular collapse following overdose, with the onset of symptoms delayed by several hours following ingestion of commonly prescribed slow-release (SR) preparations. Early signs of toxicity are bradycardia, first-degree heart block and hypotension. Hypotension results from severe peripheral vasodilation, bradycardia and decreased myocardial contractility, and typically is resistant to maximal doses of the usual inotropic agents.

In general, ingestion of 10 or more tablets causes significant haemodynamic symptoms in adults and the ingestion of 1–2 tablets of verapamil or diltiazem SR is potentially lethal in children. Advanced age and co-morbidities, such as cardiac disease, increase the risk of significant toxicity.

The other calcium channel blockers (e.g. nifedipine, felodipine, amlodipine) are dihydropyridines and tend to cause less severe hypotension, which usually responds well to volume resuscitation, rarely needing vasopressors or inotropes.

Calcium channel blockers are well absorbed, protein-bound and have a large volume of distribution. Following ingestion, peak levels occur within 1–2 hours for standard preparations and 6–12 hours for SR preparations.

Investigations and management

Early recognition of the potential for significant toxicity is vital. Ingestion of verapamil or diltiazem SR is an indication for decontamination with activated charcoal and consideration of whole-bowel irrigation. This can potentially be performed up to 4 hours after a significant ingestion; however, the risk of aspiration needs to be considered if a patient becomes systemically unwell.

Once hypotension develops, consideration should be given to early intubation and ventilation to provide secure airway control. Significant or refractory hypotension is difficult to manage and requires a logical and methodical approach.

- Volume resuscitation with sodium chloride 0.9% is first-line therapy.
- Further transient improvement in blood pressure can be seen with intravenous calcium therapy to maintain ionised calcium level above 2.0 mEq/L.
- An infusion of noradrenaline, adrenaline and/or dopamine via a central line is the next step, but patients may be resistant to maximum doses.
- High-dose insulin euglycaemic therapy is a well-accepted treatment option for inotropic therapy in severe calcium channel blocker poisoning, and may be a better choice than standard catecholamine infusions. The doses required are markedly outside usual insulin regimens, but are safe and well tolerated in a closely monitored environment. Increasingly, its early use is being advocated when severe cardiotoxicity is anticipated.[25]

Significant bradycardia can be difficult to manage. Atropine is unlikely to be effective, and it is often difficult to achieve electrical capture with ventricular pacing. In isolated cases, cardiopulmonary bypass and intra-aortic balloon pump have been successfully used as extraordinary manoeuvres.

Digoxin

Digoxin inhibits the membrane Na^+–K^+ ATPase pump, and leads to an increase in intracellular calcium and extracellular potassium. Digitalis glycosides are found in therapeutic drugs, such as digoxin and digitoxin, as well as many poisonous plants. Rhododendron, foxglove and oleander all contain glycosides and are toxic when ingested.

Acute digoxin toxicity occurs if more than 10 times the therapeutic dose is ingested. Ingestion of > 10 mg in an adult or > 4 mg in a child is potentially lethal and manifests as vomiting, hyperkalaemia and cardiovascular collapse refractory to conventional resuscitation measures.

Digoxin has a narrow therapeutic index and chronic intoxication commonly develops in elderly patients with multiple co-morbidities. The clinical features of chronic digoxin toxicity are often non-specific, but include cardiovascular (bradycardia, heart block, slow atrial fibrillation or ventricular ectopy), gastrointestinal (vomiting and abdominal pain) and neurological (confusion). Untreated, mortality within a week is 15–30%.

Investigations and management

Essential investigations include a serum digoxin level, urinalysis, electrolytes and serial 12-lead ECG. Serum digoxin levels of > 15 nmol/L (12 ng/mL) or serum potassium level > 5.5 mmol/L in the setting of acute overdose are potentially fatal.

In acute toxicity, serum digoxin levels are taken at 4 hours post-ingestion and then every 2 hours until definitive treatment is instituted. The diagnosis of chronic digoxin intoxication is based on a steady-state level 6 or more hours after the last dose. The probability of digoxin intoxication increases with the number of clinical and ECG features observed, and the measured serum digoxin level.

Prior to the availability of digoxin antibodies, significant overdose was associated with 100% mortality. Atropine and inotropes provide only temporary relief for haemodynamic instability and standard therapy for hyperkalaemia with IV calcium is *avoided* in digoxin toxicity as it may worsen cardiotoxicity. However digoxin-specific antibodies (Fab) are curative, shorten hospital length of stay and are cost-effective.[26] Following treatment, digoxin levels may be very high as most assays measure both free and Fab-bound digoxin.

In acute overdose, Fab dose is calculated on the presumption that 1 ampoule binds 0.5 mg of digoxin. For large ingestions, an initial dose of 5–10 ampoules may be required, while further stocks of antibody are sourced. Attempts at resuscitation should continue for at least 60 minutes after the administration of digoxin immune Fab (e.g. Digibind), as good outcomes have been reported even after cardiac arrest.

In chronic poisoning, empirical dosing starts with 2 ampoules. If there is no clinical improvement in 1 hour, consider giving 2 further ampoules. However, it may take up to 6 hours to detect a clinical response. It is irrational to withhold digoxin antibody from patients with chronic digoxin poisoning because of concerns about expense. The risk of death and cost of prolonged unnecessary admission to a monitored bed greatly exceed the cost of two ampoules of Fab.

Colchicine

Colchicine is derived from the autumn crocus plant (*Colchicum autumnale*), and is used to treat gout. It binds to intracellular microtubules and prevents cell division. It has a narrow therapeutic window, and is extremely toxic in overdose.

Severe gastrointestinal symptoms are the initial symptoms, and systemic features develop at doses of > 0.5 mg/kg. Ingestions of > 0.8 mg/kg are associated with multisystem organ failure, cardiovascular collapse, hepatic failure and bone marrow suppression.

Investigations and management

Early recognition of the potential severity of colchicine overdose is vital. Because there is no antidote, the mainstays of treatment are early decontamination and good supportive care. Activated charcoal should be used as soon as possible, even in delayed presentation, as decreasing the absorption of even small amounts of colchicine may be life-saving. Meticulous volume resuscitation and management in the intensive care unit is required in cases of significant poisoning.

Lithium carbonate

Lithium is a metal ion which substitutes for sodium and potassium ions; it modulates intracellular second messengers and is thought to affect neurotransmitter production (including serotonin) and release. It is available as both normal and SR preparations, and after absorption slowly redistributes to the CNS where it is most toxic. It is almost completely renally excreted.

Lithium toxicity is classified into acute and chronic.

- Significant acute lithium overdose produces acute gastrointestinal symptoms including nausea, vomiting, abdominal pain and diarrhoea. Provided adequate urinary lithium excretion is maintained, significant neurotoxicity of the type observed with chronic lithium intoxication rarely develops.

- Chronic lithium toxicity is most commonly diagnosed in older patients with renal impairment on long-term lithium therapy. Patients usually present with signs of neurotoxicity, which can cause permanent neurological sequelae or death.

Clinical features of neurotoxicity include tremor, increased tone, hyperreflexia, confusion, myoclonic jerks, convulsions and eventually obtundation. Nephrogenic diabetes insipidus and thyroid dysfunction are associated with therapeutic use and may contribute to or complicate chronic toxicity. Patients on long-term lithium therapy who have diabetes insipidus produce large amounts of urine, therefore require an increased water intake. Fluid restriction during their admission to hospital will precipitate lithium toxicity.

Investigations and management

Check urea and electrolytes following acute and chronic overdose to monitor renal function. Serum lithium levels > 5 μmol/L are not uncommon in acute ingestions, and with good management will not result in neurotoxicity. However, in chronic toxicity, clinical features of severe neurotoxicity may be present when the serum lithium level is only just above the normal range (i.e. > 1.0 μmol/L).

Management of acute poisoning depends on the dose ingested and renal function.[27] Doses <25 g rarely cause significant toxicity in the setting of normal renal function. Higher doses may cause significant gastrointestinal irritation but again, with normal renal function, can be well managed with meticulous fluid resuscitation with sodium chloride 0.9% (NaCl) to maintain a urine output of 1.5–2 mL/kg/h. The routine use of whole-bowel irrigation, which was once standard therapy, is no longer advocated. Haemodialysis is reserved for those patients who, despite the implementation of conservative measures, exhibit renal impairment, significant neurotoxicity and deteriorating clinical status.

Patients with chronic toxicity, which may be precipitated by renal failure or other drugs such as NSAIDs and angiotensin-converting enzyme (ACE) inhibitors, usually present with established neurotoxicity and dehydration. They require fluid resuscitation with NaCl and correction of renal impairment. If this fails, haemodialysis should be considered.

Signs of clinical improvement should not be expected for several days to a week post-treatment.

Herbicides

Glyphosate

Glyphosate, more commonly known by the tradename Roundup, is a widely used herbicide. Intentional ingestion of large volumes of the 'concentrate' can be life-threatening. Ingested doses of < 50 mL of concentrate cause mild gastrointestinal symptoms, but doses of > 300 mL can cause refractory shock and death. Dilute over-the-counter preparations are generally benign, but can cause mild gastrointestinal irritation or pneumonitis secondary to pulmonary aspiration.

The toxicity is thought to be due to the surfactant that is combined with the glyphosate rather than the glyphosate itself, and involves uncoupling of mitochondrial oxidative phosphorylation.[28] Dermal exposure poses no risk of systemic toxicity.

Investigations and management

Specific investigations that may be useful in these patients include baseline renal and hepatic function, arterial blood gases and a chest X-ray or assessment of pneumonitis. (See Ch 17, p. 329, for details on collecting arterial blood gases.) Worsening acidosis and isolated elevations in potassium are seen with ensuing refractory shock. Management is supportive. There is no role for decontamination or enhanced elimination, although haemodialysis may be indicated as part of supportive care.

Paraquat

N,N'-dimethyl-4,4′-bipyridinium dichloride (commonly known as 'paraquat') is a herbicide that is potentially lethal with an ingested dose of as little as one mouthful. While small accidental ingestions may be salvageable with aggressive decontamination and early dialysis, intentional ingestions of large volumes are uniformly fatal.

Paraquat toxicity is due to the production of oxygen free-radicals, which cause cellular injury and cell death. Paraquat is extremely corrosive to the gastrointestinal tract, resulting in severe upper airway and oesophageal burns. Following absorption it accumulates predominantly in the lungs, and with large ingestions patients develop hypoxia, multi-organ failure and death within days. Those patients who survive large ingestions are at risk of developing pulmonary fibrosis. Dermal exposure to intact skin poses no risk of systemic toxicity.

Investigations and management

Sodium dithionate is added to urine as a rapid qualitative test in cases of likely paraquat ingestion. Urine will turn blue in the presence of paraquat, and green in the presence of diquat, a related but less-toxic agent.[12] Serum paraquat levels may be plotted on a nomogram to predict potential lethality following ingestions, but do not contribute to the acute management. Additional investigations include serial arterial blood gases, chest X-rays and endoscopy.

Management involves immediate aggressive decontamination—this even takes priority over initial resuscitation concerns. Activated charcoal adsorbs paraquat, but any ingested substance may limit absorption of paraquat—recommendations have even including eating soil if nothing else is immediately available. Excessive or routine supplemental oxygen should be avoided, as this worsens lung damage due to increased production of reactive oxygen species, but should not be withheld if significant hypoxaemia is present.

Following decontamination, the mainstays of treatment are haemodialysis (preferably within 2 hours of ingestion) and good supportive care.

Adjunctive treatments such as N-acetylcysteine, vitamin C, dexamethasone and sodium salicylate (or aspirin) are also recommended, although their role in management has not been validated in large studies.

Insecticides

Organophosphates and carbamates[29]

Intentional ingestion of organophosphates (OPs) or carbamates is potentially life-threatening. They are used as insecticides and as 'nerve agents' in chemical warfare, and are major problems in developing countries as a preferred mode of suicide. Cross-contamination between the patient and healthcare professional is possible and every precaution should be taken. Usual PPE is enough. There have been no documented cases of significant OP poisoning in healthcare professionals caring for poisoned patients (see Ch 28). Contaminated clothing should be removed and exposed skin washed with water.

Organophosphates and carbamates both act to inhibit acetylcholinesterase (AChE) enzymes and to increase acetylcholine (ACh) concentration at cholinergic receptors. Organophosphates, if left untreated, form a permanent bond with the AChE enzyme (known as ageing); whereas carbamates do not, and hence are self-limiting in their clinical effect.

Both groups of agents are well absorbed following ingestion, have large volumes of distribution and often accumulate in lipid stores. Carbamates have less CNS absorption than organophosphates and are associated with less significant neurotoxicity.

Timing of symptom onset is dependent on the agent, dose and route of exposure and may occur within minutes of ingestion or can be delayed many hours. Clinical features are classified according to the affected receptor.

- Muscarinic effects include diarrhoea, urination, miosis, bronchorrhoea, bronchospasm, emesis, lacrimation and salivation ('DUMBBELS' mnemonic).
- Nicotinic effects include fasciculation, tremor, weakness and, most importantly, respiratory muscle paralysis.
- Haemodynamic instability and CNS effects with seizures and coma may be seen. The most common cause of death in these patients is respiratory failure.

An intermediate syndrome of muscle weakness may occur several days post-exposure, particularly in inadequately treated patients; some agents can cause organophosphate-induced delayed neuropathy (OPIDN) and chronic occupational exposure may result in neuropsychiatric sequelae.

Investigations and management

Red cell and plasma cholinesterase levels are used to confirm exposure and guide treatment after the acute resuscitation phase is completed.

Management of these poisonings requires aggressive early resuscitation, early intubation if indicated and the use of antidotes.

- Atropine is the agent of choice for treating muscarinic symptoms. Dosage is commenced at 1.2 mg IV, and doubled every 5 minutes until the patient has drying of secretions and adequate air entry. Large doses may be required in severe cases, until the desired clinical endpoints are attained.
- Pralidoxime reactivates the AChE enzyme that has been inhibited by being 'reversibly' bound to organophosphate molecules and is not effective if 'irreversible binding' (ageing) has occurred. However, as different agents age at different rates, pralidoxime administration is commenced as early as possible in all symptomatic organophosphate poisonings.

A tragic but common impediment to adequate resuscitation is the concern that staff will be 'poisoned' following exposure to these patients. This has resulted in 'Hazmat' responses being instituted in the out-of-hospital setting with delays in transport to definitive care, and patients with life-threatening toxicity being refused entry into EDs. It is the vapours of the volatile hydrocarbon diluent and *not* the non-volatile organophosphate that may cause treating staff to be aware of a strong odour and to produce mild symptoms such as headache and dizziness if exposed for long periods. This is not a significant threat to staff health. However, contact with body fluids should be avoided as per standard universal precautions, and staff should be rotated to reduce symptoms, but this should never take precedence over resuscitation of the patient.

Carbon monoxide (CO)

Carbon monoxide poisoning occurs either secondary to deliberate self-poisonings with car exhaust fumes, or accidentally, in domestic exposures to faulty gas heaters or when people try to warm themselves in winter by burning barbecue fuel inside the house. Exposure to house fires can result in both carbon monoxide and cyanide toxicity, as hydrogen cyanide is released from burning synthetic polymers used in building materials and furnishings.

Carbon monoxide has higher affinity for haemoglobin than oxygen, making haemoglobin oxygen transport less effective and thus causing hypoxia. In pregnant patients, the fetus is more susceptible to injury as carbon monoxide binds fetal haemoglobin more avidly.

Clinically poisoned patients present with headache, nausea, ataxia, confusion and poor concentration, symptoms that resolve with oxygen therapy. In more severe cases, they are found comatose, have ischaemic changes on the ECG and metabolic complications (lactic acidosis).

Deaths secondary to carbon monoxide poisoning usually occur out-of-hospital, and the large majority of patients that arrive at hospital alive survive their poisoning, but can have long-term neuropsychiatric sequelae.

Investigations and management

Carboxyhaemoglobin levels confirm the diagnosis but do not correlate with the symptoms. The presence of a metabolic acidosis with raised lactate level on arterial or venous blood gases indicate more severe poisoning, and can be a surrogate marker of toxicity if carboxyhaemoglobin levels are not available. ECG and cardiac markers are done to look for myocardial ischaemia. All female patients of child-bearing age should have a pregnancy test.

Management is along the usual lines of attention to airway, breathing and circulation, with administration of high-flow oxygen as soon as possible, and continued until all symptoms resolve. Hyperbaric oxygen should be considered for all pregnant patients and those with severe toxicity and associated end-organ damage (collapse/coma/ongoing neurological signs; myocardial ischaemia).

Iron

Iron ingestions are particularly common in children. Iron has a direct corrosive effect on the gastric mucosa and, in large doses, acts as a direct cellular toxin on the heart, liver and central nervous system.

Toxicity is determined by the dose of elemental iron ingested. Ingested doses of > 20 mg/kg of elemental iron are associated with gastrointestinal irritation; > 60 mg/kg with systemic toxicity; and > 100 mg/kg may be lethal.

Clinically poisoned patients present with vomiting and diarrhoea, which then progresses to worsening acidosis, profound shock and multi-organ failure. Those patients who survive large ingestions are prone to long-term complications including severe enteritis secondary to chronic fibrosis of the gastrointestinal tract.

Investigations and management

An abdominal X-ray can be useful to confirm ingestion, particularly in children, as the tablets are radio-opaque. Iron levels are useful at 6 hours to help determine the need for chelation therapy. These may be repeated 3-hourly until they decline. In the absence of iron levels, serial serum bicarbonate levels may be used to detect developing systemic toxicity.

Management is based around decontamination, supportive care and the use of chelating agents. Iron is not adsorbed to activated charcoal so this treatment is not indicated. For ingestions > 60 mg/kg, confirmed on X-ray, whole-bowel irrigation is the decontamination method of choice. Desferrioxamine chelation therapy is indicated where systemic toxicity (shock, metabolic acidosis, altered mental status) is present or predicted by a serum iron level greater than 90 µmol/L (500 µg/dL) at 4–6 hours post-ingestion.[30]

Hypoglycaemic agents

Insulin

Insulin stimulates the movement of glucose, potassium, magnesium and phosphate into cells. Profound refractory hypoglycaemia and clinically significant hypokalaemia may result.

Deliberate or accidental insulin overdose causes rapid onset of life-threatening hypoglycaemia. Large doses administered via subcutaneous injection create depots of insulin from which the drug is erratically released and which may cause days of hypoglycaemia.[31]

Clinical features of prolonged hypoglycaemia include seizures and depressed conscious state that, if left untreated, may lead to coma, permanent neurological injury or death.

Investigations and management

Specific investigations include serial blood sugar levels and electrolyte levels. Blood sugar should be measured every 15–30 minutes for the first few hours, then 1- to 2-hourly when blood sugar levels have been stabilised. Potassium levels should be checked 2-hourly until stabilised.

Management is centred on the IV administration of dextrose for the duration of the poisoning. Initial hypoglycaemia is treated with a bolus of IV dextrose (25–50 mL 50% in adults, and 5 mL/kg 10% in children), followed by a 10% dextrose infusion. Infusions are required for 24–48 hours, but may be longer with large ingestions. Patients with significant insulin overdose will require 50% dextrose at rates of up to 100–150 mL/h, and 10–20 mmol/h of potassium chloride. Protracted therapy with concentrated dextrose solutions must be given through a central line to prevent peripheral venous thrombophlebitis. Eight hours of euglycaemia off dextrose should be demonstrated prior to medical clearance and cessation of the dextrose infusion should take place in the morning, not overnight.

Sulfonylureas

Sulfonylureas act by increasing the release of endogenous insulin from pancreatic beta islet cells and, if taken in excess, have the potential to cause life-threatening hypoglycaemia.[32] One tablet is enough to kill a child and patients on therapeutic doses who develop renal failure are also at risk. Due to the wide range of duration of action within the sulfonylurea group, the risk of hypoglycaemia can last several days with large ingestions.

Investigations and management

Serial blood sugar levels are the most useful investigations in these patients. As the onset of hypoglycaemia can be delayed by up to 8 hours following ingestion, patients often require overnight admission for observation and serial blood glucose measurements. (See Ch 17, p. 332, for details on collecting blood glucose.) During daylight hours, conscious state can be used to guide the need for repeat blood glucose level testing, particularly for children who may find it traumatic. Insulin levels can also be performed to help confirm resolution of toxicity.

Management is based on detection and treatment of hypo-glycaemia (< 4 mmol/L in this setting). Activated charcoal may be considered < 1 hour following a large intentional ingestion in patients who are awake.

Initial hypoglycaemia is managed with IV dextrose (25–50 mL 50% in adults, 5 mL/kg 10% in children) and refractory hypoglycaemia with octreotide antidote therapy. Octreotide inhibits endogenous insulin release and is so effective in this setting that patients rarely require further IV dextrose after its administration (see Table 30.3).[33] Patients must be normoglycaemic for at least 6 hours after cessation of octreotide infusion before being considered safe for discharge.

Metformin

Metformin is a biguanide that inhibits gluconeogenesis, reduces hepatic glucose output and stimulates glucose uptake in the peripheries. It is completely renally excreted.

Unlike sulfonylurea overdose, toxicity from metformin poisoning is secondary to lactic acidosis rather than hypo-glycaemia, which is uncommon and usually benign.

The greatest risk for metformin-induced lactic acidosis is in the setting of renal failure superimposed on therapeutic use, particularly in the elderly.[32] Acidosis with acute overdose is rare, but potentially life-threatening in patients who ingest more than 10 g or who have impaired renal perfusion. Ingestion of less than 1700 mg in children is considered benign. Patients who develop lactic acidosis become clinically unwell after a few hours post-ingestion and continue to deteriorate as the lactate rises.

Investigations and management

Specific investigations include renal function and serum lactate. Patients with serum lactate levels > 12 mmol/L are at risk of cardiovascular instability, and levels > 20 mmol/L are commonly fatal without immediate definitive care. Patients

who are clinically well with a normal serum lactate at 8 hours can be medically cleared.

Management is based on good supportive care with close attention to adequate hydration and urine output. Patients with refractory acidosis or rapidly rising lactate levels > 10 mmol/L will require haemodialysis. Administration of sodium bicarbonate may be useful as a temporising measure in severe acidosis prior to dialysis.

PRACTICE TIPS

PITFALLS

- Discharging patients 'after hours'.
- Inadequate airway management of the intoxicated patient with decreased level of consciousness.
- Inappropriate decontamination of benign ingestions, the uncooperative patient or the patient at risk of aspiration.
- Failure to detect urinary retention in the agitated patient, particular if there is evidence of anticholinergic toxicity.
- Failure to administer *N*-acetylcysteine within 8 hours of ingestion in the patient at risk of paracetamol toxicity.
- Stopping *N*-acetylcysteine infusions for paracetamol overdose because of an anaphylactoid reaction. These are common and generally benign: treat symptomatically and slow the infusion rate.
- Withholding high-dose insulin-euglycaemic therapy in severe calcium channel blocker toxicity due to fear of the large insulin doses required.
- Failure to recognise that sulfonylurea overdose can result in delayed and prolonged hypoglycaemia, and should be treated with octreotide when hypoglycaemia first develops.
- Failure to recognise the high mortality of chronic digoxin toxicity. If a patient is sick and takes digoxin, check levels or treat empirically with 2 ampoules of Digibind (digoxin immune Fab).
- Compromising the care of patients with organophosphate poisoning due to unwarranted fears about nosocomial poisoning.

One pill can kill

The child presenting after eating an unknown tablet is a difficult clinical situation.

All attempts should be made to determine what tablets were accessible to the child. Should this be impossible, the child should be observed for a minimum of 8 hours, and never discharged overnight. There is no need to empirically administer activated charcoal unless a definite ingestion of a lethal dose has occurred, in which case a clinical toxicologist should be consulted for advice.

There is a group of tablets that, if ingested by a child, can be lethal with a one- or two-tablet dose (see Table 30.4), and management of a toddler who has ingested unidentified tablets must take these into consideration (see Box 30.6).

TABLE 30.3 Octreotide treatment regimen in sulfonylurea overdose		
	ADULT	CHILD
Bolus (IV)	50 µg	1 µg/kg
Infusion (IV)	25–50 µg/h	1 µg/kg/h

TABLE 30.4 Potentially lethal medications if 2 tablets are ingested by a toddler weighing 10 kg

AGENT	SEVERE TOXICITY CHARACTERISTICS
Amphetamines	Can cause confusion, agitation, hypertension and hyperthermia
Calcium channel blockers	Rapid progression to hypotension, bradydysrhythmia, shock and cardiac collapse leading to cardiac arrest
Chloroquine Hydroxychloroquine	Coma and cardiac arrest
Dextropropoxyphene	Seizure activity and cardiac toxicity leading to ventricular tachycardia
Opioids	Respiratory depression, ventricular dysrhythmias and cardio-respiratory arrest
Propranolol	Causes hypoglycaemia, ventricular tachycardia, hypothermia, seizures and coma
Sulfonylureas	Hypoglycaemia which can be slow onset up to 8 hours post ingestion
Theophylline	Vomiting, sinus tachycardia and central nervous system stimulation +/– seizures
Tricyclic antidepressants	Seizures and ventricular dysrhythmia

BOX 30.6 Management of a toddler who ingests unidentified tablets[12]

1. Admit for a minimum 12-hour observation period.
2. Ensure healthcare facility has appropriate resources to observe, resuscitate and treat patient if evidence of poisoning occurs.
3. IV access can be deferred until early evidence of toxicity is apparent.
4. Check bedside glucose level at presentation, if there is clinical evidence of hypoglycaemia, and at discharge.
5. Brief staff regarding clinical features for which the patient is being observed (see Table 30.4).
6. Monitor level of consciousness, vital signs (pulse, blood pressure and respiratory rate) and for early clinical features of hypoglycaemia.
7. Cardiac monitoring may be instituted if there is any abnormality of conscious state or vital signs.
8. Discharge patients only during daylight hours.

SUMMARY

Poisoning, whether accidental or deliberate, is an important ED presentation. The incidence differs between children and adults, with childhood presentations more likely to be accidental in nature. Although the ingestion of pharmaceuticals is common in children, the rate of poisonings from household chemicals and plants is increasing. In most cases, children do not ingest significant amounts and severe clinical symptoms are unlikely. However, the potential toxicity of some drugs such as the agents described in this chapter is high, and an accurate risk assessment and an appropriate period of observation is essential. Most importantly, one should treat the patient, not the poison. Meticulous supportive care is all that is required following most poisonings.

Adult poisonings are frequently deliberate. Self-harm attempts by drug overdose usually require hospital assessment and treatment. Emergency stabilisation and maintenance of an adequate airway, breathing and circulation is the priority. Following this, the generation of a risk assessment guides all further care and management decisions. Development of the role of ED observation wards now means that patient management, from initial assessment to final disposition, can be conducted by the same nursing team with excellent continuity of care.

CASE STUDY

A 32-year-old male presents to the emergency department (ED) after ingesting 50 × 100 mg quetiapine tablets 3 hours ago. On initial assessment he has a Glasgow Coma Scale score of 8/15, with the following vital signs:

- pulse 132 beats/minute
- blood pressure 94/67 mmHg
- respiratory rate 12 breaths/minute
- temperature 37.2°C.

He is transferred into a monitored bay where a 12-lead ECG is undertaken showing some mild QT prolongation, and a BSL is taken, returning at 6.3 mmol.

Questions
1. What is the initial risk assessment?
2. What is the initial management for this patient?
3. What other toxicological screening test should be performed?
4. What ongoing management is required for this patient?

Answers to Case Study Questions can be found on evolve
http://evolve.emergencytrauma.curtis

REFERENCES

1. McGrath J. A survey of deliberate self-poisoning. Med J Aust 1989;150(6):317–24.

2. Pond SM. Prescription for poisoning. Med J Aust 1995;162(4):174–5.

3. Hawton K, Fagg J. Trends in deliberate self poisoning and self injury in Oxford, 1976–1990. Br Med J 1992;304(6839):1409–11.

4. Royal New Zealand College of Psychiatrists Clinical Practice Guidelines Team for Deliberate Self-harm. Australian and New Zealand clinical practice guidelines for the management of adult deliberate self-harm. Aust NZ J Psychiatry 2004;38(11–12):868–84.

5. Australian Institute of Health and Welfare. Australia's health 2012. Australia's health series no.13. Cat. no. AUS 156. Canberra: AIHW; 2012.

6. Tovell A, McKenna K, Bradley C, Pointer S. Hospital separations due to injury and poisoning, Australia 2009–10. Injury research and statistics series no. 69. Cat. no. INJCAT 145. Canberra: AIHW; 2012.

7. Ministry of Health. Intentional Self-harm Hospitalisations: 2007 (provisional). Wellington: Ministry of Health; 2009.

8. Yates KM. Accidental poisoning in New Zealand. Emerg Med (Fremantle) 2003;15(3):244–9.

9. Lam LT. Childhood and adolescence poisoning in NSW, Australia: an analysis of age, sex, geographic, and poison types. Inj Prev 2003;9(4):338–42.

10. Reith DM, Pitt WR, Hockey R. Childhood poisoning in Queensland: an analysis of presentation and admission rates. J Paediatr Child Health 2001;37(5):446–50.

11. Isbister GK, Downes F, Sibbritt D et al. Aspiration pneumonitis in an overdose population: frequency, predictors, and outcomes. Crit Care Med 2004;32(1):88–93.

12. Murray L, Daly F, Little M et al. Toxicology handbook. 2nd edn. Sydney: Elsevier; 2011.

13. Daly FF, Little M, Murray L. A risk assessment based approach to the management of acute poisoning. Emerg Med J 2006;23(5):396–9.

14. Tenenbein M. Do you really need that emergency drug screen? Clin Toxicol (Phila) 2009;47(4):286–91.

15. American Academy of Clinical Toxicology/European Association of Poison Centres and Clinical Toxicologists. Position paper: single-dose activated charcoal. J Toxicol Clin Toxicol 2005;43:61–87.

16. Dart RC, Borron SW, Caravati EM et al. Expert consensus guidelines for stocking of antidotes in hospitals that provide emergency care. Ann Emerg Med 2009;54(3):386–94.

17. Megarbane B, Borron SW, Baud FJ. Current recommendations for treatment of severe toxic alcohol poisonings. Intensive Care Med 2005;31(2):189–95.

18. O'Malley GF. Emergency department management of the salicylate-poisoned patient. Emerg Med Clin North Am 2007;25(2):333–46.

19. Daly FF, Fountain JS, Murray L et al. Guidelines for the management of paracetamol poisoning in Australia and New Zealand— explanation and elaboration. A consensus statement from clinical toxicologists consulting to the Australasian poisons information centres. Med J Aust 2008;188(5):296–301.

20. Bradberry SM, Thanacoody HKR, Watt BE et al. Management of the cardiovascular complications of tricyclic antidepressant poisoning: role of sodium bicarbonate. Toxicol Rev 2005;24(3):195–204.

21. Boyer EW, Shannon M. The serotonin syndrome. N Engl J Med 2005;352(11):1112–20.

22. Burns MJ. The pharmacology and toxicology of atypical antipsychotic agents. J Toxicol Clin Toxicol 2001;39(1):1–14.

23. Love JN, Howell JM, Litovitz TL et al. Acute beta-blocker overdose: factors associated with the development of cardiovascular morbidity. J Toxicol Clin Toxicol 2000;38(3):275–81.

24. Kerns W 2nd. Management of beta-adrenergic blocker and calcium channel antagonist toxicity. Emerg Med Clin North Am 2007;25(2):309–31.

25. Nickson CP, Little M. Early use of high-dose insulin euglycaemic therapy for verapamil toxicity. Med J Aust 2009;191(6):350–2.

26. Antman EM, Wenger TL, Butler Jr VP et al. Treatment of 150 cases of life-threatening digitalis intoxication with digoxin-specific Fab antibody fragments: final report of a multicenter study. Circulation 1990;81(6):1744–52.

27. Jaeger A, Sauder P, Kopferschmitt J et al. When should dialysis be performed in lithium poisoning? A kinetic study in 14 cases of lithium poisoning. J Toxicol Clin Toxicol 1993;31(3):429–47.

28. Lee HL, Chen KW, Chi CH et al. Clinical presentations and prognostic factors of a glyphosate-surfactant herbicide intoxication: a review of 131 cases. Acad Emerg Med 2000;7(8):906–10.

29. Eddleston M, Buckley NA, Eyer P et al. Management of acute organophosphorus pesticide poisoning. Lancet 2008;371(9612):597–607.

30. Bosse GM. Conservative management of patients with moderately elevated serum iron levels. J Toxicol Clin Toxicol 1995;33(2):135–40.

31. Haskell RJ, Stapczynski JS. Duration of hypoglycemia and need for intravenous glucose following intentional overdoses of insulin. Ann Emerg Med 1984;13:505–11.

32. Harrigan RA, Nathan MS, Beattie P. Oral agents for the treatment of type 2 diabetes mellitus: pharmacology, toxicity, and treatment. Ann Emerg Med 2001;38(1):68–78.

33. McLaughlin SA, Crandall CS, McKinney PE. Octreotide: an antidote for sulfonylurea induced hypoglycaemia. Ann Emerg Med 2000;36:133–8.

34. McCoubrie D, Murray L, Daly FF et al. Toxicology case of the month: ingestion of two unidentified tablets by a toddler. Emerg Med J 2006;23(9):718–20.

CHAPTER 31
ENVENOMATION
IOANA VLAD AND KANE GUTHRIE

Essentials

- Snake bite is a rare but potentially lethal presentation in the emergency health setting, and few clinicians have managed enough cases to be completely confident of the approach to management.

- Once snake bite is considered a possibility, a standardised sequential approach to management is required, even in patients who are asymptomatic and have no obvious bite marks.

- Early effective application of a pressure-immobilisation bandage (PIB) is vital first-aid treatment for snake bite, and should always be applied.

- Observation in hospital and serial clinical and laboratory evaluation for 12 hours is required to exclude significant envenoming from snake bite.

- Appropriate antivenom therapy should be given once the diagnosis of envenoming is made. In the event of cardiac arrest from snake bite, early intravenous administration of undiluted antivenom is warranted.

- Redback spider bite is the most common medically important arachnid envenoming syndrome in Australia. Funnel-web spider envenoming is much less common, but potentially lethal. Effective antidotes are available for both species of spider.

- Marine envenomings usually cause pain and can be treated with hot-water immersion therapy and good supportive care.

- Rarer marine envenomings (box jellyfish, irukandji syndrome, blue-ringed octopus) can be lethal. Recognition of the clinical syndrome is important, and advanced life support may be required.

INTRODUCTION

Australia has a large number of deadly terrestrial and marine creatures, and every year there are thousands of presentations to emergency departments (EDs) with significant or life-threatening clinical effects related to envenomation. Snakes, spiders and marine animals, such as jellyfish, cone fish or stonefish, can all cause significant morbidity or mortality. By comparison, New Zealand has a much smaller range of poisonous creatures, and the risk of significant injury is much lower.

A standardised approach to envenoming, with appropriate first aid, clinical and laboratory evaluation and the administration of antivenom, ensures a good outcome in most cases. Early discussion with a regional Poisons Information Centre (Australia: phone 13 11 26 or New Zealand: 0800 POISON/0800 764 766) is extremely useful: these centres provide expert advice in the management of envenomation syndromes.

Venom

Venom is the poisonous secretion of an animal, such as a snake, spider or scorpion, and is usually transmitted by a bite or sting. Venom is a complex, multicomponent substance containing various enzymes and toxins. Most pathophysiological effects of envenoming can be divided into three general categories:

1. Coagulopathic
   - Procoagulant agglutinins can cause a severe venom-induced consumptive coagulopathy (VICC), due to prothrombin activation and fibrinogen consumption (defibrination). This is a feature of brown snake, tiger snake and taipan envenoming.
   - Anticoagulant toxins—for example, with black snake envenoming—cause a less severe coagulopathy.
2. Neurotoxic
   - Presynaptic inhibition of acetylcholine release results in progressive paralysis, and is a feature of tiger snake, taipan and sea snake envenomation.
   - Postsynaptic inhibition of neuromuscular activation with death adder envenoming. The first signs of paralysis are usually evident in the small, ocular muscles (diplopia, ptosis, gaze palsies) and can progress to respiratory failure. Paralysis may also result from tetrodotoxin from pufferfish ingestion or blue-ringed octopus envenoming, or due to cone-shell conotoxins.
   - Presynaptic stimulation of catecholamine release due to envenoming by funnel-web spider, or irukandji syndrome causes symptoms of sympathetic hyperstimulation, manifesting as hypertension or pulmonary oedema. Neuromuscular paralysis is not a significant clinical feature.
   - Redback spider venom also stimulates acetylcholine and catecholamine release, resulting in a constellation of symptoms known as 'lactrodectism' (described below).
3. Myopathic
   - Myotoxins are commonly found in Australian snake venom and cause significant pain and rhabdomyolysis.
   - Other effects related to venom include non-specific symptoms, such as headache, nausea and vomiting, sudden collapse and cardiac arrest, thrombotic microangiopathy (TMA) and nephrotoxicity.

Antivenom

The Commonwealth Serum Laboratory (CSL) has developed a range of antivenoms for the treatment of snake, funnel-web or redback spider, box jellyfish and stonefish envenomation.[1]

The decision to use antivenom is made once objective evidence of envenoming is obtained. All snake antivenom is administered intravenously, diluted in 500 mL of Normal saline (20 mL/kg for children) and infused over 20 minutes.

In cardiac arrest, antivenom may be given as an undiluted intravenous (IV) bolus and may be life-saving. Severe allergic reactions to these products are rare,[2] but they should always be given in an environment where full resuscitation facilities are available. Premedication with adrenaline or antihistamines to prevent anaphylactic reactions is not routinely indicated.

In the rare case of anaphylaxis to antivenom, the infusion should be stopped immediately. Give oxygen, IV fluids and administer intramuscular (IM) adrenaline 0.01 mg/kg (max 0.5 mg) to the lateral thigh, and recommence the antivenom infusion cautiously once the clinical manifestations of anaphylaxis are controlled. Rarely, ongoing administration of adrenaline by titrated infusion may be necessary to complete antivenom administration.[3] Adrenaline has to be carefully titrated to avoid hypertensive bursts in coagulopathic patients, as this could result in intracerebral haemorrhage.

Snake bite

Overview

Definite or suspected snake bite is a common emergency presentation throughout Australia. Snake bite is a time-critical emergency presentation and a simple, standardised approach is required to provide adequate treatment should envenoming occur (see Box 31.1). Early discussion with a regional Poisons Information Centre is extremely useful to aid in clinical

---

BOX 31.1 Approach to snake bite

Out-of-hospital
1. First aid
   Pressure immobilisation bandaging
2. Transport
   The patient is transported as soon as possible to a hospital that meets all of the following criteria:
   a) doctor(s) able to manage snake bite
   b) laboratory capable of performing necessary investigations on a 24-hour basis
   c) adequate stock of antivenom to provide definitive treatment.

Hospital
1. Resuscitation
2. Risk assessment
3. Determine if the patient is envenomed. Serial regular assessment and observation over a period of at least 12 hours:
   a) history
   b) serial physical examination
   c) serial laboratory investigations.
4. If envenomed, determine the type of monovalent antivenom required:
   a) geographical area (prevalent indigenous snakes)
   b) clinical and laboratory features
   c) Commonwealth Serum Laboratory snake venom detection kit (SVDK).
5. Administer the dose of monovalent antivenom required to definitively treat the envenoming.
6. Adjuvant and supportive treatment.

management decisions. Although severe envenoming is rare, it is potentially lethal.[4] Any patient bitten by a snake, whether suspected or confirmed, is eligible for inclusion in the Australian Snakebite Project (see Useful websites at end of the chapter).

First aid

The use of a pressure-immobilisation bandage (PIB) is the standard first-aid treatment used to delay the lymphatic spread of venom proximally from the bite site.[5] It is indicated for bites by all Australian snake species, as well as bites from funnel-web spiders and the blue-ringed octopus. It is not advocated for bites from the redback spider, other spiders, scorpions or stings from venomous fish.

The PIB compresses the lymphatic vessels and inhibits limb muscle movement, thus retarding venom transport and preventing venom from entering the systemic circulation. It is not definitive medical treatment but, when applied correctly, may prevent significant systemic symptoms while the patient is transferred to an appropriate medical facility. Unfortunately, PIB application can be difficult to optimise and is often performed poorly.[6] See Chapter 17, p. 349, for information on applying bandages.

The principles of adequate PIB application are:[5,6]

- Use a firm ~ 15 cm broad bandage (preferably elasticised—not crepe bandage) directly over the bite site and extend proximally to cover the whole of the affected limb.
- Use firm pressure to occlude lymphatic flow but preserve blood flow—as for supporting a sprained ankle.
- Check for distal pulse to ensure adequate blood flow.
- Include fingers and toes in the bandage to reduce limb movement.
- Splint the limb to further restrict movement.
- Immobilise the limb and the patient.
- Do not elevate the limb (as you might for a fracture).

Bites to body parts other than a limb pose a difficult problem—a pressure dressing should be applied, and efforts made to completely immobilise the patient while transportation to hospital is organised.

Useful pictorial representations of PIB application can be found on numerous websites; see the list at the end of the chapter.

Resuscitation

Most patients present with a history of possible bite and do not require immediate resuscitation. Until envenoming is excluded, all suspected snake-bite patients should initially be assessed and managed in an area equipped for cardiorespiratory monitoring and resuscitation. The priorities of care of maintaining airway, breathing and circulation remain (see Ch 15). Potential early life-threats associated with Australian terrestrial snake envenoming include:

- hypotension (brown snake, tiger snake, taipan)
- respiratory failure secondary to paralysis (taipan, tiger snake, death adder, sea snake)
- seizures (taipan)
- severe coagulopathy with uncontrolled haemorrhage (brown snake, tiger snake, taipan).

In cardiac arrest due to snake bite, undiluted antivenom administered as a rapid IV push may be life-saving.

Assessment

Once snake bite is considered a possibility, the risk assessment is straightforward: there is a risk of life-threatening envenoming and a formal process must begin, in an appropriate setting, to exclude that possibility. There is no risk stratification process that allows the clinician to identify patients who can be discharged early or without laboratory investigations. Patients with no obvious bite mark and no symptoms may still be envenomed. This is a vital step in the management pathway and ensures that life-threatening cases are not missed. It is extremely unusual for a snake to be identified with sufficient reliability to preclude further observation or investigation.[4]

Patients do not necessarily have to be transferred to tertiary urban hospitals, but they need to be observed in a medical facility with:

- laboratory facilities on site to perform serial blood tests
- antivenom available for the suspected snake genus
- a doctor who is able to deal with the life-threatening complications of snake bite or antivenom (respiratory failure secondary to neurotoxicity, anaphylaxis).

Point-of-care devices that measure INR or D-dimer should not be used as there are reports of false negative results in patients who have VICC.[8] Whole blood clotting test should not be used either, as it is not reliable when assessing snake bites.[9]

Determine if the patient is envenomed

The aim of the hospital assessment is to seek objective evidence of envenoming based on history, physical examination and laboratory data. Serial physical examination (looking for bleeding, and neurotoxicity) and investigations (full blood count [FBC], urea and electrolytes [U&Es], creatine kinase [CK] and coagulation studies) are performed until envenoming is diagnosed *or* 12 hours has expired (see Table 31.1).

There are a number of non-specific symptoms related to snake bite that by themselves do not necessitate antivenom treatment. These include nausea, vomiting, abdominal pain, malaise and mild headache. However, these symptoms *can* represent envenomation or significant underlying pathology (e.g. intracranial haemorrhage due to coagulopathy), so thorough assessment is mandatory.

Abnormalities of initial physical examination or laboratory studies consistent with snake envenoming prompt immediate antivenom therapy as outlined below (see Table 31.2). However, if the patient is clinically well and initial laboratory studies are normal, then the PIB is removed. If there is a sudden clinical deterioration, the PIB is immediately reapplied, laboratory studies repeated and antivenom administered.

If there is no discernible deterioration following removal of the PIB, the patient is observed and physical examination and laboratory studies repeated at 2, 6 and 12 hours. Twelve hours after removal of PIB the patient is reassessed and, if there is no evidence of envenoming, the patient may be discharged. Note that patients should not be discharged at night, as subtle delayed neurotoxicity may not be detected.

Antivenom administration

All snake antivenom is derived from horse serum. Monovalent antivenom is preferred to polyvalent antivenom as it is more specific, cheaper, safer and associated with a lower probability

TABLE 31.1 Assessment of snake bite[4]		
HISTORY	**PHYSICAL EXAMINATION**	**LABORATORY INVESTIGATIONS**
Geographical area where bite occurred	Vital signs	Full blood count (FBC)
Appearance of snake (usually only useful for death adders)	Mental status	renal function
	Respiratory function (PEFR/FEV₁)	creatine kinase (CK)
Anatomical site of bite	Look specifically for:	coagulation profile (aPTT, INR, fibrinogen, D-dimer, fibrin degradation products, LDH)
Number of strikes	• evidence of bite	
Use of first aid (PIB)	• lymphadenopathy	Urinalysis for blood/myoglobin
Symptoms such as collapse, nausea, vomiting, bleeding and weakness	• abnormal bleeding such as the gums	SVDK if available and indicated
	• descending symmetrical flaccid paralysis	

aPTT: activated partial thromboplastin time; FEV_1: forced expiratory volume in one second; INR: international normalised ratio; PEFR: peak expiratory flow rate; PIB: pressure-immobilisation bandage

of serum sickness. The choice of monovalent antivenom is based on:[7,10]

- knowledge of snakes found in the area
- clinical presentation
- constellation of laboratory abnormalities
- results from using CSL snake venom detection kit (Box 31.2).

Antivenom dosages are based on consensus opinion and clinical experience, but there is minimal scientific data on the antivenom dose required to neutralise venom in vivo. Recently published results from the Australian Snakebite Project[7] suggest that for all snake bites one ampoule of antivenom is enough to ensure adequate treatment of envenoming syndromes.

Polyvalent antivenom contains the equivalent of 1 ampoule of each of the monovalent antivenoms. It contains a large protein load and thus has a higher probability of causing allergic reactions. Ideally it should only be used in specific situations if it is not possible to use monovalent antivenom (Box 31.3).[10]

Adjuvant therapy

Patients who receive antivenom are counselled about the possibility of serum sickness, which can occur 4–21 days after antivenom administration. Symptoms include myalgias, fevers, malaise and arthralgias, and patients may develop a palpable non-blanching rash. Prednisone 1 mg/kg/day (up to 50 mg/day) for 5 days may attenuate the severity of serum sickness, but steroids are not routinely prescribed as prophylaxis.

Blood products such as fresh frozen plasma (FFP) or cryoprecipitate should be avoided unless there is uncontrolled and life-threatening haemorrhage.[7] Recovery of clinically acceptable coagulation appears to take longer than previously recognised[11] (about 12–18 hours rather than 4–8 hours). Snake bites are not necessarily infection- or tetanus-prone wounds, but it is reasonable to consider these risks and manage them according to standard wound care. Intramuscular tetanus toxoid should not be given to patients while coagulopathy is present due to a theoretical risk of developing intramuscular haematoma.

Snakes

Brown snake

- Eastern brown snake, *Pseudonaja textilis* (Fig 31.1)
- Western brown snake or gwardar, *P. nuchalis*
- Dugite, *P. affinis*
- Other *Pseudonaja* spp.

Brown snake envenoming is the most common cause of death from snake bite in Australia. These snakes are found in all parts of Australia, except for Tasmania, Kangaroo Island and two small islands off the coast of Perth (Carnac and Garden Islands).

Systemic envenoming may be heralded by collapse within a few minutes of the bite. The hallmark of brown snake envenoming is a severe defibrinating VICC. This may manifest clinically as bleeding gums, persistent haemorrhage at venesection or bite sites, or intracerebral haemorrhage.

Renal failure occurs in a small percentage of patients and oliguria may be present from the time of envenoming. Thrombotic microangiopathy (TMA) is a rare complication.

Rhabdomyolysis does not occur to a significant extent and neurotoxicity is rare, despite the presence of a neurotoxin in the venom. Mild diplopia and ptosis are observed occasionally, but are not predominant features of brown snake envenomation.

The VICC of brown snake envenoming is characterised by:

- elevated activated partial thromboplastin time (aPTT) and international normalised ratio (INR) (at least >3), but both usually immeasurable
- low fibrinogen (often undetectable)
- elevated D-dimer (e.g. 10 times the lower limit of normal) and fibrin degradation products

Brown snake and tiger snake envenoming may be indistinguishable early in the course, as both cause defibrinating VICC. However, in tiger snake envenoming, paralysis and rhabdomyolysis evolve over the ensuing hours.

Management

Each ampoule of brown snake antivenom contains 1000 units. Initial treatment for clinical or laboratory evidence of

TABLE 31.2 Clinical features of snake envenomation[1]

CATEGORY (GENUS)	DEFIBRINATING CONSUMPTIVE COAGULOPATHY (VICC)	NEUROTOXICITY (PRESYNAPTIC)	NEUROTOXICITY (POSTSYNAPTIC)	RHABDOMYOLYSIS	RENAL FAILURE	OTHER EFFECTS
Brown (*Pseudonaja*)	Always present with significant envenoming	Very rare	Not present	Not present	Uncommon but well recognised complication	Thrombotic microangiopathy and thrombocytopenia
Tiger (*Notechis*)	Always present with significant envenoming	Slow onset over hours	Not present	Onset over hours	Uncommon. May occur secondary to rhabdomyolysis	Thrombotic microangiopathy and thrombocytopenia
Death adder (*Acanthophis*)	Not present	Not present	Slow onset over hours	Rare	Not present	Local bite site pain often present
Black (*Pseudechis*)	Not present May have raised aPTT, but fibrinogen remains normal	Not present	Not present	Slow onset over hours/days	Secondary to rhabdomyolysis	Bite site pain may be significant Envenoming usually associated with nausea, vomiting, abdominal pain and headache Anosmia that can be irreversible
Taipan (*Oxyuranus*)	Always present with significant envenoming	May be rapid in onset	Not present	Onset over minutes/hours	Uncommon. May occur secondary to rhabdomyolysis	Thrombotic microangiopathy and thrombocytopenia
Sea snakes (*Hydrophiidae*)	Not present	May be rapid in onset	Not present	Onset over minutes/hours	Secondary to rhabdomyolysis	

aPTT: activated partial thromboplastin time

- The SVDK indicates the correct monovalent antivenom to use once a decision has been made to give antivenom.
- The SVDK is not used to determine whether or not a patient is envenomed. False-positives and false-negatives occur; so, if the SVDK does not match the clinical picture, treat the patient, not the SVDK result.
- If there is doubt about the snake responsible for the envenoming and the SVDK is not helpful (e.g. possible early tiger or brown snake envenoming in a geographical location where the two snakes co-exist), two monovalent antivenoms are superior to polyvalent antivenom.
- The SVDK is ideally performed by a meticulous and experienced technician according to the enclosed instructions.
- The SDVK is performed using a bite-site swab, which can be accessed by cutting a 'key-hole' in the PIB.
- The SVDK may also be performed on urine (second-line).
- The SVDK should not be performed on serum or blood due to the high incidence of false-positive results.
- The first positive well to turn blue within the allotted time (10 minutes) gives the result. Other wells may subsequently turn blue but are ignored. If no well turns blue within the allotted time, the test is negative and subsequent changes are ignored.

PIB: pressure-immobilisation bandage

BOX 31.3 **Indications for polyvalent antivenom**[1]

1. Appropriate monovalent antivenoms not available.
2. No SVDK result available and the range of possible snakes requires the mixing of three or more monovalent antivenoms.
3. Severe envenoming, insufficient time to wait for SVDK results, and the range of possible snakes would require the mixing of three or more monovalent antivenoms.
4. Exhausted monovalent antivenom stocks.

SVDK: snake venom detection kit

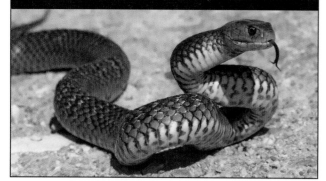

FIGURE 31.1 **Common or eastern brown snake (*Pseudonaja textilis*).**

Shutterstock/Kristian Bell

envenomation is 1 ampoule. This is lower than previous recommendations, based on emerging in vitro and in vivo data and the realisation that although antivenom may treat other components of envenoming, it does not appear to hasten recovery from VICC.[11,12]

Recheck the coagulation profile 3, 6 and 12 hours after the administration of antivenom. Marked improvements in aPTT and INR are better markers to assess recovery than fibrinogen levels,[13] and recovery is considered complete when INR < 2. Blood tests should also be performed up to 24 hours after envenomation to assess for less-common sequelae such as haemolysis or renal failure. Watch for deteriorating renal function and evidence of TMA, indicated by raised lactate dehydrogenase (LDH) and fragmented red blood cells on the blood film.

Tiger snake

- Common or eastern tiger snake, *Notechis scutatus*
- Western or black tiger snake, *N. ater*
- Copperhead, *Austrelaps* spp.
- Broad-headed snake, *Hoplocephalus bungaroides*
- Stephen's banded snake, *H. stephensi*
- Pale-headed snake, *H. bitorquatus*
- Rough-scaled snake, *Tropidechis carinatus*

Tiger snakes (Fig 31.2) are found along the coastal regions of the lower half of Australia, extending upwards into Queensland. They are the only terrestrial venomous snakes found in Tasmania and on Kangaroo Island, and Carnac and Garden Islands (Western Australia).

The features of tiger snake envenoming[14] are:

- VICC
- neurotoxicity—progressive descending flaccid paralysis
- rhabdomyolysis.

The initial stages of tiger and brown snake envenomation may be identical—the VICC is indistinguishable. However, patients with tiger snake envenoming are likely to develop a progressive paralysis over the subsequent several hours. If there is a geographical risk of a bite from either snake, and it is early in the clinical course, it may be necessary to use monovalent

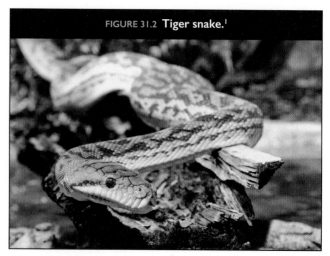

FIGURE 31.2 **Tiger snake.**[1]

Shutterstock/mroz

antivenom for both tiger *and* brown snakes to ensure adequate treatment.[4]

The neurotoxic effects of the venom initially appear as diplopia or ptosis, and can progress to diaphragmatic paralysis with respiratory failure. Antivenom does not reverse established weakness, but can prevent progression. Untreated, paralysis may persist for days before resolving. Regular assessments of peak expiratory flow rate (PEFR) or FEV_1 (forced expiratory volume) are useful objective markers of respiratory function. Refer to Chapter 17, p. 334, for techniques on obtaining these measurements.

Myotoxins in the venom can cause significant pain, muscle necrosis and rhabdomyolysis, and these symptoms can be significant features of envenomation.

Management

Each ampoule of tiger snake antivenom contains 3000 units. Initial dosage for envenomation is 1 ampoule. Recheck the coagulation profile 3, 6 and 12 hours after the administration of antivenom. Marked improvements in aPTT and INR are better markers to assess recovery than fibrinogen levels,[10] and recovery is considered complete when INR < 2.

Black snake

- Mulga or king brown snake, *Pseudechis australis* (Fig 31.3)
- Red-bellied or common black snake, *P. porphyriacus*
- Blue-bellied or spotted black snake, *P. guttatus*

Black snakes are found throughout inland and northern Australia.[15,16] They are large and aggressive snakes which inflict a painful bite. The mulga is confusingly also known as the king brown snake, but it is not a brown snake and envenoming *will not* resolve with brown snake antivenom.

Black snake venom contains myotoxins, neurotoxins and anticoagulant toxins. In contrast to the profound VICC observed in brown snake, tiger snake and taipan envenoming, black snake envenomation is associated with isolated raise in aPTT, with normal INR, fibrinogen and D-dimer levels. Envenoming by an Australian snake, associated with local pain, headache, nausea and vomiting, and a mild anticoagulant coagulopathy (increased aPTT and INR but normal fibrinogen and D-dimer), is highly suggestive of black snake envenoming.

The red-bellied black snake is found in more-coastal areas around the southeast of Australia, and envenoming is not usually lethal, even without treatment. Red-bellied and blue-bellied black snakes have less-potent toxins which usually cause minor myolysis only.

Management

Each ampoule of black snake antivenom contains 18,000 units. Initial dosage for envenoming is 1 ampoule. Antivenom prevents progression of muscle injury, but does not reverse injury that has already occurred. Indications for antivenom administration are laboratory evidence of anticoagulant coagulopathy or CK that exceeds 1000 IU/L. A much lower threshold is used if the patient has significant pain from myonecrosis, or if non-specific features of abdominal pain, vomiting or headache are severe and unresponsive to symptomatic treatment. CK is usually abnormal on arrival, but may not become grossly elevated for many hours. CK should be checked 6-hourly in the symptomatic patient or 12-hourly in the asymptomatic patient with a mild anticoagulant coagulopathy.

The red- and blue-bellied black snakes are black snakes, but can also be treated with tiger snake antivenom if necessary.

Death adder

- Common death adder, *Acanthophis antarcticus* (Fig 31.4)
- Desert death adder, *A. pyrrhus*
- Northern death adder, *A. praelongus*
- Pilbara death adder, *A. wellsii*

Death adders are found throughout most of mainland Australia and Papua New Guinea, but bites and envenoming are uncommon.[15,16] Prior to mechanical ventilation and antivenom availability, mortality was approximately 50%. The most significant venom toxin is a postsynaptic neurotoxin. Pain or stinging at the bite site is common; however, puncture wounds may not be apparent. Death adders are the only venomous Australian snakes that may possibly be identified by sight—they are short, fat snakes with a characteristic diamond-shaped head. Death adders are elusive and nocturnal. A common scenario is that the victim is bitten on the ankle after treading on the snake while walking outside with bare feet at dusk. The victim may feel little more than a sting and not see the snake.

Systemic envenoming is characterised by a progressive symmetrical descending flaccid paralysis, which usually

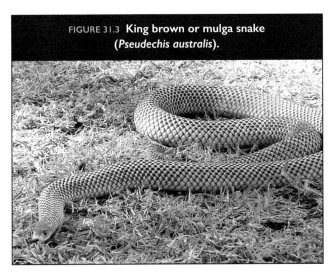

FIGURE 31.3 King brown or mulga snake (*Pseudechis australis*).

Flickr/F Delventhal/CC BY 2.0

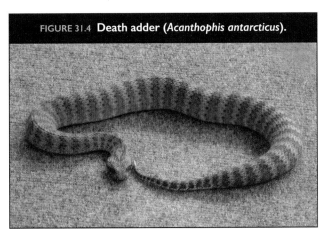

FIGURE 31.4 Death adder (*Acanthophis antarcticus*).

Flickr/Stephan Ridgway/CC BY 2.0

manifests within 6 hours, but can be delayed. Early signs include ptosis, blurred vision, diplopia and difficulty swallowing. If left untreated, generalised paralysis, respiratory failure and secondary hypoxic cardiac arrest ensue. Regular assessments of PEFR or FEV_1 are useful objective markers of respiratory function.

With airway support, paralysis resolves spontaneously after 1–2 days. Coagulopathy and renal failure are not features of death adder envenoming. Rhabdomyolysis can rarely occur. Because the toxin has a primarily postsynaptic effect, neurotoxicity may be reversed by the administration of neostigmine if antivenom is not available.[17]

Management

Each ampoule of death adder antivenom contains 6000 units. Initial dosage for envenomation is 1 ampoule. In the absence of death adder antivenom, 1 ampoule of CSL polyvalent antivenom contains 6000 units of death adder antivenom and may be administered as an alternative.

Taipan

- Coastal taipan, *Oxyuranus scutellatus*
- Inland taipan (small-scaled snake), *O. microlepidotus*
- Papuan taipan, *O. scutellatus canni*

Australian taipans are found in the northern part of Queensland and the Northern Territory. The Papuan taipan is the most lethal snake in Papua New Guinea. Taipan snake envenoming is rare and is usually lethal without antivenom treatment. It is characterised by rapid onset of VICC, neurotoxicity and rhabdomyolysis.

Taipan venom contains potent pre- and postsynaptic neurotoxins (causing paralysis), myotoxins (causing rhabdomyolysis) and procoagulants (activators of factor VII and prothrombin). The coagulopathy is similar to that caused by brown or tiger snakes. Systemic envenoming may be heralded by collapse within a few minutes of the bite and paralysis is usually apparent within 1–2 hours. Seizures have been reported as an early manifestation of envenomation.[16]

Management

Each ampoule of taipan antivenom contains 12,000 units. Initial dosage for envenoming is 1 ampoule. Recheck the coagulation profile 3, 6 and 12 hours after the administration of antivenom. Marked improvements in aPTT and INR are better markers to assess recovery than fibrinogen levels,[13] and recovery is considered complete when INR < 2. Blood tests should also be performed up to 24 hours after envenomation to assess for less-common sequelae such as haemolysis or renal failure. Watch for deteriorating renal function and evidence of TMA, indicated by raised LDH and fragmented red blood cells on the blood film.

The antivenom halts the progression of paralysis, but does not reverse established neurotoxicity.

If taipan monovalent antivenom is not available, 1 ampoule of polyvalent antivenom may be used as a substitute.

Sea snakes

There are at least 30 species of sea snake found around the coast of northern Australia. They belong to the family Hydrophiidae, and are closely related to the venomous Australian terrestrial snakes Elapidae. They are inquisitive, but rarely aggressive and bites always occur when they are handled—for example, when they are manually removed from fishing nets. Sea snakes have small fangs located in the rear of the mouth, so there is a lower risk of envenoming from a bite than with terrestrial snakes. However, it is important to realise that a snake bite at sea, on the beach or in estuarine waters *may* be from a terrestrial snake as all snakes can swim.

Sea snake venom contains postsynaptic neurotoxins (paralysis) and myotoxins (rhabdomyolysis). Most bites are superficial, relatively painless and not associated with local swelling or lymphadenitis. Rhabdomyolysis manifests as myalgia and myoglobinuria and may progress to cause renal failure. Systemic envenoming is characterised by symmetrical descending flaccid paralysis, which usually manifests within 6 hours. Early signs include ptosis, blurred vision, diplopia and difficulty swallowing. If left untreated, generalised paralysis can ensue but this is rare. Of note, the SVDK does not reliably detect sea snake venoms, but there may be cross-reactivity with tiger snake.

Management

Each ampoule of sea snake antivenom contains 1000 units. Initial dosage for envenoming is 1 ampoule. Antivenom prevents progression of muscle injury, but does not reverse injury that has already occurred. Antivenom is indicated if CK exceeds 1000 IU/L, or if there is evidence of neurotoxicity. A much lower threshold is used if the patient has significant pain from myonecrosis. CK is usually abnormal on arrival, but may not become grossly elevated for many hours. CK should be checked 6-hourly in the symptomatic patient or at 2, 6 and 12 hours after removal of PIB in the asymptomatic patient.

PRACTICE TIPS

- PIB should be applied to all patients who sustain snake bites to the limbs.
- Discuss envenoming cases with a clinical toxicologist at a Poisons Information Centre (phone 13 11 26 in Australia or 0800 POISON/0800 764 766 in New Zealand).
- Snake identification is not required to appropriately manage snake-bite envenoming.
- Obtain consent and enroll suspected snake-bite patients in the Australian Snakebite Project (http://wikitoxin. toxicology.wikispaces.net/Australian+Snakebite+Project)
- If there is a possibility of snake-bite envenoming, manage the patient as having a potentially life-threatening condition.

Spiders

Overview

Redback spider bite is the most common envenoming syndrome in Australia, with 5000 to 10,000 bites reported annually. Clinical features can be distressing and refractory to symptomatic treatment, but are not life-threatening. Funnel-web spider distribution is limited to coastal New South Wales, southern Queensland and a small area around Adelaide, and early recognition of this potentially lethal envenoming is vital.

Funnel-web spider

- Sydney funnel-web spider, *Atrax robustus* (Fig 31.5)
- Other: *Hadronyche* spp.

The funnel-web spiders comprise 40 species in two genera (*Atrax* and *Hadronyche*). These potentially lethal spiders look very similar to other, less-dangerous, big black spiders, including the trapdoor spiders (families Idiopidae and Nemesiidae) and mouse spiders (Actinopodidae family). For this reason, it is important to have a clinical approach to bite by a big black spider that occurs within the distribution area of the funnel-web species.[18]

Both genera of funnel-web spider produce venom that contains potent neurotoxins. Robustoxin (*Atrax* spp.) and versutoxin (*Hadronyche* spp.) prevent inactivation of sodium channels, leading to a massive increase in autonomic activity and neuromuscular excitation. Patients usually give a history of a bite by a big black spider with large fangs. Not surprisingly, pain is severe and fang marks are often visible. Severe systemic envenoming occurs rapidly, usually within 30 minutes and almost always within 2 hours.

Clinical features of funnel-web envenoming include:[19]

- *general*—agitation, vomiting, headache and abdominal pain
- *autonomic*—sweating, salivation, piloerection and lacrimation
- *cardiovascular*—hypertension, tachycardia, hypotension, bradycardia and pulmonary oedema
- *neurological*—muscular fasciculation, oral paraesthesia, muscle spasm and coma
- *other*—in young children, the first indication of envenoming may be sudden severe illness with inconsolable crying, salivation, vomiting or collapse.

Bites by the other big black spiders (trapdoor and mouse spiders) may be associated with significant bite-site pain, but only mild systemic symptoms, such as nausea, headache, malaise or vomiting. Significant cardiovascular, autonomic or neurological symptoms do not occur.

Management

Apply direct pressure to the bite site, secure a PIB to the affected limb and transfer patient to the nearest hospital capable of providing definitive care.

Each ampoule of funnel-web spider antivenom contains 125 units. The freeze-dried antivenom is reconstituted in 10 mL of sterile water, and the initial dose is two ampoules diluted in 100 mL of Normal saline IV over 20 minutes.

In the severely envenomed patient, the recommended initial dose is four ampoules, which can be given undiluted as an IV push in the case of cardiac arrest. Repeat doses of two ampoules are given every 2 hours until clinical features of envenoming resolve. Intramuscular injection of undiluted antivenom is a possible alternative.

Redback spider

- Redback spider (Australia), *Latrodectus hasselti* (Fig 31.6)
- Katipo spider (New Zealand), *L. katipo*

The redback and katipo spiders can both cause envenoming syndromes and are treated similarly. Whereas the redback lives in sheltered areas in close proximity to humans and bites are common, the katipo prefers grassy coastal regions and envenoming is both rare and less likely to cause significant systemic features. The venom of the redback spider contains α-latrotoxin, which acts presynaptically to open cation channels (including calcium channels) and stimulate the release of neurotransmitters.[16]

Redback spider bites are not initially painful; however, local pain usually develops 5–10 minutes after the bite and is followed by sweating and piloerection within an hour. Puncture marks are not always evident and erythema, if present, is usually

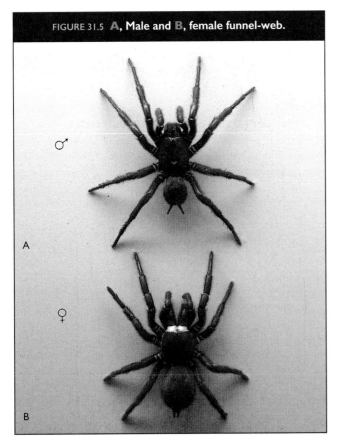

FIGURE 31.5 **A, Male and B, female funnel-web.**

A

B

Wikipedia/Sputniktilt/CC BY-SA 3.0

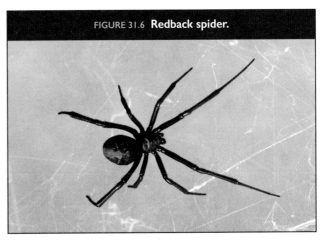

FIGURE 31.6 **Redback spider.**

Shutterstock/Peter Waters

mild. The combination of pain, piloerection and sweating is pathognomonic of redback spider bite.

Systemic envenoming (latrodectism) occurs in a minority of patients.[20] Pain typically radiates proximally from the bite site to become regional then general (e.g. pelvic, back, abdominal, chest or shoulder pain). Autonomic features include severe sweating, which may be regional (e.g. both legs) or generalised. Occasionally, priapism may develop—especially in children. Latrodectism has been mistaken for conditions such as acute surgical abdomen, acute myocardial infarction and thoracic aortic dissection.

Non-specific features of envenoming include headache, nausea, vomiting and dysphoria.

If untreated, latrodectism may follow a fluctuating course lasting 1–4 days. Rarely, patients may feel unwell for up to a week. Very rarely, untreated patients report ongoing local symptoms that last weeks or months.

Management

Treatment with simple oral analgesia and ice applied to the bite site can be enough to treat mild to moderate envenoming. Severe envenoming can cause unremitting pain requiring parenteral opiate analgesia, and/or systemic toxicity (severe abdominal pain, generalised sweating), in which case transiently improve pain, but if symptoms are significant antivenom is recommended.

Redback spider antivenom is derived from horse serum and has a low incidence of significant allergic reactions. It may be used for both redback and katipo spider envenoming. Expert recommendations have changed from IM to IV administration, which allows cessation of treatment if any allergic reactions develop. A randomised controlled trial showed no difference in pain scores between the IM and IV routes 2 hours after antivenom administration, and found that no antivenom from the IM route was measureable in the circulation.[21] This finding has raised the possibility that anecdotal experience of the clinical effectiveness of antivenom may be due in large part to a placebo effect. A more recent study suggests that antivenom provides minimally better pain relief than placebo.

Each ampoule contains 500 units (1–1.5 mL), and initial treatment is two ampoules diluted in 100 mL Normal saline, infused intravenously over 30 minutes in a monitored area. Repeat doses of two ampoules can be given, titrated according to clinical response. It is unusual for more than four ampoules to be administered in total.

Other spiders

The white-tailed spider (*Lampona cylindrata*) is ubiquitous throughout Australasia (Fig 31.7). The venom has been studied in detail, but no definite toxic components have been identified. Three local reactions to bites from *Lampona* species are reported:

- severe local pain of < 2 hours duration
- local pain and a red mark lasting < 24 hours
- a persistent and painful red lesion, which does not break down or ulcerate, and may last 5–12 days.

Mild, non-specific features may follow white-tailed spider bites, including nausea, vomiting, malaise and headache. Treatment with ice and simple analgesia such as paracetamol is effective.

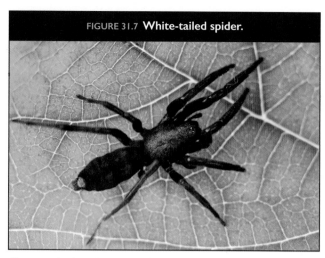

FIGURE 31.7 **White-tailed spider.**

Shutterstock/ChameleonsEye

Bites from this spider were previously suspected to cause necrotic arachnidism, a syndrome of progressive cutaneous ulceration from spider venom. A recent prospective study of 130 *Lampona* bites,[22] where the spider was caught and formally identified, showed that in every case other diagnoses (diabetic ulcers, infections or other rare conditions diagnosed on skin biopsy) were responsible for any chronic skin lesions.

PRACTICE TIPS

- Consider redback spider bite in children with inconsolable crying, acute abdomen pain or priapism.
- Administer antivenom in an environment staffed and equipped to manage anaphylaxis.
- Inform patients who receive antivenom of the potential for serum sickness in the weeks after administration.

Other terrestrial envenomations

There are a number of Australian scorpions that can cause painful stings, but there is limited knowledge about the components of the venom and their clinical effects. Pain relief with ice and simple analgesia is usually effective, and generalised symptoms are non-specific (nausea, headache and malaise) and self-limiting.

Anaphylaxis due to *Hymenoptera* spp. (honeybee and wasp stings) is a major cause of morbidity and mortality related to envenomings. In southern Australia and Tasmania, bites from native ants (*Myrmecia* spp.) can also cause anaphylaxis.[2] Standard protocols for treatment of anaphylaxis, involving adrenaline, intravenous fluids and antihistamines, are the principles of management (see 'Useful websites' at the end of this chapter).

The Australian bush tick (*Ixodes cornuatus, I. hirsti* and *I. holocyclus*) can, rarely, cause a progressive descending flaccid paralysis—almost exclusively in children. Ticks can be hidden above the hair-line or in skin folds, and a careful history and physical examination is required to confirm the diagnosis.[23] Tick removal can usually be performed using a loop of fine suture material, tightened flush to the skin surface to ensure that the mouthparts of the tick are included. Symptoms can progress up to 48 hours after a tick is removed, and symptomatic patients should be monitored in hospital to ensure resolution of muscle weakness.

Marine envenomations

Overview

Encounters with marine animals are responsible for a wide spectrum of presentations to hospital, especially in Australia. Envenoming from jellyfish can result in life-threatening reactions, and toxins from other creatures such as the blue-ringed octopus can cause fatal paralysis. Traumatic injuries from stingrays or barbed fish require meticulous wound care to ensure good outcomes.

Box jellyfish

- Multi-tentacled box jellyfish, *Chironex fleckeri*

The box jellyfish (Fig 31.8) is found in tropical Australian waters, from Queensland around to the northern border of Western Australia. Most stings occur between November and April, are benign and respond to supportive measures. Severe envenoming has been associated with at least 67 deaths in Australia, the last 12 being children.[24]

The venom components include polypeptides and enzymes, some of which are antigenic. They are thought to affect sodium and calcium channels, leading to abnormal membrane ion transport.

Stings usually occur in shallow water and are associated with immediate severe pain, typically lasting up to 8 hours. Linear welts characteristically occur in a cross-hatched pattern, and tentacles may remain adherent unless physically removed—gloves are required for this task.

Systemic envenoming is heralded by collapse or sudden death within a few minutes of the sting. Cardiovascular effects of the venom include hypotension, tachycardia or sudden cardiac arrest.[24] According to a recent study, the cardiovascular collapse that occurs after box jellyfish stings is due to hyperkalaemia, and zinc is proposed as treatment.[25] However, there are no zinc preparations available for this purpose yet and there have been no human studies evaluating its efficiency.

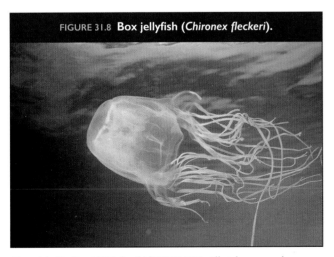

FIGURE 31.8 **Box jellyfish (*Chironex fleckeri*).**

Delayed hypersensitivity reactions occur in at least 50% of patients and manifest as pruritic erythema at the original sting site, 7–14 days after the sting.

Management

Reassure the patient, apply an ice pack and give simple oral analgesia such as paracetamol. The traditional recommendation to apply generous volumes of vinegar (5% acetic acid) to all visible sting sites to inactivate all undischarged nematocysts (sting cells) has been challenged recently in a study where in vivo application of vinegar to already discharged nematocysts is shown to promote further discharge of venom.[26,27] Do not apply a PIB as this can cause further nematocyst discharge, increased pain and may promote systemic envenoming.

Box jellyfish antivenom is indicated in the treatment of envenomed patients with evidence of cardiovascular instability, although the rapid action of the venom means that antivenom may not be effective in clinical settings.[28] Antivenom has been used in cases with ongoing severe pain refractory to opioid analgesia, but evidence for effectiveness regarding analgesia is lacking.

Each ampoule contains 20,000 units, and premedication with adrenaline is not required.

In patients with pain refractory to IV opioid analgesia, administer 1 ampoule diluted in 100 mL of Normal saline IV over 20 minutes. Further doses of 1 ampoule may be given, to a total of 3 ampoules, if pain persists.

In patients with haemodynamic compromise, administer 3 ampoules diluted in 100 mL of Normal saline IV over 20 minutes. Repeat doses of 3 ampoules are given until improvement is achieved.

Six ampoules may be given as a rapid IV push if the patient is in cardiac arrest.

Irukandji syndrome

- Irukandji jellyfish, *Carukia barnesi*
- Other jellyfish species

Irukandji syndrome is a painful sympathomimetic condition named after an Aboriginal tribe in North Queensland.[26] It is caused by envenoming by one of a number of different jellyfish species found in the coastal waters of tropical Northern Australia.[29] Best described is *C. barnesi*, a transparent thumbnail-sized carybdeid found in coastal waters of tropical Australia which can pass through stinger nets at patrolled beaches. It is one of a group of similar small jellyfish thought to cause the constellation of symptoms known as irukandji syndrome.[29] The mechanism of action of the venom has not been fully characterised, but is thought to cause massive catecholamine release.

The initial sting is usually minor and there is a short delay to the onset of systemic symptoms. Local signs such as welts, dermal markings or tentacles can be minimal or absent.[28] Multiple systemic symptoms develop from 30 to 120 minutes after contact with the jellyfish. These include a sense of impending doom, agitation, dysphoria, vomiting, generalised sweating and severe pain in the back, limbs or abdomen. Hypertension and tachycardia are common. Symptoms usually settle within 12 hours.

Severe envenoming manifests within 4 hours with ongoing significant opioid requirements. These patients are at risk of toxic cardiomyopathy, cardiogenic shock and pulmonary oedema and may require continuous positive airway pressure or intubation and mechanical ventilation (see Ch 17, p. 318, for intubation procedures). Fatal intracerebral haemorrhage has occurred in two patients, presumably due to uncontrolled hypertension.

Management

As in box jellyfish toxicity, PIB is not beneficial and topical treatment with vinegar is a priority. Management of significant pain from envenoming usually requires parenteral opioids. Fentanyl in titrated doses is recommended, and intravenous magnesium is a commonly used but unproven adjunctive therapy. Antiemetics such as promethazine are also commonly used.

If significant cardiovascular toxicity develops, treatment with intravenous nitrate infusions will help with hypertension or pulmonary oedema. ICU management is warranted for patients with respiratory compromise. There is no antivenom available for irukandji syndrome and box jellyfish antivenom is ineffective.

Other jellyfish

The bluebottle (*Physalia* spp.) is a jellyfish-like hydrozoan responsible for thousands of stings on Australian beaches (and to a lesser extent in New Zealand) each year. Clinical features include intense local pain and dermal erythema. Unlike *Physalia* stings in other parts of the world, major systemic envenoming does not occur. Stings are mild, self-limiting and respond to first-aid measures.

Management

Hot-water immersion therapy is the most effective treatment for bluebottle stings. Place the patient under a hot shower for 20 minutes (ideal temperature 45°C).[30] The shower should be hot but not scalding or uncomfortable. Administer simple oral analgesia such as paracetamol. Do not apply a PIB or vinegar, as these may worsen local symptoms. Transport to hospital is not usually required.

Other marine envenomations

The blue-ringed octopus (*Hapalochlaena* spp.) is a small brown octopus found in shallow waters around Australia. When handled or enraged, it changes colour and develops bright blue rings on its surface. The venom contains maculotoxin, a potent sodium-channel blocking agent, and the octopus delivers it via a bite from the beak, not from the tentacles. Maculotoxin is now known to be identical to tetrodotoxin found in pufferfish, and has the same neurotoxic effects. The bite of the blue-ringed octopus is not necessarily painful, and there may be minimal local signs.

Envenoming is characterised by a progressive descending flaccid paralysis, which develops rapidly over the course of minutes to hours, and can lead to respiratory compromise requiring intubation and ventilation (see Ch 17, p. 318, for intubation procedures). Usually symptoms are much less significant, and are limited to mild perioral paraesthesia. A PIB is beneficial to limit systemic absorption of the toxin. There is no antidote for maculotoxin, but with respiratory support, full recovery is expected over 24–48 hours.

A similar clinical presentation occurs after stings from the cone shell (*Conus* spp.), found in tropical waters around Australia. A barb from the end of the shell can deliver a sting containing conotoxins, which can also cause paralysis. There is no antidote, and supportive therapy is required if respiratory symptoms develop.

Stonefish (*Synanceia trachynis*) are found in the waters of northern Australia. Their dorsal spines contain venom, which is injected into the skin when the animal is stood upon. Neurotoxins, stonustoxin and enzymes in the venom cause severe debilitating pain, and remnants of the spines may remain embedded in the limb, requiring surgical debridement.

First-aid treatment for stonefish envenoming consists of hot-water immersion therapy, and can be rapidly effective in providing analgesia. It is sensible to immerse the unaffected limb in hot water also, to prevent inadvertent thermal injury if pain perception in the affected limb is impaired. If pain does not resolve with this treatment, and the geographical location is suggestive of stonefish habitat, it is appropriate to use antivenom.

Each ampoule contains 2000 units of antivenom, and one ampoule is administered for every two spine puncture wounds (to a maximum of three ampoules). It is given either undiluted by intramuscular injection, or diluted in 100 mL of Normal saline and given intravenously over 20 minutes.

A number of other barbed fish or stingrays can cause significant local tissue injury or pain. Hot-water immersion therapy is usually effective analgesia for most marine toxins, although the mechanism is unclear. Regional anaesthesia is also effective, but should not be combined with hot-water immersion due to the risk of thermal injury in an anaesthetised limb. Expert wound care (including removal of residual barbs, or formal surgical debridement), tetanus prophylaxis and antibiotic therapy are all important considerations after such traumatic injuries.

> **PRACTICE TIPS**
> ## PITFALLS
>
> - There can be pitfalls to discharging potentially envenomed patients 'after hours', so discharge should occur in daylight hours accompanied by an adult.
> - Misinterpreting venom detection kit results. Geographical location, clinical features and laboratory findings are more important in guiding snake-bite management.
> - Attempting to identify snakes. Do not rely on snake identification unless performed by a recognised expert herpetologist.
> - Administering antivenom to potentially envenomed patients in the absence of objective clinical or laboratory evidence of envenoming.
> - Treating fish stings with hot-water immersion after the administration of local anaesthetic. Severe burns may result if the onset of local anaesthesia is delayed.
> - Withholding antivenom in children, pregnant or lactating patients.

SUMMARY

Early recognition of the patient with potential envenoming is essential for paramedics and emergency nurses. An understanding of the likely causes of envenoming based on clinical presentation and geographical possibilities is an important skill to develop. This enables appropriate triage categorisation for subsequent assessment and management. Australia is home to 21 of the world's 23 most deadly snakes. Although there are few annual fatalities related to snake bite in Australia both due to antivenom availability and good supportive care, a standardised approach to managing snakebite presentations is essential to ensure that this situation continues.

This chapter provides information on the major terrestrial and marine venomous creatures in Australasia, and the management of envenoming syndromes. It should be used as a guide, in conjunction with information from services such as the Poisons Information Centres or other toxinology resources in Australia and New Zealand.

CASE STUDY

A 12-year-old boy is carried into the emergency department (ED) by his father, having suffered a witnessed snakebite to the lateral border of the left foot 20 minutes previously. The patient is mildly nauseated, but feels otherwise well. A flimsy bandage has been tied around the foot.

1. What is the most important initial intervention at triage?

A firm pressure-immobilisation bandage (PIB) is applied to the whole of the left lower limb at triage, and the patient is brought into the resuscitation area.

2. What are the important examination findings that should be sought?

His vital signs are normal, and a focused examination reveals no signs of bleeding or muscle weakness. A small window is cut through the PIB to examine the bite site, revealing two small puncture wounds with minimal dried blood and no major bruising.

3. What investigations should be performed?

An IV line is inserted, and blood sent to the laboratory for a number of haematological and biochemical assays—full blood count, urinalysis and electrolytes, creatine kinase, coagulation studies (including D-dimer and fibrinogen). A venom detection kit (VDK) is not available. Initial blood tests are all normal, including INR, aPTT, fibrinogen and D-dimer.

4. What is the ongoing management plan for this patient?

The case is discussed with the Poisons Information Centre and a definitive management plan confirmed. There are adequate supplies of antivenom available in the ED to treat envenoming from all possible snakes in the geographical region, so the PIB is removed. Ten minutes later, the patient feels increasingly unwell, with worsened nausea and a mild headache. The PIB is immediately reapplied, and repeat blood tests sent. These show marked derangement of coagulation, with an unrecordable INR and aPTT, markedly decreased fibrinogen and elevated D-dimer.

5. What further treatment is required with this new information?

In response to the clinical and laboratory abnormalities, one vial of brown snake antivenom and one vial of tiger snake antivenom are infused over 20 minutes, and the PIB removed halfway through the infusion. The patient feels better, and remains well with no ongoing headache. The coagulation abnormalities resolve over the course of 12 hours, although the D-dimer remains markedly elevated. There is no laboratory evidence of haemolytic anaemia, thrombocytopenia, renal dysfunction or rhabdomyolysis on serial blood tests, and the patient is discharged home the day after the snake bite.

 Answers to Case Study Questions can be found on evolve
http://evolve.emergencytrauma.curtis

USEFUL WEBSITES

Australian Snakebite Project, http://wikitoxin.toxicology.wikispaces.net/Australian+Snakebite+Project

Australasian Toxinology Cases, www.lifeinthefastlane.com/education/toxicology

Clinical Toxinology Resources, www.toxinology.com

Australian Venom Research Unit, www.avru.org

REFERENCES

1. White J. A clinician's guide to Australian Venomous Bites and Stings. CSL: Parkville, Melbourne, Victoria; 2013.

2. Isbister GK, Brown SG, MacDonald E et al. Current use of Australian snake antivenoms and frequency of immediate-type hypersensitivity reactions and anaphylaxis. Med J Aust 2008;188(8):473–6.

3. Brown SG, Mullins RJ, Gold MS. Anaphylaxis: diagnosis and management. Med J Aust 2006;185(5):283–9.

4. Murray L, Daly F, Little M et al. Toxicology handbook. 2nd edn. Sydney: Elsevier; 2011.

5. Australian Resuscitation Council. Envenomation: pressure immobilisation technique. Revised policy statement (8.9.1); Feb 2005.

6. Canale E, Isbister GK, Currie BJ. Investigating pressure bandaging for snakebite in a simulated setting: bandage type, training and the effect of transport. Emerg Med Australas 2009;21(3):184–90.

7. Isbister GK, Brown SGA, Page CB et al. Snakebite in Australia: a practical approach to diagnosis and treatment. MJA 2013;199(11):763–8.

8. Cubitt M, Armstrong J, McCoubrie D et al. Point-of-care testing in snakebite: an envenomed case with false negative coagulation studies. Emerg Med Australas 2013;25:372–3.

9. Isbister GK, Maduwage K, Shahmy S et al. Diagnostic 20-min whole blood clotting test in Russell's viper envenoming delays antivenom administration. QJM 2013;106:925–32.

10. O'Leary MA, Isbister GK. Commercial monovalent antivenoms in Australia are polyvalent. Toxicon 2009;54(2):192–5.

11. Isbister GK, Duffull SB, Brown SG, ASP Investigators. Failure of antivenom to improve recovery in Australian snakebite coagulopathy. Q J Med 2009;102(8):563–8.

12. Isbister GK, O'Leary MA, Schneider JJ et al. Efficacy of antivenom against the procoagulant effect of Australian brown snake (Pseudonaja spp.) venom: in vivo and in vitro studies. Toxicon 2007;49(1):57–67.

13. Isbister GK, Williams V, Brown SG et al. Clinically applicable laboratory end-points for treating snakebite coagulopathy. Pathology 2006;38(6):568–72.

14. Scop J, Little M, Jelinek GA et al. 16 years of severe Tiger snake (Notechis) envenoming in Perth, Western Australia. Anaesth Intensive Care 2009;37:613–18.

15. Currie BJ. Snakebite in tropical Australia: a prospective study in the 'Top End' of the Northern Territory. Med J Aust 2004;181(11–12): 693–7.

16. Sutherland SK, Tibballs J. Australian animal toxins: the creatures, their toxins and care of the poisoned patient. Melbourne: Oxford University Press; 2001.

17. Little M, Pereira P. Successful treatment of presumed death-adder neurotoxicity using anticholinesterases. Emerg Med 2000;12:241–5.

18. Isbister GK, Sibbritt D. Developing a decision tree algorithm for the diagnosis of suspected spider bites. Emerg Med Australas 2004;16(2):161–6.

19. Isbister GK, Gray MR, Balit CR et al. Funnel-web spider bite: a systemic review of recorded clinical cases. Med J Aust 2005;182:407–11.

20. Isbister GK, Gray MR. Lactrodectism: a prospective cohort study of bites by formally identified redback spiders. Med J Aust 2003;179(2):88–91.

21. Isbister GK, Brown SGA, Miller M et al. A randomised controlled trial of intramuscular versus intravenous antivenom for lactrodectism—the RAVE study. Q J Med 2008;101:557–65.

22. Isbister GK, Gray MR. White-tail spider bite: a prospective study of 130 definite bites by Lampona species. Med J Aust 2003;179(4): 199–202.

23. Miller MK. Massive tick (Ixodes holocyclus) infestation with delayed facial-nerve palsy. Med J Aust 2002;176(2002):264–5.

24. Currie BJ, Jacups SP. Prospective study of Chironex fleckeri and other box jellyfish stings in the 'Top End' of Australia's Northern Territory. Med J Aust 2005;183(11–12):631–6.

25. Yanagihara A et al. Cubozoan Venom-Induced Cardiovascular Collapse Is Caused by Hyperkalemia and Prevented by Zinc Gluconate in Mice. Plos ONE 2012;7(12):e51368.

26. James Cook University. Groundbreaking study: a sting in the tail for venom research http://www-public.jcu.edu.au/news/JCU_135736; accessed 16 April 2015.

27. Welfare P, Little M, Pereira P, Seymour J. An in-vitro examination of the effect of vinegar on discharged nematocysts of Chironex fleckeri. Diving and Hyperbaric Medicine 2014;44(1):30–4.

28. Nickson CP, Waugh EB, Jacups SP et al. Irukandji syndrome case series from Australia's tropical Northern Territory. Ann Emerg Med 2009;54(3):395–403.

29. Little M, Pereira P, Carrette T et al. Jellyfish responsible for Irukandji syndrome. Q J Med 2006;99(6):425–7.

30. Loten C, Stokes B, Worsley D et al. A randomised controlled trial of hot water (45°C) immersion versus ice packs for pain relief in bluebottle stings. Med J Aust 2006;184(7):329–33.

CHAPTER 32
DENTAL, EAR, NOSE AND THROAT EMERGENCIES

LUCY PATEL AND TONY SKAPETIS

Essentials

- Presentation is usually due to pain and discomfort, but serious airway compromise can occur.
- Dental emergencies are rarely life-threatening. Treatment is usually stabilisation and referral to a dentist for definitive treatment.
- Appropriate initial diagnosis and treatment can reduce future dental expenses and improve patient outcomes.
- Earache can be excruciating and early analgesia is essential.
- Taking a focused history will give clues to the diagnosis.
- The airway should be assessed and reassessed regularly as decline can be rapid.
- Patients presenting in the 'sniffing the air' position are already telling you their airway is compromised.
- Patients should never be forced to recline as this can immediately compromise their airway.
- Due to pain on swallowing, dehydration may be present. Intravenous cannulation should be attempted in an adult, but caution should be used in children as the added distress can further compromise their airway.
- Removal of a foreign body is generally most successful on the first attempt. It should not be rushed and only attempted in a controlled environment.

INTRODUCTION

With ear, nose, throat and dental emergencies, the initial presentation is usually because of pain and discomfort. Dental injuries usually occur as a result of trauma, such as a fall or an assault. Due to the close proximity of the structures in the facial area serious complications can arise, particularly if swelling of the airway is involved. Assessment of the patient's airway is a priority, along with providing adequate pain relief.

Anatomy and physiology

Mouth and throat

The oral cavity is designed for articulation in speech and mastication of food and also functions as an alternative airway.[1]

The mouth is sealed by the lips and they too are involved in articulation of speech. The oral cavity is lined by the buccal mucosa, which is rich in mucous glands. It consists of gums, alveolar bone, teeth, the hard and soft palates and the tongue. The floor of the mouth contains the openings of the submandibular and sublingual salivary glands (Fig 32.1).

The gums are adherent to the alveolus and are closely related to the teeth, whose roots are embedded into the alveolus.[2] Figure 32.2 shows the structure of a tooth. Normal primary dentition begins erupting at 6 months of age, with 20 teeth by the age of 3 years. Permanent dentition begins at 6–7 years of age with eruption of the first molar, and is usually completed by age 16–18 to a total of 32 teeth.[3]

The throat, or pharynx, consists of the upper parts of the respiratory and digestive systems. It can be divided into three parts: the *nasopharynx* lies above the soft palate and behind the nasal cavities and contains adenoid tissue and the orifices of the eustachian tubes, the *oropharynx* extends from the inferior margin of the soft palate to the level of the hyoid bone, and the *laryngopharynx* extends from the hyoid bone to the opening of the larynx anteriorly and oesophagus posteriorly[5] (see Fig 32.3).

The larynx is made up of several muscles and cartilages. It has three main functions: respiration, preventing food and saliva from entering the respiratory tract and pronation (production of sound).[2]

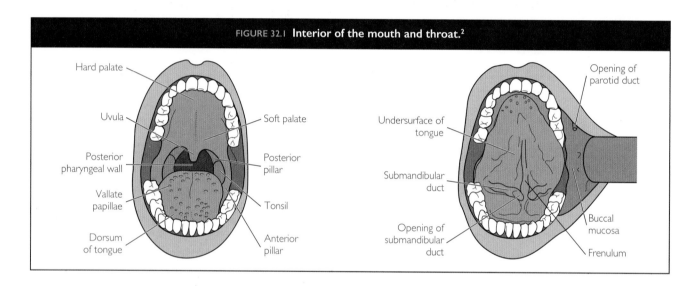

FIGURE 32.1 **Interior of the mouth and throat.**[2]

Hard palate
Uvula
Posterior pharyngeal wall
Vallate papillae
Dorsum of tongue
Soft palate
Posterior pillar
Tonsil
Anterior pillar

Opening of parotid duct
Undersurface of tongue
Submandibular duct
Opening of submandibular duct
Buccal mucosa
Frenulum

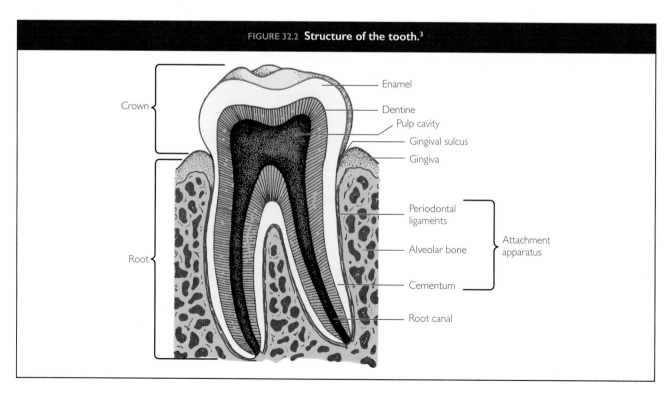

FIGURE 32.2 **Structure of the tooth.**[3]

Crown
Root

Enamel
Dentine
Pulp cavity
Gingival sulcus
Gingiva
Periodontal ligaments
Alveolar bone
Cementum
Root canal
Attachment apparatus

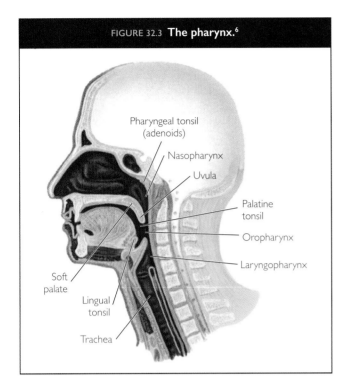

FIGURE 32.3 **The pharynx.**[6]

Pharyngeal tonsil (adenoids)

Nasopharynx

Uvula

Palatine tonsil

Oropharynx

Laryngopharynx

Soft palate

Lingual tonsil

Trachea

Ears

The ear can be divided into three parts: the *external, middle* and *inner* ear (see Fig 32.4).

The external ear consists of the pinna, external auditory canal and the lateral surface of the tympanic membrane (eardrum). The external ear serves mainly to protect the tympanic membrane, but also collects and directs sound waves.[1] Glands lining the canal secrete cerumen (earwax) to protect and lubricate the ear.

The middle ear is an air-containing space which communicates with the nasopharynx via the eustachian tube. It contains

the three ossicles and is normally sealed laterally by the tympanic membrane. Its function is to transmit and amplify sound waves from the tympanic membrane to the stapes footplate, converting energy from an air medium to a fluid medium for the membranous labyrinth.[1] The relationship of the three ossicles is depicted in Figure 32.5.

The inner ear or labyrinth communicates with the middle ear via the oval and round windows. The inner ear can be divided into two parts: the *cochlea* and the *vestibule*.[2] The cochlea converts sound waves into neural impulses with elaborate coding. The vestibule contains the utricle, the saccule and the semicircular canals which sense the position of the head and are important in maintaining the body's balance.

Nose

The nose is the air-conditioner of the body, responsible for warming and saturating inspired air, removing bacteria and particulate debris as well as conserving heat and moisture from expired air.[1] It is also responsible for the sense of smell.

The nose consists of the *external nose* and the *nasal cavity*, which is divided into right and left halves by the midline nasal septum. Each half of the cavity has olfactory, vestibular and respiratory parts depending on the type of epithelial covering.[7]

The nose is mainly constructed from cartilage, apart from the upper third where the frontal and maxillary bones form the bony ridge. The nares are separated by a membranous columella anteriorly and by the nasal septum posteriorly. The nasal septum is both cartilaginous and bony (see Fig 32.6). The lateral wall of each nasal cavity contains the inferior, middle and, sometimes, superior turbinates. These help to increase surface area and warm inhaled air.

The blood supply to the external nose is provided by the dorsal nasal artery (a terminal branch of the ophthalmic artery) and by the external nasal, lateral and septal branches of the facial artery. The main artery of the nasal cavity is the sphenopalatine. It supplies the mucosa over the turbinates and much of the septum. On the lower anterior part of the septum (Little's area), it anastomoses with the septal branch of the superior labial and the ascending branch of the greater palatine, so forming Kiesselbach's plexus, the common site for epistaxis (see Fig 32.7).[7]

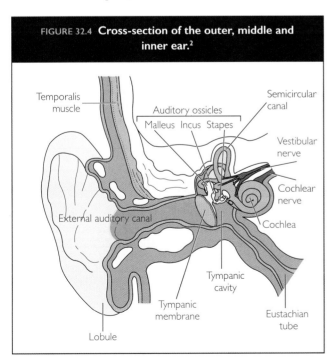

FIGURE 32.4 **Cross-section of the outer, middle and inner ear.**[2]

Temporalis muscle

Auditory ossicles
Malleus Incus Stapes

Semicircular canal

Vestibular nerve

Cochlear nerve

Cochlea

External auditory canal

Tympanic cavity

Tympanic membrane

Eustachian tube

Lobule

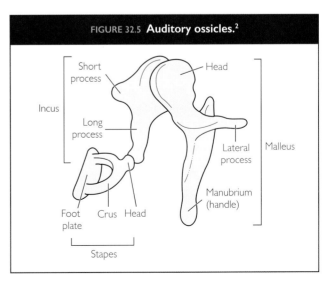

FIGURE 32.5 **Auditory ossicles.**[2]

Incus

Short process

Head

Long process

Lateral process

Malleus

Manubrium (handle)

Foot plate Crus Head

Stapes

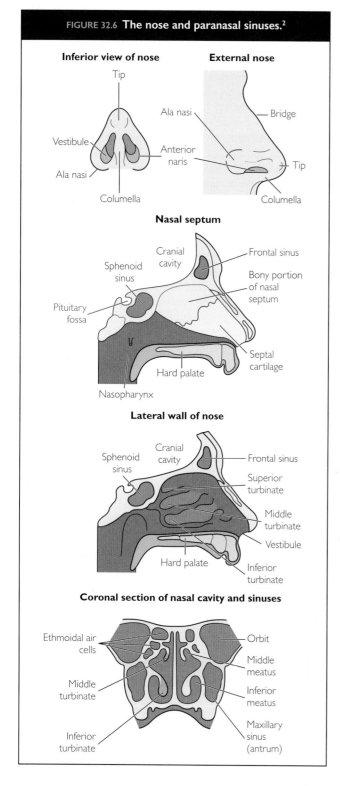

FIGURE 32.6 **The nose and paranasal sinuses.**[2]

Inferior view of nose

Tip
Ala nasi
Vestibule
Anterior naris
Ala nasi
Columella

External nose

Bridge
Tip
Columella

Nasal septum

Cranial cavity
Sphenoid sinus
Frontal sinus
Bony portion of nasal septum
Pituitary fossa
Septal cartilage
Hard palate
Nasopharynx

Lateral wall of nose

Cranial cavity
Sphenoid sinus
Frontal sinus
Superior turbinate
Middle turbinate
Vestibule
Hard palate
Inferior turbinate

Coronal section of nasal cavity and sinuses

Ethmoidal air cells
Orbit
Middle meatus
Middle turbinate
Inferior meatus
Inferior turbinate
Maxillary sinus (antrum)

Face

The face is the part of the head which lies between the eyebrow and the chin in front, and includes the ears at the side.[8] The facial skeleton is the front part of the skull, including the mandible.[7] Other important bones frequently injured include:

- the maxillae, which meet in the midline of the face and form the boundaries of the lower orbits

- the sphenoid, ethmoid, palatine and lacrimal bones, forming the basin of the orbits and conducting nerves and vessels to the eyes
- the zygoma or cheekbone
- the temporomandibular joint, the joint between upper and lower jaw.

The face also contains the paranasal sinuses (Fig 32.8), which are air-filled sacs. They lighten the weight of the skull and add resonance to the voice, and are linked to the nasal passages for fluid drainage.

Patient assessment

Approach to initial evaluation

Most presentations for a dental, ear, nose or throat problem will be due to pain. When assessing the patient, it is vital a DRSABCD approach (**D**anger, **R**esponse, **S**end for help, **A**irway, **B**reathing, **C**irculation and **D**isability) is taken due to the risk of potential complications, including airway obstruction and haemorrhage. These should be addressed before a history is taken from the patient, including relevant past medical history and medications.

Physical examination

Physical examination will vary depending on the presenting problem, and may include inspection and palpation or visualisation using an auroscope.

Identification and management of existing or impending airway obstruction takes precedence over other aspects of care.[9] A compromised patient is likely to be leaning forward with their neck extended, and on reclining their symptoms will worsen. Other signs to look for are a muffled voice and drooling due to being unable to swallow secretions. These are signs that the airway is already compromised.

Inspection

The relevant external areas should be inspected. You should note asymmetry, deformity or swelling of the face. The opening and closing of the mouth should be smooth and complete with no limitations or hesitations. Erythema, warmth or drainage is indicative of abscess, cellulitis or haematoma formation.[10]

You should be alert for signs of dehydration as patients with significant pain are unable to maintain adequate fluid intake, especially if the presenting problem is a sore throat or dental pain. General signs of dehydration include dry mucous membranes, sunken eyes, loss of skin turgor, poor capillary refill, reduced urine output and increased drowsiness or lethargy. Children may also have a lack of tears when crying.

Ears should be examined with an auroscope if available, using the largest earpiece the ear can accommodate. The patient should sit with their head facing straight ahead. The pinna should be pulled gently upwards and backwards and slightly away from the head. Children are best seated on a parent's lap and held securely with their head resting on the parent's chest. In those younger than 3 years, the pinna should be pulled down to get a good view of the tympanic membrane.[11]

The throat should be examined for erythema, exudate and swelling, and uvula placement should be noted.

FIGURE 32.7 **Arterial supply to nasal septum.**[3]

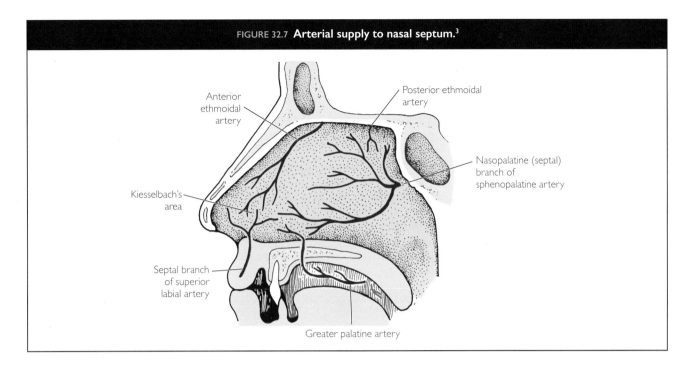

FIGURE 32.8 **Paranasal sinuses.**[61]

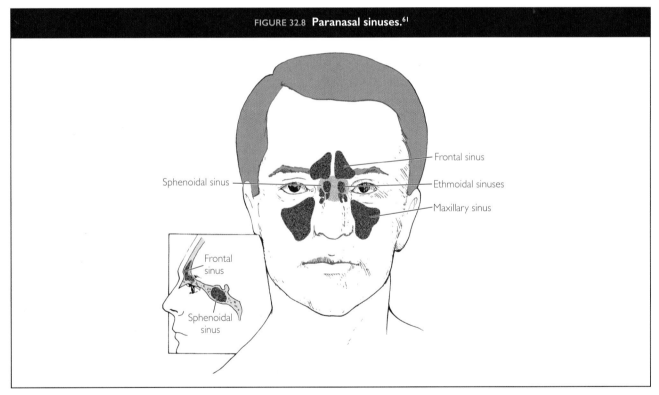

Inspection of the mouth for dental injuries should take note of how many teeth are affected and the whereabouts of any dental fragments.

Palpation

The face and neck are palpated for tenderness, crepitus or step-offs. Examination of the neck should also include palpitating the lymph nodes. Enlarged tender nodes can be an indication of infection.

Radiology

For most ear, nose, throat and dental problems, radiology is not required. There are a few notable exceptions.

A chest X-ray is used to locate missing tooth fragments if aspiration is considered likely, or a facial X-ray if they are lodged in the lip or buccal mucosa. An orthopantomogram (OPG) is also useful to assess the extent of damage to the teeth.

A computed tomography (CT) scan can be helpful in diagnosing mastoiditis, sinusitis and retropharyngeal abscess.

Initial clinical interventions

The patient should be encouraged to sit in a position of comfort. Often this is a seated or semi-erect position. Under no circumstances should a patient with signs of upper airway obstruction be forced to recline.[9] These patients should be delivered high-flow oxygen.

Patients with upper airway obstruction commonly also suffer dysphagia and may consequently also be dehydrated. Intravenous (IV) fluids should be administered, but caution should be used in children so as to not cause distress and actually worsen their condition. IV cannulation in these cases should wait until arrival at hospital where airway management equipment is readily available.

A full set of vital signs should be recorded and repeated regularly, and analgesia should be given. Pre-hospital care is an important window during which pain should be assessed and treated.[11]

Dental emergencies

Dental emergencies are not uncommon presentations in the emergency department (ED).[12] They have been noted to account for 1.3% of ED presentations overall[13] and as high as 4% by some authors.[14] They include dental pain, dental infections and dental trauma as well as complications related to dental treatment, including haemorrhage from inside the mouth and dry socket. These presentations are rarely life-threatening, and their management is usually of an empirical symptomatic basis involving stabilisation of acute conditions with appropriate referral to a dentist for more definitive treatment. Nevertheless, appropriate diagnosis and initial treatment can reduce future dental expenses as well as improve patient outcomes.

Dental pain

This type of pain can often be very acute, with dental caries being the principal cause.

Assessment

Initial symptoms include sensitivity to hot, cold and sweet stimuli, which are indicative of an inflamed pulp (reversible pulpitis).

Treatment

Symptoms are alleviated by avoiding any foods which provoke or exaggerate the pain, by covering any obvious tooth cavity using a temporary material such as Blu-Tack (is non-toxic) or a piece of chewing gum. Oral analgesics containing paracetamol are normally quite effective for such presentations.

Upon progression, the pulpitis may become irreversible with the pain intensifying and becoming more spontaneous. The addition of oral non-steroidal anti-inflammatory drugs (NSAIDs)[15] and opiates for effective analgesia is often indicated. Irreversible pulpitis requires more extensive definitive dental treatment such as root canal therapy or extraction.

Dental abscess

This condition usually results through the ingress of bacteria into the tooth pulpal tissues resulting from dental decay or as a result of trauma, and is more specifically referred to as a periapical abscess. It may also occur through bacteria progressing down the side of the tooth between the tooth root and surrounding gum, in which case it is referred to as a periodontal abscess.

Assessment

For both conditions the offending tooth or teeth become very tender to bite on, and may be associated with swelling, as well as more-systemic symptoms including fever and malaise. Assessment should include consideration of any trismus (limitation in mouth opening), tongue swelling/hardness, floor of the mouth elevation or airway obstruction.

Treatment

Treatment is usually with antibiotics, but if trismus, tongue swelling or airway obstruction is present then these would constitute a medical emergency and would require immediate surgical drainage.

> **PRACTICE TIP**
>
> Patients with suspected dental abscess should be reassessed regularly for airway compromise.

Tooth eruption

Tooth eruption is a normal developmental process beginning initially at around 6 months of age for deciduous (primary) teeth and around 6 years of age for the permanent teeth. All deciduous teeth (5 in each quadrant and 20 in total) are eventually replaced by their permanent successors, with additional permanent molar teeth (3 in each quadrant) erupting behind all the deciduous teeth. There are 32 permanent teeth in total with 16 teeth per jaw.

Assessment

During the eruption phase, the gum overlying the tooth may become slightly red and swollen and children may become irritable, salivate excessively, want to place fingers and objects into their mouth for relief or even tug on their ears at times.

Treatment

No treatment is usually necessary other than supportive care, with analgesia only indicated in more severe and persistent cases. Temporary use of such things as rusks and dummies may be of assistance.

Pericoronitis

Pericoronitis refers to inflammation of gingival tissue overlying an erupting tooth and occurs when anaerobic bacteria and/or food debris are able to penetrate from the mouth and infect the underlying tooth. It is commonly associated with erupting permanent third molars (commonly referred to as wisdom teeth) between the ages of 17 and 21 years.

Assessment

Pericoronitis may be of a mild nature consisting of only localised inflammation and intraoral swelling; at times it may be quite severe and include symptoms such as facial swelling, fever, malaise and trismus together with associated difficulty in eating.

Treatment

Treatment of mild cases involves oral analgesia as well as irrigating the site with 0.1–0.2% chlorhexidine solution (e.g Savacol) using a 5–10 mL syringe and asking the patient to maintain good oral hygiene and rinse with the same solution twice a day for the next 5 days. In the more severe pericoronitis cases, appropriate antibiotics should be administered (usually penicillin plus metronidazole), or even surgical drainage and/or extraction of the offending tooth following assessment by a dentist.

Gingivitis and periodontitis

Gingivitis refers to inflammation of the gum and periodontitis to inflammation of the deeper supporting tissues of the tooth root. Both of these conditions are bacterial in origin and usually associated with poor oral hygiene habits. Gingivitis may be exaggerated during pregnancy due to hormonal changes. Varying degrees of gingivitis are common throughout most of the general population, while periodontitis with the associated periodontal disease is more prevalent in the adult population.[16]

Assessment

Gingivitis causes the gum to become red and often bleed, with periodontitis also associated with the deepening of gum pockets surrounding the teeth, halitosis, loosening of the involved teeth due to surrounding bone loss (Figs 32.9–32.10) and even abscess formation.

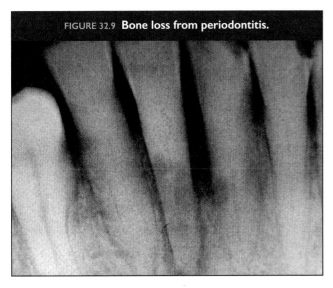

FIGURE 32.9 **Bone loss from periodontitis.**

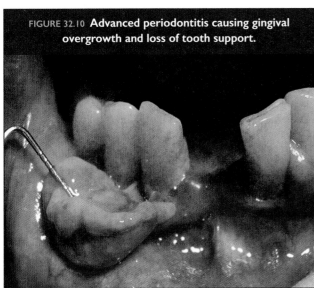

FIGURE 32.10 **Advanced periodontitis causing gingival overgrowth and loss of tooth support.**

Note the plaque and calculus surrounding the teeth due to the poor oral hygiene.

Treatment

Symptoms for both conditions may be reduced through the use of a 0.1–0.2% chlorhexidine solution as a mouthwash twice a day for the next week, together with improving oral hygiene especially through brushing. The use of analgesics may also be indicated in more-severe cases. Antibiotics are not usually indicated for either condition unless there is systemic involvement. Referral to a dentist is indicated for the longer term management of both conditions.

Maxillary sinusitis

This condition refers to an infection involving the maxillary sinus. It is usually unilateral, but may also present bilaterally at times.

Assessment

It is common for the upper back teeth to ache in such presentations and become tender to biting. This is because the roots of maxillary premolars and molars often lie in close approximation to the maxillary sinus. Other symptoms include maxillary sinus palpation tenderness, and pain worsening with changes in head position and when blowing the nose.

Treatment

Treatment involves sinus irrigation with saline, and use of antihistamines, analgesics and antibiotics.

Alveolar osteitis

This is commonly referred to as dry socket and is due to the breakdown in the granulation tissue process following a dental extraction. It occurs within a few days in at least 3%[17] of all extractions and is more commonly seen in smokers and within the mandibular dental arch.

Assessment

Symptoms include an initial improvement in the dental pain followed by a worsening of the pain several days after the extraction. Other symptoms include difficulty in chewing, with halitosis and a fetid odour commonly reported.

Treatment

This condition is self-limiting with symptoms subsiding within two weeks. Treatment involves flushing of the socket with saline, maintaining good oral hygiene and analgesics when necessary; antibiotics are not indicated.

Post-extraction haemorrhage

The causes of unexpected haemorrhage some time after an extraction include:

- damage to small blood vessels within the bony walls of the extraction socket
- soft-tissue bleeding from around the periphery of the socket
- bleeding from residual granulation tissue
- disturbance of the blood clot due to the patient eating too soon, exercising, spitting, sucking, etc.
- presence of severe gingivitis or periodontal disease
- trauma or laceration
- bleeding from soft-tissue incisions performed during the course of the extraction
- dead-space haematoma
- arterial or venous bleeding from deeper parts of the wound.

Treatment

Management of intraoral bleeds includes the use of one or more of the following:

- pressure applied with a rolled-up piece of gauze applied against the extraction site using bite pressure
- use of tranexamic acid 5% liquid solution (made up by crushing a 500 mg tranexamic acid tablet in 10 mL of saline) to soak the pressure gauze pack and promote coagulation
- packing the wound with oxidised cellulose (e.g. Surgicel), which acts as a resorbable clot matrix or alginate based products such as Kaltostat.
- use of a vasoconstrictor containing anaesthetic solution which is injected around the bleeding socket
- suturing across the wound.

Dental infections

More than 60% of odontogenic (of dental origin) infections are caused by a mix of aerobic and anaerobic bacteria, with about a third of infections attributable to anaerobes alone.[18] Aerobic pathogens typically initiate most of these infections followed by anaerobic pathogens, with a symbiosis between the two types of bacteria resulting in the more serious infections. Host factors such as age, tooth loss, diet, saliva and oral hygiene play an important role in regulating the composition and numbers of the oral flora. Dental infections will typically spread in the following ways:

- direct tissue spread
- vestibular spread with infections penetrating the dental alveolus into the vestibule (dental sulcus) of the mouth
- fascial spread with infections penetrating the dental alveolus and travelling along the tissue planes of the head and neck
- circulatory spread via blood vessels and lymphatics.

Maxillary infections typically spread to the buccal, canine and infratemporal spaces with mandibular infections spreading to buccal, submental, sublingual and submandibular spaces. Secondary spaces where odontogenic infections can spread include orbital, prevertebral, retropharyngeal, lateral pharyngeal, infratemporal, superficial and deep temporal, masseteric and pterygomandibular spaces.

Assessment

Clinical features include local symptoms such as inflammation, swelling (intra-oral and/or extra-oral), suppuration, trismus, dysphagia and dysphonia with systemic symptoms, including fever, malaise, pallor and loss of function.

Dental infections present as either a cellulitis or an abscess, or a mixture of both (see Table 32.1).

Treatment

Management of odontogenic infections should include a determination of the severity of the infection using a complete

TABLE 32.1 Signs and symptoms of facial cellulitis and abscess

CELLULITIS (SEE FIG 32.11)	ABSCESS (SEE FIG 32.12)
Acute duration	Chronic duration
Generalised pain	Localised pain
Large size	Smaller size
Diffuse borders	Well circumscribed
Indurated/doughy to palpation	Fluctuant
No pus	Pus present
Mostly aerobic	Mostly anaerobic

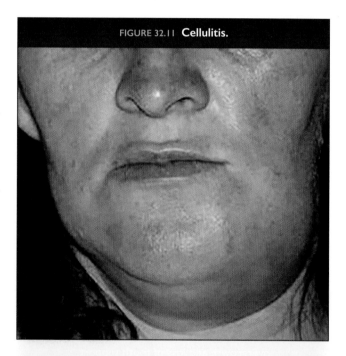

FIGURE 32.11 **Cellulitis.**

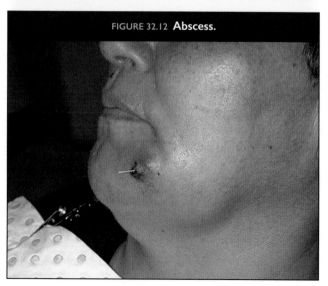

FIGURE 32.12 **Abscess.**

medical and dental history, together with a physical examination and an evaluation of the patient's host defence mechanism. Use of antibiotics is often necessary where any of the following are present:

- fever and acute infection
- infection is not well localised and is spreading
- chronic infection despite drainage/debridement
- a diminished host response (immunocompromised patient)
- inadequate response to previous antibiotics
- osteomyelitis, sialadenitis, acute ulcerative gingivitis, localised juvenile periodontitis.

Figure 32.13 summarises the appropriate management of dental infections in the ED; the shaded pathway represents the more serious odontogenic infections.[19]

Dental trauma

Trauma to the teeth falls into two broad categories:[20]

- injuries to the hard dental tissues of the mouth, including both complicated and uncomplicated crown and crown–root fractures
- injuries to the periodontal or supporting tissues of the teeth, including tooth subluxation (loosening), luxation injuries where tooth displacement has been involved and tooth avulsion.

It has been estimated that in the industrial world, by the age of 14 years 54% of children and by the age of 25 years 60% of adults have suffered some dental trauma.[21] This equates to 3 billion individuals or 60 million new injuries per year. Acute morbidity from dental injury includes pain, swelling, bleeding and infection. Long-term morbidity arises from the need for cosmetic and functional tooth replacement which may cost the patient thousands of dollars.

Dental first aid is both simple and inexpensive and can dramatically improve future dental outcomes; however, it is rarely appropriately provided. It has been documented that only 4% of emergency treatments provided by hospital doctors would be deemed appropriate for something as simple as an avulsed tooth,[22] and a recent study concluded that dentists in Australia may not be competent in providing appropriate care for traumatic dental injuries.[23] By simply covering and protecting an exposed pulp in a crown fracture or by the simple repositioning and splinting of a luxated or avulsed tooth, dental outcomes may be dramatically improved. In an effort to address the deficiency in dental trauma management, more than 120 emergency dental kits have been distributed by the NSW Rural Doctors Network in New South Wales and interstate to rural hospital EDs. These kits may be sourced at www.nswrdn.com.au/site/dental. The contents of the kit are listed in Box 32.1. These kits are to support dental education workshops (a collaboration between Western Sydney Local Health District Oral Health Network, NSW Rural Doctors Network and the University of Sydney Faculty of Dentistry), which involve 4 hours of training in the management of dental emergencies and are being delivered across several Australian states to emergency medical personnel. The effectiveness of this education has been evaluated in several publications.[24,25] Furthermore, the emergency dental kit has been shown to be useful as a resource for providing emergency

dental care, especially to rural and remote practice.[26] A more recent development by the Australian College of Rural and Remote Medicine has been the inclusion of the 'Introduction to Dental Emergencies and Odontogenic Infections' modules, delivered through their RRMEO platform and adapted for mobile devices.

Uncomplicated crown fractures

Crown fractures can be divided into two categories—uncomplicated and complicated. Uncomplicated crown fractures involve only the enamel, or the enamel in combination with the dentin.

Assessment

Patients who have damaged their dentin will complain of sensitivity to extremes of temperature, and on examination the yellow hue of the dentin will be noticed in contrast to the white of the peripheral enamel.

Treatment

If < 2 mm of tooth structure is missing, no intervention is necessary (see Fig 32.14). However, if > 2 mm of tooth structure is missing but no pulp (red centre) is exposed, either leave alone or cover with Blu-Tack as first aid or with GIC (cement) if available (Figs 32.16 and 32.19).

Complicated crown fractures

Complicated crown fractures are where the pulp has been exposed (see Figs 32.17 and 32.18).

Assessment

If the fracture site is cleaned off with gauze, a pinkish blush or bleeding can be seen. Fractures through the pulp are usually extremely painful.

Treatment

The exposed pulp and fractured tooth is covered using Blu-Tack after drying. If available, calcium hydroxide (Ca(OH)$_2$), which has bacteriocidal and remineralising properties, may be placed first over the exposed pulp followed by GIC (Figs 32.15, 32.17 and 32.18).

Luxation injuries

This is when the teeth are partially displaced from their sockets.

> **PRACTICE TIP**
>
> Loose or displaced teeth should not be manipulated unless airway intervention is required en route to the ED.

Treatment

Basic treatment principles include not repositioning deciduous teeth. Deciduous teeth are primary or baby teeth and will be replaced by their permanent counterparts which lie just below the deciduous tooth root. Repositioning or re-implanting a deciduous tooth may cause damage to the permanent successor. Displaced deciduous teeth are best left alone, or if very mobile and there is an inhalation risk, extract them.

When treating permanent-tooth injuries, give local anaesthesia when appropriate and reposition both teeth and surrounding bone (Figs 32.20 and 32.21). Splinting is done using either Blu-Tack with thick aluminium foil or with GIC if available.

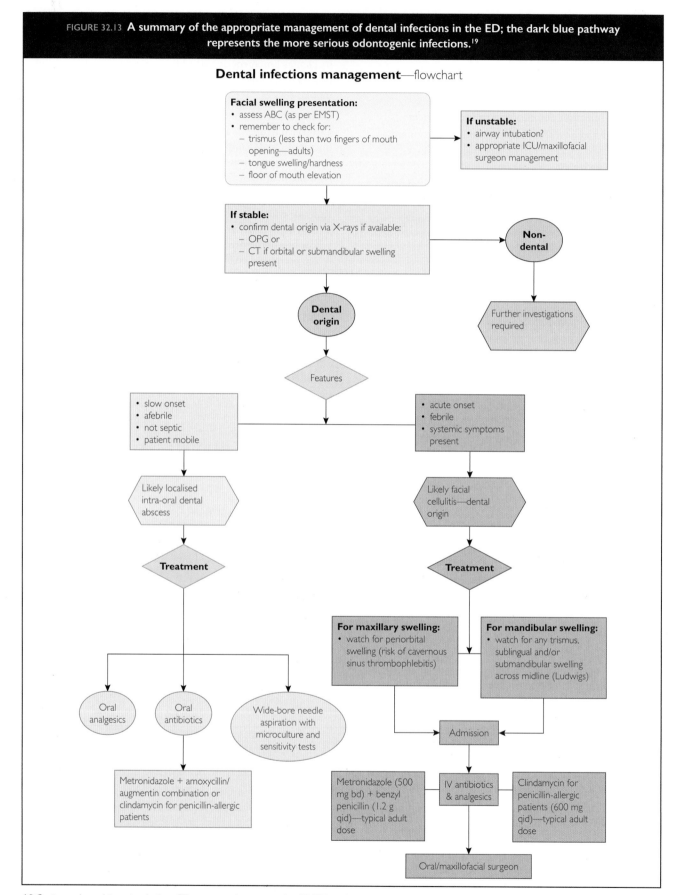

FIGURE 32.13 A summary of the appropriate management of dental infections in the ED; the dark blue pathway represents the more serious odontogenic infections.[19]

ABC: airway, breathing, circulation; CT: computed tomography; EMST: early management of severe trauma; ICU: intensive care unit; OPG: orthopantomogram.

BOX 32.1 Emergency dental kit contents

- GC Fuji IX pack (glass ionomer cement powder (GIC) + liquid + missing pad)
- Dycal (Ca(OH)$_2$ base + catalyst)
- Microbrush applicators
- Record book to record type of trauma repair, which tooth and patient details

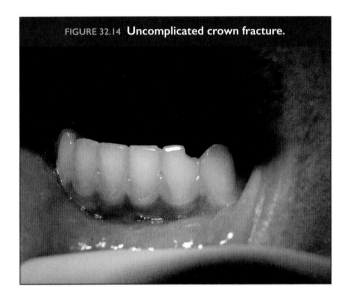

FIGURE 32.14 **Uncomplicated crown fracture.**

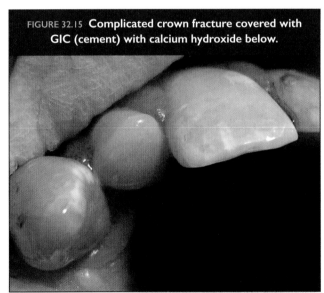

FIGURE 32.15 **Complicated crown fracture covered with GIC (cement) with calcium hydroxide below.**

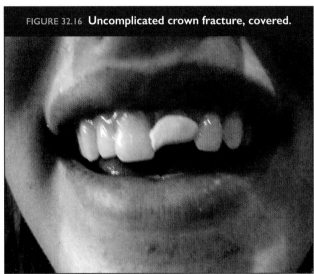

FIGURE 32.16 **Uncomplicated crown fracture, covered.**

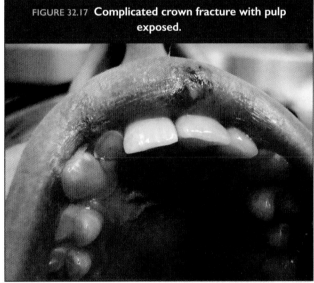

FIGURE 32.17 **Complicated crown fracture with pulp exposed.**

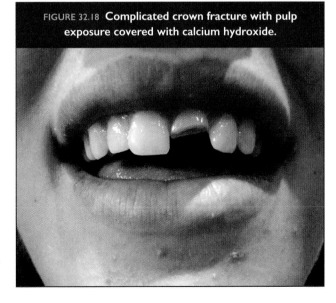

FIGURE 32.18 **Complicated crown fracture with pulp exposure covered with calcium hydroxide.**

The teeth should first be accurately repositioned, using the adjacent teeth positions as a guide. When completing the repositioning of the teeth, be sure that the patient can fully close their back teeth together and are able to chew properly. After repositioning the luxated teeth they should be splinted against adjacent sound teeth using GIC alone or GIC and fine wire (Fig 32.22). Other useful emergency splints include the use of the patient's orthodontic retainer or mouthguard if available (Fig 32.23). Alternatively a Stomahesive wafer (used

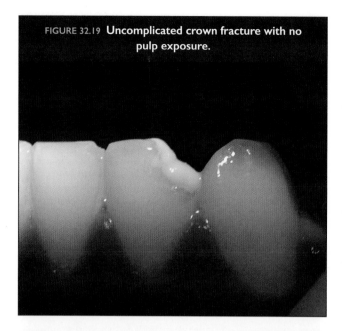

FIGURE 32.19 **Uncomplicated crown fracture with no pulp exposure.**

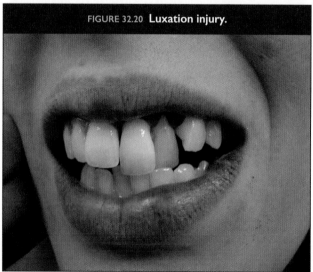

FIGURE 32.20 **Luxation injury.**

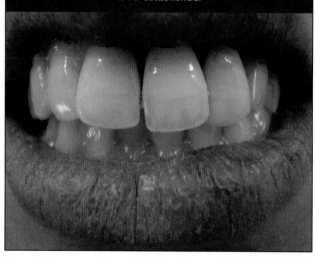

FIGURE 32.21 **Following local anaesthetic, teeth are repositioned with firm finger pressure making sure bite is re-established.**

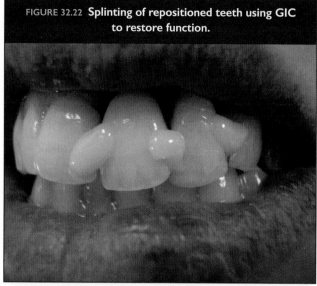

FIGURE 32.22 **Splinting of repositioned teeth using GIC to restore function.**

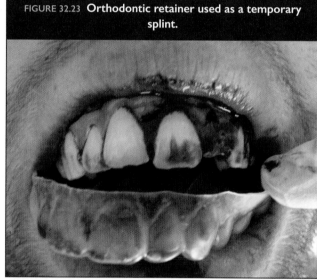

FIGURE 32.23 **Orthodontic retainer used as a temporary splint.**

to attach colostomy bags) may be cut to size and moulded over the repositioned teeth as a temporary splint.

Avulsion injuries

Avulsed teeth are a true dental emergency,[9] as time can affect the outcome. The paramedic should attempt to locate the avulsed tooth and preserve it for transport as below.

Treatment

The most ideal treatment for an avulsed tooth is immediate re-implantation. Avulsed teeth (Figs 32.24 and 32.25) should be stored in cold milk during transport and re-implanted as soon as possible. Milk has an osmolality very similar to that of human blood, and therefore helps maintain the vitality of the periodontal ligament cells which line the root of the tooth and which are critical for the tooth re-attaching back to the socket. Milk is in fact better than saliva as a transport medium as saliva carries a large bacterial load. Long-life and skim milk are equally effective. Other suitable transport media include egg albumin and physiological saline, while tap water is unsuitable because of its osmolality. An avulsed tooth is not to be placed

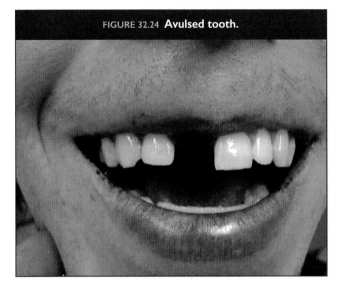

FIGURE 32.24 **Avulsed tooth.**

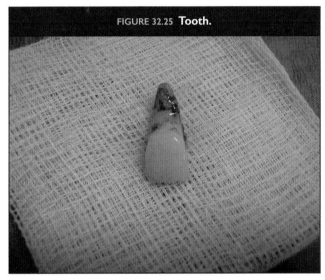

FIGURE 32.25 **Tooth.**

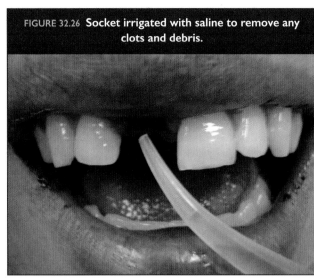

FIGURE 32.26 **Socket irrigated with saline to remove any clots and debris.**

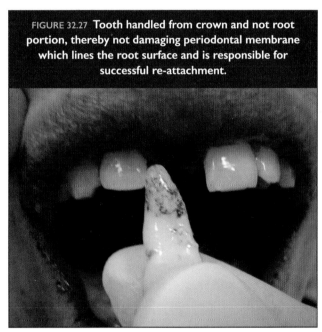

FIGURE 32.27 **Tooth handled from crown and not root portion, thereby not damaging periodontal membrane which lines the root surface and is responsible for successful re-attachment.**

Note the tooth is rinsed under running tap water for a few seconds prior to re-implantation.

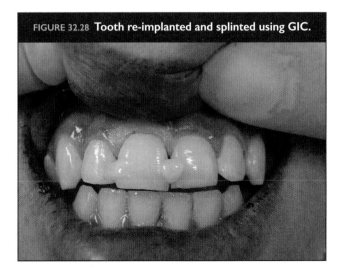

FIGURE 32.28 **Tooth re-implanted and splinted using GIC.**

in the side of the cheek, as was suggested some years ago, since several children ended up swallowing these teeth.

If an avulsed tooth has been inappropriately stored dry for more than 1 hour, re-implantation may be attempted but success is limited. It is estimated that after 1 hour of dry storage, very few if any periodontal ligament cells are still viable on the root surface to allow the tooth to reattach. In addition, an avulsed deciduous (primary) tooth should never be re-implanted. This is because in trying to replace the deciduous tooth back into the socket there is the likelihood of damage to the developing permanent tooth which lies at the base of the socket just under the deciduous tooth.

The tooth socket should first be irrigated with saline to remove any residual clot which may inhibit replantation (Fig 32.26). The avulsed tooth is handled only by the crown portion so as not to damage the periodontal ligament cells on the root surface which are essential for successful re-attachment (Fig 32.27). The avulsed tooth is rinsed under running water or saline for a few seconds to remove any gross debris, and then inserted back into the socket (Fig 32.28). It is important to avoid any aggressive cleaning as this may damage the vulnerable periodontal membrane cells. Once the tooth is correctly positioned the patient should be able to completely close their back teeth together. The tooth should then be splinted by using Blu-Tack with foil on top, or GIC if available (Fig 32.29).

An assessment of the patient's tetanus immunisation status should be done, and post re-implantation treatment/instructions should include:

- oral doxycycline 100 mg bid for 7 days if patient is > 12 years of age. If < 12 years, give penicillin V. This

FIGURE 32.29 **A,** Tooth avulsion injury. **B,** Reinsertion of the avulsed tooth. **C,** Prior to splinting, the patient should be able to completely close their teeth together. **D,** Splinting with Blu-tack. **E,** Covering the teeth with aluminium foiled paper (from a 'Jelonet' dressing package). **F,** the same patient splinted more definitively using GIC and some fishing line.

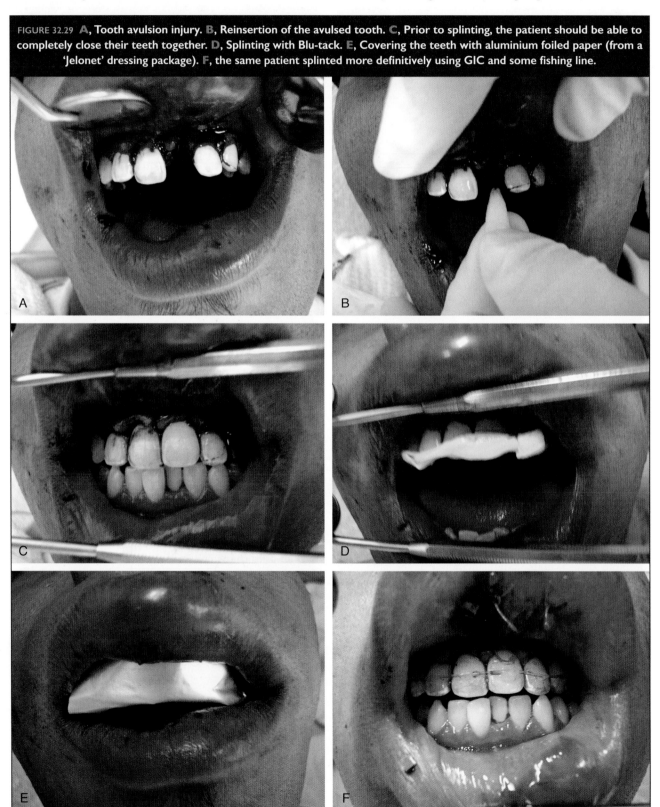

Courtesy Dr Tony Skapetis.

has been shown to help reduce post-implantation root resorption[27]

- chlorhexidine (0.1–0.2%) mouthwash twice daily for 7 days to help maintain oral hygiene
- soft diet for 2 weeks to facilitate tooth re-attachment
- follow-up by dentist as soon as practical and ideally within 2 weeks.

PRACTICE TIPS

LUXATION INJURIES

- Hold avulsed tooth by the crown only
- Transport in milk
- Rinse the root briefly under running water or saline before re-implanting
- Secure the re-implanted tooth by splinting

Ear emergencies

Most presentations to an emergency medical service are because of pain, infection or a foreign body lodged in the ear canal. Earache can be excruciating and the need for pain relief should not be underestimated.[28]

Otitis externa

Acute otitis externa is caused when the thin epithelial lining of the ear canal is damaged, primarily due to trauma (e.g. cleaning the ear with a cotton bud, or foreign-body insertion including hearing aids) or as a localised reaction to chemicals or excessive moisture. It is more common in the summer months and in humid conditions. It is also known as swimmer's ear. Patients with a pre-existing skin condition such as eczema or psoriasis may be predisposed.[29]

Otitis externa may be bacterial or fungal in nature. Fungal infection is less common and usually follows a prolonged course of topical antibacterials and/or corticosteroids.[30]

PRACTICE TIP

Otitis externa is largely preventable, so patients should be educated not to put anything into their ear canal— including cotton buds.

Assessment

Patients present complaining of itchiness, ear pain, discharge or muffled hearing. The ear canal appears red and swollen and there may be a discharge in the ear canal. On examination, tenderness may be present on moving the pinna or opening the jaw.

Treatment

The ear should not be syringed with water, but debris and exudate should be removed. This can be done either by suctioning with direct visualisation or dry-mopping using cotton wool on a thin carrier. See Chapter 17, p. 327, for a description of suctioning techniques. This should be followed with topical eardrops, which are a combination of a corticosteroid and an antibiotic, unless the patient is systemically unwell when oral antibiotics may be given.[32] Pain can usually be adequately controlled using paracetamol or ibuprofen.[31,32] The patient should also be

advised to keep the ear dry for 2 weeks and to avoid inserting anything into the ear canal, such as a cotton bud, during the course of treatment.

As otitis externa is largely preventable, patients should also be given appropriate advice about not inserting foreign objects into the ear and on using eardrops to loosen cerumen.[29]

Acute otitis media

Acute otitis media (AOM) occurs mainly in children under 10 years, but can occur at any age. AOM is an infection or inflammation in the middle ear space (behind the tympanic membrane).[32] Pain is the major symptom; in young children unable to express the location of pain, irritability, crying and tugging at the earlobes may be the presenting symptoms. AOM is often preceded by upper respiratory tract infections (URTIs) and symptoms such as cough, dysphagia and sore throat may be found.[33] The infection can enter the middle ear via the eustachian tube. Normally the middle ear is filled with air; however, after a cold or a URTI the space can be filled with mucous which can then become infected.[34]

Assessment

Patients will present with pain, which may be associated with redness and swelling over the bone behind the pinna. Other symptoms may include fever, tachycardia, headache, discharge and malaise. Diagnosis is confirmed by examining the eardrum with an auroscope. The tympanic membrane, which is usually pink, becomes a red or yellow colour and may have a lumpy appearance. It might also appear to bulge, with loss of normal landmarks. This is due to the pressure of mucous on the membrane.[34]

Treatment

Pain can usually be managed with either paracetamol or ibuprofen. Hot washcloths held over the ear can help by dilating the blood vessels and encouraging the reabsorption of fluid, and helping reduce swelling.

As most cases of AOM resolve spontaneously, antibiotics are not routinely required. However, if symptoms are not improving after 72 hours then a 5-day course of amoxicillin should be considered. Children between the ages of 6 months and 2 years should be followed up after 24 hours to see if further treatment is required. For children aged less than 6 months, Aboriginals and Torres Strait Islanders, treatment with antibiotics is recommended due to the risk of complications.[31]

PRACTICE TIP

A hot washcloth held over the affected ear can start to reduce pain while oral analgesics take effect. Ensure the temperature is not so hot as to cause a burn injury.

Labyrinthitis

Labyrinthitis is an infection of the inner ear and is thought to be associated with a viral illness.

Assessment

Sudden onset of symptoms include vertigo, nausea and vomiting, and loss of balance. Vertigo is more marked with movement of the head. Hearing loss may also be present on the affected side. Symptoms last from hours to weeks. However, vertigo can also be caused by intracranial pathology so this must be ruled out.

Treatment

Treatment includes bed rest, antiemetics and maintaining hydration (to counteract effects of vomiting).[5,35]

Furunculosis

Furunculosis is an abscess or furuncle in the ear canal. They can cause severe ear pain which is made worse by moving the tragus or opening the jaw.[28]

Assessment

Furuncles usually present similarly to otitis externa, but the pain is more severe.

Treatment

Treatment is with strong oral analgesia; the furuncle usually self-resolves.

Mastoiditis

The mastoid air-cell system is part of the middle ear cleft, so some degree of mastoid inflammation occurs whenever there is infection in the middle ear. In most cases this will not cause any problems, but in acute mastoiditis pus collects in the mastoid air cells and exerts pressure on the bony trabeculae, resulting in necrosis and formation of an abscess cavity.[36] Mastoiditis can be a complication of AOM; the symptoms usually become evident a few days after onset of AOM.

Assessment

Patients present with redness, swelling and tenderness over the mastoid process, and the pinna is displaced away from the side of the head.[29] The patient will be in severe pain and there may or may not be a discharge from the ear. Symptoms that indicate acute mastoiditis should be prioritised as urgent.[29]

> **PRACTICE TIP**
>
> Symptoms that indicate acute mastoiditis should be prioritised as urgent. Look for redness, swelling and tenderness over the mastoid process and a pinna which is displaced away from the side of the head.

Treatment

Mastoiditis can lead to a more serious intracranial infection, so treatment with IV antibiotics should begin as soon as possible and in some cases surgery is required for drainage of the abscess.

Ruptured tympanic membrane

A ruptured tympanic membrane (TM) can occur as a result of trauma or infection. Figures 32.30 and 32.31 show normal tympanic membranes. Types of trauma include penetrating trauma, such as inserting a cotton bud to clean the ear; altitude changes, such as in diving or flying; forcing air into ear canal, such as being slapped over the ear or being in the vicinity of an explosion. Infection can cause the TM to rupture due to the pressure in the middle ear.

Assessment

In the presence of trauma the patient will present complaining of severe ear pain; discharge, which may be bloody; and hearing

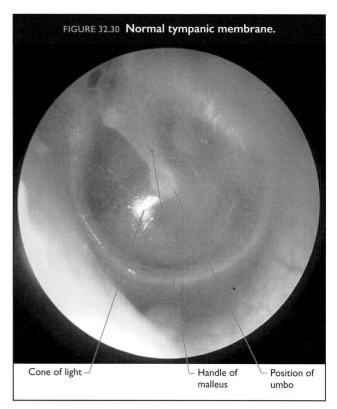

FIGURE 32.30 **Normal tympanic membrane.**

Cone of light — Handle of malleus — Position of umbo

Courtesy Mr Simon A Hickey.

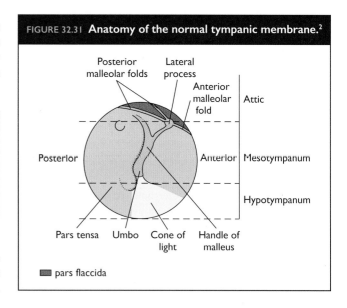

FIGURE 32.31 **Anatomy of the normal tympanic membrane.**[2]

Posterior malleolar folds — Lateral process — Anterior malleolar fold — Attic — Mesotympanum — Hypotympanum — Posterior — Anterior — Pars tensa — Umbo — Cone of light — Handle of malleus

■ pars flaccida

loss to the affected ear. In the case of infection the patient may state that the pain has gone; this is due to the release of pressure caused by the rupture of the TM. In the case of a head injury as well as a ruptured TM, the patient may also have dislocated the ossicles and damaged the inner ear. Any of these injuries can result in hearing loss, dizziness and damage to the facial nerve as it passes through the temporal bone. The resulting injury can be either permanent or temporary.[2]

Treatment

Treatment for a ruptured TM usually consists of analgesia, and patient advice to keep water out of the ear canal. They usually spontaneously heal in a few months; however, ENT department follow-up is advised. In the case of a rupture due to infection, then antibiotics may be required.[29]

Foreign body

Foreign bodies in the ear are a common presentation. The object can vary from an insect, beads and small toys to cotton buds. They prove problematic in their removal, as the area is sensitive and often the patient is a child. Removal should only be attempted by trained staff to avoid unnecessary trauma.[37] The first attempt at removal is likely to be the most successful, as repeated tries cause further swelling and bleeding and decrease patient cooperation.[38]

Assessment

An adult patient will usually be able to tell you what is stuck in the ear; however, children may be fearful of getting into trouble and may present due to secondary symptoms. Symptoms may include itching or discharge. If there is an insect in the ear, a buzzing may be heard or motion felt. The patient or parents/accompanying adult should always be asked about attempts to remove the object at home, as poorly executed attempts at foreign body removal may injure the ear canal, perforate the tympanic membrane or merely push the foreign body deeper into the canal.[39] Inspection of the ear canal should be performed using an auroscope. It is important to check that the tympanic membrane is intact.

> **PRACTICE TIP**
>
> After removing a foreign body, always re-examine the ear canal to make sure no further foreign body is present and to assess for any damage in removal of the original one.

Treatment

A patient presenting with an insect in the ear is usually very distressed due to the pain and noise associated with the insect. The first priority is to kill the insect. This can be done with olive oil, methylated spirits or lignocaine. Lignocaine has been reported to have an irritating effect that drives the insect out of the ear canal.[38] Once the insect is dead, the patient will be a lot calmer. The insect usually floats to the surface and can be easily retrieved.

Organic matter such as paper, vegetables and cottonwool cause an added problem as they swell in moist conditions, making it more difficult to retrieve them and making it difficult to flush them out. They may be grabbed onto using crocodile forceps, but the danger is that the object will be pushed further into the ear.

If the object is round and smooth, then forceps will not be able to grasp the item and other methods need to be considered. These include using gentle suction or a hook.

If the foreign body is successfully removed, then the ear canal should be inspected to ensure all matter is removed and no further damage has been caused by the removal.[29] If the object cannot be adequately visualised or retrieved, then referral to the appropriate ENT service is required and the patient should remain nil by mouth.

When approaching a child, a certain level of cooperation is required. It is helpful to gain their trust if possible by playing a few games before attempting to retrieve the object.

However, if the first attempt is not successful then the chances of cooperation for subsequent attempts is reduced. Sedation may be an option if the resources are available.[37]

Blocked ears

Cerumen or earwax, a naturally occurring substance in the ear, cleans, protects and lubricates the external ear canal. Blocked ears due to impacted wax are not something that can be dealt with in an ED. The patient should be advised to place wax-softening drops in the ear for a few days and then attend a general practitioner for syringing. The ED nurse should not perform ear syringing unless they have received formal training in the process. In the eyes of the law, you may be seen to be negligent if you do perform syringing and have not had the training or received a recent update of your skills.[39]

Trauma

A blunt force, such as a sporting injury or assault or a penetrative injury caused by a sharp object, are causes of trauma to the earlobe. An injury to the earlobe can result in a laceration to the pinna or a sub-perichondrial haematoma. Lacerations can involve the outer layer of skin or can be full-thickness involving the cartilage.

Assessment

A thorough inspection of the ear should be made and any bleeding stopped with direct pressure. The ear canal should also be inspected for injury using an auroscope. Clear fluid from the ear after trauma could be cerebrospinal fluid and brain injury should be suspected.

Treatment

Superficial lacerations can generally be treated by cleaning with normal saline and applying a non-pressure dressing. All foreign bodies should be removed to prevent tattooing or infection. Reassessment of the wound should occur in 24 hours.[39] For lacerations involving the cartilage, referral to an ENT surgeon is required. This is to ensure that the best cosmetic appearance is attained. A sub-perichondrial haematoma is a collection of blood between the cartilage and perichondrium. The blood exerts pressure on the cartilage, resulting in necrosis (leading to cauliflower ear if untreated). Treatment is evacuation of the blood followed by a pressure bandage to prevent re-accumulation.[29] See Chapter 17, p. 349, for information on applying a pressure bandage.

Nasal emergencies

Nasal problems can relate to trauma, infection or haemorrhage.

Epistaxis

Nosebleeds are a common occurrence with 60% of the population suffering a nosebleed at some time in their life.[40] Ninety per cent of nosebleeds stop spontaneously or with pinching of the soft tissue of the nose.[41] However it can be life threatening in the elderly or those with co-morbidities.[42] Epistaxis is more common in the winter months due to dry, cold air and subsequent drying of the nasal mucosa.[43] In the younger population, nosebleeds generally occur in the anterior area (Little's area or Kiesselbach's area, see Fig 32.31), due to nose-picking or insertion of a foreign body, and account for 90% of incidences. In the elderly they tend to be posterior and account for the other 10%.[45]

Assessment

When a patient presents with active bleeding, it is not always easy to obtain a history straight away. After assessing airway, breathing and circulation and acting on any life-threatening findings, attempts should be made to stop the nosebleed. Once this has been done further history can be taken. A full set of vital signs needs to be obtained and repeated regularly to monitor haemodynamic stability. A nosebleed from only one nostril is usually anterior, whereas if the patient can feel the blood running down their throat it is more likely to be posterior.[43] The history should also include asking about bleeding disorders, medications including anticoagulants, trauma and estimated blood loss. Angina and chronic obstructive airways disease can be exacerbated due to hypovolaemia or anaemia, and presence of these conditions should be considered.[45] Hypertension is not generally a cause of nosebleeds but it can prolong the course of the nosebleed and is probably a stress response to the nosebleed.[2,45]

Treatment

Pressing on the nose beneath the nasal bone for 15 minutes without interruption can usually arrest bleeding. Patients should also be advised to sit up and tilt their head forward so as to allow blood to drain out of the mouth. Swallowing can cause pressure changes in the nose that dislodge recently formed clots, and swallowed blood irritates the stomach causing the patient to vomit and again dislodge the clot. At least two adequate attempts at direct pressure should be made before more-invasive methods are considered.[43] An ice pack can also be applied to the bridge of the nose.[41] In the pre-hospital setting if the bleed cannot be arrested, a large-bore cannula should be sited and fluids given.

PRACTICE TIP

To stop epistaxis, press beneath the nasal bone (Little's area) with firm pressure for 15 minutes. Use a watch to time, as release before this time is unlikely to stop the bleeding. Consider applying an ice pack to the bridge of the nose.

Anterior management

If the bleeding site can be visualised then it may be possible to cauterise the vessel once haemostasis is achieved. This is usually done with the application of silver nitrate. Prior to its application it is important to protect the surrounding areas with a barrier cream to prevent injury to the unaffected areas. If bleeding continues then nasal packing will be required. This is usually as per department protocol and the type of packing available. Patients may be suitable for discharge if after initial treatment they maintain haemostasis. However if bleeding reoccurs nasal repacking may be required. Patients may be considered for discharge with nasal packs in situ if they live close to the hospital and have a means to return, or have access to medical review within 24 hours. However, patients with risk factors for rebleeding (on anticoagulants, hypertensive and the elderly) are more safely observed in hospital.

A recent randomised controlled trial showed applying a topical application of injectable form of tranexamic acid was better than anterior nasal packing in the initial treatment of anterior epistaxis.[40]

Posterior management

If a bleeding site is not found or bleeding continues, then a posterior bleed is the likely cause. The use of a balloon catheter is usually required. The type will depend on departmental preference. The patient should be admitted to hospital for observation, as complications can arise. The pack can become dislodged and cause an airway obstruction. There is risk of infection, particularly sinusitis due to improper draining of the sinuses. It is a painful procedure, so adequate and ongoing analgesia should be given. Some patients can also experience difficulty in swallowing, so hydration needs to be monitored.[41,45,46]

Foreign body

Foreign bodies in noses generally occur in children aged 9 months and upwards following the development of the pincer grip and an inquisitive nature to explore their surroundings.

Assessment

The presence of a nasal foreign body should be suspected in patients with unilateral discharge and unexplained pain.[38]

Treatment

In an older child it is possible to try and get them to blow the object out of the affected nostril while occluding the unaffected one; however, there is a risk that the child will inhale instead and aspirate the object. Local anaesthetic spray can be applied to the nostril and then removal by forceps performed, but in an uncooperative child sedation may be required. Always re-examine the nose after removal of the object, as other foreign matter may also be in situ.[29,37]

Trauma

Trauma to the nose is usually a result of an accident or an assault. As with all trauma, the patient should be assessed for DRSABCD first and life-threatening injuries ruled out before treatment to the nose is commenced. Nosebleeds that follow head or facial trauma may indicate cerebrospinal fluid leak or an orbital blow-out fracture.[8]

Assessment

A history should be taken. Examination of the external surface of the nose should be conducted as well as examining the internal surfaces. A nasal speculum should be used for this.

Treatment

First-aid measures include applying ice and keeping the head elevated to reduce swelling.[45] If the patient has a nosebleed, then it should be stopped using the methods described above.

Any wounds to the nose should be cleaned and dressed as appropriate; tetanus status should be ascertained and a booster given if required.

Nasal injuries are often accompanied by soft-tissue swelling and so assessment of injury is difficult initially. The patient is usually followed up after 7–10 days, once the swelling has subsided. In children the fracture heals faster, so they should be seen within 5 days.[46] This is done in an ENT clinic if deformity is still present.

A septal haematoma should also be excluded where there is suspicion of a nasal fracture. Looking up the nose with a nasal speculum, it appears as a cherry pushing down. If left untreated it can become infected and lead to an abscess and necrosis of the nasal cartilage, leading to a cosmetic deformity. An ENT specialist usually performs an incision and drainage and referral should occur as soon as possible.[29]

Sinusitis

Sinusitis is inflammation and swelling of the lining of the sinuses, causing the normal drainage mechanism of the sinus to become blocked. Acute sinusitis is diagnosed when symptoms are of less than 3 weeks duration. Viral upper respiratory tract infections and allergic rhinitis are the most common precipitants of acute sinusitis.[41] Chronic sinusitis occurs when symptoms persist for longer than 3 weeks.

Assessment

The patient will present with facial pain that increases with leaning forward, fever, yellow/green nasal discharge, nausea and headache. On palpation there may be tenderness over the sinus.

Treatment

For acute sinusitis with mild symptoms of less than 7 days' duration, symptomatic treatment is recommended. Paracetamol can be used for pain relief. Antibiotics should not be given unless symptoms persist for more than 7 days, or unless symptoms are severe.[41] Decongestants can also be used to reduce local oedema, promoting drainage and therefore helping to alleviate symptoms; but for no longer than 7 days due to rebound symptoms.[40] The patient should keep their head elevated, which can also relieve the stuffy feeling.

Throat emergencies

Patients presenting with throat problems generally experience pain and may have difficulty breathing. There is little seasonal fluctuation in the incidence of sore throat, and about 10% of the Australian population will present to a primary healthcare service annually with an upper respiratory tract infection consisting predominantly of a sore throat.[49] A bacterial or viral infection, foreign body, trauma and irritation can cause sore throat from smoke, or seasonal allergy.[50,29]

> **PRACTICE TIPS**
>
> Considerations for pre-hospital care for a child with a sore throat:
> - Do not put anything in the mouth to visualise the pharynx.
> - Do not site an intravenous line unless arrest is imminent.
> - Allow the child to be transported in a position of comfort.
> - Monitor heart rhythm for bradycardia.
> - Transport rapidly to an emergency medical service.

There are two key issues that emergency medical personnel should focus on. First is being alert for signs of respiratory compromise. In these cases, high-flow oxygen should be given and the patient transported in the position that affords the most comfort. This is usually sitting upright or semi-erect. Under no circumstances should the patient be forced to recline. If complete airway obstruction occurs, then this should be managed with bag–mask ventilation, tracheal intubation or surgical airway, depending on the skill of the paramedic.

The second issue to consider is dehydration. Many patients with severe pharyngitis are unable to maintain adequate hydration. Intravenous fluids should be administered in these cases; however, caution should be exercised in children as emotional upset from having a cannula sited could worsen the airway obstruction.[49] Do not place anything in the mouth to visualise the pharynx in a child, as this could also exacerbate the potential airway obstruction. Rapid transfer to an emergency medical service should occur, with electrocardiograph monitoring as bradycardia can be a sign of impending arrest.[50]

Epiglottitis is covered in Chapter 36.

> **PRACTICE TIP**
>
> Allow the patient to find a position which is the most comfortable for them. This may be seated or lying in a semi-recumbent position.

Pharyngitis

Pharyngitis is inflammation of the pharynx. Patients usually present complaining of a sore throat and difficulty swallowing. Pharyngitis tends to be viral, but a minority of cases are bacterial; clinically, it can be very difficult to differentiate the two. If the sore throat is accompanied by other cold-like symptoms such as a runny nose, cough and laryngitis (see below), the infection is most likely to be viral. Bacterial infection is much more likely in a patient presenting with only a sore throat. Group A beta-haemolytic *Streptococcus* (GABHS) is the most common bacteria found in bacterial pharyngitis. It can cause acute rheumatic fever and post-streptococcal glomerulonephritis, therefore the patient may be treated with antibiotics if in a high-risk group such as a child with diabetes mellitus or immunodeficiency, a history of rheumatic heart disease or features of systemic illness due to the acute sore throat.[5,51–53]

Assessment

A history should be taken. Patients may complain of soreness on swallowing, general malaise, headache and fever. Past medical history should be taken and a history of rheumatic fever should be noted.[9] The patient's voice may be hoarse or sound muffled. A set of vital signs should be taken. The presence of fever is likely and tachycardia, tachypnoea and/or hypotension may mean the patient needs more immediate attention.

Examination can help reveal if the cause is viral or bacterial. In a viral infection, you would expect to find vesicular and petechial patterns on the soft palate and tonsils, and often associated with rhinorrhoea. In a bacterial infection, there is marked erythema of the tonsils and tonsillar pillars, tonsillar exudate; and when the neck is palpated, enlarged tender anterior cervical lymph nodes are found. Uvular oedema may also be seen.[54] Diagnosis of a GABHS is based on the Centor criteria which state that the following four things must be present:

1. history of fever
2. absence of cough
3. tonsillar exudate
4. enlarged tender anterior cervical nodes.[49]

Centor criteria

1. History of fever
2. Absence of cough
3. Tonsillar exudates
4. Enlarged tender anterior cervical nodes.

Scoring:

- 4 Centor criteria = antibiotics
- 2–3 Centor criteria + positive throat swab = antibiotics
- < 2 Centor criteria and negative throat swab = no antibiotics

Treatment

For viral pharyngitis, treatment is conservative. Pain can be managed with over-the-counter analgesics like paracetamol and ibuprofen. Tablets that dissolve in water may be preferable, as they are easier to swallow.[52] Fluids should be encouraged to prevent dehydration.

For GABHS, treatment is based on how many positive Centor criteria signs are present. Those with Centor scores of 4 should be treated with antibiotics. Scores of 2–3 should have a throat swab and antibiotics given only for those where the swab comes back positive. Those who score < 2 are treated symptomatically as for viral pharyngitis.[49]

Laryngitis

Laryngitis is inflammation of the larynx and vocal cords due to viral or bacterial infection or irritation caused by allergens, chemicals or overuse. Episodes are usually self-limiting and can be influenced by weather conditions. The cords lose the ability to vibrate due to swelling and cause the voice to sound husky or to be lost altogether, breathing can be difficult and stridor may be heard. Obstruction of the airway can become serious and should be treated as soon as possible. See Chapter 36 for details on croup.

Assessment

Patients will give a history of a lowering of the normal pitch of the voice and hoarseness, which usually persists for from 3 to 8 days. They may also experience symptoms of a URTI such as sore throat, rhinorrhoea, dyspnoea, postnasal discharge and congestion. The diagnosis is often made on history alone.

Treatment

In the patient with loss of voice and sore throat, treatment consists of analgesia, steam inhalations and voice rest. Laryngitis is most often viral and antibiotics are not recommended.[52,54]

Tonsillitis

The tonsils have many crevices that seem to harbour bacteria, but tonsillitis can be either viral or bacterial and may occur in isolation or as part of a generalised pharyngitis.[56] It is more common in childhood. Rheumatic fever and acute glomerulonephritis are recognised complications of acute tonsillitis associated with GABHS. These diseases are rare in resource-rich countries, but do occasionally occur. They are still a common problem in certain populations, notably Australian Aboriginals, and may be effectively prevented in closed communities by the use of penicillin.[57]

Assessment

Patients with viral tonsillitis usually present complaining of a sore throat and may also have a blocked nose, cough and cold symptoms and general aches and pains. On examination, the tonsils will appear red, but may or may not have exudate on them. Bacterial tonsillitis tends to have more localised symptoms, such as sore throat, difficulty swallowing, referred ear pain, fever and malaise. A throat swab should be taken.

Treatment

Antibiotics are not recommended for tonsillitis; instead, the patient should rest, drink plenty of fluids and take regular analgesia for pain. However if three or more of the Centor criteria are present or the patient has had a positive throat swab or appears systemically unwell, then antibiotics should be prescribed.

Peritonsillar abscess

Peritonsillar abscess (quinsy) occurs when the bacterial infection of tonsillitis extends outside the tonsillar capsule and into surrounding tissue. The abscess is usually found in the potential space between the tonsillar capsule and the surrounding pharyngeal muscle bed. It is usually found in young adults who have a history of recurrent infections.

Assessment

The patient will usually present complaining of worsening pain, difficulty swallowing, trismus (spasm in jaw muscles causing pain on opening) and may be unable to swallow. Examination will reveal a grossly swollen tonsil deviating to the midline. Dehydration may be an issue in a patient who is unable to swallow and they should also be assessed for respiratory compromise.

Treatment

Intravenous antibiotics and fluids are commenced and referral is made to an ENT specialist who will perform an incision and drainage.

Parapharyngeal abscess

Parapharyngeal abscesses can occur as a complication of bacterial tonsillitis or pharyngitis. Patients who present with severe symptoms of trismus, pain on swallowing, hot-potato voice or muffled voice and shortness of breath should be carefully assessed to rule out this complication.

Assessment

Examination reveals asymmetric pharyngeal swelling, including the palate. Close observation of the airway is required, as it can be compromised by swelling into the neck.

Treatment

Treatment may require airway management and support if this is compromised. See Chapter 17, p. 314, for airway management techniques. Surgical drainage of the abscess is usually required along with a course of intravenous antibiotics.[53,56]

Facial emergencies

Although the facial emergencies discussed here are not life-threatening, they cause significant pain and distress to the sufferer. Facial fractures are discussed in Chapter 46.

Temporomandibular joint dislocation

The temporomandibular joint (TMJ) is a paired synovial joint capable of both sliding and hinge movements.[58] The TMJ articulates the mandibular condyle and the squamous portion of the temporal bone. The upper part of the joint allows for the sliding movement and this is separated from the lower joint by a fibrous meniscus. The lower part of the joint is responsible for the hinged movement. Young females tend to have laxer joints then males, and an unguarded yawn may take the condyle forwards and then a muscle spasm of the closing muscles holds it there.[59]

Assessment
Patients usually present with an open mouth. They may be quite distressed due to pain and anxiety.

Treatment
The dislocation can be reduced by manually pushing the mandible both backwards and downwards. Both hands are placed, with the thumbs outside the patient's teeth, on the lateral border of the mandible, which is then pushed downwards and backwards, placing the condyles back into the fossa. Gauze can be placed over the thumbs for protection. If the muscles are in spasm, then the patient may require a muscle relaxant such as diazepam. In more-severe cases a general anaesthetic may be required.[58] The patient may require anti-inflammatory medication for a few days for pain relief.

Facial cellulitis

Facial cellulitis usually occurs secondary to either odontogenic or auricular infections. Patients present with pain, swelling and redness over the affected area; treatment usually consists of antibiotics and analgesia, with no adverse outcomes. However, Ludwig's angina is a submandibular space infection involving the suprahyoid region and floor of the mouth. It elevates the tongue and pushes it posteriorly. The spaces also communicate with the parapharyngeal space and so involvement of the epiglottis is not uncommon. Therefore the main risk for this patient group is airway obstruction.[3,5,60] Dental disease, particularly of the mandibular molars, is the most common predisposing factor.[9] Other precipitating factors include poor dental hygiene, recent dental work, local trauma, tongue piercing and immunocompromise.[9,60]

Assessment
A history should include exploration for any of the predisposing factors. Patients may present complaining of dental, mouth or neck pain. Trismus and/or drooling may also be present. A set of vital signs should be recorded, as fever, chills and tachycardia are common.

Treatment
Ludwig's angina can cause airway obstruction within hours, so constant monitoring of airway patency is essential. The swelling can make endotracheal intubation difficult and it has a high failure rate. Nasotracheal intubation is the preferred method, but an advanced airway kit should be kept close at hand and ready to use. If Ludwig's angina is suspected, then rapid transfer to an emergency medical service is required.

Definitive treatment is with surgical drainage of the abscess and IV antibiotics; however, dexamethasone reduces oedema and cellulitis and can improve the airway obstruction initially. Nebulised adrenaline can also help to reduce upper airway swelling.[60]

SUMMARY

This chapter has looked at common presentations to ED involving the ear, nose throat, face and teeth. Most presentations are precipitated by pain, but due to the intimate nature of structures swelling and infection can spread to neighbouring areas. Therefore all patients should be monitored closely for airway difficulties or symptoms of intracranial infection.

CASE STUDY

You are called to attend an 80-year-old woman. On arrival at the scene you find her sitting with her head over a bucket. She has had a large epistaxis which is still actively bleeding. There is evidence of a large loss of blood. During transit the nose bleed is stopped using pressure but on arrival in the emergency department (ED) the epistaxis commences again. The site of bleeding cannot be visualised. She has a history of hypertension, atrial fibrillation and is warfarinised. Her blood pressure is 170/90 mmHg, pulse 110 beats/minute and respiratory rate 20 breaths/minute.

Questions
1. What is your first intervention?
   A. Lie the patient on her left side to prevent aspiration
   B. Obtain a full set of vital signs
   C. Insert a large-bore cannula
   D. Assess DRSABCD and apply firm pressure to the nostrils for 15 minutes.
2. What position should you get the patient into?
   A. Left lateral position
   B. Prone

C. Semi-recumbent in a position of comfort

D. Sitting up with head tilted forward

3. Which of the following treatment options would be most appropriate after your initial assessment?

A. Give antihypertensive medication to reduce blood pressure

B. Insert an appropriate nasal pack

C. Organise crossmatch blood

D. Reverse warfarin by administering vitamin K

4. What are the clinical red flags obtained during the history?

Answers to Case Study Questions can be found on evolve
http://evolve.emergencytrauma.curtis

USEFUL WEBSITES

Statref.com—suite of 3-D interactive models of human anatomy. Online ebook.

www.merckmanuals.com/professional/index.html.

REFERENCES

1. Alford B. Core curriculum syllabus: review of anatomy—the larynx; 2011. Online. www.bcm.edu/oto/core-curriculum. Accessed 7 Feb 2014.

2. Epstein O, Perkin GD, Cookson J et al. Chapter 4: Ear, nose and throat. Clinical examination. 4th edn. Sydney: Elsevier; 2008:82–104.

3. Marx J, Hockberger RS, Wallia R et al. Rosen's emergency medicine, 8th edn, Elsevier, 2014.

4. Beaudreau R. Oral and dental emergencies. In: Tintinalli JE, Stapczynski S, eds. Tintinalli's Emergency medicine: a comprehensive study guide. 7th edn. New York: McGraw-Hill; 2011.

5. Dental, ear, nose, throat and facial emergencies. In: Howard P, ed. Sheehy's emergency nursing: principles and practice. 6th edn. Elsevier; 2010:602–15.

6. Wilson SF, Thompson JM. Respiratory disorders. St Louis: Mosby; 1990.

7. Sinnatamby C. Last's anatomy. 12th edn. Sydney: Elsevier; 2011:329–454.

8. Purcell D. Minor injuries: A clinical guide. 2nd edn. Sydney, Elsevier; 2010:219–33.

9. Benko K. Acute dental emergencies in emergency medicine. Emerg Med Pract 2003;5(5):1–24.

10. Stephen T, Skillen L, Day RA et al. Canadian Bates' guide to health assessment for nurses. Toronto: Lippincott; 2009.

11. Curtis L, Morrell T. Pain management in the emergency department. Emerg Med Pract 2006;8(7):1–26.

12. Skapetis T, Curtis K. Emergency management of dental trauma. Australasian Emergency Nursing Journal 2010;13:30–4.

13. Lewis C, Lynch H, Johnston B. Dental complaints in emergency departments: a national perspective. Ann Emerg Med 2003;42(1):93–9.

14. Gibson DE, Verono AA. Dentistry in the emergency department. J Emerg Med 1987;5(1):35–44.

15. Hyllested M, Jones S, Pedersen JL et al. Comparative effect of paracetamol, NSAIDs or their combination in postoperative pain management: a qualitative review. Br J Anaesth 2002;88(2):199–214.

16. Do LG, Slade GD, Roberts-Thomson KF et al. Smoking-attributable periodontal disease in the Australian adult population. J Clin Periodontol 2008;35(5):398–404.

17. Neugebauer J, Jozsa M, Kubler A. [Antimicrobial photodynamic therapy for prevention of alveolar ostitis and post-extraction pain]. Mund Kiefer Gesichtschir 2004;8(6):350–5.

18. Storoe W, Haug RH, Lillich TT. The changing face of odontogenic infections. J Oral Maxillofac Surg 2001;59(7):739–48; discussion 748–9.

19. Skapetis T, Naim A. Dental infections management flowchart. General Practice Training Tasmania; 2012 Online. http://aci.moodlesite.pukunui.net/pluginfile.php/1581/mod_resource/content/2/Skapetis%20et%20al%202012.pdf; accessed 10 June 2015.

20. World Health Organization. Application of the International Classification of Diseases to Dentistry and Stomatology (ICD-DA). 3rd edn, Geneva: World Health Organization. 1994.

21. Glendor U. Epidemiology of traumatic dental injuries—a 12-year review of the literature. Dent Traumatol 2008;24(6):603–11.

22. Holan, G, Shmueli, Y. Knowledge of physicians in hospital emergency rooms in Israel on their role in cases of avulsion of permanent incisors. International Journal of Paediatric Dentistry 2003;13:13–19.

23. Yeng T, Parashos P. An investigation into dentists' perceptions of barriers to providing care of dental trauma to permanent maxillary incisors in children in Victoria, Australia. Aust Dent J 2007;52:210–15.

24. Skapetis T, Gerzina T, Hu W. Can a four-hour interactive workshop on the management of dental emergencies be effective in improving self reported levels of clinician proficiency? Australasian Emergency Nursing Journal 2012;15:14–22.

25. Skapetis T, Gerzina T, Hu W. Managing dental emergencies: A descriptive study of the effects of a multimodal educational intervention for primary care providers at six months. BMC Medical Education 2012;12:103.

26. Skapetis T, Gerzina T, Hu W et al. Effectiveness of a brief educational workshop intervention among primary care providers at 6 months: uptake of dental emergency supporting resources. Rural and remote health 2013;13.

27. Rawal SY, Rawal YB. Non-antimicrobial properties of tetracyclines—dental and medical implications. West Indian Med J 2001;50(2): 105–8.

28. Stevens D. Case book: earache. Pract Nurs 2008;19(4):193–6.

29. Reynolds T. Ear, nose and throat problems in Accident and Emergency. Nurs Stand 2004;18(26):47–53.

30. Clinical practice guideline. Earache; 2013. Online. www.nursing.health.wa.gov.au/docs/career/np/joondalup/CPG_Earache.pdf; accessed 7 Feb 2014.

31. Therapeutic guidelines; 2013 eTG complete. Available: on subscription to http://online.tg.org.au.

32. Leach A, Morris P, Castano R. Antibiotics for acute otitis media in children. (Protocol) Cochrane Database Syst Rev 2006;(3).

33. Scottish Intercollegiate Guidelines Network (SIGN). Diagnosis and management of childhood otitis media in primary care. Royal College of Physicians of Edinburgh. SIGN 2003;66. Online. www.sign.ac.uk/guidelines/fulltext/66/index.html: accessed 7 Feb 2014.

34. Peate I. Caring for the person with otitis media. Br J Health Care Assistants 2009;3(4):167–70.

35. Ferri F. Labyrinthitis. In: Ferri's clinical advisor. Sydney: Elsevier; 2014:640.

36. Yates P. Otitis media. In: Lalwani A, ed. Current diagnosis and treatment in otolaryngology—head and neck surgery. New York: McGraw-Hill; 2004:695–706.

37. Mackle T, Conlon B. Foreign bodies of the nose and ears in children: should these be managed in the accident and emergency setting? Int J Pediatr Otorhinolaryngol 2006;70(3):425–8.

38. Davies PH, Benger JR. Foreign bodies in the nose and ear: a review of techniques for removal in the emergency department. J Accid Emerg Med 2000;17:91–4.

39. Stubbs G. Getting to grips with the metal ear syringe. Nurs Times 2001;97(20):40–1.

40. Zahed R, Moharamzadeh P, Alizadeh Arasi S et al. A new and rapid method for epistaxis treatment using injectable form of tranexamic acid topically: a randomized controlled trial. American Journal of Emergency Medicine 2013;31:1389–92.

41. Waters TA, Peacock IV WF. Nasal emergencies and sinusitis. In: Tintinalli J, Kelen G, Stapczynski J, eds. Emergency medicine: a comprehensive study guide. 6th edn. New York: McGraw-Hill; 2004.

42. Bertrand B, Eloy P, Rombaux P et al. Guidelines to the management of epistaxis. B-ENT 2005;Suppl 1(1); 27–41.

43. Bernius M, Perlin D. Pediatric ear, nose and throat emergencies. Pediatr Clin N Am 2006;53(2):195–214.

44. Riviello RJ, Brown NA. Otolaryngologic procedures. In: Roberts JR, Hedges JR, eds. Roberts and Hedges'Clinical procedures in emergency medicine. 6th edn. Sydney: Elsevier; 2014.

45. Pfenninger J, Fowler G. Management of epistaxis. In: Pfenninger and Fowler's procedures for primary care. 3rd edn. Sydney: Elsevier; 2011.

46. Pfaff J, Moore G. Otolaryngology. In: Marx J, Hockberger R, Walls R et al, eds. Rosen's emergency medicine: concepts and clinical practice. 8th edn. Sydney: Elsevier; 2014:931–40.

47. Hasan N, Colucciello SA. Maxillofacial trauma. In: Tintinalli J, Kelen G, Stapczynski J, eds. Emergency medicine: a comprehensive study guide. 6th edn. New York: McGraw-Hill; 2004.

48. Kenealy T. Sore throat. Br Med J Clin Evid 2008;01:1509–17.

49. King BR, Charles RA. Pharyngitis in the ED: diagnostic challenges and management dilemmas. Emerg Med Pract 2004;6(5):1–24.

50. Sanders M. Mosby's paramedics textbook. 3rd edn. Toronto: Elsevier Canada; 2007.

51. Blenkinsopp A. Nurse prescribers: respiratory illness 1—Sore throat. Prim Health Care 2002;12(8):33–4.

52. Shnayder Y, Lee KC, Bernstein JM. Management of adenotonsillar disease. In: Lalwani AK, editor. Current diagnosis and treatment in otolaryngology—head and neck surgery. New York: McGraw-Hill; 2004:355–62.

53. Shores C. Infections and disorders of the neck & upper airway. In: Tintinalli J, Kelen GD, Stapczynski J, eds. Emergency medicine: a comprehensive study guide. 6th edn. New York: McGraw-Hill; 2004.

54. Reveiz L, Cardona AF, Ospina EG. Antibiotics for acute laryngitis in adults. Cochrane Database Syst Rev 2007;(2):CD004783. DOI: 10.1002/14651858.CD004783.pub3.

55. Georgalas CC, Tolley NS, Narula A. Recurrent throat infections (tonsillitis). Clin Evid 2009. Online. Available: http://clinicalevidence.bmj.com/ceweb/conditions/ent/0503/0503.jsp; accessed 7 Feb 2014.

56. Stallard T. Emergency disorders of the ear, nose, sinuses, oropharynx and mouth. In: Stone K, Humphries R, editors. Current diagnosis and treatment: emergency medicine. 7th edn. New York: McGraw-Hill; 2011.

57. The Australian Indigenous HealthinfoNet. Conditions of the respiratory tract; 2013. Online. www.healthinfonet.ecu.edu.au/print/540; 7 Feb 2014.

58. Goddard G. Temporomandibular disorders. In: Lalwani A, eds. Current diagnosis and treatment in otolaryngology: head and neck surgery. New York: McGraw-Hill; 2004:405–12.

59. Juniper RP. The temporomandibular joint. In: Yates C, ed. A manual of oral and maxillofacial surgery for nurses. Oxford: Blackwell; 2000:189–212.

60. Buckley M, O'Connor K. Ludwig's angina in a 76-year-old man. Emerg Med J 2009;26(9):679–80.

61. Barkauskas V, Pender NJ, Hayman L et al. Health and physical assessment. 2nd edn. St Louis: Mosby; 1998.

CHAPTER 33
OCULAR EMERGENCIES AND TRAUMA

JOANNA McCULLOCH

Essentials

- Never think of the eye in isolation; always compare the two eyes in assessment.
- A visual acuity of 6/6 does not necessarily exclude a serious eye injury, as both retinal detachments with the macula on and penetrating eye injuries can maintain good vision for a short period.
- No pressure should be applied to the globe if rupture or a penetrating injury is suspected. Apply a clear plastic shield to prevent pressure on the eye and loss of ocular contents.
- Do not try to open a swollen eyelid if there is a history of trauma, unless under the guidance of an ophthalmologist or senior medical officer, as a globe rupture may be present and ocular contents lost when lids are forced open.
- Slit-lamp assessment is essential if removing a corneal foreign body from the central cornea. It will provide the clinician with both depth and extent of the object. A risk of penetrating the cornea or corneal scarring can occur if the object is deeply imbedded in the cornea. This will result in vision loss.
- Do not apply drops or ointment to a patient with a penetrating eye injury.
- Chemical burns should be irrigated as soon as possible with any neutral fluid available (i.e. tap water), then irrigation continued until assessed as the cornea being clear, and no signs of limbal ischaemia.
- Do not prescribe ocular steroids unless directed by an ophthalmologist.

INTRODUCTION

Ocular-related presentations are common to the emergency department (ED). A relatively trivial traumatic presentation may mask a more serious underlying injury. Similarly, a relatively transient episode of visual loss with no abnormality found on examination may indicate potentially life-threatening cerebrovascular disease. All eye injuries presenting to the ED should be carefully evaluated with the necessary equipment and skill.[1] In relation to trauma, it must always be remembered that life-threatening injuries are managed first. The ability to identify conditions that represent a threat to the patient's vision is essential to protecting the patient's vision. The goals of managing eye injury are to prevent further injury to the intact vision, then to assess the extent of the injury and refer the patient to ophthalmology for early management and/or intervention. This chapter provides the epidemiology of ocular trauma in Australia and New Zealand, as well as a description of anatomy, ocular assessment, common ocular emergencies encountered in the ED and their management.

The availability of eye services varies widely in Australia and New Zealand. In urban centres the practitioner has greater access to ophthalmic services.

In regional Australia, the practitioner may need to rely more on their own findings and experiences.[2] The Australian rural population has an increased prevalence of pterygium, lid lesions and ocular trauma with respect to urban dwellers, and these people are more likely to have seen an optometrist, but less likely to have seen an ophthalmologist.

Anatomy and physiology

Outer eye

The eyelids fulfil two main functions: protection of the eyeball and secretion, distribution and drainage of tears (see Figs 33.1 and 33.2). The upper lid is the larger lid; it crosses over the globe to protect it. By blinking, the tear film spreads across the anterior surface of the globe to lubricate it.

Lid movement

The space between the eyelids is termed the palpebral aperture or fissure. The orbicularis oculi muscle is arranged as a ring of fibres around the palpebral aperture: contraction causes the lids to close. The blink function distributes tears across the cornea, which maintains the smooth optical surface of the cornea and displaces debris. The levator muscle in the upper lid principally performs opening of the lids, although there are some tenuous fibres which act to retract the lower lid. The levator extends from the attachments at the orbital apex to attachments at the tarsal plate and skin (forming a skin crease). The lids are securely attached at either end to the bony orbital margin by the medial and lateral palpebral (or canthal) ligaments. Trauma to the medial ligament causes the lid to flop forwards and laterally, impairing function and cosmesis. There is a brisk protective blink reflex: the afferent nerve is the optic, trigeminal (touch) or auditory; the efferent nerve is the facial nerve. The eyelashes are also protective.[3]

Skin and appendages

The skin of the eyelids is thin and only loosely attached to the underlying tissues, so that inflammation and bleeding may cause considerable swelling. The semi-rigid tarsal plate lies behind the skin and orbicularis muscle and is lined posteriorly by conjunctiva. It contains the Meibomian glands, which produce the oily lipid layer of tear film. There is a grey line (inter-marginal sulcus) as seen in Figure 33.1, an important landmark in repairing lacerations of the lid margin, which is located between the eyelashes and the Meibomian orifices (Fig 33.2).[3]

Innervation

Sensory innervation is from the trigeminal (fifth) cranial nerve, via the ophthalmic division (upper lid) and maxillary division (lower lid). The orbicularis oculi is innervated by the facial (seventh) nerve. Palsy causes an ectropion of the lower lid, but *not* ptosis. The levator muscle in the upper lid is supplied by the oculomotor (third) nerve. Palsy of the upper lid causes a ptosis. Note that all the nerves except the facial nerve reach the lids from the orbit.[3]

Blood supply and lymphatics

The eyelids are supplied by an extensive network of blood vessels, which form an anastomosis between branches derived from the external carotid artery via the face and from the internal carotid artery via the orbit. This accounts for excellent healing following trauma.

Lymphatic fluid drains into the preauricular and submandibular nodes. Preauricular lymphadenopathy is a useful sign of infective eyelid swelling (especially viral).[3]

Conjunctiva

The conjunctiva is a thin, transparent mucous membrane lining the eyelids and covering the anterior eyeball up to the edge of the cornea where it ends at the limbus. The conjunctiva folds back onto itself forming two sacs, the superior and inferior fornices. These pockets are significant for presentations of foreign bodies and contact-lens loss. It is loosely connected to the globe, therefore inflammation can cause gross swelling of the fornices and bulbar conjunctiva. The conjunctiva comprises epithelium and an underlying stroma. Within the epithelium are goblet cells, which secrete the mucin component of the tear film.[3]

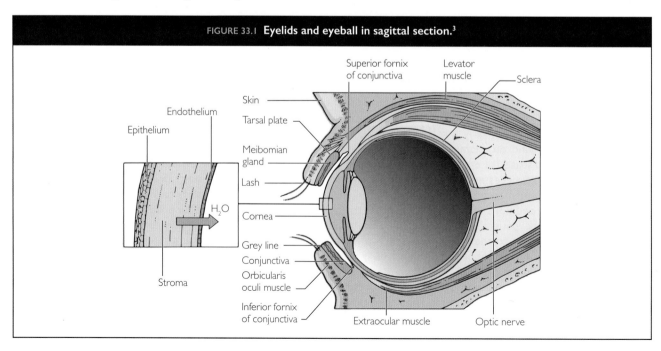

FIGURE 33.1 **Eyelids and eyeball in sagittal section.**[3]

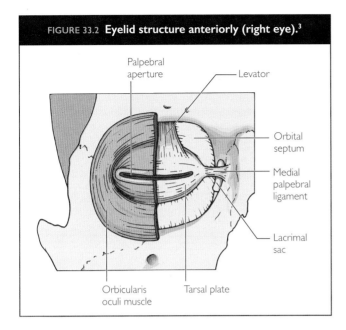

FIGURE 33.2 **Eyelid structure anteriorly (right eye).**[3]

Palpebral aperture
Levator
Orbital septum
Medial palpebral ligament
Lacrimal sac
Orbicularis oculi muscle
Tarsal plate

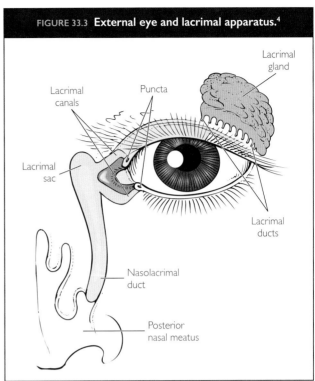

FIGURE 33.3 **External eye and lacrimal apparatus.**[4]

Lacrimal gland
Puncta
Lacrimal canals
Lacrimal sac
Lacrimal ducts
Nasolacrimal duct
Posterior nasal meatus

Tears produced in the lacrimal gland pass over the surface of the eye and enter the lacrimal canal. From there the tears are carried through the nasolacrimal duct to the nasal cavity.[4]

Cornea and sclera

The cornea and sclera form a spherical shell, which makes up the outer wall of the eyeball. Although the two are very similar in many ways, the corneal structure is uniquely modified to transmit and refract light.

The sclera is principally collagenous, avascular (apart from some vessels on its surface) and relatively acellular. It is tough despite being thin (the maximum thickness is 1 mm), and it gives attachment to the extraocular muscle, which at its thinnest point is 0.3 mm thick. It is perforated posteriorly by the optic nerve, and by the sensory and motor nerves and blood vessels to the eyeball. It has a protective function. The cornea and sclera merge at the corneal edge (the limbus).

The cornea is sensitive to touch (in contrast to the insensitive sclera) through nerve fibres from the ophthalmic division of the trigeminal nerve. The nerve endings lie under the epithelial layer. When the corneal epithelium is absent/abraded, this causes great pain.

The chief functions of the cornea are protection against invasion of microorganisms into the eye, and the transmission and focusing (refraction) of light. Refraction of light occurs because of the curved shape of the cornea and its greater refractive index compared with air. The cornea is transparent because of the specialised arrangement of the collagen fibrils within the stroma, which must be kept in a state of dehydration. This is achieved by an energy-dependent ion pump in the endothelium (direction of flow is from stroma to anterior chamber).

The cornea has five layers with the epithelium (surface layer) undergoing constant turnover with basal cells replicating, migrating to the surface and then being shed. The 'Bowman's layer', also known as the anterior limiting membrane, is not a membrane but a condensed layer of collagen; a tough layer that protects the corneal stroma. It does not regenerate when damaged. The stroma then makes up 90% of the corneal layer and is composed of parallel connective tissue. Descemet's membrane, or posterior limiting membrane, is a thin acellular layer that serves as the modified basement membrane of the corneal endothelium (the last layer). Descemet's membrane can regenerate when damaged. The endothelium is a simple squamous or low cuboidal monolayer of mitochondria-rich cells, responsible for regulating fluid and solute transport between the aqueous and the corneal stroma; in contrast to the epithelium, the cells of the endothelium do not divide This is of great clinical significance, since there is sufficient pump activity to maintain corneal dehydration. In consequence, the cornea swells and loses its transparency; this is termed corneal decompensation or bullous keratopathy. Common causes of endothelial cell loss include normal ageing and intraocular surgery (including cataract surgery).[3]

Tear production and drainage

Tears comprise water, mucous to bind the tear film to the corneal epithelium and an outer lipid layer to reduce evaporation of the water. Tears also contain some chemicals to protect against microorganisms.

The lacrimal gland secretes most of the aqueous component of the tear film. It lies in the supero-temporal part of the anterior orbit. Its anterior lobe can sometimes be seen in the upper conjunctival fornix; it is innervated by parasympathetic fibres carried by the facial nerve (Fig 33.3).

Tears collect in a meniscus on the lower lid margin, are spread across the ocular surfaces by blinking and drain into the superior and inferior puncta at the nasal end of the eyelids. Single canaliculi from the punctum unite in a common canaliculus, which ends in the lacrimal sac. This is in a bony fossa crossed anteriorly by the horizontally-directed medial palpebral ligament. Finally, tears pass down the nasolacrimal duct and reach the nasopharyngeal cavity via the inferior meatus. This accounts for the unpleasant taste which follows administration of certain eye-drops.

At birth, the nasolacrimal duct may not be fully developed, causing a watery eye. In most cases, full canalisation occurs within a year. Acquired obstruction of the nasolacrimal duct is a common cause of watery eye in adults. It may lead to an acute infection of the sac, which manifests as a cellulitic swelling just below the medial palpebral ligament.[3]

Extra ocular muscles

There are six extraocular muscles which move the globe in all positions of gaze: four rectus and two oblique. The third cranial (oculomotor) nerve controls the superior, inferior, medial rectus, while the lateral rectus muscle is controlled by the abducent sixth cranial nerve and the superior oblique trochlear muscle is controlled by the fourth cranial nerve (see Fig 33.4).

Inner eye

The internal ocular structures function primarily to refine the image formed by the cornea, and to convert light energy into electrical energy for image formation by the brain. For light to reach the retina, it must pass through a number of structures: the cornea, aqueous humour, lens and vitreous humour (Fig 33.5).

Uvea

The uvea comprises the iris and ciliary body anteriorly and choroid posteriorly.

Iris

The iris largely consists of connective tissue containing muscle fibres, blood vessels and pigment cells. A layer of pigment cells lines its posterior surface and at its centre is an aperture, the pupil. The chief functions of the iris are to control light entry to the retina and to reduce intraocular light scatter. Pupil dilation is caused by contraction of radial smooth muscle fibres

innervated by the sympathetic nervous system (trigeminal nerve). Pupil constriction occurs when a ring of smooth muscle fibres (sphincter muscle) around the pupil contract—these are innervated by the parasympathetic nervous system (oculomotor nerve).

Iris pigment (melanin) reduces intraocular light scatter. The amount of iris pigment determines eye 'colour': blue eyes have the least pigment; brown eyes have the most.

The amount of pigment can delay dilation and elongate the action of topical mydriatics.

Ciliary body

The ciliary body is a specialised structure uniting the iris with the choroid. It makes aqueous humour and anchors the lens via zonules, through which it modulates lens convexity.

Anteriorly the inner surface is folded into ciliary processes, which are the site of aqueous humour formation. Muscle fibres within the ciliary body contract, causing the inner circumference of the lens to reduce. This reduces the tension on the zonules, so that the natural elasticity of the lens causes it to become more convex to focus on near objects. This is called accommodation and is controlled by the parasympathetic system via the oculomotor nerve. Relaxation is passive, increasing tension on the zonules so that the lens is pulled flat for distance vision.[3]

Choroid

The choroid, consisting of blood vessels, connective tissue and pigment cells, is sandwiched between the retina and the sclera. It provides oxygen and nutrition to the outer retinal layers. There is a potential space between the choroid and the sclera, which can become filled with blood or serous fluid.[3]

The lens

The biconvex lens comprises a mass of long cells known as fibres. At the centre these fibres are compacted into a hard nucleus surrounded by dense fibres, the cortex. The whole

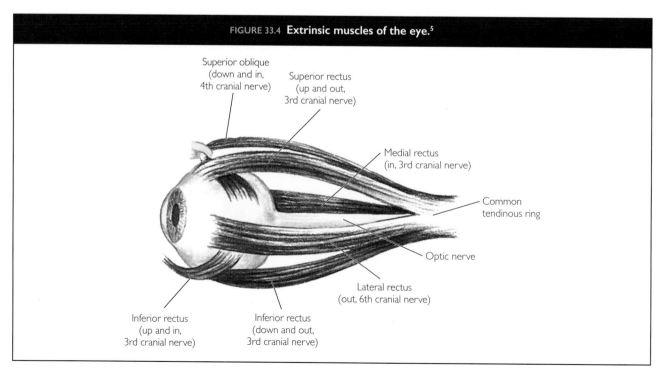

FIGURE 33.4 Extrinsic muscles of the eye.[5]

Superior oblique (down and in, 4th cranial nerve)

Superior rectus (up and out, 3rd cranial nerve)

Medial rectus (in, 3rd cranial nerve)

Common tendinous ring

Optic nerve

Lateral rectus (out, 6th cranial nerve)

Inferior rectus (up and in, 3rd cranial nerve)

Inferior rectus (down and out, 3rd cranial nerve)

Direction of movement of eyeballs is indicated in brackets.[5]

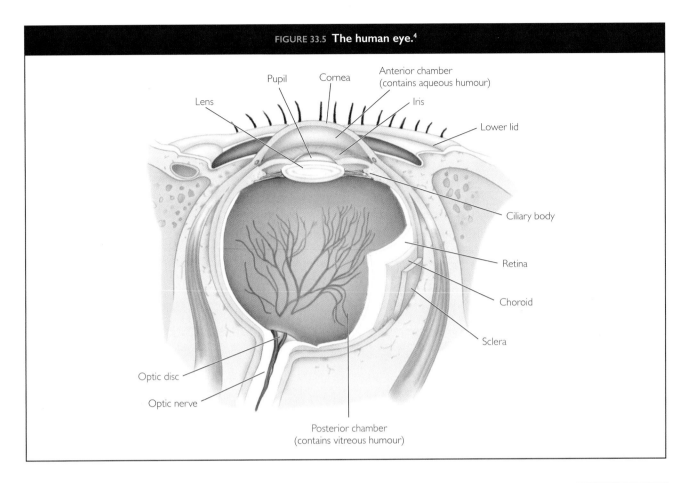

FIGURE 33.5 **The human eye.**[4]

lens is enclosed within an elastic capsule and is deformable for accommodation. The ciliary muscle is a smooth muscle that alters the shape of the lens for near or far vision. It is controlled by the parasympathetic nerve signals transmitted to the eye through the third cranial nerve (oculomotor). Stimulation of the parasympathetic nerves contracts both sets of ciliary muscle fibres, which relaxes the lens ligaments, thus allowing the lens to become thicker and increase its refractive powers. With this increased refractive power, the eye can focus on objects that are nearer. Consequently, as a distant object moves towards the eye, the number of parasympathetic impulses impinging on the ciliary muscle must be progressively increased for the eye to keep the object constantly in focus. The sympathetic stimulation has an additional effect of relaxing the ciliary muscle, but this effect is so weak that it plays almost no role in the normal accommodation mechanism.[6]

Failure of accommodation with ageing (presbyopia) occurs through loss of capsule elasticity and lens deformability. The lens is relatively dehydrated and its fibres contain special proteins. This is why it is transparent. Cataract occurs when this organisation is disrupted.[4]

Intraocular fluid

The eye is filled with intraocular fluid, which maintains sufficient pressure in the eyeball to keep it distended. Figure 33.6 demonstrates that this fluid can be divided into two portions—aqueous humour, which lies in front of the lens, and vitreous humour, which is between the posterior surface of the lens and the retina. The aqueous humour is a freely flowing fluid, whereas the vitreous humour, sometimes

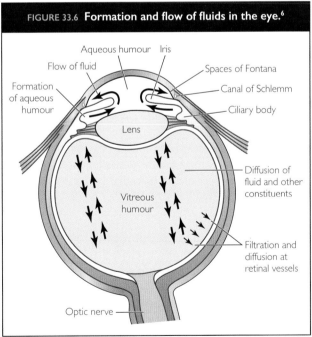

FIGURE 33.6 **Formation and flow of fluids in the eye.**[6]

called the vitreous body, is a gelatinous mass held together by a fine fibrillar network composed primarily of greatly elongated proteoglycan molecules. Both water and dissolved substances can diffuse slowly in the vitreous humour, but there is still flow of fluid.[6]

Aqueous humour

The ciliary body forms aqueous humour by ultrafiltration and active secretion. Its composition is strictly regulated to exclude large proteins and cells, but it does contain glucose, oxygen and amino acids for the cornea and lens. Neural control is via the sympathetic autonomic nervous system (beta-receptors).[3]

Aqueous humour circulates from the posterior to the anterior chamber through the pupil, leaving the eye through the trabecular meshwork, finally entering the canal of Schlemm, which empties into the intraocular veins.[6]

Aqueous production and drainage are balanced to maintain an appropriate intraocular pressure. Excess production or decreased outflow can elevate intraocular pressure above the normal 10–21 mmHg, a condition termed glaucoma.[7]

Vitreous body

The vitreous body is 99% water, but, vitally, also contains collagen fibrils and hyaluronic acid, which impart cohesion and a gel-like consistency. With increasing age, the vitreous body undergoes progressive degeneration and becomes more liquid. The vitreous humour is adherent to the retina at certain points, particularly at the optic disc and at the ora serrata. When the vitreous humour degenerates, it can pull on the retina, causing it to tear and leading to retinal detachment. The vitreous helps to cushion the eye during trauma and has a minor role as a metabolic sump.[3]

Any non-transparent substance within the vitreous humour may block light passing through the vitreous humour. The effect on vision varies, depending on the amount, type and location of the substance blocking the light. For example, in the case of haemorrhage into the vitreous humour, little light will reach the retina and vision will be severely compromised. However, cellular debris that accumulates from normal cell metabolism will cause only a relatively small shadow on the retina (a 'floater').[7]

Retina

The retina is the light-sensitive portion of the eye that contains the cones, which are responsible for colour vision, and the rods, which are mainly responsible for black-and-white vision (peripheral vision) and vision in the dark. When rods or cones are excited, signals are transmitted first through successive layers of neurons in the retina itself and finally into the optic nerve fibres and the cerebral cortex.[6]

The retina converts focused light images into nerve impulses (see Fig 33.7). It comprises the neurosensory retina and the retinal pigment epithelium (RPE). Light has to pass through the inner retina to reach photoreceptors, the rods and cones, which convert light energy into electrical energy (Table 33.1).[3] The inner retina is therefore transparent. Connector neurons modify and pass on the electrical signals to the ganglion cells. The axons run along the surface of the retina, then enter the optic nerve. An area called the macula provides for central vision. At its centre is a specialised area, the fovea, which is for high-quality vision. The rest of the retina is for peripheral vision (Fig 33.8).

Cones concentrated at the macula are responsible for fine vision (acuity) and colour appreciation. Rods are for vision in low light levels and the detection of movement. They are distributed throughout the entire retina except the fovea.

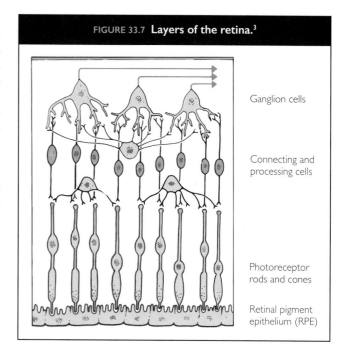

FIGURE 33.7 Layers of the retina.[3]

Ganglion cells

Connecting and processing cells

Photoreceptor rods and cones

Retinal pigment epithelium (RPE)

TABLE 33.1 Properties of rods and cones[3]

	RODS	CONES
Function	Vision in dim light, movement	Vision in bright light, colour, high resolution
Total number	> 100 million	6–7 million
Highest density	Peripheral retina	Fovea

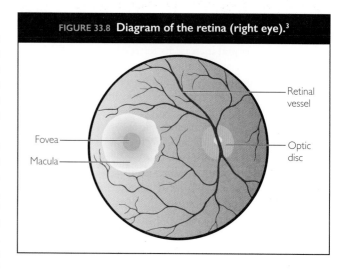

FIGURE 33.8 Diagram of the retina (right eye).[3]

Retinal vessel

Fovea

Macula

Optic disc

Photoreceptors contain visual pigments comprising retinol (vitamin A) linked to protein (opsin). Light absorption causes structural and then chemical change in visual pigments, which results in electrical hyperpolarisation of the photoreceptors.[3]

External to the neurosensory retina lies the RPE, a single layer of pigmented cells which is essential to the photoreceptor physiology. RPE cells recycle vitamin A for the formation of photopigments, transport water and metabolites, renew photoreceptors and help reduce damage by scattered light. Impairments of RPE function, which can occur with age and in many disease states, can lead to loss of retinal function and, therefore, sight.[3]

The principal blood supply of the retina is from the central retinal artery, a branch of the ophthalmic artery. The central retinal artery enters the retina at about the middle of the optic disc, an area where the optic nerve is attached and that contains no photoreceptor neurons (see Fig 33.8). After emerging through the disc, the central retina artery divides into superior and inferior branches, each of which subdivides into nasal and temporal branches. The central retinal vein drains blood from the retina through the optic disc.[8]

The blood–retinal barrier, consisting of tight junctions between the epithelial cells of the retinal vessels and between the RPE cells, isolates the retinal environment from the systemic circulation. Disruption of the barrier, as occurs in diabetic retinopathy, leads to retinal oedema and precipitation of lipid and protein, causing loss of retinal transparency and therefore loss of vision.[3]

Refraction errors

Refraction is the ability of the eye to bend light rays so that they fall on the retina. In the normal eye, parallel light rays are focused through the lens into a sharp image on the retina. This condition is termed emmetropia and means that light is focused exactly on the retina, not in front of it or behind it. When the light does not focus properly, it is called a *refractive error*.

- The individual with *myopia* can see near objects clearly (near-sightedness) but objects in the distance are blurred. A concave lens is used to correct the refraction (Fig 33.9).
- The individual with *hyperopia* can see distant objects clearly (far-sightedness) but close objects are blurred. A convex lens is used to correct the refraction (Fig 33.9).
- *Presbyopia* is a form of hyperopia, or far-sightedness, that occurs as a normal process of ageing, usually around 40 years. As the lens ages and becomes less elastic, it loses refractive power and the eye can no longer accommodate for near vision.[7]
- *Astigmatism* is caused by unevenness in the corneal or lenticular curvature, causing horizontal and vertical rays to be focused at two different points on the retina, resulting in visual distortion. It can be myopic or hyperopic in nature in relation to where the image falls.

Optic nerve

The ganglion cell axons in the retinal nerve fibre layer make a right-angled turn into the optic disc, which has no photoreceptors and corresponds to the physiological blind spot. Most optic discs have a central cavity, the optic cup, which is pale in comparison with the redness of the surrounding nerve fibres. Loss of nerve fibres as occurs in glaucoma, results in an increase in the volume of the cup.[3]

There are about 1,000,000 axons in the optic nerve. Behind the eyeball these axons become myelinated. Here the optic nerve is surrounded by cerebrospinal fluid in an anterior extension of the subarachnoid space and is protected by the same membranous layers as the brain.[3]

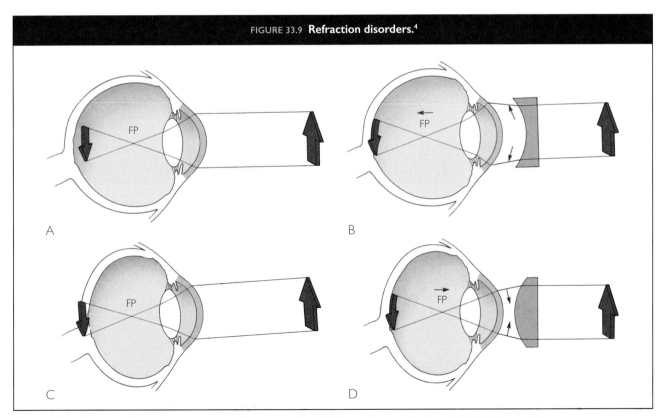

FIGURE 33.9 Refraction disorders.[4]

Abnormal and corrected refraction observed in myopia (**A** and **B**) and hyperopia (**C** and **D**).[4] *FP: focal point.*

FIGURE 33.10 The visual pathways.[4]

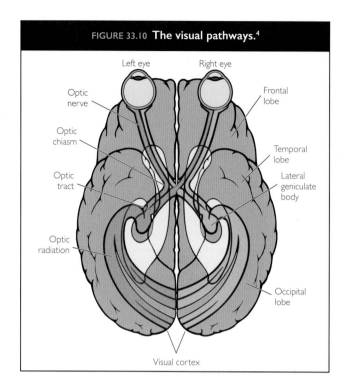

Left eye · Right eye · Optic nerve · Frontal lobe · Optic chiasm · Temporal lobe · Optic tract · Lateral geniculate body · Optic radiation · Occipital lobe · Visual cortex

Visual pathways

Once the image travels through the refractive media, it is focused on the retina, inverted and reversed left to right (Fig 33.10). From the retina, the impulses travel through the optic nerve to the optic chiasm where the nasal fibres of each eye cross over to the other side. Fibres from the left field of both eyes form the left optic tract and travel to the left occipital cortex. The fibres from the right field of both eyes form the right optic tract and travel to the right occipital cortex. This arrangement of the nerve fibres in the visual pathways allows determination of the anatomical location of abnormalities in those nerve fibres by interpretation of the specific visual field defect.[7]

Patient assessment

The vast majority of ocular injuries are minor and involve the anterior segment only. It is important, however, to bear in mind the possibility of a more major trauma and not to rule it out without a comprehensive examination. If it is assumed that the eye injury is likely to be minor, sight-threatening injuries may easily be missed.[9] Visual outcomes depend on timely management and accurate assessment. The clinician needs to recognise and manage ocular trauma effectively. Chapter 17, p. 375, contains information on some common eye emergencies and techniques on dealing with them.

The assessment of the patient with an ocular problem begins with triage and continues into the treatment area. A potential threat to vision should be triaged as emergency, triage code 2 (Ch 13), whereas a patient with a red eye and no potential loss of vision could be triaged as non-urgent if no other problems exist.

After a brief assessment to ensure that the airway, breathing and circulation (ABCs) are stable, the patient is evaluated to identify any threats to vision, for example, globe penetrating, blunt trauma, retinal artery occlusion, chemical burns and acute angle-closure glaucoma.

A focused assessment includes determination of precipitating events, duration of symptoms and identification of a worsening or improvement in signs and symptoms. Include information on the speed of onset of symptoms and when they were first noticed, and try to clarify some of the common symptoms; i.e. discriminate between soreness, irritation and stinging versus pain, itching, burning or the sensation of something in the eye, and the degree and type of any reduction in vision. Was the vision loss gradual or sudden, partial or total? Unilateral or bilateral?

A systematic approach should be used to examine the eye. Commence with lids, conjunctiva and cornea; then the anterior chamber should be examined for the presence of blood (hyphaema) or pus (hypopyon), and the pupil size, shape, position and reaction to light should be checked, as well as any photophobia and amount and type of discharge. The patient needs to be asked if there has been any previous history of eye problems or history and use of eye medication—prescribed or non-prescribed—and use of corrective lenses, past ocular surgery (including refractive) and disease such as diabetes. Document the assessment findings as per hospital policy. See Box 33.1.

The sudden presence of flashes, and explosion of floaters, web/veil like substance in field of vision suggests a retinal tear or detachment.

If the patient has a history of trauma, determine when the injury occurred and the mechanism, velocity and timing of injury. Ask whether the patient was wearing protective eyewear, glasses or contact lenses. Determine the patient's tetanus status. If the injury was a motor vehicle accident, did the airbag deploy? The alkaline powder in the airbag can cause floaters or symptoms of blunt trauma, and airbags can cause significant eye irritation.

Ophthalmic examination

The primary elements of the ocular examination are visual acuity, external features, anterior segment and extraocular motility (Box 33.1). Further examination includes a slit-lamp examination, intraocular pressure measurement and direct ophthalmoscopy.

Visual acuity

Assessment of visual acuity is the first priority and should be undertaken at triage before any other investigation or treatment (except eye irrigation) is carried out. It is impossible to allocate an accurate triage category to a patient with an ocular problem without assessment of visual acuity.[10]

It is essential to understand the principles behind vision testing and be able to perform an accurate visual acuity test. Visual acuity is a measurement of central vision only: it assesses the pathway from cornea through to occipital cortex. Vision can be tested for both near and distance, but distance is the most common test.[6,11]

Normal vision is normally defined as 6/6; it relies on the basis that both eyes are aligned (extraocular muscles functioning), cornea, lens, aqueous and vitreous humour are clear, the retina and other elements of the visual pathway are intact. The reasoning behind visual acuity is that it is one of the diagnostic tools that provides baseline data (similar to any baseline observations) and evaluates treatment while measuring the progress of any disease/condition. There may be legal implications after work-cover injuries, where a baseline vision is required.

There are numerous vision-testing tools. The Snellen chart is commonly used, and is designed to be read either at 6 or 3 metres (this is indicated on the chart). Vision charts are standardised for size and contrast and consequently are not to be photocopied or modified in any way (Fig 33.11).

Visual acuity is a measure of best-corrected distance vision. Patients should be tested with either their distance glasses on or contact lenses in. It is important to check that the glasses they are wearing were prescribed for that person, as well as being clean and scratch-free. Each eye needs to be tested separately; use an occluder or cupped hand to cover the eye which is not being tested. Avoid any pressure on the globe, especially if there is eye trauma. Ask patients to read the chart until they cannot see the line clearly and make multiple mistakes. Encourage the patient to blink, as the eye will dry and vision will blur as it dries. If the patient does not reach the 6/6 line, use a pinhole to see if it improves vision. A pinhole can be created by putting a hole in a small square of cardboard using a 19 g needle.

Visual acuity is expressed as a ratio x/y; x is the testing distance and y refers to the line containing the smallest letter the patient identifies. Record visual acuity for each eye and include vision of pinhole if used (Fig 33.12). Examples of recording of visual acuity are:

RVA (RIGHT VISUAL ACUITY)	LVA (LEFT VISUAL ACUITY)
6/9	6/6 with glasses
6/6 with pinhole	

- If the patient cannot see the top line of the Snellen chart at 6 metres, walk them forward to 3 metres—record 6/6 @ 3 metres.
- If they are still unable to read the chart, hold your hand 1 metre away and ask the patient to count how many fingers, keeping your fingers still—record CF (count fingers) @ 1 metre.

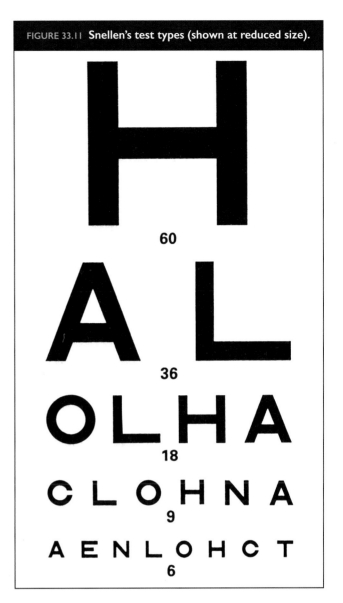

FIGURE 33.11 Snellen's test types (shown at reduced size).

- If they cannot see fingers, move your hand slowly across the eye—record HM (hand movements) @ 1 metre.
- If the patient cannot recognise hand movements, use a pen light to see if they have light perception (LP); record as NPL (no perception of light) if they are unable to see the torch going on and off.

PRACTICE TIP

VISUAL ACUITY

- Test each eye separately, using an occluder or cupped hand.
- Use distance correction if normally worn.
- Use a pinhole if the patient does not reach 6/6.

Visual field

Using a simple confrontational technique easily identifies large, dense defects of the visual field. It should be noted that this is a quick gross visual field test; the test assumes that the clinician's

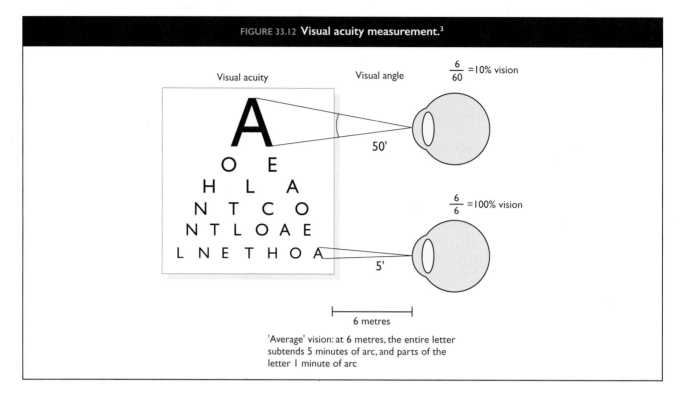

FIGURE 33.12 **Visual acuity measurement.**[3]

Visual acuity

Visual angle

$\frac{6}{60}$ =10% vision

50'

$\frac{6}{6}$ =100% vision

5'

6 metres

'Average' vision: at 6 metres, the entire letter subtends 5 minutes of arc, and parts of the letter 1 minute of arc

visual field is normal, and the patient's visual field is checked against the clinician's.

Patients should not wear glasses when having their visual field assessed. The clinician should be at the same level and 1 metre away from the patient, who covers one eye. Use a pen to test the four quadrants of the visual field. Do not bring the pen in at a vertical or horizontal position, as this will not be testing the visual field quadrants. Get the patient to look at a fixed point, such as the clinician's own eye, then slowly bring the pen in and ask the patient to say when they can see the pen tip. Repeat the test with the other eye. Document the findings.

Ocular motility

When examining ocular movement, the first step is to look for asymmetry of the corneal light reflex with a pen torch, followed by observation of the movement of the eyes as they move onto the key positions of gaze (see Fig 33.13). Impaired ocular motility may occur with an entrapped muscle secondary to a blow-out fracture, muscular injury, orbital cellulitis or underlying central nervous system problem.[1]

External features

A pen torch provides adequate illumination to examine the eyelids, conjunctiva and cornea for presence of a foreign body, discharge, loss of corneal clarity or corneal ulceration.

Fluorescein drops are a useful diagnostic aid. Fluorescein mixes into the tear film and adheres to areas of epithelial loss (ulcer or abrasion). It is best visualised using a blue light.

Inner eye

Use an ophthalmoscope or bright torch to test the pupils' reaction to light and the red reflex. Then examine the fundus (retina and optic disc) using an ophthalmoscope or a slit lamp with a 78- or 90-dioptre lens. For easier viewing, use mydriatic

eye drops to dilate the pupil, so that the fundus can be viewed effectively. At the initial assessment and before instilling dilating topical medications, the pupil should be assessed for a relative afferent pupillary defect (RAPD)—also known as the swing torch test. The test should be carried out in a dimly lit room, where the clinican can see both pupils at once. Standing slightly to the side, swing a bright light from below onto one eye and observe the response of both pupils. If normal, both pupils will constrict, meaning that there is a consensual pupil response. If there is a problem when light is shone into the affected eye, the damaged pathway will transmit less light effectively, as the occipital region senses less light entering the eye, and will cause both pupils to dilate slightly to let in more light. Document a positive RAPD.

If damage to optic nerve is 50%, then only 50% of the response will reach the Edinger-Westphal nucleus within the occipital region and only 50% return via the efferent pathway.[10]

Special investigations

The slit lamp

The slit lamp provides a highly magnified and stereoscopic view. This provides high-quality assessment, especially when assessing depth and extent of penetrating eye injury or corneal foreign body. The pen torch can assess the extent of an injury, but not the depth—this is better calculated using a slit lamp.

The basic apparatus enables only the anterior part of the eye, as far back as the lens, to be focused. A variety of supplemented lenses, both contact and non-contact, can be used to examine the inner eye (Fig 33.14).

Tonometry

Tonometry measures the intraocular pressure (IOP); normal pressures usually range from 10 to 21 mmHg. This can be performed with a device attached to the slit lamp (Goldman

FIGURE 33.13 **Visual field testing.**[3]

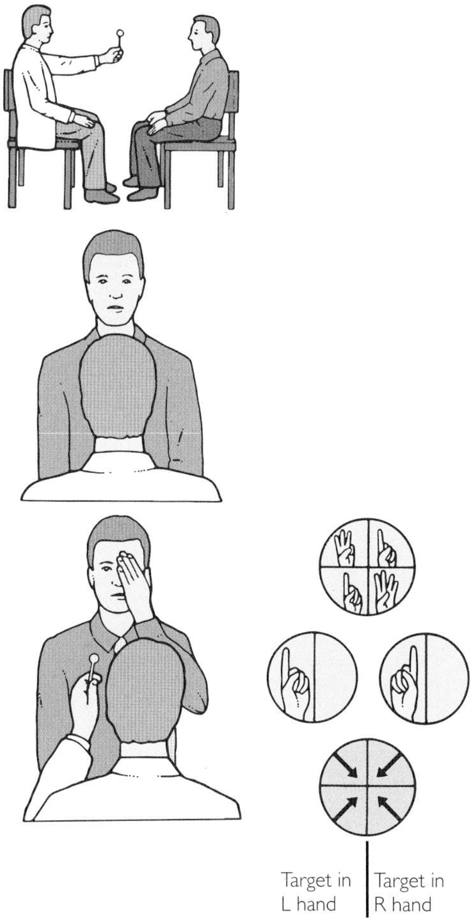

Principles
Sit at same level, faces 1 m apart.
Subject covers one eye with own hand of same side.
Compare your field with the subject's field:
– their R with your L
– their L with your R
Move target slowly, equidistant between the two of you

Steps
1. Both eyes open
   'Look at my nose. Is any part of my face missing?'
   Detects central scotoma, hemianopia

2. Each eye in turn
   a) Finger counting in quadrants
      'How many fingers do you see?'
      Detects hemianopias, quadrantanopias
   b) Compare R and L hemifields simultaneously with one finger
      'Which finger is most clear?'
      Detects less dense hemianopia
3. Each eye in turn
   Bring target in from periphery
   'Point when you first see the target'
   Detects quadrantanopias, altitudinal defects, even paracentral scotomas

Target in L hand | Target in R hand

applanation tonometry) or by using a handheld electronic gauge (Tonopen). Both require contact with the cornea; topical anaesthetic is required to perform this measurement. There are now newer devices available that measure the IOP but require no topical anaesthetic drops, i.e. ICare Tonometer.

> **PRACTICE TIP**
>
> If no device is available, ask the patient to close both eyes, and digitally touch both lids at the same time. If the intraocular pressure is very high (>30), the eye will feel really hard, like a rock/stone and urgent review by an ophthalmologist is required.

Eye emergencies

Injury or disease may cause ocular emergencies: situations encountered most often by the emergency nurse and the paramedic are discussed here (see also Ch 17, p. 375). There are four basic principles for both the nurse and the paramedic in the management of ocular trauma and other presenting ocular conditions; prevention of further injury, control of pain, control of nausea/vomiting and prevention of infection.

Red eye

A unilateral red eye has a high suspicion rate, as there is a higher incidence of more severe ocular condition (acute glaucoma, scleritis and penetrating (open) eye injury).

The ocular coat and tear film normally provides an excellent barrier to invasion of bacteria; however, if the conjunctiva or cornea is in some way compromised then bacteria may enter directly through these structures, causing a red appearance to the eye.

> **PRACTICE TIP**
>
> When a patient presents with a red eye and complains of severe ocular pain not relieved by medication (i.e. paracetamol/NSAID), this is a flag that increases triage weighting and urgency for review.

Subconjunctival haemorrhage

Subconjunctival haemorrhage is often an isolated symptom, unilateral, and caused by minor trauma such as a sneeze, anticoagulant therapy, cough or the Valsalva manoeuvre; however, it can be an indicator of a more serious intraocular and orbital trauma.[13] The haemorrhage occurs when small

FIGURE 33.14 **The slit lamp.**[12]

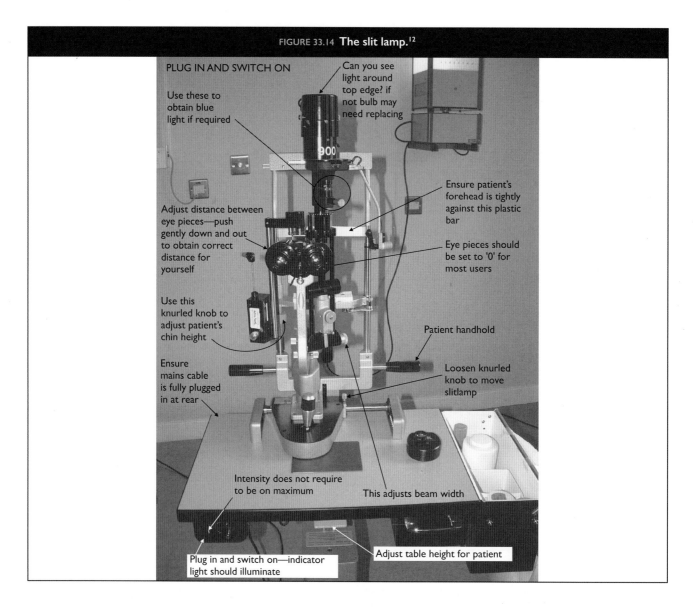

PLUG IN AND SWITCH ON

Can you see light around top edge? if not bulb may need replacing

Use these to obtain blue light if required

Ensure patient's forehead is tightly against this plastic bar

Adjust distance between eye pieces—push gently down and out to obtain correct distance for yourself

Eye pieces should be set to '0' for most users

Use this knurled knob to adjust patient's chin height

Patient handhold

Ensure mains cable is fully plugged in at rear

Loosen knurled knob to move slitlamp

Intensity does not require to be on maximum

This adjusts beam width

Plug in and switch on—indicator light should illuminate

Adjust table height for patient

blood vessels rupture and bleed, and it is painless (Fig 33.15). Check visual acuity; if reduced, suspect trauma. The typical presentation for trauma is that the haemorrhage spreads backwards, shows depth and has no clear borders. Blood pressure should also be assessed as a hypertensive patient can have spontaneous rupture of vessels.

Subconjunctival haemorrhage will spontaneously resolve within 2–4 weeks and the patient's visual acuity generally remains normal. Should healing be delayed, it is wise to check the patient's coagulation profile. There is rarely need for treatment, but in extreme cases of conjunctival drying, ocular ointments may be helpful in maintaining intact conjunctiva.[13,14]

PRACTICE TIP

History of the patient is important, assessing if patient is hypertensive, on anticoagulants or has experienced recent eye trauma. Management by the general practitioner may be the more appropriate treatment option if hypertensive or a review of anticoagulant therapy is required.

Conjunctivitis

Be aware of the diagnosis of unilateral conjunctivitis until all other more serious eye conditions are excluded.[16] Conjunctivitis

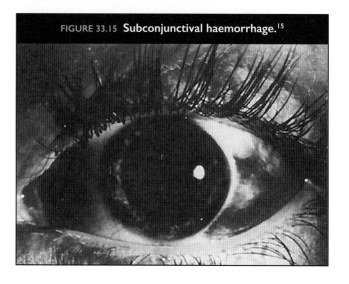

FIGURE 33.15 **Subconjunctival haemorrhage.**[15]

is a common irritation or infection of the eye due to bacteria, viruses, chemicals or allergies.[17–19]

Discharge normally appears as a relatively clear mucous membrane on the surface of the eye and, if present, can cause the eyelids to stick together in the morning.[17] Multiple aetiological factors can cause swelling (chemosis) or dilation of the blood vessels in the conjunctiva (injection).[3,20] Repeated conjunctiva infections over a number of years causes conjunctival scarring and shortening of the upper eyelid, with the lashes turning inwards and rubbing the cornea, leading to corneal abrasion, ulcers or abscesses.[17]

Not all conjunctivitis is infectious: an accurate history and assessment will identify the cases that require appropriate precautions to prevent spread (Table 33.2). Differential diagnosis includes other, more serious, forms of 'red eye', such as keratitis, uveitis, scleritis and acute angle-closure glaucoma; typically these will see a reduced visual acuity and a painful red eye. During patient assessment it is important to check for abnormalities such as injury, foreign bodies, ulceration and cellulitis and refer as appropriate (Table 33.3).

- *Allergic conjunctivitis* typically presents with an itchy, watery eye; everting the eyelid, view the conjunctival fornices which will show papillary lesions. Treatment involves identifying and eliminating the allergic agent (if possible), cool compresses and lubricating drops without preservatives; frequently this is a self-limiting condition. Children presenting with repeated episodes of allergic conjunctivitis should be referred to a paediatric ophthalmologist for further investigation.

- *Viral conjunctivitis* accounts for the majority of 'pink eye' and frequently occurs and is concurrent with viral upper respiratory tract infection, and is very contagious. Presentation may involve red, watery eyes with a gritty feeling; it may begin in one eye and spread to the other within 2 days. Symptoms often get worse within 10 days. Both eyes are diffusely red, watery discharge can occur and visual acuity is normal. Viral conjunctivitis is frequently a self-limiting condition lasting about 10 days; treatment includes cold eye packs and lubricant drops.

A particularly contagious viral conjunctivitis— *epidemic keratoconjunctivitis*—causes greater pain and redness, often with photophobia and eventual bilateral involvement. In contrast to other types of viral conjunctivitis, keratoconjunctivitis can last 3 weeks; treatment is supportive (Table 33.4).

TABLE 33.2 Comparison of types of conjunctivitis

	BACTERIAL	VIRAL (ADENOVIRAL IS COMMON)	ALLERGY
Signs	Pus-filled discharge can been seen and oedema of conjunctiva (chemosis). **Note:** in gonococcus conjunctivitis (gonorrhoea) there is a sudden onset of 12–24 hours	There is a watery mucous discharge and the eye is red with swelling of the eyelid. Involvement of the conjunctiva follicles may occur	The eye lids will be red and swollen with oedema of conjunctiva (chemosis)
Symptoms	Eye will be superficially sore and show redness, with the sensation of a foreign body present. Itching is minimal	Eye will have a sensation of a foreign body, including itching and burning. Usually starts in one eye and cross-contaminates to other eye within 2 days. There is often an association with recent upper respiratory tract infection	Eye will be itchy with a watery discharge; there will be a history of allergies
Treatment	Swab first, clean the eye, especially the lid, and administer antibiotics. **Note:** extremely important for PPE and hand-washing due to being highly contagious	Cool compress and lubricants can reduce symptoms, antibiotics may be required. **Note:** extremely important for PPE and hand-washing due to being highly contagious	Cool compress and lubricants without preservatives can reduce symptoms. If the irritant is known this must be avoided

TABLE 33.3 Differential diagnoses of eye conditions

	CONJUNCTIVITIS	IRITIS	ACUTE GLAUCOMA	KERATITIS (FOREIGN-BODY ABRASION)
Discharge	Marked	None	None	Slight or none
Photophobia	None	Marked	Slight	Slight
Pain	None	Slight to marked	Marked	Marked
Visual acuity	Normal	Reduced	Reduced	Varies with site of the lesion
Pupil	Normal	Smaller or same	Large, oval and fixed	Same or smaller

- *Bacterial infection* may involve red eyes with a gritty feeling; it may begin in one eye and spread to the other, and presents as uniformly red because of widespread engorgement of the conjunctival vessels. Visual acuity is normal and purulent discharge can occur of varying colours (grey, yellow and green) and amounts. There is minimal to no pain or preauricular adenopathy.

Antibiotic eye drops or ointment is the treatment of choice for bacterial infections (Table 33.4). Eyes should be swabbed for culture and sensitivity in high-risk populations, recurrent episodes and infants. The organism *Chlamydia trachomatis* causes repeated attacks of conjunctivitis in children, often transmitted from person to person, for example, by fingers, household cloths or by flies.[16] Large amounts of pus can indicate *Neisseria*

gonorrhoea. If present, urgent treatment to prevent corneal ulceration, corneal melting is required and consists of intramuscular ceftriaxone plus frequent eye irrigation with saline. Topical antibiotics such as erythromycin ointment should also be prescribed. Referral to an outpatient ophthalmology service and sexual health service is required if the patient is photophobic or has reduced visual acuity or persistence of symptoms.[22]

The emergency nurse should provide education, instructing the patient about hygiene—frequent washing of hands and not rubbing/touching eyes, non-sharing of towels, pillows or make-up to prevent cross-contamination. Ensure that patients and parents understand eye care and medication instructions prior to discharge and advise them to return if the patient develops pain or increased irritation.[17]

TABLE 33.4 Summary of drugs commonly used in ophthalmology[4]				
	EXAMPLES IN COMMON USE	MODE OF ADMINISTRATION	ACTION	SIDE EFFECTS
Glaucoma treatment (note that different types of glaucoma may require different therapeutic approaches)	Beta-blockers; timolol, betaxolol, levobunolol	Topical	Reduce aqueous secretion by inhibitory action on beta-adrenoceptors in the ciliary body	Ocular: irritation Systemic: bronchospasm, bradycardia, exacerbation of heartblock with verapamil, nightmares
	Muscarinic (parasympathetic) stimulants: pilocarpine	Topical	Increase aqueous outflow via trabecular meshwork by ciliary muscle contraction	Ocular: miosis (reduced vision in presence of cataract, retinal examination impaired), spasm of accommodation, brow ache Systemic: sweating, bradycardia, gastrointestinal disturbance Long term use leads to poor pupil dilation
	Alpha$_2$-stimulants: brimonidine, apraclonidine	Topical	Reduce aqueous secretion by selective stimulation of alpha$_2$-receptors and adrenoceptors in the ciliary body increase outflow by uveoscleral route	Ocular: allergy, mydriasis, eyelid retraction Systemic: dry mouth, hypotension, drowsiness, headache
	Prostaglandin derivatives: latanoprost, travoprost, bimatoprost	Topical	Increase aqueous outflow by the uveoscleral route	Ocular: iris darkening, conjunctival hyperaemia, eyelash growth
	Carbonic anhydrase inhibitors	Systemic (acetazolamide), topical (dorzolamide, brinzolamide)	Reduce aqueous secretion by the ciliary body	Ocular route: irritation, allergy Systemic (generally systemic use): malaise, paraesthesia, urea and electrolyte disturbance, aplastic anaemia

TABLE 33.4 Summary of drugs commonly used in ophthalmology[4]—cont'd

	EXAMPLES IN COMMON USE	MODE OF ADMINISTRATION	ACTION	SIDE EFFECTS
Mydriatics and cycloplegics (for retinal examination and objective refraction (retinoscopy)	Antimuscarinics: tropicamide, cyclopentolate, homatropine, atropine	Topical	Inhibit muscarinic receptors of parasympathetic nervous system to paralyse pupillary sphincter and ciliary muscle	Ocular: blurred vision (especially for near), glare, angle-closure glaucoma Systemic: tachycardia, dry mouth, confusion, tremor
	Alpha-stimulant: phenylephrine	Topical	Stimulate dilator muscle of the pupil; no cycloplegic effect	Ocular: blurred vision, glare, angle-closure glaucoma, conjunctival blanching Systemic: hypertension (with use of 10%)
Lubricants A range of preparations is available for the treatment of dry eyes	Carbomers, hypromellose, polyvinyl alcohol, liquid paraffin	Topical	Exact mechanism depends on agent	Ocular: preservative allergy/toxicity, blurred vision (especially ointments)
Anti-inflammatory agents Most important drugs in this category are corticosteroids; a variety of other agents is available, including systemic immunosuppressants	Corticosteroids: prednisolone, betamethasone, dexamethasone	Topical, periocular injection, systemic	Suppression of broad spectrum of inflammatory processes	Ocular: glaucoma (especially with local administration), cataract (especially prolonged systemic use), exacerbation of some infections e.g. herpes simplex Systemic: negligible with topical use; common and varied with systemic administration
	Mast-cell stabilisers (cromoglycate, nedocromil, lodoxamide)	Topical	Stabilise mast cells	Ocular: irritation
	Antihistamines	Topical (antazoline, azelastine, levocabastine), systemic (chlorphenamine, fexofenadine, cetirizine)	Block histamine receptor (azelastine also stabilises mast cells)	Ocular route: irritation Systemic route: drowsiness
	Non-steroidal anti-inflammatory drugs: systemic help to control ocular pain and inflammation; topical increasingly used for pain of corneal abrasion, for inflammation after cataract surgery and to maintain pupil dilation during cataract surgery	Topical (ketorolac, diclofenac, flurbiprofen)	Modulate prostaglandin production	Systemic: peptic ulceration, asthma

Continued

TABLE 33.4 Summary of drugs commonly used in ophthalmology[4]—cont'd

	EXAMPLES IN COMMON USE	MODE OF ADMINISTRATION	ACTION	SIDE EFFECTS
Anti-infective agents Topically applied antibacterial and antiviral drugs are very commonly prescribed; the use of antifungal and antiparasitic agents is much less frequent	Antibacterials: chloramphenicol, gentamicin, ciprofloxacin, neomycin, fusidic acid	Topical, occasionally intra-ocular, systemic	Range of activities and specificities	Vary with agent Ocular: allergy; corneal toxicity common with intensive use Systemic: generally only with systemic use
	Antivirals: aciclovir	Topical, systemic, intravitreal	Inhibit herpes virus DNA synthesis	Ocular: blurred vision, corneal toxicity Systemic: rashes; kidney, liver and other effects may occur with systemic use
Local anaesthetics Major uses are to relieve pain and thereby assist with clinical examination, and the facilitation of surgical anaesthesia	Oxybuprocaine, proxymetacaine, tetracaine, lignocaine	Topical, periocular injection	Block conduction along nerve fibres	Ocular: irritation, corneal toxicity Systemic: generally accidental intravascular or intrathecal (cerebrospinal fluid) injection during surgical anaesthesia: cardiac dysrhythmias, respiratory depression
Botulinum toxin: used in the management of certain ocular motility disorders and blepharospasm, and to induce ptosis for corneal protection		Injection at site of action	Prevent release of the neurotransmitter acetylcholine at neuromuscular junctions	Dependent on treatment site: e.g. unwanted ptosis or double vision

Uveitis and iritis

Uveitis is inflammation in the iris, ciliary body and choroid of the eye. Most commonly, anterior uveitis is seen, and this is known as iritis. This disorder may result from trauma, infections and autoimmune causes. Symptoms may include reduced vision, deep orbital aching, photophobia and redness. Synechiae (adhesions of the iris) may also be seen; dilating drops or heat should break this adhesion. Slit-lamp examination (slit lamp on maximum magnification) will identify flare and cells in the anterior chamber with suspended proteins causing fogginess of the slit-lamp beam.

Treatment consists of topical steroids and mydriatrics/cycloplegics (Table 33.5); steroids should only be prescribed under the direction of an ophthalmologist. The patient should be referred to an ophthalmologist outpatient service as soon as possible if in an acute phase.[22]

Trauma

Epidemiology of ocular trauma

The workplace accounts for the majority of eye injuries, followed by the home. In Australia, the rate of hospital admissions as a result of work-related injury with eye trauma as the primary diagnosis is 3% of total admissions.[23] Eye injuries are a major cause of lost working days in Australia and New Zealand, particularly in areas of production such as manufacturing plants, construction sites, factories/warehouses, mines and farms in Australia. In New Zealand during 2013 the agriculture and fishery workers (25% of all claims) accounted for the highest number of work-related claims. Males (15–64 years of age) incur the majority of eye injuries, especially boilermakers/welders, metal fitters and machinists, carpenters and plumbers. The majority of non-occupational eye injuries occur at home, predominantly in the garden or garage.[23–26] In Australia, men living in rural areas are the most likely to experience eye injury.[27,28]

The injury profile for New Zealand (2013) is similar to Australia, with overall rates showing that males aged 15–24 represent the highest group.[29] Pacific Islanders are the most likely group to be injured or report an injury, followed by Māori, European, then Asian. Over 4000 cases of eye injuries are reported yearly.[30]

Most eye injuries in industry are as a result of the eye being hit by moving parts. In New Zealand 5% of all work-related

TABLE 33.5 Nursing intervention for ocular trauma	

All patients should leave the ED having had their visual acuity checked. For some patients (corneal abrasion), topical anaesthetic may be required before checking vision.

INJURY	NURSING MANAGEMENT
Subconjunctival haemorrhage Vitreous haemorrhage	Check blood pressure Slit-lamp assessment to assess if PEI
Hyphaema Ruptured globe Scleral rupture	Pain management Head up 45° or more Movement restriction depending on grade of hyphaema Protect eye with eye shield or modified plastic cup Antiemetics Aperients Caution with the use of antithrombolytics Educate patient about avoiding activities that cause an increase in intraocular pressure: – open mouth sneezing – straining during bowel elimination – bending over – lifting heavy objects Encourage deep breathing without persistent coughing
Iris trauma Lens trauma	Pain management Eye toilet Sunglasses to reduce glare
Lacerations, abrasions	Eye toilet—irrigate wound, remove any obvious debris If full-thickness laceration suspect PEI Head up 30° Corneal abrasion—instil local anaesthetic Apply ice/cold packs Chloramphenicol eye ointment may be ordered Eye pad only if strictly necessary due to risk of further corneal disruption
Laceration to nasolacrimal system	As above
Foreign bodies	Topical anaesthetic Remove foreign body Double-pad eye if large epithelial defect, only pad if necessary due to risk of further corneal abrasion Eye toilet if required

PEI: penetrating eye injury

injuries are caused by foreign bodies and 21% are lacerations (including eyelid).[29] Tasks with the highest risk of eye injuries are grinding, welding and hammering. Other high-risk activities include cutting, drilling, spraying, smelting, sanding, chipping and chiselling.[25]

High-velocity ball and contact sports, such as squash, golf or football, also account for a proportion of eye injuries and can result in permanent loss of visual acuity.[31] Behaviour modification and addressing attitudes towards wearing eye protection in some sports is occurring.[32] Less-frequent causes include farming incidents,[23,33] self-infliction,[34] stings[35] and animal-related injuries such as falling off and being rolled on by a horse, which has resulted in several incidences of significant permanent loss of vision.[36]

Although injuries from airbag deployment do occur, in the vast majority of cases they protect rather than harm. The likelihood of sustaining an ocular injury increases significantly in cars in which the airbag did not deploy.[37–39]

Despite wearing approved and recommended eye protection and using screens, splatter burns from hot, moving particles and injury from flying metal particles continue to occur in the industrialised workplace and at home. This is partially because many models of approved protective eyewear, such as wide-vision spectacles, have gaps or fit poorly to the individual's face shape. Australian Standard/New Zealand Standard 1336:1997 states: 'wherever practicable, eye protectors should be fitted to the wearer by a person who is competent to select the correct size and type'.[25] Injuries have occurred where the gap was as small as 5 mm and as large as 20 mm.[40] Research is continuing into improving design standards, and several eye injury prevention programs are in place.

Initial assessment and management

The pre-hospital, initial or first-aid management of ocular trauma is very limited and is presented in Box 33.2. The most important aspect is protection (Fig 33.16). What is vital is at the initial assessment, whether done by an emergency nurse or paramedic, an accurate history is documented, as it provides clues to what to be identified in an examination. If the eye patient is assessed inaccurately as a low priority it may lead to long-term effects, such as a major disability of vision impairment which can also affect employment prospects.

PRACTICE TIP

- Airway and circulatory support take priority in patients with multiple injuries, but penetrating/perforated eye injuries or a globe rupture and preservation of sight warrant priority over conditions which are non-life threatening.
- If the patient has a suspected penetrating eye injury or ruptured globe do not instil any topical medications, as they are not compatible with ocular contents. If topical medications need to be used, e.g. fluorescein, to assess if there is a wound leak, use only single-use, preservative-free eye drops.
- When transporting patients, try to reduce conditions that induce vomiting; recline the patient to 10–20° angle,

reduce eye movements and get the patient to close their eyes. If a hyphaema is present, patients should sit at a 45° angle to avoid corneal staining.
- Hypoxia will worsen an eye injury as the retina has a high oxygen demand. To avoid pressure on the globe cut the top off the oxygen facemask.[21]

Clinicians should be aware there are two different classifications of eye trauma. The first is the Ocular Trauma Classification, where injuries are classified into open and closed globe injury. An open globe injury is defined as a full thickness injury of the cornea and/or the sclera, while a closed globe injury presents as a contusion injury or lamellar (partial) laceration. Open globe injuries are further categorised into penetrating injury, ruptured globe, perforated injury and injury with retained intraocular foreign body (IOFB).

The second classification is the Birmingham Eye Trauma Terminology System (BETTS), where closed globe injuries include: cornea/sclera not totally perforated through contusions from blunt trauma and partial lamellar (partial) thickness wounds in cornea/sclera. An open globe injury is defined as a full thickness wound of the globe, ruptured globe, lacerations from sharp objects, penetrating and perforating injuries with a presence of an entrance wound and IOFBs.[43]

Eye assessment should occur as part of the secondary survey. Ocular injury often occurs in conjunction with head and facial trauma (see Ch 46); thus, the patient should be carefully evaluated for an associated eye injury.[44] Eye assessment should not be withheld when periorbital oedema is present or the patient is comatose, uncooperative or combative, and it must be remembered that the extra-ocular appearance can be normal. Caution should be used when trying to open an eye with periorbital oedema when there is a history of severe trauma, as ocular contents may extrude if pressure is placed on the globe. Obtain a history and assess the patient, as previously discussed.

Check for contact lenses in the unconscious patient and remove them as soon as possible. As a result of trauma, contact lenses often become dislodged from the cornea and can be found in the superior or inferior ocular cul-de-sacs.[13] If no penetrating eye injury is present, topical fluorescein can be used to identify the contact lens position; the upper lid will need to be everted to access if contact lens is present.

Specific assessment and management for ocular injury as a result of blasts is discussed in depth in Chapter 51.

Orbital blow-out fracture

The orbital contents may be forced through the orbital floor and into the maxillary sinus; this is known as a 'blow-out' fracture and is a common presentation to EDs. The medial aspect and orbital floor are common sites for fractures. The patient's history often includes recent blunt trauma. Patients may present with pain, especially with eye movements, diplopia (double vision), eyelid swelling and crepitus after blowing their nose. Vision may be reduced secondary to having a corneal abrasion, and there may be intraocular bleeding (hyphaema), retinal bruising or detachment.

The aim of pre-hospital management is to prevent further damage or assess level of ocular damage; initial action should

---

BOX 33.2 Pre-hospital management of ocular trauma[41]

- Control haemorrhage around the eye or eyelids with direct pressure, but **no direct pressure** should be exerted on the eyeball itself.
- Ice packs may be used to reduce swelling, if no evidence or history of penetrating eye injury or lid lacerations.
- Protect the eye from pressure or rubbing with a shield or a modified polystyrene cup taped in place. The non-injured eye should not be padded as this causes needless disorientation to the patient.
- Do not remove protruding or embedded bodies.
- Do not replace an extruded eyeball. Support with a saline-moistened sterile dressing lightly taped in position.
- Do not apply any pressure to penetrating injuries and situations with extrusion of ocular contents.
- Chemical burns—clean face and hands, irrigate during transfer if able.
- Administer pain management.
- An antiemetic is usually administered and the patient kept in a sitting position if possible. Promethazine is the preferred agent for children 2–12 years and in adult patients sensitive to metoclopramide.

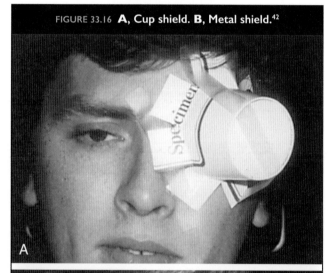

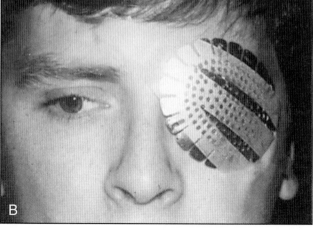

FIGURE 33.16 **A, Cup shield. B, Metal shield.**[42]

be to inspect the eye area if possible. Do not try to open the eyelid if swollen shut, as ocular contents may be lost if there is a ruptured globe. If the eye is visible, check ocular movements and observe for signs of a trapped muscle or nerve.

Icepacks can be used to reduce swelling, but only if there is no evidence of a ruptured globe or a penetrating eye injury. Instruct patients not to sneeze or blow their nose.

Clinical features

These may include restricted eye movements, especially on upwards or lateral gaze, or both; subconjunctival haemorrhage; hyperaesthesia due to a trapped infraorbital nerve—affects cheeks and upper lip; enophthalmos (displacement of the globe backwards through the orbital fracture)—this can be masked by lid swelling.

Differential diagnoses that should be excluded are orbital oedema/haemorrhage without fracture, and cranial nerve palsy.

Assessment and management

Assess extraocular muscle movement—ask the patient to look in all positions of gaze; compare both eyes looking for globe displacement. Primarily ask the patient to look up, down, left and right. To assess if there is nerve involvement, compare sensations between cheeks, top lip and front tooth. Palpate eyelids for crepitus (subconjunctival emphysema); educate patients not to blow their nose to avoid this from occurring.[3,10]

Evaluate globe patency—if no evidence of rupture, use a slit lamp to check for a hyphaema, traumatic iritis and retinal or choroidal damage. Further tests include an IOP check, testing for a relative afferent pupillary defect (RAPD). RAPD testing is a reliable way to implicate or rule out optic nerve disease. The usual response of healthy pupils to direct light is that both pupils contract equally and if the light is moved quickly from one eye to the other both pupils hold their level of contraction; if the light is moved too slowly (so that neither eye is 'dazzled'), the initial response from the first pupil is lost and both pupils dilate somewhat. With RAPD, shining the light in the good eye will cause both pupils to constrict; when the light is moved quickly to the bad eye *both* pupils will dilate. This is because a damaged optic nerve transmits light to a lesser degree, and more slowly than a healthy one; as a result, when the light is moved from the good to the bad eye, the brain interprets this as a decrease in the amount of light being shone. Colour vision testing will be performed in the ophthalmic clinic to rule out traumatic optic neuropathy.

A computed tomography (CT) scan is recommended, especially if extraocular muscles are restricted, or periorbital oedema makes assessment of the eye patency difficult.

Treatment involves ice packs to reduce swelling for 24–48 hours to enable the clinician to view the eye, and nasal decongestants for 3 days. Broad-spectrum antibiotics should be prescribed for several days as a prophylaxis against periorbital cellulitis. A surgical repair is recommended within 24 hours if the CT shows a trapped muscle or enophthalmos. Other signs may also include diplopia, non-resolving bradycardia, heart block or nausea and vomiting. A neurological consultation is recommended if the orbital roof is fractured, as there is risk of intracranial haemorrhage.

Follow-up in an ophthalmic unit is 1–2 weeks after trauma, to evaluate whether there is persistent diplopia and

enophthalmos after orbital oedema has reduced. Monitor also for secondary ocular trauma and advise patients accordingly for symptoms of orbital cellulitis and angle recession glaucoma (will present with high IOP). The patient should also be advised of the potential for retinal detachment, in which the retina peels away from its underlying layer of support tissue. Advise the patient to seek urgent medical attention if any of the following symptoms develop in the injured eye: very brief flashes of light in the extreme peripheral part of vision, a sudden and dramatic increase in floaters, a ring of floaters or hairs just to the temporal side of the central vision, a slight feeling of heaviness in the eye, a dense shadow starting in the peripheries and slowly moving to central vision, a sense of a veil or curtain being drawn over vision, straight lines that suddenly appear curved (positive Amsler grid test) or loss of central vision.

Airbag injuries

It is believed that airbag eye injury is caused by the impact of the airbag creating a shock wave through the globe and orbit, which reflects off the rear of the orbit and produces a refraction wave that tears blood vessels and nerves as it passes back towards the front of the eye.[45] The types of injuries sustained include contusion, abrasions, lacerations, retinal tears and detachments, hyphaema, haemorrhage, thermal burns (rare) and blindness. In addition, rapid deceleration due to an impact causes the ignition of a cartridge of sodium azide (an alkaline powder) which releases nitrogen gas to inflate the nylon bag, resulting in a risk of corneal–conjunctive–palpebral alkaline burns.

It must be noted that even at low speeds, airbags can deploy and cause injury and an index of suspicion should be maintained if the pre-hospital report states that the airbag was deployed. Three factors affect the severity of airbag injury:

- wearing glasses
- position and size of the driver/passenger (especially if a child)
- inflation force of the airbag.

After facial trauma from an airbag, an ophthalmological examination is necessary to assess any chemical burns of tissues exposed to the sodium azide and possible major ocular lesions.[46] Even though the majority of airbag lesions are minor and do not require hospitalisation, correct diagnosis and the choice of the most suitable treatment are necessary.[47]

Corneal foreign bodies

Working with power tools, hammering or chiselling metal, explosions and gardening are common causes of corneal foreign body (Fig 33.17).

The patient may complain of the sensation of a foreign body, mild irritation/pain and/or mild redness of eye. The use of fluorescein staining and anaesthetic drops can aid in the examination of the eye. Visual acuity is not affected unless the foreign body is lodged at the centre of the cornea. Subtarsal (evert the lid to view) or corneal foreign bodies can be removed with a moistened cotton bud after topical anaesthetic is instilled, using either a slit lamp or a pen torch, approaching the patient from the temporal aspect of the eye. Irrigation could also be tried to dislodge a foreign body.[48] As a precaution against fungal growth, patching should be avoided if the abrasive agent

FIGURE 33.17

FIGURE 33.17

Corneal foreign body.[12]

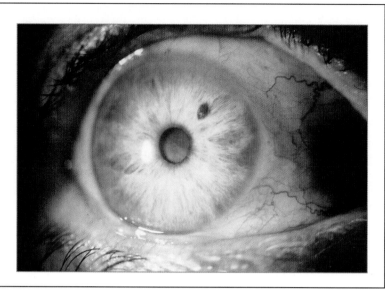

was a vegetative substance.[13] If the corneal foreign body cannot be removed within 24 hours, the patient should be referred to an ophthalmologist. If the foreign body is central and deep, do not try to remove unless assessed by a skilled clinician, due to the risk of perforation and corneal scarring. If an intraocular foreign body is suspected, the patient should be referred to an ophthalmologist immediately. Only skilled clinicians should use a 25-gauge needle to remove any foreign body.

Corneal rusting can occur as a complication following a metallic foreign body in the eye and may be loosened by the application of antibiotic ointment and padding for 24 hours, after which it is easily shelled out with the edge of a fine hypodermic needle. Use of a mechanical dental burr can result in large areas of epithelium removal.[1,13] Inflammation or ulceration can also occur as a complication. Short-acting cycloplegic eye drops (cyclopentolate 1% or homatropine 2%) can be used for pain relief, and antibiotic drops or ointments are essential if the corneal epithelium has been disrupted. Patients need daily review until any ulceration is completely healed.

Corneal abrasion

Corneal abrasions can be caused by a foreign body, explosion, traumatic facial nerve damage (poor blink reflex), airbag deployment, fingernails, inadequate tear film, prolonged wearing of contact lenses, abnormal eyelid position (entropion, ectropion) and abnormal eyelashes (trichiasis) (Fig 33.18). The patient may have a painful eye, photophobia, eye watering, blepharospasm (involuntary spasm of eyelid) and may be unable to open the eye for examination.

If the patient can open the eye, record visual acuity; instil local anaesthesia if necessary before trying to obtain a visual acuity. Treatment is the same as for corneal foreign bodies. Most corneal abrasions will heal within 24–48 hours and contact lenses can be worn 2 or 3 days after the abrasion has healed. Recurrence can occur at any time; repeated recurrent erosions should be referred to an ophthalmic outpatient department.

Hyphaema

Hyphaema is blood in the anterior chamber of the eye (Fig 33.19). It is caused by external compression, and secondary expansion of the angle with tearing of the iris root, ciliary body or pupillary margin causing blood to leak into the aqueous fluid of the anterior chamber.[50] Concurrent injuries are common, as a hyphaema is the result of severe ocular trauma. All hyphaemas need ophthalmology review.

Hyphaema is graded as follows:

- grade 1: blood level < 1/3
- grade 2: blood level > 1/3 but < 2/3
- grade 3: blood level > 2/3 but < total
- grade 4: blood level fills up the anterior chamber totally.

Visual acuity may be greatly reduced and there may be a deep aching pain, reduced vision, photophobia and a red inflamed eye. Periorbital haematoma may be present.

Initial management should be to restrict the patient's movement; have them lie down at 45 degrees and place a protective eye shield over the eye until transported to hospital.

Management of grade 1 hyphaemas can be at home if the patient is cooperative and able to return for regular check-ups. In general, all patients with hyphaema need to be examined daily for the first week to monitor intraocular pressure, corneal staining and to watch for re-bleeding. Re-bleeding, if it is going to occur, usually does so within 3–5 days of the initial injury, and can cause additional pathology.[13] Because of the risk of re-bleeding for high-grade hyphaema, strict bed rest is required for up to 5 days with elevation of bed head, 30–45° initially. An eye shield is used, not a patch. Fundal checks are required to ensure the retina is not detached or bruised. The management is variable and controversial, particularly to activity, which ranges from quiet activity to strict bed rest.[14]

Pharmacological management includes:

- topical steroids to reduce inflammation
- mydriatic—to stop ciliary spasm and to avoid accommodation
- IOP management—topical alpha$_2$-agonists, oral carbonic anhydrase inhibitor
- analgesia.

Medication, either topical or oral, can also be given to control intraocular pressure and to dilate the pupil to rest the iris and

FIGURE 33.18 **Corneal abrasion without (A, B) and with (C) fluorescein staining.**[12]

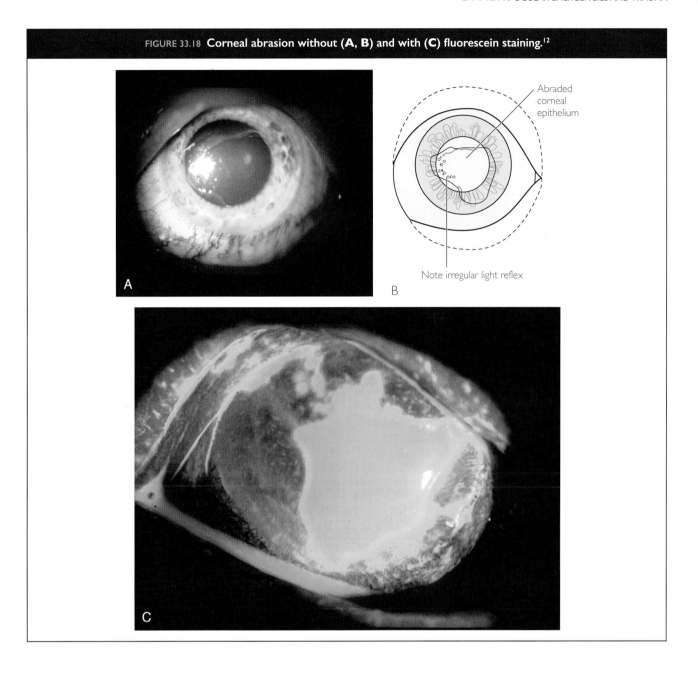

FIGURE 33.19 **Traumatic hyphaema.**[49]

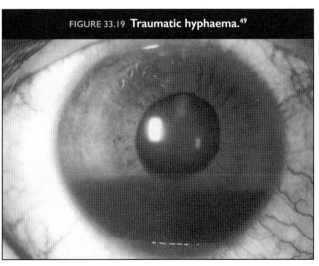

to prevent secondary bleeding. Antiemetics and aperients can also be used to prevent straining. Indications for surgery include raised intraocular pressure, unresolved clot or corneal bloodstaining. Anticoagulant therapy, salicylates and non-steroidal anti-inflammatory drugs (NSAIDs) should be avoided until reviewed by ophthalmology. Complications include the risk of re-bleeding, particularly 3–5 days after the injury, but may occur up to 14 days after the initial injury; increased intraocular pressure or corneal blood staining; and secondary glaucoma can occur acutely or months to years later.[50]

Globe injury

Severe closed globe injury involving the posterior segment may lead to permanent visual impairment and blindness through its effect on the lens, vitreous humour and retina.[51]

Initial management for any globe injury is to protect the eye and prevent further injury and vision loss. Protect the eye with a clear plastic shield if available; if not, cut down a polystyrene cup and secure. No pressure should be applied to the globe at any time. If there is bleeding around the site, irrigate with Normal saline to assess the extent of the damage. If there is an obvious penetrating injury or ruptured globe (open globe injury), or a trauma history with a high suspicion of injury, cover the eye with a shield and provide pain management. If possible, transport the patient to the nearest hospital that has eye services.

Iris and lens trauma

Tears or holes may occur with trauma to the iris, which can result in pupillary irregularities and traumatic dilation. Blunt, non-perforating ocular trauma often results in acute iritis, an inflammatory reaction involving the iris and ciliary body. Symptoms include photophobia, tearing, pain; severe inflammation will cause an IOP increase and a decrease in vision. Treatment is topical cycloplegic drops plus a topical corticosteroid, unless there is an epithelial defect until healed; steroids generally will delay healing.[13,50]

Because of the crystalline nature of the lens, cataracts may develop rapidly or over weeks to months following trauma, and cause severe visual obscuration if the opacity is within the visual pathway.[52] Lens replacement may be needed if sight is limited. If severe inflammation is associated with ocular injury, adhesions between the iris and the lens may develop. The lens may subluxate/dislocate if sufficient force has been delivered, or as the result of a corneal laceration (Fig 33.20); this may necessitate surgery for removal of the lens. Review the patient within 5–7 days, and within 1 month a check of the angle recession and fundus is recommended.

Retinal detachment

Retinal detachment is the separation of the sensory retina from the retinal pigment epithelium (RPE). It can occur following any globe injury (open and closed) where the retina breaks. In closed globe injuries, retinal detachments are known to result from enlargement in the equator region of the globe and tractions in the vitreous base that are caused by sudden compression of the eye in the anteroposterior direction.[53] These tears can take the form of small holes, horseshoe-shaped wide lesions with irregular borders, dialysis or giant tears. Retinal detachments occur immediately in 12% of patients and within 1 year after trauma in 80%.[54] The patient may have a painless loss of vision, described as a curtain or cobweb descending over vision; photopsia (flashes); or a sudden increase in floaters. If the macula is still on, the patient's vision will still be 6/6. If there is suspicion of a retinal detachment with a macula on, limit the patient's activity to lying flat on a bed until an urgent surgical repair can occur. Retinal detachments require surgical intervention. If the retinal detachment (macular off) is large a RAPD is often found.

Globe rupture (open globe injury)

A ruptured globe can be the result of either a blunt or a penetrating injury (Fig 33.21), although rupture of an old, healed large-incision cataract extraction wound is also a very common mechanism.[27] For a globe to rupture, the cornea and/or sclera must be perforated. There are anterior segment injuries, i.e. to the cornea, anterior chamber, iris and lens; and posterior segment injuries, i.e. to the sclera, retina and vitreous

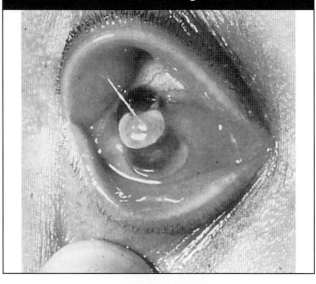

FIGURE 33.20 **Extrusion of lens through corneal laceration.**[42]

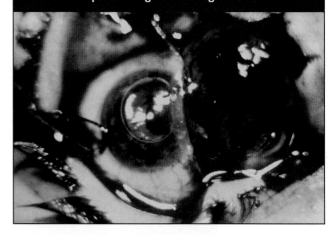

FIGURE 33.21 **Severe eyelid laceration with associated penetrating trauma to globe.**[59]

humour. Injuries of this nature usually occur with other severe injuries, in particular, facial lacerations and fractures.

Signs of a globe rupture are:

- chemosis
- restricted eye movements
- pigment under the conjunctiva
- peaked pupil
- vitreous haemorrhage
- decreased IOP.

When a ruptured globe is suspected use an eye shield, or, if this is not available, a paper cup can be modified and taped over the eye to prevent any pressure being placed on the structures around the eye or on the globe itself. This should be done before the patient is moved. Do not attempt to remove a protruding foreign body from the globe. Relevant questioning at assessment includes when it happened, where the patient thinks the entry point was, duration of pain and whether there are any actions which make symptoms reduce or increase. Ophthalmology should be contacted and the orbit imaged on CT. The patient should be kept nil by mouth.

Specialised ophthalmic operating equipment is required to surgically repair penetrating or perforating injuries, and transfer to a specialist facility should be expedited once any other more serious injuries have been managed. Activities that cause an increase in intraocular pressure must be avoided. These include:

- coughing, gagging
- lying flat
- straining at bowel movements
- bending over
- lifting heavy objects.

Appropriate analgesia should be administered, such as NSAIDs. If opiates are required, consider concurrent antiemetic as vomiting increases intraocular pressure and may cause expulsion of ocular contents. Ondansetron should be used rather than agents that may precipitate dystonic reactions.[44] Sedation may be needed to prevent persistent coughing and vomiting, and aperients may be given to prevent straining during bowel elimination.

Sympathetic ophthalmia

Following repair of a globe which has been severely injured, the major concern is to prevent sympathetic ophthalmia. This is a rare condition characterised by a severe bilateral granulomatous uveitis. It may occur from day 5 to as late as years later. If untreated, the inflammatory response may result in loss of vision in the uninjured eye.[13] It is most probably an autoimmune response that needs aggressive treatment with systemic and topical corticosteroids. Enucleation of the injured eye may need to be performed, if no useful vision and disorganisation of ocular structures is severe, within 10 days to reduce risk of sympathetic ophthalmia. The patient will need psychological and emotional support.

Scleral rupture and vitreous haemorrhage

The most common cause of scleral rupture is penetrating and perforation injury. These injuries may occur in isolation or can be associated with severe facial injuries. Failure to aggressively manage lacerations of the sclera will result in visual loss.[2] In the presence of decreased or no light perception, and/or intraocular pressure of < 10 mmHg, hyphaema and/or chemosis, scleral rupture should be considered.[56] Management is as for a ruptured globe. The vitreous is normally a clear structure. If the retinal vessels or the underlying choroid have been torn by either penetrating or blunt trauma, the severity may vary from trivial to extremely severe haemorrhage. Symptoms include floaters and dark streaks that move with the eye.[57]

Eyelid laceration

Any laceration other than superficial skin that is not involving the lid margin will need ophthalmic referral. Superficial signs may mask deeper lacerations; check for other injuries, especially in children, as they are poor historians. A full-thickness eyelid laceration is assumed to be a penetrating injury or ruptured globe until proven otherwise; consideration must be given to the possible need for tetanus prophylaxis.[16] X-rays and CT will assist in identifying foreign bodies (corneal, orbital or intraocular) and fractures. The laceration should be irrigated and

debrided—do not debride if there is suspicion of penetrating eye injury (PEI)—sutured with 6/0 non-absorbable suture and the sutures removed in 3–5 days; however, repairs can be delayed 24–48 hours with excellent results. Treatment includes regular eye care, nursing in the semi-recumbent position at 30° head up, cold pack to decrease swelling and application of chloramphenicol ointment.

Laceration to the nasolacrimal system

Epiphora (tearing) from disruption of the tear drainage system occurs in:

- 0.2% of nasal fractures
- 3% to 4% of Le Fort II or III midfacial fractures and
- 17% to 21% of nasoethmoidal fractures.[58]

The diagnosis of the condition is made when there is a daily build-up of mucopurulent discharge, or epiphora since the injury. It may take several weeks to become apparent and the injury to the nasolacrimal system may have occurred during repair of other mid-facial injuries. Where there is conjunctival infection, give topical antibiotics. If the condition worsens, warm compresses, systemic antibiotics and systemic or topical nasal decongestants are required, and occasionally a needle aspiration. If lacrimal abscess occurs, incision and drainage may be needed.

Optic nerve injury

Severe penetrating orbital injuries can result in optic nerve damage and sudden visual loss. Common causes are blunt orbital trauma (closed globe injury), objects severing the optic nerve and facial fractures.[13] The physical findings can include a pupil defect—the affected pupil is dilated and direct pupil reaction to light is absent; check relative afferent pupillary defect (RAPD) using the swing-torch test. Loss of vision can be caused by transaction, avulsion of the optic nerve, optic sheath haemorrhage, pressure on the optic nerve from bone fragments or orbital haemorrhage, direct contusion of the nerve or disruption of the blood supply to the nerve and globe. Often such injuries are irreversible; however, every effort must be made to restore vision. Fine-cut CT or MRI scans of the optic nerve and canal are important for evaluating the extent of injury. Surgical intervention and high-dose intravenous steroids are essential for managing optic nerve injuries. Steroids reduce inflammation and prevent further injury secondary to the inflammatory response.[13]

Chemical burns

Initial management at the injury site is to irrigate with running tap water for 10 minutes, for example, under a shower. Wash the patient's hands and face before commencing the irrigation. Ensure the patient's eyes are opening during the irrigation. On transporting the patient, commence an irrigation using an intravenous giving set and Normal saline/Ringer's solution on continuous flow; check with the patient what the chemical was, when did it occur? And did it enter both eyes? If both eyes are affected, rotate the irrigation between them, or set up two intravenous-giving sets and irrigate both eyes together. The quicker the irrigation starts, the better the outcome for vision.

- *Acid burns* (e.g. battery acids, sulfuric acid and hydrochloric acid) precipitate tissue proteins that set up barriers against deeper penetration. Damage is usually localised to the area of contact, with the exception of hydrofluoric acid and acids containing heavy metals, which tend to penetrate the cornea and anterior chamber.[20]

- *Alkali burns* (e.g. caustic soda, lime-plaster/cement and ammonia) penetrate the cornea rapidly because of their ability to lyse with the cell membranes. Damage is related to the alkalinity (pH) and permanent injury is determined by the nature and concentration of the chemical burn as well as the time lapsed before commencement of irrigation.[20]
- *Alcohol and solvent* burns occur from splashes while painting and cleaning. Although the corneal epithelium is frequently burnt, it regenerates rapidly.[1]

The first principle of management is copious irrigation of the eyes with running water for at least 10 minutes. On arrival at the ED, these patients need to be fast-tracked to commence eye irrigation as soon as possible, or, if irrigation commenced in the ambulance, continue the infusion for at least 30 minutes. The patient's history should include the type of chemical responsible and when it occurred. Note that acid or alkali burns have the same management, but the length of the irrigation may differ. Chemical burns are the only ocular condition where vision is not checked until after management. If patient has been sprayed with pepper spray/oleoresin capsicum gas/capsicum spray, eye irrigation will reduce some of the effects of tearing and pain.

Irrigation with saline or Ringer's solution (closer to pH of tears) should continue for another 30 minutes; topical anaesthetic is required before commencing the irrigation. At some stage during the irrigation, whether done by ED staff or paramedics, the eyelid needs to be everted to irrigate under the lid. If the department uses a Morgan lens to irrigate, again a manual irrigation with an everted lid is required to remove trapped particles. Lime/cement on contact with the tears will harden and particles will be trapped under the upper lid, causing ongoing pain and a high pH.

PRACTICE TIP

Always wait 5–10 minutes after ceasing the irrigation to check pH, otherwise the test will be of the irrigation solution. Use Universal Indicator Paper, but do not use urine pH test strips to test tear pH, as these strips can cause more trauma to the eye. Insert small strips into both the lower lid fornices. Leave in until wet (eyes become quite dry after irrigation), then after 30 seconds read the test strip. Further irrigation will be required if pH is high (alkali burns).[20] The acceptable pH range is 6.5–8.5.[16]

Visual acuity can be checked after the 30-minute irrigation. Then the eye can be examined using a slit lamp to assess damage to the ocular surface and anterior chamber.

Assessment of the chemical burn should be done using topical anaesthetic drops and fluorescein staining to determine the area of surface injury (Fig 33.22). If ischaemia is seen on limbus (if no ischaemia is present the junction of the cornea and sclera will be injected (red)), continue irrigating for

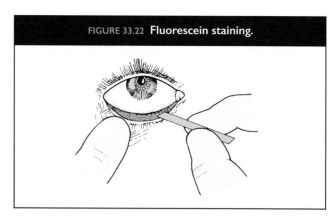

FIGURE 33.22 **Fluorescein staining.**

Touch moistened fluorescein strip to inner canthus of lower lid.

another 30 minutes. Chemical burns where the epithelium is intact or minimally disturbed can wait 24 hours to be reviewed by an ophthalmologist. Burns involving more than one-third of the epithelium and the corneal edge, with any clouding of the cornea, are potentially more serious as there may be subsequent melting of the cornea and should be referred immediately.

For more-serious alkaline burns, 10% citric and ascorbic drops 2-hourly for 48 hours over a week have shown significant outcomes, in combination with 1 g ascorbic acid daily. This regimen has an inhibitory effect on corneal melting. Topical antibiotics (chloramphenicol) and soluble steroids such as prednisolone phosphate 0.5% decrease inflammation.[1] A summary of nursing intervention for ocular trauma is provided in Table 33.5.

Glaucoma

The glaucomas are a mixed group of disorders that have some common features: optic disc cupping, visual field loss and, usually, raised intraocular pressure. Raised pressure without optic disc damage and visual field loss constitutes ocular hypertension: glaucoma in the absence of high pressure is known as normal, or low-tension, glaucoma.

Acute angle-closure glaucoma

Acute angle-closure glaucoma (AACG) (Fig 33.23) is characterised by an acute impairment of the outflow of aqueous humour from the anterior chamber. This results in a rapid and severe elevation in the IOP. In AACG, the IOP can rise to 60 mmHg and above and damages the corneal endothelium, iris, optical nerve and retina (Fig 33.24). This manifests as severe pain, blurring of vision and redness. The pain can be severe enough to cause nausea and vomiting. Diagnosis is difficult because symptoms can mimic cardiovascular and gastrointestinal processes. Visual disturbances, including transition vision loss at night, can be preceded by halos around light, and in established cases is a result of corneal oedema. Relative hypoxia of the pupillary sphincter due to elevated pressure results in the pupil being oval and non-reactive to light stimulation. Acute angle-closure glaucoma is a true ocular emergency.

Treatment is aimed at lowering the IOP and allowing aqueous humour to flow from the posterior chamber to the anterior chamber. Acetazolamide 500 mg orally or IV may be effective in acutely lowering the IOP and thereby reducing pain, with alpha$_2$-agonists topically (Iopidine,

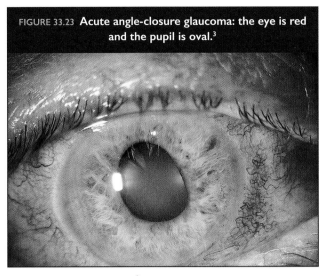

FIGURE 33.23 **Acute angle-closure glaucoma: the eye is red and the pupil is oval.**[3]

Part of the cornea is hazy.[3]

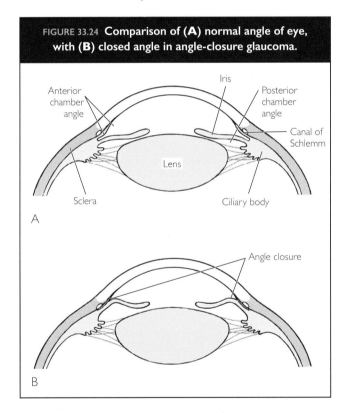

FIGURE 33.24 **Comparison of (A) normal angle of eye, with (B) closed angle in angle-closure glaucoma.**

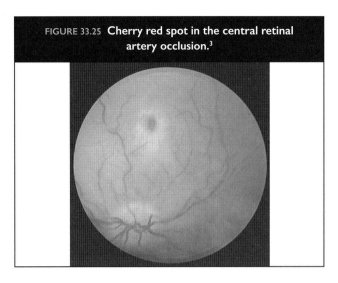

FIGURE 33.25 **Cherry red spot in the central retinal artery occlusion.**[3]

is a true ocular emergency. Retinal circulation must be re-established within 60–90 minutes to prevent permanent loss of vision. Occasionally, the patient may experience transient episodes of blindness, called amaurosis fugax, in the days prior to the occlusion. This can be equated to a transient ischaemic attack. The patient describes the episode as a shade coming down over the eye. Fundus examination shows creamy white retina oedema (cloudy swelling) with a central red fovea—the 'cherry red spot'—caused by the absence of oedema in the thinner retina at the fovea (Fig 33.25). An embolus may be seen at any point along the retinal arterioles from the disc to the periphery.

Causes include embolus (carotid and cardiac), thrombosis, giant cell arteritis or a simple angiospasm (rare) associated with migraine or atrial fibrillation. To prevent permanent loss of vision and permanent damage, treatment includes pulsed ocular compression (ocular massage), IOP-lowering drugs such as acetazolamide 500 mg and vasodilation techniques such as breathing into a paper bag. Full cardiac workup/assessment is required to exclude further embolus. No treatment has been proven effective in managing CRAO.

Central (branch) retinal vein occlusion

Central or branch retinal vein occlusion may present as a sudden painless loss of vision. Patients are usually in the older age group, often with systemic hypertension, diabetes mellitus and glaucoma. The characteristic fundus appearance is of extensive haemorrhage with a various number of cotton-wool spots. There may be disc oedema. There is no emergency management specific to vein occlusion. Gaint cell arteritis needs to be excluded as a possible diagnosis before discharge from ED. The patient should be urgently referred to an ophthalmologist.

Ocular pharmacology

The effective administration of drugs to the eyes presents unique advantages and challenges. The eye is one of the few organs to which therapeutic agents can be administered directly by non-invasive methods.

Topical anaesthetics last approximately 20 minutes; instruct the patient not to rub their eye during this time. Never send patients home with topical anaesthetic, as its repeated use is toxic to the cornea.

apraclonidine). Constriction of the pupil with 2% pilocarpine, a parasympathomimetic, 'breaks' the pupil block and re-establishes flow. The forward bowing of the iris is relieved and the angle opens to allow aqueous humour to leave the eye.[1,19,57] Re-check IOP 1 hour after initial therapy to assess effectiveness. Other agents include a hyperosmotic (mannitol) if initial therapy is not successful.

After pressure reduction, admission under the care of an ophthalmologist is required for a peripheral iridotomy or a YAG laser iridotomy.

Central retinal artery occlusion

Central retinal artery occlusion (CRAO) produces sudden, painless blindness and is usually limited to one eye. This

Mydriatic and cycloplegic drops dilate the pupil and paralyse accommodation. The patient's near vision is therefore blurred for a period of time. Patients with darker irises (dark brown/black) who have multiple mydriatics can have dilated pupils for 1–5 days. Driving is not recommended. The patient should be warned that if it is bright outside, they may find themselves dazzled by the sunlight and should wear sunglasses and take extreme care. The patient should be encouraged to have a relative take them home or to catch a taxi.[10]

Both patients and emergency nurses should be reminded about the importance of continuing topical medications for eye disease, as prescribed by the ophthalmologist. The emergency nurse should request that any already prescribed medication be brought into the ED on admission for the treating doctor to prescribe it, so that treatment can be continued.

For information on commonly used drugs in ophthalmology refer to Table 33.4.

SUMMARY

Most ocular emergencies do not represent a threat to the patient's life; however, these conditions represent a great threat to the patient's wellbeing. Once lost, vision cannot be replaced. The emergency nurse should assess patients who present with ocular problems and identify those with actual or potential threats to vision. Traumatic ocular injuries occur in many different circumstances but must always be considered in any trauma involving the face. The primary survey has precedence no matter how severe the ocular injury. Early recognition of true ocular emergencies and preventing further damage is critical for the patient's optimal visual outcome.

CASE STUDY

Paramedics are sent to the home of a 26-year-old male at 1100. On arrival they find:

- mechanism—just 30 minutes ago the patient was applying chorine powder in a swimming pool when a large volume of the substance flew up into his face. The patient washed his hands and face after the splash with tap water.
- injury—the patient is complaining of a high level of ocular pain and left eye chemical burn
- signs—lids oedematous; it is hard to view the eye as the patient has difficulty opening it; heart beat 90 beats/minute, BP 130/80, respiratory rate 22 breaths/minute

The patient is transported to hospital; paramedics have commenced irrigating the eye with Normal saline using a giving set. On arrival at hospital at 1115, the patient is triaged as a category 2, and the irrigation continues by the fast-track nurse for another 30 minutes.

His vision was checked after completion of 2 L Normal saline and found to be 6/12; pH was 8.

After examination of the eye by slit lamp, the patient was found to have no significant injury; he was treated for a corneal abrasion with Chloromycetin ointment, to be reviewed by his GP in 2 days.

1. If the patient had telephoned the emergency department (ED), what first aid advice could have been given to minimise damage to the ocular surface?
2. When a patient with a chemical eye injury arrives at the ED what triage category could be assigned?
3. Outline your immediate eye emergency management and provide clinical rationale for each action.

 Answers to Case Study Questions can be found on evolve http://evolve.emergencytrauma.curtis

---

REFERENCES

1. Kaufman DV, Galbraith JK, Walland MJ. Ocular emergencies. In: Cameron P, Jelinek G, Kelly AM et al, eds. Textbook of adult emergency medicine. 2nd edn. Edinburgh: Churchill Livingstone; 2004.

2. Manolopoulos J. Emergency primary eye care: tips for diagnosis and acute management. Aust Fam Physician 2002;31(3):233–7.

3. Batterbury M, Bowling B. Ophthalmology: an illustrated colour text. 2nd edn. Sydney: Elsevier; 2005.

4. Lewis SM, Collier IC, Heitkemper MM. Medical–surgical nursing: assessment and management of clinical problems. 7th edn. St Louis: Mosby; 2007.

5. Rudy EB. Advanced neurological and neurosurgical nursing. St Louis: Mosby; 1984.

6. Guyton AC, Hall JE. Textbook of medical physiology. 11th edn. Philadelphia: WB Saunders; 2006.

7. Brown D, Edwards H, eds. Lewis's medical–surgical nursing: assessment and management of clinical problems. Sydney: Elsevier; 2005.

8. Tortora G, Anagnostakos N. Principles of anatomy and physiology. 6th edn. New York: HarperCollins; 1990.

9. Marsden J. Ophthalmic trauma in accident and emergency. Accid Emerg Nurs 1996;4(2):54–8.

10. Marsden J. Ophthalmic trauma in the emergency departments. Accid Emerg Nurs 2002;10(3):136–42.

11. Madden AC, Simmons D, McCarty CA et al. Eye health in rural Australia. Clin Experiment Ophthalmol 2002;30(5):316–21.

12. Webb LA. Manual of eye emergencies—diagnosis and management. 2nd edn. Edinburgh: Butterworth–Heinemann; 2004.

13. Smith SC. Ocular injuries. In: McQuillan KA, Von Rueden KT, Hartsock RL et al, editors. Trauma nursing from resuscitation through rehabilitation. 3rd edn. Philadelphia: WB Saunders; 2002. p. 484.

14. Egging D. Ocular emergencies. In: Newberry L, ed. Sheehy's Emergency nursing: principles and practice. 5th edn. St Louis: Mosby; 2004.

15. Stein HA, Slatt BJ, Stein RM. The ophthalmic assistant. 7th edn. St Louis: Mosby; 2000.

16. NSW Department of Health, SOS, Agency for Clinical Innovation (ACI). Eye emergency manual. (2007) Available: to download via Apple store and Google Play.

17. Bannon A, Warrick B, Mcmurray P et al. Nurse practitioner clinical practice guidelines for the management of conjunctivitis. Sydney: Sydney West Area Health Service, NSW Department of Health; 2005. pp. 1–12. Online. www.health.nsw.gov.au/resources/nursing/practitioner/pdf/ab_np_conjunctivitis_guideline.pdf; 16 Jan 2011.

18. Sheikh A, Hurwitz B, Cave J. Antibiotics versus placebo for acute bacterial conjunctivitis. Cochrane Database Syst Rev 2003;2.

19. Royal Flying Doctor Service of Australia (Queensland section). The primary clinical care manual. Brisbane: Queensland Health; 2003.

20. Tintinalli JE, Ruiz E, Krome RL, eds. Emergency medicine: a comprehensive study guide. New York: McGraw-Hill; 1985.

21. New South Wales Health. Eye emergency modules. Online. www.health.nsw.gov.au/resources/gmct/ophthalmology/pdf/eye_manual.pdf; 16 Jan 2011.

22. Cline DM, Ma OJ, Tintinalli JE et al. Emergency medicine: a comprehensive study guide. 4th edn. Companion handbook. New York: McGraw-Hill; 2000.

23. National Occupational Health and Safety Commission. Hospitalisation due to work-related injury in Australia 2000–1. Canberra: Commonwealth of Australia; 2004.

24. Victorian Injury Surveillance System (VISS). Injury surveillance and prevention in the Latrobe Valley. Victoria: Monash University, Accident Research Centre; 1994. Online. http://monash.edu/muarc/VISU/hazard/hazspec.pdf; 16 Jan 2011.

25. WorkSafe Western Australia. Eye injuries. Perth, WA: SafetyLine on the internet; 2006. Online. www.safetyline.wa.gov.au; 9 Mar 2007.

26. Shepherd M, Barker R, Scott D et al. Occupational eye injuries. Injury Bulletin, No. 90, Queensland Injury Surveillance Unit; Mar 2006.

27. Casson RJ, Walker JC, Newland HS. Four-year review of open eye injuries at the Royal Adelaide Hospital. Clin Exp Ophthalmol 2002;30(1):15–18.

28. McCarty CA, Fu CL, Taylor HR. Epidemiology of ocular trauma in Australia. Ophthalmology 1999;106(9):1847–52.

29. Pandita A, Merriman M. Ocular trauma epidemiology:10 year retrospective study. The New Zealand Medical Journal, 2012:125(1348); www.nzma.org.nz/journal/read-the-journal/all-issues/2010-2019/2012/vol-125-no-1348/article-pandita; accessed 16 April 2015.

30. Save Sight Society NZ. http://www.savesightsociety.org.nz/htmls/eyeinjuries.html; accessed 15 April 2015.

31. Jayasundera T, Vote B, Joondeph B. Golf-related ocular injuries. Clin Experiment Ophthalmol 2003;31:110–13.

32. Eime R, McCarly C, Finch CF et al. Unprotected eyes in squash: not seeing the risk of eye injury. J Sci Med Sport 2005;8(1):92–100.

33. McAllum P, Barnes R, Dickson J. Ocular dangers of fencing wire. N Z Med J 2001;114:332–3.

34. Spencer TJ, Clark B. Self-inflicted superglue injuries. Med J Aust 2004;181(6):341.

35. Winkel KD, Hawdon GM, Ashby K et al. Eye injury after jellyfish sting in temperate Australia. Wilderness Environ Med 2002;13(3):203–5.

36. Fleming PRI, Crompton JL, Simpson DA. Neuro-ophthalmological sequelae of horse-related accidents. Clin Experiment Ophthalmol 2001;29(4):208–12.

37. Mohamed AA, Banerjee A. Patterns of injury associated with automobile airbag use. Postgrad Med J 1998;74(874):455–8.

38. Lehto KS, Sulander PO, Tervo TM. Do motor vehicle airbags increase risk of ocular injuries in adults? Ophthalmology 2003;110(6):1082–8.

39. Kenney KS, Fanciullo LM. Automobile air bags: friend or foe? A case of air bag-associated ocular trauma and a related literature review. Optometry 2005;76(7):382–6.

40. Moller J, Bordeaux S. Eye injuries in the workplace occurring while wearing recommended and approved eye protection. Adelaide: Research Centre for Injury Studies. Flinders University, South Australia; 2006. Online. www.nisu.flinders.edu.au/pubs/eyeinjury/eyeinjury.html; accessed 13 Jan 2007.

41. Ambulance Service of New South Wales. Protocols and pharmacologies. 2001. Online. www.ciap.health.nsw.gov.au/specialties/CDA/; accessed 16 Jan 2011.

42. McQuillan KA, Von Rueden K, Hartsock R et al, eds. Trauma nursing: from resuscitation through rehabilitation. 3rd edn. Philadephia: WB Saunders; 2002.

43. Kadappu S, Silverira S, Martin FJ. Aetiology and outcome of open and closed glove eye injuries in children. Clinical and Experimental Ophthalmology 2013;41:427–34.

44. Chang EL, Bernardino CR. Update on orbital trauma. Curr Opin Opthalmol 2004;15:411–15.

45. Duma SM, Kress TA, Portal DJ et al. Airbag-induced eye injuries: a report of 25 cases. J Trauma 1996;41(1):114–19.

46. Bendeddouche K, Assaf E, Emadisson H et al. Airbags and eye injuries: chemical burns and major traumatic ocular lesions—a case study. J Fr Ophtalmol 2003;26(8):819–23.

47. Corazza M, Trincone S, Virgili A. Effects of airbag deployment: lesions, epidemiology, and management. Am J Clin Dermatol 2004; 5(5):295–300.

48. Royal Children's Hospital Melbourne. Acute eye injury in children. Clinical practice guideline 2006. Online. www.rch.org.au/clinicalguide/cpg.cfm?doc_id=7955; 9 Mar 2007.

49. Abrams D. Ophthalmology in medicine: an illustrated clinical guide. St Louis: Mosby; 1990.

50. Wright KW. Textbook of ophthalmology. Baltimore: Williams and Wilkins; 1997.

51. Matthews PG, Das A, Brown S. Visual outcome and ocular survival in patients with retinal detachments secondary to open- or closed-globe injuries. Ophthalmic Surg Lasers 1998;29:48–54.

52. Moore EE, Feliciano DV, Mattox KL, eds. Trauma. 5th edn. New York: McGraw-Hill; 2004.

53. Ersanli D, Sonmez M, Unal M et al. Management of retinal detachment due to closed globe injury by pars plana vitrectomy with and without scleral buckling. Retina 2006;26(1):32–6.

54. Goffstein R, Burton TC. Differentiating traumatic from nontraumatic retinal detachment. Ophthalmology 1982;89:361–8.

55. American Academy of Ophthalmology. Eye trauma and emergencies. San Francisco: The Academy; 1985.

56. Russell SR, Olsen KR, Folk JC. Predictors of scleral rupture and the role of vitrectomy in severe blunt ocular trauma. Am J Ophthalmol 1988;105(3):253–7.

57. Sherry E, Trieu L, Templeton J, eds. Trauma. Oxford: Oxford University Press; 2003.

58. Osguthorpe JD, Hoang G. Nasolacrimal injuries: evaluation and management. Otolaryngol Clin North Am 1991;24(1):59–78.

59. Bhavsar AR. Surgical techniques in ophthalmology: retina and vitreous surgery; Philadelphia: Saunders: Elsevier; 2009.

CHAPTER 34

GYNAECOLOGICAL EMERGENCIES

DIANA WILLIAMSON

Essentials

- Any woman of childbearing age presenting with abdominal or pelvic pain should be considered pregnant until proven otherwise.
- Life-threatening conditions, e.g. hypovolaemic shock secondary to blood loss and/or sepsis secondary to an underlying infection, should always be given a high index of suspicion even in the healthy young patient.
- A detailed gynaecological and sexual health history must be undertaken for every woman presenting with pelvic and/or abdominal pain.
- Trust, rapport, sensitivity and privacy are nursing essentials when caring for women with gynaecological emergencies.
- Beware of women who present following a sudden onset of pain, with lateral pain relating to the tubes or ovaries and crampy midline pain often uterine in nature.
- Differential diagnoses must always exclude ectopic pregnancy, appendicitis and peritonitis.
- Women who have been diagnosed with a sexually transmissible infection should also be counselled about referring their sexual partners for testing and treatment (known as 'contact tracing').
- Early referral to an infectious diseases doctor and/or sexual health nurse is paramount if a sexually transmissible infection is suspected or diagnosed.
- The diagnosis of a sexually transmissible disease and the need for emergency contraception can also be an opportunity for a conversation about safe sex practices.

INTRODUCTION

Women with gynaecological problems frequently present to emergency departments (EDs). Knowledge of the normal reproductive system and functions are necessary to assess and manage women with these problems. Women may not seek care, or, despite seeking care, may not be forthcoming about all symptoms because of embarrassment or lack of knowledge. Cultural sensitivity and the need for privacy are fundamental to any discussion of problems related to the reproductive system.

This chapter focuses on gynaecological emergencies in the non-pregnant woman; obstetric trauma, obstetric emergencies and sexual assault are discussed in Chapters 35 and 40. An overview of the anatomy and physiology of the female reproductive system is provided. Principles associated with assessment for women with gynaecological emergencies are discussed. The chapter addresses common conditions seen in the emergency context, including vaginal bleeding, pelvic pain, infections, endometrial and ovarian emergencies and sexually transmitted infections (e.g. genital herpes, chlamydia, gonorrhoea, syphilis and genital warts).

Anatomy and physiology

Gynaecological emergencies affect the non-pregnant woman's ovaries, fallopian tubes, uterus, cervix, vagina and external genitalia. External genitalia include the mons pubis, labia majora and minora, clitoris, vestibular glands, hymen, urethral opening and perineum (Fig 34.1).[1] The vestibule is located between the labia minora and contains the hymen, vaginal orifice, urethral orifice, ducts of the Bartholin's glands and Skene's ducts. Bartholin's glands secrete a mucus-like fluid during excitation. The perineum is a triangular-shaped area between the posterior portion of the vestibule and anus that supports portions of the urogenital and gastrointestinal tracts.[1,2,3]

The ovaries, fallopian tubes and uterus are located inside the peritoneal cavity. Ovaries are bilateral oval structures located between the uterus and lateral pelvic wall, and diminish in size significantly after menopause. The number of ova present in the ovaries also decreases with age. During ovulation, each ovary releases a single ovum that is transported down the fallopian tubes to the uterus. The fallopian tubes transport the ovum to the uterus through muscular contractions. These bilateral tubes are not contiguous with the ovaries, which means that ova can migrate into the peritoneal cavity. This is the basic mechanism which is thought to lead to endometriosis and ectopic pregnancy in the peritoneal space (Fig 34.2).[1,3]

The uterus is a thick-walled organ shaped like an inverted pear. It is suspended in the anterior pelvis above the bladder and anterior to the rectum. A layer of peritoneum covers the superior portion of the uterus and forms the serous layer of the uterine wall. The middle layer of the uterine wall consists of smooth muscle with an inner mucous lining called the endometrium. The cervix provides entrance into the uterus.

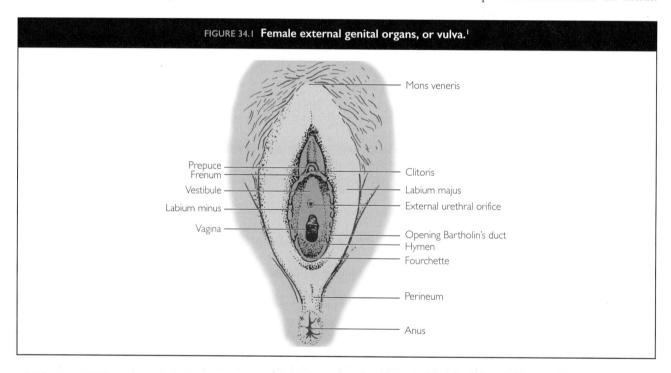

FIGURE 34.1 Female external genital organs, or vulva.[1]

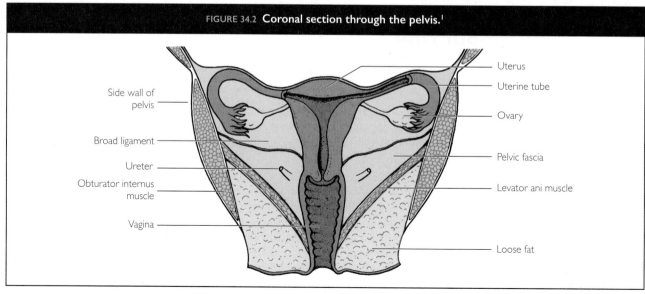

FIGURE 34.2 Coronal section through the pelvis.[1]

It is located in the vagina between the bladder on the anterior aspect and rectum posteriorly.[3]

The female sexual cycle consists of ovulation and menstruation, with each cycle regulated by hormones. Changes in hormonal levels prepare the endometrium for implantation of a fertilised ovum. If the ovum is not fertilised, the endometrium sheds the inner lining as menstrual flow. The length of each cycle ranges from 20 to 45 days, with an average of 28 days for most women. Menstrual flow lasts typically 3–7 days.[4]

Patient assessment

Pre-hospital care

Women presenting with gynaecological issues are at times transported to the ED via ambulance. Pre-hospital care for all patients, including gynaecological presentations, is performed rapidly and efficiently by assessing the patient employing the ABCDE primary survey to identify any major problems and initiate relevant management and medical interventions with the implementation of appropriate protocols and pharmacology for the emerging situation.[6]

The most commonly presenting gynaecological emergency is hypovolaemic shock secondary to blood loss and/or sepsis secondary to an underlying infection. It is important for the pre-hospital care provider to have a strong knowledge of normal female reproductive anatomy and physiology in order to treat these life-threatening disorders. Shock is discussed in further detail in Chapters 20 and 27.

The triage nurse

The role of the triage nurse is to undertake a primary assessment to detect and/or recognise potential life-threatening conditions. Only after airway, breathing and circulation (ABC) have been assessed and considered stable should the focus move onto the woman's primary gynaecological complaint (Box 34.1). In this way, the triage nurse is able to determine within a few minutes the appropriate medical urgency, the need for the allocation of a bed and initiation of first aid or appropriate interventions.[6] Refer to Chapter 13 for more detail on a focused triage patient assessment.

BOX 34.1 Triage interview information to obtain for gynaecological conditions

- Confirm the last menstrual period—whether normal, days lasted.
- If there is vaginal discharge, explore type, colour, consistency, odour and amount. Confirm if the vaginal discharge occurs around the time of normal period.
- Confirm the presence of local redness, swelling, itchiness or pain.
- If vaginal bleeding is present, determine the duration and volume.
- If bleeding is present, determine if it is associated with sexual intercourse.
- Confirm the presence or absence of other signs such as fevers, vomiting and nausea

---

The emergency nurse

The emergency nurse needs to ensure that immediate interventions take place in the presence of life-threatening conditions. Airway, breathing and circulation must be stabilised and continuous haemodynamic monitoring and interventions such as fluid resuscitation should be commenced (see Ch 17, p. 345, for haemodynamic monitoring procedures). The emergency nurse must assume that any woman of childbearing age presenting to the ED with abdominal or pelvic pain is pregnant until proven otherwise. This is important, as pregnancy expands the number of diagnoses that need to be considered, some of which are potentially life-threatening, for example ectopic pregnancy.[2]

History

A detailed gynaecological history must be undertaken for every woman presenting to an ED with pelvic or abdominal pain. The history should be undertaken in a private area and approached with sensitivity by a non-judgemental nurse or doctor, and without other family members or friends being present as many of the questions that will be asked may be of a sensitive nature. The assessment of gynaecological conditions in the non-pregnant woman needs to include the presenting complaint with associated symptomology including abnormal vaginal bleeding, discharge or fever, relevant medical and surgical history including obstetric and menstrual history, sexual history (and contraception) and pain assessment.[7]

The investigation of pain assists in discriminating between urgent and non-urgent conditions. The differential diagnoses of pain are vast and symptoms are often non-specific. Gynaecological and non-gynaecological conditions can present with referred pain to the back, buttocks, perineum or legs. Recurrent episodes of acute pain may suggest conditions such as primary or secondary dysmenorrhoea. Pain history and assessment can also provide information on the most appropriate analgesic intervention. The duration of the complaint may also be suggestive of slow leaking inflammatory mediators or an acute event such as ischaemia or ruptured cyst.[8]

The clinician should be wary of those women who present following a sudden onset of pain, with unilateral pain relating to the tubes or ovaries and crampy midline pain often uterine in nature.[8] Important associated symptoms include the presence of fever (infection), nausea/vomiting (gastrointestinal), abdominal distension (obstruction), back pain or urinary symptoms (urinary tract infection, UTI). Further information that should be elicited in a detailed history for any woman presenting with a gynaecological emergency can be found in Box 34.2.

Physical examination

The physical examination should include an assessment of the general appearance of the woman and her vital signs, including signs of anaemia. The collection of vital signs (heart rate, blood pressure, respiratory rate, temperature and oxygen saturation) provides a useful reference point to discriminate between more or less urgent cases, including signs and symptoms of hypovolaemic and/or septic shock.[2]

The extent of physical assessment undertaken initially at triage may be limited because of the triage environment, but a full abdominal assessment is desirable when possible. An abdominal examination should include inspection, auscultation

---

BOX 34.2 Detailed history-taking of presenting problem[24]

- A description of the bleeding or vaginal discharge, including onset, precipitating factors, volume (number of pads used), colour, presence of clots and duration including abdominal pain, vaginal discharge.
- Pain history including any aggravating or relieving factors: does anything make it better or worse?
- Effects of passing urine, defecation, coughing on bleeding.
- Past medical, surgical, obstetric and gynaecological history: number of pregnancies, gravida/parity; contraception methods and hormone replacement therapy.
- Menstrual cycle, including relationship of abnormal bleeding to menstrual periods, history of dysmenorrhoea, onset of menopause (if relevant).
- Sexual history, including dyspareunia, past history of sexually transmitted infection (STI) and risk factors for infection: lower abdominal pain, pelvic pain, fever, chills, vaginal discharge.
- Experience of sexual assault, trauma or domestic violence.
- Past history of abnormal cervical smears.
- Any symptoms of weakness, syncope, anaemia (tiredness/lethargy) and/or coagulopathy (easy bruising, extensive bleeding).

---

and palpation of the abdominal and pelvic cavity, assessing for tenderness, guarding, rigidity and masses.[2]

This may provide information on tumours and masses (e.g. ovarian cyst), tender areas (e.g. salpingitis) and signs of guarding suggestive of peritonitis (e.g. ruptured ovarian cyst).[2]

A careful pelvic examination is essential; ensure that privacy and a support person is provided. Inspection includes examination of the lower genital tract both externally and via speculum examination, looking for lacerations, foreign bodies, lesions/polyps, vaginal discharge, cervical os (open or closed) and bleeding from the cervical os. Bimanual pelvic examination is also generally indicated, looking for uterine and adnexal enlargement, masses, irregular contour and cervical motion tenderness (infection), masses (ovarian cyst, torsion or abscess) and to collect swabs. A rectal examination may be necessary to rule out masses, rectal bleeding and presence of haemorrhoids.[9]

This should be undertaken bearing in mind the possibility of past sexual abuse or domestic violence. Undertaking a vaginal examination in a woman who is already traumatised by sexual assault (either recently or in the past) may only exacerbate pain and trauma already experienced (see Chapter 40).

Clinical investigations

Following a complete history and gynaecological examination, pregnancy should always be excluded first in women of childbearing age who present with vaginal bleeding. Insertion of a large-bore cannula and collection of blood samples for full blood count, group and cross-match are essentials. A quantitative beta-hCG (human chorionic gonadotrophin) test and pelvic ultrasound should be performed for confirmation of pregnancy, to exclude a miscarriage or ectopic pregnancy, and a urine specimen collected for evidence of infection, diabetes and/or haematuria.[9]

Other blood tests (endocrine, clotting function, iron studies) should only be undertaken if there is evidence of other underlying disease. In postmenopausal women, referrals should be made for further investigations including a Papanicolaou (Pap) smear, hysteroscopy and histological examination of tissue via a curettage where clinically indicated.[4,9]

Psychosocial and cultural considerations

Emergency nurses must be sensitive when assessing a woman with a gynaecological condition. The public environment of many emergency areas is not always conducive to private and sensitive discussions and may prevent women from openly discussing problems.[2]

It is always preferable that the woman, if haemodynamically stable, be allocated a single room. A single room will ensure privacy, as the woman will require an abdominal palpation and, most likely, a vaginal examination. In the presence of a life-threatening event, however, the allocation of a single room may be inappropriate and unsafe. In addition, ensuring cultural safety must always be considered when discussing or assessing women in an ED.

As Australia and New Zealand is becoming increasingly multicultural, expected variations in care should be considered. In the context of gynaecological emergencies certain cultural groups will need to see female doctors only, health beliefs and health seeking behaviours may be different and clinicians need to understand the influence of the care giver's gender on the disclosure of sensitive information which may impact on the delivery of appropriate care.[10]

Female genital mutilation (FGM) is commonly performed in parts of Africa, with migrants from Somalia, Ethiopia, Sudan and Egypt, and sometimes the Middle East and Asia, comprising the majority of affected woman seen in Australia. In Somalia and Sudan more than 80% of women have undergone FGM, although in Australia and New Zealand it is unlikely that immediate complications would present to the ED. Long-term gynaecological consequences of FGM include recurrent urinary tract infection (prolonged voiding time, difficulty obtaining a mid-stream urine specimen for analysis), recurrent vaginal infections, menstrual problems: haematocolpos, retained menstrual clots as well as local scar complications (keloid, dermal cysts), local pain (chronic neuropathic pain), difficulty with even minor gynaecological procedures (e.g. Pap smear), as well as the psychological sequelae of post-traumatic stress disorder, anxiety and depression among these women.

It is important to be culturally responsive and non-judgemental in these situations and to demonstrate knowledge and respect with appropriate referral for psychological support if required.[11]

PRACTICE TIP

Understand how gender, power and cultural differences can influence the dynamics of the relationship between the patient and healthcare provider and consequent effective communication. Be sensitive to history and examination processes and, if not sure, seek appropriate advice.

Clinical presentations

Vaginal bleeding

Vaginal bleeding is a common reason for presentation to an ED and may be due to a variety of reasons. Vaginal bleeding can occur in pregnant, non-pregnant and postmenopausal women or female children. This section addresses vaginal bleeding in the non-pregnant woman. For bleeding in the pregnant woman, refer to Chapter 35.

Types and causes of bleeding

Primary dysmenorrhagia is a common presenting problem for young women, and is defined as pain and cramping during menstruation that interferes with normal activities. It is usually treated with non-steroidal anti-inflammatory drugs (NSAIDs) or the oral contraceptive pill (OCP). Some alternative therapies have also been shown to relieve or decrease pain in women suffering from primary dysmenorrhoea.

> **PRACTICE TIP**
>
> **ALTERNATIVE THERAPIES FOR PRIMARY DYSMENORRHOEA**[4]
>
> - Heating pads to the lower abdomen
> - Exercise
> - Massage
> - Acupuncture
> - Hypnosis
> - Transcutaneous electrical stimulation (TENS)

Abnormal uterine bleeding refers to any bleeding that is outside of the normal menstrual cycle, and can involve either too much or too little bleeding. *Dysfunctional uterine bleeding* (DUB) is heavy and/or irregular bleeding that cannot be attributed to another cause.[2]

> **PRACTICE TIP**
>
> **TERMS USED TO DESCRIBE ABNORMAL UTERINE BLEEDING**[4]
>
> - *Dysmenorrhoea*—the absence of a menstrual period in a woman of reproductive age
> - *Oligomenorrhoea*—infrequent (or, in occasional usage, very light) menstruation >35 days apart
> - *Menorrhagia*—abnormally heavy and prolonged menstrual period at regular intervals
> - *Metrorrhagia*—uterine bleeding at irregular intervals, particularly between the expected menstrual periods
> - *Menometrorrhagia*—a condition in which prolonged or excessive uterine bleeding occurs irregularly and more frequently than normal

Diagnosis

The typical causes of abnormal vaginal bleeding include menorrhagia, intermenstrual bleeding, metrorrhagia and postcoital bleeding. The three most common causes of meno-rrhagia are uterine fibroids, adenomyosis and DUB. Other less common causes include endometrial polyps, endometrial carcinoma, presence of an intrauterine device (IUD), pelvic inflammatory disease (PID) and some coagulation disorders.

Typical pelvic findings for the most common causes of menorrhagia are:

- an abnormal-sized uterus
- an asymptomatically enlarged uterus (fibroids)
- a symmetrically enlarged uterus (adenomyosis).[12]

Abnormal vaginal bleeding in premenopausal women is bleeding occurring outside the regular cycle. Vaginal bleeding after menopause must always be investigated because of the increased risk of malignancy. Postmenopausal causes of vaginal bleeding include atrophic endometritis, vaginitis, endometrial cancer, cervical polyps, endometrial hyperplasia and exogenous oestrogens. Vaginal bleeding usually presents pain-free and is often considered as prolonged menorrhagia.[4]

Management

Most non-pregnant women presenting with abnormal vaginal bleeding do not require immediate interventions in the ED unless they prove to be haemodynamically unstable. The treatment regimens should be aimed at the specific underlying aetiology. There are four main treatment options for women with menorrhagia:

- pharmacotherapy
- medicated IUDs
- conservative surgical management
- hysterectomy.[4]

None of these options should be commenced in the ED due to the inability to follow up these women, and they should be referred to an appropriate gynaecological practitioner for decisions about treatment.

In postmenopausal women, prolonged bleeding (more than 12 months) after the last menstrual period has ceased should be investigated. This commonly occurs in the presence of atrophic endometriosis, and hormone replacement therapy will usually control symptoms. However, any postmenopausal bleeding should be considered abnormal and be investigated, given the increased risk of reproductive cancers in women in this age group. A referral to an appropriate gynaecological practitioner for a Pap smear, endometrial biopsy and/or ultrasound is necessary to definitively rule out malignancy and allow ongoing continuity of care.[4]

Miscarriage

Miscarriage is related to early pregnancy complications. In Australia and New Zealand it is the recommended medical term for pregnancy loss of less than 20 weeks. An estimated 10–20% of post-implantation pregnancies end in spontaneous miscarriage and up to 1 in 100 in an ectopic pregnancy. Recent advances have led to earlier diagnosis and the adoption of more conservative treatment options. Hospitals can be organised to manage many of these cases on an outpatient or day-case basis to increase patient satisfaction and promote more efficient use of resources. Dedicated EPAS (Early Pregnancy Assessment Services) have been established across various locations in NSW based on international models with recognised clinical benefits associated with the service.[13]

The terminology of miscarriage has changed over the last two decades in line with research and the significant psychological impact which woman found distressing. The World Health Organization (WHO) classes miscarriage into the following categories:

- *Threatened miscarriage*: a threat of miscarriage with associated vaginal bleeding, with or without lower abdominal pain which occurs in a pregnancy of <22 weeks' gestation. The pregnancy may continue.
- *Inevitable miscarriage*: a miscarriage considered inevitable when specific clinical features indicate that a pregnancy is in the process of physiological expulsion. The pregnancy will not continue and will proceed to incomplete or complete miscarriage.
- *Incomplete miscarriage*: a miscarriage in which early products of pregnancy are partially expelled. Many incomplete miscarriages may be unrecognised missed miscarriages.
- *Complete miscarriage*: a miscarriage in which early products of pregnancy are completely expelled.[14]
- Other types of miscarriage:
  - *Missed miscarriage*: A miscarriage that is non-viable and confirmed on ultrasound, even in the absence of clinical features such as bleeding. Some women do recall a transient and/or brownish vaginal discharge, or a vague reduction in symptoms of early pregnancy.
  - *Recurrent miscarriage*: The spontaneous loss of ≥3 consecutive pregnancies before 22 completed weeks is regarded as recurrent miscarriage.[14]

Diagnosis

All women who present to the ED with a positive pregnancy test, abdominal and/or pelvic pain and bleeding require investigation for potential miscarriage. Blood is taken for a quantitative beta-hCG (beta-human chorionic gonadotrophin), which is used to confirm pregnancy and to assist the diagnose of an ectopic pregnancy. During early pregnancy, hCG levels in the blood double every 2 to 3 days, but ectopic pregnancies normally have a longer doubling time.[15]

Blood grouping is also taken to determine Rhesus type. Rhesus disease is a condition where the antibodies in a pregnant woman's blood can destroy her baby's blood cells, and occurs when the mother has rhesus-negative blood (RhD negative) and the baby in her womb has rhesus-positive blood (RhD positive). When a woman with RhD negative blood is exposed to RhD positive blood, sensitisation develops. This can occur during childbirth as their blood combines in the bloodstream impacting all subsequent pregnancies Rhesus disease is preventable by administering Rh(D) Immunoglobulin (anti-D) within 72 hours of a sensitising event.[13]

An ultrasound is necessary to confirm the diagnosis of complete miscarriage and has a positive predictive value of 98%.[13]

Management

Assessment of the woman's ABCs is critical, especially if she is unwell and is managed according to her clinical needs. All vital observations, including temperature, should be attended. In the ED the abdomen is examined for tenderness and a bimanual pelvic or speculum examination is considered if the woman is bleeding heavily or unwell. If products of conception are visible in the cervix they should be removed and consider swabs if signs of infection are evident. Any available products of conception should be sent to histology for processing.[16]

Appropriate psychological support should be offered in the ED, especially if the woman is alone as this is usually an unexpected event with psychological sequelae associated with loss. The provision of information on miscarriage should be offered to each woman or couple to ensure that they are well informed of decisions that need to be made in relation to options, referrals and the sensitive issue relating to the disposal of fetal tissue.[13]

Appropriate referral and discharge processes are important to ensure the safety and quality of patient care. Women who are stable and suitable for discharge should be referred to the most appropriate follow-up care; for example, an obstetrician, general practitioner or appropriate service as available in their locality. Women requiring inpatient care, or where there is any question regarding best management, must be referred to the obstetric and gynaecological service.

PRACTICE TIP

- Presence of pain, hypotension, tachycardia, and anaemia warrants exclusion of a life-threatening differential diagnosis such as an ectopic pregnancy.
- The experience of a miscarriage is associated with a psychological impact of varying intensity in the short or long term, or both. All women should be offered counselling or psychological support.
- Anti-D is given within 72 hours of bleeding and it is the responsibility of any doctor or nurse who has seen the patient to ensure this occurs.

Postpartum haemorrhage

Postpartum haemorrhage (PPH) is a growing concern for EDs as more women are delivering outside hospitals and the promotion of early postpartum hospital discharge programs. According to The Royal Australian and New Zealand College of Obstetricians and Gynaecologists, PPH within Australia and New Zealand remains a major cause of both maternal mortality and morbidity. It is common and in Australia the incidence is between 5 and 15%. While the majority of these cases are minor, requiring little active management and causing minimal morbidity, it must be remembered that PPH remains a leading cause of maternal death, both globally and within the Australian and New Zealand context.[17]

PPH can be classified as early, which occurs within 24 hours of delivery and is usually caused by uterine atony or retained placenta. Late PPH, which occurs from 24 hours to 6 weeks after delivery, is generally due to retained placental tissue and/or infection; 99% of all PPH is classified as early.[18]

Diagnosis

PPH is a clinical diagnosis characterised by heavy symptomatic vaginal bleeding post-delivery that makes the patient symptomatic (e.g. pallor, light-headedness, weakness, palpitations, diaphoresis, restlessness, confusion, air hunger, syncope) and/or results in signs of hypovolaemia (e.g. hypotension, tachycardia, oliguria, oxygen saturation <95%). At times, vaginal bleeding may not be abnormal as haemorrhage is internal and related to post caesarean delivery.[18]

Pre-hospital management

Ambulance protocols determine initial treatment and management plans for women who are transported with a PPH. Common to all locally authorised protocols include a primary assessment of the woman which include the 4 'T's' of Primary PPH—Tone (uterine atony), Trauma (to the genital structures), Tissue (retention of placenta or membranes) and Thrombin (coagulopathy), as well as vital signs.[19]

Immediate interventions are commenced as appropriate—gentle massage of the uterine fundus if it is not firm; fluid resuscitation and applying direct pressure to any visible lacerations. For any retained products, a pad is applied and blood loss monitored, pain is managed as per protocol and urgent transport is necessitated. PPH can be controlled by certain drugs which induce uterine contractions and should be referred to within authorised local protocols.[5]

PRACTICE TIP

- Minimal on-scene time is necessary to stabilise the mother and baby for transport to definitive care.
- The woman with a PPH should be treated like any haemorrhaging patent and resuscitation measures should be commenced accordingly.

Management

On arrival to the ED a primary assessment is undertaken to determine the woman's clinical urgency; she should be positioned flat and kept warm. Initial administration of high-flow oxygen is supported and wide-bore intravenous access should be established with blood sent for full blood count, coagulation profile and cross-match. Blood cultures must be taken if the woman is febrile or the vaginal blood/discharge is malodorous. Rapid infusion of warmed fluids is ideal and should be commenced once intravenous access is achieved. The use of group specific or group O RhD-negative blood should be given early to restore the woman's oxygen-carrying capacity and massive transfusion protocols administered where required. Facilities that provide obstetric care should adhere to massive transfusion protocols and be familiar in its use.[17,20]

Early consultation to the obstetrics and gynaecology team is crucial to encourage good transition and communication from resuscitative to definitive care.[17]

A secondary survey and a more focused examination is necessary to assess the causes of the PPH, as previously described in pre-hospital care, which specifically refers to uterine atony; uterine rupture, trauma, retained placental tissue, uterine inversion and thrombosis.[17,19] Bedside ultrasonography (FAST) is used diagnostically to identify the cause and definitive care is undertaken based on these findings.

PRACTICE TIP

The obstetrician/gynaecologist consultant should be contacted immediately as care for the patient is initiated to encourage good transition and communication from resuscitative care to definitive care.

Pelvic pain

Lower abdominal or pelvic pain is another common reason for presentation to an ED, particularly in young women. Pelvic pain can be acute, chronic or cyclic and will not always be pathological. A systematic approach will assist diagnosis and management.[2,21]

Pelvic pain may originate from the genital tract, urinary tract or bowel or may be referred from the musculoskeletal system. Physiological midcycle pelvic pain (mittelschmerz) may be present at the time of ovulation in some women who are not taking the OCP.[21]

Pain may be psychosomatic, masking a psychological issue or concern. Underlying depression, anxiety state, sexual problem or history of domestic or sexual violence should always be kept in mind as a primary or secondary reason for pelvic pain.[22]

Differentiating urgent from non-urgent causes of pelvic pain is often the main challenge faced by emergency clinicians. Pelvic pain that lasts for >6 months is considered chronic as opposed to sub-acute pain described as 3–6 month duration or acute pain which is < 3 months.[23] The common gynaecological and non-gynaecological causes of pelvic pain are summarised in the following sections.

Acute pelvic pain

The gynaecological causes of acute pelvic pain are outlined in Box 34.3. In the non-pregnant woman, the initial focus should be on differentiating abdominal pain causes from those that relate to gastrointestinal rather than pelvic causes. The non-gynaecological causes of acute pelvic pain are covered in other chapters in this text, and include:

- urological causes—cystitis, pyelonephritis, ureteric colic (see Ch 25)
- gastrointestinal causes—acute appendicitis, diverticulitis, bowel obstruction (see Ch 24)
- thrombotic causes—mesenteric thrombosis (see Ch 48).

PRACTICE TIPS[9]

- Nausea and vomiting more commonly occurs with a gastrointestinal cause.
- Cervical motion tenderness suggests pain originating from the pelvic organs.

BOX 34.3 Gynaecological causes of acute pelvic pain[4,34]

- Threatened, incomplete or septic abortion (see Ch 35)
- Ectopic pregnancy (see Ch 35)
- Acute salpingitis
- Tubal or ovarian abscess
- Endometritis
- Pelvic peritonitis
- Complications of an ovarian cyst—rupture, haemorrhage into a cyst, torsion
- Ovulation pain
- Retrograde menstruation
- Primary dysmenorrhoea
- Trauma and/or sexual assault (see Chs 40 and 42)

Chronic pelvic pain

Chronic pelvic pain is pain that is unrelated to pregnancy or the menstrual cycle and has been present for 6 months or more.[23] Common gynaecological causes of chronic pelvic pain are outlined in Box 34.4. The non-gynaecological causes of chronic pelvic pain are covered in other chapters in this text, and include:

- urological causes—bladder dysfunction, urinary tract calculi (see Ch 25)
- gastrointestinal causes—appendiceal abscess, intra-abdominal adhesions, diverticulitis, irritable bowel syndrome, inflammatory bowel disease, Crohn's disease, malignancy of the large or small intestine (see Ch 24)
- musculoskeletal causes—osteoarthritis, lumbar disc protrusion, pelvic nerve entrapment or other musculoskeletal or neurological disorder (see Ch 50).

Diagnosis

An abdominal examination should assess for tenderness, guarding, rebound, abdominal distension or masses, and a vaginal examination (bimanual and speculum) may be indicated to assess for cervical motion tenderness, masses (ovarian cyst, torsion or abscess) and to collect swabs. Watch for diffuse peritoneal signs indicating a ruptured hollow viscous, pelvic inflammatory disease (PID) or an intra-abdominal haemorrhage (ectopic or ruptured ovarian cyst).[9]

Management

The management of pelvic pain will depend on the differential diagnoses that the history and examination suggest. It will also depend on the urgent nature of the problem, i.e. how acutely unwell the woman is on presentation. It is essential that the nurse or doctor discuss the possible diagnoses with the woman and together plan the most appropriate management.[9]

Women who have long-standing chronic pelvic pain have often already seen many doctors and nurses, and often with little relief. There may be hostility towards clinical staff, especially if the woman feels that her pain is being dismissed as 'psychological'. Studies have also shown that up to 60% of woman with chronic pelvic pain have a history of sexual abuse with a significant association between physical abuse and chronic pelvic pain.[24]

It is essential to allow time to enable the woman to explore her feelings about her pain and her past care.[24] This may not always be feasible or possible in a busy ED; however, an effort should be made to ensure that the woman feels she is being listened to. Referral to a multidisciplinary pain clinic or team may enable the multifaceted nature of chronic pelvic pain to be

addressed. If violence or abuse issues are disclosed, referral to the appropriate services is indicated.

Pelvic inflammatory disease

Pelvic inflammatory disease (PID) refers to infections of the upper genital tract and includes endometritis, salpingitis, tubo-ovarian abscesses and pelvic peritonitis.[21,25]

The two most common causative organisms for PID are *Chlamydia trachomatis* and *Neisseria gonorrhoeae*.[21,25]

The major long-term consequences of unrecognised and untreated PID include scarring of the fallopian tubes leading to infertility (12%) and an increased risk of ectopic pregnancies.[4,24]

Diagnosis

The most frequent symptoms include acute pelvic pain, febrile illness, abdominal guarding and rebound tenderness, vaginal discharge and raised white cell count.[21] Postcoital or intermenstrual bleeding may also present as symptoms. During a vaginal examination the clinician should look for tenderness when moving the cervix laterally and/or adnexal or uterine tenderness.[25]

A high index of suspicion is required if the diagnosis of PID is not to be missed. The diagnosis is generally a clinical one based on signs and symptoms elicited during the examination, regardless of the results of the investigations.[21] Nonetheless, investigations should still be undertaken (Box 34.5).

Management

The management will depend on the causative organism. Common antibiotics include azithromycin, ceftriaxone, doxycycline and metronidazole. The most recent *Therapeutic Guidelines: Antibiotics, Version 15* (2014)[26] should guide management. In the majority of cases, a patient with PID can be managed as an outpatient; however, clinicians should consider hospitalisation when the woman is pregnant or there is fever >38.3°C, severe pain, tubo-ovarian abscess, concern for non-compliance and where outpatient therapy has failed.[21,25]

Ovarian emergencies

Ovarian cyst

The development of an ovarian cyst, a small sac on the ovary, usually occurs as a result of hormonal level imbalance. An ovarian cyst is likely to develop from the following condition: if the developing Graafian follicle produces insufficient levels of oestrogen, then luteinising hormone (LH) levels may be

---

BOX 34.4 Common gynaecological causes of chronic pelvic pain[24]

- Chronic pelvic inflammatory disease
- Endometriosis
- Ovarian masses, both benign and malignant
- Complications of uterine fibroids
- Pelvic vascular congestion syndrome
- Response to past sexual abuse or domestic violence

BOX 34.5 Investigations in pelvic inflammatory disease[21]

- Urine and/or serum hCG level to exclude pregnancy
- Full blood count and blood cultures
- Urine microscopy for culture
- Endocervical swab for chlamydia and gonorrhoea PCR and microscopy culture
- Pelvic ultrasound
- Screening for other STIs
- Investigation and treatment of the partner as required

hCG: human chorionic gonadotrophin; PCR: polymerase chain reaction; STI: sexually transmitted infection

inadequate to bring about ovulation. In this event the follicle-stimulating hormone (FSH) continues secretion resulting in follicle growth. Normally growth is restricted to about 2 cm. However, in this situation, growth is unrestricted and size may reach up to 8–10 cm.[2,4] Generally on presentation to the ED the woman reports significant pain usually unilaterally, delayed menstruation or menorrhagia. If the cyst has ruptured, life-threatening symptoms include acute pelvic or abdominal pain, peritonism and/or bleeding. For the most part, however, ovarian cysts are benign and asymptomatic.

Diagnosis

The differential diagnosis must exclude ectopic pregnancy, appendicitis and peritonitis. The confirmation of hCG levels is important to rule out ectopic pregnancy. The ability to palpate the ovaries is usually suggestive of rupture of an ovarian cyst with localised haemorrhage. The definitive diagnostic test is a pelvic ultrasound which can guide monitoring and treatment options.[2]

Management

The main aim of management in the ED is pain control. An NSAID is usually sufficient; however, for women with severe pain, narcotic analgesia may be necessary.[27] Close observation is necessary with regular haematocrit and haemoglobin blood testing. Gynaecological referral is needed for potential operative management; however, surgical intervention is rarely required unless hypovolaemia is present.

Ovarian torsion

In the presence of a tumour, such as a cystic teratoma, the fallopian tube or ovary can twist on itself to develop what is commonly referred to as torsion. These tumours are usually benign. Unilateral pain in the lower abdomen and possibly the flank is one of the most common presenting symptoms and fevers, dysuria and/or vomiting and nausea can be present.[27] The differential diagnosis of appendicitis must be excluded.

Diagnosis

While there may be an adnexal mass and tenderness, an ovarian torsion is notoriously difficult to diagnose. Blood tests might confirm an elevated white cell count, although this can be a nonspecific finding. The definitive test for torsion is a pelvic ultrasound with Doppler flow studies but even this is often equivocal.

Management

General management includes analgesia and appropriate resuscitation measures. If the torsion does not spontaneously resolve or the clinical diagnosis cannot be ruled out, then, despite an equivocal ultrasound, surgical intervention is necessary. If torsion is suspected, urgent gynaecological referral is needed for potential operative management.[2,28]

Ovarian hyperstimulation syndrome

Ovarian hyperstimulation syndrome (OHSS) is a known complication of ovarian stimulation occurring in 1% to 3% of patients during in-vitro fertilisation (IVF) treatment.[4] The aim of the treatment is to stimulate ovulation and produce multiple follicles without causing OHSS which can be a potentially fatal condition. To stimulate ovulation, FSH injections (e.g. Gonal-F or Puregon) are administered, followed by a second

injection of the antagonist (e.g. Cetrotide or Orgalutron) over a period of 2 weeks.[29]

Careful monitoring of women thus treated is achieved through the use of vaginal ultrasound and blood tests (serum oestradiol concentration) in order to determine the optimum number and size of developing follicles prior to egg collection. If untreated, OHSS can lead to life-threatening complications, including ascites, pleural and pericardial effusion, haemo-concentration, coagulopathy, adult respiratory distress syndrome, renal failure or even death.[4,30,31]

Diagnosis

Abdominal swelling and fluid retention is a side effect of IVF treatment, and in 1% of cases it can be severe, requiring hospital admission and treatment. If OHSS does occur, it is usually evident 2–8 days after egg collection and subsides 2–3 weeks later if a pregnancy does not occur. Where symptoms are associated with a pregnancy, then in up to 50% of cases the symptoms are more prolonged and severe.

Symptoms requiring urgent medical attention include severe nausea and vomiting, increased abdominal pain, diarrhoea, shortness of breath, increasing thirst and decreased urine output.[32]

On ultrasound the ovaries appear enlarged, sometimes greater than 10 cm, with multiple follicles and cysts; areas of haemorrhage within the ovary and free fluid may be seen surrounding the uterus or within the peritoneal cavity.[32]

Management

Mild symptoms are usually self-resolving and easily treated by rest, fluids (2–3 L per day) and mild pain relief. More severe symptoms, however, require hospitalisation with intravenous fluids, monitoring of renal function, anticoagulant therapy and sometimes drainage of fluid (ascites) from the abdominal cavity.[31,32]

Infections

Toxic shock syndrome

Toxic shock syndrome (TSS) was identified in the early 1980s and was associated largely with menses and tampon use (50–70%). The association between menses, tampon use and TSS has largely resolved in recent times with a declining annual incidence in Australia of 1–2 in 100,000 with an associated 3% case fatality[32] as a result of changes in the manufacturing of tampons.[4] Today it is known that TSS is caused by *Staphylococcus aureus* and can occur in all age groups, and is associated with a range of conditions; for example, burns, surgery, trauma or childbirth. The incidence of non-menstrual TSS remains relatively constant with a 6% case fatality rate.[32]

Of greater concern and more prominent are streptococcal infections, which clinically mimic TSS. Similarly, these infections can result in severe systemic reactions, often presenting as a life-threatening event.[4] Streptococcal TSS is more clinically relevant for the emergency nurse as the incidence of this infection is more common and not isolated to gynaecological infections. Streptococcal infection may occur from either invasive or non-invasive infections.

Diagnosis

The clinical presentation usually involves a constellation of signs and symptoms associated with a septic presentation, and many could pose a life-threatening illness. Most commonly, fever (temperature > 38.9°C) is present and associated with hypotension and a diffuse macular erythematous rash. Scaling of the palms and hands (desquamation) is often present 1–2 weeks after the acute illness. Multisystem involvement, such as renal (elevated creatinine, urea nitrogen or the presence of a urinary tract infection), neurological (altered level of consciousness) and gastrointestinal (vomiting and/or diarrhoea), can also be evident.[4]

For suspected TSS in the febrile woman, a full septic work-up is necessary. This usually includes blood cultures, swabs, urinalysis, radiological investigations and a full blood count. It must be noted, however, that blood cultures are often negative as the exotoxin is absorbed through the vaginal mucosa.[4] Hospitalisation is likely when these investigations are indicated. A septic work-up may not be indicated if a recognised source for the sepsis is identified. For further information on the management of septic shock, refer to Chapters 20 and 27.

Management

Hospital admission with supportive and antibiotic therapy is required in most cases due to the significant mortality rate, 3–6%, of this disease. If a tampon is present this must be removed.[32] For more severe cases where haemodynamic instability is evident, admission to an intensive care unit may be necessary. Supportive therapy usually involves airway management, fluids and drugs for refractory hypotension.[4]

The causative agent will determine antibiotic management. In addition, if a source for the infection can be identified then subsequent removal of this source is necessary, for example drainage of an abscess. Antibiotics are the most common treatment. However, women may get worse before they recover, even with antibiotic treatment, because of release of exotoxins. The most recent *Therapeutic Guidelines: Antibiotics, Version 15* (2014)[26] should be consulted. Usual antibiotic treatment involves a penicillin or first-generation cephalosporin. If the woman is unable to take penicillin because of allergic reactions, then clindamycin or vancomycin should be considered. Currently there is a lack of evidence to support steroid use.[4]

Tubo-ovarian abscess

Tubo-ovarian abscess (TOA) can develop from acute salpingitis and/or persistent PID and can often result from a postpartum, post-termination or post-miscarriage infection. Left untreated it can develop into a life-threatening condition (septic shock) because of rupture and contamination spilling into the peritoneal cavity.[2] This may occur as a complication of an untreated or undertreated PID. On arrival at the ED, the woman may present with pelvic or lower abdominal pain, fever, tachycardia and offensive blood-stained lochia and signs of peritonitis.[4] For further information on the management of septic shock refer to Chapters 20 and 27.

Diagnosis

The differential diagnosis of acute ruptured appendicitis must be excluded. It is important to obtain vaginal and endocervical swabs for identification and culture of organisms. Obtaining blood cultures during rigors will also assist in identification and culture of organisms. A pelvic ultrasound is usually the definitive diagnostic intervention, whereby fluid is usually identified in the pouch of Douglas. If fluid is present, signs of peritonism will usually be present on physical examination.[33]

Management

Immediate management involves correction of fluid, electrolytes and blood loss. Antibiotic management will depend on the causative organism, but urgent administration of broad-spectrum intravenous antibiotics is necessary. If the woman's condition deteriorates or fails to improve, surgical drainage of the abscess may be necessary. Urgent obstetrics and gynaecological referral is needed for potential operative management.[4,33]

Endometritis and salpingitis

Endometritis is the result of inflammation of endometrial tissue and is commonly associated with postpartum infections, including after termination or miscarriage. If this condition is allowed to spread, it can result in acute salpingitis (infection and inflammation in the fallopian tubes) and eventually widespread PID.[4,33]

Diagnosis

Common signs and symptoms associated with this condition include fever, tachycardia, abdominal tenderness, decreased bowel sounds, offensive-smelling lochia and an elevated white cell count (WCC). Vaginal swabs need to be obtained and examined for bacterial identification and antibiotic selection.[4,34]

Management

If this condition is left untreated, the woman can develop life-threatening complications such as sepsis, abscess formation and disseminated intravascular coagulopathies (DICs), and it may also affect future fertility. General management includes pain and fever control and rehydration if required. The most common antibiotics include either clindamycin or gentamycin; however, management will depend on the causative organism.[4] Admission of women who are systemically unwell, intolerant to oral antibiotics or have evidence of a TOA is warranted.[34]

Candidiasis

Candidiasis is caused by the organism *Candida albicans* and is commonly known as thrush. It is the most common vaginal infection in women and is not generally sexually transmitted. It is normal for women to have small numbers of the *C. albicans* yeast in the genital area, but a range of factors may cause it to overgrow and symptoms can develop. Some of these factors include recent antibiotics, diabetes, pregnancy, soaps and detergents used in the genital area and tight clothing that promotes excessive sweating.[17,35]

Diagnosis

The signs and symptoms in women include an abnormal white or creamy yellow vaginal discharge (cottage cheese appearance), which is thick and has a slight yeasty odour. The skin around the vagina may become red, inflamed, itchy and may extend to around the anus.[17,27] Most cases of candidiasis can be diagnosed through clinical examination and history taking for risk factors. A swab can be taken if necessary to confirm the diagnosis.

Management

The infection where uncomplicated can be treated easily with antifungal topical treatments or a one-off dose of oral fluconazole. Follow-up should be recommended for those women who have symptoms that persist or if it reoccurs within 2 months of treatment.[17,35]

Sexually transmitted infections

Sexually transmitted infections (STIs) are very common, although often underestimated. They have been called the 'hidden epidemic' because their scope and consequences are often under-recognised by both the public and healthcare professionals. The rates of STIs are gradually increasing in most countries, including Australia and New Zealand.[36]

This section reviews some of the common STIs, including their pathophysiology, signs and symptoms, diagnosis and management. Consultation and/or referral to an infectious diseases doctor or sexual health nurse or doctor is important if an STI is suspected or diagnosed. Emergency nurses must work collaboratively with other healthcare providers to ensure that STIs are recognised and treated effectively. If one STI is diagnosed, it is often wise to recommend that the woman be tested for other STIs as well as the human immunodeficiency virus (HIV). These infections often occur concurrently as the modes of transmission are similar.

The *Therapeutic Guidelines: Antibiotics, Version 15* (2014)[26] should be consulted for specific information on the most appropriate antibiotic treatment for STIs. Additional information and expanded topic advice is included based on general advice on common pathogens and contact tracings.

History-taking

Collecting a standard history from a woman who may have a risk of an STI or has presented to the ED with suggestive symptoms is no different from the standard history-taking process outlined earlier, but should incorporate the detailed points in Box 34.6.

Effective communication skills are a key building block for effective professional relationships.[8,37] Gathering a history from a woman in relation to an STI requires additional sensitivity and care. Non-verbal as well as verbal communication is particularly important when discussing these sensitive issues. Being non-judgemental, treating women and their families with respect and dignity and being aware of the cultural component of communication will assist in ensuring that women feel comfortable to tell their story to the ED nurse.[8,37] This is even more important for young women, including adolescents, who may be very reluctant to discuss these issues with someone they do not know.

Notification

In Australia, chlamydia, gonorrhoea and syphilis are notifiable conditions in all states and territories. This means that diagnoses of these infections are notified by state/territory health authorities to the National Notifiable Disease Surveillance System, maintained by the Australian Government's Department of Health and Ageing. In Australia, the population rates of diagnosis of chlamydia, gonorrhoea and syphilis continue to be substantially higher in the Northern Territory than elsewhere in the country. Substantially higher rates of diagnosis of chlamydia, gonorrhoea and syphilis have also been recorded among Indigenous peoples compared with non-Indigenous people.[35,38]

BOX 34.6 Taking a sexual history

General points:
- Ensure privacy and be non-judgemental and respectful.
- Avoid making assumptions about people, their sexual identity and their sexual practice.
- Make eye contact and have a relaxed body language.
- Provide a context for the questions that are to follow (e.g. 'I am going to ask you some questions about your sexual activity so that we can decide what tests to do.').

Terminology:
- Generally use vernacular and colloquial expressions rather than more technical expressions, but use your judgement as this may make some feel more uncomfortable.
- Adapt your language to the level of understanding of the person.
- Use the language used by the person, but be cautious as often people attempt to express issues in medical terms but may get the meaning wrong.
- It may be helpful to check back with the person that you have understood what has been said.

Questions:
- Questions should be open-ended (do not require a yes or no answer), clear and unambiguous.
- Ask 'how', 'what', 'where' type questions to explore behaviour.
- Avoid asking 'why' questions as they imply complex understanding of behaviour.
- Do not be afraid to be direct.
- Questions about sexual partners are important as they may be at risk of STIs because of their partner's sexual activity.
- Ask questions about risk-taking behaviours, e.g. What types of sexual activity do you engage in with your partner? Vaginal/oral/anal?
- Ask about knowledge and use of condoms as this provides an opportunity for further information and education.
- Finish the interview with a general open-ended request for further information, for example: 'Is there anything else that concerns you?'
- Further information on taking a sexual history can be obtained from Huffam et al (2008).[46]

Information on STIs in New Zealand is available via the Public Health Surveillance—ESR Sexually Transmitted Infections in New Zealand Annual Surveillance Report 2012.[36]

National statistics on diagnoses are not mandatory to report; however, they are collected using voluntary data from sexual health clinics, family planning clinics and diagnostic laboratories. With the exception of HIV/AIDS, STIs are not notifiable conditions.[36]

Many people have very negative feelings and stereotypes attached to STIs. Women who have been diagnosed with an STI should also be counselled about referring their sexual partners for testing and treatment. Depending on the infection, tracing partners can go back months or years. This can be a very sensitive and difficult topic and confidentiality is highly important.[38,39,40] Further information on contact tracing and management guidelines for sexually transmissible infections can be sought by accessing the website for your health department or by seeking support from a sexual health clinic or public health unit.

PRACTICE TIP

WHAT IS CONTACT TRACING?

- The term is used to describe the process of finding and notifying sexual partners when a person has been diagnosed with a sexually transmitted infection.
- It can be a very difficult and sensitive topic and confidentiality is important.
- Further information can be accessed through the *Australasian Contact Tracing Manual*, produced by the Australasian Society for HIV Medicine (2010) and available at http://ctm.ashm.org.au/
- Causative agents, signs and symptoms, diagnosis and management of common STIs can be seen in Table 34.1.

PRACTICE TIP

HIGH RISK GROUPS FOR STIs[37]

- Young men and women aged less than 25 years
- Indigenous peoples
- Gay and other homosexually active men
- People with HIV/AIDS
- Migrants from high incidence countries
- Sex workers
- People who inject drugs
- Heterosexuals with recent partner change

Genital herpes

Genital herpes is the second most common STI in Australia, with up to one in eight sexually active adults infected.[41] Genital herpes is caused by the herpes simplex virus (HSV) of which there are two types:[7]

- HSV1 (type 1)—usually found around the lips and commonly referred to as a 'cold sore'
- HSV2 (type 2)—usually found around the genitals or anus.

Genital herpes may be caused by either HSV1 or HSV2. HSV is transmitted by close skin-to-skin contact with someone who has the infection. It is a chronic, lifelong disease and usually occurs during vaginal, anal or oral intercourse. However, transmission can also occur if there is skin-to-skin contact without penetrative sex. The first attack is usually the most severe and the woman may present with fevers, malaise, myalgias, dysuria and occasionally urinary retention.[38,41,42]

Herpes is readily transmitted when blisters or ulcers are present; however, the infection is more commonly transmitted through asymptomatic shedding.[41] This is where someone infected with herpes sheds the virus from the skin without any visible signs of the herpes lesions (Fig 34.3). Similarly, transmission may occur when people are unaware they are infected with HSV because they have no symptoms, or minor ones that are unnoticed.[27,42,43]

For this reason genital herpes is not often recognised or properly diagnosed. Counselling for the patient regarding how transmission occurs, including the risk of asymptomatic viral shedding, is important to prevent further transmission of the virus to future partners. Patients with recurrent genital herpes can be treated with antiviral drugs, which can be used intermittently to treat each episode or continuously to prevent further outbreaks.[37,40,41]

There is no cure for HSV infections and patients should be referred on for counselling to a healthcare provider who is experienced in treating HSV infections and can explain the disease, answer any questions and provide treatment options for future outbreaks.[42,43]

PRACTICE TIP

Sexual partners of infected patients should be advised that they might be infected even if they have no symptoms.

Chlamydia

Chlamydia trachomatis (CT) is the most frequently reported notifiable bacterial STI condition in Australia and New Zealand.[36,37]

The prevalence of genital chlamydia infections has been reported to be unacceptably high in Indigenous Australians and in young adults. In New Zealand *Chlamydia* was the most reported STI in 2012 with a national estimation of 744 per 100,000 population based on laboratory surveillance data.[36]

In Australia 2011 data revealed 79,833 new notifications for persons aged 15 years and over or 435 cases per 100,000 population. This rate has more than tripled over the past decade, increasing from 130 notifications per 100,000 in 2001.[44]

If left untreated, *Chlamydia* infections can lead to pelvic inflammatory disease or ectopic pregnancy, and may also affect future fertility. *Chlamydia* is often referred to as 'the silent STI' because the majority of people infected do not have any symptoms. The only way the patient may discover they have the infection is if they accidentally transmit their infection to a sexual partner through unprotected sex, and/or through routine CT screening.[45,46]

Chlamydia can affect the urethra, cervix, rectum, throat and eyes and is most often transmitted through unprotected vaginal and anal sex.[37,46] *Chlamydia* in newborn babies occurs because of exposure to infected cervical fluids. The infection is most often recognised by conjunctivitis that develops 5–12 days after birth. *Chlamydia* is the most frequent identifiable infectious cause of ophthalmia neonatorum, but can also be a common cause of subacute, afebrile pneumonia at 1–3 months of age.[4,37]

Gonorrhoea

Neisseria gonorrhoea infections can infect the urethra, anus, cervix, throat and eyes of both men and women. It can be transmitted through oral, anal and vaginal sex. Condoms

TABLE 34.1 Causative agents, signs and symptoms, diagnosis and management of common STIs

	GENITAL HERPES	CHLAMYDIA	GONORRHOEA	SYPHILIS	GENITAL WARTS	TRICHOMONAS
Causative agent	Herpes simplex virus type 2	Chlamydia trachomatis	Neisseria gonorrhoeae	Treponema pallidum	Human papilloma virus (HPV) types 6 or 11	Trichomonas vaginalis
Signs and symptoms	Blistering and ulceration of the directly affected areas (may include labia majora, labia minora, clitoris and urethra; see Fig 34.3). These can be painful, tingling or itchy	In 70–90% of women, the infection is asymptomatic. When there are symptoms, these may include dysuria, abnormal vaginal discharge, abnormal vaginal bleeding, pelvic pain or pain during sex	In more than 60% of women the infection is asymptomatic. Where there are symptoms, these include cervicitis and a discoloured vaginal discharge	A primary chancre (painless sore) develops at the site (Fig 34.4) after an incubation period of approximately 21 days. In the secondary stage, a rash on the palms of the hands or soles of the feet and on other parts of the body may be seen. Second stage symptoms, if they develop, usually occur from 7 to 10 weeks after infection	Present as small swellings and can appear as single or multiple fleshy lesions (Fig 34.5). Others are flatter and harder to see	Frothy green offensive vaginal discharge
Diagnosis	A laboratory test (PCR test) is undertaken from a swab of the lesion	Detected from swabs collected from the cervix, urethra or anus or by a urine sample. PCR test or culture is undertaken	Detected by swabs collected from the cervix, urethra or anus and cultured for the organism	A sample of the chancre is taken for examination. Blood tests are used to diagnose primary and secondary syphilis	Direct examination. Confirmation by histological examination may be necessary	Detected from high vaginal swab
Management: refer to the eTG Electronic Therapeutic Guidelines: (2014) for specific information	Aciclovir in different doses and length of time depending on whether it is the first episode or a recurrence	Azithromycin, doxycycline or erythromycin are the commonly used drugs	Penicillin is most commonly used but ceftriaxone may also be prescribed. Follow-up cultures are recommended after completing treatment to ensure cultures are negative	Injections of penicillin are the most common treatment. (e.g. doxycycline)	Treatment options include topical podophyllotoxin or imiquimod, cryotherapy, hyfrecation or surgery. The option depends on number and type of the warts	Metronidazole or tinidazole

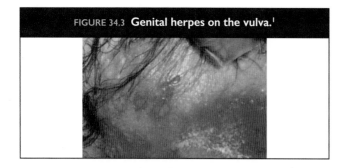
FIGURE 34.3 **Genital herpes on the vulva.**[1]

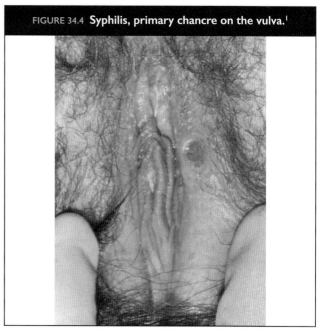
FIGURE 34.4 **Syphilis, primary chancre on the vulva.**[1]

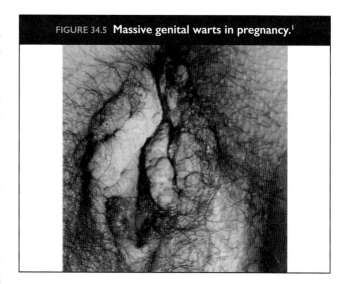
FIGURE 34.5 **Massive genital warts in pregnancy.**[1]

are highly effective in preventing gonorrhoea. Gonorrhoea is relatively uncommon in Australia and New Zealand except in certain high-risk populations; the number of reported cases is, however, on the rise.[37,38,39]

In Australia notification rates of gonorrhoea have generally increased over the past 10 years. In 2011, the national notification rate for people aged 15 years and over was 65 per 100,000 population, up from 40 per 100,000 in 2001.[39] In New Zealand 2012 data showed a national gonorrhoea rate of 89 per 100,000 population.[37]

Gonococcal infections can be asymptomatic or symptomatic and are associated with pelvic inflammatory disease, ectopic pregnancy and infertility, as well as pre-term delivery and premature rupture of membranes during pregnancy.[27] The infection may also be present in newborns if they have been exposed to infected cervical fluids. It is usually an acute illness, which presents 2–5 days after birth. The infection can cause ophthalmia neonatorum, rhinitis, vaginitis, urethritis and inflammation at sites of fetal monitoring.[4,37]

Syphilis

Syphilis is not common in Australia. Nationally, rates of diagnosis of infectious syphilis was 7 for every 100,000 in 2007. The most affected demographic was the 40- to 49-year-old age group, confined to gay men and other men who have sex with men.[47] In New Zealand there has been a steady decline in syphilis cases since a peak of 135 cases in 2009 with males comprising 93.8% of cases.[37] However, testing should still be considered if other STIs have been identified or risk factors are present.[38] Testing includes the venereal disease reference laboratory (VDRL) and the rapid plasma reagin (RPR) tests. The test specific for syphilis is the *Treponema pallidum* haemagglutination assay (TPHA). Once a person has been infected with syphilis, the infection will always show up positive on the TPHA test even when they have been successfully and adequately treated. It can arise up to 10 years after the original infection and, if left untreated, can cause serious, irreversible damage to the brain, spinal cord and other organs (see Fig 34.4).[25,37,47]

Genital warts

Genital warts are one of the most common STIs in Australia and are caused by the human papilloma virus (HPV) ('wart virus'). It is transmitted directly from skin to skin during sexual contact with an infected person. Genital warts, also known as condylomata acuminata, appear on the genitals as tiny swellings and sometimes develop into 'cauliflower-like' lumps. They are often painless and women may be unaware that they even have them.[38,45,48] Some strains of HPV infect the cervix,

causing changes to its cells. These changes can be detected on a Pap smear, and they may be present in women who have never had visible genital warts. Often these cells return to normal without any treatment, but sometimes the abnormalities persist and there may be an increased risk of developing cancer of the cervix in the future.[38,48]

Genital warts are usually an unlikely reason for presentation to an ED, but it may be worth considering testing for them in the presence of other STIs. Large genital warts, however, can be friable and bleed and may make urination difficult if they obstruct the urethra.[38,48] Women with these signs may present to the ED (see Fig 34.5).

Trichomonas

Trichomonas is caused by a tiny parasite called *Trichomonas vaginalis*, and is considered the most common curable STI in young, sexually active women. The infection mainly affects the vagina in women and the urethra of men. Most infected men are asymptomatic, whereas infected women develop symptomatic vaginitis.[49] Women who have trichomonas are at increased risk for other health consequences including PID and other STIs, particularly HIV as the infections commonly co-exist.[38,49,50]

Trichomonas during pregnancy can also lead to low-birthweight babies and prematurity.[51]

Common types of genital tumour

Many common benign genital tumours occur. Genital tumours that cause women to present to the ED include ovarian cysts, Bartholin's cyst or abscess, endometriosis of the pelvis or fibromyomata of the ovaries and/or uterus. Common malignant genital tumours include carcinoma of the cervix or endometrium, sarcoma of the uterus and serous cystadenocarcinomas of the ovary.

Bartholin's cyst or abscess

The Bartholin's gland is located within the vestibule and bilaterally at approximately 4 o'clock and 8 o'clock on the posterior lateral aspect of the vaginal orifice (Fig 34.6).[4] The Bartholin's gland provides lubrication of the vestibule through secretion of a clear fluid. This adds to the normal vaginal secretions that result from vaginal transudate, cervical mucus, uterine secretions and fallopian tube.

Diagnosis
When the Bartholin's gland is swollen (1–2 cm) the condition is usually benign and frequent sitz baths are usually sufficient treatment.[2] A sitz bath is a warm-water bath taken in the sitting position that covers only the hips and buttocks.[53]

In the presence of infection, the Bartholin's gland can obstruct which often results in abscess formation. These abscesses can become quite large, and are usually associated with severe pain and associated cellulitis. A Bartholin's abscess

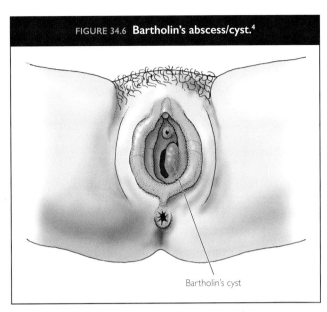

FIGURE 34.6 Bartholin's abscess/cyst.[4]

Bartholin's cyst

LifeART image, copyright 2006 Lippincott Williams & Wilkins.

can develop over 2–3 days and any pressure against the vulva, induced by activities such as walking or sitting, can cause significant pain.[4]

Management
Immediate management of a Bartholin's abscess is appropriate analgesic administration. This condition is acutely painful and requires an analgesic such as an NSAID or a short-term narcotic agent. Given that this condition is more common in sexually active women, the possibility of associated STIs should be ruled out.[2] While spontaneous rupture can occur, the abscess usually benefits from surgical intervention. A Bartholin's abscess is unsuitable for drainage in the ED as there is a high incidence of re-collection if more definitive surgical treatment is not instituted. Antibiotics are not usually required if it is drained properly; however, it is recommended that the drainage is cultured for *Neisseria gonorrhoeae* or *Staphylococcus aureus*. For women experiencing recurrent Bartholin's abscesses, the surgical procedure 'marsupialisation' can be beneficial, whereby a permanent opening is constructed to assist gland drainage.[4,53]

Endometriosis

Endometriosis is a disease of the pelvic mesenchyme where endometrial glands and stroma are found outside the uterine cavity, thus altering the peritoneal environment. It has been estimated that about 10–15% of all women have endometriosis, with higher rates in infertile women (30–40%) and in women with chronic pelvic pain (20%).[4,38]

There are a number of theories on the aetiology of endometriosis. The main theories include retrograde menstruation, coelomic metaplasia (coelomic tissue makes up the peritoneal membrane of the pelvis), and an altered immune response to blood in the peritoneal cavity; or a combination of these. Oestrogen seems to be an important facilitator of endometriosis. The condition is not seen before adolescence and settles after menopause.[4]

Diagnosis

The most common symptom is pelvic pain. This can be acute, but more frequently presents as a chronic problem. The pain is often worse 1 or 2 weeks before menses and peaks 1–2 days before the onset of menstruation. Other signs and symptoms can include dysmenorrhoea, menstrual irregularities, dyspareunia and infertility.[4]

Endometriosis is difficult to diagnose because the extent of the disease does not correlate with symptoms. The gold standard for diagnosis of endometriosis is through direct visualisation during a laparoscopy or laparotomy.[4] It is therefore essential that other causes of pelvic pain be excluded in the ED before referral for further investigation is undertaken.

Management

The overall management aim in the ED is to decrease pain, increase function, limit recurrence and maintain or ensure fertility. Acute management of endometriosis includes pain relief (NSAIDs), emotional support and appropriate gynaecological referral. Ongoing management options include medications such as oral contraceptive (progesterone), danazol and GnRH agonists and surgical diathermy or laser via laparoscopy.[4]

Emergency contraception

Emergency contraception (EC), also known as postcoital contraception, is used to prevent pregnancy after an episode of unprotected sexual intercourse or in the case of contraceptive failure. Indications for EC are failure of a barrier method or contraceptive pill, unprotected intercourse or sexual assault. The two types of EC available are emergency contraceptive pills (ECPs) or copper-releasing intrauterine contraceptive devices.[4]

Emergency contraception pills

The most common method of EC is the ECP or 'morning-after pill', which must be taken as soon as possible, but within 72 hours, to be effective. ECP consists of two regimens: the progesterone-only (levonorgestrel) formulation or a course of high-dose oestrogen and progesterone combined pills. Women accessing ECP should be given information regarding timing, dosage, side-effects, follow-up and what to expect.[34]

Primary side-effects of the combined regimen include nausea, vomiting, headaches, dizziness and breast tenderness. These side-effects are considered less severe when the progesterone-only formulation is administered.[4] The progesterone (levonorgestrel) only approach has been supported by research as the most appropriate method as it is better tolerated and more effective. Overall if taken within 72 hours of unprotected intercourse ECP has a failure rate of 0.2%–3%. The sooner it is taken the more effective it becomes.[4] In Australia and New Zealand, the ECP is available over the counter from pharmacies without a prescription. It is also available from hospital EDs, general practitioners or sexual health clinics. Information regarding specific clinical therapeutic guidelines should be consulted before administration.

Intrauterine contraceptive devices

Copper-releasing intrauterine contraceptive devices (IUCDs) are also considered highly effective with failure rate of < 1%. It functions by eliciting a sterile inflammatory response within the uterus, making the environment unsuitable for fertilisation.[4] These may be used for those women where more than 72 hours has elapsed since unprotected intercourse. Copper IUCDs can be inserted within 5 days of unprotected intercourse and can be continued for long-term contraception once in situ, but has some other disadvantages, including the potential for rare complications such as infection.[4] An IUCD must be obtained from a general practitioner and fitted by a trained professional. It is not suitable for women considered high risk for STIs or in victims of sexual assault.[4]

In cases where women present to the ED with acute salpingitis or PID, then the decision to remove the IUD must be made urgently so the infection can clear. Appropriate antibiotic therapy should be commenced before the IUD is removed. Persistent vaginal bleeding or pelvic pain related to an IUD will require removal, but not as an emergency. The woman should be referred back to the clinician who first inserted the device.[29]

PRACTICE TIPS

- Where emergency contraception has not been administered within the recommended timeframes an unplanned pregnancy is likely; women should seek immediate medical consultation.
- ECP cannot be used for long-term contraception
- The emergency contraception consultation is also an opportunity to discuss the possible risk of sexually transmitted infections, screening and unsafe sex practices.

Safe sex

Discussions around STIs and the need for emergency contraception in the ED can also be an opportunity for a conversation about safe sex. Regardless of whether the STI or pregnancy results are positive or negative, this can be an excellent time to talk about safe sex and ensure that women and their partners are aware of the risks associated with unsafe sex. Safe sex is the use of condoms and water-based lubricant during anal or vaginal intercourse. Safe sex can prevent HIV transmission, pregnancy and most STIs.[25]

PRACTICE TIP

More information on taking care of one's sexual health is available through most health department websites and specific organisations, e.g. Family Planning organisations (www.fpnsw.org.au or www.familyplanning.org.nz).

SUMMARY

Women with life-threatening and non-life-threatening gynae-cological emergencies regularly present to EDs. A woman with a gynaecological emergency may have a problem that is directly related to her sexual practices or lifestyle, and may feel embarrassed or uncomfortable discussing issues related to her problem. This presents challenging opportunities as the emergency clinician must focus on the woman in a caring, non-judgemental manner. Inability to do so can interfere with identification of potentially life-threatening gynaecological conditions and the recognition of non-life-threatening conditions. Recognition of potentially life-threatening conditions takes priority over other interventions. However, the emergency clinician must not lose sight of the long-range effect many gynaecological emergencies can have on women's fertility and sexuality.

An important part of the role of the emergency clinician is knowledge of the most appropriate referral points. In some cases this will be a specialist gynaecologist; however, it may also be women's health or family planning clinic, pain services or counselling services.

CASE STUDY

A 26-year-old woman with right-sided, lower abdominal pain and chills is seen in the emergency room. The pain began 3 days ago and is associated with vaginal discharge. Her last menstrual period was 5 days ago. She uses an IUD for contraception and had coitus 1 week ago. There is no history of nausea, vomiting or diarrhoea. Her vital signs are: blood pressure, 120/80 mmHg; pulse, 100 beats per minute; and temperature, 38°C.

Questions

1. What questions will you ask in this scenario to determine historical and clinical indicators of urgency and relevance?
2. Describe each aspect of your physical assessment, and explain each step.
3. What investigations will you perform, and why?
4. What ongoing monitoring will you provide?

Answers to Case Study Questions can be found on evolve
http://evolve.emergencytrauma.curtis

USEFUL WEBSITES

Australian Government Department of Health and Ageing—provides information on the Department's policies, programs and services, www.health.gov.au

Australian Indigenous HealthInfoNet—an excellent site for anyone interested in Indigenous health, www.healthinfonet.ecu.edu.au

Australian Women's Health Network—good resources itself and excellent links to other resources covering a wide range of women's health issues. It can be found under the section Women's Health Information Links—Women's Health Issues, www.awhn.org.au

Better Health Victoria—provides information and links that are relevant to consumers on healthy living, relationships, conditions and treatments, services and support, www.betterhealth.vic.gov.au

Bush Crisis Line—information about the 24-hour bush crisis line. It also contains resources for supporting rural and remote practitioners and their families in managing the stress associated with remote and rural practice. These resources include information sheets, links and other information on post traumatic stress disorder, surviving stress and preventing burn-out, https://crana.org.au/support/

Environmental Science and Research, New Zealand—annual reports on notifiable and other diseases in New Zealand, www.surv.esr.cri.nz

Family Planning NSW—detailed information on safe sex and emergency contraception, www.fpnsw.org.au/

Ministry of Health, New Zealand—access to publications, health education resources, data and statistics, guidelines, newsletters and online library catalogue, www.moh.govt.nz

National Centre in HIV Epidemiology and Clinical Research—here you will find the Annual Surveillance Report for HIV/AIDS, viral hepatitis and sexually transmissible infections in Australia, http://web.med.unsw.edu.au/nchecr

New Zealand Guidelines Group—evidence for practice for healthcare professionals and consumers and has information on women's health issues, www.nzgg.org.nz

NSW Health Department—information about STIs, emergency contraception and safe sex for consumers as well as healthcare professionals, www.health.nsw.gov.au/publichealth/sexualhealth/sex_factsheets.asp

Royal Australian and New Zealand College of Obstetricians and Gynaecologists—access to publications, guidelines and other information pertaining to women's health and gynaecology, www.ranzcog.edu.au

Women's Health Collaborative Core Curriculum—information and links here that are relevant to the study, teaching and practice of women's healthcare, https://ctl.curtin.edu.au/events/conferences/tlf/tlf2002/carr.html

REFERENCES

1. Fraser D, Cooper M, eds. Myles' textbook for midwives. 15th edn. Edinburgh: Churchill Livingstone; 2009.

2. Sanders Jordan K. Gynecologic emergencies. In: Howard PK, Steinmann RA, eds. Sheehy's emergency nursing: principles and practice. 6th edn. St Louis: Mosby; 2009:578–89.

3. Heitman RJ. Anatomy of the female reproductive system. In: DeCherney AH, Nathan L, Goodwin TM et al. eds. Current diagnosis and treatment obstetrics and gynecology, electronic format. 11th edn. USA: McGraw-Hill; 2013:1–37.

4. Callahan T, Caughey A. Blueprint's obstetrics and gynaecology. 6th edn. Philadelphia: Lippincott Williams & Wilkins; 2013.

5. Ambulance Service of New South Wales. NSW Ambulance Service Protocols and Pharmacology 2013.

6. Gilboy N. Unit III. Clinical foundations of emergency nursing. Chapter 7: Triage. In: Howard PK, Steinmann RA, eds. Sheehy's emergency nursing: principles and practice. 6th edn. St Louis: Mosby; 2009:59–72.

7. Lentz GM, Lobo RA, Gershenson DM, Katz VL. Comprehensive gynaecology. 6th edn. Philadelphia : Elsevier Mosby; 2013.

8. Dart R. Pelvic pain. In: Mitchell EL, Medzon R, eds. Introduction to emergency medicine. Philadelphia: Lippincott Williams & Wilkins; 2005:225–33.

9. Eliseo LJ. Abnormal vaginal bleeding in the non-pregnant patient. In: Mitchell EL, Medzon R, eds. Introduction to emergency medicine. Philadelphia: Lippincott Williams & Wilkins; 2005:201–7.

10. The Royal Australian College of General Practitioners, 2011. The RACGP Curriculum for Australian General Practice woman's health, Online http://curriculum.racgp.org.au/media/12308/womenshealth.pdf; accessed 16 April 2015.

11. The Royal Australian and New Zealand College of Obstetricians and Gynaecologists. College Statement Female Genital Mutilation (FMG). 2013 http://www.ranzcog.edu.au/college-statements-guidelines.html#gynaecology; accessed 16 April 2015.

12. Weston G, Vollenhoven B. Menstrual and other disorders. In: McDonald S, Thompson C, eds. Women's health: a handbook. Sydney: Elsevier; 2005:146–214.

13. NSW Health Maternity. Management of early pregnancy complications, 2012, Online: www0.health.nsw.gov.au/policies/pd/2012/PD2012_022.html; accessed 16 April 2015.

14. BMJ Best practice, miscarriage classifications, August 2013. Online: http://bestpractice.hmj.com.acs.hcn.com.au/best-practice/monograph/666/resources/references.html; accessed 16 April 2015.

15. AACC, Lab tests Online HCG the test, 22 June 2012. Online: http://labtestsonline.org/understanding/analytes/hcg/tab/test; accessed 16 April 2015.

16. HealthPathways Core Development Team. Miscarriage assessment, miscarriage management 2008–2014. Online http://hne.healthpathways.org.au/index.htm?toc.htm?12527.htm; accessed 16 April 2015.

17. RANZOG Management of Postpartum Haemorrhage (PPH), March 2014. Online: www.ranzcog.edu.au/doc/management-of-postpartum-haemorrhage.html PDF file; accessed 16 April 2015.

18. Maame Yaa A B Yiadom. Postpartum hemorrhage in emergency medicine. Mar 2014 Online: http://emedicine.medscape.com/article/796785-overview; accessed 16 April 2015.

19. Victorian Ambulance Service, Obstetric Emergencies CPG 2012, Online. www.ambulance.vic.gov.au/Media/docs/x03_CPG_OBSTETRIC-web-9a57627e-c340-4f99-89b9-9686f60b1d12-0.pdf; accessed 16 April 2015.

20. Belfort MA. Management of postpartum hemorrhage at vaginal delivery, July 2014. Online: www.uptodate.com/contents/management-of-postpartum-hemorrhage-at-vaginaldelivery?source=search_result&search=uterotonics&selectedTitle=1%7E11#H6; accessed 16 April 2015.

21. Cook K. Pelvic pain in females. In: Bourke S, ed. National management guidelines for sexually transmissible infections. SHSOV; 2008:35–44.

22. O'Connor V. Lower abdominal pain. In: Finn M, Bowyer L, Carr S et al. eds. Women's health: a core curriculum. Sydney: Elsevier; 2005:49–54.

23. Burgeois J, Bray M, Mathews C. Obstetrics and gynaecology—Recall. 3rd edn. Philadelphia: Woters Kluwer, Lippincott Williams & Wilkins, 2008.

24. Weston G, Vollenhoven B. Menstrual and other disorders. In: McDonald S, Thompson C, eds. Women's health: a handbook. Sydney: Elsevier; 2005:146–214.

25. Akhter S, Beckmann K, Gorelick M. Update on sexually transmitted infections. Paediatric Emerg Care 2008;25(9):608–17

26. Therapeutic Guidelines. Therapeutic guidelines: antibiotics. Version 15. Melbourne: Therapeutic Guidelines; 2010. Online. http://etg.hcn.com.au/desktop/index.htm?acc=36422; accessed 20 April 2015.

27. Platt MD, Mallory MN. Obstetric and gynaecologic emergencies and rape. In: Stone CK, Humphries R, eds. Current diagnosis and treatment emergency medicine. 6th edn. New York: McGraw-Hill; 2008.

28. IVF Australia. Your pathway of care. IVF Australia's guide to assisted reproduction. Version 8; 2009.

29. Kwan I, Bhattacharya S, McNeil A et al. Monitoring of stimulated cycles in assisted reproduction (IVF and ICSI). Cochrane Database Syst Rev 2008; 16(2).

30. Miller MA, Wirtz E, Pease J. An unusual case of tachycardia, hypotension, and intraabdominal free fluid: ovarian hyperstimulation syndrome. Am J Emerg Med 2008;26(6):736.

31. Saul T, Sonson JM. Ovarian hyperstimulation syndrome. Am J Emerg Med 2009;27(2):250e3–e4.

32. Goh J, Flynn M. Examination obstetrics and gynaecology 3rd edn. Sydney: Churchill Livingstone; 2011.

33. Dart R, Steinberg R. Pelvic infections. In: Mitchell EL, Medzon R, eds. Introduction to emergency medicine. Philadelphia: Lippincott Williams & Wilkins; 2005:216–24.

34. Brown A, Cadogan M. Emergency medicine: diagnosis and management. 6th edn. London: Hodder Arnold; 2011:376–81.

35. Chen M. The Australasian contact tracing manual. 4th edn. Australasian Society of HIV Medicine (ASHM). Canberra: Commonwealth of Australia; 2010. Online: http://ctm.ashm.org.au/Default.asp?TOC=true&PublicationID=6; accessed 16 April 2015.

36. ESR The Institute of Environmental Science and Research Ltd. Sexually Transmitted Infections in New Zealand: Annual Surveillance Report 2012 Porirua, New Zealand. Online https://surv.esr.cri.nz/PDF_surveillance/STISurvRpt/2012/2012AnnualSTIReport.pdf; accessed 16 April 2015.

37. McAllister L, Street A. Talking with colleagues, patients, clients and carers. In: Higgs J, Sefton A, Street A et al. eds. Communicating in the health and social sciences. Melbourne: Oxford University; 2005:218–29.

38. The Kirby Institute. National Blood–Borne Virus and Sexually transmissible Infections: Surveillance and Monitoring Report, 2013. The Kirby Institute, the University of New South Wales, Sydney NSW. Online. www.kirby.unsw.edu.au/sites/default/files/hiv/resources/NBBVSTI2013_0.pdf; accessed 16 April 2015.

39. Bradford D, Hoy J, Matthews G. HIV, viral hepatitis and STIs: a guide for primary care. Australasian Society for HIV Medicine (ASHM); 2008. Online: www.ashm.org.au/images/publications/monographs/HIV_viral_hepatitis_and_STIs_a_guide_for_primary_care/hiv_viral_hepatitis_and_stis_whole.pdf.

40. Thorogood C. Challenges to women's health. In: Pairman S, Pincombe J, Thorogood C et al. eds. Midwifery: preparation for practice. 2nd edn. Sydney: Churchill Livingstone; 2010.

41. Australian Herpes Management Forum (AHMF). Guidelines for clinicians: reducing the sexual transmission of genital herpes. Australia: Westmead Hospital, Westmead NSW; 2011.

42. Jaffe J, Morris JE. Infectious disease emergencies. In: Stone CK, Humphries R, eds. Current diagnosis and treatment emergency medicine. 6th edn. New York: McGraw Hill; 2008.

43. Australian Bureau of Statistics. Sexually transmissible infections 2011. Online. www.abs.gov.au/AUSSTATS/abs@.nsf/Lookup/4102.0Main+Features10Jun+2012#Intro; accessed 10 June 2015.

44. Tebb KP, Wibbelsman C, Neuhaus JM et al. Screening for asymptomatic Chlamydia infections among sexually active adolescent girls during paediatric urgent care. Arch Pediatr Adolesc Med 2009;163(6):559–64.

45. NSW Health. Sexually transmissible infections (STIs) and blood borne viruses (BBVs) factsheets. 2013. Online: www.health.nsw.gov.au/Infectious/Pages/a-to-z-infectious-diseases.aspx; accessed 10 June 2015.

46. Commonwealth of Australia Second National Sexually Transmissible Infections Strategy 2010–2013 2010. Online www.health.gov.au/internet/main/publishing.nsf/Content/ohp-national-strategies-2010-sti/$File/sti.pdf

47. Erian M, Jones I, O'Connor V. Sexually transmitted infections. In: Finn M, Bowyer L, Carr S et al. eds. Women's health: a core curriculum. Sydney: Elsevier; 2005.

48. Leaver D, Labonte G. HPV and cervical cancer. Radiation Therapist 2010;19(1):27–45.

49. Huppert JS. Trichomonosis in teens: an update. Curr Opin Obstet Gynaecol 2009;21:371–8.

50. Allsworth J, Ratner J, Peipert J. Trichomoniasis and other sexually transmitted infections: results from the 2001–2004 national health and nutrition examination surveys. Sex Transm Dis 2009;36(12):738–44.

51. Sangkomkamhang US, Lumbiganon P, Prasertcharoensook W et al. Antenatal lower genital tract infection screening and treatment programs for preventing preterm delivery. The Cochrane Collaboration: John Wiley; 2009. Online. http://mrw.interscience.wiley.com/cochrane/clsysrev/articles/CD006178/frame.html

52. Bradford D, Hoy J, Matthews G. HIV, viral hepatitis and STIs: a guide for primary care. Australasian Society for HIV Medicine (ASHM); 2008. Online: www.ashm.org.au/images/publications/monographs/HIV_viral_hepatitis_and_STIs_a_guide_for_primary_care/hiv_viral_hepatitis_and_stis_whole.pdf.

53. Stone CK, Humphries RL. Current diagnosis and treatment: emergency medicine. 6th edn. New York: McGraw-Hill; 2008.

54. Huffam S, Haber P, Wallace J et al. Talking with the patient: risk assessment and history taking. In: Bradford D, Hoy J, Matthews G, eds. HIV, viral hepatitis and STIs: a guide for primary care. Australasian Society for HIV Medicine (ASHM); 2008.

CHAPTER 35
OBSTETRIC EMERGENCIES
ALLISON CUMMINS AND CAROLINE HOMER

Essentials

- Modifications to basic and advanced basic life support approaches are appropriate for the pregnant woman in cardiac arrest because of the physiological changes that are present in pregnancy and the early postpartum period. One important modification is the necessity to tilt or wedge a pregnant woman from a supine position during ambulance transfer and cardiopulmonary resuscitation.

- Maternal collapse may be caused by thromboembolism, haemorrhage, amniotic fluid embolism, genital tract sepsis or pre-existing cardiac disease.

- Breathlessness and tachycardia are keys to the diagnosis of pulmonary embolism.

- Ectopic pregnancy should be considered in *all* women of childbearing age who present to the Emergency Department (ED) with abdominal pain.

- Women with a headache severe enough to seek medical advice or with new epigastric pain should have their blood pressure taken and urine checked for protein.

- Sepsis is often insidious in onset with a fulminating course. The severity of illness should not be underestimated.

- Trauma in pregnancy can also occur as a result of domestic violence. Domestic violence has immediate and long-term effects on the woman and her baby.

- Amniotic fluid embolism is a rare emergency, but carries a high risk of mortality. The usual scenario is that the woman experiences acute respiratory distress, then collapses often after pushing in the second stage of labour or immediately after the birth of the baby.

- A perimortem caesarean section can save the life of both the mother and baby if undertaken in the first 5 minutes after a cardiac arrest in the acute setting.

- The collapse and resuscitation of a pregnant woman is very stressful and difficult for the woman's family. They need accurate and timely information conveyed sensitively.

- Debriefing for all staff involved in obstetric emergencies should occur as soon as possible.

INTRODUCTION

For most women, pregnancy is a normal life event and most babies are born healthy without complications. Obstetric emergencies are fortunately rare; however, they can occur at home or in hospital settings. In hospital, most of these women will be in maternity units (often a birthing unit); however, some women will present through the ED or be seen first by paramedical personnel. Knowledge of the normal reproductive system and functions are necessary to care for women who have an obstetric emergency. This chapter will initially review the relevant anatomy and physiology in relation to the changes that occur during pregnancy and how these impact on emergency situations. This is followed by a description of the most acute of all obstetric emergencies, that is, a maternal collapse or cardiac arrest requiring cardiopulmonary resuscitation (CPR). This includes a discussion of the modifications that need to be made to CPR in pregnant or newly postpartum women and the requirements for a perimortem caesarean section. Caring for the family and the staff and investigating and learning from critical events such as these are also addressed. Integral to the care provided is obtaining informed consent from the woman where possible and the next of kin where the woman is unconscious. The next section of the chapter briefly describes the major obstetric emergencies that may be seen in women who present to EDs or who are admitted to intensive care units.

Obstetric emergencies are a large topic and this chapter cannot cover them all in detail. Readers are advised to access other resources, including the midwifery textbook: *Midwifery: Preparation for Practice*, which has a chapter on life-threatening emergencies and covers a number of other obstetric emergencies in more depth.[1]

Obstetric emergencies in an ED

The most recent *UK Confidential Enquiry into Maternal Deaths* reports the initial failure by many clinical staff to immediately recognise and act on the signs and symptoms of life-threatening conditions for pregnant women. A section on *Back to Basics* was included in the report to guide clinicians.[2] A recommendation from the confidential enquiries into maternal deaths in the United Kingdom[2] is the use of a modified early obstetric warning system. Observation and response charts for deteriorating patients have been introduced in Australia with some states and territories having modified the charts for pregnant women.[3]

A prior *UK Confidential Enquiry into Maternal Deaths* found that 52 of the 350 women who died from direct, indirect or coincidental causes died in the ED.[4] The majority of these women had either collapsed in the community and were already undergoing CPR on arrival or collapsed shortly afterwards. Of the women whose care was assessed in relation to ED practice, the main causes were:

- pulmonary embolism
- ectopic pregnancy
- intracerebral bleed
- sepsis
- road traffic crashes.

The other significant maternal conditions that may be seen in an ED or other critical care service are eclampsia and amniotic fluid embolism.

As there are no similar data for Australian women who present through EDs, and many of the issues will be similar to the UK context, this work has been drawn upon throughout this chapter.

Anatomy and physiology

From the onset of conception and throughout pregnancy, a woman's body undergoes many changes to allow her to accommodate and support her baby as it grows and to prepare for birth and the postnatal period. These changes occur under the influences of the hormones of pregnancy and aim to maintain and develop the women's pregnancy and the growing

baby. These changes may also increase the risk factors for some women in emergency situations.

A brief description of the main changes is presented in the next section. The section is based on a number of textbooks and reference material.[5–7] In addition, the textbook *Physiology in Childbearing*[8] provides a detailed description of the specific physiology and physiological changes.

Influence of pregnancy hormones

Oestrogen, progesterone, human chorionic gonadotrophin (hCG), human placental lactogen and relaxin are the main hormones of pregnancy, and they produce significant physiological and anatomical changes during pregnancy. Progesterone and oestrogen, produced early in pregnancy by the corpus luteum then by the placenta, work closely together for the maintenance of the pregnancy and adaptation of the mother's body in preparation for delivery and breastfeeding.

Human chorionic gonadotrophin is produced early in pregnancy as the placenta is developing and the chorionic villi embed into the uterine wall. Its main function is to maintain the corpus luteum during early pregnancy, allowing for continued secretion of oestrogen and progesterone to maintain the pregnancy, and to prevent the shedding of the endometrium, as usually occurs during the menstrual cycle. Human chorionic gonadotrophin also suppresses the maternal lymphocyte response to prevent the maternal immune system from rejecting the placenta. The hCG levels present in either urine or blood are used as indicators of pregnancy.

The placenta produces human placental lactogen (also known as human chorionic somatomammotrophin). This hormone has the primary function of promoting fetal growth. It produces a degree of maternal insulin resistance, which then alters the maternal metabolism and use of protein, carbohydrate and fat. This process changes the availability of glucose, which may be metabolised by the growing baby.

Relaxin is produced by the corpus luteum and then the placenta. It has some effects—working with progesterone—in relaxing the uterus to inhibit uterine activity during pregnancy. It also aids in the relaxation of the ligaments within the woman's pelvis and softens the cervix during labour.

Uterus

Under the influence of oestrogen and progesterone the woman's uterus relaxes and grows to accommodate the growing baby. The non-pregnant uterus weighs approximately 60 g and has a volume of approximately 10 mL. As a result of growth of the muscle fibres and increased vascular supply, the uterus increases to a weight of 1000 g and a volume of approximately 5000 mL by term.

The increase in size of the uterus and the growth of the baby produce changes in the anatomical location of the uterus. During early pregnancy, a woman's uterus is a pelvic organ; however, by the 12th week of pregnancy the uterus becomes an abdominal organ. At 20 weeks gestation the top of the uterus is at the umbilical region and by 36 to 40 weeks is at the level of the xiphisternum. The blood supply to the uterus is approximately 500 to 700 mL each minute at term, which is a significant risk factor in the reasons for haemorrhage being a leading cause of maternal death. The growth of the uterus displaces the bowel and affects how a physical assessment is performed. The pregnant or gravid uterus also poses the risk of compression of the inferior vena cava when the woman is lying supine. The inferior vena cava is compressed in the majority of pregnant women in the second trimester, and the compression may affect the uterine artery blood flow but not the fetal circulation.

As pregnancy progresses into the third trimester the uterus grows and develops an upper and lower segment. The upper segment is the ideal region for the placenta to implant as it has three layers of muscle fibres to anchor the placenta during pregnancy and to act as ligatures to the vessels of the placental site when the placenta separates at delivery. The lower segment has two layers of muscle fibres. If the placenta embeds in the lower region of the uterus it may ultimately be anchored in the lower segment. Low-lying placentas have a risk of premature separation leading to an antepartum haemorrhage and there is greater chance of a postpartum haemorrhage because of reduced ligature effects of the muscle layers.

Cervix

Under the effects of oestrogen and progesterone the cervix has increased vascularity and secretory effects. Early in pregnancy a mucus plug called the operculum develops in the cervix as a guard against ascending infection. Later in pregnancy there is a softening effect to allow for dilation and subsequent birth of the baby. There is a change to the cervical cells, which leads to a risk of bleeding directly from the cervix if the cells are disrupted, for example, during sexual intercourse or a vaginal examination.

Vagina

Under the influence of oestrogen and progesterone, vaginal changes include increased vascularity, hypertrophy of the muscle and changes to the connective tissue, which allows for the passage of the baby at birth. Secretory changes create a more acid environment as a protective mechanism against infection; this may also lead to a white discharge called leucorrhoea, which is a normal discharge during pregnancy.

Breasts

During pregnancy, oestrogen and progesterone stimulate changes to the breasts by increasing blood supply and developing the glandular tissue and the duct system in preparation for lactation. The overall hormone effects cause enlargement of the breasts, up to 5 cm and 1400 g in weight by term.

Respiratory

As the uterus enlarges and pushes up against the diaphragm and the unborn baby's need for oxygen supply and removal of carbon dioxide increases, respiratory changes occur to accommodate these demands. The woman's residual volume decreases because of the enlarging uterus; however, there is a slight flaring of the ribs to cater for the physical changes within the abdomen and thoracic cavity. There is decreased airway resistance, an increase in tidal volume, the arterial partial pressure of oxygen increases up to 105 mmHg and the maternal sensitivity to CO_2 is decreased to approximately 32 mmHg. The increased consumption of oxygen by the pregnant woman is necessary for the needs of the unborn baby.

Cardiovascular and haematological changes

As pregnancy progresses the vascular changes taking place within the uterus, cervix, vagina and breast tissue require an increase in circulating blood volume. Oestrogen and progesterone both have the effect of promoting fluid and electrolyte retention throughout pregnancy to meet these needs. Antidiuretic hormone and aldosterone also play a role in maintaining plasma volume.

Physiological effects include:

- an increase in plasma volume of approximately 45% by 32 weeks of pregnancy. The increase in blood volume predominantly supplies the uterus and helps to compensate for blood loss at delivery through an autotransfusion effect as uterine blood flow decreases and is shunted to the main circulation.
- vascular changes occur to allow for the increased blood volume. Metabolites of progesterone alter the response to the pressor action of angiotensin II, which leads to a vasodilatory effect and is evident in the normal pregnancy by a drop in blood pressure. The peak effect is usually by 28 to 34 weeks of pregnancy.
- cardiac output increases by 30–40%. This is achieved through a slight increase in heart rate, an increase in stroke volume and a decrease in systemic vascular resistance. The heart muscle increases in size to meet the increasing workload and is also slightly displaced (turned to the left) as the uterus pushes up against the diaphragm. This may be represented by a left axis deviation on a 12-lead ECG. The woman's red blood cell count increases by approximately 25% to meet the increased metabolic demands; however, since the plasma volume increases at a greater rate the woman typically experiences a physiological anaemia.
- anticoagulation components decrease, coagulation factors VII, VIII, IX and X increase; there is a slight increase in platelet numbers and there is an increased tendency to aggregate. The purpose is protective, to guard against haemorrhage; however, this does increase the risk of thromboembolism and pulmonary embolism, which is a leading cause of maternal mortality.

Gastrointestinal tract

The gastrointestinal tract plays a role in maintaining intravascular fluid volume by decreasing motility and increasing absorption. This leads to a risk of constipation and potential for mechanical obstruction. The woman's enlarging uterus also impinges on the gastrointestinal tract: as her abdomen has to accommodate the bowel and gravid uterus the stomach is displaced and emptying may be slowed due to increased intragastric pressures, which also increases the incidence of reflux.

Hepatic system

The increased metabolic demands of pregnancy increase the woman's hepatic workload. There is an increase in the viscosity of bile and the residual volume in the gallbladder, which increases the incidence of gallstone formation. The delayed bile flow can also result in mild jaundice and pruritus related to the deposits of bile salts in subcutaneous tissue—known as cholestasis of pregnancy.

Renal system

The increase in circulating volume leads to an increase in renal blood flow and glomerular filtration rate. The increase in glomerular filtration rate reduces the ability of the renal tubules to reabsorb substances such as glucose, amino acids, folic acids and some minerals.

Endocrine system

During pregnancy the woman enters into a mild hyperthyroid state which increases her basal metabolic rate to meet the increased demands of pregnancy. The increase in cardiac output and heart rate, combined with the effects of progesterone, causes vasodilation which accommodates the increased blood volume. The adrenal gland has some increase in function, in particular, increasing blood cortisol levels to meet the stressors of pregnancy and aldosterone to support the increased circulating volume. The pancreas increases the production of insulin; however, under the influence of human placental lactogen there is a decreased sensitivity to insulin, to allow for greater availability of glucose for the baby. The decreased sensitivity to insulin may also result in pregnancy-induced diabetes, which may pose risks to the woman and her unborn baby.

Immune system

During pregnancy there is a general depression of maternal immunity due to lymphocyte depressant factor and increased adrenal cortex activity. This is designed to prevent an immune response rejecting the baby which contains the father's 'foreign' DNA. Women who are Rhesus-negative and have a baby with Rhesus-positive blood are at risk of isoimmunisation which occurs when fetal blood mixes with the maternal circulation and the mother develops antibodies to the positive Rhesus factor. Exposure may occur during miscarriage, amniotic fluid sampling and placental abruption, or at delivery. Iso-immunisation is a complication for any subsequent pregnancies where the baby has a positive blood group as the mother's immune response is triggered to act against the fetal blood. Women who are Rhesus-negative should be given anti-D immunoglobulin within 72 hours of an actual or suspected exposure, to prevent isoimmunisation.

Recognition of the sick woman

One of the core skills of being a clinician is the recognition of a patient who is unwell. This is not the same as making a diagnosis. In fact the two skills are often independent of each other. Recognition of the seriously ill pregnant or postpartum woman relies on taking a complete history (listening to the cues given by her or her family) and measurement and understanding of vital signs such as heart rate, respiratory rate, temperature and pulse oximetry. It is important to reflect on the stages of shock in recognising a woman who is unwell as these basic skills will provide valuable information. It is also important to remember that pregnant women who are sick often remain looking well for longer than they would if they were not pregnant due to the physiological compensatory changes of pregnancy.

Recognition of the sick woman does not depend on complex and time-consuming tests. Recognition of illness needs to be taught to clinicians of all grades on a regular basis. It is also important to make this teaching multi-disciplinary.[9]

In recognising the sick woman, Hulbert,[9] an emergency doctor writing in the *UK Confidential Enquiry into Maternal Deaths*, stated that:

> Tachycardia is without doubt the most significant clinical feature of an unwell patient and is regularly ignored or misunderstood.

Measurements of respiratory rate and heart rate are infinitely more important than measurements of blood pressure. A normotensive patient may all too often be unwell and compensating. A tachycardic patient is hypovolaemic until proved otherwise. A patient with tachypnoea has a cardiorespiratory cause until proved otherwise. Attributing tachycardia and tachypnoea to anxiety is naïve and dangerous (p. 234).[9]

Maternal collapse

The cardiorespiratory collapse of a pregnant or postpartum woman (known as a maternal collapse) is the most dramatic of the obstetric emergencies. Cardiac arrest complicates 1 in 20,000–30,000 pregnancies, with a maternal survival rate of 6.9%.[2,10] Women are more likely to survive such an event if it happens in an acute care setting than in the community. All maternity care providers need to be adequately trained, with access to in-service education, such as emergency drill simulations to increase the survival rate for women suffering from maternal collapse.[11]

Fortunately maternal collapse and/or cardiac arrest are rare events, but they have catastrophic consequences for mother and baby. The leading cause of direct maternal deaths for the triennium 2006–08 in the UK was genital tract sepsis, preeclampsia/eclampsia followed by thromboembolism and amniotic fluid embolism.[2] Unfortunately, the early warning signs of impending maternal collapse often go unrecognised and the early detection of severe illness in pregnant women remains a challenge to all involved in their care. The relative rarity of such events, combined with the normal changes in physiology associated with pregnancy and childbirth, compounds the problem.[2]

PRACTICE TIP

The cardiovascular, respiratory and gastrointestinal changes that most affect resuscitation include:

Increased:
- plasma volume by 40 to 50%
- erythrocyte volume by only 20%
- cardiac output by 40%
- heart rate by 15–20 bpm
- clotting factors
- sequestration of blood to the uterus—30% of cardiac output flows to the uterus
- oxygen consumption by 20%
- tidal volume (progesterone-mediated)
- laryngeal angle and pharyngeal oedema

Decreased:
- arterial blood pressure by 10–15 mmHg
- systemic vascular resistance
- colloid oncotic pressure (COP) and pulmonary capillary wedge pressure
- functional residual capacity by 25%
- gastric peristalsis and motility
- effectiveness of the gastro-oesophageal (cardiac) sphincter of the stomach

The physiological changes of pregnancy alter the resuscitation of women who have a maternal collapse. These alterations need to be considered whether maternal collapse occurs in or out of hospital. The main physiological changes to consider are related to the respiratory and cardiovascular systems.[12,13]

In addition, in the supine position the pregnant uterus compresses the descending aorta and the inferior vena cava, reducing cardiac output, blood pressure and venous return. This explains the rationale for tilting the woman towards her left side during resuscitation.

These physiological changes result in a dilutional anaemia, which results in decreased oxygen-carrying capacity and increased CPR circulation demands, and also means that pregnant women are susceptible to thromboembolism. The respiratory changes mean that women are susceptible to a rapid decrease of PaO_2 with respiratory alkalosis and there are often difficulties with intubation. The gastrointestinal changes mean women have an increased risk of regurgitation and aspiration.

Modifications of basic life support in maternal collapse

Several modifications to BLS and ALS approaches are appropriate for the pregnant woman in cardiac arrest because of the physiological changes that are present in pregnancy and the early postpartum period.[13–15] Table 35.1 describes the modifications required.

TABLE 35.1 Maternal cardiac arrest algorithm[15]

MATERNAL CARDIAC ARREST

First responder

- Activate maternal cardiac arrest team
- Document time of onset of maternal cardiac arrest
- Place the patient supine
- Start chest compressions as per BLS, place hands slightly higher than usual

Subsequent responders

Maternal interventions	Obstetric interventions for patient with an obvious gravid uterus*
- Treat per BLS and ACLS algorithm - Do not delay defibrillation - Give typical ACLS drugs and doses - Ventilate with 100% oxygen - Monitor waveform capnography and CPR quality - Provide post-cardiac arrest care as appropriate	- Perform manual uterine displacement (LUD)—displace uterus to the patient's left to relieve aortocaval compression - Remove both internal and external fetal monitors if present - *Obstetric and neonatal teams should immediately prepare for possible emergency caesarean section* - If no return of spontaneous circulation by 4 minutes of resuscitative efforts, consider performing emergency caesarean section - Aim for delivery within 5 minutes of onset of resuscitative efforts

Maternal modifications

- Start IV above the diaphragm
- Assess for hypovolaemia and give fluid bolus when required
- Anticipate difficult airway; experienced staff member preferred for advanced airway placement
- If patient receiving IV/IO magnesium pre-arrest, stop magnesium and give IV/IO calcium chloride 10 mL in 10% solution or calcium gluconate 30 mL in 10% solution
- Continue all maternal resuscitative interventions (CPR, positioning, defibrillation, drugs, and fluids) during and after caesarean section

Search for and treat possible contributing factors

Bleeding

Embolism: coronary/pulmonary/amiotic fluid embolism

Anaesthetic complications

Uterine atony

Cardiac disease (MI/ischaemia/ aortic dissection/cardiomyopathy)

Hypertension/preeclampsia/eclampsia

Other: differential diagnosis of standard ACLS guidelines

Placenta abruptio/praevia

Sepsis

*An obvious gravid uterus is a uterus that is deemed clinically to be sufficiently large to cause aortocaval compression

The primary survey can be undertaken whether the woman collapses in hospital or in the community. Paramedics are often the front-line health professionals in these situations and need to consider the modifications of BLS required. It is essential that the pregnant woman is tilted using a wedge behind her back during ambulance transfer and CPR.

Life-saving surgery—caesarean section

A caesarean section is not only a last attempt to save the life of the baby, it is also an important intervention in the resuscitation of the woman in the acute care setting.[12,16] A caesarean section (known in this instance as a perimortem caesarean section) improves maternal and fetal outcomes for both mother and baby where no possibility of survival would exist in a non-perfused uterus.[13] It is recommended that perimortem caesarean section be undertaken early in the resuscitation attempt (within 5 minutes) and that equipment to facilitate this should be available on the emergency trolleys, especially in labour wards and EDs.[17,18]

PRACTICE TIP

Perimortem caesarean section is indicated when:
- personnel with appropriate skill and equipment to perform the procedure are available
- the woman fails to respond with a return of spontaneous circulation within 4 minutes
- can be performed any time the fundus is palpable above the umbilicus, as the main aim is maternal survival
- appropriate facilities and personnel are available to care for the woman and baby after the procedure.

It would be unusual for a perimortem caesarean section to be conducted in the community by paramedic staff as it is unlikely that they would have the appropriate skill and/or equipment or have on hand the facilities and personnel to care for the woman and baby after the procedure.

Survival rates for the woman and her baby are improved when perimortem caesarean section is performed within 5 minutes of ineffective maternal circulation. It may still be worthwhile to undertake a caesarean section after this period as fetal mortality is 100% if no action is taken. Some infants have survived perimortem caesarean section up to 20 minutes after maternal death. Perimortem caesarean section also increases the chance of the woman's survival. Without caesarean section, less than 10% of women suffering in-hospital cardiac arrest will survive to hospital discharge. With a caesarean section, maternal survival increases because removal of the baby results in an improvement in maternal circulation during cardiopulmonary resuscitation.[13,19] A study from the Netherlands reported a maternal case fatality rate of 83% and a neonatal case fatality rate of 58% in 55 women over a 15-year period.[17] The authors highlighted that none of the women had the caesarean section undertaken within the recommended 5 minutes after starting resuscitation and if this had been done the outcomes may have improved.

Caring for the family

The collapse and subsequent resuscitation of a pregnant woman is likely to be a very stressful and difficult time for the woman's family. Serious illness or death during pregnancy or early in the postnatal period is usually the furthest thing from any family's mind. They are likely to be shocked and express disbelief at what is going on. Particular attention needs to be paid to the woman's partner or support people who may be with her. It is likely that they will be very distressed with the situation and the resuscitation efforts that are occurring. One of the healthcare team needs to take responsibility to care for the partner and any other family or support people who are present. This may include staying with them in the room while the resuscitation takes place, but it may be that not being present may be indicated. The partner and support people need accurate and timely information and this needs to be conveyed sensitively.

Caring for the staff

A cardiac arrest or a major collapse of a pregnant woman is distressing for staff as well as the family. Pregnancy is usually surrounded with positive feelings and happiness. The collapse of a pregnant woman, which may result in one or two deaths (mother and/or baby), is one of the hardest things that health staff will have to cope with.

Debriefing for all staff involved in the event should occur as soon as possible. Often a group discussion works well in these situations where each person has a chance to talk about their experience. Often a person who was not directly involved in the event should facilitate such a group meeting as they will be more objective and can ensure the discussion remains safe and supportive. It is essential that this is undertaken in a safe and supported environment and elements of blame and recriminations are not part of this process. It is important to ensure that staff members are supported in their own shock and sadness and have the opportunity to reflect upon the event and the care provided. This is also an opportunity to reflect on the systems and assess which ones worked well and how things could be improved in the future if such an event happened again.

Investigating and reflecting

A maternal collapse, and certainly a cardiac arrest in a pregnant or postpartum woman, would be considered a serious adverse event. If the woman dies, it would be considered to be a maternal death. Maternal deaths are defined as:

> … the death of a woman while pregnant or within 42 days of termination of pregnancy, irrespective of the duration and site of the pregnancy, from any cause related to or aggravated by the pregnancy or its management but not from accidental or incidental causes.[20]

Maternal deaths are a sentinel event.[21] In most jurisdictions in Australia and in New Zealand, maternal deaths require statutory reporting to the relevant health department. Such an event would also be classified in the risk management systems as one of the most severe adverse events (for example, given a Severity Assessment Code of 1). Events assessed as being a Severity Assessment Code 1 will usually be subject to a Root Cause Analysis to determine what the root causes of the event were and whether any changes need to be made, particularly to the systems and processes, to reduce the chance of this occurring in the future.[22–26]

Summary of management

A number of key points should be remembered when confronted with a pregnant woman who has a cardiorespiratory collapse and requires resuscitation.[14,18] These are summarised in the box below. The immediate modifications to BLS are relevant to paramedic and hospital-based staff.

Clinical presentations

Supporting a normal birth

The first section provided an outline of how to support and attend a woman who unexpectedly presents to an ED in labour and looks like she is progressing quickly to give birth. A normal vaginal birth is likely in this scenario. This section is based on clinical experience of the authors and midwifery texts.[7,27]

Most of the women presenting to an ED in advanced labour will give birth to a baby who will be born head-first. Sometimes, especially if the baby is premature (that is, the woman is before 37 weeks pregnant), the baby may be born bottom-first, which is known as a breech birth. The principles for both births in an emergency situation are essentially the same—call for help (hopefully a midwife is available in the maternity unit); ensure the woman is in a safe, private space; support the woman to be upright to give birth, and have a warm space for the baby and warm blankets for both mother and baby.

Signs of an imminent birth include the woman having strong (usually painful), regular contractions. She will often describe a feeling of pressure in her vagina or rectum and an urge to push and will often be pushing involuntarily while making grunting noises. Call a midwife, if no midwife is available, then call a medical officer. Provide privacy for the woman and allow her to find a comfortable position to give birth. Invite her support person to stay with her. Ensure the room is warm and there are warm towels ready to dry the baby. Ask the woman or any support people she has with her when the baby was due as this will help determine if the baby will be premature and if this is her first second or subsequent baby (second and subsequent babies are usually born more quickly). It is important to keep calm and quiet and ensure that not too many people are in the room. Try not to disturb the woman unnecessarily.

Once the woman starts really pushing, help her into a comfortable position—being on hands and knees is the best position (Fig 35.1). Try not to have her lying on her back at any time. Ensure her underwear is removed. She may pass some blood-stained mucus from her vagina. She may also pass faeces or urine as the baby's head is descending; the area may be wiped if the woman agrees, but it may be too sensitive. The membranes (holding the waters around the baby) usually rupture at this time and fluid will be observed draining from the woman's vagina. This is all very normal.

The woman may be very vocal, crying or quiet. It is important for the staff to keep quiet and calm and encourage the woman—tell her that she is doing well and the baby will be born soon. The baby's head will gradually come into view as the labia part. Talk calmly to the woman as you see the baby's head. Place a clean sheet under the woman and put on personal protective equipment, gloves, gown and eye protection. Open a birth pack if you have one (Fig 35.2).

The woman will push involuntarily—just talk calmly to her. There is no need to tell the woman to push—her body will just take over. As the woman continues to push, the baby's head will slide over the perineum and be born. It is normal for the baby's face and head to appear bluish in colour. If faeces or meconium is present on the baby's face, wipe with a clean sponge. The birth of the head usually takes 30 to 60 minutes in a woman having her first baby, but can be just one or two contractions with a woman having her second or subsequent babies. There is no need to touch or pull on the baby it will be born with the

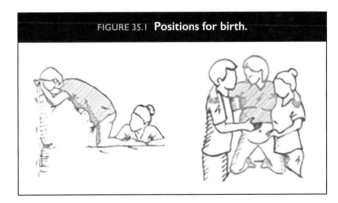

FIGURE 35.1 **Positions for birth.**

Allison Cummins

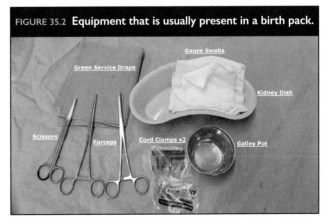

FIGURE 35.2 **Equipment that is usually present in a birth pack.**

Photograph Allison Cummins

next contraction. At the time of the next contraction, usually 2–3 minutes later, the rest of the baby will be born. Initially the baby's head will rotate and the baby's shoulders will be born. If it seems to be taking a long time, ask her to change to a more upright position so that the shoulders will be eased out.

It is not uncommon for the umbilical cord to be around the baby's neck; it will unravel as the baby is born. If the membranes are still intact over the baby's face wipe away the membrane with a clean cloth or gauze. Allow the baby to be born into the attendant's hands and immediately assist the woman to hold her baby. Assist her to place the baby on her chest and dry the baby with a warm towel while on the woman's chest. If the baby is well and crying by now, place him or her straight on to the woman's naked chest (skin-to-skin contact) and wrap both of them in a warm blanket. Congratulate the woman and her support person.

During skin-to-skin contact, continue to observe the baby's breathing, heart rate and colour. The baby may not cry, but you should be able to observe breathing patterns. The baby's colour will change from blue to pink within a minute or two. The hands and feet often remain bluish. Keep the baby on the woman in skin-to-skin contact and remove any wet or soiled linen and blankets. Place a name tag on the baby stating the mother's name and the date and time (if known) of the baby's birth. Leaving the baby on the woman's chest and breastfeeding will assist expulsion of the placenta and control bleeding.

If the baby is well and breathing, there is no rush to cut the umbilical cord. Evidence suggests that delayed cord clamping (at least 30–60 seconds) may benefit the neonate in reducing anaemia, and particularly the preterm neonate, by allowing time for transfusion of placental blood to the newborn infant, which can provide an additional 30% blood volume.[28] To cut the umbilical cord, place a cord clamp two finger breaths from the baby's abdomen on the umbilical cord and a clamp a few centimetres from the cord clamp. Cut between the clamps to separate the baby from the placenta.

The placenta and membranes are usually expelled spontaneously once the umbilical cord stops pulsating within the first hour of birth. There is no need to pull on the cord; the woman may express a feeling in her vagina that the placenta is coming or it is visible at the vulva. Have a kidney dish or a bowl available to collect the placenta in and attempt to measure the blood loss that is expelled at the time of the placenta being delivered.

If a midwife or experienced doctor is present they may recommend active management of the third stage of labour to deliver the placenta.[29] Active management of the third stage requires the use of a drug—oxytocin, usually 10 units given intramuscularly and controlled cord traction to deliver the placenta.

Keep the placenta for inspection by the midwife. Immediately after the placenta is delivered, rub the woman's fundus (this is the top of her uterus) which will now be at the level of her umbilicus. Rubbing of the fundus involves a circular massaging movement usually just above the woman's umbilicus. The uterus may initially feel soft (boggy) but usually will become contracted with the massage. It is important that the uterine fundus is firm (like a large tennis ball) and central as this will mean the bleeding is minimised. An atonic (boggy) uterus is the most common reason for a postpartum haemorrhage.

If the baby is vigorous, pink and breathing, dry thoroughly and remove the wet towel. Place the baby directly skin-to-skin on his or her mother and wrap both in a warm blanket. Skin-to-skin contact between a mother and her baby at birth reduces crying, and helps the mother to breastfeed successfully.[30] If the baby is not breathing, neonatal resuscitation will be required.

Encourage the woman to breastfeed as this assists the uterus to stay contracted and reduces excessive blood loss. Measure the woman's vital signs and vaginal blood loss. Record the details of the birth in the woman's medical record. Offer the woman and her support person something to eat and drink. Congratulate everyone on a job well done.

The next section of the chapter briefly outlines the major obstetric emergencies that may be seen in women who present to EDs or who are admitted to intensive care units. These are pulmonary embolism; ectopic pregnancy; intracerebral bleed; eclampsia; sepsis; road traffic crashes; and amniotic fluid embolism.

Pulmonary embolism

Thrombosis and thromboembolism is the third highest cause of direct maternal death in Australia and in the UK.[2,10] Delayed diagnosis, delayed or inadequate treatment and inadequate thromboprophylaxis account for many of the deaths due to venous thromboembolism.[31]

Pregnant women are at risk of venous thromboembolism because pregnancy is a hypercoagulable state.[31] Fibrin generation is increased, fibrinolytic activity is decreased, levels of coagulation factors II, VII, VIII, and X are all increased, free protein S levels are decreased and acquired resistance to activated protein C is common.[32] These changes mean that there is increased coagulation activity in women with uncomplicated pregnancies. There is also a reduction in venous flow velocity in a woman's legs by 25 to 29 weeks of gestation and this lasts until approximately 6 weeks after the birth, before it returns to the non-pregnancy state.[33,34] Health professionals must be aware that women are at risk of thromboembolism from the very beginning of pregnancy.[35]

Diagnosis

Pulmonary embolism is difficult to diagnose in pregnancy and the diagnosis is often made too late. Whilst some of the pregnant women who died from pulmonary embolism may not be able to have been saved no matter when the diagnosis was made, a small number go unrecognised, mainly because pulmonary embolism is not always considered early enough.[36]

The diagnosis of pulmonary embolism is already challenging in the non-pregnant patient but in pregnancy it becomes even more difficult.[31] The most common presentation of pulmonary embolism in pregnant women is dyspnoea and tachypnoea that may or may not be associated with chest pain.[37] Of those women who die from a potentially salvageable pulmonary embolism, many feel breathless prior to admission or presentation to hospital. Up to 75% of pregnant women will experience physiological breathlessness, which can start in any trimester.[38] It is important to remember that it is unusual to be breathless at rest in pregnancy or in the postpartum period, especially in the presence of tachycardia.[38] Obesity is the most important risk factor for thromboembolism; women at risk presenting with new chest symptoms need careful investigation.[35] It is not uncommon for a diagnosis of pneumonia to be made in a woman who ultimately is found to have a pulmonary embolism.

Diagnosis requires the use of scanning using ionising radiation. There are concerns about the use of ionising radiation in pregnancy; however, the risks of inappropriate use of anticoagulation or missing the diagnosis of PE in pregnancy far outweigh the exposure risks to the mother and baby.[39] A chest X-ray is useful to exclude diagnoses that mimic PE and to further triage patients to the most appropriate investigation. The D-dimer test is less useful in pregnancy; however, in women with a low probability of pulmonary embolism and a negative D-dimer, the diagnosis is excluded. Doppler ultrasound of both lower limbs has the benefit of being a radiation-free imaging modality. As venous thromboembolism is a continuous disease, the presence of a deep vein thrombosis can be used as a surrogate marker of PE and treatment commenced if present. The evidence to recommend either CTPA or nuclear scintigraphy is complex. There are numerous issues to consider, including effects to the mother and fetus. There is variation in scanning protocols between institutions and a decision as to the most appropriate test is best made after direct consultation with relevant specialists. MRI for the diagnosis of PE in pregnancy is a relatively new option with the distinct advantage of being a radiation-free modality. There is now promising emerging evidence supporting its use. However, availability and expertise remain the main limitations.[39]

Management

The care of the pregnant woman who has massive pulmonary embolism requires a coordinated treatment strategy by the obstetrician, intensivist, cardiothoracic surgeon, anaesthesiologist and interventional radiologist. Women who have a suspected or confirmed pulmonary embolism in late pregnancy should be treated with supplemental oxygen (to achieve an oxygen saturation of >95%) and intravenous heparin and should be transferred to a hospital that has a maternal-fetal, neonatal and cardiothoracic unit for high-risk patients. In women who are haemodynamically stable, a temporary vena caval filter should be placed once the diagnosis has been confirmed. As soon as the woman goes into active labour or a caesarean section is considered, the heparin should be stopped (and reversed with protamine if necessary). A caesarean section should not be performed while the woman is in a fully anticoagulated state; this can lead to uncontrolled bleeding and an increased risk of severe morbidity or mortality.[31]

Ectopic pregnancy

Many of the women who come into the ED with symptoms from ectopic pregnancy do not know or volunteer that they are pregnant and may not have a pregnancy test done as a routine. Ectopic pregnancy should be considered in all women of childbearing age who present with these symptoms regardless of contraceptive usage. Symptoms of an ectopic pregnancy include lower abdominal unilateral pain, light vaginal bleeding following a period of amenorrhoea, shoulder tip pain and finally shock.[40] Women may also present with less specific symptoms, including generalised abdominal pain and sometimes diarrhoea and vomiting. A negative pregnancy test can exclude ectopic pregnancy as a potential diagnosis.[41]

Mismanaging the care of women with ectopic pregnancies has always been easier than making the correct diagnosis, partly because cases present infrequently (1 in 100 pregnancies), but mainly because their presentation may not be classical. The triad of symptoms described in textbooks of emergency medicine are bleeding, abdominal pain and dysmenorrhoea, but many of the women who died, as well as some who survive, have presented with these non-specific symptoms and have not undergone a pregnancy test in the ED.

Diagnosis

As explained above, women may present to paramedics or EDs with atypical signs of ectopic pregnancy. Ectopic pregnancy is often associated with diarrhoea and vomiting and may mimic gastrointestinal disease. Fainting in early pregnancy may also indicate an ectopic pregnancy. There must be a low threshold for beta-hCG testing in women of reproductive age attending the ED with abdominal symptoms. A common practice in many departments is to undertake blood (serum) beta-hCG testing in all women of reproductive age who attend an ED with abdominal symptoms. In addition, it is recommended that pregnant women with abdominal pain should be reviewed by obstetrics and gynaecology staff, if available, or at least discussed with a specialist doctor by telephone.[36]

The diagnosis is made using beta-hCG measurements and transvaginal ultrasound.[42] Consultation and referral with an obstetrician and gynaecologist should occur as soon as possible to discuss ongoing management.

Other laboratory studies that should be obtained include:[43]

- full blood count, if significant haemorrhage is suspected
- urea, creatinine and electrolytes to rule out imbalances and hepatic or renal abnormalities
- urinalysis to eliminate urinary tract infection as a cause of pelvic pain
- blood type and Rhesus factor, if transfusion is required.

Women who are Rhesus-negative should be given anti-D immunoglobulin within 72 hours of an actual or suspected exposure, to prevent isoimmunisation.

Management

The most critical step in beginning the management is to have a high clinical suspicion for ectopic pregnancy (for example, in any woman of childbearing age). After a positive blood pregnancy test, any necessary initial resuscitation and physical examination (including pelvic examination to rule out an open cervical os or completed abortion), a transabdominal pelvic ultrasonography, followed by a transvaginal ultrasonography if needed, should be performed to identify a definitive intra-uterine pregnancy (yolk sac or fetal pole) or definitive ectopic pregnancy (extrauterine yolk sac or fetal pole).[43]

Consultation with, and referral to, an obstetric specialist is essential in the effective management of women with a suspected ectopic pregnancy. Management options include surgical and medical approaches depending on the duration of the pregnancy and the haemodynamic status of the woman. The current standard medical treatment of unruptured ectopic pregnancy is methotrexate (MTX) therapy. This decision should be made in conjunction with, if not by, the consulting obstetrician as there are a number of contraindications and cautions.[44]

PRACTICE TIP

A ruptured ectopic pregnancy is a medical emergency and needs to be managed urgently. Women may present with hypovolaemia secondary to blood loss and require urgent management to address their haemodynamic status. The insertion of two large bore intravenous cannulas and vigorous fluid resuscitation is essential.

It is important to remember that women with an ectopic pregnancy are essentially losing their pregnancy much like a miscarriage. Losing a pregnancy will be seen as actually losing a baby, with all the hopes and dreams that come with this to the great majority of women and it is likely that this will be accompanied by emotional shock, sadness and questions about this pregnancy and the future options. It is essential that the loss of this pregnancy is acknowledged and women are cared for in a sensitive manner and provided with emotional support and the amount of information they feel ready to take in at the time. Private space and time and ensuring the woman can be with her partner are also important considerations and strategies.

Intracerebral haemorrhage

Intracranial haemorrhage in pregnancy is associated with preeclampsia and hypertension. In the UK's 2011 report on maternal mortality,[2] intracranial haemorrhage and failure of effective antihypertensive therapy were a common source of substandard care. In the report, 11 women died from intracranial haemorrhage; in addition, it is recommended that all pregnant women presenting with new and potentially serious neurological symptoms must be seen promptly by a specialist doctor and neurological symptoms late in pregnancy mandate an urgent review and cerebral imaging.[45]

Diagnosis

Clinicians who work in EDs will be familiar with the means of diagnosis of an intracranial haemorrhage and the subsequent management of people with this condition. Intracranial haemorrhage is covered in Chapter 23. Paramedics may also see women with severe headaches in pregnancy or in the early postpartum period and may be the first healthcare professionals to be aware of possible diagnoses.

It is important to remember that severe headaches in pregnancy or in the early postpartum period can be indicative of intracerebral bleeding, despite it being a rare event. The following is a typical case that has direct relevance to clinicians in ED settings:[46]

> After a normal pregnancy and birth, a woman developed a severe headache with new onset hypertension early in her postnatal period. Her headache was not relieved by analgesics and was described as very severe. The midwife reassured the mother but she still had a very painful headache 2 days later: no action was taken. Her midwife had planned to review her again 4 days later but, before that, she was admitted to the Emergency Department (ED) with a fatal subarachnoid haemorrhage.

Management

Women with a headache severe enough to seek medical advice or with new epigastric pain should have their blood pressure taken and urine checked for protein as a minimum. For the most part, this will occur in the acute care setting.

Women with severe, incapacitating headaches described as the worst they have ever had should have an emergency neurological referral for brain imaging in the absence of other signs of preeclampsia. The threshold for same day referral to an obstetrician is hypertension ≥ 140 mmHg systolic and or ≥ 90 mmHg diastolic or proteinuria ≥1+ on dipstick. The systolic blood pressure is as significant as the diastolic. It is important to note that automated blood-pressure machines can seriously underestimate blood pressure in preeclampsia. Blood-pressure values should be compared with those obtained by auscultation (an anaeroid sphygmomanometer is acceptable).[47]

Eclampsia

Eclampsia (seizures) complicates 1 in 200–300 cases of pre-eclampsia in Australia. Eclampsia and preeclampsia are two of the leading causes of maternal death in the UK and in Australia.[2,10] Seizures may occur antenatally, intrapartum or postnatally, usually within 24 hours of the birth of the baby, but occasionally later. Hypertension and proteinuria may be absent prior to the seizure and not all women will have warning symptoms such as headache, visual disturbances or epigastric pain. There are no reliable clinical markers to predict eclampsia. In fact, the presence of neurological symptoms and/or signs is rarely associated with seizures.[47]

Preeclampsia generally occurs before eclampsia. Pre-eclampsia is a multi-system disorder unique to human pregnancy and characterised by hypertension and involvement of one or more other organ systems and/or the unborn baby. Raised blood pressure is commonly, but not always, the first manifestation. Proteinuria is the most commonly recognised additional feature after hypertension, but should not be considered mandatory to make the clinical diagnosis.

PRACTICE TIP

Hypertension in pregnancy is defined as:[47]

- Systolic blood pressure greater than or equal to 140 mmHg and/or
- Diastolic blood pressure greater than or equal to 90 mmHg (Korotkoff 5).

These measurements should be confirmed by repeated readings over several hours in the acute care setting. Severe hypertension in pregnancy is defined as a systolic blood pressure greater than or equal to 170 mmHg and/or diastolic blood pressure greater than or equal to 110 mmHg.[47]

A diagnosis of preeclampsia can be made when hypertension occurs after 20 weeks gestation and is accompanied by one or more of the following:

1. Renal involvement:
   - Significant proteinuria—dipstick proteinuria subsequently confirmed by spot urine protein/creatinine ratio ≥ 30 mg/mmol
   - Serum or plasma creatinine > 90 μmol/L
   - Oliguria
2. Haematological involvement
   - Thrombocytopenia
   - Haemolysis
   - Disseminated intravascular coagulation
3. Liver involvement
   - Raised serum transaminases
   - Severe epigastric or right upper quadrant pain
4. Neurological involvement
   - Convulsions (eclampsia)
   - Hyperreflexia with sustained clonus
   - Severe headache
   - Persistent visual disturbances (photopsia, scotomata, cortical blindness, retinal vasospasm)
   - Stroke
5. Pulmonary oedema
6. Fetal growth restriction
7. Placental abruption[47]

The HELLP syndrome (Haemolysis, Elevated Liver enzymes and a Low Platelet count) represents a particular presentation of severe preeclampsia, and separating it as a distinct disorder is not helpful. The guidelines from the Society of Obstetric Medicine of Australia and New Zealand (SOMANZ) provide more detail on the diagnosis of women with severe preeclampsia.[47]

Diagnosis

The diagnosis of preeclampsia is made on the basis of the level of hypertension in pregnancy and the presence of the other factors outlined in the previous section. Most commonly, women present with hypertension and proteinuria, although other renal, haematological, hepatic or neurological manifestations may occur.

Consistency in the terminology used to describe and define hypertension in pregnancy, preeclampsia and eclampsia is part of making a correct diagnosis. In the past, many different terms have been used to describe the condition, which has at times made consistent diagnosis and management more difficult.

Diagnosing a seizure as eclampsia is often a process of exclusion of other diagnoses. Most often the diagnosis of eclampsia is made in the acute care setting, even if women have the seizure outside of hospital. The further from the birth of the baby that the seizure occurs, the more carefully other diagnoses should be considered. For example, cerebral venous thrombosis may occur in the first few days of the postpartum period and can present with seizure activity. It should be remembered that eclampsia is not the most common cause of seizures in pregnancy and the differential diagnosis includes epilepsy and other medical problems that must be considered carefully, particularly when typical features of severe preeclampsia are lacking.[47]

PRACTICE TIP

The differential diagnoses of seizures in pregnancy include:
- Primary generalised epilepsy
- Subarachnoid haemorrhage
- Hypoglycaemia
- Thrombotic thrombocytopenic purpura
- Amniotic fluid embolism
- Central venous sinus thrombosis
- Water intoxication
- Phaeochromocytoma
- Local anaesthetic toxicity (e.g. epidural)
- Overdose (e.g. tricyclic antidepressants)[48]

Management

Guidelines from SOMANZ and the National Institute of Clinical Excellence (NICE) provide comprehensive information to guide the management of women with hypertensive disorders of pregnancy.[47,49] It is recommended that these are used to guide effective management and interventions. In particular, prompt treatment of severe hypertension (systolic blood pressure of 170 mmHg or higher, or a diastolic blood pressure of 110 mmHg or higher) or seizures is mandatory. The presence of severe hypertension, headache, epigastric pain or nausea and vomiting are ominous signs which should lead to urgent admission and management according to the SOMANZ Guidelines,[47] as should any concern about fetal wellbeing.

The management of eclampsia, outlined in Box 35.1, is directed towards clinicians in the acute care setting. In the out-of-hospital setting the important management strategies include the first aid management of a seizure.[50] These include keeping the woman in a safe environment, removed from danger; avoiding restraining her; placing her in the left lateral position as soon as possible; and supporting her in the immediate postictal phase. Most eclamptic seizures are self-limiting and once they are over the woman can be transported to an acute care setting.

Sepsis

Genital tract sepsis is a major cause of morbidity and mortality in pregnant and postpartum women.[51] Severe sepsis with acute organ dysfunction has a 20–40% mortality rate. Sepsis can occur in early and late pregnancy and is also commonly seen in the postpartum period. There have been reported deaths in early pregnancy often related to miscarriage or a termination of pregnancy and in later pregnancy related to the presence of a cervical suture. Infection should be suspected for women who present with pyrexia, persistent bleeding or abdominal pain,

Comprehensive protocols for the management of eclampsia (and severe hypertension) should be available in all appropriate areas.

There are four main aspects to care of the woman who sustains eclampsia in the acute care setting.

1. Resuscitation

Resuscitation requires institution of intravenous access, oxygen by mask, assuring a patent airway and removing regurgitated stomach contents from the mouth/pharynx.

The seizures are usually self-limiting. Intravenous diazepam (2 mg/minute to maximum of 10 mg) or clonazepam (1–2 mg over 2–5 minutes) may be given while the magnesium sulfate is being prepared if the seizure is prolonged.

2. Prevention of further seizures

Following appropriate resuscitation, treatment should be commenced with magnesium sulfate (4 g over 10–15 minutes) followed by an infusion (1–2 g/hr). In the event of a further seizure, a further 2–4 g of magnesium sulphate is given IV over 10 minutes. Magnesium sulphate is usually given as an intravenous loading dose, although the intramuscular route is equally effective. Monitoring should include blood pressure, respiratory rate, urine output, oxygen saturation and deep tendon reflexes. Magnesium sulphate by infusion should continue for 24 hours after the last seizure.

Magnesium sulphate is excreted renally and extreme caution should be used in women with oliguria or renal impairment. Serum magnesium concentration should be closely monitored in this situation. Magnesium is not universally successful and the recurrence rate of seizures despite appropriate magnesium therapy is 10–15%.

3. Control of hypertension

Control of severe hypertension to levels below 160/100 mmHg by parenteral therapy is essential as the threshold for further seizures is lowered after eclampsia, likely in association with vasogenic brain oedema. In addition, the danger of cerebral haemorrhage is real.

4. Birth of the baby

Arrangements for the birth of the baby should be decided once the woman's condition is stable. In the meantime, close fetal monitoring should be maintained. There is no role, with currently available treatment, for continuation of pregnancy once eclampsia has occurred, even though many women may appear to be stable after control of the situation has been achieved.

A woman in mid-pregnancy called an out-of-hours GP as she was feverish, shivery and unwell and had a sore throat, but was diagnosed as having a probable viral infection. A few hours later the GP visited again as she had developed constant abdominal pain associated with vomiting, greenish black diarrhoea and reduced fetal movements, but no vaginal bleeding. The GP suspected placental abruption, and, although she was rapidly transferred to hospital, on admission she was critically ill with marked tachycardia, breathlessness, cyanosis and confusion. The correct diagnosis of septic shock was quickly recognised, fluid resuscitation was started, senior consultants were called, advice was sought from haematology and microbiology consultants and appropriate intravenous antibiotics were commenced immediately. Despite intensive life support she died a few hours after admission to hospital.

caesarean section. As the caesarean section (CS) rate in many countries continues to rise (in 2011, the CS rate in Australia was 32.3%, with wide variations across states and territories and between public and private services, while in New Zealand it was 24.3%),[52,53] more women may be potentially at risk of infection post-caesarean section. In addition, as the hospital length-of-stay decreases in many places, more women will develop their infections outside of hospital and therefore present more readily to EDs. Genital tract sepsis related to pregnancy or childbirth can occur up to 6 weeks after the birth of the baby. Sepsis can result in septic shock, and is addressed in Chapter 29.

Pregnant women who present with a sore throat should have a throat swab collected as the cause may be community-acquired streptococcal group A and there should be a low threshold for antibiotics.[2] Deaths from sepsis, including group A streptococcus, have increased over the last 10 years. Women who have died have had children with sore throats, suggesting the infection was contracted from family members.[51]

Other risk factors for genital tract sepsis include: obesity; impaired glucose tolerance/diabetes; impaired immunity; anaemia; vaginal discharge; history of pelvic infection; history of Group B streptococcal infection; amniocentesis, and other invasive intrauterine procedures; insertion of a cervical suture; prolonged ruptured membranes (during pregnancy); vaginal trauma during birth; caesarean section; wound haematoma; and retained products of conception, either after a miscarriage or after the birth.[51]

Diagnosis

Sepsis is often insidious in onset with a fulminating course. The severity of illness should not be underestimated.[51] Many pregnant women will maintain their haemodynamic status, often appearing deceptively well until they suddenly deteriorate

following recent miscarriage or termination of pregnancy.[2] An example about sepsis in early pregnancy is taken from the report into maternal deaths from the United Kingdom. This case has specific resonance for those who work in EDs (Box 35.2).

Sepsis after the birth of the baby is often related to retained products of conception (fragments of placenta or membranes retained after the birth) or postoperative infections following

and collapse. In later pregnancy, sepsis should be considered as a differential diagnosis when a woman presents with symptoms suggestive of placental abruption. Disseminated intravascular coagulation and uterine atony are common in genital tract sepsis and often cause life-threatening postpartum haemorrhage. Treatment, including facilitating the birth of the baby, should not be delayed once septicaemia has developed because deterioration into septic shock can be extremely rapid.[51]

The most common pathogens that have been found to cause severe maternal morbidity or mortality were the beta-haemolytic *Streptococci*–Lancefield Group A, *E. coli* and *Pseudomonas*.[51]

The signs and symptoms of genital tract sepsis are often non-specific and unless genital tract sepsis is specifically considered in the differential diagnosis it may be missed until too late. The signs and symptoms are detailed in Box 35.3.

Management

In many cases of maternal mortality due to genital tract sepsis, there is a failure or delay in diagnosing sepsis, a failure to appreciate the severity of the woman's condition with resultant delays in referral to hospital, delays in administration of appropriate antibiotic treatment and late or no involvement of senior medical staff. It is essential that treatment is instigated promptly as once septicaemia develops the woman's clinical condition may deteriorate very rapidly over the course of a few hours, particularly when endotoxin-producing organisms are responsible.[51]

Women who present to out-of-hospital care providers with signs indicative of sepsis should be assessed and emergency management commenced before transfer to an acute care

setting. Usual measures in the management of sepsis or septic shock should be commenced by paramedics, including intravenous cannulation, intravenous fluid replacement to maintain pulse and BP and transport to an appropriate centre.

If pelvic sepsis is suspected, prompt early treatment with a combination of high-dose broad-spectrum intravenous antibiotics, such as cefuroxime and metronidazole, may be lifesaving. Time may be lost by waiting for microbiology results, although these results should be obtained as soon as possible.

> **PRACTICE TIP**
>
> The expert advice of a consultant microbiologist and an obstetrician should be sought at an early stage. The source of sepsis should be sought and dealt with if possible and appropriate.

Major trauma from road traffic crashes or violence

Although serious trauma during pregnancy is uncommon, it remains a major cause of maternal and fetal death and presents a variety of challenges because of the physiological changes due to pregnancy and because there are two people involved—mother and unborn baby.[54] Major trauma in pregnancy has the potential for significant maternal and fetal morbidity and mortality.[1,55] Motor vehicle crashes are by far the most common cause of serious maternal and fetal injury in the USA.[54] The latest enquiry into maternal deaths reports 17 women who died from motor vehicle crashes, either while pregnant or up to 42 days after birth.[2] A study in Sweden also found that motor vehicle crashes during pregnancy were a significant cause of maternal fatalities, fetal and neonatal deaths, responsible for almost one-third of all maternal deaths and fatalities and caused nearly three times more fetal plus neonatal deaths than maternal fatalities.[56] A study looking at the use of restraints for pregnant women involved in motor vehicle crashes found that unrestrained women were more likely to need non-obstetric surgery, suffer an abruption or fetal death.[57] Women should be advised to wear a three-point seat belt, adjusted to fit well, with the lap strap placed beneath the pregnant abdomen and the diagonal strap above the abdomen and between the breasts.[2,57,58]

Unfortunately, Australian data on major trauma from road traffic crashes or violence during pregnancy are difficult to obtain. The most recent Australian Maternal Mortality Report (2003–05)[10] reported 13 women who died as a result of motor vehicle crashes, carcinomas or infections during pregnancy or the postnatal period. These deaths were classified as 'incidental' and, as such, were seen as being outside the scope of the report and not discussed further. Deaths from road crashes were not identified separately.

Trauma in pregnancy can also occur as a result of domestic violence. Domestic violence in pregnancy is a significant issue as there are immediate and long-term effects on both the woman and her baby.[59] The prevalence of domestic violence varies depending on the context, population and measurement instruments. A review of 14 studies of violence against pregnant women reported prevalence rates between 1% and 20%.[60]

BOX 35.3 Back to basics sepsis[38]

Associated red flag signs and symptoms that should prompt urgent referral for hospital assessment, and, if the women appears seriously unwell, by emergency ambulance:

- Pyrexia >38°C
- Sustained tachycardia >100 b/min
- Breathlessness (RR > 20; a serious symptom)
- Abdominal or chest pain
- Diarrhoea and/or vomiting
- Reduced or absent fetal movements, or absent fetal heart
- Spontaneous rupture of membranes or significant vaginal discharge
- Uterine or renal angle pain and tenderness
- The woman is generally unwell or seems unduly anxious, distressed or panicky
- A normal temperature does not exclude sepsis, paracetamol and other analgesics may mask pyrexia, and this should be taken into account when assessing women who are unwell.
- Infection must also be suspected and actively ruled out when a recently delivered woman has persistent vaginal bleeding and abdominal pain. If there is any concern, the woman must be referred back to the maternity unit as soon as possible, certainly within 24 hours.

More recently, a study conducted in antenatal clinics in the UK reported prevalence rates of 2% at booking; 6% at 34 weeks of pregnancy and 5% at 10 days postpartum.[61] In the United States, a study in low-risk pregnant women reported that abuse during pregnancy was reported by 6% of women.[62]

Domestic violence in pregnancy can have catastrophic effects in relation to major trauma and death. In the most recent report of maternal mortality in Australia, there were three deaths as a result of domestic violence.[10] In the UK, of the women who died from any cause, including those unrelated to pregnancy, 14% self-declared that they were subject to domestic abuse and six women were murdered in cases of known domestic abuse.[2] In another study from the United States, women who sustained a physical assault during pregnancy experienced both immediate (uterine rupture, increased fetal and maternal mortality) and long-term sequelae (prematurity and low birth-weight infants).[63] The Australian Bureau of Statistics[64] reports that 60% of women who had experienced violence were pregnant at some time during the relationship, 36% experienced it during their pregnancy and 17% experienced it for the first time when they were pregnant.

Major trauma in pregnancy, from whichever cause, has particular deleterious effects on the unborn baby. The unborn baby is more likely to die after traumatic injury than is the woman. For example, one study over a 3-year period found that in the 240 cases of fetal death resulting from traumatic injury, just 27 of the women died.[65] Another study of more than 10,000 pregnant women hospitalised for trauma over an 8-year period found 25 fetal and 3 maternal deaths in this population.[63]

> **PRACTICE TIP**
>
> Major trauma in pregnancy can be as a result of a motor vehicle crash or from a physical assault, for example, in domestic violence. It is important to consider domestic violence as a cause when women present with trauma in pregnancy.

Diagnosis

The diagnosis of trauma in pregnancy is similar for non-pregnant patients. The additional aspects are related to consideration of the effects of the trauma on the pregnancy, particularly on the baby. One of the major complicating factors is a placenta abruptio, where the placenta separates from the uterine wall. This is the most likely cause of preterm labour in a trauma patient.

The diagnosis of the cause of other trauma or domestic violence may be difficult. Pregnant women who have experienced an assault might be reluctant to talk about it. For example, a woman presenting with vaginal bleeding might not mention that it started after she had sustained a blow to the abdomen.[54] Sensitive and careful questioning in a private and safe space is important to enable women to tell their story.[58] It is important that women have time alone with a clinician as often their partner will have accompanied her to the ED.

Paramedics will often be in an ideal position to assess a pregnant woman who has sustained trauma. Assessment will often take place outside the acute care setting and may be challenging in terms of determining the cause if family members are present. Sensitive questioning in a private environment in the home may be necessary to be able to fully understand the nature of the trauma and the possible cause.

> **PRACTICE TIP**
>
> Compression and displacement of the pelvic, abdominal and thoracic organs occur as pregnancy advances. This makes some injuries more likely and others harder to detect. The physiological changes due to pregnancy must be considered when assessing pregnant women with trauma.

Management

As with non-pregnant trauma patients, the focus of initial interventions remains the ABCs: airway, breathing and circulation.[54] Usual trauma care priorities do not change when the patient is pregnant; indeed, the baby's best chance for survival is effective resuscitation of the woman. An explanation of the physiological changes due to pregnancy and how these affect maternal resuscitation is discussed earlier in this chapter.

Identification that the woman is pregnant is the first step in effective resuscitation. Every woman of childbearing age who presents with trauma to an ED should be asked when she last menstruated and whether she could be pregnant.[54] Pregnant women with positive mechanism of injury according to time-critical guidelines should be transported to a major trauma centre. This applies even if the woman does not have evidence of physiological distress.

Early consultation with an obstetrician, midwife and neonatologist is essential in the case of these women. If the baby is likely to be born preterm, decisions need to be made about the most appropriate location for this to occur. Preterm babies are likely to require specialist care and it is generally easier to transfer the baby in utero rather than ex utero. This, of course, depends on the condition of the woman.

The pregnant woman who has experienced major trauma requires early, vigorous fluid replacement to support herself and her baby. The unborn baby will be extremely sensitive to maternal hypovolaemia: fetal hypoxia and bradycardia can develop quickly. Fetal death can occur at any gestational age and usually results from fetal hypoxia. As highlighted earlier, the changes of pregnancy can mask the signs of decompensation normally present in patients going into shock, and so vigorous fluid resuscitation is necessary. Pregnant women generally require two or more large-bore (14-to-16-gauge) intravenous catheters for fluid replacement,[54] as with most trauma patients. Resuscitation measures including the volume of fluid replacement should follow usual guidelines for patients who have experienced trauma (see Ch 15 for more detailed information on resuscitation in trauma situations).

> **PRACTICE TIP**
>
> It is important to obtain an obstetric and general medical history from the woman and/or her partner. She may also

have her antenatal record with her which will contain relevant information. This will include the patient's estimated date of birth of her baby, the numbers of previous pregnancies and births, and any complications of this or previous pregnancies. The admitting nurse should also establish whether she is currently experiencing contractions, vaginal bleeding or increased vaginal discharge (this could be amniotic fluid from around the baby), or backache or contractions, any of which could indicate that she is in preterm labour. Abdominal pain, contractions or vaginal bleeding might also indicate placental abruption where the placenta has separated from the uterine wall.[54]

Pregnant women who present with major trauma require the same diagnostic studies and interventions as non-pregnant patients. This is detailed in Chapter 48. This includes all indicated radiographic studies such as plain film X-ray, computed tomography, angiography and magnetic resonance imaging. The uterus should be shielded during radiographic procedures, except during abdominal or pelvic imaging.[54] In addition, all Rhesus-negative women should receive full dose Rhesus immune globulin (more if indicated by Kleihauer-Betke test, the blood test used to measure the amount of fetal haemoglobin transferred from a fetus to the mother's bloodstream).

Fetal monitoring is an important aspect of the care of these women. Pregnant women who experience trauma beyond 20 weeks gestation should be monitored using an electronic fetal monitor for a minimum of 4 hours.[66] Electronic fetal monitoring is usually available only in the labour ward setting, but a monitoring machine could be brought to the ED with a midwife to apply it and interpret the readings.

It is likely that women who experience trauma in pregnancy will be very anxious and concerned for the welfare of their baby. Their partner may also be present and will require support and information in a timely manner. It is important to provide as much information as possible in a caring and sensitive way. In some cases, the baby will have died before arriving at, or while in, the ED. A midwife can advise the staff about addressing this difficult and sad issue with the parents.

PRACTICE TIP

The anatomical and physiological changes of pregnancy can mask the signs of decompensation normally present in patients going into shock. Therefore, pregnant women with major trauma may not look like they are experiencing severe hypovolaemia until they collapse. Consider lower acceptable limits of vital signs as being significant in pregnant women.

Amniotic fluid embolism

Amniotic fluid embolism is a rare, but carries a high risk of mortality, obstetric emergency with reported mortality rates ranging from 16% to 86%.[67,68] It is unpredictable, often

occurring without warning and it is rapidly progressive. It occurs in about 1:8000–1:30,000 pregnancies.[1] Recent analysis from the UK suggests it is even more rare, occurring in 1.9 cases per 100,000 of women giving birth.[69] Amniotic fluid embolism is a leading cause of maternal death in the most recent maternal death reports in Australia.[10] The most recent *UK Confidential Enquiry into Maternal Deaths* states there is no change in the incidence of death from amniotic fluid embolism; however, the condition, once considered fatal, now has a reduced mortality due to improved approaches in resuscitation when the collapse occurs in a well-equipped facility.[2]

The pathophysiology and initiating event is unclear; however, usually during labour or other procedure, amniotic fluid and debris, or some as yet unidentified substance, enters the maternal circulation. This seems to trigger either a massive anaphylactic reaction, an activation of the complement cascade, or both. Progression usually occurs in two phases. Initially, pulmonary artery vasospasm with pulmonary hypertension and elevated right ventricular pressure cause hypoxia. Hypoxia causes myocardial capillary damage and pulmonary capillary damage, left heart failure and acute respiratory distress syndrome. Women who survive these events may enter the next phase. This is a haemorrhagic phase characterised by massive haemorrhage with uterine atony and disseminated intravascular coagulation (DIC). In some cases, fatal consumptive coagulopathy may be the initial presentation.[70]

The usual clinical scenario is that the woman experiences acute respiratory distress, then collapses often after pushing or immediately after the birth of the baby.[68] In many cases, women who have an amniotic fluid embolism report some or all of the following premonitory symptoms: breathlessness, chest pain, feeling cold, light-headedness, restlessness, distress, panic, a feeling of pins and needles in the fingers, nausea and vomiting.[71]

The presentation of amniotic fluid embolism can often be confused with other presentations; nevertheless prompt effective resuscitation is essential despite the underlying cause.[2]

Diagnosis

Currently no definitive diagnostic test exists for amniotic fluid embolism and often the diagnosis is only made at post-mortem examination. The diagnosis is often made by exclusion and any pregnant or newly postpartum woman who shows signs associated with pulmonary embolus, septic shock, acute myocaedia infarction, cardiomyopathy, anaphylaxis, cardiorespiratory collapse or intractable haemorrhage must be systematically evaluated to exclude a diagnosis of amniotic fluid embolism.[1]

The registries for amniotic fluid embolism in the UK and USA recommend the following four criteria, all of which must be present to make the diagnosis of amniotic fluid embolism:[72,73]

1. Acute hypotension or cardiac arrest
2. Acute hypoxia
3. Coagulopathy or severe haemorrhage in the absence of other explanations
4. All of these occurring during labour, caesarean section, dilation and evacuation, or within 30 minutes postpartum with no other explanation of findings.

The laboratory investigations to exclude amniotic fluid embolism in the acute care setting include:[74]

- full blood count with platelets
- coagulation parameters (prothrombin time, activated partial thromboplastin time, fibrinogen)
- arterial blood gases (see Ch 17, p. 329, for procedure)
- chest X-ray
- ECG (see Ch 17, p. 336, for cardiac monitoring procedures)
- V/Q scan
- echocardiogram

Management

The management of a woman with suspected amniotic fluid embolism depends on her signs and symptoms. The primary goals of management are to provide oxygen, maintain cardiac output and organ perfusion, correct coagulopathy and provide supportive therapies.[1] In the out-of-hospital setting, supportive management should occur including oxygen therapy and intravenous fluids with urgent transport to hospital. The management in the acute care setting is essentially:

- Administer oxygen to maintain normal saturation. Intubate and ventilate if necessary.
- Initiate CPR if the woman arrests. If she does not respond to resuscitation, perform a perimortem caesarean section.
- Treat hypotension with crystalloid fluids, blood products and inotropes. Consider pulmonary artery catheterisation in women who are haemodynamically unstable.
- Continuously monitor the fetus.
- Treat coagulopathy and thrombocytopenia using fresh frozen plasma, cryoprecipitate and platelet or whole-blood transfusion as appropriate.
- Additional measures in an intensive care setting may include high-dose corticosteroids, cardiopulmonary bypass, nitric oxide and inhaled prostacyclin.
- Women with symptoms suspicious of amniotic fluid embolism should be transferred to an intensive care unit as soon possible.

SUMMARY

This chapter has described the aspects of maternal physiology that affect maternal resuscitation and response to trauma during pregnancy and highlighted the modifications of BLS and ALS needed in pregnancy. Essentially, the anatomical and physiological changes of pregnancy can mask the signs of decompensation and this has implications for resuscitation and the care of women who have obstetric emergencies. The chapter also highlighted that effective resuscitation of the pregnant woman is an essential component of resuscitation of the unborn baby. This may include the undertaking of an emergency caesarean section. The chapter described the criteria for undertaking such a drastic procedure.

The diagnosis and management of pregnant or postpartum women who present to an ED with five obstetric emergency situations was addressed. The most important considerations in relation to these emergencies are:

- recognition of the women's pregnancy
- consideration of the physiological changes that will affect the diagnosis and management of the condition
- the psychological care of the women and her family
- sensitive care around the possible death of the baby and the social and emotional impact on the parents
- consideration of the impact of an obstetric emergency on the staff.

Obstetric emergencies are unique in that there are two patients to consider and care for. Fortunately, for the most part, pregnancy is a normal life event and most babies are born healthy without complications.[58] Some women will experience acute obstetric emergencies, and for those women the care discussed in this chapter is essential.

CASE STUDY

Jessica Adams, a 26-year-old woman, presented to the ED on three occasions over a 48-hour period with a history of abdominal pain and diarrhoea. She was discharged on the first two occasions with a diagnosis of gastroenteritis, even though she had a history of collapse and measured heart rates of 130 and 144 beats per minute. This is now her third presentation.

1. What questions will you ask in this scenario to determine historical and clinical indicators of urgency and relevance?

2. Describe each aspect of your physical assessment and explain each step.

3. What investigations will you perform and why?

4. What ongoing monitoring will you provide?

This case study is a real story from the UK's *Saving Mothers Lives* report.[9] Jessica (not her real name) arrested and died on this, her third, presentation. At postmortem she was found to have had an ectopic pregnancy.

This case study highlights two important issues—the importance of tachycardia and the risk of overlooking an ectopic pregnancy. Tachycardia is without doubt the most significant clinical feature of an unwell patient and is regularly ignored or misunderstood. Measurements of respiratory rate and heart rate are more important than measurements of blood pressure. A normotensive patient may all too often be unwell and compensating. A tachycardic patient is hypovolaemic until proved otherwise.

Many of the women who come into the ED with symptoms from ectopic pregnancy do not know or volunteer that they are pregnant. Occasionally these women do not have a pregnancy test done as a routine. Without a pregnancy test it is hard to include ectopic pregnancy in the differential diagnosis.

Answers to Case Study Questions can be found on evolve
http://evolve.emergencytrauma.curtis

REFERENCES

1. Thorogood C. Life threatening emergencies. In: Pairman S, Tracy S, Thorogood C, Pincombe J, eds. Preparation for practice. 2nd edn Sydney: Churchill Livingstone Elsevier; 2010: 909–70.

2. Lewis G. Saving mothers' lives: Reviewing maternal deaths to make motherhood safer—2006–08. The Eighth Report of the Confidential Enquiries into Maternal Deaths in the United Kingdom. BJOG 2011; 118(Suppl. 1):1–203.

3. ACSQHC. Recognition and response to deteriorating patients. Online. www.safetyandquality.gov.au/our-work/recognition-and-response-to-clinical-deterioration/observation-and-response-charts/; accessed 21 January 2014.

4. Lewis G, ed. Saving mothers' lives: Reviewing maternal deaths to make motherhood safer—2003–2005. London: Confidential Enquiry into Maternal and Child Health; 2007.

5. Ciliberto C, Marx G. Physiological changes associated with pregnancy. Physiology 1998; 9(2):1–3.

6. Verralls S. Anatomy and physiology applied to obstetrics. 3rd edn. Edinburgh: Churchill Livingstone; 1993.

7. Marshall J, Raynor M. Myles textbook for midwives. 16th edn. London: Churchill Livingstone; 2014.

8. Stables D, Rankin J, eds. Physiology in childbearing. 3rd edn. Edinburgh: Elsevier; 2010.

9. Hulbert D. Specific recommendations for the management of pregnant women attending Emergency Departments (ED). In: Lewis G, ed. Saving mothers' lives: Reviewing maternal deaths to make motherhood safer—2003–2005 The Seventh Report on Confidential Enquiries into Maternal Deaths in the United Kingdom. London: The Confidential Enquiry into Maternal and Child Health (CEMACH); 2007.

10. Sullivan E, Ball B, King J. Maternal deaths in Australia 2003–2005. Sydney: Australian Institute for Health and Welfare; 2008.

11. Catling-Paull C, McDonnell N, Moores A, Homer C. Maternal mortality in Australia: Learning from maternal cardiac arrest. Nursing and Health Sciences 2011;13:10–15.

12. Lipman S, Cohen S, Einav S et al. The Society for Obstetric Anesthesia and Perinatology Consensus Statement on the Management of Cardiac Arrest in Pregnancy. Online. www.soap.org/CPR-consensus-statment.pdf; accessed 23 July 2014.

13. Small K, Ruddock A. Maternal resuscitation and trauma. In: ALSO Asia Pacific, ed. Advanced Life Saving Skills in Obstetrics Manual. 3rd edn Sydney: ALSO Asia Pacific; 2013.

14. Australian Resuscitation Council & New Zealand Resuscitation Council. Guideline 11.1 Resuscitation in special circumstances. 2011. www.resus.org.au/policy/guidelines/section_11/resuscitation_in_special_circumstances.htm; accessed 23 July 2014.

15. American Heart Association. Guidelines for cardiopulmonary resuscitation and emergency cardiovascular care part 12: Cardiac Arrest in special situations. 2010. http://circ.ahajournals.org/content/122/18_suppl_3/S829.full#sec-35; accessed 1 February 2014.

16. McDonnell N. Cardiopulmonary arrest in pregnancy: two case reports of successful outcomes in association with perimortem Caesarean delivery. Br J Anaesthesia 2009;103(3):406–9.

17. Dijkman A, Huisman C, Smit M et al. Cardiac arrest in pregnancy: increasing use of perimortem caesarean section due to emergency skills training? Br J Obstet Gynaecol 2010;117(3):282–7.

18. ARC and ACCN. Standards for Resuscitation: Clinical Practice and Education. A Resource for Health Professionals. Melbourne: The Australian Resuscitation Council 2008.

19. Warraich Q, Esen U. Perimortem caesarean section. J Obstet Gynaecol 2009;29(8):690–3.

20. WHO. Maternal mortality ratio (per 100 000 live births). Online. www.who.int/healthinfo/statistics/indmaternalmortality/en/; accessed 7 August 2014.

21. Victorian Health. Sentinel event program—Annual report 2011–12 and 2012–13. Melbourne: Department of Health; 2014.

22. Ashcroft B, Elstein M, Boreham N, Holm S. Prospective semistructured observational study to identify risk attributable to staff deployment, training, and updating opportunities for midwives. BMJ 2003;327(7415):584.

23. Clinical Negligence Schemes for Trusts. Maternity Clinical Risk Management Standards. London: National Litigation Authority; 2005.

24. NSW Health. Maternity—Clinical Risk Management Program. Sydney: NSW Department of Health; 2009.

25. RCOG. Improving patient safety: Risk management for maternity and gynaecology—clinical governance advice no. 2 September 2009. 3rd edn, London: Royal College of Obstetricians and Gynaecologists; 2009.

26. Vincent C, Taylor-Adams S, Chapman E et al. How to investigate and analyse clinical incidents: Clinical risk unit and association of litigation and risk management protocol. BMJ 2000;320:777–81.

27. Pairman S, Tracy S, Thorogood C, Pincombe J, eds. Preparation for practice. 2nd edn. Sydney: Churchill Livingstone Elsevier; 2010.

28. ACOG. Timing of umbilical cord clamping after birth: Commitee Opinion No. 543. Obsterics and Gynecology 2012;120.

29. Begley C, Gyte G, Devane D et al. Active versus expectant management for women in the third stage of labour. Cochrane Database of Systematic Reviews 2011; 11:CD007412. DOI: 10.1002/14651858.

30. Moore E, Anderson G, Bergman N, Dowswell T. Early skin-to-skin contact for mothers and their healthy newborn infants. Cochrane Database of Systematic Reviews 2012; 12: CD003519. DOI: 10.1002/14651858.

31. Marik P, Plante L. Current concepts: venous thromboembolic disease and pregnancy. New England Journal of Medicine 2008; 359(19):2025–33.

32. Brenner B. Haemostatic changes in pregnancy. Thrombosis Research 2004;114:409–14.

33. Macklon N, Greer I, Bowman A. An ultrasound study of gestational and postural changes in the deep venous system of the leg in pregnancy. Br J Obstet Gynaecol 1997;104:191–7.

34. Macklon N, Greer I. The deep venous system in the puerperium: An ultrasound study. Br J Obstet Gynaecol 1997;104:198–200.

35. Drife J. Thrombosis and thromboembolism (Ch 2). In: Lewis G, ed. Saving mothers' lives: reviewing maternal deaths to make motherhood safer—2006–2008 The eighth report on confidential enquiries into maternal deaths in the United Kingdom. London: Br J Obstet Gynaecol; 2011:57–65.

36. Hulbert D. Emergency medicine (Ch 15). In: Lewis G, ed. Saving mothers' lives: Reviewing maternal deaths to make motherhood safer 2006–2008 The Eighth Report on Confidential Enquiries into Maternal Deaths in the United Kingdom: Br J Obstet Gynaecol; 2011: 167–72.

37. Gray G, Nelson-Piercy C. Thromboembolic disorders in obstetrics. Best Pract Res Clin Obstet Gynaecol 2012;26(1):53–6.

38. Oates M, Harper A, Shakespeare J, Nelson-Piercy C. Back to basics. In: Lewis G, ed. Saving Mothers' Lives: Reviewing maternal deaths to make motherhood safer—2006–08 The Eighth Report of the Confidential Enquiries into Maternal Deaths in the United Kingdom. London: Br J Obstet Gynaecol; 2011.

39. Mendelson R. Diagnostic Imaging Pathways—Pulmonary Embolism in Pregnancy. Online. www.imagingpathways.health.wa.gov.au/includes/pdf/pe_preg.pdf; accessed 15 January 2009.

40. Small K, Sneddon A. Chapter A: First trimester pregnancy complications. In: Pacific AA, ed. Advanced life saving skills in obstetrics manual. 3rd edn, Sydney: ALSO Asia Pacific; 2013.

41. O'Herlihy C. Deaths in early pregnancy (Ch 6). In: Lewis G, ed. Saving mothers' lives: Reviewing maternal deaths to make motherhood safer 2006–2008 The eighth report on confidential enquiries into maternal deaths in the United Kingdom. London: Br J Obstet Gynaecol; 2011: 80–4.

42. Kendall J, Hoffenberg S, Smith R. History of emergency and critical care ultrasound: the evolution of a new imaging paradigm. Critical Care Medicine 2007;35(5 Suppl): S126–30.

43. Chi T. Pregnancy, ectopic: differential diagnoses and workup 2009. http://emedicine.medscape.com/article/796451-diagnosis; accessed 16 Jan 2010.

44. Practice Committee of American Society for Reproductive Medicine. Medical treatment of ectopic pregnancy. Fertility and Sterility 2008;910(5 Suppl):S206–12.

45. de Swiet M, Williamson C. Other Indirect deaths (Ch 10). In: Lewis G, ed. Saving mothers' lives: Reviewing maternal deaths to make motherhood safer 2006–2008 The eighth report on confidential enquiries into maternal deaths in the United Kingdom. London: Br J Obstet Gynaecol; 2011:119–31.

46. Shakespeare J. Issues for general practitioners (Ch 14). In: Lewis G, ed. Saving mothers' lives: Reviewing maternal deaths to make motherhood safer 2006–2008. The eighth report on confidential enquiries into maternal deaths in the United Kingdom; 2011:158–66.

47. Lowe S, Bowyer L, Lust K et al. The management of hypertensive disorders of pregnancy. Society of Obstetric Medicine of Australia and New Zealand (SOMANZ). Online. www.somanz.org/pdfs/somanz_guidelines_2008.pdf; accessed 10 June 2015.

48. Munro P. Management of eclampsia in the accident and emergency department. Journal of Accident and Energency Medicine 2000;17:7–11.

49. NICE. Hypertension in pregnancy: the management of hypertensive disorders during pregnancy. London: National Institute for Health and Clinical Excellence, RCOG Press; 2010.

50. Council ARCNZR. Guideline 9.2.4—First Stage Management of a Seizure. Online. www.resus.org.au/policy/guidelines/section_9/first_aid_management_ofa_seizure.htm; accessed 23 July 2014.

51. Harper A. Genital tract sepsis (Ch 7). In: Lewis G, ed. Saving mothers' lives: Reviewing maternal deaths to make motherhood safer 2006–2008 The eighth report on confidential enquiries into maternal deaths in the United Kingdom. London: Br J Obstet Gynaecol; 2011: 85–95.

52. Li Z, Zeki R, Hilder L, Sullivan E. Australia's mothers and babies 2011. Perinatal statistics series no. 28. Cat. no. PER 59. Canberra: AIHW National Perinatal Epidemiology and Statistics Unit; 2013.

53. Ministry of Health (NZ). Maternity tables 2011. Online. www.health.govt.nz/publication/maternity-tables-2011#labourbirth; accessed 25 July 2014.

54. Criddle L. Trauma in pregnancy. AJN, American Journal of Nursing 2009;109(11):41–7.

55. Sugrue M, O'Connor M, D'Amours S. Trauma in pregnancy. ADF Health 2004;5(1):24–8.

56. Kvarnstrand L, Milsom I, Lekander T et al. Maternal fatalities, fetal and neonatal deaths related to motor vehicle crashes during pregnancy: a national population-based study. Acta Obstet Gynecol Scand 2008;87(9):946–52.

57. Luley T, Fitzpatrick B, Grotegut C et al. Perinatal implications of motor vehicle accident trauma during pregnancy: identifying populations at risk. Am J Obstet Gynaecol 2013;208(6):466.e1–5.

58. Australian Health Ministers' Advisory Council. Clinical Practice Guidelines: Antenatal Care—Module 1. Canberra: Australian Government Department of Health and Ageing; 2012.

59. Thorogood C, Donaldson C. Challenges in pregnancy. In: Pairman S, Tracy, S, Thorogood, C, Pincombe, J, eds. Preparation for practice. 2nd edn. Sydney: Churchill Livingstone Elsevier; 2010:754–818.

60. Gazmarian JA, Lazorick S, Spitz AM et al. Prevalence of violence against pregnant women. JAMA 1996;275(24):1915–20.

61. Shneyderman Y, Kiely M. Intimate partner violence during pregnancy: victim or perpetrator? Does it make a difference? BJOG 2013;120(11):1375–85.

62. Neggers Y, Goldenberg R, Cliver S, Hauth J. Effects of domestic violence on preterm birth and low birthweight. Acta Obstetricia et Gynecologica Scandinavica 2004;83(4):455–60.

63. El Kady D, Gilbert WM, Xing G, Smith LH. Maternal and neonatal outcomes of assaults during pregnancy. Obstetrics and Gynecology 2005;105(2):357–63.

64. Australian Bureau of Statistics. Personal safety survey, Australia 2012. www.abs.gov.au/ausstats/abs@.nsf/Lookup/4906.0Glossary12012; accessed 23 July 2014.

65. Weiss H, Songer T, Fabio A. Fetal deaths related to maternal injury. JAMA 2001;286(15):1863–8.

66. Mattox K, Goetzl L. Trauma in pregnancy. Critical Care Medicine 2005;33(10 Suppl):S385–9.

67. Tuffnell D. Amniotic fluid embolism. Current Opinion in Obstetrics and Gynecology 2003;15(2):119–22.

68. Avery D. Obstetric emergencies. Am J Clin Med 2009;6(2):42–7.

69. Knight M, Berg C, Brocklehurst P et al. Amniotic fluid embolism incidence, risk factors and outcomes: A review and recommendations. BMC Pregnancy and Childbirth 2012;12: 7.

70. Moore L. Amniotic Fluid Embolism. 22 Dec 2009. http://emedicine.medscape.com/article/253068-overview; accessed 15 January 2010.

71. Dawson A. Amniotic fluid embolism (Ch 5). In: Lewis G, ed. Saving mothers' lives: Reviewing maternal deaths to make motherhood safer 2006–2008 The eighth report on confidential enquiries into maternal deaths in the United Kingdom. London: Br J Obstet Gynaecol; 2011:76–80.

72. Tuffnell D. United Kingdom Amniotic Fluid Embolism Register. Br J Obstet Gynaecol 2005;112:1625–9.

73. O'Shea A, Eappen S. Amniotic fluid embolism. International Anesthesiology Clinics 2007;45(1):17–28.

74. Thorogood C. Life threatening emergencies. In: Pairman S, Tracey S et al. Preparation for practice, 2nd edn, Churchill Livingstone Elsevier, Sydney 2010; 909–70.

CHAPTER 36
PAEDIATRIC EMERGENCIES
DIANNE CRELLIN

Essentials

- Accurately assessing and appropriately managing paediatric emergencies are contingent on having a good understanding of growth and development, and of the anatomical and physiological impact of immaturity and its effect on acute illness and injury across all systems.

- Effective collaborative healthcare is contingent on developing a therapeutic relationship with the patient and their family. Gaining the trust and cooperation of children requires an understanding of cognitive and emotional development and a flexible approach to assessment and management.

- The principles of assessment and management of infants and children are the same as for adults, so this chapter should be read in conjunction with other chapters in the book addressing the topic.

- A number of tools are available to guide paediatric history-taking and examination to ensure that issues specific to children are not overlooked and that clinical findings are afforded the relevance warranted. However, the principles of assessment, triage and management for infants and children are the same as they are for adults presenting to the emergency department (ED).

- Infants may rapidly deteriorate, and frequently exhibit few or non-specific signs and symptoms of significant illness as a result of immunological immaturity. For this reason, in addition to the attention given to the signs and symptoms of the illness, particular attention should be paid to feeding, urine output, activity levels and sleeping patterns.

- Respiratory illnesses are the most common illnesses occurring in children and account for 30–40% of acute admissions to hospital. As the aetiology is most frequently viral, treatment is focused on managing the symptoms of illness.

- Infants are particularly susceptible to shock as this compensatory mechanism is easily overwhelmed, and unless aggressively treated the physiological derangements of shock rapidly become irreversible.

- Infants and young children are particularly susceptible to dehydration during episodes of illness, regardless of the type of illness, and hydration will be a focus of assessment and management of the unwell child.

- Changes in conscious state are also a feature of deterioration, regardless of the type of illness and should not be overlooked.

- Rashes can be grouped by appearance as vesicular, pustular, papular, eczematous, purpuric/vascular and erythematous, which will help determine the likely cause and therefore appropriate management.

- Trauma is a major cause of mortality and morbidity in infants, children and adolescents.

- The injuries infants and children suffer and their response to trauma is affected by their size and their level of physical and cognitive development.

- Fever is a common symptom associated with illness in children and causes great concern in the community. However, management should be focused on providing comfort. Antipyretics are not recommended to treat the temperature in the absence of signs of discomfort or to prevent convulsions.

- Children are less likely to receive analgesia than adults in the ED setting, and infants and young children are less likely to receive analgesia than older children. Management should include adequate analgesia regardless of the cause of the pain.
- Acute healthcare is the principal priority during the emergency visit; however, it is also an opportunity for emergency clinicians to provide health education and address other health and lifestyle issues such as immunisation, smoking cessation and weight management.

INTRODUCTION

Paediatrics is considered a specialty and it is often said that children are 'not little adults'. However, the majority of children assessed and treated by emergency services are not seen by paediatric specialists but by emergency clinicians, who require the skills to assess and manage both adults and children competently. Using a systematic approach to assessment and applying simple principles, it is possible to adequately assess and identify health-related problems in children presenting to emergency services and manage them effectively.

It is not intended that this chapter is an exhaustive list of potential paediatric presentations. The aim of the chapter is to address the key differences that exist between infants, children and adults and present some common and important paediatric presentations to emergency service providers. Where the presentation does not differ greatly from the adult and this is presented elsewhere in the book, these presentations have

been omitted. For those that are presented in other chapters, but where the paediatric presentation differs, discussion in this chapter will chiefly focus on these differences. A list of useful websites and additional readings has also been included at the end of the chapter.

Approach to paediatrics

Anatomy and physiology

Accurately assessing and appropriately managing paediatric emergencies are contingent on having a good understanding of growth and development and of the anatomical and physiological impact of immaturity and its effect on acute illness and injury across all systems. Children grow in size and mature anatomically and physiologically until they reach adulthood. However, this is not uniform; for example, physiological maturity of many systems is achieved by the end of infancy, while skeletal maturity is not achieved until after puberty. This means that young children may have similar physiological responses to illness and require similar management to adults, while in other circumstances their responses and management may vary greatly.

These differences and their implications will be discussed throughout the chapter in relevant sections of the text. Table 36.1 supplements this discussion and should be consulted for a more comprehensive list of the anatomical and physiological differences which exist between adults, infants and children and their clinical significance.

TABLE 36.1 The anatomical and physiological differences between infants, children and adults, and their clinical significance

DIFFERENCE	DISCUSSION	CLINICAL IMPLICATIONS
Airway differences		
Airways —smaller —more airway soft tissue	Foreign matter such as blood, mucous, vomit and teeth easily obstruct small airways Small amounts of oedema may obstruct the airway, markedly increasing airway resistance	Visualisation and clearing of the airway more difficult Suctioning of airway may be required
Tongue—larger relative to the oropharynx	Airway may be obstructed by the tongue, where there is swelling or a decrease in conscious state	In the trauma patient, open the airway using the jaw-thrust manoeuvre Repositioning may be the only intervention needed to maintain a patent airway Oropharyngeal airways may be useful in the unresponsive child
Obligate nose breathers in early infancy (< 3 months of age)	Obstructed nasal passages can produce significant respiratory distress and/or feeding difficulty	Remove secretions using saline drops or suction
Trachea—shorter in length	Increased chance of bronchial intubation Changes in head position will cause movement in ETT Flexion of the neck displaces the tube further into the trachea Extension of the neck moves the tube further out of the trachea	Ensure air-entry to both lung fields, confirm position on X-ray Secure tube carefully Record initial ETT position (centimetre mark at the gum) Maintain head in midline position and prevent extension or flexion of the neck Monitor ETT position regularly

TABLE 36.1 The anatomical and physiological differences between infants, children and adults, and their clinical significance—cont'd

DIFFERENCE	DISCUSSION	CLINICAL IMPLICATIONS
Larynx—softer and more cartilagenous	More susceptible to compression with hyperextension or hypoextension of the neck	Maintain appropriate position to ensure airway patency Use jaw thrust in the trauma patient
Larynx—positioned more anteriorly and cephalad	Increased risk of aspiration Direct visualisation of the vocal cords is more difficult during intubation	Cricoid pressure occludes airway during intubation; may also assist with visualisation of the vocal cords during intubation attempts
Cricoid cartilage—the narrowest region of the airway rather than the larynx	Cricoid ring provides a natural seal for the endotracheal tube Cuffed tubes may cause airway damage in younger children	Use uncuffed endotracheal tubes in children younger than 8 years
Epiglottis—shaped differently and relatively floppy	Epiglottis likely to 'flop' into airway obscuring view of cords during intubation	Ensure alternative laryngoscope blade (straight) available Lift epiglottis out of the way
Occiput—relatively large	Head pushed forward when lying supine, therefore neck not in neutral alignment; may result in airway compression	Place a small towel roll under the child's shoulders to maintain the appropriate airway position
Cervical spine differences		
Head—proportionately heavier Vertebral ligament—increased laxity Neck musculature—underdeveloped	Increases the risk that vertebrae may move, resulting in spinal cord injury in the absence of a fracture Pseudosubluxation of C2 on C3 Normal variant in up to 40% of children aged < 7 years and in < 20% of children aged < 16 years Secondary to ligamentous laxity Phenomenon called spinal cord injury without radiological abnormality (SCIWORA); seen predominantly in children	Normal cervical spine X-ray does not exclude cord injury Careful neurological examination needed CT scan and MRI may be useful adjuncts in the evaluation of possible spinal cord injuries Neurosurgical consultation should be obtained where extent of injury unclear
Fulcrum of flexion higher—C1–C2 in young children; C6–C7 in adults	Level of cervical spine injury occurs at fulcrum of flexion Affects outcome	Neurological deficits determined by level of injury
Growth centres in vertebrae	Increased susceptibility to shearing forces	Increases likelihood of cord injury
Ear–nose–throat		
Eustachian tubes—shorter and angle less acute	Reduced drainage of fluids	Increased number of ear infections
Respiratory differences		
Ribs —more cartilaginous —twice as compliant as those of an adult	Retractions are more common and reduce the infant's or small child's ability to maintain functional residual capacity or generate adequate tidal volume Ribs may not fracture under compression or with direct blow Provide less protection to underlying organs. Increased chest wall compliance allows traumatic forces to be transmitted to underlying thoracic structures	Work of breathing the most useful indicator of level of respiratory distress Absence of rib fracture on X-ray does not exclude possibility of injury to underlying structures Suspect pneumothoraces and/or haemothoraces in the child who has significant chest trauma with or without rib fractures

Continued

TABLE 36.1 The anatomical and physiological differences between infants, children and adults, and their clinical significance—cont'd

DIFFERENCE	DISCUSSION	CLINICAL IMPLICATIONS
Ribs—positioned more horizontally in infancy than the adults	Relatively fixed tidal volume	Dependent on rate to maintain minute volume
Mediastinum—more mobile	More likely to suffer damage due to shearing in an acceleration/deceleration injury	
Fatigue-resistant type I fibres—fewer in intercostal muscles	Become exhausted more quickly	Closely observe the child with continuous monitoring of heart rate, respiratory rate and effort, and pulse oximetry Treat respiratory distress Prevent increases to demand Allow parents to remain with child if their presence is comforting to the child Provide non-threatening environment and avoid noxious stimuli Treat pain
Diaphragm —performs most of the work of breathing —reduced role of intercostal muscles	Generation of tidal volume depends on diaphragmatic function Anything impeding diaphragm movement can lead to reduced tidal volume, e.g. distended stomach Diaphragmatic fatigue possible	Allow alert child to maintain own position of comfort to optimise respiratory effort If possible, maintain patient in upright position to support diaphragmatic function Avoid abdominal distension Smaller, more frequent feeds Nasogastric or orogastric tube insertion to decompress the stomach
Chest wall—relatively thin	Breath sounds are easily transmitted across the chest wall and over the abdomen Difficult to localise adventitious noises (including upper-airway-generated noises)	Breath sounds should be auscultated bilaterally over the anterior and posterior chest wall, and in the axillary areas, using a paediatric stethoscope Differences indicating pathology may be subtle Obtain chest X-ray films as necessary
Oxygen consumption—twice that of an adult	Higher minute volume to meet demand	Deliver highest possible concentration of oxygen to infants and children in respiratory distress
Respiratory muscles—greater oxygen and metabolite requirement	Work of breathing can account for up to 40% of the cardiac output, particularly in stressed conditions	Reduce work of breathing Mechanical ventilation to eliminate metabolic costs of work of breathing
Control of ventilation—immature	Responses to hypoxia are unpredictable	Monitor young infants closely for apnoea
Circulatory differences		
Myocardium —fewer actomysin elements and mitochondria, therefore less capacity to increase contractility —less compliant	Unable to increase stroke volume Greater reliance on increases in heart rate to increase cardiac output compared with the adult Higher atrial pressures at the same filling pressures Negative effect on preload Restricts capacity to increase stroke volume Relatively poor response to aggressive fluid resuscitation	Provide continuous cardiac monitoring with attention to trends in heart rate Larger volumes of fluid may be required to augment circulation

TABLE 36.1 The anatomical and physiological differences between infants, children and adults, and their clinical significance—cont'd

DIFFERENCE	DISCUSSION	CLINICAL IMPLICATIONS
Compensation—better able to mount compensatory response by increasing peripheral vascular resistance	May remain normotensive until 25–40% of their blood volume is lost Hypotension is a late and often sudden sign of cardiovascular decompensation	Monitor other parameters to detect hypovolaemia before hypotension apparent Aggressive resuscitation in response to earlier signs of hypovolaemia
Blood volume —larger volume per kg (child 80 mL/kg vs adult 70 mL/kg) —absolute volume much smaller	Smaller amounts of blood loss can cause volume depletion	Carefully estimate blood loss, including blood drawn for laboratory analysis Serial haemoglobin and haematocrit analysis should be obtained Consider blood replacement therapy after 40–60 mL/kg of isotonic crystalloids in the paediatric trauma patient with signs of shock or when acute blood loss totals 5–7% of the child's circulating blood volume
Vessels—smaller	Intravascular access more difficult	Cannula sizes will need to be adjusted Ensure most-competent clinician attempting access in time-critical situation Low threshold for using alternative access strategy, e.g. intraosseous administration
Systemic vascular resistance—lower	BP lower	Ensure reference range for normal BP for varying age is available
Terminal rhythm differs —children: brady/asystole; adults: VF/VT	Bradycardia often result of hypoxia Brachycardia not well tolerated in children because it significantly reduces cardiac output	Provide adequate oxygenation and ventilation Treat symptomatic bradycardia
Fluid balance		
Percentage total body water larger—infants & children: 80%; adults: 65%	Infants and young children will lose larger amounts of water through evaporation than will the adult	Calculate maintenance fluids based on each child's weight in kilograms and clinical condition
Surface area/volume ratio—larger	Children have greater potential for dehydration Maintenance fluid requirements per kilogram of body weight are higher in children	Record all sources of fluid intake and fluid loss to calculate fluid balance and adjust fluid therapy accordingly
Renal blood flow and the glomerular filtration rate—lower	Less capacity to concentrate the urine infants 2 mL/kg children 1 mL/kg adults 0.5 mL/kg	Relatively higher volumes of urine are required to indicate adequate renal perfusion
Renal system—immature	Less able to acidify urine and therefore more susceptible to hyperchloraemic acidosis with aggressive resuscitation with Normal saline	Avoid large volume resuscitation with Normal saline without close monitoring of electrolytes
Neurological differences		
Head—proportionately larger and heavier	Higher centre of gravity acts as a missile If an infant or child falls or is thrown a significant distance, the initial impact more often will be to the head, which predisposes the child to head injury	Anticipate head injury in the traumatically injured child Suggest use of preventive measures, such as seat belts, car seats and helmets, to patients and family members

Continued

TABLE 36.1 The anatomical and physiological differences between infants, children and adults, and their clinical significance—cont'd

DIFFERENCE	DISCUSSION	CLINICAL IMPLICATIONS
Skull—thinner	Provides less protection for the brain	As above
Cranial sutures —do not fuse until approximately age 16–18 months —fontanelles are junction between sutures	Fullness of fontanelle is influenced by acute changes in intracranial volume —full = intracerebral infection, haemorrhage etc —low = hypovolaemia Allow for growth of the skull and intracranial contents May allow for gradual increases in intracranial volume, i.e. hydrocephalus	Assess fontanelles for size and tension in the infant age 16–18 months or younger Measure head circumference with neurological examinations in the child up to age 16–18 months at risk for increasing intracranial pressure
Cognitive development—varies with age	Assessment of cognitive function influenced by level of development Cooperation influenced by development	Use modified GCS for neurological assessment Use age-appropriate assessment techniques Use age-appropriate management strategies

Metabolic and thermoregulatory differences

Immune system—immature	Increased susceptibility to infection Response to infection differs; often poorly localised resulting in different constellation of symptoms	Assume serious illness in babies with generalised symptoms until focus found
Surface area to body mass ratio—higher Subcutaneous fat stores—lower	Increased heat loss through radiation and evaporation, especially from the child's proportionally large head Hypothermia can cause metabolic acidosis, hypoglycaemia, coagulopathies, CNS depression, respiratory depression and myocardial irritability, making resuscitation more difficult Less-well-insulated by fat, adding to heat loss	Prevent heat loss Cover children with warm blankets or place them under warming lights if they cannot be covered Reduce draughts in clinical area Use warmed intravenous fluids or blood for volume resuscitation Warm and humidify supplemental oxygen if possible Consider placing small infants in isolettes with overbed warmers Monitor temperature in young babies in isolette with skin probe to avoid underheating or overheating and thermal injury
Heat production —infants aged < 3 months unable to rely on shivering —rely on fat stores	Increased risk of hypothermia in the small infant The burning of fat increases oxygen consumption, which can lead to hypoxia	As above
Glycogen stores—lower	Increased risk for developing hypoglycaemia	Monitor glucose frequently during and after resuscitation Administer glucose as ordered
Metabolic rate—higher	Increased oxygen and glucose consumption Increased demands associated with illness may not be met due to poor stores Results in higher nutritional needs per kilogram of bodyweight than in an adult	As above Provide supplemental oxygen to all seriously ill or injured children Consult with doctor and dietitian to provide early, adequate nutritional support to the compromised child

TABLE 36.1 The anatomical and physiological differences between infants, children and adults, and their clinical significance—cont'd

DIFFERENCE	DISCUSSION	CLINICAL IMPLICATIONS
Abdominal differences		
Diaphragm—flattened	Pushes the spleen and liver down into the abdominal cavity Unprotected by the rib cage, increasing their exposure to injury Spleen and liver are the most commonly injured abdominal organs in children	Abdominal assessment for presence of injury vital in children involved in trauma Obtain early surgical consultation as necessary Monitor serial haemoglobin and haematocrit analysis for signs of haemorrhage Abdominal girth measurements may assist assessment
Abdominal wall—less musculature and less subcutaneous tissue	Provides less protection to underlying organs	As above
Bladder position—intra-abdominal organ until approximately 2 years of age	Increased risk of bladder trauma where there is injury to the abdomen	Urine specimens can be taken suprapubically in infants and young toddlers
Musculoskeletal differences		
Bones —incomplete bone calcification —more cartilaginous —more flexible and plastic	Afford less protection to underlying structures than the stronger, more rigid bones of the adult Can absorb larger amounts of force without bone injury, transferring force to underlying structures Change the injury profile as increased cartilage weakens the bone Weakest part of the musculoskeletal system (tendon/muscle/ligament/bone) Result in plastic deformation (bowing fractures, greenstick and torus fractures) in response to trauma	Index of suspicion for organ damage should be high even in the absence of fractures where the force was significant Obtain early surgical consultation as necessary Monitor for signs of internal haemorrhage Low threshold for X-ray of limb injuries even in the absence of obvious signs of fracture as plastic deformation, torus and buckle fractures less clinically apparent
Bones growing—physeal plate and secondary ossification centres present	Physeal plate is a point of vulnerability (2–5 times weaker than other parts of the bone) Increased blood flow to physeal areas of the bone increases likelihood of vascular deposition of bacteria, e.g. osteomyelitis	Presence of secondary ossification centres and physeal plates influence interpretation of radiological images Gain paediatric orthopaedic opinion if there is any doubt about images Index of suspicion for infection should be high
Bones growing—metabolic activity higher	Healing times are substantially shorter Growing bones allow for remodeling of the bony deformity particularly in the arc of movement	

BP: blood pressure; CNS: central nervous system; CT: computed tomography; ETT: endotracheal tube; GCS: Glasgow Coma Scale; MRI: magnetic resonance imaging; VF: ventricular fibrillation; VT: ventricular tachycardia

Family-centred care and communication

In most circumstances, children present with a parent or caregiver who plays an integral role in maintaining the health and welfare of the child. Emergency care of children includes caring for the family unit, and this should be collaborative and based on a partnership. Parents and caregivers must be given the opportunity to negotiate their role in treatment decision-making and caring for their children and where children are old enough they should be included in this collaboration.

Effective collaborative healthcare is contingent on developing a therapeutic relationship with the patient and their family, and the circumstances of emergency care can make this more difficult as time is limited and patients and their families are usually anxious and worried. This challenge is magnified when communication with the patient is made more difficult because of their condition or their age. Paediatric emergency presentations require clinicians to rapidly develop rapport with adults and children whose needs may be different, and the ways that these needs can be met are likely to be different.

Parents experience a range of emotions when calling an ambulance or presenting with their children to the emergency department (ED); these may range from relief to great anxiety about the likely diagnosis and outcome, or guilt about the origins of the child's illness or injury. The parents may also have a range of concerns that they are reluctant to raise unless comfortable. Furthermore, they are likely to have had previous contact with healthcare professionals, which may even include consultation for this health concern, and their experiences may range from favourable to very unsatisfactory, which may colour their attitude towards this presentation.

Complaints about the quality of healthcare will include those where the diagnosis was missed and treatment decisions were wrong. However, a large number focus on communication and the interactions between patients, families and clinicians. Parents most frequently complain that they were not listened to or taken seriously, or that they weren't provided with sufficient information. Developing good rapport with parents and caregivers requires the clinician to listen carefully to the parents' concerns, ideally while seated, and not to interrupt. The circumstances of emergency care pre-hospital, at triage and during the diagnostic work-up and treatment phases of the emergency presentation can make this especially difficult to achieve. Simple strategies may help to overcome the limitations of the circumstances, such as using the parents' and child's names. Regardless of how minor the health problem, the parents' concerns should be acknowledged. Parents are often seeking information and reassurance, and this should be provided wherever possible. Clinicians should be aware of their own body language, the language that they use and the messages that this may convey. For example, asking a question using 'why', such as 'Why have you come today?', implies that they should have done something different.

Explanations should be provided in language that parents will understand and should not include jargon, abbreviations and acronyms. The majority of children are discharged home where parents or family members will care for them, which makes it essential that they understand the information with which they were provided. Discharge education should provide families with sufficient detail to adequately and confidently manage their child at home. It should always include a comprehensive discussion of the criteria for re-presentation. Symptomatic management of viral illness or development of secondary infection may result in deterioration. On occasions the diagnosis is difficult to make in the early stages of the illness and review is necessary to identify the specific features of illness. Parents must be given the capacity to recognise signs of treatment failure and deterioration and the confidence to return to the ED for review.

Gaining the child's confidence will improve the child's cooperation with history-taking and with the examination, and may help to reassure the parents. The strategies used to gain the confidence of the child will depend on their age and rely on showing creativity and an understanding of the cognitive development of the child and their likely fears.

Infants and young children will look to their parents for support and they should not be separated unless absolutely necessary. Age-appropriate games and toys may be used to distract and help gain the child's confidence. These strategies serve as a way of relaxing the child, but are also an excellent aid to examination. For example, an infant watching and reaching for bubbles demonstrates normal cognition. Where possible, examination should be delayed until the child has become more comfortable with the clinician. The best results are generally achieved when the child is examined in a parent's arms or on their lap with the clinician sitting on a low stool or on the ground rather than standing over the top of the child. The sequence of examination should see the more invasive and distressing techniques left until last.

As children get older, involving them as much as possible and explaining your intentions is likely to increase the child's confidence. Great care should be taken with the language used, as school-aged children can be very frightened by particular words, and can take expressions quite literally. Magical thinking can exacerbate this, but is also an excellent foundation for age-appropriate games aimed at gaining their cooperation. It may be possible to make a game out of parts of the examination: for example, explaining that you think you saw a tiger in their ear but you need to use a light to have a proper look to see if there really is one there. Reading stories and watching videos can also serve to distract the child.

Once children reach adolescence, they are usually striving for much more independence and are likely to look for this when seeking healthcare. However, this should not be assumed and clinicians will need to negotiate everyone's roles fairly early on. Generally this needn't be done formally as it becomes increasingly apparent during the consultation.

Privacy

Privacy should be provided for paediatric consultations regardless of the age of the child or the nature of the presentation. Simple health problems may be an opportunity for parents to seek assistance from healthcare professionals regarding more-sensitive issues. Adolescents are also likely to demand greater privacy and may also wish to discuss their health concerns without the presence of their parents.

PRACTICE TIPS
APPROACH TO PAEDIATRICS

- Infants and children differ from adults anatomically, physiologically and cognitively, and this must be considered when examining and managing them in the ED.
- It is essential to rapidly gain the trust of the parents and the child to assess and manage the child in the ED.
- Most complaints stem from poor communication.
- Strategies for engaging with the child and gaining their cooperation will depend on their age.
- Parents and/or caregivers must be given the opportunity to negotiate their role in clinical decision-making and caring for their children.
- Privacy for children and their families (regardless of age) should be maintained.

Assessment

The physical, cognitive and developmental differences between infants, children and adults will influence the approach to assessment and interpretation of the findings. Using a systematic approach to assessment and applying some simple principles, it is possible to adequately assess and identify health problems in infants and children. The following sections describe an approach to paediatric health assessment and highlight how the differences between adults, children and infants affect assessment.

History

The history will provide information about the chief presenting complaint, associated signs and symptoms, past medical history, family history and social history, which will identify health-related concerns and aid the diagnosis and development of a management plan for the child and their family. The focus of the history and the extent of the detail sought must also be tailored for the circumstances of the presentation (i.e. mechanism of injury where the child presents with an arm injury), the age of the patient (i.e. perinatal history where the child is < 1 month of age), the environment (i.e. pre-hospital or ED) and the urgency of the presentation.

History-taking requires significant interview skills to ensure that the history is complete regardless of the age of the patient. However, there are some unique features to paediatric history-taking where it relies on building a rapport with both patient (child) and parent, as discussed in the previous section. History-taking in paediatrics often relies on information provided by primary carers, with the child's involvement limited by their level of cognitive development and the extent of their illness.

However, it is important not to ignore the contribution that may be made by quite young children. Young children are often capable of providing important details, while parents may be less clear about the circumstances of the injury or illness of their child. For example, the mother of a 5-year-old presenting to the ED with an injury to her left arm described the injury as a fall from the monkey bars. However, discussion with the child revealed a fall which did not result in injury, followed by pulling on her arm as her friend helped her back up onto the play equipment, which resulted in a 'pulled elbow'. Alternatively, siblings may also provide valuable information, particularly descriptions of the mechanism of injury responsible for the child's presentation.

Patient history generally focuses on details about the chief presenting complaint, past medical history that includes treatments and current medication regimens, social history and family history. Paediatric history-taking may adopt this framework with details about specific paediatric health-related issues such as perinatal history collected under the relevant headings. Alternatively, mnemonics such as CIAMPEDS (see Table 36.2) have been designed to prompt clinicians to collect relevant data.[1]

Presenting complaint

Determining the nature of the presenting complaint and the associated signs and symptoms is the initial focus of history-taking. This is a detailed account of the onset of the illness or the mechanism of injury, the range and extent of signs and symptoms, the precipitating and alleviating factors and the treatment provided to date; and there are some clinical and

---

TABLE 36.2 CIAMPEDS mnemonic to guide history-taking for the paediatric presentation[1]

ELEMENT OF MNEMONIC	DESCRIPTION
Chief complaint	Identify the reason for the ED visit
Immunisation status/ Isolation	Confirm the immunisations that the child has received to date and record the reasons for delays or decisions to omit an immunisation
	Identify potential exposure to infectious diseases, e.g. parvovirus and note the source, e.g. sibling, childcare, etc
Allergies	Document a history of previous allergic or hypersensitivity reactions and include the type of reaction
Medication	Record all medications currently prescribed, those being taken and medications recently ceased. Include over-the-counter medications and herbal preparations
Past medical history/ Parent's/caregiver's impression of the child's condition	Record details of past health problems. Include prior illnesses, injuries, hospital admissions, surgical procedures and chronic physical and mental health problems. In older children include risk-taking behaviour such as: alcohol, tobacco, drug use.
	Identify the child's primary caregiver(s). Document their impression of the illness/injury, noting their specific concerns, which may be influenced by a range of factors, including: culture, previous experience of illness and healthcare
Events surrounding the illness or injury	Document the time course of the illness or time of the injury. Note the associated circumstances, precipitants and alleviating factors and the mechanism of injury for traumatic presentations
Diet and diapers (nappies)	Note recent oral intake, paying particular attention to fluids. Identify recent changes in eating patterns and consider weight changes
	Urine and stool output
Symptoms associated with the illness or injury	Identify symptoms and their pattern of progression over the course of the illness or since the time of injury

age-related factors that should be considered as they may alert the clinician to the presence of significant illness or injury.

Infants may rapidly deteriorate, and frequently exhibit few or non-specific signs and symptoms of significant illness as a result of immunological immaturity. For this reason, in addition to the attention given to the signs and symptoms of the illness, particular attention should be paid to feeding, urine output, activity levels and sleeping patterns. Research has shown that changes to any of these increases the likelihood that the infant or young child has a serious illness, and with the addition of a urine screen 90% of infants with serious illness can be detected by reviewing these simple parameters.[2,3] Furthermore, these details may also provide clues about the nature of the illness.

Poor feeding may result from shortness of breath, lethargy or general malaise, and is associated with a range of illnesses which includes serious infection, moderate to severe respiratory illness and gastrointestinal disorders. The relationship between other symptoms and feeding should also be explored. In neonates and young babies, sweating and dusky skin colour during feeding suggests cardiac disease, while projectile vomiting soon after feeding suggests pyloric stenosis. Comparison with the feeding pattern of the child or infant when well is generally the best method for determining the adequacy of feeding and this information can be provided by the carer. However, it is useful to know the average volumes consumed by infants and children at varying ages, and these can be found in Table 36.3. Similarly, changes in urine output are best estimated by comparing current output with output when well; in infants this is determined indirectly via the number of wet nappies in a day. It is generally accepted that infants will have approximately 6 wet nappies per day.

Serious illness in infants can be associated with irritability and disturbed sleep, or decreased activity and drowsiness where the infant fails to wake for feeds. Sleep may also be disturbed by respiratory illness, shortness of breath, sleep apnoea caused by enlarged tonsils, pain and a range of other circumstances.

Past history

A child's co-morbidities and the treatment received should be evaluated for the likely effect on their acute condition. This should also include the infant's perinatal history, to identify health problems resulting from prematurity, the circumstances of the delivery or congenital abnormalities. For example, the infant with congenital lung disease resulting from prematurity is at risk of more significant respiratory dysfunction associated with an acute respiratory infection.

The history should determine whether the child is showing consistent weight gain and meeting normal growth and developmental milestones. Some illnesses and abnormalities become evident as a result of failure to thrive or arrested/delayed development. For this reason, it is important to be familiar with developmental milestones and the use of growth charts to identify deviations from normal; refer to Table 36.4 for normal milestones in the first two years of life. Newborns in

TABLE 36.3 Average oral intake for neonates, infants and children

AGE	VOLUME
Infant	150 mL/kg/day
Small child	50 mL/kg/day
Older child	20 mL/kg/day

TABLE 36.4 Normal milestones in first two years of life[553]

AGE	ACHIEVEMENT—MOTOR	ACHIEVEMENT—LANGUAGE AND SOCIAL
Neonate	Lifts head Visually fixes for period	Turns to voice
6 weeks	Follows past midline	Smiles
2–4 months	Rolls over Head steady when sitting Follows objective 180 degrees	Smiles Squeals with enjoyment
5–8 months	Sits without support Transfers objects between hands	Makes babbling noises Feeds self biscuit
9–12 months	Stands holding on for support, crawls Able to use a pincer grip for small objects	Says 'mama' and 'dada' Exhibits stranger anxiety Indicates needs by gesturing
12–16 months	Walks unassisted Able to make a stack of two blocks	Says single words Drinks from a cup
17–21 months	Walks up steps Scribbles with large texta/crayon	Says several words Points to one part of the body
2 years	Runs and jumps Can copy drawing straight line	Combines words Can remove clothing

Australia and New Zealand are issued with an 'infant welfare' book (variously named in different jurisdictions) to document postnatal and maternal child health nurse examinations, including weight measurements and immunisations. There are also a number of tools available which establish growth and development norms, i.e. height and weight charts, developmental screening tools (Denver development tool), etc.

The immunisation schedule provides recommendations for the vaccination of children against a range of childhood diseases. Table 36.5 lists the Australian[4] and New Zealand[5] schedules which are government-funded. When gaining a history, it is important to ask about the immunisation status of the child. Although it is uncommon for children to be unimmunised, many children fall behind the schedule, often as a result of illness at the time vaccinations were due. A small number of families will identify themselves as conscientious objectors to immunisation or will indicate that they have had their child homeopathically immunised. Details should be obtained when vaccinations were administered overseas where the schedule may vary from the Australasian schedules.

Family history and social history

The family history will help determine whether familial or genetic disorders such as asthma, diabetes, etc, are likely. Relationships between family members and the illnesses suffered can be documented on a family tree for clarity. In some circumstances it may also be important to note consanguinity between parents, as this increases the risk of genetic and familial disorders and is common in some communities.

Siblings may also be able to contribute historical informa-tion, may be linked to the circumstances of the injury or may be a potential infectious contact. Attendance at childcare also increases the child's exposure to infectious diseases and it is important to note whether there has been a recent epidemic at the patient's childcare facility. Furthermore, childcare workers may also be able to contribute to the history.

The child's living circumstances should also be considered, in particular to identify other risks to health such as cigarette smoke exposure, which increases the risk of respiratory diseases, meningococcal disease, Perthes' disease, sudden infant death syndrome (SIDS), etc. In some circumstances, recent travel may be relevant to the current presentation.

A complete history should identify who acts as the primary carer and whether there are others who play a significant role as carer. Where a second person cares for the child for significant periods of time, this person may be able to add substantially to the history. Additionally, consideration should be given to providing this person with similar healthcare information as is provided to the parents to ensure that they are well placed to care for the child's health.

Child at risk

Mandatory reporting legislation in all jurisdictions in Australia demands that healthcare professionals report suspicions that a child has suffered physical, emotional or sexual abuse to the statutory child protection authority in that jurisdiction.[6] A summary of the legislative duties can be found on the Australian Institute of Family Studies website.[7] Child abuse is not common; however, healthcare professionals responsible for the care of children must consider the possibility and respond

TABLE 36.5 Immunisation schedules

AGE	DISEASES AND VACCINES
Australian recommended immunisation schedule (implemented 1 July 2013)*	
Birth	Hepatitis B (hepB)[a]
2 months	Hepatitis B, diphtheria, tetanus, acellular pertussis (whooping cough), *Haemophilus influenzae* type b, inactivated poliomyelitis (polio) (hepB-DTPa-Hib-IPV) Pneumococcal conjugate (13vPCV) Rotavirus
4 months	Hepatitis B, diphtheria, tetanus, acellular pertussis (whooping cough), *Haemophilus influenzae* type b, inactivated poliomyelitis (polio) (hepB-DTPa-Hib-IPV) Pneumococcal conjugate (13vPCV) Rotavirus
6 months	Hepatitis B, diphtheria, tetanus, acellular pertussis (whooping cough), *Haemophilus influenzae* type b, inactivated poliomyelitis (polio) (hepB-DTPa-Hib-IPV) Pneumococcal conjugate (13vPCV) Rotavirus[b]
6 months and over (at risk groups)	Influenza (flu) (people with medical conditions placing them at risk of serious complications of influenza) Pneumococcal conjugate (13vPCV)[e] (medically at risk)
12 months	*Haemophilus influenzae* type b and Meningococcal C (Hib-MenC) Measles, mumps and rubella (MMR)
12–18 months (at risk groups)	Pneumococcal conjugate (13vPCV) (Aboriginal and Torres Strait Islander children in high risk areas)

Continued

	TABLE 36.5 Immunisation schedules—cont'd	

AGE	DISEASES AND VACCINES
12–24 months (at risk groups)	Hepatitis A (Aboriginal and Torres Strait Islander children in high risk areas)[f]
18 months	Measles, mumps, rubella and varicella (chickenpox) (MMRV)
18–24 months	Pneumococcal polysaccharide (23vPPV) (Aboriginal and Torres Strait Islander children in high risk areas)
	Hepatitis A (Aboriginal and Torres Strait Islander children in high risk areas)
4 years	Diphtheria, tetanus, acellular pertussis (whooping cough) and inactivated poliomyelitis (polio) (DTPa-IPV)
	Measles, mumps and rubella (MMR) *Only if MMRV not given at 18 months*
4 years (at risk groups)	Pneumococcal polysaccharide (23vPPV)[e] (medically at risk)
10–15 years	Hepatitis B (hepB)[c]
	Varicella (chickenpox)[c]
	Human papillomavirus (HPV)[d]
	Diphtheria, tetanus and acellular pertussis (whooping cough) (dTpa)
15 years and over (at risk groups)	Influenza (flu) (Aboriginal and Torres Strait Islander people)
	Pneumococcal polysaccharide (23vPPV) (Aboriginal and Torres Strait Islander people medically at risk)

New Zealand national immunisation schedule (effective from 1st July 2014[#])

AGE	DISEASES AND VACCINES
6 weeks	Rotavirus (start first dose before 15 weeks)—1 oral vaccine (RotaTeq®)
	Diphtheria/Tetanus/Pertussis/Polio/Hepatitis B/*Haemophilus influenzae* type b—1 injection (INFANRIX®-hexa)
	Pneumococcal—1 injection (SYNFLORIX®)
3 months	Rotavirus—1 oral vaccine (RotaTeq®)
	Diphtheria/Tetanus/Pertussis/Polio/Hepatitis B/*Haemophilus influenzae* type b—1 injection (INFANRIX®-hexa)
	Pneumococcal—1 injection (SYNFLORIX®)
5 months	Rotavirus—1 oral vaccine (RotaTeq®)
	Diphtheria/Tetanus/Pertussis/Polio/Hepatitis B/*Haemophilus influenzae* type b—1 injection (INFANRIX®-hexa)
	Pneumococcal—1 injection (SYNFLORIX®)
15 months	*Haemophilus influenzae* type b—1 injection (Act-HIB)
	Measles/Mumps/Rubella—1 injection (M-M-R® II)
	Pneumococcal—1 injection (SYNFLORIX®)
4 years	Diphtheria/Tetanus/Pertussis/Polio—1 injection (INFANRIX™-IPV
	Measles/Mumps/Rubella—1 injection (M-M-R® II)
11 years	Tetanus/Diphtheria/Pertussis—1 injection (BOOSTRIX™)
12 years girls only	Human papillomavirus—3 doses given over 6 months (GARDASIL®)

a   Hepatitis B vaccine: should be given to all infants as soon as practicable after birth. The greatest benefit is if given within 24 hours, and must be given within 7 days.
b   Rotavirus vaccine: third dose of vaccine is dependent on vaccine brand used. Contact your State or Territory Health Department for details.
c   Hepatitis B and Varicella vaccine: contact your State or Territory Health Department for details on the school grade eligible for vaccination.
d   HPV vaccine: is for all adolescents aged between 12 and 13 years. A catch-up program for males aged between 14 and 15 years was available until December 2014. Contact your State or Territory Health Department for details on the school grade eligible for vaccination.
e   Pneumococcal vaccine:
      Medically at risk children require: a fourth dose of 13vPCV at 12 months of age; and a booster dose of 23vPPV at 4 years of age.
      Aboriginal and Torres Strait Islander children require: a fourth dose of pneumococcal vaccine (13vPCV) at 12–18 months of age for children living in high risk areas (Queensland, Northern Territory, Western Australia and South Australia). Contact your State or Territory Health Department for details.
f   Hepatitis A vaccine: two doses of Hepatitis A vaccine for Aboriginal and Torres Strait Islander children living in high risk areas (Queensland, Northern Territory, Western Australia and South Australia). Contact your State or Territory Health Department for details.
*   © Commonwealth of Australia, www.immunise.health.gov.au/internet/immunise/publishing.nsf/Content/national-immunisation-program-schedule.
#   © Ministry of Health New Zealand, www.health.govt.nz/our-work/preventative-health-wellness/immunisation/new-zealand-immunisation-schedule

appropriately where their suspicions have been aroused, as child protection is of the highest priority.

The most common concern identified by pre-hospital and ED clinicians relates to injuries where the cause is thought not to be the result of an accident. Suspicion should be aroused when there are inconsistencies in the history provided, the version of events changes over time, it is reported differently by each of the parents or does not adequately explain the presenting injuries. Less commonly, the presentation may be for an unrelated health problem and evidence of injury of potential abuse is uncovered, or the parent is disproportionately concerned about their child's condition and keen for the child to be admitted and exploration of the reason for this reveals their concern for their child's welfare while in their care. Care of the child where abuse is suspected should be handed over to a senior clinician and these suspicions raised.

Alternatively, the accompanying adult may acknowledge that there has been family services involvement with the family or this may be noted in the child's history. It is important to determine what responsibilities this places on the examining clinician; for example, reporting all injuries to state authorities, gaining consent from a state-appointed custodian, etc.

Examination

Physical examination of infants and young children and interpretation of the findings can be more difficult, as they frequently become distressed and are uncooperative when touched. Examination techniques frequently need significant adaptation and clinicians will need to rely more heavily on careful observation to elicit reliable examination data. Delaying the examination while you develop a rapport with first the parents and then the child *before* attempting to examine a potentially uncooperative child is ideal. Using strategies to increase their confidence and gain their cooperation was discussed in the previous section and is essential to make adequate examination possible.

Allowing infants to remain in their parent's arms during the examination, making a game out of parts of the examination for toddlers and providing clear explanation to older children of what is intended are examples of strategies that may help increase a child's confidence. Table 36.6 details some strategies for approaching infants and children of different ages.

Using a systematic approach to assessment ensures that priorities are addressed in order and that important features are not overlooked. Assessment conducted as a primary and secondary survey is a common approach to emergency assessment and this can be applied to children. Identifying the physical differences between adults and children where they relate to each component of the survey ensures that these differences are accounted for, and that the results of assessment are appropriately interpreted in light of these differences, while allowing the clinician to use one approach for all age groups. However, a number of other assessment tools have been designed specifically for use in children and include indicators shown to increase the recognition of serious illness in children. They will be discussed later in this section.

The following sections will address the primary survey and the collection of vital signs, highlighting the significance of immaturity. This discussion is supplemented by the details in Table 36.1.

TABLE 36.6 Age-specific approaches to physical examination during childhood[554]

POSITION	SEQUENCE	PREPARATION
Infant		
Best positioned on parent's lap, particularly for sections of the examination that are likely to be distressing	If quiet, auscultate heart, lungs, abdomen first	Clinician should sit on low chair in view of infant but out of reach while taking history, to allow infant to become more comfortable with clinician (older infant)
	Palpate and percuss same areas	
	Undress only when required to prevent babies getting cold	Gain cooperation with distraction, bright objects, rattles, talking
	Proceed in usual head-to-toe direction	Smile at infant; use soft, gentle voice
	Perform traumatic procedures last (eyes, ears, mouth [while crying])	Pacify with feeding
		Enlist parent's aid for restraining to examine ears, mouth
		Avoid abrupt, jerky movements

Continued

TABLE 36.6 Age-specific approaches to physical examination during childhood—cont'd

POSITION	SEQUENCE	PREPARATION
Toddler		
Best positioned on parent's lap, particularly for sections of the examination that are likely to be distressing	Take history first, while observing infant and allowing them to watch Use minimum physical contact initially Inspect body area through play: 'count fingers', 'tickle toes' Introduce equipment slowly Auscultate, percuss, palpate whenever quiet Examine injured limb last; start with the unaffected limb. Repeat to determine whether tenderness is reproducible Perform traumatic procedures last (same as for infant)	Clinician should sit on low chair in view of child but out of reach while taking history, to allow child to become more comfortable with clinician Ask parent to undress child well before examination attempted, to allow child to settle before attempting to examine Allow child to inspect equipment; demonstrating use of equipment is usually ineffective If uncooperative, perform procedures quickly Use restraint when appropriate; request parent's assistance Talk about examination if cooperative; use short phrases Praise for cooperative behaviour
Preschool child		
Allow child to determine where they would like to sit—on parent's lap or on the trolley Ensure parents are close	If cooperative, proceed in head-to-toe direction If uncooperative, proceed as with toddler	Request self-undressing Allow to wear underpants if shy Offer equipment for inspection; briefly demonstrate use Make up story about procedure (e.g. 'I'm seeing how strong your muscles are' [blood pressure]) Give choices when possible Expect cooperation; use positive statements (e.g. 'Open your mouth')
School-age child		
Cooperative in most positions Younger child prefers parent's presence Older child may prefer privacy	Proceed in head-to-toe direction May examine genitalia last in older child	Respect need for privacy. Expose only area to be examined Request self-undressing Explain purpose of equipment and significance of procedure, such as otoscope to see eardrum, which is necessary for hearing Teach about body function and care Use simple language for explanations as they are easily frightened by misunderstood language
Adolescent		
Same as for school-age child Offer option of parent's presence	Same as older school-age child Leave intrusive/embarrassing examinations until last	Allow to undress in private and provide gown Expose only area to be examined Respect need for privacy Explain findings during examination: 'Your muscles are firm and strong' Emphasise normalcy of anatomy and development, including genitals Examine genitalia as any other body part; may leave to end

Airway

Evaluation of the airway will concentrate on determining airway patency. A narrower airway and increased soft tissue places the infant and child at greater risk of airway obstruction, and stridor is a common paediatric presentation indicating airway obstruction. However, assessing work of breathing, which is described in the next section, should make possible evaluation of the extent of the airway obstruction.

Breathing

Infants and children tolerate respiratory distress very poorly, and respiratory dysfunction is recognised as a precursor to clinical deterioration and poor outcomes in adults.[8] It is the most common cause of paediatric cardiopulmonary arrest.[9]

The primary focus of respiratory assessment is an assessment of the work of breathing. Increased work of breathing has been shown to be an indicator of significant or serious illness in infants.[2,3] In addition, work of breathing and mental state are considered the most useful indicators of the severity of asthma.[10,11] Increased work of breathing is reliably recognised in infants and children by the presence of subcostal, suprasternal and intercostal recession (see Fig 36.1), the severity of which is defined as *mild*, *moderate* and *severe*.[12]

Secondary assessment parameters, which will contribute to the assessment of the severity of respiratory dysfunction, are:

- respiratory rate
- oxygen saturations (SpO_2)
- the presence or absence of nasal flaring.

Increasing respiratory rate suggests significant illness. However, as infants and children become more exhausted, a drop in respiratory rate may signal deterioration. It has also been shown that the respiratory rates of well infants under the age of 6 months vary considerably, from 20 to 80 breaths per minute.[13,14] For these reasons, respiratory rate should be interpreted cautiously and not in isolation. Oxygen saturations are frequently referred to as the fifth vital sign, and some evidence suggests that measurement of the SpO_2 on presentation of infants and children with respiratory illness may assist in the prediction of those likely to require admission for respiratory observation and management.

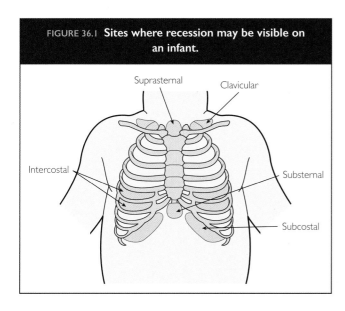

FIGURE 36.1 **Sites where recession may be visible on an infant.**

Suprasternal

Clavicular

Intercostal

Substernal

Subcostal

Finally, systemic signs such as colour, heart rate and mentation will also assist in determining respiratory adequacy. Hypoxia results in increasing pallor and in extreme circumstances cyanosis. Respiratory inadequacy results in an increasing heart rate, but infants are extremely susceptible to hypoxia and quickly respond with bradycardia. Similarly, increasing respiratory dysfunction results in deteriorating mental state and infants can progress from irritability to drowsiness very rapidly.

Infants and young children use grunting to increase airway pressure and improve functional residual capacity and therefore oxygenation in respiratory illness. This involves closing of the glottis against expiration, resulting in positive-end expiratory pressure which helps to prevent alveolar collapse. This creates the same effect as pursed-lip breathing often seen in older people with chronic lung disease. Grunting should alert the clinician to the presence of significant pathology that has the potential to impact on oxygenation.

Lung sounds contribute to diagnostic decision-making rather than an assessment of respiratory efficacy. Wheezes are an expiratory noise reflecting narrowing of the airways. They are heard in a number of common paediatric illnesses such as asthma and bronchiolitis, and less commonly with anaphylaxis and foreign-body inhalation. Other noises heard on auscultation are creps, crackles and rales, which may be widespread or localised. Adventitious lung sounds should be interpreted cautiously, as the small size of the chest and the thin chest wall results in transmission of sounds across the lung fields and even from the upper airways.

The infant or child presenting with respiratory illness and significant distress should be monitored closely for signs of deterioration, evidenced by changes in work and efficacy of breathing. Oxygen saturation monitoring is routinely used to provide continuous monitoring of these children.

Circulation

Assessment of circulatory function should rely on clinical findings, which will detect dehydration and hypovolaemia in the early stages. Even in the early stages before dehydration is severe enough to result in hypovolaemia, there is considerable overlap between the signs of each of these states. Attempts have been made to identify the most sensitive and specific signs in children, with most studies focusing on dehydration.

Simple measures are the most practical means to identify deficits in infants and children, particularly pre-hospital and at triage. Skin colour, warmth and capillary refill time (CRT) are all easily assessed without creating distress for the child. Sudden onset of pallor has been revealed by a series of studies as indicative of serious illness in infants.[2,3] Capillary refill time is an indicator of peripheral perfusion and therefore an indirect measure of cardiovascular function; 2 seconds is the accepted upper limit of normal.[15] However, clinicians are cautioned about relying exclusively on this parameter, as the evidence for its sensitivity for detecting shock in young children is not convincing, with no correlation shown between delayed CRT and bacterial infection and no correlation shown between capillary refill and invasive cardiovascular indices.[16]

The evidence for the value of capillary refill for estimating severity of dehydration is more robust, making it a useful assessment tool.[17,18] However, even in this setting clinicians are advised to interpret the results with caution, as ambient temperature and the technique and site of measurement are likely to affect the sensitivity and specificity.[18–22] In the absence of more-suitable sensitive assessment parameters, CRT is still a reasonable method for assessing peripheral perfusion and hydration for children presenting to the ED.[23]

Hypovolaemia is evidenced by signs of poor end-organ perfusion and compensatory efforts.[24] Tachycardia (see Table 36.7 for normal values for age) and signs of vaso-constriction such as skin pallor and mottling are two obvious signs of compensation aimed at improving cardiac output to secure adequate vital end-organ perfusion. As the child's condition worsens, the body initiates measures to overcome the derangements resulting from hypoperfusion, e.g. tachy-pnoea to reduce acidosis.[23] However, as the capacity to compensate deteriorates, evidence of inadequate perfusion, such as hypotension and deteriorating conscious state, become apparent.

Hypotension, defined in children as a systolic blood pressure (SBP) lower than the 5th percentile for age (see Table 36.7 for normal values),[15,25,26] occurs as a result of significant hypo-volaemia. However, in children it is a late sign, which is not apparent until approximately 30% of circulating volume is lost. There are limited data to support these values and they may even be slightly higher than the 5th percentile. However, in the absence of convincing data it is clinically rational to accept a higher threshold for the unwell child.

Measuring a child's blood pressure provides practical challenges, which may affect the accuracy of the result.[27] Young children are frequently uncooperative, are often anxious and distressed and variation in their size affects cuff selection. A cuff most closely representing 40% of the circumference of the upper arm gives a measurement closest to invasive radial blood pressure values.[28] In some circumstances the cuff is applied around the calf. However, there are no data to determine the correlation between this measurement and arterial blood pressure measurements.

As hypotension is an indicator of poor prognosis, blood pressure measurements should be recorded regularly for infants and children at risk of cardiac dysfunction and/or hypo-volaemia. However, treatment decisions should not rest solely on this parameter, particularly where the blood pressure is considered normal. The results should be considered in light of other cardiovascular findings.[24,29]

Reduced urine output is initially a mechanism to conserve fluid. However, as hypovolaemia progresses, renal perfusion deteriorates and urine output decreases further. The minimum permissible urine output for infants (2 mL/kg/h) and children (1 mL/kg/h) is much higher than the minimum volume accepted for adults (0.5 mL/kg/h).[29,30] Direct measurement of urine output in infants and children not yet toilet-trained is invasive and distressing to infants and children. To avoid catheterisation, which is common practice in adults to measure urine output, nappies are often weighed to provide an estimate of urine output. However, it has been shown that this is not an accurate measure and should not be used where the accuracy of the fluid balance assessment is critical.[31]

In summary, significant and potentially life-threatening hypovolaemia is characterised by a combination of signs such as tachycardia, prolonged CRT, hypotension, tachypnoea, altered conscious state, decreased urine output and metabolic acidosis.[23]

Disability

Conscious-state deterioration is a significant indicator of poor prognosis, and alteration in the level of activity has been shown to be an indicator of serious illness in children.[2,3] Decreased conscious state results from intracerebral pathology such as trauma and infection, but may also be an indication of inadequate oxygenation or circulation or other metabolic derangements. Children may manifest worrying changes in neurological status, such as lethargy, irritability, drowsiness, decreased activity and social interaction, including eye contact and hypotonic posturing (extended limbs and abducted hips) with a broad array of illnesses. Clinicians should be wary of the child who appears disproportionately miserable or lethargic with minor illness.

The variable developmental levels of children complicate neurological assessment and application of the Glasgow Coma Scale (GCS), a validated tool developed to standardise and quantify neurological assessment in adults. The GCS has been modified for use in children and is shown to compare favourably with the standard GCS for assessment of traumatic brain injury in older children.[32] The modified GCS is presented in Table 36.8. The Advanced Paediatric Life Support course introduces a simpler alternative as a crude way of defining conscious state in children, and this scale (AVPU) is presented in Box 36.1.[33] The AVPU scale described four levels of consciousness from alert to unconscious. It is generally accepted that 'P' (responds to painful stimuli) equates to a GCS score of 8. Finally, the value of parents and their capacity to identify

TABLE 36.7 Average vital signs by age[15]			
AGE GROUP	PULSE RATE (BEATS/MINUTE)	RESPIRATION RATE (BREATHS/MINUTE)	BLOOD PRESSURE (SYSTOLIC, mmHg)
Neonate	120–180	40–60	60–80
Infant (1 month to 1 year)	110–160	30–40	70–90
Toddler (1–2 years)	100–150	25–35	80–95
Young child (2–7 years)	95–140	25–30	90–110
Older child (7–12 years)	80–120	20–25	100–120

TABLE 36.8 The modified Glasgow Coma Scale for children[559–561]

AREA ASSESSED	INFANTS	CHILDREN	SCORE*
Eye opening	Open spontaneously	Open spontaneously	4
	Open in response to verbal stimuli	Open in response to verbal stimuli	3
	Open in response to pain only	Open in response to pain only	2
	No response	No response	1
Verbal response	Coos and babbles	Oriented, appropriate	5
	Irritable cries	Confused	4
	Cries in response to pain	Inappropriate words	3
	Moans in response to pain	Incomprehensible words or nonspecific sounds	2
	No response	No response	1
Motor response	Moves spontaneously and purposefully	Obeys commands	6
	Withdraws to touch	Localises painful stimulus	5
	Withdraws in response to pain	Withdraws in response to pain	4
	Responds to pain with decorticate posturing (abnormal flexion)	Responds to pain with flexion	3
	Responds to pain with decerebrate posturing (abnormal extension)	Responds to pain with extension	2
	No response	No response	1

A score is given in each category. The individual scores are then added to give a total score of 3 to 15. A score of < 8 is indicative of severe neurological injury.

BOX 36.1 AVPU scale[15]

Alert
Responds to **V**oice
Responds to **P**ain only
Unresponsive

deviations from normal in their child's level of function should not be underestimated.

A fontanelle is the intersection where three/four cranial bones met and create a small gap between the bones. The anterior and posterior fontanelles are palpable until, on average, 3 and 18 months of age respectively, at which time they generally close. The anterior fontanelle is the one most commonly described and palpated during an examination. Palpation of the tension of the fontanelle allows for a gross estimate of intracranial pressure (ICP; tense and bulging indicates raised ICP) or hydration status (depressed/shrunken indicates dehydration). There are limited data to support the sensitivity and specificity of these findings. In a study to determine the significance of a bulging fontanelle, 36% were associated with clinically significant abnormalities.[34] However, no attempt was made to determine the rate of abnormalities in infants without a bulging fontanelle. Fontanelle assessment findings should be considered in light of other findings and not in isolation.

Pain assessment should also be included in neurological assessment, as pain may cloud capacity for accurate assessment and interpretation of other examination findings, particularly in children.[35] Pain assessment is discussed further in Chapter 19 and in the sections on pain management and procedural sedation in this chapter.

Vital signs

Vital signs (respiratory rate, heart rate, temperature, blood pressure and oxygen saturations) and other appropriately-focused assessment parameters such as GCS, neurovascular observations, pain scores and blood glucose measurements should be recorded to provide a baseline (see Ch 17, p. 332, for information on blood glucose level sampling techniques). Values vary with age, making recognition of deviations from normal dependent on recognising normal values for the age of the child, which are presented in Table 36.7. The regularity with which these parameters are then measured will depend on the nature and severity of the illness and the treatment implemented. However, it should be recognised that the value of these parameters is usually in establishing trend data created by repeat measures, as single observations may be influenced by factors other than clinical deterioration or improvement, such as crying, sleeping, pain, etc.

Heart rate measurement in infants and young children should involve palpation of the pulse to provide other information in addition to the rate, such as strength. In infants where the carotid pulse may be difficult to locate due to their short neck, the brachial and femoral pulses provide a good alternative. Respiratory rate is most easily assessed during auscultation, but may be affected by a change in respiratory pattern brought about by the child's awareness of being observed.

Infrared tympanic thermometers (ITTs) have become the standard tool for temperature measurement for adults and children in the ED. However, there is some concern about their accuracy, particularly in infants and young children. Data supporting the sensitivity and specificity of ITTs to detect fever in febrile children are unconvincing.[36–42] However, there is some evidence to suggest that they agree more closely with core temperature than do other measurement techniques.[39–41] The authors of a 2014 systematic review conclude that available evidence does not currently support infrared thermometers for accurate and consistent temperature measurement but that further study is warranted.[43]

An oral temperature measurement, affected by hyperventilation, probe position and ingestion of hot or cold liquids, is also subject to inaccuracy and is not practical in infants and young children. Axillary temperature measurement has been advocated as a good alternative. However, studies have shown that this can be affected by ambient temperature and changes in skin perfusion;[44,45] measurements are on average likely to be from 0.4 (at low temperatures) to 1.0 degree (at temperatures over 39.0 degrees) lower than the oral or rectal temperature,[46] in contrast to tympanic and oral temperature measurements, which have been shown not to be influenced by ambient temperature in a 2012 study.[47]

The clinically rational approach is to avoid tympanic thermometers in young babies where the ear canal is not large enough to allow insertion of the probe, and to view a normal temperature reading with caution, regardless of the measurement technique. It is well recognised that septic infants may present as hypopyrexic rather than hyperpyrexic.

Weight

In paediatric emergency care, the weight of the infant and child should be measured to provide important assessment data. Fluid loss is most accurately detected by repeat weight measurements, and infants and children with actual or potential for dehydration should be weighed 6-hourly during their hospital admission. Weight is also measured to guide medication dosing and fluid volume calculations.

For infants and children too unwell to weigh, this must be estimated. On average, newborns weigh approximately 3.5 kg and reach approximately 10 kg by one year of age, having gained an average of 200 g weekly for the first few months of life followed by 100 g per week. For children between the ages of one and nine years, the most commonly-used formula for weight estimation is (Age + 4) × 2.[30] There is increasing evidence that this formula may underestimate the weight of the majority of Australian children and for this reason Australian Paediatric Life Support Australasia has recently provided a new method for calculating weight, which can be seen in Box 36.2.[15] It should be noted that the weight estimates are likely to underestimate the weight of overweight children. However, it is more appropriate to base medication doses on lean body weight making this inaccuracy unlikely to be clinically concerning. This also means that on some occasions

---

BOX 36.2 Weight estimation[15]

Age	Formula
0–12 months	(0.5 × age in months) + 4
1–5 years	(2 × age in years) + 8
6–12 years	(3 × age in years) + 7

it may be more appropriate to use an estimated weight based on age and height for markedly overweight children to prevent significant overdose.

PRACTICE TIPS

EXAMINATION

- The severity of airway obstruction is best assessed by determining the severity of the respiratory distress.
- Stridor intensity is not a useful indicator of the severity of airway obstruction.
- Work of breathing and mental state are the most useful indicators of the severity of respiratory distress.
- Respiratory noises reflect the underlying pathology, e.g. stridor is an upper airway noise and wheeze is a lower airway noise.
- Hypotension is a very late sign of hypovolaemia in infants and children.
- Capillary refill measurement is a useful adjunct to assessment, but should not be used as a single indirect measure of peripheral perfusion.
- All infants and children with an actual or potential fluid and electrolyte imbalance should be weighed naked, as weight changes are the gold-standard measure for changes in fluid balance.
- A modified Glasgow Coma Scale score for infants and children is recommended for assessment and documentation of neurological assessments.
- A single set of vital signs may be difficult to interpret. Regular observations should be made to generate trend data, which is likely to be more useful.
- Age will influence the interpretation of diagnostic images and some pathology results.

Diagnostic testing

Diagnostic testing is employed to diagnose, exclude or identify the severity of disease, guide treatment options or determine the success of treatment. It is often invasive and distressing, in particular to children. Infants and children will require a combination of procedural sedation, local anaesthetic and analgesic, or in some cases a general anaesthetic for many diagnostic procedures, increasing the potential risks to the child. Therefore, it is important to be clear about what questions will be answered by the test results and whether answers to these questions are an important part of establishing a diagnosis or selecting management strategies.

The significance of age will also need to be considered when employing many sampling and imaging techniques and when interpreting test results.

Diagnostic imaging
Diagnostic images reveal anatomical differences that exist between infants, children and adults, and this influences interpretation of many images, including chest and skeletal X-rays. For example, shape of ribs, relative size and shape of the heart, relatively flattened diaphragms and presence in infants of a prominent thymus distorting the mediastinum will all impact on what constitutes a normal chest X-ray. Skeletal immaturity is evident on skeletal X-ray with the presence of secondary ossification centres and growth plates and a higher proportion of cartilage in the bones of children, all of which influences interpretation.

Radiation safety is of particular concern for growing infants and children, and attempts are made to reduce their exposure wherever possible. There are decision rules, such as the Ottowa ankle rules (see Ch 18) and the Birmingham Children's Hospital (BCH) guidelines for computed tomography (CT)[48] validated for use in paediatrics to assist the clinician in determining whether diagnostic imaging is required.

Pathology
Diagnosis of illness in infants and children is less frequently dependent on pathology testing than it is for adults. Furthermore, paediatric presentations are less-commonly complicated by co-morbid disease, reducing the need for baseline evaluation of a range of haematological and biochemical markers.

The range of tests taken, methods for obtaining specimens and interpretation of the results are dependent on the presenting problem and the age of the patient. Smaller blood vessels and larger amounts of subcutaneous tissue make gaining intravascular access for blood sampling particularly difficult. Chapter 17, p. 339, contains information on vascular access and cathetar selection for all ages, and a section on paediatric considerations. It can also be difficult to aspirate large volumes of blood for testing, so laboratories capable of handling paediatric samples can perform these tests on much smaller samples collected in paediatric-sized blood tubes. Capillary samples from finger pricks are sometimes used as an alternative where intravenous access and larger volumes of blood are not required.

Urine specimens for microbiology and culture should be obtained from infants and young children not yet toilet-trained by urethral catheterisation or suprapubic aspirate. Urine bags applied to the skin to catch a urine specimen are not a satisfactory means to collect urine for this purpose as they are frequently contaminated.

The reference ranges for some common pathology screening tests vary with age, and this must be considered when interpreting the results: haemoglobin, serum albumin, protein (CSF) base excess, serum creatinine, erythrocyte sedimentation rate (ESR), red blood cell (RBC) count, serum potassium, etc. The reference ranges should be checked with the laboratory testing the samples.

Triage
Triage is the process used by emergency care clinicians to determine the urgency of the patient's presenting problem and allocate resources appropriate for the level of urgency of their condition. Paediatric triage assessment and decision-making, similarly to adult triage practice, relies on recognising breaches to physiology which indicate the level of urgency.[49] Triage has been formalised in the ED but the principles applied by pre-hospital clinicians to determine urgency triage category allocation for children must be based on the level of urgency of the presenting problem while considering the influence of age-related factors. Triage is discussed more extensively in Chapter 13.

Australasian EDs use the Australasian Triage Scale (formerly the National Triage Scale in Australia). Studies have repeatedly demonstrated that there is some inconsistency in the application of this scale and that the level of inconsistency may be slightly higher for paediatric triage decisions.[50-52] Infants and children are frequently allocated higher categories than adults with similar presentations.[35,53]

Guidelines recommending a standardised approach on the basis of age are often used to ensure the safety of infants and young children who may present with unrecognised serious illness. However, allocation of a higher acuity category to all infants and young children will result in many children receiving higher categories than their condition dictates, while significantly disadvantaging other, sicker patients in greater need of urgent care. These guidelines should be viewed cautiously as they corrupt the primary purpose of triage.[49]

It has been suggested that inconsistency in education contributes to inconsistency in decision-making,[54] and yet the experience and education of triage nurses in Australia varies greatly.[55,56] Similar inconsistencies exist in the preparation of nurses for undertaking paediatric triage decision-making in Australian EDs.[57] In an attempt to address this, the Australian Commonwealth government has invested in triage education by sponsoring the development of the Emergency Triage Education Kit (ETEK), which includes a section on paediatric triage. The importance of including paediatric-specific education in triage training programs is recognised nationally and internationally.[58-65]

Triage nurses must consistently and accurately identify the child requiring more-urgent attention based on the risk of mortality and morbidity, which is determined by historical data and clinical presentation and not age alone. This principle is supported by the Australasian College for Emergency Medicine, which states that 'the same standards for triage categorisation should apply to all ED settings'; 'all 5 categories should be used in all settings'; and that 'children should be triaged according to objective clinical urgency'.[66]

Triage assessment
Urgency rather than seriousness or severity of illness or injury is the foundation of the triage decision. However, appropriate triage category allocation is not possible without the recognition of the clinical features of serious illness and actual or potential deterioration, and recognition of serious illness is acknowledged as difficult in young children. A number of clinical features have been found either positively or negatively predictive of serious illness in young children; these have been discussed previously in this chapter and should be considered when determining urgency.[2,13,67-73]

It has been repeatedly shown that physiological derangements are the antecedent to deterioration and adverse outcomes, and this has also been demonstrated to be the case for children.[14,74,75] Therefore, a framework to guide triage assessment and decision-making has been developed which focuses on physiological parameters.[74,76] This was originally developed for use with adults, with a second tool for paediatrics developed at a later date.

The physiological approach directs the clinician to undertake a primary survey and therefore consider the following: the general appearance of the patient, airway, breathing, circulation and disability.[49] This assessment is supplemented with a relevant, focused secondary survey. A brief history is taken to identify from the chief complaint, past history, family and social history risk factors for rapid deterioration in condition. Identified risks should be considered in light of the physiological data collected and may result in revision of the urgency assessment.[49] The physiological approach to decision-making was developed by the Emergency Nurses Association, Victoria and was modified for paediatrics by the project team for the Department of Health, Victoria sponsored 'Consistency in Triage Project'.[74] The framework is presented in Table 36.9.

The principles of paediatric triage, the assessment framework and triage priorities are no different from those applied to adults. Identification of the physical, cognitive and developmental differences that exist between children and adults ensures that appropriate adjustments to assessment can be made and that assessment findings are appropriately interpreted in light of these differences.[30,77]

Assessment tools

The value to paediatric assessment of evidence-based indicators of serious illness in infants and children has culminated in the development of several assessment tools.[2,3,78–82] The focus of these tools is a combination of historical details and easily observable physical findings that increase the likelihood of detecting serious illness in infants and children and there are obvious similarities between them. Although none of the available tools can direct category allocation, these tools prompt assessment, thereby guiding triage decision-making. Their role is to reinforce the features that should alert the triage nurse to the increased likelihood of serious illness.[49]

The 'ABC, fluids in, fluids out' tool reflects the presenting characteristics of infants in a cohort of over 1000 babies found to have serious illness.[83] A subsequent validation study demonstrated that this tool, with the addition of urine screening for infection, has the capacity to identify 90% of seriously ill infants. The Triage Observation Tool (TOT) prompts the triage nurse to examine the clinical features listed in this tool. Despite the tool not offering a guide for triage decision-making on the basis of assessment findings, use of the TOT improved the correlation between admission rates and triage category.[78] The Pediatric Assessment Tool was designed to standardise the rapid assessment of infants and children by ED clinicians.[81] Clinicians are prompted to review the work of breathing, circulation to the skin and the appearance of the child to determine whether the child 'looks sick' or not and to broadly identify whether this reflects cardiopulmonary, cerebral or metabolic derangement. The TICLS (tone, interactiveness, consolability look/gaze and speech/cry) mnemonic provides additional guidance to clinicians unfamiliar with evaluating the appearance of infants

and children.[84] The Pediatric Observation Priority Score (POPS) is a scoring system for children aged 0–16 years based on physiological, behavioral and risk parameters,[82] which assists clinicians to assess and prioritise the needs of the child or infant and has been shown to correctly identify 85% of children safe for discharge from hospital. Descriptions of several of these tools can be found in Table 36.10.

PRACTICE TIPS

TRIAGE

- Allocate a triage category based on the level of urgency of the infant's or child's presenting problem.
- The physiological approach to triage is recommended for paediatric triage decision-making.
- Avoid standardised approaches to triage category allocation for infants and children, which may improve the safety of the child but dilute the value of triage and result in delays for other potentially sicker adult patients.

Respiratory emergencies

Respiratory failure

Respiratory failure can be defined as the inability of the respiratory system to maintain adequate oxygenation and carbon dioxide homeostasis to meet metabolic demand.[85] Broadly, respiratory failure can be seen as a result of inadequate ventilation or oxygenation or a combination of the two. Respiratory failure is often defined by arterial partial pressure of oxygen (PaO_2) and of carbon dioxide ($PaCO_2$), with arbitrary limits set. However, these values should only guide clinical decision-making and should not solely define the diagnosis as their significance will be influenced by pre-existing illness and age. For a comprehensive discussion about the physiology of respiratory failure, see Chapter 21.

Disorders of the respiratory tract are the most common illnesses in children. They are the most frequent reason for children to be seen by their general practitioner and account for 30–40% of acute medical admissions to hospital.[86] The majority of these illnesses are mild and can be safely managed at home. However, a small number of infants and children experience severe respiratory distress which may lead to respiratory failure. There are a number of age-related factors that make infants and young children more susceptible to respiratory failure than older children and adults. Table 36.1 provides a comprehensive list of the respiratory differences between infants, young children and adults.

Oxygen consumption is much higher in infants and young children than it is in adults, which helps explain a significantly higher minute volume in this age group. Tidal volume (mL/kg) is relatively fixed, and increased alveolar ventilation is achieved by an increase in respiratory rate. However, the capacity to increase the respiratory rate to meet metabolic demands can be exhausted quickly in the sick or injured infant, predisposing them to respiratory failure. Therefore, a falling respiratory rate is not always a sign of improvement, but may be a pre-terminal finding.

TABLE 36.9 Paediatric physiological discriminators developed for the Australasian (National) Triage Scale[74]

	CATEGORY 1	CATEGORY 2	CATEGORY 3	CATEGORY 4	CATEGORY 5
Airway	Obstructed	Patent	Patent	Patent	Patent
	Partially obstructed with severe respiratory distress	Partially obstructed with moderate respiratory distress	Partially obstructed with mild respiratory distress		
Breathing	Absent respiration or hypoventilation	Respiration present	Respiration present	Respiration present	Respiration present
	Severe respiratory distress, e.g. severe use accessory muscles severe retraction acute cyanosis	Moderate respiratory distress, e.g. moderate use accessory muscles moderate retraction skin pale	Mild respiratory distress, e.g. mild use accessory muscles mild retraction skin pink	No respiratory distress: no use accessory muscles no retraction	No respiratory distress: no use accessory muscles no retraction
Circulation S/S dehydration: → LOC/activity Capillary refill < 2 s Dry oral mucosa Sunken eyes → tissue turgor Absent tears Deep respirations Thready/weak pulse Tachycardia → urine output	Absent circulation Significant bradycardia, e.g. HR < 60 bpm in an infant	Circulation present	Circulation present	Circulation present	Circulation present
	Severe haemodynamic compromise, e.g. absent peripheral pulses skin pale, cold, moist, mottled significant tachycardia capillary refill > 4 s	Moderate haemodynamic compromise, e.g. weak/thready brachial pulse skin pale, cool moderate tachycardia capillary refill 2–4 s	Mild haemodynamic compromise, e.g. palpable peripheral pulses skin pale, warm mild tachycardia	No haemodynamic compromise, e.g. palpable peripheral pulses skin pink, warm, dry	No haemodynamic compromise, e.g. palpable peripheral pulses skin pink, warm, dry
	Uncontrolled haemorrhage	> 6 S/S dehydration	3–6 S/S dehydration	< 3 S/S dehydration	No S/S dehydration
Mental health emergencies[79] (used with permission from South Eastern Sydney Area Health Service)	Definite danger to life (self or others), e.g. violent behaviour possession of a weapon self-destruction	Probable danger to life (self or others), e.g. attempt/threat of self harm threat of harm to others Severe behavioural disturbance, e.g. extreme agitation/ restlessness physically/verbally aggressive confused/unable to cooperate Requires restraint	Possible danger to life, e.g. suicidal ideation Severe distress Moderate behavioural disturbance, e.g. agitated/restless intrusive behaviour bizarre/disordered behaviour withdrawn ambivalence re treatment Psychotic symptoms, e.g. hallucinations delusions paranoid ideas Affective disturbance, e.g. symptoms of depression anxiety elevated or irritable mood	Moderate distress, e.g. no agitation/restlessness irritable, not aggressive cooperative gives coherent history symptoms of anxiety or depression without suicidal ideation	No danger to self or others No behavioural disturbance No acute distress, e.g. cooperative communicative compliant with instructions known patients with chronic symptoms request for medication minor adverse effect of medication financial/social/ accommodation/relationship problem

Continued

TABLE 36.9 Paediatric physiological discriminators developed for the Australasian (National) Triage Scale[74]—cont'd

	CATEGORY 1	CATEGORY 2	CATEGORY 3	CATEGORY 4	CATEGORY 5
Ophthalmic emergencies		Penetrating eye injury Chemical injury Sudden loss of vision with or without injury Sudden-onset severe eye pain	Sudden abnormal vision with or without injury Moderate eye pain, e.g. blunt eye injury flash burns foreign body	Normal vision Mild eye pain, e.g. blunt eye injury flash burns foreign body	Normal vision No eye pain

Risk factors for serious illness or injury should be considered in the light of history of events and physiological data.
Multiple risk factors = increased risk of serious injury
Presence of one or more risk factors may result in allocation of triage category of higher acuity.

Mechanism of injury, e.g.
penetrating injury
fall > 2 × height
MCA > 60 kph
MBA/cyclist > 30 kph
pedestrian
ejection/rollover
prolonged extrication (> 30 minutes)
death same-car occupant
explosion

Co-morbidities, e.g.
history of prematurity
respiratory disease
cardiovascular disease
renal disease
carcinoma
diabetes
substance abuse
immunocompromise
congenital disease
complex medical Hx

Age < 1 month and:
febrile
acute change to feeding pattern
acute change to sleeping pattern
Victim of violence, e.g.
child at risk
sexual assault
neglect

Historical variables, for example events preceding presentation to ED:
apnoeic/cyanotic episode
seizure activity
decreased intake
decreased output
redcurrant-jelly stool
bile-stained vomiting
Parental concern

Other, e.g.
rash
actual/potential effects of drugs/alcohol
chemical exposure
envenomation
immersion
alteration in body temperature

bpm: beats/minute; HR: heart rate; LOC: loss of consciousness; MBA: motorbike accident; MCA: motor car accident; S/S: signs and symptoms

TABLE 36.10 Paediatric assessment tools		
TOOL	ASSESSMENT CRITERIA	EXPLANATION
ABC, fluids in, fluids out[83]	Activity	Reduced activity or lethargy is a significant finding
	Breathing	Increase work of breathing
	Circulation	Sudden onset of pallor is a significant finding
	Fluids in	Less than two-thirds of normal intake suggests serious illness
	Fluids out	Less than two-thirds of normal output suggests serious illness
Triage Observation Tool (TOT)[78]	**Ask**	
	Activity	Irritable, drowsy, hard to wake, not reacting to caregiver
	Feeding	> 50% reduction, fatigues, sweating, change in routine
	Dehydration	Sunken eyes, reduced urine output, dry oral mucosa
	Gastrointestinal	> 5 vomits in 24 hours, vomiting bile, > 5 watery stools in 24 hours
	Risk factors	Immune deficiency, steroids, chronic/underlying disease, neonate
	Listen	
	Cry	Persistent, weak, high-pitched, inconsolable
	Breathing	Stridor, wheeze, grunting, rapid rate, irregular
	Look/feel	
	Eye contact	No eye contact, glassy stare, unresponsive to visual stimuli
	Ventilation	Nasal flaring, tracheal tug, sternal recession, fatigued
	Skin	Rash, mottled, pallor, cyanosis
	Circulation	Reduced capillary return, hypotension/'shut-down'
	Consciousness	Lethargic, rousable to pain, unresponsive, abnormal movement
	Dehydration	Dry oral mucosa, sunken eyes, reduced urine output
	Vital signs	
	Temperature	< 35.5°C > 38.5°C (using tympanometer)
	Respiratory rate	Hypoventilation, tachypnoea
	Heart rate	Bradycardia, tachycardia
	Blood pressure	Decreased pulse pressure, hypo- or hypertension
	Oxygen saturation	< 93%

Infants and children also have a lower functional residual capacity (FRC), which is defined as the residual volume plus the expiratory reserve volume, which acts as a respiratory reserve. At FRC, the elastic recoil forces of the lungs and the chest wall are equal but opposite and there is no exertion by the diaphragm or other respiratory muscles. The smaller the FRC, the smaller the reserve and the greater the risk of hypoxia and respiratory failure. The situation is amplified in paediatric patients because of the chest-wall compliance, small thoracic cage and relatively large abdominal contents impinging on the diaphragm.[30,87]

The more compliant chest wall of the infant provides little support to the lungs. In addition to the effect that this has on FRC, increased chest-wall compliance makes it more difficult to maintain negative intrathoracic pressure, so the work of breathing is approximately three times that in the adult. However, the respiratory muscles of infants and young children are deficient in type I fatigue-resistant fibres and are therefore more susceptible to fatigue.[86,87]

Infants and young children have limited reserves to cope with respiratory illness and deteriorate rapidly once exhausted. Control of ventilation is immature in neonates and responses to hypoxic conditions are unpredictable and sometimes result in periods of apnoea.

Presentation

Respiratory assessment has been described in an earlier section of this chapter. Infants and children in respiratory failure present with varying degrees of hypoxia and hypercarbia. The infant and young child with hypoxia will become increasingly restless and confused and will initially be tachycardic. Infants are particularly sensitive to hypoxia and rapidly become bradycardic if left untreated. Infants and young children suffering hypercarbia will become increasingly drowsy, have warm, flushed diaphoretic skin and are tachycardic. Neonates tolerate hypercarbia poorly and may suffer apnoea as a result.[85]

Respiratory failure is a clinical diagnosis, which obviates the need for arterial blood gas (ABG) analysis to make the diagnosis and confirm the need for aggressive respiratory care. However, insertion of an arterial line for serial ABG analysis is justified in a child with severe respiratory illness receiving ventilatory support to monitor the effectiveness of treatments.

Management

Management of respiratory failure aims to improve ventilation, oxygenation or both. Furthermore, care should include strategies to minimise oxygen consumption such as: keeping children as calm as possible, using the parents to reduce their distress and employing appropriate distraction techniques. Antipyretics may also play a role to reduce the metabolic costs associated with fever. Strategies to improve ventilation include bronchodilators, intubation and mechanical ventilation, while strategies to improve oxygenation include oxygen therapy, non-invasive ventilation to provide continuous positive airway pressure (CPAP) or bilevel positive airway pressure (BiPAP) and intubation and mechanical ventilation to provide positive end-expiratory pressure (PEEP). Oxygen therapy and mechanical ventilation will be discussed here.

Oxygen therapy

Oxygen therapy is the mainstay of respiratory management, and yet data detailing the effectiveness of therapy or the appropriateness of different delivery systems are limited. A recent Cochrane review which aimed to determine the effectiveness of oxygen therapy and delivery methods in children found no studies comparing oxygen with no oxygen, and only four randomised controlled trials evaluating delivery devices.[88]

Nasal prongs or nasal cannulae, nasal catheters, oxygen tents and hoods and face masks are the methods used to deliver oxygen to spontaneously breathing infants and children. The choice of device is influenced by the age of the child, the oxygen flow required and the advantages and disadvantages of the available delivery systems. Ideally, oxygen is humidified. However, during pre-hospital transport and initial evaluation and resuscitation in the ED this may not be possible and should not be a priority.

The face mask is a simple device commonly used to deliver high-flow oxygen. Paediatric-sized masks are available to better fit the face of a child. The reduction in size also reduces the flow rate required to avoid carbon dioxide accumulation in the mask, and it is generally accepted that this may be as low as 4 L/min. The concentration of inspired oxygen will depend on the inspiratory flow rate of the infant and the flow into the mask.[89] Masks are not well tolerated by young children and infants and they interfere with feeding. However, they are readily available and a suitable option for older children, or temporarily in younger children until a more suitable delivery device is available.

Nasal prongs, alternatively called nasal cannulae, in smaller sizes, are an excellent alternative to the mask for oxygen delivery in young children and infants (see Fig 36.2).[90] They can be taped to the cheeks in the same way as a nasogastric tube and are well tolerated. They allow the infant to feed and are not as restrictive as an oxygen mask. Nasopharyngeal catheters are not commonly used but are another option for delivery of oxygen in children. Care must be taken when inserting a nasopharyngeal catheter to prevent oesophageal intubation and subsequent gastric distension. The disadvantages to this device is that only low-flow oxygen can be delivered and that it must

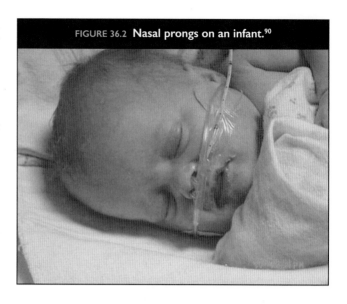

FIGURE 36.2 **Nasal prongs on an infant.**[90]

be humidified to prevent drying of nasal and nasopharyngeal secretions and membranes, making this device not ideally suited for use in pre-hospital or ED care. Furthermore, the trials summarised in the Cochrane review compared cannulae with nasopharyngeal catheters and support use of cannulae over catheters in most circumstances.[88]

Oxygen hoods are plastic boxes or domes placed over the supine infant's head; a tent is similar but covers the whole cot. A minimum flow of approximately 6 L/min is required to prevent carbon dioxide accumulation inside a hood.[91] A hood or tent is the only device which allows precise measurement of the fraction of inspired oxygen (FiO_2). However, the hood limits infant mobility, and both the hood and the tent prevent feeding, access to the infant's head and parents from nursing their child. However, tents may still be used in some inpatient areas. The value of FiO_2 measurement in emergency during the resuscitative phase of care does not outweigh the practical restrictions of these devices. They are not commonly used in the ED and are certainly not practical for pre-hospital use.

A common practice among emergency clinicians is the use a self-inflating resuscitation device to deliver oxygen to a spontaneously breathing patient. The mask is held over the patient's face but the bag is not squeezed. This practice should be avoided, as the outflow of oxygen from the bag is significantly less than the inflow of oxygen and is highly variable.[92,93]

Finally, in the absence of a well-tolerated oxygen delivery device, clinicians have used indirect means of delivery. Using a high-flow oxygen source, a stream of oxygen is aimed at the child's face. Although this practice is also not recommended, it is noteworthy that a study to determine the effectiveness of the strategy has demonstrated that 30% oxygen can potentially be delivered if a face mask is held near but not against the face,[94] while another more recent study demonstrates similar results.[95] To achieve the best results, a non-rebreather mask or the tubing with a flow rate of 15 L/min should be on the child's chest directed up towards the face.

Mechanical ventilation

Invasive ventilation is indicated when other measures to secure adequate ventilation and oxygenation have been unsuccessful. Mechanical ventilation is also used in circumstances where respiratory failure is not the primary indication, such as uncompensated shock and head trauma. However, there is evidence that bag–valve–mask (BVM) ventilation is as effective and may be safer in the pre-hospital environment, with a 4% better survival rate in children who received BVM rather than invasive ventilation.[96] These data do not necessarily support the end of pre-hospital and emergency intubation; however, they should serve as a stimulus to ensure that the likely benefits achieved from intubating and ventilating outweigh the risks.

Rapid-sequence intubation is the technique of choice for pre-hospital and ED intubations, and the principles and sequence are the same in infants and children as they are for adults. The differences in anatomy and physiology of the airway and their impact on intubation, the equipment required and the techniques used are described in the section on examination and are given in Table 36.1.

Adequate preparation is essential to ensure patient safety, and if a patient can be ventilated using a BVM device, intubation should be a controlled procedure and should not be rushed. The size of the equipment used is determined by the size of the child; Table 36.11 provides some useful formulae for calculation of tube size and insertion depth. The position of the cuff at the cricoid ring, the narrowest section of the paediatric airway, has long been used to support the use of non-cuffed endotracheal tubes in infants and children. The pressure of the cuff on the trachea was thought likely to cause trauma to the airway. Furthermore, the cricoid ring was thought to offer a natural seal and the cuff to occupy valuable airway diameter. However, a complete seal cannot be guaranteed as a tube small enough to allow for a small air leak is used to ensure that the tube is not too large. Furthermore, this can make ventilation in some circumstances difficult (e.g. poor lung compliance). There is increasing evidence that high-volume, low-pressure cuffed endotracheal tubes provide better airway protection and improve ventilation, and as there is no increase in adverse events when cuffed tubes are used in the short term, recommendations for their use are increasing.[97–99] Pre-oxygenation should occur before an intubation attempt and this should be emphasised in infants and young children who have a smaller FRC and therefore a more limited oxygen reserve.

Rapid-sequence intubation involves inducing anaesthesia followed by muscle relaxation to overcome the cough-and-gag reflex and allow intubation.[100] Induction of anaesthesia for intubation is usually achieved with a combination of medications such as benzodiazepines, anaesthetic agents such as thiopentone and propofol and opiates such as fentanyl. Cricoid pressure is applied as soon as consciousness is lost, to prevent aspiration, and is not released until tube placement in the trachea is confirmed. Succinylcholine, given once a satisfactory level of anaesthesia has been achieved, is the muscle relaxant of choice in most circumstances. Once the child is relaxed and has lost their airway protective capacity, an attempt to intubate is made. In many circumstances the tube is seen passing through the cords. Where this has not been the case clinicians must rely more heavily on other techniques to confirm placement, such as visualising the rise and fall of the chest, auscultation of bilateral breath sounds, the absence of breath sounds over the stomach and capnography. It should be noted that the correct tube size in infants and children will result in a small air leak around the tube during inspiration. A detailed discussion of the medications or the intubation technique is beyond the scope of this section and should be sought elsewhere.

Assisted ventilation pre-hospital and initially in the ED is usually achieved with a self-inflating resuscitation bag, which is available in various sizes. The relative advantages of the smaller bags are the pressure-release valve which prevents the delivery of airway pressures over 40–45 mmHg during ventilation, and the small size which prevents the inadvertent delivery of too large a tidal volume for the child. However, with vigilant monitoring of ventilation by the operator, looking for a gentle rise and fall of the chest, the adult-sized bag may be used for children of all sizes.

Once ventilation has been stabilised, a mechanical ventilator may be used to continue ventilation. The amount of dead space should be minimised when setting up a ventilator circuit by avoiding liquorice sticks, as their volume may account for a significant proportion of an infant's tidal volume. In most circumstances, infants and young children should be ventilated using synchronised intermittent mandatory ventilation (SIMV) mode or assist controlled mandatory controlled ventilation (ACMV) and pressure-controlled with the lowest pressure possible. Tidal volume is dependent on lung compliance, but is largely unaffected by the airway leak when pressure is used to control ventilation. The adjustable ventilator variables for most transport ventilators used pre-hospital and in the ED are: mode, control parameter (pressure or tidal volume), respiratory rate, inspiratory time or I : E ratio, PEEP, sensitivity and FiO_2. Some may offer the option of pressure support, which is largely unnecessary in this population as they are paralysed and sedated in most circumstances. However, where care is provided in the ED for longer periods of time, spontaneous ventilation may be appropriate and pressure support may become necessary. Alarms should also be set to alert clinicians to potential problems with ventilation. Appropriate initial ranges for the adjustable parameters and alarm limits for basic ventilation are presented in Table 36.12. For a more comprehensive explanation and advice about complex ventilation needs, a critical care text should be consulted.

There are no generally accepted guidelines for the use of non-invasive ventilation in children, and a fairly recent systematic review found very few studies evaluating efficacy.[101]

TABLE 36.11 Formulae for paediatric emergencies	
PARAMETER	FORMULA
Weight	(Age + 4) × 2
Endotracheal tube diameter	Age/4 + 4
Endotracheal tube insertion depth (at the lip)	Age/2 + 12
Endotracheal tube insertion depth (at the nose)	Age/2 + 15
Adrenaline (bolus)	0.1 mL/kg
Defibrillation energy	4 J/kg

TABLE 36.12 Appropriate initial settings for mechanical ventilation[100]

PARAMETER	VALUE
Peak inspiratory pressure	20 cmH$_2$O
Tidal volume	6–7 mL/kg
Peak end-expiratory pressure	3–5 cmH$_2$O
Respiratory rate	Age-appropriate
Inspiratory time	0.8–1 second (to maintain I:E ratio of 1:3)
Peak inspiratory pressure (alarm)	30 cmH$_2$O
Low inspiratory pressure (alarm)	15 cmH$_2$O
Low minute volume (alarm)	75% of minute volume

I:E ratio: inspiratory–expiratory ratio

However, it is used increasingly in paediatrics, including in the ED, to manage infants and children with lung disease as a means to prevent the need for invasive ventilation. High-flow nasal cannula oxygen is gaining support despite very low levels of evidence for its efficacy.[102,103] Data from a recent study show that high-flow nasal cannulae, as well as being well tolerated, improve oxygenation and that their mechanism of action, in addition to supplying oxygen, is the application of mild positive airway pressure and lung volume recruitment.[104] Robust trials comparing the efficacy of this therapy with conventional treatment are required before it can be widely recommended.[105,106]

PRACTICE TIPS

RESPIRATORY EMERGENCIES

- Infants and young children are more susceptible to respiratory failure than adults.
- Tidal volume is relatively fixed in infants; however, as a result of higher respiratory rates minute volume is much higher.
- Infants are extremely sensitive to hypoxia and rapidly develop bradycardia.
- Hypercapnia in young infants may be responsible for apnoea.
- Blood gas analysis results should be used to guide treatment but not to diagnose respiratory failure, which is a clinical diagnosis.
- Nasal prongs/cannulae are the most effective way of delivering oxygen to infants in the ED. Older children may tolerate a mask.
- Where bag–valve–mask ventilation is effective, intubation should only be attempted under ideal circumstances by a clinician experienced with paediatric intubation.

- A cuffed endotracheal tube is likely to be safe and may even be preferable in circumstances where high ventilator pressures are required.
- Endotracheal tube placement should ideally be confirmed by capnography. Auscultation of breath sounds over the lung fields and stomach may also be used to assist in confirmation of tube placement.
- Minimise dead space in the ventilator circuit.
- Pressure-controlled ventilation using the lowest pressure possible should be used in most cases.
- Appropriately-set minute volume alarms are essential for monitoring the adequacy of pressure ventilation.

Croup (laryngotracheobronchitis)

Croup is the most common cause of acute upper airway obstruction in children and accounts for approximately 15% of respiratory illness in children.[113] It is a clinical syndrome characterised by barking cough, hoarse voice and inspiratory stridor. It usually occurs in children 6 months to 6 years of age, but may occur in children aged from 3 months to 15 years. Croup is a seasonal disease and peaks in the winter when respiratory viruses are most prevalent.[113] Droplets and direct contact spread the illness and parainfluenza virus is responsible for approximately two-thirds of cases. Other viruses, such as influenza type A, respiratory syncytial virus (RSV), rhinovirus, adenovirus and enterovirus, are also known to cause croup.

Croup causes inflammation of the upper airway, the larynx, trachea and bronchi. The swelling results in narrowing of the airway, including the subglottic area, which is the narrowest section of the paediatric airway, and this is responsible for increasing difficulty in breathing as the airway lumen narrows. Increased swelling to the larynx results in a hoarse voice and the barking cough. Worsening obstruction results in stridor.[113] Increased mucous production and the generation of negative pressure on inspiration obstruct the airway further. The size of the larynx, increased loose submucosal tissues and the tight fit of the cricoid ring around the subglottic region of the trachea in the younger child are responsible for more-pronounced signs of airway obstruction.[86]

Presentation and diagnosis

Children with croup will generally present having had a prodrome featuring coryzal symptoms, a fever and a cough. The symptoms of barking cough and hoarse voice usually appear after 1–2 days and in 80% of children remain mild. Symptoms are generally worse at night and exacerbated by distress. Moderate and more-severe croup presents with inspiratory stridor and increased work of breathing.

Care should be taken during examination not to distress the child, as this will tend to worsen the airway obstruction. Children should be allowed to adopt a position of comfort and remain in a parent's arms if this alleviates distress. They should be undressed from the waist up to allow observation of respiratory effort and respiratory rate and limit the need for intrusive examination. They should also be observed for their level of activity, skin colour and the presence of stridor.

Croup severity should be assessed by evaluating the degree to which respiratory effort has increased and not the characteristics of the stridor, particularly as stridor may become progressively softer as the child deteriorates and smaller volumes of air pass through the upper airway. Saturations are also of limited value in the assessment of croup. Increasing obstruction to the airway affects the capacity to ventilate, and oxygenation will only fall once the airway is significantly obstructed and ventilation is markedly impeded. This should become clinically apparent well before a drop in oxygen saturations occurs. With increasing airway obstruction children will become increasingly tachypnoeic, tachycardic, restless and agitated.

The diagnosis is made clinically and investigations are not required unless they are intended to rule out differential diagnosis; for example, radiograph where FB aspiration is suspected.[113]

The diagnosis may, on occasions, be confused with lower airway pathology, as in some cases children will develop wheeze due to lower airway involvement and croup may precipitate wheeze in children with a history of asthma. Other differential diagnoses should be considered, in particular epiglottitis. Now rare since the introduction of the *Haemophilus influenzae* type B vaccine to the immunisation schedule, epiglottitis is a life-threatening infection which can result in complete occlusion of the airway by a swollen epiglottis. It manifests with abrupt onset of fever, pallor, signs of sepsis, drooling and a soft snore. As clinicians have less and less experience with this illness, they are at greater risk of confusing it with croup. Children with epiglottitis should be managed with great care—airway examination should *not* be undertaken to confirm diagnosis until a clinician with paediatric airway experience is prepared to intubate the airway and the resources to manage a difficult airway are available. Other presentations which may mimic croup include angio-oedema secondary to allergy, tracheitis or inhaled foreign body (FB).

Management

The mainstay of management for croup is steroids, and all children should be treated with steroids regardless of the severity of their presentation. Their effect on ameliorating the effects of airway swelling as early as 6 hours and lasting for at least 12 hours following administration is documented in a Cochrane review.[114] There is a significant improvement in severity, fewer representations to emergency and re-admissions, shorter lengths of stay and reduction in the use of adrenaline, and the number needed to treat to see one child improve is as few as five. Use of either 1 mg/kg of oral prednisolone or 0.15 mg/kg of oral dexamethasone is supported by the evidence.[115–120] Studies comparing the two steroids have used a range of dosing regimens, making it difficult to draw a conclusion about whether one is superior to the other, but there is some evidence to suggest that a single dose of oral dexamethasone is more effective than prednisolone and hence it is frequently recommended for croup treatment.

Children with mild croup—no stridor at rest and minimal increase in respiratory effort—may be discharged from the ED following a dose of steroid. Children with moderate croup, characterised by an increase in respiratory effort and stridor at rest, should be observed in the ED and if they show adequate signs of improvement within several hours they may usually be safely discharged home.[114,121] In addition to improvement in condition, the decision to discharge a child with croup is influenced by factors such as their proximity to emergency

services, the time of day (croup will predictably deteriorate overnight) and parental concern. There is currently contention about whether a second dose of steroid 12 hours later is likely to improve their condition. However, there is no published evidence to support this practice.

Children with more-severe croup, manifested by more-severe signs of respiratory distress, will need close monitoring and may require nebulised adrenaline to alleviate significant obstruction. It achieves this by temporarily reducing bronchial and tracheal secretions and airway-wall oedema. The results of a Cochrane review indicate that improvements occur within 30 minutes and that the duration of effect is between 90 and 120 minutes, after which they return to baseline severity.[122] Some data show that signs and symptoms of obstruction may improve following nebulised adrenaline by providing an opportunity for the steroids to take effect.[123] In some circumstances improvement is sufficient to allow for discharge several hours after treatment with adrenaline. However, the majority of children treated with nebulised adrenaline will require hospital admission and may need a second dose of adrenaline. A standard volume for treatment, rather than weight-based dosing, is used most consistently in Australian EDs. This is most commonly 5 mg administered as 5 mL of 1:1000 (equivalent to 0.1% solution) solution or 0.5 mL of racemic adrenaline (1% solution) diluted with saline to a total of 2–4 mL and delivered by nebuliser mask.

Supplemental oxygen should be administered to a hypoxic child with croup. However, this should serve as a stimulus to seek expert airway assistance and prepare for intubation. This should also be considered for children requiring repeated doses of adrenaline with no improvement and those with signs of exhaustion.

Traditionally, steam and inhalational therapy have been used to manage croup and are still frequently recommended for home use despite no convincing evidence of their efficacy.[124]

PRACTICE TIPS
CROUP

- A clinical syndrome characterised by fever, barking cough, hoarse voice with or without stridor.
- Diagnostic tests are not required to confirm the diagnosis of croup.
- Differential diagnoses include: epiglottitis (rare but life-threatening), angio-oedema associated with allergic reactions, tracheitis and inhaled foreign body.
- Changes in work of breathing are the most sensitive indicators of the severity of the airway obstruction.
- Oxygen saturations and the characteristics of the stridor are of limited use in assessing severity.
- Corticosteroids, such as prednisolone or dexamethasone, are recommended for all infants and children suffering croup.
- Infants and children with moderate to severe croup will require admission for airway monitoring.
- Infants and children with severe croup may require nebulised adrenaline to relieve the symptoms of airway obstruction.

Asthma

Asthma is a chronic inflammatory disorder of the lower airways where smooth muscle contraction and swelling of the airway results in airway obstruction.[125] This section should be read in conjunction with Chapter 21; it is not intended to be a comprehensive review of asthma, but will serve to highlight the ways in which paediatric asthma differs from adult asthma.

The prevalence of asthma in Australian children is one in nine,[126] and as high as one in seven in New Zealand children,[127] which is higher than in adults and significantly higher than in other parts of the world.[128] The indigenous populations of both countries have even higher rates of asthma prevalence. Children aged less than 4 years are the group most likely to visit a general practitioner or ED with asthma; and asthma is the most common long-term medical condition in children, estimated to affect approximately 20% of children aged 0–15 years.[129] There is some contention about the age at which children may be diagnosed with asthma and the European Respiratory Society Task Force suggest that the term asthma should not be used for preschool children as there is insufficient data demonstrating airway inflammation (a feature of asthma) in this age group.[130] In Australasian practice it is generally accepted that children older than 12 months may present with the features of asthma.

Presentation and diagnosis

The diagnosis of asthma in children is clinical and can be made on the basis of a history of recurrent or persistent wheeze in the absence of other causes. The wheeze is associated with viral respiratory infection, exercise or exposure to allergens such as grasses, animals and pollens. Children presenting with asthma will usually have a history or family history of atopy. Conditions such as eczema, allergic rhinitis or allergy are risk factors for persistent asthma beyond the age of six years, and over 80% of asthma sufferers have evidence of allergic sensitisation.

On examination the child with asthma will have widespread expiratory wheeze, cough, increased respiratory effort and prolonged expiration. Asymmetry on auscultation may occur as a result of mucous plugging, but FB inhalation should be considered. Cough is frequently misdiagnosed as asthma in the absence of other features of asthma. Although a common feature of asthma, it is rare for it to be the only symptom experienced in asthma. Persistent and recurrent non-specific cough frequently follows a viral respiratory infection and may not resolve for weeks to months. The cough is dry, exacerbated by exercise, is worse in the morning and is not responsive to treatment.

Severity, defined as mild, moderate, severe and critical, is primarily determined by the increase in respiratory effort and the effect of respiratory compromise on mental status. Secondary parameters, which may assist in quantifying the severity, are oxygen saturation, the ability to talk and heart rate. Other less-useful indicators, which are frequently described in texts, are wheeze intensity, arterial blood gases, pulsus paradoxus, central cyanosis, spirometry and peak flow rates.[10]

The diagnosis is often confirmed on the basis of a response to inhaled bronchodilators. Lung-function testing is not generally used to aid diagnosis as children under 7 or 8 years of age are unable to perform consistently and reliably.[125] Chest X-rays are also not of diagnostic value and do not provide evidence of severity of disease. However, a chest X-ray should be performed for infants and children with critical asthma or where the diagnosis is unclear.

Other causes of acute wheezing in children include bronchiolitis, *Mycoplasma* pneumonia, aspiration, allergy or heart failure, and should be considered when taking a history and performing an examination on the child presenting with wheeze. Preschool children frequently experience wheeze associated with a viral infection that is not responsive to asthma therapy.

Management

The management of asthma in children is similar to that of adults, and where it differs this reflects the differences in the natural history and pattern of asthma in children, the effects of the medications used and the potential for side-effects in these two populations. Guidelines recommending management for acute exacerbations are available from a number of sources; one of the most frequently used of these is the Royal Children's Hospital Asthma Management Clinical Practice Guideline.[555] Treatment recommendations based on presentation severity are clearly laid out and readers are recommended to use this or other evidence-based guidelines to guide dosing and scheduling of therapies for acute asthma management. The web address for this guideline is available in the resources section at the end of this chapter. This section will not address chronic asthma management and preventative therapy.

The evidence for inhaled bronchodilators to relieve the symptoms of acute asthma is strong. Furthermore, it has been shown that salbutamol delivered via spacer is as effective as nebulised salbutamol administered to children presenting with acute asthma.[131] There are no data about this delivery method in children with critical asthma. However, data supporting the safety of continuous undiluted (0.5%) nebulised salbutamol[132,133] and intravenous infusion of salbutamol are available.[134] Anticholinergics in combination with short-acting bronchodilators have been shown to reduce admission rates, improve lung function and clinical scores and reduce nausea and tremor.[135] Furthermore, there is a trend to improved efficacy for more severe asthma. Ipratropium bromide is advocated for use in severe and critical asthma in the first hour of management, but confers no benefit if used beyond this period.[136–138]

Corticosteroids have been shown repeatedly to result in clinical improvement in paediatric asthma,[139] and interestingly the route of administration (oral versus intravenous) appears to have minimal effect on their efficacy. Specifically, intravenous steroid administration does not result in greater efficacy.[140] Conversely, there is insufficient evidence to suggest that inhaled steroids are an efficacious alternative to systemic steroids.[141]

The use of aminophylline in critical asthma is controversial, as it carries significant risk of serious side-effects and the data to support its efficacy is not convincing. The most recent Cochrane review (2009) found evidence from a number of small trials that children receiving IV aminophylline showed improved lung function, but there was no reduction in symptoms, number of nebulised treatments or length of hospital stay when compared with children treated with placebo.[142]

Decreased oxygen saturations should not be used as an indication for the need for additional bronchodilator in the absence of other signs of bronchospasm. Ventilation–perfusion mismatch, often exacerbated by beta-agonist use, and mucous plugging are responsible for deteriorating saturations and supplemental oxygen therapy should be commenced once saturations have dropped below 92%, which is the generally accepted, although arbitrary, threshold.

There is some interest in the role of intravenous magnesium sulfate to provide additional bronchodilation; the authors of a Cochrane review examining data from seven trials, two of which were paediatric, concluded that there is not compelling evidence that magnesium has a role to play in treating asthma, but it may be of some use for those patients presenting with severe asthma.[143] Furthermore, a Cochrane review addressing the impact of inhaled magnesium sulphate also showed that they conferred no convincing benefit.[144] Ketamine has also attracted some attention as there have been anecdotal reports of its value in treating intractable asthma. However, as the results of a single study did not show benefit, authors of another Cochrane review do not recommend its use in the absence of more convincing evidence.[145]

Guidelines for admission are generally consensus-based, as there is limited evidence on which to base admission criteria. The following factors should be considered when making a decision to admit or discharge a patient from the ED:

- the severity of the attack
- the response to therapy
- the time of day
- the proximity to emergency services
- the expertise of the parents to manage at home.

Risk factors for rapid deterioration and death, such as previous near-fatal asthma, previous admissions in the last year, previous admission to paediatric ICU, heavy use of beta$_2$-agonists and repeat attendance at the ED, should also lower the threshold for admission. On discharge the family should receive a detailed action plan and advice about re-presentation.

The decision to commence a preventer is best not made in the ED but rather by a clinician who will see the child

PRACTICE TIPS
ASTHMA

- A clinical diagnosis made on the basis of recurrent wheeze in the absence of other causes.
- Responsiveness to bronchodilator may be used to confirm the diagnosis.
- Chest X-rays and other diagnostic tests are not required to confirm the diagnosis and of limited value to assess severity or determine treatment.
- Bronchodilators are used to control bronchospasm and should be given when work of breathing increases.
- Decreased oxygen saturations in the absence of other signs of bronchospasm should not be treated with bronchodilators.
- Intravenous salbutamol, aminophylline and magnesium may be used in combination to treat severe asthma in children.
- Infants and children requiring bronchodilators more frequently than 3-hourly should not be discharged home in most circumstances.

regularly and monitor their response to therapy. Referral to a paediatrician, respiratory doctor or suitable GP should be made if the child has recurrent episodes of asthma and would be likely to benefit from a preventer. This also provides an opportunity to review and update their action plan.

Bronchiolitis

In Australia and New Zealand, viral bronchiolitis occurs in infants less than 12–18 months of age, and is characterised by wheeze, cough and varying degrees of shortness of breath. It is the most common lower respiratory tract infection in infants, and approximately 3% of infants will be hospitalised with bronchiolitis in their first year of life.[146] However, most episodes are mild and can be managed at home. The aetiology includes respiratory syncytial virus (RSV), parainfluenza and influenza virus, rhinovirus and adenovirus, and as these viruses are more prevalent in winter this illness peaks during the winter.[146] Infection causes acute inflammation and oedema of the epithelial cells lining the bronchioles, increased mucous production and bronchospasm, all of which contribute to airway obstruction.

Infants with pre-existing lung disease, congenital heart disease and infants younger than 6 months, born prematurely or failing to thrive are at greater risk of increased severity of disease and more serious sequelae as a result of bronchiolitis.

Presentation and diagnosis

Bronchiolitis presents with features of upper and lower airway tract infection. There is no evidence to support the specificity or sensitivity of the clinical features of bronchiolitis for the purposes of making the diagnosis or to categorise severity. However, consensus describes the classic constellation of symptoms. Parents usually describe a prodrome of coryza, mild cough and fever lasting for 1–2 days before wheeze, crackles and increasing shortness of breath become apparent. Dyspnoea may interfere with feeding, the extent of which will be dependent on the level of respiratory distress.

Examination findings include tachypnoea, tachycardia, fever, increased respiratory effort, a prolonged expiratory phase, hyperinflation and crackles and wheeze on auscultation. Reduced oxygen saturations and dehydration may be apparent in some infants. In severe cases hypoxia and cyanosis may occur, and young infants may suffer apnoeas.

The severity of bronchiolitis, categorised as mild, moderate and severe, is not consistently defined in the literature. However, in numerous studies a number of clinical indicators are associated with more-severe disease:

- low oxygen saturation at the time of presentation
- young age
- prematurity
- cyanosis
- increased work of breathing (including individually and in various combinations: increased respiratory rate, accessory muscle use, chest wall retraction, recessions, nasal flare and/or grunting).[146]

Table 36.13 provides a consensus-based guide for defining bronchiolitis severity based on respiratory effort, oxygen saturation, feeding and the extent of dehydration.

Bronchiolitis is a clinical diagnosis, obviating the need for investigation; although for the purposes of cohorting of

	TABLE 36.13 Bronchiolitis management by severity	
SEVERITY	**CLINICAL FEATURES**	**MANAGEMENT**
Mild	Alert, pink in air Feeding well O_2 saturation > 90%	Disposition—can be managed at home Discharge advice: advise parents of the expected course of the illness, and when to return if there are problems; give parent information leaflet smaller, more-frequent feeds Follow up—review by GP within 24 hours
Moderate	Any one of: poor feeding lethargy marked respiratory distress underlying cardiorespiratory disease O_2 saturation < 90% age < 6 weeks	Disposition—admit Oxygen to maintain adequate saturation OVER 92% Fluid management: nasogastric fluids alternatively IV fluids at 75% maintenance volumes (inappropriate ADH) Monitoring—2-hourly observations
Severe	As above but with increasing O_2 requirement or signs of tiring or CO_2 retention (sweaty, irritable or apnoeas)	Consultation—involve senior staff/paediatric intensivist Disposition—admit. May require transfer to more-appropriate facility Oxygen to maintain adequate saturation Fluid management consider IV fluids at 75% maintenance (inappropriate ADH); alternatively, nasogastric fluids Monitoring—cardiorespiratory monitor

ADH: antidiuretic hormone; IV: intravenous

patients admitted to hospital to prevent nosocomial infection, a nasopharyngeal aspirate may be collected to determine the viral aetiology. Chest X-ray is of no diagnostic value unless considering an alternative diagnosis such as congestive cardiac failure which may mimic bronchiolitis, particularly if precipitated by respiratory infection. Furthermore, evidence indicates that there is no correlation between chest X-ray results and the severity of the disease.[146]

Management

The clinical presentation of bronchiolitis is very similar to asthma and it seems reasonable to assume that the treatment for asthma would be likely to be effective to treat bronchiolitis. However, this appears not to be the case. Studies summarised in a Cochrane review, which evaluated the efficacy of bronchodilators,[147] including adrenaline, beta$_2$-agonists[148] and ipratropium bromide , have not confirmed benefit of these agents to infants with bronchiolitis and cannot be recommended.[149,150] Improvement in signs in response to a salbutamol trial is at odds with the diagnosis of bronchiolitis and suggests that the infant has asthma. Steroids, although useful in the treatment of asthma and croup, have been shown in a Cochrane review[151] to have no role in bronchiolitis. The Guideline Development Group at Southern Health[146] has considered the evidence for a number of other potential treatments, such as antibiotics, ribavirin, immunoglobulin, decongestants and antitussives, and finds no convincing evidence for their inclusion in the treatment regimen for bronchiolitis. Nebulised hypertonic saline use in moderate to severe bronchiolitis (3%) has been explored in a number of studies and shows some promise.[152] However, there does not appear to be widespread acceptance of this data and treatment recommendations do not currently include hypertonic saline.

Infants with bronchiolitis are managed on the basis of severity as detailed in Table 36.14. Mild bronchiolitis can be managed safely at home. Under some circumstances, infants with moderate bronchiolitis can also be managed as outpatients, providing that regular review can be provided and admission is possible if they show signs of significant dehydration and/or hypoxia. Infants with more-severe bronchiolitis should be admitted to hospital, and the need for tertiary paediatric care considered for those with severe bronchiolitis and infants with the previously described risk factors for more-severe disease.

Inpatient management of bronchiolitis is conservative and confined to providing close observation, the provision of oxygen therapy to maintain acceptable oxygenation, and fluid management. Monitoring of respiratory parameters will depend on the severity of disease, but should occur hourly at a minimum and include continuous oxygen saturation monitoring. The threshold at which to start oxygen therapy and the saturation that should be maintained are not supported by data, but a number of educated recommendations are made varying from 90% to 95%. Administration of oxygen was described in a previous section and there is increasing support for the role of high-flow intranasal oxygen to manage severe bronchiolitis, although the quality of the evidence is low.[105]

Decisions surrounding hydration management are largely consensus-based in the absence of adequate evidence to guide clinicians. However, a multi-centred trial has recently compared nasogastric and intravenous fluid therapy for infants with bronchiolitis requiring rehydration and results support nasogastric tube rehydration as a suitable mode for fluid delivery.[153] Consensus rather than evidence supports administering 75% of maintenance fluid volumes. Fluid management is also described in more detail in a previous section.

Two studies have examined the duration of illness; the median duration of symptoms was 2 weeks, but 20% of infants had symptoms for as long as 3 weeks.[146] This should be explained to parents to ensure that their expectations for recovery are realistic.

PRACTICE TIPS

BRONCHIOLITIS

- Presents in infants less than 12–18 months of age with features very similar to asthma.
- Infants who were born prematurely, suffer a cardiac condition or are less than 6 months of age are more likely to suffer more-severe disease.
- Hydration status and oxygen saturations should be assessed in all infants with bronchiolitis, as these parameters define severity and the need for admission.
- Infants with moderate and severe bronchiolitis will require inpatient management for monitoring and may require oxygen therapy and/or rehydration.
- Although presentation is similar to asthma, steroids and bronchodilators are not helpful.

Pertussis (whooping cough)

Pertussis is a highly infectious, acute respiratory infection caused by *Bordetella pertussis* and is traditionally diagnosed in infants and toddlers, although it may affect adults. Vaccination for pertussis is included in the immunisation schedule to protect infants and young children from what potentially can be a very serious illness. Babies do not gain reliable protection from maternal antibodies and immunity from vaccination is not conferred until at least the second dose, making babies susceptible to pertussis infection in the first few months of life. This is of particular importance as very young infants are at greatest risk of severe morbidity and mortality.[154,155]

There has been a worldwide resurgence in pertussis over the last 20 years and a number of reasons for this are postulated, which include waning immunity following immunisation and improved diagnosis. The infection is usually mild in adults, so revaccination has not been routinely recommended. As adult pertussis has been increasingly implicated as the source of infection for unimmunised babies, this recommendation has more recently been challenged.[156–159] Government initiatives are beginning to target vaccination for new mothers, grandparents and others who care for young babies.[160]

Despite the availability of routine pertussis vaccination, significant numbers of infants and young children still contract

the disease and die. In Australia and New Zealand, epidemics occur every 3–4 years; there were 29,769 notifications in Australia for pertussis in 2009 compared with 34,100 notifications in 2010 and 38,602 notifications in 2011.[161] Similarly, NZ data confirms 872 cases in 2010, 1996 cases in 2011 and 5902 in 2012.[162]

Presentation and diagnosis

The classic course of pertussis can be divided into three stages of illness: the *catarrheal*, *paroxysmal* and *convalescent* stages. Infants and children usually present during the paroxysmal phase. The first stage (catarrheal), lasting 1–2 weeks, is characterised by rhinorrhoea, conjunctivitis, low-grade fever and malaise and is frequently considered insignificant by parents and clinicians.[163] Unfortunately, it is at this stage that they are most infectious. The developing cough becomes paroxysmal, marking the next stage, which can last from 2 to 6 weeks.

Pertussis is commonly known as whooping cough as a result of the characteristic 'whoop' that occurs with inspiration at the end of a coughing paroxysm. However, this is misleading as the whoop is only present in some cases. The increase in intrathoracic pressure during a paroxysm results in bulging neck veins and a reddened face, and the child may vomit. In severe cases the infant may become hypoxic, cyanosed and bradycardic during the coughing paroxysm, and some may experience apnoeas. In fact, some infants present only with apnoea and few classic symptoms. Young babies quickly become exhausted, which impairs feeding, leading to dehydration and failure to thrive. The disease is generally milder in older children, making it more difficult to recognise. Available data provide the foundation for the recommendation that where there is parental report of turning blue/purple or cyanosis, age less than 2 months and the presence of cough and rhonchi on examination, these findings should be considered to correlate with a diagnosis of pertussis and the child should be isolated and further testing completed to confirm the diagnosis.[164]

The final stage of the illness is the convalescent phase, during which the number and intensity of coughing episodes decreases. This stage may continue for many weeks.

Laboratory confirmation of the clinical diagnosis of pertussis is required and polymerase chain reaction (PCR), serology and culture are commonly used for this purpose. Isolation of *B. pertussis* from nasopharyngeal secretions is the gold standard for diagnosis. However, samples are frequently contaminated if not collected correctly and handled appropriately, lowering sensitivity. Furthermore, it takes 7–10 days before the results of the culture can be confirmed, making this test less useful clinically. The use of PCR to confirm diagnosis is increasing as it is a more sensitive test, and the Communicable Diseases Centre (CDC) and the World Health Organization (WHO) now recommend positive PCR as a diagnostic criterion for the diagnosis of pertussis infection. Pertussis infection can also be confirmed by serology and can be distinguished from a serological response to immunisation. However, this test may be less sensitive and may be of less use early in the course of the illness.

Management

The treatment of pertussis is largely conservative, as antibiotics must be commenced within a week of the onset of illness for them to be of clinical value.[165] Their role in most cases is to shorten the infectious period of the illness and reduce the risk of the spread of pertussis to vulnerable individuals. Traditionally erythromycin has been used for 14 days; however, recent evidence supports a 7-day course with newer agents such as clarithromycin or azithromycin, which have fewer side effects and are better tolerated.[166,167] An appropriate resource, such as the *Australian Medicines Handbook* or the *Therapeutic Guidelines* (see the resources section at the end of the chapter), should be consulted for doses and dosing schedules.

Infants less than 6 months of age should generally be admitted to a high-dependency area for close monitoring. These infants are likely to require oxygen and fluid management and are at risk of apnoea and other potential complications of pertussis, most commonly pneumonia. Older children will require admission if they are experiencing significant respiratory distress or hypoxia with paroxysms or apnoea. Children with suspected as well as confirmed pertussis should be isolated and infection control officers alerted to their admission. It is recommended that close contacts who are not fully vaccinated will also require treatment, and exposed children should be excluded from school for 14 days or until they have received a minimum of 5 days of antibiotic treatment although the benefits of contact prophylaxis are not clear.[165,168] Pertussis is a notifiable disease in Australia and New Zealand, so the treating clinician must inform state surveillance units of the diagnosis.

Prevention serves as one of the best management strategies for pertussis. Routine vaccination for infants includes pertussis; the immunisation schedule is discussed elsewhere in this chapter. Vaccination of adults in contact with young babies and identification and treatment of pertussis in older children and adults is vital to prevent the spread of the disease to young babies, who are at great risk of serious sequelae.

Pneumonia

Pneumonia is described in detail in Chapter 21; this discussion serves only to highlight the key differences between paediatric and adult pneumonia. Pneumonia is an inflammation of the lung tissue, the aetiology of which is to some extent age-dependent. As the causative organism is not isolated in 20–60% of cases, it is hard to accurately document their incidence, but it is estimated that viruses account for 15–35% of infections and are the most common aetiology in infants and young children, with RSV the single most-common virus. In neonates and older children, bacterial causes become a more dominant aetiology for pneumonia. Bacterial pathogens in the neonatal period include *Escherichia coli* and Group B *Streptococcus*; in infancy they include *Pneumococcus*, *Haemophilus* and infrequently *Staphylococcus*; as children get older, bacterial pathogens also include *Mycoplasma pneumoniae*.[169]

Each year the influenza virus is responsible for severe pneumonia and several paediatric deaths in Australia. In 2009 influenza A (H1N1) was responsible for an outbreak of severe pneumonia in Mexico where significant numbers of people, including children, died.[170] This pandemic soon spread to other parts of the world and large numbers of people, including children, contracted this virus in Australia and New Zealand. However, mortality was substantially lower than in Mexico where it originated.

Presentation and diagnosis

Cough, fever, dyspnoea, chest pain, vomiting, abdominal pain and anorexia are common although not specific symptoms of pneumonia.[171] Children with pneumonia frequently look unwell and are described as lethargic. Examination findings for children with pneumonia include tachypnoea, increased respiratory effort, grunting, reduced oxygen saturations and, on auscultation, crackles and decreased breath sounds.[171] Fever, tachypnoea and cough have been shown to be two of the single most-sensitive and specific signs of pneumonia.[169,171,172]

The signs and symptoms of pneumonia may vary with age, with infants presenting with more non-specific symptoms. Aetiology also varies with age. However, there appears to be limited correlation between the presenting signs and symptoms and the aetiology of pneumonia.[171,173,174] Wheeze is not characteristically present in children with pneumonia, although it may accompany viral pneumonia, and alternative diagnoses should be sought in the absence of findings, such as fever, coryza and tachypnoea, which suggest the diagnosis of pneumonia.[173,174] *Mycoplasma* is commonly associated with a more indolent pattern of illness in an older child, characterised by persistent cough. However, data are not available to support this and *Mycoplasma* cannot be reliably diagnosed.[175]

Chest X-ray (anteroposterior view) is used for confirmation of the diagnosis of pneumonia. However, the chest X-ray may be normal in the early stages of the illness. There is also no convincing evidence that viral and bacterial pneumonia can be differentiated on the basis of the X-ray findings,[169] and

---

PRACTICE TIPS
PERTUSSIS

- Can be a very serious disease, particularly in young babies who are at greatest risk of contracting the disease as immunity is not conferred until following the second vaccination at 4 months of age.
- Coughing paroxysms are the defining feature of the illness.
- The classic 'whoop' heard at the end of the coughing paroxysm is not heard in all cases and should not be relied upon to make the diagnosis.
- The diagnosis should be suspected in children with persistent cough for over 4 weeks.
- PCR (polymerase chain reaction) is recommended to confirm the diagnosis.
- Young babies should be monitored carefully as the characteristic coughing paroxysms may result in exhaustion or apnoea.
- Antibiotics are only of clinical value if commenced in the first week of illness; however, all cases should be treated to prevent community spread of the illness.
- Adults caring for infants should be revaccinated for pertussis as immunisation is unlikely to confer lifelong immunity.

routine chest X-ray has not been shown to affect the clinical outcomes.[176] Pathology does not aid diagnosis and does not usually alter management strategies, and therefore routine tests are not recommended.[169] However, the syndrome of inappropriate antidiuretic hormone (SIADH) is linked with pneumonia, and in the severely unwell urea and electrolytes should be measured. Identification of RSV may assist clinical decision-making from an infection-control perspective.

Management

Management of pneumonia is dependent on the severity of the illness and the likely aetiology. The majority of children presenting with community-acquired pneumonia will be well enough to be managed as outpatients. The evidence to support antibiotic treatment regimens (choice of agent, duration of treatment, etc.) is not strong and little has been published since this 2004 review to alter this view.[169] However, where bacterial pneumonia is suspected, empiric antibiotics are started and amoxicillin is best supported by available data.[177] Additionally, oral therapy may be used in all but those children with signs of severe disease, such as hypoxaemia and dehydration.[178] Additional robust studies evaluating the efficacy of antibiotics for the treatment of *Mycoplasma* in children are required.[179] However, in children older than 5 years, a macrolide such as roxithromycin may be commenced to cover suspected *Mycoplasma* pneumonia. Where viral aetiology is considered the most likely, infants and children are treated symptomatically and antibiotics are not prescribed. Infants and children managed as outpatients should be referred to their GP for review.

Management of infants and children with signs of more-serious illness (hypoxaemia and/or dehydration) will include admission, and focus on respiratory support and fluid management. High-flow oxygen may be required to support acceptable oxygen saturations, fluid therapy commenced to support hydration and, in a small number of cases, fluid resuscitation. Penicillin is commenced for infants and children admitted with pneumonia unless there is convincing evidence that the infection is viral. The doses and dosing schedules for all antibiotics used in the treatment of pneumonia are available from a range of sources and the agents used will be influenced by geographic resistance patterns. Paediatric tertiary hospital CPGs, prescribing resources such as the Therapeutic Guidelines website and local resistance data, should serve as treatment guides.

PRACTICE TIPS

PNEUMONIA

- Pneumonia should be suspected in children presenting with the following symptoms: cough, fever, dyspnoea, chest pain, vomiting, abdominal pain and anorexia.
- In addition to the classic features of pneumonia, it should be suspected in children with fever, tachypnoea and abdominal pain.
- Viral and bacterial causes cannot be reliably differentiated on clinical and X-ray findings in most cases.
- Most infants and children should be treated with oral amoxicillin or intravenous penicillin, depending on the severity of the illness.

Epistaxis

Epistaxis is common in children under the age of 10 years, frequently occurs recurrently and in the majority of cases is mild and self-limiting.[180] However, as the mucosa of the nose is highly vascular and supplied by branches of the internal carotid and maxillary divisions of the external carotid arteries, torrential bleeding from the nose is possible, although rare.[181]

Most uncomplicated epistaxis occurs unilaterally in the anterior part of the nose where the vessels are superficial and relatively unprotected, and therefore susceptible to nasal trauma or conditions that dry the nasal mucosa. In children this frequently involves digital trauma, the presence of a foreign body, rhinitis and exposure to allergens and cigarette smoke. The potential for epistaxis to occur secondary to systemic causes should also be considered, the most significant of which include bleeding disorders, leukaemia and thrombocytopenia.

Presentation and diagnosis

Children present to the ED with both active or recurrent bleeding and concerned parents. Serious systemic illness can generally be eliminated on the basis of the history. The likely aetiology of the bleeding may also be apparent from the history. Examination in many circumstances will identify the site of bleeding, which is most commonly in Little's area.[180] However, a general examination should also be performed to ensure that there are no signs of systemic illness present. Pathology is only warranted where an underlying systemic disorder is suspected.

Management

An attempt to control active bleeding using compression of the nostrils for between 5 and 20 minutes should be made. This is usually sufficient to stop the bleeding. However, if haemostasis has not been achieved, nasal packing and referral to ENT is indicated. Application of nasal antiseptic cream is as effective as nasal cautery for managing epistaxis,[181-183] and is less likely to result in significant complications.

PRACTICE TIPS

EPISTAXIS

- Although uncommon, epistaxis may occur in association with systemic illness such as bleeding disorders, leukaemia and thrombocytopenia.
- Most bleeding will stop using compression of the nostrils for 5–20 minutes.

Otitis media

Acute otitis media (AOM) is the most common cause of otalgia (earache) in children and is the most commonly diagnosed childhood disease. At least 90% of children will experience AOM by the age of 2 years.[184] As has been described earlier, the underdeveloped immune system coupled with the age-related differences in the Eustachian tube anatomy make the infant and young child more susceptible to ear infection than other age groups. The aetiology in Australian children is generally viral (25%), *Streptococcus* pneumonia (35%), nontypable *Haemophilus* influenza (25%) and *Moraxella catarrhalis* (15%).[185]

Childcare attendance, older siblings, younger age, dummy use and cigarette smoke exposure have all been shown by researchers and meta-analysis to increase the incidence of AOM in children.[182,186] The protective effect of breastfeeding has been debated in the literature; Uhari's meta-analysis suggĕaests that breastfeeding for 3 months is likely to have a positive effect on the incidence of AOM.[186]

Presentation and diagnosis

Infants and children with AOM present with fever, distress, interrupted sleep and complaints of earache or have been observed pulling at one or both of their ears. They may also have had discharge from the ear. There have usually been symptoms of an upper respiratory tract infection (URTI) for several days prior to the onset of more-specific symptoms. Approximately 90% of children suffering AOM will have rhinitis.

Examination usually reveals signs of URTI, such as coryza and rhinitis. The tympanic membrane (TM) shows signs of inflammation and will be red, yellow or cloudy, and is usually full or bulging with signs of effusion. Where the TM is perforated, this may be visible or the canal may be occluded by yellow mucousy discharge.

Consideration should be given to potential complications of AOM (such as mastoiditis and intracranial infection) or alternative aetiology for presenting symptoms (such as sepsis), particularly where infants or children present looking systemically unwell.

Management

Pain is a significant feature of AOM, so appropriate analgesics are essential. Paracetamol, ibuprofen or a codeine combination product should be given regularly, and stopped once the pain has resolved. Several drops of lignocaine 1% may be instilled into the ear to provide temporary (up to 30 minutes) relief for severe pain.[187] Studies summarised in a Cochrane systematic review do not support the use of decongestants and antihistamines in the treatment of AOM symptoms.[188]

A Cochrane review of the literature reports that fewer children treated with antibiotics will experience pain at 2 to 7 days or tympanic membrane perforation compared with children receiving placebo. However, 82% of children settle spontaneously by 2 days and 20 children must be treated with antibiotics to prevent one child from unnecessarily experiencing pain beyond 2 days. Furthermore, one in 14 children treated with antibiotics will experience an adverse event.[189] Children less likely to achieve resolution within several days were those under 2 years of age with bilateral AOM and those who presented systemically unwell. These results are supported by several systematic reviews describing the natural history of AOM and a number of studies conducted more recently.[190–192] This supports current recommendations that infants over the age of 1 year who are systemically well only receive antibiotics if the symptoms of ear infection persist beyond 2–3 days.

Amoxycillin is the antibiotic of first choice for the management of OM. Although there is some evidence to suggest that children less than 2 years of age gain temporary benefit from a 10-day course rather than the standard 5 days,

it is not convincing enough to merit altering dosing schedules for age-related subgroups. There is also some evidence to suggest that the dosing schedule may be reduced to once- or twice-daily doses instead of the more traditional three to four daily doses.[193] Amoxycillin and clavulanic acid may be considered in children with persistent symptoms following 48 hours of treatment with amoxycillin. Guidelines and appropriate pharmacopoeias should be used to guide the choice of agent and the dose and dosing schedule.

Persistent middle-ear effusion (OME) frequently follows an episode of AOM. These children will be largely symptom-free, although may complain of a 'blocked ear' or difficulty hearing. They should be referred to their local doctor for review in 8–12 weeks to confirm resolution of the effusion, although approximately 25% of children will have persistent effusion at 12 weeks.[192] Treatment with antibiotics during the initial infection or following development of the effusion will not alter the course, and antibiotics are not recommended.[194] There is also no evidence to support the use of antihistamines or decongestants for OME.[195] Recurrent AOM and chronic effusions, where there is hearing loss, delayed language development or failure to thrive, should be referred to ENT.

PRACTICE TIPS

OTITIS MEDIA

- Frequently associated with a viral URTI.
- Pain management is the most important focus of management of otitis media.
- Antibiotic treatment should be withheld for 2 days in children who are over the age of 1 year and systemically well, as pain will subside spontaneously in approximately 80% of these children.
- Antibiotic therapy will not reduce the incidence or aid in the management of middle-ear effusion, a common outcome of acute otitis media.

Pharyngitis

Sore throat in paediatric emergency presentations is most commonly caused by viral pharyngitis. However, the aetiology in about one-third of presentations in Australia and New Zealand will be Group A *Streptococcus* (GAS), the majority of which will occur in school-age children.[196] The complications that may occur following GAS infection, such as rheumatic fever, serve as the incentive for antibiotic treatment of presentations with a likely GAS infection. However, there is some controversy about this practice in some populations, such as non-Indigenous Australians and New Zealanders, where complication post-GAS infection is rare.[197] Conversely, the incidence of rheumatic fever in the Australian Indigenous community in the Northern Territory is the highest in the world,[198] and this is mirrored in the Māori community in New Zealand.

Presentation and diagnosis

Infants and children with pharyngitis present with fever, sore throat and/or decreased oral intake and mild irritability. Those with a viral aetiology will also present with coryza, cough and conjunctivitis, and those with Epstein-Barr infection will present with general malaise, fever and generalised lymphadenopathy and splenomegaly. The features of GAS infection are fever, pharyngotonsillitis, exudate and tender tonsillar lymph nodes. There is, however, considerable overlap between presentations of differing aetiology, making accurate diagnosis difficult. For example, exudate is present in approximately 30% of cases of non-GAS pharyngitis.[199]

Throat swabs are widely used to confirm GAS with 90–95% sensitivity.[200] They should be taken where GAS infection is suspected and prior to commencing antibiotic therapy.

Management

Non-Indigenous Australian and New Zealand children under 4 years of age and older children with viral symptoms or signs of Epstein-Barr infection and no signs of GAS should receive symptomatic management and no antibiotic therapy. These children should be given regular analgesia to ensure that they are comfortable enough to drink. Literature from the United States recommends a more cautious approach, and larger numbers of children presenting will be tested for GAS and commenced on antibiotics.

Children older than 4 years who have features of GAS infection should be treated with oral penicillin, as it has proven efficacy in eradicating the organism and preventing rheumatic fever secondary to GAS, it is safe and cost-effective[197,201] and no penicillin-resistant isolates have been reported.[199] There should be a very low threshold for treating Indigenous Australians and New Zealanders of any age with antibiotics. Pathology review in 2–3 days will confirm the need to continue the antibiotics. They can be stopped if the throat swab is negative for GAS.

There is insufficient evidence to support the role of other agents, such as steroids, in the treatment of pharyngitis in children,[202] although it should be acknowledged that vaccination for influenza and *Pneumococcus* reduces the incidence of pharyngitis.

PRACTICE TIPS

PHARYNGITIS

- Most pharyngitis, particularly in children under 4 years of age, is caused by viral infection.
- Throat swabs can be used to diagnose Group B *Streptococcus* infection and determine the need for antibiotics.
- Penicillin remains the antibiotic of choice with no resistant strains reported to date.

Cardiovascular emergencies

Shock

Shock is a complex physiological syndrome but can be most simply defined as a state where inadequate perfusion results in profound tissue hypoxia. Shock is frequently classified by pathway to shock: hypovolaemic, cardiogenic, obstructive or distributive; and may be further defined by the predominant physiological derangement: an abnormality of preload, an abnormality of contractility, an abnormality of afterload or an abnormality of vascular tone. However, it should be remembered that there is likely to be overlap between the precipitants to and the derangements of shock, and that once shock is well established a self-perpetuating inflammatory cascade, which is largely independent of the original cause, is established and is increasingly difficult to manage.[203,204] Chapters 20 and 22 describe shock in greater detail; this section will briefly focus on paediatric physiology and shock in infants and young children.

Acute illness demands an increase in cardiac output to supply oxygen and glucose to the tissues and remove waste products. Cardiac output is determined by heart rate and stroke volume, which are variable and tightly controlled to ensure adequate organ perfusion. However, infants have a relatively fixed stroke volume (see Table 36.1) and are more dependent on an increase in heart rate to increase cardiac output. Rates as high as 220 beats/minute may be seen in hypovolaemic infants.[86,205]

Infant myocardial compliance is also lower than in adults, and so for the same ventricular filling volume infants will experience higher atrial pressures. This has a negative effect on preload and also restricts capacity to increase stroke volume.[24] This also helps explain the infant's relatively poor response to aggressive fluid resuscitation.[30]

Infants are particularly susceptible to shock, as compensatory mechanisms are easily overwhelmed; unless the physiological derangements of shock are reversed, infants rapidly demonstrate a bradycardic response to deterioration, in contrast to the increasing tachycardia seen in older children and adults. This is the result of the presence of fewer beta-receptors in infant myocardium than are found in adult myocardium.[24]

Hypovolaemic shock reflects a loss of circulating blood volume; the most common causes in children are fluid loss from dehydration and blood loss from trauma. Other, less common, causes are burns, diabetic ketoacidosis, reduced intake and third-space losses. Distributive shock is most commonly caused by sepsis and in children septic shock is preceded by *E. coli*, *Staphylococcus*, *Streptococcus*, *Neisseria meningitides*, Enterobacteriaceae and other Gram-negative bacterial infections causing pneumonia, skin infections, urinary tract infections, meningitis and bacteraemia. The incidence of sepsis in US children is estimated at 0.56 cases per 1000 children, of which the majority are infants (5.6 in 1000), and mortality is approximately 10%.[206]

Presentation

Intravascular volume loss results in tachycardia to increase cardiac output, tachypnoea to increase oxygen supply and vasoconstriction with a resulting narrowing pulse pressure to increase perfusion pressure. Poor circulating blood volume results in the infant or child exhibiting pallor, mottled peripheries, delayed capillary refill and deteriorating conscious level. Hypotension is a late sign of hypovolaemic shock and has been repeatedly demonstrated to be associated with higher rates of mortality.[207,208]

Sepsis is a complex syndrome mediated by bacterial toxins and the chemical mediators of inflammation that causes vasodilation and capillary leak, myocardial depression and inhibition of cellular metabolism. The stages of septic shock are defined by different clinical findings. *Compensated* (warm) septic shock is characterised by evidence of a hyperdynamic circulation: tachycardia, tachypnoea, flushed warm skin, full pulses and widening pulse pressure. Deterioration sees this progress to *uncompensated* (cold) shock, characterised by increasing tachycardia, tachypnoea and signs more consistent with hypovolaemia such as pallor, cool to cold and mottled peripheries, delayed capillary refill and decreased conscious state.

It is noteworthy that infants and children can present with either warm or cold shock or with a combination of vasodilation and poor cardiac output, in contrast to adults, who usually present in the early stages with vasodilation and high cardiac output.[209] Immune-system immaturity is responsible for unpredictable responses to sepsis in infants, who may present with hypothermia rather than hyperthermia and a range of non-specific symptoms.

Invasive monitoring, such as arterial pressures and central venous pressures, can provide more-accurate figures for determining the extent of the cardiovascular dysfunction. However, insertion of invasive cannulae for this purpose should not be an early priority as sufficient clinical data to make an assessment, establish a treatment plan and measure its success during the resuscitation phase can be gained from non-invasive parameters. Central access will become a greater priority in the event that inotropes are required.

Biochemical markers can be used as an indirect measure of the adequacy of cardiac output and tissue oxygenation. However, they have no role in guiding immediate fluid resuscitation, given the urgency of restoring an adequate circulation in a hypovolaemic child and the potential delay in accessing laboratory results. Markers such as lactate may serve as one of the earliest predictors of mortality in sepsis.[210] Hence, biochemical markers may be better used as an indicator of the success of earlier treatment and a guide to ongoing resuscitation.[23]

Management

Management of shock must include airway and respiratory assessment and support. Children in shock will at least require high-flow oxygen and are likely to benefit from intubation and mechanical ventilation, which has been discussed previously. The focus of this section is circulatory management.

The aim of treatment, regardless of cause, is to improve organ perfusion. Potential for survival is improved by aggressive early normalisation of blood pressure values.[15,23,29,211] Initially this is achieved by administering intravenous fluids to increase the circulating blood volume. Colloids were traditionally considered likely to remain in the circulation longer than isotonic crystalloids, and for many years have been the mainstay of fluid resuscitation. However, this long-held view has been recently challenged in a Cochrane review. The authors concluded that isotonic crystalloid and colloid solutions have equivalent effects on the circulation and that adverse events following resuscitation are similar for both fluids.[212] Crystalloid fluids have gained increasing favour as the fluid of choice for circulatory resuscitation as they are widely available and inexpensive.[212,213] Normal saline is the most commonly recommended crystalloid for paediatric fluid resuscitation and there is some paediatric data to support this recommendation.[214] However, overuse can result in hyperchloraemic acidosis. Hence, alternative fluids are being considered; Hartmann's solution (contains lactate, which when converted to bicarbonate acts as a buffer) is used with increasing frequency as a resuscitation fluid of choice.[29]

Other specific fluids are recommended in certain situations to supplement initial attempts to resuscitate the circulation with crystalloids. This includes albumin in circumstances such as sepsis,[213,215] and packed cells in trauma following 40 mL/kg of crystalloid. However, as the evidence for colloids in sepsis is at best weak,[216] most clinical guidelines continue to recommend crystalloids for early resuscitation.

Guidelines for fluid resuscitation most commonly recommend fluid boluses of 20 mL/kg.[15,23,29] This volume is based on results from a study which demonstrated that the signs of hypovolaemic shock become apparent with a loss of approximately 30% of circulating blood volume, which is equivalent to about 20 mL/kg.[31] Fluid is rapidly redistributed and repeat boluses are usually required to maintain an adequate circulating volume, particularly where there is a total body fluid deficit or large volume shifts as in sepsis. Data have shown that rapid resuscitation of septic infant and children presenting to the ED with in excess of 40 mL/kg increases survival when compared with those receiving smaller volumes of fluid.[217] Infants and young children with sepsis may require volumes of up to 80–100 mL/kg over an hour to achieve adequate perfusion. There is a small body of evidence that aggressive fluid resuscitation may be associated with higher mortality.[218] However, the bulk of this work has been conducted in developing countries with children suffering diseases such as malaria. Similar effects are as yet unproven in developed countries.

Intraosseous (IO) access to the circulation for delivery of resuscitation drugs and fluids is recommended where intravenous (IV) access cannot be rapidly achieved. Insertion of an IO needle is easier than IV insertion, and is made easier with the use of insertion aids such as bone drills. Therefore, clinicians should have a low threshold for abandoning further attempts to site an IV (one or two brief unsuccessful attempts) and attempting IO access.[23]

The type of access achieved will influence the rate and methods of fluid administration. Fluids given via the IO route must be pumped under pressure as they will not run on a gravity drip set. Manual blood pump sets, syringes and pressure bags can be used for this purpose.[23] Small-bore IV cannulae also limit the flow of fluids, and higher pressures will be needed to deliver a fluid bolus. Low-volume fluid boluses can be given by 'pushing' fluids with a 20 mL or 50 mL syringe connected to a three-way tap in the fluid line, while larger volumes will require use of infusion pumps, pressure bags or pump sets.[23]

Aggressive fluid resuscitation is rarely sufficient to correct haemodynamic derangements in septic shock, and delays to inotropes and/or vasopressors are associated with increases in mortality.[219,220] Infants and children presenting with signs of high cardiac output and vasodilation, clinically manifested by warm peripheries and bounding pulses, benefit from agents that stimulate vasoconstriction, such as noradrenaline and dopamine.[182,192] Alternatively, for those presenting with evidence of 'cold' shock, which is associated with vasoconstriction and clinically manifested by cold and mottled peripheries, weak thready pulses and delayed capillary refill, inotropic agents to improve contractility such as dobutamine and adrenaline are used.[182,192] In many cases where there are features of both vasodilation and poor cardiac output, combination regimens

TABLE 36.14 Inotrope infusions commonly used for sepsis management

AGENT	PREPARATION	DOSING SCHEDULE
Adrenaline	0.3 mg/kg in 50 mL Normal saline = 6 μg/kg/mL	0.05–0.1 μg/kg/min 0.5–1.0 mL/h
	If low doses are required, 0.15 mg/kg* = 3 μg/kg/mL	0.01–0.05 μg/kg/min 0.2–1.0 mL/h
Noradrenaline	0.3 mg/kg in 50 mL Normal saline = 6 μg/kg/mL	0.05–0.1 μg/kg/min 0.5–1.0 mL/h
	If low doses are required, 0.15 mg/kg* = 3 μg/kg/mL	0.01–0.05 μg/kg/min 0.2–1.0 mL/h
Dopamine	15 mg/kg in 50 mL Normal saline = 300 μg/kg/mL	5–10 μg/min 1–2 mL/h
Dobutamine	15 mg/kg in 50 mL Normal saline = 300 μg/kg/mL	5–10 μg/min 1–2 mL/h

At very low doses, small increases in rate may generate significant changes in blood pressure

are best suited to improving perfusion. Furthermore, the haemodynamic status of children may change rapidly, requiring changes to inotropic regimens. Table 36.14 provides a guide to the dosing schedule and preparation of common paediatric inotrope infusions and Figure 36.3 provides a clinical algorithm to guide haemodynamic management in the ED of septic infants and children,[221] which is promoted by the Surviving Sepsis Campaign, an international collaboration to provide guidelines for management of sepsis and improve survival rates.[222]

PRACTICE TIPS

SHOCK

- Infants rely almost exclusively on increasing heart rate to increase their cardiac output. However, once this is exhausted they rapidly deteriorate.
- Infants may present with a low temperature associated with septic shock rather than a fever.
- Once compensatory responses are overwhelmed, infants and children may demonstrate a bradycardic response to rapid deterioration rather than the classic tachycardic response expected.
- Hypotension is a late sign of shock and is associated with poor prognosis.
- Pathology test results play no part in directing the initial fluid resuscitation of infants and children in shock.
- The aim of treatment is to improve end-organ perfusion by normalising circulating blood volume and blood pressure.
- Intraosseous access to the circulation is recommended where intravenous access cannot be rapidly achieved.

- Infants and children may require up to 80–100 mL/kg of isotonic crystalloid solutions such as Normal saline, and Hartmann's solution in boluses of 20 mL/kg to restore circulating blood volume.
- Infants and children in septic shock will usually require inotropic support to maintain end-organ perfusion.

Adjuvant therapies to treat shock, in particular septic shock, have been explored with mixed success. A Cochrane review concluded that there is sufficient evidence to support the use of low-dose long-term (> 5 days) steroids to improve sepsis mortality. A recent synthesis of the evidence has resulted in a recommendation that children with fluid refractory, catecholamine resistant shock with proven or suspected adrenal insufficiency receive steroids.[222] Two Cochrane reviews summarised the evidence for the use of human recombinant protein C in neonates[223] and in children and adults,[224] and both concluded that there is no evidence for this theoretically promising therapy.

Dehydration

Dehydration, as a result of poor oral intake and increased losses secondary to acute illness, occurs more commonly in infants than in adults, which can be explained by the physiological differences between adults and children and their responses to illness. Total body water is about 80 mL/kg at birth and falls to approximately 60–65 mL/kg by about 6 months of age, where it remains constant until adulthood. The distribution of fluids across fluid compartments also differs, evidenced by the difference in blood volume between infants (70–80 mL/kg) and adults (60–70 mL/kg); and like total body water, fluid distribution resembles that of the adult by 6 months of age.[15,24]

FIGURE 36.3

Algorithm for goal-directed time-sensitive haemodynamic management for infants and children with septic shock.

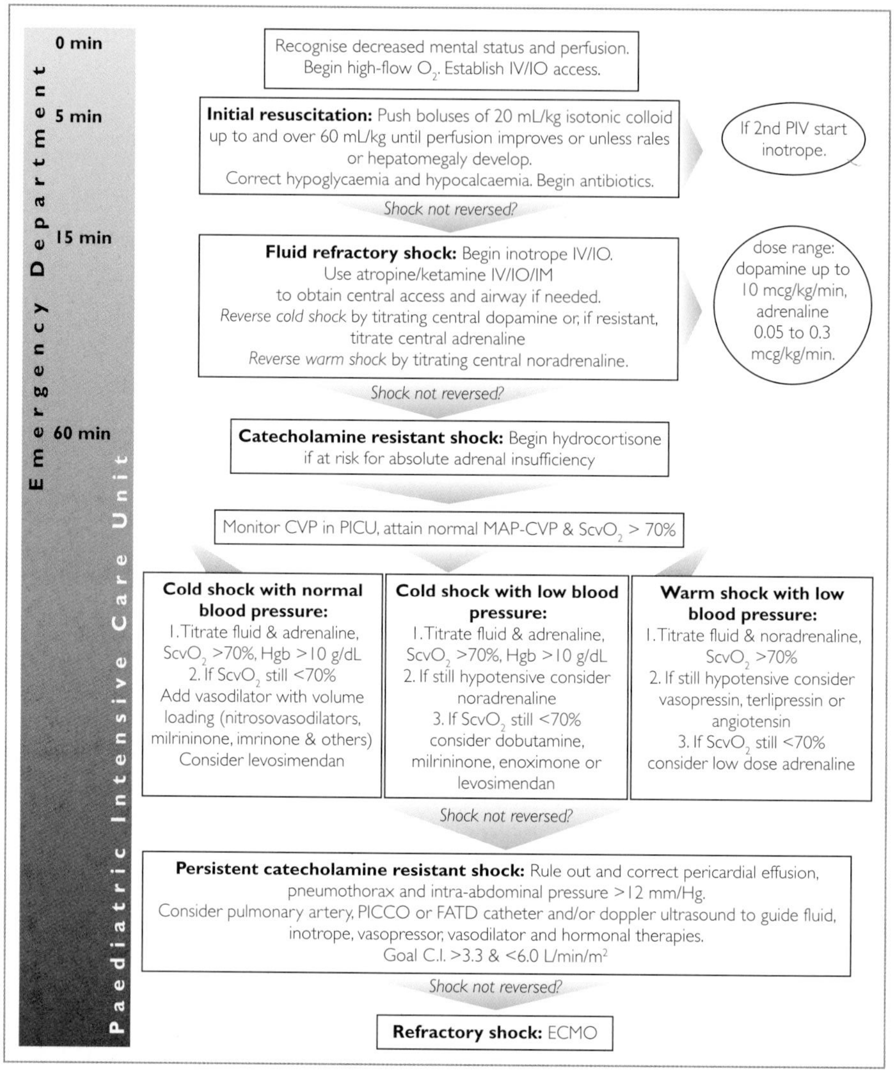

Emergency Department	**0 min**
	Recognise decreased mental status and perfusion. Begin high-flow O_2. Establish IV/IO access.
	5 min
	Initial resuscitation: Push boluses of 20 mL/kg isotonic colloid up to and over 60 mL/kg until perfusion improves or unless rales or hepatomegaly develop. Correct hypoglycaemia and hypocalcaemia. Begin antibiotics.
	Shock not reversed?
	15 min
	Fluid refractory shock: Begin inotrope IV/IO. Use atropine/ketamine IV/IO/IM to obtain central access and airway if needed. *Reverse cold shock* by titrating central dopamine or, if resistant, titrate central adrenaline *Reverse warm shock* by titrating central noradrenaline.
	Shock not reversed?
	60 min
	Catecholamine resistant shock: Begin hydrocortisone if at risk for absolute adrenal insufficiency

If 2nd PIV start inotrope.

dose range: dopamine up to 10 mcg/kg/min, adrenaline 0.05 to 0.3 mcg/kg/min.

Paediatric Intensive Care Unit

Monitor CVP in PICU, attain normal MAP-CVP & $ScvO_2$ > 70%

Cold shock with normal blood pressure:	**Cold shock with low blood pressure:**	**Warm shock with low blood pressure:**
1. Titrate fluid & adrenaline, $ScvO_2$ >70%, Hgb >10 g/dL	1. Titrate fluid & adrenaline, $ScvO_2$ >70%, Hgb >10 g/dL	1. Titrate fluid & noradrenaline, $ScvO_2$ >70%
2. If $ScvO_2$ still <70% Add vasodilator with volume loading (nitrosovasodilators, milrinone, imrinone & others) Consider levosimendan	2. If still hypotensive consider noradrenaline 3. If $ScvO_2$ still <70% consider dobutamine, milrininone, enoximone or levosimendan	2. If still hypotensive consider vasopressin, terlipressin or angiotensin 3. If $ScvO_2$ still <70% consider low dose adrenaline

Shock not reversed?

Persistent catecholamine resistant shock: Rule out and correct pericardial effusion, pneumothorax and intra-abdominal pressure >12 mm/Hg. Consider pulmonary artery, PICCO or FATD catheter and/or doppler ultrasound to guide fluid, inotrope, vasopressor, vasodilator and hormonal therapies. Goal C.I. >3.3 & <6.0 L/min/m²

Shock not reversed?

Refractory shock: ECMO

Infant renal function differs from adult renal function, further reducing infants' capacity to rapidly and aggressively respond to hypovolaemia, dehydration and low cardiac output.[24] A lower glomerular filtration rate, renal blood flow and renal immaturity explain the differences in renal function between the infant and the adult. The infant kidney has less capacity to concentrate urine, excrete a solute load or acidify urine, and is more sensitive to hyperchloraemic acidosis resulting from large-volume resuscitation with normal saline.[24,29]

Presentation

Changes in total bodyweight are considered the gold standard for assessment of dehydration.[29] It has been shown that clinicians frequently overestimate dehydration severity, with one Australian study revealing that this may be by as much as 3.2%.[17,225] This provides persuasive support for serial weight measurements for children presenting to the ED with the potential for fluid loss. All children with actual or potential fluid balance problems should have their bare weight measured as part of their initial assessment to provide a baseline for future assessments. However, accurate recent weight measurements are often not available to inform the initial hydration assessment,

and clinicians are obliged to rely on clinical features to detect dehydration and determine the severity of the fluid loss.

Identifying clinical signs and symptoms, which are sensitive and specific for dehydration and its severity, has gained significant attention from researchers. Traditionally, dehydration has been linked to a history of fluid loss (diarrhoea and vomiting), poor fluid intake and low urine output. However, data from a meta-analysis do not confirm this link, showing that these symptoms have low predictive value for moderate dehydration.[17,226–228] Conversely, parental report of normal urine output positively predicts normal hydration.[228]

Delayed capillary refill time, abnormal skin turgor and abnormal respiratory pattern have been shown to positively predict the presence of dehydration.[17,228–230] While signs such as the absence of tears, cool extremities, sunken eyes, dry mucous membranes, ill appearance and a weak pulse may be of some clinical value to the assessment of hydration, their predictive value is not as strong and results vary. Several authors have published results demonstrating that dehydration assessment tools comprised of several signs have greater predictive value than individual signs.[228,229]

Considerable variation in recommendations for the signs and symptoms most likely to predict dehydration exists, and available data do not clarify this for the clinician. In light of this, the clinically rational approach is to approximate severity of dehydration based on the number of signs of dehydration identified rather than the presence of specific individual signs and symptoms. Several tools using this approach have been developed and are shown to reliably detect dehydration and quantify severity.[228,231] Gorelick and colleagues identified a set of 11 clinical findings (Box 36.3), which in combination distinguish clinically significant levels of dehydration with high-level sensitivity and specificity.[228] The presence of any three or more of these findings demonstrates greater than 5% fluid deficit, and six or more demonstrates upwards of 7% dehydration. Friedman and colleagues have also identified a reliable method for establishing dehydration severity, and this scale has since been validated in the ED. It is based on assessments of general appearance, the extent to which the eyes are sunken, the mucous membranes and the presence or absence of tears, which are scored to provide a total from 0 to 8. The scale and scoring system are shown in Table 36.15.[231,232]

The sensitivity of laboratory tests to detect dehydration and estimate the severity is not sufficiently high to support recommendations for routine laboratory tests as a component of hydration assessment. Of those tests that are considered likely to be predictive of the severity of dehydration, bicarbonate has shown to be the most sensitive,[17,225,230,233,234] while parameters such as specific gravity of urine, the presence of ketones and urine output during rehydration show low predictive value.[227,230] Ultrasound has been tested as a means to identify severe dehydration with some success and as the use of bedside ultrasound grows there may be a role for ultrasound in the detection of dehydration.[235,236]

Management

Enteral fluids are the recommended rehydration strategy of first choice for children with dehydration in the absence of signs of hypovolaemia. Enteral fluid replacement is likely to avoid the potential fluid, electrolyte and acid–base imbalances that can occur with intravenous fluid management,[148,237] and has been shown to be potentially safer than IV rehydration,[237] and at least as effective.[148,237] The composition of the optimal solution for oral rehydration (ORS) in developed countries is a reduced osmolarity solution based on WHO recommendations, which can be seen in Table 36.16, alongside the composition of a number of other fluids commonly used for oral rehydration. Fruit juices and soft drinks require considerable dilution (1 part to 4 parts water) if they are to be used as an alternative to ORSs for children refusing to drink ORSs.[238]

Children with only mild dehydration can usually be encouraged to drink sufficient amounts of fluid to maintain adequate hydration. Frozen ORS prepared as an icy pole is increasingly used as an alternative way of providing rehydration fluids, and the authors of a small study comparing frozen ORS and standard ORS concluded that children were more likely to tolerate frozen ORS than standard ORS.[239]

A number of children will refuse to drink sufficient volumes of fluid or will not tolerate oral fluids. In the absence of signs

---

BOX 36.3 Dehydration assessment scale[228]

Features
Decreased skin elasticity
Capillary refill 0.2 s

General appearance
Absent tears
Abnormal respirations
Dry mucous membranes
Sunken eyes
Abnormal radial pulse
Tachycardia
Decreased urine output

Scoring
Presence of:

0–2 signs = nil to mild dehydration
3–5 signs = moderate dehydration
6 or more signs = severe dehydration

TABLE 36.15 Scale for establishing severity of dehydration[231,232]

CHARACTERISTIC	0	1	2
General appearance	Normal	Thirsty, restless or lethargic but irritable when touched	Drowsy, limp, cold, sweaty ± comatose
Eyes	Normal	Slightly sunken	Very sunken
Mucous membranes (tongue)	Moist	'Sticky'	Dry
Tears	Tears present	Decreased tears	Absent tears

Scoring

0 = no dehydration
1–4 = some dehydration
5–8 = moderate–severe dehydration

TABLE 36.16 Electrolyte composition of fluids commonly offered to children with diarrhoea and vomiting[556,557]

SOLUTION	SODIUM (mmol/L)	POTASSIUM (mmol/L)	CARBOHYDRATE (mmol/L)	OSMOLARITY (mOsm)
WHO recommendation	90	20	111	310
Reduced osmolarity solution	75	20	75	245
Hydralyte	55	20	80	230
Soft drink	2	0	700	750
Apple juice	3	32	690	730
Broth	250	8	0	500
Sports drink	20	3	255	340
Tea	0	0	0	5

WHO: World Health Organization

of hypovolaemia, these children can in most circumstances still be rehydrated enterally via a nasogastric (NG) tube. Australian guidelines for rehydration strongly advocate for this route, claiming that it is effective and likely to be safer than IV rehydration. However, the evidence for this contention is not overwhelming and in many countries this practice is not so common.

The decision to rehydrate enterally using an NG tube may be a pragmatic one based on the degree of procedural difficulty associated with NG tube and intravenous cannula insertion. Nasogastric tube insertion can be safely and quickly achieved in the ED to provide a route for fluid replacement,[25,29,240] and may prove to be easier than cannula placement in infants and young children with dehydration. However, although it may be easier, NG tube insertion is considered one of the most painful procedures performed in the ED,[241,242] and yet practice recommendations rarely advocate the use of analgesia or local anaesthetic. Clinicians should give consideration to the use of agents such as lignocaine spray and nebulised lignocaine prior to NG tube insertion to alleviate the discomfort associated with this procedure.

As the need for NG rehydration is most likely to be necessary in infants and young children who are rarely cooperative, restraint is usually required. A number of strategies can be used, such as wrapping their upper body in a sheet and binding hands with bandages to prevent them pulling the tube out.[23] However, the least restraint necessary for the procedure should be used. Delivery of fluids only requires the insertion of fine-bore tubes (size 8 French gauge) to allow appropriate flow rates. Continuous administration of fluid by feeding pump or manual drip set will be better tolerated than regular boluses.[23]

Where there is concern about the impact of rapid rehydration on fluid and electrolyte balance, it is recommended that replacement of losses occurs over 6 hours. The volume of fluid administered hourly is the sum of the estimated loss divided by 6 added to the hourly maintenance volume required. Table 36.17 provides an example of this calculation. Tables providing the volume of fluid administered by weight for children with moderate and severe dehydration are

available, and one, such as Table 36.17, can be found in the RCH gastroenteritis management CPG.[238] When electrolyte imbalance is not a concern, rapid rehydration regimens advocating 25 mL/kg/h to replace fluid losses over 3–4 hours are increasingly used for rehydration.[243]

> **PRACTICE TIPS**
> ## DEHYDRATION
>
> - All infants and children with actual or potential dehydration should be weighed, as short-term changes in bodyweight is the most sensitive indicator of fluid loss.
> - Pathology tests to detect and determine the severity of dehydration are not sensitive enough to be of clinical value.
> - Infants and children with dehydration (in the absence of signs of hypovolaemia) can be rehydrated enterally (orally or via a nasogastric tube) in most cases.
> - Rapid enteral rehydration via nasaogastric tube using 25 mL/kg/h over 3–4 hours may be used where electrolyte imbalance is not a concern.

Maintenance fluid management

Infants and children with acute illness often have higher losses of fluid (insensible, vomiting and diarrhoea) and drink poorly, impacting on their fluid and electrolyte balance.[23] In an attempt to overcome this, maintenance fluids are commenced as a means of providing sufficient water and electrolytes to maintain normal urine output at a similar osmolality to extracellular fluid.

Infants and children suffering fever associated with infection have been shown to secrete higher levels of antidiuretic hormone (ADH) than well children, prompting retention of water and higher rates of sodium excretion.[244] This may result in hyponatraemia and water overload. This is now defined as the syndrome of inappropriate ADH secretion (SIADH), and is linked with illnesses such as meningitis, pneumonia, bronchiolitis and gastroenteritis.[245–250] Although there is some concern that SIADH is overdiagnosed,[29] it should

TABLE 36.17 Oral and enteral rehydration fluid management for the first 6 hours: An example calculation

REPLACEMENT CALCULATION	MAINTENANCE VOLUME CALCULATION	VOLUME / HOUR
15 kg child estimated as 6% dehydrated	4 mL/hr/kg up to 10 kg	= 150 + 50
6% of 15 kg = 900	2 mL/hr/kg for each kg between 10 and 20 kg	= 200 mL/hr
Therefore:	1 mL/hr/kg for each kg over 20 kg	
Deficit = 900 mL over 6 hours	Therefore:	
= 150 mL/hr replacement	(4 × 10) + (2 × 5)	
	= 50 mL/hr maintenance	

be considered when prescribing fluid-management regimens for children and has served as a stimulus for restricting fluids in some circumstances, providing there are no signs of hypovolaemia. Furthermore, it has been recently recognised that the IV fluid composition and rates for maintenance therapy were based on data collected from well children. Acute illness results in fluid and electrolyte imbalances caused by increased fluid and electrolyte losses and, in some cases, SIADH, making the maintenance fluid regimens based on the needs of healthy children unsuitable. There is increasing data to support the use of isotonic intravenous fluids for maintenance therapy in preference to hypotonic fluids which have been repeatedly shown to increase the risk of hyponatraemia.[251,252] Recommendations for 0.9% saline as the solution of choice for maintenance therapy in hospitalised infants and children reflect this growing body of evidence.[24,29,213,253,254] For children where water retention is likely to be or would be harmful (e.g. with brain injury), Normal saline is the fluid of choice, but volumes are reduced by one-third.[24,29,213]

Maintenance fluids for infants and children should also contain glucose, as infants in particular have very limited stores of glycogen and illness will increase their glucose consumption. Addition of 5% glucose to the IV fluids will prevent hypoglycaemia in most circumstances, but will only provide about 20% of daily required calories.

PRACTICE TIPS
MAINTENANCE FLUID THERAPY

- Isotonic fluids which contain glucose are recommended for maintenance fluid management for unwell children.
- Two-thirds of maintenance volumes are recommended for children suffering illnesses where water retention is possible, such as meningitis, pneumonia and bronchiolitis.

Abnormal pulse rate or rhythm

Infants and children present to EDs with a range of cardiac dysrhythmias. Cardiac arrest rhythms are discussed elsewhere (Chs 22 and 15), and provide considerable detail about a range of dysrhythmias common to both adults and children. This section will make brief reference to those common to infants and children, and highlight the specific implications of these rhythms for infants and children. These dysrhythmias may also

occur in neonates and the principles of management will be similar. However, it is beyond the scope of this text to discuss the needs of this population specifically and clinicians would be encouraged to seek expert advice early if faced with a neonate with a dysrhythmia.

Bradyarrhythmias

Sinus bradycardia is the antecedent to most paediatric cardio-pulmonary arrests and can usually be attributed to increased parasympathetic stimulus, as occurs during intubation, metabolic derangements such as hypoxia, raised intracranial pressure caused most commonly in children by head trauma and poisoning with agents such as beta-blockers. Infants and children are particularly sensitive to these precipitants and bradycardia is poorly tolerated, as cardiac output in infants is largely rate-dependent. Infants and children quickly show signs of circulatory inadequacy, and if not treated promptly this is likely to progress to signs of circulatory collapse. Treatment should include addressing reversible causes and, if the dysrhythmia is life-threatening, basic life support is the priority (see Ch 15).

Tachydysrhythmias

Sinus tachycardia is a physiological response to a range of stimuli, and as infants rely heavily on increasing their heart rate to increase cardiac output, the extent of the tachycardia in infants and young children is proportionately much greater than in adults in similar circumstances. Tachycardia in sick infants may be as high as 220 beats/minute and in young children 180 beats/minute.[205]

Supraventricular tachycardia (SVT) is the most common tachydysrhythmia in children, occurring in 1 in 250–1000 children.[255] The pathophysiology is described in Chapter 22; in children the most common cause is atrioventricular re-entry, which involves an accessory conduction pathway between the atrium and the ventricles; and atrioventricular node re-entry, which involves a re-entry pathway within the atrioventricular node. It is usually paroxysmal, lasts on average 10 minutes and occurs recurrently.[255]

Older children present similarly to adults with SVT. However, infants will present with non-specific symptoms such as restlessness, poor feeding and lethargy. These symptoms mimic many other presentations, and, therefore, recognition of SVT in infants can be delayed. With a longer duration of SVT infants begin to show signs of respiratory distress, diaphoresis, pallor and mottling, and if prolonged for 24–48 hours signs of congestive heart failure may become apparent.[255]

Supraventricular tachycardia is usually fairly well tolerated in infants and children. However, the need for resuscitation should be considered and unstable patients will need cardioversion (see Ch 22). Stable patients with adequate perfusion should have oxygen therapy and cardiac monitoring commenced and a 12-lead ECG taken prior to attempts to revert the rhythm (Ch 17, p. 336, contains information on cardiac monitoring techniques). Vagal manoeuvres are usually attempted before pharmacological interventions. Young children may be asked to blow into a straw or blow with their thumb in their mouth. As an alternative, placing a bag containing cold water and ice across the forehead, eyes and bridge of the nose can stimulate the dive reflex. This method successfully terminates SVT in 35–60% of episodes.[256] Where vagal manoeuvres have been unsuccessful, adenosine is also the first-line treatment for SVT in infants and children and is given as a bolus every few minutes until they return to sinus rhythm, starting with 0.1 mg/kg and increasing by 0.05 mg/kg each time to a maximum of 0.3 mg/kg (see Ch 22 for further details). Cardioversion is used where adenosine fails to result in reversion.

PRACTICE TIPS
ABNORMAL PULSE RATE OR RHYTHM

- Bradycardia is a preterminal rhythm and management should focus on correcting the cause (e.g. improve oxygenation) and maintaining the adequacy of the circulation.
- Infants suffering from supraventricular tachycardia often present with non-specific symptoms, such as restlessness, poor feeding and lethargy.

Heart failure

Heart failure in neonates, infants and children occurs most commonly as a result of a congenital heart defect. It is beyond the scope of this section to detail these anomalies or the pathophysiological syndrome of heart failure. It is generally accepted as a progressive clinical syndrome caused by cardiac and non-cardiac abnormalities that result in ventricular dysfunction and a characteristic constellation of signs and symptoms.[257] For a comprehensive description of the anatomy and physiology of congenital heart disease, see the further reading list and useful websites at the end of the chapter. However, they can be grouped as those that cause a left-to-right shunt with increased pulmonary blood flow (e.g. ventricular septal defect (VSD)) and atrial septal defect (ASD), those that cause acute obstruction (e.g. aortic or pulmonary stenosis, coarctation of the aorta) and complex anomalies such as hypoplastic left heart syndrome, which cause a range of functional problems. In a small number of children, heart failure is precipitated by primary myocardial dysfunction (e.g. myocarditis), anaemia, metabolic derangements, toxins or dysrhythmias which result in a low output cardiac failure.[257,258]

Presentation and diagnosis
The age at which infants and children present with heart failure will depend on the cause. Congenital heart defects will result in heart failure in the days to months following birth, depending

on the type of defect. Primary myocardial defects and failure resulting from non-cardiac causes may present at any age.

Neonates and infants presenting with cardiac failure may have quite non-specific symptoms, most commonly lethargy, reduced feeding, sweating and tachypnoea during feeding and failure to thrive.[259] Heart failure may be precipitated by a mild respiratory infection, so signs of URTI are often present. On examination neonates and infants are usually tachypnoeic, tachycardic and show evidence of failure to thrive, hepatomegaly, a gallop rhythm and circulatory dysfunction, which may include signs of shock.[259] A murmur may also be heard on auscultation. Neonates and infants with many congenital heart defects are unresponsive to oxygen and hence this diagnosis should be considered in an infant with respiratory and circulatory dysfunction with intractable hypoxia.

Cardiomegaly is confirmed on chest X-ray and evidence of fluid overload may also be present. Older children present with more-specific signs and symptoms consistent with those found in adults.

Management
Fluid resuscitation and oxygen therapy are used to resuscitate the shocked infant regardless of the circumstances. However, in neonates and infants with a large right-to-left shunt, high-flow oxygen may worsen oxygenation. Furthermore, fluids are quickly restricted and diuretics prescribed to control preload in neonates, infants and children suffering cardiac failure. Newborns who are only days old with duct-dependent circulation will require prostaglandin to prevent duct closure and worsening of their condition.[258] Digoxin and angiotensin-converting enzyme (ACE) inhibitors remain the mainstay of heart failure treatment in neonates, infants and children.[260]

Management is complex, and advice from a specialist paediatric centre to guide treatment should be sought very early and arrangements made to transfer patients to a tertiary paediatric cardiac or intensive care unit. In the interim, the neonate or infant should be cardiac-monitored and a 12-lead ECG should be taken.

PRACTICE TIPS
HEART FAILURE

- Heart failure is often precipitated by mild respiratory infections.
- It is frequently associated with non-specific symptoms such as lethargy, decreased feeding and failure to thrive.
- Fluid resuscitation and oxygen therapy should be used to resuscitate the shocked infant.
- Treatment of heart failure is complex and expertise should be sought early.

Neurological emergencies
Seizures
Seizure is a common paediatric presentation to the ED; approximately 4–10% of children will suffer a seizure during childhood.[261] A seizure occurs where there are excessive hypersynchronous discharges from neurons, resulting in a transient, involuntary alteration of consciousness, behaviour,

motor activity, sensation or autonomic function.[261] Seizure activity prompts an increase in cerebral metabolic rate, resulting in an increase in oxygen and glucose consumption and carbon dioxide and lactic acid production. Cerebral blood flow and systolic blood pressure increases. Once metabolic demands have exceeded the supply, cerebral ischaemia, lactic acidosis, rhabdomyolysis, hyperkalaemia, hypoglycaemia, hypoxia and hyperthermia occur, all of which may lead to irreversible brain damage;[261] data show that this is likely to happen within 45–60 minutes of continuous seizure activity.[262]

Seizures are broadly classified as *generalised*, which involves the whole brain, or *partial*, which involves a region of the brain; there are many subtypes within each category. Most commonly children suffer generalised tonic–clonic seizures.[261] Seizures may result from fever, metabolic derangements such as hypoglycaemia, hyponatraemia or hypoxia, poisoning with agents such as tricyclic antidepressants, vascular or traumatic lesions, local infection, such as meningitis and encephalitis; or alternatively they may be idiopathic.[261] Fever is the most common cause of seizure in infants and children. A febrile convulsion is a benign, usually self-limiting convulsion which occurs in infants and young children in association with fever but without signs of neurological disease or infection or a history of afebrile convulsions.[263] Febrile convulsions are discussed further in the section on fever.

Epilepsy describes a condition where seizures are recurrent, and convulsive status epilepticus is defined as a continuous seizure or recurrent seizure without restoration of conscious state, lasting 30 minutes or more.[261,262,264] The majority of children experiencing status epilepticus in Australia are children with a previous history of seizures.[265]

Presentation

Infants and children may present during the seizure or in the post-ictal phase following the seizure. Infrequently they may present some time after the event, as the significance of the episode may be unrecognised by the parents. Subtle seizure activity can be difficult to detect, particularly in children with neurological deficits. Typical jerking movements may be absent and seizure activity may only result in stiffening of a limb, deviation of the eyes or an alteration in consciousness. Once a seizure has been identified, assessment of the infant or child should aim to determine the likely cause of the seizure.

Management

The priority for managing children with current seizure activity is to secure their airway, ensure adequate ventilation and perfusion, control the seizure and identify and treat where possible the underlying cause of the seizure. Blood sugar levels should be checked at the bedside and hypoglycaemia treated promptly, as this may account for a small number of seizures.[265] Furthermore, children are more susceptible to developing hypoglycaemia with prolonged seizure.

Pharmacological control of the seizure is advocated if the seizure does not spontaneously terminate within 5 minutes, and is best achieved using a benzodiazepine.[265] This may be repeated within 5 minutes if seizure activity continues. Second-line agents commonly used in Australia include phenytoin and phenobarbitone.[265] Prolonged seizure correlates with the need for airway management and ventilatory support, and this is likely in some cases to be related to respiratory depression as well as the need to control seizure activity.[265] The evidence to support the selection of one particular anticonvulsant over another is not strong.[264] However, Figure 36.4 details a commonly accepted algorithm for paediatric seizure management.[86,265]

Post-seizure management will be determined by the underlying cause of the seizure, and some children will need aggressive management of these conditions. Where the likelihood of recurrence is high, anticonvulsant infusions should also be commenced. Intravenous fluids containing glucose should be commenced to prevent hypoglycaemia. Well-looking children who have recovered from an afebrile seizure and children who have recovered from a febrile convulsion where the focus of the fever has been identified can be managed as outpatients. Parents will require considerable support, as seizures are frightening to watch. First aid should be discussed prior to discharge and clinicians should be sensitive to parental concern about their capacity to manage another seizure at home. There should be a low threshold for admission for first-time seizure if the parents are not sufficiently comfortable taking their child home.

PRACTICE TIPS
SEIZURES

- Focal seizure activity may go unrecognised.
- Benzodiazepines are the first-line treatment of seizure activity.
- Treatment should also include identifying and treating the underlying cause of the seizure.
- Check and correct hypoglycaemia, as this is a potential cause and a likely result of seizure activity in children.
- Where recurrent seizures are possible, an anticonvulsant infusion should be commenced.
- Seizures are frightening for parents and they should receive considerable support once the child is stabilised.

Febrile convulsion

Febrile convulsions warrant specific attention given their frequency of occurrence (2–4% of children worldwide),[266,267] and the concern that they generate in the community. A febrile convulsion is defined as a seizure occurring in a child aged from 6 months to 5 years, in the setting of current or recent history of fever and no signs of neurological disease or CNS infection and no history of neurological disease or previous febrile seizure.[268] They are classified as simple or complex, as follows.[268]

- A simple febrile convulsion lasts no more than 15 minutes, is generalised and occurs only once in 24 hours.
- Complex febrile seizures are either longer than 15 minutes or have focal features or occur more than once in 24 hours.

It has been suggested that the rapid rise in the temperature, rather than the height of the temperature, is responsible for febrile convulsions. However, there have been other theories postulated. Viral illnesses are usually associated with febrile convulsions and data from a number of studies have prompted a theory based on a viral aetiology (specifically human herpes virus 6B) for febrile convulsions.[269–271] Authors of a series of

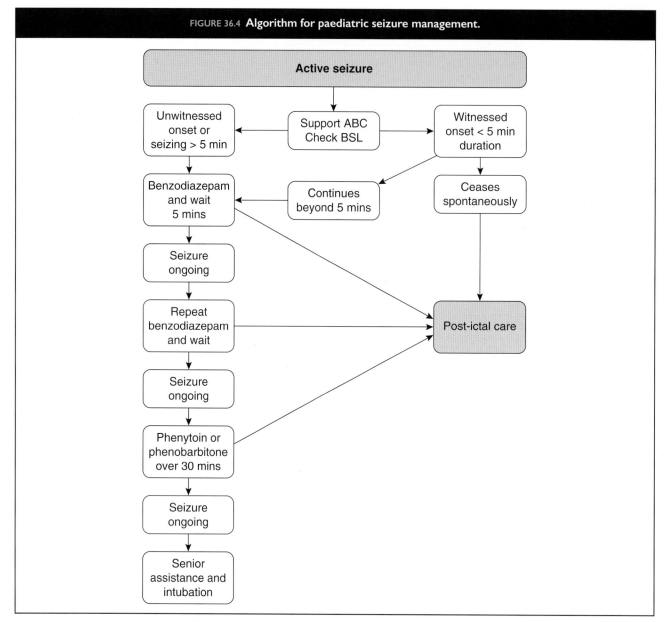

FIGURE 36.4 **Algorithm for paediatric seizure management.**

ABC: airway, breathing and circulation; BSL: blood sugar level.

population-register-based studies in Denmark suggest that genes and environmental factors may play a causal role in febrile convulsions.[272] However, the aetiology of febrile convulsions is still not well understood; it is likely to be complex and the result of multiple factors.

The rate of recurrence is 25–30%, and in 25–40% of children there will be a family history of febrile convulsion. The risk of developing epilepsy is only fractionally higher in children who have had a febrile convulsion when compared with the rest of the population (risk 1%).[267] This risk is increased to 2.4% in children who were younger than 12 months old when they had their first simple febrile convulsion or who have had multiple simple febrile convulsions, and epilepsy risk in children rises sharply to 30–50 times that in the population if the seizures are multiple and complex.[273]

Febrile convulsions are considered benign, self-limiting and unlikely to result in significant sequelae.

Presentation

Many children experiencing febrile convulsions will do so at temperatures lower than 39.0°C (and many tolerate higher fevers at a later date without seizing).[274] Febrile convulsions are usually generalised seizures and last no longer than a few minutes. In most cases they terminate spontaneously, often before the arrival of paramedics or the child is brought to the ED. However, a small number will seize for longer and a very small number will experience complex febrile seizures. Children usually recover quickly following a febrile convulsion and do not usually experience a pronounced post-ictal phase like that which generally follows seizures of alternative aetiology.

Management

Children in a convulsive state regardless of aetiology should be managed similarly. Basic life support and termination of the seizure are the first priorities of emergency service providers and ED clinicians. However, the majority of children will not present while seizing. A small number in the post-ictal phase may briefly require simple airway management. In the ED the priorities for management then become identification of the focus of the fever and parent education. The illness causing the fever is most often mild, and there is no increase in the incidence of serious bacterial infection among children who have had a febrile convulsion.[275–277] Nonetheless, a potentially serious infection should be considered.

Simple febrile convulsions are not a reason on their own for admission, so, assuming that they are otherwise well enough, these children may be discharged home. Adequate parent education prior to discharge is vital, and should include first-aid advice for seizure management and information about the likely aetiology and implications of febrile convulsions. Discussion should also include advice about fever management and febrile convulsion prevention. The parents' concern about the dangers of febrile convulsions should not be underestimated and they will require a great deal of education and support to give them confidence prior to discharge.

Studies summarised in a recent Cochrane review do not demonstrate that antipyretic therapy is effective at reducing the risk of febrile seizure in children.[278] This review failed to identify sufficient evidence to support the efficacy of paracetamol for fever clearance time and prevention of febrile convulsions.[279] The evidence summarised in the review, to support prophylactic treatment with an antiepileptic agent during a febrile illness for children who are at risk of febrile convulsion, is also not convincing,[278] particularly as the adverse side effects of these medications are substantial and outweigh any short-term benefit that may be gained from their use. Current advice to parents should state that febrile convulsions are benign, usually self-limiting, not suggestive of serious illness, do not impact on a child's cognitive outcomes and should not recommend the use of paracetamol or other agents to prevent seizure.

PRACTICE TIPS

FEBRILE CONVULSIONS

- Febrile convulsions are benign, self-limiting and very unlikely to result in significant sequelae. They are not associated with an increased risk of more-serious infection.
- Regular administration of antipyretics does not reduce the risk of febrile convulsion.

Meningitis

Meningitis is an acute inflammation of the meninges and is classified as *bacterial* or *aseptic* (viral, fungal, etc.). The bacterial aetiology is age-dependent; in neonates the predominant organisms are Group B *Streptococcus*, *E. coli* and *Listeria monocytogenes*, while in older children (and adults) the predominant organisms are *Neisseria meningitides* and *Streptococcus pneumoniae*. Since vaccination for *Haemophilus influenzae* type B (HiB) commenced over 10 years ago in Australia, the incidence of HiB meningitis is relatively rare,[280] and has been halved in New Zealand since the vaccination was introduced in 2008.[281] It is reasonable to anticipate that similar

results will be achieved for the incidence of pneumococcal meningitis following its addition to the vaccination schedule in recent years. Vaccination for *N. meninigitidis* serogroup C is also included in the schedule; however, serogroup B is responsible for approximately 85% of infections in Australia[282] and New Zealand,[283] so the effect on the incidence of *N. meningitidis* meningitis is not likely to fall significantly.

Bacterial meningitis carries significant mortality and morbidity rates; the outcomes for infants and children have steadily improved, but now remain at about 5% and 20% respectively.[284] Mortality and morbidity are highest in neonates and infants and are influenced by the organism, with rates highest for those infected with *S. pneumoniae*.[284]

Viral meningitis is most commonly caused by enteroviruses such as coxsackie and echovirus. Small numbers of cases will be caused by herpes simplex 1 and 2, which is linked with meningoencephalitis and significant mortality and morbidity if not treated early; human herpes virus 6, 7 and 8; varicella zoster; cytomegalovirus; and Epstein-Barr virus.[285]

Presentation and diagnosis

Older children may present with the classic features of meningitis, such as fever, headache, photophobia and neck stiffness, discussed in Chapter 23. However, infants and young children present with more non-specific signs and symptoms. Parents usually describe increased lethargy, irritability, poor feeding, fever and, in some cases, vomiting. On examination, these children generally look miserable and unwell but may show few classic features of meningitis. The presence of photophobia, a positive Kernig's sign (inability to flex the knee when the leg is flexed at the hip) and a positive Brudzinski sign (flexing the head forward resulting in flexing of the legs) are considered suggestive of meningitis,[286] but the sensitivity and specificity for each of these tests is not high and hence cannot be relied upon exclusively to make the diagnosis.[287] Meningeal irritation may be manifested in infants and young children by increased irritability, particularly when handled. A bulging fontanelle is often described as a feature of meningitis in infants;[286] however, the diagnosis should not be excluded if the fontanelle is found to be normal. The absence of meningeal signs and an abnormal cry reduce the likelihood of meningitis but do not exclude it.[286] Rashes may occur with some infections and meningococcal disease is linked with a petechial or purpural rash. Although there are other organisms that will also result in this rash, it should be assumed that the causative agent is *Neisseria*.

Clinicians should approach the child who has commenced antibiotic treatment in the days prior to presentation with caution. The features of serious illness, including meningitis, are likely to be subtler and easily overlooked. The diagnosis is most commonly confirmed by cerebrospinal fluid examination. The presence of cells suggests meningitis, and an increase in protein and reduction in glucose implies a bacterial organism. Gram stain will usually identify the organism, providing antibiotics have not been administered prior to specimen collection. The contraindication to lumbar puncture is raised intracranial pressure, which may be evidenced by altered conscious state, focal neurology, abnormal posturing, seizure activity or papillo-oedema. Computed tomography (CT) is not a useful guide to the risks associated with lumbar puncture and is not recommended.[288,289] Blood should also be collected for a full blood count, C-reactive protein, urea and electrolytes, glucose and culture.

Management

Resuscitation will take first priority. However, early treatment with antibiotics is also essential. The antibiotic regimen will depend on the age of the infant and local resistance patterns. *N. meningitides* is showing some decrease in susceptibility to penicillin and resistance among pneumococci is also appearing in Australia; however, this is not yet clinically significant.[282,290] Antiviral agents, such as aciclovir, should be included if viral meningo-encephalitis is suspected. Appropriate resources to guide choice of antimicrobials and the dose and schedule should be consulted to guide specific treatment. The tertiary paediatric hospitals across Australia and New Zealand offer CPGs which clearly define appropriate treatment choices.

Children with meningitis should be closely monitored, which should include neurological observations. Careful management of fluid and electrolyte balance is also an important component of meningitis management. The syndrome of inappropriate antidiuretic hormone (SIADH), which can result in hyponatraemia, is not uncommon in children with meningitis. This serves as the rationale for restricting fluids to 75% of maintenance, although evidence for this practice is not convincing and it is clear that under- or over-hydrating is linked to poor outcomes.[291]

The results from a recent Cochrane meta-analysis show that corticosteroids reduce the incidence of hearing loss, but have not been proven to improve survival.[292] These findings support the current recommendation that children with meningitis receive steroids.

PRACTICE TIPS

MENINGITIS

- Infants and young children usually present with non-specific signs of meningitis.
- The diagnosis cannot be excluded on the basis of negative Kernig's and Brudzinski signs or a normal fontanelle.
- The symptoms of meningitis may be more subtle in children who have commenced antibiotic treatment in the few days prior to presentation.
- Lumbar puncture should not be attempted where there are signs of raised intracranial pressure, such as altered conscious state, focal neurology, abnormal posturing, seizure activity or papillo-oedema.
- Following resuscitation, fluid volumes should be reduced to two-thirds of maintenance levels.
- Steroids should be given to reduce the risk of hearing impairment secondary to the infection.

Abdominal emergencies

Infectious gastroenteritis

Although death from acute gastroenteritis is relatively uncommon in developed countries, the yearly hospital admission rate for infectious gastroenteritis is second only to respiratory illness in Australia and New Zealand, at 10–12 per 1000 children.[293,294] Viruses such as rotavirus, adenovirus and norovirus cause the majority of infections. The common bacterial pathogens include *Campylobacter*, *Shigella* and *Salmonella* species; these are all communicable diseases and state health authorities should be notified of confirmed cases. Infrequently, gastroenteritis is caused by parasitic infection.[295]

It is generally accepted that childcare attendance increases the risk of contracting infectious gastroenteritis. However, in a Danish study the authors demonstrated that childcare attendance does not increase the risk of hospital admission for gastroenteritis. It is also suggested that age is a risk factor for more-significant dehydration; however, the only studies exploring the influences on severity suggest that aetiology, specifically rotavirus, rather than age is a significant risk factor.[295] Finally, breastfeeding has been shown to reduce the incidence of diarrhoeal illness but not the severity of the illness.[295]

Presentation and diagnosis

The defining feature of gastroenteritis is acute diarrhoea (defined as a decrease in the consistency of stool and/or increased frequency > 3/day) which may be accompanied by fever, general malaise and vomiting.[295] Infants and children may be intermittently irritable as a result of colicky abdominal pain. It is important to determine the extent of the child's symptoms: the number of vomits, the frequency of stools and an estimate of volume, their willingness to drink, the type of fluids offered and the volume taken (see Table 36.16). This will assist the clinician to make the diagnosis and estimate fluid loss, predict future losses and plan treatment.

Gastroenteritis presents with few specific signs. These children will usually be febrile, may look unwell and may show signs of dehydration (discussed in the section on dehydration). There will be no signs of peritonism on examination and no specific tenderness. However, they may show signs of colicky abdominal pain.

The evidence for a sign or symptom or combination that can reliably distinguish between viral and bacterial aetiology is poor. However, there is some suggestion that high fever (> 40°C), faecal blood, abdominal pain or central nervous system involvement suggest bacterial infection, whereas vomiting and respiratory symptoms are linked with viral infections.[295]

Stool cultures are not usually of clinical value.[295] In a significant proportion of samples sent for culture (estimated to be as high as 50%), the infecting organism is not isolated. For those where the causative agent is isolated, management is infrequently altered. Identifying the agent is of more interest to public health programs monitoring the spread of communicable diseases.

In the absence of a convincing history of offensive diarrhoea, an alternative diagnosis should be considered; the list of possibilities is extensive for children presenting with vomiting and scant diarrhoea.

Management

Gastroenteritis is managed symptomatically in the vast majority of cases, and the mainstay of treatment for gastroenteritis is fluid management. Intravenous fluid resuscitation is indicated for children with severe dehydration and evidence of hypovolaemia (see earlier section on dehydration). In contrast, the WHO[296] and the American Academy of Pediatrics[297] advocate oral rehydration for children who exhibit signs of mild to moderate dehydration.

The majority of children presenting to the ED do not require resuscitation and are likely to wait for medical assessment and treatment. Departments are advised to develop guidelines for commencing oral rehydration in the waiting room, as it has been shown to reduce the use of IV rehydration and admission for children with gastroenteritis.[298] This trial of oral fluids will also serve to inform clinicians about the need for more-aggressive fluid management and admission.

Where oral rehydration is not feasible, children with moderate and moderate to severe dehydration without signs of hypovolaemia can be managed with enteral fluids (e.g. via an NG tube).

Oral rehydration solution is the fluid of choice during the rehydration phase; the recommended fluid regimens are described in an earlier section and an example is provided in Table 36.17. Past guidelines have advised restriction of formula and diet for varying periods of time in the acute phase of the illness. Current evidence supports the following recommendations: maintenance of breastfeeding throughout treatment[299] and reintroduction of formula feeds and diet following the rehydration phase to decrease stool frequency and the duration of diarrhoea and improve weight gain.[237,295] The only foods to be avoided are those high in sugar. There is some evidence, although of low quality, that a lactose-free diet for infants not predominantly breast-fed may reduce the duration of the diarrhoea and reduce the risk of treatment failure.[300]

There is evidence to support the use of an oral antiemetic such as ondansetron for children who are unable to tolerate fluids due to vomiting, and this is supported by the conclusions of a recent Cochrane review.[301] However, it has been shown to increase the volume of stools and therefore it is not recommended for routine use, but rather to make successful oral rehydration possible.

Antibiotics are only used under the following circumstances: confirmed *Shigella* infection, confirmed *Salmonella* infection in infants less than 3 months of age, patients with immunodeficiency or who are systemically unwell and for those who are unwell with signs of severe invasive diarrhoea.[302] No other pharmacological agents have proven to be of benefit in the treatment of gastroenteritis.

Children with mild gastroenteritis and those with moderate dehydration who have tolerated rapid rehydration, evidenced by weight gain, may be discharged home from the ED. Parents must receive advice about the amount and type of fluid that should be offered prior to discharge and the indicators for re-presentation. Gastroenteritis is highly contagious, and infection control practices should be discussed with parents and the need for rigorous standards of hygiene reinforced. In many circumstances, review with the GP or in the ED the following day should be recommended.

Prevention is an important component of gastroenteritis management. The recently introduced rotavirus vaccine is predicted to have a significant impact on the burden of disease, and early data suggest that this is the case. Data from Queensland demonstrate a significant fall in the numbers of rotavirus notifications in 2007 (43%) and in 2008 (65%) since a publically funded vaccination program was introduced,[303] and admission rates for infants and children with rotavirus have also dropped since the introduction of this vaccine.[304]

PRACTICE TIPS
GASTROENTERITIS

- Breastfed babies may be less likely to contract gastroenteritis, but for those who do contract it the illness is no less severe.
- Gastroenteritis is characterised by diarrhoea, so an alternative diagnosis should be sought for vomiting in the absence of diarrhoea.
- Stool cultures are not routinely recommended as the infecting agent is not isolated in as many as 50% of stool cultures and the aetiology of the infection does not usually affect treatment.
- Infants and children not showing evidence of hypovolaemia can generally be rehydrated enterally; an oral rehydration solution is the fluid of choice.
- Breastfeeding should be maintained throughout the illness.
- Solids should not be withheld other than during the rehydration phase of treatment. However, foods high in sugar should be avoided.
- Ondansetron may be of some use in infants and children with significant vomiting to support enteral rehydration.
- Antibiotics are only of use in patients with confirmed *Shigella* infection, confirmed *Salmonella* infection who are less than 3 months of age or who are systemically unwell, or patients who are unwell with signs of severe invasive infection.

Constipation

Constipation is a very common problem in paediatrics and one managed regularly in the ED. It is defined as difficulty or a delay in the passage of stools causing distress and which is present for 2 or more weeks.[305] Neonates at 1 week of age have an average of 4 stools per day, which then reduces gradually to an average of 1.7 stools per day at 2 years of age and 1.2 stools at 4 years of age. There is considerable variation between individuals, particularly in breastfed infants who may pass a stool following each feed or not for many days.[305] By contrast, formula-fed infants generally have more consistent stool patterns, usually passing fewer in number than the breastfed infant but without the irregularities.

Parents are frequently concerned that constipation is a symptom of a serious physical problem. However, the most common cause of constipation in infants and children is functional and occurs in the absence of a pathological condition. Infants and children will most commonly develop withholding behaviours following painful bowel movements or other trauma which is associated with bowel habits. Fluid is reabsorbed and the stool becomes larger and harder as it is retained in the colon, increasing the child's reluctance to defecate.[305]

Presentation and diagnosis

Parents will describe large, hard stools, infrequent stools or straining and distress with attempts to pass a stool. They may also observe the child becoming restless, clenching their buttocks and wriggling in an attempt to avoid passing the stool. These children tighten their anal sphincter in response to the sensation of a full rectum rather than relaxing it, making it impossible to pass a stool. Some children may also experience faecal soiling.

A history of stool-withholding behaviour reduces the likelihood of organic disease.[305] An alternative aetiology should be sought if the presentation includes fever, weight loss or failure to gain weight, delayed passage of meconium, nausea, vomiting, abdominal distension, significant anorexia or bloody stools in the absence of a fissure.

The examination is ostensibly normal, although a faecal mass may be palpable in the abdomen and anal fissures may be visible. A diagnosis of functional constipation can in most cases be made based on the findings from the history and examination, and investigation is rarely required. Although US recommendations support occult blood testing for all children presenting with constipation[305] this is not routine practice in Australia. Abdominal X-ray may be used to exclude alternative diagnoses or demonstrate faecal loading, although data does not provide convincing evidence of its sensitivity and specificity,[306] but is not recommended to confirm a diagnosis of constipation. There is growing interest in the role that ultrasound may play in confirming and monitoring constipation but it is yet to be widely used or recommended for this purpose.

Management

Attempts have frequently been made to manage a child's constipation. However, they are often insufficient to restore regular bowel habits. Most commonly, treatments have not been used regularly or for long enough. A regimen aimed to re-establish a more suitable bowel pattern should be initiated. To achieve this, a stool-softener such as paraffin oil should be commenced at 10 mL at night and titrated to effect. A second dose in the morning may be added to achieve the desired effect. If this does not result in a normal bowel pattern within several weeks, an osmotic laxative such as sorbitol or lactulose at 3 mL/kg may be added; this should also be titrated to effect.

For children where more aggressive treatment is required, a product such as macrogol can be used to stimulate a bowel motion. There is no data to suggest that increasing fluid will resolve constipation and only limited evidence to suggest that increasing fibre will have this effect.[307] Ideally treatment should not involve the use of suppositories and enemas, which may reinforce withholding behaviours. However, they may be required where there is faecal impaction and evacuation of the rectum is needed.[305]

Education forms a significant component of the management of constipation and this should commence in the ED. Parents should be advised to expect that the child would remain on this regimen for months to years before the bowel is sufficiently well trained to maintain a regular pattern without pharmacological aid. Children will require the positive support of their parents throughout treatment. To minimise the child's embarrassment and sense of failure parents should handle faecal soiling and the other consequences of constipation sensitively.[305]

Appropriate treatment may be commenced in the ED. However, infants and children with constipation will require referral to a general paediatrician for continued management, which will involve titration of the pharmacological agents used to support regular bowel motions, identification and management of factors potentially exacerbating the constipation and behaviour modification in those children exhibiting withholding behaviours.[305]

PRACTICE TIPS
CONSTIPATION

- The most common cause of constipation in infants and children is withholding behaviours and not pathological.
- Abdominal X-rays should not be requested to confirm the diagnosis.
- The focus of treatment should be two-fold: a stool-softener to establish regular soft stools, and education to assist the child to overcome their reluctance to pass a stool.

TABLE 36.18 Common causes of abdominal pain in infants and children[558]

COMMON	UNCOMMON	RARE
Non-specific	Volvulus secondary to malrotation	Sickle cell anaemic crisis
Appendicitis	Meckel diverticulitis	Henoch-Schönlein purpura
Mesenteric adenitis	Renal colic	Pancreatitis
Constipation	Pyelonephritis	Cholecystitis
Intussusception	Acute glomerulonephritis	Acute hepatitis
Urinary tract infection	Glandular fever	Diabetes mellitus
Torsion of the testis	Drug ingestion	Haemolytic–uraemic syndrome
Gastroenteritis	Peptic ulceration	Inflammatory bowel disease
Strangulated inguinal hernia		
Pneumonia		

Abdominal pain

Abdominal pain is an extremely common non-specific symptom in children which is associated with an extensive list of conditions, some of which are presented in this chapter or in Chapter 24. Table 36.18 provides a list of likely causes of acute abdominal pain. Aetiology is influenced by age and gender, and in the vast majority of cases the problem is not surgical. However, in a significant number of cases (15%), no diagnosis is made prior to discharge from the ED. A diagnosis of non-specific abdominal pain was the fourth most frequently made diagnosis for children presenting to the ED with abdominal pain. The diagnoses made more frequently were URTI (19%), pharyngitis (17%) and viral infection (16%).[308] In a study focusing on children admitted with abdominal pain for surgical review, it was the most frequent (70%) discharge diagnosis made.[309]

Presentation and diagnosis

Abdominal pain may be the primary reason for presentation or a symptom associated with the chief complaint, and is uncommonly linked to surgical emergencies. Regardless, history-taking should be detailed to address the extensive array of possible diagnoses and the important conditions to exclude. Clues to diagnosis can be gained from the age of the child, the infant or child's past history, the pattern and characteristics of the pain and other associated symptoms. In older girls, menstrual and sexual history should also be included and it may be ideal to have parents leave during this part of the assessment. Examination should be similarly comprehensive, and include other systems to identify or exclude the signs of important differential diagnoses for abdominal pain; in boys this should include the testicles. Older children will exhibit more specific signs associated with surgical conditions consistent with those of an adult than younger children and infants.

The diagnosis of non-specific abdominal pain is one of exclusion, and it can be a diagnostic challenge to differentiate non-specific abdominal pain from more-significant pathology such as appendicitis. Diagnostic testing, including abdominal X-rays, should only be used to confirm or exclude specific diagnoses and should not be conducted for screening purposes.

Management

Management of abdominal pain will initially be directed towards resuscitation and stabilisation where necessary and pain management. A small number of infants and children will require fluid resuscitation. As noted in Chapter 19, the rationale

---

PRACTICE TIPS

ABDOMINAL PAIN

- The cause of most abdominal pain in children is not surgical. It is most commonly associated with respiratory and viral infections.
- Abdominal X-rays should not be routinely ordered for screening purposes.
- Resuscitation, stabilisation and pain management are the focus of emergency management of abdominal pain. Definitive management will depend on the aetiology of the pain.

---

for withholding analgesia to enable diagnosis is fallacious and children should receive appropriate and timely analgesia consistent with their level of pain. The diagnosis determines the definitive management of abdominal pain, which will be surgery in only a very small number of cases. Children with non-specific abdominal pain may be admitted for observation, but most can be discharged and parents provided with criteria to guide the need for review.

Intussusception

Intussusception is the invagination of a proximal segment of bowel into the distal bowel lumen.[310] This results in compression of the perfusing vessels of this section of bowel, initially causing venous congestion and bowel wall oedema. If the intussusception continues, ischaemia and finally necrosis will result.

Intussusception is the most common cause of bowel obstruction in children aged between 3 months and 6 years, with a peak incidence at 5–9 months.[311,312] However, it may occur at any age. The aetiology of intussusception is not well understood and in 90% of cases it is thought to be idiopathic. However, there is a reported association with viral illness, and the risk of intussusception increases with some conditions such as Henoch-Schönlein purpura, nephritic syndrome, Meckel diverticulum, intestinal polyps and following abdominal trauma.[313] Furthermore, a rise in the incidence of intussusception was linked with the introduction of the original rotavirus vaccine. This vaccine was withdrawn and a similar association between intussusception and the replacement vaccine has not been established.[313,314]

Presentation and diagnosis

The classic presentation for intussusception includes recent viral illness, intermittent abdominal pain demonstrated by pulling their legs up to their abdomen, redcurrant-jelly stool and a palpable abdominal mass. However, this constellation is not typical, with only 7.5–40% of presentations featuring these signs and symptoms and the redcurrant stool, when present, is a late sign.[265,315,316] Many children are pain-free, some children will present with non-specific symptoms and there is considerable overlap between the presentation associated with intussusception and other abdominal conditions in infants and children.

Vomiting is the most common feature in infants, but many will also present with unexplained distress and increasing lethargy. There may be some diarrhoea and as the illness progresses this may contain bloodstained mucous (redcurrant jelly), suggesting mucosal sloughing secondary to ischaemia. The most useful physical sign is a palpable sausage-shaped mass. The remainder of the abdominal examination may be normal. As these infants become more unwell secondary to intestinal ischaemia and necrosis, they may begin to exhibit signs of hypovolaemia.

Abdominal X-rays are frequently the imaging of first choice in the ED. However, they may be normal (up to 25%), and results are only moderately sensitive (62%) to intussusceptions.[317,318] The most sensitive (~98%) and specific (88–98%) diagnostic tool currently available for the diagnosis of intussusception is ultrasound,[317,319,320] and this replaces the more traditional air or barium enema, which is now reserved for management.

Management

Management will depend on the condition of the infant. Fluid therapy and in some instances aggressive resuscitation is the first priority of emergency management. Surgical review should be requested early. Intussusception can usually be non-operatively reduced using an enema (air or barium). However, a small number of infants will require surgical reduction of the intussusception.

PRACTICE TIPS

INTUSSUSCEPTION

- Most infants and children presenting with intussusception don't present with the classic constellation of signs and symptoms, which includes 'redcurrant-jelly stools' and drawing up of the legs towards their abdomen.
- Ultrasound is the imaging modality recommended for detecting intussusception.
- Most intussusceptions can be managed non-surgically with an air or barium enema.

Pyloric stenosis

Pyloric stenosis occurs almost exclusively in infants and is one of the most common causes of surgical emergency in this age group. The pyloric sphincter is hypertrophic and hyperplastic, causing narrowing of the pylorus and gastric outlet obstruction. The cause is unknown, but pyloric stenosis affects approximately 0.1–0.3% of infants and is more common in Caucasian infants, males (4 : 1) and infants of parents who had pyloric stenosis.[321,322]

Presentation and diagnosis

Classically, the infant presenting with pyloric stenosis is 3–6 weeks of age, but may present at between 2 and 8 weeks, is male, has a history of projectile vomiting soon after feeding and appears hungry and undernourished. Examination may reveal visible peristaltic waves and a palpable olive-shaped mass.[323,324] However, the pylorus can be difficult to palpate, particularly if the stomach is full. The infant is also likely to show signs of dehydration, the severity of which will depend on the extent of the vomiting and the delay to presentation.[322]

Identification of the enlarged pylorus is a highly specific finding. However, ultrasound is highly sensitive (~98%) and specific (100%), and is therefore used to confirm the diagnosis.[325] Blood should be collected to measure urea and electrolytes and a capillary blood gas sample sent for analysis to assess the impact of persistent vomiting and to guide treatment. The classic, but often late, finding is hypokalaemic, hypochloraemic alkalosis.[322]

PRACTICE TIPS

PYLORIC STENOSIS

- The classic presentation is of a male infant aged between 2 and 8 weeks with a history of projectile vomiting soon after feeding who looks hungry and poorly nourished.
- These infants are likely to be dehydrated and may have electrolyte and acid–base imbalances.
- Fluid resuscitation and correction of metabolic derangements are the focus of emergency management.

Management

Fluid resuscitation and correction of the metabolic derangements resulting from vomiting is the focus of the ED. Surgical consultation will guide decisions regarding the need for diagnostic tests and operative management, and this should be sought early.

Herniae

Herniae occur in all age groups, but are particularly common in infants. Inguinal herniae occur in approximately 1–4.5% of infants[326] and umbilical herniae in up to 18% of infants under 6 months of age. Inguinal herniae are more common in premature neonates, boys and twins,[322,326] and umbilical hernias are also more prevalent in premature neonates and more common in infants of Afro-Caribbean background.[309] Both hernia types can be explained by the embryological development of intra- and extra-abdominal structures, which is beyond the scope of this text but explains their prevalence in infants.

Presentation and diagnosis

Infants and neonates with an inguinal hernia will have a swelling in the inguinal region, and in some infants the swelling may extend into the scrotum or the labia majora. The swelling may only be evident when the infant is crying or straining, or may be constantly present. Where the hernia is sustained, infants will become increasingly distressed.

Umbilical herniae present with a large swelling protruding though the umbilical ring and are symptom-free.

Management

Applying gentle pressure to the mass may reduce inguinal herniae that have not reduced spontaneously. In a small number, an inguinal hernia does not spontaneously reduce and cannot be reduced by a clinician. This is a surgical emergency, as prolonged hernia increases the risk of ischaemia and necrosis. Surgical consultation at the time of the presentation should also occur for a reducible hernia if it has been appearing with increasing frequency, the infant has experienced distress with the hernia or the infant is young (< 3 months). Most infants and young children with an inguinal hernia do not require urgent treatment and can be referred to a surgeon as outpatients, but all will require surgical repair.[326]

Conversely, umbilical herniae are rarely irreducible and rarely require surgical repair unless they have not closed spontaneously by 3–5 years or the infant or child has persistent symptoms.

PRACTICE TIPS

HERNIAE

- Irreducible inguinal herniae are a surgical emergency.
- Umbilical herniae are benign and are unlikely to require correction.

Rashes and soft-tissue infections

Most rashes are not evidence of serious illness and many do not require ED management. However, the presence of a rash frequently alarms parents and prompts them to seek medical assessment for their child. A diagnosis, some simple management strategies or a referral to a specialist will usually address their concerns. Rashes are extremely common presentations to the ED and are too numerous to attempt to describe them all in this chapter. The intent of this section is to discuss some principles when assessing paediatric rashes. They can be grouped into categories based on appearance, which will help narrow the likely cause.

A careful history detailing the development of the rash (location, appearance, spread, etc), associated symptoms (e.g. itch, pain), the treatments used in an attempt to control the rash and prodromal and concurrent systemic symptoms (e.g fever, malaise) will provide vital information to assist in identifying the rash.

Rashes can be grouped by appearance as *vesicular, pustular, papular, eczematous, purpuric/vascular* and *erythematous*.[327] Furthermore, rashes can be *localised* or *widespread*. A number of terms used to describe rashes are listed in Table 36.19, and common diagnoses for each morphological category are provided in Table 36.20.

Vesicles are small, monomorphic blisters on the skin filled with clear fluid, and when ruptured they leave a small round erosion. Larger blisters are called bullae. They are most commonly caused by infection or contact dermatitis. Varicella zoster (chicken pox), herpes simplex, coxsackie (hand, foot and mouth) and herpes zoster viruses are the common viral causes of vesicular rashes. However, the frequency of varicella is declining since the introduction of routine vaccination. Bullous rashes are generally bacterial. Pustular rashes look similar to vesicular rashes. However, the raised blister-like lesions are pus-filled and the aetiology is bacterial. Pyoderma will be discussed in the next section.

The likely aetiology of papular rashes is wide and includes scabies, urticaria, molluscum, warts, acne, serum sickness and papular acrodermatitis. Papules can be red (e.g. acne) or skin-coloured (e.g. molluscum) and may be itchy (e.g. scabies); raised red rings are likely to occur with urticaria, and bruising and/or purpura may suggest an associated vasculitis (e.g. Henoch-Schönlein purpura and urticarial vasculitis). Papular acrodermatitis is classically seen in children between 1 and 3 years of age, and is a reaction to a range of infectious illnesses

\multicolumn{2}{c}{TABLE 36.19 Terms used to describe rashes}
TERM	DESCRIPTION
Lesion	Describes an area of skin disease—generally small
Eruption or rash	More-widespread skin involvement, comprised of multiple lesions
Macule	Flat area of skin with colour change
Papule	Solid raised area of skin with distinct borders less than 1 cm in diameter
Plaque	Solid, raised, flat-topped lesion with distinct borders and an epidermal change larger than 1 cm in diameter
Nodule	Raised, solid lesion with indistinct borders and a deeper portion. May be intradermal or subcutaneous. A larger nodule is called a tumour
Wheal	An area of tense oedema in the upper dermis resulting in a raised, flat-topped lesion
Vesicle	A raised, clear-fluid-filled lesion that is less than 1 cm in diameter
Bulla	A raised, clear-fluid-filled lesion that is greater than 1 cm in diameter
Cyst	A raised lesion that contains a palpable sac containing solid material
Pustule	A raised fluid-exudate-filled lesion that appears yellow
Erosion	Moist, circumscribed, slightly depressed area, e.g. base of a blister
Crusting	Dried exudate of plasma combined with blister roof which sits on the surface of the skin after acute dermatitis
Scaling	Whitish plates on the skin surface
Desquamation	Peeling of sheets of scale after acute skin injury
Excoriation	Oval or linear depression in the skin with complete removal of the epidermis exposing red dermis
Fissures	Linear, wedge-shaped cracks in the epidermis extending down to the dermis
Discrete	Distinct and discretely separated from each other
Confluent	Lesions running together
Grouped	Lesions found closely adjacent to each other
Linear	Lesions found in a straight line
Annular	Lesions found in a circular arrangement

TABLE 36.20 Differential diagnosis of rashes of varying morphology[327]			
RASH MORPHOLOGY		**DIFFERENTIAL DIAGNOSIS**	
Vesicles	Varicella zoster Coxsackie virus	Herpes simplex Contact dermatitis	Herpes zoster Impetigo
Pustular	Impetigo Scalded skin syndrome	Acne Furuncles and boils	Varicella
Papular	Moluscum contagiosum Urticaria Papular acrodermatitis	Insect bites Acne	Scabies Warts
Erythematous	Urticaria Viral exanthema Cellulitis	Tinea Intertrigo	Streptococcal perianal disease
Eczematous (red and scaly)	Eczema Dermatitis—contact	Psoriasis Dermatitis—seborrheic	Tinea
Petechial	Meningococcal disease Mechanical	Idiopathic thrombocytopenia	Viral infection

or vaccination. Scabies infestation results in a secondary reaction to the scabies antigen, manifested by a papular rash. Molluscum lesions result from a viral infection and are characterised by pearly papules localised to areas such as the face and anogential region, although they may appear anywhere.

Red scaly rashes include atopic dermatitis (eczema), seborrhoeic dermatitis (infants), contact dermatitis, psoriasis, tinea corporis and pityriasis rosea and versicolor. Redness indicates inflammation of the skin and the scale indicates epidermal involvement. These rashes can present very similarly, and although common can be misdiagnosed or poorly managed. Eczematous rashes are characterised by itch, erythema and disruption to the epidermis, and will be discussed in more detail in a following section.

Erythematous rashes are red, blanching rashes with lesions varying from small macules to large confluent areas of erythema. The most common erythematous rash is the one that accompanies a febrile illness, which is most often caused by a virus. Several of these presentations have specific features, such as measles and roseola infantum, while the majority are non-specific. Kawasaki's disease is a vasculitis, which presents with a non-specific erythematous rash in the setting of fever of over 5 days' duration, conjunctival injection, mucosal involvement and erythema of the palms of the hands and soles of the feet. It is the leading cause of acquired coronary artery disease in children, and where the diagnosis is suspected this should prompt referral to a specialist centre for further investigation (e.g. echocardiogram) and management.

Purpuric and petechial rashes should raise concern as they are linked with serious life-threatening illness. Infection with *N. meningitides*, *S. pneumoniae* and *H. influenzae* may present with fever and a non-blanching rash. Conversely, a number of relatively benign viruses are also responsible for this type of rash. These children will be relatively well, unlike those with bacterial infections. Petechiae above the nipple-line may be the result of forceful coughing or vomiting, which may be associated with a febrile illness making the presentation more difficult to differentiate from a child with a

serious bacterial infection. Henoch-Schönlein purpura (HSP) may also present with a petechial rash. The classic triad of symptoms associated with HSP are rash, abdominal pain and swollen joints. It should be assumed that serious bacterial infection is the cause of a petechial rash until proven otherwise. Other significant conditions that should be considered in the setting of a non-blanching petechial rash include coagulation disorders, thrombocytopenia secondary to leukaemia and idiopathic thrombocytopenia.

Pyoderma and cellulitis

Pyoderma is a broad term used to describe a range of bacterial skin conditions such as impetigo, folliculitis, furuncle and carbuncle, and they are one of the most common childhood skin diseases. The incidence is even higher in Indigenous children and children living in disadvantaged circumstances. It is highly contagious and spreads quickly through households and childcare centres. The most common causative organisms are Group A *Streptococcus* (GAS) *pyogenes* and *Staphylococcus aureus*; community methicillin-resistant *S. aureus* (MRSA) is appearing in increasing numbers, particularly in the Indigenous community.[328] Pyoderma frequently occurs secondarily to an existing skin disease such as eczema, scabies and molluscum. Post-streptococcal glomerulonephritis is rare in the non-Indigenous population but a significant risk for Indigenous Australians and New Zealanders.

Cellulitis occurs in the subcutaneous fat layer and mainly involves the dermis, unlike impetigo which is confined to the epidermal layers of the skin. Cellulitis may also spread to deeper layers such as the muscle and other associated structures with serious implications, such as periorbital cellulitis with spread to the structures of the eye. Cellulitis may result from a breach in the skin, which allows bacteria to colonise the wound; or alternatively it may occur with no apparent tissue injury. Cellulitis is caused by the same profile of organisms as pyoderma.

Presentation and diagnosis

Pyoderma generally presents with thick-crusted lesions, bullous lesions or the superficial ulcerations left by ruptured bullae.

There is usually surrounding erythema and the lesions may be tender or itchy. Pyoderma may be associated with fever and malaise, although this is likely to be mild.[329] Where the child appears more unwell, a more significant infection such as cellulitis should be considered.

Cellulitis manifests with an area of significant erythema, oedema, warmth and marked tenderness. The margins of the infection may be identified by the extent of the erythema, but are not palpable. Associated red streaking visible in the skin proximal to the area of cellulitis is characteristic of ascending lymphangitis. Regional lymphadenopathy and fever usually accompany cellulitis. On occasions, the macular erythema of cellulitis co-exists with areas of ulceration and frank abscess formation.

Cellulitis is frequently diagnosed in the setting of insect bite and a local allergic reaction is mistaken for cellulitis. The two can often be distinguished by their presenting features, although there is considerable overlap. An allergic reaction similarly presents with erythema, oedema and in most circumstances itch rather than pain. In those circumstances where the child complains of pain it is probably secondary to swelling, and the degree of tenderness is disproportionately low given the extent of the reaction. Cellulitis is usually tender and the child may exhibit signs of systemic illness.

Isolation of the causative organism is not always necessary in uncomplicated pyoderma and rarely possible in cellulitis.[328] Furthermore, skin swabs do not reliably differentiate between infection and colonisation.[329] However, it is generally accepted that where there are crusted or moist skin lesions, a swab for microbiology and culture should be taken. This is particularly important for impetiginous rashes secondary to chronic skin disorders where atypical and resistant bacteria may colonise and infect the skin.

Management
Pyoderma and cellulitis are treated empirically and in most cases as an outpatient with antibiotics. Topical antiseptics have not shown to be of benefit to treat pyoderma. However, data summarised in a recent Cochrane review and a separate systematic review support the use of topical antibiotics such as mupirocin.[329,330] However, the growing resistance to mupirocin should be considered when selecting an appropriate treatment. Extensive pyoderma and cellulitis should be treated with oral antibiotics to target *S. aureus* and *S. pyogenes*.[328,329] Penicillin is an effective treatment for GAS, but may be inadequate for *S. aureus*, so the antibiotic of choice is flucloxacillin or cephalexin. The frequency of dosing and the duration of therapy are not well supported by data and there may be some differences between CPG and pharmacopoeia recommendations. Hence treatment choice should be based on local recommendations that are likely to have considered local organisms and resistance patterns.

Admission and IV antibiotics should be used for periorbital cellulitis, cellulitis with associated systemic symptoms or where oral treatment has failed. The parenteral antibiotics of choice are either flucloxacillin or a first-generation cephalosporin. Where there is a collection of pus, this must be drained to ensure treatment success, regardless of whether inpatient or outpatient management is proposed.

Rest, elevation and ice should be used where the cellulitis involves a limb, in an attempt to reduce the swelling and promote comfort. Children with extensive pyoderma or cellulitis may require regular analgesia to manage the discomfort and pain associated with infection.

Prevention of pyoderma in the developing world and among Indigenous communities has been given some attention, and improved sanitation and hygiene has been identified as an important prevention strategy.[328] Parent education should include the risk of spread and infection-control practices to prevent the spread of infection to other members of the family. Children attending childcare with pyoderma should be excluded until the lesions no longer show signs of infection.

PRACTICE TIPS

PYODERMA AND CELLULITIS

- Superficial bacterial skin rashes such as impetigo are highly infectious.
- Impetigo is characterised by crusts that must be regularly washed off for antibiotic treatment to be effective.
- Cellulitis involves the dermis and may spread to surrounding structures. making it potentially more serious.
- Local allergic reactions are frequently misdiagnosed as cellulitis. Although similar, allergy is usually associated with itch and cellulitis with pain.
- Drainage is required if there is an associated collection of pus.

Atopic eczema (dermatitis)

Atopic eczema is a chronic inflammatory disease of the skin with complex pathogenesis, which includes genetic factors, immune dysregulation and skin-barrier defects.[331] In Australia and New Zealand, the incidence is higher than anywhere else in the world and 30% of children will experience eczema. It generally improves with age and many children grow out of it. However, there is no cure for eczema and most infants and young children experience recurrent episodes of varying severity. Eczema can be difficult to control and in some cases may be a debilitating illness.

Presentation and diagnosis
Eczema is characterised by dry, inflamed and itchy skin and generally develops before the age of 2 years. Classically the rash distribution is age-dependent and first appears on the cheeks of infants, then spreads to include the chin, folds of the neck, torso and limbs. In older children, eczema typically appears around the ankles and wrists and in flexures. Eczema variant, called discoid eczema, presents with round well-demarcated eczematous lesions on the limbs or trunk; there is generally a history of dry skin and either a personal or a family history of atopy. More-severe eczema will be associated with excoriation and lichenification (skin thickening), particularly where it has been poorly controlled. Eczema may be secondarily infected and show impetiginous signs suggestive of bacterial infection or vesicles, suggestive of herpes simplex infection.

Eczema is very itchy, and the itch can be one of the most difficult symptoms to manage. The itch frequently interferes with normal sleep patterns, with significant implications; for example, older children lose significant amounts of time at school. Infants with eczema become increasingly irritable and may begin to show signs of failure to thrive.

Assessment of severity is best achieved using the validated Scoring Atopic Dermatitis (SCORAD) tool developed by the European Task Force on Atopic Dermatitis.[332] The tool generates a composite score based on the extent of the following: inflammation, dryness, excoriation, crusting, lichenification, itch and the impact on sleep. A link to an education tool and a SCORAD calculator is given in the useful websites at the end of the chapter.

Eczema is a clinical diagnosis, and there are no diagnostic tests available to confirm the diagnosis. However, in certain circumstances children should be referred for allergy testing to determine the impact of allergy on their eczema.

Management

Eczema treatment is comprised of daily skin care and management of exacerbations. Daily skin care should include avoidance of aggravating factors such as soaps, perfumes, wool clothing, chlorines and other chemicals. Clothes should be rinsed a second time to remove detergents, moisturisers should be applied before swimming and the skin rinsed immediately afterwards, and products used on the skin, such as sunscreens, should be hypoallergenic. Moisturisers should be applied at least once a day following a bath in which a cleansing agent with minimal defatting activity and neutral pH is used instead of soap; and if the skin is particularly dry, moisturisers should be applied twice a day. Committed used of moisturisers will reduce the need for steroid treatment.[332,333] Furthermore, regular bleach baths have been recommended to reduce the incidence of infection. However, the data to support this to date is equivocal.[334,335]

Treatment of exacerbations will include steroids of variable potency depending on the severity of the symptoms and the area of the body affected. As a principle, the steroid with the lowest potency possible should be selected. However, this should be balanced against the likelihood that it will adequately treat the eczema. A mild-potency steroid may be commenced on affected areas of the face, axilla and groin and a mid-potency steroid on other affected areas of the body. High-potency steroids may occasionally be necessary to treat resistant eczema, but they should not be commenced without assessing the possibility of infection and ensuring that early specialist follow-up to ensure monitoring of response is available. Ointment preparations should be prescribed rather than creams, as they provide better delivery of the medication, increasing their potency, evaporate less and contain fewer additives. Concerns about the side effects of steroids are a common reason for prescription of suboptimal treatment and parental non-compliance with treatment regimens. However, evidence suggests that treatment twice daily for 4 weeks with a mild- to moderate-potency steroid is safe.[333,336–339] Treatment must weigh the likely side effects of steroid treatment against the likely outcome if treatment is withheld or is insufficient to address the problem.

As an alternative to steroids, topical calcineurin inhibitors, such as tacrolimus ointment (e.g. Protopic) 0.03% and pimecrolimus cream (e.g. Elidel) 1%, have been recommended.[340] The anti-inflammatory mechanism is different to steroids and the side-effect profile does not include skin atropy, making them ideally suited for the face. There has been some concern about the link between long-term use and neoplasms. However, more recent data do not confirm the association.[341,342] These agents are considered second-line treatments and the decision to use them is probably best made by eczema specialists.

During an exacerbation, moisturiser use should be increased and in some centres wet dressings are recommended to increase moisture in the skin and provide cooling;[343,344] other specialists consider them likely to increase skin maceration and the risk of infection.[345] They may be a useful strategy to manage moderate to severe eczema but their effect should be monitored carefully. Cool compresses may be used as an alternative to help reduce the itch.

Data suggest that there is a relationship (causation is unproven) between atopic dermatitis and immunoglobulin-E-mediated (IgE-mediated) food allergy, and that the strength of the association increases with the severity of the skin disease. Infants with moderate to severe eczema and infants and children with poorly controlled eczema, despite adequate treatment regimens, should be referred for allergy testing. Diet restrictions or other changes in lifestyle should not be implemented without allergy testing.

Many families will have sought care from a number of different clinicians and will have had varying advice about the management of their child's eczema. Despite multiple consultations, the child's eczema frequently remains a problem. The concern that this causes and the commitment required by families to manage their child's eczema should not be underestimated. These families require support and understanding.

Education is the mainstay of treatment; treatment failures can be attributed, among other things, to poor compliance, which is usually the result of inadequate education. Infants and children presenting to the ED should either be admitted for education regarding the management of the child's condition, or be provided with preliminary education in the ED with

---

PRACTICE TIPS
ATOPIC DERMATITIS

- The incidence of eczema in Australia (approx 30% of children) is higher than anywhere else in the world.
- It is characterised by dry, inflamed and itchy skin, which can be difficult to manage.
- Families presenting to the ED are often frustrated because their child's eczema is poorly controlled, despite having received advice and management from a number of professionals prior to presenting to the ED.
- Sudden increases in severity and/or crusting are likely signs of secondary infection and should be treated with antibiotics.
- Eczema management is comprised of daily skin care and management of exacerbations.
- As commitment to management plans is essential to control eczema, families should be provided with appropriate education prior to discharge from the ED.

rapid referral for review and eczema education. A number of resources are available to support emergency clinicians needing to provide education about the application of topical treatments and the use of wet dressings. Families should be provided with a written management plan to ensure adherence to the prescribed treatment regimen. The importance of maintaining daily skin care in the prevention of significant exacerbations should be stressed to parents.[346]

Urticaria

Urticaria is typically an itchy rash characterised by wheals, which may be clinically classified as ordinary urticaria (acute, chronic and episodic), physical urticaria (reproducibly induced by the same physical stimulus), angio-oedema without wheals, contact urticaria (induced by biological or chemical skin contact) and urticarial vasculitis (defined on skin biopsy).[347] This discussion will focus only on uncomplicated acute urticaria, which is defined as urticarial activity for up to 6 weeks and is not accompanied by vasculitis or angio-oedema and is not precipitated by local contact. Uncomplicated urticaria is more common in children than adults.[348] The incidence of acute urticaria is higher in children with atopic illness such as asthma, hayfever or eczema.[349–351]

Urticaria is commonly thought to be an IgE-mediated allergic reaction. However, there are likely to be a number of pathways and multiple causes for urticaria.[348] In older children with urticaria (age 6 months to 16 years), food intolerance has been found to be the precipitant in 15% of cases of acute urticaria.[352] Medications are responsible for urticaria in a few cases, but the majority of episodes of urticaria in infants and children are precipitated by viral illness.[350]

Activation of mast cells located in the skin results in rapid release of histamine, leukotriene, C4 and prostaglandin D_2, which causes vasodilation and leakage of plasma into the dermal tissues and hence the characteristic signs of urticaria. The delayed (4–8 hours) secretion of inflammatory cytokines is responsible for inflammatory infiltrate and longer-lasting lesions.[348]

Presentation and diagnosis

Acute urticaria has a fairly distinct and easily identified presentation. Parents will report the sudden appearance of a red blotchy rash, which may settle within 1–24 hours, only for new lesions to appear elsewhere. It may be described as itchy, but is not usually associated with other symptoms.[350]

The classic urticarial rash includes papules and larger wheals, which are usually surrounded by a reflex erythema. Urticaria may be associated with angio-oedema, which involves significant swelling of the lower dermis and subcutaneous tissues and may involve the mucous membranes.[347,350] Infants and children should be assessed for the presence of airway obstruction and wheeze as evidence of angio-oedema. Infrequently, urticaria with associated angio-oedema may progress to anaphylaxis.[347]

Acute urticaria is a clinical diagnosis and investigations in the ED are not indicated.[347] Where a possible precipitant has been identified, referral for allergy testing may be indicated.

Management

In the absence of angio-oedema affecting the airway or signs of anaphylaxis, acute urticaria can be managed simply with antihistamines and patient education. The role of anti-histamines in the management of urticaria is uncontroversial; loratadine and cetirizine both come in syrup preparations and are appropriate for children.[347] Conversely, the role of corticosteroids, which hold theoretical value, is debated. There are no paediatric-specific data available, but small-scale adult studies suggest that oral steroids may reduce the itch and the duration of the rash.[353] A 3-day course of oral steroid may be recommended in severe or prolonged urticaria.[354] Discharge education should include the signs and symptoms of airway involvement and anaphylaxis. Parents should also be provided with a realistic understanding of the potential prognosis (recurrent flares of rash over days to weeks).

> **PRACTICE TIPS**
> ## URTICARIA
>
> - Urticaria is characterised by the appearance of itchy wheals of varying size which settle within 1–24 hours, often with new lesions appearing elsewhere.
> - Urticaria is thought to be an allergic reaction, which may be associated with angio-oedema.
> - Antihistamines are used to manage acute urticaria. Steroids are only recommended in severe or prolonged urticaria.

Neonatal presentations

Neonates (babies aged less than 4 weeks of age) are a small cohort presenting to the ED. However, as the conditions likely to affect babies of this age can be different, their presentations very non-specific and they can deteriorate rapidly they should be assessed and managed with this in mind and their age treated as a substantial risk factor for serious illness. They should be treated with higher levels of urgency than older babies and young children for seemingly similar problems. As they are such a unique population it is beyond the scope of the text to discuss health concerns related to prematurity and congenital abnormalities. In this section excessive crying and jaundice will be discussed.

The crying baby

Infant crying generally begins in the neonatal period at 2 weeks of age, peaks at 6–8 weeks and settles at 3–4 months.[355] In a recent meta-analysis it was concluded that babies cry for an average of 110–118 minutes each day for the first 6 weeks and that this reduces to 72 minutes by 10–12 weeks of age.[356] It may be a signal that the baby is hungry, tired, requires a nappy change or is seeking comfort. Colic is a syndrome of excessive crying. However, a universally agreed definition does not exist. Most commonly, colic or excessive crying is defined as crying for more than 3 hours a day for more than 3 days a week.[357]

Crying frequently causes great concern among parents and is one of the most frequently reported problems in young babies. However, it is reported that fewer than 5% of infants have a significant organic cause for crying.[358,359] The range of possible causes is extensive, as it is a highly non-specific symptom.

Presentation and diagnosis

Parents present to the ED concerned about the wellbeing of their baby. There is either a sudden increase in crying or parents have become exhausted and are confused by the varying advice that they have received from family, friends and healthcare professionals about their baby's crying. An extensive history and examination should be undertaken to identify signs and symptoms of organic illness. This should always include urine analysis, as infants with urinary tract infections (UTIs) frequently present with non-specific symptoms and, of those babies presenting with excessive crying, a substantial number will have a UTI, despite the absence of a fever.[359] Feeding patterns, activity levels, weight gain and development should be explored to help determine the source of the crying.

Other causes of crying common to this age group which should be considered are cow's milk protein allergy, gastro-intestinal reflux, raised intracranial pressure, hair tourniquet, surgical abdomen, irreducible hernia, corneal abrasion, injury and infection, to name a few. Although not common, clinicians should be alert to risk factors for abuse. Previous presentation to a healthcare professional is a risk factor for abuse in infants.[360] Parents may be attempting to seek assistance via an ED visit for non-specific symptoms. The history and examination will guide the need for further investigation. However, it is beyond the scope of this text to explore all of the causes in detail.

Management

The priority for emergency clinicians is to determine whether the crying is associated with organic pathology or is benign. The diagnosis of colic is one of exclusion. Colic mixtures containing simethicone are of no proven benefit, while anticholinergic medications do reduce crying but have significant side effects and are therefore not recommended.[355] Having made a diagnosis of excessive crying, management centres on education, reassurance and referral for strategies to manage excessive crying. Referrals should be directed to clinicians such as: maternal child health nurses, paediatricians and social workers with particular interest and expertise in crying babies. Emergency clinicians should also be aware of the enormous stress experienced by parents of crying babies and give consideration to the potential implications of this stress. In a large study 6% of parents with crying babies admitted to physically abusive behaviours towards their babies.[361]

PRACTICE TIPS

CRYING BABY

- Crying is a normal behaviour in young babies; however, an increase in crying may be associated with significant illness or injury. Therefore, a detailed history should be taken and the baby examined carefully to detect a potential pathological cause of the crying.
- Parents presenting with a crying baby are usually very concerned about their baby and will require advice and support to manage the crying if it is determined not to be pathological.

Jaundice

Jaundice is reported as the most frequent reason for neonatal presentations to the ED.[362] It is most commonly physiological jaundice, breast-milk jaundice or secondary to sepsis. Infrequently, it is a symptom of liver disease and related congenital abnormalities such as biliary atresia. In most infants it is benign. However, unconjugated bilirubin toxicity, with neurological sequelae (kernicterus), may occur in a small number with more severe hyperbilirubinaemia.

Bilirubin is produced by the catabolism of haemoglobin. Compared with older children and adults, newborns have a high rate of haemoglobin catabolism and bilirubin production because of their elevated haematocrit and red blood cell volume per bodyweight and the shorter life span of red blood cells in the infant (70–90 days). In contrast, conjugation and clearance of bilirubin can be slow. Immaturity of hepatic glucuronosyltransferase and inadequate milk intake can cause delayed clearance of bilirubin.[363] Initially the breakdown of haemoglobin reveals lipid-soluble unconjugated bilirubin, which binds to albumin until binding sites are saturated. Free unconjugated bilirubin crosses the blood–brain barrier and is neurotoxic. Once in the liver, it is conjugated by glucuronosyltransferase to water-soluble conjugated bilirubin, which is easily excreted by the liver and biliary tract.[363] Some bilirubin may be reabsorbed in the intestine and converted back to its unconjugated form.

Physiological jaundice in neonates results from the breakdown of fetal red blood cells and the resulting increase in haemoglobin and is more common in breast-fed babies. Breast-milk jaundice is thought to be caused by a substance in breast milk that inhibits glucuronosyltransferase; reabsorption of bilirubin in the intestine is increased by breast milk, hence resulting in breast-milk jaundice.

Presentation and diagnosis

Babies with jaundice may present with no associated symptoms or with lethargy and poor feeding. More-severe jaundice, if left untreated, results in opisthotonus, seizures and eventually kernicterus which is the permanent neurological outcome of severe untreated hyperbilirubinaemia and is characterised by cerebral palsy, hearing loss and intellectual impairment.[363]

Neonates with jaundice should be evaluated for sepsis and other, more uncommon causes of neonatal jaundice. Clinicians should have a low threshold for considering full septic screening in a jaundiced neonate as the signs and symptoms of sepsis and those associated with jaundice, such as lethargy and poor feeding, are similar.

Investigation of the infant with jaundice should include a full blood count to look for anaemia, a smear for haemolysis, a reticulocyte count, bilirubin (conjugated and unconjugated) levels and a Coombs test. Babies with physiological breast-milk jaundice or jaundice secondary to sepsis have increased serum concentrations of unconjugated bilirubin, whereas conjugated bilirubin is raised in jaundice secondary to most forms of liver disease.[364]

Management

Identification of the likely cause is paramount to neonatal jaundice management. Septic neonates should be managed accordingly and referred to a neonatal unit. Babies with increased conjugated bilirubin should be discussed with a paediatric gastroenterologist.

Management of babies with increased unconjugated bilirubin will depend on the bilirubin levels, the likelihood that it will continue to rise and the associated symptoms such as lethargy and poor feeding. Most babies can be managed as outpatients with regular (daily in many cases) monitoring of bilirubin levels. However, babies requiring admission for phototherapy, or where doubt exists, should be discussed with a neonatologist. Recommendations for management of neonatal jaundice have been developed by the National Institute for Health and Clinical Excellence (NICE) and include bilirubin thresholds for treatment.[365]

PRACTICE TIPS

JAUNDICE

- Neonates presenting with jaundice should be screened for sepsis and liver disease, which, although uncommon, are a serious cause of jaundice in this age group.
- Neonates with lethargy and poor feeding, associated with increased unconjugated bilirubin, will require admission.

Fever

Fever is a symptom associated with many paediatric illnesses and is of great concern to large numbers of parents. Considerable confusion still exists in the community and among healthcare professionals about what constitutes a fever, how and when a fever should be treated and the potential consequences of fever.[366–372]

Fever is an elevated core temperature, which is usually a component of the immune response of the host to a pathogen or foreign stimuli, the most common of which is infection.[274] Immune cells release pyrogenic cytokines, cyclo-oxygenase-2 (COX-2) is induced, the arachadonic acid cascade is activated and biosynthesis of prostaglandin E_2 (PGE_2) is increased. These complex, immune-mediated reactions trigger a range of physiological events, including a rise in the hypothalamic temperature 'set point'. The physiological outcomes of these processes are increased metabolic rate resulting in increased cardiac output, which helps mobilise white cells; increased white cell activity; activation of T-lymphocytes; and stimulation of interferon production, to name a few. Moderate fever is considered to improve immune system function and potentiates the effects of antibiotics. There are few data to support the contention that fever associated with infection is harmful and increasing evidence to suggest that it may be of physiological benefit during infection.

In response to an increase in hypothalamic set point, the body will mount a response to increase heat production and reduce heat loss to raise the body temperature to the level of the set point. This is achieved by responses such as shivering and vasoconstriction. A drop in the set point will result in a reversal of these responses and vasodilation and diaphoresis will occur.

Presentation

Fever in children is defined as a temperature, measured tympanically or rectally, above 38.0°C. Infections are the most common reason for fever in children, the majority of which will be mild. However, a small number of children will have more-serious illness; occult bacteraemia rates (since the introduction of *H. influenzae* and *S. pneumoniae* vaccines) are estimated to be approximately 0.25%.[371] Fever will complicate the assessment of a range of other parameters used to assess for illness severity, such as peripheral perfusion, respiratory and heart rate and level of activity, which are all affected by high fever.

There is no convincing evidence to suggest that response to antipyretics is predictive of the severity of the illness.[372–375] Therefore, clinical decisions should not be delayed while waiting to assess response to antipyretics. There is also conflicting evidence about whether the height or duration of the fever correlates with the severity of the infection.[376–380] This data should only serve to heighten clinician suspicion for serious illness in children with high fever, but should not provide comfort where fever is low.

Management

Historically it has been practice to treat all fevers with antipyretics and a range of non-pharmacological measures based on the assumption that fever is harmful and that treating fever will eliminate its deleterious effects. However, limited evidence supports the benefits of fever to the host during infection and, conversely, has not been able to demonstrate that fever is harmful.[381–383] The decision to treat fever must weigh the benefits of fever reduction against the benefits of fever. Animal data demonstrate that treatment with paracetamol increases viral shedding and reduces immune system activity. Human data is limited and conflicting: several studies indirectly infer that antipyretic therapy may impact negatively on mortality in severe infection and on morbidity in mild infection,[383,384] while the authors of a recent meta-analysis conclude that the use of antipyretics does not delay the resolution of fever.[385] The potential toxicity of antipyretics should also be considered when weighing up the decision to treat fever. Although paracetamol is an extremely safe medication, its therapeutic use has been linked with hepatotoxicity and a small number of deaths.[383,386–388] Although causation cannot be demonstrated, a large study revealed an association between paracetamol use in infancy with later development of atopic disease.[389] Reports also show renal toxicity following therapeutic ibuprofen treatment regimens.

It is now generally accepted that the focus should be on providing comfort to the febrile child and that this may include the use of antipyretics. This is in the absence of convincing evidence to support an improvement in comfort among children receiving paracetamol for fever.[384] Antipyretic therapy is not recommended for children who remain comfortable despite their fever, and it would be reasonable to recommend that subsequent doses are not given when the first was not considered to have conferred benefit to the child. It may be useful to treat children with cardiac or respiratory failure who are febrile with antipyretics to reduce the additional metabolic demands generated by fever.[383] However, no data exist to validate this suggestion.[274]

Once the decision to treat is made, a choice must be made about the methods used to treat. A 2002 Cochrane review, aimed at assessing the effects of paracetamol for treating fever in children in relation to fever clearance time, febrile convulsions and resolution of associated symptoms, determined that there was insufficient evidence to draw conclusions on the effectiveness of paracetamol in fever management.[279] However, more recent randomised controlled trials show that paracetamol is effective against fever when compared with placebo.[390] This review focused exclusively on paracetamol, but studies comparing paracetamol and NSAIDs such as ibuprofen show equivalence.[391–393] By contrast, other studies show improved efficacy of ibuprofen[394–396] and a recent Cochrane review comparing alternating with combined or monotherapy regimens concluded that the use of both in either a combined or an alternating regimen is likely to be more effective.[396] It should be noted that the use of combined or alternating regimens may increase the risk of dosing error and should only be recommended with caution.

Non-pharmacological measures to treat fever, such as sponging, aim to overwhelm the capacity of the body to generate enough heat to maintain the febrile state. The authors of a 2003 Cochrane review concluded that a few small studies demonstrated that tepid sponging helps to reduce fever in children.[397] More-recent data also support an initial reduction in fever following sponging, which is not sustained after 2 hours and is associated with increased discomfort.[398,399] Furthermore, the body will vigorously defend the higher 'set point', potentially at considerable metabolic cost. There are no studies evaluating the risk–benefit ratio for non-pharmacological measures to treat fever. However, as fever is of benefit and unlikely to come at significant cost, unlike cooling measures, they are not recommended.

The priority of ED management of fever is to determine the source of the infection. Septic work-up in infants and children, where an obvious focus of infection has not been identified on examination, is indicated to detect serious bacterial infections such as UTI, meningitis and bacteraemia. The extent of the work-up will be determined by the symptoms at presentation, the severity of the illness and the age of the child. Table 36.21 provides a guide to the recommendations regarding appropriate diagnostic tests for febrile children of varying ages.

Accurate information should be provided to ensure that parents can make appropriately informed decisions about the care of their febrile child, including when to seek medical advice. Parents exhibit great concern about fever, but limited knowledge about its effect and management. Studies have shown that parents treating their children with over-the-counter medications, including antipyretics, are not always clear about the indications for and dosing of these medications.[400] The role of fever, the likely side effects of fever and the benefits and risks of treating fever should all be discussed with parents. The appropriate methods for treatment should be identified, which should include details about the use of antipyretics, such as the dose, the frequency and the use of other over-the-counter cold and flu preparations, which may contain paracetamol.

PRACTICE TIPS
FEVER

- Fever improves immune responses to illness and there is no evidence that it is harmful.
- The height of the fever should not be used as an indicator of the severity of the infection.
- The response to antipyretics is also not predictive of the severity of the illness.
- The focus of fever management should be to provide comfort and not to treat the temperature.
- Antipyretics, such as paracetamol and ibuprofen, are the only therapies shown to be effective at reducing fever.

Trauma

Trauma is a major cause of mortality and morbidity in infants, children and adolescents. The activities of infants, children and adolescents influence the likely mechanism of injury, which in turn can be used to predict likely injuries.[401] The size of the

---

TABLE 36.21 Recommended diagnostic workup for infants and children presenting with fever with no obvious focus

AGE GROUP	DIAGNOSTIC TESTS
Neonate	Full sepsis workup—FBE/film, blood culture, urine culture (SPA), lumbar puncture, chest X-ray
1–3 months	Full sepsis workup—FBE/film, blood culture, urine culture (SPA), lumbar puncture (may be omitted in some circumstances; should be discussed with paediatric consultant), Chest X-ray only if respiratory symptoms or signs
	Chest X-ray only if respiratory symptoms or signs
3–36 months	Looks well—urine culture if less than 6 months of age
	Looks miserable but is still relatively alert, interactive and responsive—urine culture if less than 12 months old, senior clinician review
	Looks unwell—full sepsis workup: FBE, blood culture, urine culture, chest X-ray (if respiratory symptoms or signs), consider lumbar puncture

Note: lumbar puncture should not be performed in a child with impaired conscious state or focal neurological signs

FBE: full blood examination; SPA: suprapubic aspirate

child should also be considered when predicting the likely pattern of injuries; for example, a young child hit by a car may suffer pelvic fractures, not femoral fractures like a taller adult hit by the same car. Furthermore, the proportions of the younger child increase the likelihood that they will suffer trauma to the relatively larger head.

Infants develop increasing mobility over their first year of life and accidents occur when carers underestimate the extent to which they are able to move; for example, rolling off surfaces and falling. As they become toddlers their mobility improves, but they remain clumsy and typically fall an average of four times a day—usually sustaining no injury but on occasions suffering minor trauma. As toddlers get older, parents and carers commonly provide increasingly less supervision. However, despite their improved coordination and capacity to understand simple rules, children of this age may not recognise the dangers associated with their activities, which increases their risk for accident and injury. Accidents associated with bikes, skateboards and swimming pools are not uncommon. Teenagers may engage in risk-taking behaviours such as experimenting with drugs and alcohol, sexual activity and adventurous physical activities. Many young people are involved in a range of sporting activities that also increase their risk of injury. In addition, growth and development increase the risk of some conditions related to overuse, such as Osgood-Schlatter disease.

Minor trauma is an extremely common reason for children to present to the ED. Children sustain fractures, sprains, strains and other soft-tissue injuries, burns and lacerations. However, only major trauma, fractures, pulled elbows and foreign bodies will be considered in this section.

Major trauma

Major trauma is a significant source of mortality and morbidity in children aged 1–18 years. However, presentations are much lower than for the adult population. A large paediatric trauma centre serving one Australian state reports an average of approximately 100 major trauma cases each year.[402] However, the small size of children results in transmission of force over a larger area of the body, making it more likely that they sustain multiple injuries. Motor vehicle crashes are responsible for approximately half of the fatalities in children and it is recognised that the youngest occupant in the car is the most vulnerable to injury.[403]

The priority for trauma management and the sequence of assessment and management are the same for adults and children. The differences in approach relate to the specifics of assessment and management, and are a result of different injury mechanisms and differences in anatomy and physiology between adults and children. Therefore, this section should be read in conjunction with Chapter 44, particularly the section on assessment, and Table 36.1. It is not intended to be a comprehensive review of major trauma management in children; the intent is to highlight some key areas of difference in paediatric trauma management.

Airway and circulation

Inadequate management of the obstructed airway and hypovolaemia are the main contributors to avoidable deaths in children following trauma. The sections in this chapter on respiratory failure and shock detail airway management, oxygenation and fluid resuscitation in children, and these principles can be applied to the child suffering major trauma requiring airway management, oxygenation and fluid resuscitation. Chapter 17, p. 314, also contains further information on airway management techniques for paediatric patients.

Cervical spine injury

Spinal injury is relatively rare in children, with only 10% of spinal injuries occurring in this age group. However, approximately 60–80% of spinal injuries in children involve the cervical spine, compared with 30–40% in adults.[404] A number of injury patterns occur in children: fractures, fracture and subluxation or dislocation, subluxation or dislocation without fracture, soft-tissue injury and spinal cord without radiological abnormality (SCIWORA). Subluxations and dislocations are more common in younger children, and cervical spine injuries in younger children usually involve C1 and C2 as a result of the anatomical differences that exist between young children and adults. See Table 36.1 for full details. C1 dislocation is the most common specific injury in young children.[405]

Cervical spine protection presents a clinical challenge in the uncooperative child and for toddlers and infants where available immobilisation devices don't always fit well. This is particularly problematic pre-hospital and during transport. Available evidence supports that immobilisation reduces the number and extent of spinal cord injuries, although none of this data have been derived from randomised controlled trials.[404,406,407] However, the methods for immobilisation were not consistent and included multiple techniques for immobilisation. There is insufficient evidence to guide clinicians about the optimal method for immobilising children. Therefore, in clinical practice the optimal method of immobilisation is that which best secures the spine, and this will be determined by the circumstances. Manual immobilisation may be the technique of choice until such time as an appropriately sized collar or alternative can be sourced and applied, or during examination of the neck or airway manoeuvres. However, this technique is impractical for transport. In most situations a well-fitting hard collar can achieve immobilisation for transport and management in the ED. However, alternatives may be required for some children. For example, an infant held in their mother's arms with a rolled towel tucked around their neck may be better immobilised than one lying on a trolley in a poorly fitting stiff neck collar. In some circumstances where resources allow, children may also be managed on a spinal board with blocks and straps applied to better secure the cervical spine. Where this is the case, they will also need a pad under their torso to maintain neutral alignment when lying supine. The thickness of the pad will depend on the size of the occiput (therefore, the extent to which the head is flexed forward) and hence the age of the child.

There are also limited data to support criteria for clearing the cervical spine in children. The NEXUS criteria were based on a largely adult population and did not include sufficient children younger than 9 years of age to confidently apply these criteria to young children.[408] Several studies have attempted to evaluate the capacity of cervical spine clearance protocols to detect injuries and reduce the need for imaging. However, the numbers of children in these studies with injuries is small, making it difficult to accept the results as evidence of the diagnostic accuracy of these tools. However, in the absence of evidence-based criteria specifically for children the NEXUC criteria in conjunction with the Canadian C-Spine Rule[409] serve as a reasonable basis for clearing the cervical spine in the conscious child. The UK-based National Institute for Clinical Excellence has produced criteria for radiology in children which are also based on adult guidelines.[410] They recommend as first-line investigation plain films for conscious children with risk factors for injury. To reduce radiation exposure, CT for children under 10 years of age is recommended only if the results of the plain films are unclear (review by a paediatric radiologist is advised) or there is a high suspicion of injury. These guidelines recommend CT to clear the cervical spine for unconscious children. Anatomical differences also complicate interpretation of imaging; however, this is beyond the scope of this text.

PRACTICE TIPS
CERVICAL SPINE INJURY

- Infants and children may sustain spinal cord injury without radiographic abnormalities (SCIWORA).
- Alternatives to the cervical collar should be sought where poor fitting (infants and toddlers) or lack of cooperation of the child puts the spine at risk.
- A pad should be placed under the infant's shoulders to ensure that the head does not flex forward when the infant is nursed on a spine board.
- CT to detect injury should only be used if plain films are equivocal.

Head injury

The most common single-organ-system injury contributing to mortality in children is head injury. Anatomical differences render them more susceptible to head trauma (see Table 36.1). Varying levels of cognitive development have an impact on assessment and a modified version of the Glasgow Coma Scale (GCS) has been developed, but has not been adequately validated. The original GCS has been shown to be a valid prediction of brain injury in adults. Some data suggest that the original GCS is more predictive of outcome in children than in adults,[411] while other studies have suggested that the initial presentation assessed by GCS has little or no correlation with injury.[412] The modified GCS may have overcome the limitations of the original GCS for younger children, and Holmes et al demonstrated that it compares favourably with the original GCS for assessment of traumatic brain injury in older children.[32] However, it is generally accepted that the GCS is the most appropriate way of classifying the severity of traumatic brain injury and that trend data will be of most use. Many clinicians will also advocate for the modified GCS to account for the differences in potential verbal and motor responses in different age groups.

Head injury is classified as mild, moderate and severe, and this classification system has implications for investigation and management. *Mild* is defined in Australasia as injury with an associated GCS score of 14 or 15.[413] *Moderate* head injury is defined as a head injury with an associated GCS score of 9 to 13, and a *severe* head injury as a head injury with an associated GCS score of 8 or less.

The decision to use CT in the setting of moderate and severe head injury is usually straightforward. However, the decision is more difficult where a mild head injury exists. Data support CT for all children with a GCS score less than 15 and for children with focal neurology or penetrating injury. The prognostic significance of vomiting[414,415] and the duration of the loss of consciousness is unclear, and brief seizure at the time of the injury is not significant; but seizure more than 20 minutes following the trauma is indicative of more significant injury.[416] Therefore, although available data are less conclusive, CT should be considered for children with persistent vomiting, seizure occurring at least 20 minutes after the trauma, history of loss of consciousness of at least 1 minute and post-traumatic amnesia.[403,417] A number of rules to guide the decision to CT for children with minor head injuries have been developed. To date the Pediatric Emergency Care Applied Research Network (PECARN) rule shows the highest levels of sensitivity and specificity of the available rules.[418] However, adherence to this rule may see a considerable rise in the number of CTs performed in Australasian hospitals, where practice is more conservative than in the US and Canada. Skull X-rays have a very limited role in paediatric trauma.

Head injury management adopts the same principles in paediatric patients as in adults, with few exceptions, and much of the data to support these practices are extrapolated from adult data. Therapeutic hypothermia showed some promise; however, the evidence for this practice summarised in a recent Cochrane review is unconvincing,[419] and there are very few paediatric data. However, despite this, it is practised in many paediatric intensive care units, as the theory for its value to neurological survival is credible.[420] Shann suggests that cooling did not occur early enough, at a low enough temperature or for long enough to see the likely true benefit that may be expected from therapeutic cooling.[420]

The neurocognitive outcomes of children suffering a moderate to severe head injury during their childhood are impaired when compared with a non-injured cohort. There has recently been increasing concern about the impact of mild head injury on outcomes and to date there is conflicting evidence about the likely long-term neurocognitive impact of a mild head injury.

PRACTICE TIPS
HEAD INJURY

- Parents and the modified GCS should be used when assessing the infant or child's neurological state.
- Children with a GCS score of less than 15, focal neurology or a penetrating injury should have a CT scan to determine the extent of the head injury.
- CT is also recommended for children with persistent vomiting, who suffer a seizure more than 20 minutes after the injury, have a history of loss of consciousness of greater than 1 minute and post-traumatic amnesia.
- Skull X-rays are rarely useful.
- Therapeutic hypothermia is used in many centres as it theoretically improves neurological survival.

Intra-abdominal trauma

Focused abdominal sonography for trauma (FAST) has increasingly become the standard for detecting blood in the peritoneum in adults. However, this technique remains controversial in paediatrics. The sensitivity and specificity of this tool in paediatrics is not as convincing as it is in adults and is not high enough to prompt paediatric trauma clinicians to make this a standard of care for children.[421–426] However, it may be a useful adjunct to the examination. It is also important to note that detection of free fluid is not sufficient to guide treatment in children where the majority of injuries are managed conservatively, providing that the child is haemodynamically stable. In children, more than 90% of solid-organ injuries, including hepatic and splenic injuries, are safely managed non-operatively.[427–430]

PRACTICE TIPS

INTRA-ABDOMINAL TRAUMA

- Focused abdominal sonography for trauma (FAST) is of limited value for infants and children.
- Abdominal injuries are frequently managed non-operatively in infants and children.

Fractures

Fractures are a common paediatric injury and account for over 20% of all injuries in children. Fracture is more common than other types of musculoskeletal injury, as a result of skeletal immaturity. To understand fractures in children it is essential that the anatomy of the paediatric bone is well understood; the sections of the growing bone are shown in Figure 36.5. The differences between adult and paediatric bones are highlighted in Table 36.1 and this explains their impact on the types of injuries experienced by children and the differences in assessment and management. This section serves to highlight some of the key issues in paediatric fractures, and does not detail assessment and management of specific common paediatric fractures.

Fractures in children can be categorised as either *physeal* (growth plate) or *non-physeal*. Injuries involving the physis can be further described using the Salter-Harris classification system,[431] which is shown in Figure 36.6. Salter-Harris type II injuries are the most common of these injuries. The type of fracture can also be used to describe fractures. Torus (periostium intact) and greenstick (periostium intact on one side) fractures are unique to growing bones, and reflect the softer, more malleable quality of children's bones compared with those of an adult. Fracture location is also influenced by age, with some fractures specific to paediatrics, such as supracondylar fractures, and others unlikely, such as scaphoid fractures in children < 10 years of age.

Presentation and diagnosis

Diagnosis of fracture in children can be more difficult than in adults.[432] The history may be unclear in young children, particularly where the accident has been unwitnessed. Older children may be reluctant to provide details for fear that they may get into trouble. As children are more susceptible to fracture than adults, relatively insignificant mechanisms should not be overlooked as a possible source of fracture.

Young children are often uncooperative, making examination more difficult. It can be hard to identify specific tenderness in a child distressed by examination. However, with careful palpation while watching the face of the child it is often possible to detect subtle changes suggesting specific tenderness that are reproducible each time the area is examined. Swelling can be difficult to detect in subtle injuries, particularly in toddlers, who have more subcutaneous tissue. If swelling is not visible, it may be evidenced by a slight fullness or firmness of the injured limb, which can be detected by feeling the injured and unaffected limb at the same time.

Consistent with practice in adults, neurovascular assessment should be included in injury assessment. Neurovascular injury is always a risk, but is closely linked with specific injuries such as a supracondylar fracture. The features of neurovascular injury and compartment syndrome are detailed in Chapter 50 and will not be repeated here.

The avoidance of unnecessary radiation is a high priority in paediatric emergency care, and identifying criteria to differentiate between children who require X-ray from those who do not has been attempted. The ankle and knee rules adapted from the adult Ottawa rules (Ch 18) and validated for use in paediatrics are effective decision tools to guide the decision to X-ray in children over 5 years of age.[324–331,433] However, there are no data to support the predictive value of specific clinical signs and symptoms for fractures in general.[432] In light of this and the often-subtle fractures sustained by children, it is reasonable to have a low index of suspicion for fracture and therefore a low threshold to X-ray.

Interpretation of plain films is greatly influenced by skeletal maturity and the presence of secondary ossification centres complicates interpretation. In some areas, such as the elbow,

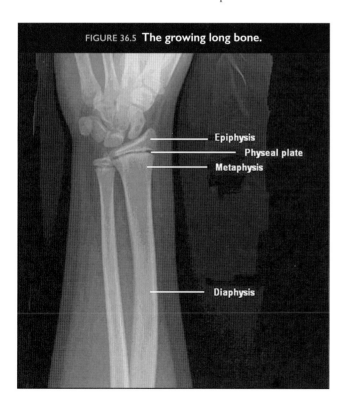

FIGURE 36.5 The growing long bone.

Epiphysis

Physeal plate

Metaphysis

Diaphysis

FIGURE 36.6 **The Salter-Harris classification system for fractures involving the growth plate.**[431]

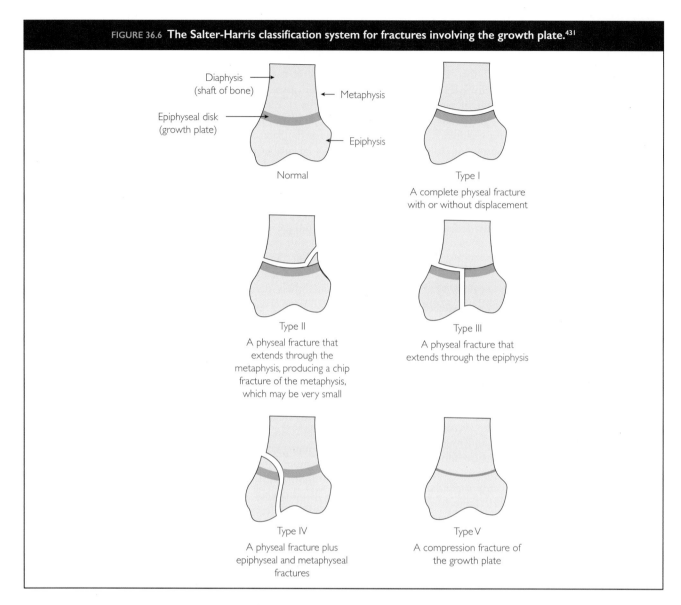

Diaphysis (shaft of bone)

Metaphysis

Epiphyseal disk (growth plate)

Epiphysis

Normal

Type I
A complete physeal fracture with or without displacement

Type II
A physeal fracture that extends through the metaphysis, producing a chip fracture of the metaphysis, which may be very small

Type III
A physeal fracture that extends through the epiphysis

Type IV
A physeal fracture plus epiphyseal and metaphyseal fractures

Type V
A compression fracture of the growth plate

these ossification centres are numerous and appear at different stages of growth, further complicating interpretation. It is also important to recognise that some subtle fractures are not always visible on X-ray, requiring the clinician to review the X-ray for the presence of other indirect indicators of fracture, such as elbow joint effusion in the setting of occult supracondylar fracture. Ideally, a clinician with paediatric expertise should review X-rays. Internationally, bedside ultrasound is also increasingly being used to diagnose fractures in children,[434–437] but is yet to be common practice in Australasia.

Management

First-aid management of fractures is no different to first-aid management in adult injury, and involves urgent reduction of the fracture if there is vascular compromise, immobilisation of the injury and analgesia. Appropriate analgesia options for children with musculoskeletal injury are discussed later in the chapter.

Specific fracture management in children does differ from management of adult injuries and will depend on the type of injury and the age of the child. Paediatric fractures

are frequently managed more conservatively than fractures of adults. Closed reduction is used more frequently, and more-significant displacement and angulation is tolerated as growth provides for significant remodelling of the injured bone with more-acceptable cosmetic and functional outcomes even if the fracture is not reduced or only partially reduced. There are no universal criteria for what degree of displacement of non-physeal injuries requires reduction; the need for reduction depends on the bone, the direction of the angulation/displacement (e.g. along the axis of movement), and the age of the child.[438] As a rule of thumb, injuries of long bones that look bent should be straightened regardless of the age of the child and the likelihood that it will remodel over time.

Displaced physeal and articular injuries require reduction (open or closed) and, in some instances, securing. Improved function and a reduction of the risk of osteoarthritis are the reasons for reduction of these injuries. Concern often centres on the possibility of growth disturbance; however, this is unlikely and can be treated if it occurs. The advice of a paediatric orthopaedic surgeon should be sought if there is any doubt about the need for reduction. Unstable fractures, such as lateral epicondylar fractures of the humerus, are also likely to require surgical management and referral should be made to a paediatric orthopaedic clinic.

Backslabs, rather than encircling casts, are frequently used to provide analgesia and protection from further injury for injuries such as torus fractures of the distal radial metaphysis.[439–442] Injuries of the elbow are also managed in backslabs rather than encircling casts, regardless of the severity of the injury, and minor injuries where the associated pain is only mild may be managed in a simple collar-and-cuff sling.[443] The outcome for some injuries, such as ankle injuries, is improved by early immobilisation and full casts are not recommended for minor ankle injuries.

Paediatric fractures heal more rapidly, so where reduction is required this may need to occur more urgently. This is significant for injuries where management is delayed while swelling resolves; for example, metacarpal fractures, nasal bone fractures. More-rapid recovery also means that young children are immobilised for shorter periods of time than adults with similar injuries. The Victorian Paediatric Orthopaedic Network provide detailed clinical guidelines to assist clinicians treating paediatric fractures in the ED, which can be accessed from either their website or the Royal Children's Hospital site.

PRACTICE TIPS
FRACTURES

- Clinicians should have a high level of suspicion for fracture in infants and children presenting with musculoskeletal injury resulting from even minor trauma.
- Growing children have open physes (growth plates), which are a potential site of bony injury.
- Torus (buckle) and greenstick fractures are unique to growing bones, and are frequently overlooked as they may present with only subtle signs.
- The Ottowa ankle and knee rules may be used in children to determine the need for ankle and knee X-rays.
- Skeletal maturity and the presence of secondary ossification centres will greatly affect interpretation of plain films.
- Management of specific fractures often differs from management of similar fractures in adults. In many cases management is more conservative and immobilisation times shorter.

Pulled elbow

A radial head subluxation, commonly known as a pulled elbow or (in US literature) a nursemaid's elbow, is an injury that typically occurs in children aged 1–5 years. The characteristic mechanism is a 'pull' on the arm and the child cries. However, in up to 50% of cases there is no history of a pull on the arm— either the mechanism was unwitnessed or the parent describes a low-velocity fall. In all cases the child refuses to use their arm and this prompts parents to seek advice.[444]

The radial head is anchored at the elbow to the capitellum of the distal humerus by the annular ligament. It is thought that under traction the ligament slips over the head of the radius and becomes trapped in the joint space. Movement pinches the ligament and causes pain. However, at rest the injury is painless, explaining the characteristic presentation.

Presentation

Children present with the affected arm hanging at their side, slightly flexed and pronated, and refuse to use the arm. There is usually no swelling or bony tenderness and no distress provided the elbow is not moved. The child is able to move the shoulder and the wrist freely but movement of the elbow, particularly supination, causes considerable distress. Radiographs are usually unnecessary. However, they may be used to rule out a fracture where the diagnosis is not clear or there have been 2–3 unsuccessful attempts at reduction.

Treatment

Treatment of a pulled elbow consists of manipulating the arm to reduce the subluxation. Two techniques have been described: forced pronation without flexion, and supination with flexion. For both techniques, the clinician places their hand under the elbow with their thumb on the radial head while the other hand holds the forearm. The forearm is either supinated and then flexed at the elbow, or while in extension the forearm is pronated. The authors of a recent Cochrane review[445] concluded that although the studies are of low quality, the pronation technique is likely to be more effective and less painful, making this the preferred technique for initial attempts and supination–flexion an alternative in the event that forced pronation is unsuccessful. A 'click' is usually felt with successful reduction, which has a positive predictive value of more than 90% in two published case series.[446] The child will usually resume normal movement of the arm within 15–30 minutes of reduction and may be discharged home. However, this may take longer where the child is older than 2 years and treatment has been delayed longer than 4 hours. Pain relief may be given prior to attempts to reduce the pulled elbow and to increase the likelihood that the child uses their arm quickly after reduction.

PRACTICE TIPS
PULLED ELBOW

- Approximately 50% of pulled elbows occur where there is no history of a pull on the arm.
- The characteristic features are: refusal to use the affected arm which hangs by their side, no swelling or bony tenderness and pain on movement of the elbow.
- Radiographs are only required to rule out an alternative diagnosis, as they are normal where there is a pulled elbow.
- Forced pronation with the arm extended should be the first technique used to resolve a pulled elbow.
- Where the 'click' is not felt and the child is still not using their arm 30 minutes following manipulation, it should be assumed that the pulled elbow has not been corrected.
- Attempts to relocate the radial head should be limited to three, at which point the child's arm can be placed in a sling and discharged home for review in 24–48 hours.

However, significant pain associated with an injury is not characteristic of pulled elbow and should prompt the clinician to question the diagnosis.

Subsequent attempts may be made if no 'click' was felt or if there is no return of movement and reduction is considered unlikely. The child's arm should be placed in a sling and discharged home after three unsuccessful attempts for review in 1–2 days. Spontaneous reduction will occur in some of these children prior to review, and the remainder will be reduced on re-presentation. Recurrence rates are about 20–25% and discharge should include education of the parents to avoid likely mechanisms for pulled elbow.

Limp/refusal to walk

Limp or refusal to walk in a young child is usually considered to be the result of trauma, and parents will frequently identify an event thought to be the cause of the limp. However, injury, transient synovitis of the hip, osteomyelitis, septic arthritis, Perthes' disease, discitis and neuromuscular disorders are among the potential causes of limp in this age group. Older children are generally able to be more specific about the onset of the limp and the precipitant. However, in this age group the limp associated with orthopaedic conditions, such as Perthes' disase and slipped upper femoral epiphysis, can be confused with limp associated with chronic injury and overuse. Furthermore, hip pain can be referred to the knee and therefore hip pathology can be overlooked.

The focus of this section is on the preschool-aged child with a limp/refusal to walk; two of the most common reasons for limp or refusal to walk in this age group are toddler's fracture and transient synovitis. The cause of transient synovitis is not clear; however, it is considered a reactive arthritis of the hip, which may be provoked by recent viral infection. A toddler's fracture was first described as a spiral fracture of the tibial shaft in a preschool-aged child, which may or may not be visible on X-ray.[447]

Presentation and diagnosis

Young children with limp/refusal to walk present to the ED with sudden onset of limp following witnessed trauma, sudden onset of limp with no witnessed trauma, or an unclear onset of limp with or without identified trauma. Careful questioning is necessary to identify the relationship between the limp and the traumatic event. Due to the subtlety of the limp or the insidious onset of the limp, the parents may attribute the limp to an unrelated trauma, when in fact the child was limping prior to this event. Examination of a child, which should include gait assessment, will provide additional clues to the likely diagnosis. An antalgic gait sees the child shorten the time that the painful limb takes weight and is linked to acute and painful conditions.

Transient synovitis

Where there is no convincing history of trauma to explain the limp, other causes need to be excluded. Classically, transient synovitis presents with a non-specific history of limp, generally following viral symptoms in the previous week or two. Commonly parents report that the child was walking normally yesterday, but was limping or refusing to walk when they got up that morning. The child may have a fever, but most commonly the temperature is normal and they appear well. The child generally presents with an antalgic gait, although a small

number of children may refuse to walk at all. However, this should increase suspicion of an alternative explanation for the limp. On examination there is some limitation to the range of motion of the hip with particular resistance to internal rotation. These signs are usually subtle and no other abnormalities are found. Significant resistance to passive movement of the hip should also prompt suspicion about the likely diagnosis.

Plain radiographs are not useful to confirm the diagnosis, and inflammatory markers are either normal or only mildly elevated. Classically, septic arthritis presents more floridly, with fever, malaise and significant joint tenderness and restricted range of motion, but at the onset of this infection limp may be the only obvious feature. C-reactive protein has been shown to be the most sensitive and specific single parameter for distinguishing between the more benign transient synovitis and the more serious septic arthritis.[448] However, it is generally accepted that the diagnosis is best made based on a constellation of signs and symptoms and a number of algorithms have been developed to support decision-making, which have been shown to have good levels of diagnostic accuracy.[449]

Transient synovitis is a diagnosis of exclusion. It is essential that alternative diagnoses such as septic arthritis, which may present similarly in the early stages, are excluded; X-ray and pathology may be used to achieve this goal.

Management

Transient synovitis generally resolves spontaneously within 2–5 days and, according to a recent systematic review, most children's symptoms will resolve within 2 weeks.[450] Improvement will be hastened by regular treatment with a non-steroidal anti-inflammatory drug (NSAID) such as ibuprofen.[451] The longer the duration of the limp without improvement, the more likely that an alternative diagnosis is the cause of the limp. Children discharged with a diagnosis of transient synovitis should be reviewed within several days and parents should be given careful instructions to return if the child develops fever, malaise, reduced range of motion or there is no improvement in 2–3 days.

Toddler's fracture

Toddler's fracture is more easily diagnosed if there is a clear history of witnessed trauma followed by limp or refusal to walk, or alternatively it can be seen on X-ray. The mechanism of injury is usually an event which exerts rotational force on the lower leg; for example, catching the foot on the slide as the child descends. However, in a small number of cases the mechanism is unclear. In these cases it is important to confirm that there was at least a clear and sudden onset of limp. Children with a toddler's fracture will usually refuse to walk and only a very small number will limp.[452] Many will resort to crawling. Point tenderness is a moderately sensitive and specific clinical finding for toddler's fracture. However, its absence is not negatively predictive.[452] Pain with dorsiflexion of the ankle has also been reported,[343] but is seen in only a few cases.[452]

Plain films are taken in the ED to confirm the diagnosis. However, normal X-rays on presentation have been reported in 13–43% of cases where a toddler's fracture was later confirmed.[447,452–455] In these circumstances the diagnosis is made clinically. Bone scan can provide a more definitive result. This may be used if confirmation of a toddler's fracture will allay concern about the potential for an alternative diagnosis.

Ultrasound and plain radiographs about a week after the injury may also reveal a toddler's fracture.[450,451]

Management

Traditional management of a toddler's fracture was application of a plaster of Paris long leg cast. However, clinicians are now applying backslabs to immobilise these fractures and increasing numbers of paediatric emergency clinicians are only using immobilisation to manage discomfort and to provide protection for the particularly active child. The evidence for the optimal way to manage these injuries is not yet available.

PRACTICE TIPS

LIMP/REFUSAL TO WALK

- Limp and refusal to walk may not always be the result of trauma, so it is essential to take a careful history to determine the relationship between limp/refusal to walk and a history of trauma.
- Transient synovitis is considered a reactive arthritis that follows a viral illness. It should be differentiated from the much more serious septic arthritis.
- Radiographs and blood results are not useful in making the diagnosis, but may assist to exclude other potential causes for the limp/refusal to walk.
- Toddler's fractures are another common cause of limp/refusal to walk that are associated with minor trauma.
- The signs are subtle and the fracture may not be visible on X-ray.
- Toddler's fractures may be managed with no immobilisation, or for pain management and protection the leg may be immobilised in a backslab.

Foreign-body aspiration

Aspiration of a foreign body (FB) occurs most commonly in infants and toddlers; the average age is between 2 and 3 years,[107] with a mortality rate of approximately 5–7%.[108] It is also one of the most common causes of accidental death in children under 1 year of age.[107] The FB is often a piece of food; nuts are the most commonly reported organic FB.[109] As children at this age have a tendency to put things in their mouths, small parts on toys and other small objects also pose a risk. Furthermore, the increasing number of toys and devices that are powered with small button batteries should prompt the clinician to consider the potential for button battery aspiration, which should be treated as an emergency.

Infants and young children are at greater risk of airway obstruction as a result of the size of their airway, the amount of soft tissue and the frequency with which they put small objects in their mouths. Furthermore, the loss of deciduous teeth throughout childhood provides a source of obstruction, as they are more easily dislodged allowing them to fall into the airway. Loose teeth should be considered a potential risk to airway patency during intubation and in trauma.

Presentation and diagnosis

The clinical presentation of infants and children following FB inhalation is highly variable, and ranges from those presenting with clear history of inhalation and obvious examination findings to those presenting with less-obvious history of inhalation and/or equivocal examination findings.

FB inhalation should be strongly suspected where the history details sudden onset of choking, coughing, dyspnoea, laboured breathing, dysphagia and gagging. Studies suggest that anywhere from 40% to 70% of children presenting with a combination of these symptoms will have a confirmed FB on bronchoscopy.[107] Depending on the size of the FB, the signs and symptoms of inhalation may be mild to absent following the initial choking episode,[109] or may only become apparent after days to weeks as the child continues to cough and develop signs of pneumonia. A choking episode may not be reported as it may not have been witnessed or was not considered significant, particularly if it was days or weeks ago. Therefore, FB inhalation should also be suspected where there is unexplained chronic cough in an infant or young child.

Examination findings may include signs of obvious upper or lower airway obstruction, such as stridor and marked increased work of breathing, decreased lung sounds or wheeze. Other respiratory signs, such as decreased oxygen saturation, are not pathognomonic for FB inhalation, but should raise suspicion.[107] Few children with FB aspiration will have normal chest auscultation. However, as this number may be as high as 5%, normal examination findings cannot be considered conclusive. Where the history and/or examination is strongly suggestive of FB aspiration or the diagnosis cannot be excluded, a chest radiograph is indicated. However, in 25–30% of cases the chest X-ray may be normal.[107,110] Therefore, chest X-ray alone cannot be used to discriminate between those who have aspirated a FB and those that have not. Where the X-ray is abnormal there will be signs of hyperinflation, mediastinal shift, localised air trapping or a radio-opaque FB.

The signs and symptoms of FB inhalation are not sufficiently sensitive or specific to support a diagnostic decision rule. In over 50% of cases, the diagnostic triad of signs and symptoms (wheeze, cough and gagging) are absent.[111] FB inhalation is unlikely in those children who present asymptomatically and have normal examination and radiological findings. All others should be considered at risk of a FB inhalation.

Management

Complete airway occlusion is an emergency and basic life support should be commenced immediately. Initial treatment involves removal of the object (if visible and safe to do so), airway opening manoeuvres, back blows and chest or abdominal thrusts, depending on the age of the child (see Ch 15 for full details).

The infant or child showing signs of partial airway obstruction but able to ventilate should be allowed to adopt a position of comfort while the adequacy of ventilation is observed. Children showing signs of significant respiratory distress will require urgent bronchoscopy to remove the FB. They should be monitored closely. However, interaction should be kept to a minimum to prevent distressing the child and increasing the risk to their airway. Clinicians with paediatric airway expertise should be immediately available or the child should be transferred to a centre with the resources to expertly manage a paediatric airway. For children presenting with less-obvious symptoms, but where there is suspicion of an inhaled FB, there should be a low threshold for performing bronchoscopy.

Parents of infants and young children should be made aware of the dangers of small parts on toys and other small objects that they may put in their mouth. Care should also be taken when giving infants and young children food, in particular, raw apple, carrot, popcorn, hard lollies, nuts and anything else that they may potentially aspirate. Children should be supervised when eating so parents can ensure that they sit quietly while eating and that they attempt one piece at a time.[112]

PRACTICE TIPS
FOREIGN-BODY (FB) ASPIRATION

- Presentation is highly variable and may include children with a less-obvious history of inhalation and/or equivocal examination findings.
- Foreign body aspiration should be suspected in young children with unexplained cough.
- Chest X-rays are normal in 25–30% of cases of FB aspiration.
- There should be a low threshold for referring infants and children to ENT with a potential FB aspiration.
- No attempts to remove the FB should be made in the ED unless there is complete airway obstruction, the FB is visible and it can be removed safely.

Foreign body

Foreign-body (FB) ingestion and FB insertion into the nose or ear are common paediatric presentations to the ED; the average age in Western countries is 2–3 years of age.[110,456,457] Food, small plastic toys, coins and other small household objects are the most common FBs.

Diagnosis is often delayed as the event is frequently not witnessed and parents are only alerted to the FB when the child or an older sibling informs them, or alternatively when they seek health advice for non-specific symptoms resulting from the FB, such as an offensive unilateral nasal discharge, bad breath or reduced hearing. Examination of a child who has inserted a FB into an ear or nostril should include both ears and nostrils, as children frequently insert FBs into multiple places.

Button batteries should be removed from the oesophagus, aural canal or nasal passages immediately as leakage of the contents and generation of external electrolytic current will result in liquefaction necrosis. It can be seen from review of the outcomes of battery lodgement that severe burns can occur within 2–2.5 hours.[458] Children with button batteries lodged in the nose, aural canal or oesophagus require urgent referral to ENT to ensure that removal occurs expediently.[456,459,460] Children must be referred for urgent follow-up, even if the battery has been rapidly and successfully removed in the ED as injuries extend after removal.[458]

Parents should be warned about the likelihood that this may occur again and the need to supervise children when eating and playing with objects small enough to swallow or insert into their ears or nose.

Ingested foreign bodies

Children frequently swallow foreign objects such as coins, causing significant alarm to their parents. Most commonly they pass into the stomach and are then rarely of concern (the exception being button batteries and magnets). Radiographs are frequently used to locate radio-opaque FBs and demonstrate that they have passed into the stomach. These children may be discharged and parents advised that it is not necessary to confirm passage of the FB through the intestinal tract by identifying the FB in the faeces or using repeat radiographs. Ingestion of magnets is a notable exception to this rule unless there is complete confidence that the child could only have swallowed one magnet. Where there is a possibility that there may be two these children should be referred to a surgeon as the two magnets may be attracted and pinch adjacent bowel loops resulting in necrosis.[461] Although radio-opaque, the magnets may sit one behind each other and therefore appear as one magnet.

Less frequently the FB, which may include a bolus of food, fish bone, coin, metal pins or pieces of plastic, becomes lodged in the pharynx or the oesophagus and this is potentially a medical emergency. Children with an FB lodged in their oesophagus may present with a history of refusal to eat, may complain of feeling that something is stuck, vomiting,[110,462,463] less commonly gagging, drooling, choking and coughing;[110,463] or alternatively they may be asymptomatic.[462,464] Uncommonly but most importantly, an FB, in particular a coin, may lodge in the oesophagus and cause airway obstruction. Airway protection is of highest priority and children should be managed in the same way as children with an FB aspiration and referred immediately to have the FB removed. Radiographs may assist in localising a radio-opaque FB. Children with an FB lodged in the oesophagus should be referred to general surgery, and where there are signs of airway obstruction, urgent referral to ENT should be made.

PRACTICE TIPS
FOREIGN-BODY (FB) INGESTION

- Most ingested FBs pass into the stomach and therefore do not require intervention (except button batteries).
- It is not necessary to confirm passage of the object by repeat X-rays or screening of the faeces.
- An FB lodged in the oesophagus or pharynx is a potential medical emergency.

Intranasal foreign bodies

Foreign bodies pushed into the nose most frequently lodge in the floor of the nasal passage below the inferior turbinate, or in the upper nasal fossa anterior to the middle turbinate, and are usually visible. They can generally be successfully removed in the ED. Alternatively, where the FB is a small lolly that will dissolve, it may be reasonable not to attempt removal and allow it to dissolve over time.

Small, round lightweight objects that are completely occluding the nostril may be removed by generating positive pressure in the nasal passage behind the object. If the child is old enough this can be achieved by asking the child to blow their nose while occluding the patent nostril, and if not old enough by having the parent blow into the child's mouth while occluding the patent nostril. Parents benefit from a demonstration of the force of the breath used for this technique. It should be a short puff of air like blowing dust off something. The child will reflexively close the glottis to protect the lungs, preventing damage.[460] Despite this, a forceful large-volume breath should not be delivered.

Prior to alternative attempts to remove the FB, phenylephrine to reduce oedema and lignocaine to provide local anaesthetic should be applied to the nasal mucosa. Techniques for removal include using suction, alligator forceps to grasp the object or a wax curette to slide behind the object and pull it forward (see Ch 17, p. 327, for suctioning techniques). Most children will require sedation to achieve sufficient cooperation to make FB removal possible (see the section on procedural sedation). However, care should be taken to ensure that they remain able to gag and cough to protect their airway during attempts to remove an intranasal FB.

Referral to ENT should be made when the FB cannot be adequately visualised, the child is not sufficiently cooperative to attempt removal or attempts to remove the FB have been unsuccessful. It is also suggested that a plain radiograph should be taken where the FB is not visible and there is suspicion that it may be a button battery, to prompt more expeditious management.[459]

Aural foreign bodies

Foreign bodies inserted into the ear are the most difficult to remove and 20–33% of children will require general anaesthetic to facilitate removal.[464-467] The external auditory canal is cartilaginous and bony, lined with only a thin layer of skin, which provides very little cushioning for the periostium. Therefore, attempts to remove the FB, in addition to being frightening to the young child, can be very painful. On occasions the FB may become impacted deep in the canal as it narrows, particularly where previous unsuccessful attempts have been made, making removal even more difficult.[460] Canal lacerations, rupture of the tympanic membrane and disruption of the ossicles are documented complications of removal attempts.[465-468]

Removal in the ED should only be attempted if the child will hold sufficiently still (see the section on procedural sedation for details), the FB can be adequately visualised, appropriate instruments for removal are available and the clinician is sufficiently skilled to remove the FB.[460] Removal attempts are less likely to be successful in younger children,[465,469] where the object is smooth and difficult to grasp,[466,467,470] has been in the ear for an extended period of time[469] and previous unsuccessful attempts have been made.[466,467] Furthermore, these factors will also increase the rate of complications resulting from removal attempts, which may be as high as 43%.[469-471] Referral to ENT without first attempting to remove the FB in ED should be strongly considered if the object is smooth and spherical or there have been previous unsuccessful attempts made by other clinicians.

The techniques most frequently used with success are water irrigation and/or suction for small, lightweight objects, or removal using small alligator forceps to grasp the object or a wax curette to lever it out from behind the object. Irrigation should not be used where the FB is likely to be a button battery

as this may increase the likelihood of the contents leaking from the battery.[460,465] Alcohol, shown to be the most effective,[465] should be used to kill live insects (found more frequently in older children) before attempts are made to remove them. However, this should not be instilled where there is tympanic perforation.[460] A light and magnification source will improve visualisation of the FB and therefore the likely success rate. Most children will require sedation to assist medical staff to make a removal attempt possible.

PRACTICE TIPS

FOREIGN BODY (FB)—INTRANASAL AND AURAL

- Most FBs in the nose are visible.
- A lightweight object which is occluding the nose may be removed using positive pressure behind the object, achieved by the child blowing the nose or by a parent blowing into their mouth while occluding the unaffected nostril.
- Most children will require sedation to make safe removal of the object possible.
- Removal of aural FBs can be difficult, therefore clinicians should have a low threshold for referring to ENT.

Pain management and procedural sedation

Pain is a frequent symptom in adult and paediatric patients presenting to the ED,[472,473] and recommendations and clinical practice guidelines consistently emphasise the importance of the adequate management of acute and procedural pain and distress.

Despite this, it is widely accepted that pain and distress is inadequately managed in EDs[474-480] and some studies even show an *increase* in pain intensity between admission and discharge for some patients.[472,481] Several subpopulations, such as children and geriatrics, are particularly vulnerable to suboptimal treatment for painful conditions and may needlessly experience pain with illness or injury.[474,482-486] Studies have shown that children are less likely to receive analgesia than adults in the ED setting, and that young children are less likely to receive analgesia than older children.[474]

A more comprehensive overview of pain and pain management strategies has been presented in Chapter 19. The following sections add to this discussion by addressing some issues in paediatric pain and distress management.

Assessment

Pain

Fundamental to adequate pain management is pain assessment, and in children this presents a significant clinical challenge to emergency service clinicians due to children's varying levels of cognitive development. Pain can be assessed in a number of ways, such as the character of the pain, the region of the body affected, radiation, the effect of pain on activity and the intensity of the pain. Assessment in emergency services usually focuses on the character and intensity of the pain. Quantifying the intensity of pain has provided a commonly accepted language to describe pain and a baseline from which to measure the impact of treatments on pain. A number of pain assessment tools are used for this purpose. However, they require adaptation depending on the child's age, i.e. behavioural tools for pre-verbal children, faces scales for early-verbal children and visual analogue scales for older children.[487,488]

Self-report is considered the gold standard for pain assessment, and the Visual Analogue Scale (VAS) is a reliable instrument for quantifying acute pain in adults;[489] there are data to support its validity in acute presentations to the ED[490] and for children.[491–495] The VAS is presented as a 100 mm horizontal line. The line is anchored on the left with 'no pain' and on the right with 'worst pain ever'. Patients are asked to indicate where on the line best represents their pain intensity. Pain intensity is rated from the left boundary as a VAS score in millimetres or centimetres.[489]

Research has cast doubt on whether the VAS is reliable when used by children 7 years of age or below.[496] To overcome the difficulty younger children have with numerical scales, scales using faces representing varying levels of pain intensity have been developed for this age group. The revised Bieri Faces Pain Scale (see Fig 36.7) has been well validated for use in children 4 years of age and older.[487,491,492,497] It is recommended

as an easy-to-use measure that allows pain intensity to be quantified in young children who may have difficulty with more cognitively demanding instruments.

Children under the age of 4 years lack the cognitive development to use self-report scales, hence observer rating scales are used for this group. The VAS Observer (VAS$_{Obs}$) appears in the literature as a proxy for self-report, where clinicians or parents perform the rating.[498,499] Reliability and validity testing shows that the scores of observers show at best only moderate correlation with those of the child.[480,500,501] Clinicians have a tendency to underestimate the child's pain, and parents in some instances may overestimate the intensity of the child's pain.

An alternative to the VAS$_{Obs}$ is the Face Legs Activity Cry Consolability (FLACC) scale (see Table 36.22), which is an observational scale[488] focusing on behaviours that research has shown are indicative of pain in infants and young children.[502] To administer FLACC, an observer looks at a young child's facial expression, leg movements, activity, if they are crying and the extent to which they can be consoled. Each of these five behaviours is given a score of 0, 1 or 2, resulting in a total score ranging from 0 (no pain/distress) to 10 (maximum pain/distress).

FIGURE 36.7 The Faces Pain Scale.

In the following instructions, say 'hurt' or 'pain', whichever seems right for a particular child.
Score the chosen face 0, 2, 4, 6, 8 or 10, counting left to right so 0 = 'no pain' and 10 = 'very much pain'.
Do not use words like 'happy' and 'sad'. This scale is intended to measure how children feel inside, not how their face looks.
Show faces only, no numbers.

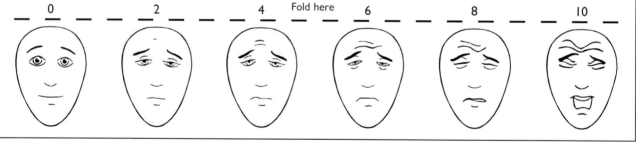

Revised from Hicks et al,[492] with permission from IASP®.

TABLE 36.22 The FLACC (Faces Legs Activity Cry and Consolability) scale[488]

	0	1	2
Face	No particular expression or smile	Occasional grimace or frown, withdrawn, disinterested	Frequent to constant frown, quivering chin, clenched jaw
Legs	Normal position or relaxed	Uneasy, restless, tense	Kicking or legs drawn up
Activity	Lying quietly, normal position, moves easily	Squirming, shifting back and forth, tense	Arched, rigid or jerking
Cry	No cry (awake or asleep)	Moans or whimpers; occasional complaints	Crying steadily, screams or sobs, frequent complaints
Consolability	Content, relaxed	Reassured by occasional touching hugging, or 'talking to'; distractible	Difficult to console or comfort

Behavioural observation scales such as FLACC have been validated predominantly in a post-operative population and more recently in cognitively impaired children.[488,503–506] However, these scales have not been well studied in the ED or in acute procedural settings, although are widely recommended for use in the ED, including in procedural circumstances.[507,508]

Sedation

Similarly to pain assessment, sedation scales have been developed to quantify the level of sedation. The University of Michigan Sedation Scale (UMSS),[509] shown in Box 36.4, is used in Australian EDs to score the level of sedation of children undergoing conscious sedation for a diagnostic or therapeutic procedure. The UMSS has been validated for children aged 6 months to 12 years of age,[509–512] and compares favourably with other scales.[511]

Sedation is defined as:

- 'mild sedation', which is equivalent to anxiolysis
- 'moderate sedation', where the patient retains the ability to respond appropriately to physical or verbal stimulation, and
- 'deep sedation', which is a level of sedation from which the patient is not easily aroused, and may include a partial or complete loss of protective airway reflexes.[513]

Using these definitions, the UMSS scores of 1, 2 and 3 represent mild, moderate and deep sedation respectively, while a score of 4 is indicative of unconsciousness.

In addition to vital signs, a baseline sedation score should be recorded before administering sedation and then at regular intervals while the patient remains sedated. The level of sedation and the agent used will determine the frequency of assessment.

PRACTICE TIPS

ASSESSMENT OF PAIN AND SEDATION

- Children as young as 4 years of age can self-report pain using the Bieri Faces Pain Scale scale.
- The FLACC (Face Legs Activity Cry Consolability) scale is recommended for children younger than 4 years of age.
- The level of sedation achieved can be assessed using the University of Michigan Sedation Scale (UMSS) (see Box 36.4).

BOX 36.4 University of Michigan Sedation Scale

Awake/alert
Minimally sedated—tired/sleepy, appropriate response to verbal conversation and/or sounds.
Moderately sedated—somnolent/sleeping, easily aroused with light tactile stimulation.
Deeply sedated—deep sleep, rousable only with significant physical stimulation
Unrousable

Acute pain management

Pain management has been described in some detail in Chapter 19, and many of the strategies described there are suitable for children. Pain relief is best achieved by using a range of strategies, both pharmacological and non-pharmacological. This section will discuss use of some of these strategies to optimally manage acute pain in children presenting to the ED.

The choice of pharmacological agent is based largely on the severity of the pain experienced by the child. However, the age of the child and their condition may play some role in influencing the agents chosen and the routes of administration. Table 36.23 provides a formulary of analgesic agents suitable for use in children with acute pain, which includes dosing regimens and the indications for use.

Mild pain is in most circumstances effectively managed with a non-opioid such as paracetamol or ibuprofen. A meta-analysis shows that there is limited evidence in children to support overall improved efficacy for one over the other.[395] However, two more recent RCTs comparing ibuprofen with paracetamol combined with codeine found that ibuprofen was at least as effective as the combination product for pain management in children with limb fractures.[514,515] A third RCT, comparing ibuprofen, paracetamol and codeine given separately, also showed improved efficacy of ibuprofen.[516] Although there is some concern about the role of prostaglandin in bone healing, there is no evidence from studies conducted in humans to confirm that NSAIDs have an effect on bone healing. Short-term use in healthy children also places them at low risk for the other side effects of NSAIDs,[517] making it reasonable to recommend their role in managing pain in children secondary to musculoskeletal injury.

Moderate and more-severe pain is most frequently controlled using opioids such as fentanyl, morphine and oxycodone. Fentanyl administered intranasally is widely used pre-hospital and in the ED as a first-line treatment for moderate to severe pain.[518] Figure 36.8 demonstrates the technique for administration. There are a number of studies which report its safety and efficacy and the role that it plays in improving time to analgesia.[519–521] These studies were conducted using a concentrated solution, which is more costly than the standard IV preparation of 100 µg/2 mL, more difficult to access and the margin for error much greater. Recent data suggest that the standard IV concentration confers adequate analgesia.[522,523] The quality of evidence remains low and there are calls for more robust studies to support current practice.[524]

Tramadol has gained some favour in ED pain management for adults with moderate to severe pain, and there are a number of studies conducted in children in postoperative models which show efficacy. However, it has yet to find a place in paediatric emergency medicine; there are no data to support its role and most emergency clinicians consider it unlikely to add any additional benefit to the agents in current use. Similarly, intravenous paracetamol has been shown to provide effective analgesia following surgery in adult ED patients, and in some studies to be as effective as morphine.[525,526] However, the data supporting safety and efficacy in children are more limited[527] and once again there are no data examining its role in the ED. Despite this, there are accepted indications for its use in

TABLE 36.23 Formulary of commonly used agents for managing acute pain and sedation in children

AGENT	DOSE	INDICATIONS	TIPS
Ibuprofen	5–10 mg/kg orally	Mild to moderate pain	May be more effective for some conditions than paracetamol, e.g. transient synovitis
Paracetamol	20 mg/kg orally (max 90 mg/kg/day)	Mild to moderate pain	Safe and effective Can be given in combination products, e.g. with codeine
Codeine	0.5–1.0 mg/kg IV	Moderate pain	Available in a range of combination products in tablet and liquid form Effect unreliable
Glucose	2 mL/procedure orally (max 5 mL/day)	Painful procedures in infants	Give several drops of glucose onto the tongue a minute or two before procedure commences and then at regular intervals throughout
Fentanyl	0.15 µg/kg intranasally	Moderate to severe pain	As effective as morphine given intranasally For larger volumes, dose can be divided and half given into each nostril
Lignocaine	1% solution	Local anaesthetic for painful conditions	Instil several drops into painful ear
Lignocaine	0.5–2% solution Bier's block: 3 mg/kg Infiltration: 3 mg/kg	Local anaesthesia for painful procedures	Can be used to infiltrate wound Used for short-term nerve block, e.g. for LAMP
Ketamine	1–1.5 mg/kg	Procedural sedation	Better results if given intravenously Give as a slow bolus (2–3 minutes) to prevent respiratory distress
Midazolam	0.5–1.0 mg/kg orally	Procedural sedation	Administer orally Intranasal administration is poorly tolerated, as it stings the nostril and runs down the back of the nose and is swallowed.
Morphine	0.05–0.1 mg/kg	Moderate to severe pain	Can be titrated intravenously until analgesia is achieved
Oxycodone	0.1 mg/kg	Moderate to severe pain	More reliable analgesia than codeine
Nitrous oxide (NO$_2$)	30–70% inhaled	Analgesia and sedation for painful procedures	Establish sedation (at least 5 minutes of NO$_2$) before commencing the procedure

IV: intravenously; LAMP: local anaesthesia, manipulation and plaster

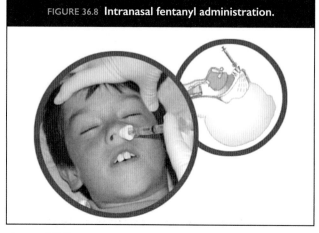

FIGURE 36.8 **Intranasal fentanyl administration.**

Courtesy Teleflex.

PRACTICE TIPS

ACUTE PAIN MANAGEMENT

- Infants and children should be treated with an appropriate agent at an appropriate dose to manage their pain.
- Intranasal fentanyl is an effective way of administering opioid analgesia quickly and without the need to insert an intravenous cannula.
- Intravenous paracetamol may be of benefit under specific circumstances.
- Local anaesthetics can be used to manage condition-specific pain, such as otalgia associated with otitis media, oropharyngeal pain secondary to stomatitis and pain secondary to fracture.

the ED and paediatric emergency clinicians are gaining some experience with its use.[528]

Local anaesthetic agents are frequently used alongside analgesics to manage condition-specific pain. Some obvious examples are nerve blocks following long-bone fracture. There are other occasions in paediatric emergency when these agents are used to manage pain and discomfort. However, data supporting their efficacy are limited. In one RCT, lignocaine used topically in the ear was shown to reduce earache in infants and children suffering otitis media.[187] Lignocaine in a viscous solution is often recommended for the pain and discomfort associated with gingivostomatitis and oral ulcers. However, a recent RCT conducted in an Australia tertiary paediatric ED has demonstrated that its use has no effect on oral intake.[529]

Procedural analgesia and sedation

Sedation is frequently used during procedures to reduce anxiety and improve cooperation. However, it is important to ensure that it is not used as an alternative to appropriate analgesics and the use of local anaesthetic agents. With few exceptions, children undergoing painful procedures should receive analgesia and/or local anaesthetic in addition to sedation. Paracetamol, ibuprofen, oxycodone, intranasal fentanyl and intravenous morphine should be considered as analgesia options for painful procedures.

Topical and infiltrated local anaesthetic agents such as lignocaine can be given prior to procedures such as intravenous cannula insertion, lumbar puncture, urinary catheter insertion, wound closure, FB removal and eye irrigation.

Nebulised lignocaine has been shown safe and effective at reducing the pain related to NG tube insertion in adults,[242,530] which has been rated as the most painful procedure performed in the ED.[480,531] Theoretically it should be of similar value in infants and young children. However, the only study to attempt to confirm this could not demonstrate similar results in young children and infants.[532] The authors question whether the considerable distress experienced by infants and children during NG tube insertion may have masked any alleviation of pain felt as a result of the lignocaine. However, delivery via a nebuliser was also a source of considerable distress for these children, making it impossible to recommend this strategy for infants and young children. Despite this, it is reasonable to consider use of nebulised lignocaine in older children who are unlikely to be distressed by a nebuliser. Furthermore, these data should prompt clinicians to consider alternatives such as a topical anaesthetic spray.

Sedation is almost universally achieved using nitrous oxide, midazolam or ketamine in Australian paediatric EDs.[533] The specifics of dose, indication and administration are detailed in Table 36.23. An increasing weight of evidence from a number of large case series demonstrates that nitrous oxide is a safe and effective way to sedate infants and children in the ED sufficiently to undergo diagnostic and therapeutic procedures.[534-538] Vomiting and desaturation are the most frequent side effects recorded, and occur at rates of approximately 6–7% and less than 1%, respectively. Published data do not record any serious adverse events. Interestingly, in a case series of 762 children the duration of fasting was shown to affect the rate of vomiting,

and deeper sedation with 70% nitrous oxide did not increase the number of adverse events.[539] Furthermore, deep sedation occurred in only 3% of children in this series, placing only a small number at risk of aspiration. The success of nitrous oxide for procedural sedation can be improved by ensuring that the child is adequately sedated before commencing the procedure, which may take 3–5 minutes. It can be difficult to achieve a satisfactory outcome where the procedure is rushed and the child becomes distressed before they have been adequately sedated.

Bone marrow toxicity and neurotoxicity are both reported with long-term use of nitrous oxide and neurotoxicity with short term use, although rarely. There are no data to guide maximum exposure, but it is recommended that alternatives are sought for patients with metabolic diseases, such as methonionine synthetase deficiency, homocystinuria and methylmalonic acidaemia. Data are not available to determine the risk, but pregnant women should also avoid exposure.[489]

Ketamine, which produces a dissociated state of sedation conferring analgesia, amnesia, sedation and immobility with preservation of airway tone, is used increasingly in procedural sedation in the ED. It is ideally suited for procedures that require the child to be completely still, such as suturing of facial lacerations, or that are likely to be particularly painful and distressing, such as fracture manipulation. Data from numerous studies and RCTs confirm that ketamine can be used effectively for procedural sedation in the ED with a low rate of side effects.[540-546]

The most common adverse events occurring in association with ketamine sedation are vomiting (12–17%), which occurs most frequently in the recovery phase, and hypersalivation (2–11%). Small numbers of children will require brief airway support such as suctioning due to hypersalivation. However, there are no reports of children requiring intubation as a result of ketamine sedation. Emergence reactions are acknowledged as a potential side effect associated with ketamine sedation. However, in a recent case series, the reported rate of emergence reactions was approximately 2%;[547] recovery in a quiet environment with minimal stimulus reduces the rate of this phenomenon. In many departments, midazolam is not routinely added to the sedation protocol to reduce the likelihood of an emergence reaction.

The prolonged recovery phase is one of the major limitations to ketamine sedation. A recent case series has demonstrated that intravenous administration of ketamine, rather than intramuscular, not only reduces the rate of some side effects but reduces the time to discharge following administration of ketamine by approximately 20 minutes.[547]

Sedation of children in the ED carries significant risk and measures should be employed to reduce the associated risks. EDs must be appropriately resourced (staffing and equipment) before attempting to sedate a patient. Staff providing sedation should be adequately trained to manage a sedated child, and should have current basic and advanced life support skills. Furthermore, children undergoing conscious sedation should have continuous monitoring and a trained clinician should be dedicated to managing the sedation and to monitor for side effects at all times until the child has recovered.

PROCEDURAL ANALGESIA AND SEDATION

- Analgesia, local anaesthesia and sedation should be used in combination for procedures likely to be painful.
- Nitrous oxide is a safe and effective way to provide sedation for a range of diagnostic and therapeutic procedures.
- Ketamine may be used where deeper sedation is required. However, greater resources will be required to provide safe and effective sedation.
- Intravenous administration of ketamine is recommended as it reduces the rate of side effects and the time to discharge.

Non-pharmacological strategies

Non-pharmacological strategies to alleviate pain and distress should also be considered for children with pain related to illness or injury and for those undergoing a painful and/or distressing procedure. There is a substantial volume of literature stressing the value of non-pharmacological measures, such as distraction and guided imagery in children with acute and chronic pain. Furthermore, there are a number of studies advocating for non-pharmacological techniques during painful procedures. However, the results from research evaluating its effectiveness are mixed.[548] A Cochrane review concentrating on the effect of these techniques for needle-related procedural pain in children concluded that there is preliminary evidence to indicate benefit.[549] However, the quality of the studies included was not ideal and additional RCTs are needed. There is a scarcity of studies focusing on use of these techniques in the ED, and what literature is available focuses on their effect during painful and distressing procedures. A recent RCT shows that distraction, the most frequently used technique, has a positive effect on the level of pain and distress experienced by children of all ages.[550]

Some paediatric EDs may have the luxury of having play therapists available to assist with distraction. However, the majority of children are seen in EDs which do not have these resources. Distraction can be provided by parents as well as staff, can be offered in the form of books, audiovisual aids, drawing and colouring-in, and should remain a priority despite limited resources. Bubble blowing, games such as 'I-spy' and storytelling can be simple ways to provide distraction.

Techniques such as immobilisation of injuries, dressing burns, hot packs, ice packs and other similar measures are useful adjuncts to pharmacological treatment. However, infants and young children may tolerate some of these measures poorly. This requires some creativity on the part of the clinician to improve compliance. Using the child's imagination and playing games can be one way of overcoming a young child's reluctance to cooperate. Involving the parents, such as having them hold a heat or cold pack in place while cuddling a child or talking to them to distract them from or to persuade them to accept a treatment, can be another way to improve compliance. Pain management should be multimodal, and this may mean that pharmacological treatments are used to make non-

pharmacological techniques possible; for example, providing nitrous oxide while a backslab for support is applied.

Administration of small volumes (0.5–1 mL aliquots) of oral glucose solutions (25–35%) to newborns and very young infants moments before a painful procedure and at regular intervals throughout has been shown to reduce the pain experienced during the procedure.[551] This should be standard practice for infants having any painful procedure performed.

NON-PHARMACOLOGICAL STRATEGIES TO MANAGE PAIN AND DISTRESS

- Employing non-pharmacological strategies to manage pain and distress should not be overlooked.
- Oral glucose (25–35%) solution should be given in small aliquots (0.5–1 mL) to neonates and infants having painful procedures.
- Distraction can be of great value to minimise the distress of procedures and improve cooperation.

Health promotion

Acute healthcare is the principal priority during an emergency contact; however, it is also an opportunity for emergency clinicians to provide health education and address other health and lifestyle issues such as immunisation, smoking cessation and weight management. Clinicians should be aware of the various primary health and social services available to support families with children to provide recommendations where appropriate. In addition to providing clinical assessment, maternal and child healthcare nurses are often an excellent support and source of local community-based, health-related information for families of neonates, infants and young children.

Opportunistic immunisation

The recommended schedule of immunisations is government-funded and is made available through local councils and other health services. The current Australian and New Zealand schedules can be seen in Table 36.5. However, for a number of reasons, significant numbers of children are inadequately vaccinated. In most circumstances, children fall behind for practical reasons such as illness at the time that they are due for their next vaccination. It is reasonable to administer the scheduled vaccines which have become due or outstanding during the ED visit for most of these children. Guidance about contraindications and likely adverse reactions and parent information sheets can be accessed from the Australian Immunisation Handbook website (see Useful websites at the end of the chapter). Children who are well behind the schedule should be referred to their GP, an immunisation clinic or a maternal child health nurse to have a 'catch-up' schedule planned. The Australian Immunisation Handbook also provides recommendations for scheduling catch-up vaccinations.[4]

It is uncommon for parents to object to immunisation for their children. However, where this is the case, the majority cite the perceived risks associated with vaccination as the reason for their objection, despite scientific evidence demonstrating that the risks to health are greater from the disease than from the vaccination. These families should be referred to an immunisation or infectious diseases clinic to have an opportunity to discuss their concerns and explore the options. A number of families will then elect to vaccinate their children.

Weight management
Obesity has become a major health concern in Australasia, and large numbers of children are now overweight. Excessive weight in childhood contributes to poor self-esteem, poor eating habits and lifelong weight-related health issues. Weight management is not the remit of the ED. However, the opportunity to address this important health problem should not be ignored.

The importance of healthy eating and exercise should be emphasised and referrals made to dietitians and other experts to address weight-management issues.

Smoking cessation
Passive smoking is a widely recognised risk to health, increasing the risk of a number of diseases, e.g. respiratory illnesses, meningococcal disease, Perthes' disease and sudden infant death syndrome (SIDS). Efforts should be made to encourage parents to quit smoking and information provided to assist them. It has been shown that parents expect to be asked about smoking and advised to stop when consulting a healthcare professional about their child's health.[552] Parents may be referred to their GP or Quit for smoking cessation advice, programs and support.

SUMMARY
The provision of emergency care to children requires that the clinician recognises the anatomical and physiological differences that exist between adults, children and infants, and understands the impact of immaturity on illness and injury, assessment and management. This chapter has provided a summary of these differences, a guide to recognition of serious illness and an overview of the presentation and management of many common paediatric presentations. This chapter should be read in conjunction with the many other chapters in this text that address presentations common in children.

CASE STUDY I

A mother brings her 4-week-old infant to the emergency department (ED), stating that the baby has been crying more than usual for 2 days. The baby is alert, there are no signs of increased respiratory effort and the baby is pink and warm.

1. Your triage assessment should identify which of the following?
   A. Airway—patent, Breathing—normal, Circulation—normal, Disability—normal, Risk factors—nil
   B. Airway—patent, Breathing—normal, Circulation—normal, Disability—normal, Risk factors—age
   C. Airway—patent, Breathing—normal, Circulation—normal, Disability—normal, Risk factors—age, increased crying
   D. Airway—patent, Breathing—normal, Circulation—normal, Disability—irritable, Risk factors—age, increased crying

2. Following more-extensive examination of the baby, it is also noted that the heart rate is 200 beats/minute. You note that:
   A. This is within normal limits for an infant of this age.
   B. This may be normal if the blood pressure is also normal.
   C. A rate this high must be caused by a dysrhythmia such as supraventricular tachycardia.

   D. This is high for this age, which may reflect significant illness.

3. The temperature is also taken rectally and found to be 36.6°C. This may be for the following reason:
   A. The room is cool and the baby is exposed.
   B. This is within the normal temperature range for young babies.
   C. The baby may be hypothermic secondary to infection.
   D. Rectal temperature measurement is unreliable.

4. If the infant's temperature had been elevated, the management should include:
   A. Fever reduction if the infant is miserable, using antipyretics
   B. Fever reduction using antipyretics, tepid sponging
   C. Fever reduction using antipyretics
   D. Fever reduction if the infant is miserable, using antipyretics, tepid sponging

5. If the baby begins to show signs of poor peripheral perfusion, treatment should include:
   A. An intravenous fluid bolus of 40 mL 4% dextrose and 1/5 Normal saline
   B. An intravenous bolus of 80 mL Normal saline

C. An intravenous bolus of 80 mL 4% dextrose and 1/5 Normal saline

D. An intravenous bolus of 40 mL Normal saline

6. The following antibiotic regimen should be given to treat likely sepsis empirically:

A. Penicillin and cefotaxime

B. Flucloxacillin and gentamicin

C. Cefotaxime and gentamicin

D. Flucloxacillin and cefotaxime

Answers to Case Study Questions can be found on evolve
http://evolve.emergencytrauma.curtis

CASE STUDY 2

A child aged 14 months with no past history has developed shortness of breath following a few days of cold symptoms. An ambulance is called by the parents and the child is transported to the ED of the local hospital.

1. As the first clinician to assess the child, your primary assessment parameter is:

   A. Work of breathing

   B. Oxygen saturations

   C. Respiratory rate

   D. Lung sounds

2. Wheeze is commonly associated with a number of conditions. Which of these sets includes one where wheeze is unlikely to be associated with this condition?

   A. Asthma, bronchiolitis, viral pneumonia

   B. Bronchiolitis, asthma, inhaled FB

   C. Asthma, croup, bronchiolitis

   D. Anaphylaxis, asthma, bronchiolitis

3. This child has moderate-marked increased work of breathing, widespread inspiratory and expiratory wheeze and his respiratory rate is 58. Therapy should commence with:

   A. A dose of adrenaline administered via nebuliser

   B. Oral steroids

   C. 5 mg salbutamol and 250 mcg ipratropium bromide via nebuliser

   D. 6 puffs salbutamol and 4 puffs ipratropium via MDI and spacer

   E. 6 puffs salbutamol via MDI and spacer

4. This child's oxygen saturations when measured are 86% in room air. The following is initially the most suitable delivery system and flow of oxygen:

   A. Nasal cannula at 6 L/min

   B. Nasal cannula at 2 L/min

   C. Face mask at 2 L/min

   D. Face mask at 6 L/min

5. Steroids are prescribed. They should be administered:

   A. Orally

   B. Intravenously

   C. Inhaled

   D. A or B—there is no significant difference in efficacy or onset

6. Children should be given a dose of salbutamol when:

   A. Wheeze can be heard (audibly or on auscultation).

   B. Wheeze can be heard and there is increased work of breathing.

   C. There is a decrease in saturations and an increased respiratory rate.

   D. Regularly to prevent deterioration.

   E. B and C.

7. There is evidence for the following agents to treat critical asthma:

   A. Aminophylline

   B. Magnesium sulphate

   C. Ketamine

   D. A and B

   E. A, B and C

8. For each of the following statements, state whether it is true or false:

   A. All children admitted with asthma should have a chest X-ray.

   B. It is unknown whether salbutamol administered via MDI and spacer is as effective as nebulised salbutamol to treat critical asthma.

   C. Children under the age of 12 months can't be diagnosed with asthma.

Answers to Case Study Questions can be found on evolve
http://evolve.emergencytrauma.curtis

USEFUL WEBSITES

Advanced Paediatric Life Support, www.apls.org.au

Australian Immunisation Handbook, www.health.gov.au/internet/immunise/publishing.nsf/Content/Handbook10-home

Auatralian Medicines Handbook, Children's Dosing Companion, https://shop.amh.net.au/products/books/2015

Blue Book, http://health.vic.gov.au/immunisation/factsheets.htm

Department of Health (Victoria), parent fact sheets, http://health.vic.gov.au/immunisation/factsheets.htm

NSW Kids and Families Policy Directives and Guidelines, www.kidsfamilies.health.nsw.gov.au/publications/policy-directives-guidelines/

DermNet NZ: the dermatology resource, www.dermnet.org.nz

New Zealand Immunisation schedule, www.moh.govt.nz/moh.nsf/indexmh/immunisation-schedule-html

Pediatric Emergency Medicine Database, www.pemdatabase.org/

Royal Children's Hospital, Melbourne, clinical practice guidelines, www.rch.org.au/clinicalguide/index.cfm?doc_id=5033

Royal Children's Hospital, Melbourne, parent fact sheets, www.rch.org.au/kidsinfo/factsheets.cfm

Sydney Children's Hospital, parent fact sheets, www.schn.health.nsw.gov.au/parents-and-carers/fact-sheets

Therapeutic Guidelines: Antibiotics, www.tg.org.au/

Westmead Hospital, parent fact sheets, www.chw.edu.au/parents/factsheets

Victorian Paediatric Orthopaedica Network www.health.vic.gov.au/vpon/

REFERENCES

1. Emergency Nurses Association. NEPC provider manual. 4th edn. Emergency Nurses Association, 2013.
2. Hewson P et al. Clinical markers of serious illness in young infants: a multicentre follow-up study. J Paediatrics Child Health 2000;36(3): 221–5.
3. Hewson PH et al. Markers of serious illness in infants under 6 months old presenting to a children's hospital. Archives of Disease in Childhood 1990;65:750–6.
4. National Health and Medical Research Council. The Australian Immunisation Handbook. 10th ed. 2013, Canberra: National Capital Printers.
5. Ministry of Health (New Zealand), Immunisation Handbook 2011. Wellington: Ministry of Health, 2011.
6. Higgins D et al. Mandatory reporting of child abuse and neglect. NCP Clearinghouse Australian Institute of Family Studies; 2009.
7. Australian Institute of Family Studies. Mandatory reporting of child abuse and neglect. 2013. Online. www.aifs.gov.au/cfca/pubs/factsheets/a141787/; accessed 12 March 2014.
8. Buist M et al. Recognising clinical instability in hospital patients before cardiac arrest or unplanned admission to intensive care. A pilot study in a tertiary-care hospital. Medical Journal of Australia 1999;171(1):22–5.
9. Rotta AT, Wiryawan B. Respiratory emergencies in children. Respiratory Care 2003;48(3):248–58; discussion 258–60.
10. Gorelick MH et al. Performance of a novel clinical score, the Pediatric Asthma Severity Score (PASS), in the evaluation of acute asthma. Academic Emergency Medicine 2004;11(1):10–18.
11. Asthma Strategy Group, Asthma Best Practice Guidelines, 2001, Royal Children's Hospital: Melbourne.
12. Yung M, South M, Byrt T. Evaluation of an asthma severity score. J Paediatr Child Health 1996;32(3):261–4.
13. Thornton AJ et al. Field trials of the Baby Check score card: mothers scoring their babies at home. Archives of Disease in Childhood 1991;66(1):106–10.
14. Thornton AJ et al. Symptoms in 298 infants under 6 months old, seen at home. Archives of Disease in Childhood 1990;65(3):280–5.
15. Advanced Life Support Group, Advanced Paediatric Life Support: The practical approach. 5th edn. London: Wiley–Blackwell; 2007.
16. Otieno H et al. Are bedside features of shock reproducible between different observers? Archives of Disease in Childhood 2004;89(10):977–9.
17. Mackenzie A, Barnes G, Shann F. Clinical signs of dehydration in children. Lancet 1989;2(8663):605–7.
18. Saavedra JM et al. Capillary refilling (skin turgor) in the assessment of dehydration. Am J Dis Child 1991;145(3):296–8.
19. Gorelick MH, Shaw KN, Baker MD. Effect of ambient temperature on capillary refill in healthy children. Pediatrics 1993;92(5):699–702.
20. Martin H, Norman M. Skin microcirculation before and after local warming in infants delivered vaginally or by caesarean section. Acta Paediatrica 1997;86(3):261–7.
21. Raju NV et al. Capillary refill time in the hands and feet of normal newborn infants. Clinical Pediatrics 1999;38(3):139–44.
22. Tibby SM, Hatherill M, Murdoch IA. Capillary refill and core–peripheral temperature gap as indicators of haemodynamic status in paediatric intensive care patients. Arch Dis Childhood 1999;80(2):163–6.

23. Crellin D. Fluid management for children presenting to the emergency department: Guidelines for clinical practice. Australasian Emergency Nursing Journal 2008;11(1).

24. Henning R. Fluid resuscitation in children. Emergency Medicine, 1995. Second Symposium on Fluid Replacement:57–62.

25. Goldstein B, Giroir B, Randolph A. International pediatric sepsis consensus conference: definitions for sepsis and organ dysfunction in pediatrics. Pediatric Critical Care Medicine 2005;6(1):2–8.

26. Haque IU, Zaritsky AL. Analysis of the evidence for the lower limit of systolic and mean arterial pressure in children. Pediatric Critical Care Medicine 2007;8(2):138–44.

27. Bailey RH, Bauer JH. A review of common errors in the indirect measurement of blood pressure. Sphygmomanometry. Archives of Internal Medicine 1993;153(24):2741–8.

28. Clark JA et al. Discrepancies between direct and indirect blood pressure measurements using various recommendations for arm cuff selection. Pediatrics 2002;110(5):920–3.

29. Hazell W, Wilkins B. Disorders of fluids, electrolytes and acid–base, in Textbook of paediatric emergency medicine, P. Cameron et al. eds. 2006, Churchill Livingstone: Edinburgh.

30. Advanced Life Support Group, Advanced Paediatric Life Support: The practical approach. 4th edn. London: Blackwell Publishing; 2005.

31. Ledbetter L. Can they or can they not? Nurses' ability to quantify stool in superabsorbent diapers. Journal of Pediatric Nursing 2006;21(4):325–8.

32. Holmes JF et al. Performance of the pediatric Glasgow Coma Scale in children with blunt head trauma. Academic Emergency Medicine 2005;12(9):814–19.

33. Advanced Life Support Committee of the Australian Resuscitation Council, Paediatric advanced life support. The Australian Resuscitation Council Guidelines. Medical Journal of Australia 1996;165:199–206.

34. Tu Y-F et al. Frequency and prediction of abnormal findings on neuroimaging of infants with bulging anterior fontanelles. Academic Emergency Medicine 2005;12(12):1185–90.

35. Whitby S et al. Analysis of the process of triage: the use and outcome of the National Triage Scale, 1997, Liverpool Health Service.

36. Craig JV et al. Infrared ear thermometry compared with rectal thermometry in children: a systematic review. Lancet 2002;360(9333):603–9.

37. Devrim I et al. Measurement accuracy of fever by tympanic and axillary thermometry. Pediatric Emergency Care 2007;23(1):16–19.

38. Dodd SR et al. In: A systematic review, infrared ear thermometry for fever diagnosis in children finds poor sensitivity. Journal of Clinical Epidemiology 2006;59(4):354–7.

39. El-Radhi AS, Barry W. Thermometry in paediatric practice 10.1136/adc.2005.088831. Arch Dis Child 2006;91(4):351–6.

40. Muma BK et al. Comparison of rectal, axillary, and tympanic membrane temperatures in infants and young children. Annals of Emergency Medicine 1991;20(1):41–4.

41. Nimah MM et al. Infrared tympanic thermometry in comparison with other temperature measurement techniques in febrile children. Pediatric Critical Care Medicine 2006;7(1):48–55.

42. Romanovsky AA et al. A difference of 5 degrees C between ear and rectal temperatures in a febrile patient. Am J Emerg Med 1997;15(4):383–5.

43. Duce SJ. A systematic review of the literature to determine optimal methods of temperature measurement in neonates, infants and children (Structured abstract). Database of Abstracts of Reviews of Effects 1996:124.

44. Benzinger M. Tympanic thermometry in surgery and anesthesia. JAMA 1969;209(8):1207–11.

45. Cusson RM, Madonia JA, Taekman JB, The effect of environment on body site temperatures in full–term neonates. Nursing Research 1997;46(4):202–7.

46. Falzon A et al. How reliable is axillary temperature measurement? Acta Paediatr 2003;92(3):309–13.

47. Chue A et al. Comparability of tympanic and oral mercury thermometers at high ambient temperatures. BMC Research Notes 2012;5(1):356.

48. Willis AP et al. Not a NICE CT protocol for the acutely head injured child. Clinical Radiology 2008;63(2):165–9.

49. Crellin D. Paediatric Triage, in Emergency Triage Education Kit. The Commonwealth Department of Health and Ageing: Canberra, 2007.

50. Crellin DJ, Johnston L. Poor agreement in application of the Australasian Triage Scale to paediatric emergency department presentations. Contemporary Nurse 2003;15(1–2):48–60.

51. Durojaiye L, O'Meara M. A study of triage of paediatric patients in Australia. Emerg Med (Fremantle) 2002;14(1):67–76.

52. LeVasseur SA, Considine J, Charles A. Consistency of triage in Victoria's emergency departments: consistency of Triage Report, 2001, Monash Institute of Health Services. Research Report to the Victorian Department of Health Services.

53. George S et al. Differences in priorities assigned to patients by triage nurses and by consultant physicians in accident and emergency departments. J Epidemiol Commun Health 1993;47(4):312–15.

54. Standen P, Dilley S. A review of triage nursing practice and experience in Victorian public hospitals. Emergency Medicine 1997;9:301–5.

55. Gerdtz M, Bucknall T. Australian triage nurses' decision-making and scope of practice. Australian Journal of Advanced Nursing 2000;18(1):24–33.

56. Gerdtz MF. Triage Nurses Clinical decision making: A multi-method study of practice processes and influences. The University of Melbourne: Melbourne, 2003.

57. Crellin DJ, Johnston L. Who is responsible for pediatric triage decisions in Australian emergency departments? A description of the educational and experiential preparation of general and pediatric emergency nurses. Pediatric Emergency Care 2002;18(5):382–8.

58. Bentley J. Facilities for children in accident and emergency departments. NT Research 1996;1:206–15.

59. Gay J. Caring for children in A & E. Paediatric Nursing 1991;3(7):21–3.

60. McMenamin C. Making A&E less traumatic for children. Paediatric nurses in accident and emergency. Professional Nurse 1995;10(5):310–12.

61. Royal College of Nursing Children, E.S.I. Group. Nursing children in the accident and emergency department 1998, London, The Royal College of Nursing of the United Kingdom.

62. Royal College of Paediatrics and Child Health, Accident and Emergency Services for Children. Report of a Multidisciplinary Working Party, 1999, Royal College of Paediatrics and Child Health, 8 June 1999.

63. Scott H. Children are receiving inadequate care in A&E. British Journal of Nursing 1997;6(13):724.

64. Seidel J. Emergency medical services for children. Emergency Medicine Clinics of North America 1995;13(2):255–66.

65. Watson S. Children's nurses in the accident and emergency department: literature review. Accident & Emergency Nursing 2000;8(2):92–7.

66. Australasian College for Emergency Medicine. Guidelines for implementation of the Australasian Triage Scale in Emergency Departments. 2013.

67. Cole TJ et al. Baby Check and the Avon infant mortality study. Archives of Disease in Childhood 1991;66(9):1077–8.

68. McCarthy PL et al. History and observation variables in assessing febrile children. Pediatrics 1980;65(6):1090–5.

69. McCarthy PL et al. Further definition of history and observation variables in assessing febrile children. Pediatrics 1981;67(5):687–93.

70. McCarthy PL et al. Predictive value of abnormal physical examination findings in ill-appearing and well-appearing febrile children. Pediatrics 1985;76(2):167–71.

71. McCarthy PL et al. Observation, history, and physical examination in diagnosis of serious illnesses in febrile children less than or equal to 24 months. Journal of Pediatrics 1987;110(1):26–30.

72. Stanton AN, Downham MA, Oakley JR. Terminal symptoms in children dying suddenly and unexpectantly at home. BMJ 1978;2:1249–51.

73. Waskerwitz S, Berkelhamer JE. Outpatient bacteremia: Clinical findings in children under two years with intial temperatures of 39.5°C or higher. Journal of Pediatrics 1981;99(2):231–3.

74. Considine J, LeVasseur S, Charles A. Consistency of triage in Victoria's emergency departments: literature review, 2001, Monash Institute of Health Services Research. Report to the Victorian Department of Human Services: Melbourne.

75. Kumar N et al. Triage score for severity of illness. Indian Pediatrics 2003;40(3):204–10.

76. Emergency Nurses Association Victoria, Position statements: triage and educational preparation of triage nurses, 2000, Emergency Nurses Association, Victoria.

77. Crellin D. How are children different?, in Paediatric trauma manual, Bevan C, Officer C, eds. Melbourne; 2004.

78. Browne GJ, Gaudry PL, Lam L. A triage observation scale improves the reliability of the National Triage Scale. Emergency Medicine 1997;9:283–288.

79. Cain P, Waldrop RD, Jones J, Improved pediatric patient flow in a general emergency department by altering triage criteria. Acad Emerg Med 1996;3(1):65–71.

80. Wiebe RA, Rosen LM. Triage in the emergency department. Emergency Medicine Clinics of North America 1991;9(3):491–505.

81. Dieckmann, RA, Brownstein D, Gausche-Hill M. The pediatric assessment triangle: a novel approach for the rapid evaluation of children. Pediatric Emergency Care 2010;26(4):312–15.

82. Kelly J et al. The Paediatric Observation Priority Score (POPS); A useful tool to predict the likelihood of admissions from the emergency department. Emergency Medicine Journal 2013;30(10):877–8.

83. Hewson PH, Gollan RA. A simple hospital triaging system for infants with acute illness. J Paediatr Child Health 1995;31(1):29–32.

84. American Academy of Pediatrics. Pediatric education for prehospital professionals: PEPP textbook. Sudbury, MA: Jones & Bartlett Publishers, 2006.

85. Henning R. Respiratory failure. In: Care of the critically ill child, Macnab A, Macrae D, Henning R, eds. Churchill Livingstone: Edinburgh, 1999.

86. Aung K, Htay T. Vasopressin for cardiac arrest: a systematic review and meta-analysis. Archives of Internal Medicine 2005;165(1):17–24.

87. Milner AD, Greenough A. Applied respiratory physiology. Current Paediatrics 2006;16:406–12.

88. Rojas, MX, Granados Rugeles C, Charry-Anzola LP. Oxygen therapy for lower respiratory tract infections in children between 3 months and 15 years of age. Cochrane Database of Systematic Reviews 2009(1):CD005975.

89. Frey B, Shann F. Oxygen administration in infants. Archives of Disease in Childhood Fetal & Neonatal Edition 2003;88(2):F84–8.

90. Cambridge University Hospitals. Infant with nasal cannula [image]. www.cuh.org.uk/resources/images/rosie/neonatal/nicu/how_we_care/vital_needs/nasal_cannula_131008.jpg.

91. Myers TRC. American Association for Respiratory, AARC Clinical Practice Guideline: selection of an oxygen delivery device for neonatal and pediatric patients—2002 revision & update. Respiratory Care 2002;47(6):707–16.

92. Carter BG et al. Oxygen delivery using self-inflating resuscitation bags. Pediatric Critical Care Medicine 2005;6(2):125–8.

93. Tibballs J, Carter B, Whittington N. A disadvantage of self-inflating resuscitation bags. Anaesthesia & Intensive Care 2000;28(5):587.

94. Davies P et al. The efficacy of noncontact oxygen delivery methods. [Erratum appears in Pediatrics. 2006 Sep;118(3):1325]. Pediatrics 2002;110(5):964–7.

95. Blake DF et al. The efficacy of oxygen wafting using different delivery devices, flow rates and device positioning. Australasian Emergency Nursing 2014;17(3):119–25.

96. Gausche M et al. Effect of out-of-hospital pediatric endotracheal intubation on survival and neurological outcome: a controlled clinical trial.[see comment][erratum appears in JAMA 2000 Jun 28;283(24):3204]. JAMA 2000;283(6):783–90.

97. Khine HH et al. Comparison of cuffed and uncuffed endotracheal tubes in young children during general anesthesia. Anesthesiology 1997;86(3):627–31; discussion 27A.

98. Newth CJ et al. The use of cuffed versus uncuffed endotracheal tubes in pediatric intensive care. Journal of Pediatrics 2004;144(3):333–7.

99. Weiss M et al. Prospective randomized controlled multi-centre trial of cuffed or uncuffed endotracheal tubes in small children. British Journal of Anaesthesia 2009;103(6):867–73.

100. Henning R. Assisted ventilation. In: Care of the critically ill child, Macnab A, Macrae D, Henning R, eds. Churchill Livingstone: Edinburgh, 1999.

101. Loh LE, Chan YH, Chan I. Noninvasive ventilation in children: a review. Jornal de Pediatria 2007;83(2 Suppl):S91–9.

102. Schibler A et al. Reduced intubation rates for infants after introduction of high-flow nasal prong oxygen delivery. Intensive Care Medicine 2011;37(5):847–52.

103. Brink FT, Duke T, Evans J. High-flow nasal prong oxygen therapy or nasopharyngeal continuous positive airway pressure for children with moderate-to-severe respiratory distress? Pediatric Critical Care Medicine 2013;14(7):e326–31.

104. Spentzas T et al. Children with respiratory distress treated with high-flow nasal cannula. Journal of Intensive Care Medicine 2009;24(5):323–8.

105. Beggs S et al. High-flow nasal cannula therapy for infants with bronchiolitis. Cochrane Database of Systematic Reviews 2014;DOI: 10.1002/14651858.CD009609.pub2.

106. Mayfield S et al. High-flow nasal cannula therapy for respiratory support in children. Cochrane Database of Systematic Reviews 2014;DOI: 10.1002/14651858.CD009850.pub2.

107. Cohen S et al. Suspected foreign body inhalation in children: what are the indications for bronchoscopy? Journal of Pediatrics 2009;155(2):276–80.

108. Foltran F et al. Inhaled foreign bodies in children: A global perspective on their epidemiological, clinical, and preventive aspects. Pediatric Pulmonology 2013;48(4):344–51.

109. Foltran F et al. Foreign bodies in the airways: A meta-analysis of published papers. International Journal of Pediatric Otorhinolaryngology 2012;76, Supplement 1(0):S12–19.

110. Reilly J et al. Pediatric aerodigestive foreign body injuries are complications related to timeliness of diagnosis. Laryngoscope 1997;107(1):17–20.

111. Wiseman NE. The diagnosis of foreign body aspiration in childhood. Journal of Pediatric Surgery 1984;19(5):531–5.

112. Rider G, Wilson CL. Small parts aspiration, ingestion, and choking in small children: findings of the small parts research project. Risk Analysis 1996;16(3):321–30.

113. Leung AKC, Kellner JD, Johnson DW. Viral croup: a current perspective. Journal of Pediatric Health Care 2004;18(6):297–301.

114. Russell K et al. Glucocorticoids for croup. Cochrane Database of Systematic Reviews 2011;DOI: 10.1002/14651858.CD001955.pub3.

115. Fifoot AA, Ting JY. Comparison between single-dose oral prednisolone and oral dexamethasone in the treatment of croup: a randomized, double-blinded clinical trial. Emergency Medicine Australasia 2007;19(1):51–8.

116. Geelhoed GC. Budesonide offers no advantage when added to oral dexamethasone in the treatment of croup. Pediatric Emergency Care 2005;21(6):359–62.

117. Geelhoed GC, Macdonald WB. Oral dexamethasone in the treatment of croup: 0.15 mg/kg versus 0.3 mg/kg versus 0.6 mg/kg. Pediatric Pulmonology 1995;20(6):362–8.

118. Geelhoed GC, Macdonald WB. Oral and inhaled steroids in croup: a randomized, placebo-controlled trial. Pediatric Pulmonology 1995;20(6):355–61.

119. Geelhoed GC, Turner J, Macdonald WB. Efficacy of a small single dose of oral dexamethasone for outpatient croup: a double blind placebo controlled clinical trial [see comments]. BMJ 1996;313(7050):140–2.

120. Port C. Towards evidence based emergency medicine: best BETs from the Manchester Royal Infirmary. BET 4. Dose of dexamethasone in croup. Emergency Medicine Journal 2009;26(4):291–2.

121. Parker R, Powell CV, Kelly A-M. How long does stridor at rest persist in croup after the administration of oral prednisolone? Emergency Medicine Australasia 2004;16(2):135–8.

122. Bjornson C et al. Nebulized epinephrine for croup in children. Cochrane Database of Systematic Reviews 2013;DOI: 10.1002/14651858.CD006619.pub3.

123. Walker DM. Update on epinephrine (adrenaline) for pediatric emergencies. Current Opinion in Pediatrics 2009;21(3):313–19.

124. Moore M, Little P. Humidified air inhalation for treating croup: a systematic review and meta-analysis. Family Practice 2007;24(4):295–301.

125. National Asthma Council Australia. Asthma management handbook. South Melbourne: National Asthma Council Australia Ltd, 2006.

126. Australian Centre for Asthma Monitoring. Asthma in Australia 2011: with a focus chapter on chronic obstructive pulmonary disease, AIHW: Canberra, 2011.

127. Ministry of Health. The Health of New Zealand Children: Key findings of the New Zealand Health Survey 2011/12, 2012, Ministry of Health: Wellington.

128. Lai CKW et al. Global variation in the prevalence and severity of asthma symptoms: phase three of the International Study of Asthma and Allergies in Childhood (ISAAC). Thorax 2009;64(6):476–83.

129. Australian Centre for Asthma Monitoring. Asthma in Australian children: findings from Growing up in Australia, the longitudinal study of Australian children, 2009, Cat. no. ACM 17. AIHW: Canberra.

130. Bousquet J et al. Uniform definition of asthma severity, control, and exacerbations: document presented for the World Health Organization Consultation on Severe Asthma. Journal of Allergy and Clinical Immunology 2010;126(5):926–38.

131. Cates CJ, Welsh EJ, Rowe HB. Holding chambers (spacers) versus nebulisers for beta-agonist treatment of acute asthma. Cochrane Database of Systematic Reviews 2013;DOI: 10.1002/14651858.CD000052.pub3.

132. Katz RW et al. Safety of continuous nebulized albuterol for bronchospasm in infants and children. [Erratum appears in Pediatrics 1994 Feb;93(2):A28]. Pediatrics 1993;92(5):666–9.

133. Singh M, Kumar L. Continuous nebulised salbutamol and oral once a day prednisolone in status asthmaticus. Archives of Disease in Childhood 1993;69(4):416–19.

134. Browne GJ, Trieu L, Van Asperen P. Randomized, double-blind, placebo-controlled trial of intravenous salbutamol and nebulized ipratropium bromide in early management of severe acute asthma in children presenting to an emergency department. [Summary for patients in J Fam Pract. 2002 Jul;51(7):596; PMID: 12160489]. Critical Care Medicine 2002;30(2):448–53.

135. Griffiths B, Ducharme FM. Combined inhaled anticholinergics and short-acting beta2-agonists for initial treatment of acute asthma in children. Cochrane Database of Systematic Reviews 2013;DOI: 10.1002/14651858.CD000060.pub2.

136. Plotnick LH, Ducharme FM. Combined inhaled anticholinergic agents and beta-2-agonists for initial treatment of acute asthma in children. (Cochrane Review), in The Cochrane Library John Wiley & Sons, Ltd: Chichester, UK. 2000:CD000060.

137. Qureshi F et al. Effect of nebulized ipratropium on the hospitalization rates of children with asthma. New England Journal of Medicine 1998;339(15):1030–5.

138. Zorc JJ et al. Ipratropium bromide added to asthma treatment in the pediatric emergency department. Pediatrics 1999; 103(4 Pt 1):748–52.

139. Rowe BH et al. Early emergency department treatment of acute asthma with systemic corticosteroids. Cochrane Database of Systematic Reviews, 2001.

140. Barnett PL et al. Intravenous versus oral corticosteroids in the management of acute asthma in children. Annals of Emergency Medicine 1997;29(2):212–17.

141. Edmonds M et al. Early use of inhaled corticosteroids in the emergency department treatment of acute asthma. Cochrane Database of Systematic Reviews, 2003.

142. Mitra Andrew AD et al. Intravenous aminophylline for acute severe asthma in children over two years receiving inhaled bronchodilators. Cochrane Database of Systematic Reviews, 2005.

143. Rowe BH et al. Magnesium sulfate for treating exacerbations of acute asthma in the emergency department. Cochrane Database of Systematic Reviews 2000;DOI: 10.1002/14651858.CD001490.

144. Powell C et al. Inhaled magnesium sulfate in the treatment of acute asthma. Cochrane Database of Systematic Reviews 2012;DOI: 10.1002/14651858.CD003898.pub5.

145. Jat Kana R, Chawla D. Ketamine for management of acute exacerbations of asthma in children. Cochrane Database of Systematic Reviews 2012;DOI: 10.1002/14651858.CD009293.pub2.

146. Southern Health, Ensuring infants and children with bronchiolitis receive the best possible care. Evidence-based practice guideline for the management of bronchiolitis in infants and children. 2006: Online. www.mihsr.monash.org/hfk/pdf/hfkbronchguideline.pdf.

147. Gadomski AM, Brower M. Bronchodilators for bronchiolitis. Cochrane Database of Systematic Reviews 2010; DOI: 10.1002/14651858.CD001266.pub3.

148. Hartling L et al. Oral versus intravenous rehydration for treating dehydration due to gastroenteritis in children. Cochrane Database of Systematic Reviews 2006;DOI: 10.1002/14651858.CD004390.pub2.

149. Hartling L et al. Epinephrine for bronchiolitis. Cochrane Database of Systematic Reviews 2011;DOI: 10.1002/14651858.CD003123.pub3.

150. King V et al. Pharmacologic treatment of bronchiolitis in infants and children: a systematic review. Archives of Pediatrics & Adolescent Medicine 2004;158(2):127–37.

151. Fernandes RM et al. Glucocorticoids for acute viral bronchiolitis in infants and young children. Cochrane Database of Systematic Reviews 2013;DOI: 10.1002/14651858.CD004878.pub4.

152. Zhang L et al. Nebulised hypertonic saline solution for acute bronchiolitis in infants. Cochrane Database of Systematic Reviews 2013;DOI: 10.1002/14651858.CD006458.pub3.

153. Oakley E et al. Nasogastric hydration versus intravenous hydration for infants with bronchiolitis: a randomised trial. The Lancet Respiratory Medicine 2013;1(2):113–20.

154. Munoz FM. Pertussis in infants, children, and adolescents: diagnosis, treatment, and prevention. Seminars in Pediatric Infectious Diseases 2006;17(1):14–19.

155. Tanaka M et al. Trends in pertussis among infants in the United States, 1980–1999. JAMA 2003;290(22):2968–75.

156. Bisgard KM et al. Infant pertussis: who was the source? Pediatric Infectious Disease Journal 2004;23(11):985–9.

157. Centers for Disease, C, Prevention, Pertussis—United States, 2001–2003. Morbidity & Mortality Weekly Report 2005;54:1283–6.

158. Edwards KM. Overview of pertussis: focus on epidemiology, sources of infection, and long term protection after infant vaccination. Pediatric Infectious Disease Journal 2005;24(6 Suppl):S104–8.

159. Elliott E et al. National study of infants hospitalized with pertussis in the acellular vaccine era. Pediatric Infectious Disease Journal 2004;23(3):246–52.

160. Crowcroft NS et al. Severe and unrecognised: pertussis in UK infants. [Erratum appears in Arch Dis Child. 2006 May;91(5):453]. Archives of Disease in Childhood 2003;88(9):802–6.

161. NNDSS Annual Report Writing Group, Australia's notifiable disease status, 2011: Annual report of the National Notifiable Diseases Surveillance System, 2011: Online. www.health.gov.au/internet/main/publishing.nsf/Content/cda-pubs-annlrpt-nndssar.htm; accessed 15 June 2015.

162. Ministry of Health, New Zealand Public Health Observatory, 2012.

163. Crowcroft NS, Pebody RG. Recent developments in pertussis. Lancet 2006;367(9526):1926–36.

164. Mackey JE et al. Predicting pertussis in a pediatric emergency department population. Clinical Pediatrics 2007;46(5):437–40.

165. Altunaiji Sultan M et al. Antibiotics for whooping cough (pertussis). Cochrane Database of Systematic Reviews 2007;DOI: 10.1002/14651858.CD004404.pub3.

166. Langley JM et al. Azithromycin is as effective as and better tolerated than erythromycin estolate for the treatment of pertussis. Pediatrics 2004;114(1):e96–101.

167. Lebel MH, Mehra S. Efficacy and safety of clarithromycin versus erythromycin for the treatment of pertussis: a prospective, randomized, single blind trial. Pediatric Infectious Disease Journal 2001;20(12):1149–54.

168. Royal Children's Hospital. Pertussis. Clinical Practice Guidelines 2004 [cited 2010 16 February]; Online. www.rch.org.au/clinicalguide/cpg.cfm?doc_id=5236; accessed 15 June 2015.

169. Kumar P, McKean MC. Evidence based paediatrics: review of BTS guidelines for the management of community acquired pneumonia in children. Journal of Infection 2004;48(2):134–8.

170. Chowell G et al. Severe respiratory disease concurrent with the circulation of H1N1 influenza. New England Journal of Medicine 2009;361(7):674–9.

171. Korppi M et al. The value of clinical features in differentiating between viral, pneumococcal and atypical bacterial pneumonia in children. Acta Paediatrica 2008;97(7):943–7.

172. Palafox M et al. Diagnostic value of tachypnoea in pneumonia defined radiologically. Archives of Disease in Childhood 2000;82(1):41–5.

173. Mathews B et al. Clinical predictors of pneumonia among children with wheezing. Pediatrics 2009;124(1):e29–36.

174. Starr M. Community acquired pneumonia. In: Textbook of paediatric emergency medicine, P. Cameron et al, eds. 2006, Elsevier: Edinburgh.

175. Wang K et al. Clinical symptoms and signs for the diagnosis of *Mycoplasma pneumoniae* in children and adolescents with community-acquired pneumonia. Cochrane Database of Systematic Reviews 2012;DOI: 10.1002/14651858.CD009175.pub2.

176. Cao AMY et al. Chest radiographs for acute lower respiratory tract infections. Cochrane Database of Systematic Reviews 2013;DOI: 10.1002/14651858.CD009119.pub2.

177. Lodha R, Kabra SK, Pandey RM. Antibiotics for community-acquired pneumonia in children. Cochrane Database of Systematic Reviews 2013;DOI: 10.1002/14651858.CD004874.pub4.

178. Rojas-Reyes MX, Granados Rugeles C. Oral antibiotics versus parenteral antibiotics for severe pneumonia in children. Cochrane Database of Systematic Reviews, 2006.

179. Mulholland S et al. Antibiotics for community-acquired lower respiratory tract infections secondary to *Mycoplasma pneumoniae* in children. Cochrane Database of Systematic Reviews 2012;DOI: 10.1002/14651858.CD004875.pub4.

180. Loughran S et al. A prospective, single-blind, randomized controlled trial of petroleum jelly/Vaseline for recurrent paediatric epistaxis. [see comment]. Clinical Otolaryngology & Allied Sciences 2004;29(3):266–9.

181. Kubba H et al. A prospective, single-blind, randomized controlled trial of antiseptic cream for recurrent epistaxis in childhood. Clinical Otolaryngology & Allied Sciences 2001;26(6):465–8.

182. Murthy P et al. A randomised clinical trial of antiseptic nasal carrier cream and silver nitrate cautery in the treatment of recurrent anterior epistaxis. Clinical Otolaryngology & Allied Sciences 1999;24(3):228–31.

183. Ruddy J et al. Management of epistaxis in children. International Journal of Pediatric Otorhinolaryngology 1991;21(2):139–42.

184. Daly K, Scott Giebink G. Clinical epidemiology of otitis media. Paediatr Infect Dis J 2000;19(5):S31–6.

185. Massa H, Cripps A, Lehmann D. Otitis media: viruses, bacteria, biofilms and vaccines. Med J Aust 2009;191(9):S39–43.

186. Uhari M, Mantysaari K, Niemela M. A meta-analytic review of the risk factors for acute otitis media. Clinical Infectious Diseases 1996;22(6):1079–83.

187. Bolt P et al. Topical lignocaine for pain relief in acute otitis media: results of a double-blind placebo-controlled randomised trial. Archives of Disease in Childhood 2008;93(1):40–4.

188. Coleman C, Moore M. Decongestants and antihistamines for acute otitis media in children. Cochrane Database of Systematic Reviews 2011;DOI: 10.1002/14651858.CD001727.pub5.

189. Venekamp Roderick P et al. Antibiotics for acute otitis media in children. Cochrane Database of Systematic Reviews 2013;DOI: 10.1002/14651858.CD000219.pub3.

190. Spiro DM et al. Wait-and-see prescription for the treatment of acute otitis media: a randomized controlled trial 10.1001/jama.296.10.1235. JAMA 2006;296(10):1235–1241.

191. Rovers MM et al. Day-care and otitis media in young children: a critical overview. European Journal of Pediatrics 1999;158(1):1–6.

192. Rosenfeld RM, Kay D. Natural history of untreated otitis media. Laryngoscope 2003;113(10):1645–57.

193. Thanaviratananich S, Laopaiboon M, Vatanasapt P. Once or twice daily versus three times daily amoxicillin with or without clavulanate for the treatment of acute otitis media. Cochrane Database of Systematic Reviews 2013;DOI: 10.1002/14651858.CD004975.pub3.

194. van Zon A et al. Antibiotics for otitis media with effusion in children. Cochrane Database of Systematic Reviews 2012;DOI: 10.1002/14651858.CD009163.pub2.

195. Griffin G, Flynn CA. Antihistamines and/or decongestants for otitis media with effusion (OME) in children. Cochrane Database of Systematic Reviews 2011;DOI: 10.1002/14651858.CD003423.pub3.

196. Danchin MH et al. Burden of acute sore throat and group A streptococcal pharyngitis in school-aged children and their families in Australia. Pediatrics 2007;120(5):950–7.

197. Del Mar CB, Glasziou PP, Spinks AB. Antibiotics for sore throat. Cochrane Database of Systematic Reviews, 2006(4):CD000023.

198. Carapetis JR, Currie BJ, Mathews JD. Cumulative incidence of rheumatic fever in an endemic region: a guide to the susceptibility of the population? Epidemiology & Infection 2000;124(2):239–44.

199. Danchin MH et al. Treatment of sore throat in light of the Cochrane verdict: is the jury still out? Medical Journal of Australia 2002;177(9):512–15.

200. Gerber MA. Diagnosis and treatment of pharyngitis in children. Pediatr Clin North Am 2005;52(3):729–47.

201. Lan A, Colford J. The impact of dosing frequency on the efficacy of 10-day Penicillin or Amoxicillin therapy for Streptococcal Tonsillopharyngitis: A meta-analysis. Pediatrics 2000;105(2).

202. Bulloch B, Kabani A, Tenenbein M. Oral dexamethasone for the treatment of pain in children with acute pharyngitis: a randomized, double-blind, placebo-controlled trial. Annals of Emergency Medicine 2003;41(5):601–8.

203. Bochud P-Y, Calandra T. Pathogenesis of sepsis: new concepts and implications for future treatment. BMJ 2003;326(7383):262–6.

204. Seear MD. Shock. In: Care of the critically ill child. Macnab A, Macrae D, Henning R, eds, Churchill Livingstone: Edinburgh: 1999.

205. NSW Department of Health. Recognition of a sick child in the emergency department, NSW Health: Sydney 2005:1–5.

206. Watson RS et al. The epidemiology of severe sepsis in children in the United States. American Journal of Respiratory & Critical Care Medicine 2003;167(5):695–701.

207. MacLeod J et al. Predictors of mortality in trauma patients. American Surgeon 2004;70(9):805–10.

208. Shapiro NI et al. Isolated prehospital hypotension after traumatic injuries: a predictor of mortality? Journal of Emergency Medicine 2003;25(2):175–9.

209. Ceneviva G et al. Hemodynamic support in fluid–refractory pediatric septic shock. Pediatrics 1998;102(2):e19.

210. Duke TD, Butt W, South M. Predictors of mortality and multiple organ failure in children with sepsis. Intensive Care Medicine 1997;23(6):684–92.

211. Rivers EP et al. Early and innovative interventions for severe sepsis and septic shock: taking advantage of a window of opportunity. CMAJ Canadian Medical Association Journal 2005;173(9):1054–65.

212. Perel P, Roberts I, Ker K. Colloids versus crystalloids for fluid resuscitation in critically ill patients. Cochrane Database of Systematic Reviews 2013;DOI: 10.1002/14651858.CD000567.pub6.

213. Wilkins B, Goonasekra CDA, Dillon MJ. Water, electrolyte and acid–base disorders and acute renal failure, in Care of the Critically Ill Child, A Macnab, D Macrae, R Henning, Eds. Churchill Livingstone: Edinburgh, 1999.

214. Upadhyay M et al. Randomized evaluation of fluid resuscitation with crystalloid (saline) and colloid (polymer from degraded gelatin in saline) in pediatric septic shock. Indian Pediatrics 2005;42(3):223–31.

215. Finfer S et al. A comparison of albumin and saline for fluid resuscitation in the intensive care unit.. New England Journal of Medicine 2004;350(22):2247–56.

216. Akech S, Ledermann H, Maitland K. Choice of fluids for resuscitation in children with severe infection and shock: systematic review. BMJ 2010;341:c4416.

217. Carcillo JA, Davis AL, Zaritsky A. Role of early fluid resuscitation in pediatric septic shock. JAMA 1991;266(9):1242–5.

218. Maitland K et al. Mortality after fluid bolus in African children with severe infection. New England Journal of Medicine 2011;364(26):2483–95.

219. Ninis N et al. The role of healthcare delivery in the outcome of meningococcal disease in children: case–control study of fatal and non-fatal cases. BMJ 2005;330(7506):1475.

220. Thompson MJ et al. Clinical recognition of meningococcal disease in children and adolescents. Lancet 2006;367(9508):397–403.

221. Brierley J et al. Clinical practice parameters for hemodynamic support of pediatric and neonatal septic shock: 2007 update from the American College of Critical Care Medicine.[Erratum appears in Crit Care Med. 2009 Apr;37(4):1536 Note: Skache, Sara [corrected to Kache, Saraswati]; Irazusta, Jose [corrected to Irazuzta, Jose]]. Critical Care Medicine 2009;37(2):666–88.

222. Dellinger RP et al. Surviving Sepsis Campaign: International Guidelines for Management of Severe Sepsis and Septic Shock 2012; Intensive Care Medicine 2013;39(2):165–228.

223. Kylat Ranjit I, Ohlsson A. Recombinant human activated protein C for severe sepsis in neonates. Cochrane Database of Systematic Reviews, 2006.

224. Martí-Carvajal AJ, Salanti G, Cardona-Zorrilla AF. Human recombinant activated protein C for severe sepsis. Cochrane Database of Systematic Reviews, 2008.

225. Vega RM, Avner JR. A prospective study of the usefulness of clinical and laboratory parameters for predicting percentage of dehydration in children. Pediatric Emergency Care 1997;13(3):179–82.

226. Porter SC et al. The value of parental report for diagnosis and management of dehydration in the emergency department. Annals of Emergency Medicine 2003;41(2):196–205.

227. Steiner MJ, Nager AL, Wang VJ. Urine specific gravity and other urinary indices: inaccurate tests for dehydration. Pediatric Emergency Care 2007;23(5):298–303.

228. Gorelick M, Shaw K, Murphy K. Validity and reliability of clinical signs in the diagnosis of dehydration in children. Pediatrics 1997;99:E6.

229. Duggan C et al. How valid are clinical signs of dehydration in infants? Journal of Pediatric Gastroenterology & Nutrition 1996;22(1):56–61.

230. English M et al. Signs of dehydration in severe childhood malaria. Tropical Doctor 1997; 27(4):235–6.

231. Friedman JN et al. Development of a clinical dehydration scale for use in children between 1 and 36 months of age. Journal of Pediatrics 2004;145(2):201–7.

232. Goldman RD, Friedman JN, Parkin PC. Validation of the clinical dehydration scale for children with acute gastroenteritis. Pediatrics 2008;122(3):545–9.

233. Teach SJ, Yates EW, Feld LG. Laboratory predictors of fluid deficit in acutely dehydrated children. Clinical Pediatrics 1997;36(7):395–400.

234. Yilmaz K et al. Evaluation of laboratory tests in dehydrated children with acute gastroenteritis. Journal of Paediatrics & Child Health 2002;38(3):226–8.

235. Chen L et al. Use of bedside ultrasound to assess degree of dehydration in children with gastroenteritis. Academic Emergency Medicine 2010;17(10):1042–7.

236. Levine AC et al. Ultrasound assessment of severe dehydration in children with diarrhea and vomiting. Academic Emergency Medicine 2010;17(10):1035–41.

237. Fonseca BK, Holdgate A, Craig JC. Enteral vs intravenous rehydration therapy for children with gastroenteritis: a meta–analysis of randomized controlled trials. Archives of Pediatrics & Adolescent Medicine 2004;158(5):483–90.

238. Royal Children's Hospital. Clinical practice guideline: Gastroenteritis. 2013. Online: www.rch.org.au/clinicalguide/guideline_index/Gastroenteritis/; accessed 15 June 2015.

239. Santucci KA et al. Frozen oral hydration as an alternative to conventional enteral fluids. Archives of Pediatrics & Adolescent Medicine 1998;152(2):142–6.

240. Stock A, Gilbertson H, Babl FE. Confirming nasogastric tube position in the emergency department: pH testing is reliable. Pediatric Emergency Care 2008;24(12):805–9.

241. Ducharme J, Matheson K. What is the best topical anesthetic for nasogastric insertion? A comparison of lidocaine gel, lidocaine spray, and atomized cocaine. Journal of Emergency Nursing 2003;29(5):427–30.

242. Wolfe TR, Fosnocht DE, Linscott MS. Atomized lidocaine as topical anesthesia for nasogastric tube placement: A randomized, double-blind, placebo-controlled trial. Annals of Emergency Medicine 2000;35(5):421–5.

243. Powell CVE et al. Randomized clinical trial of rapid versus 24-hour rehydration for children with acute gastroenteritis. Pediatrics 2011;128(4):e771–8.

244. Sharples PM et al. Plasma and cerebrospinal fluid arginine vasopressin in patients with and without fever. Archives of Disease in Childhood 1992;67(8):998–1002.

245. Dhawan A, Narang A, Singhi S. Hyponatraemia and the inappropriate ADH syndrome in pneumonia. Annals of Tropical Paediatrics 1992;12(4):455–62.

246. Kanakriyeh M, Carvajal HF, Vallone AM. Initial fluid therapy for children with meningitis with consideration of the syndrome of inappropriate anti-diuretic hormone. Clinical Pediatrics 1987;26(3):126–30.

247. McJunkin JE et al. La Crosse encephalitis in children. New England Journal of Medicine 2001;344(11):801–7.

248. Neville KA et al. High antidiuretic hormone levels and hyponatremia in children with gastroenteritis. Pediatrics 2005;116(6):1401–7.

249. Poddar U et al. Water electrolyte homeostasis in acute bronchiolitis. Indian Pediatrics 1995;32(1):59–65.

250. von Vigier RO et al. Circulating sodium in acute meningitis. American Journal of Nephrology 2001;21(2):87–90.

251. Foster BA, Tom D, Hill V. Hypotonic versus isotonic fluids in hospitalized children: a systematic review and meta-analysis. The Journal of Pediatrics 2014(0).

252. Wang J, Xu E, Xiao Y. Isotonic versus hypotonic maintenance iv fluids in hospitalized children: a meta-analysis. Pediatrics 2014;133(1):105–13.

253. Duke T, Molyneux EM. Intravenous fluids for seriously ill children: time to reconsider. Lancet 2003;362(9392):1320–3.

254. Mathur A et al. Hypotonic vs isotonic saline solutions for intravenous fluid management of acute infections. Cochrane Database of Systematic Reviews, 2004(2):CD004169.

255. Manole MD, Saladino RA. Emergency department management of the pediatric patient with supraventricular tachycardia. Pediatric Emergency Care 2007;23(3):176–85; quiz 186–9.

256. Muller G, Deal BJ, Benson DW Jr. 'Vagal maneuvers' and adenosine for termination of atrioventricular reentrant tachycardia. American Journal of Cardiology 1994;74(5):500–3.

257. Hsu DT, Pearson GD. Heart failure in children: part I: history, etiology, and pathophysiology. Circulation: Heart Failure 2009;2(1):63–70.

258. Choong R. Heart Failure. In: Textbook of paediatric emergency medicine. Cameron et al, eds. Elsevier: Edinburgh; 2006.

259. Macicek SM et al. Acute heart failure syndromes in the pediatric emergency department. Pediatrics 2009;124(5):e898–904.

260. Beggs S et al. Cardiac failure in children. In: 17th Expert Committee on the Selection and Use of Essential Medicines 2009: Geneva.

261. Friedman MJ, Sharieff GQ. Seizures in children. Pediatric Clinics of North America 2006;53(2):257–77.

262. Riviello JJ Jr et al. Practice parameter: diagnostic assessment of the child with status epilepticus (an evidence-based review): report of the Quality Standards Subcommittee of the American Academy of Neurology and the Practice Committee of the Child Neurology Society. Neurology 2006;67(9):1542–50.

263. American Academy of Pediatrics. Provisional Committee on Quality Improvement, Practice parameter: the neurodiagnostic evaluation of the child with a first simple febrile seizure. Pediatrics, 1996;97(5):769–72; discussion 773–5.

264. Appleton R, Macleod S, Martland T. Drug management for acute tonic–clonic convulsions including convulsive status epilepticus in children. Cochrane Database of Systematic Reviews, 2008.

265. Lewena S et al. Emergency management of pediatric convulsive status epilepticus: a multicenter study of 542 patients. Pediatric Emergency Care 2009;25(2):83–7.

266. Berg AT et al. A prospective study of recurrent febrile seizures [see comments]. New England Journal of Medicine 1992;327(16):1122–7.

267. Verity CM, Golding J. Risk of epilepsy after febrile convulsions: a national cohort study. [Erratum appears in BMJ 1992 Jan 18;304(6820):147]. BMJ 1991;303(6814):1373–6.

268. American Academy of Paediatrics. Seizures, febrile seizures: guideline for the neurodiagnostic evaluation of the child with a simple febrile seizure. Pediatrics 2011;127(2):389–94.

269. Dewhurst S et al. Human herpesvirus 6 (HHV-6) variant B accounts for the majority of symptomatic primary HHV-6 infections in a population of U.S. infants. J Clin Microbiol 1993;31:416–18.

270. Epstein L et al. The role of primary human herpes virus 6, 7(HHV-6, HHV-7) infection in febrile status epilepticus. Ann Neurol 2005;58(Suppl 9):S79–S80.

271. Hall C et al. Human herpesvirus-6 infection in children: a prospective study of complications and reactivation. N Engl J Med 1994;331:432–8.

272. Vestergaard M, Christensen J. Register-based studies on febrile seizures in Denmark. Brain & Development 2009;31(5):372–7.

273. Annegers JF et al. Recurrence of febrile convulsions in a population-based cohort. Epilepsy Research 1990;5(3):209–16.

274. Plaisance KI, Mackowiak PA. Antipyretic therapy: physiologic rationale, diagnostic implications, and clinical consequences. Archives of Internal Medicine 2000;160(4):449–56.

275. Seltz LB, Cohen E, Weinstein M. Risk of bacterial or herpes simplex virus meningitis/encephalitis in children with complex febrile seizures. Pediatric Emergency Care 2009;25(8):494–7.

276. Shah SS et al. Low risk of bacteremia in children with febrile seizures. Archives of Pediatrics & Adolescent Medicine 2002;156(5):469–72.

277. Trainor JL et al. Children with first-time simple febrile seizures are at low risk of serious bacterial illness. Acad Emerg Med 2001;8(8):781–7.

278. Offringa M, Newton R. Prophylactic drug management for febrile seizures in children. Cochrane Database of Systematic Reviews 2012;DOI: 10.1002/14651858.CD003031.pub2.

279. Meremikwu M, Oyo-Ita A. Paracetamol versus placebo or physical methods for treating fever in children. Cochrane Database of Systematic Reviews 2002; 2 CD003676. DOI: 10.1002/14651858.CD003676.

280. Moore HC, Lehmann D. Decline in meningitis admissions in young children: vaccines make a difference. Medical Journal of Australia 2006;185(7):404.

281. Kids Health. Immunisation Overview. 2014 [cited 2014 15th September]; Available from: http://www.kidshealth.org.nz/immunisation–overview; accessed 15 June 2015.

282. Australian Meningococcal Surveillance Programme, Annual report of the Australian Meningococcal Surveillance Programme 2006;Communicable Diseases Intelligence 2007;31(2):185–94.

283. Health K. Meningococcal disease. 2014. Online. http://www.kidshealth.org.nz/meningococcal-disease; accessed 15 June 2015.

284. Baraff LJ, Lee SI, Schriger DL. Outcomes of bacterial meningitis in children: a meta-analysis. Pediatric Infectious Disease Journal 1993;12(5):389–94.

285. Starr M. CNS infections, meningitis and encephalitis, in Textbook of paediatric emergency medicine. Cameron et al. eds. Elsevier: Edinburgh; 2006.

286. Curtis S et al. Clinical features suggestive of meningitis in children: a systematic review of prospective data. Pediatrics 2010;126(5):952–60.

287. Bilavsky E et al. The diagnostic accuracy of the 'classic meningeal signs' in children with suspected bacterial meningitis. European Journal of Emergency Medicine 2013;20(5):361–3. 10.1097/MEJ.0b013e3283585f20.

288. Rennick G, Shann F, de Campo J. Cerebral herniation during bacterial meningitis in children. BMJ 1993;306(6883):953–5.

289. Shetty AK et al. Fatal cerebral herniation after lumbar puncture in a patient with a normal computed tomography scan. Pediatrics 1999;103(6 Pt 1):1284–7.

290. Roche P et al. Annual report Invasive pneumococcal disease in Australia, 2006. Pneumococcal Working Party of the Communicable Diseases Network Australia; 2006.

291. Maconochie IK, Baumer JH. Fluid therapy for acute bacterial meningitis. Cochrane Database of Systematic Reviews 2008;DOI: 10.1002/14651858.CD004786.pub3.

292. Brouwer MC et al. Corticosteroids for acute bacterial meningitis. Cochrane Database of Systematic Reviews 2013;DOI: 10.1002/14651858.CD004405.pub4.

293. Hall GV et al. Frequency of infectious gastrointestinal illness in Australia, 2002: regional, seasonal and demographic variation. Epidemiology & Infection 2006;134(1):111–18.

294. Hellard M, Fairley CK. Gastroenteritis in Australia: who, what, where, and how much? Australian & New Zealand Journal of Medicine 1997;27(2):147–9.

295. Guarino A et al. European Society for Paediatric Gastroenterology, Hepatology, and Nutrition/European Society for Paediatric Infectious Diseases evidence-based guidelines for the management of acute gastroenteritis in children in Europe. Journal of Pediatric Gastroenterology & Nutrition 2008;46 Suppl 2:S81–122.

296. World Health Organization Dept. of Child and Adolescent Health and Development, Reduced osmolarity: oral rehydration salts (ORS) formulation: a report from a meeting of experts jointly organised by UNICEF and WHO, 2002, World Health Organization, Geneva.

297. American Academy of Pediatrics, Committee on Quality Improvement, and Gastroenteritis, Practice parameter: the management of acute gastroenteritis in young children. Pediatrics 1996;97:424–35.

298. Craven JA, Campbell L, Martin CT. Waiting room oral rehydration in the paediatric emergency department. Irish Medical Journal 2009;102(3):85–7.

299. Faruque AS et al. Breast feeding and oral rehydration at home during diarrhoea to prevent dehydration. Archives of Disease in Childhood 1992;67(8):1027–9.

300. MacGillivray S, Fahey T, McGuire W. Lactose avoidance for young children with acute diarrhoea. Cochrane Database of Systematic Reviews 2013;DOI: 10.1002/14651858.CD005433.pub2.

301. Fedorowicz Z, Jagannath VA, Carter B. Antiemetics for reducing vomiting related to acute gastroenteritis in children and adolescents. Cochrane Database of Systematic Reviews 2011;DOI: 10.1002/14651858.CD005506.pub5.

302. Sirinavin S, Garner P. Antibiotics for treating salmonella gut infections. (Cochrane Review), in The Cochrane Library, John Wiley & Sons, Ltd: Chichester, UK. 2000:CD001167.

303. Lambert SB et al. Early evidence for direct and indirect effects of the infant rotavirus vaccine program in Queensland. Medical Journal of Australia 2009;191(3):157–60.

304. Buttery JP et al. Reduction in rotavirus-associated acute gastroenteritis following introduction of rotavirus vaccine into Australia's national childhood vaccine schedule. The Pediatric Infectious Disease Journal 2011;30(1):S25–9 10.1097/INF.0b013e3181fefdee.

305. North American Society for Pediatric Gastroenterology Hepatology and Nutrition. Evaluation and treatment of constipation in children: summary of updated recommendations of the North American Society for Pediatric Gastroenterology, Hepatology and Nutrition. Journal of Pediatric Gastroenterology & Nutrition 2006;43(3):405–7.

306. Reuchlin-Vroklage LM et al. Diagnostic value of abdominal radiography in constipated children: A systematic review. Archives of Pediatrics & Adolescent Medicine 2005;159(7):671–8.

307. Tabbers MM et al. Constipation in children. LID – 0303 [pii]. (1752–8526 (Electronic)).

308. Scholer SJ et al. Clinical outcomes of children with acute abdominal pain. Pediatrics1996;98(4 Pt 1):680–5.

309. Holland A, Gollow IJ. Acute abdominal pain in children: an analysis of admissions over a three-year period. Journal of Quality in Clinical Practice 1996;16(3):151–5.

310. Royal Children's Hospital. Intussusception. 2005 [cited 2010 5 Jan]; Online. www.rch.org.au/clinicalguide/cpg.cfm?doc_id=5216; accessed 15 June 2015.

311. Newman J. Intussusception in babies under 4 months of age. CMAJ 1987;136:266–9.

312. Turner D, Rickwood AM, Brereton RJ. Intussusception in older children. Archives of Disease in Childhood 1980;55(7):544–6.

313. Waseem M, Rosenberg HK. Intussusception. Pediatric Emergency Care 2008;24(11):793–800.

314. Soares-Weiser K et al. Vaccines for preventing rotavirus diarrhoea: vaccines in use. Cochrane Database of Systematic Reviews 2012;DOI: 10.1002/14651858.CD008521.pub3.

315. Klein EJ, Kapoor D, Shugerman RP. The diagnosis of intussusception. Clinical Pediatrics 2004;43(4):343–7.

316. Mackay AJ, MacKellar A, Sprague P. Intussusception in children: a review of 91 cases. Australian & New Zealand Journal of Surgery 1987;57(1):15–7.

317. Henderson AA et al. Comparison of 2-View Abdominal radiographs with ultrasound in children with suspected intussusception. Pediatric Emergency Care 2013;29(2):145–50. 10.1097/PEC.0b013e3182808af7.

318. Smith D et al. The role of abdominal x-rays in the diagnosis and management of intussusception. Pediatr Emerg Care 1992;8:325–7.

319. Hryhorczuk A, Strouse P. Validation of US as a first-line diagnostic test for assessment of pediatric ileocolic intussusception. Pediatric Radiology 2009;39(10):1075–9.

320. Verschelden P et al. Intussusception in children: reliability of US diagnosis—a prospective study. Radiology 1992;184:741–4.

321. MacMahon B. The Continuing Enigma of Pyloric Stenosis of Infancy: A Review. Epidemiology 2006;17(2):195–201. 10.1097/01. ede.0000192032.83843.c9.

322. Louie JP. Essential diagnosis of abdominal emergencies in the first year of life. Emergency Medicine Clinics of North America 2007;25(4):1009–40.

323. Gotley LM et al. Pyloric stenosis: A retrospective study of an Australian population. Emergency Medicine Australasia 2009;21(5):407–13.

324. Taylor ND, Cass DT, Holland AJA. Infantile hypertrophic pyloric stenosis: Has anything changed? Journal of Paediatrics and Child Health 2013;49(1):33–7.

325. Niedzielski J et al. Accuracy of sonographic criteria in the decision for surgical treatment in infantile hypertrophic pyloric stenosis. Arch Med Sci 2011;7(3):508–11.

326. Wang KS et al. Assessment and Management of Inguinal Hernia in Infants. Pediatrics 2012;130(4):768–73.

327. Phillips R, Orchard D, Starr M. Dermatology, in Textbook of Paediatric Emergency Medicine, P. Cameron et al. Editors. 2006, Churchill Livingstone: Edinburgh.

328. Andrews RM et al. Skin disorders, including pyoderma, scabies, and tinea infections. Pediatric Clinics of North America 2009;56(6):1421–40.

329. George A, Rubin G. A systematic review and meta-analysis of treatments for impetigo. British Journal of General practice 2003;53(491):480–7.

330. Koning S et al. Interventions for impetigo. Cochrane Database of Systematic Reviews 2012;DOI: 10.1002/14651858.CD003261.pub3.

331. Ong PY, Boguniewicz M. Atopic dermatitis. Primary Care; Clinics in Office Practice 2008;35(1):105–17.

332. Kunz B et al. Clinical validation and guidelines for the SCORAD index: consensus report of the European Task Force on Atopic Dermatitis. Dermatology 1997;195(1):10–19.

333. Lucky AW et al. Use of an emollient as a steroid–sparing agent in the treatment of mild to moderate atopic dermatitis in children. Pediatric Dermatology 1997;14(4):321–4.

334. Kaplan SL et al. Randomized trial of 'bleach baths' plus routine hygienic measures vs routine hygienic measures alone for prevention of recurrent infections. Clinical Infectious Diseases, 2013.

335. Bath-Hextall FJ et al. Interventions to reduce Staphylococcus aureus in the management of atopic eczema: an updated Cochrane review. British Journal of Dermatology 2010;163(1):12–26.

336. Callen J et al. A systematic review of the safety of topical therapies for atopic dermatitis. British Journal of Dermatology 2007;156(2):203–21.

337. Eichenfield LF et al. Effect of desonide hydrogel 0.05% on the hypothalamic–pituitary–adrenal axis in pediatric subjects with moderate to severe atopic dermatitis. Pediatric Dermatology 2007;24(3):289–95.

338. Eichenfield LF, Miller BH, Cutivate G. Lotion Study, Two randomized, double-blind, placebo-controlled studies of fluticasone propionate lotion 0.05% for the treatment of atopic dermatitis in subjects from 3 months of age. Journal of the American Academy of Dermatology 2006;54(4):715–17.

339. Friedlander SF et al. Safety of fluticasone propionate cream 0.05% for the treatment of severe and extensive atopic dermatitis in children as young as 3 months. Journal of the American Academy of Dermatology 2002;46(3):387–93.

340. Boguniewicz M et al. A randomized, vehicle-controlled trial of tacrolimus ointment for treatment of atopic dermatitis in children. Pediatric Tacrolimus Study Group. Journal of Allergy & Clinical Immunology 1998;102(4 Pt 1):637–44.

341. Arellano FM, Arana WC et al. Risk of lymphoma following exposure to calcineurin inhibitors and topical steroids in patients with atopic dermatitis. J Invest Dermatol 2007;127(4):808–16.

342. Margolis D, Hoffstad O, Bilker W. Lack of association between exposure to topical calcineurin inhibitors and skin cancer in adults. Dermatology 2007;214(4):289–95.

343. Goodyear HM, Spowart K, Harper JI, Wet-wrap dressings for the treatment of atopic eczema in children. British Journal of Dermatology 1991;125(6):604.

344. Mallon E, Powell S, Bridgman A. 'Wet-wrap' dressings for the treatment of atopic eczema in the community. Journal of Dermatological Treatment 1994;5:97–8.

345. Pei AY, Chan HH, Ho KM. The effectiveness of wet wrap dressings using 0.1% mometasone furoate and 0.005% fluticasone proprionate ointments in the treatment of moderate to severe atopic dermatitis in children. Pediatric Dermatology 2001;18(4):343–8.

346. Staab D et al. Evaluation of a parental training program for the management of childhood atopic dermatitis. Pediatric Allergy & Immunology 2002;13(2):84–90.

347. Grattan C, Powell S, Humphreys F. Management and diagnostic guidelines for urticaria and angio-oedema. British Journal of Dermatology 2001;144:708–14.

348. Amar SM, Dreskin SC. Urticaria. Primary Care; Clinics in Office Practice 2008;35(1):141–57.

349. Simons FE. Prevention of acute urticaria in young children with atopic dermatitis. Journal of Allergy & Clinical Immunology 2001;107(4):703–6.

350. Zuberbier T. Urticaria. Allergy 2003;58:1224–34.

351. Zuberbier T et al. Acute urticaria: clinical aspects and therapeutic responsiveness. Acta Dermato–Venereologica 1996;76(4):295–7.

352. Kauppinen K, Juntunen K, Lanki H. Urticaria in children. Retrospective evaluation and follow-up. Allergy 1984;39(6):469–72.

353. Poon M, Reid C. Oral corticosteroids in acute urticaria. Emergency Medicine Journal 2004;21:76–7.

354. Zuberbier T et al. Dermatology Section of the European Academy of Allergology Clinical, Immunology Global, Allergy Asthma European, Network European Dermatology, Forum World Allergy, Organization Guideline: Management of Urticaria. Allergy 2009;64(10):1427–43.

355. Hiscock H. The crying baby. Australian Family Physician 2006;35(9):680–4.

356. Wolke D, Samara M. Meta-analysis of fuss/cry durations and colic prevalence across countries in 11th International Infant Cry Research Workshop. 2011. Netherlands.

357. Herman M, Le A. The crying infant. Emergency Medicine Clinics of North America 2007;25(4):1137–59.

358. Barr RG. Crying in the first year of life: good news in the midst of distress. Child: Care, Health & Development 1998;24(5):425–39.

359. Freedman SB, Al-Harthy N, Thull-Freedman J. The crying infant: diagnostic testing and frequency of serious underlying disease. Pediatrics 2009;123(3):841–8.

360. Evanoo G. Infant crying: a clinical conundrum. Journal of Pediatric Health Care 2007;21(5):333–8.

361. Reijneveld SA et al. Infant crying and abuse. The Lancet 2004;364(9442):1340–2.

362. Calado CS et al. What brings newborns to the emergency department?: a 1-year study. Pediatric Emergency Care 2009;25(4):244–8.

363. Moerschel SK, Cianciaruso LB, Tracy LR. A practical approach to neonatal jaundice. American Family Physician 2008;77(9):1255–62.

364. Hartley JL, Davenport M, Kelly DA. Biliary atresia. Lancet 2009;374(9702):1704–13.

365. National Institute for Clinical Excellence. Recognition and treatment of neonatal jaundice. 2010 [cited 2014 19 March]; Online. www.nice.org.uk/CG98; accessed 15 June 2015.

366. Chiappini E et al. Parental and medical knowledge and management of fever in Italian pre-school children. BMC Pediatrics 2012;12(1):97.

367. Betz M, Grunfeld A. 'Fever phobia' in the emergency department: a survey of children's caregivers. Eur J Emerg Med 2006;13:129–33.

368. Rupe A, Ahlers-Schmidt C, Wittler R. A comparison of perceptions of fever and fever phobia by ethnicity. Clin Pediatr 2010;49:172–6.

369. Walsh A, Edwards H, Fraser J. Influences on parents' fever management: beliefs, experiences and information sources. J Clin Nurs 2007;16:2331–40.

370. Poirier MP, Collins EP, McGuire E. Fever phobia: a survey of caregivers of children seen in a pediatric emergency department. Clinical Pediatrics 2010;49(6):530–4.

371. Wilkinson, M, Bulloch B, Smith M. Prevalence of occult bacteremia in children aged 3 to 36 months presenting to the emergency department with fever in the postpneumococcal conjugate vaccine era. Academic Emergency Medicine 2009;16(3):220–5.

372. Baker MD, Fosarelli PD, Carpenter RO. Childhood fever: correlation of diagnosis with temperature response to acetaminophen. Pediatrics 1987;80(3):315–18.

373. Mackowiak PA. Diagnostic implications and clinical consequences of antipyretic therapy. Clinical Infectious Diseases 2000;31 (Suppl 5):S230–3.

374. Mazur LJ, Kozinetz CA. Diagnostic tests for occult bacteraemia: temperature response to acetaminophen versus WBC count. American Journal of Emergency Medicine 1994;12(4):403–6.

375. Weisse ME, Miller G, Brien JH. Fever response to acetaminophen in viral vs. bacterial infections. Pediatric Infectious Disease Journal 1987;6(12):1091–4.

376. Elshout G et al. Duration of fever and serious bacterial infections in children: a systematic review. BMC Family Practice 2011;12(1):33.

377. Bonadio WA et al. Correlating changes in body temperature with infectious outcome in febrile children who receive acetaminophen. Clin Pediatr (Phila) 1993;32(6):343–6.

378. McCarthy PL, Dolan TF. The serious implications of high fever in infants during their first three months. Six years' experience at Yale–New Haven Hospital Emergency Room. Clinical Pediatrics 1976;15(9):794–6.

379. Stanley R, Pagon Z, Bachur R. Hyperpyrexia among infants younger than 3 months. Pediatric Emergency Care 2005;21(5):291–4.

380. Trautner BW et al. Prospective evaluation of the risk of serious bacterial infection in children who present to the emergency department with hyperpyrexia (temperature of 106 degrees F or higher). Pediatrics 2006;118(1):34–40.

381. Mackowiak PA. Fever: blessing or curse? A unifying hypothesis. Annals of Internal Medicine 1994;120(12):1037–40.

382. Mackowiak PA, Boulant JA. Fever's glass ceiling. Clinical Infectious Diseases 1996;22(3):525–36.

383. Shann F. Antipyretics in severe sepsis. Lancet 1995;345(8946):338.

384. Russell FM et al. Evidence on the use of paracetamol in febrile children.[see comment]. Bulletin of the World Health Organization 2003;81(5):367–72.

385. Purssell E, While AE. Does the use of antipyretics in children who have acute infections prolong febrile illness? A systematic review and meta-analysis. Journal of Pediatrics 2013;163(3):822–7.e1–2.

386. Heubi, JE, Barbacci MB, Zimmerman HJ. Therapeutic misadventures with acetaminophen: hepatoxicity after multiple doses in children. Journal of Pediatrics 1998;132(1):22–7.

387. Hynson JL, South M. Childhood hepatotoxicity with paracetamol doses less than 150 mg/kg per day. Medical Journal of Australia 1999;171(9):497.

388. Ranganathan SS et al. Fulminant hepatic failure and paracetamol overuse with therapeutic intent in febrile children. Indian Journal of Pediatrics 2006;73(10):871–5.

389. Beasley R et al. Association between paracetamol use in infancy and childhood, and risk of asthma, rhinoconjunctivitis, and eczema in children aged 6–7 years: analysis from Phase Three of the ISAAC programme. Lancet 2008;372(9643):1039–48.

390. Gupta H et al. Role of paracetamol in treatment of childhood fever: a double-blind randomized placebo controlled trial. Indian Pediatrics 2007;44(12):903–11.

391. Autret-Leca E, Gibb IA, Goulder MA. Ibuprofen versus paracetamol in pediatric fever: objective and subjective findings from a randomized, blinded study. Current Medical Research & Opinion 2007;23(9):2205–11.

392. Kramer LC et al. Alternating antipyretics: antipyretic efficacy of acetaminophen versus acetaminophen alternated with ibuprofen in children. Clinical Pediatrics 2008;47(9):907–11.

393. Vauzelle-Kervroedan F et al. Equivalent antipyretic activity of ibuprofen and paracetamol in febrile children. Journal of Pediatrics 1997;131(5):683–7.

394. Hay AD et al. Paracetamol plus ibuprofen for the treatment of fever in children (PITCH): randomised controlled trial. [Erratum appears in BMJ. 2009;339:b3295]. BMJ 2008;337:a1302.

395. Perrott DA et al. Efficacy and safety of acetaminophen vs ibuprofen for treating children's pain or fever: a meta-analysis. Archives of Pediatrics & Adolescent Medicine 2004;158(6):521–6.

396. Wong T et al. Combined and alternating paracetamol and ibuprofen therapy for febrile children. Cochrane Database of Systematic Reviews 2013;DOI: 10.1002/14651858.CD009572.pub2.

397. Meremikwu M, Oyo-Ita A. Physical methods for treating fever in children (Cochrane Review), in The Cochrane Library2003, John Wiley & Sons, Ltd: Chichester, UK. p. CD004264.

398. Alves JGB, Almeida NDC, Almeida CDC. Tepid sponging plus dipyrone versus dipyrone alone for reducing body temperature in febrile children. Sao Paulo Medical Journal = Revista Paulista de Medicina 2008;126(2):107–11.

399. Thomas S et al. Comparative effectiveness of tepid sponging and antipyretic drug versus only antipyretic drug in the management of fever among children: a randomized controlled trial. Indian Pediatrics 2009;46(2):133–6.

400. Simon HK, Weinkle DA. Over-the-counter medications. Do parents give what they intend to give? Arch Pediatr Adolesc Med 1997;151(7):654–6.

401. Department of Human Services (Victoria), Review of trauma and emergency services 1999: Final Report, 1999, Department of Human Services (Victoria): Melbourne.

402. Trauma Service Royal Children's Hospital, Trauma Statistics. unpublished data, 2009.

403. Avarello JT, Cantor RM. Pediatric major trauma: an approach to evaluation and management. Emer Med Clin North Am 2007;3:803–36.

404. Hutchings L et al. Developing a spinal clearance protocol for unconscious pediatric trauma patients. Journal of Trauma, Injury Infection & Critical Care 2009;67(4):681–6.

405. Hutchings L, Willett K. Cervical spine clearance in pediatric trauma: a review of current literature. Journal of Trauma–Injury Infection & Critical Care 2009;67(4):687–91.

406. Chandrasekhar A, Moorman D, Timberlake G. An evaluation of the effects of semi rigid cervical collars in patients with severe closed head injury. The American Surgeon 1998;64(7):604.

407. Viccellio P et al. A prospective multicenter study of cervical spine injury in children. Pediatrics 2001;108(2).

408. Hoffman J et al. Validity of a set of clinical criteria to rule out injury to the cervical spine in patients with blunt trauma. N Engl J Med 2000;343:94–9.

409. Chung S et al. Trauma Association of Canada Pediatric Subcommittee National Pediatric Cervical Spine Evaluation Pathway: Consensus Guidelines. Journal of Trauma and Acute Care Surgery 2011;70(4):873–84. 10.1097/TA.0b013e3182108823.

410. National Institute of Health and Clinical Excellence. Clinical Guideline CG56. Head injury: triage, assessment, investigation and early management of head injury in infants, children and adults. 2007. Online. www.nice.org.uk/guidance/CG56; accessed 15 June 2015.

411. Lieh-Lai MW et al. Limitations of the Glasgow Coma Scale in predicting outcome in children with traumatic brain injury. Journal of Pediatrics 1992;120(2 Pt 1):195–9.

412. Falk A-C et al. Are the symptoms and severity of head injury predictive of clinical findings three months later? Acta Paediatrica 2006;95(12):1533–9.

413. Neurological Society of Australasia and Royal College of Surgeons, The management of acute neurotrauma in rural and remote locations. 2nd edn. East Melbourne: Neurosurgical Society of Australasia Inc; 2002.

414. Quayle KS, Minor head injury in the pediatric patient. Pediatric Clinics of North America 1999;46(6):1189–99.

415. Thiessen ML, Woolridge DP. Pediatric minor closed head injury. Pediatric Clinics of North America 2006;53(1):1–26.

416. Ghajar J, Hariri RJ. Management of pediatric head injury. Pediatric Clinics of North America 1992;39(5):1093–125.

417. Swaminathan A, Levy P, Legome E. Evaluation and management of moderate to severe pediatric head trauma. Journal of Emergency Medicine 2009;37(1):63–8.

418. Pickering A et al. Clinical decision rules for children with minor head injury: a systematic review. Archives of Disease in Childhood 2011;96(5):414–21.

419. Sydenham E, Roberts I, P Alderson. Hypothermia for traumatic head injury. Cochrane Database of Systematic Reviews 2009;Issue 2. Art. No.: CD001048. DOI: 10.1002/14651858.CD001048.pub4.

420. Shann F. Hypothermia for traumatic brain injury: how soon, how cold, and how long? Lancet 2003;362(9400):1950–1.

421. Fox JC et al. Test Characteristics of focused assessment of sonography for trauma for clinically significant abdominal free fluid in pediatric blunt abdominal trauma. Academic Emergency Medicine 2011;18(5):477–82.

422. Benya E et al. Abdominal sonography in examination of children with blunt abdominal trauma. AJR Am J Roentgenol 2000;174:1613–16.

423. Coley B et al. Focused abdominal sonography for trauma (FAST) in children with blunt abdominal trauma. J Trauma 2000;48:902–6.

424. Emery K et al. Absent peritoneal fluid on screening trauma ultrasonography in children: a prospective comparison with computed tomography. J Pediatr Surg 2001;36:565–9.

425. Holmes J et al. Emergency department ultrasonography in the evaluation of hypotensive and normotensive children with blunt abdominal trauma. J Pediatr Surg 2001;36:968–73.

426. Soudack M et al. Experience with focused abdominal sonography for trauma (FAST) in 313 pediatric patients. J Clin Ultrasound 2004;32:53–61.

427. Deluca JA et al. Injuries associated with pediatric liver trauma. American Surgeon 2007;73(1):37–41.

428. Gaines BA. Intra-abdominal solid organ injury in children: diagnosis and treatment. Journal of Trauma–Injury Infection & Critical Care 2009;67(2 Suppl):S135–9.

429. Giss S et al. Complications of nonoperative management of pediatric blunt hepatic injury: diagnosis, management, and outcomes. J Trauma 2006;61:334–9.

430. Landau A et al. Liver injuries in children: the role of selective nonoperative management; A large, single-institution study demonstrating the success of nonoperative management for blunt hepatic trauma. Injury 2006;37:66–71.

431. Merck. Merck Manual for Health Care Professionals; Fractures. 2010; Online. www.merckmanuals.com/professional/injuries_poisoning/fractures_dislocations_and_sprains/fractures.html?qt=salter&sc=&alt=sh; accessed 15 June 2015.

432. Al-Adhami AS et al. Clinical diagnosis of fractures in a paediatric population. European Journal of Emergency Medicine 2005;12(2):99–101.

433. Dowling S et al. Accuracy of Ottawa Ankle Rules to exclude fractures of the ankle and midfoot in children: a meta-analysis (Structured abstract). Academic Emergency Medicine 2009;16(4):277–87.

434. Cho K-H et al. Ultrasound diagnosis of either an occult or missed fracture of an extremity in pediatric-aged children. Korean J Radiol 2010;11(1):84–94.

435. Chaar-Alvarez FM et al. Bedside ultrasound diagnosis of nonangulated distal forearm fractures in the pediatric emergency department. Pediatric Emergency Care 2011;27(11):1027–32. 10.1097/PEC.0b013e318235e228.

436. Eckert K et al. Ultrasound diagnosis of supracondylar fractures in children. European Journal of Trauma and Emergency Surgery 2013:1–10.

437. Rabiner JE et al. Accuracy of point-of-care ultrasonography for diagnosis of elbow fractures in children. Annals of Emergency Medicine 2013;61(1):9–17.

438. Laine JC, Kaiser SP, Diab M. High-risk pediatric orthopedic pitfalls. Emergency Medicine Clinics of North America 2010;28(1):85–102.

439. Davidson JS et al. Simple treatment for torus fractures of the distal radius.[see comment]. Journal of Bone & Joint Surgery—British Volume 2001;83(8):1173–5.

440. Firmin F, Crouch R. Splinting versus casting of 'torus' fractures to the distal radius in the paediatric patient presenting at the emergency department (ED): a literature review. International emergency nursing 2009;17(3):173–8.

441. Plint AC et al. A randomized, controlled trial of removable splinting versus casting for wrist buckle fractures in children 10.1542/peds.2005–0801. Pediatrics 2006;117(3):691–7.

442. Plint AC, Perry JJ, Tsang JLY. Pediatric wrist buckle fractures: Should we just splint and go? Canadian Journal of Emergency Medicine 2004;6(6):397–401.

443. Oakley E, Barnett P, Babl FE. Backslab versus nonbackslab for immobilization of undisplaced supracondylar fractures: a randomized trial. Pediatric Emergency Care 2009;25(7):452–6.

444. Macias CG, Bothner J, Wiebe R. A comparison of supination/flexion to hyperpronation in the reduction of radial head subluxations. Pediatrics 1998;102(1).

445. Krul M et al. Manipulative interventions for reducing pulled elbow in young children. Cochrane Database of Systematic Reviews 2012;DOI: 10.1002/14651858.CD007759.pub3.

446. Schutzman SA, Teach S. Upper-extremity impairment in young children. Annals of Emergency Medicine 1995;26(4):474–9.

447. Dunbar JS et al. Obscure tibial fracture of infants—the toddler's fracture. Journal of the Canadian Association of Radiologists 1964;15:136–44.

448. Singhal R et al. Septic arthritis vs transient synovitis in children in a tertiary health care centre study. Journal of Bone & Joint Surgery, British Volume 2012;94–B(Supp XXXVI):11.

449. McCanny PJ et al. Implementation of an evidence based guideline reduces blood tests and length of stay for the limping child in a paediatric emergency department. Emergency Medicine Journal 2013;30(1):19–23.

450. Asche SS et al. What is the clinical course of transient synovitis in children: a systematic review of the literature. Chiropractic & manual therapies 2013;21(1):39.

451. Kermond S et al. A randomized clinical trial: should the child with transient synovitis of the hip be treated with nonsteroidal anti-inflammatory drugs? Annals of Emergency Medicine 2002;40(3):294–9.

452. Halsey MF et al. Toddler's fracture: presumptive diagnosis and treatment. Journal of Pediatric Orthopedics 2001;21(2):152–6.

453. Lewis D, Logan P. Sonographic diagnosis of toddler's fracture in the emergency department. Journal of Clinical Ultrasound 2006;34(4):190–4.

454. Shravat BP, Harrop SN, Kane TP. Toddler's fracture. Journal of Accident & Emergency Medicine 1996;13(1):59–61.

455. Tenenbein M, Reed MH, Black GB. The toddler's fracture revisited. American Journal of Emergency Medicine 1990;8(3):208–11.

456. Higo R et al. Foreign bodies in the aerodigestive tract in pediatric patients. Auris, Nasus, Larynx 2003;30(4):397–401.

457. Stone J et al. GI Nurses' retrospective look at foreign body ingestions in children. Gastroenterology Nursing 1996;19(2):70–1.

458. Litovitz T et al. Emerging Battery–Ingestion Hazard: Clinical Implications. Pediatrics, 2010.

459. Glynn F, Amin M, Kinsella J. Nasal foreign bodies in children: should they have a plain radiograph in the accident and emergency? Pediatric Emergency Care 2008;24(4):217–18.

460. Heim, SW, Maughan KL. Foreign bodies in the ear, nose, and throat. American Family Physician 2007;76(8):1185–9.

461. A-Kader HH. Foreign body ingestion: children like to put objects in their mouth. World Journal of Pediatrics 2010;6(4):301–10.

462. Cheng W, Tam PKH. Foreign-Body ingestion in children: experience with 1,265 cases. Journal of Pediatric Surgery 1999;34(10):1472–6.

463. Wai Pak M et al. A prospective study of foreign body ingestion in 311 children. International Journal of Pediatric Otorhinolaryngology 2000;58:37–45.

464. Caravati EM, Bennett DL, McElwee NE. Pediatric coin ingestion. A prospective study on the utility of routine roentgenograms. American Journal of Diseases of Children 1989;143(5):549–51.

465. Ansley JF, Cunningham MJ. Treatment of aural foreign bodies in children. The American Academy of Pediatrics 1998;101(4):638–41.

466. Marin JR, Trainor JL. Foreign body removal from the external auditory canal in a pediatric emergency department. Pediatric Emergency Care 2006;22(9):630–4.

467. Thompson SK, Wein RO, Dutcher PO. External auditory canal foreign body removal: Management practices and outcomes. The Laryngoscope 2003;113:1912–15.

468. DiMuzio J Jr, Deschler DG. Emergency department management of foreign bodies of the external ear canal in children. Otology & Neurotology 2002;23(4):473–5.

469. Schultze S, Kerschner J, Beste D. Pediatric external auditory canal foreign bodies: a review of 698 cases. Otolaryngol Head Neck Surg 2002;127:73–8.

470. Di Muzio J, Deschler DG. Emergency department management of foreign bodies of the external auditory canal in children. Otology & Neurotology 2002;23:473–5.

471. Balbani AP et al. Ear and nose foreign body removal in children. International Journal of Pediatric Otorhinolaryngology 1998; 46(1–2):37–42.

472. Tcherny-Lessenot S et al. Management and relief of pain in an emergency department from the adult patients' perspective. Journal of Pain & Symptom Management 2003;25(6):539–46.

473. Zempsky WT et al. Relief of pain and anxiety in pediatric patients in emergency medical systems. Pediatrics 2004;114(5):1348–56.

474. Alexander J, Manno M. Underuse of analgesia in very young pediatric patients with isolated painful injuries. Annals of Emergency Medicine 2003;41(5):617–22.

475. Ducharme J, Barber C. A prospective blinded study on emergency pain assessment and therapy. Journal of Emergency Medicine 1995;13(4):571–5.

476. Innes G et al. Procedural sedation and analgesia in the emergency department. Canadian Consensus Guidelines. Journal of Emergency Medicine 1999;17(1):145–56.

477. McCarthy C, Hewitt S, Choonara I. Pain in young children attending an accident and emergency department. Journal of Accident & Emergency Medicine 2000;17(4):265–7.

478. Petrack EM, Christopher NC, Kriwinsky J. Pain management in the emergency department: patterns of analgesic utilization. Pediatrics 1997;99(5):711–14.

479. Rupp T, Delaney KA. Inadequate analgesia in emergency medicine. Annals of Emergency Medicine 2004;43(4):494–503.

480. Singer AJ et al. Comparison of patient and practitioner assessments of pain from commonly performed emergency department procedures. Annals of Emergency Medicine 1999;33(6):652–8.

481. Ducharme J, Gutman J. Pain management in the emergency department. Academic Emergency Medicine 1995;2(9):850–2.

482. Beyer JE et al. Patterns of postoperative analgesic use with adults and children following cardiac surgery. Pain 1983;17(1):71–81.

483. Chan L, Russell TJ, Robak N, Parental perception of the adequacy of pain control in their child after discharge from the emergency department. Pediatric Emergency Care 1998;14(4):251–3.

484. Cimpello LB, Khine H, Avner JR, Practice patterns of pediatric versus general emergency physicians for pain management of fractures in pediatric patients. Pediatric Emergency Care 2004;20(4):228–32.

485. Friedland LR, Pancioli AM, Duncan KM. Pediatric emergency department analgesic practice. Pediatric Emergency Care 1997;13(2):103–6.

486. Liebelt EL. Reducing pain during procedures. Current Opinion in Pediatrics 1996;8(5):436–41.

487. Bieri D et al. The Faces Pain Scale for the self-assessment of the severity of pain experienced by children: development, initial validation, and preliminary investigation for ratio scale properties. Pain 1990;41(2):139–50.

488. Merkel SI et al. The FLACC: a behavioral scale for scoring postoperative pain in young children. Pediatric Nursing 1997;23(3):293–7.

489. Australian and New Zealand College of Anaesthetists and Faculty of Pain Medicine. Acute pain management; scientific evidence. 2nd edn. Melbourne: Australian and New Zealand College of Anaesthetists; 2005.

490. Bijur PE, Silver W, Gallagher EJ, Reliability of the visual analog scale for measurement of acute pain. Academic Emergency Medicine 2001;8(12):1153–7.

491. Goodenough B et al. Pain in 4- to 6-year-old children receiving intramuscular injections: a comparison of the Faces Pain Scale with other self-report and behavioral measures. Clinical Journal of Pain 1997;13(1):60–73.

492. Hicks CL et al. The Faces Pain Scale–Revised: toward a common metric in pediatric pain measurement. Pain 2001;93(2):173–83.

493. Polkki T, Pietila A-M, Vehvilainen–Julkunen K. Hospitalized children's descriptions of their experiences with postsurgical pain relieving methods. International Journal of Nursing Studies 2003;40(1):33–44.

494. Stinson JN et al. Systematic review of the psychometric properties, interpretability and feasibility of self-report pain intensity measures for use in clinical trials in children and adolescents. Pain 2006;125(1–2):143–57.

495. van Dijk M et al. Observational visual analog scale in pediatric pain assessment: useful tool or good riddance? Clinical Journal of Pain 2002;18(5):310–16.

496. Shields BJ et al. Pediatric pain measurement using a visual analogue scale: a comparison of two teaching methods. Clinical Pediatrics 2003;42(3):227–34.

497. Belville RG, Seupaul RA. Pain measurement in pediatric emergency care: A review of the Faces Pain Scale–Revised. Pediatric Emergency Care 2005;21(2):90–3.

498. Lawrence J et al. The development of a tool to assess neonatal pain. Neonatal Network 1993;12(6):59–66.

499. McGrath PJ et al. CHEOPS: A behavioural scale for rating postoperative pain in children. In: Advances in pain research and therapy, Fields HL, Dubner R, Cervero F, eds. Raven Press: New York; 1985:395–402.

500. Kelly AM, Powell C, Williams A. Parent visual analogue scale ratings of children's pain do not reliably reflect pain reported by child. Pediatric Emergency Care 2002;18(3):159–162.

501. Singer AJ, Gulla J, Thode HC Jr. Parents and practitioners are poor judges of young children's pain severity. Academic Emergency Medicine 2002;9(6):609–12.

502. Buttner W, Finke W. Analysis of behavioural and physiological parameters for the assessment of postoperative analgesic demand in newborns, infants and young children: a comprehensive report on seven consecutive studies. Paediatric Anaesthesia 2000;10(3):303–18.

503. Malviya S et al. The revised FLACC observational pain tool: improved reliability and validity for pain assessment in children with cognitive impairment. Pediatric Anesthesia 2006;16(3):258–65.

504. Manworren, RC, Hynan LS. Clinical validation of FLACC: preverbal patient pain scale. Pediatric Nursing 2003;29(2):140–6.

505. Merkel S, Voepel-Lewis T, Malviya S. Pain assessment in infants and young children: the FLACC scale. American Journal of Nursing 2002;102(10):55–8.

506. Willis MHW et al. FLACC behavioural pain assessment scale: A comparison with a child's self–report. Pediatric Nursing 2003;29(3):195–8.

507. Crellin D et al. Analysis of the validation of existing behavioral pain and distress scales for use in the procedural setting. Paediatric Anaesthesia 2007;17(8):720–33.

508. von Baeyer CL, Spagrud LJ. Systematic review of observational (behavioral) measures of pain for children and adolescents aged 3 to 18 years. Pain 2007;127(1–2):150.

509. Malviya S et al. Depth of sedation in children undergoing computed tomography: validity and reliability of the University of Michigan Sedation Scale (UMSS). British Journal of Anaesthesia 2002;88(2):241–5.

510. Malviya S et al. Can we improve the assessment of discharge readiness?: A comparative study of observational and objective measures of depth of sedation in children. Anesthesiology 2004;100(2):218–24.

511. Malviya S, Voepel-Lewis T, Tait AR. A comparison of observational and objective measures to differentiate depth of sedation in children from birth to 18 years of age. Anesthesia & Analgesia 2006;102(2):389–94.

512. McDermott NB et al. Validation of the bispectral index monitor during conscious and deep sedation in children. Anesthesia & Analgesia 2003;97(1):39–43.

513. American Academy of Pediatrics et al. Guidelines for monitoring and management of pediatric patients during and after sedation for diagnostic and therapeutic procedures: an update. Pediatrics 2006;118(6):2587–602.

514. Drendel AL et al. A randomized clinical trial of ibuprofen versus acetaminophen with codeine for acute pediatric arm fracture pain. Annals of Emergency Medicine 2009;54(4):553–60.

515. Friday JH et al. Ibuprofen provides analgesia equivalent to acetaminophen–codeine in the treatment of acute pain in children with extremity injuries: a randomized clinical trial. Academic Emergency Medicine 2009;16(8):711–16.

516. Clark E et al. A randomized, controlled trial of acetaminophen, ibuprofen, and codeine for acute pain relief in children with musculoskeletal trauma.[see comment][erratum appears in Pediatrics. Pediatrics 2007;119(3):460–7.

517. Southey ER, Soares-Weiser K, Kleijnen J, Systematic review and meta–analysis of the clinical safety and tolerability of ibuprofen compared with paracetamol in paediatric pain and fever. Current Medical Research & Opinion 2009;25(9):2207–22.

518. Herd D, Borland M. Intranasal fentanyl paediatric clinical practice guidelines. Emergency Medicine Australasia 2009;21(4):335.

519. Borland M et al. A randomized controlled trial comparing intranasal fentanyl to intravenous morphine for managing acute pain in children in the emergency department. Annals of Emergency Medicine 2007;49(3):335–40.

520. Borland ML et al. Intranasal fentanyl is an equivalent analgesic to oral morphine in paediatric burns patients for dressing changes: a randomised double blind crossover study. Burns 2005;31(7):831–7.

521. Borland ML, Jacobs I Geelhoed G. Intranasal fentanyl reduces acute pain in children in the emergency department: a safety and efficacy study. Emergency Medicine 2002;14(3):275–80.

522. Borland M, Milsom S, Esson A. Equivalency of two concentrations of fentanyl administered by the intranasal route for acute analgesia in children in a paediatric emergency department: a randomized controlled trial. Emergency Medicine Australasia 2011;23(2):202–8.

523. Crellin D, Ling RX, Babl FE. Does the standard intravenous solution of fentanyl (50 microg/mL) administered intranasally have analgesic efficacy? Emergency Medicine Australasia 2010;22(1):62–7.

524. Hansen MS et al. Intranasal fentanyl in the treatment of acute pain—a systematic review. Acta Anaesthesiologica Scandinavica 2012;56(4):407–19.

525. Serinken M et al. Intravenous paracetamol versus morphine for renal colic in the emergency department: a randomised double-blind controlled trial. Emergency Medicine Journal 2012;29(11):902–5.

526. Bektas F et al. Intravenous paracetamol or morphine for the treatment of renal colic: a randomized, placebo-controlled trial. Annals of Emergency Medicine 2009;54(4):568–74.

527. Palmer GM et al. Introduction and audit of intravenous paracetamol at a tertiary paediatric teaching hospital. Anaesthesia & Intensive Care 2007;35(5):702–6.

528. Babl FE, Theophilos T, Palmer GM. Is there a role for intravenous acetaminophen in pediatric emergency departments? Pediatric Emergency Care 2011;27(6):496–9. 10.1097/PEC.0b013e31821d8629.

529. Hopper SM et al. A double blind, randomised placebo controlled trial of topical 2% viscous lidocaine in improving oral intake in children with painful infectious mouth conditions. BMC Pediatrics 2011;11:106.

530. Cullen L et al. Nebulized lidocaine decreases the discomfort of nasogastric tube insertion: a randomized, double-blind trial. Annals of Emergency Medicine 2004;44(2):131–7.

531. Babl FE et al. Procedural pain and distress in young children as perceived by medical and nursing staff. Paediatric Anaesthesia 2008;18(5):412–19.

532. Babl FE et al. Does nebulized lidocaine reduce the pain and distress of nasogastric tube insertion in young children? A randomized, double-blind, placebo-controlled trial. Pediatrics 2009;123(6):1548–55.

533. Borland M et al. Procedural sedation in children in the emergency department: a PREDICT study. Emergency Medicine Australasia 2009;21(1):71–9.

534. Annequin D et al. Fixed 50% nitrous oxide oxygen mixture for painful procedures: A French survey. Pediatrics 2000;105(4):E47.

535. Babl FE et al. High-concentration nitrous oxide for procedural sedation in children: adverse events and depth of sedation. Pediatrics 2008;121(3):e528–32.

536. Babl FE, Oakley E, Sharwood LN. The utility of nitrous oxide. Emergency Medicine Journal 2009;26(7):544–5.

537. Frampton A et al. Nurse administered relative analgesia using high concentration nitrous oxide to facilitate minor procedures in children in an emergency department. Emerg Med Journal 2003;20:410–13.

538. Zier JL et al. Sedation with nitrous oxide compared with no sedation during catheterization for urologic imaging in children. Pediatric Radiology 2007;37(7):678–84.

539. Babl FE et al. Preprocedural fasting state and adverse events in children receiving nitrous oxide for procedural sedation and analgesia. Pediatric Emergency Care 2005;21(11):736–43.

540. Acworth JP, Purdie D, Clark RC. Intravenous ketamine plus midazolam is superior to intranasal midazolam for emergency paediatric procedural sedation. Emerg Med J 2001;18:39–45.

541. Brown JC et al. Emergency department analgesia for fracture pain. Annals of Emergency Medicine 2003;42(2):197–205.

542. Green SM et al. Predictors of emesis and recovery agitation with emergency department ketamine sedation: an individual-patient data meta-analysis of 8,282 children. Annals of Emergency Medicine 2009;54(2):171–80.e1–4.

543. Krauss B, Green SM. Procedural sedation and analgesia in children. Lancet 2006;367(9512):766–80.

544. McQueen A et al. Procedural sedation and analgesia outcomes in children after discharge from the emergency department: ketamine versus fentanyl/midazolam. Annals of Emergency Medicine 2009;54(2):191–7.e1–4.

545. Roback MG et al. Adverse events associated with procedural sedation and analgesia in a pediatric emergency department: a comparison of common parenteral drugs. Academic Emergency Medicine 2005;12(6):508–13.

546. Roback MG et al. A randomized, controlled trial of i.v. versus i.m. ketamine for sedation of pediatric patients receiving emergency department orthopedic procedures. Annals of Emergency Medicine 2006;48(5):605–12.

547. Ramaswamy P et al. Pediatric procedural sedation with ketamine: time to discharge after intramuscular versus intravenous administration. Academic Emergency Medicine 2009;16(2):101–7.

548. Kleiber C, Harper DC. Effects of distraction on children's pain and distress during medical procedures: a meta-analysis. Nursing Research 1999;48(1):44–9.

549. Uman LS et al. Psychological interventions for needle-related procedural pain and distress in children and adolescents. Cochrane Database of Systematic Reviews, 2006(4):CD005179.

550. Sinha M et al. Evaluation of nonpharmacologic methods of pain and anxiety management for laceration repair in the pediatric emergency department. Pediatrics 2006;117(4):1162–8.

551. Stevens B et al. Sucrose for analgesia in newborn infants undergoing painful procedures. Cochrane Database of Systematic Reviews 2013;DOI: 10.1002/14651858.CD001069.pub4.

552. Sheahan SL. Documentation of health risks and health promotion counseling by emergency department nurse practitioners and physicians. Journal of Nursing Scholarship 2000;32(3):245–50.

553. Starte D, Meldrum D. Developmental surveillance and assessment. In: Practical paediatrics, Roberton MD, South M, eds. Churchill Livingstone: Edinburgh; 2006.

554. Hockenberry M, Wilson D. Wong's Nursing care of Infants and children 2007, St Louis: Mosby.

555. Fitzgerald DA, Kilham HA. Bronchiolitis: assessment and evidence-based management. Med J Aust 2004;180(8):399–404.

556. Gastanaduy AS, Begue RE. Acute gastroenteritis. Clinical Pediatrics 1999;38(1):1–12.

557. Hahn S, Kim S, Garner P. Reduced osmolarity oral rehydration solution for treating dehydration caused by acute diarrhoea in children. Cochrane Database of Systematic Reviews, 2002(Issue 1):Art No:CD002847.

558. Beasley S. Abdominal pain and vomiting in children, in Practical paediatrics, Roberton DM, South M, eds, Churchill Livingstone: Edinburgh; 2007.

559. Davis RJ et al. Head and spinal cord injury. In: Rogers MC, ed. Textbook of pediatric intensive care. Baltimore: Williams & Wilkins; 1987.

560. James H, Anas N, Perkin RM. Brain insults in infants and children. New York: Grune & Stratton; 1985.

561. Morray JP et al. Coma scale for use in brain-injured children. Crit Care Med 1984;12:1018–20.

CHAPTER 37

MENTAL HEALTH EMERGENCIES
NICHOLAS PROCTER AND MONIKA FERGUSON

Essentials

- Incorporate the needs of consumers and their family/carers into clinically informed responses. People with mental health concerns have better outcomes when clinical judgement is combined with the 'voice' of the consumer and carer.
- Seek help from specialist mental health/drug and alcohol workers to intervene early to prevent an escalation of crisis or recurrence of mental illness.
- Provide a positive, supportive response without further increasing the risk of stigmatising mental illness or enforcing excessive surveillance and scrutiny, which may increase distress and further alienate the consumer.
- Provide a comprehensive mental state examination with all consumers experiencing mental health problems/mental illness. Active engagement with the consumer, carers and other emergency personnel will help ensure that a comprehensive assessment is possible.
- Continue to conduct regular observations and communicate with the consumer, ensuring that their concerns are listened to.
- Use an accredited interpreter whenever assessing a person who does not speak English. Non-accredited interpreters (such as family members and friends) should only be used in cases of extreme emergency.
- Be alert to the dangers of self-interest when working with a person who is acutely mentally unwell. Seek help and assistance and make decisions as a team. This is not the time to be a hero.

INTRODUCTION

This chapter guides the practitioner through the considerable challenges of working with mental health consumers pre-hospital and on arrival at an emergency department (ED). It encapsulates the best of current practice in mental health care relevant to a range of emergency settings and across the life span. Comprehensive discussion of mental health emergencies is beyond the scope of this chapter; therefore the material presented here focuses on those conditions seen frequently within the paramedic and ED scope of practice. It is a compilation of practice thinking and innovation in the care of consumers who have symptoms of anxiety, panic, depression, mania, schizophrenia, eating conditions, Münchausen's syndrome, serotonin syndrome and neuroleptic malignant syndrome.

A focus is also placed on dual diagnosis, and suicide, parasuicide and self-harm, as well as to legal considerations, managing violence and aggression, seclusion and restraint and cultural considerations. This chapter concludes by highlighting the importance of interprofessional collaboration and the prevention of communication breakdown and clinical pathway deadlock between individual practitioners and organisations.

Background

The 2010 announcement of psychiatrist Patrick McGorry as Australian of the Year has brought mental health into the spotlight, representing a significant public acknowledgement of mental health as a growing national concern across Australia. Results from the 2007 National Survey of Mental Health and Wellbeing, conducted by the Australian Bureau of Statistics,[1] indicate that one in five people aged between 16 and 85 years experience at least one of the highly prevalent forms of mental illness (anxiety, affective conditions and substance-use conditions) in any one year. Prevalence rates vary depending upon age and are highest during the early adult years. It is estimated that almost 64,000 Australians (aged 18–64 years) have a psychotic illness and are in contact with public specialised mental health services each year, with prevalence rates being highest for males aged 25–34 years.[2]

Hickie and colleagues[3] identify the following trends in mental health in Australia:

- People aged between 25 and 49 years account for 56% of all suicides in Australia, and rates are highest in men aged 25–29 years (31.1 per 100,000).
- More than half of all health-related disability costs in 15- to 34-year-olds are attributable to mental health problems.
- 27% of all years lived with disability in Australia are attributable to mental conditions.
- Less than 40% of consumers with mental conditions receive any mental health care in a 12-month period compared with almost 80% for other common physical health problems.
- 75% of mental health care is provided in the primary care sector, with limited access to specialist support.
- Almost 50% of consumers with mental conditions are not recognised by their general practitioner as having a psychological problem.
- Over 50% of psychotic conditions commence before age 25, often with a delay of 2–8 years before first presentation for treatment.
- Up to 60% of cases of alcohol/other substance use could be prevented by earlier treatment of common mental health problems.

Although current rates of mental illness among Aboriginal and Torres Strait Islander people are undetermined, data from the 2008 Health and Welfare of Australia's Aboriginal and Torres Strait Islander Peoples Survey[4] outline that Indigenous Australians are twice as likely than non-Indigenous Australians to report either high or very high levels of psychological distress.

There are also indications for the future of mental health care in Australia. There is an increasing incidence of mental conditions in young people, increased numbers of presentations for care, and more disturbed behaviour, often in association with alcohol or other substance misuse problems. Most likely, the incidence of mental illness across Australia will continue to increase, particularly among younger consumers, partly because of the adverse effects of current social and environmental factors (including increased family breakdown, decreasing participation in and sense of belonging to community-based structures such as churches, sporting and recreational associations and social clubs, and increased exposure to substances such as cannabis and illicit stimulants), as well as ineffectiveness of current treatment modalities.[5] The prevalence of mental conditions among older adults will also continue to rise as the ageing of Australians is accompanied by an increased incidence of vascular, degenerative and other brain conditions.[3]

There are similar concerns in New Zealand. The Te Rau Hinengaro or New Zealand Mental Health Survey, undertaken between 2003 and 2004, was a nationwide face-to-face household survey of residents aged 16 years and over. It aimed to estimate the prevalence and severity of anxiety, mood, substance and eating conditions in New Zealand, and associated disability and treatment. There were 12,992 participants (including 2595 Māori and 2236 Pacific Island people). Compared with other World Mental Health survey sites, New Zealand has relatively high prevalences, although almost always a little lower than for the USA.[6] Key findings of the survey were as follows:[7]

- 46.6% of the population are predicted to meet criteria for a condition at some time in their lives, with 39.5% having already done so and 20.7% having a condition in the past 12 months.[8]
- Younger people have a higher prevalence of mental illness in the past 12 months and are more likely to report having ever had a mental illness.
- Females have higher prevalences of anxiety conditions, major depression and eating conditions than males, whereas males have substantially higher prevalences of substance-abuse conditions.
- Prevalence is higher for people who are disadvantaged, whether measured by educational qualification, equivalised household income or living in more-deprived areas.[9]

Prevalence is higher for Māori and Pacific Islanders than for the other composite ethnic group. The 12-month prevalence is 29.5% and 24.4% respectively for Māori and Pacific Islanders (compared to 20.7% for the total New Zealand population). This appears to largely be attributed to the youthfulness of these populations and their relative socioeconomic disadvantage.[10]

People with more serious mental condition in the past 12 months are more likely to have visited the healthcare sector for mental health reasons, including for problems with their use of alcohol/other drugs. However, the proportion making a visit is low—only 58.0% of those with serious mental illness, 36.5% of those with moderate mental illness and 18.5% of those with mild mental illness.[10]

Co-morbidity of mental illness (the experience of more than one condition/disease by an individual) is common, with 37.0% of those experiencing 12-month mental illness having two or more conditions (most frequently mood and anxiety conditions). Co-morbidity is associated with suicidal behaviour and increased service use.

There is also co-morbidity between mental and physical conditions. People with mental illness have a higher prevalence of several chronic physical conditions compared to people without mental illness of the same age. People with chronic physical conditions are also more likely to experience mental illness compared with those without physical conditions.

In the New Zealand mental health survey, 15.7% reported having thought seriously about suicide (suicidal ideation), 5.5% had made a suicide plan and 4.5% had made an attempt. The risk of suicidal ideation in the past 12 months was higher in females, younger people, people with lower educational qualifications and people with low household income, and among people living in more-deprived areas.[11]

Various Australian mental health policies[12–14] acknowledge that many of the determinants of good mental health, and of mental illness, are influenced by factors beyond the health system. The Fourth National Mental Health Plan 2009–2014[13] explicitly outlines the need for services being developed and delivered in a way that reduces the risk of people falling through the gaps, reduces unnecessary duplication and complexity and promotes collaboration between services at all levels. This is particularly important to paramedical and other health personnel working in the context of significant efforts being made to combine mental health services within the general health system and a community-based system of assessment, treatment and support. A whole-of-government, cross-sectorial approach is based upon principles of human rights and equity, and the belief that integrated mental health and community services could and should provide holistic care to consumers in a manner that contributes to the prevention of illness and the reduction of stigma.[15]

> **PRACTICE TIP**
>
> People who live with mental illness are also more at risk of physical health problems (e.g. cancer, cardiovascular illness or diabetes) and average life expectancy is shorter. Be equally alert to physical and mental health. Apply this knowledge to the consumer's assessment and treatment.

Prevalence of mental health admissions in emergency departments

As indicated by the prevalence of mental illness in Australia and New Zealand, mental health in emergency situations is also a growing concern, with increasing numbers of distressed consumers presenting in mainstream hospital and community settings.[15] Certain mental health presentations are more common in EDs than others. In Australia, it was estimated that there were almost 250,000 ED visits with a mental-health related principal diagnosis during 2010–2011.[16] The most common principal diagnoses were: neurotic, stress-related and somatoform conditions (28%); mental and behavioural conditions due to psychoactive substance use (25%); and affective conditions (15%). Schizophrenia, schizotypal and delusional conditions accounted for a further 13% of visits. Individuals aged 15–54 accounted for a higher proportion of mental-health-related visits (78%) compared to all ED visits (51%).

Pathways to the ED

Mental health consumers experiencing significant distress can come to the attention of emergency mental health services in a number of ways. They may present to an ED via their own mode of transport, or that of a family member/carer. They may

also be transported by a community mental health team, or by police officers. Alternatively, paramedics may transport the individual via ambulance. Whatever the pathway, the safety of the person in distress, the attending professionals, family members and bystanders are major priorities.

Transport to the ED via ambulance

Guidelines for the transport of an individual to hospital via ambulance vary from state to state. The details here use current Victorian protocol[17] as an example (it is recommended that readers use this as a guide only, in conjunction with specific legislation and protocols within their state/territory). The Victorian protocol recognises the need to provide a person-focused approach, in which the consumer, their family/carer and other health/mental health professionals are involved in the transport decision. Where a decision has been made that a person requires admission to an approved mental health service, the decision about the most appropriate form of transport should include assessing the following:

- the individual's physical and mental state
- the individual's immediate treatment needs
- risk of harm the individual poses to themselves and others
- the likely effect on the individual of the proposed mode of transport
- expressed wishes of the individual and/or their carer(s), where practicable
- availability of the various modes of transport, including non-emergency patient transport vehicles
- the distance to be travelled
- the individual's need for support and supervision during the period of travel.

In certain circumstances, consideration should first be given to non-ambulance transport (other options include private vehicle, mental health professional agency vehicle, non-emergency patient transport vehicle). Transport via police vehicle should be seen as a last resort (used only when absolutely necessary, such as when an individual is in police custody), due to the potential to give the impression that the person is suspected of having committed a crime, which could cause unnecessary distress and anxiety, and perpetuate stigma. Where an individual is detained under the relevant Mental Health Act (see Ch 4), the police must maintain their custody and therefore will remain until the conclusion of the person's mental health assessment, even if the person is transported by ambulance to the ED.

If it is decided that an ambulance is the preferred mode of transport, the ambulance responses are categorised into the following three codes: emergency, urgent and routine (see Table 37.1). Generally, people experiencing a mental illness who may require transport to hospital need to be assessed by a health/mental health professional first, to determine whether hospitalisation is required, as well as what form of transport is needed. Sometimes, such as in cases of an overdose, a consumer/family member/carer will need to contact ambulance services directly. In these instances, a judgement will be made by the ambulance service to categorise the request in accordance with Table 37.1. If, upon ambulance arrival, the person appears to have a mental illness but does not require hospitalisation, then the local mental health service triage must be contacted

TABLE 37.1 Categories of ambulance response[17]		
AMBULANCE CATEGORY AND ACUITY	RESPONSE	DESCRIPTION
Code 1—emergency	Emergency response using lights and sirens, with person being transported to nearest appropriate ED for treatment/stabilisation.	There is an actual or potential risk that the person's life is immediately threatened (e.g. suicide attempt or overdose of harmful substance)
Code 2—urgent	A response (no lights and sirens) where the person is transported to the nearest ED or nearest appropriate mental health service.	The person: • exhibits evidence of acute mental illness, accompanied by agitation, distress, impulsivity, unpredictability and/or propensity to destructive acts • has attempted/threatened suicide but their life is not immediately threatened • is unable to be contained safely in a care or support situation in the community and has been sedated to enable safe transport • requires approved mechanical restraint for safe transport, or • is in crisis and has been apprehended by police under the Mental Health Act.
Code 3—routine	In some circumstances (e.g. in rural areas), a person will need to be transported to the nearest appropriate approved mental health service for admission (rather than the catchment area service the person should normally be admitted to). This may occur where either: • the person's wellbeing may be adversely affected by a long-distance transfer, or • a long-distance transfer at that time might adversely affect the provision of acute ambulance care in the rural community from which the ambulance would need to be dispatched.	Adequate care is currently being provided, but the person requires transport to an approved mental health service (e.g. inter-hospital transfers). Other forms of transport have been considered and deemed unsuitable by the mental health professional.

to arrange appropriate management. If the person requires hospital treatment but refuses ambulance transport, the paramedics must contact the local area mental health service triage to organise a more urgent response.

Pre-hospital assessment and management

Mental health conditions can be a common response for paramedics and therefore paramedics play a crucial role in pre-hospital assessment, treatment and care, particularly in instances when assistance from mental health services is not present (for example, when an ambulance has been requested by a member of the community, rather than by a community mental health team). Paramedics are well placed to undertake a screening mental state examination (mental health assessment) to determine if the person is at risk of self-harm or harm to others, is becoming aggressive and whether action is required to reduce this risk. A screening mental state examination involves enquiring about the individual's current circumstances and any recent changes in their life, as well as understanding their present thought processes and content, actions, emotions

and feelings.[18] Consultation with family/friends present can further assist with understanding the individual's current behaviour and experiences. Conducting screening risk and mental state assessments at first contact can also help build a clinical picture over time, documenting any significant change in behaviour, suicidal ideation or clinical presentation.

Prior to transfer (and if time permits), paramedics are well placed to inquire about and document the immediate home or living environment and all collateral contacts, including any efforts to obtain collateral information from them. Other documentation to be completed by paramedics includes the use of mechanical devices or pharmacological agents for restraint and any adverse events that compromise safety to paramedics, the person being transported, family members or bystanders. In many instances there will be no mental health professional present or available to assess or assist with the person. In severe cases paramedics may be required to administer pharmacological interventions such as lorazepam (1–2.5 mg orally) or midazolam (5–10 mg intramuscularly) and provide physical restraints—sometimes without the need to consult a mental health practitioner.

ED triage assessment

Upon arrival at the ED, the first step in the care process is triage assessment. In mental health emergencies, the screening and classifying of distressed persons to determine priority needs and actions calls for sharp assessment skills and efficient use of human resources, equipment and other resources. If appropriate resources are not available for urgent cases, then steps should be taken to bring these to the consumer as soon as possible. Table 37.2 has been adapted from best-practice principles currently used in New South Wales[19] (again, it is important to ensure that readers also access protocols from their own state/territory). It outlines some key markers for determining mental health triage categories and the typical presentations observed or reported by secondary (non-consumer) sources. While these categories differ in their degree of risk, complexity and cross-cultural applicability, they do offer a consistent approach to decision-making following

initial screening of all incoming referrals and admissions to the ED. It is worth noting that of the total mental health-related emergency visits in Australia during 2010–2011, over 80% of these were classified as either semi-urgent or urgent; less that 10% were classified as emergencies and approximately 1% required resuscitation.[16]

For each presentation the assessor should answer the following questions:

- Can I safely interview this consumer on my own, or do I need backup?
- Is the consumer going to be safe where they are?
- Can they be left alone and/or with others safely?
- What degree of observation do they need and can it be provided in the ED?
- Where is the most appropriate place to interview the consumer given their level of arousal and agitation?

TABLE 37.2 Mental health triage assessment in the emergency department[19]

TRIAGE CATEGORY AND TREATMENT ACUITY	DESCRIPTION	TYPICAL PRESENTATION OBSERVED AND/OR REPORTED
1 Immediate	Definite danger to life (self or others)	Observed: • Violent behaviour • Possession of a weapon • Self-harm in ED • Displays extreme agitation/restlessness • Bizarre/disoriented behaviour
2 Emergency Within 10 minutes	Probable risk of danger to self or others AND/OR Individual is physically restrained in ED AND/OR Severe behavioural disturbance	Observed: • Extreme agitation/restlessness • Physically/verbally aggressive • Confused/unable to cooperate • Hallucinations/delusions/paranoia • Requires restraint/containment • High risk of absconding and not wanting treatment Reported: • Attempt/threat of self-harm • Threat of harm to others • Unable to wait safely
3 Urgent Within 30 minutes	Possible danger to self or others Moderate behaviour disturbance Severe distress	Observed: • Agitation/restlessness • Intrusive behaviour • Confused • Ambivalent about treatment • Not likely to wait for treatment Reported: • Suicidal ideation • Situational crisis • Presence of psychotic symptoms: • Hallucinations • Delusions • Paranoid ideas • Thought disordered • Bizarre/agitated behaviour Presence of mood disturbance: • Severe symptoms of depression • Withdrawn/uncommunicative • And/or anxiety • Elevated/irritable mood

Continued

TABLE 37.2 Mental health triage assessment in the emergency department[19]—cont'd

TRIAGE CATEGORY AND TREATMENT ACUITY	DESCRIPTION	TYPICAL PRESENTATION OBSERVED AND/OR REPORTED
4 Semi-urgent Within 60 minutes	Moderate distress	Observed: • No agitation/restlessness • Irritability without aggression • Cooperative • Gives coherent history Reported: • Pre-existing mental health condition • Symptoms of anxiety or depression without suicidal ideation • Willing to wait
5 Non-urgent Within 120 minutes	No danger to self or others No acute distress No behavioural disturbance	Observed: • Cooperative • Communicative • Compliant with requests Reported: • Known consumer with chronic psychotic symptoms • Pre-existing non-acute mental health condition • Known consumer with chronic unexplained somatic complaints • Request for medication • Minor adverse effect of medication • Seeking assistance with financial/social problems

Answering these questions will help make the fullest and safest triage assessment possible, to benefit the consumer, their family/carers and the treatment team. The assessment must be recorded clearly and, if decisions are made, reasons given. In many instances the assessment will involve formulation of a differential diagnosis—most commonly for episodic referrals. It will be teamwork and interdisciplinary consultation, collaboration on the need for further investigations and active involvement of sub-specialties in clinical cases that will help determine an appropriate clinical pathway. The names of other colleagues who are consulted or involved in the decision must also appear in the clinical record.

After triage

Once the triage assessment has been made, a brief mental state assessment will be conducted, usually by a general nurse and/or medical officer. The purpose of the mental health assessment is to obtain information about specific aspects of the individual's mental health experiences and behaviour at the time of interview (see Box 37.1).[20] If necessary, the individual will then be referred to the mental health team for a further interview, with an assessment conducted by a mental health liaison nurse consultant. Following this assessment, the mental health nurse, in consultation with the mental health team and the referring medical officer, will make a decision about the next course of action. In instances where immediate care is needed, the individual will then be admitted to hospital. Alternatively, if it is deemed safe and in the best interests of the individual to go home, the mental health nurse will provide them with information regarding support services in the community. These services should be as specific to the concerns experienced by the individual as possible. In instances where it is clear that additional community support

---

BOX 37.1 Important items for mental state assessment[21]

- *Appearance*—attire, cleanliness, posture (sitting and/or standing) and gait
- *Behaviour*—facial expression, relaxed or cooperative or aggressive. Describe in detail activity, agitation, level of arousal (including physiological signs)
- *Speech*—form and pattern, language spoken, volume and rate. Is it coherent, logical and congruent with questioning?
- *Mood*—apathetic, irritable, labile, optimistic or pessimistic, thoughts of suicide. Do reported experience and observable mood agree?
- *Thought*—particular preoccupations, ideas and beliefs. Are they rational, fixed or delusional? Do they concern the safety of the consumer or other consumers? Do they relate to the person's attire, speech or mood and, if so, how?
- *Perception*—abnormalities including hallucinations occurring in any modality (auditory, visual, smell, taste, touch)
- *Intellect*—brief note of cognitive and intellectual function. Is the consumer orientated in time, place and person? Is the consumer able to function intellectually at a level expected from their history?
- *Insight*—how does the consumer explain or attribute their symptoms? What is the consumer's understanding of the factors contributing to their current situation? How does the consumer perceive their need for care and/or treatment and support?

The full mental state examination may be built up over several interviews by elaboration of these topics using increasingly direct, closed questioning, as well as collateral information provided by friends and family members.

is needed, the nurse will make a referral to a community mental health team.

Referral and care continuity

Crucial to the practice of effective mental health interventions is the way that an assessment is communicated, the way in which symptoms are described and the language used by both practitioners and consumer in this process. The formulation of a succinct summary of a consumer's history, current circumstances and main problems will help set the diagnosis in context.[22] It is particularly useful in conveying essential information upon discharge, when making a referral to a specialist mental health service or when referring for other specialist intervention. The time and trouble taken to communicate assessment findings will go a long way to helping ensure continuity of information and, if more than one provider is involved, continuity of the therapeutic relationship and timely referral for additional assessment or care (Box 37.2).

The role of ED mental health liaison nurse consultants

In some Australian states and territories, general hospitals have employed mental health liaison nurse consultants to assist with clinical assessment and treatment of people experiencing mental health problems/mental illness. The role is developed and defined by the needs of the hospital/health service. The main workload is assessment and support for consumers with new or pre-existing mental illness, management of emotional complications of physical illness or trauma, management of the behavioural disturbance, assessment of abnormal social behaviour, management of behavioural and emotional consequences of intoxication and drug use, and clinical assessment following attempted suicide and self-harm. High consumer satisfaction with the role has been found, particularly in terms of the service provided, information offered and improvements to consumer health outcomes.[24] Similarly, recent evidence indicates that this role can play an important part in ED-based outpatient services, particularly regarding improved consumer access to specialised metal health care.[25]

Psychiatric Emergency Care Centres

Extending the role of liaison nurse consultants, many hospitals now have Psychiatric Emergency Care Centres (PECC), which have been developed alongside EDs. These centres serve to provide timely, specialist mental health assessment on-site in the ED.[26] Generally, these services offer 24-hour mental health staff presence. PECC also provide high-level observation/immediate care for people requiring short-term mental health care (usually up to 48 hours). While the nature of work undertaken within a PECC may vary across jurisdictions, there is usually a protocol for fast-tracking mental health assessments of ED presentations. The PECC environment should be one that is constantly monitored, providing appropriate use of sedation and restraint, in line with local policies and clinical protocols.

Mental health conditions

This section outlines various mental health conditions that may be seen in emergency situations. The symptoms and diagnostic characteristics described are based on the American Psychiatric Association's *Diagnostic and Statistical Manual of Mental Disorders*.[27] The WHO International Classification of Diseases[28] can also be used for diagnosis. It is important to note that while these descriptions are important, each individual will experience mental health conditions differently, and so presentations of the same diagnosis might differ from person to person. Additionally, many consumers will experience comorbidity—that is, a diagnosis of more than one condition. At all times, care should be tailored to the individual as much as possible.

By their very nature, mental health conditions must be assessed holistically, taking account of psychosocial, cognitive, biological and interpersonal domains. Assessment therefore requires the practitioner to have an understanding and recognition of the symptoms of mental health conditions, and to be able to distinguish these from physical health diagnoses. Assessment is primarily made through talking to the individual and, where possible, their family/carers/friends and any other professionals involved in their care. Various assessment tools can be used for the different conditions, and typically these will be in a questionnaire-type format, addressing the experience of various symptoms. However, a richer and deeper understanding will come from listening to the individual sharing their story, as well as from observations of the individual's behaviour.

Anxiety conditions

Anxiety is the most commonly experienced mental health condition, affecting approximately 15% of Australians and New Zealanders aged between 16 and 85 years, with a higher prevalence in women than men.[1,7] Some of the anxiety conditions include generalised anxiety, obsessive compulsive conditions, social phobia, panic condition, agoraphobia, specific phobia and post-traumatic stress. Common to all of these is excessive fear and anxiety, as well as related physical/behavioural symptoms; often this experience is so overwhelming that it can interfere with a person's day-to-day functioning.

While the causes of anxiety are not fully understood, it is likely that a particular anxiety condition is a result of several interacting factors and is affected by stressful life events and personality traits such as:[29]

- excessive or unrealistic worries (generalised anxiety condition)

BOX 37.2 Important items for referral to additional services[23]

- Description of the presenting complaint, its intensity and duration.
- Relevant current and past medical history and medication.
- A note of mental state examination results with key or contradictory findings highlighted.
- An estimate of degree of urgency in terms of risk to the consumer and others.
- Indication of referrer's expectations (assessment, advice, admission).
- The most urgent requests should be reinforced by telephone or email.

- compulsions and obsessions which the consumer cannot control (obsessive compulsive condition)
- intense excessive worry about social situations (social anxiety condition)
- panic attacks (panic condition)
- an intense, irrational fear of everyday objects and situations (phobia).

Generalised anxiety condition

Generalised anxiety is one of the more commonly experienced anxiety conditions. Many individuals diagnosed with this condition report having experienced feelings of anxiety and nervousness throughout their lives.[26]

Symptoms and diagnostic criteria

The symptoms of generalised anxiety involve excessive anxiety or worry, about particular life domains, which is perceived to be difficult to control by the individual. Symptoms are both psychological and physical (see Box 37.3 for diagnostic criteria).

Management

Treatment can help people manage, reduce or even eliminate anxiety symptoms. Diagnosis is generally made by a psychiatrist. Clinical psychologists, social workers or counsellors often manage ongoing treatment. Effective treatments include medication, cognitive behavioural therapy and community support and recovery programs. During cognitive behaviour therapy, a person learns new and effective ways to cope with their symptoms. The skills of the nurse will include cognitive behavioural interventions, understanding the nature of the concern, offering reassurance and focusing on the positive abilities of the person to take control of the situation, to overcome the limitations of their thinking.

Panic

Due to the associated physical symptoms of a panic attack, people experiencing this condition might present to the ED. Panic condition has a high co-morbidity with other anxiety and depressive conditions.[30]

Symptoms and diagnostic criteria

Panic condition is signified by recurrent, unexpected panic attacks. The acute panic attack usually begins with a sudden onset. Key diagnostic criteria are described in Box 37.4.

Management

The skills needed to manage panic are to be calm and reassuring and to reduce unnecessary or distressing stimulation. The practitioner should speak in a calm and controlled voice, asking the consumer to focus on their breathing, talking to them in such a way that they are helping to de-escalate the situation, letting the consumer know that they are in a safe and protective environment and that they will feel better once they regain control of their situation. Actively helping the consumer to relax, and educating other practitioners to take a similar stance, will greatly enhance the consumer's ability to reduce the intensity of the panic. It may be necessary to have a relative or friend sit with the consumer, working closely with the practitioner to reinforce that they are safe and that no one intends to make their situation worse or bring harm. Aspects of communication with a person in the acute phase of panic are discussed in Box 37.5.

BOX 37.3 Criteria for diagnosing generalised anxiety

People diagnosed with generalised anxiety describe excessive anxiety or worry for the majority of the week for at least 6 months. The person may be preoccupied about work and work relationships, performing well at school or at some other activity. Despite their best efforts, the person struggles to control or block out their worries and preoccupations. At the same time they may experience motor restlessness, irritability, difficulty in concentration, feeling highly strung and an inability to process everyday information. The physical effects of generalised anxiety include tense and sore muscles and disturbed sleep. Where sleep is possible, it may be only for short periods and unsatisfying. The change in the person's behaviour is not attributable to the physiological effects of a substance or to another medical condition.

BOX 37.4 Criteria for diagnosing a panic condition

People diagnosed with a panic condition experience an overwhelming and abrupt surge of intense fear and discomfort that reaches a peak usually within a short time-frame (usually minutes). The person is visibly distressed, often sweating, with a rapid and thumping heartbeat. They may also be trembling and describe a sense of impending doom. Additional feelings and sensations include shortness of breath and a feeling that the person is not breathing in adequate amounts of air. The person may also feel as if they are suffocating or choking. The strength of emotions and feelings of dizziness and/or light-headedness may be accompanied by a fear of losing control or 'going crazy', or perhaps a fear of dying. For the diagnostic criteria to be met, the panic attack itself must have been followed by at least 30 days of at least one of the following: (a) persistent concern/worry about additional panic attacks or their consequences; or (b) a significant maladaptive change in behaviour related to the panic attacks. The change in thought, feeling and behaviour is not attributable to the physiological effects of a substance or to another medical condition.

PRACTICE TIP

Be alert to the contagion effects of anxiety and panic, and guard against them. Front-line workers working in high-stress environments must initiate self-care to reduce the impact of mental health presentations on their own health and wellbeing.

Affective conditions

Affective conditions involve a change in affect or disturbance in mood. Affective conditions are experienced by women more than men (7.1% versus 5.3% in Australia; 9.5% versus 6.3% in New Zealand).[1,7] Some affective conditions include major depression, mania (as a feature of bipolar condition) and post-natal depression.

BOX 37.5 Aspects of communication with a person in the acute phase of panic[31]

- *Foster trust and confidence*—stay with the consumer; ensure continuity of practitioners; reassure the consumer that they are not dying, will not lose consciousness, that you are working with others to help resolve the situation and restore calm. This will help counter feeling out of control, a fear of having a heart attack or losing one's mind.
- *Model calmness and reassurance*—have the consumer follow you in the taking of long, deep breaths. Breathing with the consumer will help encourage teamwork and joint problem-solving. Slow, deep breathing can help reduce panic to a manageable level of anxiety. Consumers in a panic state may take their physiological symptoms as an indication that they are going to die.
- *Self-monitor your own reactions to acute panic*—do some deep breathing, use quiet pauses and seek out support from colleagues to maintain self-confidence and clear thinking. Acute anxiety can be transmittable from one person to another and this can create a roller-coaster of emotions.

BOX 37.6 Criteria for diagnosing a major depressive condition

People diagnosed with a major depressive condition often experience a feeling of depressed mood for most of the day, nearly every day for the week just past. There may be a markedly diminished interest or pleasure in most or a majority of activities for several days during the past 14-day period. The marked diminished interest in pleasure is often indicated by a subjective account or observation from others (for example, work colleagues or family members). At the same time there may be significant weight loss (when the person is not actively dieting) or weight gain, or a decrease in appetite nearly every day. They may have difficulty sleeping (either getting to sleep or staying asleep) or hypersomnia reported nearly every day. The subjective impression of the person is that they are 'not the same', with noticeable psychomotor agitation/retardation nearly every day (observable by the person, and noticeable to others, and not merely subjective feelings of restlessness or being slowed down). An overwhelming feeling of fatigue and/or loss of energy nearly every day may leave the person in a distressed and unsettled state of mind. There may also be impairment in family, social, employment or other important areas of daily functioning. The change in thought, mood and behaviour is not attributable to the physiological effects of a substance or to another medical condition.

Major depression

Depression affects the way someone feels, causing a persistent lowering of mood. Annually, it is estimated that more than 800,000 Australian adults and 95,000 children/young people are affected by depression.[32] Globally, depression is the third leading contributor to the disease burden.[33]

Symptoms and diagnostic criteria

Depression is often accompanied by a range of physical and emotional symptoms that can impede the way a person is able to function at home, at work and in their everyday life. Key diagnostic criteria are outlined in Box 37.6.

Management

Management of depression can involve medication, individual therapy or community and social support programs—or a combination of all three. Medications assist the brain to restore its usual chemical balance, helping to control the symptoms of depression. Individual therapy involving a doctor, psychologist or other healthcare professional talking with the person about their symptoms, and discussing alternative ways of thinking about and coping with them, can be effective, particularly in building confidence and self-esteem. Similarly, community support programs are most helpful when they include information about the condition, accommodation support and options and help with finding suitable employment, training and education, psychosocial rehabilitation and mutual support groups. Understanding and acceptance by the community—including the therapeutic community in the ED—is also very important.

Postnatal depression

Postnatal depression is a significant clinical condition occurring in 10–15% of women within 6 months postpartum. The risk factors for postnatal depression include a personal or family history of depression, severe 'baby blues', ambivalence towards or unwanted pregnancy, and poor social and/or partner support. Postnatal depression is much less common than the postnatal blues and, if left untreated, may become a chronic condition.

Symptoms

The clinical features of postnatal depression are similar to those of major depression, although during mental state assessment there may be thought content that includes worries about going outside the home, and worries and concerns about the baby's health or the ability to cope adequately with the baby.

Management

Management of postnatal depression is largely supportive, educative and interactive between practitioner and consumer. Providing an explanation of the condition and education about treatment can provide a certain amount of relief. This can help women and their partners give meaning to their experience and prevent unhelpful worry that they are 'going crazy' or that their situation is one of personal failure because they are unfit to be a mother. Explaining what postnatal depression is, how it is not related to personal shortcomings and giving ample opportunity for the mother to talk openly and freely about such things as her relationship with her own mother, her partner, her disappointments, frustrations or stressors can generate trust and informed awareness of the situation. The emergency nurse can assist with organising help with childcare or respite, placing the woman in touch with support organisations and peer support workers, helping the woman recruit ongoing help and support from her general practitioner, family and friends and referring the woman to professional mental health care.

Depression in later life

Consistent with global estimates,[34] it has been predicted that the number of people aged over 65 years will exceed one million by 2030 in New Zealand[35] and will comprise 25% of the Australian population by 2050.[36] While many people can age well, growing older also presents certain challenges, including increased isolation and loneliness, deaths of partners and/or friends, as well as the development of medical conditions and cognitive decline,[37] all of which can contribute to feelings of alienation, hopelessness and lowered self-esteem.[38] Not surprisingly, depression is one of the most common mental health concerns in later life and can have severe effects on physical health and social relationships.

Management

Treating depression in older people requires flexibility and sensitivity, such as working at a slower pace and being prepared for the potential need to repeat conversations when interacting with older adults.[39] In addition, the use of pharmacological treatment needs to be considered with caution, as such treatments can place older people at increased risk of injury as a result of adverse effects.[40] The emergency nurse can support a person with depression in later life by promoting activities that improve nutrition, social interaction and social support and family relationships. While this might seem difficult to do in a busy ED, the initial naming of these interventions in the presence of family, for example, can go a long way as similar messages are given by others (general practitioner, community nurse) who will also have contact with the consumer. Some consumers may have a negative view of themselves as people, of their contribution to family and society and of their future. Family members, social support networks and others important in the life of the consumer should be reminded that depression is not a weakness or a failure and that family education and social support and, in some instances, antidepressant medication can bring considerable benefit.

Manic episode

A manic episode is a period of unusually elevated mood and irritability which affects occupational and social functioning. Such an episode is typically experienced by individuals with a diagnosis of bipolar I condition.

Symptoms and diagnostic criteria

A manic episode is primarily marked by symptoms of elevated mood and a tendency to engage in behaviour that could have serious social or financial consequences.[41] Diagnostic criteria are listed in Box 37.7.

Management

The specific management of a manic episode will include administration of medication (usually a benzodiazepine or antipsychotic in acute behaviour disturbance), keeping the environmental stimuli to a minimum, allowing the person to move yet remain under constant observation and providing physical supports as continuous motor activity, sleeplessness and overactivity may lead the patient to physically stop without much warning. The combined elements of this approach are designed to decrease the prospect of behaviour escalating and becoming out of control, and help restore calm at a time when the consumer does not have adequate internal control. This will

---

> **BOX 37.7 Criteria for diagnosing a manic episode**
>
> At the time of a manic episode people experience a distinct period of abnormally and persistently elevated, expansive or irritable mood and out-of-character and persistently increasing goal-directed activity or energy. These combined experiences last at least 7 days and are present most of the day, nearly every day. The symptoms at this time are such that immediate hospitalisation may be required. During the episode the person displays disturbed mood and increased energy or physical activity and there is a noticeable change from their usual behaviour, incorporating the following symptoms: a feeling of overstated self-esteem/grandiosity; a decreased need for rest or sleep; being extravagant and overly more talkative than usual, with a pressure to keep talking. There is a discernible rapid thinking—sometimes described as a 'flight of ideas'. The subjective experience at this time is that thoughts are racing and the person is easily distracted, giving rise to attention being too easily drawn to insignificant or immaterial external stimuli. Disturbance in mood is so severe as to cause marked impairment in functioning in social, family and work-related activity. The change in behaviour is not attributable to the physiological effects of a substance or to another medical condition.

also help promote physical safety for the consumer, staff and others present.

Schizophrenia

Schizophrenia affects the regular functioning of the brain, interfering with a person's ability to think, feel and act. In Australia, schizophrenia is the most commonly experienced psychotic condition, with two-thirds of consumers experiencing their first episode prior to the age of 25 years.[2] Some individuals do recover completely from this illness, and, with time and appropriate medication, community support and acceptance, most find that their symptoms improve. However, for many, schizophrenia is a prolonged illness which can involve years of distressing symptoms and disability. Family and social relationships may be fragmented or broken and, as a result of the episodic nature of the illness, stigma and other social factors, there may be an inability to maintain contact with consumers over prolonged periods. This situation is made more challenging when the causes of schizophrenia are not fully understood by both the scientific community and wider society. Recently it has been accepted by a range of professionals that stress, for example, or use of drugs such as marijuana, LSD or speed can trigger the first episode of the illness. Consumers affected by schizophrenia have one 'personality', just like everyone else. It is a myth and totally untrue that those affected have a so-called 'split personality'.

Symptoms and diagnostic criteria

Schizophrenia is often character*istised* by a range of cognitive, behavioural and emotional dysfunctions. Diagnostic criteria are shown in Box 37.8.

BOX 37.8 Criteria for diagnosing schizophrenia

People diagnosed with schizophrenia experience at least two of the following symptoms for a majority of days during a 30-day period: delusions (fixed false beliefs that are not amenable to change in light of contradictory evidence); hallucinations (often in the form of hearing or visual perception-like experiences that occur without external stimulus); disorganised and often incoherent speech; grossly disorganised/catatonic behaviour (may be expressed in a range of ways, such as childlike silliness or unexpected agitation); negative symptoms (i.e. reduced emotional expression and avolition). For a significant portion of the time since the onset of the condition, the level of functioning in one or more major areas, such as work, day-to-day interpersonal relations or self-care, is distinctively below the level achieved prior to the start of the condition. The changes in behaviour are not attributable to the physiological effects of a substance or other known physical condition.

BOX 37.9 Criteria for diagnosing anorexia nervosa

The overall clinical picture for people diagnosed with anorexia nervosa is marked by a restricted energy intake comparative to daily requirements, leading to a significantly lower body weight (defined as weight that is less than minimally normal/expected for age and gender, developmental stage and pre-existing physical condition). People experience an intense fear of gaining weight/becoming fat, or express dogged behaviour that interferes with putting on weight, even though they are at a notably low weight. There are conspicuous changes in the way in which they describe and experience their body weight and shape, and this may be expressed in words or drawings. There is also a steadfast lack of personal recognition of the risk and potential seriousness of the current low body weight.

Management

When a person experiencing schizophrenia requires emergency mental health care, they are likely to be encountering severe symptoms of psychosis. It is important to encourage the individual to feel safe, and to de-escalate their stress as much as possible. The management of such consumers involves the following key features:[31]

- *Clarity and congruence*—ensure that communication is congruent between verbal and non-verbal messages. This is because some consumers may be very sensitive to non-verbal behaviour and whether the non-verbal supports the verbal message. Where possible use 'I' and 'you' rather than 'we' and 'us' to avoid confusing the consumer.
- *Model desired behaviours*—model expression of thought and feeling by interacting with other practitioners in the presence of the consumer with an inclusive fashion, then, where possible, openly discuss, repeat and reassure the core messages from the healthcare workers. Consumers with schizophrenia may take additional time to reach a level of trust where they can accept actions directed from healthcare professionals towards them.
- *Foster trust and relationship-building*—follow through on commitments made, inform the consumer when you will be talking to them, give careful explanations for treatments and medications and allow the consumer to control the amount of self-disclosure that takes place in the interaction. Such actions demonstrate trust by making the healthcare worker accessible to the consumer both physically and emotionally.

Eating conditions

An eating condition is characterised by persistent thoughts and disturbance regarding eating, eating-related behaviour and body weight. There is no single cause for eating conditions; a number of factors are involved to varying degrees in different people, including genetic inheritance, personal and

psychological factors related to adolescence or family issues, for example, and social factors such as media representation of body image. It is estimated that approximately 2 in every 100 people will develop some kind of eating condition at some time in their lives. More females than males tend to be affected, particularly young women. Typically, there is a high prevalence of co-morbidity with other mental illnesses, particularly major depression.[42] While eating conditions can include limited food intake (anorexia nervosa), food intake followed by purging (bulimia nervosa) or overeating (compulsive overeating),[43] anorexia nervosa is likely to be the greatest concern in emergency situations, due to the physical effects of extreme weight loss.

Symptoms and diagnostic criteria of anorexia nervosa

Anorexia nervosa is characterised by restricted food (energy) intake. This condition commonly begins in adolescence or early adulthood. Diagnostic criteria are described in Box 37.9.

Management

Due to the physical manifestations associated with anorexia nervosa, management requires a multi-disciplinary approach involving psychiatrists, dietitians, psychologists, nurses and others. In some instances, the associated medical implications will be severe, particularly when major organs are affected by prolonged reduced energy intake.[27] It is essential that these physical impairments are treated along with the psychological impacts. For example, initiating cardiovascular monitoring is important, considering the risk of profound bradycardia and electrolyte abnormalities associated with this condition (see Ch 17, p. 336, for cardiac monitoring techniques). Since many individuals will also experience depression, anxiety and/or bipolar condition, this co-morbidity needs to be considered in the individual's management. Once the immediate physical implications are managed, some individuals may require admission to specialist eating condition wards for treatment.

Münchausen's syndrome

Münchausen's is a complex condition that centres upon the intentional production or feigning of physical or psychological signs or symptoms, often to gain attention or the 'sick role'.[44] An alternative presentation, Münchausen's syndrome by proxy, is a form of child abuse, usually by the mother, in which there is the deliberate production of physical or psychological signs or symptoms in a child, in the absence of an external incentive (see Ch 40).[45]

Symptoms

Symptoms of this condition vary and can include a range of physical or psychological complaints (from abdominal complaints through to pseudo-seizures). Other characteristics of individuals who exhibit this condition include: a dramatic style of presentation (that is, the individual presents in significant distress and is demanding in their requests); a background that provides the individual with enhanced medical knowledge; and vaguely presented histories or reluctance to provide answers regarding medical history/prior hospitalisations.[44]

Management

Munchausen's syndrome requires careful assessment and observations of symptoms, generalised illness behaviour and hospitalisations over the years. Skills required of the nurse will include careful assessment and history taking, good observation skills to be able to differentiate true illness behaviours and understanding of the family functioning dynamic.

Serotonin syndrome

Serotonin syndrome is a relatively rare yet dangerous condition associated with the introduction of or increase in a serotonin agent (commonly selective serotonin re-uptake inhibitors).

Symptoms

Serotonin syndrome is characterised by altered mental state, racing thoughts and agitation, tremor, shivering, diarrhoea, hyperreflexia, myoclonus (spasm of a muscle or group of muscles), ataxia, hypertension and hyperthermia. It can occur as a result of overdose or drug combinations and, rarely, with therapeutic doses.[46] The onset is usually rapid and most acute cases resolve with appropriate treatment within 24–36 hours.

Management

First actions include making sure that offending agent(s) is/are ceased immediately. If the condition is due to overdosage, activated charcoal should be considered (see Ch 30). For the treatment of agitation, seizures and myoclonus, benzodiazepines may be considered. Treatment for respiratory distress and dehydration should be accompanied by close monitoring of the consumer. If there is concern for dangerous medical complications, the consumer should be provided with close nursing supervision.

Neuroleptic malignant syndrome

Neuroleptic malignant syndrome (NMS) is seen in consumers who have recently commenced neuroleptic medications, or for whom the dosage of a neuroleptic has increased, either intentionally or unintentionally. It may also be seen in individuals for whom a dopaminergic agent has been rapidly withdrawn. Risk factors are listed in Box 37.10.

Symptoms

NMS is characterised by fever, muscular rigidity, pallor, dyskinesia, altered mental status, unstable blood pressure and pulmonary congestion. Death is usually due to respiratory failure, cardiovascular collapse or myoglobinuric renal failure.[48] There can be a latent period of several days and the condition can be difficult to clinically distinguish from serotonin syndrome.[47]

BOX 37.10 Risk factors for NMS*[47]

Consumer factors:
- male sex (male:female = 2:1)
- dehydration
- agitation
- organic brain disease.

Drug-dosing factors:
- high initial neuroleptic dose
- high-potency neuroleptic (e.g. haloperidol)
- rapid dosage increase
- depot neuroleptics.

* Duration of drug exposure and toxic overdose are not related to risk of developing NMS.

Management

Clinical management of NMS begins with stopping the agents thought to be causing it. In critical cases supportive measures such as oxygen, steps to reduce temperature such as cooling blankets, antipyretics, cooled IV fluids and ice packs should be considered. If the consumer has acute behavioural disturbance, oral benzodiazepines can be helpful. The condition may last 7–10 days if secondary to oral antipsychotics, and up to 21 days for depot antipsychotics.

Substance misuse and dual diagnosis

Substance misuse conditions (dependency or harmful use of alcohol or other drugs) are slightly less prevalent than other forms of mental illness, affecting 5.1% and 3.5% of Australian[1] and New Zealand adults[7] respectively. These conditions are more frequently experienced by younger men (aged 16–24 years) and are commonly experienced by people with another mental health condition.[1] Consumers experiencing a mental illness and a co-existing alcohol and other drug condition are referred to as having a dual diagnosis. There is considerable concern among paramedics and ED staff that consumers with a dual diagnosis may receive less-than-optimal treatment, in part because:

- these consumers often present as a diagnostic challenge as each condition may complicate the other
- the separation of drug and alcohol and mental health services may allow some consumers to 'fall down the gaps'.

Lack of early identification and treatment increases the cost for the consumers, the family, healthcare systems and the community. As consumers with dual diagnosis are often seen in an emergency context, it is important to ensure coordination of services for this consumer group. Access would have to be ensured to drug and alcohol agencies, either by the location of a dual-diagnosis practitioner in the service or by the availability of a designated worker within the integrated mental health service.

The outcome indicators of good clinical management include:

- improved alliances between drug and alcohol services and the ED, bringing coordination of all matters pertaining to drug (including alcohol) issues, including prevention, treatment, health promotion, education and evaluation, into a coherent framework for action

- seriously mentally ill consumers are treated by the psychiatric services, with the drug and alcohol services using their allocated worker for those who do not meet the criteria for case management in the psychiatric service.[48]

The combined effect of the above is improved connectedness with consumer preferences,[49] stigma reduction and improved teamwork and collaboration across disciplines. For more detail regarding use of alcohol, tobacco and other drugs, and management of overdose, see Chapter 41.

Suicide, parasuicide and self-harm

Although suicide, parasuicide and self-harm are typically considered behaviours, not mental health conditions, there exists an elevated risk for engagement in these behaviours among those diagnosed with a mental condition.[26] Encountering suicidal and self-harming behaviours is a common experience for paramedics and emergency nurses, and these will often be displayed by consumers who present with dual diagnosis (that is, drug/alcohol misuse and another mental health condition) and who have recently experienced a situational crisis, such as relationship breakdown.

Suicide

The WHO defines suicide as 'the act of killing oneself … deliberately initiated and performed by the person concerned in the full knowledge, or expectation of, its fatal outcome'.[50] In many countries, suicide is among the 10 leading causes of death for all ages.[59] Rates of suicide are thought to be underreported, with 522 deaths by suicide recorded in New Zealand in 2010,[51] and 2273 in Australia in 2011,[52] typically with higher rates in males and those living in rural areas.[51,53] The ED is central to any strategy for reducing the incidence of suicide, particularly because a key predictor of eventual suicide is a history of depression and a previous suicide attempt.[11,54] It is hoped that opportune intervention in the ED may prevent some suicides. Training specifically aimed at recognising, assessing and managing consumers with suicidal ideation is needed.

Parasuicide and self-harm

Many suicide attempts do not end in death and the incidence of parasuicide (the performance of suicidal behaviour with a non-fatal outcome) and self-harm ('deliberate damage to the body without suicidal intent'[55]) is much higher than that of suicide, occurring more frequently in females than males.[51,56] There were 2825 reported incidents of intentional self-harm hospitalisations in New Zealand in 2010,[51] and an estimated 26,062 in Australia during 2010–2011.[56] Of those in Australia, 82% were accounted for by intentional self-poisoning and 13% by intentional self-harm by sharp object.[56] Other examples of self-harming behaviours include: jumping from heights, attempted hanging, high-speed motor vehicle crashes that are deliberate and burning of flesh. While some people will only engage in these behaviours once, or for a short duration of time, others will continue for many years. There is a connection between suicide, parasuicide and self-harm, with previous attempts and expressions of self-harming

behaviour being common among those who have completed suicide.[55,57,58]

Immediate care following parasuicide and self-harm

Paramedics and ED nurses are often some of the first responders when a person has engaged in suicidal/self-harming behaviours, and therefore both play a crucial role in providing immediate care. Due to the nature of suicidal and self-harming behaviours, there is likely to be an immediate need to tend to the medical aspects of the behaviour[59] (e.g. wound suturing). Ensuring the safety of the individual and others present is also essential. This involves checking whether the individual is in possession of any items that could be used to cause further harm (e.g. sharp objects). Once these needs have been met, specific psychological care can begin.

Suicide assessment and management

The best course of action when managing an individual who is believed to be suicidal is to raise the topic with the individual, either directly or indirectly, with the view to understand risk and protective factors for suicide. It is preferable to do so knowing something of the framework and/or system supports available to the practitioner if indeed suicide is a very real option for the consumer. This is particularly the case with migrants and refugees who are alienated by a range of cultural and linguistic barriers.[60] Warning signs are listed in Box 37.11.

While the approach taken must be non-threatening, open and confidential, confidentiality cannot always be unconditionally assured. A careful balance must be maintained between preserving confidentiality as a fundamental aspect of clinical practice and the need to breach it on rare occasions in order to promote the consumer's optimal interests and care, and/or the safety of others.[62] There will, however, be many professional situations that call for the sharing of information between practitioners. On occasions, consumers or relatives may be asked to provide a considerable amount of personal information, especially when consumers are first assessed or admitted. When this happens, it should be explained in a sensitive manner that other staff will have access to some of the information. Employees therefore have a duty of care to ensure

---

BOX 37.11 Warning signs of suicidal intentions[61]

The majority of people give warning signs about their suicidal intentions. Some of these warning signs are:

- expression of hopelessness or helplessness
- written or spoken notice of intention, saying goodbye
- dramatic change in personality or appearance
- irrational, bizarre behaviour
- overwhelming sense of guilt, shame or reflection
- changed eating or sleeping patterns
- severe drop in school or work performance
- giving away possessions or putting affairs in order
- lack of interest in the future
- self-harming actions, such as overdoses, which can be lethal to the person.

that they are aware of the implications of any legislation relevant to their particular role, and follow the statutory requirements of legislation and the requirements of their employer.[62]

Nevertheless, empathy and a genuine interest in the inner life of the person involved must be apparent during the clinical interview. In this way, it may be possible to motivate the consumer to come around to the idea that suicide is no longer a viable alternative. The following biopsychosocial approach, based on the International Association for Suicide Prevention guidelines,[64] is essential to promote an individual approach. Although interactions can be constrained by time in the ED, this process highlights the importance of adopting a narrative approach—a process where the consumer is encouraged to share their story with the clinician, and where the consumer and clinician can identify the needs of the individual.[65]

> **PRACTICE TIP**
>
> Be alert to behaviours that indicate a possible increased risk of suicide, such as giving away possessions, talking about suicide or the withdrawal from family, friends and normal activities. Document and communicate this knowledge to others as part of the consumer's assessment.

First contact: a positive, supportive response
Initial contact with suicidal persons is particularly important, but it often occurs in less than ideal circumstances, such as on the street, in a busy ED, in the person's home or on the telephone.

Managing people with suicidal thoughts and actions in crisis situations hinges upon ensuring safety for all concerned. This means scanning the environment for potential risks, speaking in a calm voice and favourably shifting risk as far as possible. Many people in suicidal crisis are at high imminent risk of suicide/self-harm, and require constant one-to-one monitoring and secure support. In the ED it is not always realistic or desirable for the primary support person to constantly be at the side of and interacting with someone while simultaneously recording observations. The important point here is for human contact with the distressed person, attending to any immediate health concerns following assessment. This is an opportunity for the clinician to generate trust with the person, maintaining support and facilitating appropriate expressions of anger.

Clinical engagement with people who are suicidal can evoke mixed feelings in everyone and paramedic/ED staff are not immune to having thoughts and feelings which could be anti-therapeutic. It is important that the first response is not primarily defensive. It is critical to realise that not everybody has to take on the responsibility of treating those with suicidal thoughts/actions, but at the very least those who are in the situation where such persons may present should have the basic skills to make a general assessment of suicidal persons (even though they should not feel obliged to continue management). Indeed, any potential therapist should be aware of their limitations, and be willing to seek the assistance of colleagues with appropriate referral.

It is important to recognise that often suicidal persons have recently perceived rejection, and a considerable degree of

expertise and patience may be required in order to establish rapport. This can be achieved by communicating the wish to understand what is happening to that person and that time has been set aside to do so.

Having established a reasonable environment in which to assess the person, that person should be allowed to present their history in as full a manner as possible. When attempting to elicit information from suicidal persons it should be remembered that challenging or direct questions which could be interpreted as critical will rarely help. Rather, open-ended and non-judgemental comments, such as: 'Things seem to be difficult for you right now' or 'You must have been feeling pretty upset about that', can encourage people to talk about their difficulties, and the open-ended question: 'Can you tell me more about it?' is often useful.

Some consumers may remain resistant, but by stressing that it is important to try to understand what is happening and by the therapeutic use of silence, which further indicates a willingness and openness to listen, most will respond and rapport can be achieved.

Assess the degree of suicidal intent
Assessment must recognise the basic human need for autonomy as well as safety, and this means creating strategies to enable disclosure and trust wherever possible. More direct questions may be necessary in order to elucidate the degree of suicidal intent. Suicidal thoughts and behaviour usually revolve around interpersonal phenomena, and the role of persons of significance to the consumer should be sought. This may necessitate a systematic enquiry about the person's relationship with family members and friends. More specifically, suicidal intent can be determined on the basis of the degree of planning, knowledge of the lethality of the intended suicidal act, the degree of isolation of the person and also by asking open-ended questions, such as: 'What are your feelings—right now—about living and dying?' Such a question permits those with suicidal thoughts to express their feelings in a way that is not provided for by direct questions such as: 'Do you really want to kill yourself?', which may be too confronting and does not allow for the ambivalent feelings which are almost invariably present in these consumers.

> **PRACTICE TIP**
>
> Reassure consumers that no matter how challenging their situation is right now, the way forward is best achieved by working together. Where possible use a conversational-style risk-assessment approach to create interactive dialogue and trust.

Commence initial management
The most important initial decision is based on assessment of the safety of the suicidal person. It may be that the opportunity of ventilating thoughts and feelings to a concerned person has been sufficient for some suicidal consumers. In the absence of a mental condition, or if suicidal thoughts and actions have resulted in positive changes in personal relationships, further contact may be unnecessary, although the opportunity for further follow-up should be left open, particularly if there are inadequate social supports.

For those who are profoundly suicidal with a severe mental illness, detention under the relevant Mental Health Act and hospitalisation may be necessary (see Ch 4). Indeed, sometimes compulsory hospitalisation in order to reduce the likelihood of danger to the person or to others is required. If so, it must be emphasised to the consumer and their relatives/carers/friends that it has been done in order to protect, not punish, the person. If this should happen, try to bring the relative and/or friend in with you to help ensure that this is the best solution for the problem at hand.

Suicide, parasuicide and self-harm in Aboriginal, Māori and Pacific Island people

The subject area of suicide, parasuicide and self-harm among Aboriginal Australians is one of persistent and overwhelming tragedy, marked by expressions of pain, disconnection and despair. Based on data from NSW, Qld, WA, SA and the NT, during the period 2006–2010, the third leading cause of death among Aboriginal and Torres Strait Islander peoples was external causes (15%, compared to 6% of non-Indigenous deaths), of which 30% were caused by suicide.[66] Rates are typically higher for men in rural communities,[58,67–69] and often the death results from violent means, particularly hanging or firearms.[69] Self-harm is thought to be equally common among males and females.[69]

Several writers warn against a narrow focus on either non-suicidal or suicidal behaviour in the Aboriginal context.[70] All self-harming behaviour, they argue, should be seen as a drastic response to certain stressful experiences (risk factors) and violence in the broader social and emotional context of cultural meaning, cultural identity, historical and current socio-economic conditions.[71] Additionally, threats towards death by hanging may have significant historical messages of hurt, injustice, tyranny and domination for Aboriginal people.[71]

Rates of suicide, parasuicide and self-harm are also more prevalent among Māori and Pacific Islanders. In 2010, there were 104 Māori deaths by suicide, a rate 53.6% higher than the non-Māori rate.[51] There were also 21 Pacific Islander deaths by suicide in this period. These elevated rates can be attributed to higher rates of social deprivation and disadvantage, as well as acculturative stress, resulting from colonisation in the 1800s;[7] much like those factors faced by Aboriginal Australians.

Suicide, parasuicide and self-harm in refugees and asylum seekers

Suicide, parasuicide and self-harm are common issues for refugees and asylum seekers, with suicide thought to be the leading cause of premature death for individuals in immigration detention in Australia.[72] A refugee is someone who, 'owing to a well-founded fear of being persecuted on account of race, religion, nationality, membership of a particular social group, or political opinion, is outside the country of their nationality, and is unable to or, owing to such fear, is unwilling to avail him/herself of the protection of that country'.[73] An asylum-seeker is someone who has left his or her country of origin in search of protection—whether or not their claim for refugee status has been determined.

A recent study exploring the use of one ED by immigration detainees in Darwin during 2011 found that the most common primary diagnosis of all attendances was psychiatric problems (24% of 770 total attendances).[74] Of these attendances, 138 were associated with self-harm, more commonly among men. Twenty of the total attendances were by children (9–17 years), of which 75% were related to self-harm.

Suicidal and self-harming behaviour among these populations may be associated with the considerable uncertainty for the individual, which can contribute to anxiety, mental distress and uncertainty for the future. Such factors are thought to be linked to depression, post-traumatic stress and other mental health concerns among these individuals.[75] Specifically, these behaviours might be associated with rejected visa applications and claims for permanent protection being refused, as well as being linked to past trauma and/or torture issues.

The acts of suicide and self-harm by asylum seekers are widely regarded by practitioners as among the most common and stressful emergency issues encountered by health and human service professionals. Emergency workers may feel overwhelmed and be left feeling unsure what to do by the complexity and the unusual depth of personal feeling they confront. For this reason there is a real need for emergency workers to work together with advocate, migration, refugee and trauma services so that all concerned can be supported in managing their own feelings and reactions while making themselves available to the consumer. As with any individual engaging in these behaviours, it is important to ensure the safety of the consumer and to encourage them to feel listened to and validated.

Other considerations when providing emergency mental health care

Legal considerations

It is important to be reminded of the legal considerations when providing emergency mental health care. In particular, not all people come to the attention of emergency health services voluntarily. In some instances, a person may be treated without their consent or against their will. This situation arises when a person requires urgent treatment to save the person's life or to prevent serious harm to the individual's health, or when the individual is in need of urgent treatment but is incapable of giving consent. Involuntary treatment orders can take the form of specific 'licence conditions', Community Treatment Orders or a legal order for care by an authorised officer for immediate detention under relevant legislation. For more detail and the Mental Health Acts for each state and territory, see Chapter 4.

In addition to involuntary detention, some Mental Health Acts also contain regulations for the administration of sedatives. For example, the New Zealand Mental Health Act contains a provision that enables a medical practitioner, in certain circumstances, to administer an appropriate sedative to a person (Section 110A). If a medical practitioner administers urgent sedation, they must do so in accordance with relevant guidelines and standards of care and treatment issued by the Director-General of Health under Section 130 of the Act.

Occasionally, issues will arise when people with mental illnesses come into contact with the criminal justice system. There is much publicity of critical incidents involving mentally disturbed people, which gives rise to the popular belief that a high proportion of people with mental illness commit crimes. This is generally not the case. Most people with a mental illness, including those with major illnesses, do not commit crimes; but people with mental illness nevertheless are over-represented in the criminal justice system.[76]

Managing an aggressive or violent consumer pre-hospital and in the ED

Aggression and violence in healthcare is a growing concern. For example, a recent South Australian Ambulance Service report indicated a 74% increase in incidents of physical and verbal abuse directed at paramedics in the past 2 years (from 57 incidents in 2012 to 99 incidents in 2013).[77] In addition to their role in dealing with the aftermath of pre-hospital aggression and violence, EDs are also faced with occurrences of aggression and violence within the hospital setting.[78] ED nurses are frequently subjected to verbal abuse (e.g. swearing or obscenity, shouting and sarcasm) and physical abuse (e.g. pushing, hitting, use of a weapon and punching).[79] Risk factors thought to be associated with these incidences include a past history of violence, substance and alcohol misuse, medical diagnoses (including mental illness), long waiting times and time of day (with increased incidents in the evenings). Some researchers play down the linkages between violence and mental illness.[80] While some have found that those individuals who experience co-morbid schizophrenia/other psychoses and substance misuse are at a greater risk of violent behaviour,[81] others have found that this risk is no greater than that for those individuals who have a substance-use condition only.[82]

Robust and assertive practice of early identification and early intervention of aggression and violence are the first steps in any de-escalation process. Where the prospect of violence is real, staff must act in a defensive and anticipatory manner, at all times ready for the level of violence to escalate.[83] Early detection of the potential signs of aggression is the first step towards prevention and de-escalation. Some signs of potential aggression and general pre-hospital and ED management guidelines are listed in Box 37.12 (see also Ch 10 for pre-hospital scene assessment and management). The primary concern in the management of violent or aggressive people (and of the impact of their behaviour on those present) is positive engagement and safety leading to de-escalation of the consumer's behaviour in the least restrictive environment. This is not a time to be a hero. Rather, it is a time to ensure personal safety and for all involved to work using exemplary communication, teamwork and strategic use of medication and physical interventions.

PRACTICE TIP

Be alert to warning signs of aggression—behaviours that indicate an increased risk of aggression include intense staring, yelling, intoxication, threatening gestures. Use de-escalation techniques and seek support. This is not the time to be a hero.

BOX 37.12 Detection and management of aggression[83]

Early detection of the potential signs of aggression:
- Being under the influence of alcohol or other drugs, particularly psychostimulants
- Having slurred speech, being sarcastic, abusive, threatening, using foul language
- Intruding personal space; defiant and uncooperative
- Hostile facial expression with prolonged eye contact and staring
- Bloodstained clothing, dishevelled appearance
- Possession of a weapon (actual or potential)
- Obvious motor restlessness, pacing, tapping feet (exclude akathisia), clenching of fists or jaws, twisting of neck.

Pre-hospital and ED management guidelines for aggression:
- Consider personal safety at all times
- Avoid an argumentative, confrontational response
- Show you are listening—paraphrase back a summary of what is being said to you and communicate that you are trying to solve the problem
- Calm the person as much as possible, encouraging them to slow down prior to solving the problem
- Show concern through verbal and non-verbal responses. Avoid patronising their concerns
- Adopt a non-threatening body posture, voice tone and disposition more broadly
- Consider the safety of other consumers and their visitors at all times
- Avoid an audience or crowd forming around the consumer
- Place the person in a quiet and secure area and let staff know what is happening and why
- Never turn your back on the individual
- Don't walk ahead of the individual and ensure adequate personal space
- Avoid sudden movements or elevation of voice that may startle or be perceived as a threat, danger or attack
- Provide continuous observation and record behaviour changes in consumer notes
- Wear a personal duress alarm at all times
- Let the person talk
- Never block off exits and ensure you have a safe escape route.

Seclusion and restraint

As discussed earlier in the chapter, certain situations (i.e. when an individual is behaving in ways that put them at risk to themselves or others) will require paramedics to implement processes of physical and/or chemical restraint in order to safely provide care and/or transport of the individual. For these same reasons, restraint is sometimes required in the ED. Each state, territory and emergency care provider will have different regulations regarding seclusion and restraint (see Ch 4), including which professionals (for example, paramedics and nurses) are able to provide these responses.

In instances where chemical restraint may be necessary, some of the more common agents used in this situation include diazepam, midazolam and haloperidol. While clinical observations after administration of intravenous medications will vary, depending upon local protocols, close monitoring after chemical restraint will involve recording vital signs every 15 minutes for the first hour, every 30 minutes for the second hour and then hourly for 4 hours (see Ch 29).

There are, however, some concerns about the use of these practices. For example, the primary concerns about ED seclusion rooms are three-fold. First, there is a danger that people *out of sight* are also *out of mind*, meaning that staff may be less concerned with acts of self-harm, physical distress or injury. Second, such a setting may exacerbate mental distress by removing any capacity that the individual has to make decisions or take control of their situation. Removing personal control and freedom in this can be a traumatising and possibly re-traumatising effect. Third, the person may perceive that being placed in a room against their will is the direct result of disclosing their distress and thoughts of self-harm to a health worker, resulting in the individual feeling punished for speaking honestly about their predicament. Each of these factors can hinder an individual's future encounters with the mental health care system.

Opposing this stance is the view that the consumer is unable to take control and it is the right of staff to have a safe, predictable and protected environment. Viewed this way, seclusion and restraint can, when used properly, be a life-saving and injury-sparing measure designed to protect consumers in danger of harming themselves or others.[84] To be effective, seclusion must be supported by adequate policies and procedures which are periodically reviewed for determining when, why and how measures will be used and evaluated. Even in the most secure environments risk cannot be eliminated completely. Mental health support does not stop when a person is secluded. A clinically informed response means that staff continue to advocate for the consumer. Staff must scrutinise the seclusion area so that it is, as far as possible, supportive and calming. It is imperative that the area is critically assessed so that it is free of hanging and other self-harm points.

Cultural considerations when providing an emergency mental health response

As outlined in Chapter 5, Australia and New Zealand are increasingly becoming multicultural nations, and being aware of cultural differences when providing mental health care is essential to good practice, regardless of the setting.

The importance of culture

'Culture' gives meaning and context to the way people communicate thinking, action and events. Culture also allows people to make assumptions about social and emotional life, illness and death and how they should be understood within a particular context or setting. When individuals from one culture find themselves living in a different cultural context, there may be differences in the way that they communicate distress and suffering. In mental health emergencies it is important to look beyond taken-for-granted assumptions regarding the way that symptoms of mental distress are communicated and the

personal meaning that people from culturally and linguistically diverse cultures give to diagnosis, treatments and outcomes. Consequently, people from culturally and linguistically diverse backgrounds remain a population group requiring special attention to their mental health status.[85] The challenges of a diverse population—of developing a culturally inclusive mental health assessment—remain.

Cultural and language considerations

Below are some cultural and language considerations relevant to the assessment of emergencies in mental health:

- It is not uncommon for stress to increase the likelihood that a person from a culturally and linguistically diverse culture will revert to their language of origin.
- If a person speaks a language other than English at home, it may be helpful to use an accredited interpreter service. Family members should only be used in emergency situations.
- Be aware that a prior relationship between the patient and an interpreter can be a problem in small ethnic groups— in particular, new and emerging communities—where there tend to be fewer accredited interpreters and where individuals might have concerns about the confidentiality of involving an interpreter.

Cultural differences can result in markedly variable mental health presentations. Cultural differences can influence the way in which symptoms are presented, what is considered a good outcome, acceptance of prescription medication and help-seeking behaviour more generally.

Refugees and asylum seekers

During 2012, Australia and New Zealand received 16,110 asylum application claims (a 36% increase in the number of claims received in 2011), primarily from individuals originating from Afghanistan, Sri Lanka, the Islamic Republic of Iran, Pakistan and China.[73] The media pays heavy attention to the health and wellbeing of those in immigration detention, and it is not uncommon for these individuals to present to EDs. Having an awareness and understanding of the ongoing impacts of uncertainty, isolation and trauma experienced by these individuals is essential to providing culturally appropriate care.

> **PRACTICE TIP**
>
> Mental health assessment must be culturally competent. Ask the person about how their situation would be understood and responded to by people from their own cultural group. This may mean asking about how their experiences would be expressed or explained in their cultural context.

Collaboration and teamwork between mental health professionals

Irrespective of practice setting, clinical conflict in mental health care is inevitable because of the episodic nature of mental illness, differing approaches to care and availability of resources. Consequently, service provision for consumers with mental health problems can be hindered due to a breakdown of communication and deadlock between individual service providers, consumers and organisations. The solution to these problems is deadlock prevention and promotion of partnership. Also important is a commitment by managers, codified in formal policy, to deal with escalated conflict directly with their counterparts.

It is acknowledged that a formal policy and process may seem cumbersome, especially when the issue (e.g. consumer admission to hospital) is time-sensitive. But resolving the problem early on is ultimately more desirable in a health service where many issues have significant implications for numerous parts of the service. Unilateral responses to unilateral escalations of conflict are a recipe for inefficiency, ill-feeling and a sense of 'we'll win next time' taking hold, making future conflict even more difficult to resolve.[86]

When consumers and healthcare professionals collaborate more freely they are more likely to trust each other. When consumers trust their organisations, they are more likely to give of themselves now in anticipation of future change and reward.

The benefits of creatively preventing and resolving conflict include:

- conflict resolution, which reduces individual and organisational ambiguity, and increases transparency and efficiency of healthcare
- new lines of communication and professional relationships, which facilitate timely access to appropriate mental health resources and supports
- a decrease in the number of problems that are pushed up the management chain.

SUMMARY

Paramedic and emergency health worker assessment and care of consumers in mental health emergencies is dependent on a range of factors within the individual and the environment. The practitioner who takes a holistic approach to care will take account of social, psychological and medical interventions, which are essential if we are to address the many myths about the practice of mental health care. The 17th-century philosopher René Descartes conceptualised the distinction between the mind and the body when he viewed the 'mind' as completely separable from the 'body'. And, as we have seen in this chapter, mental health practitioners and advocates have been trying to put them back together. This separation between so-called 'mental' and 'physical' health has no real relevance to the scientific understanding of health in the 21st century, yet the myths and misinformation persist. It will be the skills of practitioners in their formulation of diagnosis and treatment of symptoms that can be bewildering to consumers and their relatives, the reassurance that they are working with others to improve quality of life and continuity of information about treatment that will help diffuse crisis and reduce suffering in some of the most vulnerable people in our society.

Mental health emergencies found pre-hospital and in the ED are varied and challenging for both the consumer and the emergency health worker. There is a range of factors that must be considered to make the fullest and most informed assessment possible, including the nature of presenting problem, cultural considerations, quality of information available and interdisciplinary collaboration. Regardless of the presenting problem, it is important for the emergency practitioner to treat the consumer and their family with respect and empathy, while simultaneously operating within a human rights framework protecting the consumer and others from harm.

CASE STUDY

Troy is a 19-year-old male who recently broke up with his girlfriend of two years. He was told by his former girlfriend that she had found someone new and 'wanted nothing more to do with him'. Troy's girlfriend had grown tired of Troy's mood changes and brooding. Some days he seemed fine, while at other times he was irritable and had ongoing difficulties at work and in his family.

Troy had been out drinking with his mates and had tried to call his former girlfriend several times by phone. She had refused to take his calls. He wanted to see if he could get back together with her. When his calls went unanswered, Troy went to his former girlfriend's house by taxi. He tried to see her, to tell her 'he could not live without her' and that 'his life would soon be over'. His former girlfriend refused to come to the door. The police were called and Troy was removed from the property.

Troy returned home and continued drinking alone. He went out to his back shed, and with some rope strung a noose up across the central beam of the shed. He also bound his legs together with electrical tape. He then called his mate Phil and told him that he was 'going away for a while'. Troy was in an intoxicated state. He told Phil that he no longer needed his car and that Phil could now use it. Phil said that he would come over to see him, but Troy insisted that everything was now sorted and that he was fine and did not need any help. After the phone call, Phil drove to Troy's house. Troy was found hanging and barely alive. Phil grabbed Troy's legs to ease the strain of the rope. He also managed to attract a neighbour's attention. The neighbour came running to assist and with the aid of a ladder, both men removed the noose and lowered Troy's body to ground level. Police and ambulance were called.

Questions

1. What principles of mental health triage are important on arrival at Troy's house? Why are they important?

2. What mental health-related questions and observations might be useful at the first point of contact with Troy?

Troy arrives at the accident and emergency department (ED).

3. What is the goal of initial contact and treatment for someone like Troy, and how might it be achieved?

4. What might be the purpose of a mental state assessment of Troy on arrival at the accident and ED?

 Answers to Case Study Questions can be found on evolve
http://evolve.emergencytrauma.curtis

USEFUL WEBSITES

ABC 7.30 Report, Why are mentally-ill children tied up and tormented? www.abc.net.au/news/2013-12-10/why-are-mentally-ill-children-tied-up-and-tormented/5148180

Beyondblue, www.beyondblue.org.au/

Mental Health Foundation of New Zealand, www.mentalhealth.org.nz/

Mental Health in Multicultural Australia, www.mhima.org.au/

Mental Health Services in Australia, mhsa.aihw.gov.au/home/

National Eating Disorders Collaboration, www.nedc.com.au/

Refugee Council of Australia, www.refugeecouncil.org.au/

SANE Australia, www.sane.org/

Suicide and self-harm crisis interview, www.youtube.com/watch?v=fLXfDepZ-o0

Suicide Prevention Australia, http://suicidepreventionaust.org/

REFERENCES

1. Australian Bureau of Statistics (ABS). National survey of mental health and wellbeing: Summary of results (No. 4326.0). Canberra: 2007.

2. Morgan VA, Waterreus A, Jablensky A et al. People living with psychotic illness 2010: Report on the second Australian national survey. Canberra, Australia: Department of Health and Ageing, 2011.

3. Hickie IB, Groom GL, McGorry PD et al. Australian mental health reform: time for real outcomes. Med J Aust 2005;182(8):401–6.

4. Australian Bureau of Statistics (ABS) and Australian Institute of Health and Welfare (AIHW). The health and welfare of Australia's Aboriginal and Torres Strait Islander Peoples (No. 4704.0). Canberra, Australia, 2008.

5. Andrews G. The crisis in mental health: the chariot needs one horseman. Med J Aust 2005;182(8):372–3.

6. Wells JE, Browne MA, Scott KM et al. Prevalence, interference with life and severity of 12 month DSM-IV disorders in Te Rau Hinengaro: the New Zealand mental health survey. Aust N Z J Psychiatry 2006;40(10):845–54.

7. Oakley Browne MA, Wells JE, Scott KM, eds. Te Rau Hinengaro: the New Zealand mental health survey: summary. Wellington: Ministry of Health; 2006.

8. Wells JE, Oakley Browne MA, Scott KM et al. Te Rau Hinengaro: the New Zealand mental health survey: overview of methods and findings. Aust N Z J Psychiatry 2006;40(10):835–44.

9. Oakley Browne MA, Wells JE, Scott KM et al. Lifetime prevalence and projected lifetime risk of DSM-IV disorders in Te Rau Hinengaro: the New Zealand mental health survey. Aust N Z J Psychiatry 2006;40(10):865–74.

10. Foliaki SA, Kokaua J, Schaaf D et al. Twelve-month and lifetime prevalences of mental disorders and treatment contact among Pacific people in Te Rau Hinengaro: the New Zealand mental health survey. Aust N Z J Psychiatry 2006;40(10):924–34.

11. Beautrais AL, Wells JE, McGee MA et al. Suicidal behaviour in Te Rau Hinengaro: the New Zealand mental health survey. Aust N Z J Psychiatry 2006;40(10):896–904.

12. Council of Australian Governments. Roadmap for national mental health reform 2012–2022. Online. www.coag.gov.au/node/482; 2 Dec 2013.

13. Australian Health Ministers. Fourth National Mental Health Plan: an agenda for collaborative government action in mental health 2009–14. Canberra: Australian Government; 2009.

14. Australian Health Ministers. Framework for the implementation of the National Mental Health Plan 2003–8 in multicultural Australia. Canberra: Australian Government; 2004.

15. Kalucy R, Thomas L, King D. Changing demand for mental health services in the emergency department of a public hospital. Aust N Z J Psychiatry 2005;39(1–2):74–80.

16. Australian Institute of Health and Welfare. Mental health services—in brief 2013. Cat. no. HSE 141. Canberra: AIHW, 2013.

17. Victorian Government Department of Health. Ambulance transport of people with a mental illness protocol 2010. Melbourne: Author; 2010. Online. www.health.vic.gov.au/mentalhealth/publications/amb-transport0910.pdf; accessed 5 Feb 2014.

18. NSW Health, Ambulance Service of New South Wales, and NSW Police Force. Memorandum of Understanding: Mental health emergency response July 2007. Online. www.police.nsw.gov.au/__data/assets/pdf_file/0009/98469/mou_mental_health_emergency_response_nsw_health_ambulance_police200707.pdf; accessed 23 Jul 2014.

19. Mental Health and Drug and Alcohol Office. Mental Health for Emergency Departments—A Reference Guide. Sydney, Australia: NSW Department of Health, 2009. Online. www0.health.nsw.gov.au/resources/mhdao/pdf/mhemergency.pdf; accessed 27 Nov 2013.

20. Treatment Protocol Project. Management of mental disorders. 2nd edn. Sydney: World Health Organization Collaborating Centre for Mental Health and Substance Abuse; 1997.

21. Davies T. ABC of mental health: mental health assessment. Br Med J 1997;314(7093):1536–9.

22. American Psychiatric Association, American Psychiatric Nurses Association, National Association of Psychiatric Health Systems. Learning from each other: success stories and ideas for reducing restraint/seclusion in behavioral health. Arlington, VA: American Psychiatric Association; 2003. Online. www.aha.org/content/00-10/learningfromeachother.pdf; accessed 5 Dec 2013.

23. Paquette M, Rodemich C. Psychiatric nursing diagnosis care plans for DSM-IV. Sudbury: Jones and Bartlett; 1997.

24. ACT Health (2002). The ACT Nurse Practitioner Project. Final Report of the Steering Committee. Canberra: ACT Department of Health, 2002. Online. acnp.org.au/sites/default/files/docs/act_np_project_0.pdf; 10 Feb 2014.

25. Wand T, White K, Patching J et al. Outcomes from the evaluation of an Emergency Department based mental health nurse practitioner outpatient service. J Am Acad Nurse Pract 2012;24:149–59.

26. NSW Ministry of Health. Emergency department models of care. Online. www0.health.nsw.gov.au/pubs/2012/pdf/ed_model_of_care_2012.pdf; accessed 23 Jul 2014.

27. American Psychiatric Association. Diagnostic and statistical manual of mental disorders. 5th edn. Arlington, VA: Author; 2013.

28. World Health Organization. International statistical classification of diseases and related health problems. 10th edn. Geneva: Author; 2010. Online. Available: http://apps.who.int/classifications/icd10/browse/2010/en; 5 Feb 2014.

29. SANE Australia Factsheet 12. Anxiety disorders. Online. www.sane.org/images/stories/information/factsheets/1007_info_12anxiety.pdf; accessed 08 Jan 2011.

30. Judd LL, Kessler RC, Paulus MP et al. Comorbidity as a fundamental feature of generalised anxiety disorders: results from the national comorbidity study (NCS). Acta Psychiatr Scand 1998;98(suppl 393):6–11.

31. Paquette M, Rodemich C. Psychiatric nursing diagnosis care plans for DSM-IV. Sudbury: Jones and Bartlett; 1997.

32. Hickie IB. Preventing depression: a challenge for the Australian community. Med J Aust 2002;177(suppl):S85–6.

33. Collins PY, Patel V, Joestl SS et al. Grand challenges in global mental health. Nature 2011;475:27–30.

34. World Health Organization. Global Health and Aging. NIH Publication no 11-7737. 2011. Online. www.who.int/agein g/publications/global_health/en/; accessed 28 Nov 2013.

35. Office for Senior Citizens. Briefing to the incoming minister. New Zealanders: Getting older, doing more. 2012. Online. www.msd.govt.nz/documents/about-msd-and-our-work/publications-resources/corporate/bims/osc-bim-2008.pdf; 10 Dec 2013.

36. Australian Bureau of Statistics. Who are Australia's older people? Reflecting a nation: Stories from the 2011 census, 2012–2013. Online. www.abs.gov.au/ausstats/abs@.nsf/Lookup/2071.0main+features752012–2013; accessed 10 Dec 2013.

37. Hamer HP, Lampshire D, Thomson S. Mental health of older people. In: Procter N, Hamer HP, McGarry D et al, eds. Mental health: A person-centred approach. Melbourne, Australia: Cambridge University Press, 2014:262–86.

38. Butterworth P, Gill SC, Rodgers B et al. Retirement and mental health: Analysis of the Australian national survey of mental health and well-being. Social Science & Medicine 2006;62(5):1179–91.

39. Lenze EJ, Loebach Wetherell J. State of the art: A lifespan view of anxiety disorders. Dialogues in Clinical Neuroscience 2011; 13(4):381–99.

40. Peron EP, Gray SL, Hanlon JT. Medication use and functional status decline in older adults: A narrative review. American Journal of Geriatric Pharmacotherapy 2011;9(6): 378–91.

41. Semple D, Smyth R, Burns J et al. Oxford handbook of psychiatry. Oxford: Oxford University Press; 2005.

42. Silberg JL, Bulik CM. The developmental association between eating disorders symptoms and symptoms of depression and anxiety in juvenile twin girls. J Child Psychol Psychiatry 2005;46(12):1317–26.

43. SANE Australia Factsheet 20. Eating disorders. Online. www.sane.org/information/factsheets-podcasts/179-eating-disorder; accessed 08 Jan 2011.

44. Huffman JC, Stern TA. The diagnosis and treatment of Munchausen's syndrome. Gen Hosp Psych 2003;24:358–63.

45. McNicholas F, Slonis V, Cass H. Exaggeration of symptoms of psychiatric Münchausen's syndrome by proxy. Child Psychol Psychiatr Rev 2000;5:69–75.

46. Tinetti ME, Bogardus Jr ST, Agostini JV. Potential pitfalls of disease-specific guidelines for patients with multiple conditions. N Engl J Med 2004;351(27):2870–4.

47. Rogers I, Williams A. Heat related illness. In: Cameron P, Jelinek G, Kelly AM et al, eds. Textbook of adult emergency medicine. 3rd edn. Edinburgh: Churchill Livingstone; 2009; 848–51.

48. Deans C, Soar R. Caring for clients with dual diagnosis in rural communities in Australia: the experience of mental health professionals. J Psychiatr Ment Health Nurs 2005;12(3):268–74.

49. Procter NG. Providing emergency mental health care to asylum seekers at a time when claims for permanent protection have been rejected. Int J Ment Health Nurs 2005;14(1):2–6.

50. World Health Organization. Primary prevention of mental, neurological and psycho-social disorders. Geneva: Author; 1998. Online. whqlibdoc.who.int/publications/924154516X.pdf; accessed 5 Feb 2014.

51. Ministry of Health. Suicide facts: Deaths and intentional self-harm hospitalization 2010. Wellington: Ministry of Health, 2012.

52. Boyce P, Carter G, Penrose-Wall J et al. Summary of Australian and New Zealand clinical practice guideline for the management of adult deliberate self-harm. Australas Psychiatr 2003;11:150–5.

53. Australian Bureau of Statistics. 2209.0—Suicides, Australia, 2010. Online. www.abs.gov.au/ausstats/abs@.NSF/Latestproducts/8D157E15E9D912E7CA257A440014CE53?opendocument; accessed 10 Dec 2013.

54. Beautrais AL. National strategies for the reduction and prevention of suicide. Crisis 2005;26(1):1–3.

55. Martin G, Swannell SV, Hazell PL et al. Self-injury in Australia: A community survey. Med J Aust 2010;193:506–10.

56. Pointer S. Trends in hospitalised injury, Australia, 1999–00 to 2010–11. Injury research and statistics series, no. 86. Cat. no. INJCAT 162. Canberra: Australian Institute of Health and Welfare, 2013.

57. McAllister M. Multiple meanings of self harm: a critical review. Int J Ment Health Nurs 2003;12(3):177–85.

58. Cantor C, Neulinger K. The epidemiology of suicide and attempted suicide among young Australians. Aust N Z J Psychiatry 2000;34(3):370–87.

59. Wand T. Duty of care in the emergency department. Int J Ment Health Nurs 2004;13:135–9.

60. Procter N. Mental health crisis intervention for asylum seekers in the emergency department. Aust Emerg Nurs J 2006;9(3):113–17.

61. SANE Australia Factsheet 14a. Suicidal behaviour and self harm. Online. www.sane.org/information/factsheets-podcasts/211-suicidal-behaviour-and-self-harm; 08 Jan 2011.

62. Bloch S, Pargiter R. Developing a code of ethics for psychiatry. In: Coady M, Bloch S, eds. Code of ethics and the professions. Melbourne: Melbourne University Press 1996; 193–225.

63. Tadd GV. Ethics and values for care workers. Oxford: Blackwell Science; 1998.

64. International Association for Suicide Prevention. Guidelines for suicide prevention. Online. www.iasp.info/suicide_guidelines.php; accessed 20 Jan 2011.

65. Procter N, Baker A, Grocke K et al. Introduction to mental health and mental illness: human connectedness and the collaborative consumer narrative. In: Procter N, Hamer HP, McGarry D et al, eds. Mental health: A person-centred approach. Melbourne, Australia: Cambridge University Press, 2014:1–24.

66. Australian Health Ministers' Advisory Council (AHMAC). Aboriginal and Torres Strait Islander Health Performance Framework 2012 Report. Canberra: AHMAC.

67. Hunter E, Reser J, Baird M et al. An analysis of suicide in indigenous communities of North Queensland: the historical, cultural and symbolic landscape. Canberra: Commonwealth Department of Health and Aged Care; 2001.

68. Kosky RJ, Dundas P. Death by hanging: implications for prevention of an important method of youth suicide. Aust N Z J Psychiatry 2000;34(5):836–41.

69. Hunter E, Harvey D. Indigenous suicide in Australia, New Zealand, Canada and the United States. Emerg Med (Fremantle) 2002;14(1):14–23.

70. Aoun S. Deliberate self-harm in rural Western Australia: results of an intervention study. Aust N Z J Ment Health Nurs 1999;8(2):65–73.

71. Harrison J, Miller E, Weeramanthri T et al. Information sources for injury prevention among Indigenous Australians: status and prospects for improvement. Injury Research and Statistics series 8. Adelaide SA: Australian Institute of Health and Welfare; 2001.

72. Procter NG, De Leo D, Newman L. Suicide and self-harm prevention for people in immigration detention. Med J Aust 2013;199(11):730–2.

73. United Nations High Commission for Refugees (UNHCR). Convention Relating to the Status of Refugees 2012. Online. www.unhcr.org/pages/49da0e466.html, accessed 26 Nov 2013.

74. Deans AK, Boerma CJ, Fordyce J et al. Use of Royal Darwin Hospital emergency department by immigration detainees in 2011. Medical Journal of Australia 2013;199(11):776–8.

75. Procter N, Babakarkhil A, Baker A et al. Mental health of people of immigrant and refugee backgrounds. In: Procter N, Hamer HP, McGarry D et al, eds. Mental health: A person-centred approach. Melbourne: Cambridge University Press, 2014:197–216.

76. Victorian Institute of Forensic Mental Health. Consolidating and strengthening clinical programs: addressing dual diagnosis and offending behaviour in forensic services. Melbourne: Victorian Institute of Forensic Mental Health; 2004. p. 9

77. ABC. SA Ambulance Service report shows attacks against paramedics on rise. Online. www.abc.net.au/news/2014-07-18/sa-ambulance-violent-attacks-against-paramedics-are-on-rise/5606988?WT.ac=statenews_sa; accessed 23 Jul 2014.

78. Kennedy, MP. Violence in emergency departments: under-reported, unconstrained, and unconscionable. Med J Aust 2005;183(7):362–5.

79. Pinch J, Hazelton M, Sundin D et al. Patient-related violence against emergency department nurses. Nursing and Health Sciences 2010;12:268–74.

80. Walsh E, Fahy T. Violence in society. Br Med J 2002;325(7363):507–8.

81. Fasel S, Gulati G, Linsell L et al. Schizophrenia and violence: Systematic review and meta-analysis. PloS Medicine 2009;6(8).

82. Short T, Thomas S, Mullen P et al. Comparing violence in schizophrenia patients with and without comorbid substance-use disorders to community controls. Acta Psychiatrica Scandinavia 2013. Online. onlinelibrary.wiley.com/doi/10.1111/acps.12066/pdf; accessed 12 Dec 2013.

83. Brooks JG. The violent patient. In: Cameron P, Jelinek G, Kelly AM et al. eds. Textbook of adult emergency medicine. 2nd edn. Edinburgh: Churchill Livingstone; 2004:590.

84. American Psychiatric Association, American Psychiatric Nurses Association, National Association of Psychiatric Health Systems. Learning from each other: success stories and ideas for reducing restraint/seclusion in behavioral health. Arlington, VA: American Psychiatric Association; 2003. Online. www.aha.org/content/00-10/learningfromeachother.pdf; accessed 5 Dec 2013.

85. Australian Health Ministers. Framework for the implementation of the national mental health plan 2003–8 in multicultural Australia. Canberra: Australian Government; 2004.

86. Weiss J, Hughes J. Want collaboration? Accept and actively manage conflict. Harv Bus Rev 2005;83(3):92–101.

CHAPTER 38
PEOPLE WITH DISABILITIES
DAVID FOLEY

Essentials

- People with a disability are more likely to receive inadequate assessment and care, probably because of historically based assumptions.
- The number of people with an intellectual disability seeking both primary healthcare and emergency healthcare is increasing because of de-institutionalisation and longer life expectancy.
- Carers and personal support workers must be involved in the care of those with a disability.
- Carers who are family members may be able to provide consent; however, personal support workers cannot act as the person responsible.
- The presence of pain is very likely but difficult to assess, and it is better to assess distress based on prior observations of contentment and distress.
- The person with an intellectual disability may have difficulty in speaking, but they may be able to understand what is said to them.
- Use the communication strategies described by the Centre for Developmental Disabilities Studies.
- Touch should be avoided until after discussion with the carer or personal support worker.
- People with an intellectual disability are likely to have several undiagnosed health problems.
- Syndromes associated with intellectual disability are associated with particular health problems.
- Seizures are prevalent in people with an intellectual disability.
- Anxiety is very disabling for most people with an intellectual disability and can adversely affect emergency care.
- Injury from falls is common.

INTRODUCTION

Definition of disability

Disability is a multifaceted perception of:
- the way people function
- their ability to participate in the activities of daily living, and
- the environment that restricts their capacity to join in.

The disabilities that people live with are often categorised as intellectual, psychiatric, sensory, speech, physical and diverse.

Disability used to be defined as a health condition; however, this medical approach placed 'the problem of disability' in the individual, and the answer to 'their problem' was to treat them. This failed to recognise how people fit into society. Disability is now acknowledged as a barrier that exists between a person and their social, legal and physical surroundings. Often the way to overcome these barriers is to change the environment. For example, instead of just trying to give someone back the ability to walk the solution is to improve their mobility with easier access to public locations with ramps and lifts.

The International Classification of Functioning, Disability and Health describes 'disability' as including impairment, activity limitation and participation restriction effected by environment. Activity limitation refers to restrictions in 'core activities' of self-care, mobility and communication.

The level of assistance a person requires classifies a person's activity limitation as:[5]

- *profound*—unable to perform the activity or always needs aid
- *severe*—sometimes needs help
- *moderate*—has difficulty but doesn't need assistance
- *mild*—uses equipment because of disability but without difficulty.

More particularly, intellectual disability—the preferred Australian term—is defined as being present in a person when all three of the following criteria are met:[6–8]

- Intelligence that is significantly below average as measured with an intelligence quotient assessment.
- Considerable difficulties with the personal skills needed to live and work in the community.
- Limitations in intelligence and living skills that are evident before the person is 18 years old.

Historical context

The history of how people with disabilities have been considered is important, as it reveals how beliefs about disability began, which subsequently determines how people act towards people with disability. It is important to understand this history in order to appreciate the present treatment of people with disabilities. (For further resources, see Useful websites at the end of this chapter.)

Aristotle, believed to be the father of logic and influential in modern thought, supported the Greek practice of leaving 'deformed' babies to die of exposure. He is also supposed to have alleged that those 'born deaf become senseless and incapable of reason'.[1] While this Greek custom was not universal, it continues to influence current thinking, that people with disabilities have a lesser value which may influence how healthcare professionals treat people with a disability.

During the medieval era, people with an intellectual disability (ID) were labelled generically as *natural fools* and *idiots*. They were cared for with others from the edges of society in charitable religious institutions, beginning the practice of institutional care, which continued and was developed during the Industrial Revolution with 'asylums'.[2] Asylum institutionalisation shaped public opinion so that people housed in these places were believed to be 'unable, unworthy, or unfit to contribute to society and who were therefore best housed apart from society'.[2] It was not until the 1970s and '80s that the trend towards person-centred care and recognition of the rights of people with disabilities was recognised in

---

BOX 38.1 Historical views of people with an intellectual disability[3]

Wolf Wolfensberger, an American academic who developed *social role valorisation* and who was very influential in the development of disability policy, claimed (1972) that there have been eight ways in which people with intellectual disabilities have been regarded:

- A subhuman menace that is animal- or vegetable-like.
- A menace and a genetic threat to civilisation.
- An object of dread sent as God's punishment.
- An object of pity who deserves charity.
- A holy innocent, incapable of sin, sent by God for a special purpose.
- A diseased, incurable organism.
- An object of ridicule, such as jester, court fool or village idiot.
- An eternal child in a state of arrested development.

Many of these views have their roots in the Middle Ages, but they persist into the current time and form the opinions of many people in our society. Wolfensberger claimed that these are roles that are given to people with an intellectual disability because these people do not have an obvious role expectation.

---

legislation (Box 38.1), leading to de-institutionalisation. In Western countries, adults with intellectual disabilities mostly live in community houses, supported independent living or in families that receive additional support. These improved living conditions, together with better medical care, mean that people with an ID are living longer. Not only are people living longer, but they are also using community health services rather than healthcare delivered within an institution. This means that the percentage of people with IDs attending emergency departments (EDs) is increasing.

Nature of problem in emergency care

The increasing number of people with disabilities who are using emergency services creates several issues that can arise with the care of this group of people, in particular, difficulties with communication, management of pain, recognition of co-morbid conditions and challenging behaviour. It is also not clear to emergency health workers what role carers and personal support workers should adopt when accompanying a person with a disability. When pain is not recognised or communication is impaired and carers are not involved, outcomes can be calamitous—as illustrated by the death of a young man in an ED from peritonitis caused by swallowing a plastic drink-bottle lid.[4] The purpose of this chapter is to address these issues and to suggest a strategy that includes carers in more-effective emergency care.

National Disability Insurance Scheme

The Australian National Disability Insurance Scheme (NDIS), now known as DisabilityCare Australia, commenced in July 2013 and is designed to improve healthcare for people with disabilities by increasing individualised services that should reduce reliance on emergency services. It is hoped that the NDIS will be able to fund the daily support that people with a disability need, consequently reducing unplanned ED visits through early intervention. This may also mean that when people do attend an ED their visit will be better supported. Full implementation of the NDIS is not expected to be complete until after 2016 (see Useful websites at the end of this chapter).

Broader implications

The predicament of people with an intellectual disability highlights issues that are common to many who seek emergency care. These problems can include having:

- difficulty making themselves understood
- undiagnosed health problems
- pain that is difficult to assess
- behaviour that is threatening or frightening.

Better delivery of care to people with an intellectual disability will therefore lead to better ways to deliver emergency care to people who share these problems, and this could include people who are intoxicated, have dementia or delirium or have a mental health problem.

> **PRACTICE TIP**
>
> Problems with communication, undiagnosed health problems, pain and confronting behaviour need to be considered and planned for when dealing with people who have an intellectual disability.

Aetiology and epidemiology of intellectual disability

Aetiology

Intellectual disability may be caused by genetic abnormalities, environmental factors, or a combination of both. For disorders such as Down syndrome, the diagnosis may be made clinically at birth and confirmed with genetic testing within days. However, some diagnoses take years to establish and some may never have a genetic or environmental cause identified. There are up to 7000 genetic disorders known to be associated with cognitive disability.[9] For 50–70% of people who have an ID, the cause of their disability is not known. This is particularly so for people with a mild impairment. For people with a profound disability the cause is usually genetic and identifiable.[9]

Preventable environmental causes, such as fetal alcohol syndrome, iron-deficiency anaemia and iodine deficiency, contribute to a large proportion of ID. Accidents causing brain injury are another preventable cause.[9]

Epidemiology

In Australia those with an ID make up 3% of the population, according to Wen.[10] However, a review that included Australian, New Zealand and North American studies on the demographics of people with an ID concluded that the prevalence of ID is very difficult to measure, but is probably between 0.7% and 1.3%.[11] Based on these prevalence rates, there are between 155,000 and 288,000 people—or, if Wen[10] is correct, there are approximately 650,000 people—with an ID in Australia in 2014. In New Zealand it is estimated that there are between 30,500 and 56,600 people with an ID.

Most people with an ID have a mild disability and are aged between 5 and 64 years.[11,12] There are very few people over the age of 65 who have an intellectual disability; however, with better healthcare and accommodation numbers in this group are expected to increase.

Intellectual disability morbidity

People with an ID are likely to have more than one disability-linked condition not found to the same degree in the general population. There have been several studies reporting on the occurrence of morbidity that may be linked to ID; while not necessarily caused by ID, these morbidities are certainly more prevalent in people who have an ID. In a frequently cited Australian study it was reported that each intellectually disabled person had between four and five medical conditions, half of which were undiagnosed at the time of the investigation.[13]

It has been suggested that behaviour or other factors, such as sedentary lifestyle, contribute to the morbidity associated with intellectual disability, in addition to problems directly linked to the disability.[14]

In a Swedish study into the prevalence of chronic diseases, 80% of individuals with ID had at least one chronic disease and half of them had more than two.[15] This 1989 study continues to be supported by more recent research; however, definitive Australian studies are still lacking, although the Donald Beasley Institute of New Zealand reported on prevalence in 2003.[11] Epilepsy is the most common morbidity found in individuals with an ID; blindness is 20 times more common than in the general population, deafness 12.5 times more common and psychiatric illness 4.5 times more common in these people.[16] As the presence of ID in people is associated with an increased morbidity, it is therefore likely that this group of people have an increased mortality.

> **PRACTICE TIP**
>
> Consider disability-linked health problems for all people with a disability who present for emergency care.

Particular health problems

Particular health problems occur with greater frequency in people with an ID. These include epilepsy and low-velocity injuries such as occur with falls. These injuries are found more commonly when particular behavioural characteristics are present, often as a result of inadequate coping skills and an inability to understand consequences. In addition, diseases associated with particular syndromes, such as congenital heart disease and endocrine disorders associated with Down syndrome, should be expected. Furthermore, lifestyle diseases associated with a sedentary lifestyle occur with greater frequency.

There have been few studies that have reported what the increased risk of disease is for people with an intellectual disability; however, the most recent attempt to quantify this through a methodical review of the research literature was undertaken by Jansen and colleagues.[17] A summary of their findings, with relative risks calculated, is given in Table 38.1.

Grossman and colleagues[19] have also tabulated medical conditions commonly associated with particular intellectual disability causes, and these are summarised in Table 38.2.

In particular, the most common health problems in the general population of people with an ID are:

- seizures, often intractable and difficult to manage
- chronic serous otitis media associated with anatomical alterations of the face and decreased immune function
- congenital heart disease
- viral myocarditis
- constipation and faecal impaction caused by medication and hypothyroidism
- gastro-oesophageal reflux disease (GORD), particularly in people with cerebral palsy
- chronic aspiration associated with GORD and dysphagia

- most musculoskeletal disorders occur in people with cerebral palsy and are usually a result of joint contractures, which result in limited mobility, osteoarthritis, pressure ulcers, discomfort, hip subluxation and scoliosis
- in about 20% people with Down syndrome, the atlanto-axial joint of the spine is unstable due to lax ligaments and variations in bone morphology
- hypothyroidism, a particular problem in people with Down syndrome
- diabetes mellitus
- leukaemia has an increased incidence in people with Down syndrome
- dental disease.

PRACTICE TIP

Particular health problems should be considered when assessing people with known disability syndromes.

TABLE 38.1 Prevalence of health problems[17]			
HEALTH PROBLEM	PREVALENCE IN PEOPLE WITH AN ID (%)	PREVALENCE IN GENERAL POPULATION (%)	RELATIVE RISK INCREASE
Seizures	23.8	1.7	14.0
CNS conditions	24.9	5	5.0
Sensory loss	13.7	3.4	4.0
Hypothyroidism	5.7	3.2	1.8
Endocrine conditions	5.2	1.9	2.7
Chronic skin disease	17.2	7.1	2.4
Increased risk of fracture*	Low bone mass BUA: male: 52 ± 4 dB/MHz female 34 ± 3 dB/MHz	Low bone mass BUA: male: 89 ± 2 dB/MHz female: 68 ± 2 dB/MHz	Approx 4
Sleep problems	35.7	7.1	5.0
Hepatitis A (in institutionalised people)	54	22	2.5
Congenital disorders	5.0	0.4	12.5
Musculoskeletal impairment	6.0	0.5	12.0
Strabismus	5.3	1.1	4.8
Other disorders of the CNS	4.4	1.1	4.0
Deafness	6.3	2.3	2.7
Fracture lower leg	5.0	1.9	2.6
Congenital anomalies, musculoskeletal system	3.1	1.3	2.4
STI (males)	2.6	0.4	6.5

BUA: broadband-ultrasound attenuation; CNS: central nervous system; ID: intellectual disability; STI: sexually transmitted infection

*A fall of about 20 db/MHz is associated with a relative risk of fracture of 1.95 (95% CI 1.50–2.52, p < 0.0001)[18]

TABLE 38.2 Syndrome-associated conditions[17]

ID CAUSE	MEDICAL CONDITION	PREVALENCE BY CAUSE OF ID (%)
Cerebral palsy	Gastro-oesophageal reflux	8–10%
	Hearing loss	10%
	Hip dislocations, scoliosis, contractures, gait disorder	10%
	Seizures	33%
	Strabismus	50%
Down syndrome	Acquired hip dislocation	6%
	Atlanto-axial instability	14–22%
	Cataracts	15%
	Congenital heart disease	50%
	Deafness	75%
	Diabetes mellitus	1.4–10%
	Early Alzheimer's disease	near 100% > age 40 years
	Gastrointestinal atresias	12%
	Hirschsprung disease	1%
	Leukaemia	1%
	Psychiatric disorders	22%
	Seizure disorders	12–15%
	Severe refractive errors	50%
	Serous otitis media	50–70%
	Thyroid disease	15%
Fetal alcohol syndrome	Hearing loss	66%
	Heart defects	29–41%
	Recurrent serous otitis media	93%
	Renal hypoplasia, duplication of the kidney and collecting system, and bladder diverticula	10%
	Vision problems	94%
Fragile X syndrome	Autism	16%
	Mitral valve prolapse	22–77%
	Recurrent serous otitis media	60%
	Seizures	14–50%
	Strabismus	30–56%
Irradiation-induced intellectual disability	Microcephaly, leukaemia	2%
Trisomy 18	Congenital heart disease	99%

ID: intellectual disability

Injury mechanism

The incidence of falls, burns, foreign-body aspiration, drowning and poisoning is higher in people with an ID.[20]

Falls are a particular issue for people with an ID; over a 12-month period it was found that 10% of a population of people with ID had experienced a fall, resulting in tissue damage and that 30% of the group had been to an ED within that period for some form of injury.[14]

The incidence of injury for individuals with an ID is twice as high as for the general population.[21] This has been more recently supported in a Canadian study that found injury to be the most common reason for emergency presentation.[21] It is also interesting to note that males with an ID are just as likely to be injured as females with an ID, a pattern quite different to the general population.[22] Thus, emergency staff dealing with people who have an ID can expect to see just as many men as women, and to see proportionally more injuries as a result of falls, drowning, foreign-body aspiration and poisoning. Greater awareness of the likelihood of injury should raise the index of suspicion for these injuries when someone with an ID presents to the ED. Emergency staff also need to be aware that this group of people has an increased chance of being moderately or severely injured. As a consequence, they are more likely to be hospitalised; accordingly, admission rates from trauma were found to be almost double that of the general population.[22]

Of particular note is the risk of cervical nerve damage in people with Down syndrome who have atlanto-axial instability. This is more of an issue in children with Down syndrome, as the instability resolves in many adults.

> **PRACTICE TIP**
>
> Be suspicious that injury may be the result of foreign-body aspiration, drowning or poisoning.

Major emergency care issues for people with an ID

Not only is the person with an ID at increased risk of injury and prone to particular health problems, but their treatment, including emergency care, is also more complex and yet neglected. There have been many studies[13,23–27] investigating the medical care of people with an ID, and they have identified the following issues.

- Common problems such as hearing and visual loss are often not managed with corrective lenses or hearing aids. Thus a person with an ID may have an uncorrected sensory loss, threatening communication that is already difficult.
- Screening tests such as blood pressure measurement, Pap smears and prostate examinations are performed less frequently than in the general population, and so easily detected problems remain undiagnosed.
- Health problems are under-investigated, consequently more tests need to be conducted to establish the extent of the health problem.
- Known risk factors associated with particular syndromes are frequently neglected. For example, people with Down syndrome are more likely to have thyroid, cardiac and coeliac disease; therefore people with Down syndrome presenting with vague symptoms need to be investigated for these diseases.
- Atypical behaviours are often expressed when a person is suffering a serious health disorder, and this can mask the problem. In particular, irritability, inactivity, loss of appetite, disturbed sleep, speech which is more difficult to understand, self-injuring behaviour or loss of daily living functioning are all possible signs of a health problem.
- Not only might behaviours be atypical, but people with an ID who are usually able to communicate their needs also may not complain of discomfort or pain, and even people who know them well may not suspect that they are not well.
- Significant health problems will be found in people who present with psychiatric problems or behavioural difficulties if they are carefully assessed.

In addition to these issues, there are extra barriers to the provision of quality emergency care that need to be overcome. Table 38.3 summarises these barriers.

TABLE 38.3 Barriers to effective emergency care[28]

BARRIER ENVIRONMENT	BARRIER TO EFFECTIVE EMERGENCY CARE
Healthcare provider barriers leading to inadequate patient information	Knowledge, training and experience with people who have an ID
	Communicating with the person who has an ID
	Physical examination of the person with an ID
	Lack of time
	Consent for examination and treatment
Associated with patient and carer	Lack of understanding of the role and function of emergency services
	Explaining the problem
	Difficult past experiences with emergency care
	Unable to cooperate
	Atypical pain behaviour
Associated with the healthcare system	Long waiting exacerbates anxiety and consequent challenging behaviour
	Failure of preventative care, resulting in avoidable emergency visits
	Failure to recognise and account for issues associated with intellectual disability

ID: intellectual disability

Assessment of pain

In a review of clients of a Victorian disability service, it was found that over half were not able to communicate in an easily understood way that they were in pain; and even though it is highly likely that they had pain, their pain was not documented.[28] This finding is consistent with people who have an ID and who present for emergency care. These people with pain need to be carefully assessed as they are more likely to have a pre-existing health problem that increases the likelihood of significant morbidity.[13] It is also an imperative to reduce pain, and detect and treat its cause in all people. However, in many people who have an ID it is difficult to determine the presence of pain and often it is not possible to use self-reporting pain-scale tools. It is therefore important that other means of pain assessment are used.[29]

People with mild or moderate communication impairments may be able to self-report pain. However, they are less able to describe the location of the pain, take longer to respond to it and often do not demonstrate decipherable signs of pain.[31] For these patients, emergency workers need to prudently assess the pain, consider its pathological cause and confirm observations with the person's carer.[29] This is important, as the patient's description is likely to be vague, poorly localised and possibly misleading.

Before assessing pain in people with an ID, emergency staff need to briefly assess cognitive and communication abilities, as people with more-profound ID are usually unable to indicate that they are in pain.[32] Pain assessment tools that rely on patients describing or grading their pain will not succeed. In people where communication is non-verbal, other methods of pain assessment need to be used and the best available form of pain assessment is skilled clinical assessment combined with a familiarity and understanding of the person.[33] For emergency staff, paramedics and first-responders, this is also unlikely to succeed as they probably do not know the patient. As communication with people who have profound communication impairment relies on the skill of carers to interpret behavioural, facial and verbal cues, carers become essential for pain assessment. In addition, each person will have an individual language of pain that cannot be generalised.[29]

Although carers and people who know the patient well seem to intuitively identify signs of distress consistent with being in pain, they are usually unsure of their assessment.[34] In response, a tool developed from palliative care, supplements and validates carer assessment. DisDAT (Disability Distress Assessment Tool) is a method that could be used by emergency staff to assess distress in people with an ID. It is likely to be most effective if a carer who knows the patient has completed the 'The Distress Passport' on the front page. However, the authors assert that anyone who cares for patients with severe communication difficulties will be able to use this tool to effectively detect distress.

DisDAT is not a pain scale, as it does not score pain, but instead describes the context of distress and possible causes of distress. 'In people with severe communication difficulties, there is no evidence that pain produces any specific or unique pain behaviours or signs. This has profound implications, since it means that pain cannot be an assessment goal in such patients. However, assessing distress can be, after which its cause must be determined.'[34] The goal of this tool is to reduce the signs of distress and associated behaviours as indicators that pain has been reduced.[34] The tool and its instructions for use are shown in Figure 38.1.

Assessment of the person with an ID

First assessment considerations for first-responders, paramedics and emergency staff

Emergency staff, paramedics and first-responders need to make a concerted effort to assess the patient in an area with as few distractions as possible, as many people with an ID are easily distracted and anxiety is a common experience for people with an ID.[35]

Before beginning assessment, gather as much pertinent information as possible. In particular, attempt to discover usual functional abilities and communication strategies. It is also important to identify co-morbid conditions, medical history medications and allergies.[19] The person from an institutional setting is likely to have a care plan with them; this will describe much of this detail and is usually current.

When first meeting the person with an ID, it is important that first-responders, paramedics and emergency staff introduce themselves by name and role. It is a frequent occurrence for this formality to be omitted, and this distresses many emergency patients. On introduction it is imperative that emergency staff do not assess the person's communication on visual appearance alone. Many people with significant communication difficulties do not have obvious physical deformities; alternatively, many people with obvious ID-associated syndromes have minimal communication difficulties. For example, a person with Down syndrome with obvious distinguishing features may be adept at understanding spoken language and may also have an extensive vocabulary. It is therefore important to attempt to gain a health history from the patient; this should then be confirmed with the carer or personal support worker. These accompanying people may be required to provide the history of the presenting complaint and relevant health information if the patient has severe communication impairment.

The occurrence of an acute illness or injury in the person with an ID can be accompanied by atypical responses. Any evidence of change in motor activity, irritability, refusal to eat, change in bowel habit, loss of weight or decrease in cognition should be investigated further.[19] There are numerous documented occurrences of behavioural change that are likely to be misleading. In one illustrative case, 'Ray' was 'cured' of his obsessive–compulsive behaviour when five ribs were found to be fractured.[36]

> **PRACTICE TIP**
>
> In order to most effectively assess the person with an ID and to preserve their dignity the following principles are recommended:
> - Assume the person is able to understand what you are asking.
> - Adapt your assessment communication style to the person's communication ability.
> - If a carer accompanies a person, include them in your assessment.

FIGURE 38.1 DisDAT (Disability Distress Assessment Tool).[35]

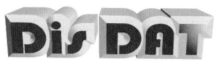

Disability Distress Assessment Tool

v19

Individual's name:	
DoB:	**Gender:**
NHS No:	
Your name:	
Date completed:	
Names of others who helped complete this form:	

THE DISTRESS PASSPORT
Summary of signs and behaviours when content and when distressed

---

Appearance when CONTENT

Face   Eyes

Tongue/jaw

Skin

Appearance when DISTRESSED

Face   Eyes

Tongue/jaw

Skin

Vocal signs when CONTENT

Sounds

Speech

Vocal signs when DISTRESSED

Sounds

Speech

Habits and mannerisms when CONTENT

Habits

Mannerisms

Comfortable distance

Habits and mannerisms when DISTRESSED

Habits

Mannerisms

Comfortable distance

Posture & observations when CONTENT

Posture

Observations

Posture & observations when DISTRESSED

Posture

Observations

Known triggers of distress (write here any actions or situations that usually cause or worsen distress)

This tool relies on observed signs and behaviours to identify distress in people of any age with severe communication difficulties of any cause, and has features which help with monitoring and assessing the cause of the distress. For a full-size version of the tool in colour, see www.disdat.co.uk.[33]

FIGURE 38.1 DisDAT (Disability Distress Assessment Tool).[35]—cont'd

v19

Disability
Distress Assessment Tool

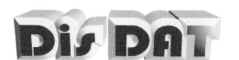

Please take some time to think about and observe the individual under your care, especially their appearance and behaviours when they are both content and distressed. Use these pages to document these.

We have listed words in each section to help you to describe the signs and behaviours. You can circle the word or words that best describe the signs and behaviours when they are content and when they are distressed.

Your descriptions will provide you with a clearer picture of their 'language' of distress.

COMMUNICATION LEVEL *

This individual is unable to show likes or dislikes	Level 0
This individual is able to show that they like or don't like something	Level 1
This individual is able to show that they want more, or have had enough of something	Level 2
This individual is able to show anticipation for their like or dislike of something	Level 3
This individual is able to communicate detail, qualify, specify and/or indicate opinions	Level 4

* This is adapted from the Kidderminster Curriculum for Children and Adults with Profound Multiple Learning Difficulty (Jones, 1994, National Portage Association).

FACIAL SIGNS

Appearance

Information / instructions	Appearance when content	Appearance when distressed
(Ring) the words that best describe the facial appearance	Passive Laugh Smile Frown Grimace Startled Frightened Other:	Passive Laugh Smile Frown Grimace Startled Frightened Other:

Jaw movement

Information / instructions	Movement when content	Movement when distressed
(Ring) the words that best describe the jaw movement	Relaxed Drooping Grinding Biting Rigid Other:	Relaxed Drooping Grinding Biting Rigid Other:

Appearance of eyes

Information / instructions	Appearance when content	Appearance when distressed
(Ring) the words that best describe the appearance	Good eye contact Little eye contact Avoiding eye contact Closed eyes Staring Sleepy eyes 'Smiling' Winking Vacant Tears Dilated pupils Other:	Good eye contact Little eye contact Avoiding eye contact Closed eyes Staring Sleepy eyes 'Smiling' Winking Vacant Tears Dilated pupils Other:

SKIN APPEARANCE

Information / instructions	Appearance when content	Appearance when distressed
(Ring) the words that best describe the appearance	Normal Pale Flushed Sweaty Clammy Other:	Normal Pale Flushed Sweaty Clammy Other:

Continued

FIGURE 38.1 DisDAT (Disability Distress Assessment Tool).[35]—cont'd

VOCAL SOUNDS (NB. The sounds that a person makes are not always linked to their feelings)

Information / instructions	Sounds when content	Sounds when distressed
(Ring) the words that best describe the sounds *Write down* commonly used sounds (write it as it sounds; 'tizz', 'eeiow', 'tetetetete'):	**Volume**: high medium low **Pitch**: high medium low **Duration**: short intermittent long **Description of sound / vocalisation**: Cry out Wail Scream Laugh Groan / moan Shout Gurgle Other:	**Volume**: high medium low **Pitch**: high medium low **Duration**: short intermittent long **Description of sound / vocalisation**: Cry out Wail Scream Laugh Groan / moan Shout Gurgle Other:

SPEECH

Information / instructions	Words when content	Words when distressed
Write down commonly used words and phrases. If no words are spoken, write NONE (Ring) the words which best describe the speech	Clear Stutters Slurred Unclear Muttering Fast Slow Loud Soft Whisper Other, e.g. swearing	Clear Stutters Slurred Unclear Muttering Fast Slow Loud Soft Whisper Other, e.g. swearing

HABITS & MANNERISMS

Information / instructions	Habits and mannerisms when content	Habits and mannerisms when distressed
Write down the habits or mannerisms, e.g. "Rocks when sitting"		
Write down any special comforters, possessions or toys this person prefers.		
Please (Ring) the statements which best describe how comfortable this person is with other people being physically close by	Close with strangers Close only if known No one allowed close Withdraws if touched	Close with strangers Close only if known No one allowed close Withdraws if touched

BODY POSTURE

Information / instructions	Posture when content	Posture when distressed
(Ring) the words that best describe how this person sits and stands.	Normal Rigid Floppy Jerky Slumped Restless Tense Still Able to adjust position Leans to side Poor head control Way of walking: Normal / Abnormal Other:	Normal Rigid Floppy Jerky Slumped Restless Tense Still Able to adjust position Leans to side Poor head control Way of walking: Normal / Abnormal Other:

BODY OBSERVATIONS

Information / instructions	Observations when content	Observations when distressed
Describe the pulse, breathing, sleep, appetite and usual eating pattern, e.g. eats very quickly, takes a long time with main course, eats puddings quickly, "picky".	Pulse: Breathing: Sleep: Appetite: Eating pattern:	Pulse: Breathing: Sleep: Appetite Eating pattern:

FIGURE 38.1 **DisDAT (Disability Distress Assessment Tool).**[35]—cont'd

Information and Instructions

DisDAT is

Intended to help identify distress cues in individuals who have severely limited communication.

Designed to describe an individual's usual content cues, thus enabling distress cues to be identified more clearly.

NOT a scoring tool. It documents what many carers have done instinctively for many years thus providing a record against which subtle changes can be compared.

Only the first step. Once distress has been identified the usual clinical decisions have to be made by professionals.

Meant to help you and the individual in your care. It gives you more confidence in the observation skills you already have, which in turn will give you more confidence when meeting other carers.

When to use DisDAT

When the team believes the individual is NOT distressed

The use of DisDAT is optional, but it can be used as a
– baseline assessment document
– transfer document for other teams

When the team believes the individual IS distressed

If DisDAT has already been completed it can be used to compare the present signs and behaviours with previous observations documented on DisDAT. It then serves as a baseline to monitor change.

If DisDAT has not been completed:

a) When the person is well known DisDAT can be used to document previous content signs and behaviours and compare these with the current observations

b) When the person is new to a carer, or the distress is new, DisDAT can be used to document the present signs and behaviours to act as a baseline to monitor change.

How to use DisDAT

1. **Observe the individual** when content and when distressed—document this on the inside pages. *Anyone* who cares for them can do this.
2. **Observe the context** in which distress is occurring.
3. **Use the clinical decision distress checklist** on this page to assess the possible cause.
4. **Treat or manage** the likeliest cause of the distress.
5. **The monitoring sheet** is a separate sheet, which may help if you want to see how the distress changes over time.
6. **The goal** is a reduction in the number or severity of distress signs and behaviours.

Remember

- Most information comes from several carers together.
- The assessment form need not be completed all at once and may take a period of time.
- Reassessment is essential as the needs may change due to improvement or deterioration.
- Distress can be emotional, physical or psychological. What is a minor issue for one person can be major to another.
- If signs are recognised early then suitable interventions can be put in place to avoid a crisis.

Clinical decision distress checklist
Use this to help decide the cause of the distress

Is the new sign or behaviour:

- Repeated rapidly?
Consider pleuritic pain (in time with breathing)
Consider colic (comes and goes every few minutes)
Consider: repetitive movement due to boredom or fear.

- Associated with breathing?
Consider: infection, COPD, pleural effusion, tumour

- Worsened or precipitated by movement?
Consider: movement-related pains

- Related to eating?
Consider: food refusal through illness, fear or depression
Consider: food refusal because of swallowing problems
Consider: upper GI problems (oral hygiene, peptic ulcer, dyspepsia) or abdominal problems.

- Related to a specific situation?
Consider: frightening or painful situations.

- Associated with vomiting?
Consider: causes of nausea and vomiting.

- Associated with elimination (urine or faecal)?
Consider: urinary problems (infection, retention)
Consider: GI problems (diarrhoea, constipation)
- Present in a normally comfortable position or situation?
Consider: anxiety, depression, pains at rest (e.g. colic, neuralgia), infection, nausea.

If you require any help or further information regarding DisDAT please contact:
Lynn Gibson   01670 394 260
Dorothy Matthews   01670 394 808
Dr. Claud Regnard   0191 285 0063 or e-mail on
claudregnard@stoswaldsuk.org

For more information see
www.disdat.co.uk

Further reading

Regnard C, Matthews D, Gibson L, Clarke C, Watson B. Difficulties in identifying distress and its causes in people with severe communication problems. *International Journal of Palliative Nursing* 2003;9(3):173–6.

Regnard C, Reynolds J, Watson B, Matthews D, Gibson L, Clarke C. Understanding distress in people with severe communication difficulties: developing and assessing the Disability Distress Assessment Tool (DisDAT). *J Intellect Disability Res* 2007;**51(4)**:277–292.

**Distress may be hidden,
but it is never silent**

Physical examination

The physical examination is more important in this population of people, as a detailed history may be difficult to obtain. It is also likely that the patient with an ID has other undiagnosed problems that complicate the presentation.[13] It is important that emergency staff consider that people with an ID are more likely to be injured and more likely to have some particular chronic diseases, and therefore need to be more carefully assessed. In addition to undiagnosed problems, people with a disability are more likely to have been prescribed one or more medications. Consequently, the paramedic and ED staff need to identify what pharmacotherapy the person is receiving and to consider polypharmacy as a contributing factor.

In people with a disability, physical findings may be misleading or confusing; for example, a person with spastic quadriplegia is likely to have a stiff neck which may be confused with significant CNS pathology. There are also documented cases of people with 'acute intestinal obstructions but few physical signs'.[28]

During the examination a family member or personal care worker should be present; this will reduce anxiety in the patient and they may also be able to explain or interpret physical assessment findings.

An explanation of what is going to be done in the physical examination with short, single-concept sentences using simple words must occur. The accompanying person must also receive an explanation; also check with this person for consent to perform the examination. They may be able to provide consent or indicate if the patient is able to consent.

It may also be appropriate to sedate the person for a thorough examination, and this should not be ruled out because the emergency worker fears causing offence.

Ethical care and consent to medical treatment

When a person with a disability is able to understand the proposed treatment, the reason it is being given and how it will be administered, then that person is able to consent to the proposed treatment. If a person with a disability cannot give informed consent, then their legal guardian will need to provide consent; however, this should not preclude paramedics and emergency staff from obtaining the permission of the person prior to any procedure, investigation or assessment. This is part of supported decision-making, which should be guided by the following principles so that people with disability:[29]

- are notified and encouraged to exercise their fundamental human rights
- have the right to live free from neglect
- 'have the right to be respected for their worth, dignity, individuality and privacy'
- have the right to access appropriate assistance and support that will enable them to maximise their capacity to exercise choice and control
- are allowed and encouraged to determine their own best interests, including the right to exercise informed choice and take calculated risks
- have procedures and investigations conducted unobtrusively, with the smallest infringements on the fewest rights

- are provided with services and support based on best evidence, best practice and with a strong focus on person-centred care.[29]

Inspection

Observe the patient for signs of particular syndromes, for example Down syndrome, fetal alcohol syndrome, fragile X, chromosome 22q11.2 deletion syndrome (formerly Catch-22 syndrome), and many others that have particular facial characteristics. See Table 38.4 for a summary of the more prevalent syndromes and their physical features. Having some idea of the likely syndrome will help identify more-common risk factors.

- Observe for signs of distress as described in DisDAT (Fig 38.1); also watch the part of the body that the person avoids touching or continually touches and rubs.
- Inspect teeth and gums, as more than half of all people with an ID have untreated dental caries.[39]
- Check for signs of dehydration, particularly dry mucosa.
- Obesity is prevalent in people with mild to moderate ID; however, lack of nourishment is more widespread in those with more-profound ID.
- Assess respiratory rate, breathing pattern, skin colour and oxygen saturation; this is particularly important as respiratory disease is the major cause of death.[40] This is because of reflux, aspiration pneumonia, poor thoracic expansion and frequent asthma.

Inspection is arguably the most important part of the assessment of a person with an ID, since a history may be difficult to obtain and the person may be unable to describe any symptoms. It is also possible that inspection is the only means available because touching the patient could be difficult, producing alarming behaviour. This is particularly so in people with autism spectrum disorder who may be averse to touch; it is also likely where anxiety is prominent. Before touching the patient, check with the carer for the best approach.

Auscultation

Using a stethoscope may be difficult if the patient does not like to be touched. Interpretation of breath sounds may also be difficult, as patients with an ID may not respond to requests to breathe deeply. Breathing may also be shallow. Despite these complexities, respiratory auscultation should be performed because of the high risk of respiratory problems.

The assessment of indirect blood-pressure measurement with a sphygmomanometer or electronic non-invasive blood-pressure machine is often difficult. Many people with an ID do not like the sensation of increasing pressure as the bladder inflates. The assessment of indirect blood pressure may have to be omitted if it causes undue distress and is not vital.

Palpation

As described previously, touch may be difficult because of behavioural responses; findings may also be misleading because of increased muscle tone that may mimic an acute abdomen. However, bowel obstruction, perforation and peritonitis are all causes of avoidable death in people with an ID.[4,27]

	TABLE 38.4 Syndrome features[39]	
SYNDROME	FACIAL FEATURES	OTHER PHYSICAL FEATURES
Down syndrome	Short broad head Epicanthal folds (upper eyelid covers inner corner) Flat nasal bridge Open mouth	Short fingers Broad hands Reduced muscle tone Lax ligaments with mobile joints Short stature Gap between first and second toes
Fragile X syndrome (features more prominent with age and in males)	Long face Prominent jaw and ears Strabismus	Flat feet Mobile joints
Fetal alcohol syndrome	Flat mid face Short palpebral fissures Indistinct philtrum (vertical groove in the upper lip) Thin upper lip Low nasal bridge Minor ear anomalies Small jaw	
Angelman syndrome	Wide and smiling mouth Pointed chin Prominent tongue Wide-spaced teeth Large jaw Deep set blue eyes Small head	Frequent and inappropriate laughing Wide-based gait
Catch-22 (22q11.2 deletion) syndrome	Microcephaly Cleft palate Round face Almond-shaped eyes Bulbous nose Malformed large ears	Vision loss Congenital heart disease Severe intellectual and physical disability
Congenital hypothyroidism	Thick neck Puffy face Large tongue	Short stature Dry, swollen skin Jaundice Large abdomen Umbilical hernia Cold, mottled arms and legs
Prader-Willi syndrome	Blue eyes 'Unusual facial features'	Fair, sun-sensitive skin Poor muscle tone Obesity Short stature Small hands and feet Cryptorchidism Scoliosis
Turner syndrome (female only)	Webbing of the neck Low posterior hairline Small mandible Prominent ears Epicanthal folds	Broad chest Cubitus valgus (elbows turned in) Hyperconvex fingernails Short stature

Particular clinical presentations

Seizures and epilepsy

Seizure activity in a person with an intellectual or physical disability such as cerebral palsy may be very difficult to recognise. Seizures may present as a behaviour change. Carers will usually be able to describe how a seizure might be recognised; however, there is a tendency for some carers to classify the seizure rather than describe it and this can lead to an inaccurate diagnosis.[41]

The cause of ID is often also the cause of epilepsy, and for some people this can mean that seizure activity contributes to cognitive decline. It is more prevalent in disorders such as tuberous sclerosis. A seizure in people with Down syndrome may indicate the onset of Alzheimer's disease.[42]

Phenobarbitone and phenytoin, drugs often used in the general population, are to be avoided in people with an ID. Both of these agents can cause a decline in intellectual function, and phenytoin toxicity may result in enduring CNS injury. Furthermore, a small change in dose of phenytoin can produce a large alteration in the serum level (i.e. a narrow therapeutic range). The clinical manifestations of toxicity are subtle and are frequently overlooked, especially if the person is unable to describe any side effects they may be experiencing.[28,42] For paramedics who encounter a person in an active seizure the usual recommendation is to administer midazolam if the duration of seizure is greater than 5 minutes. For further information on the diagnosis and management of epilepsy, see Chapter 23.

Neuroleptic malignant syndrome

Neuroleptic drugs are frequently prescribed for people with an ID, because of the severity of neuroleptic malignant syndrome (NMS) and the risk of death. It is important to assess for hyperthermia, muscle rigidity and hypertension. See Chapter 23 for management of this condition.

Alzheimer's disease

Almost all people with Down syndrome over the age of 40 years have the characteristic amyloid plaques of Alzheimer's disease, and this group of people is likely to develop dementia 20–30 years earlier than the general population.[43] The most important factor in the assessment of a person with Down syndrome who appears to have dementia is the exclusion of treatable or self-limiting health problems that produce a change in cognition.[43]

Musculoskeletal injury

Reduced weight-bearing, poor dietary intake of calcium, diminished vitamin D levels and the use of anticonvulsants all increase the risk of fractures in people with an ID.[28] As already indicated, many people with the disabilities described in this chapter are also prone to falls because of poor balance and risky behaviour. Furthermore, people with cerebral palsy are more likely to develop joint problems associated with contractures. It is therefore important that the presence of musculoskeletal injury should not be ruled out until properly assessed.

Atlanto-axial instability

The occiput, the atlas (C1) and the axis (C2) form a unit that is very mobile, allowing rotation of the head around the odontoid bone; however, the joint is not stabilised with bone: instead structures are kept in place with ligaments. This joint also allows flexion and extension, but this can be excessive in some individuals with Down syndrome who have lax ligaments. In particular, laxity of the transverse atlantal ligament or possibly malformations of the odontoid bone lead to instability.[44]

Children with Down syndrome can be screened radiologically, although this is not recommended.[46] It is not usual to find atlanto-axial instability as a result of clinical symptoms; however, there have been rare fatalities as a result of this problem and so it needs to be considered.[47] It appears that this is mostly a problem in children with Down syndrome, with up to 20% affected;[45] in adulthood, the joint stabilises for most individuals. When there are clinical manifestations of spinal cord compression, they are rare with only about 1% affected and they usually occur slowly over weeks.[45]

The presence of the following signs and symptoms could be a result of spinal cord compression:

- neck stiffness or torticollis—an important sign
- unexplained behaviour change
- refusal to participate in usual activities
- changing hand preference
- neck pain
- ataxic gait
- increased reflexes
- clonus
- upgoing plantars
- urinary incontinence
- progressive spasticity in the legs.

PRACTICE TIP

Care should be exercised with procedures that involve hyperextension of the neck in people, particularly children with Down syndrome (such as intubation and instillation of eye drops).

Communication with the person with an ID

Advice on communication with a person with an ID is given in Box 38.2.

Other care issues

Intrathecal baclofen pumps

In order to reduce generalised hypertonia that occurs with cerebral palsy and spinal cord injuries, baclofen is inserted directly into the thecal sac surrounding the spinal cord and continuously infused using a pump.[48,49] If coma or signs of respiratory depression occur, overdose should be suspected and the pump should be stopped immediately. This requires a specialised device, and until it can be turned off or the reservoir emptied, airway, breathing and circulation need to be supported. If the pump fails or the infusing tube becomes blocked, then signs of withdrawal may become evident; these include tachycardia, blood pressure changes, hyperthermia, increased spasticity and rhabdomyolysis that may proceed to multisystem failure.[50]

BOX 38.2 **Communication with the person who has an intellectual disability[48]**

Due to the high frequency of communication difficulties in people with intellectual disability, communication may take more time and the use of non-verbal communication may be necessary. The following are useful communication strategies to use with people with cognitive and/or communication difficulties.

- Always try to speak directly with the person with a disability, rather than a family member/carer or support worker. Find out if the person wishes the carer or support worker to stay for the consultation, and if they are happy for them to speak on their behalf.
- Be aware that while the person with a disability may have difficulty in speaking, he or she may be able to understand what is said to them.
- Find out how the person communicates, e.g. how do they indicate 'yes' or 'no', before asking questions.
- If a person uses a communication device, ask them to show you how to use it.
- Before you start, explain what will happen in the consultation, using brief, simple and direct sentences. Some people may be anxious, and not know what to expect or how to participate.
- Before examining the person, tell or show them what you are going to do and why you are doing it. Check they understand what you have said, and that they agree. Supplement verbal communication with pictures and gestures such as pointing to parts of the body.
- When giving advice or instructions, check that the person has understood by asking them to repeat what you have said in their own words. Let the person know you understand them. If you have trouble understanding, ask them to repeat. Don't pretend that you understand.
- Don't ask questions in a way that suggests an answer. Check responses to your question by asking again in a different way.
- Some people may take time to answer your questions. A good rule of thumb is to wait at least 10 seconds for a response.
- Some people may not be able to read letters, make appointments, tell the time or read instructions on medications. Family members, other carers or support workers can assist here.
- Understanding the concept of time may be difficult. Use examples from their daily routines, e.g breakfast, lunch and dinner, rather than three times a day. Try to relate questions to familiar routines or events in their life.

Ventriculoperitoneal shunts

Ventriculoperitoneal (VP) shunts are catheters used to treat hydrocephalus; they are placed into the ventricles of the brain where they collect cerebrospinal fluid (CSF), which is then transported to the peritoneum. An obstruction in this drainage system causes a rise in intracranial pressure (ICP). Signs and symptoms are consistent with rising ICP and are likely to include irritability; headache; nausea and vomiting; reduced cognition; ataxia; changes in respirations, blood pressure and pulse; and a bulging fontanelle in infants. Emergency management should include elevating the person's head and managing their airway, breathing and circulation. If stable, the patient should have a computed tomography scan of the head and a neurosurgical consultation should be arranged for surgical shunt revision.[50]

If a child presents with signs of raised ICP and infection (fever, ill appearance, redness over the site, tenderness over the tubing, abdominal pain and tenderness), then the shunt may be infected. In these circumstances a lumbar puncture with CSF collection for culture and sensitivity should occur, followed by appropriate broad-spectrum antibiotics.[50]

Gastrostomy tubes

An increasing number of people with feeding difficulties are having enterostomy devices inserted. They are implemented to avoid aspiration and where nutritional intake is inadequate because of difficulty swallowing. These devices can be inserted via the nasogastric route or, for longer-term use, via a stoma.

Percutaneous endoscopic gastrostomy tubes (PEGs or buttons) terminate in the stomach (Fig 38.2), whereas jejunostomy tubes (J tubes) terminate in the jejunum of the small bowel (Fig 38.3). PEGs are more routinely used for feeding, whereas J tubes are used for people with gastro-oesophageal reflux.

People with feeding tubes are likely to present for emergency care if the tube leaks gastric contents, becomes obstructed or is dislodged. The first assessment priority in all these circumstances is the person's level of hydration, as they may have a significantly reduced fluid intake. For the person who is unable to safely swallow fluids, intravenous hydration may be required to maintain fluid intake. Medication may also have been missed.[50]

PEG tubes that are blocked with food or medication can sometimes be cleared with a carbonated cola or a proteolytic enzyme solution; if this fails, replacement will be necessary. Tubes that have come out need to be replaced quickly to prevent constriction and closure of the stoma; however, this should be attempted by an experienced and suitably trained person. In particular, jejunostomy tubes need to be guided back into position under fluoroscopy. Attempts by inexperienced practitioners can result in false tracts being created. If there is going to be some delay, an indwelling urinary catheter may be used to keep the stoma open.

When PEG tubes have been reinserted in the ED, their position needs to be confirmed radiologically. Patients should not be discharged until definitive tube placement has been achieved.

Challenging behaviour and anxiety

A change in behaviour is often a reason a person with an ID is brought to an ED. Often the abnormal behaviour is a result of distress, illness or pain.[51] Once a pathological cause has been ruled out or treated, only then can the behaviour be managed with a pharmacological, psychiatric or behavioural intervention.[47]

Two particularly difficult forms of challenging behaviour are 'stereotypical or self-stimulatory' and 'self-injurious'.

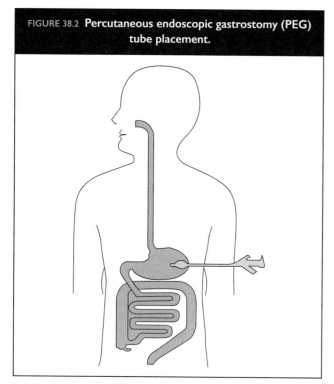

FIGURE 38.2 **Percutaneous endoscopic gastrostomy (PEG) tube placement.**

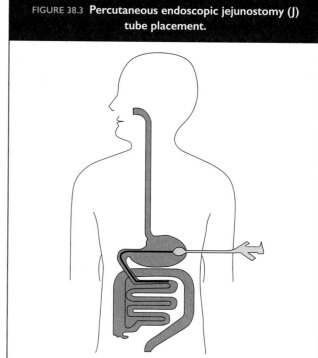

FIGURE 38.3 **Percutaneous endoscopic jejunostomy (J) tube placement.**

Stereotypical behaviour is characterised by repeated stimulation of a sense or senses. In the emergency setting it may be triggered by the unfamiliar and frightening surroundings that cause anxiety. As a result, the person may begin to rock, to tap or repeatedly taste things. If this behaviour is a result of anxiety, it may be managed with the help of the carer who may effectively soothe the person; or a socially acceptable alternative could be provided, such as a piece of rubber to chew on.[52] Self-injurious behaviour results in physical injury and may also be the result of anxiety; however, it may be more difficult to manage and be less socially acceptable, and so chemical or physical restraint may need to be used.[52] For all forms of behaviour the patient may have a healthcare plan that details the causes and describes management strategies and, in consultation with the accompanying carer, these strategies should be used.

Anxiety is a very common experience for people with an intellectual disability and this can be manifested as a diagnosable psychiatric disorder that may cause greater impairment than diminished cognitive abilities.[53] Carers and personal support workers must be involved in the prevention and management of anxiety in the emergency setting. Touching the patient in an effort to calm them is likely to exacerbate the problem. The person who knows the patient best should be the individual to use soothing techniques. However, once the patient becomes uncontrollably anxious there may be little that can be done apart from the administration of suitable pharmacological agents, restraint or removal from the area.

The role of carers and personal support workers

Carer is the term used for a person who lives with a person who has a disability; usually this will mean that they are a parent or sibling. *Personal support workers* (PSWs) are employed to perform this role. The term 'carer' is sometimes used for both roles. These people are integral to the delivery of effective care for the person with a disability. Some PSWs have known their clients for more than 20 years and may be more familiar with their health issues than many parents. It is therefore essential to involve carers and PSWs in the emergency care of patients with a disability.

PRACTICE TIP

Personal support workers cannot act as the 'person responsible' to provide consent.

SUMMARY

People with an ID who seek emergency care are at increased risk of particular disorders such as epilepsy and anxiety. People with an ID are most likely to die of a respiratory disorder. Having an ID predisposes to particular health conditions, many of which are related to the syndrome that caused their ID. Depending on the communication ability of the person, assessing their emergency needs and level of pain or distress is difficult, and needs to be carefully performed with the assistance of the person who normally cares for them. Failure to acknowledge behavioural changes and signs of distress can result in inadequate assessment of serious pathologies. Generalisations cannot be applied when assessing pain, as people with ID may display their distress in idiosyncratic ways.

CASE STUDY

A 36-year-old intellectually disabled man is brought to the emergency department (ED) by ambulance. His personal support worker (PSW) accompanies him from his residential accommodation. He was brought in because the staffing at his community house noticed that he was not his usual self and he had lost his appetite.

Questions

1. After introducing yourself to the patient and their PSW with your name and role, it is then important that you ask:
   A. the PSW to remain outside so that the patient answers without fear of disclosing private details to the PSW.
   B. the PSW to remain with your patient and direct all questions to the PSW.
   C. the patient a simple question, such as 'Where does it hurt?' to determine their communication ability.
   D. the PSW what the patient's communication abilities are.

2. Your patient with an intellectual disability has a PSW at all times in his residential accommodation and a registered nurse visits when he needs assistance with his healthcare needs. How would you triage the patient?
   A. He needs to be urgently assessed and closely monitored.
   B. He can wait in the waiting room with his PSW.
   C. He should be moved to a quieter area.
   D. His triage priority should be determined on physiological parameters as for every other patient seeking emergency care.

3. You notice that your patient is slim, of short stature, has an extended face, enlarged ears and that he sits on the bed with widely abducted legs. These observations are important because:
   A. His elongated face and ears indicate that he may have Marfan's syndrome, indicating that he is at risk of aortic dissection and cardiac ischaemia.
   B. His facial features, short stature and mobile joints indicate that he may have fragile X syndrome, indicating that he is more at risk of seizures and mitral regurgitation with congestive heart failure.
   C. His hypermobile hips indicate that he probably has Down syndrome, indicating an increased risk of thyroid disease, congenital heart disease and dislocated hips.
   D. These physical appearance findings, while informative, are unlikely to have much bearing on his emergency care.

4. You determine that your patient is unable to indicate that he has pain, as he has no language abilities. How will you best determine if he has any pain or discomfort?
   A. Ask his carer if he has pain.
   B. Use a tool to assess facial expression as an indicator of distress.
   C. If he appears in distress to you, he is likely to be in pain.
   D. Use information provided in his healthcare plan or from his carer to determine his appearance when content in comparison to when distressed.

 Answers to Case Study Questions can be found on evolve
http://evolve.emergencytrauma.curtis

USEFUL WEBSITES

Australasian Society for Intellectual Disability, www.asid.asn.au

Australian National Disability Insurance Scheme (NDIS), www.ndis.gov.au

Centers for Disease Control and Prevention, Developmental disabilities, www.cdc.gov/ncbddd/dd/ddmr.htm

Centre for Developmental Disability Health Victoria (CDDHV), www.cddh.monash.org

Centre for Disability Studies, www.cds.med.usyd.edu.au/index.php

Donald Beasley Institute, www.donaldbeasley.org.nz

Intellectual disability mental health elearning, www.idhealtheducation.edu.au

National Council on Intellectual Disability, http://www.ncid.org.au

Queensland Centre for Intellectual and Developmental Disability, www2.som.uq.edu.au/som/Research/ResearchCentres/qcidd/Pages/default.aspx

Understanding Intellectual Disability and Health, St George's, University of London, www.intellectualdisability.info

Understanding Intellectual Disability and Health, Changing Values, www.intellectualdisability.info/changing-values

Disability Services Australia, history of disability, www.dsa.org.au/Pages/BeInformed/History-Of-Disability.aspx

REFERENCES

1. Merriam G. Rehabilitating Aristotle: a virtue ethics approach to disability and human flourishing. In: Ralston DC, Ho J, editors. Philosophical reflections on disability. Dordrecht: Springer; 2010:133–54.

2. Brown I, Radford JP. Historical overview of intellectual and developmental disabilities. In: Brown I, Percy M, editors. A comprehensive guide to intellectual and developmental disabilities. 2nd edn. Baltimore: Paul H Brookes; 2007:17–34.

3. Radford JP, Park DC. Historicial overview of developmental disabilities in Ontario. In: Brown I, Percy M, editors. Developmental disabilities in Ontario. 2nd edn. Toronto: Ontario Association on Developmental Disabilities; 2003:3–18.

4. Chivell WC. An inquest taken on behalf of our Sovereign Lady the Queen at Adelaide in the state of South Australia, on the 2nd and 3rd and 17th of July 2001 and the 24th of August 2001, before Wayne Cromwell Chivell, a Coroner for the said State, concerning the death of Saverio Gadaleta. Adelaide: Coroners Court, South Australia; 24 Aug 2001.

5. Australian Network on Disability. What is a disability? Online. www.and.org.au/pages/what-is-a-disability.html; accessed 24 Feb 2014.

6. Australian Institute of Health and Welfare. Disability in Australia: intellectual disability. Bulletin no. 67. Cat. no. AUS 110. Canberra: AIHW. Online. Available: www.aihw.gov.au/publications/index.cfm/title/10582; 24 Feb 2014.

7. Department of Human Services. Intellectual disability Better Health Channel. Online. www.betterhealth.vic.gov.au/bhcv2/bhcarticles.nsf/pages/Intellectual_disability?open; accessed 24 Feb 2014.

8. Disability Information Service. Intellectual disability: the facts. Disability SA. Fullerton, SA: Department for Families and Communities; 2009.

9. Percy M. Factors that cause or contribute to intellectual and developmental disabilities. In: Brown I, Percy M, editors. A comprehensive guide to intellectual and developmental disabilities. 2nd edn. Baltimore: Paul H Brookes; 2007:125–48.

10. Wen X. The definition and prevalence of intellectual disability in Australia. AIHW catalogue no DIS 2. Australian Government Publication. Canberra: Australian Institute of Health and Welfare; 1997.

11. Bray A. Demographics and characteristics of people with an intellectual disability: review of the literature prepared for the National Advisory Committee on Health and Disability to inform its project on services for adults with an intellectual disability. Wellington: National Health Committee and Donald Beasley Institute; 2003.

12. Larson SA, Lakin KC, Anderson L et al. Prevalence of mental retardation and developmental disabilities: estimates from the 1994/1995 National Health Interview Survey Disability Supplements. Am J Ment Retard 2001;106(3):231–52.

13. Beange H, McElduff A, Baker W. Medical disorders of adults with mental retardation: a population study. Am J Ment Retard 1995;99(6):595–604.

14. Janicki MP, Davidson PW, Henderson CM et al. Health characteristics and health services utilization in older adults with intellectual disability living in community residences. J Intellect Disabil Res 2002;46(Pt 4):287–98.

15. Asberg KH. The need for medical care among mentally retarded adults: a 5-year follow-up and comparison with a general population of the same age. Br J Ment Subnormality 1989;35(68):50–7.

16. Beange H, Taplin JE. Prevalence of intellectual disability in northern Sydney adults. J Intellect Disabil Res 1996;40(Pt 3):191–7.

17. Jansen DE, Krol B, Groothoff JW et al. People with intellectual disability and their health problems: a review of comparative studies. J Intellect Disabil Res 2004;48(2):93–102.

18. Khaw KT, Reeve J, Luben R et al. Prediction of total and hip fracture risk in men and women by quantitative ultrasound of the calcaneus: EPIC—Norfolk prospective population study. Lancet 2004;363(9404):197–202.

19. Grossman SA, Richards CF, Anglin D et al. Caring for the patient with mental retardation in the emergency department. Ann Emerg Med 2000;35(1):69–76.

20. Sherrard J, Tonge BJ, Ozanne Smith J. Injury risk in young people with intellectual disability. J Intellect Disabil Res 2002;46(Pt 1):6–16.

21. Lunsky Y, Balogh R, Khodaverdian A et al. A comparison of medical and psychobehavioral emergency department visits made by adults with intellectual disabilities. Emerg Med Int 2012; 427407.

22. Sherrard J, Tonge BJ, Ozanne Smith J. Injury in young people with intellectual disability: descriptive epidemiology. Inj Prev 2001; 7(1):56–61.

23. Howells G. Are the medical needs of mentally handicapped adults being met? J R Coll Gen Pract 1986;36(291):449–53.

24. Lennox NG, Diggens J, Ugoni A. Health care for people with an intellectual disability: general practitioners' attitudes, and provision of care. J Intellect Dev Disabil Res 2000;25(2):127–33.

25. van Schrojenstein Lantman-De Valk HM, Metsemakers JF, Haveman MJ et al. Health problems in people with intellectual disability in general practice: a comparative study. Fam Pract 2000;17(5):405–7.

26. Wilson DN, Haire A. Health care screening for people with mental handicap living in the community. BMJ 1990;301(6765):1379–81.

27. Ziviani J, Lennox N, Allison H et al. Meeting in the middle: improving communication in primary health care consultations with people with an intellectual disability. J Intellect Dev Disabil Res 2004;29(3):211–25.

28. Cheetham T, Lovering JS, Telch J et al. Physical Health. In: Brown I, Percy M, eds. A comprehensive guide to intellectual and developmental disabilities. 2nd edn. Baltimore: Paul H Brookes; 2007:629–44.

29. Koutoukidis G. Health planning: an organisational approach to meeting the needs of individuals with a disability. Ageing and Disability Conference. Adelaide: National Disability Services; 2007.

30. Policy and Planning Disability SA. Safeguarding people with disability: overarching policy. Department for Communities and Social Inclusion. Adelaide, Government of South Australia. 2013; Policy number: DIS/366 – POL-SER-002-2013

31. Foley DC, McCutcheon H. Detecting pain in people with an intellectual disability. Accid Emerg Nurs 2004;12(4):196–200.

32. Hennequin M, Morin C, Feine JS. Pain expression and stimulus localisation in individuals with Down's syndrome. Lancet 2000;356(9245):1882–7.

33. Biersdorff KK. Incidence of significantly altered pain experience among individuals with developmental disabilities. Am J Ment Retard 1994;98(5):619–31.

34. Davies D, Evans L. Assessing pain in people with profound learning disabilities. Br J Nurse 2001;10(8):513–16.

35. Regnard C, Reynolds J, Watson B et al. Understanding distress in people with severe communication difficulties: developing and assessing the Disability Distress Assessment Tool (DisDAT). J Intellect Disabil Res 2007;51(Pt 4):277–92.

36. Cheetham TC, Challenges in medical care for persons with developmental disabilities: An Illustrative case: 'Ray'. Clinical Bulletin of the Developmental Disabilities Program. 2001;12(3) Online. www.ddd.uwo.ca/bulletins/2001Sept.pdf; accessed 25 April 2015.

37. Gibbs SM, Brown MJ, Muir WJ. The experiences of adults with intellectual disabilities and their carers in general hospitals: a focus group study. J Intellect Disabil Res 2008;52(12):1061–77.

38. Cheetham TC. Challenges in medical care for persons with developmental disabilities: an illustrative case: 'Ray'. Clinical Bulletin of the Developmental Disabilities Program. London: The University of Western Ontario 2001;12(3):1–9.

39. Brown I, Percy M, eds. A comprehensive guide to intellectual and developmental disabilities. 2nd edn. Baltimore: Paul H Brookes; 2007.

40. Cumella S, Ransford N, Lyons J et al. Needs for oral care among people with intellectual disability not in contact with Community Dental Services. J Intellect Disabil Res 2000;44(Pt 1):45–52.

41. Durvasula S, Beange H, Baker W. Mortality of people with intellectual disability in northern Sydney. J Intellect Develop Disabil 2002;27(4):255–64.

42. Bernal J. Epilepsy. Understanding intellectual disability and health. Online. www.intellectualdisability.info/physical-health/epilepsy; accessed 19 Jan 2010.

43. Prasher V, Percy M, Jozsval E et al. Implications of Alzheimer's disease for people with Down syndrome and other intellectual disabilities. In: Brown I, Percy M, eds. A comprehensive guide to intellectual and developmental disabilities. 2nd edn. Baltimore: Paul H Brookes; 2007:681–700.

44. Trumble S. Dementia in Down syndrome. Untangling the threads. Aust Fam Physician 1999;28(1):49–53.

45. Ali FE, Al-Bustan MA, Al-Busairi WA et al. Cervical spine abnormalities associated with Down syndrome. Int Orthop 2006;30(4):284–9.

46. Down's Syndrome Medical Interest Group. Cervical spine instability. Basic medical surveillance essentials for people with Down's syndrome. Nottingham: DSMIG; 1996.

47. Saad KF. A lethal case of atlantoaxial dislocation in a 56-year-old woman with Down's syndrome. J Intellect Disabil Res 1995; 39(Pt 5):447–9.

48. Centre for Developmental Disability Studies. Health care in people with intellectual disability—guidelines for general practitioners. North Sydney: CDDS for NSW Health; 2006.

49. Fehlings D, Hunt C, Rosenbaum P. Cerebral palsy. In: Brown I, Percy M, eds. A comprehensive guide to intellectual and developmental disabilities. 2nd edn. Baltimore: Paul H Brookes; 2007:279–86.

50. Shirley KW, Kothare S, Piatt Jr JH et al. Intrathecal baclofen overdose and withdrawal. Pediatr Emerg Care 2006;22(4):258–61.

51. Adirim TA, Rosenman ED. Evaluation of the developmentally or physically disabled patient. In: Marx J, Hockberger R, Walls R, eds. Rosen's Emergency medicine: concepts and clinical practice. 8th edn. Philadelphia: Mosby; 2013.

52. Percy M, Brown I, Lewkis SZ. Abnormal behavior. In: Brown I, Percy M, eds. A comprehensive guide to intellectual and developmental disabilities. 2nd edn. Baltimore: Paul H Brookes; 2007:309–34.

53. Davis E, Saeed SA, Antonacci DJ. Anxiety disorders in persons with developmental disabilities: empirically informed diagnosis and treatment. Reviews literature on anxiety disorders in DD population with practical take-home messages for the clinician. Psychiatr Q 2008;79(3):249–63.

CHAPTER 39
THE OLDER PERSON
DAVID FOLEY

Essentials

- The ageing process affects human physiology.
- Emergency care must account for individual ageing processes particular to each person.
- The functional, cognitive and emotional status of the older person must be assessed and managed.
- Particular attention must be paid to the assessment and treatment of pain, which is often not assessed or treated.
- Polypharmacy is such a significant cause of morbidity that it must be considered as a contributing risk factor for all older people.
- It is essential to include the carer in emergency management of the older person.
- An assessment of activities of daily living and instrumental activities of daily living is required.
- Mental status testing is an important part of assessment.
- Falls are the most common cause of injury.
- Expected physiological responses to stress are delayed.
- Resuscitation after injury needs to be aggressive and prompt.
- Rapid functional decline is a sign of a potentially life-threatening illness.
- Malnutrition affects older people who seek emergency care.
- Skin care is essential and where injury occurs, keep the wound moist.
- A serious infection can present with vague signs and symptoms.
- Carefully consider functional decline before discharging home.
- Accurately and carefully complete standardised discharge or transitional care forms.
- It is particularly useful for ambulance staff to assess the living arrangements of older people and to bring in their medications in order to assist with discharge planning.

INTRODUCTION

Definition of older person

People in Australia and New Zealand are termed 'older' or 'elderly' at the age of 65 years. This is an arbitrary value, historically based on the age at which a pension could be received. Otto von Bismarck, in his role as German Chancellor, set a limit of 70 years in 1889, but this was reduced to 65 years in 1916.[1] Countries that provided an 'old age pension' adopted this age, and it has entered the lexicon as the beginning of older age. This was reinforced by Eric Erikson, who defined his eighth stage of psychosocial development as beginning at 65 years.[2]

As a consequence of improved healthcare and a large increase in the birth rate from 1946 to 1964 (demographic birth boom), more people are entering older age than at any other time in history.[3]

Ageing population

In Australia, New Zealand and other developed countries the ageing of the population has meant a steady increase in the number and proportion of older people using emergency services. This has been occurring, for example, in the UK, Belgium, Sweden and the USA.[4–8] In Melbourne during 2008–09, 60% of the population aged over 85 years presented for emergency care and they comprised 4.7% of all ED presentations.[9]

Together with a decreasing birth rate, increasing life span has meant that the average age of Australians is increasing, so that by 2020 18% of the population will be over 65, a proportion that will have tripled since 1901.[10] In 1976, 8.8% of the New Zealand population were 65 years or over; in 2006 this had risen to 12.3% and by the late 2030s one-quarter of New Zealand's population is projected to be in this age group.[11] For New Zealand women, life expectancy has risen from 73 years in 1955 to 81.9 in 2006. For men it has increased in the same period from 68.2 to 77 years.[11]

The increase in life expectancy has significant implications for paramedics and emergency department (ED) staff, not only because of the increasing numbers of older people but also because they need to be aware of the different emergency care requirements of this age group. For many years children have been recognised as requiring different emergency care, with most Australian capital cities providing specialised paediatric care; however, specialised emergency care is not typically available to older people. This is despite their very specific and often complex requirements for emergency care that reflects the physiological, psychological and social changes that occur with ageing.[5] Consequently, older people presenting to the ED are more likely to arrive by ambulance, have higher acuity problems, and will take more time to evaluate. One-third of these patients are admitted, many to the intensive care unit.[12] Box 39.1 summarises older patient ED patterns.[13–18]

While acute medical problems of the older patient may be similar to those of younger adults, the presentation of older people is often different and the presence of co-morbidities of ageing complicates the presentation.[19] It is therefore crucial that emergency care providers understand how the ageing process can complicate presentations and also exacerbate the severity of the presenting complaint. In addition, elder abuse and neglect take different forms: these are discussed in Chapter 40.

Assessment
Pathophysiology

The assessment of the older person requires an understanding of age-related changes. Without knowledge of normal ageing

> **BOX 39.1 Patterns of older person ED use**
>
> Compared with younger adults, older people:
> - are over-represented in the ED population
> - have an increased probability of being admitted
> - have a longer length of stay in the ED
> - will have more tests done on them; and will use more time and resources
> - are prescribed more medications
> - are more severely ill and their medical outcomes are worse
> - are more likely to be inaccurately diagnosed
> - use ambulances more often
> - are more likely to arrive during daytime hours
> - when discharged are more compliant with follow-up care
> - are more dependent after discharge
> - are more likely to be discharged without their presenting complaint resolved
> - have less time spent on resuscitation
> - are less likely to understand discharge instructions
> - are not asked about their self-care ability
> - endure worse standards of care
> - are more likely to return to an ED for treatment of the same or another problem.

changes, pathology may be confused with normal physiology. However, the ageing process is particular to individuals and dependent on genetics, nutritional status, level of fitness, lifestyle and presence of disease.[20]

> **PRACTICE TIP**
>
> Ageing is individual and is not predicted by a person's age.

Bodily change results from cellular alterations; cells die and are not replaced, leaving fewer working cells. Muscle mass decreases; however, adipose tissue increases, so that the proportion of total body fat increases.[21] Bone mass decreases, as does intracellular fluid; although extracellular fluid remains mostly unchanged. As a result, total body fluid is diminished, which increases the risk of dehydration. Age-related changes and associated clinical manifestations are listed in Table 39.1.

Familiar noticeable effects include greying hair that thins and is lost from the scalp, wrinkles and a more pronounced bony appearance as body fat diminishes. This is associated with

TABLE 39.1 Gerontological differences in assessment: age-related changes and associated clinical manifestations[22]

SYSTEM	EXPECTED AGEING CHANGES	CLINICAL MANIFESTATIONS
Cardiovascular		
Cardiac output	Force of contraction decreased	Myocardial oxygen demand increased
	Fat and collagen increased	Stroke volume and CO decreased
	Heart muscle decreased	Fatigue, shortness of breath, tachycardia occur
	Ventricular wall thickened	Blood flow to vital organs and periphery decreased

TABLE 39.1 Gerontological differences in assessment: age-related changes and associated clinical manifestations[22]—cont'd

SYSTEM	EXPECTED AGEING CHANGES	CLINICAL MANIFESTATIONS
Cardiac rate and rhythm	Dependence of atrial contraction increased Loss of fibres from bundle of His Mitral valve stretching Ventricles slow to relax Sinus node pacemaker cells decreased	HR slow to increase with stress Decrease in maximum HR (e.g. 80-year-old person, 120 beats/minute; 20-year-old person, 200 beats/minute) Possible AV block Recovery time from tachycardia prolonged Premature beats increased
Structural changes	Aortic valves sclerotic and calcified Baroreceptor sensitivity decreased Mild fibrosis and calcification of valves	Diastolic murmur present in 50% of older patients Heart position landmarks change
Arterial circulation	Elastin and smooth muscle reduced Vessel rigidity increased Vascular resistance increased Aorta becomes dilated	Modest increase in systolic BP Rigid arteries contribute to coronary artery and peripheral vascular disease
Venous circulation	Tortuosity increased	Inflamed, painful or cord-like varicosities
Peripheral pulses	Arteries rigid	Pulses weaker but equal Circulation slowed to periphery Cold feet and hands
Respiratory		
Structures	Cartilage degeneration Vertebrae rigid Strength of muscles decreased Respiratory muscles atrophy Thoracic wall rigidity increased Ciliary action decreased	Kyphosis Anterior–posterior diameter increased Use of accessory muscles decreased Chest rigid and barrel-shaped Respiratory excursion decreased Cough and deep breathing diminished Lung compliance decreased
Change in ventilation and perfusion	Pulmonary vascular bed decreased Alveoli decreased Alveolar walls thickened Elastic recoil decreased	Total lung volume not changed Vital capacity decreased Residual lung volume increased Mucus thickens PaO_2 and O_2 saturation decreased Hyperresonance
Ventilation control	Response to hypoxia and hypercarbia decreased	Ability to maintain acid–base balance decreased Respiratory rate 12–24 breaths/minute
Integumentary		
Skin	Collagen and subcutaneous fat decreased Sweat glands decreased Epidermal cell turnover slowed Skin tissue fluid decreased Capillary fragility increased Pigment cells decreased Sebaceous gland activity decreased Sensory receptors decreased Thresholds for touch, vibration, heat, pain increased	Skin less elastic Wrinkles and folds increased Extremity fat lost; fat on trunk increased Skin heals slowly Skin dry Skin tears and bruises easily Skin colour uneven Normal skin lesions increased Ability to respond to heat and cold decreased Ability to feel light touch decreased Cutaneous pain sensitivity declines

Continued

TABLE 39.1 Gerontological differences in assessment: age-related changes and associated clinical manifestations[22]—cont'd

SYSTEM	EXPECTED AGEING CHANGES	CLINICAL MANIFESTATIONS
Hair	Melanin decreased	Grey or white hair
	Germ centre and hair follicle decreased	Hair quantity decreased and thinner
		Scalp, pubic, axillary hair decreased
		Facial hair on men decreased
		Facial hair on women increased
		Growth slowed
Nails	Blood supply to nail bed decreased	Nails thickened and brittle
	Longitudinal striations increased	Nails split easily
		Potential for fungal infection increased
Urinary		
Kidney	Renal mass decreased	Protein in urine increased
	Number of functioning nephrons decreased	Potential for dehydration increased
	Glomerular filtration rate decreased	Creatinine clearance decreased
	Renal plasma flow decreased	Serum creatinine and urea increased
		Excretion of toxins and drugs decreased
		Nocturia increased
Bladder	Bladder smooth muscle and elastic tissue decreased	Capacity decreased
		Less control; stress incontinence
Micturition	Sphincter control decreased	Frequency, urgency and nocturia increased
Reproductive		
Male structures	Prostatic enlargement	Sexual response less intense
	Testicular volume decreased	Longer to achieve erection
	Sperm count decreased	Erection maintained without ejaculation
	Seminal vesicles atrophy	Force of ejaculation decreased
	Serum testosterone constant	
	Oestrogen level increased	
Female structures	Oestradiol, prolactin, progesterone diminished	Responses to changing hormone levels altered
	Size of ovaries, uterus, cervix, fallopian tubes, labia decreased	Cervical, vaginal secretions decreased
	Associated glands and epithelium atrophied	Intensity of sexual response gradually decreased
	Elasticity in the pelvic area decreased	Potential for vaginal infections increased
	Breast tissue decreased	Potential for vaginal and uterine prolapse increased
	Vaginal pH becomes alkaline	
Gastrointestinal		
Oral cavity	Dentine decreased	Taste changes
	Gingival retraction	Potential loss of teeth
	Bone density lost	Gingivitis
	Papillae of tongue decreased	Bleeding gums and dry mouth
	Taste threshold for salt and sugar increased	Oral mucosa dry
	Salivary secretions decreased	
Oesophagus	Lower oesophageal sphincter pressure decreased	Epigastric distress
	Motility decreased	Dysphagia
		Potential for hiatal hernia and aspiration

TABLE 39.1 Gerontological differences in assessment: age-related changes and associated clinical manifestations[22]—cont'd

SYSTEM	EXPECTED AGEING CHANGES	CLINICAL MANIFESTATIONS
Stomach	Gastric mucosa atrophy Blood flow decreased	Decreased gastric emptying
Small intestine	Intestinal villi decreased Enzyme secretions decreased Motility decreased	Slowed intestinal transit Absorption of fat-soluble vitamins delayed
Large intestine	Blood flow decreased Motility decreased Sensation to defecation decreased	Potential for constipation and faeces impaction
Pancreas	Pancreatic ducts distend Lipase production decreased Pancreatic reserve impaired	Impaired fat absorption Decreased glucose tolerance
Liver	Number and size of cells decreased Hepatic protein synthesis impaired Ability to regenerate decreased	Lower border extends past costal margin Decreased drug metabolism
Musculoskeletal		
Skeleton	Intervertebral disc narrowed Cartilage of nose and ears increased	Height diminished by 2.5–10 cm Nose and ears lengthen Kyphosis Pelvis wider
Bone	Cortical and trabecular bone decreased	Bone resorption exceeds bone formation Potential for osteoporotic fractures
Muscles	Number of muscle fibres decreased Muscle fibres atrophy Muscle regeneration slowed Contraction time and latency period prolonged Flexion of joints increased Ligaments stiffening Sclerosis of tendons Tendon flexor reflexes decreased	Strength decreased Agility decreased Rigidity in neck, shoulders, hips and knees increased Potential restless legs syndrome
Joints	Cartilage erosion Calcium deposits increased Water in cartilage decreased	Mobility decreased Range of motion limited Osteoarthritis
Nervous		
Structure	Loss of neurons in brain and spinal cord Brain size decreased Dendrites atrophy Major neurotransmitters decreased Size of ventricles increased	Conduction of nerve impulses slowed Peripheral nerve function lost Reaction time decreased Response time slowed Potential for altered balance, vertigo, syncope Postural hypotension increased Proprioception diminished Sensory input decreased EEG alpha waves decreased

Continued

TABLE 39.1 Gerontological differences in assessment: age-related changes and associated clinical manifestations[22]—cont'd

SYSTEM	EXPECTED AGEING CHANGES	CLINICAL MANIFESTATIONS
Sleep	Deep sleep decreased	Difficulty falling asleep
	Rapid eye movement (REM) sleep decreased in old-old adults	Period of wakefulness increased
		Sleep time averages 6 hours
Visual		
Eye structure	Orbital fat lost	Eyes sunken
	Eyebrows and eyelashes grey	Eyes dry
	Elasticity of eyelid muscles decreased	Potential ectropion and entropion
	Tear production decreased	Potential conjunctivitis
		Potential corneal abrasion
Cornea	Corneal sensitivity decreased	
	Corneal reflex decreased	
	Arcus senilis	
Ciliary	Aqueous humour secretion decreased	Ability of lens to accommodate declines
	Ciliary muscle atrophy	Presbyopia
		Peripheral vision decreased
Lens	Less elastic, more dense	Lens yellow and opaque
		Less ability to adapt to light and dark
		Tolerance to glare decreased
		Incidence of cataracts increased
		Night vision impaired
Iris and pupil	Pigment lost	Visual acuity decreased
	Smaller pupil	Pupils appear constricted
	Vitreous gel debris increased	Floaters
Auditory		
Structure	Hairs in external auditory canals of men increased	Potential conductive hearing loss
	Ceruminal glands decreased	Cerumen more dry
Middle ear	Middle ear bone joints degenerate	Sound conduction decreased
	Eardrum thickens	
Inner ear	Vestibular structures decline	Sensitivity to high tones: 's', 't', 'f', 'g' decreased
	Hair cells lost	Understanding of speech decreased
	Cochlea atrophies	Discrimination of background voice decreased
	Organ of Corti atrophies	Equilibrium–balance deficits
		Potential for tinnitus
Immune		
	Secretory immunoglobulin (IgA) declines	Increased potential for infection on mucosal surfaces
	Thymus gland involuted	Impaired cell-mediated immune response
	Lymphoid tissue decreased	Malignancy incidence increased
	Antibody production impaired	Response to acute infection reduced
	Decreased proliferative response of T and B cells	Potential recurrence of latent herpes zoster and tuberculosis
	Autoantibodies increased	Autoimmune disease increased

AV: atrioventricular; BP: blood pressure; CO: cardiac output; EEG: electroencephalogram; HR: heart rate

the hollow of the axilla becoming deeper and the ribs becoming more prominent as intercostal spaces deepen. The ears elongate, a second chin is acquired and wrinkles develop around the eyes.[20] These are changes caused by structural changes of the skin in which the epidermis flattens as a result of the loss of papillae leading to a decrease in adhesion between the layers of the skin, making it prone to peel off with shearing forces.[19]

> **PRACTICE TIP**
>
> Take more care to avoid applying shearing forces to an older person's skin.

The cause of wrinkles remains unexplained, but it is likely to be the result of collagen and elastin degradation.[19] The thickness of the skin also decreases because of the loss of subcutaneous fat, resulting in poorer insulation and an increase in cold-sensitivity.

> **PRACTICE TIP**
>
> Keep older people warmer.
>
> There is an average decrease in height of 5 cm by the age of 80 and this is due to a loss of body fluid, cartilage atrophy, vertebral thinning, increased kyphosis and curvature of hips and knees.

Cardiovascular system

Change in the cardiovascular system occurs as a result of ageing processes in the myocardium and vasculature. The myocardium loses contractility, resulting in decreased cardiac output, particularly when stressed. There are also changes that are dependent on the properties of connective tissue and muscle, thus elasticity and muscle mass reduce, leading to decreased heart weight relative to bodyweight. Mild left ventricular hypertrophy develops as a result of the stiffening of the aorta due to collagen changes. These collagen changes also make the heart less pliable. As a result of these changes, myocardial work reduces and total peripheral resistance increases, resulting in decreased organ perfusion and a diminished ability to increase blood flow in response to an increase in demand; consequently, hypoxia occurs more rapidly. This is compounded by a reduction in maximal heart rate that is directly related to age, so that a 75-year-old would have an approximate maximal heart rate of 162 beats/minute.[19] Tachycardia in the older person is sustained for longer and blood pressure increases to a more marked degree. The vasculature thins and stiffens with ageing, increasing peripheral resistance, which increases systolic pressure, and baroreceptors become less sensitive so that postural hypotension becomes more pronounced.[21,22] As a result, the older person responds more slowly to insults to their cardiovascular system, and treatment aimed at restoring blood pressure and pulse rate may be less effective. Thus it is important that these effects are taken into consideration when assessing the older person. It is not unusual to find that the hypovolaemic older patient does not have the expected tachycardia, so other signs of poor perfusion, such as skin colour, urine output and conscious state, must be considered.

> **PRACTICE TIP**
>
> Hypoxia is more likely and cardiovascular insults are less well tolerated, therefore be more careful when assessing perfusion, paying particular attention to skin colour, urine output and level of consciousness.

In the older person, dysrhythmias and conduction disturbances are more prevalent, harder to diagnose and not tolerated as well.[23] Pharmacological treatment is also more complex. In particular, the prevalence of atrial fibrillation (AF) exceeds 10% for people over the age of 80 years, especially in the presence of hypertension or ischaemic heart disease.[23] Antidysrhythmic drugs are associated with an increased risk of adverse reaction and therefore need to be used with care.[23]

Respiratory system

As cartilage becomes stiffer because of increased calcium deposits, the trachea and rib cage become less flexible. A developing kyphosis increases the anterior–posterior chest diameter. The muscles of inspiration also become weaker. Cumulatively, these effects reduce ventilation. Cough and gag reflexes diminish, complicated by hypertrophy of mucous glands and loss of cilia, leading to an increase in the retention of respiratory secretions. Alveoli reduce in number; the lungs shrink and lose elasticity, resulting in a loss of vital capacity. The combined effects of decreased ventilation, retention of secretions and loss of vital capacity reduce oxygen saturation. Thus it is quite common to have a reduction in the arterial partial pressure of oxygen (PaO_2) in older people; however, it is probably not a linear relationship as some have suggested.[24] With less-effective gas exchange and a decreased ability to clear mucus and debris, there are increased risks for older people and they should be carefully assessed for respiratory compromise; any threat to respiratory function should be carefully monitored as compensatory mechanism will be reduced. Older people will, for these reasons, have increased rates of chest infections. It is important to note that arterial oxygenation does decrease with age, so that the median PaO_2 for a person over the age of 70 will be about 80 mmHg; however, $PaCO_2$ does not change with age,[24] so an abnormal CO_2 level will indicate pathology.

> **PRACTICE TIP**
>
> Respiratory infections are more likely and less well tolerated and $PaCO_2$ is one of the most reliable laboratory indicators of diminished function; clinically—confusion and other signs of hypoxia must be considered.

Gastrointestinal system

Gastric emptying, splenic blood flow and gastrointestinal motility all decrease with age. The lumen of the intestine becomes more alkaline; the wall thins and decreases its absorptive surface, which results in decreased absorption. The overall decrease in subcutaneous fat allows abdominal organs to be more easily palpated. Auscultation of the bowel will not usually reveal a change in bowel sounds despite the reduced motility of the gut.[25]

As people become older the liver becomes more fibrous and smaller. In addition, blood flow to the liver decreases. Older people usually cope well with these changes; however, drug metabolism that depends on liver function will often decrease. Consequently usual drug dosages can result in dose-related side effects, and so smaller doses need to be considered.

Abdominal pain

One of the most difficult ED presenting complaints for older people is abdominal pain. It is a very important symptom, as up to 63% will be admitted and 20% will require urgent surgery to investigate and treat their acute abdomen. The rate of surgery for abdominal pain in the older patient is about double that of younger people and the mortality rate is 10 times higher.[25] Unfortunately, the older person may present to the ED with vague abdominal pain, but have a life-threatening problem. Classic signs of guarding and rebound may be absent, even when the bowel may have perforated. Perforation is more common with appendicitis and cholecystitis because of the decreased blood flow and a thinner gut wall. For these reasons it is important that the older patient is more carefully assessed and extra laboratory and radiographic tests are usually indicated.[25] Abdominal assessment is discussed in Chapters 24 and 25.

> **PRACTICE TIP**
>
> Carefully assess abdominal pain as it is more likely to be associated with serious pathology.

Renal system

As people age there is a decrease in the number and size of nephrons, resulting in a 20% decrease in the size of the kidney by the age of 80. Total renal blood flow also diminishes. This loss of nephrons and decrease in blood flow results in a decrease in the glomerular filtration rate (GFR). A decrease in GFR increases the chance of adverse drug reactions and drug-induced renal failure. The older person is also more susceptible to renal damage caused by episodes of hypotension.[24] Diminished tubular function of the nephron predisposes the older person to metabolic acidosis, loss of fluid and increased serum chloride levels. This decreased ability to maintain water homeostasis predisposes older people to dehydration, but it can also mean that they are less able to excrete excessive water, so they are also less able to excrete metabolic waste products of creatinine, urea and nitrogen.[25] The implications of this for all paramedics and emergency staff are that fluid overload is a real risk and fluid resuscitation must be titrated to central venous pressure and urine output. In addition, it is important to commence fluid balance charts and monitor vital signs, keeping in mind the potential for fluid overload.

> **PRACTICE TIP**
>
> - Take care with renally cleared medications, as they are more likely to produce adverse effects.
> - Dehydration and metabolic acidosis is more likely.
> - There is an increased risk of fluid overload.

Endocrine system

Fibrotic changes to the thyroid gland lead to decreased thyroid hormone release, resulting in a reduced metabolic rate. The adrenal glands secrete less as a result of diminished adreno-corticotrophic hormone release from the pituitary. Insulin secretion also falls and this is exacerbated by a decreased sensitivity to insulin. This leads to impaired glucose metabolism with hyperglycaemia in the non-diabetic person.[21]

The senses

Decreasing sensory function can affect the older person's ability to remain safe. Visual loss with presbyopia is very common. This is an inability to focus on near objects, which is a result of reduced lens elasticity. Peripheral vision is also diminished concurrently, with less-light-responsive pupils making vision in dim light more difficult. The lens also becomes more opaque as cataracts form: this is more likely in individuals who have been exposed to more ultraviolet light.[21]

Inner-ear changes result in hearing loss in which high-frequency sound is lost first. This can be exacerbated by the accumulation of cerumen that becomes harder with age.[21] The sense of smell and taste can also diminish with age.[21] The ability to sense pressure, pain, cold and heat become reduced with ageing.[21] The older person's decreased ability to detect damage as a result of pressure or temperature increases the need for vigilance to ensure that damage as a result of prolonged pressure is prevented by frequent turning. This is usually achieved by turning older patients every 2 hours if they are immobile, and using specialised mattresses. Care also needs to be taken to prevent exposure to excessive cold or heat. See Chapter 14.

> **PRACTICE TIP**
>
> When talking to an older person speak clearly, facing them, and make sure that hearing aids are in place and working. Also ensure that any glasses are worn.

Nervous system

There is a decline in cognitive functioning after the age of 20 years, which is usually evident in the performance of timed tests; however, intelligence is stable until the ninth decade. Any significant deterioration in cognitive abilities is not part of normal ageing. Acute causes of cognitive loss include electrolyte disturbance, infection or medications. The most common chronic aetiologies for cognitive loss in older people include multi-infarct dementia and Alzheimer's disease.[25]

The size of the brain decreases after the age of 25 by about 20% over the next 70 years. This may be partly due to a loss of neurons and atrophy of the cortex. Neurotransmitter function is also affected by changes in receptors and the ability to produce neurotransmitters.[25] Blood flow to the brain also decreases, and this is related to the reduced metabolic demands of the brain. The blood–brain barrier in the older person becomes less effective, increasing the chance of meningitis and exaggerating responses to medications that cross this barrier.[26] Consequently, narcotic analgesia is more likely to produce respiratory depression as a result of its central nervous system (CNS) effects. For this reason narcotics need to be given in smaller aliquots. However, it also means that analgesia can be produced with smaller doses.[26]

The nervous system is also less able to effectively respond to changes in external temperature, predisposing the older person to hypothermia and hyperthermia.

Neurotransmitters of the CNS are also altered, resulting in slowed mental functioning.[26] It is therefore important that when assessing the older person in the ED they should have a mental status examination, and assessment of functional status.

PRACTICE TIP

- Give narcotic analgesia in small doses.
- Routinely perform a mental status examination.

Musculoskeletal system

The atrophy of tissue as people age extends to muscle and bone. Muscle fibres decrease in number, being replaced by fibrous tissue. This atrophy of muscle results in decreased muscle strength and movement. The rate of atrophy appears to be activity related, so that more-sedentary individuals will lose muscle tone and function more quickly. Tendons also shrink and harden. Bone mass decreases, resulting in more brittle bones, particularly in women. Calcium absorption from the gut decreases, the interior surfaces of long bones are reabsorbed and new production of bone slows. These changes greatly increase the risk of fractures and when a fracture occurs it will heal more slowly.[21]

PRACTICE TIP

Carefully assess for fractures, as they are much more likely to occur, even for usually innocuous mechanisms of injury such as a fall from a height below 1 metre.

Functional assessment

'Elderly patients may view their health in terms of how well they can function rather than in terms of disease alone'.[12] The presence of disease may therefore be less important than the loss of function that results. Many authors agree that functional assessment of older people in the ED should be mandatory.[11,12,27–32] It is important to assess an older person's ability to perform the usual tasks of independent living: this is what constitutes a functional assessment. It is important because these abilities will often change with age, and a visit to the ED may be the first indication that there is a developing functional deficit at home. In a screen of older ED patients, it was found that:

- 79% had activities of daily living (ADL) or instrumental activities of daily living (IADL) deficits
- the ED may play a key role in assessing older persons
- 49% had hazards in their home environment.[29]

Functional assessment includes an appraisal of independence with fundamental ADL, social activities or IADL. It should also include an evaluation of how much assistance is needed to accomplish these tasks of daily living with measurements

BOX 39.2 ADL and IADL scales[33,34]

The activities of daily living (ADL) scale assesses:
- bathing
- dressing
- toileting
- transfer
- continence
- feeding.

The instrumental activities of daily living (IADL) scale assesses:
- telephone use
- walking
- shopping
- preparing meals
- housework
- handiwork
- laundry
- taking medicines
- managing finances.

of sensory ability, cognition and ambulatory competence (Box 39.2).[12]

Functional assessment may indicate some loss of cognitive function; however, this also needs to be assessed. Saunders suggests that where functional decline is noted or is the reason for ED attendance, an algorithm should be used to guide admission or discharge (see Fig 39.1).[31]

The functional assessment will occur after a primary and secondary survey has been completed.

Confusion, dementia and Alzheimer's disease in the emergency health setting

As Australasia's population ages, it is recognised that an increasing number of confused older people, and older people who are at risk of becoming confused, present to EDs. EDs are excessively stimulating and disorientating for older unwell patients and it is difficult to achieve a normal sleep/wake cycle in this environment. These factors contribute to the challenges of providing high-quality nursing care to this group of patients.[36]

Impaired cognition occurs in up to 40% of all people over the age of 70 who present for emergency care.[37,38] In assessing and managing the older patient with impaired cognition it is important to distinguish between delirium and dementia. Delirium is an acute state of confusion, whereas dementia is a permanent loss of memory and intellectual ability.[39] The mental status exam enables detection of cognitive impairment and also some differentiation between delirium and dementia. It is evident that delirium is frequently not detected in over 70% of cases[40] and should therefore be screened for. Figure 39.2 summarises the assessment process and basic principles for nurses caring for older patients who are confused.

Mental status exam

The mental status exam is an important component of assessment of the older patient. Investigations into its use revealed

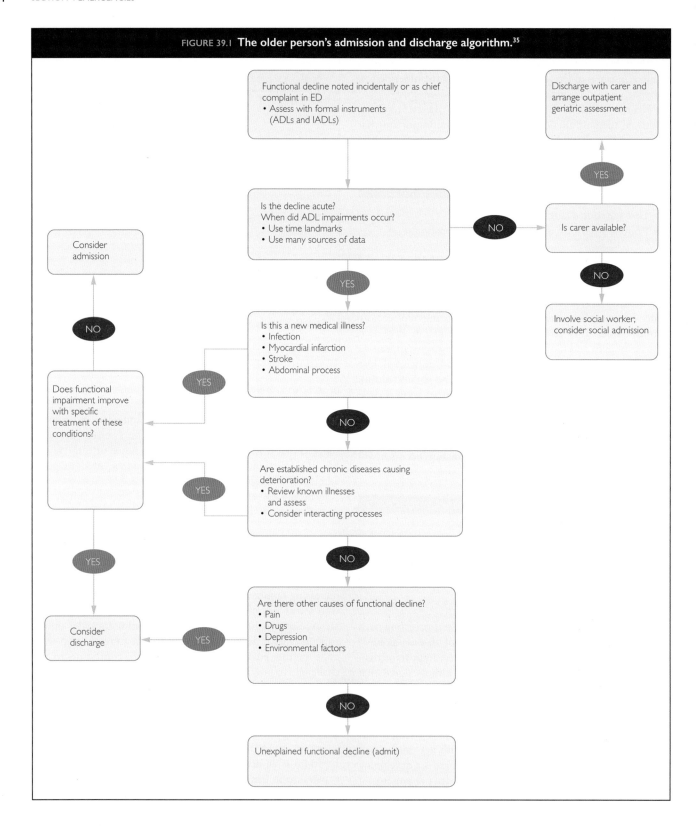

FIGURE 39.1 The older person's admission and discharge algorithm.[35]

a high incidence of impairment in older patients and the fact that delirium and dementia are often missed in the ED.[28] In a screen of 385 patients 65 years or older, 10% of patients met the criteria for delirium and 38% of patients with delirium were discharged from the ED, with an unexplained fall as the most common diagnosis.[41] In a cognitive screen of patients over 65 who had no known history of dementia, 34% had moderate or

severe impairments that had not been previously diagnosed.[27] It is therefore important to assess cognitive ability.

PRACTICE TIP

Routinely assess cognitive function.

FIGURE 39.2 Assessment and management of older patients with confusion.[36]

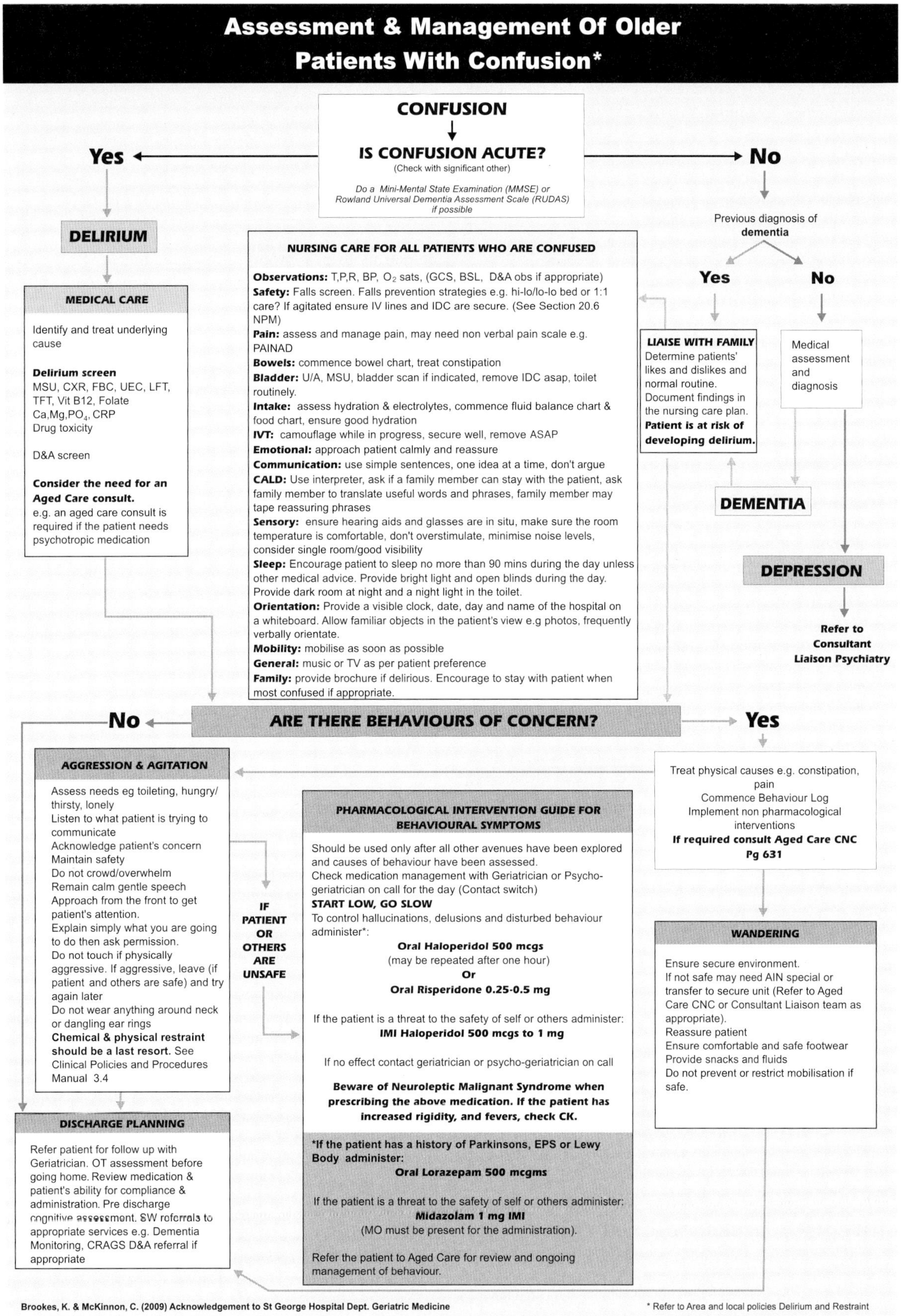

Assessment & Management Of Older Patients With Confusion*

CONFUSION
↓
IS CONFUSION ACUTE?
(Check with significant other)

Do a Mini-Mental State Examination (MMSE) or Rowland Universal Dementia Assessment Scale (RUDAS) if possible

Yes ← → **No**

DELIRIUM

MEDICAL CARE

Identify and treat underlying cause

Delirium screen
MSU, CXR, FBC, UEC, LFT, TFT, Vit B12, Folate Ca,Mg,PO₄, CRP
Drug toxicity

D&A screen

Consider the need for an Aged Care consult.
e.g. an aged care consult is required if the patient needs psychotropic medication

NURSING CARE FOR ALL PATIENTS WHO ARE CONFUSED

Observations: T,P,R, BP, O₂ sats, (GCS, BSL, D&A obs if appropriate)
Safety: Falls screen. Falls prevention strategies e.g. hi-lo/lo-lo bed or 1:1 care? If agitated ensure IV lines and IDC are secure. (See Section 20.6 NPM)
Pain: assess and manage pain, may need non verbal pain scale e.g. PAINAD
Bowels: commence bowel chart, treat constipation
Bladder: U/A, MSU, bladder scan if indicated, remove IDC asap, toilet routinely.
Intake: assess hydration & electrolytes, commence fluid balance chart & food chart, ensure good hydration
IVT: camouflage while in progress, secure well, remove ASAP
Emotional: approach patient calmly and reassure
Communication: use simple sentences, one idea at a time, don't argue
CALD: Use interpreter, ask if a family member can stay with the patient, ask family member to translate useful words and phrases, family member may tape reassuring phrases
Sensory: ensure hearing aids and glasses are in situ, make sure the room temperature is comfortable, don't overstimulate, minimise noise levels, consider single room/good visibility
Sleep: Encourage patient to sleep no more than 90 mins during the day unless other medical advice. Provide bright light and open blinds during the day. Provide dark room at night and a night light in the toilet.
Orientation: Provide a visible clock, date, day and name of the hospital on a whiteboard. Allow familiar objects in the patient's view e.g photos, frequently verbally orientate.
Mobility: mobilise as soon as possible
General: music or TV as per patient preference
Family: provide brochure if delirious. Encourage to stay with patient when most confused if appropriate.

Previous diagnosis of dementia

Yes   **No**

LIAISE WITH FAMILY
Determine patients' likes and dislikes and normal routine. Document findings in the nursing care plan. **Patient is at risk of developing delirium.**

Medical assessment and diagnosis

DEMENTIA

DEPRESSION

Refer to Consultant Liaison Psychiatry

No ← **ARE THERE BEHAVIOURS OF CONCERN?** → **Yes**

AGGRESSION & AGITATION

Assess needs eg toileting, hungry/thirsty, lonely
Listen to what patient is trying to communicate
Acknowledge patient's concern
Maintain safety
Do not crowd/overwhelm
Remain calm gentle speech
Approach from the front to get patient's attention.
Explain simply what you are going to do then ask permission.
Do not touch if physically aggressive. If aggressive, leave (if patient and others are safe) and try again later
Do not wear anything around neck or dangling ear rings
Chemical & physical restraint should be a last resort. See Clinical Policies and Procedures Manual 3.4

IF PATIENT OR OTHERS ARE UNSAFE

Treat physical causes e.g. constipation, pain
Commence Behaviour Log
Implement non pharmacological interventions
If required consult Aged Care CNC Pg 631

PHARMACOLOGICAL INTERVENTION GUIDE FOR BEHAVIOURAL SYMPTOMS

Should be used only after all other avenues have been explored and causes of behaviour have been assessed.
Check medication management with Geriatrician or Psycho-geriatrician on call for the day (Contact switch)
START LOW, GO SLOW
To control hallucinations, delusions and disturbed behaviour administer*:

Oral Haloperidol 500 mcgs
(may be repeated after one hour)
Or
Oral Risperidone 0.25-0.5 mg

If the patient is a threat to the safety of self or others administer:
IMI Haloperidol 500 mcgs to 1 mg

If no effect contact geriatrician or psycho-geriatrician on call

Beware of Neuroleptic Malignant Syndrome when prescribing the above medication. If the patient has increased rigidity, and fevers, check CK.

*If the patient has a history of Parkinsons, EPS or Lewy Body administer:
Oral Lorazepam 500 mcgms

If the patient is a threat to the safety of self or others administer:
Midazolam 1 mg IMI
(MO must be present for the administration).

Refer the patient to Aged Care for review and ongoing management of behaviour.

WANDERING

Ensure secure environment.
If not safe may need AIN special or transfer to secure unit (Refer to Aged Care CNC or Consultant Liaison team as appropriate).
Reassure patient
Ensure comfortable and safe footwear
Provide snacks and fluids
Do not prevent or restrict mobilisation if safe.

DISCHARGE PLANNING

Refer patient for follow up with Geriatrician. OT assessment before going home. Review medication & patient's ability for compliance & administration. Pre discharge cognitive assessment. SW referrals to appropriate services e.g. Dementia Monitoring, CRAGS D&A referral if appropriate

Brookes, K. & McKinnon, C. (2009) Acknowledgement to St George Hospital Dept. Geriatric Medicine

* Refer to Area and local policies Delirium and Restraint

Performing a mental status exam is not only important to detect the presence of altered cognition, but it also helps to establish the reliability of a person's history of their presenting complaint. Changes in the mental status exam can also be a symptom of a medical emergency that may have a reversible cause. Performing this exam early also allows for more effective discharge planning. Many clinicians advocate the use of the Mini-Mental State Examination (MMSE), developed by Marshall and Folstein in 1975, and the six-item Cognitive Impairment Test.[42]

Treatment of delirium

Identifying and treating the cause is the usual method for managing delirium; for example, hypoxia treated with oxygen is effective. However, a few patients will need their symptoms managed.[38] Physical restraints should be avoided as this increases agitation and is likely to worsen the delirium. Effective management may involve simple interventions such as ensuring patients have their glasses and hearing aids, having familiar people beside them and turning off the lights to aid sleep.[42] If drug therapy is to be used, haloperidol in smaller doses (0.5–1.0 mg) is the agent of choice and benzodiazepines should be avoided.[42]

Pain management

Untreated pain in older adults is associated with poorer outcomes; in particular, it is evident that the pain associated with a fractured hip will increase length of stay and increase the risk of delirium by 900%.[43,44] Despite this, pain care is often inadequate in EDs, so that there are minimal decreases in pain intensity scores.[45] For older ED patients, the situation is worse as they have the greatest possibility of not receiving adequate analgesia;[46] and for those with hip fractures, 28.6% receive no analgesia.[47]

PRACTICE TIP

- It is essential that paramedics and emergency nurses formally assess all older people for the presence of pain.
- Pain assessment should be repeated frequently to document efficacy of analgesia and trends in the patient's condition.[48]

If pain is detected it must be documented, treated and reassessed.[48] Treatment must occur if the person reports their pain as being moderate or worse. Prior to transfer, paramedics need to consider the administration of methoxyflurane or intranasal fentanyl with the dose adjusted for age above 60 years.[49] If an opioid is required pethidine should not be used, as it is associated with a higher risk of delirium and norpethidine toxicity.[50] Paramedics are guided to use intravenous morphine.[49] When an opioid has been administered, then prophylactic treatment of constipation needs to be implemented.[51]

Skin integrity, pressure-area care

As people age all layers of the skin atrophy, subcutaneous fat diminishes and papillae that give skin its texture flatten out. These papillae normally help to adhere the layers of skin together: the loss of skin texture and papillae allow the

---

BOX 39.3 Assessment of skin tears[52]

- Volume of blood loss
- Foreign bodies
- Cleanliness of the wound
- Signs of infection
- Tetanus status
- Presence of skin tags to be removed with sterile scissors
- Approximation of wound edges for closure
- Suitability for use of clear film dressing

---

epidermis to peel away more easily, increasing the likelihood of skin tears. Blood vessels under the skin become more fragile and are easily damaged, leading to bruising. It is therefore important to carefully assess the skin of the older person in the ED to look for damage and to assess for risk of damage in the ED. Skin damage in the ED tends to be acutely traumatic as a result of invasive procedures, movement around the bed, poor lifting technique and hard cot sides; or chronic with the development of pressure ulcers. Pressure-area care is discussed in Chapter 14.

Skin tears

Skin tears can be divided into two categories:

- those that are caused by a clean laceration resulting in a gaping wound without bruising
- those that are caused by abrasions that result in irregular superficial wounds which are painful and prone to infection.

Refer to Box 39.3 for assessment of skin tears.

Inexperienced practitioners should not attempt to treat skin tears, and plastic surgery consultation should be sought before attempting to close with sutures or adhesive tape or with clear film dressings. While awaiting advice, cover with a sterile moist dressing to prevent drying, but also avoid maceration by the excessive use of water (see Ch 18).

PRACTICE TIP

Only experts in wound care should treat skin tears.

Pressure ulcers

Unfortunately, older people can be left to lie on hard foam mattresses or ambulance stretchers for long periods of time, predisposing them to pressure ulcers. In addition, patients who have required extrication, for example, from a motor vehicle crash, are often transported on hard plastic or timber backboards, which further contributes to prolonged pressure. It is recommended that backboards be removed from trauma patients as soon as possible during initial patient assessment (see Ch 44). In an older person with reduced mobility, poor skin, inadequate nutrition, dehydration and incontinence, periods of 1 hour or more in one position on wet sheets can lead to the development of a pressure ulcer, which may not be noticed for another 24 hours. It is therefore essential to assess for pressure ulcer susceptibility and provide pressure area care by turning

- Sensory perception
- Mobility
- Moisture
- Nutrition
- Activity
- Friction and shear

This scale uses six categories. There is a maximum possible score of 23, indicating little or no risk; a score < 17 indicates that the person is at risk of developing a pressure ulcer and needs to be routinely turned to relieve the pressure on the skin and underlying tissues. For example, a person who is unresponsive (sensory perception = 1), constantly moist (by perspiration or urine) (moisture = 1), confined to bed (activity = 1), immobile (mobility = 1), has less than 2 servings of protein a day (nutrition = 1) and requires assistance in moving (friction and shear = 1) will have a Braden score of 6. There are many emergency patients who would score similarly.

the patient every 2 hours and, where available, using specialised air mattresses. This needs to be a routine component of the care of all older patients. The Braden Scale (Box 39.4) is routinely used to assess for the risk of pressure ulcer development.

Older people and trauma

Increased incidence of trauma

Diminished vision, hearing and touch expose older people to increased risk of injury. Loss of peripheral vision, decreased hearing and slowed reaction times increase the risk of older pedestrians being struck by vehicles; poorer vision in dim light predisposes older people to falls in their home; decreased touch increases the chance of burns. These changes of ageing contribute to the increase in the rate of trauma in older people. The rate of hospital separations increases exponentially,

becoming extremely high in the 85+ age group (Fig 39.3).[53] This increased rate of injury and hospitalisation will translate to even more presentations as the proportion of older people in the population increases.

Falls

Falls are the main cause for injury-related hospital separations (admissions or episodes of care) in people over 65 years of age.[53]

Falls in older people are not necessarily a direct consequence of the ageing process and it is important that the cause of the fall be investigated. Predisposing conditions such as cardiac-induced loss of consciousness must be accounted for. The reason for the fall is likely to be complex, despite a simple explanation. It is unlikely to be accidental and without a precipitating factor.[54] Common contributing factors include gait disturbance, syncope, CNS lesions, postural hypotension and dizziness.[55]

The National Injury Prevention Plan identified four priority injury aetiologies that require attention from Australian health authorities: falls in older people (65+ years) were listed as the primary concern.[56] 'In 2010 the estimated number of hospitalised injury cases due to falls in people aged 65 years and over was 83,800; an increase of over 20,000 in the last 10 years'.[57]

In New Zealand, falls 'are the leading cause of injury hospitalisation and one of the top three causes of injury-related deaths. Between 1993 and 2002, more than 160,000 people were hospitalised for fall-related injuries, accounting for 43 per cent of all unintentional injury-related hospital admissions'. Falls in New Zealand account 'for 21 per cent of unintentional injury-related fatalities'.[58] Falls in older people are therefore a critical public health concern and a major issue for first-responders, paramedics and ED staff.

- 'Mortality after a hip fracture remains significant, being 11–23% at 6 months and 22–29% at 1 year from injury.'[59]
- 20–30% of older people who fall suffer moderate to severe injuries.[60]

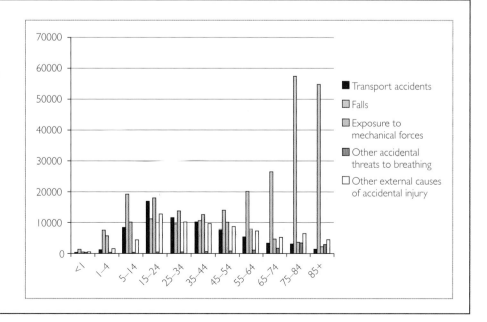

FIGURE 39.3

Separations (admissions or episodes of care) by external cause in ICD-10-AM groupings and age group, all hospitals, Australia, 2007–2008.[53]

- Falls are a major cause of traumatic brain injury in older people.[61]
- Approximately 3–5% of falls cause fractures.[62]
- The most common injury sustained from a fall is an isolated fracture.[55]

It is therefore important to assess for significant injury in all older patients who present with a fall. On assessment, the most common injury associated with a fall was fractures to the hip and femur.[63] This injury has a significant mortality of 11–23% at 6 months post fall and as high as 29% a year after the injury.[59]

It is important that if no injury is found that requires hospitalisation following a fall, the older person should be referred to a multidisciplinary team that is able to provide suitable interventions in the home environment. Emergency medical services are beginning to develop and implement health screening programs[64] and falls assessment and referral programs for those patients who may not require immediate hospitalisation.[65] Where admission occurs, discharge planning must begin early with appropriate referral, as it is important to prevent future injuries from falls. Injury prevention activities are listed in Box 39.5.[66]

PRACTICE TIP

Assess for injury in all older people who have fallen over.

Complications and morbidity

Trauma in older people has been documented to result in significant morbidity such that only 8% of survivors returned to independent living 1 year post polytrauma; although another longer-term study found that 89% of survivors of blunt multiple trauma were independent and living at home after 3 years.[67] It is evident that mortality in older patients correlates with their injury severity and is influenced by blood and fluid requirements and by Glasgow Coma Scale (GCS) score.[68] Therefore, resuscitation needs to be individualised and account for pre-existing pathology.[65]

Resuscitation

The process of resuscitation in the older patient is conducted in the usual manner of prioritising care of the airway, breathing and circulation. However, the older person is more vulnerable and less adaptable to homeostatic changes, partly because of reduced reserves. These changes can be difficult to predict, as they are a result of loss of function that is variable among older persons. It is vitally important that rapid, aggressive resuscitation is commenced in the unstable older trauma patient and that careful informed and expedient assessment of the apparently stable patient occurs.[65]

Hypertension in the older person is common and this may mask hypovolaemia, which can be compounded by the slower resting heart rate that occurs with ageing or from the use of negative chronotropes such as beta-blockers used to treat hypertension. The presence of these common changes leads to a widespread belief that older patients have significantly impaired cardiac function and therefore need less fluid resuscitation: this results in untreated hypovolaemia. However, disregard of reduced cardiac function will lead to fluid overload. It is

BOX 39.5 Injury prevention activities for the older person

- Remove or tack down all scatter rugs.
- Check staircases for stability; install handrails whenever possible.
- Apply non-slip strips to stairways.
- Carpet areas that are prone to spills or slipperiness.
- Reduce clutter and open clear pathways through all rooms.
- Pad wooden or metal furniture edges.
- Install bright lights in hallways and entrances.
- Place non-slip mats in the bathtub and shower.
- Install grab bars near all bathrooms.
- Install smoke detectors, and check them at regular intervals.
- Obtain assistance with cooking, as needed. Extra care is required when using gas stoves.
- Use assistive cooking devices, such as burner shields, long-handled utensils and protective hand gear.
- Do not wear loose-fitting garments while cooking.
- Use rear stove burners rather than front ones, and avoid storing goods you may need over the stove.
- Check central furnaces and space heaters frequently to ensure proper functioning.
- Reduce thermostat settings on water heaters and clearly label all hot water taps.
- Annually review the directions for operating major appliances.
- Wear short-sleeved, non-synthetic shirts and pyjamas.
- Do not smoke, especially while resting.
- Keep easy-to-operate fire extinguishers readily accessible.
- Use hot water bottles and heating pads only at low temperatures.
- Know how to access emergency help.
- Eliminate night driving if patient is affected by night blindness.
- Wear seat belts.
- Drive only in familiar locations, avoiding highly congested areas and roadways under construction.
- Contact your vehicle licensing agency to inquire about an 'over 75 refresher course'.

therefore important that all older patients be carefully assessed and continually monitored for adequate fluid replacement and overload. There is evidence that although poorly perfused, older patients may appear haemodynamically stable, and invasive haemodynamic monitoring should be considered earlier than is usual for younger patients.[68]

PRACTICE TIP

Very carefully assess and monitor fluid replacement.

Infection

There are many factors that lead to infection in the older person but, combined with a diminished immune function, the risk of infection is very high.[69] Consequently, older patients are more likely to die because of bacteraemia and sepsis.[68] Older people with respiratory tract, abdominal, CNS and multiple infections are at highest risk. Alternatively, patients with urinary tract infections have the lowest sepsis mortality risk.[69] The reasons that age contributes to an increase in susceptibility to infection are summarised in Box 39.6.

In addition to the increased susceptibility and mortality from infection, older people may present atypically so that the expected signs of infection are absent. These patients may present with weakness, fatigue and functional decline, perhaps combined with anorexia. These are not specific, making infection recognition difficult. Fever may be present in isolation or the older person with an infection may present with hypothermia. It is therefore important to suspect infection in the older person who presents with non-specific signs.

Polypharmacy

Polypharmacy is the use of several drugs together in the treatment of disease, suggesting arbitrary, unempirical prescriptions or superfluous medications for one person. The definition also includes the prescribing of more medications than is clinically indicated, or at excessive dosages, or prescribed at too frequent intervals.[70] However, it may be appropriate to prescribe and administer multiple medications for older people who are more likely to have chronic conditions that require a range of medications. In Australia, up to 22% of all emergency presentations in older people are related to medication use.[70] This is related to the complexity of drug use, as 21% of people 65 years and over were taking four or more different medications (see Fig 39.4).[71] The incidence of multiple medications is very similar in New Zealand.[72]

Underlying medical problems, changing pharmacokinetics of ageing and treating side effects with more medications exacerbate the problems of polypharmacy.[25] It is therefore important to assess for the presence of polypharmacy as a cause of or contributing factor in emergency presentations. Medications that are more likely to cause problems in the older patient include narcotics, sedative-hypnotics, antidepressants, diuretics, non-steroidal anti-inflammatory drugs (NSAIDs) and angiotensin-converting enzyme (ACE) inhibitors.[25] Narcotics and sedative hypnotics alter consciousness, increase the risk of falls and depress respiration. Electrolyte imbalances and dehydration may result from diuretics. Uraemia, hypertension, cardiac failure and sodium retention can all result from NSAID use as well as the generally expected problem of gastrointestinal bleeding.[25]

Polypharmacy implications will extend beyond contributing to an emergency presentation; it may also complicate analgesia administration, as narcotics, sedative-hypnotics and NSAIDs are common and effective medications for controlling pain in the emergency health setting. When administering these agents, particularly narcotics, consider the effects by providing

---

BOX 39.6 **Age-related infection risks**[39]
• Decreased pulmonary function and cough reflex
• Decreased gastric acidity and gastrointestinal motility
• Invasive devices (urinary catheters, nasogastric tubes)
• Thin, easily traumatised skin
• Decreased activity secondary to motor problems
• Atherosclerosis and decreased capillary blood flow
• Inadequate nutrition and hydration
• Lack of immunisation
• Neuropsychological diseases
• Chronic use of medications
• Chronic diseases (diabetes, cardiac disease, renal disease, alcoholism)
• Previous exposures to hazardous materials (asbestos, chemicals, dusts)
• Impaired host defence mechanisms
• Hospitalisation or long-term care facilities

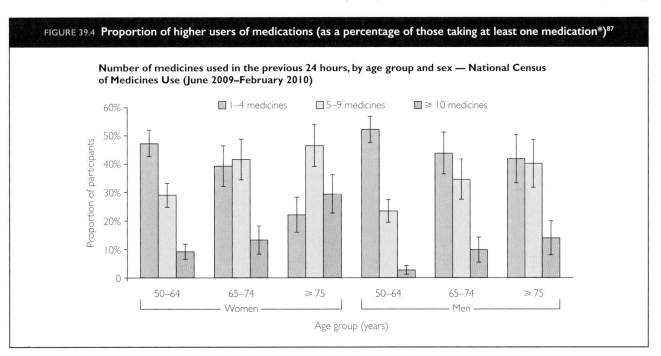

FIGURE 39.4 **Proportion of higher users of medications (as a percentage of those taking at least one medication*)**[87]

low doses slowly titrated. However, this is not a reason to withhold adequate analgesia, which can also be supplemented by the use of paracetamol and has a high safety profile in older people.[25] Figure 39.5 demonstrates the effects of ageing upon drug metabolism and Box 39.7 describes common causes of medication errors made by older people.

Toilet care, feeding, privacy

The restriction in mobility, increased likelihood of incontinence and risk of skin damage make toilet care an important component of older patient care. Both older men and older women are more prone to urinary incontinence. Thirty per cent of older people at home have been found to have urinary incontinence, and this rises to 50% for people in nursing homes.[75,76] Urinary incontinence in men increases with age, but women are twice as likely to suffer from incontinence. Eliopoulos[20] recommends that the person with incontinence should be checked 2-hourly for wetness and, when present, all clothing and linen affected should be changed, then the skin should be cleansed and dried. Failure to do this will result in skin breakdown and a continual odour of urine, which is embarrassing for the patient.

Increased lengths of stay in the ED have meant that it is now more important to consider the nutritional needs of all ED patients. For older people the problems are compounded by an increased incidence of chronic poor nutritional intake. Malnutrition or risk of malnourishment exists in 80% of older people who present to Australian hospitals.[77] For many older

---

BOX 39.7 Common causes of medication errors by older adults[74]

- Poor eyesight
- Forgetting to take medications
- Use of non-prescription over-the-counter drugs
- Use of medications prescribed for someone else
- Use of medications that are out of date (expired)
- Failure to understand instructions or the importance of drug treatment
- Refusal to take medication because of undesirable side effects, such as nausea and impotence
- Doubling-up of generic equivalents

FIGURE 39.5 Effects of ageing on drug metabolism.[74]

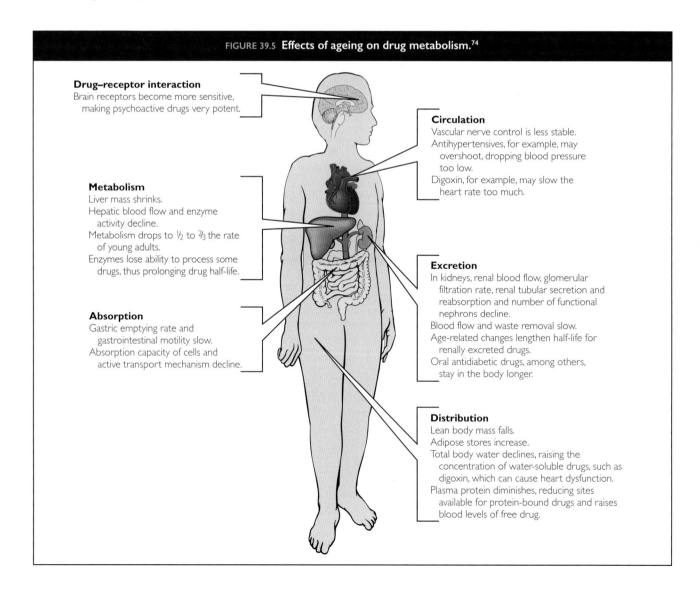

Drug–receptor interaction
Brain receptors become more sensitive, making psychoactive drugs very potent.

Metabolism
Liver mass shrinks.
Hepatic blood flow and enzyme activity decline.
Metabolism drops to ½ to ⅔ the rate of young adults.
Enzymes lose ability to process some drugs, thus prolonging drug half-life.

Absorption
Gastric emptying rate and gastrointestinal motility slow.
Absorption capacity of cells and active transport mechanism decline.

Circulation
Vascular nerve control is less stable.
Antihypertensives, for example, may overshoot, dropping blood pressure too low.
Digoxin, for example, may slow the heart rate too much.

Excretion
In kidneys, renal blood flow, glomerular filtration rate, renal tubular secretion and reabsorption and number of functional nephrons decline.
Blood flow and waste removal slow.
Age-related changes lengthen half-life for renally excreted drugs.
Oral antidiabetic drugs, among others, stay in the body longer.

Distribution
Lean body mass falls.
Adipose stores increase.
Total body water declines, raising the concentration of water-soluble drugs, such as digoxin, which can cause heart dysfunction.
Plasma protein diminishes, reducing sites available for protein-bound drugs and raises blood levels of free drug.

people, food may become less appetising and small, frequent amounts of high-calorie, high-protein foods should be offered to them. Since mobility is often restricted because of arthritis or other problems, food should be delivered in a manner that allows older people to consume it without difficulty. Assistance may often be required to remove lids and wrapping, food should be within reach and vision deficits need to be accommodated for by indicating where the food is. While incontinence may be embarrassing for the patient and increase the work of the nurse or paramedic, this is not a reason to withhold fluids; drinks should be readily available. The carbohydrate and sugar content of food and drinks should be considered for older patients who have diabetes. Many older patients who present with a problem that is likely to require surgery are fasted, exacerbating already existing poor nutrition. The withholding of food and fluids in these circumstances should be carefully considered. For example, a person with a fractured wrist may not need to be fasted as the treating procedure may be performed under a regional block, not a general anaesthetic, or the procedure delayed until the following day.

The ED is an impersonal crowded space; it is not uncommon for patients to be cared for in the aisles. This is not an appropriate way to care for people and threats to privacy will frequently occur in such an environment. For older people these issues are compounded by hearing loss causing emergency staff to raise their voices. Any discussion of a personal nature should occur in areas where privacy is ensured; in Australia this is mandated by federal legislation in the Privacy Act.[78] Toileting of people in aisles is never appropriate. In a busy ED, one strategy to overcome these issues of privacy is always to keep a cubicle free even when there are people in the aisles. This cubicle can be used when privacy is required.

Communication

When people present with a health emergency, their care is expedited when they are able to describe their presenting complaint and the history of this complaint. For a patient without the ability to do this, healthcare professionals rely more heavily on physical examination and information from anyone accompanying the person. For many older people the ageing process affects communication by causing hearing loss, and speech can also be impaired by conditions that increasingly occur with ageing. Many older people are non-English-speaking, which will also affect communication. However, it must never be assumed that the older patient cannot communicate and every attempt should be made to understand their concerns. Discomfort can be assessed from body position and facial expressions. The partner or spouse, if present, is likely to understand their requirements and should be included in attempts to communicate.

> **PRACTICE TIP**
>
> Always include the older person in all interactions.

End-of-life care

A large number of elderly patients at end of life die in the ED or before being transported to an ED and many of them

are admitted to hospital knowing that they are dying and that modern interventional medicine has little to offer.[85] For paramedic and ED staff managing the patient who is reaching the end of life is complex and at times difficult. Decisions and conversations with relatives and carers of patients about resuscitation status, advance care plans and patient wishes should be handled in a sensitive, compassionate and professional manner.[86] If the older patient is aware, conversations should occur with them and with their family. An important discussion will be around the older person's right to refuse active treatment of their disease or injury and instead concentrate on palliative goals of comfort care. For the most part, a decision should be clinical, but a delicately handled conversation can relieve anxiety and avoid misunderstandings or unrealistic expectations further along the clinical path. It is imperative to ensure medical staff make a clear decision and communicate it to all treating clinicians as well as document it clearly in the notes. Limitations must be clearly spelt out and consistent with information that has been communicated.[86]

In order to most effectively manage spiritual, social, psychological and physical concerns a multidisciplinary team approach should be used. As part of this approach it is also important to perform a comprehensive assessment of symptoms that the person is experiencing. As the palliative patient begins to deteriorate their regular medications may not need to be administered. The important medications to remember charting before the patient leaves the ED are for pain, anxiety/sedation, increased secretions and nausea/vomiting.[86] Pain and dyspnoea are two very frequent symptoms that can often respond well to medication.[79] Additional guidelines are available from the Australian and New Zealand Society for Geriatric Medicine and the NSW Emergency Care Institute (see also Ch 53).

Care of the partner/spouse

The partner or spouse of an older person may have been their partner for decades and should be included in any decisions about their care. It is also likely that the older patient may be the carer for another person in their home, and this needs to be investigated further before discharge. If the older patient is very ill, the frail partner at home needs to be included in care decisions, notified of what has occurred and, where possible, brought to the ED. Sadly, it is not uncommon for an older person to die in the ED and at these times partners must be involved in decisions about care and resuscitation. The presence of partners during resuscitation needs to be considered, and while there continues to be debate about this issue, health organisations need to develop policy and strategies to include partners in all resuscitation efforts. At other times people may be brought to the ED from nursing homes, places separate from their spouse, and in these circumstances it is important to ensure that the older person's partner is aware of their presence in the ED.

Discharge from the ED and transitional care

One of the most difficult aspects of emergency care of older people is their discharge from the ED. The culture of the ED is usually one in which discharge as soon as possible is an objective of care, in order to prevent overcrowding. This is a situation not conducive to careful discharge and emergency staff need to be aware that a hasty, unplanned discharge can have dire consequences and will result in return ED visits.[79] For the older person it is very important that, prior to any attempts at discharge, a functional assessment has been completed to determine suitability of out-of-hospital living arrangements. Often where there is a mild cognitive impairment it has never been previously recognised,[28] thus cognitive and functional assessments become essential before discharge in order to prevent marginal coping abilities becoming a failure to cope at home.

Establishing a functional and socioeconomic profile enables a strategy for better management of the patients discharged by the ED.[28] This should be a nursing and paramedic responsibility. Ambulance staff can provide vital information about living arrangements of older people and the medications they are prescribed. This is achieved by taking careful note of the premises and by bringing in the prescribed medications.

When an ED nurse plans discharge there is a reduction in the proportion of unscheduled ED return visits and the transition back home into the community healthcare network is improved.[79] Therefore, EDs should consider employing a discharge nurse, particularly if the department frequently cares for older people. While care needs to be taken to ensure that older people are not inappropriately returned to their home, it is still possible to reduce acute admissions by identifying patients suitable for short-term home support in an attempt to maintain previous levels of independence. This can be accomplished without reducing quality of care or patient satisfaction.[80]

Older patients who are discharged with prescriptions should have the prescription filled within the hospital, to prevent any barriers to script-filling such as immobility or distance.[81] It is also important that proper instructions are provided, as it has been found that of 'patients for whom narcotic analgesics were prescribed, 7% drove vehicles while taking these medications'.[81] In a cohort of interviewed patients who had been discharged home with new medications:

- 44% did not know dosages
- 32% did not know the dosing schedules
- 36% could not identify the purpose of the medication.[82]

Proper medication instructions need to include information about the adverse effects, interactions, dosage amount and frequency. This information needs to be in both written and oral form and presented in a manner that the patient understands.

Ideally the patient should be followed up to check that they have understood the medication instructions.[83,84]

PRACTICE TIP

Discharging older patients to a nursing home needs to include a consideration of changes in functional and cognitive abilities. Nursing homes are staffed and arranged to cater for different needs. It is important, therefore, that the older person's requirements for care are carefully assessed, documented and communicated to the relevant person in charge of receiving nursing home admissions. Most nursing homes have standardised hospital transfer forms, and these must be used and accurately completed.

Box 39.8 lists the important principles of emergency care of older people (based on work done for the Society for Academic Emergency Medicine [SAEM]).[31] These principles need to be considered when caring for older patients.[31]

The ED encounter is an opportunity to assess important conditions in the patient's personal life.

BOX 39.8 Principles of emergency care for the older person[31]

- The older patient's presentation is frequently complex.
- Common diseases present atypically in the older person.
- The confounding effects of co-morbid diseases must be considered.
- Polypharmacy is common and may be a factor in presentation, diagnosis and management.
- Recognition of the possibility of cognitive impairment is important.
- Some diagnostic tests may have different normal values.
- The likelihood of decreased functional reserve must be anticipated.
- Social support systems may not be adequate, and patients may need to rely on caregivers.
- A knowledge of baseline functional status is essential for evaluating new complaints.
- Health problems must be evaluated for associated psychosocial adjustment.

SUMMARY

The older person has a physiology affected by the ageing process that will be unique, and each person will have different diseases and psychosocial needs to be considered. Therefore, optimal emergency care of older patients requires comprehensive care that can account for this individuality. Pain is often poorly managed and in all older people it must be assessed and treated. Assessment, treatment and discharge of the older person must also account for the functional, cognitive and emotional status of the patient.

When interviewing the older person, it is essential that the carer is included. A functional evaluation is also essential and must include an assessment of ADL and IADL. When assessed, decreases in cognitive function are prevalent in older patients who seek emergency care. It is therefore important that mental status testing occurs to help determine the need for further investigations. Where rapid functional decline is found, this must be seen as a sign of a potentially life-threatening illness.

However, for the older person, a serious infection can present with vague signs and symptoms. Discharge to home must account for functional decline and transfers to a nursing home require communication of information in standardised forms.

CASE STUDY

Mrs Brown is a widowed 86-year-old woman who collapses while shopping at her local supermarket at 9.30 am. As a first-responder on the scene, you make certain that the area is safe. You check that Mrs Brown responds to your questions; you assess her airway, preserve her cervical spine, verify breathing effectiveness, check for presence of a pulse and ensure that she is not bleeding. She tells you that she is at the movies and that it is 10 pm. Her radial pulse is 62 beats/minute; her respiratory rate is 16 breaths/minute. You notice an abrasion on her left leg and she complains of pain in her left hip.

Questions

1. As the paramedic who receives the hand-over from the first-responder, you assess the severity of Mrs Brown's complaint of pain by:
   A. Asking her to rate her pain on a 10-point scale, with 10 being the worst pain imaginable and 0 being no pain.
   B. Asking her to show you on a line from no pain to worst pain imaginable what her pain level is.
   C. Assessing her level of cognitive impairment and, based on this, using an appropriate tool, such as the Abbey Pain Scale.

2. It is important that you assess Mrs Brown's confusion further. What should you consider in your paramedic assessment to more accurately ascertain the nature and possible cause of her diminished cognitive state?
   A. Assess for causes of delirium.
   B. Assess for closed head injury.
   C. Assess for pain.
   D. Assess for dementia.

3. Your assessment of the patient's medical history and medications reveals that she is a type II diabetic and has a list of her regular medications in her handbag. The handwritten list includes the following:
   - Frusemide 40 mg in the morning
   - Potassium chloride 600 mg in the morning
   - Digoxin 0.25 mg in the morning
   - Atenolol 50 mg in the morning
   - Metformin 300 mg three times a day
   - Diclofenac 50 mg twice a day
   - Warfarin 2 mg in the morning

   From this list of medications you conclude that:
   A. This is a very typical list of medications prescribed to many older people.

   B. She has a diagnosed cardiac problem that is appropriately medicated.
   C. She is at risk of a drug interaction.
   D. This is a case of polypharmacy.
   Given these medications and clinical symptoms, what injuries or illness could Mrs Brown have? What type of hospital should she be transported to, and why?

4. Mrs Brown is transported to the nearest emergency department (ED). She continues to be confused and on arrival at the ED she is making very little sense. Her monitored rhythm is a controlled atrial fibrillation; her blood pressure is measured at 126/84 mmHg; her other observations have not significantly altered (pulse 64 beats/minute, respiratory rate 16 breaths/minute, Glasgow Coma Scale score 12 [E4 V3 M5]). Which of the following is the most appropriate assessment to perform next?
   A. Severity and location of pain.
   B. Presence of lower limb deformity.
   C. Blood glucose level.
   D. Assessment of left leg abrasion.

5. Mrs Brown is hypoglycaemic and is appropriately treated; however, an hour later she is still confused: pulling leads, tugging at the IV line and wanting to get off the bed. Which of the following actions could be implemented initially to manage her symptoms of confusion?
   A. Physically restrain her.
   B. Administer 10 mg of IV diazepam.
   C. Administer 1.0 mg of IV haloperidol.
   D. Make sure she has her glasses and hearing aid.

6. A radiograph reveals an intertrochanteric fracture of the left hip and Mrs Brown is scheduled for an open reduction and internal fixation after admission to an orthopaedic ward. The surgery is booked to begin in 8 hours and so Mrs Brown is fasted. Given these circumstances, which of the following is the *LEAST* important to consider as part of her care in the ED?
   A. Requirement for analgesia.
   B. Possible presence of malnutrition.
   C. Planning for transitional care.
   D. Skin care.

7. What nursing considerations should you ensure are performed and in place prior to transport to the ward?

USEFUL WEBSITES

Acute Aged Care Interface, Victorian Government health information, www.health.vic.gov.au/acute-agedcare

Acute Care Geriatric Nurse Network (ACGNN), www.acgnn.ca

American College of Emergency Physicians, Geriatric emergency medicine, www.acep.org/ACEPmembership.aspx?id=25112

Australian and New Zealand Society for Geriatric Medicine (ANZSGM), www.anzsgm.org

Geriatric Education for Emergency Medical Services, www.gemssite.com

Geriatrics: a basic review for emergency health care providers, http://faculty.washington.edu/dgruen/table_of_contents.htm

Policy on the care of elderly patients in the emergency department, Australasian College for Emergency Medicine, www.acem.org.au/
getattachment/1b47b3b9-0643-4860-b3c9-52435d8cf8d0/Policy-on-the-Care-of-Elderly-Patients-in-the-Emer.aspx

Royal Australian College of General Practitioners, Medical care of older persons in residential aged care facilities, www.racgp.org.au/
your-practice/guidelines/silverbook/

REFERENCES

1. Social Security Online. History—Otto von Bismarck. Online. www.socialsecurity.gov/history/ottob.html; accessed 5 Feb 2010.

2. Erikson EH. Eight stages of man. In: Childhood and society. 2nd edn. New York: WW Norton; 1963:247–74.

3. National Center for Health Statistics. Health, United States, 2005, with chartbook on trends in the health of Americans. Hyattsville: Centers for Disease Control and Prevention; 2005.

4. Caplan GA, Williams AJ, Daly B et al. A randomized, controlled trial of comprehensive geriatric assessment and multidisciplinary intervention after discharge of elderly from the emergency department—the DEED II study. J Am Geriatr Soc 2004;52(9):1417–23.

5. Downing A, Wilson R. Older people's use of accident and emergency services. Age Ageing 2005;34(1):24–30.

6. Grief CL. Patterns of ED use and perceptions of the elderly regarding their emergency care: a synthesis of recent research. J Emerg Nurs 2003;29(2):122–6.

7. Kihlgren AL, Nilsson M, Sorlie V. Caring for older patients at an emergency department—emergency nurses' reasoning. J Clin Nurs 2005;14(5):601–8.

8. Moons P, Arnauts H, Delooz HH. Nursing issues in care for the elderly in the emergency department: an overview of the literature. Accid Emerg Nurs 2003;11(2):112–20.

9. Lowthian JA, Curtis AJ, Jolley DJ et al. Demand at the emergency department front door: 10-year trends in presentations. Med J Aust 2012;196(2):128–32.

10. Australian Bureau of Statistics. Population projections 1997–2051. Cat. no. 3222.0. Canberra: ABS; 2000.

11. Statistics New Zealand Tatauranga Aotearoa. New Zealand's 65+ population: a statistical volume. Wellington: Statistics NZ; 2007.

12. Birnbaumer DM. The elder patient. In Marx JA, Hockberger RS, Walls RM, Eds. Rosen's emergency medicine: Concepts and clinical practice. 8th edn. London: Elsevier Health Sciences 2013.

13. Roberts DC, McKay MP, Shaffer A. Increasing rates of emergency department visits for elderly patients in the United States, 1993 to 2003. Ann Emerg Med 2008;51(6):769–74.

14. Salvi F, Morichi V, Grilli A et al. The elderly in the emergency department: a critical review of problems and solutions. Intern Emerg Med 2007;2(4):292–301.

15. Yim VW, Graham CA, Rainer TH. A comparison of emergency department utilization by elderly and younger adult patients presenting to three hospitals in Hong Kong. Int J Emerg Med 2009;2(1):19–24.

16. Ong TJ, Ariathianto Y, Sinnappu R, Lim WK. Lower rates of appropriate initial diagnosis in older emergency department patients associated with hospital length of stay. Australasian Journal on Ageing. 2014 Mar 13.

17. Kessler C, Williams MC, Moustoukas JN, Pappas C. Transitions of care for the geriatric patient in the emergency department. Clin Geriatr Med 2013;29(1):49–69.

18. Lowthian J, Curtis A, Stoelwinder J et al. Emergency demand and repeat attendances by older patients. Internal Medicine Journal 2013;43(5):554–60.

19. Lawson P, Richmond C. 13 emergency problems in older people. Emerg Med J 2005;22(5):370–4.

20. Herbert RA. The biology of human ageing. In: Redfern SJ, Ross FM, eds. Nursing older people. 3rd edn. Edinburgh: Churchill Livingstone; 1999:55–78.

21. Eliopoulos C. Gerontological nursing. 8th edn. Philadelphia: Lippincott Williams and Wilkins; 2013.

22. Wooding Baker M, Heitkemper MM, Chenoweth, L. Older adults: Age-related physiologic changes. In: Brown D, Edwards H, et al eds. Medical-surgical nursing: assessment and management of clinical problems. 3rd edn. Chatswood: Elsevier Australia; 2012:69–71.

23. Guize L, Piot O, Lavergne T, et al. Cardiac arrhythmias in the elderly. Bull Acad Natl Med 2006;190(4–5):827–41; discussion 873–6.

24. Blom H, Mulder M, Verweij W. Arterial oxygen tension and saturation in hospital patients: effect of age and activity. Br Med J 1988;297(6650):720–1.

25. Urden L, Stacy KM, Lough ME. The older adult patient. In: Thelan's critical care nursing: diagnosis and management. 7th edn. St Louis: Elsevier. 2014:1072–94.

26. Kresevic DM. Assessment of physical function. In: Boltz M, Capezuti E, Fulmer T, Zwicker D, eds. Evidence-based geriatric nursing protocols for best practice. 4th ed. New York (NY): Springer Publishing Company; 2012. p. 89–103. [revised guidelines (2012) online. www.guideline.gov/content.aspx?id=43918; accessed 26 Feb 2014].

27. Adams JG, Gerson LW. A new model for emergency care of geriatric patients. Acad Emerg Med 2003;10(3):271–4.

28. Chiovenda P, Vincentelli GM, Alegiani F. Cognitive impairment in elderly ED patients: need for multidimensional assessment for better management after discharge. Am J Emerg Med 2002;20(4):332–5.

29. Gerson LW, Rousseau EW, Hogan TM et al. Multicenter study of case finding in elderly emergency department patients. Acad Emerg Med 1995;2(8):729–34.

30. Rutschmann OT, Chevalley T, Zumwald C et al. Pitfalls in the emergency department triage of frail elderly patients without specific complaints. Swiss Med Wkly 2005;135(9–10):145–50.

31. Sanders AB. The elder patient. In: Tintinalli JE, Kelen GD, Stapczynski JS, eds. Emergency medicine: a comprehensive study guide. 6th edn. McGraw-Hill; 2004: 1896–900.

32. Voyer P, Sych-Norrena L. Gerontology. Challenges in emergency room care for the elderly. Can Nurse 2003;99(1):22–4.

33. Katz S, Ford AB, Moskowitz RW, et al. Studies of illness in the aged: the index of ADL: a standardized measure of biological and psychosocial function. JAMA 1963;185:914–19.

34. Lawton MP, Brody EM. Assessment of older people: self-maintaining and instrumental activities of daily living. Gerontologist 1969;9(3):179–86.

35. Lach MS. Functional decline. In: Sanders AB, ed. Emergency care of the elder person. St Louis: Beverly Cracom Publications; 1996. pp. 143–52.

36. Department of Human Services Victoria. Clinical practice guidelines for the management of delirium in older people. Victorian Government; 2006. Online. www.health.vic.gov.au/acute-agedcare; 26 Feb 2014.

37. Hustey FM, Meldon SW. The prevalence and documentation of impaired mental status in elderly emergency department patients. Ann Emerg Med 2002;39(3):248–53.

38. Wilber ST. Altered mental status in older emergency department patients. Emerg Med Clin North Am 2006;24(2):299–316, vi.

39. Sanders AB, ed. Emergency care of the elder person. St. Louis: Beverly Cracom Publications; 1996.

40. Han JH, Zimmerman EE, Cutler N et al. Delirium in older emergency department patients: recognition, risk factors, and psychomotor subtypes. Acad Emerg Med 2009;16(3):193–200.

41. Lewis LM, Miller DK, Morley JE et al. Unrecognized delirium in ED geriatric patients. Am J Emerg Med 1995;13(2):142–5.

42. American Psychiatric Association. Practice guideline for the treatment of patients with delirium. Am J Psychiatry 1999;156(5 Suppl):1–20.

43. Morrison RS, Magaziner J, Gilbert M et al. Relationship between pain and opioid analgesics on the development of delirium following hip fracture. J Gerontol A Biol Sci Med Sci 2003;58(1):76–81.

44. Morrison RS, Magaziner J, McLaughlin MA et al. The impact of post-operative pain on outcomes following hip fracture. Pain 2003;103(3):303–11.

45. Rupp T, Delaney KA. Inadequate analgesia in emergency medicine. Ann Emerg Med 2004;43(4):494–503.

46. Jones JS, Johnson K, McNinch M. Age as a risk factor for inadequate emergency department analgesia. Am J Emerg Med 1996; 14(2):157–60.

47. Holdgate A, Shepherd SA, Huckson S. Patterns of analgesia for fractured neck of femur in Australian emergency departments. Emerg Med Australas 2010;22(1):3–8.

48. Terrell KM, Hustey FM, Hwang U et al. Quality indicators for geriatric emergency care. Acad Emerg Med 2009;16(5):441–9.

49. Ambulance Victoria. Clinical practice guidelines for ambulance and MICA paramedics: pain relief. CPG A0501. Doncaster: Ambulance Victoria; 2013. pp. 68–70.

50. Australian Medicines Handbook. Pethidine—analgesics. (2014) Online. http://amh.hcn.net.au/view.php?page=chapter3/monographpethidine.html; 26 Feb 2014.

51. Williams RE, Bosnic N, Sweeney CT, et al. Prevalence of opioid dispensings and concurrent gastrointestinal medications in Quebec. Pain Res Manag 2008;13(5):395–400.

52. Garratt S. Assessment of patterns of body defence and healing. In: Koch S, Garratt S, eds. Assessing older people: a practical guide for health professionals. Sydney: Maclennan and Petty; 2001:127–39.

53. Australian Institute of Health and Welfare. Australian hospital statistics 2007–08. Health services series no. 33. Cat. no. HSE 71. Canberra: AIHW; 2009.

54. Nelson RC, Amin MA. Falls in the elderly. Emerg Med Clin North Am 1990;8(2):309–24.

55. Bell AJ, Talbot-Stern JK, Hennessy A. Characteristics and outcomes of older patients presenting to the emergency department after a fall: a retrospective analysis. Med J Aust 2000;173(4):179–82.

56. Helps Y, Cripps R, Harrison J. Hospital separations due to injury and poisoning, Australia 1999–2000. Injury Research and Statistics Series, No. 15. Adelaide: Australian Institute of Health and Welfare; 2002.

57. Australian Institute of Health and Welfare. Hospitalisations due to falls by older people, Australia: 2009–10. Injury Research and Statistics Series No. 70. Cat. no. INJCAT 146. Canberra: AIHW; 2013.

58. Accident Compensation Corporation. Preventing injury from falls: the national strategy 2005–15. Online. www.acc.co.nz/PRD_EXT_CSMP/groups/external_ip/documents/guide/wcm2_020951.pdf; accessed 26 Feb 2014.

59. Haleem S, Lutchman L, Mayahi R et al. Mortality following hip fracture: trends and geographical variations over the last 40 years. Injury 2008;39(10):1157–63.

60. Sterling DA, O'Connor JA, Bonadies J. Geriatric falls: injury severity is high and disproportionate to mechanism. J Trauma 2001; 50(1):116–19.

61. Thomas KE, Stevens JA, Sarmiento K, et al. Fall-related traumatic brain injury deaths and hospitalizations among older adults—United States, 2005. J Safety Res 2008;39(3):269–72.

62. Wilkins K. Health care consequences of falls for seniors. Health Rep 1999 Spring;10(4):47–55(Eng); 47–57(Fre).

63. Australian Institute of Health and Welfare. Hospitalisations due to falls by older people, Australia 2005–2006. Canberra: AIHW; 2008.

64. Shah MN, Clarkson L, Lerner EB et al. An emergency medical services program to promote the health of older adults. J Am Geriatr Soc 2006;54(6):956–62.

65. Snooks H, Cheung WY, Halter M et al. Support and assessment for fall emergency referrals (SAFER 1) trial protocol. Computerised on-scene decision support for emergency ambulance staff to assess and plan care for older people who have fallen: evaluation of costs and benefits using a pragmatic cluster randomised trial. BMC Emerg Med 2010;10(1):2.

66. Newberry L, Criddle LM, eds. Sheehy's manual of emergency care. 6th edn. St Louis: Mosby; 2005. p. 794.

67. Young L, Ahmad H. Trauma in the elderly: a new epidemic? Aust N Z J Surg 1999;69(8):584–6.

68. Callaway DW, Wolfe R. Geriatric trauma. Emerg Med Clin North Am 2007;25(3):837–60, x.

69. Girard TD, Ely EW. Bacteremia and sepsis in older adults. Clin Geriatr Med 2007;23(3):633–47, viii.

70. Lim WK, Woodward MC. Improving medication outcomes in older people. Aust J Hosp Pharm 1999;29(2):103–7.

71. Bolton G, Tipper S, Tasker J. Medication review by GPs reduces polypharmacy in the elderly: a quality use of medicines program. Aust J Primary Health 2004;10(1):78–82.

72. Martin I, Hall J, Gardner T. Prescribing for patients aged 65 years and over in New Zealand general practice. N Z Med J 2002;115(1164):U221.

73. National Prescribing Service. What is polypharmacy? National Prescribing Service Newsletter 13. Sydney: NPS; 2000.

74. Brown D, Edwards H, eds. Lewis's medical–surgical nursing: assessment and management of clinical problems. Sydney: Elsevier; 2005:74.

75. Durrant J, Snape J. Urinary incontinence in nursing homes for older people. Age Ageing 2003;32(1):12–18.

76. Landi F, Cesari M, Russo A et al. Potentially reversible risk factors and urinary incontinence in frail older people living in community. Age Ageing 2003;32(2):194–9.

77. Bolin T, Bare M, Caplan G et al. Malabsorption may contribute to malnutrition in the elderly. Nutrition 2010;26(7–8):852–3.

78. Australian Government: Attorney–General's department. Privacy Act 1988. Act No. 119 of 1988 as amended. Canberra: Office of Legislative Drafting and Publishing; 2010.

79. Australian and New Zealand Society for Geriatric Medicine. Position Statement 16, Palliative Care for the Older Person; 2009 www.anzsgm.org/documents/PS16PalliativeCarefinalendorsed3june09.doc

80. Guttman A, Afilalo M, Guttman R et al. An emergency department-based nurse discharge coordinator for elder patients: does it make a difference? Acad Emerg Med 2004;11(12):1318–27.

81. Hardy C, Whitwell D, Sarsfield B et al. Admission avoidance and early discharge of acute hospital admissions: an accident and emergency based scheme. Emerg Med J 2001;18(6):435–40.

82. McIntosh SE, Leffler S. Pain management after discharge from the ED. Am J Emerg Med 2004;22(2):98–100.

83. Maniaci MJ, Heckman MG, Dawson NL. Functional health literacy and understanding of medications at discharge. Mayo Clin Proc 2008;83(5):554–8.

84. Raynor DK. Medication literacy is a 2-way street. Mayo Clin Proc 2008;83(5):520–2.

85. Forero R, McDonnell G, Gallego B et al. A literature review on care at the end-of-life in the emergency department, Emergency Medicine International, 2012: 486516, doi:10.1155/2012/486516

86. NSW Emergency Care Institute. End of Life. www.ecinsw.com.au/end_of_life accessed 22 May 2014.

87. Morgan TK, Williamson M et al. A national census of medicines use: a 24-hour snapshot of Australians aged 50 years and older. Med J Aust 2012; 196(1):50–3.

CHAPTER 40
VIOLENCE, ABUSE AND ASSAULT

MARIE GERDTZ

Essentials

General

- The hidden nature of family violence has multiple damaging psychological and behavioural effects: these may span a lifetime and can affect present and future generations.
- Children and women are particularly vulnerable to exposure to family violence.
- The complex nature of family violence demands a team-based approach that often involves police, paramedics, nurses, doctors, social workers and counsellors, who need to work collaboratively towards providing immediate and longer-term care and social support to an individual and a family.

Child abuse and neglect

- In Australasia, any person who holds concerns about the physical or emotional safety of a child may make a report to the statutory child protection service; healthcare professionals are mandated to report suspected child abuse in a number of jurisdictions.
- Paramedics and emergency nurses must be aware of the processes for responding to suspected child abuse and neglect and understand the way in which organisational policies and procedures articulate with their legal responsibilities to report cases of suspected abuse and neglect.

Domestic violence by intimate partners

- Violence between intimate partners is not influenced by socioeconomic status or other demographic factors; in most cases of intimate partner abuse the perpetrators are men.
- There is no predictable pattern of illness or injury that brings someone who has experienced intimate partner abuse to the attention of emergency medical services or to seek emergency department (ED) care: however, victims of intimate partner abuse have significantly more psychiatric presentations and a greater incidence of attempted suicide and alcohol-related problems than other people who use emergency health services.
- The collection of evidence from victims of sexual assault must be performed by an experienced emergency doctor or nurse who has received specific training in the care of persons who have been sexually assaulted.

Elder abuse and neglect

- Elder abuse and neglect take different forms: the common feature is harm or potential harm to the health and wellbeing of an older person.
- A competent elder has the right to make his or her own personal care decisions.
- An elder may choose to stay in the abusive situation despite all efforts to effect a change.
- Victims of abuse often have both positive and negative feelings towards their abusers; this makes separation from the abuser difficult.
- In responding to cases of elder abuse, the aim of any intervention is to protect the older person from immediate harm and break the cycle of mistreatment.

INTRODUCTION

Violence is a major public health issue: for people in all age groups, it is one of the leading causes of mortality and morbidity worldwide.[1]

In 2002, the World Health Organization's (WHO) report into violence and health sought to raise awareness among members of the general public about interpersonal violence and to highlight it as a problem that is amenable to preventative intervention. The important work of the WHO emphasises the crucial role that public health services have to play in helping society as a whole to address the causes and consequences of all types of violence.

Violence is defined as:

> The intentional use of physical force or power, threatened or actual, against oneself, another person, or against a group or community, that either results, or has a high likelihood of resulting in injury, death, psychological harm or maldevelopment.[2]

Currently, the definitions for different kinds of violence are based on the characteristics of the perpetrator.[2] Box 40.1 contains definitions for different types of violence based on the key characteristics of the perpetrator.

Hostility within families and intimate relationships are, by far, the most prevalent form of violence documented in developed countries. Injuries arising, either directly or indirectly, from this form of violence and abuse are frequently encountered by paramedics in the field and by emergency department (ED) staff. Paramedics and nurses play an essential role in assessment and first-line management of both physical and psychological injuries.

Mostly the victims of interpersonal violence will come to the attention of emergency medical services or ED staff because of obvious physical injuries; however, a substantial number of cases will also go unrecognised and unreported. The hidden nature of family violence exerts powerful, multiple, damaging and psychological and behavioural effects on a person. These effects may span a lifetime and permeate present and future generations.

BOX 40.1   Definitions for different types of violence based on the characteristics of the perpetrator

Self-directed violence involves acts that are inflicted against oneself (deliberate self-harm).

Interpersonal violence includes acts inflicted by another individual or a small group on a person (assault).

Collective violence involves acts perpetrated by larger groups such as states or organised political groups towards individuals or groups (assault).

Interpersonal violence involves family and intimate partner violence (child, intimate partner and elder abuse—assault).

Community violence—violence among unrelated individuals, who may or may not be known to each other (assault which generally takes place outside the home).

To effectively identify, intervene and prevent violence and abuse, paramedics and emergency nurses must work collaboratively as part of a multidisciplinary and multiprofessional team. In Australia, nurses, doctors and police have statutory obligations to report family violence involving child abuse or neglect.[3] Paramedics do not typically have a statutory reporting obligation. However, this does not restrict the paramedic's ability to report cases of suspected abuse. An ethical obligation to report such cases may exist where no clear legal obligation is present.

The child at risk

All children have the right to grow up nourished and supported in homes that are consistently loving and caring. Illness and injury resulting from suspected child maltreatment evokes strong emotional responses among healthcare professionals and the wider community. In recent years the levels of child neglect and abuse in Australia have increased and have rightly become an issue of national concern.[4]

Child abuse and neglect can affect the health status of a person over the course of an entire lifetime. Research shows that the psychosocial experiences of childhood abuse may be transmuted into a spectre of physical disease states and cause ongoing psychosocial problems well into adulthood.[5–12] The mechanism underlying this theory of transmutation appears to be related to the increased involvement in behavioural risk factors such as drug and alcohol abuse, poor diet and lack of exercise among children who have been abused.[7] Research also shows that abused children are at greater risk of growing into abusive adults when compared with non-abused children.[8]

Child abuse and neglect also impose financial burdens on society and the healthcare system. Direct costs associated with child abuse and neglect include multiple episodes of hospitalisation, and involvement of the child welfare and judicial systems. Indirect costs linked to child abuse and neglect include, but are not limited to, the increased need for special education among abused children and higher rates of juvenile delinquency and criminality in adulthood.[12]

Data from the Australian Institute of Health and Welfare (AIHW)[3] shows that:

- the number of children who are subject to a notification of child abuse or neglect, the number of children under care and protection orders and the number in out-of-home care are all on the rise in Australia
- Aboriginal and Torres Strait Islander children are over-represented in all of the above areas.

In 2009, the Council of Australian Governments endorsed the National Framework for Protecting Australia's Children 2009–2020.[4] This structure is important to health policy and planning because it acknowledges that child protection is a shared responsibility, for families, communities, the professions, services and governments. Under the national framework, state and territory governments maintain their statutory responsibilities for child protection. Reforms to state and territory systems are geared towards a shared model that is built on a foundation of prevention, early intervention and the development of targeted services for at-risk families and children.

Neglect

The AIHW defines neglect as:

> Any serious omissions or commissions by a person having the care of a child which, within the bounds of cultural tradition, constitute a failure to provide conditions which are essential for the healthy, physical and emotional development of a child.[3]

Neglect may be physically apparent in a child who is unkempt, left unattended, not dressed appropriately for the weather or malnourished. Failure to provide adequate physical protection, nutrition or healthcare is also considered neglect, but neglect can also include lack of human contact and love. Notwithstanding these definitions, the lack of visible bruises or broken bones belies the fact that ongoing child neglect represents a silent, serious and pervasive attack on children, which can leave lasting mental and physical health problems throughout a lifetime.

Recognising neglect is often difficult in pre-hospital and emergency health settings because of the limited, one-time contact staff have with families. Health professionals need to be alert for behaviours that are suggestive of neglect. Be aware that neglect can be physical, emotional or educational.

Failure to thrive

Failure to thrive is defined as the condition in children younger than age 5 years whose growth persistently and significantly deviates from norms for age and sex based on national growth charts. Measurements for height, weight and head circumference are plotted against normal childhood growth patterns. Failure-to-thrive children will normally score below average in all three areas.

Although the cause of failure to thrive may be medical, for example, *Giardia* organism infection, coeliac disease, lead poisoning or malabsorption, psychosocial causes are often linked to and reported as child neglect. Poor parenting practices, chronic family illnesses, parental depression and substance abuse among caregivers are often linked to failure to thrive. The consequences of untreated failure to thrive include developmental and behavioural difficulties secondary to nutritional deprivation of the nervous system and other systems.

Accordingly, a multidisciplinary approach to treating failure to thrive provides the best opportunity for success. Family assessment, nutritional counselling, medical intervention and family support are needed to correct failure to thrive.

Physical abuse (non-accidental injury)

The AIHW defines physical abuse as:

> Any non-accidental physical act inflicted upon a child by a person having the care of a child.[3]

Physical abuse of a child typically entails a repeated pattern of behaviour, but may also include a single episode. Physical abuse involves an unreasonable level of force, and includes injury, torture and maiming. In Australasia, corporal punishment of children is also considered physical abuse.

Non-disclosure of physical abuse is common among children, who may harbour feelings of shame or confusion. In addition, it is not uncommon for children to be unaware that physical abuse is not only inappropriate but also unlawful. A further difficulty in identifying physical abuse is the number of conditions that may mimic abuse. For this reason, all possible physiological or pathological causes for any physical findings must be considered as part of the assessment of a child who presents to the ED with an injury.[13] Box 40.2 shows examples of some conditions that mimic physical abuse. It is important to rule out these conditions before attributing the presentation to abuse.

In addition to situations where physical signs may mimic abuse, two substantive patterns of physical abuse are particularly relevant to emergency presentations. These syndromes are shaken baby syndrome and Factitious Disorder Imposed on Another (previously known as Münchausen's syndrome by proxy).

Shaken baby syndrome

Vulnerability to child abuse is significantly influenced by age,[1] and fatal causes of physical abuse are largely found among young infants.[14] Shaken baby syndrome (SBS) occurs when infants are shaken vigorously. According to the American Academy of Pediatrics, SBS is a violent form of abuse that occurs in infants younger than 2 years, but can involve children as old as 5 years.[15]

The mechanism underlying SBS is acceleration–deceleration of the head, which creates a triad of injuries: subdural haemorrhage, retinal injury and altered level of consciousness. Importantly, there may be no external signs of trauma. Babies

---

BOX 40.2 Some examples of conditions known to mimic physical abuse

- **Sudden infant death syndrome (SIDS)**. This can appear as child abuse because of pooling of blood, mottling and other discolouration associated with death. The definitive cause of death can only be determined by autopsy.
- **Clotting disorders**, such as Wiskott-Aldrich syndrome, haemophilia and thrombocytopenia purpura, cause bruises in varying stages of healing.
- **Mongolian spots** are birthmarks found predominantly in people with dark pigmentation. Mongolian spots do not change colouration or size over time and have a greyer appearance than bruises.
- **Multiple petechiae and purpura** of the face can occur when vigorous crying, retching or coughing increases vena cava pressure. Unlike intentional choking, there are no marks around the neck.
- **Bullous impetigo** may appear as an infected wound or burn. This condition may reflect neglect if caregivers are apathetic about care of lesions.
- **Cultural or ethnic practices**, such as coining or cupping, are used to treat pain, fever or poor appetite. Coining—rubbing a coin over bony prominences—causes a striated 'pseudoburn'. Cupping (warming a cup, spoon or shot glass in oil and then placing it on the neck, back or ribs) can result in a petechial or purpuric rash over the affected area.
- **Osteogenesis imperfecta** is an inherited disease that can result in multiple fractures with minimal trauma and causes a tendency to bleed easily.

shaken into unconsciousness are often put to bed in the hope that the injuries will resolve. In these cases, the window for therapeutic intervention is lost.

The spectrum of symptoms arising from SBS vary; they may include vomiting and irritability in mild shakings and range to unconsciousness, convulsions and even death in severe shakings.

To rule out SBS, healthcare workers should look for any external signs of injuries such as bruises. A fundoscopic examination of the pupils should be performed to look for retinal haemorrhages. Pupil dilation may be required in some patients. A computed tomography (CT) scan should be obtained to identify brain haemorrhages. Magnetic resonance imaging (MRI), when available, is extremely helpful for detection of subdural haematoma. A skeletal survey should be obtained to rule out fractures, especially in the area of the ribs.

Factitious Disorder Imposed on Another

Factitious Disorder Imposed on Another, previously referred as Münchausen's syndrome by proxy, represents a complex multi-factorial form of child abuse deliberately perpetrated against a child.[16,17] The secondary gain associated with the child's condition is the motivator for abuse, and for this reason the caregiver will seek medical attention for the condition and therefore may be encountered in the emergency setting. The outcomes for children involved are known to be poor, as the abuse is typically sustained and may go undetected for many years.[17] The *Diagnostic and Statistical Manual of Mental Disorders*, 5th edition (DSM-V)[17] specified four key features of the syndrome:

1. Falsification of physical or psychological signs or symptoms or the induction of injury or disease in another associated with identified deception.
2. The individual presents another individual to others as ill, impaired or injured.
3. The deceptive behaviour is evident even in the absence of obvious external rewards.
4. The behaviour cannot be explained by another mental disorder.

In Factitious Disorder Imposed on Another, the child is subjected to illnesses perpetuated by caregivers who may administer drugs to induce symptoms, introduce pathogens or otherwise contribute to a child's illness. Caretakers may also falsify medical histories and symptoms. In this context caregivers typically have little insight into their abusive patterns of behaviour. In extreme cases, caretakers have caused the death of a child.

In terms of management, the paramedic and nurse should attempt to project an objective, non-judgmental attitude. Despite their abusive behaviour, the parent has a right to nursing care that is provided respectfully and sympathetically. Communication with the parent is best focused on addressing initial concerns and the wellbeing of the child, rather than on confrontation about the behaviour or labelling. Because of the clinical features of the disorder, the treatment team should plan to confront the parent in a unified manner, and communication around protection of the child must follow standardised procedures for mandatory reporting as per other types of abuse and neglect.[17]

Emotional abuse

Emotional abuse is defined by the AIHW as:

> Any act by a person having the care of a child that results in the child suffering any kind of significant emotional deprivation or trauma.[3]

Emotional abuse encompasses psychological harm, mental injury and verbal abuse. This can be defined as acts or the lack of acts that cause or could possibly cause serious cognitive, behavioural, emotional or mental disorders.[3] Caregivers who use extreme measures of discipline such as locking a child in a cupboard, or less-severe acts, such as habitual belittling, are sufficient to warrant notification to protective services.

Although emotional abuse is almost always found with every form of child maltreatment, this type of abuse is often very difficult to identify, as cultural factors appear to strongly influence the non-physical techniques that parents may choose to discipline their children.[2] Verbal abuse is one of the most common forms of emotional abuse.[18]

Sexual abuse

Sexual abuse is defined by the AIHW as:

> Any act by a person having the care of the child which exposes a child to, or involves a child in, sexual processes beyond his or her understanding or contrary to accepted community standards.[3]

Child sexual abuse—involvement of children in sexual activities that violate social taboos—is usually done for gratification or profit of a significantly older person. Developmentally, children do not have the capacity to understand these acts and, as such, are not able to give informed consent. Types of sexual abuse include, but are not limited to: fondling, digital manipulation, exhibitionism, pornography and actual or attempted oral, vaginal or anal intercourse.

Legal and social systems that are designed to protect children from abuse in Australasia depend heavily on data from the medical examination to provide evidence that can withstand intense scrutiny. The integrity of this evidence is vital because of its potential to protect children from further abuse and to prosecute the offender/offenders. Consequently, emergency care professionals must be able to recognise sexual abuse and be skilled in examinations with medical and forensic strength. Screening and treatment protocols specifically addressing child sexual abuse are recommended for all EDs.

Assessment and management

The priorities in the assessment and management of a child presenting with suspected abuse or neglect must follow a clear and comprehensive process. Clinical practice guidelines for medical and nursing staff have been developed to streamline the process and set priorities for the assessment and management of physical and sexual abuse.[18] Although there is no Australasia-wide guideline for paramedic management of cases of suspected child abuse, the UK Ambulance Service Clinical Practice Guidelines provide detailed guidance for paramedics who encounter cases of child abuse or neglect.[19]

Regardless of the type of abuse that is suspected, the assessment priorities remain unchanged:

- to diagnose, treat and document injuries
- to interpret the injury and/or behavioural patterns that have led to suspicion of abuse

- to notify the hospital social worker
- to comply with legislation governing the reporting of abuse.

Diagnose, treat and document injuries

In all types of suspected abuse, assessment and treatment of urgent medical problems remain the priority. This should be done according to resuscitation principles, with care to collect any clothing that is removed during this process. Care of injury is the primary medical concern.

Infants and children who are brought to the ED with an injury that appears as though another person might have deliberately inflicted it require a full physical assessment. This needs to be carried out by an experienced medical officer. A complete physical examination will contain height and weight measures and examination of the head, mouth, eyes, ears, chest, abdomen, back and limbs.

After immediate physical needs are resolved, further assessment is then initiated. Query the child and caregivers, avoiding judgments of possible perpetrators or reasons why the injury occurred. Healthcare providers must remember that investigation of child abuse allegations is the responsibility of police and protective services.

Reassure the child and caregiver that you are there to help. Establish trust, allay fears and lay groundwork for expression of concerns. Give the child some degree of control by providing choices. 'Which colour gown do you want—blue or green?' 'May I listen to your heart, or do you want to listen to it first?' Be clear and explain what you are doing. Be honest: if something will hurt, say so.

Obtain a detailed history, paying close attention to the sequence of events.

Interpret the injury and/or behavioural pattern

In cases of suspected physical abuse, a full physical assessment is required. Height and weight must be included, along with examination of the head, mouth, eyes, ears, chest, abdomen, back and limbs. Contact with the nominated hospital social worker early in the presentation is recommended, and will assist with the overall evaluation and liaison with family and protective services.[20]

In order to perform a physical examination and provide a report to protective services, consent is required from the child's parent or legal guardian. In an ED, the physical examination should be performed by an appropriately qualified and experienced medical practitioner and should only be performed once.

Preparing the child for medical evaluation is extremely important. Give the child lots of decisions to make, such as what colour of gown to wear, who he or she wants in the examination room and if he or she wants to sit on the right or left side of the table. Always tell the truth and promise only what you can control. While the child is fully clothed, explain the purpose of the examination. Explain actions with a soft, reassuring voice throughout the examination to keep children informed and to decrease anxiety. Remind children that they are in charge, so if anything hurts, the examiner will stop and together they will decide on a different way to do things. When the examination is over, reassure them and then give them a chance to ask questions.

Investigations should include a clotting profile and X-ray if fractures are suspected. A bone scan or skeletal survey may be used to diagnose clinically unsuspected recent or old fracture sites.

In cases where sexual abuse is suspected, examination and the collection of evidence must be performed by appropriately trained and skilled medical practitioners. However, very limited inspections to determine the amount of bleeding or the extent of a rash are sometimes necessary and can be done with the cooperation of the child.

In the case of acute sexual assault, rapid evaluation is indicated and should occur within 72 hours of the assault. The primary responsibility of the ED nurse in such circumstances is to notify the appropriate staff (medical and social worker), and to ensure that the child is comfortable and receiving the appropriate level of emotional support and privacy.

Comply with local policy and legislation governing the reporting of abuse

Australia does not have a single child protection service, but rather eight separate child protection systems. The departments responsible for managing child protection across jurisdictions and the legislation under which it is governed also differ.[3] In Australia, any person who holds concerns about the physical or emotional safety of a child may make a report to the statutory child protection service. Nurses are specifically named as one of a group of professionals in child protection legislation in a number of jurisdictions. The AIHW provides a helpful summary of mandatory reporting requirements by jurisdiction.[3]

Currently, mandatory reporting does not exist in New Zealand; however, the law protects anyone who, out of concern for a child, reports suspected abuse and neglect to the New Zealand Department of Child Youth and Family Services.[23]

Because of the complex nature of child abuse and neglect, the issues surrounding its management require the expertise of many professionals. With the advent of mandatory reporting and the development of protective services for children in all Australian states, most acute care services have developed a streamlined and multidisciplinary approach to assessment and reporting.[4] Emergency nurses must be aware of these processes locally and understand the way in which organisational policies and procedures articulate with their legal responsibilities to report abuse and neglect.

Domestic violence by intimate partners

Intimate partner violence (IPV) is defined as actual or threatened physical or sexual violence or psychological or emotional abuse.[1] This may manifest as acts of physical aggression, psychological abuse, forced intercourse and other forms of controlling behaviour, such as isolating a person from family or friends, monitoring their movements or limiting access to assistance or information.

Different types of IPV commonly co-exist in the same relationship: the defining factors in all cases are power and control. The perpetrator creates fear in the victim to exert control. Other terms that have been used to describe IPV include spouse abuse, courtship violence and wife beating. In Australasia, the term 'domestic violence' is most commonly used to describe violence between intimate partners, including heterosexual and same sex partners.

Prevalence

Violence between intimate partners exists in all countries and is believed to be independent of social, economic or religious factors.[1]

- The overwhelming burden of abuse is borne by women and perpetrated by men.[1]
- Notwithstanding these statistics, there is little data in Australia to describe the rates of domestic violence in gay and lesbian relationships.[24]

At every age in the life span, females are more likely to be sexually or physically assaulted by their father, brother, family member, neighbour, boyfriend, husband, partner or ex-partner than by a stranger or an anonymous assailant.[1]

Descriptive reports suggest that there may be substantial barriers to the reporting of intimate partner abuse in same sex relationships due to community attitudes. Furthermore, lesbians are believed to experience much higher levels of fear about intermate partner abuse and sexual assault than gay men or other women.[24]

A landmark study describing the prevalence of domestic violence in Australia was conducted by Roberts et al in 1996.[25] Of 1223 ED attendances included in this study, the researchers found a lifetime prevalence rate of 15.5% (8.5% of men, 23.9% of women). In line with international literature, the study also found that women were at greater risk than men for abuse as adults. In this study, women were also found to be at greater risk than men for being doubly abused (first as a child and subsequently as an adult). From the study data, 2% of women were current victims of domestic violence. It was noted that these women commonly presented to the ED between the hours of 5 pm and 8 am, when no social-work services were available for referral of victims. Other surveys of Australian EDs suggest similar statistics, based on self-disclosure, and estimate a lifetime prevalence of between 19% and 24% of women and 8% of men.

The abused partner

Those who are exposed to domestic violence tend to visit EDs more often than non-victims do; however, most often their visits will be for complaints other than those directly related to domestic violence. Research indicates that many people who experience abuse fear being blamed, judged or humiliated and are reluctant to discuss their situation—let alone undergo painful examinations and answer questions about the abuse.[25] This reluctance is typically strong among those who may abuse drugs or alcohol, and who may be trying to avoid contact with police.

There is often no predictable pattern to the complaints that bring someone who has experienced domestic violence to the ED. The only difference in diagnostic disorders between victims and non-victims is that victims have significantly more psychiatric presentations and a greater incidence of attempted suicide and alcohol-related problems.[26] In particular, women in violent relationships may come to the ED with complaints related to depression or gastrointestinal disorders.

Some women do not experience physical violence in a relationship until they become pregnant. In such situations, the unborn child may be perceived as a threat to the abuser, as someone coming between the partners; someone who takes away the woman's attention. Spontaneous abortions and preterm deliveries can also be related to physical abuse. Indicators of domestic violence in the context of midwifery and obstetric practice include late bookings, poor attendance at check-up clinics, attendance at the ED with depressions, anxiety, self-harm or somatic symptoms, and repeat ED attendances for any problem. In addition, the abused woman may be evasive or reluctant to speak about her injuries or issues in front of her partner.

Despite reasons given by a woman for ED presentation, or the presence or absence of risk factors, all people who repeatedly seek medical care in an ED should be screened for family violence.

The abusive partner

Factors associated with a man's risk of abusing his partner are diverse, and include:

- individual factors—for example, young age, heavy drinking, depression, personality disorders, low income and having witnessed abuse as a child
- relationship factors—for example, marital conflict, economic stress
- community factors—poverty
- societal factors—for example, traditional gender norms or social norms supportive of violence.

Alcohol and other drugs of abuse also play a role in many cases of domestic violence. In some instances, both partners may be substance abusers.[26] In fact, the strongest predictor for acute injury from domestic violence is a history of alcohol or other drug abuse by the abuser.[26] Alcohol decreases impulse control. A person inclined to violence finds it easier to commit aggressive acts while intoxicated. Methamphetamines and, to a lesser degree, cocaine can alter thought processes and cause paranoia, which may be aimed at the partner. Despite this, mind-altering substances are not an excuse for violent behaviour. Many people who use drugs do not abuse their spouses; the tendency for violence must already exist.

In the pre-hospital and ED setting, the stereotype of an abuser is the man who will not allow his partner to answer any questions, and will not allow her to be alone with the nurse. However, it is just as likely that the abuser will be very cooperative with nursing staff and appear compassionate towards his spouse, allowing her to interact normally. Importantly, control may be subtly communicated to the spouse with very discrete gestures and expressions that only the victim can perceive.

The role of the emergency nurse

The role of the emergency nurse in the management of people who have experienced domestic violence must initially focus on ensuring that the physical needs of the individual are met. In addition to attending to these needs, the emergency nurse has the responsibility to screen, document and refer people who have been exposed to violence in order to optimise outcomes.

In the provision of care for women who have experienced domestic violence, it is essential to understand that the ability to leave an abusive relationship is a complex social, psychological and economic process. Importantly, this decision can involve substantial risk to the individual, and for this reason must be managed as an ongoing process in which the emergency team provides non-judgmental support and access to services until the woman is living safely and without fear.

Research shows that people who have experienced domestic violence typically move through a series of phases in the process of leaving an abusive relationship. These phases include:

- pre-contemplation, where there is little conscious awareness of the violent behaviour as abuse
- contemplation, where the person is unsure whether leaving is possible or if she will, in fact, decide to leave
- preparation, where plans are made to leave and action is subsequently taken.

It is important to note that progression through each of these phases is not linear and that relapses involving returning to the relationship might occur.

For the nurse, understanding where the person is in terms of the various phases of leaving a violent relationship can provide a useful framework for listening, providing supportive care and informing decisions with respect to making referrals and determining the woman's readiness for change.

Throughout all phases of thinking and acting to stop violence, the role of the healthcare team is to empower the individual to make decisions that will improve her personal safety and that of any of her dependants. In addition to informing the delivery of supportive care, knowledge of the phases of abuse in domestic violence can also act to inform risk assessment. It is essential to note that 70% of murders that take place in the context of domestic violence occur as the women has left or is leaving home.

Screening

Routine screening will increase identification of domestic violence, and some EDs use this approach; however, there is no evidence that carrying out screening improves health outcomes for women. One study found that before implementing routine screening, only 0.4% of emergency patients were identified as victims of domestic violence. After screening was implemented, 14.2% of patients were identified as victims. Only 1.3% of emergency patients questioned refused to answer.[27]

Privacy is essential for the screening interview. Questions should not be asked in a public place, such as a centrally located triage desk or waiting room. The patient should never be questioned in the presence of a possible abuser.

Three questions have been very effective in identifying victims of domestic violence.[28] These questions are listed in Box 40.3. Positive answers can be investigated further.

The emergency nurse may become suspicious of domestic violence because of specific physical and behavioural findings.

These observations should form the basis for a more-focused assessment, which might include the following questions:

- I notice you have bruises on your face. Has someone hit you?
- Your partner seems very anxious. Did he hurt you?

As with all interpersonal communication, the emergency nurse should assess the woman in a manner that is appropriate to her level of education and to the rapport the nurse has established with the woman. Consideration must also be given to her cognitive and emotional state, and her levels of anxiety.

Surveys of women in violent relationships and those not in violent relationships show that most are grateful to healthcare providers who enquire about violence and abuse in relationships and do not consider this line of enquiry offensive or intrusive. Victims have been interviewed regarding their experiences in the ED. Half of the women interviewed reported negative experiences in the ED, such as feeling humiliated, being blamed for their abuse, having abuse minimised and not being identified as victims of domestic violence.[29]

The emergency nurse must have a high index of suspicion and be alert for physical and behavioural clues. Many behavioural clues related to domestic violence are the same as those for child abuse. The patient may wait several hours or days before seeking help for her injuries. She may hope to avoid embarrassment or the need to lie about her injuries, or the perpetrator may prevent her from leaving home. The patient may have a history of several injuries, telling the nurse that she is clumsy or stupid and frequently falls or bumps into things. She may bypass closer EDs so that personnel do not get suspicious of her frequent visits. The given mechanism of injury may not fit physical findings.

As with child abuse, the victim may have bruises, fractures and other injuries in various stages of healing. Most victims of domestic violence do not present for treatment of their injuries.

Documentation

Documentation on the medical record can be very helpful to an abused person, as it can be used as evidence in court. The notes should be very specific. The clearer the information, the less likely the nurse will have to appear in court to explain them.

Photographic evidence may also be collected with the person's permission, if possible; photographs are valuable evidence. Documentation should include as much as is possible. Quotes from the abused person need to be correctly identified in the record using quotation marks. This approach should be used to record the person's description of the incident. The name of the abuser should be asked and documented in direct quotation. Injuries should be recorded on a body map. Documentation should also note whether the incident was reported to the police.

Documentation should include all standard nursing data, including time of arrival, preferred language, history of event, type and severity of injuries sustained and the nature of the examination that is conducted. In addition, the nurse should note whether the injuries are consistent with the history given, and if there have been previous episodes of domestic violence. It is vital that the nurse determines the age and whereabouts of any children in the family, to ensure that they are in safe care. Treatment and referrals should also be noted. If the patient

---

BOX 40.3 Questions to ask to identify victims of domestic violence

1. Have you been hit, kicked, punched or otherwise hurt by someone within the past year? If so, by whom?
2. Do you feel safe in your current relationship?
3. Is there a partner from a previous relationship making you feel unsafe now?

identifies the perpetrator of the abuse by name, then this should also be included in the notes. Because of the often recurring nature of domestic violence, it is essential that all agencies (such as police, drug and alcohol services or child protection services) involved in the event be noted. Even if a patient denies physical abuse, the nurse should chart findings and the suspicion that the findings do not fit the history and may indicate abuse.

Alerting other agencies and referrals

In Australia, many agencies are available to assist people who have experienced domestic violence. The availability of these services is determined by where a person lives. The network of community supports for victims of domestic violence includes telephone counselling and helplines, emergency shelters and accommodation, child protection agencies, police and legal services. In the ED setting, a decision of referral needs to consider the immediate safety of the person who has experienced abuse to return home. Alternative arrangements for safe accommodation and absolute confidentially are of utmost importance.

Policies and procedures for referral

Due to variability in the location and availability of support services, clearly written protocols and procedures for managing the care and referral of people who have experienced domestic violence are necessary in the ED setting.[30] On discharge from the ED, the abused person will require specific information about domestic violence resources that exist within the community; these resources vary between jurisdictions and each ED should become proactive by compiling and maintaining an up-to-date list of local refuges, and counselling and support services for people who have experienced domestic violence. Local domestic violence support groups can provide a great deal of information for emergency nurses.

The nurse may offer pamphlets or cards with phone numbers. Some people may refuse cards or phone numbers because it might not be safe to take home material that deals with domestic violence. If the patient will not take any material, give the number of the ED or the name of a local domestic violence support organisation for the person to look up in the phone book.

Education of the public

The best places to display posters and provide pamphlets on domestic violence are the treatment room and bathroom. The waiting room is too public, and the victim may have to walk in front of several people, including the perpetrator, to get the information. Treatment rooms and bathrooms provide the patient with a chance to read a pamphlet in private, even if he or she is not able to take it home.

Patient education

While most abused people are aware that battering a partner is against the law, they may not realise that more-subtle acts, such as threats of bodily harm, false imprisonment, harassment or forcing someone to perform acts against his or her will, are also against the law. Frequently, discussion of these issues is the first step in providing the patient information on domestic violence.

Reassure the patient that he or she is not to blame for the abuse. Many patients incorrectly believe that they have done

something to incite a beating and are sure they can prevent further beatings if they simply behave in the appropriate manner. However, this is untrue; the pattern of abuse will continue until an outside intervention stops it.

If the patient is receptive, discuss the effect partner abuse is likely to have on children. Many women may not be motivated to leave for themselves, but may be willing to leave for the sake of their children. Much research has shown that violence travels in family lines. If children witness abuse or are victims of abuse, they are much more likely to become abusers. If the abuser is not already hitting the children, chances are very good that he or she will soon do so.

Reporting domestic violence

After a person decides to seek treatment for injuries as a result of violence, the next decision is whether to report the crime. The ED nurse can assist in this process by facilitating police contact.

When intervening in domestic violence, the nurse must not use the 'did she leave him?' factor as a determinant of effectiveness. Most patients do not leave after the first few episodes. Years later, the patient may use the information the nurse provided. Survivors report that simple acknowledgment and a non-judgmental attitude helped them enormously in the emergency setting.

If the patient has decided not to go home, the nurse should help him or her explore resources. Most shelters do not automatically accept all comers if they have safe alternatives. Does the patient have relatives or friends who will accept them? Do they have financial resources for travelling to friends or relatives out of town? Are there children still at home who must be protected?

The immediate plan usually involves protection for the patient and children. After the patient has formed a plan, he or she needs access to a phone to implement it. Long-term needs for an abused person include legal assistance, employment and housing. The ED is not the best place to make plans for meeting these needs.

Sexual assault

Sexual assault occurs in many contexts, including families, instances where the perpetrator is known to the victim and within the wider community where the perpetrator is unknown.

Sexual assault is a crime of power and control: sex is used as a way of controlling and humiliating the victim. It involves a wide range of behaviours with the common characteristic of unwanted sexual contact. Coercion encompasses a whole spectrum of degrees of force and may include psychological intimidation and threats.

The survivor

'Survivor' is a common term used for people who have been sexually assaulted. The person who has experienced sexual assault has lived through a life-threatening event. Use of the term 'victim' denotes helplessness and hopelessness. The term 'survivor' has more of a positive, empowering connotation. In addition, the use of 'survivor' as an identifying term can be helpful when counselling people who have experienced sexual assault. However, some professionals working in the area of sexual assault treatment do not use the term because it is felt that it may minimise or take away from the devastation of the actual event.

Pre-hospital management

Paramedic management of survivors of sexual assault is detailed in practice guidelines developed by the Joint Royal Colleges Liaison Committee.[21] Although these inform practice in the UK, they are relevant to paramedic practice in Australia and New Zealand. Paramedics should be cautious about disturbing evidence, but this should not constrain the primary and secondary survey or management of significant threats to health. Paramedics should be non-judgmental and should not elicit details about the alleged assault, other than information immediately relevant to the care of the individual. The sexual assault victim should be transported to an appropriate hospital and the hospital notified to assist in the early triage so that triage does not occur in a public space.

Initial ED management

Evaluation of the sexual assault survivor in the ED requires planning, development of specific policies and procedures and education of staff. The goal of ED management is to provide sensitive, individualised care for each person in a manner that ensures adherence to legal and regulatory requirements. Attention in the first instance is to address the physiological needs of the survivor and the simultaneous preservation of evidence. Where it is possible, care of survivors of sexual assault should be managed in conjunction with appropriately skilled and resourced sexual assault teams.

Following triage, the patient should immediately be placed in a safe, secure room. It is never acceptable for a survivor of sexual assault to wait in the waiting room. A medical screening examination will be conducted by a senior ED doctor. The purpose of the examination at this stage is to rule out an emergency medical condition. A nurse should be instructed to remain with the patient throughout the ED visit to provide continuity and decrease repetition of data. The patient should be allowed a support person, such as a family member, friend or representative from a rape crisis centre.

Detailed assessment

The examination of a sexual assault survivor has been called 'another rape'. The goal of ED care is to cause as little additional stress as possible. All interactions should be handled with sensitivity and understanding. Every effort should be made to ensure that the patient has the opportunity to make informed choices about medical care.

Police are generally well-prepared to deal sensitively with survivors of sexual assault. The nurse should ensure that the patient is well-informed and understands the examination process. Consent should be obtained for medical treatment, including evidentiary examination and photographs. The patient must understand that the evidence collected will be used for prosecution of the accused rapist if a report is made. Many patients are not ready to file a report with law enforcement, even with treatment in the ED.

Examinations performed within 72 hours of the assault are more likely to yield evidence of assault; however, this timeframe should not negate performing examinations on individuals assaulted beyond the 72-hour timeframe. When questioning the patient, the patient does not need to describe the assault in specific minute-by-minute detail. Translate medical terms into everyday language. History-taking may be delayed when the patient's emotional response to questioning makes it impossible to ascertain the information. Documentation should be completed legibly and clearly. If the case is called to court, the nurse may be asked to discuss what was written in the record. The nurse must be able to understand what he or she wrote months or even years after it was written, so the nurse should write it in such a manner that it can be explained to a jury.

Potential use of various date-rape drugs (e.g. flunitrazepam (Rohypnol), gamma-hydroxybutyrate (GHB) and ketamine) should be assessed while obtaining other historical data. This data helps the medical or nursing professional or other examiner to determine the need for drug screening. Assaults with these agents are referred to as drug-facilitated sexual assaults.

Collection of evidence

The collection of evidence should be performed by an experienced emergency doctor or nurse who has received specific training in the care of people who have been sexually assaulted.

Collection of various laboratory tests should be accomplished early in the presentation to allow for pregnancy test results. A negative pregnancy test is needed to administer medication for prevention of pregnancy. The patient's clothing is collected and placed in paper rather than plastic bags for evaluation at the local crime laboratory. Use of plastic allows body fluids and other trace evidence to deteriorate more quickly.

A head-to-toe physical assessment is completed to assess for all injuries. Documentation of any injuries should include colour and size of injuries, such as bruises, abrasions, lacerations or avulsions. Use of body figures on the documentation tool can assist in recording this data. A Wood's lamp or other ultraviolet light is used to identify semen on the patient's skin. Semen appears as an orange or blue-green colour on the skin. The fluorescent area should be swabbed with a moistened cotton-tipped applicator. A control swab should then be taken from an area of the body adjacent to where the swab was taken. Caution should be taken when reporting Wood's lamp findings because other materials such as lint also fluoresce.

Oral swabs are taken for evidence of semen and as a reference sample. Reference samples include saliva, blood, semen, pubic hair and body hair. These reference samples are compared with specimens from potential suspects.

For the female patient, the pelvic examination begins with a gross visual examination. Photographs are then used to detect and document genital trauma. Colposcopic photographs have become standard as part of the pelvic or genital evaluation. The colposcope provides binocular vision, magnifies the area by 5–30 times and can take photographs. Documentation should indicate whether the injury is apparent without use of the colposcope. Injuries should be described by size, appearance and location.

Pubic hair is combed to look for foreign hairs. A representative number of the patient's pubic hairs are cut close to the skin for comparison. During the pelvic examination, swabs and slides are taken from the vaginal pool.

Historically, baseline testing for chlamydia and gonorrhoea has also been performed. Recently, some established programs have stopped performing these tests because each patient is offered prophylactic antibiotic treatment.

Rectal examination includes colposcopy, swabs, slides and baseline testing for sexually transmitted infections (STIs) (as indicated by local policy). The perianal area should be cleansed after taking vaginal/penile specimens to avoid contamination from vaginal or perianal drainage.

All swabs and slides must be labelled to identify the patient and the source. After they are collected, swabs or slides should be placed in a drying box with cool airflow. Drying swabs and slides also prevents deterioration of evidence.

The testing of swabs and slides is done by a forensic laboratory in the hope of linking evidence to potential suspects. DNA testing methods allow detection of semen donor type beyond the 72-hour timeframe (detection has occurred as many as 5–6 days after a sexual assault).

Care must be taken by the clinical staff to prevent any contamination of evidence collected. All equipment that comes in contact with evidence must be clean. The nurse should limit handling of evidence and take care not to leave any of his or her own DNA on the evidence. This can be facilitated by using gloves and by not talking over the evidence.

To maintain validity of evidence collected, the ED staff must be able to verify the whereabouts of all evidence. All transfers of evidence must be carefully documented. The best practice is to keep transfers of evidence to a minimum.

A shower and clean clothing should be available for the patient after the sexual assault examination. Ideally, the hospital will maintain a store of clean new or used clothing. If desired by the patient, medication should be provided for prevention of pregnancy and STIs. Consent for pregnancy prevention should be obtained after a negative pregnancy test result and after the patient is informed of associated risks. Prophylaxis for human immunodeficiency disease (HIV) is not yet routine for all sexual assault victims, but may be considered.

Patients should be re-checked within 2 weeks. Referral to a gynaecologist or nearby clinic is essential—cultures for *Chlamydia* and *Neisseria gonorrhoeae* can be obtained at this time. At the follow-up appointment, timelines for HIV testing can be discussed. Many established specialised teams include follow-up care as part of their overall program.

Elder abuse and neglect

Elder abuse and neglect take different forms; however, the common feature is harm or threatened harm to the health or welfare of an older person.[31] The emergency nurse should always remember that despite rising concerns about elder abuse, there are no uniform comprehensive definitions of the term. Indeed, positive identification of elder abuse is easy only in cases where outright battering is visible.[32]

Origin of the problem

Four main theories have been used to explain elder abuse: role theory, transgenerational theory, psychopathology theory and stressed caregiver theory.

Role theory

As the parent ages and becomes more childlike, the child must assume a parental role. The elder who once helped the child must now take orders from that child. The psychological impact of this role reversal is significant for both generations. When role conflicts are present, the potential for abuse increases substantially.

Transgenerational theory

The underlying philosophy of transgenerational theory is that violence is a learned behaviour. If a child grows up in a family in which aggressive behaviour is a part of life, the child exhibits similar behaviour. If the parent abused the child, then the child as the caregiver abuses the parent in retribution.

Psychopathology theory

Altered impulse control caused by psychological problems such as mental illness or drug or alcohol dependence places the elder at greater risk for abuse. The typical abuser is a middle-aged, white woman who lives with the victim, is an alcohol or drug addict and has long-term financial problems and high stress levels. The abuser perceives the victim as the source of this stress.

Stressed caregiver theory

This is one area in which the nurse providing long-term care for the elderly person can abuse the elderly person as easily as the family caregiver. Caregivers under stress have limited amounts of internal resources. Stress associated with the health-care environment and stress in the individual's personal and family life may lead the caregiver to express stress through mistreatment of the elderly. Women may also find themselves in the caretaker role for their spouse's parents.

Signs and symptoms

Elder abuse cannot be assessed quickly or easily from a cluster of signs and vague presenting symptoms. Keen awareness when performing the physical examination is essential to identify elder abuse.

Each category of abuse or neglect is associated with distinct diagnostic and clinical findings. Almost half of the cases of substantiated abused and neglected older people were individuals who were not physically able to care for themselves. The elder person's history should be obtained from several sources whenever possible. Interactions between the caregiver and the elder person should be carefully observed. The patient may be fearful or agitated in the presence of the caregiver, or may appear passive and compliant. The caregiver may use harsh words and tone when speaking to the patient or say demeaning things to the elder person. Assess the patient's mental status carefully.

When assessing the patient, observe carefully for signs of malnourishment. Note the presence of old and new bruises. Bruises on the upper aspects of both arms suggest that the patient has been held tightly and shaken. Bruises on the trunk suggest beating with fists. Bruises on the wrists or ankles occur when the patient has been tied down. Cigarette burns on the skin may be present. Old, healed burns appear as skin discolourations. (Photographs of bruises, lacerations and other injuries should be obtained to document type and extent of injuries.)

Blows to the eyes can cause dislocation of the lens, subconjunctival haemorrhage or retinal detachment. Whiplash injuries are seen after repeated, violent shaking. Consider the possibility of sexual abuse. Difficulty walking or sitting may be a subtle sign, whereas bruises or lacerations of the inner thighs or genitalia are more-overt signs. Pain or itching in the genital area may indicate a sexually transmitted disease. Multiple decubiti without interventions suggest neglect.

Screening

When screening for elder abuse, the patient and suspected abuser should be interviewed separately. Begin with general questions about the patient's perception of safety in the home:

- Do you feel safe where you live?
- Do you need help taking care of yourself?
- Who prepares your meals?
- Who makes decisions about your finances?
- How many people are living in your home?

More-specific questions about maltreatment might include the following:

- Do you have any disagreements with your caregiver—if so, what are these disagreements about?
- When you disagree, what happens?
- Are you ever physically hurt or confined to your room?
- Do you ever have to wait long periods for food or your medicine?
- Has anyone ever failed to answer your requests for help?

When talking with the suspected abuser, empathy and an understanding approach go a long way in obtaining information about the patient's care environment. Try to identify specific issues that may present problems resulting from the patient's diagnosis. For example, close monitoring for skin breakdown in a patient with dementia and frequent episodes of incontinence is a challenge. In talking with this patient's caregiver, you might say, 'Caring for your father in this stage of his dementia must be a real challenge at times. Do you ever feel overwhelmed with the responsibility? How do you deal with it?' It is essential to avoid confrontation in this phase of the assessment.

Interventions

The competent elder person has the right to make his or her own personal care decisions. He or she may choose to stay in the abusive situation, despite all efforts to effect a change. Victims of abuse often have both positive and negative feelings towards their abusers. Such ambivalence makes separation from the abuser difficult for the abuse victim.

The primary goal of intervention is to protect the patient from immediate and future harm. A secondary—and equally important—goal of intervention is to break the cycle of mistreatment. The wellbeing of the abused individual must be considered concurrently with the coping ability of the abuser. Elder abuse is divided into two broad categories with regard to intervention in family-mediated abuse and neglect. First are cases in which the elder person has physical or mental impairment and is dependent on the family for daily care needs. The second group comprises individuals with minimal needs or care needs overshadowed by pathological behaviour of the caregiver. Potential intervention strategies include referrals to community agencies for continual monitoring of the situation, support services to decrease caregiver stress, close healthcare follow-up to prevent switching to another healthcare provider, reports to adult protective services with removal of the individual from a harmful environment or use of 24-hour supervision through a home health agency.

Care needs of older people in the home increase over time; however, resources of the family in terms of psychosocial and financial reserves do not always increase at the same rate. Intervention requires a multidisciplinary team approach. Such a team is able to assess aspects of the situation such as physical injury, mental status, competency, financial irregularities, legality, treatment, assistance, protection or prosecution. When there is a high degree of suspicion for elder abuse, consult social services or the responsible agency in your area. When appropriate, contact a home health agency to make an initial home assessment. In acute situations, the elder person may require shelter or protective care.

SUMMARY

Interpersonal violence is a pervasive, multi-factorial problem that affects the health and wellbeing of people in all countries and occurs across the life span. In every case of abuse, violence stems from the need to exert power and control over another person. The perpetrator of any form of violence transgresses the basic human rights of another for their own gain. Women and children are most often affected by violence, but men may also fall victim to sexual assault.

Paramedics have an important role in identifying cases of suspected abuse in individuals living in the community, and in referring these individuals to appropriate health agencies. As part of the multidisciplinary healthcare team, the emergency nurse is in a position to detect and manage the consequences of all types of interpersonal violence. In addition to their clinical role, emergency nurses have a responsibility to promote opportunistic self-disclosure of abuse among vulnerable populations when they are seeking emergency care for unrelated health problems.

Nurses also have statutory requirements to report child abuse and neglect in Australia, and it is vital that clinicians become familiar with the organisational and jurisdictional process for mandatory reporting of this type of abuse.

CASE STUDY

Child's history

Charlie is an 18-month-old boy. He was found by a neighbour at approximately 1900 hours crawling in his front yard, wearing only a nappy and a light T-shirt. The neighbour could not find his mother inside the house or yard, so contacted the police. The police attended the home and in turn called an ambulance. Charlie was assessed for evidence of injury by paramedics who comforted and warmed him before he was transported to the emergency department (ED) for further assessment and management.

On arrival in the ED, Charlie was found to be slightly dehydrated, cold and hungry. He was wrapped in a warm blanket and given a bottle, which he took well. At no time was he upset and was noted by the treating emergency doctor to be a happy and interactive child.

Charlie's medical records indicate that he was born via normal vaginal delivery at 32 weeks gestation; he was of low birth weight and was substance-affected. He spent three months in the neonatal intensive care unit. Due to his prematurity, low birth weight and substance withdrawal, he had some initial feeding and attachment problems with his mother. Concerns of a mild developmental delay were raised by the maternal and child health nurse at 12 months and were to be followed up in the paediatric clinic of the outpatient department; however, Charlie's mother did not attend the scheduled appointment.

Family history

Charlie is of Aboriginal descent and the youngest child in his family. He has two siblings (aged 3 and 4 years). His sister is currently living with his maternal grandmother; his brother is being cared for by his aunty. Charlie's mother Zoe is 20 years old and has a history of drug abuse, but has not used any illicit substances in the past 6 months.

Recently Zoe secured casual work and things were generally progressing very well for her and Charlie until she received a summons to attend court on the same day Charlie was taken to the ED. It was for this reason that Zoe needed to attend an urgent meeting with her solicitor and so left Charlie in the care of her boyfriend.

Charlie's father visits him one weekend per month. He currently lives approximately 2 hours away.

Questions

1. What are Charlie's actual and potential health problems?

2. Develop a care plan that addresses each of the problems you identify. In the plan include aims/goals, interventions and expected outcomes.

3. Outline the legal responsibilities of the nurse within your jurisdiction with regard to any protective concerns you have for Charlie.

 Answers to Case Study Questions can be found on evolve
http://evolve.emergencytrauma.curtis

REFERENCES

1. Krug EG, Dahlberg LL, Mercy JA et al. World report on violence and health. Geneva: World Health Organization; 2002.

2. World Health Organization. Global consultation on violence and health. Violence: a public health priority. Geneva: WHO; 1996.

3. Australian Institute of Family Studies. Child protection Australia 2010–2012. Canberra: Australian Institute of Health and Welfare; 2013. Online. www.aihw.gov.au/publication-detail/?id=60129542755; accessed 21 January 2014.

4. Commonwealth of Australia. Protecting children is everyone's business: national framework for protecting Australia's children 2009–20. Canberra: Australian Council of Governments; 2009.

5. Dube SR, Felitti VJ, Dong M et al. The impact of adverse childhood experiences on health problems: evidence from four birth cohorts dating back to 1900. Prev Med 2003;37(3):268–77.

6. Dube SR, Felitti VJ, Dong M et al. Childhood abuse, neglect, and household dysfunction and the risk of illicit drug use: the adverse childhood experiences study. Pediatrics 2003;11(3):564–72.

7. Felitti VJ. The relationship of adverse childhood experiences to adult health: turning gold into lead. Psychosom Med Psychother 2002;48(4):359–69.

8. Hillis SD, Anda RF, Felitti VJ et al. The association between adverse childhood experiences and adolescent pregnancy, long term psychosocial consequences, and fetal death. Pediatrics 2004;113(2):320–7.

9. Dong M, Dube SR, Felitti VJ et al. Adverse childhood experiences and self-reported liver disease: new insights into the causal pathway. Arch Intern Med 2003;163(16):1949–56.

10. Whitfield CL, Anda RF, Dube SR et al. Violent childhood experiences and the risk of intimate partner violence in adults: assessment in a large health maintenance organization. J Interpersonal Violence 2003;18(2):166–85.

11. Dube SR, Anda RF, Felitti VJ et al. Childhood abuse, household dysfunction, and the risk of attempted suicide throughout the lifespan: findings from the adverse childhood experiences study. JAMA 2001;286(24):3179–80.

12. United States Department of Health and Human Services. Sexual assault—nurse examiner development and operation guide. Office for Victims of Crime. Washington DC: U.S. Government Printing Office; 2000.

13. Kirschner RH, Wilson H. Pathology of fatal child abuse. In: Reece RM, Ludwig S, eds. Child abuse medical diagnosis and management. 2nd edn. Philadelphia: Lippincott Williams and Wilkins; 2001;467–516.

14. Reece RM, Ludwig S, eds. Child abuse: medical diagnosis and management. 2nd edn. Philadelphia: Lippincott Williams and Wilkins; 2001.

15. American Academy of Paediatrics: Committee on Child Abuse and Neglect. Shaken baby syndrome: rotational cranial injuries—technical report. Pediatrics 2001;108(1):206–10.

16. Barber MA, Davis PM. Fits, faints or fatal fantasy? Fabricated seizures and child abuse. Arch Dis Child 2002;86(4):230–3.

17. American Psychiatric Association. Diagnostic and statistical manual of mental disorders (DSM-V). 5th edn. Washington, DC: American Psychiatric Association; 2013;324–6.

18. Emergency Nurses Association USA, Centers for Disease Control and Prevention. Intimate partner violence: fact sheet. Emergency nursing core curriculum. 5th edn. 2000. Des Plaines: The Association; 2001.

19. The Royal Children's Hospital. Child Abuse Guideline. Melbourne: Royal Children's Hospital. Online. www.rch.org.au/clinicalguide/guideline_index/Child_Abuse_Guideline/; accessed 20 January 2014.

20. Joint Royal Colleges Ambulance Liaison Committee (JRCALC). UK Ambulance Service clinical practice guidelines. (2006). Coventry: JRCALC. Online. www2.warwick.ac.uk/fac/med/research/hsri/emergencycare/prehospitalcare/jrcalcstakeholderwebsite/guidelines.

21. Bromfield L, Higgins D. National comparison of child protection systems. In: Child abuse. Prevention Issues No. 22. Melbourne: Australian Institute of Family Studies.

22. Kelly P, MacCormick J, Strange R. Non-accidental head injury in New Zealand: the outcome of referral to statutory authorities. Child Abuse Negl 2009;33(6):393–401.

23. World Health Organization. Violence against women: a priority health issue. Geneva: WHO; 1997.

24. Bartels L. Emerging issues in domestic/family violence research Australian Institute of Criminology. 2010. Online. www.aic.gov.au/publications/current%20series/rip/1-10/10.html; accessed 15 June 2015.

25. Roberts GL, O'Toole BI, Raphael B et al. Prevalence study of domestic violence victims in an emergency department. Ann Emerg Med 1996;27(6):741–53.

26. de Vries Robbe, M, March L, Vinen J et al. Prevalence of domestic violence among patients attending a hospital emergency department. Aust N Z J Public Health 1996;20(4):364–8.

27. Laurie L. Violence against women: nurses lead the way in research and intervention for female assault victims. Am J Nurs 2005;105(9):72.

28. Morrison LJ, Allan R, Grunfeld A. Improving the emergency department detection rate of domestic violence using direct questioning. J Emerg Med 2000;19(2):117–24.

29. Taft A. Violence against women in pregnancy and after childbirth. Australian Domestic and Family Violence Clearinghouse Issues Paper 6. Sydney: University of NSW; 2002.

30. Ramsden C, Bonner M. An early identification and intervention model for domestic violence. Aust Emerg Nurs J 2002;5(1):15–20.

31. Feldhaus KM, Houry D, Kaminsky R. Lifetime sexual assault prevalence rates and reporting practices in an emergency department population. Ann Emerg Med 2000;36(1):23–7.

32. Collins KA, Bennett AT, Hanzlick R. Elder abuse and neglect. Autopsy Committee of the College of American Pathologists. Arch Intern Med 2000;160(11):1567–8.

CHAPTER 41
ALCOHOL, TOBACCO AND OTHER DRUG USE
CHARLOTTE DE CRESPIGNY AND JANICE ELLIOTT

Essentials

There are essential considerations regarding the safe care of people who may be affected by psychoactive substances such as alcohol, sedatives, opioids, psycho-stimulants or inhalants. These are:

- Never assume that the patient is merely affected by a psychoactive substance. All patients have the right to high-quality clinical assessment and treatment whether or not they are affected by psychoactive substances.
- A patient who is intoxicated or similarly incapacitated and cannot safely manage their environment, thinking, problem-solving or physical functions adequately is at serious risk of injury, misjudging situations or other people's behaviour and communication, and is unlikely to be able to give informed consent.
- A patient who is apparently intoxicated may *instead* have (for example) head or other serious injury, acute infection, stroke, hypoglycaemia or other medical crises.
- A patient who is intoxicated can *also* have a serious injury or other medical condition (which may or may not be obvious).
- A patient who is intoxicated and has a concurrent mental health condition may present as a result of the intoxication, which may or may not exacerbate a concurrent mental health condition.
- A patient may present moderately intoxicated, but still be at risk of imminent over-dose due to the amount (dose) of a substance recently consumed still taking effect—e.g. excessive binge-drinking.
- A patient may be at imminent risk of toxicity or overdose due to recent consumption of *more than one* substance such as alcohol and sedatives or opioids.
- A patient may present with an injury or other medical emergency and also be at risk of alcohol withdrawal—which can be life threatening.
- A person may have ceased or significantly reduced their usual level (dose) of consumption of a substance before presentation and withdrawal.
- Alcohol withdrawal alone or in combination with other depressants can be life threatening.
- Always err on the side of caution until satisfied that the patient is medically safe to leave.

INTRODUCTION

It is essential for the emergency clinician to have knowledge and understanding with regard to alcohol, tobacco and other drug (ATOD)-related presentations. Developing an understanding of the physiological and psychological effects of ATODs enable the anticipation, monitoring and early intervention and treatment of complications associated with ATOD use. Furthermore, developing an understanding of the clinical manifestations assists us to provide care in a humane and compassionate manner.

This chapter provides an overview of common ATOD use and likely emergency presentations. Several case studies are referred to throughout to assist your learning. The common substances are summarised, the likely clinical features of each group are presented and for a large number the specific care required for each overdose or withdrawal state is also presented.

An awareness and understanding of the physiological and psychological effects of ATOD is essential for the paramedic and emergency clinician. It enables clinicians to anticipate and monitor for potential complications and deterioration, commence assessment and treatment in the pre-hospital setting and further assist with assessment, diagnosis and ongoing treatment in the ED environment. As points of first contact emergency clinicians are uniquely placed to screen for ATOD use and detect risk factors and potential health problems. This provides an opportunity for early assessment, intervention and treatment.

Overview and background

Psychoactive substances: alcohol, tobacco and other drugs (ATODs)

The term 'drugs' is often used in reference to illicit drugs; however, in this chapter we are referring to all psychoactive substances, whether they be legal or illegal. These include alcohol, tobacco (nicotine) and other drugs. They also include pharmaceuticals, alternative preparations and various substances. In Australia, fewer people overall use illicit drugs compared with legal drugs such as alcohol, caffeine and nicotine, and prescribed and over-the-counter pharmaceuticals.[1,2]

ATODs have dose-related psychoactive effects on the central nervous system (CNS/brain), resulting in the person's altered physical function, mood and cognition. ATODs affect the CNS's (brain's) core body functions, such as respiration, temperature regulation, blood pressure, heart rate, conscious-ness and neural responses to external stimuli, including balance, movement, coordination and fine motor skills. ATODs can induce serious and often unpredictable adverse effects, including acute intoxication, overdose, toxicity and drug-induced psychosis. These effects can occur with first time use, occasional use or regular dependent use. These are commonly used ATODs:[1,2]

- Depressants, such as alcohol, sedatives, anaesthetics, ketamine, GHB, inhalants, opioids
- Psychostimulants, such as nicotine, caffeine, ephedrine, pseudoephedrine, adrenaline, methamphetamine, amphetamines, cocaine, mephedrone
- Hallucinogens, such as lysergic acid diethylamide (LSD), ecstasy (MDMA) *which also has psychostimulant effects*, magic mushrooms (psilocybin) and datura (angel trumpet plant)
- THC (Cannabis)—now in a category of its own due to its multiple effects on mood and cognition including CNS depression, thought and perceptual distortion, mild paranoia and hallucinations.

Regular use of most psychoactive drugs develops tolerance due to the CNS adapting its functions so as to maintain homeostasis. Tolerance requires the person to use increasing amounts/doses

to achieve the desired, original effect. Withdrawal can occur with cessation or rapid reduction in amount/dose of the ATOD use. The time of onset and length of the withdrawal symptoms depend on the type, action and half-life of the particular ATOD involved.

Note: alcohol withdrawal can be life threatening. ATOD-related problems are global. The World Health Organization (WHO) reports these to be within the top 20 risk factors for ill-health worldwide.[1]

While harmful ATOD consumption is preventable, risky use is associated with high rates of morbidity and mortality, representing a significant public and individual health and economic burden. More than 80% of Australians consume alcohol at some time, many from the age of 15 years. Many use prescribed and non-prescribed pharmaceuticals, and 'alternative' medicine; fewer people are now smoking tobacco in Australia. However, whether smoked, sniffed or chewed tobacco still causes the highest drug-related morbidity and mortality in Australian society. According to the 2010 National Drug Strategy Household Survey (2011):[3]

> … the proportion of people aged 14 years or older smoking daily (15.1%) declined, continuing a downward trend that began in 1995. The decline in daily smoking was largest for those aged in their early-20s to mid-40s, while the proportion of those aged over 45 years who smoked daily remained relatively stable or slightly increased between 2007 and 2010. Despite the decline in the proportion of people in Australia smoking tobacco, the number of smokers has remained stable between 2007 and 2010, at about 3.3 million.

Thus though tobacco use is declining, its longer term medical consequences are still impacting on continuing smokers, new smokers and those who have smoked.

Similarly, according to the same 2010 survey above, alcohol remains second to tobacco for morbidity and mortality.[3]

> As the Australian population has increased, the number of people drinking at risky levels increased between 2007 and 2010.

The risk of alcohol-related death or injury for healthy adult men and women is below 1 in 100 if they consume 2 or fewer standard drinks per day, i.e. up to two 10-gram beverages (10 to 20 grams of pure alcohol) in 24 hours. Caution is needed if drinking increases above this level due to risks of short- and longer-term alcohol-related injury, illness and death. This is incrementally more rapid for women than for men.[4] Alcohol-related injury and illnesses greatly impact on ambulance, emergency units, hospitals and various healthcare services.

Importantly, while there is decline in use of illicit drugs, non-medicinal use of pharmaceuticals (e.g. analgesics, opioids, anxiolytics) has increased. Legal and socially sanctioned drugs (e.g. tobacco and alcohol) are those most likely to cause serious injury, acute and chronic medical conditions and death to more people than those using illicit drugs (e.g. methampheta-mines and heroin) and resultant deaths and health problems overall.[3,4]

There are related, significant social and economic costs to individuals and the wider community from non-medical use of all psychoactive substances. Costs to the Australian economy are above several billion dollars per annum.[5]

Harmful ATOD use seriously affects individuals, families, communities and healthcare systems. In a New Zealand study of more than 1200 25-year-olds, 77% of the cohort had tried illicit drugs, with cannabis dependence accounting for the majority of illicit drug dependence.[6] The latest New Zealand survey[7] reported:

> In 2012/13, 0.2% of New Zealand adults aged 16–64 years reported having used amphetamines at least monthly … which equates to about 6000 New Zealanders … [with] no significant difference in self-reported 'at least monthly' amphetamine use between men (0.3%; 0.1–0.7) and women (0.1%; 0.1–0.3) … At least monthly amphetamine use declined with increasing age.

This indicates that younger people are more likely to use amphetamines and thus are at greater risk of emergency events.

The 2010 Australian National Drug Strategy Household Survey reported similar trends in methamphetamine and amphetamine use in Australia:[8]

> Between 1998 and 2010, there was a small decrease in the recent use of meth/amphetamines. Males aged between 20 and 29 years were the only age group to record a statistically significant decrease in recent meth/amphetamines use in 2010 (from 9.8% in 2007 to 6.8%). But they remain the age group most likely to have recently used meth/amphetamines in 2010. Meth/amphetamines use was high among unemployed.

Clinicians at the 'front-line' report that they regularly encounter people acutely affected by methamphetamine and amphetamines:[8]

> Recent [amphetamine] users were more than twice as likely as non-users to have been diagnosed with or treated for a mental illness in the previous 12 months (25.6% compared with 11.7%). And this proportion increased between 2007 and 2010 (from 20.3% in 2007 to 25.6%).

In 2009 the National Health and Medical Research Council reported that alcohol consumption accounted for 3.3% of the total burden of disease and injury in Australia in 2003.[4] Due to reporting anomalies, the actual number of alcohol-related emergency department (ED) presentations is unknown; it is likely to account for a large proportion of all presentations. For example, alcohol accounted for 13% of all deaths in 2006 among Australians aged 14–17 years and it is estimated that one Australian teenager dies and more than 60 are hospitalised weekly from alcohol-related causes.[4] Alcohol is a major contributor to premature death and hospitalisation of older Australians—among 65- to 74-year-olds, almost 600 die and a further 6,500 are hospitalised due to alcohol-related diseases.[4]

Understanding ATOD problems

Humans have used psychoactive substances for thousands of years. It should be stated that ATOD use always serves a purpose, no matter how risky or harmful. For example, ATOD use may serve ceremonial, medicinal, social or personal purposes. Each person's ATOD experience, and any associated problems, is always influenced by the dynamic interrelationship between the:

- environment in which the use occurs
- type of drug and its effects, and
- individual's physical and psychological characteristics, personal history, life experiences and cultural beliefs.[9]

All staff involved in healthcare delivery need to have an understanding of how a particular patient's life context and history, mental health, physical health, family and socioeconomic situation may influence their current pattern of ATOD use, and related health issues. For example, a person may have only used a particular drug once or they may use regularly. It should be considered whether a person has been living in an unsafe or violent family situation. Has the person been sexually or otherwise abused as a child or in their adult lives? Often but not exclusively, people with substance-use issues have poor life opportunities and experiences.

Terminology

As with any health condition, the professional language used to describe ATOD problems, including *dependence* (often referred to as addiction), needs to reflect the actual nature of the problem and related diagnosis. It is important that all paramedics and nurses, wherever they practise, use objective, accurate terms to describe a person's actual ATOD problem, and do not use stereotypical language or incorrect terms. Well-described conditions reliably convey a relevant diagnosis and related problems. For example, 'intoxication and short-term risk' and 'regular excessive use and long-term risk' are preferable to vague and less-precise terms such as 'alcoholism'. It is important not to stereotype and label people by using negative terms such as 'druggie', 'user', 'addict' or 'alcoholic', but rather to refer to them as the 'person', 'client' or 'patient', which humanises them and their problem. The terminology currently recommended in describing ATOD use is listed in Box 41.1.

Spectrum of ATOD problems

As well as understanding the dynamic interrelationship between the drug, the person and their environment, we must also understand that there is no 'one size fits all' single ATOD-related problem.[9] Rather, there is a spectrum of varying health and social problems. For some, these problems may be a single episode and never repeated. For others, the problems may be sporadic and occur from time to time. For yet others, their issues may be complex and more enduring. A person may vary their pattern of use according to circumstance, and be at risk of different problems over their lifetime. They may move in and out of various patterns of use, or cease ATOD use at some stage.[11] A minority of people develop complex co-existing mental illness (comorbidity) involving ATOD dependence and mental illnesses. They can be stabilised if consistently offered integrated assessment and treatment, and social support. Many, typically if untreated or undertreated, frequently relapse and have general and mental health complications requiring paramedic and emergency care.[9,12] Comorbidity is as a complex chronic illness.[12]

Take the case of a young person seriously injured while intoxicated with amphetamines (speed). He did not resume any speed use once he had recovered. When he was older, in response to the grief of losing his best friend, he started binge drinking, which quickly accelerated to daily drinking and dependence. His alcohol dependence was relatively short-lived, as he sought counselling and was assisted in working through his grief. He stopped drinking for 6 months as advised by his general practitioner. He did resume drinking later on, but within low-risk levels as a healthy adult male.

BOX 41.1 **Terminology of various patterns of ATOD use**

Experimental drinking or drug use

Drinking alcohol or another drug for the first time to experience the effects, or consuming unfamiliar types of alcoholic drinks or using other drugs. The person's experience of experimental drinking often determines whether or not they decide to drink again, or what type of alcohol they are likely to prefer. This pattern of drinking may be at low risk, or high risk to acute intoxication.

Social and recreational drinking or drug use

Drinking or using a drug to enhance personal pleasure in a social setting, and at levels which may or may not have harmful results. This term implies that the person is not dependent on the alcohol or other drug used.

Intoxication

Results from the acute pharmacological action of psychoactive drugs on the brain, in which the chemical (alcohol or other drug) changes brain function, perception and mood. The level of intoxication increases with *dose over time* (amount of drinks or drug consumed in a session), resulting in increasing levels of physical and behavioural changes and diminishing capacity.

Risky drinking or drug use

Drinking or using a drug at a level and frequency that increases the short-term risk of harm to health and safety, for example injuries or overdose from acute intoxication, such as can happen from experimental or occasional use; binge-drinking or binge drug use. If the person regularly drinks alcohol or uses drugs at a risky level, this is also referred to as *regular excessive use*.

High-risk drinking or drug use

Drinking or using a drug at a level and frequency that will cause harm to longer-term health, for example, physical (e.g. heart, liver or pancreatic disease) and mental health problems such as suicidal thoughts, depression, anxiety and/or sleep disturbances. High-risk drinking or drug use often has serious adverse family and social consequences. Again, this pattern of drinking is also referred to as *regular excessive use*.

Symptomatic drinking or drug use

Drinking to change or reduce unpleasant feelings, pain, thoughts or experiences, or to avoid certain situations or responsibilities. The person may drink to get a feeling of emotional or physical numbness or temporary happiness.

Tolerance

Alcohol or other drug tolerance occurs after a person has regularly consumed a psychoactive substance such as alcohol, and higher amounts of alcohol are then required to produce the same feelings of intoxication. The National Health and Medical Research Council explains this as:

> People who drink [alcohol] regularly at a given level gradually show less immediate and apparent effects of alcohol at this level of drinking. This tolerance has a metabolic element, whereby the liver becomes faster and more efficient at breaking down alcohol; and a functional element, whereby the person learns to cope with and compensate for the deficits induced by alcohol.[10]

Figure 41.1 illustrates how such problems may manifest, be interlinked and can resolve. Expanding on Thorley's model, the three major patterns of problems are discussed below.[13]

Depending on the nature and problems associated with a patient's ATOD use, and whether or not they want to have information or further assistance, an appropriate aftercare plan is required. This may include health information regarding ATOD use; information on access to local health and community services; and where to seek specialist services if needed.

Offer the patient and/or their family up-to-date written material and phone numbers where they can get reliable ATOD information and advice.

ATOD presentations

Intoxication

Intoxication is the acute action of psychoactive substances on the CNS (brain). The level of intoxication is according to dose and duration of continued consumption.[4,12] Intoxication may be a 'once-off' event, occasional or frequent. Intoxication can impact seriously on people's health, safety and social and personal situations. Importantly, the mood-altering effect and diminished cognitive capacity of an intoxicated person may place them at risk of self-harm, suicide or violence. Drug interactions may occur from concurrent use of other psychoactive drugs (poly-drug use). Accidental overdose may occur due to the ATOD itself.

Regular excessive use

Regular excessive use is the impact of regular excessive consumption of alcohol or another psychoactive substance such as a benzodiazepine or opioid; in other words, 'too much too often' but not at reliant levels (dependence). This has risks for both their short-term health and their longer-term health.[3,4,12]

While the person will not be psychologically dependent, they may have become physically tolerant (neuro-adapted) to the drug or alcohol. They need to consume more to feel the original intoxicating effects.

Tolerance

Tolerance is the response of the brain (central nervous system, CNS) to ensure that all normal brain functions are maintained in the presence of regular effects of a psychoactive drug such as a depressant like alcohol. The brain adapts to the regular amount of alcohol or drug in the body. The person may experience social or health problems associated with their ATOD use, such as financial problems, family or work problems, hypertension, heart disease, pancreatic or liver disease, hepatitis C, memory and other cognitive problems, injury or cancer, and so on.[12]

Dependence

What we mean by *dependence* is when a person is physically tolerant to, and psychologically dependent on (addicted to), the ATOD they are using. The following characteristics are common in people who are ATOD-dependent—the person:

- uses more of the drug than they intend to
- has made a number of unsuccessful attempts to cut down or control their use
- spends most of their time acquiring and using the drug—giving up or reducing time spent doing other important things (work, friends or family)

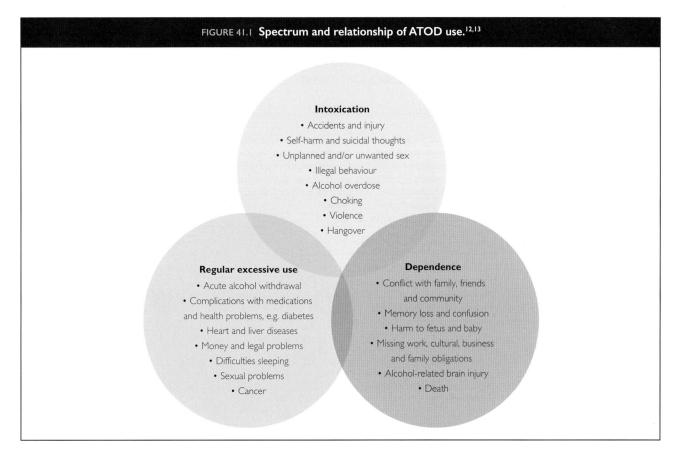

FIGURE 41.1 **Spectrum and relationship of ATOD use.**[12,13]

- continues to use despite knowing that there are associated medical, psychological or financial problems associated with using
- acquires physical tolerance (i.e. needs more of the drug to achieve the same effect)
- experiences psychological or physical withdrawal (often both) when they reduce or stop using the drug.

People who are dependent generally require medical, psychological and social support based on a comprehensive physical and mental health assessment, integrated co-morbidity management as required and intensive multidisciplinary interventions. This approach is required to assist them in managing this chronic condition, and its social and emotional consequences.[12,14] It is important to understand that despite the complexity of this condition, many people experiencing dependence can be successful in overcoming their ATOD dependence and go on to live optimal lives.[12]

ATOD emergency assessment and screening

Careful overall physical and ATOD assessment and monitoring are required, regardless of the environment, whether in a home, public place in transit or at the ED.

Physiological and neurological

Signs and symptoms related to ATOD effects are known to cause and complicate injuries and many serious illnesses.[12] The patient may be experiencing any one of a number of serious clinical problems associated with ATOD use, such as those outlined in Box 41.2.

BOX 41.2 Serious problems associated with ATOD use[12]

- Head or other serious injury
- Acute intoxication
- Complications from alcohol withdrawal
- Infection
- Overdose
- Psychosis
- Acute illness
- Unstable chronic illness.

The effects of frequently used ATOD are listed in Table 41.1. As with the assessment and management of any patients, first and foremost is safety of staff and patients, particularly with the angry or aggressive patient. Useful strategies to minimise risk are outlined in Box 41.3.

ATOD screening and assessment are crucial to making an accurate diagnosis and deciding on and delivering safe and appropriate care.[12] It is very important for paramedic and emergency staff to feel confident and competent in identifying and intervening effectively in these patients' acute ATOD problems according to the particular context of care delivery.

Some diagnoses can be masked or confused by the presence of AOD intoxication or withdrawal.[12] This can lead to medical problems being wrongly diagnosed or overlooked. Examples of such problems are summarised in Box 41.4.

It is therefore very important to remember that what *may appear* to be an ATOD presentation *may not be*. It could be a

TABLE 41.1 Effects of frequently abused substances[15]

SUBSTANCE	PHYSIOLOGICAL AND PSYCHOLOGICAL EFFECTS	EFFECTS OF OVERDOSE	WITHDRAWAL SYMPTOMS
Stimulants			
Nicotine	Increased arousal and alertness; performance enhancement; increased heart rate, cardiac output and blood pressure; cutaneous vasoconstriction; fine tremor, decreased appetite; antidiuretic effect; increased gastric motility	Rare: nausea, abdominal pain, diarrhoea, vomiting, dizziness, weakness, confusion, decreased respirations, seizures, death from respiratory failure	Craving, restlessness, depression, hyperirritability, headache, insomnia, decreased blood pressure and heart rate, increased appetite
Cocaine Amphetamines: amphetamine, chlorphentermine, dextroamphetamine, methamphetamine, methylphenidate	Euphoria, grandiosity, mood swings, hyperactivity, hyperalertness, restlessness, anorexia, insomnia, hypertension, tachycardia, marked vasoconstriction, tremor, dysrhythmias, seizures, sexual arousal, dilated pupils, diaphoresis	Agitation; increased temperature, pulse, respiratory rate, blood pressure; cardiac dysrhythmias, myocardial infarction, hallucinations, seizures, possible death	Severe craving, severely depressed mood, exhaustion, prolonged sleep, apathy, irritability, disorientation
Caffeine	Mood elevation, increased alertness, nervousness, jitteriness, irritability, insomnia; increased respirations, heart rate and force of myocardial contraction; relaxation of smooth muscle, diuresis	Rare: hyperstimulation, nervousness, confusion, psychomotor agitation, anxiety, dizziness, tinnitus, muscle twitching, elevated blood pressure, tachycardia, extrasystoles, increased respiratory rate	Headache, irritability, drowsiness, fatigue
Depressants			
Alcohol Sedative–hypnotics: *barbiturates*: phenobarbitone, pentobarbitone *benzodiazepines*: diazepam, alprazolam *non-barbiturates–non-benzodiazepines:* chloral hydrate zolpidem zopiclone	Initial relaxation, emotional lability, decreased inhibitions, drowsiness, lack of coordination, impaired judgment, slurred speech, hypotension, bradycardia, bradypnoea, constricted pupils	Shallow respirations; cold, clammy skin; weak, rapid pulse; hyporeflexia, coma, possible death	Anxiety, agitation, insomnia, diaphoresis, tremors, delirium, seizures, possible death
Opioids			
Heroin Morphine Opium Codeine Fentanyl Hydromorphone Dextropropoxyphene Pentazocine Pethidine Oxycodone Methadone	Analgesia, euphoria, drowsiness, detachment from environment, relaxation, constricted pupils, constipation, nausea, decreased respiratory rate, slurred speech, impaired judgment, decreased sexual and aggressive drives	Slow, shallow respirations; clammy skin; constricted pupils; coma; possible death	Watery eyes, dilated pupils, runny nose, yawning, tremors, pain, chills, fever, diaphoresis, nausea, vomiting, diarrhoea, abdominal cramps

TABLE 41.1 Effects of frequently abused substances[15]—cont'd

SUBSTANCE	PHYSIOLOGICAL AND PSYCHOLOGICAL EFFECTS	EFFECTS OF OVERDOSE	WITHDRAWAL SYMPTOMS
Cannabis			
Marijuana Hashish	Relaxation, euphoria, lack of motivation, slowed time sensation, sexual arousal, abrupt mood changes, impaired memory and attention, impaired judgment, reddened eyes, dry mouth, lack of coordination, tachycardia, increased appetite	Fatigue, paranoia, panic reactions, hallucinogen-like psychotic states	None except for rare insomnia, hyperactivity
Hallucinogens			
Lysergic acid diethylamide (LSD) Psilocybin (mushrooms) Dimethyltryptamine (DMT) Diethyltryptamine (DET) 3,4-Methylenedioxy-methamphetamine (MDMA) Mescaline (peyote) Phencyclidine (PCP)	Perceptual distortions, hallucinations, delusions (PCP), depersonalisation, heightened sensory perception, euphoria, mood swings, suspiciousness, panic, impaired judgment, increased body temperature, hypertension, flushed face, tremor, dilated pupils, constricted pupils (PCP), nystagmus (PCP), violence (PCP)	Prolonged effects and episodes, anxiety, panic, confusion, blurred vision, increases in blood pressure and temperature	None
Inhalants			
Aerosol propellants Fluorinated hydrocarbons Nitrous oxide (in deodorants, hair spray, pesticide, whipped cream spray, spray paint, cookware coating products) Solvents (petrol, kerosene, nail polish remover, typewriter correction fluid, cleaning solutions, lighter fluid, paint, paint thinner, glue) Anaesthetic agents (nitrous oxide, chloroform) Nitrates (amyl nitrate, butyl nitrate)	Euphoria, decreased inhibitions, giddiness, slurred speech, illusions, drowsiness, clouded sensorium, tinnitus, nystagmus, dysrhythmias, cough, nausea, vomiting, diarrhoea, irritation to eyes, nose, mouth	Anxiety, respiratory depression, cardiac dysrhythmias, loss of consciousness, sudden death	None

---

BOX 41.3 Clinical tips for the angry or aggressive intoxicated patient[12]

Remember: your safety comes first. Try to:
- work in pairs
- stand slightly side-on, at least half an arm's length away, and with your feet slightly apart
- use space for self-protection—ensure that you have easy access to the open door
- give them space too—do not crowd them; keep furniture between yourself and them if feeling unsafe, etc
- speak in a calm, reassuring way
- avoid raising your voice. Keep your own emotions in check

- avoid challenging or threatening them by your tone of voice, eyes or body language
- let them air their feelings and acknowledge these
- determine the source of their anger and, if possible, alleviate it
- be flexible with their care, within reason
- be aware of workplace policies on preventing and managing aggression
- use available security measures or carry a personal duress alarm.

> **BOX 41.4 Examples of medical conditions at risk of being misdiagnosed or overlooked in the presence of ATOD intoxication or withdrawal[12]**
>
> - Head injury
> - Cerebrovascular accident (CVA)
> - Infection
> - Hypoxia
> - Hypoglycaemia
> - Other metabolic imbalances
> - Liver disease
> - Impending overdose
> - Adverse drug reaction
> - Psychosis.

condition that mimics intoxication or withdrawal and yet be disguising an acute injury or medical condition. Alternatively, it may be that intoxication or withdrawal is complicating another serious condition.

Due to the high and frequent occurrence of serious injury and illness among people presenting with intoxication and other ATOD conditions to the emergency setting, two key concepts need to be kept in the forefront of clinicians' minds. These are *'think pathology first'* and consider the possibility of *other or multiple co-existing diagnoses*. Through developing an understanding of what the behavioural and physical manifestations are for each stage of intoxication or withdrawal, the clinician will be able to confidently develop a clinical 'index of suspicion' for the patient presenting with behavioural or physical symptoms secondary to ATOD use.[12]

Alcohol (or what seems to be) intoxication is commonly associated with trauma and serious medical conditions. Detecting whether alcohol is present, and subsequently measuring concentration, is critical in discerning the apparent effect. This can assist differential diagnosis. Is intoxication the single condition, or is there the risk of concurrent injury, toxicity or medical emergency?[12]

Engaging with the patient with ATOD problems

A person may present to the usually busy ED for a number of reasons. It is always an ideal setting to screen them for ATOD problems. This not only offers the emergency staff the means to better understand their patient's immediate requirements, but it is a timely opportunity to provide:

- early and brief intervention
- access to community services
- referral to specialist treatment if needed.

This is as important for this patient as it is for a patient with any other serious health problem. All of these activities can be delivered quickly, with little difficulty and to good effect by emergency clinicians. These are not time-consuming and can be implemented while attending to the patient's general healthcare requirements. Importantly, they are known to be effective.[12]

Showing concern about how you may help the person will increase the likelihood of their engagement with the conversation about their recent ATOD intake and current concerns. It is of primary importance to be aware of your own beliefs about people's ATOD use, and to promote a non-judgmental manner. Patients need to be assured that this is usual practice for all patients, as ATOD use is a genuine health issue. Similarly, patients need to understand that in order to help the patient it is important to know what ATODs they use and any problems related to this.

Opening questions can be as simple as:

- 'Can you tell me if you currently use alcohol, tobacco or other drugs?'
- 'Can you tell me what you have been taking recently?'
- 'Was there anything different about what you chose to take today?'
- 'Can you tell me what you have taken today?'
- 'What time did you last take your alcohol, tobacco or other drug/s?'

It is essential that the questioning be empathetic in tone. Emergency staff want to help the patient by understanding the patient's circumstances and accurately assessing their needs. An interrogative tone by staff will only result in the patient becoming defensive and evasive. However, it should be noted that the highly pressured and time-constrained pre-hospital and ED environments might provide challenges to a consistently empathetic approach.

Screening for risk

The first step to identifying the patient who is at risk from immediate or longer-term ATOD problems is to screen for patterns of use and risk of harm. To do this well, it is necessary to use valid, reliable screening instruments that are easy to use and not time-consuming. The result of a screening is an assessment of the patient's ATOD history and its impact on their current condition and overall health.[12] This forms the basis of a good diagnosis and informs which interventions may be required in the ED, as well as longer-term strategies. While the ED is usually very busy, it is necessary to remember the immediate and life-threatening risks a patient may present with. The screening process is not prolonged. However, the nurse or doctor may feel they do not have enough time because of competing demands and may have difficulty maintaining patient focus. Nonetheless, screening is necessary for:

- duty of care of the patient
- making an accurate diagnosis of the current problem
- raising patients' awareness of risky practices
- longer-term benefits through referral and support mechanisms.

Failure to adequately screen may have lethal consequences.

A recently validated screening tool to identify alcohol, tobacco and other drug risk is the Alcohol, Smoking and Substance Involvement Screening Test (ASSIST).[15] ASSIST is designed for busy generalist clinicians. It is an easy-to-use questionnaire that takes between 5 and 8 minutes to administer, and from which the patient score will indicate their level of risk. It screens for risky and high-risk use of alcohol, tobacco, cannabis, cocaine, amphetamines, sedatives, hallucinogens, inhalants and opiates. It also includes a guide for delivery of a brief intervention, which can be applied in any healthcare setting.[12,16]

If screening reveals there is risk due to the person's alcohol consumption or other drug use, they then need to be fully assessed. This involves taking the ATOD-use history in a safe, confidential place with sensitivity towards the patient (and their family). As always, respect for the patient's cultural identity and associated needs is paramount.[17]

Assessment for diagnosis

Assessment should be carried out in a timely manner. The patient must not be intoxicated, acutely ill or incapacitated. In the ED it may be that their assessment is relatively brief so as to determine the most pressing risk factors and how these may affect their condition. If time and the patient's condition allows, and depending on the resources available, then a more extensive assessment can be undertaken by an ED clinician, specialist ATOD liaison nurse or medical officer. Importantly, the findings from the ATOD assessment need to be communicated to the whole ED team and, if the patient is admitted, the ward team. This will form the basis of further diagnosis and the type of interventions required for the patient's particular condition. The wider multidisciplinary team may need to undertake more-detailed investigations and utilise specialist input as available.

Full assessment can be undertaken once the patient has been transferred to a ward or other relevant facility. Early referral within the hospital or to a community service is important if the patient is likely to have a serious ATOD problem.

Dependence, with tolerance influencing risk of withdrawal, is a critical issue for ATOD assessment. Similarly, identification of any co-existing mental health or related physical problems is crucial. Figure 41.2 offers a systematic way of undertaking the ATOD assessment. If assessment has revealed problems associated with the person's recent and longer term ATOD use, then selections of key medical and psychological therapies need to be employed when appropriate.

Taking the ATOD history

When taking a patient's ATOD history, *show the patient you are concerned about their health and drug use without judging or rejecting them*—any drug use, including illicit drug use, is a legitimate health issue in the ED, not a moral issue. Again, it is about being aware of your own personal beliefs in order to ensure that you have strategies to combat these. Many patients feel embarrassed and ashamed, and have had bad experiences in the past with healthcare professionals who have refused help or been judgmental. Offer high-quality health information about ATOD use for them to take home. Invite them to talk to a professional that you can refer them to. Alternatively, suggest they phone their local alcohol and drug information service (you can give them the phone number or even make the call for them at the time). If the patient is resistant or becomes anxious or angry, do not persist—rephrase the questions, leave the conversation to another time or desist altogether.[12]

For general assessment guidance, see Section 2.2 in *Alcohol, Tobacco and Other Drugs: Clinical Guidelines for Nurses and Midwives 2012*, and for information about accessing validated assessment tools, see Section 4.[12]

Some specific concerns
Mental health problems
It is important to recognise the need for mental health assessment and psychosocial support. If significant problems

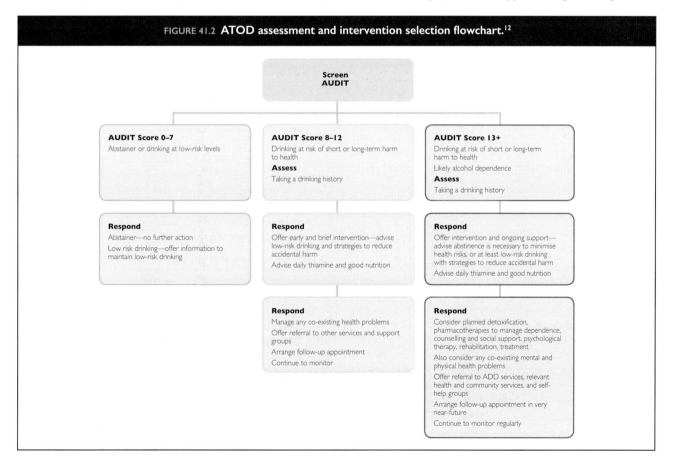

FIGURE 41.2 ATOD assessment and intervention selection flowchart.[12]

exist at this time ensure that a comprehensive mental health examination is undertaken once the patient is stable and able to be interviewed.

Transmission of blood-borne viruses

There may be a risk that serious medical complications are associated with the patient's injecting drug use; for example, if they have injected amphetamines or heroin and shared any of the injecting equipment, including needles, syringes, tourniquets, spoons and water when mixing the drug, etc. Any of these items can spread bacterial infections causing septicaemia, cellulitis, endocarditis and pericarditis, and blood-borne viruses such as human immunodeficiency virus (HIV) and hepatitis B and C. Other serious complications can occur from injecting drugs, including damage to blood vessels at injection sites, abscesses, thromboses, kidney or liver damage, electrolyte abnormalities and dysrhythmias.[12]

Physical signs of non-medical injecting drug use and thus risks of viral or bacterial infection:[12]

- abnormal but even pupil size (uneven pupil sizes are associated with serious medical conditions) in association with:
  - puncture marks in cubical fossa, or other accessible veins
  - cellulitis associated with possible injection sites
  - phlebitis associated with possible injection sites
  - endocarditis.

Concealment of illicit drugs

The process of swallowing or inserting illegal packets of drugs for the purpose of evading law enforcement can be fatal. Individuals engaged in such activities are frequently labelled in the media as 'body packers' or 'mules'. The most frequent cause of death among people concealing drugs is acute drug intoxication, overdose or toxicity from rupture of the package(s) within the gastrointestinal tract.[18] In EDs near airports, people who may have concealed drugs internally are often brought in by police and, less commonly, may self-present, because the drugs they have concealed have begun to be absorbed which is extremely dangerous and likely to cause rapid overdose or toxicity. Heroin, cocaine, methylenedioxymethylamphetamine (MDMA or ecstasy) are drugs known to be concealed during importation, usually in swallowed or rectally inserted plastic bags, packets or condoms (Fig 41.3).[1,3,4,7,19]

The perforation of a concealed package is life threatening. Each patient should be assessed immediately for signs of increasingly acute intoxication (discussed later in the chapter), treated accordingly, observed and monitored closely. Any patient that does not pass a primary survey (ABCD) at any time during their presentation must have the assessment halted and life-saving measures implemented. These patients should all have an abdominal examination and a non-contrast abdominal computed tomography (CT) scan. No investigations can be undertaken without their consent. No CT should be performed on a woman who may be pregnant. If there is a possibility that she is pregnant, a beta-hCG (human chorionic gonadotropin) test should be performed prior to CT to confirm whether or not she is pregnant. CT scans should be reported by an emergency or radiology registrar/consultant prior to discharging the patient. If there is a high clinical index of suspicion and the CT findings are equivocal, consent must

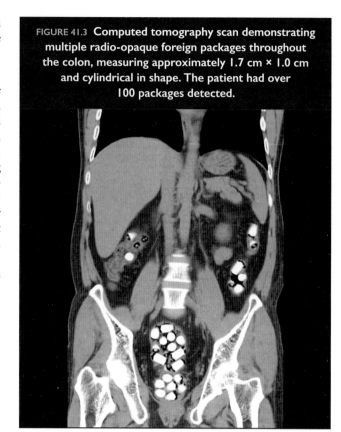

FIGURE 41.3 Computed tomography scan demonstrating multiple radio-opaque foreign packages throughout the colon, measuring approximately 1.7 cm × 1.0 cm and cylindrical in shape. The patient had over 100 packages detected.

Courtesy Department of Radiology, St George Public Hospital, Sydney.

be gained for an oral liquid bowel evacuation stimulant to be administered. The nursing staff and police must sight the resulting motions.

If concealment is confirmed, the patient should be observed closely and treated with privacy. Continue to observe for signs of drug intoxication and any physical signs and symptoms of overdose. With consent from the patient, an oral liquid bowel preparation solution should be given to accelerate evacuation. Enemas and suppositories should not be used because of the risk of package perforation. If the patient refuses to take the preparation, they should be admitted and observed until all packages are passed. An estimate of the number of packages on initial CT should be made and a check CT carried out to confirm absence of further packages. The patient should remain in hospital under police supervision until the repeat CT is clear and all packages are accounted for.

ATOD *and* mental illness (comorbidity)

It is recognised that people experiencing a serious ATOD problem, particularly dependence, are very likely to experience co-existing mental health conditions (co-morbidity).[12,14] A significant number of these people present to EDs in crisis because they are seriously affected by their ATOD use and/or their mental health condition. Most commonly, these are anxiety disorders, particularly post-traumatic stress disorder or depression, and patients are at risk of self-harm or suicide. The less common disorders are psychotic conditions, such as bipolar disorder or schizophrenia. All of these patients require specialist assessment, monitoring and individualised treatment once their emergency crisis is resolved (Ch 37). Such patients will respond best if they are assessed and treated using an integrated, shared-care approach involving the medical team, nursing team, specialist ATOD and mental health teams. It is now well recognised that these patients can and will respond better to this combined approach to treatment being delivered simultaneously rather than sequentially, even though the latter still occurs in some areas. It is recognised that trying to treat one disorder before the other is far less effective, and also runs the serious risk of exacerbating relapse and worsening health overall.[1,12,14,20,21]

Drug-induced psychosis

The acute effects of some psychoactive drugs may induce acute psychosis, which is very likely to resolve, providing no further use of that drug occurs. These drugs are predominantly THC (cannabis), psychostimulants (e.g. amphetamine, methamphetamine, cocaine) and occasionally alcohol. Which people are vulnerable to drug-induced psychosis is poorly understood. It may occur with 'once off' or irregular use or regular longer-term use. The patient needs to feel safe and protected from self-harm or endangering others. They may experience suicidal ideation.

Duration of drug-induced psychosis

The duration is variable due to the pharmacological properties of the drug and its action on the CNS and half-life. It is important to note that while psychostimulant-induced psychosis can resolve following cessation of psycho-stimulant use, this may take from days to weeks to settle fully.[12,22]

Acute medical management

This patient requires pharmacological management typically involving a combination of benzodiazepines and antipsychotics.[12,22–23]

Benzodiazepines directly sedate the patient, while antipsychotics take time (for example, 2–3 weeks to take the required antipsychotic effect), so they have the benefit of producing immediate, short-term sedative effect. Pharmacological interventions are usually necessary to adequately assess the patient for their mental health, ATOD and physical health condition/s. The patient will also need to be admitted as a hospital inpatient. They are likely to be detained under the appropriate Mental Health Act (Ch 37), under which you must practise.

Major ATOD groups

To access the major categories and subgroups of commonly used ATODs within each group, see Section 3 in *Alcohol, Tobacco and Other Drugs: Clinical Guidelines for Nurses and Midwives 2012*.[12]

Depressants

Alcohol

Alcohol is absorbed rapidly across the wall of the small intestine and carried to the brain by the blood. It travels to every organ of the body, having a potentially toxic effect on all physiological systems.[4,12,24] While the rate of absorption is delayed slightly in the presence of food, especially proteins and fats, within only a short time (minutes), it is carried to the brain and intoxicates the person according to the amount consumed. Faster absorption occurs when alcohol is mixed with carbonated liquids. Metabolism of alcohol is predominantly by the liver, and occurs at a rate of about one standard drink (10 g of

pure alcohol) per hour. This cannot be accelerated by drinking water, juice, coffee or other means.

The concentration of alcohol in the body can be determined by assessing the breath or blood alcohol concentration (BAC). Alcohol may be measured in the blood within 15–20 minutes of ingestion, peaks in 60–90 minutes and is excreted in 12–24 hours. BAC is affected by the amount consumed, drinking rate, body size and composition, drink concentration, gender and hormones. For the healthy adult drinker who has not developed CNS tolerance, the BAC is generally predictable of the effects of alcohol. Importantly for the emergency clinician, a patient's BAC may still be rising for some time after presentation, depending on when they last drank.

It is important to know that for healthy adult men who regularly drink more than 60 g or more (6 standard drinks) most days and healthy adult non-pregnant women who regularly drink more than 40 g or more (4 standard drinks) most days, there is an associated and significant additional risk of long-term physical conditions. These risks increase rapidly with further drinking above these limits.[4] Cancer, cardiovascular disease, stomach, pancreatic, liver and kidney disease, blood dyscrasias, osteoporosis, malnutrition, neurological and other serious conditions can all be caused or acutely and chronically exacerbated by alcohol.[4,12,24]

There is a high likelihood of co-morbidity of mental health problems with alcohol dependence, particularly depression and anxiety disorders, as well as a range of serious physical illnesses. Alcohol can interact with, or alter the effect of, many over-the-counter and prescribed medications, as well as other drugs.[24,25]

Drugs that interact with alcohol in an additive or synergistic manner include opioids, anti-hypertensive, antibiotics, antihistamines, anti-anginal medications and salicylates (aspirin). Alcohol taken with aspirin may cause or exacerbate gastrointestinal (GI) bleeding. Alcohol taken with paracetamol can increase the risk of liver damage. Potentiation and cross-tolerance of alcohol with other CNS depressants is a serious risk when another CNS depressant is taken with alcohol, increasing the depressant effect and possibility of overdose; for example, benzodiazepines and opioids.

Effects

Alcohol has complex effects on the neurons in the brain. It increases the levels of dopamine, and depresses all areas and functions of the CNS. The effects of alcohol are related to the concentration of alcohol consumed (dose), how much is consumed over time and the person's age, gender, health status and individual susceptibility to the drug.[12]

High blood ethanol levels are associated with respiratory depression and an increased risk of vomiting and aspiration leading to pulmonary oedema.[26] Aspiration is the most significant cause of death in non-injury ethanol-related deaths, due mainly to depression of the gag-reflex. Ethanol is a vasodilator, especially of cutaneous vessels, partly due to a depressant effect on the central vasomotor centre, but also due to a direct effect on peripheral blood vessels.[27] This results in a small reduction in systolic blood pressure and stroke volume and a compensatory increase in heart rate and cardiac output. In addition, as ethanol directly irritates the lining of the oesophagus and stomach and induces vomiting, especially with large ingestion, a 9-Weiss tear causing haematemesis may result.[28] Minor effects include oesophagitis, gastritis and symptoms similar to those associated with gastro-oesophageal reflux disease.

The effects of ethanol on the elderly are often multi-factorial and additive. A combination of reduced lean body mass and liver enzyme function, together with decreased gastric motility, may lead to higher blood alcohol levels and an exacerbation of effects. In addition, because of altered pharmacokinetic parameters, especially metabolism and elimination, concurrent pharmacotherapy may be affected, particularly those drugs with a narrow therapeutic window such as digoxin, warfarin and potassium supplements and those relying on renal clearance such as opiate analgesics, e.g. codeine.

It is important for ED clinicians to be aware of the harmful organic effects that can be caused by harmful alcohol use and how this may affect the patient's current condition, including differential diagnosis and co-morbidities, and increased risks of complications including toxicity, haemorrhage, thrombosis or hypertension.

Intoxication

Intoxication is potentially lethal and may be associated with accidental injury or overdose. It can also exacerbate many health conditions. When a patient presents to the ED in an intoxicated state, it is often not appropriate to try to educate or suggest to them that they stop drinking or offer them complex health information. They are unlikely to be able to understand or remember what you have said. What is important is not to assume they are 'just intoxicated'—*always assume* that there may be an underlying injury or serious medical condition.[12,25] Alcohol intoxication increases the likelihood of head injury, which is the predominant medical risk for intoxicated people and should always be the first consideration when assessing an intoxicated person or someone who appears intoxicated.

The acute effects of alcohol intoxication involve depressed respiration, diminished cough, diminished gag reflexes (potential for aspiration and asphyxiation) and cardiovascular dysfunction inducing various dysrhythmias. As with other depressant drugs, people are also at risk of accidental overdose from excessive alcohol, and there is a strong link between intoxication of alcohol and suicide.[4,15,25] Binge-drinking excessive amounts of alcohol over a brief period of time (hours not days) can lead to sudden cardiac dysrhythmias, shortness of breath, changes in blood pressure and sudden death. Older or frail people have an increased risk of falls and serious injury from drinking even small amounts. They may also experience serious drug interactions if they drink when taking medicines or other substances. Young people who drink to intoxication are often at greater risk because they lack experience and skills in managing drinking and can become very acutely intoxicated, leading to overdose.

Intoxication is evidenced with increasing BAC, increasingly diminished capacity of the person to manage their environment, their mood, behaviour and physical changes. Effects include an initial sense of relaxation, euphoria, loss of inhibitions; then impaired judgment, poor concentration and mood swings. For example, a person may transition from elation to depression, possible aggression, irritability and emotional lability. Box 41.5 lists the common signs of alcohol intoxication.

The person who is alcohol-tolerant will have a higher BAC than expected from their observed behaviour, and an apparent lower level of intoxication. That is, they do not seem as

BOX 41.5 Signs of alcohol intoxication[12]

- Positive blood alcohol concentration
- Flushing—dilation of peripheral blood vessels
- Altered cognition
- Inappropriate emotional responses
- Smell of alcohol
- Slurred or incoherent speech
- Mood swings
- Increasing sedation
- Ataxia
- Analgesic effect despite injury/illness
- Altered behaviour
- Decreasing consciousness.

intoxicated as one would expect looking at their clinical signs. This explains why some people who are tolerant to alcohol, as evidenced by high BAC (e.g. well over the legal driving limit for adults of 0.05% in Australia and 0.08% in New Zealand), genuinely believe that they are safe to drive or undertake other complex tasks. It is a complex issue.

Be aware that an intoxicated person whose first language is not English may revert to their native tongue at this time and therefore have difficulty communicating or understanding instructions, and so on.

Figure 41.4 illustrates the signs according to level of alcohol intoxication as detected by BAC in the non-alcohol-tolerant adult. This can be reliably obtained by blood or breath measurement.

Out-of-hospital and ED management

As with all patients, management includes monitoring and responding appropriately to the patient's vital signs and level of consciousness. Guidelines for the level of observation and intervention for different levels of intoxication are outlined in Table 41.2. Like other depressants, alcohol can cause overdose if a person has consumed high doses over a short period of time. Alcohol-induced CNS depression leads to respiratory and circulatory failure manifested by depressed respirations, hypotension, hypothermia, decreasing level of consciousness and high BAC. This can occur with binge-drinking or drinking alcohol while taking other CNS depressants.

Priorities include maintenance of a patent airway and gas exchange (primary survey—ABCD). Interventions will be dependent on the individual clinician's scope of practice; in the pre-hospital setting, this may include the insertion of supraglottic devices or the insertion of an endotracheal tube; in the ED the nurse should be prepared to assist with intubation if required and be proficient in the administration of oxygen. See Chapter 17, p. 314, for airway management techniques. The establishment of intravenous (IV) access should be considered when possible, as hypotension can be corrected with IV fluids. Hypothermia can be corrected with either passive or active warming, dependent upon the available resources. It is essential to conduct a thorough health examination of the physical state, specifically assessing for any signs of injury. Exclude medical conditions other than alcohol intoxication (e.g. head injury, CVA, drug overdose, hypoglycaemia, psychosis, severe

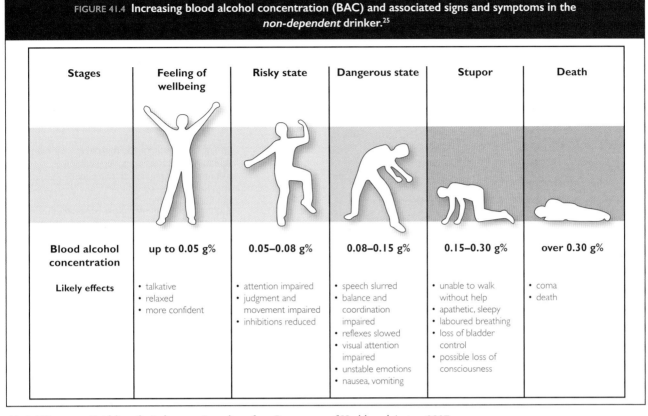

FIGURE 41.4 Increasing blood alcohol concentration (BAC) and associated signs and symptoms in the *non-dependent* drinker.[25]

Stages	Feeling of wellbeing	Risky state	Dangerous state	Stupor	Death
Blood alcohol concentration	up to 0.05 g%	0.05–0.08 g%	0.08–0.15 g%	0.15–0.30 g%	over 0.30 g%
Likely effects	• talkative • relaxed • more confident	• attention impaired • judgment and movement impaired • inhibitions reduced	• speech slurred • balance and coordination impaired • reflexes slowed • visual attention impaired • unstable emotions • nausea, vomiting	• unable to walk without help • apathetic, sleepy • laboured breathing • loss of bladder control • possible loss of consciousness	• coma • death

Alcohol Treatment Guidelines for Indigenous Australians from Department of Health and Ageing, 2007.

liver disease), using blood tests, X-rays, scans and so on, as appropriate.

The management of the patient with an altered level of consciousness is discussed in Chapter 23. Because of the risk of vomiting and subsequent aspiration, offer ice chips rather than water. IV fluids are required to maintain hydration if the patient is not well enough to drink water safely after 12 hours. The administration of parenteral thiamine is required for those patients considered to be at risk of thiamine deficiency due to poor nutritional status (and this includes those who are regular drinkers). If the patient requires ongoing IV glucose in order to establish normal blood glucose levels, thiamine must be administered in order to prevent Wernicke's encephalopathy. Previously the recommendations have been for administration of IV thiamine prior to administration of glucose in order to prevent Wernicke's encephalopathy. There are no clear guidelines in relation to this, and current literature suggests that a single dose of glucose is unlikely to cause this effect. The urgent treatment of hypoglycaemia with glucose should not be delayed in order for thiamine to be administered.[29]

Ascertain the patient's mental status (e.g. confusion, suicidal ideation, disorientation, panic, hallucinations, paranoia and psychosis). The intoxicated patient is at an extreme risk of falling: take all precautions to prevent this. For example, lower the bed, put padded bed rails up, do not ever leave them unaccompanied in the toilet, assist them to stand and walk if required and ensure the patient is closely observed. If the patient is to be admitted, the ED nurse should ensure that regular TPR and BP observations are undertaken concurrently

once commencement of monitoring with the CIWAR-Ar withdrawal chart has begun.[12]

It is important to have as accurate information as possible about the amount and frequency of drinking, and particularly *time of the last drink*. Document this clearly in the case notes and hand-over to team members in the ED and receiving ward. When taking a drinking history, do not accept or use phrases such as 'social drinker' or 'occasional drinker'. If the person cannot give exact amounts initially, ask in a non-judgmental manner questions such as:

'How many drinks have you had today?'

'What type of container was the alcohol in?'

'Is this how much you usually drink in a day?'

'How long have you been drinking like this?'

The intoxicated patient may present in various emotional states; Tables 41.2 and 41.3 shows how the clinician can best respond and support them, taking into consideration possible risks.[12]

Thiamine deficiency: Wernicke's encephalopathy

Thiamine carries glucose across the brain barrier. Chronic alcohol consumption affects thiamine in the body in at least two ways: it decreases the absorption of thiamine from the GI tract and changes the structure of thiamine. The alteration of thiamine molecules prevents their utilisation in the cells. Insufficient thiamine leads to Wernicke's encephalopathy, which is an acute inflammatory haemorrhagic condition of the brain, and an acute medical crisis.

Thiamine (vitamin B_1) deficiency is common in people who are malnourished and/or regularly drink alcohol at high-risk levels.[12] It is precipitated by the intake of glucose by the

TABLE 41.2 Observations and actions required to care for the intoxicated patient[12]

PATIENT OBSERVATIONS/STATUS	ACTIONS REQUIRED
Opens eyes spontaneously	Conduct BAC test and record
Is orientated	Conduct and record vital signs
Makes appropriate verbal responses	Observe hourly for first 3 hours, then 2-hourly if condition does not worsen
Obeys simple commands	Follow normal procedures for admission
Stands without support	Ensure patient lies in recovery position on very low bed if not requiring spinal immobilisation. If so, have suction readily available and the patient in a very closely supervised area and be ready to log-roll the patient if they feel like or commence vomiting. An antiemetic should be administered prophylactically.
BAC as expected in relation to observed intoxication	Consider a high risk for falls—put bed rails up, assist with walking, follow hospital guidelines for patients at high risk of falling
	Do not offer food or drink until patient has woken, is more sober and alert
Opens eyes spontaneously	Conduct, monitor and record vital signs, including oxygen saturations and GCS score
Is orientated	Conduct BAC test and record
Makes appropriate verbal responses	Observe no less than every 15 minutes
Obeys simple commands	Ensure patient can stand unaided at least 3 hours after admission
Cannot stand without assistance	Ensure patient lies in recovery position on very low bed, or as above for the trauma patient
Level of intoxication and BAC as expected	Do not shower or offer food or drink until fully alert and able to stand and walk unaided
	Follow hospital guidelines for patients at high risk of falling
	Consult medical officer
Opens eyes to simple stimuli (touch, voice)	Conduct, monitor and record vital signs, including oxygen saturations and GCS score
Obeys simple commands	Conduct BAC test if possible
Not able to make appropriate answers	Observe continually—if not possible, no less than every 5 minutes
	Keep patient in recovery position, or as above for the trauma patient
Is disorientated or	Ensure immediate medical assessment
Behaviour is of concern, particularly if not consistent with BAC	Keep patient on at least half-hourly (30 minutes) observation until they are alert, are able to respond fully and can safely manage their environment
	Follow hospital guidelines for patients at high risk of falling
	This situation is serious—there may be acute illness, injury and/or intoxication from other drugs
Does not open eyes to simple stimuli	Emergency—notify medical officer. Do not leave patient alone or unobserved
	Keep in recovery position, or as above for the trauma patient
Does not respond to painful stimuli and/or	Check and maintain airway
	Administer oxygen
Is disorientated and unsure of who they are	Ensure has patent IV cannula
	Commence CPR as necessary

BAC: blood alcohol concentration; CPR: cardiopulmonary resuscitation; GCS: Glasgow Coma Scale; IV: intravenous

thiamine-deficient patient.[12] *If untreated*, it is likely to cause memory impairment and may lead to Korsakoff's syndrome, a form of amnesia characterised by permanent inability to learn, loss of short-term memory and dementia. In the clinical setting, if diagnosed quickly, accurately and treated appropriately, this condition can resolve. However, there may be some residual cognitive deficits in some patients.

Acute Wernicke's encephalopathy can occur in adult males who drink 80 grams or more of pure alcohol (8 standard drinks) daily or most days, and females or older/frail people

TABLE 41.3 Behavioural states and care of the intoxicated patient[31]

PATIENT BEHAVIOUR	CARE
Anxious, agitated, panicky	Ensure close observation and supervision
	Approach them respectfully, calmly and confidently
	Move and speak in an unhurried way
	Ensure a simple, uncluttered environment
	Try to offer a quiet environment
	Provide frequent reassurance, e.g. 'It won't take much longer'
	Remain with them and calm them down
	Explain all interventions in simple, short sentences; repeat if needed
	Protect them from injury. Do not leave them unattended on a chair, in a bathroom or outside
	Consider whether you might need an interpreter
	Enable their family member or friend to sit with them, if possible
Confused or disorientated	Medical review is necessary
	Protect them from injury
	Settle them on a very low bed to prevent injury from falls
	Do not leave unattended
	Undertake frequent observation and close supervision
	Maintain an uncluttered environment; remove unnecessary equipment/furniture
	Do not disturb them unnecessarily once settled
	Provide well-lit surroundings to avoid strange/unusual perceptions
	Use a private area if possible
	Advise and explain to them what you need to do before touching them, when and why this is necessary
	Address them by their preferred name
	Help them to lie on their side in the recovery position
	Enable them to wear their own clothes if possible
	Regularly orientate—explain what is happening and where they are, who you are and your role, what day/time it is
	Use/display object(s) familiar to them such as their possessions they have with them
	Accompany them to any other place e.g. bathroom
Altered perception and/or hallucinations	Medical review is necessary
	Ensure continual or very frequent observation and close supervision
	Explain perceptual errors; explain to them that they may be seeing things differently due to the acute effects of alcohol
	Continue to protect them from risk of injury
Angry, aggressive	Stand to the side of the patient, at least half an arm's length away
	Make sure you are not positioned in a corner or area that you cannot move from quickly
	Wherever possible, clear the area of other patients and staff not directly involved in the patient's care
	Speak calmly, reassure, use short sentences, be reasonably flexible with requests and actions
	Remind them that you want to help them and keep them safe. Keep your own emotions in check
	Do not challenge or threaten by tone of voice, eyes or posture
	Advise and explain to them before you touch them, when and why this is necessary
	Let them vent their feelings, and acknowledge their feelings
	Check what may be the possible source of anger, e.g. untreated pain, fear, psychosis
	Continue to protect them from injury, however possible
	If you feel unsafe, you *are* unsafe: get assistance and do not approach the patient unless there are skilled staff with you
	Call security

who drink 60 grams or more of alcohol daily or most days.[12] This condition is largely preventable requiring 100 mg thiamine daily throughout the person's drinking career.[12,24,25,27]

For acute management of thiamine deficiency and possible onset of encephalopathy, see Section 3 in *Alcohol, Tobacco and Other Drugs: Clinical Guidelines for Nurses and Midwives 2012*.[12]

All patients assessed as being at high risk of alcohol dependence should be examined for ocular abnormalities, including nystagmus (an involuntary eye movement), paralysis of the lateral rectus muscles (muscles of the eye), ataxia (abnormal gait) and a global confusion state. Signs and symptoms are summarised in Box 41.6.

Importantly, symptoms of Wernicke's encephalopathy can be difficult to distinguish from intoxication or withdrawal, and it is potentially reversible.[12]

Patients who drink at the levels cited above or who are withdrawing from alcohol may be hypoglycaemic from poor food intake, malabsorption or excessive vomiting, exacerbating thiamine deficiency.

Glucose solutions may precipitate Wernicke's encephalopathy. Therefore, 100 mg IM or IV thiamine should be administered when considering ongoing glucose products administration.[13,30] Note that if IV thiamine is administered, there is a risk of anaphylactic shock and resuscitation equipment should be available nearby. The person will require at least three 100–200 mg doses of thiamine three times a day for the first 3 days while acutely ill or withdrawing from alcohol, and should then continue with 100 mg oral thiamine daily (plus other essential vitamins and minerals) for the time they continue to drink alcohol.[12,24,25,27,30] It is critical to continue monitoring, assessment and intervention as needed until the patient is medically safe.

The patient should be reassured and re-orientated regularly. This patient group is particularly at risk of injury due to poor coordination and impaired judgment, and their safety must be a priority.[12]

Alcoholic hallucinosis

Alcohol hallucinosis is rare. It is a cluster of psychotic symptoms that appears during or following a period of heavy alcohol use, but is not due to acute intoxication alone and is not a symptom of the withdrawal syndrome. The disorder is

---

BOX 41.6 **Signs and symptoms of Wernicke's encephalopathy***[21,25,30]

- Ophthalmoplegia (reduced eye movements or nystagmus)
- Ataxia—unsteady gait
- Acute disorientation
- Neuropathy—altered/lost sensation in extremities
- Confusion
- Poor concentration
- Impaired memory
- Labile mood.

Wernicke's encephalopathy may co-exist with intoxication and withdrawal.

---

characterised by hallucinations (typically auditory, but often involving other senses), perceptual distortions (usually visual, tactile or auditory), paranoid or other delusions, psychomotor disturbances and abnormal affect (ranging from intense fear to ecstasy). The sensorium is usually clear, although some degree of clouding of consciousness may be present. Supportive care and close supervision to prevent injury are the major focus of intervention. This includes withdrawal observations in order to identify and manage symptoms of the withdrawal syndrome that may also emerge.[12,24,25]

Alcohol withdrawal

Alcohol withdrawal can emerge in people who are physically dependent (tolerant) if they cease or drastically reduce their consumption level. This may have life-threatening effects. While people can experience uncomplicated withdrawal, a significant number will experience serious complications, particularly if injured or otherwise ill.[12,24,25] A patient may call for assistance or present to the ED after trying to 'detox' at home, and be 1 or 2 days into withdrawal with serious complications arising.

Withdrawal is due to the falling BAC and starts between 6 and 12 hours *after the last drink and before the BAC reaches zero*; e.g. it may start at 0.1% BAC. This is due to CNS tolerance and neuro-adaptation. The severity of alcohol withdrawal ranges from mild through moderate to severe. It is unpredictable in terms of which person will experience complications, except when it is known that the person has a history of complications such as withdrawal seizures or hallucinations, in which case these are highly likely to recur.[12,24,25]

Signs and symptoms of alcohol withdrawal (Fig 41.5) occur between 6 and 24 hours after the last drink. The usual course is 5 days, but can be up to 14 days. Further delays in onset may be caused by administration of other CNS depressants; for example, opioid analgesia or anaesthetics.[12]

Symptoms range from mild (nausea, insomnia, mild sweating) to severe (hypertension, electrolyte imbalance, hallucinations, fevers, dehydration and electrolyte imbalances). Severe withdrawal may occur within 24 hours or may be delayed until 48 hours or more after the last drink. The presence and severity of each of these symptoms varies with the level of severity of withdrawal. Presence of concomitant illness, infection, injury or other physical trauma and recent surgery increases the likelihood of complicated alcohol withdrawal.

See Box 41.7 for clinical index of suspicion of alcohol withdrawal and Table 41.4 for levels of severity.

Refer to Table 41.4 for the features of alcohol withdrawal, and these are characterised as features of mild, moderate or severe withdrawal.

It is important to note that any seizure can be life threatening and all seizures should be investigated to establish a cause. Alcohol withdrawal seizures are preventable in people with a known history by use of prophylactic diazepam-loading regimens.

Approximate time of onset of alcohol withdrawal complications after the last drink is:

- seizures 6–48 hours
- disorientation 48 hours
- confusion 48 hours
- hallucinations 48 hours
- delirium tremens 2–6 days.

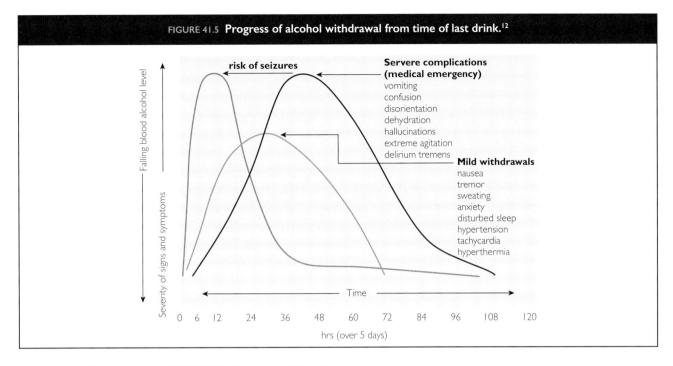

FIGURE 41.5 Progress of alcohol withdrawal from time of last drink.[12]

BOX 41.7 Clinical index of suspicion of alcohol withdrawal[12]

- History of adult male regularly drinking 80 grams or more (8 standard drinks) over several weeks or more.
- History of adult woman or older/frail person regularly drinking 60 grams (6 standard drinks) or more.
- The person is alcohol dependent.
- Symptoms occur less than 10 days since the last drink.
- Person is regularly drinking even smaller amounts of alcohol with other depressants, e.g. benzodiazepines or opioids.
- Previous episodes of alcohol withdrawal.
- Person has had alcohol withdrawal seizures or other serious symptoms before.
- The current presentation is alcohol related.
- Previous history of an alcohol-related condition (e.g. alcoholic hepatitis, alcoholic cardiomyopathy, pancreatitis, oesophageal varices, liver disease).
- Person's physical appearance indicates excessive drinking, e.g. facial vascularisation, reddened eyes, signs of liver disease (e.g. ascites, jaundice), muscle wasting, spider naevi, palmar erythema, previous injuries.
- Pathology results show raised serum gamma-glutamyl transpeptidase (GGT) and/or raised mean cell volume (MCV).
- Person is displaying or reporting symptoms such as hypertension, anxiety, sleep disturbance, agitation, tremor, sweatiness, nausea/vomiting or retching, possibly due to alcohol withdrawal.

Delirium tremens

Delirium tremens ('the DTs') is the most serious complication of alcohol withdrawal syndrome and is a *medical emergency*. It usually develops 2–5 days after the last drink, but may take 7 days to develop.[12,31] Dehydration, infection, dysrhythmias, hypotension, renal failure and pneumonia can be precipitating factors of delirium tremens, which can lead to death in 20% of cases. If recognised and treated effectively, the mortality rate reduces to < 5%. Symptoms include exaggerated features of alcohol withdrawal; autonomic instability (e.g. fluctuations in blood pressure, or pulse may be hypertensive and tachycardic); disturbance of fluid balance and electrolytes; hyperthermia and sweating; extreme agitation, restlessness or disturbed behaviour—this may be to the extent where the person needs restraint or to be detained under the Mental Health Act for their protection; gross tremor; confusion and disorientation; paranoid ideation, typically of delusional intensity; and hallucinations affecting any of the senses, but typically visual (highly coloured, animal form).[12,25,27,31] The usual course is 3 days, but can be up to 14 days.

Clinical management of alcohol withdrawal

The most systematic and effective way to monitor and measure the severity of withdrawal is to use a validated and reliable withdrawal scale. A *withdrawal scale is not a diagnostic tool*, but merely guides in the identification and monitoring of symptoms indicative of the severity of the alcohol withdrawal syndrome. Used as a baseline, and then repeated regularly according to severity of symptoms, any changes in the patient's condition are measured and scored over time, assisting diagnosis and prescribing and administering medications—generally diazepam to prevent seizures. Other symptomatic medications may be required to reduce and contain alcohol withdrawal symptoms, and other complications.

The Clinical Institute Withdrawal Assessment for Alcohol—Revised Version (CIWA-Ar)[12,24,25] should be started as soon as the risk of withdrawal is suspected, either before or in the ED. It should be conducted hourly if scoring 8 or above (requires immediate medical examination), or 4-hourly if scoring less than 8. It is useful to include the Glasgow Coma Scale (GCS) score; temperature, pulse and respiration (TPR);

TABLE 41.4 Features of alcohol withdrawal[12]

MILD WITHDRAWAL	MODERATE WITHDRAWAL	SEVERE WITHDRAWAL
Mild pyrexia, e.g. 37°C (no infection suspected)	Mild pyrexia, e.g. 37°C (no infection suspected)	Fever
Mild anxiety	Moderate sweating	Excessive sweating
Slight tremor	Mild tremor	Dehydration
Mild sweating	Restlessness/agitation	Marked tremor
Nausea	Dyspepsia	Nausea/vomiting
Vomiting	Nausea/vomiting	Diarrhoea
Mild dehydration	Diarrhoea	Hyperventilation and panic
Headaches	Headache	Tachycardia
Mild hypertension	Weakness	Hypersensitivity to stimulation
Tachycardia	Loss of appetite	Acute anxiety (may/may not respond to reassurance)
Dyspepsia	Mild to moderate hypertension (diastolic reading of 100–110 mmHg)	Extreme agitation
Malaise	Dehydration	Moderate/severe hypertension
	Moderate anxiety (will respond to reassurance)	Seizures (see note)
	Hyperventilation and panic attacks	Hallucinations (auditory, tactile, visual)
	Insomnia/nightmares	Disorientation/confusion (time, place)

Note: any seizure can be life-threatening. All seizures should be investigated for cause. Alcohol withdrawal seizures are preventable in people with a known history by use of a prophylactic diazepam-loading regimen.

---

and blood pressure assessment on the same case-note form as the CIWA-Ar to allow concurrent monitoring of health status, identifying other problems through objective clinical signs. The CIWA-Ar uses a 10-item scale for assessing and monitoring the clinical course of alcohol withdrawal. The scale allows a quantitative rating from 0 to 7—with a maximum possible score of 67—for withdrawal symptoms.

For more information on alcohol withdrawal management, see Section 3.1.1 in *Alcohol, Tobacco and Other Drugs: Clinical Guidelines for Nurses and Midwives 2012*, and for a CIWA-Ar alcohol withdrawal instrument see Section 4 Appendix 9.[12]

> **PRACTICE TIP**
>
> The Clinical Institute Withdrawal Assessment for Alcohol—Revised Version (CIWA-Ar) is copyright-free. To become familiar with using the CIWAR-Ar and to learn how to apply the CIWAR-Ar, the Center for Health Care Evaluation has developed an online case study learning application.[32]

Withdrawal

The goal of treatment is to prevent any complications associated with alcohol withdrawal. Complications are more likely if there is co-existing injury, infection or serious illness. Monitoring, early recognition and effective management of the initial, milder stages of withdrawal are therefore crucial in preventing progression to severe, life-threatening stages. It is important to administer 100 mg parenteral as soon as possible during ongoing glucose/dextrose supplementation and then three times a day during acute illness and withdrawal. It is

also essential to treat any concurrent conditions, and provide withdrawal symptom relief with medication, including antiemetics and analgesics. Hydration and electrolyte balance are critical and intravenous fluids are likely to be required.

The medical officer may prescribe pharmacological treatment to prevent seizures and combat acute withdrawal symptoms, without over-sedating the patient. The most commonly prescribed pharmacological treatment, known to be most effective for alcohol withdrawal, is diazepam. This is because it belongs to the only drug group that prevents alcohol withdrawal seizures, is long-acting and has cross-tolerance with alcohol.

Clinical specialist advice about alcohol withdrawal and recommended medication regimens may be available from specific drug and alcohol services in your area. The ED nurse should inform the treating doctor if dosing is inadequate to control withdrawal symptoms. Haloperidol may be required in addition to diazepam to control symptoms of alcohol withdrawal, especially when psychotic symptoms such as hallucinations or paranoid ideation (particularly if acted upon with aggression) are pronounced. Multivitamin and mineral preparations are also required. A daily fluid balance chart should be commenced and fluids need to be encouraged, as dehydration from sweating, nausea, vomiting and diarrhoea may cause an exacerbation of the withdrawal syndrome. Electrolytes may be monitored as a component of medical management, including magnesium. To access advice on current best-practice alcohol withdrawal management, see relevant references and websites at the end of this chapter.

Benzodiazepines

The benzodiazepine group of sedative–hypnotics (sometimes referred to as minor tranquillisers) are commonly prescribed, and may be used problematically.[12,30] Benzodiazepines replaced barbiturates in the late 1980s for medical treatment of anxiety and poor sleep because they are far safer, having a wider therapeutic range than barbiturates, thus reducing risk of overdose and causing less toxicity.[12,31]

Effects

Benzodiazepines have a general CNS-depressant effect that is dose dependent, and includes decreased anxiety, sedation and anticonvulsant effects. Even after taking therapeutic doses as prescribed, tolerance can develop quickly, even after only 2–3 weeks. Although there is a wide therapeutic margin of safety, rendering them relatively safe, benzodiazepines can have adverse reactions if tolerance has developed. These can include rebound anxiety and insomnia with short-acting benzodiazepines, and confusion and memory loss with longer acting drugs, causing the person to take increasing doses to get the original effect.[12,31]

Excessive doses cause initial euphoria; increasing intoxication; impaired cognition, judgment and fine motor coordination; slurred speech; loss of inhibitions and motor coordination; then progression from sedation to hypnosis and then stupor. Benzodiazepines can cause respiratory depression, but this effect is minimal unless other CNS depressants are used concurrently (e.g. alcohol and opioids), whereby a synergistic action may occur resulting in respiratory depression that can be life-threatening. In rare cases there may be agitation, hostility and bizarre, uninhibited behaviour.[12,31]

These drugs are usually taken orally, but the capsule or tablet form may be injected intravenously, often causing serious vascular damage, cellulitis and tissue damage. Other complications from injecting these drugs include thrombosis, transmission of hepatitis B and C and HIV, and bacterial infections causing abscesses, necrosis, septicaemia and endocarditis.[12]

Overdose

Overdose of a major sedative–hypnotic such as a barbiturate can cause death from respiratory depression. This is far less likely with benzodiazepines than with barbiturates and opioids. Overdose of benzodiazepines is treated with flumazenil, a specific benzodiazepine antagonist. There are no known antagonists to counteract the effects of other sedative–hypnotic drugs. Emergency life-support measures must be taken in cases of overdose.[12] Table 41.5 presents emergency management of CNS depressants.

Withdrawal

If a therapeutic dose is prescribed, and continued for longer than 6 weeks, tolerance, physical dependence and withdrawal on cessation or rapid reduction will affect 15–50% of people (studies vary). Common, less frequent and uncommon symptoms of benzodiazepine withdrawal are listed in Box 41.8.

Acute withdrawal can last for up to 6 weeks, and longer-term use may result in withdrawal symptoms lasting from 6 months to 1 year, with intensity of symptoms gradually diminishing. Not everyone will experience symptoms, and of those who do, the symptoms are not always disabling. Use of higher doses is more likely to produce a withdrawal syndrome with more severe symptoms. Withdrawal from short-acting benzodiazepines (e.g. oxazepam, temazepam, alprazolam and

---

TABLE 41.5 Emergency management of overdose of depressant drug[15]

AETIOLOGY	ASSESSMENT FINDINGS	INTERVENTIONS
Ingestion, inhalation or injection of CNS depressants—accidental or intentional	Aggressive behaviour Agitation Confusion Lethargy Stupor Hallucinations Depression Slurred speech Pinpoint pupils Nystagmus Seizures Needle tracks Cold, clammy skin Rapid, weak pulse Slow or rapid shallow respirations Decreased oxygen saturation Hypotension Dysrhythmia ECG changes Cardiac or respiratory arrest	*Initial* Ensure patent airway Anticipate intubation if respiratory distress evident Establish IV access Obtain temperature Obtain 12-lead ECG Obtain information about substance (name, route, when taken, amount) Obtain specific drug levels or comprehensive toxicology screen Obtain a health history including drug use and allergies Administer antidotes as necessary Perform gastric lavage if necessary Administer activated charcoal and cathartics as appropriate *Ongoing* Monitor vital signs, temperature, level of consciousness, oxygen saturation, cardiac rhythm

CNS: central nervous system; ECG: electrocardiogram; IV: intravenous

---

BOX 41.8 Benzodiazepine withdrawal symptoms[12]

Common withdrawal symptoms
- Anxiety
- Agitation
- Depression
- Insomnia
- Irritability
- Increased muscle tension
- Restlessness
- Poor concentration
- Sweating
- Headache
- Poor memory
- Muscle ache and twitching
- Less-frequent symptoms
- Nightmares
- Panic attacks
- Decreased appetite
- Increased sensory perception (e.g. metallic taste)
- Gastric upset
- Agoraphobia

- Nausea
- Weight loss
- Palpitations
- Increased temperature
- Feelings of unreality
- Dry retching
- Sweating
- Tremor
- Ataxia
- Depersonalisation
- Light-headedness/dizziness
- Lethargy
- Blurred vision

Uncommon symptoms
- Delusions
- Seizures (more common with concurrent alcohol withdrawal)
- Paranoia
- Persistent tinnitus
- Hallucinations
- Confusion

---

lorazepam) typically produces a faster and more severe onset of symptoms than withdrawal from long-acting benzodiazepines (e.g. diazepam and nitrazepam), and may be more difficult to endure.

People can experience withdrawal seizures and other serious complications, and so benzodiazepine use should never be ceased abruptly.[12,31]

Clinical management of benzodiazepine withdrawal

While paramedical or emergency staff may not typically see benzodiazepine withdrawal, onset may occur in the presence of another acute condition if a patient has been ill and unable to access the benzodiazepine or have been trying to withdraw at home and presents with symptoms. If the patient presents for other reasons, their potential for withdrawal needs to be assessed and appropriate observation, monitoring and treatment implemented.

Pharmacological management of benzodiazepine withdrawal typically involves converting to longer-acting diazepam (maximum 80 mg per day) from the average daily dose of their particular benzodiazepine (e.g. a shorter-acting oxazepam). This is with the intent of implementing a gradual diazepam reduction regimen.[12,31] Diazepam is to be used with extreme caution or is contraindicated in certain conditions e.g. chronic airways disease, respiratory failure, liver disease. In such cases a shorter-acting benzodiazepine may be considered.[12,31] Other symptomatic medications can be used to prevent and reduce severity of withdrawal symptoms, providing this is safe in the presence of a current injury or illness.

Regular observations and monitoring are required to identify and effectively treat withdrawal symptoms, and prevent severe withdrawal. There is also the need to provide a safe, non-stimulating and non-judgmental therapeutic environment. Complementary therapies, such as warmth and massage for muscle tension, cramping and aching, can be helpful. The patient requires support and reassurance if they are experiencing any distortion of sensory stimuli.

Opioids

Opioids are either naturally derived such as morphine, codeine and heroin,[33] or made synthetically. Opioids are CNS depressants that relieve strong pain.[12] Opioids *decrease spontaneous activity* of neurons in the CNS involving inhibition of adenyl cyclase activity and decrease in cellular concentrations of cyclic adenosine monophosphate (cAMP).[34] This produces the effects listed in Box 41.9.

Intravenous administration causes rapid absorption and CNS effects. Illicit morphine, codeine and heroin are consumed in Australia and New Zealand. As with any illicit drug, it is not possible to determine the dose or purity of heroin, although

---

BOX 41.9 Effects of opioids[12]

- Analgesia
- Drowsiness
- Sense of tranquillity
- Sense of detachment from external environment
- Miosis (constriction of pupils)
- Slowed peristalsis
- Constipation
- Orthostatic hypotension
- Slurred speech
- Decreasing consciousness
- Respiratory depression
- In rare cases: delirium
- Respiratory arrest.

it is more possible to assess the doses used of the non-medical (illicit) pharmaceutical opioids.

In Australia and New Zealand, non-medical use of slow-release morphine, non-prescription and prescription codeine (often from branded medicines such as Nurofen Plus and Panadeine) has become relatively common. According to availability and price, use of illicit opioids is higher than that of heroin.[3]

Intoxication

The acute clinical manifestations of opioid intoxication are listed in Box 41.10.

Caution: Opioid intoxication can rapidly progress to overdose, depending on the half-life and dose of opioid and the route of administration.[12,35]

Additionally, the person may have also used another depressant, such as alcohol or benzodiazepine, which greatly increases risk.

Tolerance

Daily or almost daily opioid use results in tolerance, neuro-adaptation and lowering of pain threshold, within weeks or months.[12] The resultant hypersensitivity to even mild pain[12] can be problematic and increases the likelihood of continued use in greater doses as the person attempts self-medication. Where there is illness, surgery or injury, poorly assessed and managed pain can result in poor healing and extreme discomfort, and in frequent requests for pain relief, patient distress and possibly angry outbursts and premature self-discharge. This situation is often misinterpreted as drug-seeking behaviour rather than poorly relieved pain.

Pain in the opioid-tolerant patient therefore requires comprehensive assessment and additional pain relief, which may include larger doses of opioids, more-frequent or con-tinuous administration of opioids and patient-controlled analgesia (PCA), possibly boosted by complementary analgesia such as non-steroidal anti-inflammatory medications and/or local block anaesthesia (Ch 19).

Providing opioid analgesia and combinations of varying medications for analgesia will not make the patient relapse or become more drug dependent.[12] In fact, withholding opioids or under-dosing of opioid analgesia will more than likely exacerbate existing drug problems, precipitate relapse and inhibit optimal healing from their current medical condition.[33,36] Both out-of-hospital emergency personnel and emergency nurses can play a significant role in ensuring patient comfort and therefore compliance by ensuring that adequate analgesia is administered and that their care is delivered in a non-judgmental manner.[12,37]

Overdose

Accidental overdose is not uncommon, and may be associated with use of pharmaceutical opioids or 'street' heroin. It can occur with occasional use whereby tolerance is low or in dependent use and higher levels of tolerance. This is typically due to unknown doses or concurrent use of other depressants such as alcohol or benzodiazepines.

Overdose is unpredictable due to unknown dose (potency) and purity of 'street' heroin. It can also be unpredictable when pharmaceutical opioids are used for medical or non-medical reasons. It is essential to try and view packaging or ask about what brand/type of opioids, and any other depressants, the person has taken—ideally identify trade name and dose.

Some additional overdose risks:

- Reduction in tolerance after period of abstinence (e.g. following release from prison, discharge from rehabilitation or hospital)
- Leakage and ingestion from packaged illicit heroin trafficking ('body stuffers')[12,36]

Signs of overdose are included in Box 41.11.

Clinical management of overdose

Overdose of opioids is a **medical emergency**. The patient's airway and oxygenation should be established immediately and a narcotic antagonist such as naloxone should be given as soon as life support is instituted. The patient should be monitored closely because narcotic antagonists have a shorter duration of action (half-life) than most opioids and may need to be re-administered owing to the short half-life compared with that of the opioid used. A toxicological blood or urine screen is extremely helpful to identify the specific drug or combination of drugs used. Because the longer plasma half-life of methadone is 24–48 hours compared with the much shorter half-life of heroin or morphine (2–3 hours), people who overdose from methadone and require emergency treatment with naloxone may seem to recover initially but can lapse into respiratory depression and coma if not adequately monitored and treated.[12,31]

The effects of methadone or buprenorphine overdose can persist for up to 72 hours, even in cases where people have been resuscitated. Depending on the magnitude of the overdose, they should be closely observed for a period of up to 72 hours, and medical assessment will determine the need for additional naloxone administration.[12]

BOX 41.10 Acute effects of opioid intoxication[12]

- Euphoria
- Orthostatic hypotension
- Constricted pupils (miosis)
- Respiratory depression
- Decreased level of consciousness
- In rare cases: delirium.
- Constipation
- Appears tranquil

BOX 41.11 Signs of an opioid overdose[12]

- Increasing drowsiness (may be sudden)
- Decreasing level of consciousness
- Increasingly slowed respiration
- Cyanosis
- Subnormal temperature
- Miosis
- Weak pulse
- Bradycardia
- Pulmonary oedema.

Pharmacological management of opioid overdose

Note that maintenance of airway and breathing are most important in overdose management—follow CPR protocol. See Chapter 17, p. 314, for a discussion of airway management techniques.

Naloxone (Narcan), an opioid antagonist, is used as a reversal agent and will reverse the effect of opioid overdoses. If used incorrectly, people who were previously sedated may become agitated, aggressive and difficult to manage due to sudden precipitated withdrawal syndrome. It is important to titrate the dose of naloxone to ensure the client improves their respiration but does not go into opioid withdrawal. The aim is a state of semi-consciousness with adequate respiration.

If the patient becomes fully conscious they may experience precipitated withdrawal and refuse further care. It is not uncommon practice to administer naloxone IM prior to giving the IV dose in case the patient does experience precipitated withdrawal syndrome and absconds after the IV dose. This strategy improves the wellbeing of the patient outside of the ED, but does not guarantee it. The naloxone may still 'wear off', leading to decreased respiration and depressed conscious state due to the long-acting nature of the opioid.

Naloxone is a first-line treatment and should always be given in the case of respiratory depression.[16]

In particular:

- Naloxone hydrochloride (naloxone) is available as 1 mL ampoules of 400 μg and as a 'Min-I-Jet' containing 2 mg in 5 mL.

- A dose of 0.8–2 mg by IV injection should be administered, repeated at intervals of 2–3 minutes to a maximum of 10 mg. If respiratory function does not improve, other diagnostic options, such as other drug intoxication or other organic causes of loss of consciousness, including hypoglycaemia, should be considered.

The subcutaneous (SC) or IM injection route should be used if an IV route is not accessible. The same regimen should be employed as for IV use, but the clinician should expect a slower response.

Naloxone is a short-acting drug. Therefore, repeated injections or IV infusion may be needed if a longer-acting opiate such as methadone or buprenorphine has been taken. Following naloxone administration, patients may seem to recover initially. However, as a consequence of the long half-life of methadone or buprenorphine, patients may then lapse into respiratory depression. Naloxone can be given as a continuous intravenous infusion of 2 mg diluted in a 500 mL IV titrated at a rate determined by the clinical response.

The effects of methadone or buprenorphine overdose can persist for up to 72 hours, even in circumstances where people have been resuscitated. Depending on the magnitude of the overdose, they should be observed for a period of up to 72 hours. For high-dose intoxication, naloxone infusion should be considered.[37]

CASE STUDY 1—OPIOID OVERDOSE

A 22-year-old female (Sue) was attended by paramedics at 4 am outside a nightclub. She was not breathing. Her friends said she had been at the club since 11 pm, and was reportedly happy, drinking alcohol and seemingly not too intoxicated. Finding her unresponsive, and following the initial primary survey, the paramedic crew administered an opioid antagonist (naloxone) from which she was roused. She appeared slightly intoxicated with alcohol but otherwise alert. She was transported to the nearest emergency department (ED). Once in the ED she was medically examined and put in an observation area. About 20 minutes after her arrival a nurse walking past the cubicle saw that Sue was unconscious.

Questions

1. Why might this have happened?
2. How could this have been avoided?
3. What risks were there to her safety and wellbeing?
4. What advice would you give to other out-of-hospital emergency personnel, nurses and medical staff?

Answers to Case Study Questions can be found on evolve
http://evolve.emergencytrauma.curtis

Withdrawal

Opioid withdrawal has a characteristic group of symptoms (syndrome) resulting from sudden cessation or reduction in daily prolonged use of an opioid drug (Box 41.9). People who use opioids regularly can experience a moderate to severe withdrawal, which, while distressing, is not life threatening.

Time of onset and intensity of withdrawal is associated with the half-life of the opioid used (Table 41.6). Objective and subjective symptoms of opioid withdrawal can be seen in Box 41.12.[12]

Withdrawal from a shorter-acting opioid such as morphine or heroin can begin 4–12 hours after the last dose and last for between 4 and 10 days. Withdrawal from methadone, with its longer half-life, has a later onset, starting 24–48 hours after the last dose and lasting from 10 to 20 or more days. It is important for the clinician to know the half-life of each opioid drug so as to more accurately predict likely time of onset of symptoms from the time of last dose, likely duration of withdrawal and identifying and effectively managing the withdrawal symptoms.[12,31]

Clinical management of withdrawal

Cessation or rapid reduction of opioids will precipitate withdrawal due to tolerance and neuro-adaptation. The opioid withdrawal syndrome has a characteristic group of symptoms ranging from moderate to severe, but these are not life threatening.

- Lacrimation
- Rhinorrhoea
- Yawning
- Sweating
- Piloerection
- Hot and cold flushes
- Mydriasis
- Tremor
- Restlessness
- Anxiety
- Muscle twitches
- Nausea/vomiting
- Abdominal cramps
- Muscle and joint aches
- Craving
- Hypertension.

Providing calm, non-stimulating, supportive and safe environment while undertaking adequate monitoring and assessment of withdrawal symptoms, and timely administration of medication and necessary treatments, can ensure the patient manages with fewer risks of complications. It is useful, if possible, to involve the patient in their own assessment, experience and management of severity of their withdrawal symptoms and pain. Considering and respecting the efficacy of their self-report of symptoms, and effectiveness (or not) of their current treatment, can greatly assist in reducing any anxiety they may have about being under-medicated or not believed.[12,37,38]

Buprenorphine is the preferred prescribed medication for a significant number of people experiencing opioid withdrawal symptoms (unless there is a risk of contraindications). It comes in sublingual tablets or film that dissolve under the tongue in about 5 minutes, and is absorbed directly through the lining of the mouth into the bloodstream. Crushing the tablets does not seem to have much impact on absorption. If it is swallowed whole, most of the drug will be metabolised by the liver before reaching the general circulation, and is therefore ineffective. The therapeutic effect lasts from 1 to 2 days.[12,39,40]

Symptomatic medications should be provided to relieve symptoms such as nausea, painful muscle cramps, diarrhoea, etc.

Naltrexone as well as opioid withdrawal

The possibility of naltrexone-precipitated withdrawal should be considered if a patient presents with signs of opioid withdrawal in conjunction with *delirium or intractable vomiting*. If the patient has a recent history of opioid dependence, they need to be carefully assessed, examined for signs of self-administered naltrexone or other drug use and questioned about the time of their last dose/use, particularly of opioids. An absence of track marks should not exclude this diagnosis.

The administration of an opioid agonist such as naltrexone is unhelpful, and patients should be warned that taking heroin or other opioids would not alleviate their symptoms. Antagonist-induced withdrawal is extremely traumatic, and the patient should be given appropriate nursing care and repeated assurance.

Treatment is therapeutically supportive based on symptoms.[12,39,41] The most important part of management is reassurance that symptoms, although severe, will be short-lived. There is a risk of delirium and agitation for approximately 4 hours with naltrexone-precipitated withdrawal. Symptomatic medications are likely to be required to relieve discomfort and anxiety.

Pharmacotherapy for opioid-dependent patients in a general hospital

If a patient is already receiving opioid dependence treatment with prescribed methadone, buprenorphine or combined buprenorphine and naltrexone, their *usual prescribed dose must be continued* during their stay in the ED and if admitted to hospital. This is to maintain their pharmacotherapy regimen and ensure psychological and physical stability. This regimen will prevent withdrawal *but will not* provide pain relief. It is important that the ED clinician identify and communicate this to the medical team, especially as this patient will experience hypersensitivity to pain, particularly after-hours, so that arrangements can be made to obtain their usual pharmacotherapy medications, and that appropriate pain relief is also prescribed and administered. The continuation of the prescribed pharmacotherapy is essential to maintain the patient's regimen, prevent relapse and any other complications and ensure their maximum comfort and safety. Importantly, this will also influence effectiveness of pain management and healing.[12,37,39]

For more information on pain management for opioid tolerant people, see Section 3.1.3 in *Alcohol, Tobacco and Other Drugs: Clinical Guidelines for Nurses and Midwives 2012*.[12]

TABLE 41.6 Signs of opioid withdrawal[12]		
TYPE OF OPIOID	TIME AFTER LAST DOSE SYMPTOMS APPEAR (HOURS)	DURATION OF WITHDRAWAL SYNDROME (DAYS)
Heroin/morphine	6–12 hours	5–7 days
Pethidine	3–4 hours	4–5 days
Methadone	24–48 hours	10–21 days
Morphine sulfate (e.g. Kapanol, Contin) (intravenously)	8–24 hours	7–10 days
Codeine (orally)	8–24 hours	5–10 days
Buprenorphine, naloxone	Variable, but generally around 48 hours	Can be prolonged, as with methadone; generally 10–14 days
Tramadol	12–20 hours	7 days or longer

Solvents

Solvents (inhalants or volatile substances) include gases (e.g. nitrous oxide) and highly volatile compounds or mixtures of compounds; for example, petrol, paint, aerosols (anti-perspirants, flyspray, hydrocarbon-based adhesives and lighter fluid).[42] These products vaporise causing a 'high' feeling when inhaled. The commonly used term 'sniffing' relates to nasal or oral inhalation. It may be inhaled from a plastic bag or pre-soaked cloth or directly from a container; for example a product container, soft drink can or drink bottle.[12]

How much has been used?

Quantification of solvent use is extremely difficult. Ask about and record the type of solvent used, and the frequency, quantity, date and time of last use. It may be possible to ask the patient why they are using this, any positives and negatives of use and if they intend to continue or stop use at this stage. Medical and social assessment should be undertaken and health monitored to ensure physical and mental health is supported even if sniffing continues.

Note: a common perception is that inhalant use is an exclusively 'Aboriginal' issue, which *is not the case*. Youth and adults of many cultural and socio-economic backgrounds are known to have used inhalants.

Effects

Solvent intoxication resembles alcohol intoxication. Onset of action is very quick, with CNS impairment generally clearing within a few hours of inhalation. High doses can cause coma and death. People may harm themselves (accidentally or intentionally) or become aggressive due to the intoxicating and hallucinating effects.[12,42]

While individual components of various compounds may differ, the overall effect of most solvents is CNS depression. People may experience acute problems associated with inhalant-induced malnutrition caused by the appetite-suppressant effects.

- Solvents induce respiratory depression and cardiac dysrhythmias, which can be fatal with '*sudden sniffing death*' being recorded.[42]
- Sudden death can also result if the person is startled such as when another person approaches and tries to remove the inhalant container from them.[12]
- Very high doses can result in convulsions.[42]
- Hallucinations and delusions can occur.
- Repeated use can result in, for example, rash and excoriation around nose and mouth; weight loss and malnutrition due to lost appetite; respiratory problems; liver damage.[42]
- There can be serious damage to the nervous system, causing brain damage with cognitive and neurological disabilities. Some people may recover while others remain permanently disabled.[42]
- Self-harm may occur accidentally or intentionally.

Note: Removal of lead from all petrol has reduced the devastating impact from lead on short and longer-term health; however, inhaling petrol is still dangerous.[12] In some remote Australian communities OPAL fuel has replaced other petrol with success. A story about OPAL from the community perspective can be viewed on YouTube.[43]

For more information on the acute effects of solvent inhalants, see Section 3.5.2 in *Alcohol, Tobacco and Other Drugs: Clinical Guidelines for Nurses and Midwives 2012*.[12]

Cannabis

Delta 9 tetra hydrocannabinol (THC) is the active ingredient that causes the psychoactive effects of cannabis. It is difficult to classify THC in cannabis due to its mixture of mood, cognitive, motor and perceptual affects. It therefore does not clearly belong to any particular class of drugs, and is presented here separately.[12,44]

THC effects include: perceptual changes which can include frank hallucinations, psychomotor changes with slowed reaction time, distance judgment and impaired coordination, cognitive impairment with sedation, slowed thinking, difficulty concentrating and impaired memory. Toxicity, tolerance, withdrawal and psychosis can occur. Psychosis may co-exist or be triggered by cannabis (THC) use in some individuals.[12,20,31,44]

Effects

At low to moderate doses, THC produces fewer immediate physiological and psychological effects than other classes of psychoactive drugs, including alcohol. Although its mechanism of action is uncertain and multi-faceted, THC affects dopamine and other neurotransmitter activity and a variety of receptors in the brain. When smoked, THC rapidly enters the blood-stream with plasma concentrations peaking within 30 minutes and effects lasting for up to 4 hours. If ingested, onset is about an hour and effects are milder, often experienced in waves.[12,31,44]

The psychoactive (intoxicating) effects of THC comprise a combination of stimulation and depression in low doses and, for some people, hallucinogenic and depressant effects in high doses. It can cause slight increase in heart rate to about 20 beats/minute above baseline. Because it is stored in body fat, it is eliminated slowly, resulting in a half-life of 2–7 days. Its metabolites can be measured in blood or urine and are inactive, merely confirming that cannabis has been used at some time recently (e.g. in the last few weeks), and this does not confirm or refute intoxication.[12,31]

For more information on cannabis (THC) acute effects and withdrawal, see Section 3.2 in *Alcohol, Tobacco and Other Drugs: Clinical Guidelines for Nurses and Midwives 2012*.[12] See also Table 41.1 for the effects of frequently abused substances. It includes a list of cannabis withdrawal symptoms.

Psychostimulants

A range of symptoms and behaviours are associated with psychostimulant intoxication. These can vary in intensity according to people's individual differences and the actual drug consumed. Some useful tips for the clinician are given in Boxes 41.13 and 41.15.

The clinical team should have a high degree of suspicion of acute intoxication from a psychostimulant in any patient who has dilated pupils, tachycardia, agitation, hyperactivity, fever and/or behavioural abnormalities. The possibility of cocaine or other psychostimulant use should be considered in a young person with unexplained myocardial ischaemia or infarction, dysrhythmias, myocarditis or dilated cardiomyopathy.[12,45] For detailed information see Section 3 in *Alcohol, Tobacco and Other Drugs: Clinical Guidelines for Nurses and Midwives 2012*.[12]

BOX 41.13 Clinical tips for interacting with the psychostimulant-intoxicated patient[12]

Generally

- Wherever possible, provide a quiet environment to reduce unnecessary CNS stimulation.
- Approach the patient in a quiet, calm and confident manner.
- Move and speak in an unhurried way.
- Introduce yourself and explain to them your role and what you are doing.
- Use their proper name when speaking to them.
- Remain with the person to calm them if anxious or frightened.
- Stand beside them rather than face to face.
- Control your body language so you do not appear aggressive or intrusive.
- Minimise how many clinicians are attending to them.
- Reassure the person frequently (e.g. 'It won't take much longer', 'I am just going to do … because …').
- Explain any interventions needed, no matter how simple— such as moving the pillow, taking their TPR (explain what you mean by 'TPR').
- Protect them from injury, e.g. do not leave them unattended or on a bed without safeguards; lower the bed as close to the floor as possible.
- Brief and frequent attendances can reassure them that they are being cared for and prevent unnecessary agitation.

Confusion/disorientation

- Explain in simple terms what is happening.
- Provide frequent reality orientation.
- Reduce amount of unnecessary equipment and furniture nearby.
- Reduce amount of unnecessary noise.
- Display familiar objects for the person, e.g. personal belongings.
- Ensure frequent observation and close supervision.
- Accompany them to and from places (e.g. bathroom, lounge, X-ray).

Altered perception and hallucinations

- Explain their perceptual errors; tell them that you understand what is happening but what is real (e.g. that the curtain does not have snakes on it).
- Provide care for them in well-lit surroundings to avoid perceptual ambiguities from poor light.

Common psychostimulants

Nicotine

Nicotine is a short-acting psychostimulant that results in rapid development of tolerance and physical dependence after a short period of use.[12,45] The CNS stimulation occurs for a short time then reduces quickly, resulting in withdrawal and craving. Smoking one nicotine cigarette immediately raises blood pressure and heart rate, and decreases blood flow to

body extremities and brain. It is important for the clinician to understand the acute physiological effects of nicotine, and nicotine withdrawal, as they will alter the patient's physiological and psychological response to illness and create numerous risk factors for others. Note that nicotine consumption is measured by the strength in mgs, and actual number of cigarettes smoked per day (not the number of packets).

Withdrawal management

A patient who is dependent on nicotine and in hospital will experience withdrawal symptoms because they have had to stop smoking. They will require clinical intervention and support during their admission, and this may be a time when they actually consider giving up, or, if they have relapsed, restarting their cessation program. Nicotine withdrawal starts 1–2 hours after the last cigarette and peaks at between 24 and 72 hours, due to the short half-life of nicotine. While not life-threatening, it is characterised by distressing symptoms, including increased tension and agitation, disturbed sleep, muscle spasm, headache and loss of concentration (Table 41.1).

Acute nicotine withdrawal is associated with craving which often leads to relapse.[12,31,45] The patient needs support and self-help information and should be put in touch with the Quitline free telephone support line as soon as they are able. They may wish to use nicotine replacement patches or gum as pharmacological assistance in managing their withdrawal while in acute care, and later for gradual cessation (if it is medically safe to administer). A combination of nicotine replacement therapies (NRTs) in the form of patches, spray or nicotine gum or lozenges decreases withdrawal symptoms more than any NRT alone.[12,30,45] ED nurses are ideally situated to help patients consider giving up smoking. Educating them about NRTs and how to use them (e.g. patches, gum and nasal spray), and how to contact the local QUIT service to get support, can boost their potential for success.[12,45]

It is *very important* to assess for immediate and longer term harms associated with psychostimulants, including risk of withdrawal. People may present having been on a 3- or 4-day binge of any of these psychostimulants. If this occurs regularly, it is very likely that they have become tolerant and will go into withdrawal.

Onset and duration of acute effects
Amphetamine

- Onset of action when taken orally is about 30–60 minutes, with peak cardiovascular effect at 60 minutes and CNS effects about 2 hours.
- Duration of effect is about 4–6 hours. Intranasal intake (snorting) produces effects within a few minutes; smoking and intravenous use produces even faster effects.[12]

Ecstasy (MDMA) *also hallucinogenic*

- Onset of action when taken orally is 30–60 minutes with peak effect at 90 minutes.
- Duration of effect is about 4–6 hours.

Cocaine

- Cocaine is a powerful psychostimulant on the CNS derived from the coca plant. This action on the brain reward system magnifies pleasure and can quickly lead to tolerance and dependence.

- Cocaine increases levels of dopamine in the brain, producing euphoria and increasing energy and alertness.
- Onset of action when snorted is within minutes. When 'crack' is inhaled or cocaine is taken intravenously, action is within seconds.
- There is an immediate and marked 'rush' that is highly pleasurable with heightened cognitive awareness, energy and euphoria lasting for about 30 minutes.
- Rapidly diminished effects due to short half-life.[12,45]
- Symptoms of cocaine intoxication[12] are outlined in Box 41.14.

Withdrawal

Repeated binges over a timeframe of weeks can lead to marked tolerance, neuro-adaptation and physical dependence, and withdrawal on cessation or rapid reduction. In the first 9 hours to 14 days after last cocaine use there is extreme exhaustion, hunger, a strong need to sleep, strong craving, marked agitation and mood swings which may extend to serious depression and suicidal ideation. The three-phase pattern of cocaine withdrawal is very similar to amphetamine withdrawal.[12]

For more information on cocaine see Section 3.3.3 in *Alcohol, Tobacco and Other Drugs: Clinical Guidelines for Nurses and Midwives 2012.*[12]

Amphetamines

Amphetamine is a synthetic psychoactive drug that stimulates the CNS, peripheral nervous systems and cardiovascular system. Peripherally, amphetamines stimulate the release of noradrenaline from stores in adrenergic nerve terminals, as well as directly stimulating adrenaline receptors. Centrally, amphetamines have a stimulating effect on several cortical centres including the cerebral cortex, medullary respiratory centre and reticular activating system. Amphetamines slow down catecholamine metabolism by inhibiting monoamine oxidase. The sum total of these effects can result in a clinical state of vasoconstriction, hypertension and tachycardia associated with hyperactivity and agitation.[12,31,45] There are medically prescribed psychostimulants for treatment of narcolepsy, attention deficit disorders and serious weight control, as well as illicit amphetamines.

Amphetamine (speed) and methamphetamine crystals ('crystal', 'ice') are illegal and are in increasing demand and availability worldwide.

Toxicity

Acute toxicity may be manifested by cardiac palpitations, tachycardia, increased respiratory rate and fever. At high levels of overdose, seizures, hypertension and dysrhythmias or myocardial ischaemia can occur. The patient experiences restlessness, paranoia, agitated delirium, confusion and repetitive stereotyped behaviours. Death is usually related to stroke, fatal dysrhythmias or myocardial infarction.[12,45]

As with any illicit drug, the manufacture of illicit amphetamines lacks quality control, with unknown purity, dose and ingredients resulting in extreme variability in nature, quality and chemical composition of these drugs. These factors place people who use amphetamines at a very real risk of being exposed to lethal adulterants, unknown doses, unpredictable side effects and toxicity.[45]

The acute toxic effects are due to increased stimulation and sympatho-mimetic activity of the CNS, possibly resulting in a drug-induced psychosis, paranoia and seizures. The toxic effects are 'an extension of the pharmacological properties of the drug, being determined by dose, route of administration', as well as by the mental state of the person.[45] Without immediate medical intervention, death may occur from dysrhythmia, myocardial infarction, hyperthermia or cerebral haemorrhage (stroke). Any young person presenting with any of these conditions needs to be assessed for acute psychostimulant toxicity.[12]

People who use psychostimulants may experience persecutory delusions, feeling hostile and violent towards others, as a response to the intoxicated experience. Panic may result in irrational behaviour, causing harm to self or others.[12]

Amphetamine-induced psychosis may progress to perceptual disturbances, delirium, paranoid delusions and aggressive or violent behaviour, and may be difficult to differentiate from acute paranoid schizophrenia. Psychotic symptoms generally subside soon after the drug use ceases, although some people may experience persistent symptoms for weeks or months.[12,45]

Chronic toxicity can be manifested by depression, anxiety and panic attacks (suicidal ideation has been reported), nutritional deficits and weight loss. Neuropsychiatric complications include poor concentration and attention, memory impairment, sleep disturbances, hallucinations and flashbacks (vivid sense of reliving the past drug-use experience). Rhinorrhoea, nasal ulcers, epistaxis, sinusitis and perforation of the nasal septum often manifest chronic intranasal use.[45]

Complications of amphetamine use

Complications are directly related to the route of administration, rapidity with which the brain is affected, dose and the person's individual vulnerabilities. Chronic cocaine or amphetamine use may lead to impairment of concentration and memory, irritability, mood swings, paranoia and depression. With intranasal use, the nasal septum and mucosa may be damaged, and frequent sniffing and rhinitis are common signs of intranasal use. Unsafe injecting may result in collapse and scarring of

---

BOX 41.14 Symptoms of cocaine intoxication[12]

- Pupils may be enlarged
- Increased BP and TPR
- Dry mouth
- Suppressed appetite
- Hyper-alertness and level of activity
- Pressured speech
- Increased self-confidence
- Euphoria
- Exhilaration
- Rapid mood swings
- Repetitious behaviour
- Panic
- Inability to sleep
- Paranoia
- Aggression
- Dysphoria and delirium.

BP: blood pressure; TPR: temperature, pulse and respiratory rate

the veins, thrombosis, cellulitis, bacterial infections, wound abscess, septicaemia, pericarditis, endocarditis and transmission of bacteria and blood-borne viruses—hepatitis B and C, and HIV.[12]

Psychostimulant-induced psychosis

A psychostimulant-induced psychosis can arise from once-off, occasional or regular use of psychostimulants. This form of psychosis is typically temporary. It generally progresses from paranoid delusions to visual hallucinations of 'snow lights', and tactile hallucinations of 'bugs' crawling under the skin. This drug-induced psychosis will settle with abstinence, usually within days or weeks. The acute phase is treated as for any other psychotic state. As well as good assessment and history taking, skin excoriations from scratching and needle marks, and elevated blood pressure, heart rate and temperature may help differentiate a stimulant psychosis from other psychoses.[12,45]

When the person presents they may be very agitated, irritable and aggressive. Management involves careful 'first line' assessment and treatment to ensure they can be safely treated. This may involve sedation and physical restraint.

Note: physical restraint alone is not enough to ensure patient safety and can result in elevation of the patient's agitated and aggressive state. Treatment is focused on 'safety first'. However consideration that underlying pathology is a cause or exacerbation of the severe behavioural change is considered, until excluded.[12,21-23]

Psychostimulant withdrawal

People who are dependent on psychostimulants rarely use 7 days a week, but rather in 'runs' of 3–4 days, due to exhaustion. Nevertheless, tolerance soon develops and withdrawal occurs with sudden cessation or reduction in amounts used.

Duration of acute withdrawal symptoms is associated with the type of psychostimulant drug used and its half-life, as well as duration of use, amount used and level of tolerance (e.g. 1–4 days for cocaine, up to about 3 weeks for amphetamines). Cessation results in what is often referred to as the immediate phase ('crash'), whereby the person experiences intense CNS-depressant-like symptoms, with a craving for sleep and feelings of exhaustion replacing the craving for the drug.[12,40] Withdrawal from psychostimulants is not life-threatening, but severe depression can be a symptom of withdrawal and may lead to suicidal ideation, self-harm and possibly death. People also report subtle muscular aches and pains. Eventually mood can settle, but intense craving for the drug may remain for some time, similar to what happens with nicotine cessation. The three phases of withdrawal and cessation are outlined in Box 41.15.

Clinical management of withdrawal

To date there is little reliable evidence of which prescribed medication regimen is most effective for treating psychostimulant withdrawal. Tailored symptomatic treatment and good nursing care in a supportive and safe environment are essential. The following need to be attended to:

- Observe at least 4-hourly.
- Monitor stages of withdrawal and adapt care to changing needs.
- Monitor depressed mood to identify and prevent risk of self-harm.

BOX 41.15 Phases of psychostimulant cessation[12,45]

Phase I—crash

The 'crash' (hangover) following cessation of psychostimulant use such as amphetamines begins about 9 hours after the last dose, and can last up to 2 days. This may be associated with a binge, and may or may not progress to the phase II withdrawal.

Crash symptoms include:

- extreme lethargy
- hunger
- formication
- headache
- anxiety
- insomnia
- irritability
- agitation
- aggression
- confusion
- mood lability.

Phase II—withdrawal

If neuro-adaptation and dependence have developed, the crash will be followed by the second phase—withdrawal. This will be associated with a period of normal moods, little craving for the drug and normal sleep pattern for 1–4 days. However, dysphoria and craving for the drug then start to increase again, in conjunction with:

- flattened mood
- disturbed sleep
- agitation
- anxiety
- lack of energy.

Possible aggressive outbursts may return, and delusional (paranoid) thinking with hallucinations may occur. Craving for the drug can be intense.

Phase III—extinction (prolonged withdrawal)

'Extinction' of withdrawal is characterised by gradual diminishing of the acute symptoms, and may last for weeks or several months. There can be episodic craving in response to environmental stimuli (cues) to use, and a feeling of anhedonia (inability to respond to pleasant events). The frequency of craving and the anhedonia does decrease over time, but likelihood of relapse is high.

- Ensure adequate food and fluid intake—expect variations, including hunger or poor appetite.
- Support during angry outbursts.
- Provide self-help information (e.g. *Getting through amphetamine withdrawal* from Turning Point in Victoria).
- Offer tips for coping with cravings, improving sleep, relaxation, coping with mood swings, aches and pains, nutrition and strange thoughts by focusing on the present.[12,45]

Methylphenidate

Methylphenidate (MPH, e.g. Ritalin) is a centrally-acting sympathomimetic psychostimulant. It is prescribed to children and adolescents, and occasionally adults, diagnosed with attention deficit hyperactivity disorder (ADHD). This assists in reducing their over-active, impulsive behaviours and improves concentration. It is also prescribed for people with diagnosed narcolepsy. Some people use illicit MPH and ingest or inject crushed, diluted tablets which places them at risk of systemic toxicity.[46] Methylphenidate tablets are chalky in consistency, and if not filtered well prior to injecting can cause emboli in vessels of the eyes and lungs.

For more information on amphetamines see Section 3.3.2 in *Alcohol, Tobacco and Other Drugs: Clinical Guidelines for Nurses and Midwives 2012.*[12]

Ecstasy—hallucinogenic with psychostimulant effects

Ecstasy is 3,4-methylenedioxymethylamphetamine (MDMA). It is a psychostimulant with hallucinogenic properties that cause pleasant emotional effects, euphoria and increased energy. Illicit production of ecstasy has increased significantly in Australia.[3,12]

As with other psychostimulants, MDMA has created concern about the safety of its use because of large variations in quality, and frequent substitution of what is sold as MDMA for other highly toxic drugs. While the chemical process of production is not very complicated for those with the expertise, impurities and poor technical expertise often lead to highly toxic products being sold. Like amphetamine and methamphetamine, MDMA is smuggled in from South East Asia and elsewhere, as well as produced locally in clandestine 'factories', resulting in large quantities being sold in both Australia and New Zealand.

Effects

As MDMA is related to mescaline and amphetamine, it has hallucinatory and stimulant properties. It induces pleasant emotional effects, euphoria and increased energy, although it is associated with potentially lethal complications such as hyperthermia.[12,45,47,48,56]

Autonomic effects:

- hypertension
- tachycardia
- poor temperature regulation—hyperthermia
- possible toxicity to serotonergic neurons.[31]

Quite common emergency MDMA presentations involve people with hyperthermia syndromes (see Ch 28). MDMA appears to decrease heat loss through constriction of blood vessels near the skin, and possibly through increased heat production by muscles and the brain. These effects may be amplified by dehydration and a poor ability to cool by sweating. MDMA can mask the body's normal thirst and exhaustion responses, particularly if the person is dancing or otherwise physically active for long periods of time without hydration. Because of its effects, MDMA can temporarily reduce the body's ability to regulate core temperature; so in high-temperature surroundings (for example, clubs) combined with physical exertion, hyperpyrexia can occur when the person cannot stay cool. Sustained hyperpyrexia can lead to rhabdomyolysis (muscle breakdown), which may rapidly progress to renal failure and death.

While dehydration is undesirable, people can experience water intoxication and hyponatraemia (dilution of the blood causing swelling of the brain) from drinking large amounts of water without salt replacement, causing water retention. There are also cases with no evidence of excessive water consumption, possibly due to MDMA inducing release of anti-diuretic hormone (vasopressin) by the pituitary gland.[45,47]

The use of ecstasy can exacerbate depression and may produce temporary depression as an after-effect for some people. Some people may also experience unexpected mood swings 1 or 2 days after using MDMA. MDMA use can be very dangerous when combined with other drugs (particularly monoamine oxidase inhibitors (MAOIs) and antiretroviral drugs, in particular ritonavir). Combining MDMA with MAOIs can precipitate a hypertensive crisis.[47]

Clinical management

The clinical management of acute MDMA (ecstasy) intoxication involves immediate treatment of symptoms and any complications as they emerge, as with other psychostimulants. There is a view that the drug dantrolene may be useful in the treatment of hyperthermia induced by the use of MDMA, but care needs to be taken in its use.[47,49,50]

For more information on MDMA see Section 3.4.5 in *Alcohol, Tobacco and Other Drugs: Clinical Guidelines for Nurses and Midwives 2012.*[12]

Some other drugs

Gamma-hydroxybutyrate (GHB)

GHB is a **depressant** neurotransmitter found naturally in the human CNS. GHB is not a true GABA agonist, but it is found naturally in the CNS where it acts as an inhibitory neurotransmitter. Medical use of GHB as an IV anaesthetic agent in the mid to late 1960s became unpopular due to its lack of analgesic effect, and risk of large doses causing seizures.[47]

GHB also has dopaminergic activity, increasing acetylcholine with endogenous opioids.[12,31,51–54] More recently, it has been used in the treatment of narcolepsy and alcohol dependence.

GHB is used as a 'street drug' with similar action to benzodiazepines, and known to be highly dose-dependent. It is mainly used for its euphoric effect. In high doses, profound sedation and seizures can occur; the short- and long-term effects of GHB can be seen in Box 41.16.

GHB, and similar agents (gamma-butyrolactone and -butanediol), have been known to be used illicitly. Street names include 'grievous bodily harm', 'scoop', 'liquid x' and 'liquid E'. GHB can be masked when added to alcoholic beverages, causing drowsiness and eventual stupefaction at higher doses. It has been known to be used to 'spike' alcoholic drinks by perpetrators intent on sexual assault (rape).[12,51,54]

GHB is usually ingested as a liquid and is rapidly absorbed by the GI tract, with peak plasma levels occurring within 15–45 minutes. Most GHB is metabolised prior to excretion via the kidneys within 8–10 hours of ingestion.

Due to its rapid absorption and excretion (about 9 hours), it is difficult to substantiate cases of drug rape by the time a victim reports the crime.[52,53] It is strongly advised that for anyone presenting to ED with a report of unexplained memory loss and/or signs of rape and alcohol consumption a urine and/or blood drug screen test is taken as soon as possible (and

BOX 41.16 GHB effects[12]

Low-dose short-term effects
- A state of euphoria
- Feeling calm, relaxed or tranquil
- Dizziness
- Disinhibition
- Nausea
- Placidity
- Visual disturbance—usually blurred vision
- Hot/cold flushes
- Drowsiness
- Increasingly sociable
- Increased levels of confidence
- Talkative
- Diaphoresis

High dose—short-term effects
- Rapid onset drowsiness +++
- Impaired movement and speech
- Confusion/disorientation
- Vomiting and nausea
- Muscular stiffness
- Short episodes of unconsciousness
- Aggression when stimulated despite being near respiratory arrest
- Uncontrollable twitching (tics)
- Agitation
- Visual disturbances—hallucinations
- Seizures
- Respiratory depression, arrest
- Death

BOX 41.17 GHB overdose symptoms[12,55]

- Decreased level of consciousness/coma
- Acute delirium
- Severe respiratory depression
- Hypothermia
- Respiratory acidosis
- Vomiting
- Hypotension (occasionally)
- Bradycardia.

For more information on GHB go to Section 3.1.5 in *Alcohol, Tobacco and Other Drugs: Clinical Guidelines for Nurses and Midwives 2012.*[12]

Ketamine

Ketamine is a dissociative anaesthetic with **stimulant properties** when taken in low doses. Ketamine is mainly used non-medically for its euphoric effect. Ketamine may be swallowed, snorted, smoked or injected, and is often called 'K' or 'Special K'. It has multiple mechanisms of CNS action.[12,56]

Onset of action varies with route of administration, and ranges from 30 seconds (IV) to 10–20 minutes (oral). Typical duration of action is 1–3 hours, with a half-life of 3 hours. Potential dangers of ketamine use are drug-induced psychosis, violence, accidents and marked psychomotor and cognitive impairment.[12,56]

It can produce a range of schizophrenia-like symptoms, including:
- flattened affect
- thought disorders
- depersonalisation
- catatonia.

Intoxication

Symptoms of ketamine intoxication are listed in Box 41.18. Ketamine overdose leads to:
- respiratory depression
- hyperthermia
- seizures—these can occur in people with known seizure disorders (literature reports that ketamine use may induce or terminate seizures).[12,57]

For more information on ketamine, see Section 3.5.1 in *Alcohol, Tobacco and Other Drugs: Clinical Guidelines for Nurses and Midwives 2012.*[12]

Hallucinogenics

Hallucinogens (psychedelics) include naturally-occurring and synthetic substances. They distort thinking, mood and perception—typically inducing illusions or hallucinations. They are most commonly used 'once off' or occasionally.

The acute effects of hallucinogens are due to the disrupted interaction between nerve cells and the neurotransmitter serotonin in the CNS. Distributed throughout the brain and spinal cord, the serotonin system is involved in the control of behavioural, perceptual and regulatory systems, including mood, hunger, body temperature, sexual behaviour,

other necessary forensic evidence) to assist early diagnosis and medical management and investigation of this crime. The effects of GHB intoxication are associated with the dose of the substance, and are grouped together as short-term effects (low dose) and short-term effects (high dose) (Box 41.16).[12] The more serious effects are associated with higher doses of GHB.

Overdose

Concurrent use of alcohol or other CNS depressants is common in GHB overdose. Overdose should be considered in any case of unexplained sudden coma, i.e. without any evidence of head injury, intake of coma-inducing drugs or increasing intracranial pressure. People typically regain consciousness spontaneously within 5 hours of ingestion. GHB overdose symptoms are listed in Box 41.17.[55]

Recovery from GHB toxicity is normally uneventful, although interim management of airway and respiration may be required.

Close observation is always required, as ingestion of GHB can cause rapid onset of CNS and respiratory depression and, in severe cases, coma—the incidence of directly related deaths in Australia is increasing.[54] Management is supportive and based on symptoms. A recent study undertaken in Australia identified that out of 170 emergency presentations, airway compromise (51%) and respiratory alterations (44%) were common manifestations of GHB intoxication requiring intervention.[53]

- Initial rush
- Nausea and vomiting
- Slurred speech
- Blurred vision
- Numbness and ataxia
- Cardiovascular and respiratory stimulation
- Dissociative 'out of body' sensations (flying or floating), detachment from immediate environment
- Muscle rigidity
- Reduced response to pain
- Risk of respiratory collapse and failure
- Feelings of aggression
- Overstimulation
- Temporary paralysis
- Hallucinations
- Euphoria

muscle control and sensory perception. Under the influence of hallucinogens, people can experience various forms of hallucinations, some of which produce rapid, intense mood swings from euphoria to paranoia and panic.[56,57]

Substances in this category include: lysergic acid diethylamide (LSD), phencyclidine (PCP), psilocybin and datura. These substances are not usually associated with tolerance, dependence or withdrawal.[12,57]

Intoxication
Symptoms include:
- altered perception, thought, emotions
- unusual and vivid perception of shapes, colour, sounds
- blurred boundary between self and surroundings
- feeling of detachment
- dizziness
- weakness
- nausea.

For further information on hallucinogenics, see Section 3.4.1 in *Alcohol, Tobacco and Other Drugs: Clinical Guidelines for Nurses and Midwives 2012.*[12]

Anabolic androgenic steroids (AAS)

In Australia and New Zealand AAS substances are available illegally through the 'black' market, internet and are commonly veterinary preparations.[12,50] AASs can synthesise body tissue and increase muscle mass and promote development of male sexual characteristics.

AASs are synthetically modified derivatives of testosterone available in oral or parenteral form.

People commonly use AAS substances for increased physical stamina, sexual or sporting performance, muscle strength and definition and possibly 'health'.[12,58,59]

AASs can be injected intramuscularly and those injecting may not consider that they can be at risk of contracting bacterial or viral infections including HIV and hepatitis B or C.[12]

People using AASs may also use other substances; for example, growth or reproductive hormones, diuretics, beta-2-

AASs, thyroxin, insulin, creatinine monohydrate.[12,58] People seeking the effect of AAS usually prefer the high anabolic effects.

Examples of AAS
- Water based. Stanazol is rapidly absorbed and more rapidly excreted then oil-based steroids, which may need to be administered twice a week. It is often injected with a 23-gauge or 21-gauge needle, as the powder in suspension can clog a narrower needle.
- Oil-based Deca 50 takes longer to absorb and take effect, and has a longer effect than water-based steroids, e.g between 2 and 3 weeks, although some people may use these more frequently. Oil-based steroids are usually injected with a 25-gauge needle.
- Anapolon 50 tablets are swallowed and the effects are short-acting. These tablets are taken twice a day.[12]
- AAS tablets are associated with more-adverse side effects due to the pharmacokinetics of substance during its 'first pass' through the digestive system. This causes the substance to lose some of its potency and can cause liver damage. Some AAS tablets have a coating designed to prevent it from being destroyed by acids in the stomach, and are categorised as C-17 alpha alkylated, and the coating used is also toxic to the liver.[12,31]

Note: Anapolon may be more toxic than injectable steroids, but this remains unclear.

AAS use—serious risks[12,58,69]
- abscesses, cellulitis, endocarditis etc (blood-borne viruses, bacterial infections)
- tendon or ligament damage.
- adenocarcinoma of prostate
- adenocarcinoma of colon
- Wilms tumour
- testicular atrophy
- gynaecomastia in men
- irregularities or cessation of menstruation
- hypokalaemic-induced dysrhythmia (due to concomitant diuretic use)
- hypertension
- oedema
- insulin resistance or impaired glucose tolerance
- diabetes
- increased low-density lipid proteins and decreased high-density lipid proteins
- salt and fluid retention
- cancer of liver, kidneys, prostate
- liver damage, e.g. jaundice, cirrhosis, tumours
- immunological changes
- sleeping difficulties
- acne
- loss of body hair
- aggression
- irritability
- labile mood
- depression
- mania
- psychosis.

AASs are often taken in combination with other substances and may potentiate or enhance the effects of other substances; therefore, it is important when assessing the patient who is using AAS to ensure a complete substance and medication history is gathered in order to anticipate and treat the more serious side effects. Box 41.19 lists some of the clinical features likely to be noted and their association with other substances and medications.

BOX 41.19 Clinical manifestations of anabolic androgenic steroid use in combination with other substances

AAS and psycho-stimulants
- Increased body temperature
- Increased heart rate
- Increased blood pressure
- Masked pain
- Increased cardiac pressure resulting in convulsions and cardiac arrest
- Increased aggression
- Euphoria

AAS and depressants, e.g. benzodiazepines, opiates, alcohol
- Reduced responsiveness to pain

AAS and diuretics
- Increases sodium levels causing fluid retention
- Altered sodium/potassium balance (kidney damage, muscle weakness, cardiac arrest)

AAS and clonidine
- Increased risk of kidney and liver disease

AAS and insulin
- Risk of insulin-related death

SUMMARY

An awareness and understanding of the physiological and psychological effects of ATOD is essential for the paramedic and emergency clinician. It enables clinicians to anticipate and monitor potential complications and deterioration, commence assessment and treatment in the pre-hospital setting and further assist with assessment, diagnosis and ongoing treatment in the ED environment. Screening for ATOD use can detect risk factors and potential health problems, and is the first step towards assessment, early intervention and treatment.

High-quality care ensures that the health needs of individual patients are kept to the fore, and the patient is respected, well informed and provided with holistic care. Even in busy emergency environments or during assessment, stabilisation and transportation to hospital, clinical management needs to be focused on attending to this patient's immediate needs, and empowering the person to better manage their own lives. Some people take longer than others to trust healthcare professionals and services, and to change their risky health behaviours, such as poor diet, smoking or risky drinking or drug use. If emergency staff can engage the patient and make them feel valued, they may consider taking up a suggestion for follow-up, return for treatment as required and move towards reducing or stopping harmful drinking or drug use.[12,59]

CASE STUDY 2—BRIAN

Part 1

You (the paramedic) have been sent to the rear entrance of a local wine bar, to attend a man who has reportedly fallen and is unable to get up. It is 0200 on a cold winter Sunday morning. On your arrival, Mike, the manager of the wine bar, meets you, and he points you towards a man sitting upright against the fence, and tells you that this is Brian, his business partner. Brian is apparently asleep, with what looks like a handkerchief wrapped around his left hand. It is stained with blood. His shirt is vomit-stained, and he appears to have been incontinent. Brian rouses intermittently and becomes agitated and verbally aggressive. Mike says they finished work just before midnight, and had a 'few drinks' after closing for the night. Mike also tells you that Brian had been drinking steadily throughout the evening, and has probably consumed about 2–3 bottles of red wine. Brian was last seen taking a crate of empty bottles to the bin. Mike heard the sound of breaking bottles, and when he went to investigate found Brian lying amongst the broken glass. He had tried to stand but was unable to get to his feet. Brian told Mike that he had slipped and fallen.

Questions

1. How will you ensure your safety and the safety of others while assessing Brian?
2. How will you assess Brian?
3. What do you think has happened? And why?
4. What would you do first?
5. What interventions and resources would you consider using?

Part 2

Brian allows you to examine him. The hand laceration is deep. You bandage the wound, knowing that it will require suturing. You tell Brian that he needs to go to hospital. While Brian is not happy, with Mike's help he agrees to go in the ambulance to the hospital.

Brian arrives at emergency. You are now the triage nurse. The paramedic gives you a detailed hand-over and describes his behaviour at the scene. The paramedic explains that once the patient had been loaded into the ambulance he seemed to settle down. The paramedic had also ascertained from Mike that when Brian drinks as he did tonight, he becomes aggressive. He has been drinking heavily for the last month and a half.

Brian appears to be asleep, and is snoring loudly with slow respirations. He is pale and his skin is cool. He has a weak radial pulse and is tachycardic. When you attempt to rouse him, he opens his eyes to painful stimuli only. He has a dressing on his left hand and smells strongly of alcohol.

He rouses temporarily and tries to sit on the side of the wheeled barouche.

Questions (continued)

6. What are treatment priorities of care for Brian?
7. Where is the most appropriate place for Brian to be nursed in the emergency department (ED)?
8. What interventions and resources might you anticipate using during Brian's stay in the ED?
9. Are there any other conditions that could mimic Brian's condition and behaviour? How would you assess for these?
10. What observations and interventions will Brian require?
11. Assuming that Brian is medically cleared and his hand sutured, what discharge advice could Brian be given?
12. What support services could be offered to Brian while he is in the ED, and for when he is ready to go home?

 Answers to Case Study Questions can be found on evolve
http://evolve.emergencytrauma.curtis

CASE STUDY 3—NATALIE

Part 1

As a paramedic, you attend a 25-year-old woman (Natalie) whose neighbour reported as behaving bizarrely.

When you arrive at the front door you hear shouting. You are met by a woman (Sandra) who says she called you because she is so worried about her friend. She tells you that Natalie had been 'partying' 5 days ago and only came home about an hour ago. She has been behaving erratically ever since. When you try to enter the house, Natalie starts throwing plates at you and threatens you with a knife. She shouts that you are from the devil's army.

Natalie appears frightened and disorientated. She is unkempt, and while her clothes are intact they are dirty and very creased. Sandra tells you that it is common for Natalie to go out for a couple of days at a time, and take 'speed and ecstasy'. She does not know what Natalie has taken this time.

Questions

1. How can you ensure that you can safely assess Natalie?
2. What interventions and resources do you anticipate will be required?
3. What do you suspect has occurred? And why?

Part 2

The police are called and have arrived, and with Sandra's reassurance, Natalie allows you to assess her. She is still talking about the 'devil's army' in between incoherent, rambling speech. When asked, she tells you her name and

date of birth, but does not know what day it is. Her attention span is brief but she responds to instructions intermittently.

Her pupils are enlarged, and react to light. She is tachypnoeic with a respiratory rate of 36 breaths/minute, and tachycardic at 140 beats/minute; her blood pressure is 90/60 mmHg. She has dry oral mucosa, and her skin is hot and dry to the touch. Sandra tells you that Natalie takes an injection for her diabetes, but doesn't know when she last injected. Natalie is unable to recall.

Questions (continued)

4. What assessments will you need to perform on Natalie?
5. What interventions will you initiate?
6. How will you ensure that Natalie can be safely transported to hospital?

Part 3

On arrival at the emergency department (ED), the paramedic provides you, the triage nurse, with a hand-over, which includes Natalie's condition, recent events, assessments and interventions undertaken prior to arriving at the ED. The police are also in attendance.

Natalie's airway is clear; she continues to be tachypnoeic and tachycardic with a weak pulse. The paramedic has established an intravenous line, and she is currently receiving Normal saline. The paramedic also informs you of her known medical history and reports that a blood sugar level result read 'high'. Natalie continues talking in rambling sentences, is agitated and intermittently verbally aggressive.

Questions (continued)

7. What is the safest environment in which to assess and treat Natalie?

8. What do you think has happened?

9. How does this explain her clinical signs and symptoms?

10. Once you are able to assess Natalie safely, what will the priorities of her care be?

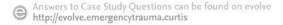

Answers to Case Study Questions can be found on evolve
http://evolve.emergencytrauma.curtis

USEFUL WEBSITES

Alcohol, Smoking and Substance Involvement Screening Test (ASSIST), www.who.int/substance_abuse/activities/assist/en/

Alcohol, Tobacco and Other Drugs: Clinical Guidelines for Nurses and Midwives. 2012. http://www.sahealth.sa.gov.au/wps/wcm/connect/9087368041793eefa6e1ef67a94f09f9/ATOD+Clinical+Guidelines+for+Nurses+and+Midwives+V3+2012-DASSA-Oct2013.pdf?MOD=AJPERES&CACHEID=9087368041793eefa6e1ef67a94f09f9

Drug and Alcohol Nurses of Australasia (DANA), www.danaonline.org

South Australian Department of Health: Substance Misuse and Dependence, http://www.sahealth.sa.gov.au/wps/wcm/connect/Public+Content/SA+Health+Internet/Clinical+resources/Clinical+topics/Substance+misuse+and+dependence/Drug+and+alcohol+publications+and+resources+for+heath+professionals

NSW Health, best-practice alcohol withdrawal management, www.health.nsw.gov.au/policies/gl/2008/pdf/GL2008_011.pdf

Royal Australasian College of Physicians—Australasian Chapter of Addiction Medicine (AChAM), www.racp.edu.au/page/australasian-chapter-of-addiction-medicine/

REFERENCES

1. World Health Organization (WHO). Lexicon of alcohol and drug terms. Geneva: WHO; 1994. Online. www.who.int/substance_abuse/terminology/who_lexicon/en/print.html; accessed 2 Mar 2010.

2. National Centre for Education and Training on Addiction Consortium, ed. Alcohol and other drugs: a handbook for health professionals. Canberra: Australian Government Department of Health and Ageing; 2004.

3. Australian Institute of Health and Welfare 2011. 2010 National Drug Strategy Household Survey Report. Drug statistics series no. 25. Cat. no. PHE 145 Canberra: AIHW.

4. National Health and Medical Research Council. Australian guidelines to reduce health risks from drinking alcohol. Canberra: Commonwealth of Australia; 2009.

5. Collins DJ, Lapsley HM. The costs of tobacco, alcohol and illicit drug abuse to Australian society in 2004/05. Canberra: Commonwealth Department of Health and Aged Care; 2008.

6. Boden JM, Fergusson DM, Horwood LJ. Illicit drug use and dependence in a New Zealand birth cohort. Aust N Z J Psychiatry 2006;40(2):156–63.

7. Ministry of Health 2013. Amphetamine Use 2012/13: Key findings of the New Zealand Health Survey. Wellington: Ministry of Health.

8. Australian Institute of Health and Welfare. 2010 National Drug Strategy Household Survey Report. Drug statistics series no. 25. Cat. no. PHE 145; Canberra: AIHW; 2011: 126.

9. Zinberg N. Drug, set and setting. New Haven: Yale University Press; 1984.

10. National Health and Medical Research Council. Australian drinking guidelines. Health risks and benefits. Canberra: NHMRC; 2001. Online. https://www.nhmrc.gov.au/_files_nhmrc/publications/attachments/ds9.pdf; accessed 15 June 2015.

11. Ritter A, King T, Hamilton M. 2013. Drug use in Australian society. Melbourne: Oxford University Press.

12. de Crespigny C, Talmet J (eds). Alcohol, tobacco and other drugs: clinical guidelines for nurses and midwives; 2012. Version 3. The University of Adelaide School of Nursing and Drug and Alcohol Services SA. Online. www.sahealth.sa.gov.au/wps/wcm/connect/9087368041793eefa6e1ef67a94f09f9/ATOD+Clinical+Guidelines+for+Nurses+and+Midwives+V3+2012-DASSA-April2014.pdf?MOD=AJPERES&CACHEID=9087368041793eefa6e1ef67a94f09f9

13. Thorley A. The effects of alcohol. In: Plant M, ed. Drinking and problem drinking. London: Junction Books, 1982.

14. Cooper DB. Introduction to mental health-substance use. Radcliffe Pub, Oxford; New York, 2011.

15. Lewis SM, Collier IC, Heitkemper MM. Medical–surgical nursing: assessment and management of clinical problems. 7th edn. St Louis: Mosby; 2007:169–70.

16. Smoking and Substance Involvement Screening Test (ASSIST), www.who.int/substance_abuse/activities/en/Draft_The_ASSIST_Guidelines.pdf; accessed 29 April 2015.

17. Clancy C, Coyne P. Specialist assessment in a multidisciplinary setting. In: Rassool H, Gaffoor M, eds. Addiction nursing: perspectives on professional and clinical practice. Gloucester: Stanley Thornes; 1997.

18. Koehler S, Ladham S, Rozin L et al. The risk of body packing: a case of a fatal cocaine overdose. Forensic Sci Int 2005;161(1):81–4.

19. Low VH, Dillon EK. Agony of the ecstasy: report of five cases of MDMA smuggling. Australas Radiol 2005;49(5):400–3.

20. de Crespigny C, Emden C, Drage B et al. Missed opportunities in the field: caring for clients with co-morbidity problems. Collegian 2002;9(3):29–34.

21. Baker A, Lee NK, Jenner L, eds. Models of intervention and care for psychostimulant users. 2nd edn. National Drug Strategy Monograph Series No 51. Commonwealth of Australia. Canberra: Australian Government Department of Health and Ageing; 2004.

22. Chow F, Wodak A, Graham R. Poisonings, overdosage, drugs and alcohol. In: Fulde G, editor. Emergency medicine: the principles of practice. 6th edn. Sydney: Elsevier; 2014:536–81.

23. Hoggett K. Drugs of abuse. In: Cameron P, Jelinek G, Kelly AM et al, eds. Textbook of adult emergency medicine. 4th edn. Sydney: Elsevier; 2009:943–52.

24. Haber P, Lintzeris N, Proude E et al. Guidelines for the treatment of alcohol problems. Canberra: Australian Government Department of Health and Ageing; 2010.

25. Australian Department of Health and Ageing. Alcohol treatment guidelines for indigenous Australians. Canberra: Department of Health and Ageing; 2007.

26. Patel VB, Why HJ, Richardson P et al. The effects of alcohol on the heart. Adverse Drug React Toxicol Rev 1997;16(1):15–43.

27. Johnstone RE, Reier CE. Acute respiratory effects of ethanol in man. Clin Pharmacol Ther 1973;14(4):501–8.

28. Leiber CS. Hepatic, metabolic and nutritional disorders of alcoholism: from pathogenesis to therapy. Crit Rev Clin Lab Sci 2000;37(6):551–84.

29. Donnino MW, Vega J, Miller J, Walsh M. Myths and misconceptions of Wernicke's Encephalopathy: What every emergency physician should know. Annals of Emergency Medicine 2007;50(6):715–21.

30. Allison MG, McCurdy MT. Alcoholic metabolic emergencies. Emergency Medicine Clinics of North America 2014;32(2):293–301.

31. South Australian Drug and Alcohol Services Council material. Parkside: DASC; 1996.

32. Center for Health Care Evaluation. Clinical Practice Guidelines Online Course: CIWA-Ar Case Study #1; www.chce.research.va.gov/apps/PAWS/content/4.htm

33. Fawcett P. Conversion of morphine to heroin with acetic anhydride. Report to the Dunedin Intravenous Organisation. Dunedin: DIO; 1996.

34. Connor M, Christie MD. Opioid receptor signalling mechanisms. Clin Exp Pharmacol Physiol 1999;26(7):493–9.

35. Haber PS, Dermikol A, Lange K et al. Management of injecting drug users admitted to hospital. Lancet 2009;374(9697):1284–93.

36. Farquhar S, Fawcett J, Fountain J. Illicit intravenous use of methylphenidate (Ritalin) tablets: a review of four cases. Australas Emerg Nurs J 2002;5:25–9.

37. Compton P, Althanasos P, de Crespigny C. Opioid tolerance and the management of acute pain. Workshop presented at the Drug and Alcohol Nurses of Australasia 2006 Conference: bridging evidence and practice. Sydney; 21–23 June 2006.

38. Department of Health (England) and the devolved administrators. Drug misuse and dependence. UK Guidelines on Clinical Management. London: Department of Health (England), Scottish Government, Welsh Assembly Government and Northern Ireland Executive; 2007. Online. www.nta.nhu.uk/uploads/clinical_guidelines2007.

39. Athanasos P, de Crespigny C. Specific nursing strategies for the pain management of opioid dependent patients. Paper presented at the Drug and Alcohol Nurses of Australasia 2006 Conference: bridging evidence and practice, 21–23 June 2006. Sydney; 2006.

40. Young R, Saunders J, Hulse G. Opioids. In: Hulse G, White J, Cape G, eds. Management of alcohol and drug problems. Melbourne: Oxford University Press; 2002.

41. Gowing L, Proudfoot H, Henry-Edwards S et al. Evidence supporting treatment: the effectiveness of interventions for illicit drug use. Canberra: Australian National Council on Drugs; 2001.

42. Beasley M, Frampton L, Fountain J. Inhalant abuse in New Zealand. N Z Med J 2006;119(1233):U1952.

43. BP Australia. BP helps tackle petrol sniffing: the 10 year journey of Opal. Youtube. www.youtube.com/watch?v=9EjcA6tlFmE; accessed 29 April 2015.

44. Frei M, Berends L, Kenny P et al. Cannabis withdrawal. In: Alcohol and other drug withdrawal: practice guidelines, 2nd edn, Turning Point Alcohol and Drug Centre. A Victorian Government project; 2012.

45. Latt N, White J, McLean S et al. Central nervous system stimulants, In: Hulse G, White J, Cape G, eds. Management of alcohol and drug problems. Melbourne: Oxford University Press; 2002.

46. Parran TV Jr, Jasinski DR. Intravenous methylphenidate abuse: prototype for prescription drug abuse. Arch Intern Med 1991;151(4):781–3.

47. Denborough MA, Hopkinson KC. Dantrolene and 'ecstasy'. Med J Aust 1997;166(3):165–6.

48. Hahn H. MDMA Toxicity. Medscape. Online. http://emedicine.medscape.com/article/821572-overview; accessed 29 April 2015.

49. Hall AP1, Henry JA. Acute toxic effects of 'Ecstasy' (MDMA) and related compounds: overview of pathophysiology and clinical management. Br J Anaesth 2006;96(6):678–85. Epub 2006 Apr 4.

50. Mason PE, Kerns WP 2nd. Gamma hydroxybutyric acid (GHB) intoxication. Acad Emerg Med 2002;9(7):730–9.

51. Karch S. Karch's pathology of drug abuse. 3rd edn. Florida: CRC Press; 2002.

52. Munir VL, Hutton JE, Harney JP et al. Gamma-hydroxybutyrate: a 30-month emergency department review. Emerg Med Australas 2008;20(6):521–30.

53. Caldicott DG, Chow FY, Burns BJ et al. Fatalities associated with the use of gamma-hydroxybutyrate and its analogues in Australasia. Med J Aust 2004;191(6):310–13.

54. National Institute on Drug Abuse. NIDA Infofacts: LSD Revised 05/06. Online. www.nida.nih.gov/infofacts/lsd.html; 9 Mar 2010.

55. Hulse G, White J, Cape G, eds. Management of alcohol and drug problems. Melbourne: Oxford University Press; 2002.

56. White J, Martin J, Krum H et al. Hallucinogens. In: Hulse G, White J, Cape G, eds. Management of alcohol and drug problems. Melbourne: Oxford University Press; 2002

57. Larance, B, Degenhardt L, Dillon P, Copeland J. 2005. Use of performance and image enhancing drugs among men. A review. National Drug and Alcohol Research Centre. University of NSW. NDARC Technical Report No. 232. Sydney.

58. New South Wales Department of Health. Anabolic androgenic steriods: information for medical practitioners, NSW Department of Health. Sydney; 2002.

59. Jarvis TJ, Tebbutt J, Mattick RP, Shand F. 2005. Treatment approaches for alcohol and drug dependence. An introductory guide. 2nd edn. John Wiley and Sons Ltd, Chichester.

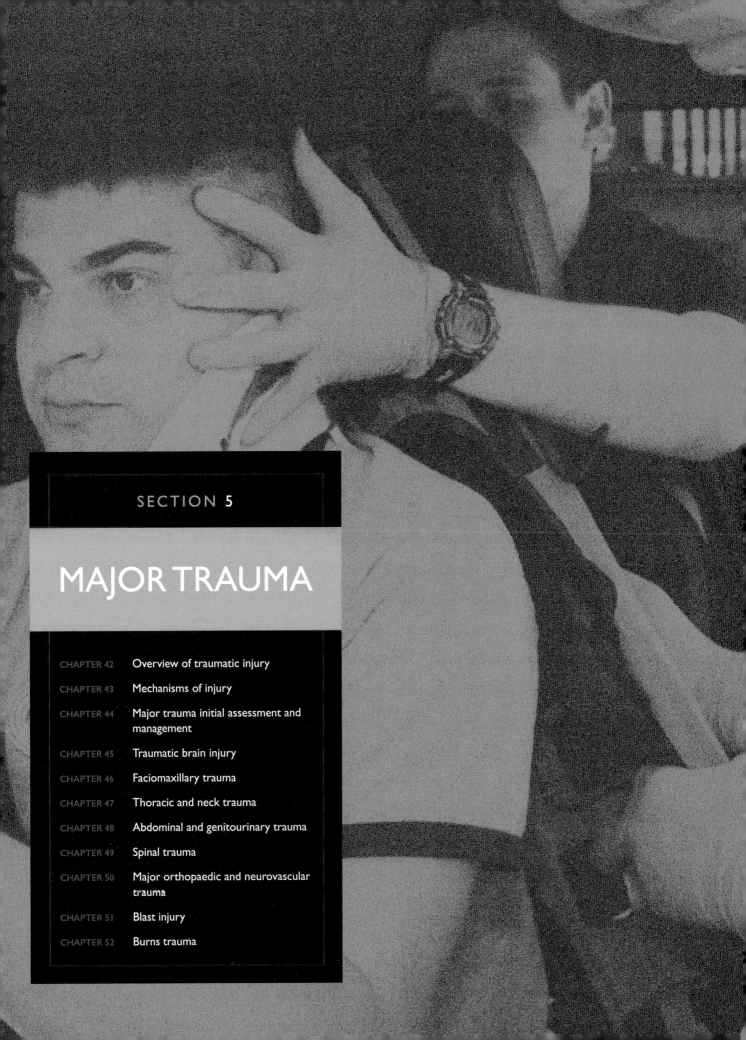

CHAPTER 42

OVERVIEW OF TRAUMATIC INJURY

ERICA CALDWELL, ANDREA HERRING (DELPRADO) AND KATE CURTIS

Essentials

- Epidemiology is an essential instrument in understanding trauma as both a clinical and a public health problem, because of its implications for clinical practice, social policy, public policy, legislation, injury prevention programs and as a source of data for trauma research.
- Injury is the fourth most common cause of death in Australia and accounts for more years of lost life up to 65 years of age than cardiovascular disease and cancer combined. Male injury death rates are, on average, about twice those of females.
- Falls are the most commonly reported external cause of admission for both males and females. Although fall rates were concentrated in the older age groups, our understanding of contributing factors is limited by a lack of information about the nature of the falls.
- While the rate of male suicide has fallen since its peak in 1997, men are still almost four times more likely to commit suicide than women.
- Aboriginal and Torres Strait Islander suicide rates are nearly double the rate for other Australians, and the transport injury death rate almost three times as high.
- The relationship between alcohol and an increased risk of injury or death is demonstrated in many settings, including accidents, violence and self-harm.
- Worldwide, the predominant cause of early death after trauma continues to be central nervous system (CNS—brain) injury, followed by exsanguination.
- Australian and New Zealand firearm-related injuries are low in comparison with the rest of the world. Firearms are used in 8% of assaults in New Zealand compared with 50% in the USA.
- One per cent of the population of Australia and New Zealand suffers from burns each year. Children under 5 years of age made up the largest single group of burns victims, followed by males aged 10–29 years. The vast majority occurred in the kitchen (40%), while about 15% involve the workplace.
- The perception of injuries as preventable events rather than acts of random unexpectedness is fundamental to the success of any injury prevention program.

INTRODUCTION

This chapter gives an overview of trauma management that provides clinicians with a context for trauma care and their role in trauma management systems. It provides an overview of the epidemiology of trauma in Australia and New Zealand, examines patterns of injury, injury prevention, standardisation of clinical trauma management and the development of organised trauma systems in Australia and New Zealand. The first step in framing the context of trauma is to understand the nature, extent and distribution of the problem.

Trauma incorporates a large spectrum of ailments, ranging from minor injury requiring little medical intervention through to severe multisystem trauma, requiring complex treatments from a multidisciplinary team. Of the many public health challenges facing pre-hospital and in-hospital clinicians on a daily basis, traumatic injury is one of the most significant as a cause of mortality and morbidity. This is on a global scale, whether from large-scale disasters (both natural and man-made) or the day-to-day non-intentional injuries and intentional interpersonal violence. The sources cited in this chapter were the most recent available at the time of publication and currency varies across specific areas of injury.

Globally, although the number of deaths from injury has risen by 24% since 1990, death rates following injury were only marginally higher in 2010 (9.6%) compared with two decades earlier (8.8%).[1] In 2000, injuries accounted for 10.3% of all disability-adjusted life-years (DALY),[16] but the number of injuries, and hence DALY, has increased to 10.7%.[2] This global increase is demonstrated in Figures 42.1

and 42.2. DALY is defined as years of healthy life lost and is the sum of years lived with disability (YLD) and years of life lost (YLL). DALYs are a powerful tool for priority setting as they measure disease burden from non-fatal as well as fatal conditions.

Since 1990, deaths due to road crashes grew by 46%, and road injuries now rank as the world's eighth-leading cause of death and the number-one killer of young people ages 15 to 24.[4] Road crashes result in 1.3 million deaths annually and 78.2 million nonfatal injuries warranting medical care. Approximately 90% of all road crashes now happen in low- and middle-income countries; yet they account for only half of the world's motor vehicles. More than half of global deaths are among pedestrians (35%) and operators of motorised two-wheeled vehicles (16%). The increasing use of vehicles over time has led to more air pollution, which also negatively impacts health via emissions and decreased physical activity. Deaths attributable to air pollution, to which motor vehicles are an important contributor, grew by 11% in 2010. In May 2011, the UN Decade of Action for Road Safety 2011–2020

FIGURE 42.1 Global death ranks with 95% UIs for the top 25 causes in 1990 and 2010, and the percentage change with 95% UIs between 1990 and 2010.[1]

1990		2010		
Mean rank (95% UI)	Disorder	Disorder	Mean rank (95% UI)	% change (95% UI)
1·0 (1 to 2)	1 Ischaemic heart disease	1 Ischaemic heart disease	1·0 (1 to 1)	35 (29 to 39)
2·0 (1 to 2)	2 Stroke	2 Stroke	2·0 (2 to 2)	26 (14 to 32)
3·0 (3 to 4)	3 Lower respiratory infections	3 COPD	3·4 (3 to 4)	−7 (−12 to 0)
4·0 (3 to 4)	4 COPD	4 Lower respiratory infections	3·6 (3 to 4)	−18 (−24 to −11)
5·0 (5 to 5)	5 Diarrhoea	5 Lung cancer	5·8 (5 to 10)	48 (24 to 61)
6·1 (6 to 7)	6 Tuberculosis	6 HIV/AIDS	6·4 (5 to 8)	396 (323 to 465)
7·3 (7 to 9)	7 Preterm birth complications	7 Diarrhoea	6·7 (5 to 9)	−42 (−49 to −35)
8·6 (7 to 12)	8 Lung cancer	8 Road injury	8·4 (5 to 11)	47 (18 to 86)
9·4 (7 to 13)	9 Malaria	9 Diabetes	9·0 (7 to 11)	93 (68 to 102)
10·4 (8 to 14)	10 Road injury	10 Tuberculosis	10·1 (8 to 13)	−18 (−35 to −3)
10·8 (8 to 14)	11 Protein–energy malnutrition	11 Malaria	10·3 (6 to 13)	21 (−9 to 56)
12·8 (11 to 16)	12 Cirrhosis	12 Cirrhosis	11·8 (10 to 14)	33 (25 to 41)
13·2 (9 to 18)	13 Stomach cancer	13 Self-harm	14·1 (11 to 20)	32 (8 to 49)
15·6 (12 to 20)	14 Self-harm	14 Hypertensive heart disease	14·2 (12 to 18)	48 (39 to 56)
15·8 (13 to 19)	15 Diabetes	15 Preterm birth complications	14·4 (12 to 18)	−28 (−39 to −17)
16·1 (12 to 20)	16 Congenital anomalies	16 Liver cancer	16·9 (14 to 20)	63 (49 to 78)
16·9 (13 to 20)	17 Neonatal encephalopathy*	17 Stomach cancer	17·0 (13 to 22)	−2 (−10 to 5)
18·3 (14 to 22)	18 Hypertensive heart disease	18 Chronic kidney disease	17·4 (15 to 21)	82 (65 to 95)
21·1 (6 to 44)	19 Measles	19 Colorectal cancer	18·5 (15 to 21)	46 (36 to 63)
21·1 (12 to 36)	20 Neonatal sepsis	20 Other cardiovascular and circulatory	19·7 (18 to 21)	46 (40 to 55)
21·3 (19 to 26)	21 Colorectal cancer	21 Protein–energy malnutrition	21·5 (19 to 25)	−32 (−42 to −21)
21·6 (18 to 26)	22 Meningitis	22 Falls	23·3 (21 to 29)	56 (20 to 84)
23·2 (21 to 26)	23 Other cardiovascular and circulatory	23 Congenital anomalies	24·4 (21 to 29)	−22 (−40 to −3)
23·7 (20 to 28)	24 Liver cancer	24 Neonatal encephalopathy*	24·4 (21 to 30)	−20 (−33 to −2)
23·8 (20 to 27)	25 Rheumatic heart disease	25 Neonatal sepsis	25·1 (15 to 35)	−3 (−25 to 27)
	27 Chronic kidney disease	29 Meningitis		
	30 Falls	33 Rheumatic heart disease		
	35 HIV/AIDS	62 Measles		

☐ Communicable, maternal, neonatal and nutritional disorders
☐ Non–communicable diseases
☐ Injuries

—— Ascending order in rank
---- Descending order in rank

UI=uncertainty interval. COPD=chronic obstructive pulmonary disease.

*Includes birth asphyxia/trauma. An interactive version of this figure is available online at http://www.healthdata.org/gbd/data-visualizations

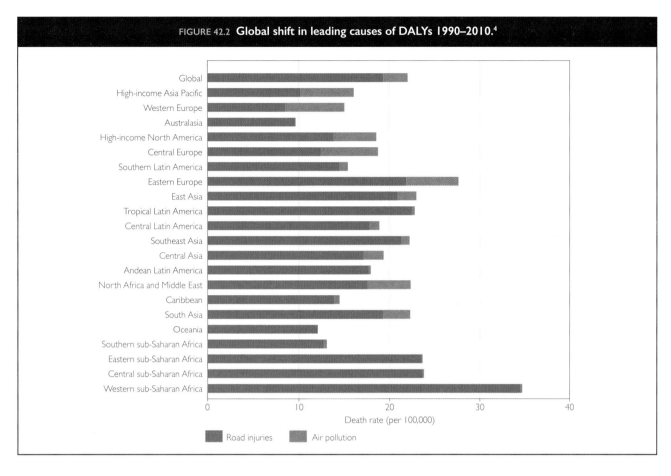

FIGURE 42.2 Global shift in leading causes of DALYs 1990–2010.[4]

was launched in more than 100 countries with the goal of preventing 5 million road traffic deaths and 50 million serious injuries.

In 2010, injury was estimated to account for 6.5% of the total burden of disease in Australia and remains the leading cause of death in those aged 1 to 45 years. Injuries account for more potential years of life lost than cancer and heart disease combined.[5] In New Zealand, injuries are the fifth leading cause of health loss and the third leading cause of premature mortality.[6] Injury (unintentional and intentional) is the leading cause of death for ages 1 to 34 years, and the second leading cause of hospitalisation. The injury List Of All Deficits (LOAD) framework conceptualises the full range of deficits and adverse outcomes following injury and violence (Figure 42.3).[7]

In view of the magnitude of this problem, the role of trauma clinicians is pivotal. Trauma clinicians require not only an in-depth understanding of the mechanism of injury, physiological responses to trauma and structured approaches to injury management; they also need to understand the determinants and extent of traumatic injury as a significant and burgeoning public health issue. As well as a working knowledge of trauma systems, trauma clinicians also need to understand their role within these systems and how this role can optimise patient outcomes through the continuum of trauma care.

History

Death and disability resulting from injury have been embedded in the evolution of Australian and New Zealand societies. Death and injury resulting from falls or tribal conflict and as sequelae of nomadic life are an integral part of Indigenous Australian Aboriginal Dreamtime.[8] During European colonisation of Australia and New Zealand, traumatic injury was a common cause of death among convicts and settlers alike. Indeed, trauma was once considered an inevitable part of life in terms of how often it occurred and how likely it was to result in death. However, present-day expectations of trauma management and injury outcomes have changed substantially.

Contemporary understanding of patterns of injury and physiological responses to trauma were accelerated through periods of military conflict. An improved understanding of the mechanism of injury during World War II meant that countless lives were saved through the simple actions of splinting and immobilisation of major fractures.[9] The Vietnam War saw a significant improvement in our understanding of the physiology of shock[9]—the importance of haemostasis and fluid resuscitation resulted in the emergence of surgical field hospitals. Consequently, soldiers were surviving long enough to return home to deal with permanent physical disabilities and post-traumatic stress that resulted from their injuries.

In Australia, injury was first recognised as a national health priority in 1996[5] and the subject of three national prevention plans: the National Injury Prevention and Safety Promotion Plan: 2004–2014; the National Falls Prevention for Older People Plan: 2004 Onwards; and the National Indigenous Safety Promotion Strategy.[10–12]

Despite the acknowledged importance of injury as an issue, and injury prevention as a solution, progress towards a

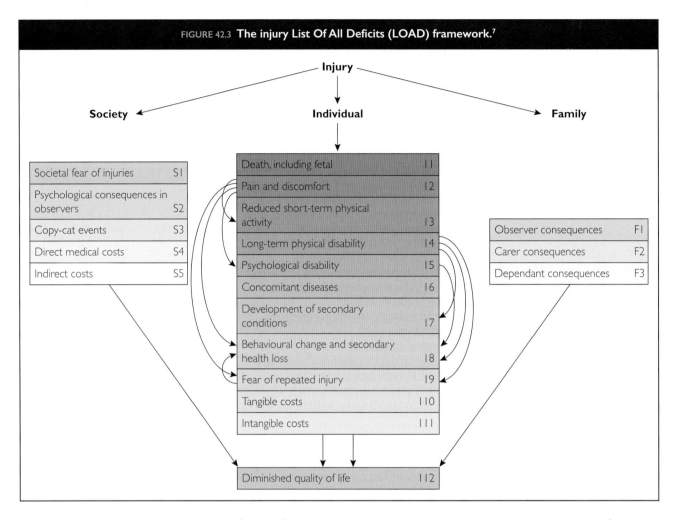

FIGURE 42.3 **The injury List Of All Deficits (LOAD) framework.**[7]

systematic response has been slow. Further, funding for injury research has consistently remained less than half that for cancer research, and less than diabetes, mental health, cardiovascular and obesity research.[13]

Epidemiology of trauma in Australia and New Zealand

Epidemiology is an essential instrument in understanding trauma as both a clinical and a public health problem because of its implications for clinical practice, social policy, public policy, legislation, injury prevention programs and as a source of data for trauma research. Data elements, such as incidence, prevalence, rates, risk, age, sex, ethnicity, geographical distribution, morbidity and mortality, are rich sources of information for both clinicians and public health researchers alike.

In Australia in 2010–11, injury admissions to hospital were more common in males than females for all age groups up to 64 years; the largest difference being for ages 15–24. After age 65, injury rates were higher for females. About 1 in 6 injury cases were classified as high threat to life. Two main causes of injury in 2010–11 were falls (39%) and transport incidents (12%). Over 170,000 people were hospitalised as a result of falls in 2010–11, 53% of the cases occurring at ages 65+. Transport injuries were more common in males than females and rates highest for the 15–24-year-old age group.[5] Most injuries occur in settings such as car crashes, interpersonal violence, sporting

and recreational activities and work. More than half the most severe injuries in Australia are also caused by road trauma.[14]

In New Zealand, males account for nearly three-quarters of injury-related health loss, with self-inflicted and transport injuries the leading causes. Falls account for more than half of all injury-related health loss in older age groups and self-inflicted injury rates are highest in young people. Māori experience twice the rate of injury-related health loss compared to non-Māori, with health loss from assault four times higher in Māori. A third of all injury-related health loss results from traumatic brain injury and spinal cord injury. Alcohol and mental illness each contribute towards a quarter of all injury-related health loss.[6] For adolescent males injury is the leading cause of hospitalisation (43%), while for females it is the second leading cause of hospitalisation (10%), after complications of pregnancy and childbirth (43%).

Trauma mortality in Australia

The four most prevalent causes of injury death in Australia are suicide (30%), transport incidents (24%), falls (19%) and assault (4%).[15] Prior to 1991 the leading cause of death from external causes was motor vehicle collisions. It is important to recognise the limitations of the various data sources for injury mortality data. Information from several sources indicates that some estimates of numbers of injury deaths in 2004–05, based on Australian Bureau of Statistics (ABS) mortality data, are falsely low. Comparisons between the number of deaths obtained using the ABS mortality unit record data collection and the number of deaths obtained using data supplied by the National Coroners Information System (NCIS) confirmed underestimation of road traffic injury and homicide.[16] Despite this, overall injury mortality in Australia has declined from the period from 1997–98 to 2005–06 (most recent data at time of publishing).[17] More children die from injury in Australia (36%) than from cancer (19%) and diseases of the nervous system combined (11%).[18] There are approximately 250 deaths and more than 50,000 child hospitalisations due to injury each year in Australia. The injury causes vary by age groups, with infants most likely to die of assault and suffocation, toddlers of drowning and teenagers through car crashes (Fig 42.4).[19,20]

In 2012, 9275 people died from external causes—the fourth most common cause of death in Australia following cardiovascular, respiratory disease and cancer. Injury accounts for more years of lost life up to 65 years of age than cardio-vascular disease and cancer combined. Rates of injury mortality are consistently higher in males than in females. Injury is the leading cause of death in those aged under 45 years.[19]

Suicide

Suicide became a national public health concern in Australia during the 1990s. Prevention strategies and re-investment in mental health services at both state and federal levels have meant that the male suicide rate in 2002 was the lowest since 1985, and was 20% lower than in 1997. There were 2191 deaths from suicide registered in 2008 and this increased to 2535 in 2012, resulting in a ranking as the 14th leading cause of all deaths. Three-quarters (75.0%) of people who died by suicide were male, making suicide the tenth leading cause of death for males, continuing the trend since 1999. In 2012, over a quarter of male deaths in the 20–24, 25–29 and 30–34-year age groups were due to suicide. Similarly, for females, suicide deaths comprise a higher proportion of total deaths in younger age groups compared with older age groups (32.6% of deaths of 15–19-year-olds and 25.2% of deaths of 20–24-year-olds).[19] Men are still almost four times more likely to commit suicide than women, regardless of age category.[5]

In 2012, the most frequent method of suicide was hanging, a method used in half (54%) of all suicide deaths. Poisoning was used in 23%, followed by firearms (6.8%). The remaining methods were jumping from a high place, contact with sharp object and other.[19]

Mortality data from the ABS are the main source of suicide statistics in Australia. The ABS is part of a complex process that generates these statistics. The two other main contributors are coroners and the National Coroners Information System (NCIS). Coding rules that form part of the International Classification of Diseases (ICD), which the ABS is required to apply, also affect the statistics.[16] In recent years the ABS has cautioned that suicide data may be underestimated, and that observed changes over time are likely to have been affected by delays in coroners finalising a cause. Changes over time in the number of recorded suicides by method might reflect changes in suicidal behaviour in the Australian population, perhaps because of specific influences. For example, it has been suggested that decreases in suicide using firearms could be the result of the stricter gun laws introduced in 1996. However, part of the observed change could be due to alterations in case ascertainment or coding of the data. Under-enumeration of suicide cases could have more effect in some external-cause groups than in others; for example, suicide deaths from drowning can be difficult to distinguish from unintentional deaths by the same mechanism.[21]

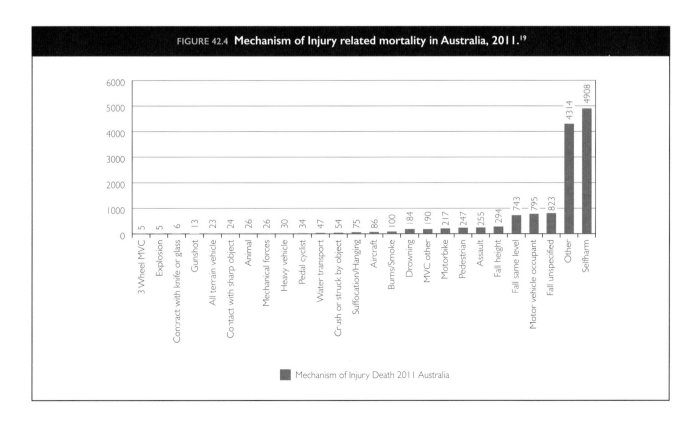

FIGURE 42.4 Mechanism of Injury related mortality in Australia, 2011.[19]

Transport-related deaths

Between 1950 and 2005, rates of transport-related deaths in Australia more than halved.[22] In the last decade to 2011, transportation deaths continued to decline, although at a much slower rate (*n* = 129). In 2011, there were 1627 road deaths (rate 8.0 per 100,000 population) and 30,574 people were seriously injured (rate 14.8 per 100,000).[22] The largest proportion of motor vehicles involved in crashes were cars (94%).[15] Further details of transport-related injuries are provided later in the chapter.

Falls deaths

In 2007–08 in Australia, falls were the most commonly reported external cause of hospital admission for both males and females. Queensland, Tasmania, the ACT and NT all had falls death rates above the national average, while falls deaths in South Australia were significantly lower than the national average. Although fall rates were concentrated in the older age groups, our understanding of contributing factors is limited by a lack of information about the nature of the falls. In 81% of deaths related to falls, the cause of the fall was unknown or not documented. Of the known factors contributing to falls-related deaths, tripping, slipping or stumbling on the same level was the most common (*n* = 75), followed by falling from a building or structure (*n* = 51), stairs or steps (*n* = 39) and on or from ladders (*n* = 25).[15]

Falls injury is responsible for a significant burden on the community which is equivalent, in economic terms, to 5% of health budget. In order to reduce the impact of fall-related injury among older people on the health system, significant resources need to be directed towards the promotion of evidence-based falls prevention programs at the local level across the state. Residents of aged care facilities are significantly over-represented in the hospital data.[22] Falls prevention is an integral part of injury prevention strategies in Australia and there is evidence to support injury prevention group and home-based exercise programs, and home safety interventions to reduce the rate of falls and risk of falling. Multifactorial assessment and intervention programs reduce the rate of falls and it has been shown that doing Tai Chi reduces the risk of falling.[23]

Work-related fatalities

Between 2002 and 2012, 2596 workers were killed while working. Analysis of data derived from workers' compensation claims (National Data Set for compensation-based statistics—NDS), notifications under occupational health and safety legislation (Notified Fatalities Collection—NFC) and coronial data (NCIS) identified that in 2012, 223 workers (1.93 deaths per 100,000 workers) died due to an injury incurred at work. This is similar to the previous 2 years and represents a significant fall from the 311 deaths recorded in 2007. This is the lowest fatality rate since the series began 10 years ago.[24]

The majority (96%) of the workers killed were male. Workers aged 65 years and over experienced a fatality rate of 6.2 deaths per 100,000 workers in 2009–10, more than three times the rate for all workers. Workers aged 25–34 years experienced the lowest fatality rate of all age groups.

Between 2002 and 2012, two-thirds of fatalities involved vehicles, with half of the vehicle-related incidents occurring on public roads. Trucks were the vehicle most often involved in fatalities. In 2012, 40 truck drivers were killed on public roads and 26 workers in cars. In other fatalities, 29 workers (13%) were killed when they fell from a height, 8 of whom fell from the roof of a building; 26 workers (12%) were killed when hit by a falling object. Of these workers, 5 were hit by falling trees and 4 by metal objects. Sixty-two per cent of fatalities occurred within three industries: (1) transport, postal and warehousing; within this industry the road freight transport sector recorded 29.09 deaths per 100,000 workers—15 times the all industries rate; (2) agriculture, forestry and fishing; and (3) construction. Between 2002 and 2012, 523 truck drivers were killed while working, equating to 20% of all fatalities. In 2012, 25 farm managers and 17 farm labourers were killed. In 2012, 63 bystanders were killed, the highest since 2007.[24]

Trauma mortality in New Zealand

In New Zealand—as reported in the NZ Burden of Disease, Injuries and Risk Factors Study 2006–2016—injury is the third leading cause of premature death and, like Australia, suicide, followed by transport, falls and interpersonal violence, are the predominant causes (Fig 42.5). In infants and children, the major causes of injury-related health loss vary depending on the age of the child or young person. Transport injuries were the predominant cause of health loss in children and young people, accounting for 45% of injury-related health loss. In infants, interpersonal violence accounted for over 40% of injury-related health loss. Drowning was an important cause of health loss in children under 9 years of age, with self-inflicted injury increasing in importance from the age of 10.[6]

Trauma morbidity in Australia and New Zealand

For every trauma patient who dies from their injuries, there are nearly six who survive to hospital discharge. For patients with severe injuries (Injury Severity Score (ISS) > 15), the Australian Trauma Registry Report 2010–2012 shows that 53% of these patients are admitted to intensive care for a median of 4 days. The median length of hospital stay for this cohort of seriously injured patients varies from 7 to 11 days.[14] Not all morbidities resulting from trauma are severe or fulminantly disabling. Some result in significant dysfunction, pain, cost and other sequelae, while many minor injuries heal, leaving little or no residual dysfunction. In a significant proportion of more-serious injury, recovery is incomplete, and injury results in a degree of ongoing dysfunction or the onset of secondary conditions (such as osteoarthritis in injured joints). In the 2012 Survey of Disability, Ageing and Carers, nearly one in five people in Australia (18.5%) had a reported disability. Of these, 7% reported injury was the underlying cause of their main disabling condition.[35] The link between major trauma and mental health sequelae is well recognised, but early identification and intervention methods are areas of ongoing exploration.[26]

Trauma risk factors

Whether intended or accidental, most physical injuries can be prevented by identifying their causes and removing them. Understanding some of the risk factors for injury may have predictive value in anticipating patterns of trauma in certain

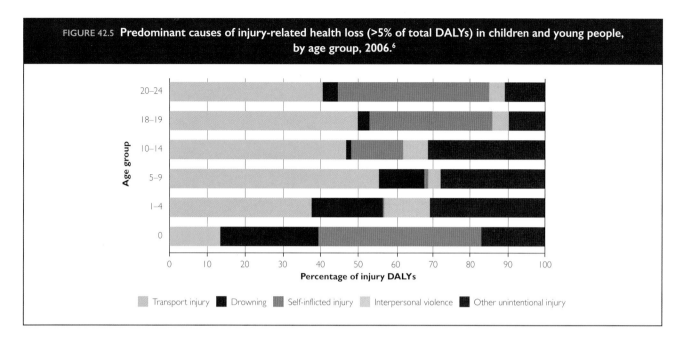

FIGURE 42.5 **Predominant causes of injury-related health loss (>5% of total DALYs) in children and young people, by age group, 2006.**[6]

populations and/or informing and evaluating injury prevention strategies. While examining the multitude of trauma risk factors is beyond the scope of this text, age, gender, cultural background, alcohol and other drugs, geography, temporal variations and the complex issue of driver distraction may all contribute to injury risk.

Age

Age has a bimodal influence on risk of death from injury across the human life span. In Australia, injury and poisoning are the most common causes of death from early childhood through to middle age, but the rate of injury deaths is highest in the age group 75 years and older.[5]

Similarly, age influences risk in trauma morbidity and mortality in two main ways. The first is increased exposure to risk of traumatic injury. For example, among the seriously injured who survived to hospital admission in Australian between 2010 and 2012, the 15–24-year age group was the most represented.[14] However, a comparison of the age-specific death rates for all injuries for the same period showed that people aged 75 years and older had the highest death rates for all injuries. Therefore, while injury is generally associated with the younger age groups, actual death rates from trauma among the older population are proportionally greater.[5] Types of injury mechanism vary with age. Suffocation and burns are prominent in the early childhood years, transport and sport-related injury in adolescents, suicide among young adults and falls in the elderly.

The second influence age has on morbidity and mortality risk is physiological response to trauma. In children, the high ratio of body mass to surface area means that they are less able to absorb high-impact energies in trauma. Combined with their limited ability to physiologically compensate for traumatic injuries, this means that children are at high risk of death and permanent disability from a given mechanism of injury. At the other end of the chronological scale, older person trauma is gaining increasing recognition as a subgroup requiring specialist attention.[27] People over the age of 55 years have a limited ability to compensate for physiological derangements induced by traumatic injury. Co-morbidities and common medications taken in this age group, such as anticoagulants and antihypertensives, further complicate trauma resuscitation and rehabilitation. See Chapters 36 and 39 for detailed discussion of paediatric and elderly physiological differences.

Gender

The difference in risk of injury between men and women is perhaps the most striking of all trauma risk factors. In Australia, male injury rates are, on average, about twice those of females.[5] This disparity between the genders is also reflected across most categories of injury death. In Australia, men are also almost four times more likely to commit suicide[5] or be severely injured, regardless of mechanism.[14]

It has been well established that men are over-represented in road trauma in Australia and New Zealand (72%). However, the percentages of men and women surviving to hospital discharge are similar (men 85%, women 82%).[28] Despite females having an overall higher rate of hospital admissions from falls, males required admission more frequently than females, with injuries from mechanical forces (e.g. sport) and assault.[5] The differences between the sexes in the number of presentations, the type of injury mechanism and activities performed at the time of the injury illustrate gender differences found in many common social practices. Injury prevention messages need to take into account the complexity and inter-active character of gender.[29]

Indigenous Australians

Indigenous Australians consistently have an injury mortality rate 3.4 times higher than other people in Australia.[30] In a 2012 report by the National Public Health Partnership it was found that the Aboriginal and Torres Strait Islander suicide rate was nearly twice as high, and the transport injury death rate almost three times as high, as for other Australians.[12,19] Although not a common cause of injury, fatal assault (homicide) was over seven times higher for Aboriginal and Torres Strait Islander males than for other males, with the rate for Indigenous females more than 11 times higher than that for other females.[12]

Even remoteness of residential location does not alter this trend. Death rates for Aboriginal and Torres Strait Islander people living in metropolitan cities are about twice those of other residents. In view of the high level of trauma morbidity and mortality risk among Indigenous Australians, a National Aboriginal and Torres Strait Islander Injury Prevention Plan has been developed. Through a consultative process with awareness of the sensitivities of Indigenous communities, this plan aims to complement the National Injury Prevention Plan and address the specific issues faced by the Aboriginal and Torres Strait Islander communities (see Ch 5).[12,31]

Alcohol and other drugs

Alcohol and other substances impair cognitive function, attention span, judgement and reaction time, often well after they have been metabolised and excreted. The relationship between alcohol and an increased risk of injury or death has been demonstrated in many settings, including road trauma, violence and self-harm.[32] Similarly, a study in New Zealand demonstrated a strong significant association between habitual marijuana use and car-crash injury.[33] More than 40% of alcohol-related crash injuries in New Zealand are suffered by people who have not been drinking; most innocent victims are car passengers, and this includes almost all children who are injured through drink-driving.[33]

The influence of other types of substance use on risk of injury remains unclear due to a paucity of data and larger-scale epidemiological studies.[34] However, the introduction of legislation to support large-scale roadside saliva testing for substances other than alcohol across Australia will provide public health researchers with a unique opportunity to more accurately assess the influence of substance use on injury risk (although the sensitivity of these tests has been questioned). There is a dose-related increase in violent behaviour when an individual uses methamphetamine compared to when they are not. This risk of violent behaviour is also increased by psychotic symptoms and/or alcohol consumption.[35]

Co-intoxication with alcohol and other drugs is a risk factor for increased in-hospital complications.[36] The collection of accurate data on drinking patterns of these patients would therefore be useful in determining whether ED can be used for these hard-to-reach population groups (see Ch 41).[32]

Geography—the tyranny of distance and terrain

Both Australia and New Zealand have many communities in remote and rural regions. This means that there are large distances between medical facilities, and these may have varying levels of medical care available. In 2009–10, the age-standardised rate of hospitalised injury cases increased with remoteness of the person's place of usual residence; the lowest rate was for residents of major cities (1728 per 100,000 population) and was highest for residents of very remote areas (4299 per 100,000 population) (Fig 42.6). This pattern was observed for males and females and is partly attributed to the higher rates of injury among Indigenous people, who comprise a higher proportion of the population in more remote areas.

The designated trauma centres are situated in the metropolitan areas and therefore many trauma patients are assessed, stabilised, admitted or treated in non-trauma centres. In NSW, approximately 40% of seriously injured (ISS > 15) patients are initially managed outside a major trauma centre each year.[14] For the major trauma patients, distance from definitive care can have life-threatening consequences and a person suffering major injury in rural Australia is three times as likely to die from

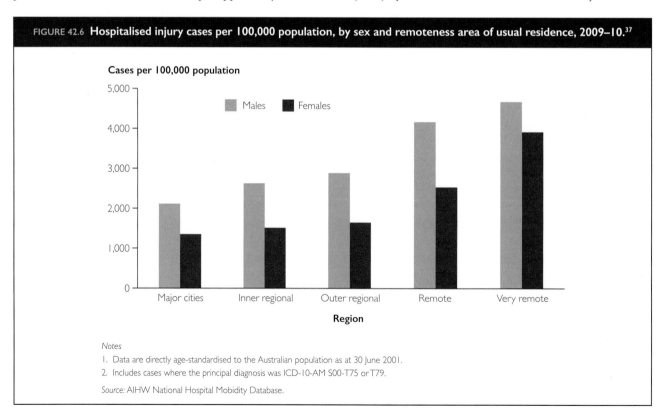

FIGURE 42.6 **Hospitalised injury cases per 100,000 population, by sex and remoteness area of usual residence, 2009–10.**[37]

Cases per 100,000 population

Notes
1. Data are directly age-standardised to the Australian population as at 30 June 2001.
2. Includes cases where the principal diagnosis was ICD-10-AM S00-T75 or T79.

Source: AIHW National Hospital Mobidity Database.

injury than those in a major city.[38,39] It is for this reason that education for pre-hospital and ED personnel is so important. Box 42.1 further illustrates some of the more practical issues around rural trauma.

Driver behavioural factors

Certain behavioural factors continue to be implicated in many serious road crashes. The most significant are identified in Table 42.1.

Awareness of the injury risk posed by driver distraction has been raised through increasing research and media attention over the last decade. Driver distraction occurs 'when a driver is delayed in the recognition of information needed to safely accomplish the driving task because some event, activity, object or person within or outside the vehicle compelled or tended to induce the driver's shifting attention away from the driving task'.[41] Driver distraction is considered by road-crash researchers as a subgroup of the broader problem of driver inattention.[41,42]

Visual distraction occurs when drivers focus their attention on another visual target, such as an in-car navigation system, for an extended period of time, shifting their attention away from the road. Auditory distraction occurs when drivers focus on auditory signals such as conversation on a mobile phone. Removal of one or both hands from the steering wheel to physically manipulate an object results in biomechanical distraction from the physical tasks required to drive safely, such as steering or changing gears. Cognitive distraction includes any thoughts or cognitive processes that absorb a driver's attention to the point where they are unable to navigate safely through the road network (Box 42.2).[42]

External-to-vehicle driver distractions, for example, billboard advertising, are also known major contributors to road crashes; however, the incidence of these distractions is likely to be under-reported.[42]

The full impact of driver distraction on the incidence of road crashes in Australia and New Zealand has yet to be systematically investigated;[42] however, there is evidence that a majority of serious injury crashes in Australia involve driver inattention and that most forms of inattention and distraction observed are preventable.[43] Driver distraction is involved in approximately 10% of police-reported crashes in New Zealand,[44] and a nationwide survey found that over 50% of respondents reported sending or reading between 1 and 5 text messages while driving in a typical week, despite the majority agreeing that text messaging while driving impairs driving performance.[45]

Using a mobile phone results in the driver being four times more likely to be involved in a crash that results in hospital attendance and that using a hands-free adjunct is no safer.[46] Between 1% and 7% of drivers have been observed using mobile phones at any given moment during the day in Australia, more so the younger driver.[47] For pedestrians and drivers, more injuries are related to talking than texting, although for drivers, reaching for the phone accounts for the most injuries. These rates do not mean that texting is less distracting, but probably reflect a lower amount of texting while driving or walking.[48] More systematic collection of mobile phone use in crash data is needed.

BOX 42.1 Characteristics of and problems associated with rural trauma[38,143]

By comparison with metropolitan areas, in rural trauma there are:

- greater distances travelled
- higher speed of travel—more severe injuries
- poorer road quality
- older age and poorer condition of vehicles
- poor seatbelt compliance
- fatigue and alcohol issues
- delays in discovery times as a result of remoteness/longer transport times
- rural ambulances less well-equipped to deal with multiple trauma
- lower levels of rural practitioner trauma experience (less frequent)
- hospitals less well-equipped to deal with major road crashes and multiple people.

TABLE 42.1 Deaths and serious injuries by main behavioural factor[40]

	PROPORTION OF TOTAL DEATHS (%)	PROPORTION OF TOTAL SERIOUS INJURIES (%)
Speeding	34	13
Drink driving	30	9
Drug driving	7[a]	2
Restraint non-use	20	4
Fatigue	20–30[b]	8

Note: categories are not mutually exclusive

a. Estimate excludes fatalities involving both alcohol and other drugs, which are included in the drink driving estimate.

b. Estimates of fatigue involvement in serious casualty crashes vary considerably. However, it is widely recognised as a significant contributing factor.

BOX 42.2 Inside-vehicle distraction sources[44]

- Passengers
- Telecommunications
- Entertainment systems
- Emotional upset or preoccupation
- Personal effects
- Vehicle controls
- Food/drink
- Smoking
- Animal/insect inside vehicle
- Sneezing/coughing/itching

Research has demonstrated that reaction times are slower among drivers talking on a phone than among those talking to a passenger; however, this does not mean that a conversation with a passenger does not have distraction potential. Young drivers' crash risk is significantly increased by the presence of similarly-aged passengers in the vehicle,[47] particularly emotionally difficult conversations, which have been demonstrated to be more disruptive to driving with the passenger present than those conducted using a handsfree telephone.[49]

The effects of fatigue on serious road casualties are difficult to quantify. Fatigue is a contributing factor in crashes which involve long trips and extensive periods of continuous driving, and also in short trips when the driver has previously been deprived of sleep. Shift workers are particularly at risk. There is evidence that sleep deprivation can have similar hazardous effects to alcohol consumption. Studies have found that people driving after being awake for 17 to 19 hours perform more poorly than those with a BAC of 0.05.[50]

Patterns of injury in Australia and New Zealand

International trauma literature reports a reduction in the mortality rate from exsanguinations, yet rates of the other causes of death appear to be unchanged. The predominant cause of early death after trauma continues to be CNS brain injury (21.6–71.5%), followed by exsanguination (12.5–26.6%), while sepsis (3.1–17%) and multi-organ failure (MOF) (1.6–9%) continue to be predominant causes of late death. These improvements might be explained by developments in the availability of multislice computed tomography (CT), implementation of standardised trauma management concepts and logistics of emergency rescue.[51]

In 2003, the vision for a national approach to injury data collection took shape in the form of the National Trauma Registry Consortium (Australia and New Zealand) (NTRCANZ). The NTRCANZ was a joint initiative between the Royal Australasian College of Surgeons, the Australasian Trauma Society and the University of Queensland Centre of National Research on Disability and Rehabilitation (CONROD—which has now been disbanded).[28] In November 2010 the Alfred Hospital/National Trauma Research Institute in Melbourne and the National Critical Care and Trauma Response Centre in Darwin announced an agreement to jointly fund the development of the Australian National Trauma Registry by each contributing A$350,000.[52] Efforts to obtain federal government support for this important program continue, and it released its inaugural national trauma report in October 2014.[14] The data presented below in each category are the most recent available at time of publication.

Blunt injuries

In Australia and New Zealand over 95% of all major trauma is blunt.[14,53] The majority of blunt trauma in Australia is related to road trauma (52%), falls (31%) and violence (6%).[24] Of all major trauma patients admitted to designated trauma centres, approximately two-thirds have sustained injuries to the head, approximately half chest injuries, one-third had each of face, spine, upper limb and lower limb injuries, and one-fifth had abdominal injuries. Patients with isolated head injuries alone

have a higher mortality rate (34%) than other isolated body regions (11%) combined, or those with isolated spine injuries (2%). Polytrauma patients, defined as patients with two or more significantly injured body regions, have the highest mortality rate (57%).[14]

Violence and penetrating injuries

Assaults have grown by 5% each year from 1995 to 2007; four times the annual growth of the Australian population in the same period. Assault is seasonal. The number of assaults peaks in the spring and summer months of October to February and is lowest from April to July.[54] Conversely, the rates of homicide have decreased (a 4-year low) to 1.9 victims per 100,000 persons in 2013 (or 430 people).[55] Penetrating injuries include firearm injuries, stabbing and impalement. Australasian firearm-related injuries are low in comparison with the rest of the world,[56–58] but increased by 6% between 2009 and 2013.[55] There has been a dramatic increase in the use of knives in murder (28% to 36%), and a more gradual increase in relation to attempted murder from 2001 to 2009.[59] Firearms are used in 8% of assaults in New Zealand compared with 50% in the United States.[60] Patients are overwhelmingly males in their second and third decades of life, and in New Zealand apprehensions for possession of an offensive weapon have increased over the 1999–2008 period, from 23.0 to 31.9 per 10,000 population, particularly in the 14- to 20-year-old male age group.[61] The use of alcohol and other drugs, gang membership, unemployment and firearm ownership are often identified as patient characteristics in victims of penetrating trauma.[57,62] Most penetrating injuries are minor, with only a small proportion of trauma admissions to major trauma centres sustaining severe injury (4%).[14]

Specific patterns of injury

Road traffic crash trends in serious injury

In Australia over the 9-year period from 2000–01 to 2008–09, age-standardised rates for persons seriously injured due to a road traffic crash increased from 138.3 to 156.7 per 100,000 population, an average annual increase of 1.6%. All jurisdictions, except for the ACT,[63] Victoria and NT, showed statistically significant increases in age-standardised rates of serious injury due to road vehicle traffic crashes.[64] Rates of life-threatening cases involving drivers of motor vehicles, motorcyclists and pedal cyclists all rose significantly over this period. Motorcyclists show an average annual rate of increase of 6.9%. Age-specific rates for males in all age groups increased significantly with the largest average annual increases in the 45–64 years and 65 years and over age groups with increases of 14.7% and 13.9% respectively. For females injured as motorcyclists there were significant increases for those aged 25–44 years and 45–64 years. Persons living in remote areas recorded the highest average annual rate of increase of 5.8%, while persons living in major cities, inner and outer regional areas recorded smaller, but significant average, annual rates of increase.[64]

Cyclists have a number of risk factors that do not affect car drivers such as decreased stability, a much lower level of protection and being less visible to other road users than a car or truck. These factors combined give cyclists a high level of risk per time unit travelled, although this risk is significantly lower than the risk carried by motorcyclists. In New Zealand between 2008 and 2012, over 1500 cyclists required hospitalisation due to injuries received from crashes involving motor vehicles on public roads in New Zealand. In the same 2008–12 period, 45 cyclists died in crashes involving motor vehicles on public roads. An additional 893 cyclists were hospitalised in 2012 for traffic incidents not involving a motor vehicle. Nearly a quarter of cyclists killed or injured in motor vehicle crashes are aged 10–19 years old and 74% of cyclists involved in police-reported crashes are male.[65] Similarly, in Australia, the majority (81.1%) of hospitalisations occurred in males. Of hospitalisations, 47.6% were for people aged 0–14 years. Three-quarters of cycling-related deaths were due to head injury and > 90% were caused by collisions with motor vehicles.[66] It has been shown that cycle helmets are effective in reducing head injury, with those not wearing a helmet 5.5 times more likely to sustain a severe head injury, and three times higher treatment costs.[67] Mandatory helmet legislation has resulted in a sustained decline in bicycle-related head injuries in NSW in the past two decades (1991–2010).[68] Accurate data on cycling participation, use of injury prevention strategies and injury profiles will assist in reducing bicycle-related injury.

Pedestrian injuries recorded a significant annual rate of decrease of 1.8% over the period. In 2000–01, 31% of all high threat to life road injuries sustained by males aged 45–64 years occurred while they were riding motorcycles or pedal cycles. This had risen to over 51% in 2008–09.

Serious injury involving a railway train or level-crossing incidents

Approximately one rail user was seriously injured per 100 million passenger kilometres travelled in Australia in 2008–09. The risk of serious injury, based on kilometres travelled, is more than 10 times as high for passengers travelling by car than for passengers travelling by train.[69]

For the 5-year period 2004–05 to 2008–09, 868 persons were seriously injured in Australia due to transport accidents involving a train, an average of 174 per year. Rail users made up two-thirds (66.5%) of all serious injury cases, most commonly occurring while boarding or alighting from trains.

Over the same 5-year period, 248 persons were seriously injured in Australia due to a level-crossing incident, an average of 50 per year; serious injury rates were highest among young adults (20–24 years of age). Most common circumstances involved car occupants (42.3%) and pedestrians (29.6%) injured in a collision with a train. Mean length of stay in hospital was 9.2 days, more than double that of non-rail-related injuries (4.0 days).[69] In New Zealand in 2013 there were 11 deaths and 126 injuries related to railways. This includes 5 deaths and 15 injuries in level crossing incidents, 6 deaths where a person was on a track and 109 injuries in operating and other accidents.[70]

Major railway disasters

Major railway disasters are uncommon; however, they do occur. They often involve a number of fatalities and persons seriously injured. These incidents are widely reported in the media, such as the Granville train disaster in 1977 (83 fatalities), Glenbrook, NSW in 1999 (7 fatalities), Waterfall in 2003 (7 fatalities) and the level-crossing crash near Kerang in Victoria in 2007

(11 fatalities). These disasters are expensive; the estimated cost of rail accidents that occurred in Australia in 1999 was A\$133 million. During 1999, rail-related suicides and attempted suicides were estimated to have cost A\$53 million.[69]

Sporting injury

Exercise is important in promoting health and wellbeing. However, sport and recreation injuries are common and, although predominantly minor, can lead to people dropping out of sport.[56] Nearly two-thirds of the Australian population aged 15 years and over (11.7 million people) reported that they had participated in sport and physical recreation at least once during 2011–12. Sports injuries cost Australians \$1.5 billion annually.[71] Walking for exercise remained the most popular activity over time with a similar participation rate from 2009–10 to 2011–12 (23% and 24% respectively). The participation rate for cycling or BMXing increased from 6.5% to 7.6%. Similarly, the rate of people participating in jogging or running increased from 4.3% in 2005–06, to 6.5% in 2009–10, to 7.5% in 2011–12.[72] Sports injuries are a major source of emergency department (ED) presentations, and the leading cause of child injury ED visits.[73] The rate of major trauma, inclusive of deaths, due to participation in sport and active recreation, has increased over recent years; in Victoria, and likely across Australia, much of it can be attributed to cycling and off-road motor sports.[74]

Football injury

Several codes of football are played in Australia and New Zealand. These include football (soccer), Australian Rules, rugby league and rugby union. Of the four main football codes, soccer (outdoor) is the most popular. Participation shows strong regional differences, with Australian Rules being played in Victoria and South Australia and rugby predominantly played in NSW and Queensland.[71] In Queensland, 15.3% of football-injury-related presentations to ED were due to rugby league, 14.3% to soccer, 4.5% rugby union, 3.7% Australian rules, 3.1% touch football and 21.3% football unspecified. The injuries occur as a result of falls, or striking or colliding with another person or an object.[75]

Burns

One per cent of the population of Australia and New Zealand (220,000) suffers from burns each year. From 1 July 2011 to 30 June 2012 there were 2772 cases that required admission to a burns unit in Australia and New Zealand; however, only 15 of the 17 burns units entered data.[76] Fortunately, Australia and New Zealand has a lower percentage of major burns, with 82% of both paediatric and adult cases being less than 10% when compared to 70% in the United States. Over half of these burn admissions (57%), however, occurred in rural and remote areas with significant implications for transport and pre-hospital care.[76]

Over the past 20 years, the survival rate for patients with a severe burn injury has improved dramatically. Early surgical intervention, skin substitutes, nutrition and advances in intensive care have improved the survival and outcomes for patients with burns to > 80% of total body surface area. Burns are a common reason for children under 5 years of age to present to an ED, currently accounting for 4% of all injury presentations in this age group.[77] Burns in children in this age group made up the largest single group of burns victims (33%) across all ages.[77] The vast majority occurred at home (89%) and in the kitchen (47%). Burns injuries can result from scalds, hot objects, chemical, fire and flames and sun or friction. Trend estimates over the seven-year study period showed no evidence of decline (see Ch 52).

Spinal cord injury

Australia was the first country to implement a national population-based register for surveillance of spinal cord injury (SCI) cases.[78] In 1986, data collection on SCI was initiated by John Walsh, based on cases reported by the six Australian spinal units (SUs), and is now continued by the AIHW National Injury Surveillance Unit, a unit of the Flinders University Research Centre for Injury Studies. Cases of spinal cord damage from traumatic causes, as well as from non-traumatic causes (e.g. from disease processes such as cancer), that were treated by the SUs are registered.[78] The SCI population has been estimated to number in excess of 6000, with ongoing costs associated with the long-term care estimated to be about A$200 million per year.

In Australia in 2007–08, the main causes of traumatic SCI were land transport involving motor vehicle occupants and unprotected road users, i.e. motorcyclists, pedal cyclists, pedestrians; high and then low falls.[79] This was inversely the case in New Zealand from 2007 to 2009, where falls accounted for the highest percentage of SCI, followed by medical causes such as spinal abscess, Guillain-Barré and metastatic lesions, then motor vehicle and then motorbike collisions (see Ch 49).[79,80]

Effects of injury on society

To understand the magnitude of trauma as a public health issue, collecting data on the prevalence and types of trauma alone is insufficient. The effect of injury on society needs to be considered in order to monitor its impact on acute health and rehabilitation services, the workforce and families and significant others. Ongoing measurements of the impact of trauma in these areas are necessary to inform public policy, legislation, funding, resource allocation and distribution. An understanding of the effects of injury on society is therefore essential for clinicians, from pre-hospital to rehabilitation.

Psychological/personal

In an effort to reduce trauma mortality, the focus of trauma management has been predominantly physiological. However, improved survival has resulted in a growing awareness of the problem of the psychological impact of traumatic injury. Two areas identified in the trauma literature include post-traumatic stress and impact of trauma on cognitive function and personality.

Post-traumatic stress

As times of military conflict accelerated our understanding of physiological responses to traumatic injury, the problem of emotional sequelae stress reactions among trauma survivors has also emerged. After World War I, post-traumatic stress was called shell shock; during World War II, it was referred to as combat fatigue; following the Vietnam War, it was labelled the post-Vietnam syndrome; and after the Gulf War, Gulf War syndrome emerged, although its physiological and/or psychological origins remain a topic of intense debate.

According to the American Psychiatric Association,[81] post-traumatic stress disorder (PTSD) is defined as an anxiety disorder that persists for a period > 1 month following the occurrence of a traumatic event involving actual or threatened death, serious injury or threat to the physical integrity of oneself or others. Symptoms of PTSD include physiological (impaired memory, sympathetic hyper-arousal, sleep disturbance, headaches, gastrointestinal disturbances, chest pain, dizziness, etc), psychological (depression, anxiety disorders, conduct disorders, dissociation and eating disorders), social (interpersonal problems, alcohol and substance use, employment problems, trouble with the law and homelessness) and self-destructive behaviours (suicide attempts, risky sexual behaviour, reckless driving, self-injury).

Some studies have reported an incidence of up to 51% of patients who had sustained traumatic injuries meeting diagnostic criteria for PTSD,[26] yet psychological consequences such as PTSD are currently neglected in burden-of-injury calculations.[82] While there is little evidence for the efficacy of early debriefing on post-traumatic injury, there is some evidence that early cognitive behavioural therapy may lessen the psychological impact of injury and help prevent progression to PTSD.[83]

According to the American Psychiatric Association's practice guidelines for the treatment of patients with acute stress disorder (ASD) and PTSD, ASD was added to the established list of psychiatric diagnoses in 1995 to distinguish individuals with PTSD-like symptoms that lasted < 1 month from persons who experienced milder or more-transient difficulties following a traumatic event. While the relationship between ASD and the development of PTSD remains controversial,[84] recognition of ASD or PTSD symptoms in trauma patients who re-present to the ED can assist clinicians in appropriate triage and referral to psychiatric support services for injured patients. In addition to post-traumatic stress, there are a range of cognitive and behavioural changes that can result from neurotrauma. Further, trauma centres (while the patient is in hospital), outpatient clinics and general practitioners should screen patients for symptoms of ASD to assist with early intervention. Research in 2012 demonstrated that the majority of trauma patients experience high levels of anxiety and stress in hospital, and patients who score highly in Depression, Anxiety and Stress scales at 3 months post injury are likely to continue to have symptoms at 6 months post injury.[85]

Cognitive/behavioural changes

Cognitive and behavioural changes arising from traumatic brain injury vary according to the mechanism of injury and resultant focal or diffuse damage to cerebral tissue. In general, cognitive disorders result from disorders of attention, concentration and memory, problems with communication, difficulty with reasoning and judgement and difficulties with planning and initiating daily activities. Behavioural sequelae may include impulsivity, irritability, agitation, aggression, depression and egocentrism in interpersonal relationships. Even in minor head injuries, these changes can have a significant impact on work performance and safety, subsequent workplace absence and on relationships with family and significant others. These effects represent an enormous hidden impact of trauma on individuals and their functioning in society.

As with other psychological sequelae of traumatic injury, clinicians have an important role to play in recognising symptoms of cognitive disorders and behavioural change in trauma patients and in initiating early/appropriate referrals; for example, by conducting the abbreviated post traumatic amnesia score (AWPTAs) in minor head injury patients being discharged from the ED. For a more detailed examination of traumatic brain injury, see Chapter 45.

Legislation

Australia and New Zealand have been world leaders in introducing legislative changes to improve road and workplace safety. Subsequent improvements in the rates of trauma-related morbidity and mortality have demonstrated the important contribution of legislation in addressing trauma as a public safety issue. The Australian Government released the National Road Safety Strategy 2001–2010, followed by the 2011–2021 strategy, which identifies the main issues expected to affect road trauma levels in the foreseeable future and sets out the priority areas for action.[51] The mix of measures adopted in individual jurisdictions, and the details of specific measures, will vary to reflect local circumstances and priorities.

Seatbelts, child restraints

Wearing seatbelts and using child restraints in motor vehicles and helmets by motorcyclists and their passengers was made compulsory by legislation in all Australian states and territories by 1973.[86,87] This legislation led to a consistent decline in road trauma deaths over the subsequent three decades. By 2004, the number of road trauma deaths had dropped to less than 1600 deaths per year in Australia, with a slight increase in 2005.[37] The risk of fatal injury can be reduced by 45% and the risk of serious injury by 50% through the use of seatbelts alone.[87] New legislation regarding child restraints was introduced in Australia in 2010. The Australian Transport Council (comprising transport ministers from across Australia) approved new laws which introduced a mandatory, size-appropriate restraint system for all children up to the age of seven years in order to significantly improve the safety of children when travelling in vehicles. Seating children from age four to under seven years of age in an appropriate booster seat reduces their risk of injury in a crash by almost 60% when compared with a child sitting in an adult seatbelt without a booster seat. However, up to 79% of children are not always restrained appropriately.[86]

Speed limits, drink-driving laws, improved law enforcement technology

Reduced speed zoning has been used as a strategy to modify driver behaviour and reduce the risk of accidents in areas prone to motor vehicle crashes or pedestrian injury. By the end of 2001, the speed limit in all Australian streets was reduced from 60 kph to 50 kph (unless otherwise signed), and is linked to a 20% reduction in casualty crashes, with greater reductions for crashes involving serious injuries and fatalities. Some evaluation studies identified particular benefits for pedestrians and other vulnerable groups.[51,88,89] Similarly, speed zoning near schools has been reduced to 40 kph during before and after school times; this has resulted in a 23% reduction in casualty crashes and a 24% reduction in all pedestrian and bicyclist crashes outside schools in Victoria.[51]

Random breath-testing for alcohol was initiated on a wide scale in Victoria in 1976. Speed and/or red-light cameras were first introduced in Victoria in 1983. The success of these law-enforcement initiatives led to their subsequent dissemination to other Australian states and territories. More recently, these technologies have further developed to include more-accurate laser-based speed-detection devices, digital imaging, red-light cameras and point-of-testing tools for the detection of illicit substances. Research demonstrates that the contribution of these technologies to the reduction in serious injury and road trauma mortality is often hampered by the multifactorial nature of the research context. However, these technologies have proved to be effective strategies in addressing the issue of legislative compliance.[90]

Vehicle safety

'Design Rules for Motor Vehicle Safety' were introduced to Australian legislation through the Motor Vehicles Standards Act in 1989. This brought Australian vehicle design standards into line with many international standards. Design standards include improved tyres, windscreens, head restraints, lights, indicators and brakes; vehicle impact resistance in cars; increased occupant protection and roll-over strength in buses; mandatory fitting of seatbelts in new passenger vehicles from 1970; use of retractable belts and progressive extension of seatbelt requirements to other motor vehicles; mandatory use of anchorage points for child restraints; and installation of speed limiters in heavy vehicles.

Licensing restrictions for inexperienced drivers

It is well established in road crash data in Australia and New Zealand, and worldwide, that young drivers, under the age of 20 years, are over-represented in crash mortality statistics.

Graduated driver licensing (GDL) systems are regarded as the primary means of ensuring that novice drivers (typically young drivers) are introduced to the use of motor vehicles in a safe, controlled and low-risk manner. Some real-world effectiveness in the reduction of teenager accidents through the use of graduated driver licensing has been shown in the USA: after introducing a GDL system, the state of Texas, where more teenage drivers were involved in fatal car accidents on the state's roads than any other demographic group, saw a 32.5% drop in teenager road fatalities between 2002 and 2009.

The first GDL systems involving a learner licensing phase, an intermediate, provisional or probationary licensing phase and full licensing were developed in Australia in the 1960s. North American GDL systems emerged in the late 1980s and 1990s, heavily influenced by a revamped graduated licensing system introduced in New Zealand in the 1980s, and have now been adopted in almost all US and Canadian jurisdictions. These systems place particular emphasis on passenger restrictions and night-time driving curfews for young drivers.

The Australian approaches to GDL combines restrictions on young drivers with intensive training requirements, but also adds significant enforcement (zero tolerance with regard to speeding, driving while impaired by alcohol or other drugs and the use of mobile telephones by young drivers) and penalty components (particularly the suspension of a driver's licence for offences, the impoundment of motor vehicles and opportunities to attend traffic offender intervention programs as part of the penalty process).

The risk of death for a teenage passenger is greater when a

teenager is driving. In Australia, where the age of passengers is not reliably recorded, studies of provisionally licensed drivers have shown that their odds of crashing increase between 1.4 and 1.5 times when carrying one passenger (of any age), and between 2.3 and 2.6 times when carrying three or more passengers.[91]

Prior to the introduction of passenger restrictions in Victoria, carrying more than one passenger increased the fatal crash risk of first-year provisional-licence driver to four times the level of driving alone or with only one passenger. More than a quarter of these drivers involved in fatal crashes were carrying multiple passengers at the time of the crash. Risk of crash is reduced when:

- the passenger is an adult aged 25 year or more
- the passenger is a child aged 12 years or under.

In Australia,[86] different states have introduced different requirements for carrying peer passengers for first-year provisional-licence drivers:

- In Victoria, no more than one passenger aged 16–21 years can be carried at any time of day.
- In Queensland and NSW, no more than one passenger aged 21 years and under can be carried between 11 pm and 5 am.
- In Western Australia, no more than one passenger can be carried between midnight and 5 am for the first 6 months.

Other passenger restrictions apply in several states when returning to driving after a licence suspension or at night-time. A landmark study in North Carolina, USA by Foss et al in 2001[93] found that the introduction of a night-time curfew was linked to a reduction in night-time crash rates by 43%. Night-time curfews were subsequently introduced into 37 states in the United States by 2004. This stimulated intense public debate on the issue in Australia. In 2007 NSW introduced passenger laws for provisional drivers under the age of 25 and night-time driving passenger laws (no passengers from 11 pm to 5 am). Since July 2014, in South Australia P1 licence holders under the age of 25 are not allowed to drive between midnight and 5 am, and are not allowed to have more than one passenger at any time. Similar laws are being introduced across Australia. In New Zealand, however, provisional/restricted drivers are permitted to drive between 10 pm and 5 am, and can carry passengers only if accompanied by a supervisor. Research from New Zealand and the USA has clearly shown that strong passenger restrictions—restriction to *none or only one* passenger at *all times*, not just at night—is a feature of the most effective graduated licensing models.[91]

Workplace injury legislation

Stronger workplace legislation has been developed to enforce work safety standards in both Australia and New Zealand. In the 1980s, Australia followed the legislative trend of the UK after the recommendations of a parliamentary inquiry into occupational health and safety were mandated by law. Consequently, Australia has the seventh lowest workplace fatality rate among 20 similarly developed economies.[93] Workers' compensation data suggests that the Australian workplace has become safer, with workplace fatalities having almost halved since the mid-1990s, with a significant decrease in the number of compensated claims in the same period.[94]

However, employer and employee compliance remains a problem and a burden. The model Work Health and Safety (WHS) Regulations are made under the *Work Health and Safety Act* and outline a wide range of matters relating to work health and safety, including: managing risks to health and safety and general workplace management; hazardous work involving noise, hazardous manual tasks, confined spaces, falls, demolition work, electrical safety and energised electrical work; construction work; hazardous chemicals; mines and asbestos. They are model provisions only. To be legally binding they need to be enacted or passed by Parliament in each jurisdiction. In New Zealand, *The Health and Safety in Employment Act 1992* (the HSE Act) and the *Hazardous Substances and New Organisms Act 1996* (the HSNO Act) provide similar regulations.

The burden of injury

The burden of injury is documented in different ways depending on mechanisms of injury. Road injury, for example, uses mortality as a key indicator; whereas sports injury focuses more on hospitalisation and medical care. Costing models also vary sector by sector. Road injury costs include property damage, long-term disability costs and insurance administration costs in a full-cost model. Work-related-injury costing models include time off work, lost production, equipment damage cost, compensation costs and insurance administration costs. Outside these areas, cost of injury data is limited. This makes comparisons difficult.

In an attempt to weave together the different patterns of injury and make meaningful comparisons of injuries with different mixes of death, hospitalisation and non-hospital treatment, Monash University Accident Research Centre (MUARC) developed a method of estimating the lifetime cost of injury for Victoria.[95] Lifetime costs include treatment costs (direct) and loss of productivity (indirect), but do not include property damage. The lifetime cost of falls exceeds that of motor vehicle crashes and suicide and self-harm, despite the importance of the latter two in terms of mortality. When age distribution is considered, adolescent and young adults, especially males, account for a disproportionate portion of the cost of injury in Australia.

Australia-wide, the burden of trauma is immense, responsible for 522,330 hospitalisations in 2008–09 and the second highest cause of hospital admissions expenditure, following cardiovascular disease.[96] In 2004–05, injury accounted for A\$3.4 billion (7%) of allocated health expenditure in Australia—an increase of 22% since 2001—the greatest proportion of which was spent during hospital admission.[96] In New Zealand, injury (unintentional and intentional) is the second leading cause of hospitalisation. Injuries account for more potential years of life lost than cancer and heart disease combined.[97] In 2013 the social costs of road trauma alone were estimated to be \$3.29 billion.[98] NSW-based research demonstrated that higher treatment costs are associated with severity of injury, intensive care admission and traumatic brain injury. Once a patient had more than two body regions injured (i.e. polytrauma), their median costs increased exponentially to \$7,419 for three regions injured and \$16,703 for four or more regions injured.[99] The complex nature of the trauma patient does not allow accurate funding prediction using the activity-based funding models currently employed in Australia.[100] Strategies to decrease in-hospital cost and improve quality include multidisciplinary rounds, case management, trauma coding strategies[100] and trauma pathways,[101] as well as the development and implementation of trauma clinical practice guidelines.[27,101] Compensation schemes in Australia and New Zealand vary between state, territory and country and depend on injury mechanisms.

Human cost

The cost to society is significant. For those who do not survive injury, there is a net loss of their contribution to society. On average, each fatal injury before the age of 75 years results in the loss of 32 years of potential life, compared with 9 years for cancer and 5 for cardiovascular disease.[15] The subsequent grief and loss experienced by families and significant others has an impact on their mental health, and leads to secondary healthcare costs, loss of productivity and subsequent economic burden. For those who survive traumatic injury, recovery periods and long-term disabilities result in a reduced economic contribution and/or long-term economic liability imposed on health and social systems. These costs have underpinned the development of highly organised and outcome-focused systems of trauma management and prevention.

Injury prevention

In view of the realisation of the incidence of trauma and its cost to society, there has been an increasing emphasis on prevention strategies. However, trauma care professionals are yet to convince policy-makers and the public that injuries can be controlled.[102] Clinicians who care for trauma patients clearly recognise the need for prevention and control strategies to curb trauma mortality and morbidity. In contrast, there is some evidence to suggest that trauma clinicians have a poor understanding of the principles of injury prevention.[103] To initiate or participate in injury prevention programs, clinicians need to be aware of the principles that underlie injury prevention, and understand accepted models of injury control. This role is seen to be part of the role of the trauma coordinator, but competing priorities and time restraints see injury prevention consuming only 4.8% of their time in 2011. This has increased from 0% in 2007.[104]

Principles of injury prevention

The perception of trauma as preventable events rather than acts of random unexpectedness is fundamental to the success of any injury prevention program. There are a number of principles that underpin effective injury prevention and safety promotion—these are listed in Box 42.3.[10] Understanding these principles empowers clinicians to involve themselves in preventing injury rather than being limited to dealing with the physical, emotional and psychological sequelae of traumatic injury. Paramedics are ideally placed to be a significant contributor to injury prevention, as they see the actual scenes where people are injured.

Models of injury control

Given the complex nature of injury and the multitude of contexts in which injury can occur, systematic and comprehensive approaches to controlling injury are required. In 1949, William Haddon began developing the most widely used epidemiological model of injury prevention: the Haddon matrix.

- The first axis of the Haddon matrix likens injury to a disease, such as cancer or an infection, by applying the elements of the epidemiological triad—host, vector and environment. Fundamental to understanding injury as a disease, Haddon defined injury as the uncontrolled release of energy, including kinetic, thermal, chemical, electrical or ionising radiation.[105]
- The second axis is made up of three time intervals: pre-event, event and post-event.

Haddon[106] described 10 strategies for injury prevention, with an emphasis on reducing the transfer of energy through reduction of environmental hazards.[102] These strategies are listed and applied in Box 42.4. Runyan[107] applied the principles of policy analysis to create a three-dimensional Haddon matrix. These principles include effectiveness, cost, freedom, equity, stigmatisation, preferences of the affected community or individuals and feasibility. Runyan's approach[107] reflects a more holistic approach to decision-making that is often a necessary part of clinical practice. Nevertheless, translation into action remains an assumption of this model rather than being an integral part of its approach.

Australia and New Zealand have achieved some significant gains in the prevention of a number of different types of injuries where concerted efforts have been made. The vision for the Australian National Injury Prevention and Safety Promotion Plan[10] is for governments, the private sector and communities to all work together to ensure that people have the greatest opportunity to live in a safe environment free from the impact of injuries. The plan embraces a number of other national strategies for areas such as Kidsafe, falls prevention, alcohol, mental health, youth suicide, Aboriginal and Torres Strait Islanders, road safety and improvements to rural and regional health. However, the National Injury Prevention

BOX 42.4 The Haddon strategies applied[142,142]

1. Prevent creation of the hazard
   Do not manufacture three-wheeled all-terrain vehicles (ATVs), certain types of ammunition and certain poisons; ban human pyramids.
2. Reduce amount of the hazard
   Limit pills per container, decrease water temperature in homes, limit contact drills in football.
3. Prevent release of the hazard.
   Provide handrails for the elderly, improve braking capability of vehicles, reduce alcohol use by drivers.
4. Alter release of the hazard
   Develop blister packaging of pills, child safety seats and seatbelts to control deceleration forces, release bindings on skis.
5. Separate person and hazard in time and space
   Create bike and pedestrian paths, remove trees near roadways, evacuate hurricane paths.
6. Place barrier between the person and the hazard
   Build bike helmets, childproof closures, four-sided pool fencing, use protective goggles, insulate electric cords.
7. Modify basic qualities of the hazard
   Use breakaway poles near roadways, energy-absorbing surfacing, shatterproof glass in windscreens.
8. Strengthen resistance to the hazard
   Prevent osteoporosis, promote muscle conditioning in athletes, apply earthquake and hurricane building codes.
9. Begin to counter damage done
   Use early detection systems: smoke detectors, road-side phones, early warning systems, emergency response systems.
10. Stabilise, repair damage and rehabilitate
    Undertake treatment, rehabilitation, vocational and self-care retraining, modification of environment for disabled.

Working Group, which led the development of strategies for this plan, no longer exists and, as a result, there is no clear governance and leadership for this national health priority in Australia. Similarly, the New Zealand Injury Prevention Strategy (NZIPS) was disestablished in December 2013.

Trauma registries

Trauma registries in Australia and New Zealand were established as part of emerging organised systems of trauma management. While the data collected can vary, most trauma registries collate information on injury types and severity, health information coding, patient demographics, injury event data, details of ambulance transfer and treatment, ED or trauma centre treatment and details of interhospital transfer of trauma patients. This information serves to quantify the extent and sequelae of injury for the purpose of monitoring patterns of injury, improving quality of trauma management, planning of trauma services and comparing treatment across centres, and it can be used to promote injury prevention. Trauma registries also provide an excellent source of data to determine the financial costs of injury. There is no standardisation of data

collected by trauma registries; however, the establishment of a national Australian trauma database, with plans to extend this to include New Zealand, holds the potential to develop a more coherent understanding of traumatic injury, to respond to national policy in relation to trauma and develop nationally consistent strategies and research to tackle the problem.[14]

Trauma scores—measuring injury, its impact and outcomes

Several trauma scores have been developed in an attempt to quantify injury severity and mortality prediction. Many of these trauma scores were developed using data from the Major Trauma Outcome Study (MTOS) undertaken in North America in the early 1980s. Aims of the MTOS were to refine methods for injury severity scoring, to establish national normative outcomes for trauma and to provide trauma care institutions with objective evaluations of quality assurance and outcome.[108]

The Trauma Score and Revised Trauma Score

The Trauma Score (TS) is a physiological score based on the Glasgow Coma Scale, as well as on assessments of cardiovascular status (capillary return and systolic blood pressure) and respiratory status (rate and effort). Weighted values assigned to the variable are added to obtain the TS. Although the TS has been widely used, capillary refill and respiratory expansion are difficult to assess in the field at night and are often open to broad interpretation among trauma clinicians. To address these issues, the Revised Trauma Score (RTS) was developed. The RTS is based on the Glasgow Coma Scale, systolic blood pressure and respiratory rate. Assessed at patient admission and other times, the RTS provides physiological information that can be used for pre-hospital and interhospital triage. When combined with ISS (see below), patient age and type of injury, the resulting indices can be used for quality assurance and comparisons of outcome between or among hospitals of groups of patients.

Abbreviated Injury Scale

The Abbreviated Injury Scale (AIS) is an anatomical injury rating. Early work characterising the severity of individual injuries was conducted by De Haven at Cornell in the 1950s. This early scale was used primarily by crash-investigation teams to quantify injury as part of their testing programs. The Association for the Advancement of Automotive Medicine (AAAM) became the parent organisation of the AIS in 1973. The AIS forms the underlying system for a number of commonly-derived injury severity and outcome scores, including the Injury Severity Score (ISS), New Injury Severity Score (NISS) and Trauma and Injury Severity Score (TRISS).

The first AIS dictionary was published in 1976 with more than 500 injury descriptions. The AIS is a 'consensus derived, anatomically based system that classifies individual injuries by body region on a 6-point ordinal severity scale ranging from AIS 1 (minor) to AIS 6 (currently untreatable)'.[109] In addition to the severity score, a numerical injury identifier is allocated to assist in computerisation of data: a five-digit code is associated with each unique description of injury, similar in function to ICD-10-CM codes. The AIS is used to calculate the ISS. Subsequent revisions were published in 1980, 1985 (when penetrating injury scores were introduced), 1990, 1998 (updated), 2005 (revised) (AIS05), with minor updates in 2008 and 2014.

Injury Severity Score

The Injury Severity Score (ISS) is the most commonly used injury score to reflect overall severity and probability of survival, and is used to undertake epidemiological research, trauma centre studies, patient outcome evaluation and healthcare systems research. To determine the ISS, the body is divided into six regions. The ISS is the sum of the squares of the three highest AIS scores in three different body regions.[110] ISS scores range from 1 to 75; an ISS of > 12 or >15 is considered severe, depending on local policy. An acknowledged limitation of the ISS is the inability to account for multiple serious injuries within the one body region; for example, a patient who has bilateral fractured femurs has only one fractured femur counted in the calculation of ISS, as both these injuries are in the same body region (extremities). Despite these limitations, the ISS remains the most widely used injury severity scoring system, largely because alternative methods have not yet been found that both increase the accuracy of mortality predictions and justify an industry-wide switch to a new system.

New Injury Severity Score

The New Injury Severity Score (NISS)[111] is a modification of the ISS.[110] Since its introduction in 1997, the NISS has been found to be more accurate than the ISS at predicting mortality and post-injury multiple-organ failure.[111] The NISS simplifies the process and allows more than one injury from the same region to count by taking the three highest AIS scores regardless of location. NISS has yet to be widely tested and adopted as a replacement for the ISS.

Alternative methods of quantifying injury severity have been suggested, including A Severity Characterisation of Trauma (ASCOT), which uses the anatomical profile (AP) to provide the anatomical element of the scoring system. Systems based on International Classification of Diseases coding have also been put forward (ICISS),[112] but none has yet achieved widespread acceptance.

Standardised clinical trauma management

Since the introduction of the Advanced Trauma Life Support (ATLS) guidelines by the American College of Surgeons in 1978, there have been attempts by many countries with organised systems of health to standardise approaches to the clinical management of trauma.[113] After importing and adapting the ATLS guidelines under licence, the Early Management of Severe Trauma (EMST) guidelines were introduced to Australia and New Zealand by the Royal Australasian College of Surgeons in 1988. EMST guidelines are the same as the ATLS, with a few minor adaptations to the nuances of medical practice in this region. EMST provides a common language and general approach to managing trauma for all emergency healthcare clinicians. The problem of error in trauma management contributes significantly to preventable or potentially preventable morbidity and mortality.[114] Indeed, most preventable errors occur not because of ignorance or lack of resources, but because the correct therapeutic and diagnostic

measures are not performed at the right time, in the right amount or in the right order.[115]

A standardised trauma management environment holds the potential to ensure effective and coordinated trauma team response (trauma call), defined roles for trauma team members with clear leadership, shared goals and priorities in trauma management, evidence-based interventions, standard time-frames for trauma management (according to resource availability) and a systems approach to managing trauma that extends beyond primary and secondary survey. However, variability in resources and distribution of trauma patients across trauma systems mean that a one-size-fits-all solution to standardising trauma care is doomed to fail. To meet the changing demands of resource variability, a principles approach to developing standardised trauma care is recommended.

Principles of standardising trauma management

In addition to EMST guidelines, standardising trauma management is heavily dependent on local resources, the frequency and type of trauma received, the experience level of clinicians and the role of the facility in an organised trauma system. Similarly, standardising trauma management is also determined by the developed nature of the surrounding trauma system, including pre-hospital triage guidelines and systems for transferring patients to major trauma centres.

Pre-hospital trauma triage, using a series of protocols and guidelines, aims to get the right patient to the right hospital. With a common understanding and goals to work towards, all levels of trauma care within a system need to develop standardised approaches to managing trauma that meet and evolve with changing local resource constraints and demands for trauma services.

The principles in Table 42.2 offer a guide for emergency and trauma healthcare professionals involved in trauma management to develop locally relevant approaches to trauma management that articulate with larger trauma systems.

Organised trauma systems in Australia and New Zealand

Not unlike comparable countries in the developed world, organised trauma systems in Australia and New Zealand vary in their level of development. The aim of a trauma system is to facilitate treatment of the injured patient at the right hospital, resulting in optimal care for all trauma patients. Particular emphasis is placed on the development of a trauma system that encompasses pre-hospital care, acute care in the hospital setting, recovery and rehabilitation, in both hospital and home settings (Box 42.5).

Trauma systems are required to provide an organised and coordinated response to injury and there is a significant body of evidence that a systems approach to trauma management reduces trauma morbidity and mortality.[116–118] Fundamental to the trauma system infrastructure is a network of hospitals committed to treating individuals with injuries that span the spectrum of severity.[119] Being part of a trauma system requires hospitals to be 'designated' at a prescribed level of care. The level of designation most commonly used is that promulgated by the American College of Surgeons Committee on Trauma, which has been adapted to the Australasian context (Box 42.6).[120]

Having an inclusive trauma system, where all hospitals with 24-hour ED access are classified at different levels of trauma

TABLE 42.2 Principles of standardising trauma management[10,138,139]

STANDARDISATION PRINCIPLE	RATIONALE
Use EMST guidelines as a beginning point	EMST guidelines offer a common language and understanding of the overall approach to trauma management, and are therefore a good beginning point and overall structure for standardising trauma management.
Gather an evidence base	Knowledge and practice in trauma management is changing rapidly. To ensure best practice in trauma management, and therefore optimal trauma patient outcomes, it is important that standards of practice are based on current research and best practice in trauma management. Systematic approaches to reviewing literature and determining best practice in trauma management can seem like an overwhelming task for many hospitals already struggling with burgeoning clinical workloads. However, much of this sort of work is often undertaken by governmental bodies, such as NSW ITIM and major trauma services. The role of major trauma services and larger teaching hospitals that receive trauma is to share this sort of information. However, it is up to committed groups of clinicians at smaller hospitals to adapt this information for their own local resources.
Maintain a focus of the elements of care known to influence outcome	The multitude of tasks in trauma management demands that trauma clinicians prioritise what they do. It is therefore important that standardised approaches to trauma care maintain a clear focus on what improves patient outcome. For example, many sizeable hospitals in country regions have the resources available to perform CT scans on trauma patients. However, many of these facilities do not include an in-house or even on-call neurosurgeon. Trauma systems research suggests that trauma patients are more likely to survive the sooner they are transferred to a major trauma service. Clearly, the focus of smaller regional hospitals needs to be to stabilise the trauma patient and transfer them to the nearest major trauma facility as soon as possible. Delays incurred by unnecessary procedures, such as CT scans (which are usually repeated at major trauma services), only threaten the trauma patient's chances of survival.
Develop a clear and transparent process for calling in a trauma team	Trauma management is clearly a team effort. Even in smaller country hospitals where resources are scarce, a clear and efficient means of calling in the additional resources required to manage trauma patients needs to be developed in institutions. Communications technology makes this easier, including long-range pagers and mobile phones, often already used by these smaller hospitals for other purposes.
Develop clinical practice guidelines, protocols and algorithm-based approaches to trauma management	Standardised approaches to trauma management require the development of clinical practice guidelines, trauma protocols or trauma algorithms to delineate team roles, ensure effective use of available resources, time-efficient management of the trauma patient and transfer to the appropriate level of care as soon as the trauma patient is sufficiently stable for transfer.
Develop clinical pathways for post-initial resuscitation, single-system-injured patients	Receiving trauma hospitals, both big and small, need to have clear clinical pathways to guide the post-initial resuscitation management of patient with isolated or single-system injuries.

service, facilitates these hospitals being included in ongoing aspects of trauma care, education and patient management. These hospitals are also supported by having a well-defined transfer protocol in place and written agreements regarding the acceptance of transfers, in the event that trauma patients require treatment at a higher level of care within the system.

Australia

In 1993 the National Road Trauma Advisory Council (NRTAC)[120] published a report of the working party on trauma systems. This report formed the blueprint for the development of state-based, regionalised trauma systems in Australia. In NSW, a system of trauma care was first proposed in 1988; in 1991, designation of trauma centres occurred, level 3 being the highest. March 1992 saw the introduction of pre-hospital trauma bypass via a trauma triage tool. The NRTAC report of 1993 contained some 23 recommendations for trauma system structure. In 1994, in line with the NRTAC recommendations, the NSW trauma system was again reviewed and the labelling of trauma hospitals was changed to the currently accepted major, regional and urban trauma centres. In 1997 the NSW Rural Trauma Plan was released and the Early Notification of Severe Trauma—Rural Trauma Triage and Bypass was introduced. The Greater Metropolitan Transitional Taskforce again reviewed trauma in NSW in 2000, and in 2002 the NSW Institute of Trauma and Injury Management was established. At this stage there was a recommendation to reduce the number of designated major trauma centres in the greater metropolitan area of Sydney. The most recent New South Wales State Trauma plan was released in March 2010. In this plan, the number of major trauma centres (level 1) is reduced to five in greater metropolitan Sydney and one in Greater Newcastle.[121] Another review was undertaken in late 2014. The NSW Ambulance Pre Hospital Trauma Triage Protocol T1 mandates that major

---

BOX 42.5 Phases of trauma care

Pre-hospital
- Injury scene
- Ambulance
- Retrieval
- Acute care

Emergency department
- Operating suite
- Intensive care
- Acute care wards
- Rehabilitation and recovery
- Rehabilitation:
  - inpatient/acute care
  - outpatient
  - community

Other
- Injury prevention
- Education
- Performance/quality programs

BOX 42.6 Levels of trauma centres and model resource criteria[130]

Level I—provides 24-hour full spectrum of care for the most critically injured patient, from initial reception and resuscitation through to discharge and rehabilitation, and, ideally, a surgical trauma admitting service (bed card). Also research, education and fellowship training, quality improvement program, prevention and outreach programs and the principal hospital for reception of interhospital transfer of major trauma patients.

Level II—can be either metropolitan- or rural-based; provides comprehensive 24-hour clinical care identical to that of a Level I service without the additional leadership, research and education components.

Level III—provides prompt assessment, resuscitation, 24-hour on-call emergency general surgical and anaesthetic service, and stabilisation of a small number of seriously injured patients while arranging for their transfer to the responsible major trauma service. A Level III service can provide some definitive care for non-major-trauma patients according to patient needs and available resources.

Level IV—a resuscitating hospital where the major trauma patient is transferred out as soon as possible. A medical doctor needs to be in attendance within half an hour. Level IV services are not intended to care for major trauma patients, but are recognised because they participate in the care of minor trauma, and because, on occasions, individual patients may self-present with major trauma, or in rural situations there may be an occasional need for resuscitation of a major trauma patient, with rapid transfer on. Guidelines should exist for this management and transfer process.

Level V—may be large, mature tertiary institutions, which are not designated for trauma care specifically. In the rural setting, these institutions will usually be very small and isolated hospitals or medical centres, with no immediately available medical practitioner.

---

trauma patients be transported directly to a major trauma centre if within 1 hour of transport.[122]

In Victoria, the *Review of Trauma and Emergency Services* (ROTES) report was published in 1999 and led to the development of a comprehensive and integrated system of trauma management, with a strong research element. There are two adult and one paediatric Major Trauma Services designated in Victoria. Other components of the Trauma System include statewide system organisation and management of trauma response with trauma triage and transfer protocols, enhanced retrieval and transfer services, education and training, research, service and technology developments and a quality management program. Since 2000, a marked improvement in patient management and reduction in preventable or potentially preventable deaths[116] has occurred, largely due to the increase in admissions to expanded major trauma services after the introduction of the Victorian State Trauma System.

In South Australia, a state trauma system was established in 1997 and demonstrated a significant reduction in trauma mortality among patients attending major trauma services after four years of system implementation.[117]

Following recommendations of the report *A Healthy Future for Western Australians—Report of the Health Reform Committee: March 2003*,[123] WA began developing its own trauma system. These recommendations focused on hospital role delineation and networking of trauma services across the state. The 2007 report *Trauma System and Services: Report of the Trauma Working Group* contained 52 initiatives to form the framework of the WA Trauma System. Through 2008 and 2009 these initiatives were endorsed by the State Health Executive. In 2010 Royal Perth Hospital was designated the Major Trauma Service, and in 2012, the Clinical Cluster Lead process determined there be a single Adult Major Trauma Service situated at Royal Perth Hospital and a Paediatric Major Trauma Centre be situated at the Princess Margaret Hospital for Children. The

Clinical Services Framework 2010 included the further role delineation of designated trauma services from level 3–6 as part of the ongoing development of an integrated trauma system for WA.[123] This process continues to the time of publication.

A trauma system was established in the NT in 2007 with the Royal Darwin Hospital designated as the Major Trauma Service for the Territory. The Australian Government committed $65.8 million to establish the National Critical Care and Trauma Response Centre at the Royal Darwin Hospital as a key element of its disaster and emergency medical response. There is no pre-hospital protocol or overarching tasking authority/coordination. Due to geographical isolation, distance and time there is not the ability to over-fly any locations; all are transported to the closest facility. Decisions if via road or air transport are dependent on location (i.e. within a 150 km radius of Darwin) and environmental considerations (limited access during wet vs dry season weather). Queensland has implemented a State Trauma Plan with a coordinating body and three designated level 1 trauma centres.[124] The Royal Hobart Hospital is the major trauma centre for Tasmania. The ACT has no formal system of trauma management outside their established system of health, although Canberra Hospital is the designated trauma centre.

New Zealand

Despite efforts to coordinate trauma care in NZ in the decade leading up to 2010, no effective trauma system and no nation-wide trauma data collection process was established.[125] Recognising that deficiency, in 2011 the National Health Board established the Major Trauma National Clinical Network.[126] The terms of reference of the Network include:

- development and implementation of an annual Network work plan to address service quality and delivery issues
- promoting a nationally coordinated and consistent approach to the delivery of major trauma services including the identification and implementation of appropriate sector-wide communication strategies
- clinical leadership that facilitates collaborative and inclusive relationships with all stakeholders
- providing expert clinical advice on specific areas; for example, existing clinical effectiveness, service improvement and development and treatment
- providing advice on monitoring and auditing of major trauma services to inform continuous quality improvement.

While not directly funded to achieve all these objectives, the Network has facilitated revision of the NZ Optimal Care Guidelines, encouraged the formation of trauma services in each hospital and described a major trauma minimum data set. It was anticipated that by July 2015 all trauma-receiving hospitals would have established a process to collect the minimum data set on all major trauma admissions and submit that data to a National Trauma Registry.[126] By describing a system of care, requiring the appointment of trauma clinicians and mandating the collection and submission of major trauma data it is expected that the quality of trauma care in New Zealand will be measurable and be able to be improved in the coming years.[126]

Trauma verification

The Australasian Trauma Verification Program is a multi-disciplinary intercollegiate process, developed through the Royal Australasian College of Surgeons (RACS) to assist hospitals in analysing their system of care for the injured patient. The review covers the process of care from pre-hospital through to discharge from acute care, and identifies the strengths and weaknesses of the hospital's trauma service.[127] It has been demonstrated that the trauma verification process results in significant improvements in patient care, enhancement of institutional pride and commitment to care of the injured patient.[128] Yet it remains voluntary and unmandated by government authorities, and significant resource and outcome variance exists between trauma centres.[14,129]

There are four different levels of trauma centre as defined by the RACS.[130] Part of the verification process defines resource-level criteria and capabilities for each level (Box 42.6). For example, a level 1 trauma centre must be capable of providing the full spectrum of care for the most critically injured patient, from initial reception and resuscitation through to discharge and rehabilitation. By contrast, a hospital designated level 4 is one where the major trauma patient is resuscitated and transferred out as rapidly as possible to definitive care. A trauma system ensures that guidelines are in place to facilitate this process. Full criteria can be found on the RACS website (www.racs.edu.au).

Multidisciplinary approach

An organised multidisciplinary team approach to the care of the injured patient is essential to the successful development of injury management services. Within trauma centres the multidisciplinary team is developed, led and evaluated by the trauma service. At a minimum, the trauma service should consist of the trauma medical director, trauma coordinator, trauma data manager and administrative support. The trauma service may also include trauma fellows, trauma registrars and case managers. The trauma service coordinates the larger multidisciplinary team, tailored to the needs of each patient, and typically consists of various medical and nursing specialties, allied health and rehabilitation clinicians. Direct communication between pre-hospital and in-hospital care providers is of paramount importance and is facilitated when there is a dedicated ambulance liaison person. The trauma service is responsible for the education of the multidisciplinary team and the overall care rendered by the team (Fig 42.7).

The provision of trauma care in Australia and New Zealand is uniquely multidisciplinary, from the composition of trauma teams to the heavy reliance on subspecialty surgical care. The patient is generally admitted to a ward under the duty surgeon, and any specialty medical team as required; for example, orthopaedics or neurosurgery. The bulk of the operative management is performed by orthopaedic surgeons (66%). The remainder of surgery is performed by plastic and maxillofacial

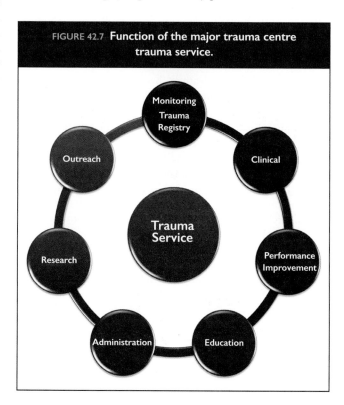

FIGURE 42.7 Function of the major trauma centre trauma service.

(10%), neurosurgery (10%), cardiothoracics, vascular, ear–nose–throat and urology surgeons.[131] This is one area where coordination and communication problems can arise in trauma patient care, and using trauma case management or a dedicated trauma surgical team that admits all trauma patients, rather than multiple individual surgical services, alleviates these problems and has been demonstrated to improve patient outcomes.[132–135]

Trauma nursing

The field of trauma encompasses a large variety of nursing specialties, such as injury prevention, emergency, perioperative, intensive care, high-dependency and ward surgical roles through to rehabilitation. However, the trauma case manager or trauma nurse specialist has additional knowledge and expertise in the complex care required of the traumatically injured patient throughout the whole span of trauma care. Trauma nurses work to ensure that all injured patients and their families are provided with complete physical and emotional care.

The roots of trauma nursing developed in wartime experiences, including those of Florence Nightingale in the Crimean War in 1854, military nurses in the Spanish–American War of 1898, in World Wars I and II and then in the Korean and Vietnam Wars. These nurses established the first principles for nursing management of devastating traumatic injuries: triage, rapid evacuation, surgical intervention, stabilisation and early rehabilitation. The civilian population recognised that an organised trauma system was essential in the United States in 1961, and the first trauma research nurse was employed in Maryland in 1961. It is asserted by Beachley et al[136] that Elizabeth Scanlan, Nursing Director of the Center for the Study of Trauma when it opened in 1969, was visionary in her approach to developing a competent nursing staff specific to trauma and resuscitation. The first trauma nurse coordinator was appointed in 1972 in Illinois, United States.[136]

In Australia, the role of trauma nurse coordinator (TNC) has evolved over the past 30 years. In the mid-1980s, two emergency nurses in large teaching hospitals in Sydney were appointed as trauma nurses. This was congruent with trauma system development in NSW and with progression of the concept of designated trauma centres. These nurses pioneered the specialty of trauma nursing in Australia. Along with their respective trauma medical directors, each was responsible for organising their institutions to receive and care for trauma patients.[137]

Currently in Australia, there are two main roles for trauma nurse specialists:

- First, the trauma coordinator or trauma program manager who, in conjunction with their trauma medical directors, oversees trauma care delivery. The role includes educating staff in the concept of trauma teams and systems, general trauma management, data collection, maintenance of a trauma database and evaluation and performance improvement of trauma care. As it becomes more and more evident that the coordination of the hospital trauma system results in improved patient outcomes, the number of nurses performing this role in Australia is increasing.

- Second, the role of trauma case manager.[101,137] The trauma case manager is supervised by the trauma coordinator and is responsible for the day-to-day clinical coordination of trauma patient care and informal bedside staff education and patient advocacy. The case managers highlight any system problems or performance indicator violations, and pass them on to the trauma coordinator for follow-up.

In 2010 in Canberra, ACT, the first trauma nurse practitioner position was introduced. It is likely this role will slowly be adopted across Australia and New Zealand. The roles of the trauma specialist are summarised in Table 42.3.[140]

TABLE 42.3 Specialist trauma nurse role responsibilities identified[140]

CLINICAL ACTIVITIES	EDUCATION	PERFORMANCE IMPROVEMENT	ADMINISTRATION	DATA COLLECTION	RESEARCH
• Direct patient care • Assessment and initial resuscitation • Ward rounds • Facilitation of medical team referrals • Allied health referrals • Multidisciplinary team reviews • Management of outpatient clinics • Advanced clinical skills	• Staff education and bedside teaching • Implementation of policy • Patient and family education • Maintenance of continued professional development • Presentation at conferences • Community outreach–injury prevention • Tertiary teaching	• Review of patient care for complications/adverse events • Audits • Policy/strategy development • Trauma committee meetings • Implementation of policy	• Management of staff • Rosters • Ordering stock • Attending meetings • Typing minutes • Budget preparation • Recruitment	• Trauma data collection • Maintenance of trauma registry • Report generation	• Initiating/participating in research programs • Implementation of research into practice

SUMMARY

Some trauma systems in Australia and New Zealand are well established, but others have yet to reach maturity. The problem of injury in society is of a magnitude that demands the attention of healthcare providers on a daily basis, regardless of how organised or lacking the surrounding trauma systems are. An improved understanding of the incidence and prevalence of trauma can empower clinicians of all levels of experience to contribute to improving the trauma system they work in at a local level. It also helps them to reflect on how their respective departments fit into a wider trauma system, and to work towards improving trauma networks and approaches to trauma management at a regional level.

Predominant patterns of injury mean that trauma clinicians in Australia and New Zealand are relative experts in the management of blunt trauma. However, knowledge and skill in managing penetrating trauma and special patterns of injury need to be maintained if the trend towards increasing numbers of patients being injured by these mechanisms continues. The risk factors that help identify who is most likely to be injured can help clinicians comprehend and further develop their knowledge and skills bases in line with the diversity of injured patients they are likely to care for.

An in-depth knowledge of the nature and outcomes of traumatic injury means that trauma clinicians are in a unique position to contribute to injury prevention and interdisciplinary trauma research. Standardising clinical trauma management holds the potential to reduce error and foster inter-organisational trauma research to improve trauma patient outcomes.

USEFUL WEBSITES

The Institute for Health Metrics and Evaluation (IHME) is an independent global health research center at the University of Washington that provides rigorous and comparable measurement of the world's most important health problems and evaluates the strategies used to address them. The Global Burden of Disease: Generating Evidence, Guiding Policy provides an overview of the reasons why the Global Burden of Disease (GBD) is an essential tool for evidence-based health policymaking. Data GBD Compare is new to IHME's lineup of visualisations and has countless options for exploring health data:

www.healthmetricsandevaluation.org/sites/default/files/policy_report/2014/IHME_T4H_Full_Report.pdf

www.healthmetricsandevaluation.org/gbd/publications/policy-report/global-burden-disease-generating-evidence-guiding-policy

Trauma.org is an independent, non-profit organisation providing global education, information and communication resources for professionals in trauma and critical care, www.trauma.org

The National Trauma Research Institute, www.ntri.org.au/

REFERENCES

1. Lozano R, Naghavi M, Foreman K et al. Global and regional mortality from 235 causes of death for 20 age groups in 1990 and 2010: a systematic analysis for the Global Burden of Disease Study 2010. Lancet. 2012;380(9859):2095–128.

2. Institute for Health Metrics and Evaluation. The global burden of disease: generating evidence, guiding policy. Seattle, WA: IHME; 2013.

3. Institute for Health Metrics and Evaluation. GDB data visualisations. Online. http://healthmetricsandevaluation.org/gbd/visualizations/regional; acccessed 30 April 2015.

4. Global Road Safety Facility (GRSF), Institute for Health Metrics and Evaluation (IHME). Transport for health: the global burden of disease from motorized road transport. GRSF & IHME; 2014.

5. Australian Institute of Health and Welfare (AIHW): Pointer S. Trends in hospitalised injury, Australia 1999–2000 to 2010–11. Canberra: AIHW; 2013.

6. Ministry of Health and Accident Compensation Corporation. Injury-related health loss: A report from the New Zealand Burden of Diseases, Injuries and Risk Factors Study 2006–2016. Wellington: New Zealand Ministry of Health; 2013.

7. Lyons RA, Finch CF, McClure R et al. The injury List of All Deficits (LOAD) Framework—conceptualizing the full range of deficits and adverse outcomes following injury and violence. Int J Inj Contr Saf Promot 2010;17(3):145–59.

8. Berndt RM, Berndt CH. The speaking land: myth and story in Aboriginal Australia. Vermont: Inner Traditions; 1994.

9. Kirkup J. Foundation lecture. Fracture care of friend and foe during World War I. ANZ J Surg. 2003;73(6):453–9.

10. National Public Health Partnership (NPHP). The National Injury Prevention and Safety Promotion Plan: 2004–2014. Canberra: NPHP; 2004.

11. National Public Health Partnership (NPHP). The National Falls Prevention for Older People Plan: 2004 Onwards. Canberra: NPHP; 2004.

12. National Public Health Partnership (NPHP). The National Aboriginal and Torres Strait Islander Safety Promotion Strategy. Canberra: NPHP; 2004.

13. National Health and Medical Research Council. Research funding statistics and data. 2014; www.nhmrc.gov.au/grants/research-funding-statistics-and-data.

14. Alfred Health. Caring for the severely ill in Australia: Inaugural report of the Australian Trauma Registry 2010 to 2012. Melbourne, Victoria: Alfred Health; 2014.

15. Kreisfeld R, Newson R, Harrison J. Injury deaths, Australia 2002. Adelaide: AIHW; 2004.

16. Henley G, Harrison JE. Injury deaths, Australia 2004–05. Adelaide: AIHW; 2009.

17. Australian Institute of Health and Welfare. Australia's Health 2012. Canberra: AIHW; 2012.

18. Australian Bureau of Statistics. 3303.0—Causes of Death, Australia, 2004. 2007; www.abs.gov.au/AUSSTATS/abs@.nsf/allprimarymainfeatures/3AA156BFD4C7E1E0CA25729D0010CB69?opendocument; accessed 16 June 2015.

19. Australian Bureau of Statistics. Causes of Death, Australia, 2012. 2014; www.abs.gov.au/ausstats/abs@.nsf/Lookup/by%20Subject/3303.0~2012~Main%20Features~Key%20Characteristics~10009; accessed 16 June 2015.

20. Mitchell RJ, Curtis K, Chong S et al. Comparative analysis of trends in paediatric trauma outcomes in New South Wales, Australia. Injury 2013;44(1):97–103.

21. Harrison JE, Pointer S, Elnour AA. A review of suicide statistics in Australia. Adelaide: AIHW; 2009.

22. Watson W, Clapperton A, Mitchell R. The incidence and cost of falls injury among older people in New South Wales 2006/07. Sydney: NSW Department of Health; 2010.

23. Gillespie LD, Robertson MC, Gillespie WJ et al. Interventions for preventing falls in older people living in the community. Cochrane Database Syst Rev. 2012(9).

24. Safe Work Australia (SWA). Work-related Traumatic Injury Fatalities Australia 2012: SWA; 2013.

25. Australian Bureau of Statistics. 4430.0—Disability, Ageing and Carers, Australia: Summary of Findings, 2012. 2014; www.abs.gov.au/AUSSTATS/abs@.nsf/Lookup/4430.0Main+Features12012?OpenDocument. accessed 03/10/14.

26. Wiseman T, Foster K, Curtis K. Mental health following traumatic physical injury: an integrative literature review. Injury 2013;44(11):1383–90.

27. Scheetz LJ. Differences in survival, length of stay, and discharge disposition of older trauma patients admitted to trauma centers and nontrauma center hospitals. J Nurs Scholarsh 2005;37(4):361–6.

28. National Trauma Registry Consortium (Australia and New Zealand) (NTRCANZ). The national trauma registry (Australia and New Zealand) 2003 report. Herston: NTRCANZ; 2005.

29. Mitchell R, Curtis K, Fisher M. Understanding trauma as a men's health issue: sex differences in traumatic injury presentations at a level 1 trauma center in Australia. J Trauma Nurs 2012;19(2):80–8.

30. Australian Indigenous HealthInfoNet. Overview of Australian Indigenous health status 2013. Perth, Western Australia: Australian Indigenous HealthInfoNet; 2014.

31. Helps YLM, Harrison JE. Reported injury mortality of Aboriginal and Torres Strait Islander people in Australia, 1997–2000. Adelaide: AIHW; 2004.

32. Chikritzhs T, Evans M, Gardner C et al. Australian Alcohol Aetiologic Fractions for Injuries Treated in Emergency Departments. Perth: National Drug Research Institute, Curtin University;2011.

33. Connor J, Casswell S. The burden of road trauma due to other people's drinking. Accid Anal Prev 2009;41(5):1099–103.

34. Sheridan J, Bennett S, Coggan C et al. Injury associated with methamphetamine use: a review of the literature. Harm Reduct J 2006;3:14.

35. McKetin R, Lubman DI, Najman JM et al. Does methamphetamine use increase violent behaviour? Evidence from a prospective longitudinal study. Addiction 2014;109(5):798–806.

36. Rootman DB, Mustard R, Kalia V, Ahmed N. Increased incidence of complications in trauma patients cointoxicated with alcohol and other drugs. J Trauma 2007;62(3):755–8.

37. Australian Institute of Health and Welfare. Figure 6.11 Australia's Health 2012. Canberra: AIHW. 2012;295. Online www.aihw.gov.au/WorkArea/DownloadAsset.aspx?id=10737422169; accessed 4 May 2015.

38. Danne PD. Trauma management in Australia and the tyranny of distance. World J Surg 2003;27(4):385–9. Australian Transport Safety Bureau (ATSB). Road crash casualties and rates, Australia, 1925 to 2005. Canberra: ATSB; 2007. Online. Available: www.infrastructure.gov.au/roads/safety/publications/2008/pdf/1925_05_casualties.pdf.

39. Australian Bureau of Statistics. Australian Social Trends March 2011: Health outside major cities. Canberra: ABS; 2011.

40. Australian Transport Council. National Road Safety Strategy 2011–2020; 2011:25.

41. Stutts JC, Reinfurt DW, Rodgman EA. The role of driver distraction in crashes: an analysis of 1995–1999 Crashworthiness Data System Data. Annu Proc Assoc Adv Automot Med 2001;45:287–301.

42. Young K, Regan M. Road safety implications of driver distraction: Australasian road safety handbook. Sydney: Austroads; 2003.

43. Beanland V, Fitzharris M, Young KL, Lenné MG. Driver inattention and driver distraction in serious casualty crashes: data from the Australian National Crash In-depth Study. Accid Anal Prev 2013;54:99–107.

44. Gordon C. Driver distraction: An initial examination of the 'attention diverted by' contributory factor codes from crash reports and focus group research on perceived risks. Paper presented at: Institute of Professional Engineers Technical Conference 2005; Auckland: New Zealand.

45. Hallett C, Lambert A, Regan MA. Text messaging amongst New Zealand drivers: Prevalence and risk perception. Transport Res F-Traf 2012;15(3):261–71.

46. McEvoy SP, Stevenson MR, McCartt AT et al. Role of mobile phones in motor vehicle crashes resulting in hospital attendance: a case-crossover study. BMJ 2005;331(7514):428.

47. World Health Organization (WHO). Mobile phone use: a growing problem of driver distraction. Geneva, Switzerland: WHO; 2011.

48. Nasar JL, Troyer D. Pedestrian injuries due to mobile phone use in public places. Accid Anal Prev 2013;57:91–5.

49. Lansdown TC, Stephens AN. Couples, contentious conversations, mobile telephone use and driving. Accid Anal Prev 2013;50:416–22.

50. Australian Transport Council (ATC). National Road Safety Strategy 2011–2020: ATC; 2011.

51. Pfeifer R, Tarkin IS, Rocos B, Pape HC. Patterns of mortality and causes of death in polytrauma patients—has anything changed? Injury 2009;40(9):907–11.

52. Delprado A. President's message, December 2010, Trauma Talk. I. Civil. Australasian Trauma Society 2010. 2010;12:1–7.

53. Cameron P, Dziukas L, Hadj A et al. Major trauma in Australia: a regional analysis. J Trauma 1995;39(3):545–52.

54. Australian Institute of Criminology. Violent crime statistics—Assault. 2009; www.aic.gov.au/statistics/violent%20crime/assault.html.

55. Australian Bureau of Statistics. 4510.0—Recorded Crime—Victims, Australia, 2013. 2014; www.abs.gov.au/ausstats/abs@.nsf/mf/4510.0.

56. Chambers AJ, Lord RS. Management of gunshot wounds at a Sydney teaching hospital. Aust N Z J Surg 2000;70(3):209–15.

57. Wong K, Petchell J. Severe trauma caused by stabbing and firearms in metropolitan Sydney, New South Wales, Australia. ANZ J Surg 2005;75(4):225–30.

58. Hsee L, Civil I. Management of low-velocity, non-gunshot-wound penetrating abdominal injury: have we moved with the times? NZ Med J 2008;121(1287):26–31.

59. Bartels L. 'Knife crime' in Australia: Incidence, aetiology and responses. Canberra: Australian Instititue of Criminology; 2011.

60. Alatini M. Analysis of Unintentional Child Injury Data in New Zealand: Mortality (2001–2005) and Morbidity (2003–2007). Auckland: Safekids New Zealand; 2009.

61. New Zealand Ministry of Justice. Regulatory Impact Statement: Reducing knife crime: New Zealand Ministry of Justice; 2011.

62. Reed JA, Smith RS, Helmer SD et al. Rates of unemployment and penetrating trauma are correlated. South Med J 2003;96(8):772–4.

63. Ogilvie R, Curtis K, Palmer C et al. Incidence and outcomes of major trauma patients managed in the Australian Capital Territory. ANZ J Surg 2014;84(6):433–7.

64. Henley G, Harrison JE. Trends in serious injury due to land transport accidents, Australia 2000–01 to 2008–09. Canberra: AIHW; 2012.

65. New Zealand Ministry of Transport. Cyclists—Crash statistics for the year ended 31 December 2012: New Zealand Ministry of Transport; 2013.

66. Thompson DC, Patterson MQ. Cycle helmets and the prevention of injuries. Recommendations for competitive sport. Sports Med 1998;25(4):213–19.

67. Dinh MM, Curtis K, Ivers R. The effectiveness of helmets in reducing head injuries and hospital treatment costs: a multicentre study. Med J Aust 2013;198(8):415, 417.

68. Olivier J, Walter SR, Grzebieta RH. Long term bicycle related head injury trends for New South Wales, Australia following mandatory helmet legislation. Accid Anal Prev 2013;50:1128–34.

69. Henley G, Harrison JE. Serious injury due to transport accidents involving a railway train, Australia 2004–05 to 2008–09. Canberra: AIHW; 2012.

70. Transport NZMo. Rail level crossing statistics. 2014; www.transport.govt.nz/research/roadcrashstatistics/raillevelcrossingstatistics/; accessed 16 June 2015.

71. Australian Bureau of Statistics. 4156.0.55.001—Perspectives on Sport, May 2009 www.abs.gov.au/AUSSTATS/abs@.nsf/Lookup/4156.0.55.001Feature+Article1May%202009#PARALINK0; accessed 15 June 2015.

72. Australian Bureau of Statistics. 4177.0—Participation in Sport and Physical Recreation, Australia, 2011–12. 2013; www.abs.gov.au/AUSSTATS/abs@.nsf/Lookup/4177.0Main+Features12011-12?OpenDocument; accessed 16 June 2015.

73. Australian Institute of Health and Welfare (AIHW). A picture of Australia's children. Canberra: AIHW;2005.

74. Andrew NE, Gabbe BJ, Wolfe R, Cameron PA. Trends in sport and active recreation injuries resulting in major trauma or death inadults in Victoria, Australia, 2001–2007. Injury 2012;43(9):1527–33.

75. Hockey R, Knowles M. Sports Injuries. Injury Bulletin. 2000. www.qisu.org.au/ModCoreFilesUploaded/Bulletin_59131.pdf. Accessed 03/10/14.

76. Bi-National Burns Registry Project Team. Bi-National Burns Registry Annual Report. Melbourne, Victoria: Australian and New Zealand Burn Association (ANZBA) & Monash University Department of Epidemiology and Preventive Medicine; 2013.

77. Barker R, Scott D, Hockey R, Spinks D, Pitt R. Burns and scalds in Queensland toddlers. Injury Bulletin. 2005. www.qisu.org.au/ModCoreFilesUploaded/Bulletin_89100.pdf; accessed 16 June 2015.

78. Cripps RA. Spinal cord injury, Australia 2004–05. Adelaide: AIHW; 2006.

79. Norton L. Spinal cord injury, Australia 2007–08. Canberra: AIHW; 2010.

80. Canterbury District Health Board. Burwood Spinal Unit admissions statistics 2007–2009. Christchurch: Canterbury DHB; 2010.

81. American Psychiatric Association (APA). Diagnostic and Statistical Manual of Mental Disorders, 4th Edition. Washington, DC: APA; 2000.

82. Haagsma JA, Polinder S, Toet H et al. Beyond the neglect of psychological consequences: post-traumatic stress disorder increases the non-fatal burden of injury by more than 50%. Inj Prev 2011;17(1):21–6.

83. Bisson JI, Shepherd JP, Joy D et al. Early cognitive-behavioural therapy for post-traumatic stress symptoms after physical injury. Randomised controlled trial. Br J Psychiatry 2004;184:63–9.

84. Ursano RJ, Bell C, Eth S et al. Practice guideline for the treatment of patients with acute stress disorder and posttraumatic stress disorder. Am J Psychiatry 2004;161(11 Suppl):3–31.

85. Wiseman T, Curtis K, Lam M, Foster K. Depression anxiety and stress following traumatic injury: a longitudinal study. Scandinavian Journal of Trauma, Resuscitation and Emergency Medicine 2015;23:29.

86. Koppel S, Charlton JL. Child restraint system misuse and/or inappropriate use in Australia. Traffic Inj Prev 2009;10(3):302–07.

87. Conybeare JAC. Evaluation of automobile safety regulations: The case of compulsory seat belt legislation in Australia. Pol Sci 1980;12(1):27–39.

88. Kloeden CN, Woolley JE, McLean AJ. A follow-up evaluation of the 50 km/h default urban speed limit in South Australia. Paper presented at: 2007 Road Safety Research, Education and Policing Conference; 17–19 October, 2007; Melbourne, Australia.

89. Hoareau E, Newstead S, Cameron M. An evaluation of the default 50 km/h speed limit in Victoria: Monash University Accident Research Centre; 2006.

90. Corben B, Lenné M, Regan M, Triggs T. Technology to enhance speed limit compliance. Paper presented at: Road Safety Research, Policing and Education Conference; 18–20 November, 2001; Melbourne, Australia.

91. Williams AF, Ferguson SA, McCartt AT. Passenger effects on teenage driving and opportunities for reducing the risks of such travel. J Safety Res 2007;38(4):381–90.

92. Foss RD, Feaganes JR, Rodgman EA. Initial effects of graduated driver licensing on 16-year-old driver crashes in North Carolina. JAMA 2001;286(13):1588–92.

93. National Occupational Health and Safety Commission (NOHSC). Fatal Occupational Injuries—How does Australia compare internationally? Canberra: NOHSC; 2004.

94. Safe Work Australia (SWA). Guide to the model work health and safety regulations: SWA; 2011.

95. Watson WL, Ozanne-Smith J. The cost of injury to Victoria. Melbourne: Monash University Accident Research Centre; 1997.

96. Australian Institute of Health and Welfare (AIHW). Health system expenditure on disease and injury in Australia, 2004–05. Canberra: AIHW; 2010.

97. Accident Compensation Corporation (ACC). New Zealand Injury Prevention Strategy. Five-year Evaluation—Final report May 2010: ACC; 2010.

98. New Zealand Ministry of Transport. The Social Cost of Road Crashes and Injuries 2013 update: New Zealand Ministry of Transport; 2013.

99. Curtis K, Lam M, Mitchell R et al. Acute costs and predictors of higher treatment costs of trauma in New South Wales, Australia. Inury 2014;45(1):279–84.

100. Curtis K, Lam M, Mitchell R et al. Major trauma: the unseen financial burden to trauma centres, a descriptive multicentre analysis. Aust Health Rev 2014;38(1):30–7.

101. Sesperez J, Wilson S, Jalaludin B et al. Trauma case management and clinical pathways: prospective evaluation of their effect on selected patient outcomes in five key trauma conditions. J Trauma 2001;50(4):643–9.

102. Lett R, Kobusingye O, Sethi D. A unified framework for injury control: the public health approach and Haddon's Matrix combined. Inj Control Saf Promot 2002;9(3):199–205.

103. Knudson MM, Vassar MJ, Straus EM et al. Surgeons and injury prevention: what you don't know can hurt you! J Am Coll Surg 2001;193(2):119–24.

104. Curtis K, Leonard E. The trauma nurse coordinator in Australia and New Zealand: demographics, role, and professional development. J Trauma Nurs 2012;19(4):214–20.

105. Haddon W Jr. The changing approach to the epidemiology, prevention, and amelioration of trauma: the transition to approaches etiologically rather than descriptively based. 1968. Inj Prev 1999;5(3):231–5.

106. Haddon W Jr. Energy damage and the ten countermeasure strategies. J Trauma 1973;13(4):321–31.

107. Runyan CW. Using the Haddon matrix: introducing the third dimension. Inj Prev 1998;4(4):302–7.

108. Champion HR, Copes WS, Sacco WJ et al. The Major Trauma Outcome Study: establishing national norms for trauma care. J Trauma 1990;30(11):1356–65.

109. Association for the Advancement of Automotive Medicine (AAAM). Abbreviated Injury Scale 2005–Update 2008. Barrington, Illinois: AAAM; 2008.

110. Baker SP, O'Neill B, Haddon W Jr, Long WB. The injury severity score: a method for describing patients with multiple injuries and evaluating emergency care. J Trauma 1974;14(3):187–96.

111. Osler T, Baker SP, Long W. A modification of the injury severity score that both improves accuracy and simplifies scoring. J Trauma 1997;43(6):922–6.

112. Rutledge R, Hoyt DB, Eastman AB et al. Comparison of the Injury Severity Score and ICD-9 diagnosis codes as predictors of outcome in injury: analysis of 44,032 patients. J Trauma 1997;42(3):477–89.

113. Carmont MR. The Advanced Trauma Life Support course: a history of its development and review of related literature. Postgrad Med J 2005;81(952):87–91.

114. Ministerial Taskforce on Trauma and Emergency Services & The Department of Human Services Working Party on Emergency and Trauma Services. Review of Trauma and Emergency Services Victoria 1999. Melbourne: Acute Health Division, Victorian Government, Department of Human Services; 1999.

115. Chua WC, D'Amours SK, Sugrue M et al. Performance and consistency of care in admitted trauma patients: our next great opportunity in trauma care? ANZ J Surg 2009;79(6):443–8.

116. Cameron PA, Gabbe BJ, Cooper DJ et al. A statewide system of trauma care in Victoria: effect on patient survival. Med J Aust 2008;189(10):546–50.

117. Brennan PW, Everest ER, Griggs WM et al. Risk of death among cases attending South Australian major trauma services after severe trauma: the first 4 years of operation of a state trauma system. J Trauma 2002;53(2):333–9.

118. Curtis KA, Mitchell RJ, Chong SS et al. Injury trends and mortality in adult patients with major trauma in New South Wales. Med J Aust 2012;197(4):233–7.

119. MacKenzie EJ, Hoyt DB, Sacra JC et al. National inventory of hospital trauma centers. JAMA 2003;289(12):1515–22.

120. National Road Trauma Advisory Council (NRTAC). Report of the working party on Trauma Systems. Canberra: Commonwealth Department of Human Services and Health; 1993.

121. New South Wales Health. Selected specialty and statewide services plans. Number six. NSW Trauma Services Plan. North Sydney: NSW Health; 2009.

122. Ambulance Service of New South Wales. T1 Protocol Major Trauma. Sydney, 2012.

123. State Trauma Office. Western Australia State Trauma Registry Report 2011. Perth, Western Australia: Department of Health; 2011.

124. Queensland Health. A trauma plan for Queensland: Queensland Government; 2006.

125. Civil I, Christey G. Personal Communication, 28/05/14.

126. Royal Australasian College of Surgeons & Health Quality and Safety Commission New Zealand. Quality and Safety Challenge 2012 Final Project Report: Health Quality and Safety Commission New Zealand; 2012.

127. Royal Australasian College of Surgeons (RACS). Trauma verification 2006: RACS; 2006.

128. Ehrlich PF, Rockwell S, Kincaid S, Mucha P Jr. American College of Surgeons, Committee on Trauma Verification Review: does it really make a difference? J Trauma 2002;53(5):811–16.

129. Leonard E, Curtis K. Are Australian and New Zealand trauma service resources reflective of the Australasian Trauma Verification Model Resource Criteria? ANZ J Surg 2014;84:7–8.

130. Royal Australasian College of Surgeons (RACS). Model Resource Criteria For Level I, II, III & IV Trauma Services in Australasia: RACS; 2009.

131. Balogh Z. Traumatology in Australia: provision of clinical care and trauma system development. ANZ J Surg 2010;80(3):119–21.

132. Ursic C, Curtis K, Zou Y, Black D. Improved trauma patient outcomes after implementation of a dedicated trauma admitting service. Injury 2009;40(1):99–103.

133. Curtis K, Lien D, Chan A et al. The impact of trauma case management on patient outcomes. J Trauma 2002;53(3):477–82.

134. Dutton RP, Cooper C, Jones A et al. Daily multidisciplinary rounds shorten length of stay for trauma patients. J Trauma 2003;55(5):913–19.

135. FitzPatrick MK, Reilly PM, Laborde A et al. Maintaining patient throughput on an evolving trauma/emergency surgery service. J Trauma 2006;60(3):481–6.

136. Beachley M. The evolution of trauma nursing and the Society of Trauma Nurses: a noble history. J Trauma Nurs 2005;12(4):105–15.

137. Curtis K, Donoghue J. The trauma nurse coordinator in Australia and New Zealand: a progress survey of demographics, role function, and resources. J Trauma Nurs 2008;15(2):34–42.

138. Cooper DJ, McDermott FT, Cordner SM, Tremayne AB. Quality assessment of the management of road traffic fatalities at a level 1 trauma centre compared to other hospitals in Victoria, Australia. J Trauma 1998;45(4):772–9.

139. Sampalis JS, Denis R, Frechette P et al. Direct transport to tertiary trauma centers versus transfer from lower level facilities: impact on mortality and morbidity among patients with major trauma. J Trauma 1997;43(2):288–96.

140. Walter E, Curtis K. The role and impact of the specialist trauma nurse: An integrative review. J Trauma Nursing 2015;22:153–69.

141. Baker SP, O'Neill B, Ginsburg MJ et al. The injury fact book. 2nd edn. New York: Oxford University Press; 1992.

142. Haddon W Jr. The basic strategies for preventing damage from hazards of all kinds. Hazard Prevent 1980;16:8–12.

143. Australian Transport Safety Bureau (ATSB). Road crash casualties and rates, Australia, 1925 to 2005. Canberra: ATSB; 2007. Online. www.infrastructure.gov.au/roads/safety/publications/2008/pdf/1925_05_casualties.pdf; accessed 20 July 2015.

CHAPTER 43

MECHANISMS OF INJURY
JACINTA STEWART AND TRISH ALLEN

Essentials

- Each mechanism of injury generates specific biomechanical forces which act on the body. The type of force, duration and the surface area over which the force is applied determine the pattern of injury.
- The forces that result in blunt trauma are most commonly due to rapid deceleration or acceleration.
- Penetrating injury causes damage as it passes through the body or tissue, and with sufficient force may also affect surrounding tissues.
- Safety devices, such as restraints and air bags, have reduced injuries associated with some motor vehicle collisions. However, if these devices are worn incorrectly, injuries may occur.
- Bombs and explosions can cause unique patterns of injury rarely seen outside combat areas.

INTRODUCTION

Understanding mechanism of injury is a vital part of trauma management. Knowing the mechanism of injury can assist in determining types of injury and in identifying common injury patterns with blunt and penetrating trauma. It is essential that paramedics and nurses develop sound knowledge and assessment skills in this area to accurately evaluate potential and actual injuries. This chapter provides an overview of the kinematics involved in trauma and describes the pattern of injuries that can be sustained with common mechanisms of injury, including blunt, penetrating, blast and inhalation injury.

However, while knowledge of injury patterns is useful, and raises the index of suspicion for certain injuries, it is essential that each trauma patient is assessed systematically and thoroughly using the primary and the secondary surveys, as discussed in Chapter 44.

Kinematics

It is important to appreciate the laws of physics in order to understand the mechanism of injury. Kinematics is the process of evaluating an event and determining the injuries that are likely to occur, given the motion involved. This includes evaluation of aspects such as position, angle and speed, and how these affect the body in motion. Physics is the foundation on which kinematics is based. There are four particular laws of physics that are relevant to mechanism of injury.

1. *Newton's first law of motion* states that a body at rest remains at rest and a body in motion remains in motion unless acted on by an outside force.[1] Some examples of stationary objects set in motion by energy forces are pedestrians hit by a vehicle, and blast and gunshot victims. Moving objects interrupted or acted on to stop their motion include people falling from a height, vehicles hitting a stationary object or vehicles braking to a sudden stop.

2. The *law of conservation of energy* states that energy is neither created nor destroyed, but changes form. As a car decelerates slowly, the energy of motion (acceleration) is converted to friction heat in braking (thermal energy).[2]

3. *Newton's second law of motion* states that the force that an object exerts on another object is equal to the mass of the object multiplied by its acceleration. Multiplying an object's acceleration by its mass gives the force of impact absorbed by the object stopping it.

4. The *law of moving objects* states that kinetic energy (E_k) is the energy associated with motion, and reflects the connection between weight (mass) and speed (velocity).[3] The equation to calculate kinetic energy is $E_k = \frac{1}{2}mv^2$, where m is mass and v is velocity. Consequently, doubling the weight of the moving object doubles the impact, but doubling the speed *quadruples* the impact.

PRACTICE TIP

If two vehicles were travelling at the same speed and collide, the total energy would be evenly distributed between the two vehicles. There is a common myth that implies that if a vehicle was travelling at 50 km/hr and collided head-on with another vehicle of the same size travelling at 50 km/hr the total collision impact would be estimated to be 100 km/hr. In fact, there is no distinguishable difference between the damage caused by the above-mentioned scenario and a single vehicle impact of a vehicle travelling at 50 km/hr and hitting a stationary object, such as a brick wall. The theoretical basis for this is Newton's Third Law of Motion, which states that for every action there is an opposite and equal reaction.[4]

Injury concepts

Injury occurs when an external source of energy dissipates more rapidly than the body's ability to tolerate it. Energy originates from several sources, including kinetic (motion or mechanical), chemical, electrical, thermal and radiation sources. Absence of heat and oxygen may cause injury also; for example, frostbite,

BOX 43.1 Essential concepts for mechanisms of injury

Acceleration—increase in velocity or speed of a moving object

Acceleration/deceleration—increase in velocity or speed of object followed by decrease in velocity or speed

Axial loading—injury occurs when force is applied upwards and downwards with no posterior or lateral bending of the neck

Cavitation—creation of temporary cavity as tissues are stretched and compressed

Compression—squeezing inward pressure

Compressive strength—ability to resist squeezing forces or inward pressure

Deceleration—decrease in velocity or speed of a moving object

Distraction—separation of spinal column with resulting cord transection, seen in legal hangings

Elasticity—ability to resume original shape and size after being stretched

Force—physical factor that changes motion of body at rest or already in motion

High velocity—missiles that compress and accelerate tissue away from the bullet, causing a cavity around the bullet and the entire tract

Inertial resistance—ability of body to resist movement

Injury—trauma or damage to some part of the body

Kinematics—process of looking at an accident and determining what injuries might result

Kinetic energy—energy that results from motion

Low velocity—missiles that localise injury to a small radius from centre of the tract with little disruptive effect

Muzzle blast—cloud of hot gas and burning powder at the muzzle of a gun

Shearing—two oppositely directed parallel forces

Stress—internal resistance to deformation, or internal force generated from application load

Tensile strength—amount of tension tissue can withstand and ability to resist stretching forces

Tumbling—forward rotation around the centre; somersault action of the missile can create massive injury

Yaw—deviation of bullet nose in longitudinal axis from straight line of flight

drowning or suffocation.[5] A basic component in producing injury is absorption of kinetic energy. Box 43.1 defines essential concepts for understanding mechanisms of injury.

Blunt trauma

Blunt trauma results from acceleration, deceleration, compression, shearing or direct forces.

Acceleration injuries occur when a moving object strikes a stationary or slower-moving body (e.g. a blow from a blunt object). Deceleration injuries are the reverse and occur when a moving body hits a solid or slower-moving object. Compression injuries occur with a squeezing inward pressure applied to tissues. Shearing injuries occur when two oppositely directed parallel forces are applied to tissue. Shearing forces can cause organs such as the liver and heart to pull away or fold around muscles and ligaments that secure them in position.[6] This type of injury results in severe internal bleeding. Multiple injuries are common with blunt trauma. Lungs, bowel and other air-filled structures are subject to explosion injuries. Compression injuries to solid organs, such as liver and spleen, may present with minimal external signs of injury. Hollow organs move out of the way more easily than solid organs, therefore solid organs take the brunt of the force resulting in contusions and tears. Blunt energy is transmitted in all directions, resulting in organs or tissues being susceptible to rupture if pressure is not released.[7]

The most common causes of blunt trauma are unintentional falls, and motor vehicle collisions (MVCs). Other causes include motorbike and bicycle collisions, pedestrian injuries, interpersonal violence, sporting and recreational injuries. It is also important to note that blunt trauma can also be associated with penetrating injury; for example, an impalement of an object during an MVC.

Falls

The mechanism of injury associated with falls is vertical deceleration. The severity and type of injury prevalence is often associated with the distance or height of the fall, the area of body impact, the landing surface and whether the fall is broken by objects on the way down.[6] Falls of > 3 metres are considered significant, as the person is subjected to gravitational potential energy which converts to kinetic energy, resulting in a great amount of energy transferred to the person. The greater the change in momentum on impact the larger the force applied to the person.[7,8] In addition to this it is important to consider the increasingly elderly population in Australasia: increased fragility and co-morbidities lead to a greater risk associated with relatively minor falls (see Ch 39).[9,10] The majority of falls in the elderly involve 'same height' falls. Of equal concern is falls in children: children have a relatively large head in comparison to body size and a less-well-developed neck musculature which, during falls, increases momentum and results in increased risk of head injury.[11] Head injuries may result from impulsive loading, which leads to movement of the brain within the skull; subsequent rotational movement may result in tearing of blood vessels, subdural bleeding and axonal injury. Impact loading may also occur, which may result in skull fracture or scalp lacerations. This force may create a pressure wave in the brain and skull, and cause brain contusions.[12]

If a person lands on their feet, they have the potential for Don Juan syndrome: a trio of injuries including bilateral calcaneous fractures, compression fractures of the vertebrae and bilateral Colles' fractures. The energy transferred from deceleration into the feet causes the calcaneous fractures. This energy then travels vertically upwards through the femurs, vertebral column and into the skull base, causing compression fractures in any of these areas.[6]

A fall that causes a person to place their hands out on impact will result in the transfer of energy up through the person's wrists, forearms and shoulders. This type of injury is common in falls from scooters or bicycles. Spinal injuries are another injury associated with falls. This is particularly common when the point of impact is the head, such as happens when diving head-first into water. With this impact, injuries occur because the weight and force of the torso, pelvis and legs bear down on the head and cervical spine. This type of injury is known as a compression injury or axial loading injury. Vertebral bodies are compressed and wedged, producing vertebral fragments that can pierce the spinal cord (see Ch 49). However, it is important to remember that even simple falls, such as tripping, have the potential for people to hit their head, leading to significant head or spinal injury, or both.

Motor vehicle collisions

With a motor vehicle collision, there are multiple phases that occur during deceleration.

1. Before a collision occurs, the occupant and vehicle are moving at the same speed. The first phase occurs when the vehicle impacts with another object—the motion of the vehicle continues until the kinetic energy is dissipated through damage to the vehicle or until the restraining force of the object is removed.

2. The next phase is deceleration of the occupant, which can result in compression or shearing trauma to the occupant. Injuries sustained will depend on the mass of the occupant and the protective devices within the vehicle. In addition, children have greater skeletal compliance, which allows diffusion of energy, resulting in the reduced likelihood of fractures.[11]

3. The third phase occurs when internal structures continue to move until they collide with another internal structure, or vasculature, muscles or ligaments suddenly restrain them.

Different damage occurs with each point of impact; therefore, they must be considered separately to avoid missed injuries.[2] Figure 43.1 illustrates the three points of impact with sudden deceleration forces. The size of the occupant also deserves consideration. Due to the smaller size of children, any blunt-force impact will affect a larger portion of their body, potentially resulting in multisystem trauma.[11] Modern vehicles have been adapted with safety devices such as seatbelts, airbags and crumple zones, which can dissipate the force of impact and reduce the severity of injuries that may occur.[6]

Paramedics should provide detailed information to emergency staff regarding the nature of the incident, as this will assist in determining possible injuries. This information is summarised in Box 43.2. An example of questions to ask is outlined in Box 43.3.

Different impacts can have an effect on the types of injuries that occur with MVCs. For more detail on injury to specific regions of the body, please refer to later chapters.

Frontal impact

This type of impact occurs when the front of the vehicle impacts another object, which may be moving or stationary, resulting in damage to the front of the vehicle. Depending on the levels of energy involved and the speed, multiple injuries can occur, especially if the occupant is unrestrained and driving an older-model vehicle without airbags. Interior structures, such as the windscreen, steering wheel, steering column, dashboard or instrument panel, injure the occupant when contact is made with them. After the vehicle stops, unrestrained occupants in

FIGURE 43.1 The three phases of a motor vehicle collision.

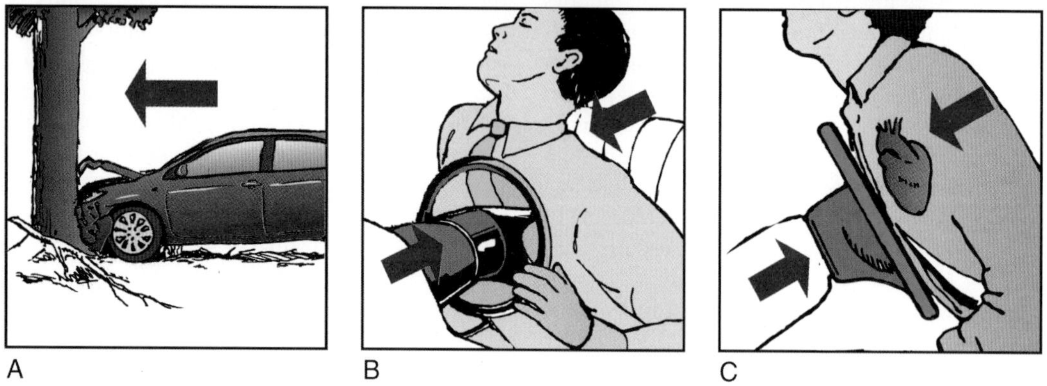

A, Car hits tree. B, Body hits steering wheel, causing fractured ribs and sternum. C, Heart strikes chest wall, causing myocardial contusion.

BOX 43.2 Pre-hospital information for road collisions

- Patient position in vehicle
- Restraint device/s
- Vehicle characteristics—model/year
- Area of impact, e.g. front, side, rear end
- Details of impact, e.g. stationary object or moving vehicle
- Damage evident, e.g. steering wheel, windscreen
- Vehicle trajectory following impact
- Other occupants in vehicle—position, condition

BOX 43.3 Additional considerations for blunt and penetrating mechanism of injury information[13]

- What is the event type? (e.g. falls, motor vehicle collision)
- What was the estimated energy exchange?
- What protective devices were used? (e.g. seatbelt, helmet)
- What clues are evident from the scene?
- What are the obvious and potential injuries?
- Does the patient have any past medical history or take any medications that may affect their management?
- Is the patient under the influence of drugs and alcohol and what is the significance of this?
- What treatment has been initiated prior to hospital?
- How have they responded to any treatments given?

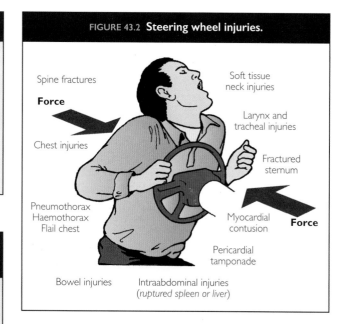

FIGURE 43.2 Steering wheel injuries.

---

the front seat continue to move down and under, or up and over, the dashboard (Fig 43.2).

Down and under

The first path an occupant may travel after frontal impact is down and under. With this path, the occupant continues forward movement downwards and into the steering column or dashboard. The knees impact the dashboard; however, the upper legs absorb most energy. This mechanism causes patella dislocations, midshaft femur fractures and posterior dislocations or fractures of acetabulum or femoral head. The transfer of energy causes the classic knee–femur–hip injury from the knee through the femur into the hip, as shown in Figure 43.3. When one of these injuries is identified, the patient should be carefully evaluated for the other injuries.

Up and over

Continued forward motion from frontal collision carries the unrestrained body up and over, so that the chest and abdomen hit the steering wheel. Head injuries, such as contusions and scalp lacerations, skull fractures, facial fractures, cerebral haemorrhage or cerebral contusions can occur when the head or face strikes the steering wheel or dashboard. The skull stops suddenly after striking the steering wheel, windscreen or another stationary object, but the brain continues to move

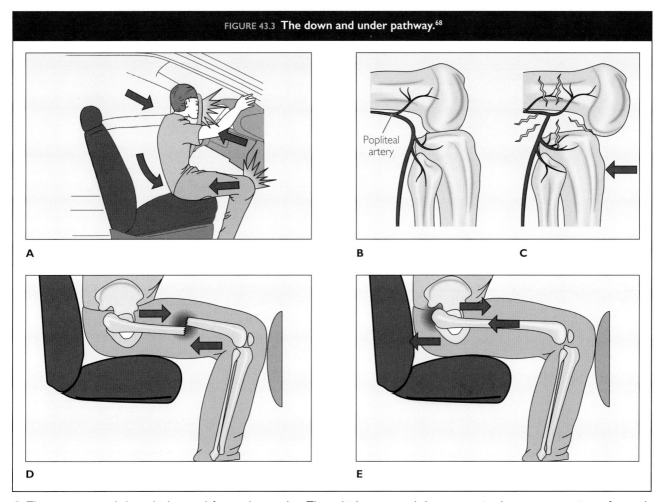

FIGURE 43.3 The down and under pathway.[68]

A. The occupant and the vehicle travel forwards together. The vehicle stops and the unrestrained occupant continues forwards until something stops that motion. **B.** The knee has two possible impact points in a motor vehicle collision: the femur and tibia. **C.** The popliteal artery lies close to the joint. Separation of the femur and tibia stretches, kinks and tears the artery. **D.** When the femur is the point of impact, the energy is absorbed along the bone shaft, which may result in fracture. **E.** The continued forward motion of the pelvis onto the femur can override the femur head, resulting in a posterior dislocation of the acetabular joint.

forwards and strikes the inside of the skull. This area of the brain is compressed and may sustain bruising, oedema or contusion. The other side of the brain continues to move forwards and may be disrupted and shear away from tissue and vascular attachments (Fig 43.4).

This impact can cause two separate injuries—shear injury and compression injury—to the same organ. When the head collides with an object, injury to the cervical spine can also occur. The spider-web effect of a damaged windscreen suggests the possibility of cervical spine injury and head injury (see Chs 45 and 49).

Chest injuries occur when the thorax is compressed against the steering wheel. Injuries include fractured ribs and sternum, anterior flail chest, blunt cardiac injury and lung contusion. The abdomen may also collide with the steering wheel, causing compression and shearing injuries. Thoracic vertebral injuries occur as energy travels along the spine; however, these injuries are less common because the thoracic vertebrae are so well protected.

If steering-wheel deformity is reported, the index of suspicion for neck, face, thoracic or abdominal injuries increases significantly. Injuries caused by colliding with the steering wheel may be visible as abrasions on the anterior chest; however, the absence of visible markings does not exclude injury (see Ch 47).

Rear impact

Rear-impact collision occurs when a stationary or slower-moving vehicle is struck from behind. Initial impact accelerates the vehicle and may force it into a frontal collision. When the vehicle suddenly accelerates, hyperextension of the neck may occur, especially when head-rests are not properly positioned. Strained and torn neck ligaments also may occur. Figure 43.5 demonstrates how these injuries occur. The collision commonly involves two points of impact, rear and frontal, which increases the chance for occupant injuries.

Side impact

When a vehicle is struck on either side, most injuries are dependent on vehicle deformity and intrusion into the interior compartment. With side impact, occupants generally receive

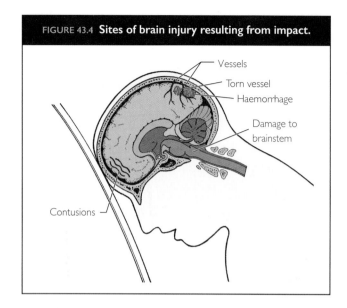

FIGURE 43.4 Sites of brain injury resulting from impact.

most injuries on the same side of their body as the vehicle impact, and are subjected to compression and deceleration forces. A second collision may occur between occupants if another passenger is in the vehicle. The head and shoulder of one occupant may impact the other occupant's head and shoulder. Injuries that may occur are flail chest, pulmonary contusion and rib fractures. Thoracic aortic tear may occur, as the inertia of the heart may produce traction on the aorta.[15] Numerous musculoskeletal injuries can occur. Strain on the lateral neck can cause cervical spine fractures or ligament tears (Fig 43.6).

Rotational impact
When the corner of one vehicle strikes another stationary vehicle, a vehicle travelling in the opposite direction or a slower vehicle, a rotational impact occurs. The part that is hit on the second vehicle stops forward motion, whereas the rest of the vehicle rotates around until all energy is transformed. As the vehicle is hit, the occupant's forward motion continues until it impacts with the side of the vehicle as the vehicle begins rotating. Injuries that occur in rotational impacts are a combination of those seen in frontal and lateral impacts.

Vehicle rollover
Rollover is when a car flips, regardless of whether the motion is end-over-end or side-over-side. In rollovers, injuries are sometimes difficult to predict. Occupants frequently have injuries in the same body areas where damage occurs to the vehicle. Just as the vehicle impacts at different angles, several times, so do the body and internal organs of the occupant. In the rollover mechanism, the chance for axial loading injuries is increased.

Ejection
Ejection occurs when an occupant is thrown from the vehicle. Occupants who are ejected may sustain injuries at initial point of impact, during flight or at the final resting point. Increased mortality is associated with ejection, and those at greatest risk of ejection are unrestrained occupants.

Restraints
Restraint systems are designed to prevent injuries and decrease the severity of injuries by allowing occupants to decelerate at the same rate as the vehicle, rather than being thrown against interior structures or being ejected from the vehicle. The most effective restraint system is the three-point seatbelt—a shoulder harness and lap belt—because it reduces facial, head and abdominal injuries and long-bone fractures. Seatbelt bruising patterns on the abdomen or chest imply significant energy exchange (see Ch 48).

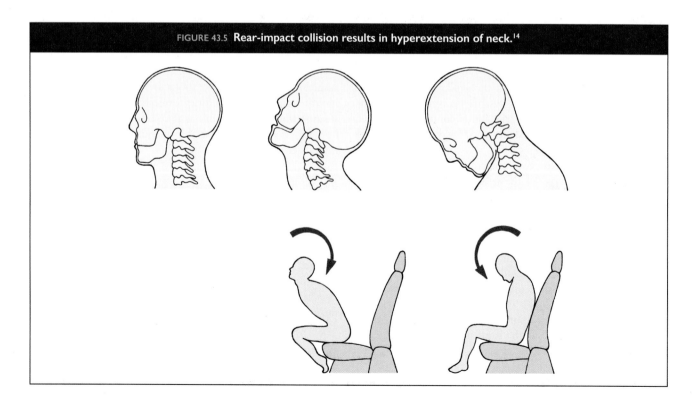

FIGURE 43.5 Rear-impact collision results in hyperextension of neck.[14]

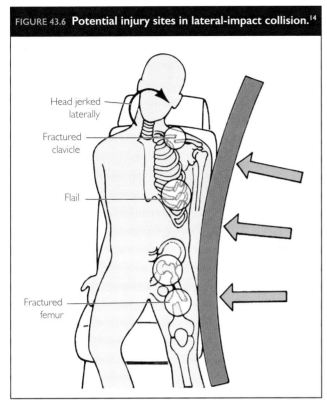

FIGURE 43.6 **Potential injury sites in lateral-impact collision.**[14]

Head jerked laterally

Fractured clavicle

Flail

Fractured femur

Injury is still possible in lateral collision with airbag inflation; however, injuries are usually fewer with airbag inflation than without.

Box 43.4 describes injuries that occur with proper seat belt usage,[2] and Figure 43.7 illustrates injuries associated with improper wearing of seatbelts.

PRACTICE TIP

The direction of impact assists with determining the potential for injury and may guide decision-making regarding bypass protocols.

Child restraints

The introduction of mandatory child restraints are highlighted as being a major public health development reducing injury and fatality of children in motor vehicle collisions.[16] In Australia motor vehicle collisions are the leading cause of death in children aged 1–14 years and are considered one of the top three causes of serious injury in children of this same age group.[16] Child restraints are effective as they distribute the force of the collision over the child's strongest body region and protect the child from hitting the interior of the vehicle. The main principle in reducing force involves restraining the child from moving downwards in a collision. The most common injuries of restrained children involved in motor vehicle collisions are head injuries where their head collides with the internal structures of the vehicle. Injuries to the child occupant are substantially increased when child restraints are inappropriately used or fitted.[17] Some of the common forms of misuse include harness straps being poorly adjusted or

BOX 43.4 **Injuries with appropriate restraint systems**[2]

Spinal
Cervical vertebral fractures from flexion forces
Neck sprains secondary to hyperextension
Lumbar vertebral fractures secondary to flexion–distraction forces

Thoracic
Soft tissue injuries of the chest wall associated with belt placement
Sternal fractures with or without myocardial contusion
Fewer than three rib fractures if restrained; more than four if unrestrained
Trauma to breast in females

Abdominal
Soft-tissue injuries (contusions, abrasions, ecchymosis)
'Seat belt' friction burns or abrasion where seat belt rests
Injuries to small bowel secondary to crushing and deceleration
Ruptured aorta secondary to longitudinal stretching of the vessel
Injuries to the liver, pancreas, gallbladder and duodenum secondary to crushing forces

FIGURE 43.7 **A seatbelt that is positioned above the rim of the pelvis allows the abdominal organs to be trapped between the moving posterior wall and the belt.**[68]

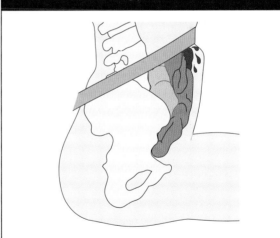

Injuries to the pancreas and other retroperitoneal organs, as well as blowout ruptures of the small intestine and colon, result.

incorrectly positioned, seatbelts being incorrectly routed or twisted and incorrect fitting of locking clips.[18] Figure 43.8 illustrates the correct fitting for child restraints.

Australian law requires that children up to the age of seven must be secured in an age-appropriate child restraint approved by Standards Australia.[16] Additional to this, children seven years and younger must be seated in the rear of the vehicle when there are at least two rows of seats. If all the rear seats are occupied by children 7 years and younger a child of 4 years of age or older may be secured by an age appropriate device in

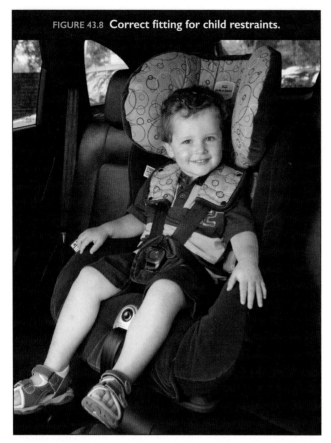

FIGURE 43.8 **Correct fitting for child restraints.**

Courtesy Kidsafe WA.

the front seat. For more specific guidelines of age appropriate restraint please refer to Table 43.1.

Vehicle safety devices
Airbags are not mandatory in all Australian or New Zealand vehicles; however, most recent-model cars are equipped with dual front, side and head impact airbags. Further, in Victoria, since January 2011 new vehicles must be fitted with electronic

stability control to be registered, and curtain airbags are mandatory in all new cars manufactured from 2012. The use of airbags in new vehicles is supported by the Australasian New Car Assessment Program (ANCAP), which in turn is supported by all New Zealand and Australian motoring clubs, the New Zealand government, Australian state governments and the FIA (Fédération Internationale de l'Automobile) Foundation.[21,22]

Airbags are a supplementary restraint and are most effective when used in conjunction with seatbelts. Airbags are designed to protect occupants in frontal and lateral deceleration collisions by inflating on impact, cushioning the head and chest, then rapidly deflating. Australian airbags are triggered to deploy at higher-impact speeds compared with airbags in the United States; this reduces the likelihood of injury resulting from 'unnecessary' airbag deployment.[23]

Injuries reported from airbag deployment include facial soft-tissue injury, facial and forearm bruising and corneal abrasions. Serious injuries have been seen in small drivers who adjust the seat closer to the steering wheel. Injuries to children from airbags have been reported in the United States; however, Australian and New Zealand standards for child restraints means that properly tethered restraints can only be mounted in the rear seats, where appropriate anchorage is provided (Ch 42).[21]

> **PRACTICE TIP**
>
> A photograph taken at the scene can provide hospital staff with an appreciation of the injury mechanism.

Vulnerable road users

Motorbike collisions
The extent of injury from motorbike collisions is dependent on the amount and type of kinetic energy and the body part that sustains impact, but this mechanism has a high potential to cause severe injuries. The size of motorbikes, the irregular outline and low contrast with background environment are factors that make riders less visible to other road users.[24] Motorcyclists are more likely to sustain severe thoracic injury,[25] and head, neck and extremity injuries. Clues to the amount of force sustained during a collision include length of tyre skid marks, deformity of the motorbike, deformity of the helmet and stationary objects impacted. The condition of a motorbike driver is often similar to an occupant ejected from a vehicle.

Three types of motorbike impacts with predictable injuries are head-on impact, angular impact and ejection. During a head-on impact, the motorbike impacts an object that stops the bike's forward motion. The bike flips forwards, so the rider strikes or travels over the handlebars. As the rider strikes the handlebars, abdominal and chest injuries and shearing fractures of the tibia can occur. Bilateral femur fractures occur if the rider's feet are trapped at the time of impact. Neck injuries may occur as the helmet does not provide neck protection. Angular impact may occur when the rider collides with signs, mirrors on cars or other such objects. When a motorbike is hit at an angle and collapses on the rider, the angular impact injures

TABLE 43.1 Age-related restraint recommendations[20]	
AGE OF CHILD	**REQUIRED RESTRAINT**
<6 months	Rearward-facing approved child restraint
6 months– <4 years	Rearward-facing approved child restraint or A forward-facing approved child restraint with an inbuilt harness
4 years– <7 years	A forward-facing approved child restraint with an inbuilt harness or An approved booster seat, restrained by a seatbelt that is properly adjusted and fastened
7 years– <16 years	A suitable approved child restraint or Wear a seatbelt that is properly adjusted and fastened

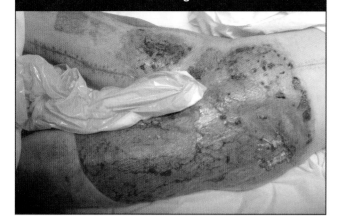

FIGURE 43.9 **Extensive degloving to abdomen and left thigh from friction sustained during a motorbike collision.**

The patient was dragged along the road for 50 metres.

the side that is crushed between the rider and ground. Injuries tend to occur in lower extremities such as open fractures of the tibia or fibula, crushed legs, ankle dislocation and soft-tissue injuries. Abrasions and surface burns may occur if protective clothing such as boots, leather garments and helmets are not worn (Fig 43.9). When a rider is thrown or ejected off the motorbike, injuries occur to whatever body part is struck by another vehicle or object at the time of impact and at the point of impact when the body lands. The rest of the body absorbs energy from the impact.[2] Riders are at significant risk of head injury and the use of helmets reduces this risk by about 72%.[26]

Bicycle injuries

Common mechanisms of injury for bicycle injury are through falls, and collisions with stationary or moving objects. Most fatalities result from on-road collisions with other traffic.[27] The rider generally falls as a result of losing control of the bicycle, which may be due to uneven ground surfaces, performing stunts, speeding or rider error. Bicycle collisions have certain common patterns of injuries. The spokes of a cycle wheel can fracture the feet when feet are caught in the wheel. These injuries may cause the person to be thrown and sustain other injuries. The rider can be thrown over the handlebars as a result of impact, which can cause head, neck and chest injuries. Seat or straddle injuries can occur if there is impact with the middle bar or seat. This can lead to injuries such as vaginal tears, scrotal injuries and perineal contusions. Bicycle-mounted child seats are another cause of injuries with bicycle use. The child may fall from the seat, the seat can detach from the bicycle, the bike can tip over or an extremity of the child may be caught in wheel spokes.[2] Helmets provide a 63–88% reduction in the risk of head, brain and severe brain injury for all ages of bicyclists, and injuries to the upper and mid-facial areas are reduced by 65%.[28]

Pedestrian trauma

In addition to the nature of the impact and vehicle size and speed, the height and age of the pedestrian will have an effect on the type of injuries sustained. Children tend to face the approaching vehicle; however, adults tend to protect themselves by turning sideways.[29] There are three phases of injury in pedestrian trauma.

1. The initial impact occurs when the bumper of the vehicle impacts with the lower extremity of the pedestrian.
2. Following this, head, chest and abdominal injuries occur as the pedestrian hits the bonnet or windscreen.
3. The pedestrian may then fall to the ground, resulting in further head, chest and upper extremity injuries.[29]

Very small children are rarely thrown clear of the vehicle because of their low centre of gravity, size and weight. A child may be knocked down and under the vehicle, then run over. Multisystem trauma should be suspected in any child hit by a car. A combination of injuries referred to as Waddell's triad often occurs when a child is struck by a car (Fig 43.10). Waddell's triad is characterised by injuries to the chest, head and femurs.[30] Musculoskeletal injuries are more common than head and neck injuries in the adult population; however, in the child population head and neck injuries predominate, with musculoskeletal injuries being the second most prevalent.[31]

Crush injuries

The most common mechanism of crush injury is blunt trauma in which there is sudden or severe compression of the chest or upper abdomen; for example, on being wedged between a truck and a wall, or having a vehicle roll onto the patient and, most commonly, children being reversed over in the driveway. Crush injuries can cause traumatic asphyxia, which is a clinical condition characterised by cyanosis and oedema of the neck and face, subconjunctival haemorrhage and petechial haemorrhage of face, neck and upper chest.[32] Mortality increases significantly with prolonged compression.[33] It is important to consider the amount of force applied and the period of time it has been applied. Some patients have survived large compression forces for short periods of time, while others have died from relatively small forces being applied for a prolonged period. Crush injury to limbs is discussed in Chapter 50.

Interpersonal violence

Interpersonal violence occurs between individuals and is often divided into intimate partner, acquaintance and stranger violence.[34] Patterns of assault injuries differ between communities due to cultural and social factors. Injuries resulting from assault will vary according to the force and object used. The most common injury sites are head, neck or face, and vary from minor abrasions to multisystem trauma. Bodily force or use of sharp or blunt objects are the most common methods used. Males are more likely to be injured by kicks, head butts or broken drinking glasses. Females are predominantly exposed to blunt violence. Defensive injuries are commonly found on the upper limbs, hands and back.[35] One type of interpersonal violence that is increasingly being reported in the media is the 'Coward's punch' (previously known as 'king hit'). The 'coward's punch' is generally characterised by a single blow to the head, causing the person to fall to the ground with a period of unconsciousness. The unconsciousness may result from the punch or as a result of the impact between the head and the ground. Shock waves from the rapid acceleration and deceleration involved in this mechanism are likely to cause tissue damage, swelling, inflammation, nerve disruption and skull fractures. Subarachnoid haemorrhage may also result from torsional injury to the vertebral artery due to rapid

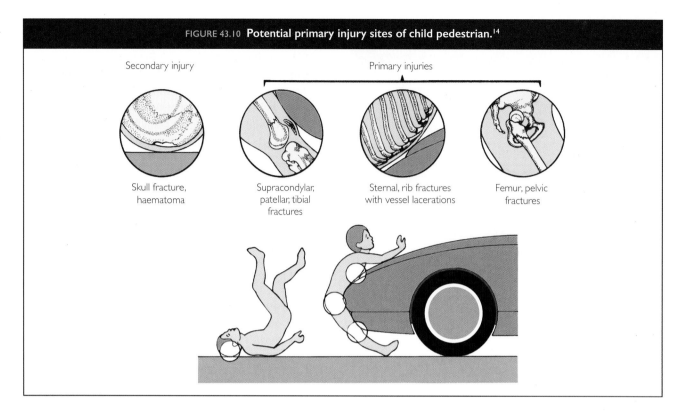

FIGURE 43.10 **Potential primary injury sites of child pedestrian.**[14]

Secondary injury

Skull fracture, haematoma

Primary injuries

Supracondylar, patellar, tibial fractures

Sternal, rib fractures with vessel lacerations

Femur, pelvic fractures

cranio-cervical rotation.[36] Interpersonal violence is particularly hard to assess because of the stigma connected to its reporting and the lack of non-healthcare epidemiological data available. See Chapter 40.

Hanging and strangulation

Self-inflicted strangulation is one of the most common forms of successful suicide methods wordwide.[37] The severity of injuries associated with hanging are dependent on the height of the fall, the type and position of the neck ligature used and whether the body is fully or partially suspended. Paramedics should consider these aspects at the scene and communicate to clinical staff during hand-over. The most common form of injuries are minor abrasions, bruising (with potential to increase swelling) and lacerations. More-serious associated injuries are hypoxic brain injury, and vascular, vertebral and/or spinal injuries.[38] The mechanisms of injury include venous obstruction leading to hypoxia and unconsciousness, arterial spasm due to carotid pressure, arterial dissection due to hyperextension of the neck and vagal collapse due to pressure on the carotid sinuses. Cervical spine and spinal cord injuries are rare, reported to occur in 0.6% of near hanging cases; however, these injuries should be considered, particularly if the drop height is greater than the height of the person.[39,40] It is important to remember that not all hanging incidents are self-inflicted; some may result from accidents or experimental activities, such as window blind cords.

Watercraft/boating

Boating accidents can occur from colliding with another boat, explosions, capsizing or an obstruction in the water. Occupants of boats are not routinely provided with restraint systems, and the boats are not built to absorb the energy associated with impacts. There is potential for drowning or hypothermia when

occupants are thrown into the water and water temperatures are cold, in addition to severe injuries from motorised propellers. Other injuries may be similar to those seen in people ejected from a vehicle.

In recent years, personal watercraft such as wave-runners and jet-skis have become popular recreational vehicles.[2] Different styles allow the driver to sit, stand or kneel while operating the vehicle, with some vehicles allowing up to three passengers. Mechanisms of injury include collisions (with other watercraft, boats, swimmers or objects in the water), falls from the watercraft, handlebar straddle injuries, axial loading and hydrostatic injuries.[41] The potential for injury is very similar to the injury patterns seen with motorcycle collisions and all-terrain vehicles. Spinal fractures at the thoracolumbar region may occur from collisions or hard landing on the seat after the craft has been airborne.[42] Rectal, vaginal and perineal trauma may occur when passengers or drivers hit the water or seat at high speed. Drowning is another complication associated with these types of incidents and is discussed in Chapter 28.

All-terrain vehicles

All-terrain vehicles, also commonly known as 'quad bikes', were traditionally designed for use on unpaved off-road terrain such as farms. Capable of speeds up to 100 kilometres per hour these vehicles have low pressure tyres and a high centre of gravity, making them more prone to rollover. Injuries associated with all-terrain vehicle use generally occur when the occupant is ejected from the saddle or as a result of collision with a stationary object.[1] Other mechanisms include rollover, crush injury and burns from contact with the exhaust.[43] The three broad groups of injury are head injury, musculoskeletal/orthopaedic injury and abdominal-thoracic injury.[44] Clothesline or wire fence injury to the neck and face has been reported as an injury pattern associated with all-terrain vehicle use, particularly in children and adolescents, when striking a fence while the vehicle is moving.[45]

Sports- and recreation-related injuries

Injuries associated with sports are generally caused by compressive forces or sudden deceleration. Twisting, hyperflexion or hyperextension can cause other injuries. Factors that affect injury include lack of protective equipment, lack of conditioning and inadequate training of the participant. Mechanisms associated with sports and recreational activities are similar to those involved in MVCs, motorcycle collisions and bicycle collisions. Potential mechanisms associated with individual sports are numerous; however, the general principles are the same as with falls and MVCs:

- What energy or forces impact on the victim?
- Which parts of the body are affected by the energy or force?
- What are the obvious injuries?
- Which injuries are associated with the involved energy or force?

Damaged equipment, such as a broken or cracked helmet or buckled bicycle wheel, can help establish impact. Table 43.2 describes injuries associated with the common sporting and recreational activities in Australia and New Zealand.

PRACTICE TIP

There is mixed evidence on the routine application of cervical spine immobilisation for patients with blunt trauma (see Ch 49). Clinicians should be familiar with the clinical decision rules available to guide decision-making on the application of cervical spine immobilisation and clearance process.

Penetrating trauma

Penetrating trauma refers to injuries caused by a foreign object penetrating or entering the body. The penetrating object creates energy that dissipates into the surrounding tissue. The extent of damage caused will be dependent on the object that is used to cause the injury, the amount of energy or force behind the object, the distance from the victim to the weapon and the type of tissue that is penetrated. Penetrating trauma may be divided into low- and high-velocity injuries. Low-velocity injuries most commonly include stab wounds and impalements, whereas high-velocity injuries refer to gunshot wounds.

Penetrating trauma can be caused by numerous objects, including knives and guns. Although penetrating injuries are

---

TABLE 43.2 Sports- and recreation-related injuries[2,46–50]

SPORT/RECREATIONAL ACTIVITY	POTENTIAL INJURIES
Boxing	Cumulative brain damage, ocular injuries, lacerations, nasal fractures, hand fractures
Cycling/bicycle riding	Head injuries, spinal cord injuries, abdominal injuries, vaginal tears, scrotal injuries, perineal contusions, facial lacerations, upper extremity injuries, lower extremity injuries
All-terrain vehicles	Head injuries, spine injuries, chest injuries involving rib and sternum, clavicle fractures, burns from exhaust
Gymnastics	Spinal cord injuries, extremity fractures, sprains, strains
Football/rugby/soccer	Spinal cord injuries, head injuries, knee strains, fractures, lacerations, dislocations
Basketball/netball/hockey	Lower extremity sprains, strains, fractures, lacerations, contusions
Cricket	Groin injuries, upper and lower extremity sprains and strains, ball impact injuries
Skiing/snowboarding	Head injuries, lower extremity fractures, exposure to elements
Bungee jumping	Major impact-related injuries, intraocular haemorrhages, spinal cord injuries, perineal nerve injuries, soft-tissue injuries
Running	Lower extremity injuries, strains, sprains
Horse riding	Head injuries, spinal cord injuries, bite wounds, crush wounds, lower extremity injuries, upper extremity injuries
Skateboarding/scooter riding	Lower extremity injuries, upper extremity injuries, lacerations, head injuries, contusions, facial injuries, sprains, strains
Play equipment	Upper and lower extremity injuries, spinal cord injuries, head injuries
Body-boarding/surfing	Lacerations, spinal cord injuries, abdominal injuries
Springboard and platform diving	Head injuries, spinal cord injuries, respiratory complications associated with near-drowning and drowning

a significant cause of severe injury and death in some other countries, deaths from stabbings and firearms constitute only a small proportion in Australasia.[51] However, in Australasia it is important to consider other objects such as industrial and farming equipment and those objects causing penetrating injuries due to secondary mechanisms, such as in MVCs or falls.

Low-velocity penetrating wounds

Stab wounds

Stab wounds are categorised as low-velocity injuries as the energy exerted behind them is low. Damage results from the penetration of the object through the skin into the tissue and/or body cavity. Damage to surrounding tissue is usually kept to a minimum, and as such is isolated to the area of penetration (Fig 43.11).

In assessing patients with low-velocity penetrating trauma, it is beneficial to have insight into the object used and hence the size and length of the object. The position of the attacker and the victim will indicate the projected path of the object; the gender of the attacker is also useful, as women tend to stab in a downwards motion, whereas men tend to stab upwards.[51] It is important to consider the victim's position at the time of penetration. If the victim is hunched over or leaning forward in an attempt to ward off the attacker, the actual entrance point of the object when the patient is lying on a hospital bed may not correspond with the extent or location of the underlying tissue injury. In addition to this, the wound track may not be straight, making it difficult to determine the extent of the wound and where the wound track ends.[53]

Although stab wounds are considered low-velocity injuries, exerting minimal energy, a single stab wound can penetrate several body cavities with the potential to cause lethal injuries. For example, the object can enter both the chest and the abdominal cavity with one single penetration and may cause damage to more than one body organ.

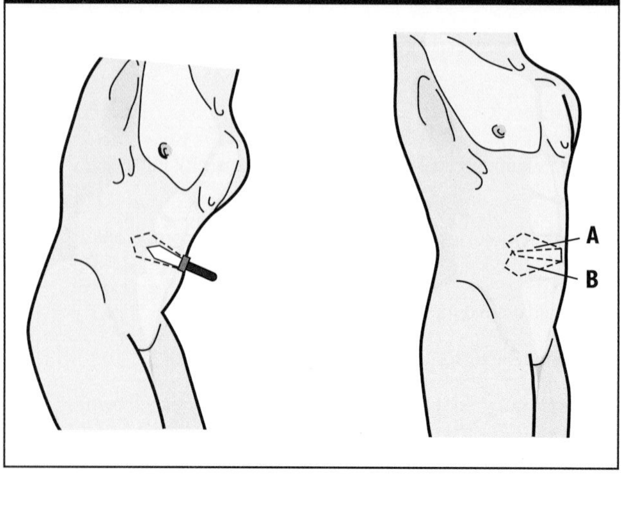

> **PRACTICE TIP**
>
> Remember that small wounds may be deceptive: they may hide extensive internal damage caused by the attacker moving the object once penetration occurs.[2]

> **PRACTICE TIP**
>
> Establishing a wound trajectory is beneficial but should never override a thorough clinical examination.

Impalements

Impalements are also generally classified as low-velocity injuries and can result from a multitude of factors, including falls, MVCs or secondary to flying or falling objects. In Australasia, it is important to consider secondary mechanisms from industrial and farming equipment as well as simple, everyday household and garden items, such as lawn-mower blades. Removal of impaled objects may result in extensive haemorrhage and hence an unstable patient.

> **PRACTICE TIP**
>
> Impaled objects should be secured in position until the patient is in a controlled environment where surgical support is immediately available.[2] Figure 43.12 displays the use of dressings to secure a foreign object prior to transport.[54]

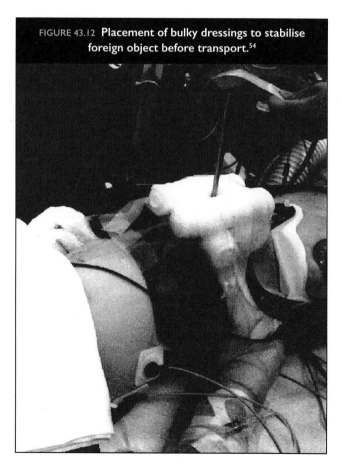

FIGURE 43.12 **Placement of bulky dressings to stabilise foreign object before transport.**[54]

FIGURE 43.11 **Damage produced by a knife blade inside victim depends on the movement of the blade internally.**[52]

High-velocity penetrating wounds

Gunshot wounds

Injuries and deaths from gunshot wounds account for only a small percentage of traumatic deaths and hospitalisations within Australasia.[55] Statistics collected in 2012 by the Australian Bureau of Statistics reported that firearm use was used for criminal activity in 34.6% of attempted murders, 17.3% of murders and 8.3% of robbery offences.[56] However, overall injury resulting from firearm use is relatively low.[51] As a result, experience in managing patients with gunshot injuries is limited in comparison to the United States and some other countries.

Gunshot wounds fall under the category of high-velocity injuries. The most common penetrating wounds caused by firearms in Australasia are from handguns, shotguns, small-calibre rifles and air rifles.[57] Although gunshot wounds are generally considered to produce high-velocity injuries, they can be further categorised by the type of weapon used—either low-velocity or high-velocity. The law of moving objects states that kinetic energy (E_k) = $\frac{1}{2}mv^2$, where m is mass and v is velocity. This indicates that the *velocity* at which an object strikes a person, rather than the mass/size of the object, will determine the severity of patient injuries.[6]

The transfer of energy from a weapon to the object it strikes causes particles to be moved out of position. This is referred to as *cavitation*, and can be permanent or temporary depending on the amount of energy transferred and the elasticity of the object it hits.[6] Permanent cavitation causes a hole that remains after the energy has dissipated, whereas in temporary cavitation the tissue particles may return to their original location. Temporary cavitation may become permanent depending on

the amount of energy transfer from the weapon to the tissue.[6] The size of permanent cavitation is affected by tissue elasticity. For example, cavitation through bone will result in greater permanent cavitation than that through more-elastic tissue.[58]

Low-velocity weapons include handguns and some short-barrel rifles. Bullets fired from these types of guns travel at 300 to 900 m/s, limiting the amount of tissue disruption to a temporary cavity of 3–6 times the diameter of the bullet. Low-velocity bullets cause tissue in the path of the bullet to be pushed aside, causing tissue damage to be relatively localised to the centre of the bullet tract.

High-velocity weapons include hunting and long-barrel assault rifles. Bullets travel at a speed > 900 m/s and, as a result, are responsible for greater tissue damage. High-velocity bullets can create a temporary cavitation of 30–40 times the diameter of the bullet. The high velocity of the bullet creates the cavity by compressing and displacing tissue around the bullet.

Figure 43.13 shows the cavitational differences between high-velocity and low-velocity bullets.

In addition to the velocity, bullet profile (and hence the shape of its nose) and the yaw, tumble and fragmentation of the bullet are important factors in determining the extent of damage. The *yaw* of the bullet refers to the deviation of the nose of the bullet from a straight path, causing it to hit the target at an angle (Fig 43.14). *Tumbling* refers to the change in rotation of the bullet as it hits the body, causing the bullet to somersault in a forward motion through the tissue and leading to extensive tissue destruction.[6] Bullets such as hollow-point bullets are designed to mushroom or expand on impact, causing the bullet to tumble. This increases the frontal surface area, providing maximum energy transfer, reducing penetration with a hard

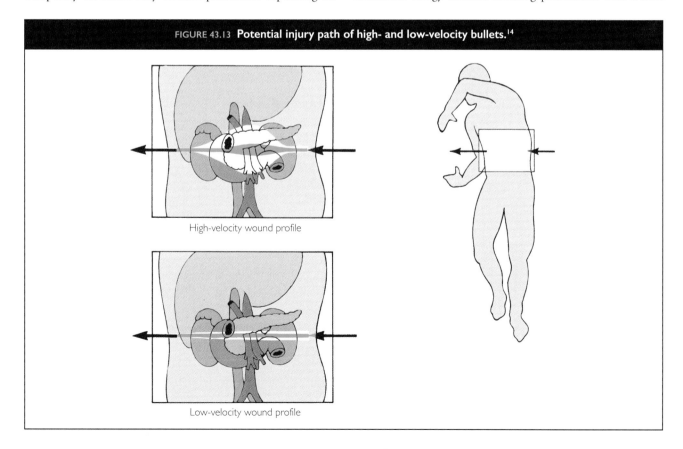

FIGURE 43.13 Potential injury path of high- and low-velocity bullets.[14]

High-velocity wound profile

Low-velocity wound profile

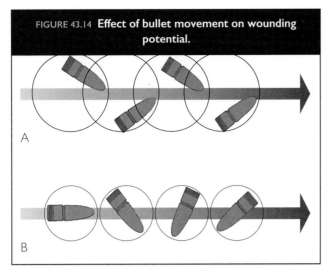

FIGURE 43.14 **Effect of bullet movement on wounding potential.**

A, Yawing. **B,** Tumbling.

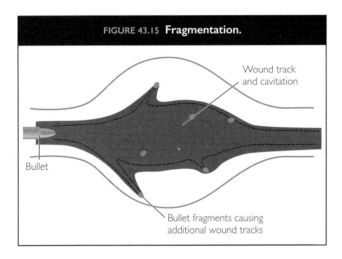

FIGURE 43.15 **Fragmentation.**

Wound track and cavitation

Bullet

Bullet fragments causing additional wound tracks

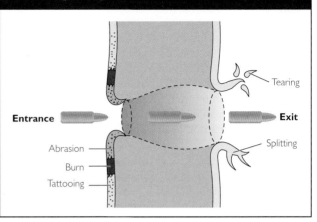

FIGURE 43.16 **A spinning missile produces a 1–2 mm abraded edge along the wound if it enters straight.**

Entrance | Exit

Tearing

Splitting

Abrasion
Burn
Tattooing

target but increasing the damage when it strikes a soft target (Fig 43.14).[59] Both yawing and tumbling increase the surface area of body tissue that the bullet comes into contact with, resulting in greater temporary and permanent cavities.

Some bullets, such as high-velocity jacketed and semi-jacketed bullets, are designed to fragment.[59] *Fragmentation* occurs when the bullet breaks apart on impact. This means that the bullet fragments will spread out over a wider area of tissue, causing damage to more areas (Fig 43.15). Both hollow-point and semi-hollow-point bullets are used by Australian police to quickly disable offenders using the least number of bullets necessary.[60]

Identifying entry and exit wounds may help determine the pathway of the bullet and therefore indicate potential organs and bones the bullet may have come in contact with. Entrance wounds are usually round or oval in shape, whereas exit wounds are stellate or starburst in shape. Figure 43.16 compares entrance and exit wounds.

If the gun has been fired within close range—less than 25 cm away—the entrance wound may also be accompanied by a graze or a small burning tattoo. The exit wound will not exhibit these features. Exit wounds may not always be found, as it is possible for the bullet to lodge itself within dense tissue or bone.

If it enters at an angle, the abraded side is on the bottom of missile, with more skin contact, and covers a much wider area. Differences in entrance and exit wounds are also depicted. Exit wounds are generally longer and more explosive.

> **PRACTICE TIP**
>
> It is important not to wash around the patient's wound area or the patient's hands as these may contain gunpowder traces essential for forensic investigations.[61]

> **PRACTICE TIP**
>
> When assessing a patient with a penetrating injury, it is useful to tape a metal object such as a paper clip to each wound prior to radiological imaging. This will assist with identifying trajectories.

Blast injuries

Blast injuries are uncommon in Australasia; however, the potential exists, especially with hazardous explosions within industrial settings such as oil refineries, mines, shipping docks and chemical plant sites. The potential for blast injuries has also heightened with increased terrorist activity, and paramedics and nurses working with the defence forces have recently had significant exposure to these injuries in conflict-ridden areas. An explosive refers to any substance that has the ability to cause decomposition by the sudden release of gas and thermal energy in a limited space.[62] The effects or injuries associated with blasts may occur in three main phases: primary, secondary and tertiary.[59] Figure 43.17 illustrates how injuries occur from an explosive blast.

Primary injuries

Primary injuries are associated with the effects of the pressure waves. The nature of expanding gas causes equal amounts of air to be displaced, known as a shock wave or 'overpressure'. The shock wave lasts several milliseconds and causes damage at the interface of tissues. The degree of damage is directly related to the power behind the blast and the duration of the shock

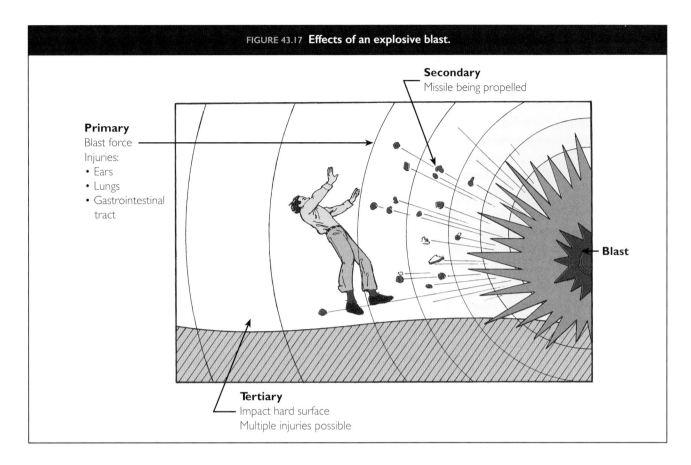

FIGURE 43.17 Effects of an explosive blast.

wave.[63] Following the shock wave, a vacuum is generated at the explosion site, which creates a negative pressure wave. It has a duration of up to three times that of the shock wave, and is commonly associated with barotrauma injury.

Other injuries commonly associated with primary blasts include myocardial contusion, shearing of large cardiac vessels, detachment and tearing of the bowel, rupturing of the eardrum, pulmonary haemorrhage and rupture.[59]

Secondary injuries

Secondary blast injuries involve the projection of bomb fragments and nearby debris through the air, often at enormous speeds comparable to those of missiles. This occurs as a result of the blast wind that immediately follows the shock wave. The blast wave causes a mass displacement of air and is responsible for avulsion, amputation and shrapnel injuries.[62] Other injuries include lacerations, abrasions, contusions, fractures and penetrating injuries.

Tertiary injuries

Tertiary blast injuries result from the person being displaced either onto the ground or into other objects. Injuries from tertiary blasts are similar to those of being ejected from a vehicle or a fall.

Quarternary injuries

Miscellaneous injuries, also known as quarternary blast injuries, may result from, but are not limited to, building collapse leading to crush injuries, burns from fire, hypothermia associated with prolonged extrication or toxic effects from chemicals, or psychological trauma, all occurring after the explosion.[59,60]

Quinary injuries

An additional injury phase, quinary blast pattern, has recently been defined. This is associated with hyperinflammatory states manifested by hyperpyrexia, diaphoresis, low central venous pressure and a positive fluid balance.[59] This area requires further research for increased understanding of the mechanisms involved. The mechanism and management of blast injury is discussed in more detail in Chapter 51.

Additional weapons

The increasing terrorist activity around the world has not only heightened the interest in blast injuries, but also those of nuclear/radiological, chemical and biological weapons. The risk of nuclear weapons being used to cause mass destruction and casualties is much less than the risk of the use of chemical or biological weaponry because of the difficulties in gaining access to the agent.[62] Chemical weapons contain chemicals with the potential to kill, injure or incapacitate humans. The extent of damage is dependent on the chemical used, its physical properties including vapour pressure, density and boiling point and the environmental conditions of wind speed, temperature and rain.[62] Biological weapons contain organisms that cause disease or deterioration of material. Such weaponry is easily produced in large quantities, is relatively stable, may be transferred quickly and is difficult to identify.[62] As such, biological agents have the potential for high lethality. The mechanism and management of chemical biological radiological injury is discussed in more detail in Chapter 12.

Inhalation/pulmonary injuries

Inhalation or pulmonary injury is a major contributing factor in early mortality following a burn trauma.[64] Inhalation injury may be a result of three mechanisms: carbon monoxide poisoning, thermal injury and chemical damage. These may occur singularly or in combination, and may lead to broncho-constriction and respiratory distress.[65] The three distinct categories of inhalation injury are carbon monoxide (CO) poisoning, upper airway injury and lower airway injury.[66] These are discussed in detail in Chapters 21 (CO) and 52 (burns).

Carbon monoxide is a colourless, odourless and tasteless gas produced during combustion. When inhaled it combines with haemoglobin, for which its affinity is more than 200 times greater than that of oxygen, reducing oxygen-carrying capacity. This results in hypoxia and asphyxiation.[67] Upper airway injury may be caused by direct heat or chemical damage of the pharynx, larynx, glottis, trachea and large bronchi.[66] Both of these mechanisms lead to erythema, oedema and ulceration of the airway above the vocal cords. Lower airway injury refers to injury below the vocal cords, and usually results in death. All inhalation injuries predispose the patient to pneumonia and acute respiratory distress syndrome requiring ventilatory support.[66] Management of inhalation injury is discussed in more detail in Chapter 21.

SUMMARY

Understanding the mechanism of injury is important for determining the types and patterns of injury that occur in trauma patients. Laws of physics and kinematics provide a way of understanding the impact of certain forces on the human body. This chapter has summarised the possible effects of blunt and penetrating trauma, outlining the various types of impact that can occur and potential injuries that may result. Treatment of trauma patients relies on rapid and accurate assessment to locate possible injuries. Rapid intervention is required to ensure optimal outcomes.

CASE STUDY 1

A 50-year-old man has fallen from a cherry-picker platform onto concrete, predominantly landing on his right side. His work colleagues report he had a brief loss of consciousness and has no recollection of the incident. He has an obvious contusion on the right side of his head, a painful right scapula, an iron rod penetrating from a wound in his right thigh and a puncture wound plus deformity at his right elbow. On arrival, he appears confused and restless; his heart rate is 105 beats/minute, respiratory rate 22 breaths/minute (shallow) and he appears moderately distressed with pain.

Questions

1. What questions would you ask to gather a greater understanding of the event?
2. Given the mechanism involved in this case, what type of injuries would you observe for?
3. How should the impaled object in his right thigh be managed?
4. Describe your plan of care for this patient based on the anticipated injuries.
5. Consider a similar case from your practice; what injuries are similar and dissimilar to this case?

 Answers to Case Study Questions can be found on evolve
http://evolve.emergencytrauma.curtis

CASE STUDY 2

An 18-year-old female is involved in an altercation with her partner. During the event she sustains stab wounds to the abdomen and upper extremities. Prior to arrival at the emergency department (ED), police have covered the abdominal wound with cling wrap and paramedics have applied manual pressure to control bleeding. On arrival, the patient is conscious but distressed with pain.

Questions

1. What information should be included in the handover from paramedics to ED staff?
2. Describe the body regions where you might expect to observe defensive injuries.
3. Based on the mechanism of injury described in this case, outline the potential injuries for each body region.

 Answers to Case Study Questions can be found on evolve
http://evolve.emergencytrauma.curtis

REFERENCES

1. Janik M, Straka L, Krajcovic J et al. All-terrain vehicle related crashes among children and young adults: A systematic review of the literature with illustrative case report. Rom J Leg Med 2012;20:263–8.

2. Revere CJ. Mechanism of injury. In: Newberry L, ed. Sheehy's emergency nursing principles and practice. St Louis: Mosby; 2003; 215–30.

3. Venes D, ed. Taber's encyclopedic medical dictionary. Philadelphia: FA Davis; 2001.

4. Kieser J, Taylor M, Carr M. Forensic biomechanics. Hoboken: Wiley Blackwell; 2013.

5. World Health Organisation. Injury prevention and control: a guide to developing a multisectoral plan of action, surveillance and research. Online. www.emro.who.int/dsaf/dsa730.pdf; 10 Sep 2010.

6. Dickinson M. Understanding the mechanism of injury and kinetic forces involved in traumatic injuries. Emerg Nurse 2004;12(6):30–5.

7. McQuillan KA, Von Rueden KT, Hartsock RL et al. Trauma nursing: from resuscitation through rehabilitation. 3rd edn. Philadelphia: WB Saunders; 2002.

8. Aunon-Martin I, Doussoux PC, Baltasar JLL et al. Correlation between pattern and mechanism of injury of free fall. Strat Traum Limb Recon 2012;7:141–5.

9. Hill K, Schwarz J. Assessment and management of falls in older people. Intern Med J 2004;34(9–10):557–64.

10. Young L, Ahmad H. Trauma in the elderly: a new epidemic? Aust N Z J Surg 1999;69(8):584–6.

11. Moloney-Harmon PA, Czerwinski SJ. Nursing care of the paediatric trauma patient. St. Louis: Saunders; 2003; 107–17.

12. Goldsmith W, Plunkett J. A biomechanical analysis of the causes of traumatic brain injury in infants and children. Am J Forensic Med Pathol 2004;25:89–100.

13. Cole E. Trauma Care: Initial assessment and management in the emergency department. Oxford: Blackwell; 2009.

14. Neff JA, Kidd PS. Trauma nursing: the art and science. 2nd edn. St Louis: Mosby; 1993.

15. Echemendia Fuentes C. Inertia effect of the heart as a contributing factor in aortic injuries in near-side impacts. The George Washington University: ProQuest Dissertations Publishing; 2008.

16. Lennon AJ, Darvell M, Edmonston CJ et al. Evaluation of the 2010 child restraint legislation in Queensland. Queensland University of Technology: Brisbane; 2011. Online. http://eprints.qut.edu.au/48812/; 30 January 2014.

17. Bulger EM, Kaufman R, Mock C. Childhood restraint injury patterns associated with restraint misuse: Implications for field triage. Prehosp Dis Med 2008;23(1):9–15.

18. Koppel S, Charlton JL, Rudin-Brown CM. The impact of new legislation on child restraint systems (CRS) misuse and inappropriate use in Australia. Traffic Inj Prev 2013;14:387–96.

19. Roads and Traffic Authority. Choose right buckle right. 2010. Online. http://roadsafety.transport.nsw.gov.au/downloads/choose_right_buckle_right.pdf

20. Australian Road Rules. Part 16: Rules for persons travelling in or on vehicles. National Transport Commission, February, 2009. Online. www.ntc.gov.au/filemedia/Reports/ARR_February_2009_final.pdf; 30 January 2014.

21. Australasian College of Road Safety. Policies of the college. Mawson: ACT 2607; 2002.

22. Land Transport New Zealand. 2005. Online. www.nzta.govt.nz/resources/results.html?catid=2

23. Australian Government Department of Infrastructure and Transport. Vehicle standards: airbags 2009. Online. www.infrastructure.gov.au/roads/vehicle_regulation/vehicle/index.aspx; 5 Dec 2009.

24. Wells S, Mullin B, Norton R et al. Motorcycle rider conspicuity and crash related injury: case control study. Br Med J 2004;328(7444):857–62.

25. Tham K-Y, Seow E, Lau G. Patterns of injuries in helmeted motorcyclists in Singapore. Emerg Med J 2004;21:458–82.

26. Liu B, Ivers R, Norton R et al. Helmets for preventing injury in motorcycle riders. Cochrane Database Syst Rev 2008;1:CD004333.

27. Jacobson GA, Blizzard L, Dwyer T. Bicycle injuries: road trauma is not the only concern. Aust N Z J Public Health 1998;22(4):451–5.

28. Thompson DC, Rivara F, Thompson R. Helmets for preventing head and facial injuries in bicyclists. Cochrane Database Syst Rev 1999;4:CD001855. DOI: 10.1002/14651858.

29. Hotz J, Kennedy A, Lutfi K et al. Preventing pediatric pedestrian injuries. J Trauma 2009;66(5):1492–9.

30. Merrell GA, Driscoll JC, Degutis LC et al. Prevention of childhood pedestrian trauma: a study of interventions over six years. J Bone Joint Surg 2002;84-A(5):863–7.

31. Chakravarthy B, Lotfipour S, Vaca FE. Pedestrian injuries: emergency care considerations. Cal J Emerg Med 2007;8(1):15–21.

32. Richards CE, Wallis DN. Asphyxiation: a review. J Trauma 2005;7:37–45.

33. Hurtado TR, Della-Giustina DA. Traumatic asphyxia in a 6-year-old boy. Pediatr Emerg Care 2003;19(3):167–8.

34. Ranney ML, Odero W, Mello MJ et al. Injuries from interpersonal violence presenting to a rural health center in Western Kenya: characteristics and correlates. Inj Prev 2009;15(1):36–40.

35. Shah Jainik P, Mangal HM, Vora Dipak H et al. Profile of defensive injuries in homicidal deaths. Ind J For Med & Path 2012; 5(3):115–19.

36. Pilgrim J, Gerostamoulos D, Drummer OH. 'King hit' fatalities in Australia, 2000–2012: The role of alcohol and other drugs. Drug Alcohol Depend 2014;135:119–32.

37. Harrison J, Pointer S, Elnour A. A review of suicide statistics in Australia. Australian Institute of Health and Welfare; 2009. Online. www.aihw.gov.au/publication-detail/?id=6442468269

38. Martin MJ, Weng J, Demetriades D et al. Pattern of injury and functional outcome after hanging: analysis of the national trauma data bank. Am J Surg 2005;190(6):836–40.

39. Nichols SD, McCarthy MC, Ekeh AP et al. Outcome of cervical near-hanging injuries. J Trauma 2009;66:174–8.

40. Adams N. Near hanging. Emerg Med 1999;11:17–21.

41. Gill RS, Whitlock K, Jawanda AS et al. Epidemiology of personal watercraft injuries. J Trauma Treatment 2012;1(2):112–15.

42. Carmel A, Drescher MJ, Leitner Y et al. Thoracolumbar fractures associated with the use of personal watercraft. J Trauma 2004;57(6):1308–10.

43. Soundappan S, Holland A, Roy G et al. Off-road vehicle trauma in children: A New South Wales Perspective. Pediatr Emer Care 2010;26(12):909–13.

44. Concannon E, Hogan, A, Lowery A et al. Spectrum of all-terrain vehicle injuries in adults: A case series and review of the literature. Int J Surg Case Rep 2012;3(6):222–6.

45. Graham J, Dick R, Parnell D et al. Clothesline injury mechanism associated with all-terrain vehicle use by children. Ped Emer Care 2006;22(1):45–7.

46. Choo KL, Hansen JB, Bailey DM. Beware the boogie board: blunt abdominal trauma from body boarding. Med J Aust 2002;176(1):326–7.

47. Fong CP, Hood N. A paediatric trauma study of scooter injuries. Emerg Med Australas 2004;16(2):139–44.

48. Orchard J, James T, Alcott E et al. Injuries in Australian cricket at first class level 1995/1996 to 2000/2001. Br J Sports Med 2002;36(4):270–5.

49. Pringle RG, McNair P, Stanley S. Incidence of sporting injury in New Zealand youths aged 6–15 years. Br J Sports Med 1998;32(1):49–52.

50. Falvey EC, Eustace J, Whelan B et al. Sport and recreation-related injuries and fracture occurrence among emergency department attendees: implications for exercise prescription and injury prevention. Emerg Med J 2009;26(8):590–5.

51. Wong K, Petchell J. Severe trauma caused by stabbing and firearms in metropolitan Sydney, NSW, Australia. Aust N Z J Surg 2005;75(4):225–30.

52. National Association of Emergency Medical Technicians (US) Prehospital Trauma Life Support Committee in cooperation with the Committee on Trauma of the American College of Surgeons. PHTLS: Prehospital trauma life support. 7th edn. Burlington: Jones & Bartlett; 2011.

53. Bird J, Faulkner M. Emergency care and management of patients with stab wounds. Nurs Stand 2009;23(21):51–9.

54. Riggle A, Bollins J, Konda S et al. Penetrating pediatric trauma owing to improper child safety seat use. J Ped Surg 2010; 45(1):245–8.

55. Chambers AJ, Lord RS. Management of gunshot wounds at a Sydney teaching hospital. Aust N Z J Surg 2000;70(3):209–15.

56. Australian Bureau of Statistics. Recorded crime-victims Australia 2012. ABS; 2013. Online. www.abs.gov.au/ausstats/abs@.nsf/Lookup/4510.0Chapter42012

57. Kreisfeld R. Firearm deaths and hospitalizations in Australia. NISU Briefing Adelaide: NISU; 2005; 1–22. Online. www.nisu.flinders.edu.au/briefs/firearm_deaths_2005.pdf; 26 Jan 2007.

58. Hunt J, Weintraub S, Marr A. Kinematics of trauma. In: Feliciano D, Mattox K, Moore E, eds. Trauma. 6th edn. New York: McGraw-Hill; 2008: 105–15.

59. Wolf S, Bebarta V, Bonnett C et al. Blast injuries. Lancet 2009;374(9687):405–15.

60. Roach S. 2001 interview, unpublished. Cited in Stewart J, Curtis K. Missed oesophageal injury in gunshot wounds: a case presentation. Australas Emerg Nurs J 2002;5(3):28–34.

61. Taylor I. Emergency care of patients with gunshot wounds. Emergency Nurse 2009;17(4):32–9.

62. Caldicott DG, Edwards NA. The tools of the trade: weapons of mass destruction. Emerg Med (Fremantle) 2002;14(3):240–8.

63. Frykberg ER. Medical management of disasters and mass casualties from terrorist bombings: how can we cope? J Trauma 2002;53(2):201–12.

64. Rehberg S, Maybauer MO, Enkhbaatar P et al. Pathophysiology, management and treatment of smoke inhalation. Expert Rev Respir Med 2009;3(3):283–97.

65. Hilton G, Kearney K. Thermal burns: the ABCs are crucial, since the major threat is often inhalation injury. Am J Nurs 2001;101(11):32–4.

66. Urden LD, Stacy KM, Lough ME. Thelan's Critical care nursing: diagnosis and management. 4th edn. St Louis: Mosby; 2002.

67. Schwartz S, Pantle H, McQuay N. Inhalation injuries. ICU Dir 2011;4(6):163–71.

68. McSwain NE, Paturas JL. The basic EMT: comprehensive prehospital patient care. 2nd edn. St Louis: Mosby; 2001.

CHAPTER 44

MAJOR TRAUMA INITIAL ASSESSMENT AND MANAGEMENT

KELLIE GUMM

Essentials

- Emphasis in the pre-hospital phase of care should be on the primary survey and include airway maintenance, control of external bleeding and shock, immobilisation and immediate transfer to the nearest highest level of care.
- Emphasis at the scene should be on obtaining and reporting information to the receiving hospital (time of injury, events and patient's history).
- Optimal patient outcomes require early trauma centre notification.
- Advanced planning for the trauma patient's arrival is essential and the trauma team should be assembled and ready to treat the patient.
- The mechanism of injury and patient history form the fundamental information that help anticipate the care required for potential injuries and their severity.
- Primary and secondary surveys provide the standard sequence of priorities for the assessment of patients with multiple injuries.
- Primary and secondary surveys should be repeated frequently to remain vigilant to deterioration and to identify any new treatments required.
- Repeat tertiary survey > 24 hours to assist in identifying any missed injuries.

INTRODUCTION

Major trauma is a time-critical emergency and successful management results from prompt diagnosis of injuries, appropriate resuscitation and stabilisation and prevention of secondary injury. While trauma care is ideally provided in institutions that specialise in trauma,[1,2] the incidence of traumatic injury is not limited to densely populated areas where there are short transport times and the majority of designated trauma centres are located. It is therefore incumbent on paramedics and emergency nurses to realise that, wherever they practise, essential clinical competencies and a sound knowledge base in trauma management is necessary to provide the highest-quality care to this fragile patient population. Although specialised trauma centres have designated trauma treatment areas and multidisciplinary staff allocated to trauma management from resuscitation through to rehabilitation, most emergency departments (EDs) must be able to provide trauma care while also dealing with innumerable other patients presenting with an assortment of ailments from sore throats to cardiac events.[3] In the rural setting, the number of trauma patients may not be as great as in trauma centres, but the seriousness of the situation faced by pre-hospital providers and emergency nurses and their requisite knowledge is similar.

This chapter focuses primarily on trauma patient assessment, which is applicable in any clinical situation and the preparation for and management of the trauma patient during the resuscitative phase of ED care. Pre-hospital trauma management in the context of decision-making, equipment and extrication is discussed in Chapters 10 and 11.

In Victoria the State Trauma System (VSTS) was established in 1999 and ensures a coordinated approach to the management of the severely injured patient. Now up to 85%[4] of Victoria's major trauma patients receive definitive care at a major trauma service. In Victoria, South Australia and New South Wales this is linked to better patient outcomes.[2,5,6] The primary survey is a valuable framework for the initial evaluation of the trauma patient. It is, however, important to consider carefully all that occurs prior to the initial assessment and management in the pre-hospital environment and on admission. Careful preparation and planning are needed.

Preparation

Trauma patients may arrive in the ED by private vehicle, ambulance, helicopter or on foot. The amount of time it takes a trauma patient to reach an ED or trauma centre after injury varies by location, length of time to report the injury, availability of emergency medical services (EMSs), length of rescue and many other variables. Time has been a major influence in the development of world trauma systems and centres, especially the 'golden hour'.[5,7] This term was coined by R. Adams Cowley using research from World War I which demonstrated that the mortality and morbidity of injured patients increased with the amount of time to resuscitation and definitive care: there was an increase of 10% with a 1-hour delay and an increase of 75% with a 10-hour delay. Thus, it was determined that the worst enemy of a trauma patient immediately after an injury was time.[8,9] However, in today's more-sophisticated trauma systems and EMSs, the concept of the 'golden hour' can be interpreted as meaning the window of opportunity in which emergency staff can save a patient's life or limb. This could be a few minutes for some (threatened airway) or hours for others (vascular limb injury).[1,8,9] The golden hour may only be applicable to urban centres, whereas the 'silver day' is more appropriate and realistic for the remote areas of Australia and New Zealand. Increasingly, government health agencies are focusing on finding a balance between delivering effective pre-hospital medical services and retrieving appropriate patients in a timely fashion, and ensuring their delivery to the highest level of care available.

To decrease mortality and morbidity a coordinated approach with pre-hospital care providers can assist in expediting care in the field and allow the receiving hospital advance notice to ensure mobilisation of the trauma team and hospital set-up. ED preparation is essential to maintain the principle of 'do no further harm' cited in the *Advanced Trauma Life Support Course Manual* (2012)[7] and to expedite care. Preparation includes facility design for the trauma bay or resuscitation area cubicle, trauma team presence on patient arrival and necessary drugs and equipment to handle potentially complicated injuries. The first thing to consider is where the resuscitation will take place. Each ED has architectural strengths and weaknesses which require creative solutions for maximum use of space and efficiency of personnel.

Resuscitation room and equipment

The primary objective of a trauma resuscitation area is to facilitate rapid assessment of a severely injured patient supported by adequate lighting, space and equipment. This will allow the identification and treatment of life-threatening injuries and to seamlessly integrate the paramedic staff into the department.[10]

Most centres now have trauma guidelines to assist all practitioners in the identification, prioritisation and treatment of patient injuries. These guidelines should be readily available in various forms such as posters, laminated cards, desktop icons or online, to ensure easy access at all times.[3,11] Box 44.1 illustrates some of the essential equipment required to carry out the procedures mentioned above. This is not an exhaustive list; however, it covers the essentials.

Figure 44.1A shows the typical layout of a trauma bay and is an example of a single-patient resuscitation area that can accommodate two patients if necessary. This example provides a more sophisticated arena for trauma care in a larger-volume ED than may be found in most facilities.

Staff trauma education

Managing today's complex hospital environment requires skilled nursing leaders, who both understand and can manage

---

BOX 44.1 Essential supplies, instruments and trays[3,7]

Airway
Intubation supplies with various-sized blades, handles and tubes easily accessible
Tracheostomy and cricothyroidotomy supplies

Breathing
Chest tube insertion trays with underwater-seal drains and chest tubes
Rapid-sequence induction medications
Laerdal bag and various size masks
Ventilator
Oxygen

Circulation
Thoracotomy tray including rib spreaders, vascular clamps, long-handled instruments, pledgets and cardiac sutures
Autotransfusion supplies
Blood and fluid warmer (preferably high-volume devices)
Venous access supplies for peripheral, interosseous and central access with range of sizes
Defibrillator with paediatric and internal paddles

Miscellaneous
Resuscitation trolley containing ACLS drugs
Transport monitor with ECG, NIBP, pulse oximetry and end-tidal CO_2
Dressings, suture supplies, splinting material
Gastric tubes, urinary drainage system
FAST ultrasound machine
Warming devices—convection blankets (e.g. Bair Hugger)

ACLS: advanced cardiac life support; CO_2: carbon dioxide; ECG: electro-encephalogram; FAST: focused abdominal sonography in trauma; NIBP: non-invasive blood pressure

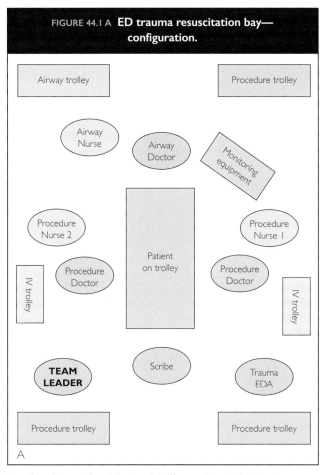

FIGURE 44.1 A **ED trauma resuscitation bay—configuration.**

Based on diagram from The Royal Melbourne Hospital, Victoria.

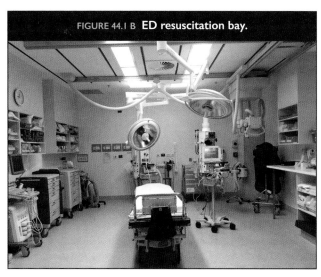

FIGURE 44.1 B **ED resuscitation bay.**

Courtesy of The Royal Melbourne Hospital, Melbourne, Victoria.

the complex needs of high-acuity patients and the ward environment to ensure safe outcomes for patients and staff.

Gabbe,[2] Atkin[6] and Duffield[12] all demonstrated that there are better patient outcomes when there is a higher volume of patients, greater clinical experience, i.e. nurses who have a higher education and more experience caring for the patient population ensure better patient outcomes.

Paramedic training in most states of Australia is two-tiered. The first tier is a three-year Bachelor degree of advanced life support paramedic training; this includes airway/ventilation skills (not including intubation or cricothyroidotomy), IV skills and a range of drug and fluid therapy options, principally aimed at treating hypovolaemia and managing pain in trauma. Standard training for all paramedics includes casualty extrication, spinal care and packaging and pelvic and limb trauma splinting, with a variety of equipment options available to facilitate each intervention. Paramedics receive annual training updates in trauma patient management and are expected to follow practice guidelines and trauma time-critical guidelines that are both consensus-based and substantially similar to those used in trauma centres. The second tier is a postgraduate certificate or diploma for intensive-care paramedics. This adds skills such as advanced airway management (use of rapid sequence induction (RSI) in Victoria) and tension pneumothorax decompression.

The most sophisticated pre-hospital and in-hospital trauma systems are ineffective without a well-trained and organised trauma team. It is essential that all hospitals, no matter the size, have a multidisciplinary trauma team available in the ED whenever called.[13] All team members should have a minimum skill set and knowledge base consisting of trauma patient triage, primary and secondary survey assessment and adjuncts including airway and spinal immobilisation, breathing and circulation skills. Roles can be interchangeable, with each role filled by the most experienced clinician present at the time.[11,14] This is especially relevant for the non-trauma centre where staff may have to rely on paramedics to fill roles out of hours.

Trauma-team training with scenarios executed before receiving critically injured patients is an effective way to achieve an advanced level of communication. The literature is now beginning to show the impact of the various courses, with trauma patient outcomes improving after completion of the Advanced Trauma Life Support (ATLS) course worldwide.[15] Trauma education in many settings is moving into the future with a wide range of learning modalities available. These include online, low-fidelity (models) and high-fidelity (human patient simulators with heartbeats and constricting pupils) courses, making the simulation environment more realistic and hence improving the education outcomes.

In Australia and New Zealand, a variety of trauma training is available for paramedics and nurses, including:

- postgraduate degrees
- short courses offered by local trauma centres
- the Trauma Nursing Program (TNP) hosted by the College of Emergency Nursing Australasia
- the Trauma Nursing Core Course (TNCC) from the Australian College of Emergency Nursing
- Advanced Trauma Care for Nurses (ACTN), USA Society for Trauma Nurses
- Early Management of Severe Trauma (EMST) paramedic/nurse observers course held by the Royal Australasian College of Surgeons—derived from the American College of Surgeons Advanced Trauma Life Support (ATLS) course
- Course in Advanced Trauma Nursing (CATN): course in advance trauma nursing run by the Australian College of Emergency Nurses

- Definitive Perioperative Nursing Trauma Care (DPNTC)
- Emergency Management of Severe Burns (EMSB), run by the Australian and New Zealand Burn Association (ANZBA)
- International Trauma Life Support (ITLS) course, run by the Australian College of Emergency Nursing
- Pre-Hospital Trauma Course (PHTC), run by CareFlight
- Pre-Hospital Trauma Life Support (PHTLS), from the Committee of the National Association of Emergency Medical Technicians (NAEMT) in cooperation with the Committee on Trauma of the American College of Surgeons
- Managing Obstetric Emergencies and Trauma Course (MOET)
- Interactive web-based scenarios as well as information on upcoming trauma conferences and links to other web-based trauma resources such as trauma management guidelines, e.g. those available on www.trauma.org.

There are many locally run courses available at local major trauma services. Further information on trauma courses can be provided by the trauma nurse coordinator at your nearest trauma centre.

The trauma team

Nurses who care for trauma patients are required to have specific advanced skills and knowledge to enable them to fulfil their role in the trauma team (TT). In large metropolitan centres, there will be numerous medical and nursing staff members to make up the team; however, in regional or rural areas the nurse may be the only healthcare professional available and will be required to have a more-developed skill set.[16] Table 44.1 illustrates the roles of the TT and the multidisciplinary team members who could fulfil each role. Team-member responsibilities are identified by the procedures they are required to conduct, such as establishing IV access or focusing on a specific anatomical area for assessment (e.g. head, left side of the patient's body). Responsibilities should be clearly defined, whether the trauma resuscitation is accomplished in a level 1 trauma centre or a small rural ED.[17,18]

As illustrated in Figure 44.1B, at major trauma centres most TTs would consist of other staff in addition to this list. Such teams would include the core group of:

- Team leader: ED consultant or surgeon
- Airway: nurse (airway competency) and doctor (anaesthetic fellow or consultant)
- Procedure: one nurse and one doctor (trauma registrar or emergency registrar) team for each side of the patient, for IV line insertion, indwelling catheters, FAST exam and to assist with log roll
- Scribe: nursing team leader (also helps direct nursing care of less-experienced nurses in the procedure role)[19]
- Emergency Department Assistant (EDA), also called Orderly or Health Care Assistant: trained assistant can help with removing clothes, applying warm blanket, log rolls, equipment, transport, blood delivery and collection, external cardiac massage
- Radiographer: available to perform X-rays within 5 minutes

- Consultant general surgeon and intensivist: available in the hospital and within a short time of the patient arriving at the ED
- Surgical registrar.

In addition to the core TT, other medical and allied health personnel who provide valuable background support are also notified through a trauma paging system. Not all of these need be immediately present at the trauma, but they can be notified of the arrival of the trauma patient by the trauma call page:

- blood bank
- biochemistry
- haematology
- operating theatre floor coordinator
- bed management
- trauma service.

There must be the capacity to directly communicate with other relevant specialists, such as neurosurgeons, orthopaedic surgeons, cardiothoracic surgeons, plastic surgeons and interventional radiologists, to assist in the ongoing management and definitive care of these patients.

It may be worthwhile to enlist the assistance of other personnel such as social and/or pastoral care workers to support the family from the time of the patient's admission. Peer-support teams can provide any debriefing or peer support to staff involved in particularly distressing trauma resuscitation.

Trauma protocols and guidelines for care throughout the patient continuum are recommended to ensure ongoing quality and standard of care, and to delineate staff responsibilities from the scene through to before, during and after patient arrival at the trauma service. The guidelines assist in maintaining consistency of patient care throughout their journey. Refer to Chapter 42 for information on trauma algorithm development.

Trauma team notification

Trauma team activation criteria ensures early identification of a severely injured patient who requires specialised resources from the hospital to form the TT, including personnel from ICU; surgery; anaesthetics and ED, while also notifying radiology, blood bank, theatre and bed management about the patient's impending arrival. EMSs play a large role in the pre-notification of the TT by providing essential information about the patient's condition that will help in the decision to activate a TT or not. Notification of team members can be via overhead paging and/or a dedicated paging system. A degree of over-triage is required to ensure capture of all severely injured trauma patients.[18,20,21]

Designated trauma centres enhance communication to the team by establishing 'trauma call-out' criteria to notify the TT of a potentially major trauma patient's impending arrival. Trauma team activation has traditionally been based on physiological criteria; specific high-risk injuries and mechanism of injury (see Box 44.2). There is consensus that mechanism of injury alone as a criterion for TT activation is not predictive of severity of injury or outcome, and that physiological measurements are highly sensitive. Major trauma presentations comprise an extremely small percentage of overall ED presentations in the majority of smaller hospitals; however, it could be asserted that over-triage in these smaller centres might be a good process as they may benefit from TT training.[18,20–23]

TABLE 44.1 Core multidisciplinary trauma team[3,12]

ROLE	CORE COMPETENCIES/SKILLS
Team leader GP/surgeon Anaesthetist Emergency doctor	Competencies Competent and experienced in assessment and management of the trauma patient according to EMST principles Skills *Supervision* of the team Appropriate *allocation* of team members Assessment of priorities and making team aware of these • overseeing of resuscitation • listening to hand-over from EMS Prioritising treatment and investigation procedures Directing the performance of a range of invasive procedures, including: • endotracheal intubation and mechanical ventilation • prescription and administration of anaesthesia and analgesia • intercostal catheter insertion • intravenous cannulation and fluid resuscitation • arterial blood gas sampling • environmental control (i.e. temperature/safety) • diagnostic peritoneal lavage Making appropriate referrals early in the treatment of the patient. Ensuring that plans for *definitive management* are formulated at appropriate *pivotal points in resuscitation.* Arranging for the transfer of patient to a place of definitive care
Airway nurse and doctor GP/anaesthetist MICA paramedic RN/paramedic	Competencies Competent and experienced in airway management Skills Maintenance of airway, application of O_2, immobilisation of cervical spine Checking respiratory status and performing or assisting in endotracheal intubation and mechanical ventilation Administration of anaesthesia and analgesia as necessary Insertion of nasogastric tube Talking to patient, assessment of GCS, checking pupil reaction, seeking information on next of kin, relaying information to scribe Management of cervical spine
Procedure nurse and doctor GP/surgeon ED doctor RN/paramedic	Competencies Competent and experienced in the invasive procedures to be performed or in assisting the setup and assistance in insertion Skills Assistance with or performance of a range of invasive procedures, not limited to: • intercostal catheter insertion • intravenous cannulation and fluid resuscitation • arterial blood gas sampling • diagnostic peritoneal lavage • urinary catheterisation Attachment of monitoring equipment (ECG, NIBP, SaO_2) Application of splints and dressings, performance of log roll Performance of 12-lead ECG Performance of procedures as directed by the team leader
Scribe Supervisor/RN	Skills Recording and documenting vital signs at frequent intervals Documenting the time of performance of procedures including the hand-over from EMS Documenting the time of administration of drugs Ensuring that procedures suggested by the team leader are carried out in a timely manner In conjunction with the team leader, controlling the access of personnel to resuscitation bay

ECG: electroencephalogram; EMS: emergency medical services; EMST: early management of severe trauma; MICA: mobile intensive-care ambulance; NIBP: non-invasive blood pressure; RN: registered nurse; SaO₂: oxygen saturation of arterial blood

---

BOX 44.2 MIST—mechanism of injury mnemonic[7]

M Mechanism of injury—time of the event, events related to the accident, patient's medical history
I Injuries—known or suspected injuries
S Signs—vital signs taken at the scene, including blood pressure
T Treatment—any treatment conducted at the scene or en route

BOX 44.3 Trauma team activation criteria[22–27]

Vital signs
Systolic blood pressure < 90 mmHg
Pulse rate > 124 beats/minute
Respiratory rate < 12 or > 24 breaths/minute
Glasgow Coma Scale score ≤ 9
Oxygen saturation < 90%

Injuries
All penetrating injuries to head, neck, torso or groin
All blunt injuries to a single region or to two or more regions comprising head, neck, torso or groin

Specific injuries
Suspected spinal cord injury
Limb-threatening injuries and/or amputations
Burns > 20% or suspected respiratory tract involvement
Major compound fracture/open dislocation of limb
Fractures of two or more of: humerus, femur, tibia
Fractured pelvis

Mechanism of injury
Ejection from vehicle
Motor/cyclist impact > 30 kph
Fall from height (> 3 m)
Struck on head from objects falling > 3 m
Explosion
High-speed motor vehicle collision (60 kph or over)
Pedestrian impact
Prolonged extrication (> 30 minutes)

And
Pregnancy > 20 weeks with ruptured membranes/PV (per vaginal) bleeding/fetal heart rate < 100 beats/minute
Age > 55 years
Significant underlying medical condition

While it is necessary to mobilise the entire TT to manage multi-trauma patients with critical injuries, it is neither practical nor economically sound to mobilise the entire team for every patient. Unnecessary TT activations divert resources away from other hospital activities, which could potentially compromise patient care.[18] Thus, most centres use a tiered response to trauma to enable them to differentiate between the severely injured patients who have a higher likelihood of an increased mortality and those with a lower mortality.[21,22] Preventing under-triage is important. Under-triage can result in treatment delays and serious injuries may not be diagnosed quickly enough, leaving the patient to clinically deteriorate and contributing to secondary complications.[1] Optimal triage systems can provide an appropriate balance of triage and resource allocation. Each hospital should have its own activation criteria based on its individual patient population to ensure that all major trauma patients and those with complex injuries receive adequate reception by the appropriately trained multidisciplinary team. While it may be difficult to minimise under- and over-triage rates,[21,22] it is essential that the triage system is monitored and changes implemented as required.

Clinician judgement and the manifestation of delayed trauma call criteria should be considered in addition to pre-hospital TT activation. For example, not all serious injuries meeting TT activation criteria may fall under one of the categories in Box 44.3. Thus, a senior clinician should be able to decide to activate the trauma team based on clinical judgement. And, if trauma criteria are not identified or evident on initial presentation, the TT should be activated immediately on recognition, regardless of time after presentation.

PRACTICE TIP

Trauma call-out or upgraded trauma call-out should be activated in the event of patient deterioration, or at the time it is recognised that the patient fulfills trauma call-out criteria—regardless of time after presentation.

Preparation

Preparation begins before the patient arrives; Box 44.4 gives a summary of preparation measures. As stated previously, preparation includes an organised area within the scope of the facility's resources to accommodate resuscitation of a severely injured patient. The team should be called as soon as possible prior to the patient arriving, and information should be disseminated to all members in the moments available before the resuscitation begins, so as to prioritise tasks. This communication can clarify confusion about responsibilities, but also helps individual members focus as a team on anticipated injuries. The effectiveness of EDs and trauma centres depends on the entire team working together with a common vision of efficient, skilled and organised management.

In most instances, some prior notification is provided by the ambulance service. The person receiving the notification should elicit as much information as possible without compromising rapid transport of the patient. Knowing in advance the mechanism of injury and patient acuity facilitates set-up of special equipment. Being aware, for example, that a patient in a vehicle rollover in winter was found in a paddock will help the TT anticipate and intervene early for hypothermia. Knowing that a patient has a penetrating abdominal injury and is hypotensive will enable early notification of the consultant surgeon, anaesthetist and operating suite. It is not financially prudent to open a large number of supplies and trays before patient arrival; however, it is wise to secure necessary equipment ahead of time and have it readily accessible.

BOX 44.4 Preparation for the arrival of a trauma patient

Notification of trauma patient meeting the trauma call-out criteria
Trauma call-out dispatched (on-call medical officers in rural areas notified)
Standard room preparation—the trauma bay should be checked daily and then prior to patient arrival (ensuring all equipment is in working order and stock lists are adequate)

Equipment
Oxygen and suction
Airway trolley, including preparation of intubation drugs
Monitors, fixed and transport
Defibrillator—ensure enough paper and battery charged
Procedure and IV trolleys
Multipurpose packs and trays (1–2)
Blood tubes for baseline blood and cross-match
Priming of fluid warming devices
Turning on ultrasound machine
IV fluid bag and line primed ready to go
O-negative blood

Forms
Pathology and X-ray
Trauma flow sheet
Wrist bands and labels

Trauma team arrival
Donning of lead gowns and standard precautions
Allocation of staff roles and discussion of expected patient
Notification of blood bank and pathology

Documentation

The ambulance patient care record (PCR) should be filed in the inpatient medical record. This record contains patient details that can assist in monitoring trends in the patient's condition, providing details of clinical events and describing the initial findings at the scene that may not be evident to those who subsequently care for the patient. Accurate, succinct and timely documentation of the trauma resuscitation is essential to patient management, giving the scribe a pivotal role in the TT. The scribe's record captures the efforts of the paramedics at the scene to the first moments of a patient's arrival. It also provides data on the patient's physiological response to treatment, and may be used as evidence in police investigations or the Coroner's Court (see Ch 4). In addition, these records are used for case reviews and quality-assurance activities locally and nationally.

Accurate documentation is paramount for good trauma management. Documentation of vital-sign changes, decreased urinary output and amounts and types of fluid administration quickly identifies indicators that alert the astute nurse to physiological compromise in the patient's condition. These indicators should be used to regularly update the TT leader. Tools used for documentation vary, but generally involve formatted trauma charts. Many institutions use trauma flow sheets rather than a narrative script. Flow sheets are usually more efficient and user-friendly, and accommodate rapid documentation in the stressful atmosphere of trauma resuscitation. The flow sheet may also help guide the primary survey and ensure that all procedures are carried out.

Initial resuscitation

All trauma patients should be assessed from the time of their trauma through to hospital admission using the primary and secondary surveys; however, any life-threatening condition identified during assessment must be treated immediately before proceeding to the next phase of care. Initial resuscitation is performed at the scene by the paramedics who conduct an initial primary survey, and assess and treat any life-threatening injuries. Emphasis is placed on airway maintenance, haemorrhage control, fluid resuscitation and immediate transport with a focus on minimising scene time.[7,12]

Once the primary survey is completed, patient assessment continues with the secondary survey, which includes anticipating plans for transport to a major trauma service or the closest most appropriate service. Prehospital triage guidelines enable identification of patients who should be immediately triaged to the highest level of trauma centre. The guidelines typically require assessment of physiological parameters, region or type of injury and mechanism of injury. The current time-critical guideline used by paramedics in Victoria is shown in Figure 44.2.

Once the patient arrives at the ED or trauma centre the process is repeated, beginning with the paramedic team handing over. Utilisation of the MIST acronym (see Box 44.2) ensures that the most pertinent information is handed over in a timely manner. It is vital that the TT listens to the paramedic hand-over, as the paramedics were the first to conduct the primary survey in the pre-hospital environment and en route to the facility. This hand-over will provide valuable information on the mechanism of injury and the patient's injuries, treatment and vital signs (MIST).[3,7]

The MIST framework provides the structure necessary to ensure that the TT remains focused in a very distracting environment by any member of the TT in any situation to rapidly identify and treat immediate life-threatening injuries. The initial medical response does not usually allow for the more detailed patient history that can be made available later. A team member can then seek out the paramedic soon after for a more detailed history.

Once handover is complete the initial resuscitation commences with the TT conducting the primary survey, and assessing and treating any life-threatening injuries. Once the primary survey is completed, patient assessment continues with the secondary survey, which includes anticipating plans for

FIGURE 44.2 Pre-hospital major trauma criteria for Victoria.[88]

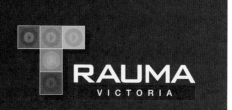

Victorian State Trauma System
Pre-hospital Major Trauma Triage

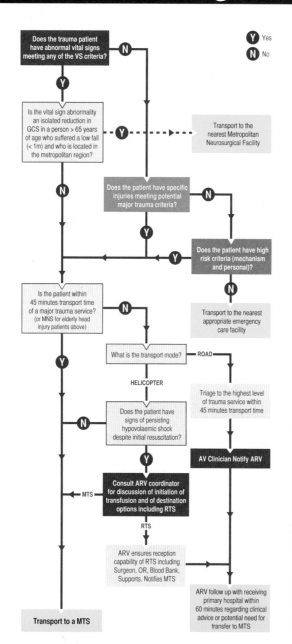

Y Yes
N No

Pre-hospital Vitals Signs Major Trauma Criteria

Age	Term - 3 mths	4-12 mths	1-4 yrs	5-12 yrs	12+ yrs	Adult
HR	<100 or >180	<100 or >180	<90 or >160	<80 or >140	<60 or >130	<60 or >120
RR	>60	>50	>40	>30	>30	<10 or >30
BP sys	<50	<60	<70	<80	<90	<90
SpO₂			<90%			<90%
GCS			<15			<13

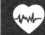

Specific injuries meeting potential major trauma criteria

All penetrating injuries
(except isolated superficial limb injuries)

Blunt injuries:

- Serious injury to a single body region such that specialised care or intervention may be required, or such that life, limb or long term quality of life may be at risk
- Significant Injuries involving more than one body region

Specific Injuries:

- Limb amputation
- Suspected Spinal Cord Injury
- Burns > 20% BSA or suspected respiratory tract burns
- Serious crush injury
- Major compound fracture or open dislocation
- Fracture to two or more of: femur, tibia, humerus
- Fractured Pelvis
- Spinal Fracture

High Risk Criteria for Major Trauma

- Ejection from vehicle
- Motor / cyclist impact > 30 kph
- Fall from height > 3 m
- Struck on head by object falling > 3 m
- Explosion
- High speed MCA > 60 kph
- Pedestrian impact
- Prolonged extrication

AND:

- Age > 55 / Age < 16
- OR Pregnant
- OR Significant comorbidity

Adult Retrieval Victoria
ARV   1300 36 86 61
Coordinators of Critical Care Services

PIPER   1300 13 76 50
Paediatric Infant Perinatal Emergency Retrieval

Version 1.0 | 22-10-2014

transfer or transport to another unit or major trauma service. The tertiary survey must be conducted after 24 hours, when a patient leaves the ICU and/or prior to patient transfer to assist in identifying missed or overlooked injuries.

Primary survey

Multi-trauma patients suffer from many and varied life-threatening injuries. If these injuries are not addressed in a clinically appropriate sequence, a potentially non-fatal threat can quickly escalate and become fatal.[27] It is essential that the initial systematic primary survey is prioritised and followed, in both the pre-hospital and the hospital phases of care.

The primary survey should be conducted in the following sequence:[7]

A. Airway maintenance with cervical spine control
B. Breathing and ventilation
C. Circulation with haemorrhage control
D. Disability: neurological status
E. Exposure and temperature control.

During the primary survey, life-threatening conditions are identified and treated. In this chapter, the prioritised assessment and management will be discussed in sequence for the purposes of clarity; however, these steps are frequently accomplished simultaneously.[3,7,12]

Airway and cervical spine stabilisation

Assessment of the trauma patient's airway and ventilatory status is the *top priority*. Patients at high risk of airway compromise include the unconscious, those with an altered level of consciousness, head injuries or blood loss and those affected by alcohol and other drugs.

The goals of airway and ventilation assessment are to:

1. Secure a patent airway
2. Ensure adequate oxygenation
3. Provide adequate ventilation
4. Monitor ongoing status of airway patency and ventilatory status
5. Maintain in-line spinal immobilisation.

Airway, breathing and circulation assessment should be conducted using 'look, listen and feel' techniques.

The best way to assess the airway is to speak to the patient. If they are able to verbalise in a comprehensible orientated way, this is evidence that the airway is clear. If orientated, the patient's brain is being perfused and there is no immediate evidence of brain injury. On the other hand, no speech or incomprehensible or disorientated speech will reveal a compromised airway and/or potential traumatic brain injury.

Look for the presence of airway compromise: close examination of the patient may reveal obvious injuries that can cause airway obstructions, such as:

- foreign bodies (vomitus or blood)
- evidence of airway burns (see Ch 52)
- fractures or lacerations to the face, larynx, neck or maxillofacial region.

At this stage, pallor or cyanosis can help confirm the presence of an airway obstruction, with cyanosis being a late sign.

Listen for abnormal sounds such as:

- snoring, gurgling
- stridor
- hoarseness
- inability to talk in sentences.

These sounds are all associated with a partial occlusion of the airway.

Feel for tracheal position and diminished air movement.

While assessing the airway, it is paramount that the cervical spine remains immobilised. There should be no hyperflexion, hyperextension or rotation. The patient should be nursed in neutral position with a cervical collar on. If the collar is removed for any manoeuvres, then manual in-line stabilisation is necessary. The American College of Surgeons Committee on Trauma[7] has reported that 5% of trauma patients develop new neurological symptoms or worsening of existing symptoms once they reach the ED, strongly suggesting that inadequate spinal immobilisation has the potential to exacerbate spinal injury. Paramedics and nurses need to have a heightened awareness of the vulnerability of the spine, and all management must be aimed at preventing spinal cord injury or exacerbating a pre-existing injury.[3,12,28,29] See Chapter 17, p. 323, for further information on cervical spine immobilisation techniques, and p. 314 for airway management.

> **PRACTICE TIP**
>
> Be aware of the patient with maxillofacial trauma who refuses to lie down flat! This patient may have such severe injuries that they can only manage their secretions and maintain a patent airway while sitting up.[7]

Table 44.2 illustrates life-threatening airway problems—which must be treated immediately—their signs and symptoms, and the interventions to manage these problems.

Breathing and ventilation assessment

A breathing problem may have already been identified during the assessment of the airway. It is important to remember that adequate ventilation requires optimum functioning of the lungs, chest and diaphragm; during initial assessment of the patient's breathing, each of these must be examined individually.

Look closely and examine the patient's chest wall integrity for:

- fractures, lacerations and/or bruising
- paradoxical chest movements
- tachypnoea and/or abnormal respiratory rate
- use of accessory and/or abdominal muscles
- further assessment of patient colour.

Listen for absent or decreased breath sounds and unequal air entry.

Feel for:[3,7,12]

- subcutaneous air
- chest wall instability and/or crepitus
- position of trachea
- dullness and/or hyperresonance.

If the patient is already intubated, confirm appropriate endotracheal tube (ETT) placement by visualising symmetrical chest rise and fall, and auscultating over the stomach then the lung fields and end-tidal carbon dioxide ($EtCO_2$) monitoring

TABLE 44.2 Life-threatening airway problems[3,7]

PROBLEM	SIGNS AND SYMPTOMS	INTERVENTIONS
Airway obstruction (complete or partial)	Dyspnoea, laboured respirations Decreased or no air movement Presence of foreign body in airway Trauma to face or neck Breathlessness Agitation Combativeness Cyanosis Stridor Drooling	Airway opening manoeuvres: • jaw thrust • chin lift • suction Airway adjuncts: • nasal airway • oral airway • endotracheal tube • laryngeal mask airway (LMA) Surgical airway:
Inhalation injury	History of enclosed-space fire, unconsciousness or exposure to heavy smoke Dyspnoea Wheezing, creps, crackles Hoarseness Singed facial or nasal hair Carbonaceous sputum Burns to face or neck Blisters in the oral cavity	• cricothyroidotomy • tracheostomy Provide high-flow oxygen (100%) via non-rebreather mask or bag–valve–mask device Prepare for endotracheal intubation as soon as possible

if available (see Ch 17, p. 323, for ETCO$_2$ monitoring techniques). These techniques should be performed after intubation and then whenever a patient is moved; for example, from stretcher to bed. Patients intubated by paramedics may be moved several times, increasing the potential for ETT displacement. Where equipment in use by paramedics differs from hospital equipment, continue to use that of the paramedics until ready to change over in an orderly fashion. Once ETT placement is confirmed, further diagnostic studies should be obtained, such as chest X-ray, ongoing EtCO$_2$, oxygen saturation measurements and arterial blood gases (see Ch 17, p. 329, for information on collecting arterial blood gases).[7] During this time the paramedic who intubated the patient should be questioned as to the reason for intubation, how it was performed, a description of the patient prior to the procedure, what was used to secure the ETT and a description of the airway and any difficulties that were encountered. Pre-hospital airway procedures are usually governed by guidelines and protocols, although these may differ from what individual trauma hospital practitioners are used to.

Table 44.3 illustrates some of the life-threatening breathing problems a multi-trauma patient may be faced with, their signs and symptoms and interventions required.

Circulation with haemorrhage control

Haemorrhage is the principal cause of preventable death after traumatic injury.[31] It is essential that all hypotension is considered hypovolaemic until proven otherwise. Uncorrected haemorrhagic shock will lead to inadequate cellular perfusion, anaerobic metabolism and the production of lactic acid. This leads to profound metabolic acidosis, which also interferes with blood-clotting mechanisms, and promotes coagulopathy and blood loss. Hypothermia, acidosis and the consequences of massive blood transfusion all lead to the development of coagulopathy; mortality for these patients is three to four times higher than those without coagulopathy.[31] Even if control of mechanical bleeding is achievable, patients may continue to bleed from all lacerated surfaces. This leads to the worsening of haemorrhagic shock, and so to a worsening of hypothermia and acidosis, prolonging the vicious cycle.[32] For details on the physiology of shock see Chapter 20.

The goals of circulation and haemorrhage control assessment are to:

- identify signs and sources of haemorrhage
- assess mental status
- assess pulses
- assess skin colour, temperature and moisture.

PRACTICE TIP

An easy way to remember all the potential chest injuries is A–J:[30]

A. Airway transection or tear
B. Bronchial tear or rupture
C. Cord (spinal) injury
D. Diaphragmatic rupture
E. Esophageal (oesophageal) injury
F. Flail chest or rib fracture
G. Gas in the chest or abdomen
H. Haemothorax
I. Infarction from AMI
J. Jugular venous distension from cardiac tamponade.

TABLE 44.3 Life-threatening breathing problems[3]

PROBLEM	SIGNS AND SYMPTOMS	INTERVENTIONS
Tension pneumothorax	Dyspnoea, laboured respirations Decreased or absent breath sounds on affected side Unilateral chest rise and fall Tracheal deviation away from affected side Cyanosis Jugular venous distension Tachycardia and hypotension History of chest trauma or mechanical ventilation Chest pain Decreased oxygen saturation	Requires immediate intervention without radiological confirmation Provide high-flow oxygen (100%) via non-rebreather mask or bag–valve–mask device Perform rapid chest decompression by needle thoracotomy on affected side Place chest tube on affected side
Pneumothorax	Dyspnoea, laboured respirations Decreased or absent breath sounds on affected side May have unilateral chest rise and fall May have visible wound to chest or back Bruising or abrasions on chest Pain May have decreased saturations History of chest trauma	Provide high-flow oxygen (100%) via non-rebreather mask or bag–valve–mask device Place chest tube on affected side Place occlusive dressing over any open chest wound and secure on three sides with tape
Haemothorax	Dyspnoea, laboured respirations Decreased or absent breath sounds on affected side May have unilateral chest rise and fall May have visible wound to chest or back History of chest trauma (often penetrating) Tachycardia Bruising or abrasions on chest Pain May have decreased saturations	Provide high-flow oxygen (100%) via non-rebreather mask or bag–valve–mask device Consider autotransfusion Prepare for urgent transport to operating theatre for massive haemothorax
Sucking chest wound (open pneumothorax)	Dyspnoea, laboured respirations Decreased or absent breath sounds on affected side Visible, sucking wound to chest or back Chest pain May have decreased saturations	Provide high-flow oxygen (100%) via non-rebreather mask or bag–valve–mask device Cover wound with occlusive dressing and secure on three sides with tape Watch for signs of tension pneumothorax and remove dressing during exhalation if they are noted Place chest tube on affected side
Flail chest	Dyspnoea, laboured respirations Paradoxical chest wall movement Chest pain Tachycardia May have decreased saturations	Provide high-flow oxygen (100%) via non-rebreather mask or bag–valve–mask device Prepare for intubation and mechanical ventilation in compromised patients
Full-thickness circumferential burn of thorax	Dyspnoea, laboured respirations Shallow respirations Obvious circumferential burns to thorax	Provide high-flow oxygen (100%) via non-rebreather mask or bag–valve–mask device Prepare for immediate escharotomy

Key signs of significant blood loss are altered consciousness, poor perfusion, skin pallor, weakened or thready pulses and signs of external bleeding. When assessing a trauma patient, it is essential to consider that the shocked state may not be haemorrhagic and the patient could be suffering from cardiogenic or neurogenic shock. During the hand-over, the paramedic can provide a description of the amount of blood loss at the scene; this may help differentiate between the types of shock. However, paramedics' estimation of external blood loss has been shown to be unreliable.[33] Cardiogenic shock in the trauma patient may be due to a diaphragm injury, pericardial tamponade, blunt myocardial injury or tension pneumothorax. Pericardial tamponade should be suspected when there is hypotension unexplained by other findings, i.e. tension pneumothorax, haemothorax, abdominal or other haemorrhage.

PRACTICE TIP

The signs and symptoms of pericardial tamponade and tension pneumothorax are similar, thus careful assessment of the patient is paramount.[12] For example, distended neck veins are a sign of cardiogenic shock and can be hidden by the cervical collar.[17]

Neurogenic shock results from spinal cord injury. This profound shock is due to loss of sympathetic tone and is characterised by hypotension with no tachycardia or vasoconstriction and a normal pulse pressure. Multi-trauma patients with suspected or confirmed spinal cord injury should always be treated initially as if hypovolaemic (see Ch 49).

Assessment

Look for:

- level of consciousness
- obvious signs of external bleeding
- skin colour for pallor and/or cyanosis
- neck veins (collapsed or distended)
- abnormalities underneath the hard collar.

Key changes in the patient's condition can indicate ongoing blood loss (see Table 44.4). Capillary refill time is a good measure of perfusion in children, but its usefulness decreases with patient age and diminishing health status, and is affected by environmental temperature, making this test less reliable in the field.

Listen for muffled heart sounds that indicate pericardial tamponade.

Begin basic and advanced life support measures for pulseless patients. Patients who are in traumatic cardiopulmonary arrest at the scene have an overall mortality rate of 95%, especially following blunt trauma (97%).[33] The National Association of Emergency Services Physicians (NAEMSP) and the American College of Surgeons Committee on Trauma have established guidelines regarding the termination or withholding of out-of-hospital resuscitation in cardiopulmonary arrest cases in response to the low survival rates, although adoption of these guidelines is controversial. They advise that providers may cease efforts in patients with witnessed cardiopulmonary arrest who have had 15 minutes of unsuccessful resuscitation attempts.[3,34–36]

In the trauma patient population, always consider tension pneumothorax and cardiac tamponade as potential causes of pulselessness. These quickly reversible conditions can be managed with needle thoracentesis and pericardiocentesis, respectively.

Feel:

- assess skin for moisture and temperature
- palpate pulses for presence, quality, rate and rhythm.

Peripheral pulses may be absent following direct injury, hypothermia, hypovolaemia or vasoconstriction. For decreased systolic blood pressure, assess central pulses (femoral or carotid) bilaterally for quality, rate and regularity. Box 44.5 lists approximate minimal systolic blood pressures palpable in adults at various sites.

Consider that tachycardia precedes hypotension, and that patients may be on medications that regulate heart rate. Table 44.5 outlines the life-threatening circulatory problems, signs and interventions.

Focused abdominal sonography in trauma (FAST) is a quick method to detect occult abdominal bleeding in shocked patients, and form part of the primary survey if the patient is haemodynamically unstable and the source of bleeding unknown; otherwise, they are adjuncts to the secondary survey. The indications for FAST are altered sensorium, altered sensation, ambiguous physical examinations, those with a seatbelt sign (see Fig 44.3) and patients who will require prolonged sedation or anaesthesia (radiological investigations or operative procedures) and thus are unable to have a full abdominal examination.

FAST is also low-cost, safe, quick and accurate in the diagnosis of intraperitoneal bleeding, haemopneumothoraces and pericardial tamponade, and is now more than ever accepted as an integral adjunct to the primary survey. FAST scanning is now being trialled in the pre-hospital environment by paramedic crews, with some studies finding that paramedics could achieve a high level of accuracy with a 1-day hands-on training course. FAST scanning in this environment has been found to be a challenge, having to deal with movement, combative patients, difficult access and short timeframes. NSW established the world's first FAST course for nurses; the benefits of this are increased numbers of staff available to enable consistent efficient and immediate care, which can be particularly advantageous to smaller centres without many medical resources. Many ultrasound machines now are more compact, easily usable and thus can be kept so that they are readily available. FAST has the advantage of being able to be completed at the bedside in the trauma bay, it is non-invasive and has the additional benefit of being able to be easily repeated; FAST provides early, accurate information and has no side effects, proving it to be a useful adjunct when considering management options. However, FAST is very operator-dependent and requires training and practice; scans can be distorted by gas; and it is not sensitive to diaphragm, bowel and pancreatic injuries. It is unreliable in patients with ascites and subcutaneous air.[7,12,37–39]

Disability (neurological)

During the primary survey, only a brief, focused neurological assessment is performed. This assessment is conducted at the end of the primary survey using the Glasgow Coma Scale score

TABLE 44.4 Classes of haemorrhagic shock, assessment and interventions[7,11,12,31]

CLASS	ASSESSMENT	INTERVENTIONS
Class I haemorrhage—up to 15% blood loss (up to 750 mL) Exemplified by the condition as if a patient had donated blood	Slightly anxious Pulse < 100 beats/minute Skin warm and dry Normal blood pressure Normal pulse pressure or increased Normal respirations: 14–20 breaths/minute Urine output > 30 mL/h	Administer oxygen Control obvious bleeding Establish large-bore IV access (14–16-gauge) Administer IV crystalloid fluid (3:1 rule) Warm fluids and patient
Class II haemorrhage—15–30% blood (750–1500 mL) Uncomplicated haemorrhage managed with crystalloid resuscitation	Mildly anxious Tachycardia: 100–120 beats/minute Slightly cool skin Normal systolic blood pressure Pulse pressure narrows Respirations 20–30 breaths/minute Urine output decreased slightly: 20–30 mL/h	Administer oxygen Establish large-bore IV access (14–16 gauge) Administer IV crystalloid fluid (3:1 rule) May require blood products Warm fluids and patient Identify and control bleeding source Surgical intervention may be needed
Class III haemorrhage—30–40% blood loss (1500–2000 mL) Complicated haemorrhagic state requiring blood producte and crystalloid	Confusion, agitated Tachycardia: 120–140 beats/minute Cool, diaphoretic and pale Decreased systolic blood pressure Narrow pulse pressure Respirations 30–40 breaths/minute Urine output 5–15 mL/h	Administer oxygen Establish 2 or more large-bore IV access (14–16 gauge), continue rapid infusion of blood and crystalloid, titrating to patient response Warm fluids and patient Identify and control bleeding source Prepare for surgical intervention
Class IV haemorrhage—greater than 40% blood loss (2000 mL or more) Preterminal event, patient requires aggressive resuscitation measures	Confused, lethargic, decreased GCS Tachycardia: > 140 beats/minute, thready pulse Pale, cool, diaphoretic Severely decreased blood pressure Respirations > 35 breaths/minute Narrowed pulse pressure Urine output negligible ABGs: metabolic acidosis and respiratory alkalosis	Administer oxygen Place multiple large-bore IV lines (14–16 gauge), continue rapid infusion of blood and crystalloid, titrating to patient response Warm fluids and patient Identify and control bleeding source Surgical intervention required

Initial warm fluid bolus of 1–2 L for adults (including that given in the pre-hospital environment), absolute fluid boluses should be based on patient responses.

ABG: arterial blood gas; GCS: Glasgow Coma Scale; IV: intravenous

---

BOX 44.5 Estimating adult systolic blood pressure (BP)[3]

If the pulse is palpable, systolic BP is at least:

- radial: 80 mmHg
- femoral: 70 mmHg
- carotid: 60 mmHg

(GCS) (see Ch 14 for detailed discussion) and the AEIOU mnemonic (Box 44.6). A decrease in the GCS is evidence of decreased cerebral perfusion and oxygenation; this could be due to hypovolaemia, brain injury, hypoxia or drug use. At this point, the oxygenation, ventilation and perfusion of the patient should be re-evaluated (ABC). Absence of spontaneous movement in the extremities and poor respiratory effort are early signs of spinal trauma.[7,12,41,42] If the patient is exhibiting

TABLE 44.5 Life-threatening circulation problems, signs and interventions[7]

PROBLEM	SIGNS AND SYMPTOMS	INTERVENTIONS
External haemorrhage	Obvious bleeding site	Elevation where able
		Direct pressure
Shock	Tachycardia	Provide high-flow oxygen (100%) via non-rebreather mask or bag–valve–mask device
	Weak, thready pulses	
	Cool, pale, clammy skin	Place two large-bore IV lines and infuse with warm isotonic crystalloid solution (Hartmann's or 0.9% NaCl); early administration of blood components
	Tachypnoea	
	Altered mental state	Administer fluid bolus (1 L in adults or 20 mL/kg in children)
	Delayed capillary refill	Prepare to administer blood
	Oliguria or anuria	
Pericardial tamponade	Tachycardia	Pericardiocentesis
	Muffled heart sounds	
	Distended neck veins	
	Hypotension	
	ECG showing electromechanical dissociation	
	Signs of hypovolaemic shock	

ECG: electrocardiogram; IV: intravenous; NaCl: sodium chloride

---

FIGURE 44.3

A and **B**, Seatbelt signs.

Courtesy of The Royal Melbourne Hospital, Victoria.

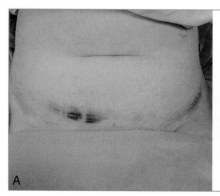
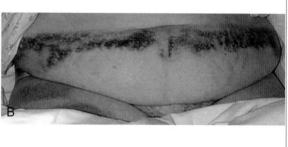

BOX 44.6 AEIOU mnemonic[40]

A Alcohol and drugs
E Endocrine, encephalopathy
I Insulin
O Opiates and oxygen
U Uraemia

If one of the above is not the cause of the decreased Glasgow Coma Scale score, it should be considered traumatic.

---

motor posturing, or has gross pupillary dilation or asymmetry, consider mannitol infusion, manoeuvres to maximise cerebral venous outflow, brief hyperventilation or emergent surgical intervention.

Any decreased level of consciousness or pupil abnormality will be investigated further during the secondary survey.[3,7,41,42] It is important to consider the patient's conscious state from the time of injury until the time of assessment; if the patient was brought in by ambulance, the paramedic will be able to provide information regarding the patient's conscious state, trends and changes during their management and any treatments provided that may have had some contributory impact.

Exposure and temperature control

Exposure of the trauma patient is the final step of the primary survey, and prepares the patient for the secondary survey. Completely and rapidly remove the patient's clothing to assess for injuries, haemorrhage or other abnormalities; however, this step should not be completed until the patient reaches an environment where active warming can replace the patient's clothing, unless exposure is needed to diagnose or treat an injury. Observe the patient's overall general appearance, noting body appearance, asymmetry, guarding or the presence of odours such as alcohol, petrol and urine. Collection, securing and preserving of all patient clothing and belongings should be done.

Trauma-induced coagulopathy (TIC) and the triad of death

Acute traumatic coagulopathy (ATC) is an early endogenous coagulopathy that is characterised by systemic anticoagulation and fibrinolysis exacerbated by hypothermia, acidosis and haemodilution, which contribute collectively to the established trauma-induced coagulopathy (TIC). Trauma-induced coagulopathy (TIC) is defined as a hypercoagulable state that occurs after a traumatic injury and exacerbates blood loss. It is an imbalance of the dynamic equilibrium between procoagulant factors, anticoagulant factors, platelets, endothelium and fibrinolysis.[43] *Coagulopathy* is present in up to a quarter of major trauma patients, and these patients are four times more likely to die than those patients who present with normal coagulation.[30–36,43,44]

Haemorrhage and resuscitation induce cellular changes that are characteristic of ischaemia and/or reperfusion injury (Fig 44.4). This response is immune-inflammatory and compromise both intrinsic and adaptive immunity. When blood loss is severe a range of inflammatory mediators, cytokines and oxidants are almost immediately produced in large quantities and released. This disregulation is the presumed cause of organ failure and death.[45] The introduction of damage control resuscitation has been shown to improve haemostasis, achieve better haemorrhage control, limit haemodilution and hypothermia and improve outcomes of bleeding trauma patients.[43] Patients who develop TIC have an increased likelihood of multi-organ failure (MOF), Acute Lung Injury (ALI) infection, prolonged ventilation hours, ICU admission and increased early and late mortality.[43,45] TIC can occur within

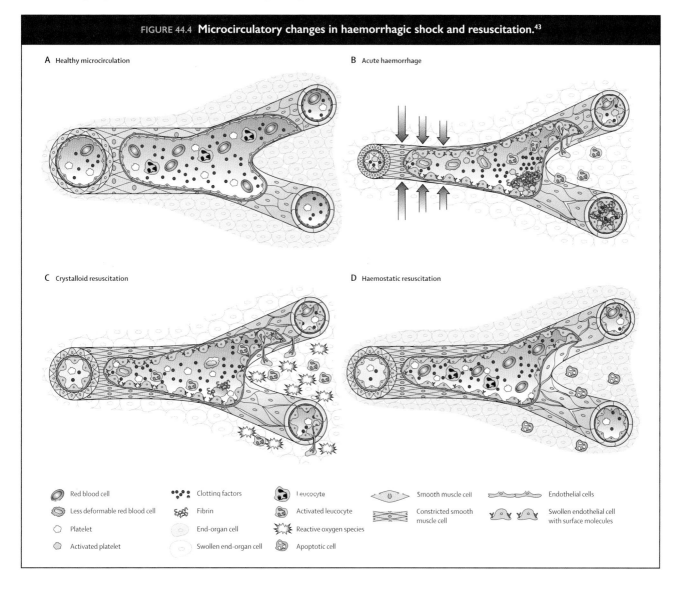

FIGURE 44.4 Microcirculatory changes in haemorrhagic shock and resuscitation.[43]

A Healthy microcirculation

B Acute haemorrhage

C Crystalloid resuscitation

D Haemostatic resuscitation

Red blood cell

Less deformable red blood cell

Platelet

Activated platelet

Clotting factors

Fibrin

End-organ cell

Swollen end-organ cell

Leucocyte

Activated leucocyte

Reactive oxygen species

Apoptotic cell

Smooth muscle cell

Constricted smooth muscle cell

Endothelial cells

Swollen endothelial cell with surface molecules

minutes of an injury and is present in up to 25% of patients admitted to hospital. It is imperative that the paramedic and ED nurse mitigate progression of TIC as much as possible.

Hypothermia exacerbates TIC and is an indicator of severe injury. Hypothermia is associated with an increase in post-trauma complications such as multi-organ failure, systemic inflammatory respiratory sepsis (SIRS) and sepsis.[43,46] The majority of major trauma patients are hypothermic on arrival in the ED because of environmental conditions at the scene. Inadequate protection, intravenous fluid administration and ongoing blood loss worsens the hypothermic state.[30,46–49] Haemorrhagic shock leads to decreased cellular perfusion and oxygenation, and inadequate heat production. Hypothermia has dramatic systemic effects on the body's functions, but most importantly in this context it exacerbates coagulopathy and interferes with blood homeostatic and platelet mechanisms.[30,32]

Hypothermia is defined as a temperature below 36.5°C, and can be classified as mild (34–36°C), moderate (32–34°C) and severe (< 32°C).

Acidosis is caused by inadequate tissue perfusion, hypoxia and tissue injury and is another contributing factor that is worsened by the presence of hypothermia and coagulopathy. Acidosis has several negative effectors on haemostasis and includes platelet and coagulation dysfunction especially in a pH < 7.2.[30,45,48] It can be an independent predictor of mortality and morbidity in major trauma; an increased base deficit increases transfusion requirements, causes multi-organ failure and increases major trauma patient mortality and morbidity.[30,46–49]

Figure 44.5 illustrates some of the multifactorial conditions that contribute to the potentially lethal complication of hypothermia in a traumatic injury.

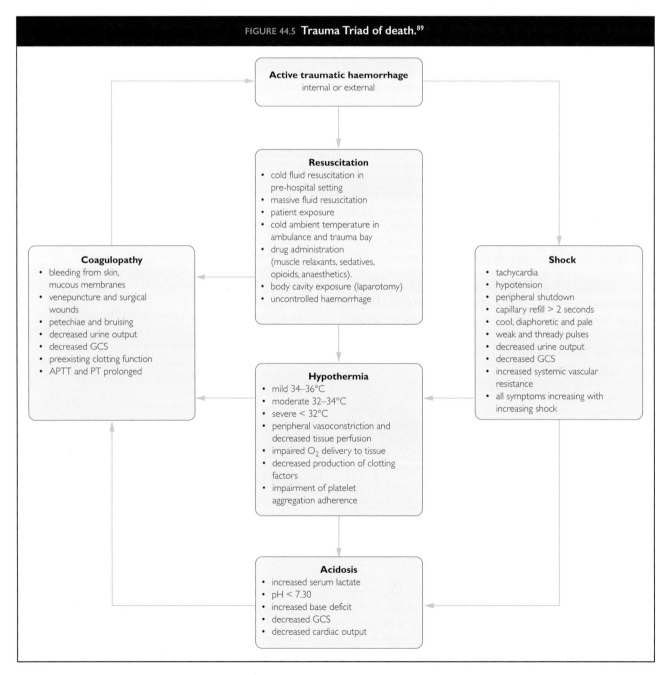

FIGURE 44.5 **Trauma Triad of death.**[89]

Active traumatic haemorrhage
internal or external

Resuscitation
- cold fluid resuscitation in pre-hospital setting
- massive fluid resuscitation
- patient exposure
- cold ambient temperature in ambulance and trauma bay
- drug administration (muscle relaxants, sedatives, opioids, anaesthetics).
- body cavity exposure (laparotomy)
- uncontrolled haemorrhage

Coagulopathy
- bleeding from skin, mucous membranes
- venepuncture and surgical wounds
- petechiae and bruising
- decreased urine output
- decreased GCS
- preexisting clotting function
- APTT and PT prolonged

Shock
- tachycardia
- hypotension
- peripheral shutdown
- capillary refill > 2 seconds
- cool, diaphoretic and pale
- weak and thready pulses
- decreased urine output
- decreased GCS
- increased systemic vascular resistance
- all symptoms increasing with increasing shock

Hypothermia
- mild 34–36°C
- moderate 32–34°C
- severe < 32°C
- peripheral vasoconstriction and decreased tissue perfusion
- impaired O_2 delivery to tissue
- decreased production of clotting factors
- impairment of platelet aggregation adherence

Acidosis
- increased serum lactate
- pH < 7.30
- increased base deficit
- decreased GCS
- decreased cardiac output

Once the patient enters the ED, all modalities of care should be implemented while trying to maintain or increase the patient's temperature (see Box 44.7).

During the course of the primary survey, the five most important rules to remember are:[3,7,12,17,41–44,50]

1. The patient should be repeatedly reassessed, particularly if clinical signs change.
2. Any immediately life-threatening condition diagnosed should be rectified without delay.
3. Penetrating wounds and implements must be left for formal surgical exploration.
4. Any external bleeding should be stopped by using direct pressure.
5. The patient must be kept warm.

Primary survey interventions

Primary survey interventions are implemented as they are identified in the clinical setting; they are outlined in this text according to priority.

Airway

Simple manoeuvres in the pre-hospital environment and ED can improve the patency of the patient's airway; interventions begin simply, then move to the more complex (see also Table 44.2). An experienced paramedic, ED or critical-care-trained nurse can implement many of the following simple manoeuvres.

1. Chin lift or jaw thrust.
   - Chin lift can be accomplished by placing two fingers under the mandible and gently lifting it upwards, moving the chin anteriorly; caution should be exercised in patients with known or suspected spine injuries.
   - Jaw thrust is useful to assist with maintaining a seal on a bag–valve–mask device if the patient is requiring ventilation assistance and for those with a potential spinal injury. The angles of the lower jaw are grasped with one hand each side and the jaw is displaced forwards.
2. Clear the airway.
   - This can be accomplished with a suction device or a manual scoop. If patients are required to be turned on their side to clear the airway, this must be done with a log-roll (see Ch 49).

BOX 44.7 Hypothermia prevention and management[30,48,49]

- Remove all wet, blood soaked clothes, linen and covers.
- Keep patient covered.
- Apply blankets (external active rewarming temperature-regulated blankets).
- Warm all fluids and blood products before transfusion.
- Increase room temperature.
- Humidify inspired gases.
- Control haemorrhage.
- Reverse shock.
- Be aware of causes of heat loss such as drugs, long operative events such as exploratory laparotomies, ongoing exposure.

---

3. Insert nasopharyngeal or oropharyngeal airway.
   - The nasopharyngeal airway is passed into the posterior oropharynx by gently sliding it into one nostril. This airway may be better tolerated in the conscious patient, as it is less likely to induce gagging and vomiting.
   - Nasophyargeal insertion is contraindicated in any significant maxillofacial injury or suspected basal skull fracture. In these cases an oropharyngeal airway should be used. The oropharyngeal airway is inserted into the mouth behind the tongue, and in adults it is best inserted upside down and turned 180° once it touches the soft palate. Caution needs to be exercised in the conscious patient (GCS ≥ 9) as oropharyngeal airways may cause gagging, vomiting and aspiration (see Ch 21).[7,50]

PRACTICE TIP

Gagging in the neurological patient (trauma or otherwise) has a negative impact on intracranial pressure and the oro-/nasopharyngeal airway and laryngoscopy should all be used if this problem is suspected.

---

4. Definitive airway
   - An endotracheal or nasotracheal airway is inserted if the above methods have failed to adequately maintain a patent airway. Other indications for a definitive airway in the trauma patient include patients with a GCS < 9, apnoeic patients, patients unable to protect their own airways from secretions or foreign matter or those with airway burns. The paramedic and ED nurse should anticipate the need for a cricothyroidotomy (Fig 44.6). Indications include failure to intubate, airway swelling/burns and severe facial or neck trauma.[7,50] Ensure that all equipment, including laryngoscope globes, endotracheal tube cuff and pulse oximetry, has been thoroughly checked and is in working order prior to intubating the patient. A failure to secure an airway as a result of equipment failure can have a catastrophic conclusion.
5. Maintain cervical spine immobilisation.
   - Trauma patients should be treated as having a spinal injury until proven otherwise. Cervical spine immobilisation is achieved by utilising a stiff cervical collar while keeping the spine in neutral alignment. If unable to apply a hard collar in uncooperative patients, small infants or babies or child with traumatic torticollis, manual inline stabilisation should be maintained.[7,52] See Chapter 17, p. 323 for cervical spine immobilisation techniques. If the collar is to be removed at any time, or the patient needs to be moved, one person should be allocated as the team leader and be responsible for immobilising the spine with manual traction and coordinating any patient movement. Log-rolling a spinal immobilised patient requires the assistance of at least three people. In regional and rural areas, the paramedic and other support staff can assist with log-rolling should there not be enough nursing and medical staff available.

FIGURE 44.6

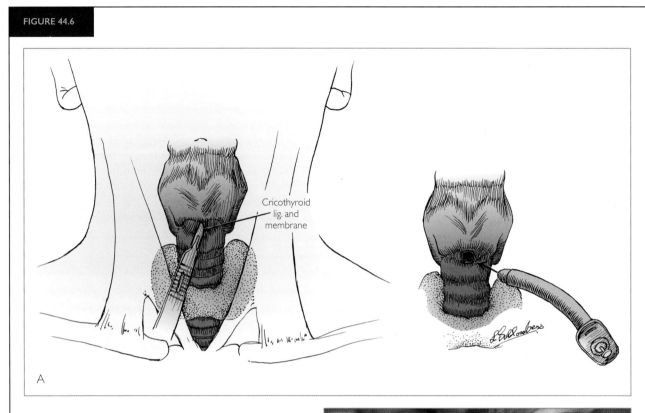

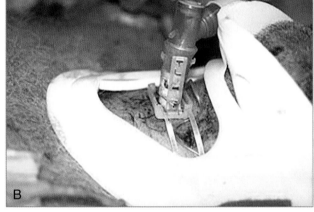

A, Cricothyroidotomy technique.[90] **B**, Completed cricothyroidotomy.

B, Courtesy of Liverpool Hospital Trauma Service, Sydney, NSW.

- Airway management techniques can cause cervical spine movement. In particular, the chin lift/jaw thrust can increase disc space by > 5 mm despite the presence of either a hard or a soft collar. Likewise, oral endotracheal intubation produces a 3–4 mm increase in disc space. By contrast, oral/nasal airway insertion can be responsible for 2 mm posterior subluxation.[53] The spinal board should be removed on admission or at the first log-roll, to prevent pressure-related complications from prolonged spinal board use.[28,29]
- To maintain cervical spine alignment in children, a folded towel can be placed under the child's shoulders as this prevents their relatively large head forcing their neck into flexion (Fig 44.7).

Breathing and ventilation

In the trauma patient, breathing and ventilation can be compromised for a variety of reasons, such as decreased GCS (caused by head injuries, drugs or hypotension), mechanical failure (spinal injury), ventilation failure (generally caused by multiple rib fractures, flail segment, pulmonary contusion, pneumothorax, tension pneumothorax or large haemothorax) or airway obstruction. A more detailed thoracic assessment is described in Chapter 47. However, the key interventions in breathing and ventilation are described below, and are also listed in Table 44.3.

1. Oxygen administration.
   - All treatment should be aimed at correcting hypoxia— oxygen administration is the simplest intervention, and should be titrated to the patient's needs.

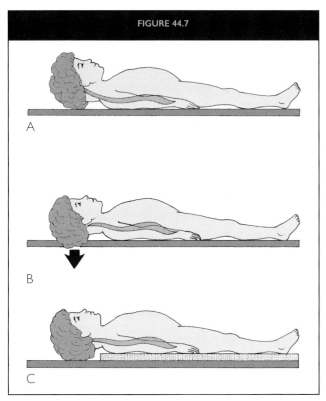

FIGURE 44.7

A, Young child immobilised on a standard backboard; note how the large head forces the neck into flexion. Backboards can be modified by an occiput cutout (**B**) or a double mattress pad (**C**) to raise the chest.[91]

- All spontaneously breathing trauma patients should have high-flow (15 L/min) oxygen delivered by a non-rebreather mask. If the patient requires some assistance or ventilation, then a bag–valve–mask device with a reservoir can be used. If inadequate respiratory effort continues, the patient will require intubation.
- An oxygen saturation of >95% is optimum (see Ch 21). Oxygen saturation monitoring can be conducted by the ED nurse as an adjunct to the look, listen and feel techniques, using a SpO_2 device which estimates the peripheral arterial oxygen saturation. Be aware of SpO_2 inaccuracies in the presence of carboxyhaemoglobin, hypothermia, anaemia and hypovolaemia (mean arterial pressure [MAP] < 50 mmHg).
- Patients require continuous assessment to monitor for improvements and deterioration in their condition.

2. Needle decompression.
- Chest decompression via needle or finger thoracostomy is indicated in patients with profound respiratory distress, unilateral breath sounds, subcutaneous emphysema and any time that a tension pneumothorax is suspected. This should be conducted immediately without waiting for radiological confirmation.
- The signs and symptoms of a tension pneumothorax include respiratory distress, neck vein distension, tachycardia, hypotension, trachea deviation and decreased breath sounds to the affected side. Assessment is more difficult in the intubated patient as some of these

signs are altered due to the intubation, and the risk of tension pneumothorax is increased in those receiving positive-pressure ventilation.

PRACTICE TIP

Tension pneumothorax and pericardial tamponade signs and symptoms are very similar; therefore care must be taken in patient assessment to differentiate between the two.

- *Tamponade*—distended neck veins, hypotension, muffled heart sounds, pulsus paradoxus, narrowing pulse pressure.
- *Tension pneumothorax*—respiratory distress, neck vein distension, tachycardia, hypotension, tracheal deviation, absent breath sounds on the affected side.

- A 14-gauge angio catheter (needs to be at least 45 mm long) is inserted into the pleural space above the 5th rib, mid-axillary line, or over the 2nd rib, mid-clavicular line. Needle or finger decompression converts a tension pneumothorax into a simple pneumothorax; the catheter should be left in place until an intercostal chest tube is in place.

3. Intubation.
- Nasal/oral intubation or a surgical airway provides the ultimate definitive airway. The ED nurse or paramedic at the scene plays an important role in intubation, and must monitor the patient carefully throughout the procedure.
- Rapid-sequence intubation (RSI) is a widely used and recommended airway technique (see Box 44.8). The patient's breathing must then be maintained with manual bagging or, preferably, by attaching the patient to a ventilator. Ventilator observations which regularly assess air entry, ETT secretions, SaO_2 and ventilator settings should then be commenced, and ventilator settings adjusted accordingly.
- If intubation fails, the paramedic and/or ED nurse should be ready to assist/manage the airway by anticipating the equipment needed and the procedure to be followed, given in the failed intubation algorithm shown in Figure 44.8.

4. Sucking chest wounds.
- Seal sucking chest wounds (open pneumothorax) with a three-sided occlusive dressing followed by chest tube insertion. This creates a one-way valve; the dressing is sucked to the chest on inspiration, and then allows the air to escape on expiration.
- If the dressing was to completely seal off and the air became trapped, a tension pneumothorax or further barotrauma is possible.

5. Intercostal catheter insertion and management.
- Indications for intercostal catheters (ICCs) in the trauma setting include both pneumothorax and haemothorax. If haemothorax is visualised on chest X-ray it should be treated with ICC. In addition, an

---

BOX 44.8 Rapid-sequence induction procedure[7]

- Check all equipment is in working order, especially globe for laryngoscope and cuff on endotracheal tube.
- Preoxygenate patient and administer rapid-sequence medications.
- Apply cricoid pressure if requested by the intubator, and do not remove until advised by the intubator.
- Monitor the patient's vital signs—especially blood pressure, heart rate and SpO$_2$.
- Perform intubation.
- Inflate cuff to provide seal—be careful not to over-inflate.
- Secure endo/nasotracheal tube.
- Resume/continue with ventilation.
- Check tube placement:
  - listen at epigastrium for absence of sounds
  - listen for breath sounds bilaterally in lung fields
  - look for equal chest expansion
  - look for colour and level of consciousness
  - monitor oxygen saturation and end-tidal carbon dioxide levels
  - chest X-ray for radiological confirmation of placement.

SpO$_2$: oxygen saturation of blood pressure

ICC should be placed in all patients following needle decompression and should be considered in those even with small pneumothoraces requiring positive-pressure ventilation or transport in an air ambulance (helicopter or fixed-wing aircraft), as pressure changes can lead to tension pneumothorax. The ICC in a haemothorax evacuates blood and reduces the risk of clotted haemothorax; in pneumothorax the ICC facilitates removal of air and fluid, allows expansion of the lung and prevents tension pneumothorax.

- The standard ICC should be a large 32-French gauge placed into the intercostal space above the 5th rib in the mid-axillary line. The nurse's role is not only to assist with set-up and insertion where necessary, but also to carefully monitor the ICC and underwater-seal drainage (UWSD) unit (see Ch 17, p. 332, for techniques on attaching a USWD unit). An ICC is normally inserted in emergency conditions; however, an aseptic technique needs to be adhered to to reduce infection risks. The ICC should be sutured close to the skin and dressed with a secure, occlusive dressing to prevent any air leaving from the insertion site and any back-and-forth movement of the tube into the chest, which can increase the risk of infection.
- Drainage of 200 mL/h for 2 to 4 hours is an indication for exploratory thoracotomy. The patency of the tube is also important to monitor, as a tension pneumothorax can develop if the tube becomes blocked or kinked, removed or disconnected.[7,12] Troubleshooting ICC problems are discussed in Chapters 21 and 47.

Patients with large blood loss may require fluid and early blood transfusion.[7]

Circulation and haemorrhage control

The primary survey thus far has already provided clues to the sufficiency of the circulation, such as respiratory rate, skin pallor, level of consciousness and severe external bleeding. Haemorrhage control is the next primary goal, followed by fluid resuscitation.

1. Haemorrhage control
   - All signs of external haemorrhage must be identified and direct pressure applied to stop the bleeding. Fractures to the long bones and pelvis can result in large-volume blood loss and should be splinted in the pre-hospital environment. Most ambulances carry a range of splints suitable for the pelvis and the long bones; these should be applied at the scene without causing time delays, or on arrival at the ED.
   - Patients who are haemodynamically unstable with a pelvic fracture have a high mortality rate, thus haemorrhage control should include early non-invasive pelvic stabilisation.[55] This can be achieved with a specially designed pelvic sling or with a sheet wrapped as tightly as possible around the patient's greater trochanters and symphysis pubis regions. The sling should be tightened to 180 newtons, which is equivalent to lifting an 18 kilo weight.[52] If a splint has not been applied prior to admission this can be done on arrival, either on transfer from the ambulance trolley or at the time of log-rolling (see Ch 17, p. 352, for an explanation of different splinting techniques). Splints and slings fitted in the pre-hospital stage should not be removed, even during the initial assessment, until the patient has been stabilised (see Fig 44.9).
   - FAST should be conducted as part of the primary survey if the patient is shocked, as a means of identifying the source of blood loss. These tests are not organ-specific, but can identify free fluid in the peritoneum.[40] The nurse needs to be aware that a positive result will mean that the patient will need to go to theatre, as ultimately haemorrhage control must be attended to in the operating suite. Therefore, the nurse should anticipate and prepare the patient for rapid transport to the operating or angiography suite.

2. IV access
   - Insert two large-bore IV (16-gauge or larger) to allow for rapid fluid transfusion if required. The preferred site for these lines in the adult is the forearm's antecubital vein. If cannula insertion is unsuccessful, the patient may require central venous intraosseous or a peripheral cutdown procedures to gain access.
   - IV access gained by paramedics may be poorly sited or of a less desirable gauge. IV cannula placement in the field is often compromised by poor light, poor patient positioning, restlessness, pain or hypotension and inadequate skin cleaning prior to insertion. Therefore additional or alternative access should be sited at an appropriate time.
   - Intraosseous (I/O) needles are an effective alternative for IV access and are appropriate for all ages when venous access is not possible or after two failed attempts.[7,56] Intraosseous devices can be quickly inserted within

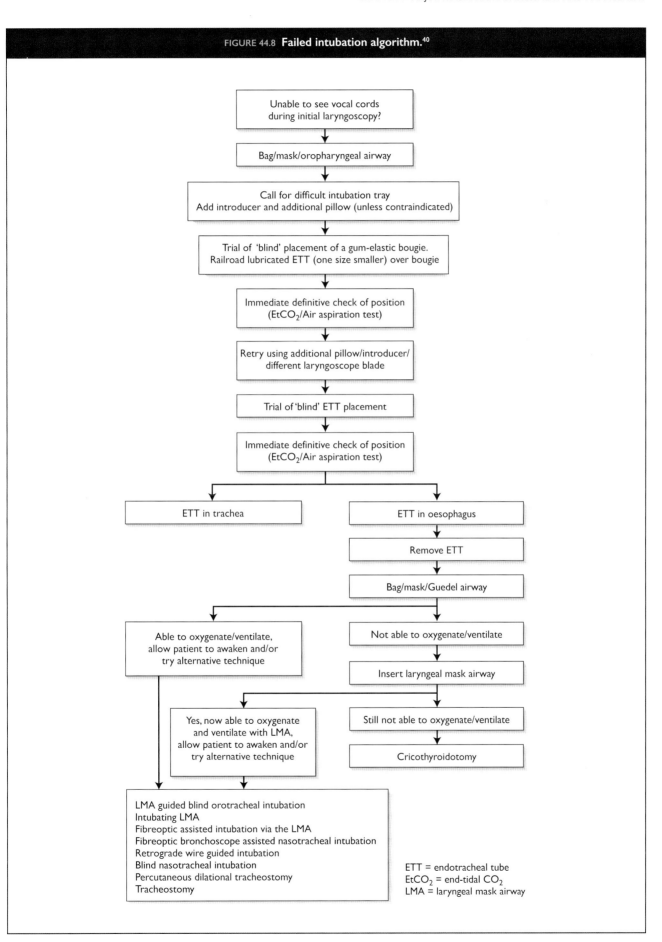

FIGURE 44.8 **Failed intubation algorithm.**[40]

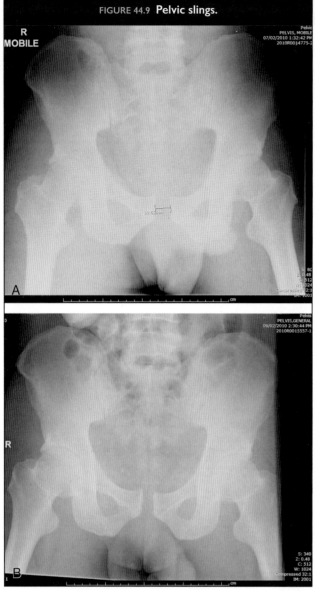

FIGURE 44.9 Pelvic slings.

A, Separated sacroiliac joint prior to sling application: pubic symphysis diastases with widening up to 1.9 cm. **B,** SI joint reduction post application of sling, to 15 mm.

1 minute and flow rates of up to 125 mL/min obtained. Insertion sites include the proximal tibial, distal tibia and proximal humerus. I/O infusions should be limited to emergency resuscitation and discontinued as soon as venous access is obtained.[7,56,57]

- I/O infusions can be painful when fluid in infused—if this is the case then lignocaine can be administered to assist with pain control in the hospital setting. I/O must be closely monitored for other complications such as extravasation of fluids and medication which could occur if not monitored closely and can cause compartment syndrome. Other complications are fractures caused by insertion and osteomyelitis which is more common when I/O used for greater than 24 hours is associated with either multiple attempts or aseptic technique (see Fig 44.10).[7,55,56]

3. Fluid resuscitation
   - There is much controversy in the literature concerning the type of fluid to use in trauma resuscitation.[7,51,58–60] One Australian study[60] demonstrated that there is no significant difference in critically injured patients' outcomes when resuscitated with either a colloid or a crystalloid solution. However, the head-injured subset of trauma patients resuscitated with a colloid solution had higher rates of mortality and poorer functional outcomes than those resuscitated with a crystalloid solution. This has led to a change in practice and a recommendation that trauma patients, especially those with head injuries, should not be resuscitated with colloid solutions.
   - There are complications related to the rapid infusion of large volumes of fluid in the trauma patient, especially for those with penetrating trauma. Aggressive resuscitation using crystalloid fluids also has other hazardous and reproducible physiological consequences. After approximately 750 mL of administered crystalloid solution has been infused, cytokines are activated and an iatrogenic dilutional coagulopathy occurs; platelets, prothrombin time, partial thromboplastin time and thromboelastograph evaluations demonstrate statistically abnormal differences compared with normal values in patients who have post-traumatic hypotension and have received no or limited fluid resuscitation.[1]

Damage control resuscitation

Damage control resuscitation (DCR) has resulted in a change in resuscitation practice over the last 10 years. This is a multi-pronged approach to resuscitation that aims to prevent and manage acidosis, hypothermia and TIC. The DCR strategies include active warming and heat loss prevention, aggressive early blood product administration, aimed at preventing and reversing coagulopathy, restoring blood volume and hence oxygen delivery to the tissues. DCR typically is a temporising procedure and the patient will more than likely require life-saving surgical or radiological intervention for ongoing management of these bleeding sources.[31–32]

- Permissive hypotension is a concept of tolerating a lower blood pressure, which may prevent any clot that has formed at bleeding sites from being dislodged. Research on animals and in humans has shown that a systolic blood pressure of > 80 mmHg is enough to dislodge clots. This has contributed to the trend towards limiting fluid resuscitation until haemorrhage is controlled.[31,32,58] In the patient with a penetrating injury, limiting fluid resuscitation improves outcome due to platelet aggregation inhibition and dilution of clotting factors. An increase in blood pressure can cause a clot to be disrupted, reverse vasoconstriction and increase blood loss.[1,7]

- In the presence of uncontrolled haemorrhage in a patient with a known or suspected traumatic brain injury, one of the important goals is prevention of secondary brain injury from hypotension. Therefore, a systolic blood pressure (SBP) of at least 90 mmHg should be maintained, using fluid resuscitation and/or inotropic support,[41,42,58] while the optimal blood pressure in those without a traumatic brain injury with uncontrolled haemorrhage is an SBP of

FIGURE 44.10 Intraosseous access.

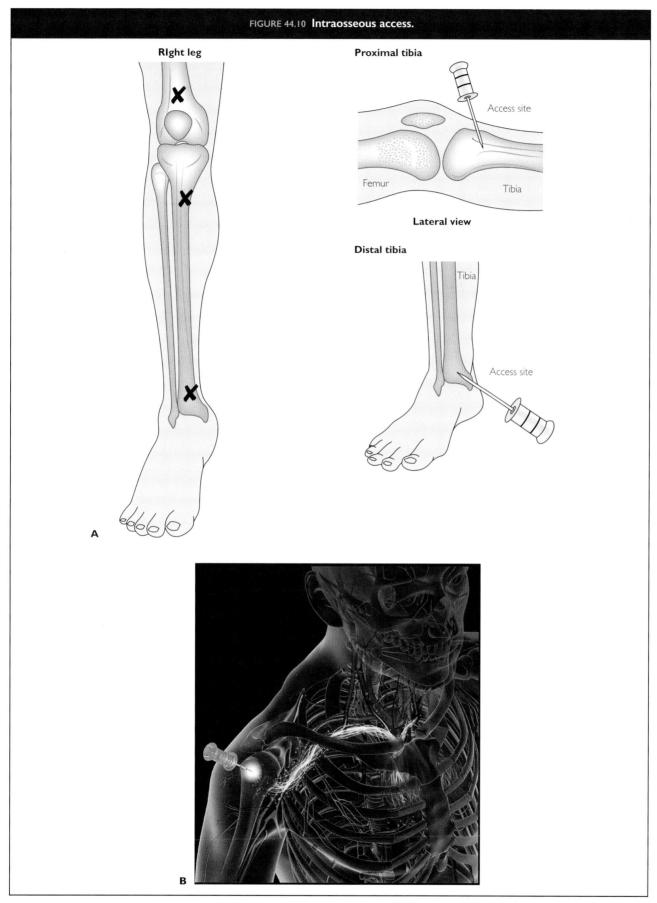

A. The Royal Children's Hospital, Melbourne.[57] B. Courtesy Teleflex Incorporated.

80–90 mmHg. Treatment in the pre-hospital environment may differ from these guidelines; for example, Victorian paramedics administer fluid in blunt and penetrating cases in much smaller doses and to an SBP ≥ 100 mmHg, and in NSW it is done to a radial pulse.

- It is essential that paramedics and ED nurses monitor and titrate the amount and type of fluid being administered against the patient's response, and keep the treating medical staff constantly updated. In the pre-hospital and ED environment, keeping track of fluid resuscitation volumes can be challenging in stressful situations; keeping the empty fluid and blood bags aside can assist in keeping track of volumes administered. Fluid given in the pre-hospital environment should also be taken into consideration when blood products are administered.

PRACTICE TIP

PERMISSIVE HYPOTENSION

- Transfuse to systolic blood pressure of 80–90 mmHg (be wary of head injury).
- Use small fluid boluses of 200 mL crystalloid initially.
- Early blood product administration, 1:1:1:1 packed red blood cells, fresh frozen plasma, platelets and cryo-precipitate, with a focus on fibrinogen replacement.
- Fluid and patient warming.

---

4. Blood administration
- Blood transfusion is fundamental to the care of the trauma patient. The main purpose of transfusing red blood cells is to restore the oxygen-carrying capacity of the intravascular volume. The circulating blood is often depleted of essential clotting products and the coagulation functions may also be affected. Essential blood products, such as platelets, fresh frozen plasma and cryoprecipitate, may need to be given, along with the red blood cells.
- Haemorrhagic shock, as graded by the American College of Surgeons, falls into four classifications (see Table 44.4). Class III or IV signifies the need for haemorrhage control and triggers the need for a liberal transfusion strategy or damage control resuscitation[51] using a 1:1:1:1 transfusion strategy of packed red blood cells, fresh frozen plasma, cryoprecipitate, and platelets. Early administration of clotting products and blood is intended to reduce coagulopathy and thrombocytopenia.[7,31,58] The estimated volume needed for transfusion is based on the percentage loss of circulating blood volume and the patient's ability to compensate. Estimated blood volume for an adult is 70 mL/kg.[3]
- Massive blood transfusion is defined as either replacement of 100% of the patient's total blood volume in < 24 hours or administration of 50% of the patient's blood volume in 1 hour. Complications of massive transfusion include thrombocytopenia, coagulation factor depletion, hypocalcaemia, hyperkalaemia, acid–base disturbance, hypothermia, adult respiratory

distress syndrome (ARDS) and multi-organ failure. The patient's clinical condition must be closely monitored, with early involvement of the Blood Bank for transfusion support.[1] A massive transfusion protocol should exist in each centre receiving trauma patients.

- Artificial haemoglobin and blood replacements, as well as coagulation drugs such as recombinant factor VIIa (rFVIIa), are becoming more readily available. However, to date there is no empirical evidence to support their use in trauma. Factor VIIa has been shown to lower the prothrombin time and to reduce visible coagulopathic haemorrhage following trauma. It also reduces blood transfusion requirements in blunt trauma patients and there is a similar trend in penetrating injury. An outcome benefit in terms of mortality, morbidity, ICU stay and cost has not been demonstrated, although there is a trend in the reduction of multi-organ failure, TRALI (transfusion-related acute lung injury) and ARDS. Additionally, evidence is emerging that the coagulant and metabolic milieu must be favourable, or made favourable, for the drug to work.[34]
- Since 2010, massive transfusion protocols have begun to include tranexamic acid. In 2010 the results were published of a study entitled CRASH-2, a large, multinational, randomised placebo-controlled trial which trialled the use of the antifibrinolytic tranexamic acid (Txa) in trauma patients with or at risk of significant haemorrhage.[62] The study found that the administration of intravenous tranexamic acid in adult trauma patients with significant haemorrhage, within 8 hours of injury, can be used safely as an adjunctive therapy and may decrease bleeding and mortality. Further, Txa costs dramatically less than rFVIIa (less than one-tenth).

Emergency department thoracotomy

There is much controversy in the literature surrounding the indications for emergency department thoracotomy (EDT), with survival rates quoted as anything from 2% to 31%.[34,51,63,64] In addition to the controversy, EDT is a costly procedure that can pose a risk to healthcare workers. The aim of an EDT is to evacuate haematomas, repair injuries and control haemorrhage, and in doing so prevent or treat air embolism.[11,51]

The indications for EDT are listed in Table 44.6. EDT is suggested mostly for penetrating chest trauma, as the survival rate and neurological outcomes from blunt trauma in cardiac arrest are very poor.[64] EDT is not commonly performed, and as it is usually done for patients in extremis in the trauma environment, it is usually a very stressful procedure. ED nurses need to be familiar with the emergency thoracotomy instruments. It is also prudent to anticipate EDT in those patients receiving cardiopulmonary resuscitation, as these patients usually require large volumes of fluid and urgent transfer to the operating theatre once haemorrhage control has been attained. Early notification to blood bank, haematology and theatre is essential.

The patient's pre-morbid state, age and co-morbidities and the logistics of the procedure (available operating theatre, cardiothoracic surgeon, scrub staff) must be taken into consideration before going ahead with EDT.[65]

TABLE 44.6 Indications for emergency department thoracotomy (EDT)[51,63–65]

PENETRATING TRAUMA PRESENTING TO ED	
Extremis with signs of life—pupillary response to light, respiratory effort, response to pain, cardiac activity on ECG	Non-intubated patients: CPR < 5 minutes before admission
	Intubated patients: CPR < 10 minutes before admission
Witnessed cardiac arrest	
Persistent post-injury hypotension (systolic blood pressure < 60 mmHg) unresponsive to fluid resuscitation	
Refractory moderate post-injury hypotension (systolic blood pressure < 80 mmHg)	
BLUNT TRAUMA	
Witnessed cardiac arrest with vital signs present	

CPR: cardiopulmonary resuscitation; ECG: electrocardiogram

Adjuncts to the primary survey

All life-threatening injuries identified in the primary survey must be treated before progressing to the secondary survey. In the clinical setting with a full TT present, many of the following adjuncts can be completed in sequence with assessment and resuscitation. In a less-well-resourced setting, they should occur after life-threatening injuries have been addressed.

Monitoring

Monitoring should be applied in the pre-hospital environment and maintained until the patient's condition is considered stable. This includes continuous monitoring of the patient's vital signs, GCS and neurovascular status, which enables the paramedic at the scene and en route and the TT to identify the patient's injuries and titrate the patient's response to resuscitation. Cardiac and ventilatory monitoring leads, pulse oximetry, core body temperature monitoring and $EtCO_2$ should be commenced as soon as practical in the primary survey.[7,12]

Once the patient has arrived at the treating hospital and patency of the airway is established, venous (VBG) or arterial blood gases (ABG) should be taken to enable assessment of ventilation and to monitor the patient's transfusion state (see Ch 17, p. 329, for information on collecting arterial blood gases). Changes in pH and the base deficit can prompt not only ventilation changes but also transfusion requirements. Close monitoring of the $EtCO_2$ will assist in assessing the efficacy of ventilator settings and in confirming placement of the ETT at the time of intubation. Any deterioration should be immediately communicated with medical staff.

Urinary catheters and gastric tubes

An indwelling urinary catheter (IDC) is a vital adjunct, as urine output is a sensitive sign of the volume status in the patient and can give an indication of the patient's renal perfusion.[67] Urethral injury is a contraindication for IDC insertion, and and should be suspected in the presence of blood at the urethral meatus, perineal bruising, swelling, a high-riding prostate and

in patients with a straddle or maligned pelvic fracture. In a female, additional signs such as lower abdominal tenderness and macroscopic haematuria are also contraindications.[66,67] See Chapter 48 for urinary catheter insertion guidelines in pelvic trauma.

Gastric tubes are indicated to assist in stomach decompression, decreasing the risk of aspiration, especially in the patient who cannot protect their own airway, and to prevent obstruction of diaphragmatic motion in the paediatric patient. Patients with extensive faciomaxillary and/or suspected basal skull fractures should have their gastric tube placed orally. Orogastric tubes are not routinely placed in the pre-hospital setting, although orogastric tubes, particularly in children, may be placed in unconscious patients.

Laboratory tests

It is essential that, as an adjunct to the primary survey, baseline bloods are taken: this can be at the time of peripheral or central line insertion. Blood tests should include group and hold, coagulation studies, full blood count and biochemistry. All female patients of childbearing age will require a beta-hCG (pregnancy) test; this can be done on a urine dipstick and confirmed with blood test. It is essential that the blood samples are correctly labelled and signed, as significant delays in obtaining cross-matched blood can occur with simple labelling errors. Table 44.7 lists the most common tests and their clinical implications. Massive transfusion protocols are moving towards goal-directed transfusion therapy, using viscoelastic haemostatic assays, such as ROTEM and TEG. These tools measure clot formation and breakdown in whole blood, enabling rapid and timely identification of coagulopathy and product replacement needs.[68]

Primary survey X-rays

The 'trauma series' X-rays include lateral cervical spine, chest and pelvis. Diagnostic studies should not delay or interfere in any way with ongoing patient resuscitation. The chest and pelvic X-ray can quickly identify large sources of blood loss and help to guide resuscitation and early blood transfusion.[7] The lateral cervical spine X-ray can identify a significant cervical spine fracture; however, if it is negative, this does not rule out cervical spine injury and spinal immobilisation must be maintained until formal assessment of the entire spine is conducted.[29,69] See Chapter 49 for spinal clearance guidelines.

Do not avoid diagnostic tests in the pregnant patient. Radiation risk in pregnancy is related to the fetal radiation dose and the stage of pregnancy, being most significant during organogenesis (up to 9 weeks gestation). Most diagnostic radiology procedures pose no substantial risk to the mother or fetus when compared with other risks throughout the pregnancy.[12,69,70] The pregnant woman presents two patients for care, but the principle of care is to provide trauma care to the mother. Optimal resuscitation of the mother will allow the optimal chance of fetal survival. Table 44.8 outlines the common radiology studies and their clinical implications.

Unique patient groups

The paediatric, elderly, obstetric and obese patient should have the primary survey conducted systematically as for other patients; however, there exist special criteria in each group which need to be considered. Each of these groups also has increased

TABLE 44.7 Common laboratory tests[8,71]	
LABORATORY TEST	CLINICAL IMPLICATIONS
Full blood count (FBC)	Haematocrit and haemoglobin may be normal or above normal despite acute haemorrhage; normal values do not exclude haemorrhagic shock
Electrolytes	Baseline data
	Rule out electrolyte imbalance
Coagulation profile	Baseline data
	Rule out coagulopathies
	Include activated partial thromboplastin time (APTT) and international normalised ratio (INR)
	Fibrinogen
Amylase/lipase levels	Baseline data
	Elevated value may indicate possible intraabdominal injury
Lipase	Baseline data
	Elevated value may indicate possible intraabdominal injury; has higher sensitivity for pancreatic injury
Lactate	Baseline data
	Elevated level correlates with acute haemorrhage, shock and increased anaerobic metabolism
Arterial blood gas (ABG)	Assess ventilatory and respiratory status
	Acidosis, especially in the presence of normal or decreased $PaCO_2$ level, correlates with shock
	Base deficit of −6 or greater correlates with acute haemorrhage and shock
	Decreased PaO_2 and SaO_2 and an elevated $PaCO_2$ may indicate an airway or breathing emergency
Liver function tests (LFTs)	Baseline data
	Elevated values may indicate liver damage
Type and cross-match	Prepare for administration of blood and blood products
Urinalysis	Dip for blood; gross haematuria suggests injury

$PaCO_2$, partial pressure of carbon dioxide in arterial gas; PaO_2, alveolar-arterial difference in partial pressure of oxygen; SaO_2, arterial oxygen saturation

TABLE 44.8 Primary survey X-rays[3]		
EXAMINATION	INDICATION	CLINICAL IMPLICATIONS
Chest X-ray	Blunt trauma	Should be taken immediately upon arrival if possible
	Chest trauma or pain	Anteroposterior examination with patient in supine position if immobilised
	Shortness of breath	Do not delay treatment of a suspected tension pneumothorax for a chest X-ray
	Abnormal breath sounds	
Pelvic X-ray	Blunt trauma	Anteroposterior examination with patient in supine position
	Pelvic pain or instability	Should be taken early in the resuscitation
	Blood at urethral meatus	
Cervical spine X-ray	Blunt trauma	Cross-table lateral film usually obtained early in resuscitation, with three views required to complete the series which include C1 to T1
	Trauma above nipple line	
	Neck tenderness	Immobilisation should be maintained until spine is radiographically and clinically cleared
	Neurological deficit	

TABLE 44.9 Paediatric, elderly and pregnant patient group considerations[1,3,7,11,12,70,72,73]			
PAEDIATRIC (CH 36)	ELDERLY > 65 (CH 39)	PREGNANT (CH 35)	BARIATRIC
Special Considerations			
Include the carer in emergency management Infants may rapidly deteriorate	Physiological effects of ageing Include the carer in emergency Ensure early cognitive assessment Will sustain a more significant injury than those younger with the same amount of force Higher index of suspicion Impact of pre-existing medical conditions	Consider pregnancy in all females 10–50 years of age Best treatment for the fetus is optimal care of the mother 12 weeks: uterus intrapelvic organ Uterus is thick-walled, of limited size and sits in bony pelvis 20 weeks: uterus at umbilicus Enlarged fetus is protected by amniotic fluid 34–36 weeks: uterus at costal margins If vertex presentation, fetal head is in the pelvis	Large size Significant increase in adipose tissue Oedematous limbs
Airway			
Be aware of anatomical differences Place padding beneath infant's and young child's shoulder to ensure neutral alignment of cervical spine Oropharyngeal airway not turned 180° Anticipate intubation	Require early intubation due to decrease in cardiopulmonary reserves Fragile tissues in oropharyngeal and nasopharyngeal airways Degenerative changes to laryngeal cartilage increases risk of fracture with neck trauma Arthritic changes to jaw and spine	Pregnant patients may have a normal $PaCO_2$ in respiratory failure due to changing tidal volume 8 times to risk of failed intubation due to mucosal oedema	Lack of landmarks and increased adipose tissue increase difficulty for intubation and cricothyroidotomy Be aware of airway obstruction when patient supine due to increase in adipose tissue Increase risk of aspiration caused by gastro-oesophageal reflux, hiatus hernia and increased abdominal pressure Regular O_2 mask to small Co-morbidities of sleep apnoea V/Q mismatching due to reduced lung volumes
Breathing			
Difficult for children to increase tidal volume Children use abdominal muscles for respiration Signs of pneumothorax are less obvious in a child Ensure gastric tube in intubated patient Bradycardia a sign of hypoventilation	Decreased respiratory reserve and increase in chronic diseases (COPD) Caution with CO_2-retaining patients Decreased ability to increase work of breathing Pain control and physiotherapy essential Less tolerant of pulmonary injuries	BP falls by 5–15 mmHg in 2nd trimester Minute ventilation increases due to increased progesterone Decreased residual volume Beware of pregnant patient with $PaCO_2$ of 35–45 mmHg	Oxygen consumption and carbon dioxide production increases Breathing effort increases and efficiency of air exchange decreases Decreased functional residual capacity Decreased lung and chest wall compliance SpO_2 may not work on periphery due to increased adipose tissue Difficulty auscultating breath sounds

Continued

TABLE 44.9 Paediatric, elderly and pregnant patient group considerations[1,3,7,11,12,70,72,73]—cont'd

PAEDIATRIC (CH 36)	ELDERLY > 65 (CH 39)	PREGNANT (CH 35)	BARIATRIC
Circulation			
Heart rate assessed using brachial and femoral pulses	Decreased total blood volume	Cardiac output increase 1.0–1.5 L/min by week 10	Metabolic and cardiac demands increase
Decreased BP ominous sign in a child	Decreased cardiac function	Beware that pregnant patient in supine position can compress vena cava and decrease cardiac output	Cardiac output, stroke volume increase
Bradycardia a hallmark of impending cardiac arrest	Predisposed to dysrhythmias	Heart rate increase 15 beats/minute	Hypoxia and hypercarbia leads to pulmonary hypertension and right-sided heart failure
Small surface area makes children very prone to hypothermia	More dependent on atrial filling to drive cardiac output	34 weeks: increase in plasma volume and decreased haematocrit	Risk for venous thromboembolism
	Decreased glomerular filtration rate and renal blood flow	Blood loss of 1200–1500 mL before signs of shock	Vascular access poor due to loss of landmarks, greater skin-to-blood vessels distance and short neck
	Decreased creatinine clearance rates	Increase in white blood cells	BP cuffs may not fit
	Beware of normal BP in a elderly patient	Increase in clotting times	May need Dopplers for pulses due to oedematous limbs
	Prone to anaemia	Anaemia	FAST scan useless
	Be cognisant of cardiac medications (beta-blockers)		Inability to CT scan or X-ray due to weight restrictions

BP: blood pressure; COPD: chronic obstructive pulmonary disease; CT: computed tomography; FAST: focused abdominal sonography in trauma; PaCO$_2$: partial arterial pressure of carbon dioxide; SpO$_2$: oxygen saturation; V/Q: ventilation–perfusion

psychosocial needs. Table 44.9 illustrates the differences in priorities for paediatric, pregnant, elderly and bariatric (obese) patients.

For paediatric patients the quantities of blood, fluids and medications vary with the size of the child, as does the degree and rapidity of heat loss. Injury mechanisms and patterns are also different.[7,11,12] These are discussed in Chapter 36.

The elderly patient will sustain more significant injury than will a younger patient from the same amount of force. The ED nurse should have a higher index of suspicion, as the elderly trauma patient has a significantly increased mortality and morbidity rate. For the elderly patient, special consideration needs to be given based on the physiological body changes of the older person, mechanisms of injury, pre-existing medical conditions and response to injury (see also Ch 39).[6,11,74,75]

Pregnant trauma patient presentations are not frequent, but pregnancy must be considered in any female patient aged 10–50 years. The best treatment for the fetus is the provision of optimal treatment of the mother. It must be considered that the anatomical and physiological changes in pregnancy may modify the patient's response to the injury.[7,11,72,73] Early recognition of pregnancy by palpation of the abdomen for a gravid uterus, laboratory testing (beta-hCG), patient history of menstrual cycle and early fetal assessments and monitoring with early liaison with an obstetrician are important for maternal and fetal survival.

The pregnant or gravid uterus also poses the risk of compression of the inferior vena cava when the woman is lying supine. The inferior vena cava is compressed in the majority of pregnant women in the second trimester, and the compression may affect the uterine artery blood flow. To overcome this, manual manipulation of the uterus is required in emergency situations when clinicians are unable to place the pregnant female in the lateral position because of injury or treatment such as cardiopulmonary resuscitation. Manual manipulation is achieved by placing one hand on either side of the pregnant abdomen and lifting the uterus and fetus off the vena cava and spine, and repositioning it to the lateral side of the abdomen. This relieves pressure on the vena cava, reinstating maternal circulation. A pillow can be placed under the left buttock, repositioning the pregnant female into the lateral position. Placental abruption and other obstetric emergencies and physiology are discussed in Chapter 35.

Obesity worldwide is rapidly becoming a significant public health issue, with more than 1 billion adults and 22 million children under 5 years of age being overweight, and 300 million adults being obese;[76] this equates to 23.2% of the world's population being overweight and 9.8% being obese. As in other developing countries, Australia is seeing rapid growth in this population. It is estimated that worldwide by 2030 there will be 2.6 billion overweight individuals with 1.12 billion suffering from obesity.[77]

Obesity affects every body system and results in the patient being in a chronic inflammatory state. The patient's sheer physical size also increases the challenges involved in both the pre-hospital and the in-hospital environments, making every procedure more challenging. The mortality rate for the obese trauma patient is increased eight times when compared with a trauma patient in the normal weight range. Injury mechanisms also affect the obese patient differently. The increased adipose tissue means that there is an increased force when a traumatic mechanism is sustained; obese patients have an increased incidence of thoracic, pelvic and lower extremity injuries and a lower incidence of head injuries.[77–79]

In the pre-hospital environment there are particular challenges in this group, mainly due to the physical size of the patient. Standard equipment carried in ambulances often is not suitable in managing the obese patient and there may be time delays in sourcing equipment such as spine boards or ambulance trolleys suitable for a weight over 230 kg. In some instances, alternative methods may need to be implemented for splinting and spinal immobilisation. Restrictions on air ambulances may also have impacts on triage and transfer decisions, potentially extending scene times and increasing transportation times. This could be fatal in a time-critical case. It is imperative that paramedics take as comprehensive a history as possible from the patient as early as possible so that the hospital can be prepared for the patient. This may be the only time that these details can be obtained.[77–79]

Secondary survey

The secondary survey is not performed until the primary survey and its adjuncts have been completed. Many major trauma patients require transport to the operating suite for treatment of life-threatening injuries such as damage control surgery/laparotomy (Ch 47), and thus the secondary survey would need to be completed postoperatively.[1,7] The secondary survey is a complete physical examination using the 'head-to-toe' method. The aim is to identify all injuries and the interventions required. Table 44.10 outlines the secondary survey assessment guidelines and interventions, and Figure 44.11 shows specific body region assessments.

Tertiary survey

Exit block exists in many hospitals and can result in considerable delays in transferring the trauma patient to the ward. If the patient has an extended length of stay in the ED, they require the performance of the tertiary survey in the ED rather than in the ward. The trauma tertiary survey, as defined by the American College of Surgeons,[7] is an evaluation that identifies and catalogues all injuries and operative interventions after the initial resuscitation. It encompasses a repeated primary and secondary survey, including a head-to-toe assessment. This should consist of a comprehensive review of the patient's medical records with emphasis on mechanism of injury and

---

TABLE 44.10 Secondary survey interventions[3,12]

ASSESSMENT	INTERVENTIONS
F = Full set of vital signs/five interventions	In addition to obtaining a complete set of vital signs, consider the five interventions: • Cardiac monitor • Pulse oximeter (SpO$_2$) • Urinary catheter if not contraindicated • Gastric tube (oral or naso) • Laboratory studies Facilitate family presence
G = Give comfort measures	Verbal reassurance Touch Pain control
H = History Should include mechanism of injury (see Ch 43). Can be obtained from family. AMPLE is a useful pneumonic to ensure all essential information is obtained: **A**llergies **M**edications currently used **P**ast illnesses/**P**regnancy **L**ast meal **E**vents leading up to accident	
H = Head-to-toe assessment	
Head, skull and face	
Look for lacerations, ecchymosis, deformities, contusions, bleeding, drainage from nose and ears, and check pupil size and reactivity, ocular bleeding swelling, crepitus Feel for tenderness, note bony crepitus, deformity, bony step-offs and midface instability	Pain control Maintain airway patency Remove contact lenses Haemorrhage control

Continued

TABLE 44.10 Secondary survey interventions[3,12]—cont'd	
ASSESSMENT	INTERVENTIONS
Cervical spine and neck (see Ch 49)	
Remove the anterior portion of the cervical collar to inspect and palpate the neck. Maintain manual stabilisation of cervical spine while collar is removed. Look for wounds, ecchymosis, deformities and distended neck veins Feel for tenderness, note bony crepitus, deformity, swelling, subcutaneous emphysema and tracheal position	Maintain spinal immobilisation Ensure correctly fitting cervical collar, consider changing from hard collar (extrication collar) to a soft collar (Philadelphia) Use direct pressure if haemorrhage control required
Chest (see Ch 47)	
Look for breathing rate and depth, wounds, deformities, ecchymosis, use of accessory muscles, paradoxical movement, expansion and symmetry Listen to breath and heart sounds Feel for tenderness, note bony crepitus, subcutaneous emphysema and deformity including clavicles and shoulders	Prepare for needle decompression to relieve tension pneumothorax Prepare for chest tube insertion to follow needle decompression or for pneumothorax or haemothorax Prepare for pericardiocentesis as needle for relief of pericardial tamponade
Abdomen and flanks (see Ch 48)	
Look for sounds, distension, ecchymosis or seatbelt sign and scars Listen for bowel sounds in each quadrant Feel four quadrants for tenderness, rigidity, guarding, masses and femoral pulses	Anticipate FAST or Assist with DPL Insert gastric tube and urinary catheter Anticipate transportation to CT scanner Maintain high index of suspicion of a lumbar spine fracture or hollow viscus injury if seatbelt sign present
Pelvis and perineum (see Chs 48 and 50)	
Look for wounds, deformities and lacerations; ecchymosis, priapism, blood at the urinary meatus or in the perineal area Feel the pelvis for instability or crepitus and anal sphincter tone, prostate position, rectal wall integrity or vaginal wall integrity	Apply external pelvic immobilisation (i.e. pelvic sling or sheet) if not done already in patients with suspected pelvic fracture Assist with urethrogram if bladder trauma suspected
Extremities (see Ch 50)	
All four limbs and hands and feet should be examined Look for deformity, open wounds, ecchymosis and swelling, rotation, shortening Feel for ecchymosis, abnormal bony movement, joint instability wounds and deformities Assess motor and sensory deficits, circulation and capillary refill Compartment syndrome pulses, pain, paralysis, paraesthesia, pallor	Check pulses in all limbs Apply splints to extremity fractures and elevate effected limbs Administer analgesia followed by pain assessment Assist with radiography studies Dress all open wounds with sterile dressings Administer antibiotics as required
I = Inspect posterior surfaces	
Maintain cervical spine stabilisation and support injured extremities while the patient is log-rolled Look at posterior surface for wounds, deformities and ecchymosis Feel posterior surfaces for tenderness and deformities, pain, anal sphincter tone (if not performed previously)	Maintain spinal precautions Control external haemorrhage

CT: computed tomography; DPL: diagnostic peritoneal lavage; FAST: focused assessment with sonography in trauma; SpO₂: oxygen saturation

FIGURE 44.11 Secondary survey assessments.

SECONDARY SURVEY

HEAD-TO-TOE ASSESSMENT

Continuously reassess ABCD

Face
• lacerations
• faciomaxillary fractures
• check for broken teeth
• check for contact lenses
• check eye vision and pupils
• inspect for ecchymosis around the eyes

Neck and Cervical Spine
Immobilise until injury has been excluded.
Inspect and palpate for:
• tenderness
• penetrating wounds
• subcutaneous emphysema
• tracheal deviation
• laryngeal fracture
• observe appearance of neck veins

Head
• Examine and palpate scalp for swellings, depressions and lacerations
• examine ear canals, mouth and nose for leakage of CSF

Thorax
Examine entire chest
• palpate clavicle and ribs
• apply gentle sternal compression to check for sternal fracture or flail segments
• auscultate breath and heart sounds
• do ECG
• consider cardio/pulmonary contusion:
  –cardiac dysrhythmias
  –ruptured aorta/diaphragm
• perforated oesophagus
• think abdominal injuries if lower ribs injured

Musculoskeletal
Inspect all limbs:
• bruising
• wounds
• soft tissue injuries
• deformities
• pain/tenderness
• vascular/neurological deficits
• pelvic mobility

Spine and Neurological
Includes motor and sensory evaluation of the extremities
Re-evaluation of:
• conscious level
• pupil size and response
• full GCS
Signs of spinal injury:
• hypotension
• relative bradycardia
• decreased motor power and sensation below level of lesion
• decreased sphincter tone
• priapism

Abdomen
Inspect, auscultate and palpate for:
• presence of free intra-peritoneal fluid
• bowel sounds
• guarding
Look for bruising/pain/tenderness
Consider signs of renal injury:
• flank pain
• bruising
• haematuria

Pelvis and Perineum
Inspect for:
• haematoma/bleeding
• contusion/lacerations
• scrotal haematoma
• tampon
• consider pregnancy test
• consider pelvic fractures

Rectum
Inspect and palpate for:
• sphincter tone
• prostate
• blood in faeces

Insert—if time permits
Insert tubes as necessary
NGT
• decompress stomach
• consider orogastric tube, if base of skull suspected
• protect cervical spine
IDC
• only insert if pelvis stable and no blood at urethral meatus
• monitor urinary output
• urinalysis attended—blood
• consider suprapubic catheter

Other considerations
• Danger to self
• Completely undress the patient for examination. Remember privacy and warmth during examination
• Get a complete set of vital signs
• Ensure clear, accurate and concise documentation
• Obtain history
  •Pre-hospital information
  M Mechanisims of injury
  I Injuries sustained
  S Signs and symptoms
  T Treatment
  •Patient-generated history
  A Allergies
  M Medications
  P Past history
  L Last ate and drank
  E Events leading up to incident
• Tetanus
• Analgesia
• Antibiotics

Trauma Advice & Referral Line: 1800 700 001
OR
Victorian Adult Emergency Retrieval
& Coordination Service: (03) 9417 3800
Prepare patient for definitive care
Complete forms for transfer and photocopy all documentation X-rays, ECG, Obs, GCS, Ambulance Case sheet
If time does not allow for comprehensive notes consider reporting after patient leaves and fax to receiving hospital
Consider telephoning receiving hospital to hand over to nursing staff
Communicate with and support family/friends

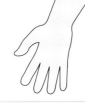
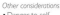

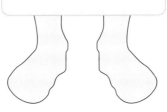

Adapted from Victorian Department of Human Services

relevant co-morbidities, and examination of all blood tests, radiology and procedures.

The recommended time-frame for the tertiary survey is ≥ 24 hours, and once the patient regains consciousness post injury.[80] The trauma tertiary survey is a vital part of the trauma patient's assessment: it provides continuity of care, promotes communication among the multidisciplinary trauma caregivers to meet the needs of the patient, strengthens the plan of care and maximises patient outcomes. Regular tertiary surveys have also been shown to decrease the mortality and morbidity in the multi-trauma patient and can be conducted by the ED nurse or medical staff members.[8]

Ongoing nursing care in the ED

After the initial resuscitation, patients not requiring urgent operative intervention may spend significant time in the ED. There are several key aspects of nursing care that will contribute to improved patient outcome and experience.

IV fluids and medication administration

A fluid balance chart must be commenced or continued, ensuring that all fluids administered are recorded from the time of admission; this includes all fluid outputs, including estimations of blood and fluid loss. This is essential to assist in the monitoring not only of fluid resuscitation but also to allow you to monitor for any signs of kidney injury post contrast administration or from trauma. Ensure that there are adequate fluids prescribed for the ongoing care of the patient, and if the patient is able to eat and drink, ensure that this is documented and that the patient is commenced on diet and fluids as soon as they are able.

Observations and progress notes

All essential details of patient admission should be documented, including any interventions and/or treatment, a list of valuables, next of kin details and any additional history.

Ensure that frequent observations are ordered and commenced, including vital signs, GCS, fluid balance chart, monitoring of ICCs and ventilation observations.

Analgesia

Ensure that the patient's pain score is recorded and measured, and that appropriate analgesia is prescribed and dosed according to the patient's response. If the patient is a child, record their weight for calculation of drug dosing. Paediatric patients present special challenges related to their age and development; it is key to all family/carers to be available to assist/nurse infants and toddlers during pain assessments for reassurance and assistance with assessment (see Ch 36, Table 36.6). If the patient has complex pain needs, referral to the acute pain service may be appropriate.

Venothromboembolism prophylaxis

Early commencement of venothromboembolism (VTE) prophylaxis can prevent early development of deep vein thrombosis (DVT) and/or pulmonary embolism (PE); this should be discussed with the treating team. Nurses should be aware of the contraindications for pharmacological prophylaxis and, if one of these exists, ensure that the patient has alternative VTE prophylaxis measures in place, such as compression stockings and/or electronic sequential calf compressors or foot pumps. Patient education regarding VTE prevention is also fundamental to the care of a trauma patient.

Spinal care

If the patient requires spinal immobilisation for a suspected or confirmed spinal cord or column injury, ensure that regular 4-hourly log-rolling and collar care is attended to. This will enable visual inspection of the patient's skin surfaces, hygiene and also assist in chest physiotherapy (see Ch 14 for pressure-area and other essential nursing care).

Criteria for early transfer

All members of the TT must know their hospital's capabilities and limitations in caring for patients. The vast majority of patients will be easily cared for at a local level and will not require transfer; however, it is essential that those patients who do need to be transferred be referred early. In Australia and New Zealand, triage to a major trauma service should be within 15–30 minutes.[13] The major trauma service has the resources to provide expert treatment throughout the span of trauma care. Each hospital should have established interhospital trauma transfer guidelines specific to their territory, region or state readily available to all staff. The ED nurse should be aware of these guidelines and aim to expedite transfer to definitive care if required within 30 minutes of arrival.[1] Table 44.11 defines major trauma patient characteristics which indicate transfer is required to a major trauma service.

Family presence

Family presence in trauma resuscitations is a highly controversial topic, with wide-ranging opinions offered.[81–83] Historically, both medical and nursing staff viewed family as guests rather than an integral part of the patient's illness, recovery and/or death.[81] Substantial research[81–82] has demonstrated that there are benefits for families in being present, such as allowing a shared experience between patient and family, helping to facilitate grieving if death occurs, assisting with closure and decreasing family fear and anxiety. Some researchers believe that these benefits far outweigh the risks, such as the effect that witnessing the resuscitation may have on the family, increasing stress on the trauma team, interference from family, lack of support for the family during the resuscitation, as well as an increased risk of medico-legal action. In fact, many family members only recall the pain of the resuscitation and have no real memory of specific procedures and events.[82,83] It should be remembered that 'family' not only pertains to those related by blood or marriage, but also to significant others who share an established relationship with the patient.

The success of the family presence depends on all TT members, particularly the nursing staff—who are usually responsible for preparing the family to enter the resuscitation— guiding and supporting them throughout and being able to answer their questions.[82,83] Considerations for family presence are discussed further in Chapters 15 and 53. Most hospitals, especially trauma centres, will have as part of the TT a social worker or pastoral care worker who can be available to support the family throughout the resuscitation and throughout the patient's hospital stay in the case that a member of the TT team

TABLE 44.11 Criteria for early transfer of trauma patients[14,92]

VITAL SIGNS (MAJOR TRAUMA IF ANY ONE OF THE FOLLOWING PRESENT)	ADULT > 15 YEARS	NEWBORN < 2 WEEKS	INFANT < 1 YEAR	CHILD 1–8 YEARS	LARGE CHILD 9–15 YEARS
Respiratory rate (breaths/minute)	< 10 or > 30	< 40 or > 60	< 20 or > 50	< 20 or > 35	< 15 or > 25
Cyanosis	Present	Cool/pale clammy	Cool/pale clammy	Cool/pale clammy	Cool/pale clammy
Hypotension (mmHg)	< 90	—	< 60	< 70	< 80
Glasgow Coma Scale	< 13	< 15	< 15	< 15	< 15

Injuries

Serious or suspected serious penetrating injuries:

- to head/neck/chest/abdomen/pelvis/axilla/groin

Blunt injuries:

- patient with a significant injury to a single region head/neck/chest/abdomen/pelvis/axilla/groin
- patient with injury to two or more of the above body regions

Specific injuries:

- limb amputations/limb-threatening injuries
- suspected spinal cord injury
- burns > 20% or suspected respiratory tract
- serious crush injury
- major compound fracture or open dislocation
- fracture to two or more of the following: femur/tibia/humerus
- fractured pelvis

(medical or nursing) is not available to support families in this situation.

Post-traumatic stress

Traumatic injury and mental health disorders are co-associated.[84] Patients with traumatic injury report a substantial reduction in health-related quality of life compared to other patients, including long-term psychological and physical disability.[85] The psychological impact of injury includes the development of acute and long-term mental health problems, such as post-traumatic stress, depression and anxiety. ASD occurs in up to 45% of injury survivors[85] and, similar to PTSD, involves an anxiety response that includes re-experience of the traumatic event, intrusive memories, dreams and strong emotional distress on exposure to triggering events.[86,87] Early identification of depression, anxiety and stress symptoms and associated prevention may reduce long-term symptoms and negative impacts. Intensive care unit admission and high levels of depression, anxiety and stress at 3 months post injury are predictors for high levels of depression, anxiety and stress at 6 months.[84] Low levels of depression, anxiety and stress during hospital admission are correlated with low levels of depression, anxiety and stress at 3 and 6 months. It is recommended that using a validated tool such as the DASS-21, which takes 2 minutes to complete, should be used as a screening tool in admitted trauma patients to identify patients at risk of long-term symptoms and facilitate preventive intervention.[84]

SUMMARY

The importance of thorough and accurate initial assessment and management of the trauma patient at all phases of care cannot be overstated. System, staff and departmental preparation minimises confusion and decreases the time to definitive care. A systematic approach to assessment and intervention improves patient outcomes through early recognition of potentially life-threatening injuries and intervention for identified problems.

The paramedic and ED nurse must advocate for trauma patient protection and prevent secondary insult as much as possible, while assisting with necessary life-saving interventions. They should have solid trauma management knowledge and be able to assess the trauma patient, be aware of the patient's physiological status and treatment received and expedite the patient to definitive care.

CASE STUDY

Part 1—pre-hospital

Mechanism

A 22-year-old male, the single occupant of a ute driven at high speed on a wet and cold night, crashes into a tree. He is entrapped in the vehicle upside down by his legs for approximately 1 hour. He has been drinking since 6 pm, and there is a strong smell of alcohol on his breath. He is found by passers-by who call the major trauma service (MTS). He is transferred to hospital via helicopter. The scene is attended by the fire brigade who assist with the extrication.

Time-frame is:

- 2100 hours—ambulance called
- 2145 hours—arrival at scene
- 2230 hours—departure from scene
- 2310 hours—off stretcher.

Injuries

Altered conscious state, swollen and bruised left eye, seat-belt abrasion to chest and abdomen, complaining of pain to chest, abdomen and numbness and pain in lower legs. Query spinal cord injury, obvious open lower leg fracture with large blood loss.

Signs—2150 hours

- Systolic blood pressure 90 mmHg
- Pulse rate 110 beats/minute
- Oxygen saturation unknown
- Glasgow Coma Scale (GCS) score 13 (eye 3, verbal 4, motor 6)
- Temperature 34°C.

Treatment

- Spinal immobilisation: head held in pouring rain, clothing removed from around neck and cervical collar applied.
- Extrication using spine board, patient initially upside down in vehicle held by seat-belt.
- Patient's wet clothing removed.
- Intravenous (IV) access 16G to right bicep, patient flailing around, very hard to cannulate and get blood pressure, SpO$_2$ not sensing as peripherally shut down.
- Pelvis wrap applied with sheet.
- Palpable surgical emphysema on the left chest wall, with decreased air entry, chest decompressed with pneumocath, audible hiss, intercostal catheter (ICC) inserted.
- Splint to heavily bleeding lower leg and gauze pads applied.
- Oxygen applied 8 L/min.

Questions

1. What are the priorities of care by the emergency medical service staff?
2. Is the patient's treatment conducted according to the primary survey?
3. What alternatives to IV access could have been utilised in this case?
4. Why is the mechanism of injury important information in diagnosing injuries?

Part 2—emergency department

The paramedic calls the MTS and provides hand-over to the receiving consultant. Based on this information a trauma alert is initiated and the patient is given a triage category 1.

- Mechanism—high-speed motor vehicle collision versus tree, then roll-over, entrapped possibly 60 minutes.
- Injuries—possible closed head injury, chest, abdomen and spine, open tibia fracture large.
- Signs—heart rate 130 beats/minute, blood pressure 100 mmHg, respiratory rate 24 breaths/minute, oxygen saturation unknown, GCS 12 with loss of consciousness and retrograde amnesia.
- Treatment—1 × IV cannula, IV fluids, oxygen, pelvic splint and ICC inserted.

The trauma team assemble to meet the patient and primary and secondary surveys are performed.

Primary survey

- Airway—patent, trachea midline, cervical spine collar in situ
- Breathing—oxygen via non-rebreather 15 L/min, air entry, unequal, increased work of breathing, obvious chest deformity on right side, possible flail.
- Circulation—1 × IV cannula noted, unable to insert any others due to vasoconstriction and hypovolaemia, intraosseous catheter inserted into left tibial plateau. Commence uncrossed O-negative red blood cell transfusion immediately and 1 unit fresh frozen plasma, 1 unit platelets.
- Disability—patient eye opening to voice, not obeying commands or verbalising, GCS 8 (eye 3, verbal 1, motor 4); patient's temperature was 34°C, hypothermia guideline was implemented, remaining wet clothes removed and warm fluids and blanket applied.

Signs—2310 hours

- Blood pressure 100/60 mmHg
- Pulse rate 110 beats/minute
- Respiratory rate 20 breaths/minute

- Oxygen saturation 92%
- Temperature 34°C
- GCS score 8
- Pupils PEARL 4+.

Treatment

- A decision is made to intubate, additional IV access is gained and infusion of red blood cells is commenced and a pelvic sheet replaced with a pelvic binder.

Adjuncts to primary survey

- Chest X-ray—multiple right-sided rib fractures, haemopneumothorax.
- Pelvis X-ray—open-book pelvic fracture.
- FAST: negative.

Secondary survey

- HEENT—bruising and abrasions to left eye, external auditory canal NAD (no abnormalities detected), no crepitus or bony step-offs. Cervical collar in situ.
- Chest—seat-belt bruising, visible flail segment, reduced breath sounds to right side.
- Abdomen/pelvis—seat-belt abrasion to abdomen, pelvic sling in situ, abdomen soft, and pelvis not manipulated, blood at the external meatus.
- Extremities—NAD; obvious left leg tibial fracture ?
- Neurological examination—patient sedated, unable to assess sensation and/or motor, was moving all limbs on arrival.
- Back/spine—nil bruising or deformity, step or abrasions, anal tone NAD.
- History—unable to attain past medical history as patient GCS 3 and intubated

Adjuncts to secondary survey

- Trauma bloods—ethanol; full blood count; coagulation profile; urea, electrolytes, creatinine; liver function; cross-match.
- Insertion of arterial line.
- Arterial blood gases: pH 7.30; PCO_2 45 mmHg, PO_2 100 mmHg, lactate 3.3 μ/L
- Computed tomography (CT) trauma series.
- X-ray right leg.
- Emergency trauma urethrogram.
- Indwelling catheter (IDC).
- Nasogastric tube.
- Splint to open tibial fracture.
- ICC for haemopneumothorax.

Initial treatment plan

The patient undergoes an emergency trauma urethrogram which is normal and an IDC is inserted. He has an ICC inserted into his right chest which drains 200 mL of haemoserous fluid. He has a nasogastric tube inserted which drains bile-stained fluid. Once stabilised, he has a CT trauma series (head, neck, chest, abdomen and pelvis) with CT angiography of chest. Emergency theatre is booked for open reduction internal fixation of his open tibial fracture and external fixation of his pelvis; spinal precaution is maintained and the pelvic sling is maintained.

The patient remains haemodynamically stable during transfer to CT, his blood pressure is maintained at 90–100 mmHg with blood products and crystalloid solution. He is commenced on morphine and midazolam infusions for sedation and analgesia. He remains intubated for the management of his chest injuries; he is admitted to the intensive care unit post-theatre for ongoing stabilisation, rewarming and resuscitation.

CT results

- Brain—closed head injury; isolated small frontal cerebral contusion.
- Cervical spine—NAD.
- Chest—fractured right ribs 1–9 with flail, pulmonary contusion and haemopneumothorax.
- Abdomen—grade 2 liver lacerations.
- Pelvis: open-book pelvic fracture with 5 cm diastases of symphysis pubis and extremity fractures.
- Thoracolumbar spine—transverse processes of T5–9 level.
- Extremity—open, comminuted and displaced midshaft tibia and fibula fractures.

Questions (continued)

5. What level of trauma team activation does this case meet?
6. What would the indications for intubation be in this case?
7. What are the indications for activating a massive blood transfusion guideline?
8. What would impede the assessment of the patient's abdomen?
9. Outline the acute trauma coagulopathy and the steps in this case that may have prevented and/or worsened this condition.
10. How would a liberal transfusion strategy be managed in this case?
11. What steps would need to be taken to deem this patient's cervical spine injury-free?

USEFUL WEBSITES

Australian and New Zealand Burns Assciation, www.anzba.org.au

Australian Emergency Nurses Association, www.acen.com.au

CareFlight NSW, www.careflight.org

Prehospital Trauma Life Support, www.sdc.qld.edu.au/phtls.htm

Trauma Nursing Program (College of Emergency Nursing Australasia), www.tnp.net.au

Trauma.org, www.trauma.org

REFERENCES

1. Moore EE, Feliciano DV, Mattox KL. Trauma. 7th edn. New York: McGraw-Hill; 2012.

2. Gabbe B, Simpson P, Sutherland A et al. Improved functional outcomes for major trauma patients in a regionalized, inclusive system. Annals of Surgery 2012;255(6):1009–15.

3. Newberry L, ed. Sheehy's emergency nursing: principles and practice. 5th edn. St Louis: Mosby; 2003.

4. Victorian State Trauma Registry 1 July 2011 to June 2012: Summary Report. Melbourne, Victoria: Monash University: Victorian State Trauma Outcome Registry and Monitoring Group; 2012.

5. Cameron PA, Gabbe BJ, Cooper DJ et al. A state-wide system of trauma care in Victoria: effect on patient survival. Med J Aust 2008;189(10):546–50.

6. Atkin C, Freedman I, Rosenfeld J et al. The evolution of an integrated state trauma system in Victoria, Australia. Injury 2005; 36(11):1277–87.

7. ATLS manual. American College of Surgeons, Committee on Trauma. Initial assessment and management. In: Advanced Trauma Life Support® for Doctors. 9th edn. Chicago, Illinois: 2012.

8. Newgard CD, Schmicker RH, Hedges JR et al. Emergency medical services intervals and survival in trauma: assessment of the 'golden hour' in a North American prospective cohort. Ann Emerg Med 2010; 55(3):235–46.

9. Morrison CA, Carrick MM, Norman MA et al. Hypotensive resuscitation strategy reduces transfusion requirements and severe postoperative coagulopathy in trauma patients with hemorrhagic shock: preliminary results of randomized controlled trial. J Trauma 2011; 70(3):652–62.

10. Australian College of Emergency Medicine. Guidelines on emergency department design. (2007). Online. www.acem.org.au/media/policies_and_guidelines/G15_ED_Design.pdf; accessed 20 Jan 2014.

11. McQuillan KA, Makic MB, Whalen E, eds. Trauma Nursing: from resuscitation through rehabilitation. 4th edn. Philadelphia: WB Saunders; 2008.

12. Hotz H, Henn R, Lush S et al. Advanced trauma care for nurses. Instructor manual. Sante Fe: Society of Trauma Nurses; 2003.

13. Duffield C, Roche M, O'Brien-Pallas L et al. Glueing it together: nurses, their work environment and patient safety. Centre for Health Services Management. NSW Health: UTS; 2007.

14. ROTES. Review of trauma and emergency services: Victoria 1999. Final report of the Ministerial Taskforce on Trauma and Emergency Services and the department Working Party on Emergency and Trauma Service. Melbourne: Department of Human Services; 1999.

15. Collaborative Health Education and Research Centre annual report. A collaborative regional trauma management model: II. Melbourne: CHERC; 2008; 25–6.

16. Hogan MP, Boone DC. Trauma education and assessment. Injury 2008;39(6):681–5.

17. Hardwood-Nuss AL, Wolfson AB, Linder CH et al. Clinical practice of emergency medicine. 5th edn. Philadelphia: Lippincott; 2010.

18. Bell K, Edington J et al. Trauma team composition policy. Bendigo: Bendigo Healthcare Group Trauma Committee; 2004

19. Bevan C, Officer C, Crameri J et al. Reducing 'cry-wolf'—changing trauma team activation at a pediatric trauma centre. J Trauma 2009;66(3):698–702.

20. Clements A, Curtis K, Horvat L, Shaban R. The effect of a nurse team leader on communication and leadership in major trauma resuscitations. International Emergency Nursing 2014.

21. Curtis K, Olivier J, Mitchell R et al. Evaluation of a tiered trauma call system in a level 1 trauma centre. Injury 2011;42(1):57–62.

22. DiDomenico PB, Pietzsch JB, Paté-Cornell ME. Bayesian assessment of overtriage and undertriage at a level 1 trauma centre. Philos Transact A Math Phys Eng Sci 2008;336(1874):2265–77.

23. Cox S, Currell A, Harris L et al. Evaluation of the Victorian State adult pre-hospital triage criteria. Injury 2012;42(5);573–81.

24. Advisory Committee on Trauma. TRM08.03 Trauma Team Activation: Trauma Call, Version 6.0. The Royal Melbourne Hospital; 2013. http://clinicalguidelines.mh.org.au/brochures/TRM08.03.pdf

25. Advisory Committee on Trauma. TRM08.02 Trauma Team Activation: Trauma Alert, Version 6.0 The Royal Melbourne Hospital; 2013. http://clinicalguidelines.mh.org.au/brochures/TRM08.02.pdf

26. Victoria State Trauma Committee. Adult pre hospital major trauma criteria. About the VSTS. Online. www.health.vic.gov.au/trauma/about.htm.

27. Teixeira PG, Inaba K, Hadjizacharia P et al. Preventable or potentially preventable mortality at a mature trauma center. J Trauma 2007;63(6):1338–46.

28. Kwan I, Bunn F, Roberts I. Spinal immobilisation for trauma patients. Cochrane Database Syst Rev 2001; (2):CD002803.

29. Morris CG, McCoy EP, Lavery GG. Spinal immobilisation for unconscious patients with multiple injuries. BMJ 2004;329(7464):495–9.

30. Cohen SS. Trauma nursing secrets: questions and answers reveal the secrets to safe and effective trauma nursing. Philadelphia: Hanley and Belfus; 2003.

31. Curry, N. Davis, P. What's new in resuscitation strategies for patients with multiple trauma? Injury 2012;43(7):1021–8.

32. Grottke O, Henzler D, Rossaint R. Use of blood and blood products in trauma. Best Pract Res Clin Anaesthesiol 2007;21(2):257–70.

33. Williams B, Boyle M. Estimation of external blood loss by paramedics: is there any point? Prehosp Disaster Med 2007;22(6):502–6.

34. Willis CD, Cameron PA, Bernard SA et al. Cardiopulmonary resuscitation after traumatic cardiac arrest is not always futile. Injury 2006;37(5):448–54.

35. Ambulance Victoria. Clinical practice guidelines for ambulance and MICA paramedics. Melbourne: Victoria; 2009.

36. Hopson LR, Hirsh E, Delgado J et al. Guidelines for withholding or termination of resuscitation in prehospital traumatic cardiopulmonary arrest: Joint Position Statement of the National Association of EMS Physicians and the American College of Surgeons Committee on Trauma. J Am Coll Surg 2003;196(1):106–12.

37. Walcher F, Kirschning T, Muller MP et al. Accuracy of prehospital focused abdominal sonography for trauma after a 1-day hands-on training course. Emerg Med J 2010;27(5):345–9.

38. Melanson SW, McCarthy J, Stromski CJ et al. Aeromedical trauma sonography by flight crews with a miniature ultrasound unit. Prehosp Emerg Care 2001;5(4):399–402.

39. Cox M, Forrest-Horder S. Training the FAST nurse in trauma care. Building a sustainable psychiatry workforce. NSW Health Expo; 2008.

40. Cameron P, Jelinek G, Kelly AM et al, eds. Textbook of adult emergency medicine. 3rd edn. Edinburgh: Churchill Livingstone; 2009.

41. Brain Trauma Foundation. Guideline for the Management of Severe Traumatic Brain Injury. J Neurotrauma 2007;(24) Supp 1–2.

42. Reed D. Initial management of closed head injuries. Sydney: NSW Institute of Trauma and Injury Management; November 2011.

43. Gruen RL, Brohi K, Schreiber M et al. Haemorrhage control in severely injured patients. The Lancet 2012;380(9847):1099–108.

44. Brohi K, Cohen MJ, Ganter MT et al. Acute traumatic coagulopathy: initiated by hypoperfusion: modulated through the protein C pathway? Ann Surg 2007;245(5):812.

45. Frith D, Brohi K. The pathophysiology of trauma-induced coagulopathy. Current Opinion In Critical Care 2012;18(6):631–6.

46. Mommsen P, Andruszkow H, Frömke C et al. Effects of accidental hypothermia on posttraumatic complications and outcome in multiple trauma patients. Injury 2013;44(1):86–90.

47. Moore K. Hypothermia in trauma. J Trauma Nurs 2008;15(2):62–6.

48. Kirkpatrick AW, Chun R, Brown R et al. Hypothermia and the trauma patient. Can J Surg 1999;42(5):333–43.

49. Lewis AM. Trauma triad of death: emergency! Nursing 2000;30(3):62–4.

50. Ollerton J. Emergency airway management in the trauma patient. Sydney: NSW Institute of Trauma and Injury Management; January 2007.

51. Boffard K. Manual of Definitive Surgical Trauma Care. London: Hodder Arnold; 2011.

52. The Royal Children's Hospital Melbourne. 2014 Clinical Practice Guidelines Cervical Spine Assesssment. Online. www.rch.org.au/clinicalguide/guideline_index/Cervical_Spine_Injury/; accessed 25 August 2014.

53. Zunder I. Initial trauma assessment: the anaesthetist's role. Trauma.org; 2002. Online. www.trauma.org/archive/anaesthesia/initialassess.html; accessed 17 June 2015.

54. Gumm K, Liersch K, McDonald D, Judson R, ACT. TRM06.02 Pelvic binder guideline V2 Melbourne: The Royal Melbourne Hospital Trauma Service July 2012.

55. Heetveld M. Management of haemodynamically unstable patient with a pelvic fracture. Sydney: NSW Insitute of Trauma and Injury Management; January 2007.

56. Day M. Intraosseous devices for intravascular access in adult trauma patients. American Association of Critical Care Nurses 2011; 31(2):76–90.

57. Melbourne TRCH. Intraosseous access. Online. www.rch.org.au/clinicalguide/guideline_index/Intraosseous_Access/. accessed March, 2014.

58. Pascoe S, Lynch J. Adult trauma clinical practice guidelines: management of hypovolaemic shock in the trauma patient. Sydney: NSW Institute of Trauma and Injury Management; 2007.

59. Cochrane Injuries Group Albumin Reviewers. Human albumin administration in critically ill patients: systematic review of randomised controlled trials. Br Med J 1998;317(7153):235–40.

60. Finfer SR, Boyce NW, Norton RN. The SAFE study: a landmark trial of the safety of albumin in intensive care. Med J Aust 2004;181(5):237–8.

61. Zalstien S, Pearce A, Scott DM et al. Damage control resuscitation: a paradigm shift in the management of haemorrhagic shock. Emerg Med Australas 2008;20(4):291–3.

62. Olldashi F, Kerçi M, Zhurda T et al. Effects of tranexamic acid on death, vascular occlusive events, and blood transfusion in trauma patients with significant haemorrhage (CRASH-2): a randomised, placebo-controlled trial. Lancet 2010;376(9734):23–32.

63. Wise D, Davies G, Coats T et al. Emergency thoracotomy: 'how to do it'. Emerg Med J 2005;22(1):22–4.

64. Doll D, Bonanno F, Smith MD et al. Emergency department thoracotomy (EDT). Trauma 2005;7:105–8.

65. Hopson LR, Hirsh E, Delgado J et al. Guidelines for withholding or termination of resuscitation in pre-hospital traumatic cardiopulmonary arrest: a joint position paper from the National Association of EMS Physicians Standards and Clinical Practice Committee and the American College of Surgeons Committee on Trauma. Prehosp Emerg Care 2003;7(1):141–6.

66. Cullinane D, Schiller H, Zielinski M et al. Eastern Association for the Surgery of Trauma Practice Management Guidelines for Hemorrhage in Pelvic Fracture—Update and Systematic Review. Journal of Trauma 2011;71(6):1850–68.

67. Holevar M, Edbert J, Luchette F et al. Practice management guidelines for the management of genitourinary trauma. Chicago: Eastern Association for the Surgery of Trauma; 2004.

68. Stensballe J, Ostrowski SR & Johansson PI (2014): Viscoelastic guidance of resuscitation. Current Opinion in Anesthesiology 27, 212–18.

69. Hoffman JR, Mower WR, Wolfson AB et al. Validity of a set of clinical criteria to rule out injury to the cervical spine in patients with blunt trauma. National Emergency X-radiography Utilization Study Group. N Engl J Med 2000;343(2):94–9.

70. Einsiedel P, Gumm K, Judson R, Trauma TACo. TRM 08.07 Xray imaging during pregnancy V3. Melbounre: The Royal Melbourne Hospital Trauma Service; March 2014.

71. Kidd PS, Sturt PA, Fultz J. Mosby's emergency nursing reference. 2nd edn. St Louis: Mosby; 2000.

72. Gumm K, Kennedy M, Oats J et al. TRM05.01 The pregnant trauma patient guideline V3.0 3.14: The Royal Melbourne Hospital Trauma Service; March 2014.

73. Mendez-Figueroa H, Dahlke J, Vrees R, Rouse D. Trauma in pregnancy: an updated systematic review. American Journal of Obstetrics & Gynecology 2013;209(1):1–10.

74. Gabbe B. Special focus report: elderly major trauma patients. Melbourne: Victorian State Trauma Registry and Monitoring Group (VSTORM); 14 August 2012.

75. Stevenson J. When the trauma patient is elderly. J Perianesth Nurs 2004;19(6):392–400.

76. WHO. The SuRF report 2: surveillance of chronic disease risk factors. Geneva: WHO; 2005.

77. Kelly T, Yang W, Chen CS et al. Global burden of obesity in 2005 and projections to 2030. Int J Obes (Lond) 2008;32(9):1431–7. Epub 8 Jul 2008.

78. Ziglar MK. Obesity and the trauma patient: challenges and guidelines for care. J Trauma Nurs 2006;13(1):22–7.

79. VanHoy SN, Laidlow VT. Trauma in obese patients: implications for nursing practice. Crit Care Nurs Clin North Am 2009;23(3):377–89.

80. Biffl WL, Harrington DT, Cioffi WG et al. Implementation of a tertiary trauma survey decreases missed injuries. J Trauma 2003; 54(1):38–44.

81. Jabre P, Belpomme V, Azoulay E et al. Family presence during cardiopulmonary resuscitation. The New England Journal of Medicine 2013;368(268):1008–18.

82. Holzhauser K. Family presence during resuscitation: A randomised controlled trial of the impact of family presence. Australasian Emergency Nursing Journal 2006;8(4):139–47.

83. Aldridge MD, Clark AP. Making the right choice: family presence and the CNS. Clin Nurse Spec 2005;19(3):113–16.

84. Wiseman T, Foster K, Curtis K. Mental health following traumatic physical injury: An integrative literature review. Injury 2013; 44(11):1383–90.

85. Sluys K, Häggmark T, Iselius L. Outcome and quality of life 5 years after major trauma. Journal of Trauma 2005;59(1):223–32.

86. Advisory Committee on Trauma. TRM 01.01 Post Traumatic Amnesia screening and management, Version 1.0. The Royal Melbourne Hospital; 2014. http://clinicalguidelines.mh.org.au/brochures/TRM01.01.pdf; accessed 2 May 2015.

87. Bryant B, Knights K. Pharmacology for Health Professionals. 3rd edn; Elsevier; 2011.

88. Victoria State Trauma Committee. Adult pre-hospital major trauma criteria. About the VSTS. Online. http://health.vic.gov.au/hospitalcirculars/circ02/adult_circ2902.pdf; accessed 17 June 2015.

89. Curtis K, Fraser M, Grant N et al. Adding insult to injury, hypothermia in the trauma patient: a trauma centre's experience in monitoring temperature. Achiev Nurs 2004;6:30–5.

90. Zuidema GD, Rutherford RB, Ballinger WF, eds. The management of trauma. 4th edn. Philadelphia: WB Saunders; 1985.

91. Roberts J, Hedges J, eds. Clinical procedures in emergency medicine. 3rd edn. Philadelphia: WB Saunders; 1998.

92. Bevan C. Pre-hospital criteria for paediatric major trauma patients. Melbourne: The Royal Children's Hospital; 2005.

CHAPTER 45
TRAUMATIC BRAIN INJURY
BRONTE MARTIN, JACQUI MORARTY AND MANOJ SAXENA

Essentials

- Traumatic brain injury is a significant cause of mortality and morbidity in our society.
- The primary injury is due to the effect of mechanical traumatic effects on the central nervous system.
- Secondary insults (such as hypoxia, hypotension and hypercarbia) have the potential to significantly worsen the initial primary injury and are potentially preventable if recognised and treated.
- Close observation, monitoring and targeted interventions to mitigate against secondary insults are important.
- Guidelines for severe traumatic brain injury recommend maintenance of systolic blood pressure > 90 mmHg, partial arterial oxygen pressure > 60 mmHg, intracranial pressure < 20 mmHg and cerebral perfusion pressure between 50 and 70 mmHg.
- A Glasgow Coma Scale score < 9 may suggest a severe traumatic brain injury.
- Computed tomography plays an important role in diagnosis and management of traumatic brain injury.

INTRODUCTION

Traumatic brain injury (TBI) is defined as an injury to the brain (cerebrum and brainstem) produced by mechanical forces that cause damage to neurological structures. The effects range between mild TBI, with no apparent lasting effects, through to permanent severe TBI, which can result in irreversible, permanent changes to the victim's life. Such changes can often negatively affect both family and interpersonal relationships, thus representing the significant social burden and cost associated with this injury. An important challenge in the emergency treatment of patients who have sustained TBI is the prevention of the injury from progression of the primary injury and preventing secondary insults from exacerbating the primary injury. The principles for preventing secondary injury are the avoidance of hypoxia, hypo/hypercapnoea and hypotension.[1] Paramedics and emergency nurses have major roles in preventing or ameliorating these potential secondary injuries. Improving the recovery of patients with TBI is dependent on a coordinated healthcare system that ensures comprehensive multidisciplinary management from the point of injury through to rehabilitation and post-discharge care.[2]

Epidemiology

Traumatic brain injury is a major source of death and disability worldwide.[3] In Australia, there were an estimated 22,710 hospitalisations involving traumatic brain injury in 2004–05.[4] The true incidence of TBI is unknown and is thought to be highly underreported, as many people with mild TBI are not admitted to hospital. TBI permanently changes the lives of not only the victim and their family, but also their productivity in society. The estimated cost of TBI in Australia in 2008 was $A8.6 billion, and lifetime costs per TBI patient are estimated to be $A2.5 million and $A4.8 million for moderate and severe TBI respectively.[5]

TBIs occur most frequently as a result of motor vehicle collisions, violence and falls.[6] Changes in momentum cause stress and deformation of brain tissues, including neuronal, axonal and vascular structures.[7] Alcohol is recognised as a contributing factor in the incidence of TBI, placing the victim at greater risk for injury and making assessment of the head-injured patient more complex.[8] Causes of TBI differ by age: falls are most common for people older than age 65 years, whereas motor vehicle crashes remain the prevalent cause for people 5–64 years of age, with the 15- to 24-year-old age group at greatest risk.[4] Traumatic brain injuries caused by firearms have a high association with fatality, with a 90% mortality rate.[9] The high incidence, cost and loss of productive years associated with TBI reinforces the need to develop more-effective prevention strategies.[6]

This chapter begins with a brief review of anatomy and physiology. It also provides an overview of assessment techniques for adult patients with acute head injuries. Current management options for TBI are also discussed. Refer to Chapter 36 for discussion of paediatric trauma, Chapter 39 for trauma in the elderly and Chapter 35 for obstetric trauma.

Injury mechanism

Traumatic brain injury occurs as a consequence of two principal insults—primary brain injury and secondary brain injury.

- Primary brain injury is that caused by the external forces on the brain structures at the time of injury.

- Secondary brain injury is the damage to the brain that results both from the natural history of the evolution of the primary brain injury and from acute disorders of the respiratory and cardiovascular system that are associated with both the brain injury directly and extracranial trauma.

Common examples of the natural evolution of primary brain injury include cerebral swelling, ischaemic and hypoxic damage, hydrocephalus, infection and the effects of raised intracranial pressure.[10,11] The consequences of extracranial trauma may manifest as episodes of systemic hypoxia or hypotension. Preventing secondary injury is an important goal of pre-hospital and hospital care.

Traumatic brain injury is a complex mixture of primary and secondary injury insults. For example, the blow to the head that lacerates a cerebral blood vessel and causes haemorrhage into the brain (intracerebral contusion) is a primary brain injury. Secondary injury is caused by the associated local tissue oedema and hypoperfusion which results in ischaemic damage

---

BOX 45.1 Classification of traumatic brain injuries[77]

Primary injury
1. Extra-axial:
   - Epidural haematoma
   - Subdural haematoma
   - Subarachnoid haemorrhage
   - Intraventricular haemorrhage
2. Intra-axial:
   - Axonal injury
   - Cortical contusion
   - Intracerebral haematoma
3. Vascular:
   - Dissection
   - Carotid cavernous fistula
   - Arteriovenous dural fistula
   - Pseudoaneurysm
   - Secondary injury
4. Acute:
   - Diffuse cerebral swelling
   - Brain herniation
   - Infarction
   - Infection
5. Chronic:
   - Hydrocephalus
   - Encephalomalacia
   - Cerebrospinal fluid leak
   - Leptomeningeal cyst

---

to the affected area.[10] The swelling itself may additionally cause respiratory-centre depression (resulting in hypoxia and hypercarbia), and this may potentially be further complicated in the setting of additional extracranial trauma by chest injuries and by reduced brain perfusion as a consequence of shock (commonly hypovolaemic/haemorrhagic). Box 45.1 shows the classification of TBIs.[12]

Anatomy and physiology

The hair, scalp, skull, meninges and cerebrospinal fluid (CSF) protect the brain from injury. The scalp consists of five layers of tissue: skin, subcutaneous tissue, epicranial aponeurosis, ligaments and periosteum. The skull is composed of many bones, including the frontal, parietal, temporal and occipital bones (Fig 45.1).

Cranial bones join with facial bones to form the cranial vault, a rigid cavity that can hold 1400–1500 mL of material. Internal bony structures of importance are depressions at the base of the skull called the anterior, middle and posterior fossae. The frontal lobe is located in the anterior fossa; parietal, temporal and occipital lobes in the middle fossa; and brainstem and cerebellum in the posterior fossa.

Three layers of meninges surround the brain and provide additional protection. The outermost is the dura mater (meaning 'tough mother'), which consists of two layers of tough fibrous tissue. The inner layer of the dura mater forms the falx cerebri and tentorium cerebelli. Potential spaces located above the dura mater (epidural) and below the dura mater (subdural)

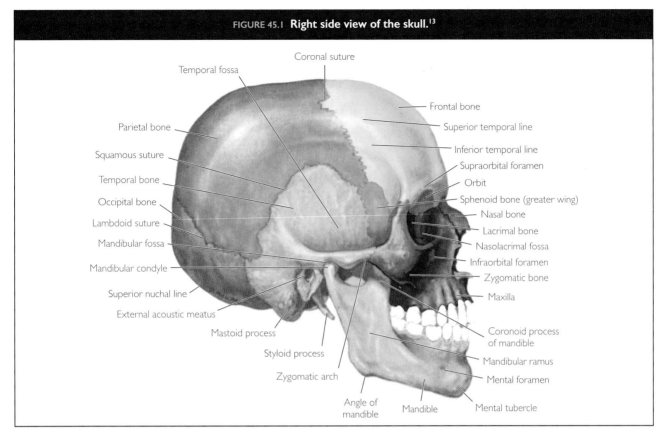

FIGURE 45.1 **Right side view of the skull.**[13]

Labels (clockwise from top):
Coronal suture
Temporal fossa
Frontal bone
Superior temporal line
Inferior temporal line
Supraorbital foramen
Orbit
Sphenoid bone (greater wing)
Nasal bone
Lacrimal bone
Nasolacrimal fossa
Infraorbital foramen
Zygomatic bone
Maxilla
Coronoid process of mandible
Mandibular ramus
Mental foramen
Mental tubercle
Mandible
Angle of mandible
Zygomatic arch
Styloid process
Mastoid process
External acoustic meatus
Superior nuchal line
Mandibular condyle
Mandibular fossa
Lambdoid suture
Occipital bone
Temporal bone
Squamous suture
Parietal bone

are at risk for haematoma formation because the middle meningeal artery lies in the epidural space, and veins are located within the subdural space. The middle meningeal layer is the arachnoid mater (meaning 'spiderlike'), a fine, elastic layer. Below the arachnoid mater, the subarachnoid space contains arachnoid villi, finger-like projections that form channels for CSF absorption. Adhering to the surface of the brain is the pia mater (meaning 'tender mother') (Fig 45.2). More-detailed anatomy of the brain is presented in Chapter 23.

Although the average brain accounts for only 2% of the total bodyweight, it consumes approximately 20% of the body's resting oxygen consumption. It is a highly metabolic and active organ whose main energy source is oxygen and glucose. Cerebral blood flow is vital to maintaining cerebral function.

Cerebral autoregulation is an important concept in healthy brain tissue (although its utility in pathological states such as TBI is unclear). Cerebral autoregulation may be defined as the intrinsic ability to maintain a constant cerebral blood flow over a range of blood pressures. In health, cerebral autoregulation maintains cerebral blood flow at an average of 50 mL/100 g brain tissue/minute between mean arterial blood pressures of 50 and 150 mmHg. This phenomenon protects the brain against ischaemia at low blood pressures and against oedema and potential haemorrhage at very high blood pressures. Cerebral autoregulation is thought to be mediated through a combination of myogenic, neurogenic and metabolic mechanisms acting at the level of the vascular endothelium.[14]

In addition, oxygen, carbon dioxide and pH all exert an influence on cerebral blood flow. Hypoxia, hypercarbia and acidosis cause vasodilation that increases cerebral blood flow, cerebral volume and intracranial pressure (ICP). Lower levels of carbon dioxide cause vasoconstriction and lower cerebral blood volume. As such, brain tissue is very susceptible to hypoxia and hypoglycaemia.[11,15]

Secondary injuries limit the ability of the injured brain to adapt to minor variations in physiology and maintain adequate cerebral blood flow. Cerebral autoregulation is thought to be impaired after TBI, and cerebral blood flow may be pressure-dependent. Therefore, a decrease in cerebral perfusion pressure (CPP) may lead to ischaemia, while, conversely, increases in CPP can increase blood flow and raise ICP as a result (see Fig 45.3).

Excitotoxic changes increase cerebral metabolism and may predispose ischaemia, even in the presence of normal or increased cerebral blood flow. The release of neurogenic factors from damaged brain cells can also affect the cerebral vasculature. The resultant impact on the injured brain can be severe, with exacerbation of cerebral swelling. In some cases systemic effects, such as coagulopathy, will ensue.[11,13] As a result of these effects, clinicians may manipulate metabolic parameters in the management of patients with severe TBI.[11,13] The pathway of CNS injury and ischaemia is shown in Figure 45.4.

Major traumatic brain injuries

Traumatic brain injury may be grouped into focal injuries or diffuse injuries. *Focal injuries* have an identifiable area of involvement, whereas *diffuse injuries* involve the entire brain. Examples of focal injuries include skull fractures and haematomas, often occurring after a focal injury or fall; diffuse injuries generally occur after rapid deceleration from high speeds (diffuse axonal injury). Head injuries can be classified according to severity as minimal, mild, moderate or severe.

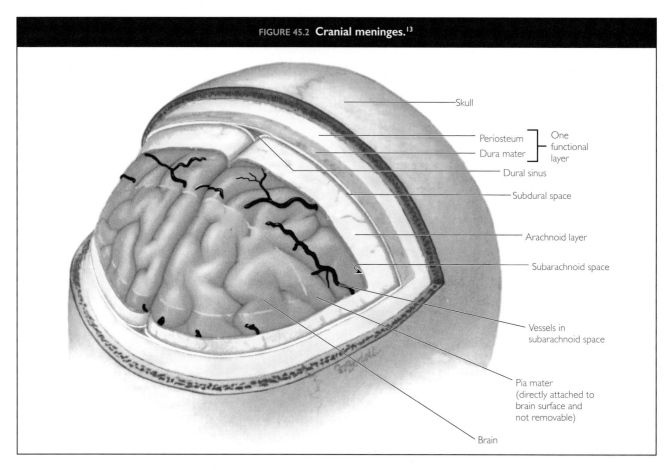

FIGURE 45.2 **Cranial meninges.**[13]

Skull

Periosteum
Dura mater
} One functional layer

Dural sinus

Subdural space

Arachnoid layer

Subarachnoid space

Vessels in subarachnoid space

Pia mater (directly attached to brain surface and not removable)

Brain

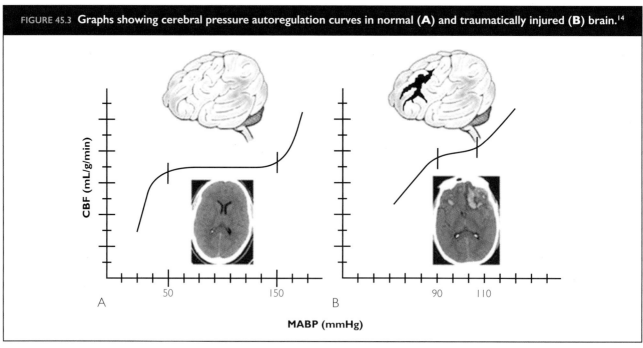

FIGURE 45.3 **Graphs showing cerebral pressure autoregulation curves in normal (A) and traumatically injured (B) brain.**[14]

Focal head injuries

Scalp lacerations

The scalp protects the brain from injury by acting as a cushion to reduce energy transmission to underlying structures. Excessive force applied to the scalp often causes a laceration; the scalp has an extensive vascular supply with poor vasoconstrictive properties, causing lacerations to bleed profusely. Bleeding should be controlled with direct pressure to the affected area, followed by wound repair and tetanus prophylaxis as indicated. It is important to note that patients can exsanguinate from profusely bleeding scalp lacerations, and therefore must be regarded as a surgical emergency if haemorrhage is unable to be

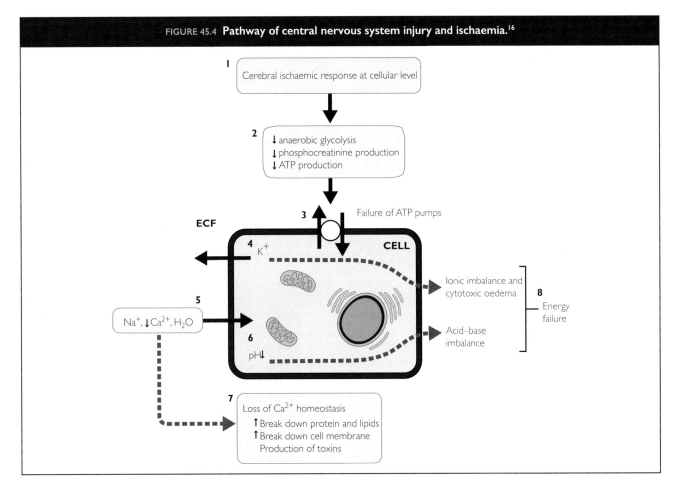

FIGURE 45.4 Pathway of central nervous system injury and ischaemia.[16]

controlled. The application of staples or clips may also be used for rapid closure and can be life-saving.[17]

Skull fractures

Skull fractures occur when energy applied to the skull causes bony deformation. Clinical presentation of skull fractures is directly correlated to the type of fracture, area involved and damage to underlying structures.

- A *linear skull fracture* is non-displaced and associated with minimal neurological deficit. Supportive care is usually all that is required.[18]
- When energy displaces the outer table of bone below the inner table of the adjoining skull, a *depressed skull fracture* occurs (Fig 45.5). Surgical elevation is required when depressed bone fragments become lodged in brain tissue.
- An *open skull fracture* requires urgent neurosurgical referral because of the risk of underlying injury and infection.[18,20]
- A *basilar (base) skull fracture* develops when enough force is exerted on the base of the skull to cause deformity. The base of the skull includes any bony area where the skull ends, and is not limited to the posterior aspect of the skull. Portions of the facial bones comprise the base of skull, such as the roof of the orbit. The occipital condyles are also part of the base of the skull and fractures of these may cause cervical spine instability.

A basilar skull fracture may be visualised on diagnostic imaging (Fig 45.6); however, this is not always true, and diagnosis may therefore also be made on the basis of clinical findings. Basilar skull fractures that overlay the middle meningeal artery are the cause of more than 75% of epidural haematomas. A basilar skull fracture may also cause intracerebral bleeding.

Neurological changes that occur with a basilar skull fracture can range from mild changes in mentation to combativeness and severe agitation. Combative behaviour is often considered a hallmark of a basilar skull fracture. Clinical manifestations of basilar skull fracture include periorbital ecchymoses (raccoon eyes) (Fig 45.7) from intraorbital bleeding, and Battle's sign (bruising over the mastoid process seen behind the ears) (Fig 45.8) 12–24 hours after initial injury. Other clinical manifestations include haemotympanum (blood behind the tympanic membrane caused by a fracture of the temporal bone), and CSF leak from the nose or ear caused by temporal bone fracture. If the tympanic membrane is intact, fluid drains through the eustachian tube and appears as CSF rhinorrhoea. However, absence of visible CSF does not eliminate the possibility of a basilar skull fracture.

If a clear fluid leak from the nose or ear is suspected of being CSF, formation of two distinct rings when the fluid drips onto filter paper, called the 'halo' or 'ring' sign, suggests the presence of CSF (Fig 45.9). The fluid should also be tested for glucose as this is a normal finding in CSF. Suspicion of a CSF leak can be reliably conformed by laboratory testing for beta-2-transferrin—a protein that is highly specific to CSF. The reference range is 10.0–19.2 mg/L.[18,22] CSF rhinorrhoea or otorrhoea should be permitted to drain freely and not be obstructed. Nasal packing is not recommended for CSF

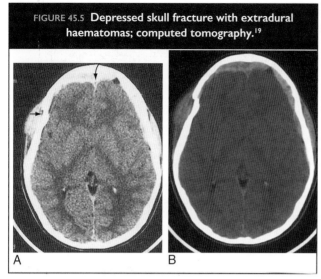

FIGURE 45.5 **Depressed skull fracture with extradural haematomas; computed tomography.**[19]

A, B, Axial 'brain and bone windows' demonstrate the right temporal bone depressed several millimetres with an evident fracture line (arrow) anteriorly. Soft-tissue contusion overlying the fracture is also noted. A large extradural collection (curved upper arrow) anteriorly crosses the midline and displaces the falx posteriorly, and there is a second contiguous left frontal extradural collection as well. Other images (not shown) demonstrated bilateral skull fractures. Note the generalised cerebral swelling with complete effacement of the frontal horns.

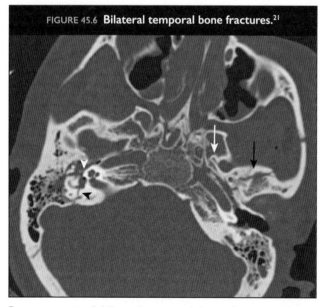

FIGURE 45.6 **Bilateral temporal bone fractures.**[21]

Patient sustained bilateral temporal bone fractures after a motor vehicle collision. On the right, non-displaced transverse temporal bone fracture, lateral subtype (black arrowhead), and associated air in the vestibule of the semicircular canals (white arrowhead) were identified. Non-displaced fracture through the left temporal bone perpendicular to the carotid canal (black arrow) was also identified.

rhinorrhoea, but may be required for haemorrhage control in the setting of complex facial fractures. To promote patient comfort, a nasal bolster is useful for CSF rhinorrhoea.

A diagnosis of skull fracture is usually made by a combination of clinical examination and computed tomography (CT)

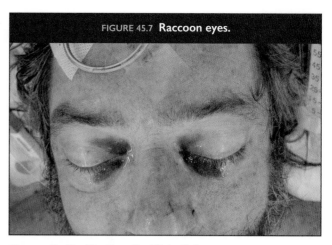

FIGURE 45.7 **Raccoon eyes.**

Courtesy Dr Ken Harrison, CareFlight, Sydney.

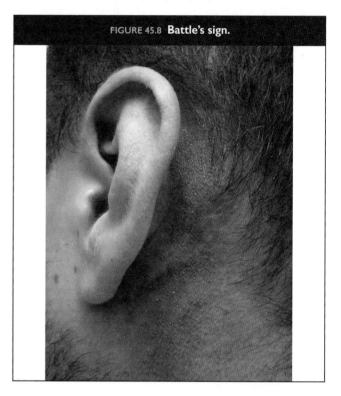

FIGURE 45.8 **Battle's sign.**

scan that includes base-of-skull views. Nasogastric or nasal endotracheal intubation and nasal temperature probes should be avoided, as there is a risk of these lodging intracranially.

Contusion

Cerebral contusion is a bruise on the surface of the brain that occurs from movement of the brain within the cranial vault (Fig 45.10). When an acceleration or deceleration injury occurs, two contusions may result: one at the initial site of impact (coup) and one on the opposite side of the impact (contra-coup).[7,23] Common areas affected include the temporal and frontal lobes. On CT, contusions will appear as areas of high density within superficial grey matter. Areas of low density from associated vasogenic oedema may often surround them.[12] The clinical presentation varies with size and location of the contusion. Commonly occurring symptoms include altered level of consciousness, nausea, vomiting, visual disturbances, weakness and speech difficulty.

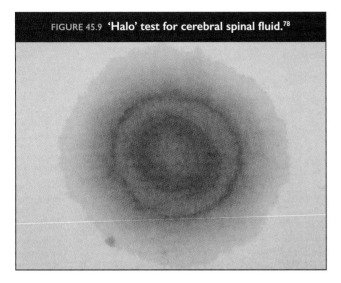

FIGURE 45.9 'Halo' test for cerebral spinal fluid.[78]

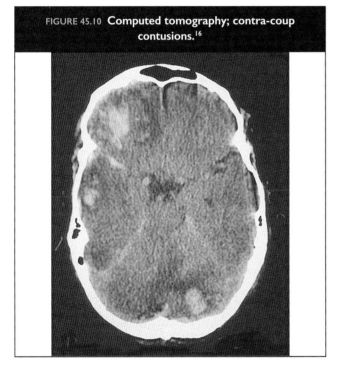

FIGURE 45.10 Computed tomography; contra-coup contusions.[16]

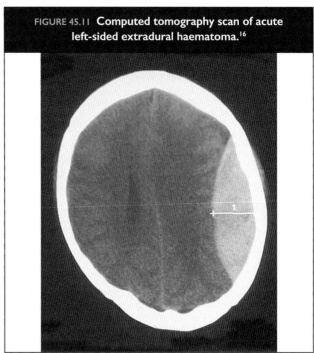

FIGURE 45.11 Computed tomography scan of acute left-sided extradural haematoma.[16]

Epidural/extradural haematoma

Extradural haematoma (EDH) is bleeding between the inner surface of the skull and the dura mater (Fig 45.11). Commonly, a torn middle meningeal artery (caused by an accompanying skull fracture) leads to a rapidly forming haematoma; however, some patients may have no evidence of skull fracture. An acute EDH appears on CT as a well-defined, hyperdense, biconvex extra-axial collection. Mass effect, sulcal effacement and midline shifts can also often be seen on CT as a result of EDH.[12]

A rapidly expanding EDH is a neurosurgical emergency. Signs and symptoms include a brief period of unconsciousness followed by a lucid period, then another loss of consciousness. This brief lucid period is considered a hallmark of an EDH; however, it does not occur in all patients. If alert, the patient with an EDH complains of severe headache and may exhibit hemiparesis and a dilated pupil on the side of injury. Surgical intervention will be guided by the neurosurgeon.

Note that extra-axial haematoma is a term that may be used to describe an EDH or a subdural haematoma (SDH).

Subdural haematoma

Subdural haematomas occur more frequently than any other intracranial injuries and have concurrently the highest morbidity and mortality of all haematomas. A subdural haematoma may be acute, subacute or chronic. Traumatic SDH usually results from dissipation of energy, usually sudden deceleration that ruptures bridging cortical veins in the subdural space. This causes bleeding into the subdural space between the dura mater and arachnoid, and leads to development of a haematoma (Fig 45.12). An acute SDH appears on CT as hyperdense, homogenous, crescent-shaped extra-axial collection. Most occur supratentorially and are often seen along the falx and tentorium.[12] SDH are frequently associated with parenchymal injury and associated mass effect. Clinical features are loss of consciousness, hemiparesis and fixed, dilated pupils.

Subacute subdural haematomas develop 48 hours to 2 weeks after injury. The clinical presentation is progressive decline in level of consciousness as the haematoma slowly expands. The brain compensates as a result of slow blood collection over time, so decline in neurological function occurs gradually. After the subdural is drained, the patient improves quickly with little or no lasting neurological deficit.

Chronic subdural haematomas are seen frequently in the elderly, and progress slowly. Blood collects over 2 weeks to several months; by the time a person is examined, the causative mechanism may have been forgotten. Chronic subdural haematomas are initially tolerated because of brain atrophy associated with ageing. As the brain decreases in size, the space within the cranial vault increases. A haematoma collects over time without obvious changes in neurological status until its size is sufficient to produce a mass effect. Subdural haematomas may be managed either surgically or conservatively, dependent on size and clinical presentation.

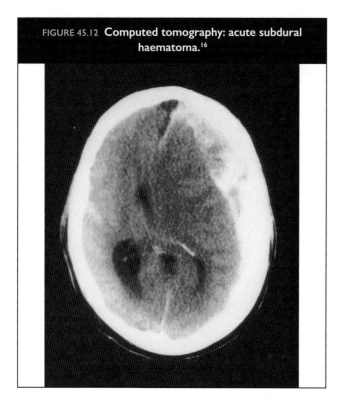

FIGURE 45.12 Computed tomography: acute subdural haematoma.[16]

Traumatic subarachnoid haemorrhage

Bleeding into the subarachnoid space is a common clinical finding in TBI patients. Traumatic subarachnoid haemorrhage (SAH) can develop from the disruption of small pial vessels, extension of contusion or haematoma into the subarachnoid space or transependymal diffusion of intraventricular haemorrhage. Common sites for SAH include sylvian and interpeduncular cisterns, often seen occurring contralateral to site of impact (as seen in contra-coup injuries). On CT, acute SAH appears as linear, serpentine areas of high density conforming to cerebral sulci and cisterns (Fig 45.13).[12] The major clinical associations with SAH are acute hydrocephalus, cerebral vasospasm and fibrous scarring. Management is largely geared to minimising secondary brain injury and monitoring for sequelae.[10]

Other focal injuries

Intraventricular haemorrhage and intracerebral clots (Fig 45.14) are types of focal injuries. Management depends on the size of the clot and the source of bleeding. Surgical evacuation may be necessary in concert with medical management of increased ICP. Firearms or other projectiles frequently cause penetrating injuries to the head. These injuries typically result in significant focal injuries along the path of entry (Fig 45.15).

Diffuse brain injuries

Concussion

A concussion can occur as a result of a direct blow to the head or from an acceleration or deceleration injury in which the brain collides with the inside of the skull. Brief interruption of the reticular activating system may occur, causing transient amnesia. A classic concussion is characterised as loss of consciousness followed by transient neurological changes such as nausea, vomiting, temporary amnesia, headache and possible

FIGURE 45.13 Computed tomography: acute traumatic subarachnoid haemorrhage (SAH).[24]

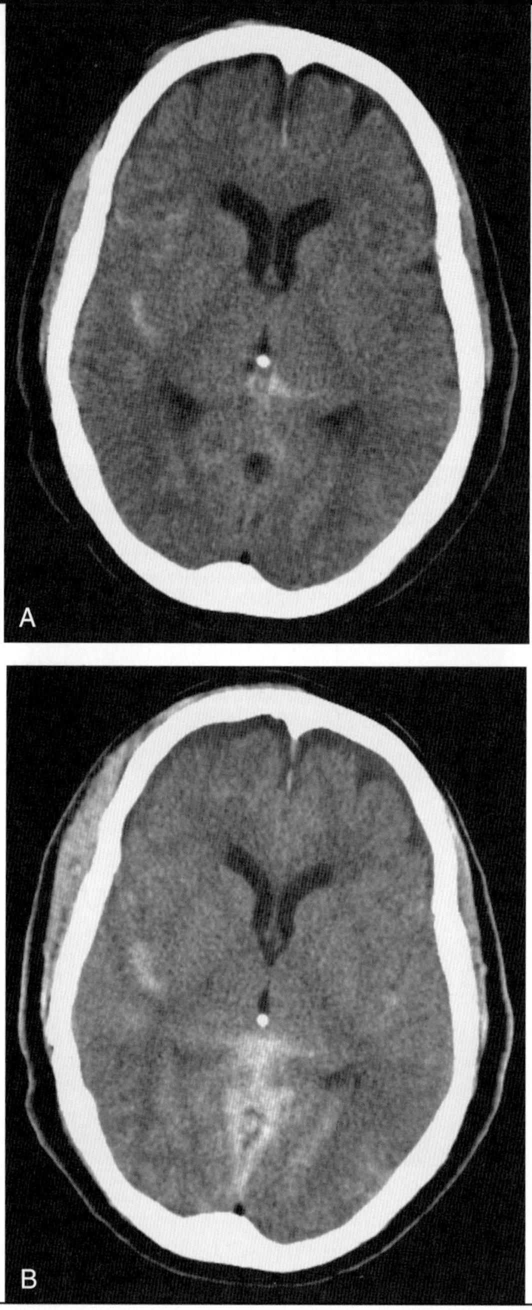

A, Initial scan demonstrates haemorrhage in the quadrigeminal plate cistern posterior to the pineal gland and in the right sylvian fissure.
B, Follow-up scan performed 7 hours later reveals increasing hyperattenuation along the tentorium. The presence of contrast in vascular and meningeal structures limits assessment for progression of SAH.

brief loss of vision. (See also the section on mild traumatic brain injury later in this chapter.)

Diffuse axonal injury

The phrase 'diffuse axonal injury' (DAI) illustrates the major pathophysiological event associated with the most severe form

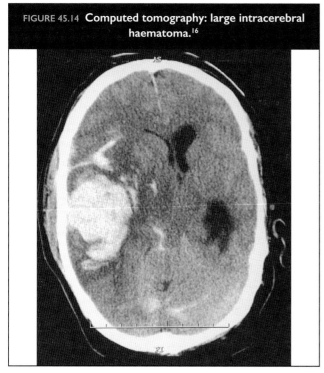

FIGURE 45.14 **Computed tomography: large intracerebral haematoma.**[16]

Note mass effect.

of TBI. This injury is almost always the result of blunt trauma that causes rotational acceleration and deceleration forces, resulting in shearing and disruption of neuronal structures, predominantly white matter. DAI is most commonly seen in the frontal and temporal lobe white matter (mild), corpus callosum (moderate) and midbrain (severe). On CT, DAI lesions appear as small petechial haemorrhages; however, only a small percentage of DAIs are associated with haemorrhage (Fig 45.16A). Magnetic resonance imaging (MRI) is more sensitive in detecting DAIs, appearing as multiple small foci of increased signal on T2 images (Fig 45.16B).[12] Prognosis for diffuse axonal injuries depends on the degree of injury (mild, moderate or severe) and the severity of damage from any associated secondary injury.

- Mild DAI is characterised by loss of consciousness for 6–24 hours. Initially the patient may exhibit decerebrate or decorticate posturing, but improves rapidly within 24 hours. Return to baseline neurological status may occur over days, but periods of amnesia may be present.

- Moderate DAI is a coma lasting longer than 24 hours, possibly extending over a period of days. Brainstem dysfunction (decorticate/decerebrate posturing) is evident almost immediately and may continue until the patient begins to wake. Patients with moderate DAI usually recover, but rarely return to full pre-injury neurological function.

- Severe DAI is characterised by brainstem impairment that does not resolve. Victims of severe DAI remain comatose for days to weeks. Autonomic dysfunction may also be present. Overall prognosis for severe DAI is extremely poor. Early CT scans may be unremarkable; magnetic resonance imaging (MRI) will show DAI early (Fig 45.16).

Patient assessment and management

The assessment of the patient with TBI follows the same systematic primary and secondary survey approach to trauma as discussed in Chapter 44.

Primary survey and resuscitation

In the primary survey, cardiopulmonary stabilisation is imperative for patients with severe brain injury. Airway patency, maintenance of optimal oxygenation and tissue perfusion are vital, as the brain is adversely affected by secondary insults, particularly hypotension and hypoxia.[11] See Chapter 17, p. 314, for airway management techniques. While hypotensive resuscitation is a contemporary concept for the bleeding trauma patient, it is recommended that patients with head injuries are maintained with a systolic blood pressure of > 90 mmHg, prior to ICP monitoring. As the level of consciousness is affected by both hypoxia and hypotension, any neurological assessments undertaken in the presence of these abnormalities need to be concurrently recorded. The neurological findings need to be interpreted within the context of these vital sign abnormalities and ideally neurological examination should be repeated after the correction of the abnormalities. Alcohol, sedatives and recreational drugs may all also impact on initial neurological evaluation. A Glasgow Coma Scale (GCS) score during the pre-hospital and early management is an important assessment of neurological status and allows evaluation of neurological progress over time, may be a helpful prognostic tool and also is a useful guide for predicting the intensity of early management; A complete GCS includes eye opening, motor response, verbal response and pupillary reaction.[26]

Pre-hospital considerations

The pre-hospital phase of care for the patient with TBI is an important component of optimising subsequent recovery for patients.[27] The period that immediately follows a TBI is when cerebral tissue is at its highest risk for secondary injury related to cerebral ischaemia, disruption of cerebrovascular autoregulation and cerebral oedema. Once on-scene, emergency medical service providers must make decisions on immediate treatment, transport modality and destination. Although evidence is limited, outcomes for TBI appear to be improved for patients with shorter pre-hospital times.

Pre-hospital management should be directed towards prevention and/or limitation of secondary brain insults, while facilitating rapid transport to an appropriate facility (where applicable) capable of providing neurocritical care evaluation and intervention.[27,28] Interventions in the pre-hospital setting should be directed towards maintaining adequate oxygenation, ventilation, blood pressure and monitoring oxygen saturations, end-tidal carbon dioxide ($ETCO_2$), non-invasive blood pressure and neurological status, including pupillary status.[27,28] Emphasis is placed on regular, repeated observations and meticulous attention to basic supportive care in the field, as these areas have shown the greatest impact on outcomes associated with TBI.

Key concepts of pre-hospital TBI management are given in Box 45.2.[27] Chapter 17, p. 323, contains information on $ETCO_2$ monitoring techniques.

Secondary survey and assesment

After ensuring adequate control of airway, breathing and circulation (ABC) and a brief neurological assessment, the next

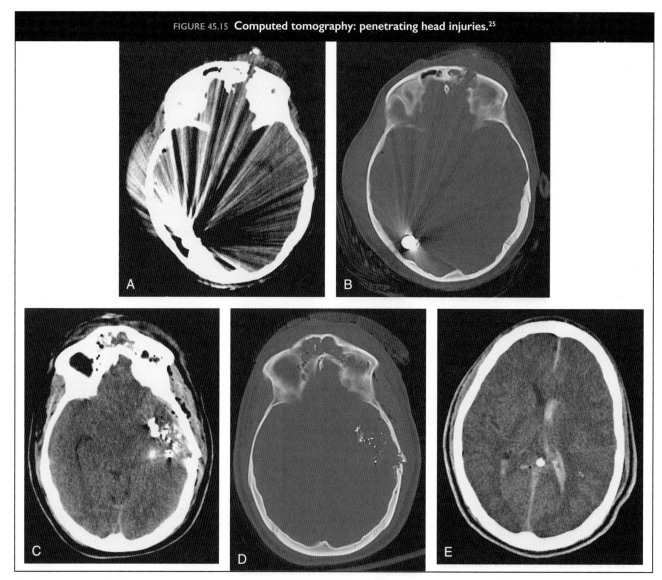

FIGURE 45.15 **Computed tomography: penetrating head injuries.**[25]

A, Gunshot wound. There is a large bullet fragment in the right parietal lobe causing extensive streak artifact.
B, Bone window shows entry site in the left frontal bone with bevelled edges.
C, D, Different patient with entry wound in the left orbit demonstrates blood, bullet and bone fragments along the bullet trajectory in the left temporal lobe. Left temporal bone fracture represents a ricochet injury.
E, In a third patient, diffuse intraventricular haemorrhage and displaced fracture fragment in the splenium of the corpus callosum is evident.[25]

priority should be to perform a complete, concise neurological assessment. Assessment should include:

- history and mechanism of injury
- vital signs
- GCS
- pupils examination
- full neurological examination
- external head and neck examination.

Taking a history and mechanism of how the head trauma was sustained is important. It can assist in determining immediate acute management strategies and likely pathways; it can also be suggestive of prognostic outcome.[16] Assessment of the level of consciousness should be directed towards acquiring the highest-level response with the least stimulus. Subtle changes in level of consciousness are the earliest indication of deterioration in the patient with a head injury. A blood glucose level should always be taken, preferably in conjunction with the initial vital-sign measurements (see Ch 17, p. 332, for blood glucose sampling techniques).

Time to definitive care and patient disposition

All patients with TBI need careful consideration regarding their disposition. Ideal management of severe TBI patients begins with rapid transport to a definitive trauma centre with neurosurgical capabilities, and early, aggressive resuscitation, with particular attention paid to meticulous airway and blood-pressure management.[29] In rural or urban settings, the emphasis should be on airway protection and maintenance of adequate ventilation and circulation while awaiting rapid transfer/transport to a definitive centre.[29]

Early administration of tranexamic acid should be

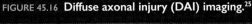

FIGURE 45.16 **Diffuse axonal injury (DAI) imaging.**[25]

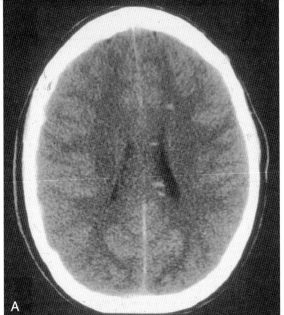

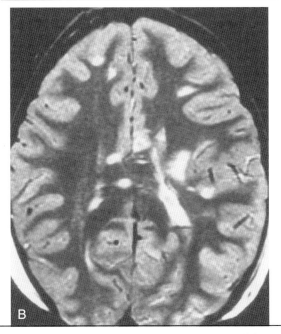

A, Computed tomography scan demonstrates small haemorrhagic DAIs in the deep white matter and corpus callosum.
B, Axial T2-weighted (2500/80) magnetic resonance image demonstrates typical locations of DAI: subcortical white matter, corpus callosum and corona radiata.

BOX 45.2 **Key concepts of pre-hospital traumatic brain injury management**[27]

Assessment
Pulse oximetry
Blood pressure
Glasgow Coma Scale (GCS)
Pupils

Decision-making
Minimise out-of-hospital time
Transport direct to a centre with neurosurgical capability (where possible)
Transport paediatric patients direct to paediatric trauma centre (where possible)

Airway
Maintain pulse oximetry > 90%
Avoid hypoxia
Use airway adjuncts (intubate, guedels, LMA) if unable to maintain adequate airway, pulse oximetry > 90% or if GCS < 9

Breathing
Apply supplemental oxygen
Avoid hyperventilation (unless signs of imminent herniation)
Bag–valve–mask ventilation can be as effective as intubation

Circulation
Avoid hypotension
Maintain systolic blood pressure with small crystalloid bolus if required

considered for all trauma patients at risk of significant bleeding and this medication should be administered as early as possible after injury,[30] ideally within 3 hours. Further clinical trials are planned to understand the safety and efficacy of tranexamic acid specifically in high-income countries and further explore the role of tranexamic acid for patients with head injury.[31,32]

Following resuscitation and early CT imaging, it is the role of the emergency nurse to ensure that the patient goes to an appropriate inpatient clinical area for ongoing acute management. In many moderate and severe TBI cases this may be an intensive care or high-dependency unit; in time-critical injuries such as EDH, the patient will go directly to theatre.

Essential nursing care

The first priority of care for the head-injured patient is rapid resuscitation. Initial stabilisation of the head-injured patient is directed towards maintenance and support of oxygenation and ventilation, restoration of circulating volume and blood pressure. Current recommendations for treatment of severe head injury specify that interventions to reduce an increased ICP should be considered in the presence of clinical signs of transtentorial herniation such as unilateral or bilateral pupillary dilation, asymmetric pupillary reactivity, motor posturing or continued neurological deterioration after physiological stability has been restored.[33] Figure 45.17 illustrates the mechanism that causes herniation.

Frequently, concomitant cervical spine trauma can be associated with TBI; therefore cervical spine stabilisation should be maintained until adequate radiographical examinations have ruled out cervical spine trauma. Appropriate fitting of cervical collars (see Chapter 17) is essential to reduce the contribution of a collar to increasing ICP, as a response to distortion of venous drainage.[34,35]

Prevention of secondary brain injury begins with recognition of factors that correlate with further brain injury, such

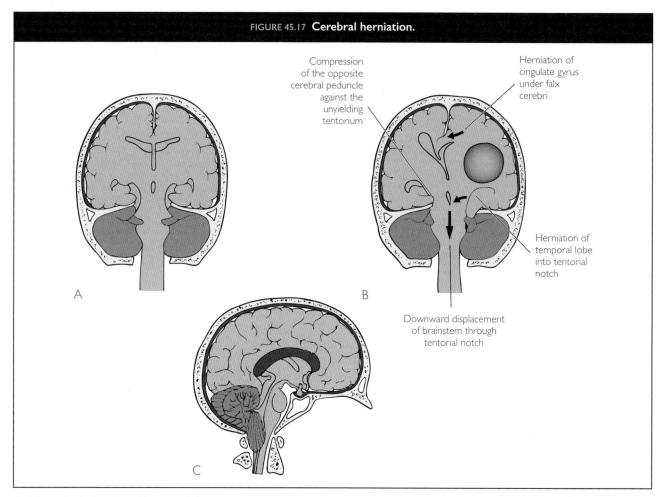

FIGURE 45.17 **Cerebral herniation.**

Compression
of the opposite
cerebral peduncle
against the
unyielding
tentorium

Herniation of
cingulate gyrus
under falx
cerebri

Herniation of
temporal lobe
into tentorial
notch

Downward displacement
of brainstem through
tentorial notch

A, Normal relationship of intracranial structures.
B, Shift of intracranial structures.
C, Downward herniation of the cerebellar tonsils into the foramen magnum.

as hypoxia, hypercapnia, hypotension and cerebral ischaemia secondary to increased ICP. Hypoxia and hypotension during the immediate post-injury period substantially increase the rate of morbidity and mortality associated with head injury.[28] Presence of a secure airway, adequate ventilatory rate/inspired oxygen and correction of hypovolaemic shock by fluid/blood product resuscitation can decrease the incidence of hypoxia, hypercapnia and hypotension. Evaluation of the severity of a head injury by CT scanning generally occurs after stabilisation.

After initial stabilisation, the emergency nurse should consider other interventions that promote return of optimal neurological function. General guidelines for care of the patient with a head injury include ensuring a patent airway, ventilatory support as indicated, haemodynamic stability (systolic blood pressure [SBP] above 90 mmHg), ongoing neurological assessment, administration of pharmacological agents as needed (i.e. neuromuscular blocking agents, anticonvulsants) and other interventions based on patient condition.

Table 45.1 outlines a number of key elements in the care of the patient with TBI. These elements are in addition to those important for the care and resuscitation of the critically injured. These elements also relate to those patients who are not critically injured but who still require close observation and vigilance regarding early signs of deterioration.

An integral component of caring for head-injured patients is inclusion of the family or significant others in the plan of care. Head injuries can be overwhelming for the family; psychosocial support and education regarding the injury cannot be overemphasised.

Glasgow Coma Scale

Completing the GCS allows assignment of numerical values to clinical findings and assists in recognition of trends in neurological changes, facilitates prognostication and is a component to evaluating the severity of the head injury. Interpretation of the GCS must be correlated with other clinical assessment findings. Presence of other physiological conditions, such as hypotension, hypothermia, abnormal blood glucose level, alcohol or intoxication, may artificially lower the total GCS score. In the absence of previously identified physiological conditions, patients with a total GCS < 9 suggests a severe head injury. The Paediatric GCS is an adapted version of the adult scale and is described in Chapter 36.

An abnormal pupillary response to light can indicate intracranial pathology. Normal pupillary response to direct light examination is constriction. Consensual reaction (constriction of the opposite pupil) should occur with direct light examination. Unilateral pupil dilation may indicate

TABLE 45.1 Essential nursing care of the patient with a traumatic brain injury[79,80]		
NURSING CARE ELEMENT	INTERVENTION	RATIONALE
GCS assessment	Half-hourly GCS monitoring for at least 4 hours after any TBI, then as ordered by the doctor	Enables early detection of deterioration in neurological status
	The GCS should be done together with the nurse to whom the patient is being handed over, to ensure consistency in assessment and documentation	Inter-rater reliability in GCS assessments by nurses is problematic: this is a mitigation strategy
Head of bed elevation	Elevate to 30° where MAP > 60 mmHg	Promotes venous drainage of brain and reduces ICP
Temperature monitoring; core temperature often rises in response to injury	Intubated patients should have continuous thermal monitoring and maintenance of normothermia	Avoid hyperthermia—as the core temperature rises, CO_2 production increases.
	Note: avoid hypothermia as part of the trauma triad in the resuscitative phase	High $PaCO_2$ can cause raised ICP
Cervical collar	Ensure not too tight—watch closely, especially with facial swelling. In consultation with medical staff, remove in intubated patients if patient well sedated and not at risk of moving	The neck can swell over the first 24 hours, and the collar can become constrictive and impair cranial venous return and cause a raised ICP
Adequate analgesia and sedation	Careful patient monitoring for signs of pain and agitation	Maintain normal ICP
	Use sedation scales and depth of neuromuscular blockade (train of four)	Optimise mechanical ventilation
Clustering of care	Group nursing interventions to provide a longer episode of rest, i.e. suctioning/washes/turns, mouth/eye care, etc	Reduces noxious stimuli

CO_2, carbon dioxide; GCS, Glasgow Coma Scale; ICP, intracranial pressure; MAP: mean arterial pressure; $PaCO_2$, partial arterial pressure of carbon dioxide; TBI: traumatic brain injury

early compression of the third cranial nerve. Anisocoria, or unequal pupils, is a normal finding in 20–25% of the population, so assessment of reactivity in the dilated pupil is critical. Bilateral fixed and dilated pupils are indicative of impending transtentorial herniation. Figure 45.18 illustrates pupil reactions at different levels of consciousness. Focal lesions such as EDHs or SDHs can cause pupil dilation as a result of compression of the third cranial nerve. Unequal pupils or bilaterally dilated pupils suggest severe intracranial pathology and urgent neurosurgical intervention needs to be considered in a time-critical manner.

Abnormal motor responses include inequality in movement from side to side, and posturing.

- Decorticate posturing is rigid flexion with arms flexed towards the core and lower extremities extended. This type of posturing is associated with lesions above the midbrain.
- Rigid extension of the arms with wrist flexion and rigid extension of lower extremities is decerebrate posturing. This type of posturing is associated with an insult to the brainstem.

The distinction between these two postures is important, as the decerebrate posture indicates a deeper level of coma. Figure 45.19 illustrates decerebrate and decorticate posturing. If a patient's motor component of the GCS changes

from decorticate to decerebrate, the need for neurosurgical intervention needs to be considered immediately, as it may indicate a rising ICP. Lateralisation occurs when patients with TBI have clinical signs of unilateral decorticate and decerebrate posturing. Posturing may be spontaneous or elicited by verbal or painful stimuli.

Intracranial pressure

In the adult patient, the skull is a closed box containing the brain, CSF and blood. For ICP to remain within normal limits (0–15 mmHg), an increase in blood, CSF or brain mass must be accompanied by a reciprocal decrease of one of the other components. This is referred to as the Monro-Kellie doctrine.[37] Sustained ICP > 20 mmHg is a neurosurgical emergency associated with increased mortality and morbidity in TBI.[29] Failure to reduce ICP may subsequently cause additional ischaemia and necrosis of brain tissue.

An ICP monitoring device is inserted via a burr hole into the brain using an intraventricular, parenchymal or subdural catheter (Fig 45.20). ICP monitoring aids the detection of intracranial mass lesions, guides adjunctive therapies to control ICP and, with certain monitoring devices such as an external ventricular drain, may facilitate a reduction in ICP by CSF drainage.[39] A further function of ICP monitoring is to allow a derived calculation of cerebral perfusion pressure.

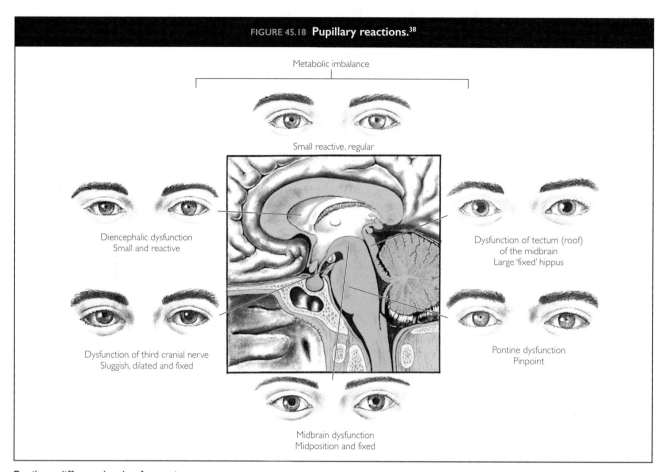

FIGURE 45.18 **Pupillary reactions.**[38]

Metabolic imbalance

Small reactive, regular

Diencephalic dysfunction
Small and reactive

Dysfunction of tectum (roof)
of the midbrain
Large 'fixed' hippus

Dysfunction of third cranial nerve
Sluggish, dilated and fixed

Pontine dysfunction
Pinpoint

Midbrain dysfunction
Midposition and fixed

Pupils at different levels of consciousness.

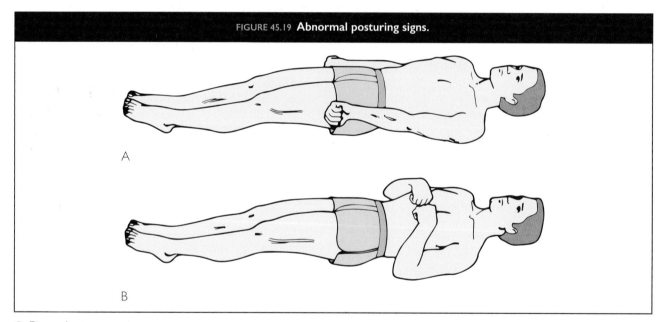

FIGURE 45.19 **Abnormal posturing signs.**

A

B

A, Decerebrate posturing.
B, Decorticate posturing.

Cerebral perfusion pressure

The cerebral perfusion pressure (CPP) is the difference between the mean arterial pressure (MAP) and the ICP (CPP = MAP − ICP). Evidence suggests that maintaining CPP above 50 mmHg is necessary to prevent cerebral ischaemia and associated secondary injury.[11,29] Vasopressor agents such as noradrenaline are used to augment the MAP to maintain a CPP between 50 and 70 mmHg; however, care must be taken in the context of trauma to ensure that the underlying causative factor for hypotension is not hypovolaemia.[11]

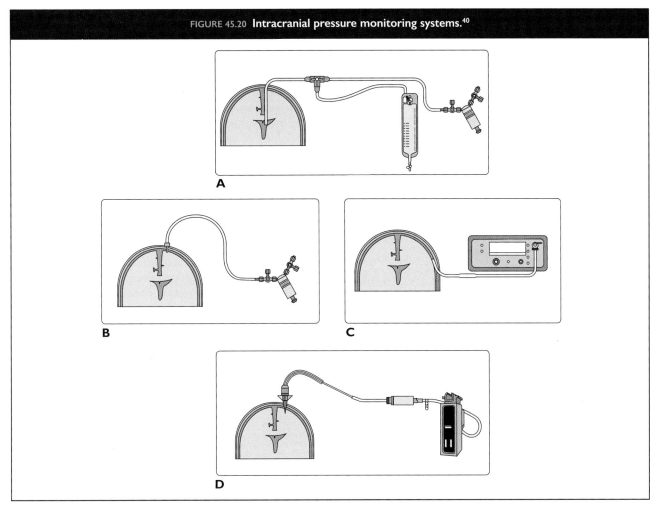

FIGURE 45.20 Intracranial pressure monitoring systems.[40]

A, Ventricular pressure monitoring system.
B, Subarachnoid pressure monitoring system.

C, Epidural pressure monitoring system.
D, Intraparenchymal pressure monitoring system.

A key factor in monitoring the CPP is accurate placement of the arterial transducer. When the patient is in the head-elevated position, the arterial transducer should be level with and zeroed to the foramen of Monro. Failure to do this will result in either an under- or an over-estimation of CPP, which has the potential of being deleterious to patients.[36,40,41]

Hyperventilation

Hyperventilation to a $PaCO_2$ of 30 mmHg (25–30 mmHg in extreme cases) lowers ICP by causing cerebral vasoconstriction and reducing cerebral blood flow. The effect usually peaks within 30 minutes and diminishes over the next 1–3 hours. It is important to note that cerebral blood flow has been shown to be significantly decreased (up to half that of a non-injured brain) in the first 24 hours post-injury and therefore the additional use of hyperventilation may induce additional cerebral ischaemia.[29] In resuscitated patients with unequivocal signs of raised ICP or impending cerebral herniation (witnessed neurological deterioration or lateralising signs or pupillary dilation) hyperventilation may be instituted as a temporising measure while neurosurgical intervention is considered.[29,37]

Thermoregulation

In the pre-hospital setting, hypothermia, when combined with acidosis and coagulopathy, has been associated with poor long-term outcomes.[10,15,42] Preventing hypothermia in this context may be important, particularly if control of haemorrhage is difficult to achieve.

A raised body temperature is common in the first few days of hospital admission after TBI. The systemic inflammatory response to injury and direct damage to the hypothalamic control centres for thermoregulation often result in a raised temperature during intensive care and hospital stay. A rising core temperature can result in increased CO_2 production. Additionally, an elevated temperature may be associated with exacerbation of injury with intracellular derangements and increased blood–brain permeability, which adds to cerebral oedema.[42] Data from animal studies and observational case series in humans support the practice of avoiding fever and maintaining a normal body temperature; however, to date there have been no studies demonstrating that maintaining a normal temperature after TBI improves patient-centred outcomes. Some studies have, however, shown that reducing temperature is an effective method of controlling raised ICP.[43] A suggested definition for normothermia for use in clinical practice may be to maintain core body temperature at 37°C, although temperatures as high as 38°C have been accepted in clinical trials.[44]

Induced hypothermia is a potential therapeutic strategy that remains controversial.[45] The hypothesis is that induced hypothermia may have neuroprotective properties, preventing or altering the biological cascade that causes secondary brain injury. Several cooling strategies are available and rapid, safe onset of hypothermia in intubated patients may be obtained by the intravenous injection of 30 mL/kg (approximately 2 L of a crystalloid solution such as 0.9% saline) that has been refrigerated at 4°C.[46] Alternatives include the use of surface-cooling devices (water-circulating cooling blankets[47] or ice packs in the axilla or groin) or intravenous cooling catheters.[48] When cooling strategies are implemented, careful attention needs to be taken to prevent shivering, which is a physiological mechanism to aid the body to increase temperature. Neuromuscular blockade and deep sedation are generally required for inducing and maintaining hypothermia, but this combination of the need for these pharmacological agents and hypothermia has the effect of altering drug metabolism (e.g. prolonging the action of sedative and analgesic drugs). Therefore, the intervention of hypothermia may indirectly prolong the duration of mechanical ventilation and length of stay in hospital and this may be associated with acquired complications due to delayed mobilisation (e.g. pressure sores, pneumonia, catheter-related blood stream infection). The depth of hypothermia (ranging between 33°C and < 36°C)[37,42] and duration of hypothermia are also not clearly defined at present. Continuous monitoring of core temperature for TBI patients requiring mechanical ventilation is recommended.[42]

Osmotherapy

The use of intravenous solutions that exert an osmotic diuretic effect have been the mainstay of treatment for an elevated ICP. The two most common agents used are mannitol 20% and hypertonic saline (> 1.5% saline).[49]

- Mannitol 20% solution is an osmotic diuretic that reduces ICP by changing the osmotic gradient, causing fluid to leave cerebral extracellular tissues and move to intravascular beds. Movement of fluid reduces total brain mass, therefore decreasing ICP. Mannitol should be administered at doses of 0.25–1 g/kg when signs of transtentorial herniation are present or progressive neurological deterioration is evident. The patient's overall volume status should be assessed before administration of mannitol. The effect of mannitol begins within 10–20 minutes and peaks between 20–60 minutes, with a therapeutic duration of 4–6 hours.[49]

- Hypertonic saline solutions of various concentrations may also be used for the interim treatment of raised ICP. Hypertonic saline has been shown to decrease cerebral water content and ICP with at least the same efficacy as mannitol. Hypertonic saline infusion causes plasma expansion via redistribution of fluid from the intravascular space. The resultant increase in MAP is achieved with less volume required than with isotonic fluids. Suggested doses of hypertonic saline to achieve effective reduction in ICP are 5 mL/kg of a 3% solution given as a bolus or, alternatively, rapid infusion.[49]

There are number of side effects associated with the use of osmotic agents and these include hypotension as a consequence of an induced diuresis and accumulation of the agent in the central nervous system (which may paradoxically increase ICP) in the context of disruption of the blood–brain barrier.

In summary, as with hyperventilation, in resuscitated patients with unequivocal signs of raised ICP or impending cerebral herniation (witnessed neurological deterioration or new lateralising signs or pupillary dilation), osmotic diuretics may be used as a temporising measure while neurosurgical intervention is considered.

Miscellaneous therapies

Barbiturate therapy may be considered for patients with refractory intracranial hypertension. Haemodynamic stability should be confirmed before induction of barbiturate coma. Early seizure activity should be treated with appropriate anticonvulsants. Side effects include complications related to prolonged sedation and acquired infections.

Prophylactic anticonvulsants are often used for the prevention of seizure-induced secondary injury, and possibly reduce late post-injury seizure activity.[50] Paralytics in conjunction with sedation may help control ICP. High-dose corticosteroids have been shown to increase mortality when administered to hospitalised patients after head injury,[51] and are considered to be contraindicated for TBI.

PRACTICE TIP

ICP AND PATIENT POSITIONING

Instigate a 'head-up' bed tilt while maintaining a neutral spine alignment to facilitate a decrease in ICP. Alternatively, if the patient is deemed suitable, elevate the head of the bed 30–45° to facilitate venous drainage.[40]

Instigating a 'head-up' bed tilt while maintaining a neutral spine alignment may facilitate a decrease in ICP; alternatively, if cervical spine injury has been ruled out (or deemed stable for particular positioning by the treating neurosurgeon) and the patient is haemodynamically stable, elevating the head of the bed 30–45° may also facilitate venous drainage.

There are a number of other monitoring and protocol-driven interventions, including the following adjuncts to monitoring: jugular venous oxygen saturation monitoring, brain-tissue oxygen monitoring, brain temperature monitoring and cerebral microdialysis. The near future will bring multimodal monitoring where multiple parameters can be successfully monitored via the one catheter. For the latest news on traumatic brain injury research see the Australian-driven EvidenceMap.org website.

Analgesia in traumatic brain injury

There are no specific guidelines or evidence pertaining to the use of specific pharmacological agents to manage pain associated with minor head injury. Head injury alone can result in headache which does require the use of analgesia. The drug of choice will be dependent on clinical signs, need and clinical context. Where CNS-depressant analgesics are used, such as those containing opiates, careful attention must be paid to monitoring the patient's neurological status. Managing pain in the patient with TBI is a clinical challenge. This is particularly important for patients with multiple injuries, including fractures. Importantly, analgesia should not be withheld from the patient with headache or other pain sources if the clinical need is present.[20]

There are a number of non-pharmacological methods for treating pain, including reducing noxious stimuli by providing a quiet and dark environment, and allowing family to comfort the patient (providing they are not causing overstimulation). The intermittent use of cold packs can also provide an analgesic effect.

PRACTICE TIP

NON-PHARMACOLOGICAL ANALGESIA ADJUNCTS

Beneficial adjuncts to analgesia and improving patient comfort include intermittent use of cold packs and reduction of noxious stimuli by providing a quiet and dark environment.

Nursing the patient in a head-elevated position reduces swelling and thereby mitigates pain. These are all difficult to achieve in a busy ED, so expediting the patient's disposition to a ward bed is a priority.

Radiology

X-ray

Skull X-rays have limited application in the management of TBI.[12] They may be of use in rural and remote centres that have no access to more-definitive CT examinations as a precursor for possible referral for neurosurgical advice. The presence of a skull fracture increases the probability of intracranial pathology and, therefore, increased risk of deterioration.[20,52]

BOX 45.3 Imaging options for traumatic brain injury (TBI)[52,77]

Skull X-ray:
- as a screening tool in rural and remote settings in absence of CT availability

Computed tomography (CT):
- acute setting
- moderate and severe TBI; GCS < 13
- mild TBI with concurrent risks
- suspected skull fracture

Magnetic resonance imaging:
- acute setting with neurological findings unexplained on CT
- suspected DAI

Angiography:
- suspected vascular injury or infarction

DAI: diffuse axonal injury; GCS: Glasgow Coma Scale

Computed tomography

Computed tomography scan remains the modality of choice for the initial assessment of acute head injury. CT is widely available in most urban centres and is a fast, highly accurate investigation for the detection of skull fractures and acute intracranial haemorrhage, and easily accommodates critical-care support equipment. CT is recommended for all patients with moderate to severe TBI (GCS < 12). Additionally, CT is recommended for patients with mild TBI who have concurrent signs such as headache or vomiting, loss of consciousness > 5 minutes, amnesia, persistent neurological deficit, depressed skull fracture or penetrating injury, or are aged over 60 years or have known coagulopathy.[12,52]

CT angiography can be performed in addition when vascular injury or involvement is suspected. Traumatic vascular injuries are most commonly associated with skull-base fractures.[12]

Magnetic resonance imaging

Magnetic resonance imaging is recommended for patients with acute TBI whose neurological findings are unexplained by CT. MRI is more sensitive to extra-axial smear collections, nonhaemorrhagic lesions, brainstem injuries and SAH than is conventional CT. The use of fluid-attenuated inversion recovery (FLAIR) imaging in conjunction with MRI improves the detection of focal cortical and white matter shearing injuries, such as diffuse axonal injuries (DAIs). Note that limited critical-care support and equipment can be used on patients while in the MRI suite due to magnetic field limitations.[12]

Summary of imaging options

A summary of imaging options for TBI is given in Box 45.3.[12,52]

Mild traumatic brain injury

Mild traumatic brain injury (mTBI) is a major public health concern, given the large number of patients affected each year. It represents approximately 80% of all head injuries sustained. Mild traumatic brain injury is defined by the American Congress of Rehabilitation Medicine as a traumatically induced physiological disruption of brain function as manifested by at least one of the following:

- any period of loss of consciousness
- any loss of memory for events immediately before or after the accident
- any alteration in mental state at the accident, such as feeling dazed, disorientated or confused
- focal neurological deficits that may or may not be transient but where the severity of the injury does not exceed the following:
  - a loss of consciousness of approximately 30 minutes or less
  - after 30 minutes, an initial GCS of 13–15, and
  - post-traumatic amnesia not greater than 24 hours.[53]

Many patients admitted with an mTBI will exhibit subacute cognitive deficits, particularly in attention, memory, reasoning and thought-processing, which will generally resolve over a period of 1–3 months.[54] However, approximately 15–25% of cases experience ongoing symptoms, which can include headaches, dizziness, visual disturbance, memory difficulties, poor concentration, difficulty dividing attention, alcohol intolerance, fatigue, irritability, depression and anxiety.[55] The difficulty associated with the assessment of these patients is that the cognitive deficits associated with mTBI are too subtle to detect by routine neurological examination and require cognitive screening[56] such as the Standardized Assessment of Concussion,[57] although even cognitive measures such as the ImPACT Test Battery for Concussion have been demonstrated to not predict post-concussive symptoms at 1 week or 3 months.[55]

The presence of mTBI-predicted postconcussional symptoms 1 week post-injury is associated with female and premorbid psychiatric history.[55,58] At 3 months, pre-injury physical or psychiatric problems, but not mTBI, most strongly predicted continuing symptoms, along with concurrent anxiety, PTSD symptoms, other life stressors and pain.[55] Recovery from cognitive deficits has been shown to be adversely affected by advancing age.[59]

Assessment of mild traumatic brain injury

As the impact of deficits following mTBI can cause a disruption in a person's ability to perform the activities of daily life, it is essential that all patients who present with mTBI have a thorough assessment, including both a cognitive and a functional assessment. Patients and their families should be educated about the impact such deficits could have on the patient's functional abilities and should be provided with strategies to manage such deficits, in an attempt to reduce the impact that mTBI has on the patient's ability to perform functional activities.

The Abbreviated Westmead Post Traumatic Amnesia Scale (A-WPTAS) was developed to assist with the early identification of cognitive impairment following mTBI, and in particular to assess patients' ability to lay down new memories over a 24-hour period.[60] The A-WPTAS is based on the original Westmead Post Traumatic Amnesia Scale and incorporates the GCS. The A-WPTAS consists of the 15 questions from the GCS plus assessment of new learning through the addition of three Westmead PTA picture-recall questions. If the patient has a GCS of 13–15 the revised A-WPTAS is commenced

hourly or until a score of 18 is achieved in the first 24 hours following injury. If the patient does not pass the A-WPTAS after 4 hours post-injury time, they should be considered for admission and commencement of the Westmead PTA scale. The tool is designed for use with patients who have a GCS ≥ 13 to assist in the measurement of post-traumatic amnesia in this MTBI group.[61] If the patient has a GCS of <13 at the time of injury, or emerged from coma after 24 hours after injury, the Westmead PTA scale should be commenced.[62] Outcomes of preliminary research conducted on the use of A-WPTAS suggest that patients who achieve 18/18 on the A-WPTAS could be considered to have emerged from post-traumatic amnesia; however, further research is required to validate this finding and to further study the use of A-WPTAS.[62] For further information see the A-WPTAS education and screening tools webpage (listed under Useful websites).

Sports concussion

Concussion head injuries are common in many sporting and recreational activities and are often referred to as concussion. The section will deal with sports concussion, which is defined as a complex pathophysiological process affecting the brain, induced by traumatic biomechanical forces.[61]

Symptoms may manifest immediately, hours or days post-impact.[62] It is important to be aware of the signs of a concussion, as it can result in distressing symptoms and clear declines in cognitive abilities, which need to be managed.[63] There are a number of changes that may indicate a concussion. Symptoms include headache, dizziness or balance issues and feeling slowed down.[64] Other cognitive impairments include amnesia and slowed reaction times.[61] Concussion may or may not involve loss of consciousness and can also cause sleep disturbance and fatigue.[61]

There are a number of assessments that can be used to determine concussion, which can be completed at the location of the sports event on the sideline, but should be followed up with further review. An assessment of concussion must involve evaluation of the individual's cognitive function, assessing memory, attention/concentration, orientation and amnesia. It should be noted that standard assessment of orientation alone has shown to be unreliable in the sporting situation when compared with assessment of memory and delayed recall.[65] Furthermore, this initial, often sideline, assessment should be used to initially assist identification of concussion but should not replace comprehensive neuropsychological assessment that will detect the more subtle deficits that may exist beyond acute episodes.[4] Individuals who exhibit other physical symptoms, such as balance issues, should also undergo further assessment.

An example of an assessment tool is the Sports Concussion Assessment Tool (SCAT), originally developed at the International Symposium on Concussion in Sport and recently further developed at a 2008 symposium into the SCAT2.[61] The tool enables healthcare professionals to complete an assessment of concussion; however, it is still being validated.

The majority (80–90%) of concussions will resolve in a short period, generally 7–10 days, although the recovery time may be longer in children and adolescents.[66] Concussion should be managed individually, with general trends and expectations used as a framework for considering an individual's unique symptoms, problems and experiences.[67] The science of concussion is evolving, and therefore management and return-to-play decisions remain in the realm of clinical judgement on an individual basis.[66] Individuals should be encouraged to rest—both physically and cognitively—with the expectation that injuries will recover spontaneously over the following few days.[61] If individuals do not rest, activities such as returning to work may exacerbate symptoms and may delay recovery. Advice should be provided to individuals and their families, including the signs and symptoms to watch for in the first 24–48 hours.

While the literature remains divided on the occurrence of second-impact syndrome, it should be discussed. *Second-impact syndrome* is defined as occurring when an athlete who has sustained an initial head injury, most often a concussion, sustains a second injury before the symptoms of the first have fully resolved.[68] Second-impact syndrome will present as diffuse cerebral swelling that results in increased ICP.[68] Given the chance that this may occur, despite the controversy mentioned, it needs to be considered, given what evidence does exist in the literature.

Guidelines have been provided by the American Academy of Neurology[69] of not allowing an individual to return to sports until post-concussion symptoms have resolved. Premature return could also result in further injury, especially if the individual is experiencing slowed reaction times as they may be unable to respond appropriately and thus risk future injury.[70] Education is required to ensure that athletes are aware of this potential risk, as they remain reluctant to report an incidence of concussion and the associated symptoms.[71] It is, however, reported that individuals who have sustained a previous concussion are more likely to report the second impact, which may indicate that a previous history of concussion seems to increase the athlete's injury susceptibility. In addition, those with a history of concussion have worse clinical outcomes, including more severe acute signs and symptoms and longer periods of acute recovery following the second impact.[72]

Post-concussion symptoms

The International Statistical Classification of Diseases and Related Health Problems, 10th edition (ICD10), defines post-concussion syndrome (PCS) as 'a syndrome that occurs after head trauma (usually with some loss of consciousness) and [which] may be accompanied by feelings of depression and anxiety resulting in fear of permanent brain damage'.[72] The ICD10 recognises that neurological abnormalities are often not associated with the syndrome and are not required for diagnosis. The ICD10 criteria for PCS is three or more of the following symptoms: headache, dizziness, malaise, fatigue, noise intolerance, irritability, insomnia, depression, anxiety, emotional lability, subjective concentration, memory or intellectual difficulties and reduced alcohol tolerance.[72]

Impact on resuming functional activities

Kay believes that when the primary deficits of an mTBI go undetected or a patient is not aware of the deficits, their ability to cope and adapt to the deficits will result in greater psychological deficits.[73] Functional outcome can be affected by a number of factors. Patients should be educated about detected cognitive deficits and possible symptoms that may occur as a result of the mTBI.[74] Patient discharge advice is summarised in Box 45.4. Waiting for patients to fail will prolong their symptoms and reduce their ability to cope.

Provision of information booklets informing the patient about their injury and suggested coping strategies has been shown to reduce the anxiety in patients and subsequently lower the incidence of ongoing problems to some degree.[76] Kay advocates advising the patient's family or significant other of the symptoms and involving them in strategies to assist in managing the deficit.[73]

BOX 45.4 Patient advice following head injury[75]

General advice

1. The patient should read and understand these instructions.
2. Rest comfortably at home in the company of a responsible adult for the next 12–24 hours.
3. Resume normal activity after feeling recovered.
4. Drink clear fluids and consume a light diet only for the first 6–12 hours (a normal diet may be commenced as desired after that).
5. Mild painkillers (such as paracetamol) may be taken for headache as directed by the doctor.
6. Following head injury, a small number of patients develop ongoing symptoms, such as recurrent mild headache, concentration difficulties, difficulty with complex tasks, mood disturbance, etc. If you notice such problems, consult your local doctor for appropriate outpatient brain injury referral.
7. Avoid exposure to activities that may create risk of further head injury within the next 2 weeks.

8. If you do not understand these instructions and advice, check with emergency department staff before your discharge or consult your local doctor.
9. If you require a certificate for work, please make this clear to emergency department staff.

Report immediately the following problems:

1. Persistent vomiting (more than twice).
2. Persistent drowsiness—unable to be woken up completely.
3. Confusion or disorientation or slurred speech.
4. Increased headache (not relieved by standard doses of paracetamol).
5. Localised weakness or altered sensation or incoordination.
6. Blurred or double vision.
7. Seizures, fits or convulsions.
8. Neck stiffness.

SUMMARY

Head injuries are a major cause of traumatic deaths and cause significant long-term disability. Presentations to hospital for management of TBI are frequent, and this patient group will continue to confront emergency medical service providers and emergency nurses with multiple challenges. Recognition and prevention of secondary injuries related to ischaemia, increased ICP and hypoxia are essential for these challenging patients. Additionally, the increasing use of illicit intoxicating substances will continue to make the patient assessment and management process problematic. Preventing the injury from becoming worse, particularly from secondary brain injury, by having systems in place to recognise, report and action a deteriorating neurological state early, are the mainstays of clinical practice for this patient group. Nurses are a vital part of the acute care of patients with TBI.

CASE STUDY

A 28-year-old male patient presents with periorbital bruising and confusion post assault, with a fluctuating level of consciousness.

Questions

1. Describe the immediate assessment.

2. What is his most likely injury, and why?

3. Describe the rationale for maintenance of normal arterial blood gas values for the ventilated patient with signs of traumatic brain injury.

4. Describe clinical strategies to minimise secondary brain injury.

5. Describe the rationale and transfer criteria for referral to a trauma centre with neurosurgical services.

6. Differentiate between focal and diffuse traumatic brain injury.

7. Explain the rationale for the frequency of head injury nursing observations.

8. What is the earliest sign of a deterioration in the patient with a head injury?

9. Explain the Munro-Kellie doctrine as it relates to raised intracranial pressure in the patient with traumatic brain injury.

Answers to Case Study Questions can be found on evolve
http://evolve.emergencytrauma.curtis

USEFUL WEBSITES

American College of Surgeons trauma programs, www.facs.org/trauma/index.html

Brain Foundation, Australia, www.brainaustralia.org.au

Brain Trauma Foundation, www.braintrauma.org

Emergency Care Institute—AWPTAS education and screening tools www.ecinsw.com.au/awptas

NSW Institute of Trauma Injury and Management, www.itim.nsw.gov.au/index.cfm

The management of acute neurotrauma in rural and remote locations: A set of guidelines for the care of head and spinal injuries, 3rd edn, 2009, www.nsa.org.au/documents/pub_neurotrauma.pdf

Trauma.org, www.trauma.org

Victorian State Trauma System, www.health.vic.gov.au/trauma

World Health Organization Collaborating Centres for Neurotrauma, www.who.int/violence_injury_prevention/about/collaborating_centres/en/

EvidenceMap.org, http://neurotrauma.evidencemap.org/

REFERENCES

1. Caulfield EV, Dutton RP, Floccare DJ et al. Prehospital hypocapnia and poor outcome after severe traumatic brain injury. J Trauma 2009;66(6):1577–82.

2. Riggio S, Jagoda A. Traumatic brain injury: from bench to bedside to home. Mt Sinai J Med 2009;76(2):95–6.

3. Smith M. Critical care management of severe head injury. Anesthetic and Intensive Care Medicine 2014;15(4):164–7.

4. Helps Y, Henley G, Harrison JE. Hospital separations due to traumatic brain injury, Australia 2004–05. Injury research and statistics series number 45. Cat no. INJCAT 116. Adelaide: Australian Institute for Health and Welfare; 2008.

5. Access Economics. The economic cost of spinal cord injury and traumatic brain injury in Australia. Report by Access Economics Pty Limited for the Victorian Neurotrauma Initiative. Melbourne: VNI; 2009.

6. Myburgh JA, Cooper DJ et al. Epidemiology and 12-month outcomes from traumatic brain injury in Australia and New Zealand. J Trauma Injury Infect Crit Care 2008;64(4):854–62.

7. Bandak FA. On the mechanics of impact neurotrauma: a review and critical synthesis. J Neurotrauma 1995;12(4):635–49.

8. Crocker P, Zad O et al. Alcohol, bicycling, and head and brain injury: a study of impaired cyclists' riding patterns RI. Am J Emerg Med 2010;28(1):68–72.

9. Sosin DM, Sniezek JE, Waxweiler RJ. Trends in death associated with traumatic brain injury, 1979 through 1992: success and failure. JAMA 1995;273(22):1778–80.

10. Reilly PL, Bullock R. Head injury—pathophysiology and management. 2nd edn. London: Hodder Education; 2005.

11. Halliday J, Absalom AR. Traumatic brain injury: from impact to rehabilitation. Br J Hosp Med (Lond) 2008;69(5):284–9.

12. Potapov A, Pronin I, Kornienko V, Zakharova N. Neuroimaging of traumatic brain injury. Springer International Publishing; 2014.

13. Lindsay DT. Functional human anatomy. St Louis: Mosby; 1996.

14. Rangel-Castilla L, Gasco J, Nauta HJ et al. Cerebral pressure autoregulation in traumatic brain injury. Neurosurg Focus 2008;25(4):E7.

15. McQuillan KA, Von Rueden KT, Hartsock RL et al. Trauma nursing: from resuscitation through rehabilitation. 4th edn. Missouri: WB Saunders; 2009.

16. O'Shea RA. Principles and practice of trauma nursing. Edinburgh: Churchill Livingstone; 2005.

17. Turnage B, Maull KI. Scalp laceration: an obvious 'occult' cause of shock. South Med J 2000;93(3):265–6.

18. Qureshi NH, Harsh IV G. Skull fractures. Emedicine. Continuing education; 2002. Online. www.emedicine.com/med/topic2894.htm; 26 Jan 2007.

19. Adam A, Dixon AK. Grainger and Allison's diagnostic radiology. 5th edn. New York: Churchill Livingstone; 2008.

20. The Neurosurgical Society of Australasia. The management of acute neurotrauma in rural and remote locations: a set of guidelines for the care of the head and spinal injuries. 3rd edn. 2009. Online. www.nsa.org.au/documents/item/44; accessed 4 May 2015.

21. Soto JA, Lucey BC. Emergency radiology: the requisites. Philadelphia: Mosby; 2009.

22. Welch KC, Stankiewicz J. CSF rhinorrhea. Emedicine. Continuing education; 2002. Online. Available: www.emedicine.com/ent/topic332.htm; 29 Jan 2007.

23. Ropper A. Neurological and neurosurgical intensive care. 5th edn: Lippincott, Williams & Wilkins; 2012.

24. Jallo J, Loftus CM, eds. Neurotrauma and critical care of the brain. New York: Thieme Medical Publishers; 2009.

25. Haaga J, Dogra VS, Forsting M et al. eds. CT and MRI of the whole body. 5th edn. Philadelphia: Mosby; 2009.

26. American College of Surgeons Committee on Trauma. Advanced trauma life support. 9th edn. Chicago: American College of Surgeons Committee; 2012.

27. Minardi J, Crocco TJ. Management of traumatic brain injury: first link in chain of survival. Mt Sinai J Med 2009;76:138–44.

28. Badjatia J, Carney N, Crocco TJ et al. Guidelines for prehospital management of traumatic brain injury. 2nd edn. Brain Trauma Foundation (USA); 2008.

29. Robert J, Appleby I. Traumatic brain injury: initial resuscitation and transfer. Anesthetics & Intensive Care Medicine. 2014;15(4):161–3.

30. CRASH-2 Trial Collaborators. Effects of tranexamic acid on death, vascular occlusive events, and blood transfusion in trauma patients with significant haemorrhage (CRASH-2): a randomised, placebo-controlled trial. Lancet 2010; 376:23–32.

31. P Perel, Al-Shahi Salman R, Kawahara T et al. CRASH-2 (Clinical Randomisation of an Antifibrinolytic in Significant Haemorrhage) intracranial bleeding study: the effect of tranexamic acid in traumatic brain injury—a nested, randomised, placebo-controlled trial. Journal of Health Technology Assessment 2012;16(13).

32. Dewan Y, Komolafe EO, Mijia-Mantilla JH et al. CRASH-3—tranexamic acid for the treatment of significant traumatic brain injury: study protocol for an international randomized, double-blind, placebo-controlled trial. CRASH-3 Trials 2012;13;87.

33. Fortune JB, Feustel PJ, Graca L et al. Effect of hyperventilation, mannitol, and ventriculostomy drainage on cerebral blood-flow after head injury. J Trauma 1995;39(6):1091–9.

34. Davies G, Deakin C, Wilson A. The effect of a rigid collar on intracranial pressure. Injury 1996;27(9):647–9.

35. Stone MB, Tubridy CM, Curran R. The effect of rigid cervical collars on internal jugular vein dimensions. Acad Emerg Med 2010;17(1):100–2.

36. Gill M, Martens K, Lynch E, Salih A, Green S. Interrater reliability of 3 simplified neurologic scales applied to adults presenting to the ED with altered levels of consciousness. An Emerg Med 2007;49(4):403–7.

37. Helmy A, Vizcaychipi M, Gupta A. Traumatic brain injury: Intensive care management. Br J Anaesth 2007;99(1):32–42.

38. Huether SE, McCance KL. Understanding pathophysiology. 5th edn. St Louis: Mosby; 2011.

39. Brain Trauma Foundation and American Association of Neurological Surgeons Joint Section on Neurotrauma and Critical Care. Guidelines for the management of severe head injury. 3rd edn. The American Association of Neurological Surgeons; 2007.

40. Thelan LA et al. Critical care nursing: diagnosis and management. 7th edn. St Louis: Mosby; 2013.

41. Kirkman M, Smith M. Intracranial pressure monitoring, cerebral perfusion pressure estimation and ICP/CPP guided therapy: a standard of care or optional extra after brain injury? Br J Anaesth 2014;112(1):35–46.

42. Kirkman M, Smith M. Therapeutic hypothermia and acute brain injury. Anaesthesia & Intensive Care Medicine 2014;15(4):171–5.

43. Saxena MK, Taylor CB, Hammond NE et al. Temperature management in patients with acute neurological lesions: an Australian and New Zealand point prevalence study. Critical care and resuscitation: Journal of the Australasian Academy of Critical Care Medicine 2013;15(2):110–18.

44. Sydenham E, Roberts I, Alderson P. Hypothermia for traumatic head injury. Cochrane Database of Systematic Reviews. (2):CD001048. PubMed PMID: 19370561.

45. Bernard SI, Buist M, Monteiro O, Smith K. Induced hypothermia using large volume, ice-cold intravenous fluid in comatose survivors of out-of-hospital cardiac arrest: a preliminary report. Resuscitation 2003;56(1):9–13.

46. Carhuapoma JR, Gupta K, Coplin WM et al. Treatment of refractory fever in the neurosciences critical care unit using a novel, water-circulating cooling device. A single-center pilot experience. J Neurosurg Anesthesiol 2003;15(4):313–18. PubMed PMID: 14508172.

47. Broessner G, Beer R, Lackner P et al. Prophylactic, endovascularly based, long-term normothermia in ICU patients with severe cerebrovascular disease. Bicenter Prospective, Randomized Trial Stroke 2009;40(12):e657–65.

48. Maas A, Stocchetti N, Bullock R. Moderate and Severe Traumatic Brain injury in adults. Prophylactic, Lancet Neurology 2008;7(8):728–41.

49. Wakai A, Roberts IG, Schierhout G. Mannitol for acute traumatic brain injury. Cochrane Database of Systematic Reviews 2007;1: CD001049. DOI: 10.1002/14651858.CD001049.pub4.

50. American Academy of Neurology. Practice parameter: Antiepileptic drug prophylaxis in severe traumatic brain injury. Report of the Quality Standards Subcommittee. Neurology 2003;60(1):10–16.

51. CRASH Trial Collaborators. Effect of intravenous corticosteroids on death within 14 days in 10008 adults with clinically significant head injury: randomised placebo-controlled trial. Lancet 2004;364(9442):1321–8.

52. Reed D. Adult trauma clinical practice guidelines: initial management of closed head injury in adults. NSW Institute of Trauma and Injury Management; 2011.

53. Committee of the Head Injury Interdisciplinary Special Interest Group of the American Congress of Rehabilitation Medicine. Definition of mild traumatic brain injury. J Head Trauma Rehabil 1993;8(3):86–7.

54. Levin H, Mattis S, Ruff R et al. Neurobehavioral outcome following minor head injury: a three centre study. J Neurosurg 1987;66:234–43.

55. Ponsford J, Cameron P, Fitzgerald M et al. Predictors of postconcussive symptoms 3 months after mild traumatic brain injury. Neuropsychology 2012;26(3):304–13.

56. Cammermeyer M, Evans JE. A brief neurobehavioral exam useful for early detection of post-operative complications in neurosurgical patients. J Neurosci Nurs 1988;20(5):314–23.

57. Naunheim RS, Matero D, Fucetola R. Assessment of patients with mild concussion in the emergency department. J Head Trauma Rehabil 2008;23(2):116–22.

58. Dischinger PC, Ryb GE, Kufera JA, Auman KM. Early predictors of postconcussive syndrome in a population of trauma patients with mild traumatic brain injury. Journal of Trauma—Injury, Infection and Critical Care 2009;66(2):289–96.

59. Kibby MY, Long CJ. Minor head injury: attempts at clarifying the confusion. Brain Inj 1996;10(3):159–86.

60. Shores EA, Lammel A, Hullick C et al. The diagnostic accuracy of the Revised Westmead PTA Scale as an adjunct to the Glasgow Coma Scale in the early identification of cognitive impairment in patients with mild traumatic brain injury. J Neurol Neurosurg Psychiatry 2008;79(10):1100–6.

61. McCrory P, Meeuwisse W, Johnston K et al. Consensus statement on concussion in sport: the 3rd international conference on concussion in sport held in Zurich, November 2008. Br J Sports Med 2009;43(Suppl. 1):i76–90.

62. Aubry M, Cantu R, Dvorak J et al. Summary and agreement statement of the First International Conference on Concussion in Sport, Vienna 2001. Recommendations for the improvement of safety and health of athletes who may suffer concussive injuries. Br J Sports Med 2002;36(1):6–10.

63. Iverson GL, Gaetz M, Lovell MR et al. Cumulative effects of concussion in amateur athletes. Brain Inj 2004;18(5):433–43.

64. Guskiewicz KM, McCrea M, Marshall SW et al. Cumulative effects associated with recurrent concussion in collegiate football players: the NCAA concussion study. JAMA 2003;290(19):2549–55.

65. McCrea M, Kelly JP, Kluge J et al. Standardized assessment of concussion in football players. Neurology 1997;48(3):586–8.

66. McCrory P, Johnston K, Meeuwisse W et al. Summary and agreement statement of the 2nd International Conference on Concussion in Sport, Prague 2004. Br J Sports Med 2005;39:i78–86.

67. Iverson GL, Brooks BL, Collins MW et al. Tracking neuropsychological recovery following concussion in sport. Brain Inj 2006;20(3):245–52.

68. Cantu RC, Voy R. Second impact syndrome: a risk in any contact sport. Physician Sports Med 1995;23:27–34.

69. American Academy of Neurology. Practice parameter update: Evaluation and management of concussion in sports. Report of the Quality Standards Subcommittee. Neurology 2013;80(24):2250–7.

70. McCrory PR, Berkovic SF. Second impact syndrome. Neurology 1998;50(3):677–83.

71. Mansell JL, Tierney RT, Higgins M et al. Concussive signs and symptoms following head impacts in collegiate athletes. Brain Inj 2010;24(9):1070–4.

72. Mittenberg W, Strauman S. Diagnosis of mild head injury and the post-concussion syndrome. J Head Trauma Rehabil 2000;15(2):783–91.

73. Kay T. Neuropsychological treatment of mild traumatic brain injury. J Head Trauma Rehabil 1993;8(3):74–85.

74. Kay T, Newman B, Cavallo M et al. Toward a neuropsychological model of functional disability after mild traumatic brain injury. Neuropsychology 1992;6:371–84.

75. Cameron P, Jelinek G, Kelly A et al. Textbook of adult emergency medicine. 2nd edn. Edinburgh: Churchill Livingstone; 2004.

76. Ponsford J, Willmott C, Rothwell A et al. Impact of early intervention on outcome following mild head injury in adults. J Neurol Neurosurg Psychiatry 2002;73(3):330–2.

77. Le TH, Gean AD. Neuroimaging of the traumatic brain injury. Mt Sinai J Med 2009;76(2):145–62.

78. Sunder R, Tyler K. Basal skull fracture and the halo sign. Fig. 1. CMAJ. JAMC

79. Heron R, Davie A, Gillies R et al. Interrater reliability of the Glasgow Coma Scale scoring among nurses in sub-specialties of critical care. Aust Crit Care 2001;14(3):100–5.

80. Mayer SA, Chong JY. Critical care management of increased intracranial pressure. J Intensive Care Med 2002;17(2):55–67.

CHAPTER 46
FACIOMAXILLARY TRAUMA
JENNIFER LESLIE

Essentials

- Patients with faciomaxillary injuries will be concerned about returning to normal function (eating, breathing and communicating) and appearance.
- Initial assessment and management follows trauma principles, and the paramedic and emergency nurse must not be distracted by the sometimes horrific appearance of facial injuries.
- Airway problems from faciomaxillary injuries can occur due to swelling of injured tissues in the oropharynx and/or haemorrhage from lacerated facial vessels. Be prepared for the possibility of a difficult intubation.
- Life-threatening haemorrhage from faciomaxillary trauma is rare. Haemodynamic compromise may result from other bleeding sources and a thorough patient assessment is essential.
- Haemorrhage from faciomaxillary trauma can usually be controlled by packing of the nasopharynx. Uncontrolled bleeding may require angiographic embolisation and/or emergency surgical reduction of fractures.
- During repair of soft-tissue injuries to the face, ensure that normal contours of the face are followed.

INTRODUCTION

Assessment and management of facial injuries—regardless of severity and gruesome appearance—does not take priority over recognition and treatment of life-threatening injuries. Rapid assessment using a systematic approach, beginning with airway and cervical spine stabilisation, breathing, circulation (ABCs) and neurological assessment, is essential. Faciomaxillary trauma may result in airway obstruction and management problems, respiratory distress and haemorrhage. Faciomaxillary injuries have the potential for undesirable functional and cosmetic outcomes. The aim of treatment is to ensure return of function and cosmetic repair.

Anatomy and physiology

Facial skeleton

The principal facial bones are the frontal bone, nasal bone, maxilla, zygoma and mandible (Fig 46.1). Figure 46.2 outlines the overlying facial contours. The inferior portion of the frontal bone articulates with the frontal process of the maxilla and nasal bone and laterally with the zygoma. The orbit has a complex anatomy composed of the frontal bone superiorly, zygoma laterally, maxilla inferiorly and processes of the maxilla and frontal bone medially. Paired nasal bones that form the bridge of the nose articulate with the frontal bone above and maxilla laterally (Fig 46.3) forming the nasal cavity divided by the nasal septum. The zygoma forms the cheek and the lateral wall and floor of the orbital cavity. Articulations with the maxilla, frontal bone and zygomatic process of the temporal bone form the zygomatic arch.

The maxilla forms the upper jaw, anterior hard palate, part of the lateral wall of the nasal cavity and part of the orbital floor. Below the orbit the maxilla is perforated by the infraorbital foramen to allow passage of the infraorbital vessels and nerves. The inferior portion of the maxilla forms the alveolar process which joins the left and right sides of the maxilla. The alveolar processes together form the alveolar arch, which houses the upper teeth.

The mandible is a horizontal horseshoe body with two rami, anterior coronoid processes and posterior condyloid processes. The mandibular notch lies medial to the zygomatic arch and separates the two processes. The mandible articulates with the temporal bone to form the temporomandibular joint, whereas the upper body of the mandible, called the alveolar ridge, contains the lower teeth.

Sinus cavities are found within the maxilla (also referred to as the maxillary antrum), frontal bone and the ethmoid and sphenoid bones of the skull. Consider the midface as vertical buttresses that resist functional forces such as biting and horizontal buttresses that house the facial organs such as the eyes, and give the face shape. It is thought that sinuses and the facial skeleton have evolved to provide a 'crumple zone' that protects the brain and eyes from injury, and also to reduce cranial weight, enhance the voice and humidify the breath, among other functions.[1] However, patients with facial fractures may still sustain severe head injuries and should be assessed accordingly.[2]

Nerves, glands and blood supply

The facial nerve (cranial nerve VII) provides motor, parasympathetic and sensory and motor innervation to the face. It originates in the brainstem, emerges on the face near the parotid gland, then divides into five branches (Fig 46.4). Specific functions for each branch are listed in Table 46.1.

Other cranial nerves that may be affected by facial trauma are the oculomotor, trochlear and the three branches of the trigeminal nerve. Function and testing for each nerve are described in Table 46.3.

The parotid gland, one of the salivary glands, is located adjacent to the anterior ear and drains into the oral cavity through the parotid duct (Fig 46.5).

Blood supply to the face arises from the external carotid artery. The principal vessels supplying the face are the lingual,

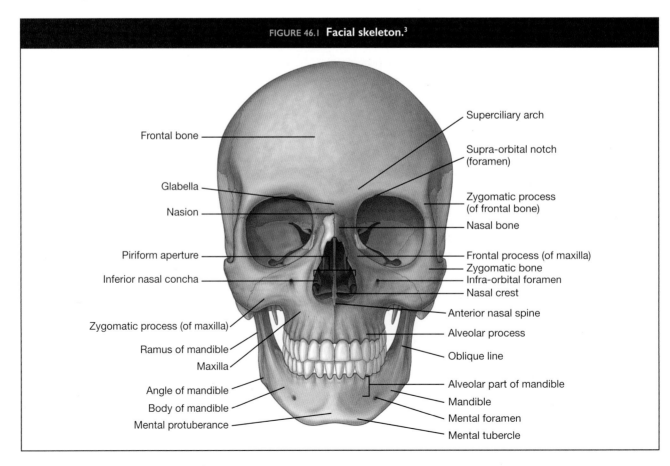

FIGURE 46.1 Facial skeleton.[3]

Frontal bone

Glabella

Nasion

Piriform aperture

Inferior nasal concha

Zygomatic process (of maxilla)

Ramus of mandible

Maxilla

Angle of mandible

Body of mandible

Mental protuberance

Superciliary arch

Supra-orbital notch (foramen)

Zygomatic process (of frontal bone)

Nasal bone

Frontal process (of maxilla)

Zygomatic bone

Infra-orbital foramen

Nasal crest

Anterior nasal spine

Alveolar process

Oblique line

Alveolar part of mandible

Mandible

Mental foramen

Mental tubercle

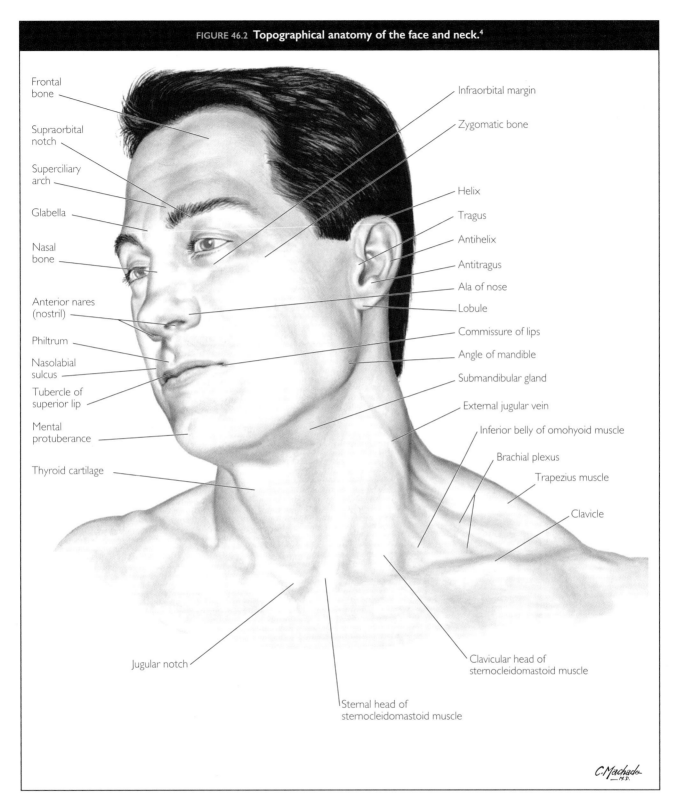

FIGURE 46.2 **Topographical anatomy of the face and neck.**[4]

Frontal bone

Supraorbital notch

Superciliary arch

Glabella

Nasal bone

Anterior nares (nostril)

Philtrum

Nasolabial sulcus

Tubercle of superior lip

Mental protuberance

Thyroid cartilage

Jugular notch

Sternal head of sternocleidomastoid muscle

Infraorbital margin

Zygomatic bone

Helix

Tragus

Antihelix

Antitragus

Ala of nose

Lobule

Commissure of lips

Angle of mandible

Submandibular gland

External jugular vein

Inferior belly of omohyoid muscle

Brachial plexus

Trapezius muscle

Clavicle

Clavicular head of sternocleidomastoid muscle

C.Machado
M.D.

facial, posterior auricular, superficial temporal, ophthalmic and maxillary arteries. Blood supply to the face is excellent; collateral supply is plentiful with several anastomoses existing between the carotid system of either side (Fig 46.6).

Injury mechanism

Motor vehicle collisions (MVCs), falls and assaults are the most common cause of facial fractures and occur most frequently in young men.[5–12] Since the latter years of the 20th century assault has overtaken MVCs as the main cause of facial fractures in many populations; however, injuries from MVCs remain more severe due to higher-velocity trauma.[5,9,10] Facial injury from falls is common among the elderly[13–16] and children under five,[17–19] and the most common presenting problem in patients suffering domestic violence injuries.[20] Sporting injuries and work injuries account for most of the remainder.[9] In the elderly,

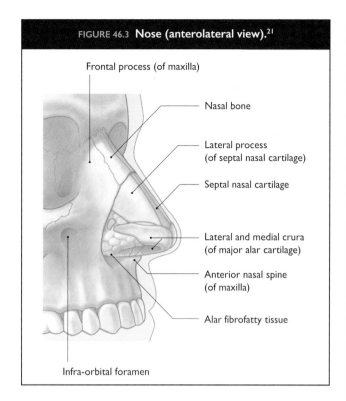

FIGURE 46.3 **Nose (anterolateral view).**[21]

Frontal process (of maxilla)

Nasal bone

Lateral process
(of septal nasal cartilage)

Septal nasal cartilage

Lateral and medial crura
(of major alar cartilage)

Anterior nasal spine
(of maxilla)

Alar fibrofatty tissue

Infra-orbital foramen

TABLE 46.1 Facial nerve branch functions

BRANCH	FUNCTION
Buccal	Wrinkle nose
Cervical	Wrinkle skin of neck
Mandibular	Purse and depress lips
Temporal	Raise eyebrows, wrinkle forehead
Zygomatic	Close eyelids

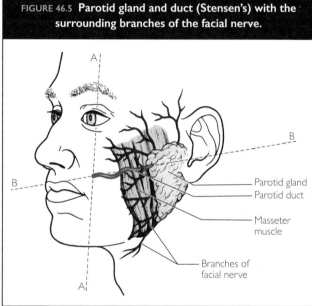

FIGURE 46.5 **Parotid gland and duct (Stensen's) with the surrounding branches of the facial nerve.**

Parotid gland
Parotid duct

Masseter
muscle

Branches of
facial nerve

Line B approximates the course of the duct, which enters the mouth at the junction of lines A and B.[36]

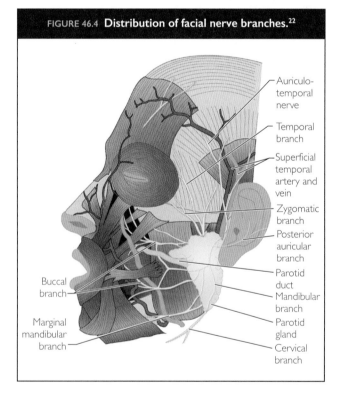

FIGURE 46.4 **Distribution of facial nerve branches.**[22]

Auriculo-temporal nerve

Temporal branch

Superficial temporal artery and vein

Zygomatic branch

Posterior auricular branch

Parotid duct

Mandibular branch

Parotid gland

Cervical branch

Buccal branch

Marginal mandibular branch

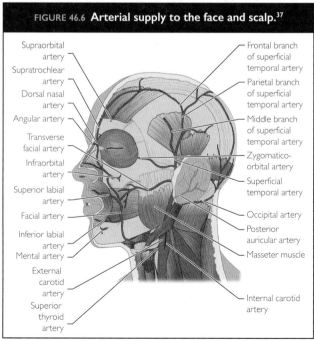

FIGURE 46.6 **Arterial supply to the face and scalp.**[37]

Supraorbital artery

Supratrochlear artery

Dorsal nasal artery

Angular artery

Transverse facial artery

Infraorbital artery

Superior labial artery

Facial artery

Inferior labial artery

Mental artery

External carotid artery

Superior thyroid artery

Frontal branch of superficial temporal artery

Parietal branch of superficial temporal artery

Middle branch of superficial temporal artery

Zygomatico-orbital artery

Superficial temporal artery

Occipital artery

Posterior auricular artery

Masseter muscle

Internal carotid artery

osteoporosis increases the risk of multiple facial fractures.[23] In children, bone flexibility and fat pads around the jaw, combined with underdeveloped facial skeleton and paranasal sinuses, help absorb energy and reduce the frequency of facial fractures.[24] Table 46.2 identifies gravitational forces required to fracture various facial bones.

TABLE 46.2 Force of gravity impact required for facial fracture[36]	
BONE	FORCE OF GRAVITY (g)
Nasal bones	30
Zygoma	50
Angle of mandible	70
Frontal-glabellar region	80
Midline maxilla	100
Midline mandible (symphysis)	100
Supraorbital rim	200

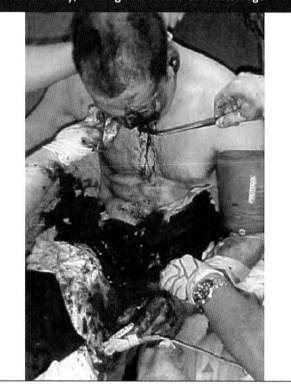

FIGURE 46.7 **Patient leaning forward to clear and maintain own airway, allowing flow of severe haemorrhage.**[45]

Seatbelts, airbags and laminated windscreens reduce the severity of facial injuries/fractures in road trauma;[25–27] however, as a result of airbag deployment, facial injuries, such as lacerations, abrasions and chemical burns, are common.[8,28–30] Intracranial injuries, ocular injuries,[31] cervical spine injuries and pulmonary contusions are the most frequent injuries that occur with faciomaxillary fractures.[25,32–34] The greater the force of the trauma, the more likely concomitant injuries are to occur; hence the need for a thorough history of the trauma event.[32] Alcohol intoxication is often associated with faciomaxillary trauma in those patients injured in MVCs and assaults.[8,10–12,35] Penetrating injuries to the face can occur from shotguns, gunshots, knives and numerous other impaling objects. The prevalence of the mechanism of faciomaxillary injury varies between and within countries.

Patient assessment

As with all trauma care, an organised approach to patient assessment is essential, ensuring life-threatening injuries are identified and the patient stabilised. Facial injuries not threatening the airway or causing life-threatening haemorrhage can be assessed as part of the secondary survey, no matter how disfiguring the injuries appear.[38]

Initial evaluation

Asphyxia due to upper airway obstruction from various causes is the major cause of death from facial trauma.[39] When performing a primary survey of the airway, the paramedic and emergency nurse must maintain cervical spine precautions and the cervical spine should remain protected until injury is excluded, according to institutional protocol (see Ch 44 for more detail on primary survey and Ch 17, p. 323, for cervical spine immobilisation).

The initial assessment is to open the patient's mouth. Foreign objects (e.g. dentures or avulsed teeth) can obstruct the airway and need to be removed with a finger sweep or Magill forceps (see Ch 17). Suctioning of blood and vomitus is also essential.

Once the mouth and upper airway is clear, the paramedic and emergency nurse need to assess for airway compromise. The airway may be opened using chin lift or jaw thrust techniques. If the mandible is displaced, the tongue loses anatomical support and occludes the airway, and may need to be manually held forward. In the pre-hospital setting it may be necessary to place the patient in the lateral position, or in life-threatening situations place the patient prone. In the ED, a towel clamp or heavy suture may be used to achieve this by providing stability to the tongue.[40] Altered mental status from alcohol, drugs or head injury can diminish the patient's gag reflex, increase risk of vomiting and leave the airway unprotected. Severe fractures of the midface compromise the airway secondary to maxillary prolapse, haemorrhage, swelling and haematoma formation.[40] It may be necessary for the paramedic and emergency nurse to place manual anterior traction on the maxilla to relieve obstruction from posteriorly displaced midface fractures.[41,42] Frequent suctioning of the oropharynx is required when bleeding or excessive secretions are present (see Ch 17, p. 327, for suctioning techniques). Be aware that anterior traction of fractured facial bones may increase haemorrhage.[42] Allow the patient to sit upright, or elevate the head of bed to promote drainage if the cervical spine has been cleared. Cervical spine clearance following institutional protocol is a priority in the awake patient with faciomaxillary trauma for this reason. Alternatively, place the patient in the recovery position to protect the airway while maintaining cervical spine precautions.[43] It is appropriate to allow the patient to find a position of comfort if they are awake and talking and are driven to sit up due to impending airway obstruction or vomiting, or are actively resisting spinal immobilisation and their conscious state is compatible with the appreciation of cervical spine pain (Fig 46.7).[44]

An oropharyngeal airway can be used in an unconscious patient to prevent obstruction from the tongue; however, nasopharyngeal airway use is not recommended in patients with faciomaxillary trauma because of the risk of intracerebral malpositioning via the cribriform plate.[32] For the same reason, orotracheal intubation is preferred in patients with facial injuries. If an airway cannot be maintained utilising the previously mentioned techniques, the paramedic qualified to do so will perform insertion of an endotracheal tube or a laryngeal mask airway (LMA) or Combitube following local service guidelines.[40,46] The LMA does not provide complete protection of the airway, so there is still the risk of aspiration (see Ch 17, p. 320, for LMA insertion techniques).[42] On arrival at the emergency department (ED) the airway needs to be assessed again for the need to intubate and the emergency nurse will assist as per institutional protocol. The success rate of emergency oral intubation in patients with oral swelling and haemorrhage can be as low as 80%, so a specific difficult airway algorithm and equipment is important.[47] In situations where intubation is not available, the emergency nurse will manage the airway using the safest patient position. Again, this may be the recovery/lateral position (or sitting up, leaning forward if the patient is alert) if haemorrhage and secretions are likely to block the airway or cause aspiration. If the patient is maintaining their oxygen saturation, an awake fibre-optic intubation in the operating theatre avoids potential airway emergencies.[40]

Rarely, intubation is required and cannot be accomplished due to excessive swelling or massive haemorrhage obscuring the vocal cords. In this situation a surgical airway such as a cricothyroidotomy needs to be performed.[40] Paramedics with sufficient training in the technique may perform this procedure following local service protocol. Cricothyroidotomy may also be performed in the ED (see Ch 17, p. 322). A needle cricothyroidotomy is recommended in children less than 12 years of age to prevent damage to the cricoid cartilage.[39] A tracheostomy will usually be required to provide a definitive airway once the patient is stabilised.[48] Due to the difficulties in airway management of the severely facially injured patient a treatment algorithm will be useful (Fig 46.8).

High-flow supplemental oxygen is required by all trauma patients, aiming to maintain oxygen saturation >95%. If needed, assisted ventilations can be accomplished with a bag–valve–mask (BVM). However, swelling and facial fractures can make use of a BVM difficult with some patients. A two-person bagging technique may assist in this situation.

See Chapters 17 (p. 314) and 44 (p. 1127) for more detail on airway assessment and management.

PRACTICE TIP

The airway should be constantly monitored for increasing oedema and haemorrhage, which may block the airway at a later stage.

Once a patent airway and satisfactory ventilation are established, the next priority is haemorrhage control. Massive blood loss causing haemorrhagic shock after facial bleeding is rare, and the paramedic and emergency nurse must search for alternative haemorrhage sites in the haemodynamically unstable patient (see Ch 44 for more detail on haemorrhage assessment and management). However, exsanguination can rarely occur

from bleeding facial vessels.[38,49,50] Due to the rich arterial blood supply to the face from internal and external carotid arteries, and the multiple anastomoses of the facial vessels, control of bleeding can be difficult. Haemorrhage needs to be controlled swiftly.[42] Blood transfusion is likely to be required in most cases of severe facial fractures.[51] The nose, supplied by a complex group of vessels arising from the maxillary and ophthalmic arteries, is the most likely source of extensive bleeding.[49,50] Blood clots are removed from the nose and throat to visualise the site of bleeding. When the bleeding is anterior (epistaxis), the nose is pinched between the fingers and thumb while applying icepacks to the nose and forehead. Petroleum-impregnated gauze, foam-rubber packs, nasal balloons or a nasal tampon may be inserted to control anterior bleeding (Fig 46.9).[52] If bleeding is arising from posterior vessels, pharyngeal packing or a Foley catheter or Epistat tube *with the balloon inflated within the nasopharynx* can be used to tamponade posterior bleeding.[39,49,50,52] Be aware that intracranial insertion is a risk of this technique. If a base of skull fracture is suspected, a large gauge catheter may be inserted by an experienced doctor, checking placement after 10 cm of catheter inserted.[53] Any packing should be securely taped to the face.

Severe haemorrhage from facial trauma may also be controlled by manual reduction of the facial bones.[41] In some situations, angiography and transcatheter arterial embolisation of bleeding vessels may be necessary,[49,50] and can also be performed prior to surgical fixation of fractures.[42] Ligation of arteries and veins may be necessary to control blood loss in institutions where angiography is not available or embolisation is unsuccessful. It is important for the emergency nurse to anticipate the need for the patient to be transferred for definitive care to a tertiary centre with angiography or operating suites and to expedite the process. Once haemorrhage is controlled repair of fractures can be delayed while more urgent problems are managed.[42]

PRACTICE TIP

An ENT tray or trolley containing examination and packing equipment will expedite treatment of facial haemorrhage.

Once cervical spine injury has been ruled out, epistaxis is best managed with the patient in a sitting position. Due to the rich blood supply to the face, simple lacerations can bleed profusely. Direct digital pressure with sterile gauze or pressure applied with a large cotton-tipped swab applied to external sources of bleeding is usually effective, although infiltration with adrenaline solution (e.g. lignocaine 1% with adrenaline 1:100,000) or suturing of large vessels may be required.[52] Care must always be taken to ensure underlying structures such

PRACTICE TIP

Blood loss may go unnoticed in the awake patient swallowing blood. Paramedics and emergency nurses need to encourage the patient to spit out blood and secretions to avoid nausea and vomiting. The patient may be given the opportunity to perform their own suction when necessary.

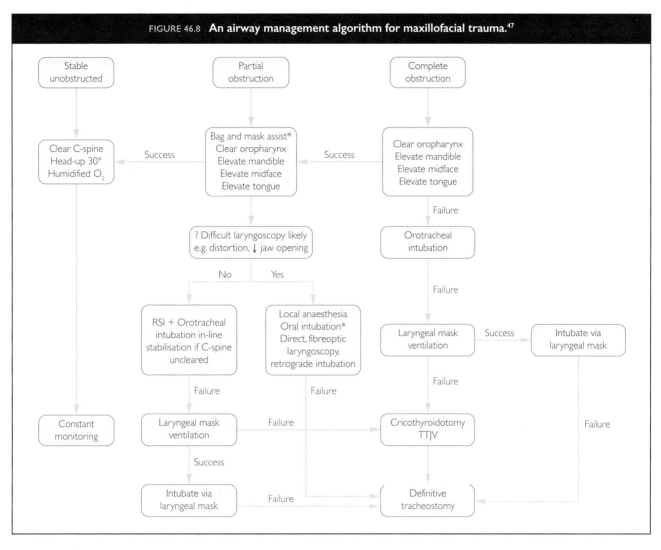

FIGURE 46.8 **An airway management algorithm for maxillofacial trauma.**[47]

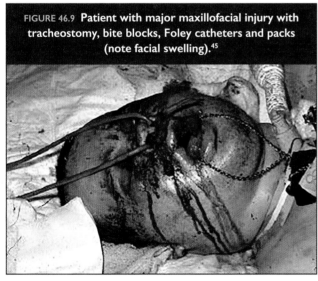

FIGURE 46.9 **Patient with major maxillofacial injury with tracheostomy, bite blocks, Foley catheters and packs (note facial swelling).**[45]

as nerves and glands are not damaged during assessment and treatment of bleeding vessels.

Bleeding in the oral cavity can often be controlled by direct pressure. The paramedic and emergency nurse can identify the bleeding source and ask the awake patient to apply direct pressure with gauze. If the patient is unconscious and intubated, the paramedic and emergency nurse need to pack the oral cavity laceration until the wounds can be sutured.

History should include whether anticoagulants have previously been prescribed.

Physical examination

Assessment for deformity should occur as soon as possible, prior to swelling obstructing any bony deformities (Fig 46.10).

Assessment of vision-threatening injuries is also a priority. Observe for eyelid ecchymosis, assess eyes for loss of vision, visual acuity, pupillary reactivity and symmetry, extraocular movements and diplopia (double vision). More detail on eye assessment is presented in Chapter 33, and on ear and dental assessment in Chapter 32.

Inspection

The paramedic or emergency nurse begins inspection of the face by looking down on the face from the vertex of the head to compare height of malar eminences (cheek bones), then inspects the face from below the chin again to compare both sides of the face for symmetry. Observe for proptosis (protruding eye) and enophthalmos (sunken appearance of the eye). Observe for widening of the distance between the medial canthus (called telecanthus). Observe for injuries to structures

TABLE 46.3 Cranial nerves involved in facial trauma

NERVE	NAME	FUNCTION	DESCRIPTION	ASSESSMENT
III	Oculomotor	Motor	Eyeball movement; supplies 5 of 7 ocular muscles	Pupil response; ocular movement to four quadrants
IV	Trochlear	Motor	Eyeball movement (superior oblique)	As above
V	Trigeminal	Motor and sensory	Facial sensation; jaw movement	Assessing pain, touch, hot and cold sensations, bite, opening mouth against resistance
VII	Facial	Motor and sensory	Facial expression; taste from anterior two-thirds of tongue	Zygomatic branch: have patient close eyes tightly
				Temporal branch: have patient elevate brows, wrinkle forehead
				Buccal branch: have patient elevate upper lip, wrinkle nose, whistle

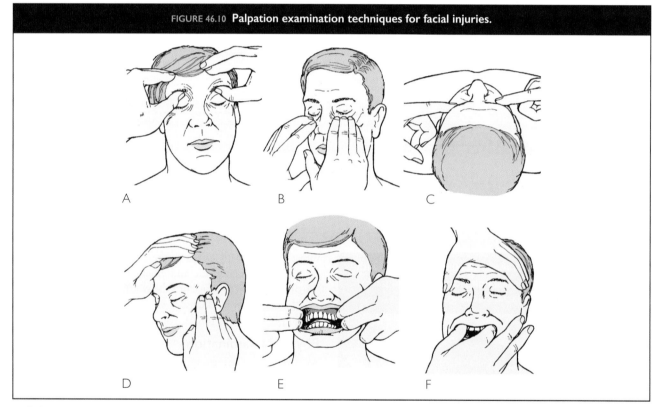

FIGURE 46.10 **Palpation examination techniques for facial injuries.**

A, Palpation for irregularities of supraorbital ridge. **B**, Palpation for irregularities of infraorbital ridge and zygoma. **C**, Comparing height of malar eminences. **D**, Palpation for depression of zygomatic arch. **E**, Visualisation of gross dental occlusion. **F**, Manoeuvre to ascertain motion in maxilla.

around the eyes, such as to tear-duct apparatus and muscles of the eyelid.[54] Inspect all wounds for the presence of foreign bodies, such as avulsed teeth.

Raccoon eyes or periorbital ecchymosis suggest anterior basilar skull fracture, LeFort fracture or nasoethmoid injury, whereas nasal or ear drainage positive for cerebrospinal fluid (CSF) occurs with cribriform plate fracture or basilar skull fracture. Appearance of a bull's eye or halo when bloody drainage from the nose or ear is placed on white paper indicates the presence of CSF. Clear fluid positive for glucose also indicates CSF.

Deep lacerations of the cheek and over the jaw should be carefully evaluated for injury to the parotid gland, parotid (Stensen's) duct and branches of the facial nerve. Look intranasally for septal haematoma and lacerations to the mucosa. Block one nostril at a time to assess whether the patient can breathe through both. Ask the patient if teeth close and fit together properly, then observe for limitations in the patient's ability to completely open the jaw, pain on biting down and loss of bite strength, which may indicate fracture and displacement of the mandible or alveolar ridge.

Inspect inside the mouth cavity and intraoral wounds for loose teeth, dentures, oropharyngeal bleeding and swelling. Observe for injury to the tongue and sublingual haematomas. Rigid collars will restrict mouth opening; it is necessary to re-inspect the oral cavity after the cervical spine is cleared.

Palpation

Using a systematic approach with both hands simultaneously, palpate for tenderness, step-off irregularities and crepitus of supraorbital ridge and zygoma. Gently palpate nasal bones and palpate laterally for depressions in the zygomatic arch. Visualise the mouth and palpate for loose, broken and missing teeth, gross dental malocclusion, soft-tissue lacerations and haematomas. Palpate the temporomandibular joint in the open and closed positions to assess for dislocation. Check midface stability by attempting to move the upper teeth and hard palate with one hand while stabilising the forehead with the other (Fig 46.11). Palpate for subcutaneous emphysema, which may indicate injuries within the oral, orbital or nasal cavity and resultant filling of the soft tissues with air.

Evaluate the cranial nerves, including the facial nerve and branches for motor and sensory function (Table 46.2). Loss of sensation over the lower lip may indicate injury to the inferior alveolar nerve and possible mandibular fracture. Numbness over the upper lip occurs with fracture in the maxilla and injury to the infraorbital nerve. Inspect and palpate the ear and external ear canal.

Clinical interventions

Lacerations

The aim of treatment of soft-tissue trauma is complete closure of the wound to ensure functionality and cosmesis. Repair of facial lacerations should occur as quickly as possible, unless surgical repair to underlying structures is necessary.[54] Simple lacerations can be cleaned, debrided and sutured by primary intention within 24 hours of injury, with best effect before

8 hours. The wound needs to be assessed for consideration of how it should be repaired, and whether specialist advice and treatment needs to be requested, such as in damage to underlying structures (e.g. glands, nerves, ducts, eye injuries); avulsed tissue injury; and wounds to the nose and ears. It is especially important to consider the cosmetic outcome of soft-tissue injuries to the face, as this will be of high priority to the patient.[55] Deeper lacerations and lacerations associated with fractures are conservatively debrided, irrigated and closed by the treating specialist. Pulse irrigation is best performed with Normal saline solution,[56] and wounds covered with saline-soaked gauze. Avulsed and degloved tissue is considered viable due to the face's vascular nature, so excessive debridement should be avoided.

Repair of facial lacerations in uncooperative patients is extremely difficult and may injure other important structures. Delaying repair until the patient is more cooperative usually results in a better outcome. Use of povidone–iodine solution and hydrogen peroxide solutions should be avoided as they may delay tissue healing (see Ch 18).[56,57]

Lacerations of eyebrows and eyelids should be repaired before swelling occurs, so that borders can be matched. The eyebrows should never be shaved because landmarks are eliminated and the brow is unlikely to grow back.[56] When suturing the brow, hairs are aligned so that they slant in a downward and outward direction. Vermilion–cutaneous and vermilion–mucosal margins are important anatomical landmarks in repair of lip lacerations. Ensure borders are perfectly aligned to prevent development of step-off deformity of the lip.[56] Figure 46.12 illustrates closure of this type of laceration. Tissue loss from the lip requires reconstruction by a plastic surgeon.[56]

Intraoral injuries should be meticulously cleaned and irrigated. Superficial tongue, buccal mucosa and gingival lacerations do not need suturing.[56] Gaping intraoral and tongue lacerations should be sutured, as should the thin tissue overlying the mandibular and maxillary ridge.[56] Reanastamosis of amputated tongue can be achieved.[58] The amputated tongue should be kept moist by wrapping in saline-soaked gauze.

Tissue adhesives can play a part in repair of low-tension facial lacerations in children and adults because of the speed of

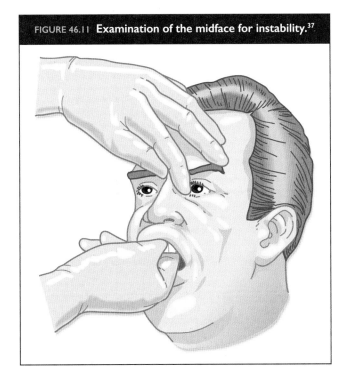

FIGURE 46.11 Examination of the midface for instability.[37]

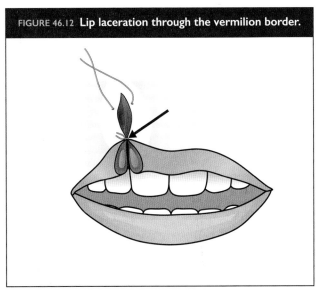

FIGURE 46.12 Lip laceration through the vermilion border.

application, reduction in pain and anxiety of repair, resistance to bacterial growth and the lack of need to remove sutures.[59] Day-1 tensile strength is only about 10–15% of that of a suture-repaired wound. It cannot be used over joints. Tissue glue typically adheres for 7–14 days and then sloughs off with the epidermis. Petroleum-based ointments, including antibiotic ointments, should not be used on the wound after gluing as these substances can weaken the tissue glue.[60] Simple, small, non-gaping facial lacerations that are not over a joint or on hairy skin surfaces may also be repaired with wound tape (e.g. Steristrips).[56]

Discharge planning should include instructing the patient to apply emollient to facial laceration repairs: daily massage with an emollient cream has been shown to improve appearance of the scar.[60] The patient should avoid spending time in the sun so that post-inflammatory hyperpigmentation does not occur, and they should be advised to use sunscreen on the wound after it is healed. Wounds to the oral cavity must be rinsed clean after meals.[56] The patient should be made aware of when sutures are to be removed, signs and symptoms of infection, pain relief strategies and wound care. Further information regarding wound care can be found in Chapter 18.

Mammalian bite wounds

Bite wounds include scratches, punctures, lacerations and avulsions. Initially, these wounds may look innocuous; however, they can lead to serious infections and complications. Lacerations caused by animal or human bites are highly contaminated because of the bacteria and debris in the mouth. Facial bites, especially those in children, require meticulous

management. Most patients do well with careful debridement, ample irrigation and cleansing and loose closure by suture. Close follow-up is required for at least 5 days. Because subsequent plastic reconstruction may be needed, it may be useful to consult with a plastic surgeon at the time of initial repair. Extensive facial animal bites frequently require surgical exploration and repair, and in children may involve fractures to the face or skull.[56,61] Detailed discussion on the types of bacterial transmissions and management of mammalian wounds is found in Chapter 18.

Friction injuries

Bitumen rash and other friction injuries to the face present a unique problem because of potential tattooing or epidermal staining.[62] Gunpowder can cause permanent discolouration of skin and should be removed by using a local anaesthetic and scrubbing with a hard brush or hard-bristle toothbrush in the first hour, if possible, taking into consideration forensic implications. Early removal will also reduce the amount of burning from gunpowder to the epithelial and collagen layers of the skin. Moist wound healing is recommended for abrasions.[56] Visible glass fragments can be lifted with tape applied gently to the face.

Radiology

X-ray

Plain radiography remains useful in the assessment of minimally displaced single injuries to the facial skeleton that are suspected on initial assessment (Table 46.4). Terminology describing certain views may differ between institutions.

TABLE 46.4 Radiographical examination for maxillofacial injury

TEST	DESCRIPTION
Water's view (posteroanterior)	Single most useful X-ray in maxillofacial injury
	Delineates orbital rim and floor
	Detects blood in maxillary sinus
Towne's view	Mandible condyles–subcondylar regions of orbital floor
Anterior, posterior and lateral	Skull
	Sinus, roof of orbit
Submental vertex (jug handle)	Zygomatic arch
	Details base of skull
AP and lateral oblique mandible	Condylar, coronoid, body and symphysis
Occlusal and apical	Palate, symphysis, roots of teeth
CT scan	Provides definitive diagnosis in cervical spine injury
	Standard for assessing soft-tissue injuries
	Standard for assessing complex facial fractures; should be ordered when concomitant brain and facial injuries are identified
MRI	Useful for identifying soft-tissue injuries in optic nerve
	Muscle herniation, infraocular and intraocular haematomas, entrapment

AP: anteroposterior; CT: computed tomography; MRI: magnetic resonance imaging

Isolated mandibular fractures are routinely assessed using orthopantomogram (OPG) and mandibular views.[63] Suspected fractures of the alveolar process, zygomatic body or Le Fort I fractures can be performed using paranasal sinus view (Water's view), mandibular views, occlusal view or OPG.[63] Isolated suspected zygoma fractures can be assessed utilising axial cranial projection, also known as submental vertex or bucket/jug handle view.[63]

Ultrasound

Ultrasound is helpful in identifying foreign bodies,[64] effusion in the temporomandibular joint,[63] and carotid–cavernous sinus fistula.[63] Ultrasound has also been found to be useful in identifying orbital and zygomatic fractures.[63]

Computed tomography scan

Computed tomography using multidetector CT scanning (MDCT) has made rapid CT of the face possible at the same time as other body parts. It is important to ensure that the patient is not overexposed to radiation, and the emergency nurse should ensure that a facial CT is requested with other CTs in the multiple-trauma patient, if one is indicated. This will prevent the patient from requiring additional radiology at a later stage. CT scan with multiplanar reconstructions in the sagittal and coronal plains is the radiology of choice in all obviously displaced facial fractures, allowing the most precise diagnoses. CT is particularly useful in scanning the orbital fractures, Le Fort II and III, panfacial fractures, nasoethmoidal fractures and mandibular condyles.[63,64] 3-D imaging assists in preoperative planning, model surgery and fabrication of custom implants, saving operating time.[64]

Angiography

Angiographical embolisation of bleeding facial vessels unable to be controlled utilising direct pressure is being practised more frequently where facilities are available. Multiple bleeding points can be identified and the technique can be repeated as necessary.[64]

Magnetic resonance imaging

Magnetic resonance imaging (MRI) may be useful in assessing injury to the soft tissue of the temporomandibular joint.[64]

The choice of which imaging modality to use is based on availability, physical findings and the cost and usefulness of particular studies.[65]

Clinical presentations

Soft-tissue trauma

Abrasions, contusions and lacerations to the face, oral mucosa and nasal mucosa need to be assessed and treated as mentioned in the section on clinical interventions. Bleeding, swelling and subsequent airway compromise may occur in the absence of facial fractures, particularly in those patients taking anticoagulants or those with clotting disorders.[64]

Nerve and gland injuries

Assessment

Effects of trigeminal nerve (V) injury depend upon the branch that is injured. V1 is injured at the supraorbital notch, with complete transection resulting in anaesthesia of the nose, eyebrow and forehead. V2 is usually injured by faciomaxillary fractures with resultant sensory deficits of the ipsilateral cheek, upper lip, gums and hard palate. V3 is associated with injury to the mandible and results in anaesthesia of the chin. Incomplete transection or scarring of the branches of cranial nerve V may result in intractable pain and neuroma formation.[66]

Temporal bone fractures and deep cheek lacerations can cause damage to branches of the facial nerve, resulting in changes to facial expression. Injury to the temporal branch causes forehead asymmetry because the patient cannot wrinkle the forehead on the affected side. With injury to the temporal or zygomatic branch, the patient is unable to fully close the eyelids on the affected side. Buccal branch injury keeps the patient from pursing the lips to whistle, and injury to the mandibular branch causes inability to lower or depress the lower lip. At rest, elevation of the lower lip occurs on the affected side. Injury to the facial nerve can be easily missed if the patient is unconscious or has numerous facial dressings. Temporal bone fractures and deep cheek lacerations can damage the parotid gland and parotid duct. Lacerations of the parotid duct or the parotid gland are a rare occurrence.

Management

Nerve lacerations need to be repaired within 72 hours. Most patients with traumatic facial paralysis after blunt facial trauma have a good prognosis for complete recovery.[66] Figure 46.13 indicates the poor outcome of significant damage to facial muscles and nerves.

Duct cannulisation is used to determine patency when injury is suspected, and either re-anastamosed or the duct ligated.

Nasal injuries

Assessment

Nasal fractures are the most common facial fracture because the nose is the most prominent facial bone and offers the least resistance (Fig 46.14). Nasal fractures occur most commonly in assaults, MVCs and sports. They can occur in isolation or associated with other fractures to the midface. Fractures to the nose can occur from lateral, frontolateral, frontal and caudal impacts, resulting in different fracture patterns. Overlooked nasal injury can lead to permanent deformity and airway obstruction from septal deviation, and abnormal bone growth in children.

Clinical findings include swelling, deformity, bleeding (epistaxis), contusion, periorbital bruising, pain and crepitus. In children, the nose is more elastic and resistant to fractures; however, dislocations are common. Nasal bones are lined with mucoperiosteum, which creates an open fracture when overlying tissue is lacerated. Careful examination of each naris can identify septal haematomas, lacerations and ability of the patient to breathe through their nose. A septal haematoma appears as a bulging, tense bluish mass that feels doughy when palpated (Fig 46.15). Bleeding may be intranasal or in the pharynx. A plain X-ray is generally unreliable in the assessment of undisplaced nasal fractures. A CT scan provides better information, particularly of the position of the nasal septum and patency of the airway, if available and appropriate. If palpation indicates deformity and mobility, a referral should be made, otherwise permanent disfigurement may result.

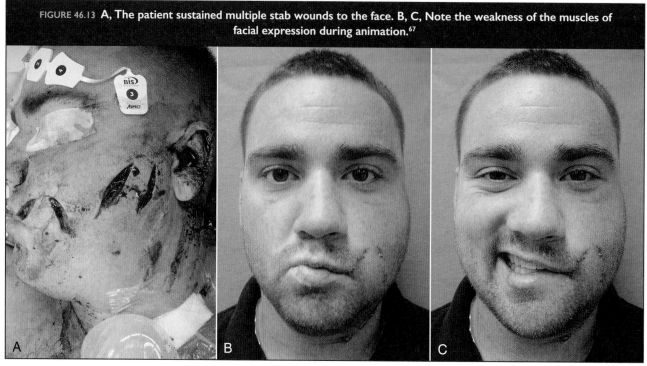

FIGURE 46.13 **A,** The patient sustained multiple stab wounds to the face. **B, C,** Note the weakness of the muscles of facial expression during animation.[67]

Courtesy Dr Daniel Plank.

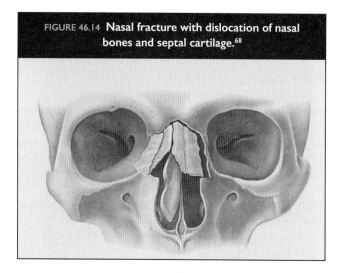

FIGURE 46.14 **Nasal fracture with dislocation of nasal bones and septal cartilage.**[68]

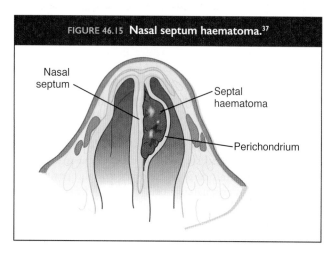

FIGURE 46.15 **Nasal septum haematoma.**[37]

Nasal septum

Septal haematoma

Perichondrium

Management

Initial interventions focus on controlling bleeding with direct pressure. Ice packs and direct nasal pressure for about 10 minutes usually stop bleeding and help relieve pain from simple nasal fractures. Once epistaxis is controlled and the patient can breathe from each nostril and there is no septal haematoma, no further emergency treatment is needed. Encourage the patient to seek further review a few days later.

Open repair of nasal fractures is often required when the septum is damaged. In many cases, surgical fixation of the fracture may not take place until the swelling subsides to ensure adequate cosmesis. Ongoing epistaxis or CSF leak requires specialist referral. Septal haematomas should be emergently drained to prevent airway obstruction and necrosis of septal cartilage. After draining, the nasal cavity requires packing.

Naso-orbito-ethmoid fractures

Assessment

Naso-orbito-ethmoid fractures are more complicated and are generally caused by a severe frontal blow. The bones involved may include nasal bones, frontal process of maxilla, medical orbit, lacrimal bone, ethmoid and cribriform plate. They cause damage to ethmoid sinuses, lacrimal ducts, canthus ligaments and orbital contents. The patient will have swelling, periorbital haematoma, subconjunctival haemorrhage and possible loss of olfactory function. Intercanthal distance may be increased—called traumatic telecanthus (Fig 46.16).[54] If the cribriform plate is affected and the dura torn, CSF rhinorrhoea occurs. CT scan is required to identify the extent of this complicated injury.

Management

Anterior or posterior nasal packing may be required to control bleeding. When the fracture involves the nasal mucosa of the

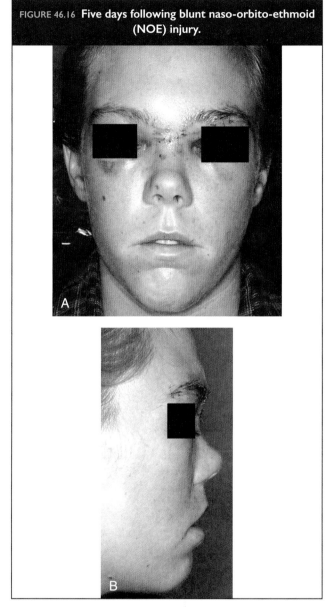

FIGURE 46.16 **Five days following blunt naso-orbito-ethmoid (NOE) injury.**

This patient has a typical appearance following NOE injury. Note the telecanthus, depression of the nasal bridge and dorsum, vertically shortened nose, and upturned nasal tip.[69]

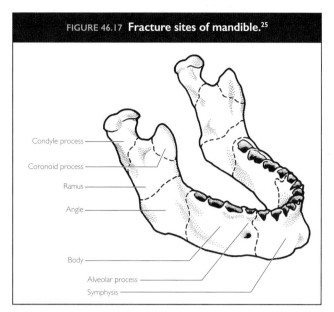

FIGURE 46.17 **Fracture sites of mandible.**[25]

lacrimal system, blowing the nose may cause intracranial air or subcutaneous emphysema that can later cause localised infection or meningitis, so noseblowing needs to be discouraged. Naso-orbito-ethmoid fractures require open fixation.

Mandibular fractures

Assessment

Mandibular fractures are the second most-common facial fracture. Blunt force, such as a severe blow to the face during personal assault, MVCs, contact sports or falls is the usual mechanism of injury. Mandibular fractures are classified according to the region of the jaw injured. The most common sites for fracture are the condyle, angle of the mandible, symphysis, body and ramus (Fig 46.17). Direct fall onto the chin will often result in mandibular condyle fractures. Reciprocal fractures often occur on the side opposite the point of impact.

A orthopantomogram (OPG) is best for radiographical imaging of the entire mandible at once (Fig 46.18A) and posteroanterior readiograph will give an indication of displacement (Fig 46.18B). CT may be performed with 3-D reconstruction useful for planning future surgery, or if a suspected fracture is not evident on plain X-ray (Fig 46.19). Mandibular fractures can be a significant life-threatening injury if loss of bony support displaces the tongue posteriorly and obstructs the airway.[54]

Due to the mobility of the jaw mandible fractures are very painful. Malocclusion is the cardinal sign of mandible fracture (Fig 46.20). Signs and symptoms vary with fracture site; however, point tenderness and crepitus may be palpated and step-off deformity found. Trismus (spasm of jaw muscles) and decreased range of motion, i.e. jaw opening, are usually noted. The face may be asymmetric with swelling and contusion. Paraesthesia in the lower lip and chin imply injury to the inferior alveolar nerve (see Table 46.5). The oral cavity should be assessed for broken or loose teeth, lacerations or contusion.[54] Ears require inspection for tears in the external canal and a ruptured tympanic membrane from mandibular condyle fractures. A fracture of the mandible is considered to be compound if it is within a tooth-bearing segment.[54] Temporomandibular joint dislocation may also occur following direct trauma to the face and in whiplash injuries. Patients may complain of being unable to close their mouth.

Management

Treatment consists of surgical intervention with open reduction and internal fixation or, less frequently, wiring of jaws, depending on the location of the fracture. Some Australian sites prefer to use endoscopic access surgery.[42] Repair occurs soon after injury, first because the patient's nutritional status is quickly impaired due to jaw immobility,[54] and second because movement at the fracture site increases the risk of infection to the bone, especially if there are tears to the gingival mucosa. If repair is delayed prophylactic antibiotics are recommended.[42] Condylar fractures in children are often treated conservatively. Sublingual haematoma can compromise the airway and

FIGURE 46.18

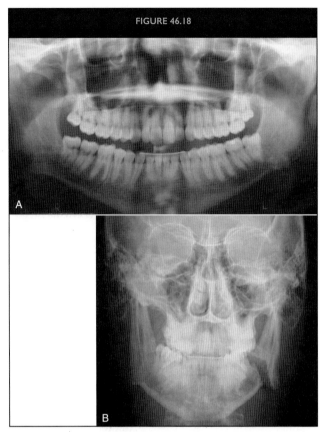

A, Panoramic radiograph demonstrating fracture at the left angle and right parasymphysis area. **B**, Posteroanterior radiograph of the skull showing severe lateral displacement of the mandible angle on the left. The fracture at the right parasymphysis is also evident.[70]

FIGURE 46.19 **Three-dimensional CT reconstructions of minimally displaced mandibular fractures.**[25]

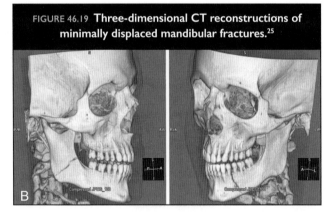

needs to be drained. Paramedic and emergency nursing care includes applying ice compresses to the face to minimise swelling and relieve pain, administering analgesia and allowing the patient to sit upright as soon as a cervical spine injury is excluded. A soft cervical collar will help stabilise mandibular fractures temporarily.[52] Mouth rinses may also be commenced. Intravenous antibiotics are indicated for open fractures, and repair of intraoral lacerations should occur as soon as possible.

Temporomandibular joint dislocations require treatment in the ED. Sedation is given and the dislocation reduced in the ED. Post-reduction X-rays are taken to ensure successful reduction.

FIGURE 46.20 **Malocclusion caused by fracture.**[71]

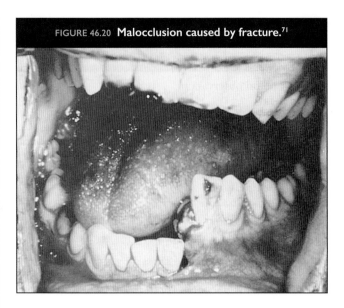

Maxillary and alveolar fractures
Assessment

Maxillary, or midface, fractures, caused by significant force, are usually a combination of fractures involving several facial structures. Again the most common cause is assaults and MVCs. Maxillary fractures are rarely seen in children because of the flexibility and pliable nature of their faciomaxillary structures. Maxillary fractures are classified as Le Fort I, II and III as shown in Figure 46.21E (i.e. lower third, middle third and orbital complex) maxillary antrum (maxillary sinus) fractures. However, fractures do not always follow these patterns and are often a combination of two classifications, or occur only on one side of the face. Fractures of the alveolar process of the maxilla often occur in association with dental injuries. Plain radiographs of the face can be used to confirm diagnosis, although CT scan is generally used to substantiate the extent of the fractures if clinically suspected (Fig 46.21A–D).

Patients with maxillary fractures complain of severe facial pain, anaesthesia or paraesthesia of the upper lip and perhaps some visual disturbances (see Table 46.5). Clinically, the patient has severe facial swelling, contusions, periorbital or orbital swelling, subconjunctival haemorrhage, elongation and flattening of the face, facial asymmetry, epistaxis, crepitus and malocclusion, and may occasionally exhibit airway obstruction. CSF may leak from the nose.

Le Fort I, or lower third fracture, is a horizontal fracture in which the body of the maxilla is separated from the base of the skull above the palate but below the zygomatic process attachment (Fig 46.21A). Separation may be unilateral or bilateral. Paranasal sinus X-rays and OPGs are useful in diagnosis. Swelling of the upper lip and cheek is often present. There is a free-floating segment of the upper teeth and lower maxilla; however, the fracture may not be displaced. The hard palate and upper teeth are mobile when moved by grasping the alveolar process and anterior teeth[55]—a technique used to assess for maxillary mobility.

Le Fort II, or middle third fracture, involves the pyramidal area including the central maxilla, nasal area and orbito-ethmoid bones, and the pterygoid process is pulled from the base of skull (Fig 46.21B). This portion of the face is a

TABLE 46.5 Facial fractures: clinical and radiographical findings, and complications for specific facial fractures[72]

FRACTURE	CLINICAL PRESENTATION	RADIOGRAPHICAL FINDINGS	COMPLICATIONS
Naso-orbital	Symptoms: pain, visual abnormalities Signs: massive periorbital and upper facial oedema and ecchymosis, epistaxis, traumatic telecanthus, foreshortening of nose with telescoping; associated intracranial injuries	Views: CT scan Findings: disruption of interorbital space and comminution of nasal pyramid; frontal, zygomatic, orbital, maxillary fractures common	Residual upper midface deformity ('dish face'); telecanthus; frontal sinus–nasolacrimal system pathology with mucocoele, mucopyocoele, dacryocystitis
Zygoma			
Arch	Symptoms: pain in lateral cheek, inability to close jaw Signs: swelling, crepitus over arch, obvious asymmetry	Views: Water's submentovertex Findings: depression of arch, comminution	Contour irregularities of arch area, flattening of arch
Body 'tripod fracture'	Symptoms: pain, trismus, diplopia, numb upper lip, lower lid, bilateral nasal area Signs: swelling, ecchymosis of malar and periorbital areas; palpable infraorbital rim 'step-off'; entrapment of extraocular muscles with disconjugate gaze; scleral ecchymosis, displacement of lateral canthal ligament	Views: Water's submentovertex, CT scan Findings: clouding, air/fluid level maxillary sinus, separation of zygomaticomaxillary, zygomaticofrontal and zygomaticotemporal suture lines	Residual malar deformity, enophthalmos, diplopia, infraorbital nerve anaesthesia, chronic maxillary sinusitis
Orbital floor	Symptoms: diplopia, orbital pain Signs: periorbital oedema, ecchymosis, enophthalmos, extraocular muscle entrapment, disconjugate gaze; hyphaema, subluxation of lens, retinal detachment, rupture of globe with direct eye trauma	Views: Water's, CT scan, tomograms Findings: air/fluid level maxillary sinus, herniated adnexa and/or orbital floor fragments in maxillary sinus	Enophthalmos, diplopia; recurrent orbital cellulitis with implant (alloplastic) extrusion
Mandible			
Condyle	Symptoms: pain at fracture site, referred pain to ear Signs: crepitus, excessive salivation, swelling of condylar region, deviation of jaw towards fracture, cross-bite or open-bite deformity	Views: AP, oblique, Water's, OPG Findings: nondisplaced, or displaced anteriorly and medially	Ankylosis of TMJ; chronic TMJ
Angle	Symptoms: pain at fracture site, inability to close mouth Signs: swelling at angle of jaw, ecchymosis, crepitus, malocclusion	Views: OPG, mandibular series Findings: non-displaced (favourable) or posterior fragment displaced upwards and medially (nonfavourable)	Non-union, malunion, osteomyelitis
Body	Symptoms: pain at fracture site, limitation of movement Signs: swelling, ecchymosis, crepitus, malocclusion	Views: OPG, mandibular series Findings: non-displaced (favourable), or posterior fragment displaced upwards and medially, anterior fragments rotated lingually (nonfavourable)	Osteomyelitis, infection (tooth in fracture line)

Continued

TABLE 46.5 Facial fractures: clinical and radiographical findings, and complications for specific facial fractures[72]—cont'd

FRACTURE	CLINICAL PRESENTATION	RADIOGRAPHICAL FINDINGS	COMPLICATIONS
Symphysis	Symptoms: pain Signs: malocclusion, frequent association with soft tissue wounds of lower lip, tongue	Views: mandibular series, submentovertex Findings: non-displaced or lingual rotation or anterior fragments, may be associated with angle or condyle fractures	Residual malocclusion, loss of chin projection, asymmetry; osteomyelitis
Maxilla			
Le Fort I (transverse)	Symptoms: pain upper jaw, numb upper teeth Signs: midfacial oedema and ecchymosis, epistaxis, malocclusion, mobility of maxillary dentition	Views: Water's, OPG, CT scan Findings: opaque maxillary sinus, displacement of fragments of alveolus if comminuted; fracture through maxillary sinus and pterygoid plates	Loss of teeth, infection, malocclusion
Le Fort II (pyramidal)	Symptoms: pain midface, numb upper lip, lower lid, lateral nasal area Signs: midfacial oedema and ecchymosis, epistaxis, malocclusion, mobility of midface, nasal flattening, anaesthesia infraorbital nerve territory	Views: Water's, CT scan Findings: opaque maxillary sinuses, separation through frontal process, lacrimal bones, floor of orbits, zygomaticomaxillary suture line, lateral wall of maxillary sinus and pterygoid plates	Non-union, malunion lacrimal system obstruction, infraorbital nerve anaesthesia, diplopia, malocclusion
Le Fort III (craniofacial dysjunction)	Symptoms: pain face, difficulty breathing Signs: 'donkey-face' deformity, malocclusion, mobile face, marked facial oedema and ecchymosis, epistaxis, CSF rhinorrhoea	Views: Water's, CT scan Findings: separation of midthird of face at zygomaticofrontal, zygomaticotemporal and nasofrontal sutures, and across orbital floors; opaque maxillary sinuses	Non-union, malunion, malocclusion, lengthening of midface, lacrimal system obstruction

CT: Computed tomography; CSF: cerebrospinal fluid; AP: anteroposterior; TMJ: temporomandibular joint

tripod shape with the apex at the nose. Grasping the front teeth and palate causes movement of the nose and upper lip, with no movement of the orbital complex. Significant force is required to fracture this area so the patient should be carefully evaluated for other injuries. The nose, lips and eyes are usually oedematous with subconjunctival haemorrhage and periorbital contusions. Double vision and sensory disturbances may be present. Haemorrhage from the nose and mouth is frequently noted. The presence of CSF rhinorrhoea suggests an open base of skull fracture.

Le Fort III, or orbital complex fracture, causes total cranial facial separation (Fig 46.21C). The face is mobile, with frontal bone involvement. Massive oedema, contusion, periorbital haematomas, anterior and posterior haemorrhage and malocclusion are present with a spoonlike appearance of the face noted in side profile. Swelling occurs quickly so that fractures may be difficult to palpate.

Management
Management of severe maxillary fractures includes aggressive airway control. Endotracheal intubation may be difficult

because of haemorrhage, oedema and loss of normal anatomical contour. Ensure that difficult airway, cricothyroidotomy or tracheostomy equipment is readily available. Once the airway is managed and satisfactory ventilation is occurring, bleeding needs to be controlled. Initially, packing of posterior nasal cavity and anterior nasal cavity is necessary, as is suturing of lacerations in the oral cavity.[49] Ongoing haemorrhage after following these measures requires emergency angiogram and embolisation and/or ligation.[46,49] In less-life-threatening maxillary injuries, excessive secretions and bleeding may require ice compresses and nasal packing to control bleeding and frequent suctioning to ensure airway patency and patient comfort. The alert patient may benefit from being provided with a Yankauer sucker to use as required to remove oral secretions and blood. The patient should be positioned upright and leaning forwards (as soon as the cervical spine is cleared) to promote drainage of blood and decrease swelling. Alert patients tend to assume this position themselves without prompting. Ice compresses aid pain relief and decrease swelling; prophylactic antibiotics and analgesia should be administered as prescribed. Airway assessment should be continued regularly.

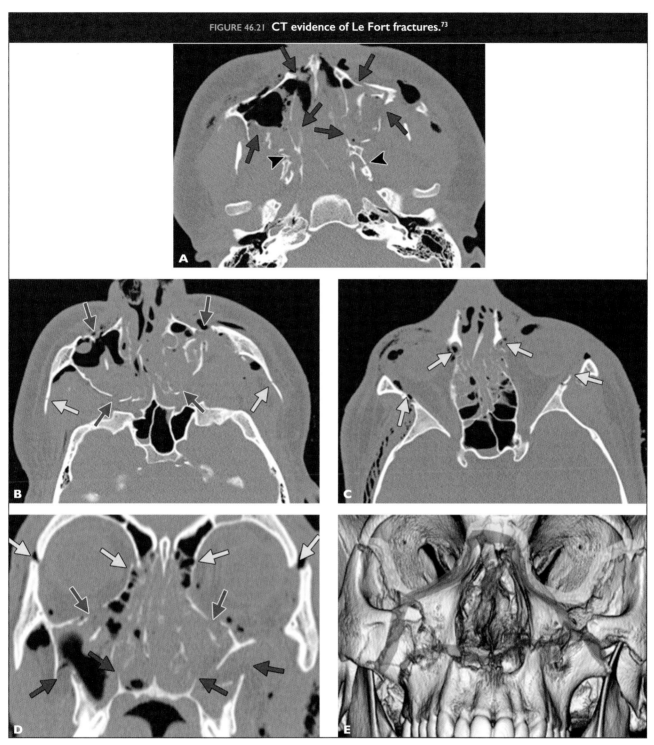

FIGURE 46.21 CT evidence of Le Fort fractures.[73]

Multiple Le Fort fractures in the same patient. (Colour keys correspond to the region affected by the fracture type described in E.) **A**, Axial unenhanced CT image at an inferior level of the maxillary sinuses demonstrating bilateral fractures through the pterygoid plates (arrowheads) and maxillary sinus walls (red arrows); findings indicative of type I Le Fort fractures. Pterygomaxillary dissociation due to fracture extension through the pterygoid plate is a criterion for Le Fort classification. **B**, Axial unenhanced CT image at a superior level of the maxillary sinuses depicting fractures through the medial margins of the anterior and posterior maxillary walls, which are characteristic of type II Le Fort fractures (blue arrows), and nondisplaced fractures through the zygomatic arch, which are a component of type III Le Fort fractures (yellow arrows). **C**, Axial unenhanced CT image at the level of the orbits showing fractures through the nasal bridge, medial orbital walls and lateral orbital walls (yellow arrows); findings indicative of type III Le Fort fractures. **D**, Coronal unenhanced CT image demonstrating type I Le Fort fractures of the inferior aspect of the maxillary sinus walls (red arrows), type II Le Fort fractures of the inferomedial orbital walls (blue arrows), and type III Le Fort fractures of the medial and lateral orbital walls (yellow arrows). **E**, Three-dimensional CT image in frontal orientation delineating type I (red), II (blue), and III (yellow) Le Fort fractures.

Zygomatic fractures

Assessment

Fractures of the zygoma usually occur in two patterns: zygomatic arch fracture and tripod fracture (Fig 46.22). Fractures of the orbital floor may also be present with zygomatic fractures. Injury is usually caused by blunt trauma to the front and side of the face. With a tripod fracture, the zygoma fractures in three places: zygomatic arch, posterior half of the infraorbital rim, and frontozygomatic suture. A step deformity is palpated at the infraorbital rim and frontozygomatic suture area with flattening or asymmetry of the cheek, periorbital oedema, circumorbital or subconjunctival ecchymosis, trismus and pain exacerbated by mouth opening (see Table 46.5). Entrapment of the inferior rectus muscle may occur, and causes double vision and asymmetry of ocular levels and anaesthesia of the upper lip, cheek, teeth and gums. The patient may have unilateral epistaxis. A thorough ocular assessment should be performed (see Ch 33).

The mnemonic TIDES is helpful in determination and description of assessment of zygomatic fractures (Box 46.1). Plain radiographs with a 'jughandle' view demonstrate zygomatic arch fracture, whereas CT scans are generally needed to demonstrate the extent of the fracture.

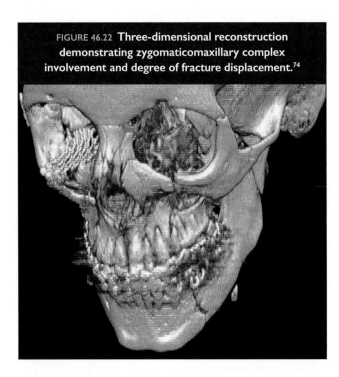

FIGURE 46.22 **Three-dimensional reconstruction demonstrating zygomaticomaxillary complex involvement and degree of fracture displacement.**[74]

BOX 46.1 TIDES mnemonic for zygomatic fractures

T   Trismus—tonic contracture of muscles of mastication
I   Infraorbital—hypoaesthesia or anaesthesia
D   Diplopia—double vision
E   Epistaxis—nosebleed
S   Symmetry absence—flatness or depression of cheek

Management

Interventions focus on pain control and decreasing swelling. Patients with a single injury can usually be discharged from the ED for review by the appropriate specialist as an outpatient. Fractures of the zygoma may not require surgery if the fracture is undisplaced.

Orbital fractures

Assessment

The orbital bones are made up of the facial bones surrounding the orbital space. Orbital fractures frequently result from sports, such as a cricket ball thrown at the eye and altercations involving punches to the face. Golf balls can extend past the protective orbital rim and rupture the globe. Three basic patterns of fractures have been described:

- orbital-zygomatic
- naso-orbito-ethmoid (see under nasal injury)
- internal orbital or blow-out fractures.

Different combinations of these basic patterns can occur.

Orbital-zygomatic fractures and orbital blow-out fractures can occur independently, but are often found in combination. There are two theories as to the cause of orbital blow-out fractures:

- The buckling theory, which suggests that direct pressure on the orbital rim transmits force to the weaker orbital floor causing fracture.
- The hydraulic hypothesis, which suggests fracture occurs when blunt trauma to the globe causes abrupt rise in orbital pressure, causing the orbital floor to fracture and forcing orbital contents to prolapse into the maxillary sinus (Fig 46.23).[29]

Inferior rectus muscle, inferior oblique muscle, infraorbital nerve, orbital fat and connective tissue become entrapped in the orbital floor, so extraocular movements, especially upward gaze, should be carefully evaluated. Palpation of the orbital rim may identify an irregularity. The globe may also become entrapped. Blow-out fracture of the medial orbital wall can also occur with prolapse of medial orbital contents into the ethmoidal sinus (Fig 46.24). Subcutaneous orbital emphysema suggests fracture in the sinus arch. Proptosis or bulging of the eye and limitation of extraocular motion suggest orbital involvement (Fig 46.25A and B). Double vision, pupil asymmetry, enophthalmos (sunken appearance), anaesthesia of the cheek and upper lip, ptosis or drooping of the lid and a sunken appearance are clinical manifestations of blow-out fracture (see Table 46.5). Nausea and vomiting are an indication of a trapdoor orbital fracture that may indicate muscle entrapment in the orbital floor, especially in the paediatric population.[33] CT scan and specialist referral are required. Orbital roof fractures are highly associated with ocular and neurological injuries. A thorough ocular assessment is required (see Ch 33).

Management

If the globe is perforated, manipulating the eyes or noseblowing can lead to intraorbital air. Nose-blowing, coughing, sneezing, vomiting and straining can force air from sinuses through the fracture into the orbital space. Ice compresses and elevating the head of the bed decrease swelling and relieve pain. The patient should be reminded to avoid straining and nose-blowing.

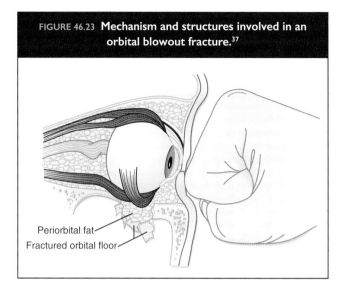

FIGURE 46.23 **Mechanism and structures involved in an orbital blowout fracture.**[37]

Periorbital fat
Fractured orbital floor

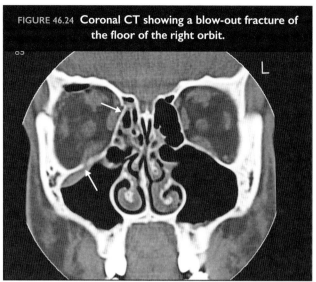

FIGURE 46.24 **Coronal CT showing a blow-out fracture of the floor of the right orbit.**

Fractures of the lamina papyracea (with blood within the ethmoid complex) and orbital floor (with herniation of orbital contents and air within orbital cavity) are arrowed.[75]

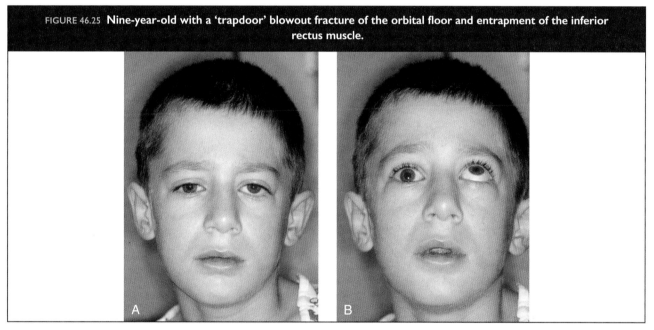

FIGURE 46.25 **Nine-year-old with a 'trapdoor' blowout fracture of the orbital floor and entrapment of the inferior rectus muscle.**

This injury represents a surgical emergency; the orbit must be explored and the muscle released expeditiously. **A**, Frontal gaze. **B**, Upward gaze.[76]

Surgical intervention is usually postponed until swelling diminishes, usually between 5 and 10 days post-fracture,[29] but earlier with children, CSF leakage and penetrating objects.[33] The aim of surgery is to reconstruct the contours of the orbit and release soft tissues that have prolapsed. Indication for repair is generally based on the degree of enophthalmos and diplopia.[29,33] The most common complications of orbital fractures relate to the globe. In addition, strabismus, enophthalmos, eyelid retraction, lacrimal duct obstruction and telecanthus are common after fracture of the orbit, especially in midface trauma.[29] Patients with single injury can usually be discharged from the ED for review by the appropriate specialist as an outpatient. Fractures of the orbit may not require surgery if the fracture is undisplaced.

PRACTICE TIP

Many patients with facial injuries smoke and drink alcohol, behaviours that will adversely affect healing. Discharge planning from the ED should include advice not to smoke or drink whilst healing takes place.

SUMMARY

Faciomaxillary injuries are a common occurrence in the ED. Special attention should be given to stabilising the cervical spine, clearing and maintaining a patent airway and controlling haemorrhage. Ongoing airway assessment is essential. The goal of treatment is to manage life-threatening airway problems and haemorrhage, return function and provide cosmetic repair.

CASE STUDY

The police have called the emergency medical services to attend a semiconscious male involved in an alleged assault with a baseball bat. The police report he smells of alcohol and has been struck across the jaw and to the bridge of the nose. There is bleeding from the nose and mouth. He is already developing massive swelling across the middle of his face. He is drowsy but rousable and is able to tell the police who he is and can move all his limbs on command. He complains of jaw pain and difficulty opening his mouth and severe pain across the bridge of his nose.

Questions

1. On arrival at the scene, what is your initial assessment?
2. What is your initial management plan?
3. On arrival at the ED, what is your initial assessment?
4. What is your initial management plan?
5. What radiology will be required?
6. What is the likely definitive treatment for this patient?

 Answers to Case Study Questions can be found on evolve
http://evolve.emergencytrauma.curtis

REFERENCES

1. Kellman R, Schmidt C. The paranasal sinuses as a protective crumple zone for the orbit. Laryngoscope 2009;11:1682–90.
2. Martin RC II, Spain DA, Richardson JD. Do facial fractures protect the brain or are they a marker for severe head injury? Am Surg 2002;68(5):477–81.
3. Drake R, Vogl A, Mitchell A. Gray's basic anatomy. Churchill Livingstone; 2012.
4. Netter FH. Atlas of human anatomy. 5th edn. Philadelphia: Saunders; 2011.
5. Allareddy V, Allareddy V, Nalliah R. Epidemiology of facial fractures. J Oral Maxillofac Surg 2011;69:2613–18.
6. Alvi A, Doherty T, Lewen G. Facial fractures and concomitant injuries in trauma patients. Laryngoscope 2003;113(1):102–6.
7. Shere JL, Boole JR, Holtel MR et al. An analysis of 3599 midfacial and 1141 orbital blowout fractures among 4426 United States Army soldiers, 1980–2000. Otolaryngol Head Neck Surg 2004;130(2):164–70.
8. Hogg NJ, Stewart TC, Armstrong JE et al. Epidemiology of maxillofacial injuries at trauma hospitals in Ontario, Canada between 1992 and 1997. J Trauma 2000;49(3):425–32.
9. Erdmann D, Follmar KE, Debruijn M et al. A retrospective analysis of facial fracture etiologies. Ann Plast Surg 2008;60(4):398–403.
10. Lee KH, Snape L, Steenberg LJ et al. Comparison between interpersonal violence and motor vehicle accidents in the aetiology of maxillofacial fractures. Aust N Z J Surg 2007;77(8):695–8.
11. Lee K. Epidemiology of mandibular fractures in a tertiary trauma centre. Emerg Med J 2008;25:565–8.
12. Elledge R, Elledge R, Aquilina P et al. The role of alcohol in maxillofacial trauma—comparative retrospective audit between two centres. Alcohol 2011;45:239–43.
13. Gerbino G, Roccia F, De Gioanni PP et al. Maxillofacial trauma in the elderly. J Oral Maxillofac Surg 1999;57(7):777–83.
14. Velayutham L, Sivanandarajasingam A, O'Meara C, Hyam D. Elderly patients with maxillofacial trauma: the effect of an ageing population on a maxillofacial unit's workload. British Journal of Oral and Maxillofacial Surgery 2013;51:128–32.
15. Wade C, Hoffman G, Brennan P. Falls in elderly people that result in facial injuries. 2004. British Journal of Oral and Maxillofacial Surgery 2004;42:138–41.
16. Kloss F, Tuli T, Hachl O et al. The impact of ageing on craniomaxillofacial trauma—a comparative investigation. Int J Oral Maxillofac Surg 2007;36:115–63.
17. Kotecha S, Scannell J, Monaghan A et al. A four year retrospective study of 1,062 patients presenting with maxillofacial emergencies at a specialist paediatric hospital. Br J Oral Maxillofac Surg 2008;46(4):293–6.

18. Imahara S, Hopper R, Wang J, Rivara F. Patterns and outcomes of pediatric facial fractures in the United States: A survey of the National Trauma Data Bank. J Am Coll Surg 2008:207:710–16.

19. Eggensperger-Wymann N, Holzle A, Zachariou Z, Iizuka T. Pediatric craniofacial trauma. J Oral Maxillofac Surg 2008;66:58–64.

20. Le BT, Dierks EJ, Ueeck BA et al. Maxillofacial injuries associated with domestic violence. J Oral Maxillofac Surg 2001;59(11):1277–84.

21. Moses K. Atlas of clinical gross anatomy. 2nd edn. Philadelphia: Saunders; 2013.

22. Bogart B. Elsevier's integrated anatomy and embryology. St Louis: Mosby; 2007.

23. Werning JW, Downey NM, Brinker RA et al. The impact of osteoporosis on patients with maxillofacial trauma. Arch Otolaryngol Head Neck Surg 2004;130(3):353–6.

24. Ferreira PC, Amarante JM, Silva PN et al. Retrospective study of 1251 maxillofacial fractures in children and adolescents. Plast Reconstr Surg 2005;115(6):1500–8.

25. Marx J, Hockberger R, Walls R. Rosen's emergency medicine. 7th edn. St Louis: Mosby; 2010.

26. Brookes CN. Maxillofacial and ocular injuries in motor vehicle crashes. Ann R Coll Surg Engl 2004;86(3):149–55.

27. Cruz AA, Eichenberger GC. Epidemiology and management of orbital fractures. Curr Opin Ophthalmol 2004;15(5):416–21.

28. Major MS, MacGregor A, Bumpous JM. Patterns of maxillofacial injuries as a function of automobile restraint use. Laryngoscope 2000;110(4):606–11.

29. Stacy D, Doyle J, Gutowski K. Safety device use affects the incidence patterns of facial trauma in motor vehicle collisions: An analysis of the National Trauma Database from 2000 to 2004. Plast Reconstr Surg 2008; 121:2057–64.

30. American Society of Anesthesiologists. Practice guidelines for management of the difficult airway: An updated report by the American Society of Anesthesiologists Task Force on Management of the Difficult Airway. Anesthesiology 2013;118:251–70.

31. Chang EL, Bernardino CR. Update on orbital trauma. Curr Opin Ophthalmol 2004;15(5):411–15.

32. Mithani SK, St-Hilaire H, Brooke BS et al. Predictable patterns of intracranial and cervical spine injury in craniomaxillofacial trauma: analysis of 4786 patients. Plast Reconstr Surg 2009;123(4):1293–301.

33. Follmar KE, Debruijn M, Baccarani A et al. Concomitant injuries in patients with panfacial fractures. J Trauma 2007;63(4):831–5.

34. Mulligan R, Friedman J, Mahabir R. A nationwide review of the associations among cervical spine injuries, head injuries, and facial fractures. J Trauma 2010;68(3):587–92.

35. Laverick S, Patel N, Jones DC. Maxillofacial trauma and the role of alcohol. Br J Oral Maxillofac Surg 2008;46(7):542–6.

36. Rosen P et al. Emergency medicine. 6th edn. St Louis: Mosby; 2010.

37. Burton J, Kuehl K. Emergency medicine. 2nd edn. Philadelphia: Saunders 2013.

38. Tung TC, Tseng WS, Chen CT et al. Acute life-threatening injuries in facial fracture patients: a review of 1,025 patients. J Trauma 2000;49(3):420–4.

39. Ceallaigh P, Ekanaykaee K, Beirne C, Patton D. Diagnosis and Management of common maxillofacial injuries in the emergency department. Part 1: advanced trauma life support. Emerg Med J 2006;23:796–7.

40. Kellman RM, Losquadro WD. Comprehensive airway management of patients with maxillofacial trauma. Craniomaxillofac Trauma Reconstruction 2008;1:39–48.

41. Perry M, ed. Head, neck and dental emergencies. Oxford: Oxford University Press; 2005.

42. Tuckett J, Lynham A, Lee G et al. Maxillofacial trauma in the emergency department. The Surgeon 2014:12:106–14.

43. Berlac P, Hyldmo PK, Kongstad P et al. Prehospital airway management: guidelines from a task force from the Scandinavian Society for Anaesthesiology and Intensive Care Medicine. Acta Anaesthesiol Scand 2008;52(7):897–907.

44. Perry M, Morris C. Advanced trauma life support (ATLS) and facial trauma: can one size fit all? Part 2: ATLS, maxillofacial injuries and airway management dilemmas. Int J Oral Maxillofac Surg 2008;37(4):309–20.

45. Perry M, Dancey A, Mireskandari K et al. Emergency care in facial trauma—a maxillofacial and ophthalmic perspective. Injury 2005;36:875–96.

46. Schade K, Borzotta A, Michaels A. Intracranial malposition of nasopharyngeal airway. J Trauma 2000;49(5):967–8.

47. Edibam C, Robinson H. Faxiomaxillary and upper-airway injuries. In: Berston A, Soni N. Oh's intensive care manual 7th edn. Elsevier; 2014.

48. American Society of Anesthesiologists. Practice guidelines for management of the difficult airway: An updated report by the American Society of Anesthesiologists Task Force on Management of the Difficult Airway. Anesthesiology 2013;118: 251–70.

49. Shimoyama T, Kaneko T, Horie N. Initial management of massive oral bleeding after midfacial fracture. J Trauma 2003;54(2):332–6.

50. Yang WG, Tsai TR, Hung CC et al. Life-threatening bleeding in a facial fracture. Ann Plast Surg 2001;46(2):159–62.

51. Cogbill T, Cothren C, Ahearn M et al. Management of maxillofacial injuries with severe oronasal hemorrhage: a multicenter perspective. J Trauma 2008;65:994–9.

52. Lynham AJ, Hirst JP, Cosson JA et al. Emergency department management of maxillofacial trauma. Emerg Med Australas 2004;16(1):7–12.

53. Veeravagu A, Joseph R, Jiang B et al. Traumatic epistaxis: Skull base defects, intracranial complications and neurosurgical considerations. Int J Surg Case Rep 2013;4(8):656–61.

54. Ochs MW, Tucker MR. Management of facial fractures. In: Peterson LJ, editor. Contemporary oral and maxillofacial surgery. 4th edn. St Louis: Mosby; 2003. pp. 527–58.

55. Singer AJ, Mach C, Thode HC et al. Patient priorities with traumatic lacerations. Am J Emerg Med 2000;18(6):683–6.

56. Dulecki M, Piper B. Irrigating simple acute traumatic wounds: a review of the current literature. J Emerg Nurs 2005;31(2):156–60, 220–6.

57. Wilson JR, Mills JG, Prather ID et al. A toxicity index of skin and wound cleansers used on in vitro fibroblasts and keratinocytes. Adv Skin Wound Care 2005;18(7):373–8.

58. Egozi E, Faulkner B, Lin KY. Successful revascularization following near-complete amputation of the tongue. Ann Plast Surg 2006;56(2):190–3.

59. Farion K, Osmond MH, Hartling L et al. Tissue adhesives for traumatic lacerations in children and adults. Cochrane Database Syst Rev 2002;(3):CD003326.

60. Brinker D, Hancox JD, Bernardon SO. Assessment and initial treatment of lacerations, mammalian bites, and insect stings. AACN Clin Issues 2003;14(4):401–10.

61. Mitchell RB, Nanez G, Wagner JD et al. Dog bites of the scalp, face and neck in children. Laryngoscope 2003;113(3):492–5.

62. Ellis III E. Soft tissue and dentoalveolar injuries. In: Peterson LJ, Ellis E, Hupp JR et al. eds. Contemporary oral and maxillofacial surgery. 4th edn. St Louis: Mosby; 2003.

63. Ernst A, Herzog M, Seidl R. Head and neck trauma—an interdisciplinary approach. Stuttgart: Georg Thieme Verlag, 2006.

64. Perry M. Maxillofacial trauma—developments, innovations and controversies. Injury 2009;40(12):1252–9.

65. Bagheri S, Jo C. Clinical review of oral and maxillofacial surgery 2nd edn. St Louis: Mosby 2014.

66. Katzen JT, Jarrahy R, Eby JB et al. Craniofacial and skull base trauma. J Trauma 2003;54(5):1026–34.

67. Cunningham LL, Khader R. Oral and maxillofacial trauma. 3rd edn. Saunders, Elsevier; 2013.

68. Reddy L V. Nasal fractures. In: Fonseca RJ. Oral and maxillofacial surgery. 2nd edn. Saunders, Elsevier; 2009.

69. Engelstad M. Current therapy in oral and maxillofacial surgery, Philadelphia: Saunders 2012.

70. Steed, MB, Bagheri SC. Clinical review of oral and maxillofacial Surgery: A case-based approach.; Mosby, Elsevier; 2014: 239.

71. Sheehy SB, Jimmerson CL. Manual of clinical trauma care. 2nd edn. St Louis: Mosby; 1994.

72. Trunkey DD, Lewis FR. Current therapy of trauma. 2nd edn. Toronto: BC Decker; 1986.

73. Winegar B, Murillo H, Tantiwongkosi B. Spectrum of critical imaging findings in complex facial skeletal trauma. Radiographics 2013;33:3–19.

74. Papageorge MB, Oreadi D. Oral and maxillofacial trauma. Saunders Elsevier; 2013.

75. Adam A, Dixon AK. Grainger and Allison's diagnostic radiology. 5th edn. New York: Churchill Livingstone; 2008.

76. Bell RB, Al-Bustani SS. Current therapy in oral and maxillofacial surgery. Saunders, Elsevier; 2012: 304–23.

CHAPTER 47
THORACIC AND NECK TRAUMA

MARY LANGCAKE, KATE CURTIS AND ELIZABETH WALTER

Essentials

- Simple manoeuvres, such as needle decompression of the chest, may be lifesaving.
- One of the earliest signs of clinical deterioration in patients with chest trauma is tachypnoea. If a patient cannot complete a sentence on one breath, this is a warning sign of incipient respiratory failure.
- Early and effective analgesia is key.
- Do not delay definitive management in life-threatening chest trauma waiting for a chest X-ray.
- Oxygen saturation is unreliable in determining the degree of hypoxaemia, but is useful for monitoring changes in patient condition.
- The presence of pain, chest-wall tenderness and subcutaneous emphysema indicates underlying lung or airway injury, which may require intervention.
- Patients with blunt chest trauma will have lung contusions. Severe contusions:
  - evolve over time
  - may cause deterioration in respiratory status
  - require constant monitoring to detect deterioration.
- Multidisciplinary management involving physiotherapy, pain team, nursing and medical staff reduces morbidity and mortality in patients with blunt chest injury.
- Neck trauma presents challenges because of the concentration of critical structures in a confined space.
- CT angiography is the key to assessment of penetrating neck trauma.

INTRODUCTION

Injuries to the thorax and its contents encompass some of the most life-threatening situations in trauma care, and require rapid assessment and management. Autopsy reports of patients dying from motor vehicle collisions (MVCs) in Australia demonstrate that serious thoracic injuries occur in 84% of deaths, and are second in incidence only to major head injuries.[1] Analysis of 2013 data from New South Wales shows that among severely injured patients admitted to trauma centres in the Sydney metropolitan area, the chest is the third most frequently injured body region.[2] Even in parts of the world such as Australasia, with relatively low prevalence of civilian firearm injuries, the incidence of penetrating thoracic trauma is second only to that of abdominal injury, and potentially just as lethal.[3] First-responders need to know how to perform life-saving interventions at the scene, since thoracic trauma resulting in such conditions as tension pneumothorax may be rapidly fatal unless managed appropriately. All staff caring for patients with major thoracic trauma must be familiar with the proper management of thoracic injuries to minimise potential mortality and morbidity.

Since the thoracic outlet extends into the root of the neck and contains major vascular and neural structures, any of which may be injured, it is reasonable to consider thoracic and neck trauma together.

The aim of this chapter is to review the anatomy of the thorax and neck, to consider mechanisms of injury as they relate to these structures and to consider approaches to assessment and management of the most common injuries associated with trauma to the thorax and neck.

Anatomy and physiology

The thorax extends from the supraclavicular fossae at the base of the neck inferiorly to the diaphragm, which is highly mobile. Diaphragmatic excursion may extend the limits of the thoracic cavity anteriorly down to and even slightly below the costal margins, and posteriorly to the 12th thoracic vertebra. As the diaphragm moves down, negative pressure is generated within the thoracic cavity causing an influx of air via the nose or mouth, and expansion of the lungs.

The thoracic wall is comprised of the back and chest musculature, as well as the bony skeleton formed by the sternum, ribs and spine. It affords protection to the contents of the thoracic cavity. Within the thoracic cavity proper lie the thoracic viscera: the lungs and associated tracheobronchial tree, the oesophagus, the heart and major vascular structures (Fig 47.1). Penetrating injuries of the torso, even beyond the defined anatomical boundaries of the thorax, may still damage intrathoracic structures.

The thoracic pleura cover both the inner aspect of the chest wall (parietal pleura) and the surface of the lungs (visceral pleura). These two layers fuse centrally at the pulmonary hilum to envelop the major vascular and bronchial structures. A thin film of clear pleural fluid separates and lubricates these two surfaces, keeping them in close apposition so that the interpleural space under normal circumstances, is only a 'potential space'. A mechanical breach of either pleural surface may result in influx into this space of air (pneumothorax), blood (haemothorax) or both (haemopneumothorax).

Injury mechanism

Mechanisms of thoracic injury fall into two main categories: blunt and penetrating. Other, less common mechanisms include burns (Ch 52) and blast (Ch 51). Blunt trauma may be sustained following the sudden application of force over a broad surface area of the body, whether from a direct blow by moving solid objects (e.g. fists, cricket bats, falling rocks), sudden rapid deceleration (e.g. motor vehicle collisions, falls) or crushing (e.g. entrapment between wall and vehicle bumper). Penetrating injuries result from piercing or cutting of tissues from bullets, knives, shrapnel, glass shards or other implements. Mixed patterns of injury may be seen where combined mechanisms of energy transfer occur, such as blasts where blunt injury may result from the patient being thrown against a wall, penetrating injury occurs via the shrapnel generated by the blast and burns result from the direct thermal effects of the explosion.

Significant injury to most of the intrathoracic structures can be immediately life-threatening. Death may occur secondary to exsanguination, severe respiratory failure with concomitant hypoxia, obstructive shock (tension pneumothorax) with resultant cardiac failure or direct cardiac injury. Oesophageal injuries can lead to significant morbidity and mortality from overwhelming mediastinal sepsis if missed but the course is usually more protracted.

Patient assessment

Approach to initial evaluation

Patients with thoracic injuries may present dramatically with profound shock or severe respiratory distress, but some may demonstrate only subtle physiological changes initially. An understanding of the history and mechanism of injury permits prediction of the likelihood of thoracic injury. Primary survey will assess and secure an airway, and should identify immediately life-threatening thoracic injuries, such as tension pneumothorax, which must be managed promptly before further assessment is undertaken. In the field, ask the patient with chest trauma to tell you their name and what happened. If the patient can answer and complete the sentence in one breath it gives a rapid indication of not only a patent airway, but also adequate respiratory status at that point in time. But remember to repeat the exercise regularly since respiratory failure can occur progressively and rapidly in patients with significant thoracic trauma. Noise in the environment may make it difficult for the paramedic to hear breath sounds on auscultation, therefore direct and continuous observation of the patient is paramount. Detailed secondary survey is essential to detect the presence of potentially life-threatening injuries, such as simple pneumothorax, haemothorax or flail chest. Selective use of radiology, coupled with careful examination, should reveal even subtle thoracic injuries.

> **PRACTICE TIP**
>
> A rapid screening tool is to ask the patient their name and what happened. If the patient can answer, this indicates that their airway is clear. If they can complete the sentence in one breath it gives a rapid indication of respiratory status, and a lucid answer confirms adequate cerebral perfusion.

In the patient with thoracic trauma, assessment of the respiratory system follows the sequence of inspection, palpation and auscultation. Measurement of vital signs including pulse and respiratory rate should be undertaken, and oxygen saturation should be recorded. In a cold, shocked patient or one who is agitated or combative, pulse oximetry may not provide an accurate indirect measure of arterial blood oxygen, and should not be relied upon solely as an indicator of the physiological status of the patient. However, it is a useful gauge of any change in the patient's condition. Tachypnoea or respiratory distress may indicate direct injury to the thoracic wall or underlying lungs, but can also be an early and sensitive indicator of severe circulatory shock.[4] Furthermore, severe brain injury can produce abnormalities of the respiratory system through impairment of brainstem function. Thus, any patient presenting in a confused or agitated state after sustaining a major mechanism of injury should first be presumed to be in either haemorrhagic shock or hypoxic shock (or both) until proven otherwise.

FIGURE 47.1 Anatomy of the thorax and its contents.

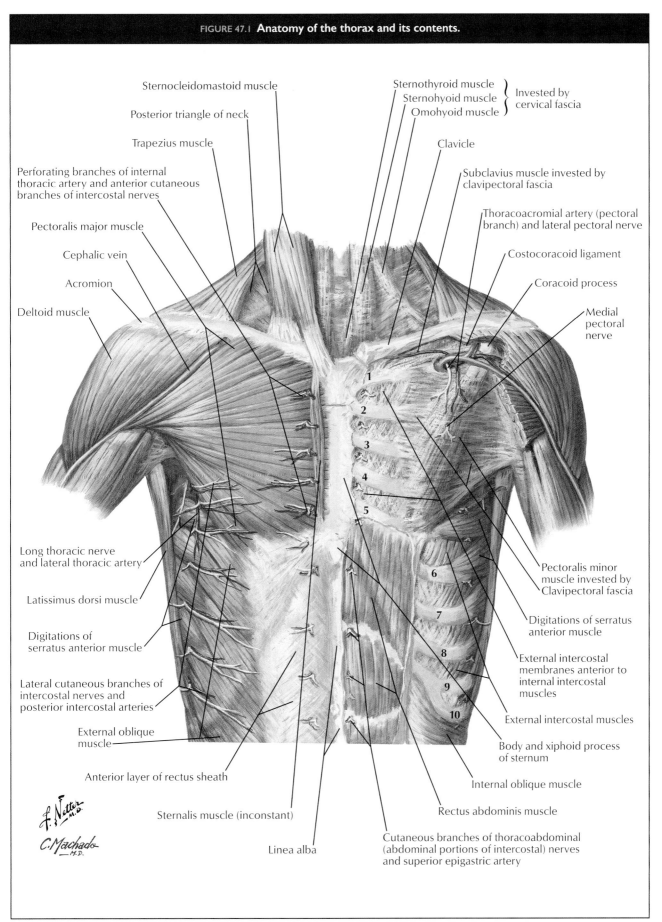

Sternocleidomastoid muscle

Posterior triangle of neck

Trapezius muscle

Perforating branches of internal
thoracic artery and anterior cutaneous
branches of intercostal nerves

Pectoralis major muscle

Cephalic vein

Acromion

Deltoid muscle

Sternothyroid muscle
Sternohyoid muscle   Invested by
Omohyoid muscle   cervical fascia

Clavicle

Subclavius muscle invested by
clavipectoral fascia

Thoracoacromial artery (pectoral
branch) and lateral pectoral nerve

Costocoracoid ligament

Coracoid process

Medial
pectoral
nerve

Long thoracic nerve
and lateral thoracic artery

Latissimus dorsi muscle

Digitations of
serratus anterior muscle

Lateral cutaneous branches of
intercostal nerves and
posterior intercostal arteries

External oblique
muscle

Anterior layer of rectus sheath

Sternalis muscle (inconstant)

Linea alba

Pectoralis minor
muscle invested by
Clavipectoral fascia

Digitations of serratus
anterior muscle

External intercostal
membranes anterior to
internal intercostal
muscles

External intercostal muscles

Body and xiphoid process
of sternum

Internal oblique muscle

Rectus abdominis muscle

Cutaneous branches of thoracoabdominal
(abdominal portions of intercostal) nerves
and superior epigastric artery

Continued

FIGURE 47.1 **Anatomy of the thorax and its contents.—cont'd**

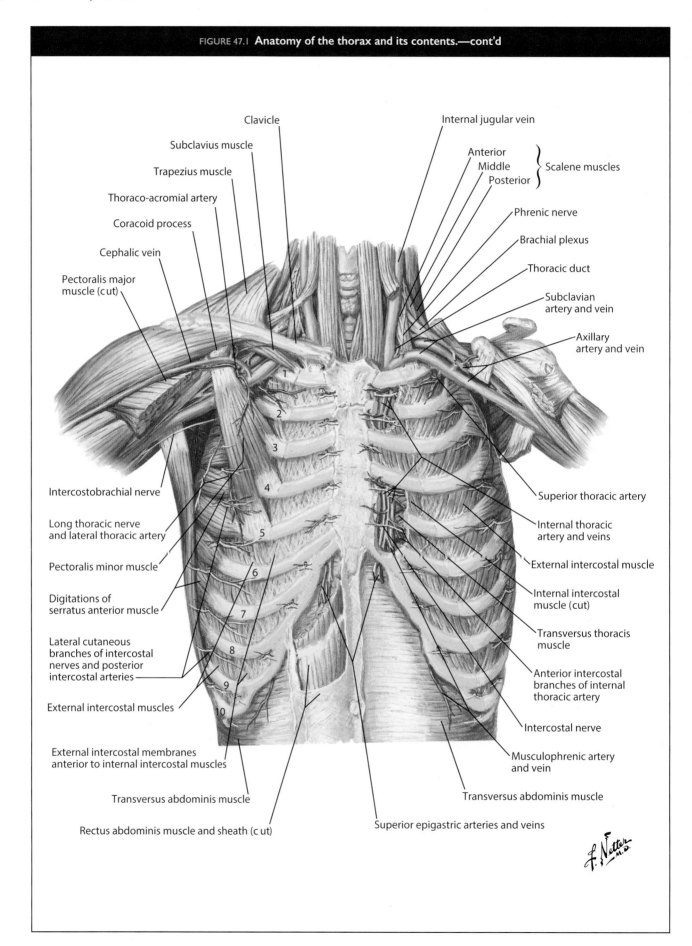

Inspection

Visual inspection of the chest should occur first, paying particular attention to less-visible areas that could easily be ignored, such as the axillae. The patient should be fully exposed to facilitate thorough inspection and minimise the risk of missed injury, but hypothermia must be prevented, and the dignity of the patient preserved. When expedient, a log-roll must be performed to inspect the back, especially when there is a history of penetrating trauma. Relevant findings include ecchymoses (bruising), haematomas or abrasions that might indicate significant blunt force trauma. Discrete breaks in the skin, such as lacerations, incised wounds or punctures, are the hallmarks of penetrating injury. Do not overlook entry and exit wounds of projectiles. Where possible, haemorrhage should be controlled by direct pressure. Be aware that dried blood may hide underlying wounds, therefore detailed inspection is essential. Photographs of wounds should be taken with an indicator of size (such as a tape measure), for forensic purposes. In some centres, digital photographs can be linked to the radiology system, allowing easy access.

Observation of the mechanics of breathing is essential. Segmental chest wall motion abnormalities may indicate a flail chest and highlight the presence of lung injury. Use of the accessory muscles of respiration such as the intercostals and sternocleidomastoids, indicates increased work of respiration, which may rapidly lead to fatigue and respiratory failure. Respiratory rate and rhythm should be recorded since this may provide evidence of underlying physiological derangement.

Palpation

Palpation of the thorax and back will provide evidence not only regarding the underlying integrity of the thoracic wall and rib cage, but also about the possibility of underlying lung injury.[5] Subcutaneous emphysema, typically felt as a fine crackling, indicates the presence of an air leak from either pneumothorax or tracheobronchial injury. Coarse crepitus felt over the ribs is caused by fractured rib ends grating against each other. In the awake, alert patient this will be associated with significant pain. Chest wall movement can be assessed by placing the hands on either side of the chest and noting their motion. Asymmetry indicates a major difference in air entry, suggesting the presence of pneumothorax, haemothorax or haemopneumothorax.

Auscultation

Although detailed description of specific auscultatory findings is not really possible in the typically noisy pre-hospital or emergency department (ED) setting,[6] auscultation of the chest walls laterally will confirm the presence or absence of breath sounds, and permit comparison of right and left sides. Absence of breath sounds is a sinister sign indicating either tension pneumothorax or massive haemothorax, both of which may prove rapidly fatal unless urgent management is undertaken. The typical muffled heart sounds of pericardial tamponade may be difficult to distinguish due to ambient noise, and the diagnosis should be made based on associated clinical signs, which will be discussed below.

Clinical interventions

In the pre-hospital environment the patient may exhibit severe respiratory distress coupled with worsening shock.

Auscultation of the chest may reveal a unilateral absence of breath sounds. This is an emergency since these signs indicate a strong likelihood of tension pneumothorax, a condition that rapidly progresses to loss of consciousness and death if not treated. Urgent intervention to decompress the thoracic cavity is required which may be achieved via needle thoracostomy, the placement of a large bore cannula in the second intercostal space, in the midclavicular line on the affected side. A hiss of air not only confirms the diagnosis, but also relieves the intrathoracic pressure. Tube thoracostomy may be performed in the field or in the ED prior to any radiological investigation.

When the patient subsequently reaches the trauma centre and haemodynamic status has been reviewed, fluid administration should be prescribed by the trauma team leader. This might be crystalloid initially, but should be replaced by blood and blood products in the haemodynamically unstable patient. The trauma nurse must be familiar with the use of a fluid warmer, as it is essential to correct or prevent hypothermia.

The trauma nurse should ensure that oxygen is administered, preferably via face mask. In some trauma centres high-flow nasal prong (HFNP) oxygen is applied to patients with thoracic injury. The benefits of HFNP include that the oxygen is warmed and moist, facilitating clearance of secretions, and a small amount of post end-expiratory pressure (PEEP) is maintained, which is thought to diminish the work of breathing.[7] A full set of vital signs, including temperature, should be obtained and regularly repeated and, as above, pulse oximetry should be measured continuously to monitor changes in patient condition.

While the medical team are conducting the primary survey, a manual non-invasive blood pressure (NIBP) should be attended prior to the application of an automatic NIBP device, as automatic NIBP can be unreliable in the acute trauma setting.[8] The nurse should then place standard chest leads for continuous cardiac rhythm monitoring. Abnormalities on a full 12-lead electrocardiogram (ECG) may indicate either pre-existing cardiac disease or the presence of possible blunt cardiac injury. Subsequent ECG changes, including the development of dysrhythmias, may indicate either ischaemia or evolving cardiac injury. Venous blood should be taken for measurement of electrolytes, full blood count and coagulation studies. Remember, initial haemoglobin levels *do not* correlate with the extent of blood loss as it can take 8–12 hours before accurate blood levels are measurable once the interstitial fluids are redistributed into the blood plasma.[9] Initial abnormal changes observed can be due to haemodilution from resuscitative efforts. Venous blood gas gives information about pH and lactate levels, which will indicate whether the patient is acidaemic due to anaerobic metabolism (see Ch 17, p. 332). These parameters are also useful for monitoring response to resuscitation. Interpretation of venous blood oxygen content provides useful information about ventilation and perfusion. Where there is associated blunt abdominal trauma, measurement of liver enzymes and amylase and lipase may help reveal visceral injury.

Prompt, adequate analgesia in patients with significant blunt thoracic trauma may make the difference between survival and death, particularly in the elderly patient. Pre-hospital personnel may be concerned about administering narcotic analgesia in shocked trauma patients due to the vasodilatory response that may occur. If in doubt it is advisable either to contact the receiving hospital for advice or to use methoxyfluorane (Penthrane) inhalational anaesthesia, which is known to have relatively mild haemodynamic effects, and does not predispose the heart to rhythm disturbances.[10] The trauma nurse should not hesitate to request that the patient receive pain relief in a timely manner. A patient whose pain is well controlled will more easily be able to cooperate with the remainder of the examination process. Furthermore, the psychological stress of major trauma may be diminished if pain is controlled early in the presentation.[11,12] Haemodynamically stable patients may receive parenteral narcotics initially, but subsequently specialised pain team consultation should be obtained to determine the optimal analgesic regimen for the patient during the admission. Options include patient-controlled analgesia (PCA), with or without ketamine infusion, paravertebral blocks or, in some patients, the placement of a thoracic epidural may be indicated.

Clear documentation is essential, noting the initial assessment and management, plans for investigation or treatment and the times when observations or interventions are undertaken, including drug administration. Response to treatment should be recorded, including the time at which the observations are made. This allows trends in the patient's condition to be determined. Any deterioration in the patient's status should be documented and reported to the trauma team leader.

Communication is an important part of the trauma nurse's role in caring for an injured patient. This is especially so with the patient with thoracic trauma. By constantly checking in with the patient it may be the trauma nurse who first notes increasing shortness of breath or an inability to complete a sentence in one breath that presages deterioration in the patient's condition.

In a rural or regional centre, where the facilities may not be available to manage the patient with significant thoracic injury, transfer to a major trauma centre may be required. The trauma nurse will be responsible for expediting 'packaging' of the patient for safe transport. This may involve securing endotracheal tubes and intravenous lines to prevent dislodgement, and ensuring the patient's belongings accompany them. Preparation for transfer is discussed in detail in Chapter 16.

Radiology

Radiological studies are helpful in the initial evaluation of the patient with thoracic injuries. These tests vary not only in their availability, but also in their sensitivity and specificity for the diagnosis of particular injuries. The haemodynamic status of the patient must be taken into account when determining which radiological investigations to perform.[13] In the unstable patient not responding to resuscitation, treatment decisions must be made using clinical judgement without waiting for radiology or moving the patient out of the ED to obtain further investigations. Any transport of such a patient should only be to a location where definitive management of the underlying life-threatening injury can be performed, be this the operating theatre or the interventional radiology suite.

The chest X-ray

The single-view chest X-ray (CXR) is by far the most useful radiographic study that can be obtained during the initial

evaluation of patients with suspected or confirmed chest injuries (Table 47.1). The bony structure of the chest wall and musculature are shown in Figure 47.2. A portable, supine CXR is quite sensitive for diagnosing the most common life-threatening thoracic injuries. It may be sufficient to indicate the need for major therapeutic interventions, such as urgent thoracotomy in massive haemothorax, or be useful in planning management, such as the need for tube thoracostomy. Furthermore, plain CXR may provide evidence of injury to the mediastinal structures such as the thoracic aorta, which will be discussed further below. The importance of CXR in the initial evaluation of the patient with known or suspected thoracic injury is such that the radiographer should be a member of the multidisciplinary trauma team responding to all newly arrived major trauma patients.

As an adjunct to primary survey a normal initial CXR will rule out the thoracic cavity as a source of major occult haemorrhage in the patient presenting in shock. Conversely, life-saving procedures should never be delayed until a CXR is obtained in patients with high clinical suspicion of major thoracic injury.[14] For example, a patient with respiratory distress, haemodynamic shock, tracheal deviation and unilateral absence/decrease of breath sounds has a tension pneumothorax and should undergo urgent chest decompression before a CXR is performed. In this situation any delay in definitive treatment may prove fatal.

Most patients with significant thoracic injury will undergo computed tomography (CT) as part of their workup. This will be discussed further below. As a consequence of the increased use of CT, formal upright, two-view CXR (i.e. posterior–anterior and lateral projections), which must be obtained in the radiology department, is now seldom used. This is important since thoracic cage injuries may be accompanied by bony spinal injuries, which would preclude the upright views.

In patients with penetrating injuries, all missile or knife entrance or exit wounds should be identified with a radio-opaque marker such as an open paperclip prior to CXR to

TABLE 47.1 Supine chest X-ray findings and correlating intervention	
FINDING ON SUPINE PLAIN CHEST X-RAY	INTERVENTIONS
Large pneumothorax	Tube thoracostomy
Large haemothorax	Tube thoracostomy
Rib fractures	Analgesia; ensure physiotherapy; monitor for respiratory failure; suspect lung contusion or thoracic vascular injury
Elevated left diaphragm or viscera seen in lower left chest or nasogastric tube coiled in left lower chest	Suspect left diaphragm rupture
Pneumomediastinum	Suspect oesophageal injury
Widened/indistinct mediastinum	Search for thoracic aortic disruption

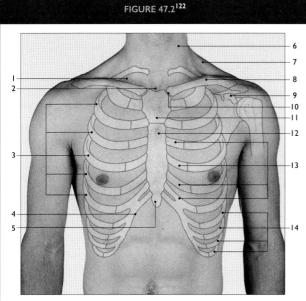

FIGURE 47.2[122]

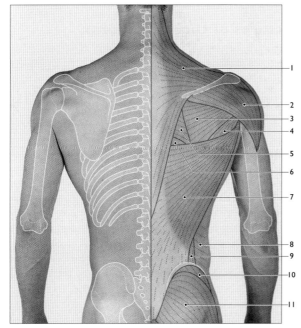

A, Frontal view of the trunk demonstrating bony and soft tissue structures. 1. Supraclavicular fossa. 2. Jugular notch. 3. True ribs. 4. Costal margin. 5. Xiphisternum. 6. Sternocleidomastoid. 7. Trapezius. 8. Clavicle. 9. Coracoid process. 10. Sternoclavicular joint. 11. Manubrium. 12. Body of sternum. 13. Costal cartilages. 14. False ribs.
B, Posterior view of the trunk demonstrating surface anatomy, bony and soft tissue structures. 1. Trapezius. 2. Deltoid. 3. Infraspinatus. 4. Teres major. 5. Rhomboid major. 6. Auscultatory triangle. 7. Latissimus dorsi. 8. External oblique. 9. Lumbar triangle. 10. Gluteus medius. 11. Gluteus maximus.

facilitate determination of likely trajectories, and thus identify possible zones of major injury.

Ultrasound

Focused assessment sonography in trauma (FAST) was principally developed as an extension of normal ultrasound to determine the presence of free fluid in the abdominal cavity. Most major trauma centres now include FAST as part of the primary survey. Extended FAST (e-FAST) is now used to assess the thoracic cavity. A skilled operator can detect both fluid (haemothorax) and air (pneumothorax), and published reports indicate high sensitivity, in some instances more sensitive that plain X-ray.[15–18] In the pre-hospital setting it can indicate the need for chest decompression in the shocked polytrauma patient in whom the classic signs of tension pneumothorax (distended neck veins, absent breath sounds, tracheal deviation) may be difficult to elicit.

Computed tomography (CT) scan

Compared to other imaging modalities, CT has a high degree of sensitivity and specificity for the detection of subtle injuries in the chest.[19] While pneumothoraces or haemothoraces too small to be seen on plain CXR are readily detected by the CT the clinical significance of such subtle findings remains unclear. However, most Australian trauma centres do not have CT facilities co-located in the ED, thus requiring patients to be some distance away. The dedicated trauma bay is a relatively controlled and safe environment for a seriously injured patient. During transport, transfer and time in the CT suite the ability of the trauma team to respond to acute deterioration in the patient's condition is limited by both space and resources.

While haemodynamic instability is an absolute contra-indication to moving a patient to the CT scanner, the concept of 'metastability' has been described. This term was coined to describe patients who have evidence of ongoing volume loss that can be controlled with higher than normal volume infusion of crystalloid and/or blood products.[20] It is possible to maintain a certain level of stability, even if the haemodynamic parameters are not normal. With modern multidetector computed tomography (MDCT) scanners being able to perform 'pan scans' in minutes, important information can be achieved in the metastable patient that may assist in planning the management course and appropriate interventions (Table 47.2).

In the assessment of thoracic aortic trauma, MDCT spiral technology with three-dimensional reconstruction has allowed CT scanning to catch up to angiography in terms of image quality; 64- or 256-slice scanners can image with submillimetre-section thicknesses and an image matrix rivalling Digital Subtraction Angiography (DSA). CT scanning is ideal for evaluating the non-arterial injuries in patients with polytrauma, such as patients with brain, spinal, pelvic, spleen, liver and/or kidney injuries. A single intravenous administration of contrast material can be used for a combined vascular and nonvascular evaluation. Thus MDCT scanning may eventually become the new criterion standard, especially in the detection of blunt thoracic aortic disruptions (Fig 47.3), and in the evaluation of stable patients with gunshot wounds traversing the mediastinum where such scanning has been shown to be not only faster, but also just as sensitive and specific as contrast aortography.[21,22]

Angiography

Historically, biplanar DSA has been considered the gold standard in the diagnosis of vascular injuries in stable patients,

TABLE 47.2 Use of computed tomography as a diagnostic tool in thoracic trauma

MECHANISM	CLINICAL SCENARIO	UTILITY
Penetrating	Mediastinal missile traverse	Evaluate integrity of mediastinal vascular and aerodigestive structures
Blunt	'Abnormal' mediastinum on CXR	Indicate presence of mediastinal haematoma/thoracic aortic disruption
Blunt	Suspected diaphragmatic tear (elevated diaphragm or viscera overlying lower lungs fields on CXR)	Diagnose ruptured diaphragm
Blunt or penetrating	Persistent thoracic opacification on CXR	Differentiation between undrained/clotted haemothorax, lung contusion, atelectasis and lung consolidation

CXR: chest X-ray

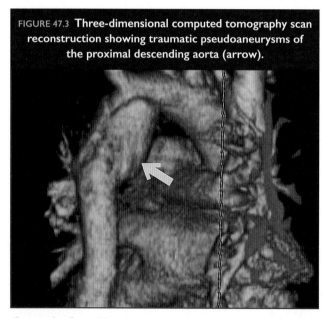

FIGURE 47.3 **Three-dimensional computed tomography scan reconstruction showing traumatic pseudoaneurysms of the proximal descending aorta (arrow).**

Courtesy Dr Caesar Ursic.

and was for some time the only modality available to accurately delineate blunt and penetrating injuries to the thoracic aorta and its branches. However, as described above, significant improvements have occurred in CT technology over the last two decades, with MDCT scanners now producing superb images of the vascular tree in three dimensions and at sub-millimetre resolutions rivalling those derived from angiography. As MDCT resolution continues to improve, its non-invasive nature and ability to assess other injuries in the polytrauma patient are likely to convert those vascular surgeons who still routinely require angiography to confirm thoracic vascular injuries, and to decide between operative or endoluminal repair.

Magnetic resonance imaging

There is as yet no convincing evidence to support the use of magnetic resonance imaging (MRI) in the evaluation of the patient with acute thoracic trauma. The MRI scanner is usually not easily or rapidly accessible and requires considerable patient preparation prior to use, making it an inconvenient and danger-ous destination for the newly injured patient. Additionally, the

more widely available CT scan provides sufficiently detailed images of the thorax to make the use of MRI's slightly greater resolution of negligible value in these patients.

Fractures of the bony thorax

Managing patients with significant blunt chest wall trauma requires adequate and effective analgesia coupled with physio-therapy to permit clearance of secretions. Failure to combine these approaches increases the risk of the patient developing severe pulmonary dysfunction which may progress to pneumonia and respiratory failure. Adequate oxygen therapy, to prevent hypoxia, assists in reducing the work of breathing, thus minimising the risk of fatigue.[23]

Rib fractures and pulmonary contusion

Rib fractures are the most common sequelae of blunt thoracic trauma, and may also follow some penetrating injuries. They cause severe pain, which results in decreased inspiratory effort and ineffective cough. Failure to clear respiratory secretions, with occlusion of small airways, contributes to a further decline in pulmonary function. If analgesia is inadequate, this can lead to alveolar collapse and consolidation. The presence of rib fracture in more than one anatomical region doubles the incidence of respiratory failure.[24] If the decline in pulmonary function is not reversed, then pneumonia and respiratory failure may supervene with the need for mechanical ventilation in severe cases. In patients with pre-existing pulmonary disease, or in the elderly, this may prove fatal.[25–27] Fractured ribs may result in haemothorax, most commonly as a result of damage to intercostal arteries which lie along the inferior border of each rib. Furthermore, the sharp edges of fractured ribs can lacerate the adjacent lung parenchyma, potentially causing both pneumothorax and haemothorax. It should be remembered that rib fractures imply the transfer of a significant amount of energy to the thoracic cage, and that the underlying lung suffers injury as a result.

Pulmonary contusion associated with multiple rib fractures may lead to delayed-onset respiratory failure. The three components of pulmonary contusions are oedema, atelectasis and haemorrhage into the pulmonary interstitium and alveoli. The ensuing mismatch in pulmonary ventilation/perfusion leads to hypoxaemia (Fig 47.4). Pulmonary contusions often do not manifest early on, so the presence of one or more rib fractures

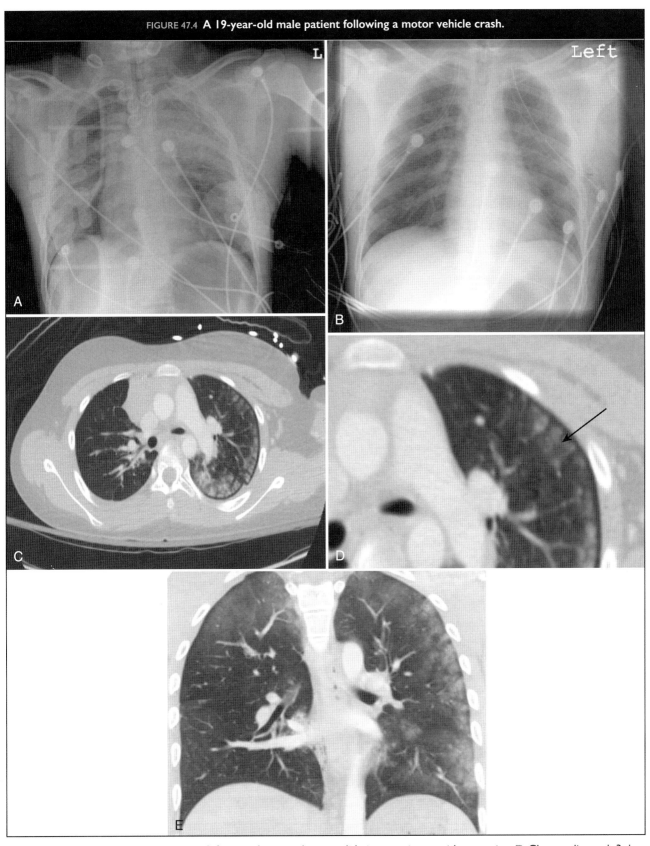

FIGURE 47.4 **A 19-year-old male patient following a motor vehicle crash.**

A, Initial chest radiograph demonstrates left upper lung patchy consolidation consistent with contusion. **B,** Chest radiograph 3 days later demonstrates rapid resolution of pulmonary contusion. **C,** Axial section through a CT scan demonstrates left-sided contusion affecting both the upper and the lower lobes, not confined to a single lobe. **D,** There is sparing of 1–2 mm of subpleural space (arrow). **E,** Coronal image demonstrates extent of lung contusion.[28]

in a recently injured patient must lead to early prediction and management with adequate analgesia, chest physiotherapy and supplemental oxygen. There is an almost linear relationship between the number of ribs fractured in any given patient and patient mortality.[29–31] Furthermore, where pulmonary contusions are present on initial scanning, this indicates that the patient has sustained severe thoracic trauma and they are at risk of rapid deterioration in their respiratory status.

Assessment

Any patient complaining of pain and tenderness over one or more ribs after a blunt injury to the chest should be considered to have at least one fractured rib, regardless of X-ray finding. Crepitus may be present, and if lung parenchymal or tracheobronchial tree injury has occurred, subcutaneous emphysema may be palpated. This results from entrapment in the muscles and subcutaneous tissues of air under pressure that has escaped from lacerated lung pleura.

It has been reported that screening CXRs miss rib fractures more than 50% of the time.[24] Treatment of the patient suspected of having fractured ribs should not be delayed pending radiological confirmation (Fig 47.5). Dedicated rib views, i.e. X-rays taken at various oblique angles, are more sensitive in detecting fractured ribs, but they rarely change the management of the patient and therefore should be discouraged.[32] Finally, these fractures may be seen incidentally on chest CT scans, but CT performed purely to diagnose rib fractures in the absence of other indications is a costly and unnecessary investigation. In most cases, the diagnosis of rib fractures should be a clinical one based on the history and physical examination of the patient. Should CXR reveal fracture of the first or second ribs, careful examination of the ipsilateral arm should include assessment of neurovascular status due to the close proximity of major neural and vascular structures, such as the brachial plexus and subclavian artery and vein.

Management

The mainstay of treatment for fractured ribs is adequate analgesia permitting effective inspiratory effort and coughing.

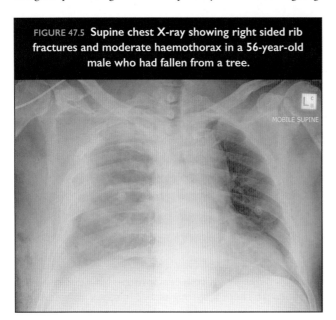

FIGURE 47.5 Supine chest X-ray showing right sided rib fractures and moderate haemothorax in a 56-year-old male who had fallen from a tree.

Courtesy Radiology Department, St George Hospital, Sydney.

Supplemental oxygen should be administered where required. In patients with multiple rib fractures, and especially in the elderly, inpatient admission will be necessary to allow for administration of parenteral narcotics and close monitoring of respiratory function. Pain team review should be obtained since invasive techniques for analgesia delivery may be required. Thoracic epidurals have been shown to be superior to simple narcotic administration, but are time-consuming to establish and may be associated with complications.[33–35] If the location of the rib fractures is high in the thorax the use of epidural anaesthesia can result in severe haemodynamic compromise. For unilateral rib fractures paravertebral block may be useful using a catheter infusion of local anaesthetic.[120] Intercostal nerve blocks afford satisfactory analgesia, but the effect is short-lived, so that the procedure must be repeated frequently, making it impractical in most cases.[121] The advantage of analgesia using local anaesthetic is it is narcotic sparing, which is particularly important in the elderly or patients with renal impairment.

Aggressive chest physiotherapy with encouragement of deep breathing and coughing is essential, and incentive spirometry provides a visual scale of respiratory effort and is useful for monitoring progress. If respiratory fatigue occurs with progressive hypoxaemia or hypercarbia, then the use of non-invasive ventilatory assistance, such as continuous positive airway pressure (CPAP) or bi-level positive airway pressure (BiPAP), may prove beneficial in conjunction with adequate analgesia. More recently, high-flow nasal prong (HFNP) delivery of humidified, high concentrations of oxygen is being used prophylactically in this group of patients.[36] This has the added benefit of providing a small amount of positive end-expiratory pressure (PEEP), which not only prevents collapse by 'splinting' the alveoli (when the patient keeps their mouth closed), but may also recruit new alveoli, thus resulting in improved gas exchange. The benefits of this approach are that humidification of secretions facilitates clearance, the mechanical splinting of the alveoli reduces the work of breathing, thereby decreasing the risk of respiratory fatigue, and patient comfort is increased since they are able to talk, thus increasing compliance.

In certain cases of severe blunt thoracic trauma the above multidisciplinary approach fails and respiratory failure appears imminent. The nurse caring for these patients must be alert to the warning signs: worsening tachypnoea, use of accessory muscles and inability to complete a sentence in one breath. Do not wait for changes in oxygen saturation before calling for assistance as this is an unreliable indicator of hypoxaemia. These patients will require intubation (see Ch 17, p. 318) and mechanical ventilation until pulmonary contusions abate, respiratory mechanics improve and pain control is optimised. Signs of pneumonia, such as fever, purulent sputum and progressive changes on chest X-ray, should be treated with appropriate intravenous antibiotics. Finally, the patient should be cautioned that rib fractures can and do cause pain for many weeks, if not months.

PRACTICE TIP

To assess the effectiveness of analgesia in the patient with rib fractures, ask them to take a deep breath and cough. It is essential that they are able to do so.

Sternal fractures

Fractures of the sternum occur almost exclusively as a result of direct blows to the anterior chest. This can occur as a result of an MVC where the driver strikes the steering wheel when airbags are not employed, following a fall from height or as a result of interpersonal violence. Sternal fractures are among the most painful of the thoracic-wall injuries and in 10% of cases are associated with multiple rib fractures and lung contusions. They may also be a predictor of blunt cardiac injury.[37–39] While they are not intrinsically life-threatening, the painful nature of these fractures may lead to significant short-term disability with reduced respiratory effort. As with rib fractures, this in turn can soon progress to pulmonary atelectasis, bacterial pneumonia and respiratory failure, unless early and adequate analgesia is ensured.

Assessment

Patients with sternal fractures complain of severe pain and tenderness over the central chest wall. Palpation may reveal an irregularity of the fracture site if significant displacement and overlap of the bone ends has occurred, and crepitus may be felt on palpation and during deep inspiration and expiration. Displaced fractures may be visible on the anteroposterior (AP) CXR and fracture lines will be visible on chest CT scan. There is little need for a dedicated lateral sternal view since this will rarely influence management if a clinical suspicion of sternal fracture exists (Fig 47.6).

Management

Treatment of sternal fracture follows the same pathway as that for rib fractures. Hospital admission may be required to

FIGURE 47.6

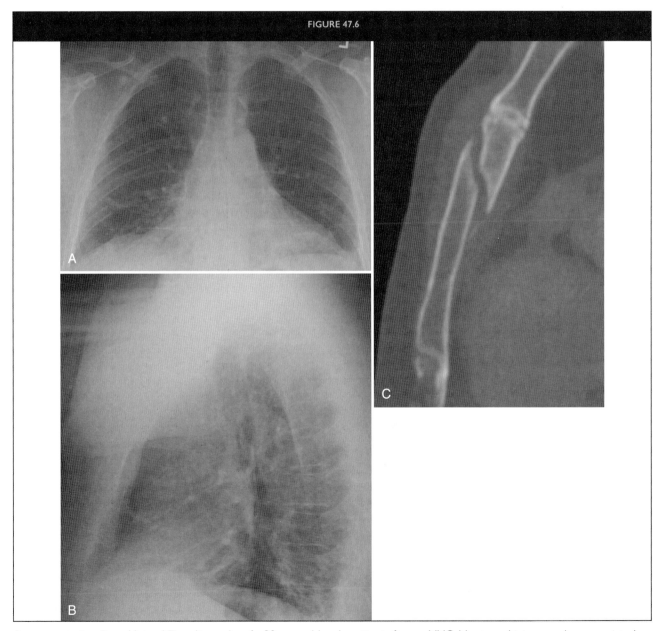

Anteroposterior **A**, and lateral **B**, radiographs of a 32-year-old male patient after an MVC. No sternal injury can be appreciated on these images. **C**, Sagittal reconstructed images through the sternum clearly show the minimally displaced sternal fracture that was not seen on plain radiographs.[28]

establish an effective analgesic regimen and to ensure that the patient has adequate respiratory function prior to discharge. Weaning to oral analgesics, narcotics or other regimens may proceed once pain control is deemed adequate and the patient is able to maintain adequate inspiratory effort and clear secretions. As above, monitoring for the early signs and symptoms of respiratory failure is essential to allow for timely intervention. In rare circumstances, the fracture segments will require surgical stabilisation if they fail to fuse over the ensuing months or if they override each other to such an extent that they produce significant cosmetic deformity.[40]

Clavicular fractures

Fractures of the clavicle are common after blunt thoracic trauma. The usual site of injury is at the junction of the middle and proximal third of this S-shaped bone. Although the fracture itself is neither life- nor limb-threatening, its presence should alert the clinician that a considerable amount of force has been applied to the chest and that underlying thoracic injuries may be present.

Assessment

Patients with fractured clavicles generally complain of localised pain and tenderness over the fracture site which is aggravated by motion of the ipsilateral shoulder joint, and deformity or bruising of the soft tissues overlying the fracture may be noted. The standard AP CXR is very sensitive in demonstrating these fractures (Fig 47.7), even though the diagnosis will be apparent clinically in patients who can cooperate with the physical examination.

A careful vascular examination of the arm is important in order to detect injury to vascular structures since injury of the subclavian artery by the sharp bony ends of the clavicle may occur. Absent or diminished distal pulses may indicate vascular thrombosis or occlusion by an intimal flap; a pulsatile mass, palpable thrill or audible bruit in the supraclavicular fossa may signal an underlying traumatic arteriovenous fistula. Furthermore, neurological examination is essential to detect injury to the brachial plexus.

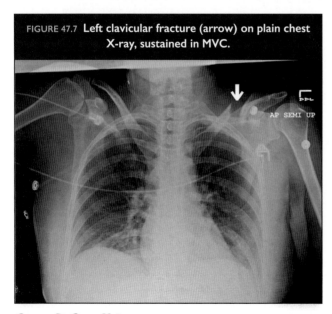

FIGURE 47.7 **Left clavicular fracture (arrow) on plain chest X-ray, sustained in MVC.**

Courtesy Dr Caesar Ursic.

Management

The vast majority of clavicular fractures are treated non-operatively with oral analgesics. A sling to support the arm for a few weeks serves to decrease motion at the fracture site and can help diminish discomfort. Surgical fixation is generally only required for the treatment of open or compound fractures, while delayed operation may be indicated for fractures that fail to heal (non-union) after several months. Occasionally, fractures that are cosmetically unacceptable due to extreme displacement and overlapping of the two fracture segment ends may require surgical intervention for correction.[41,42] Acute vascular injuries will also require urgent intervention when present.

Scapular fractures

The scapula, one of the thickest bones of the human body, is not easily fractured. When fractures do occur, they indicate that great force has been transferred to the upper torso. Thus a high index of suspicion should exist regarding the presence of underlying thoracic injury, notably pulmonary contusion. Rarely, scapulothoracic dissociation may result with severe and sometimes life-threatening consequences.

Assessment

These fractures manifest clinically with significant pain of the shoulder region, tenderness on palpation of the posterior shoulder, limited range of shoulder motion (due to pain) and occasional overlying soft-tissue haematomas and bruises. They are often visible on the plain CXR (Fig 47.8A), but the full extent of the fracture, including any involvement of the glenohumeral joint, is best seen on CT scan (Fig 47.8B). Distal radial and ulnar pulses should be documented. If there is suspicion of vascular injury, angiography should be considered.

As mentioned above, a serious variant of the scapular fracture is the scapulothoracic dissociation, which includes separation of the scapular articulation from the thoracic wall and is accompanied by frequent injury to the brachial plexus and the underlying axillary or proximal brachial artery.[43] These patients present with abnormal vascular, motor and sensory examinations of the involved extremity, and may have massive haemorrhage in and around the shoulder joint which can become life-threatening. If scapulothoracic dissociation is suspected based on the clinical examination, an emergency arteriogram of the involved upper extremity is indicated to diagnose vascular injuries and stage their surgical repairs.

Management

The majority of scapular fractures will not require operative intervention and can be treated with analgesics and temporary shoulder immobilisation with an arm sling to allow the fracture to stabilise. Only fractures involving the glenohumeral joint which are significantly displaced will benefit from open reduction and stabilisation, and this procedure may be delayed for several days until the patient's overall condition improves. Scapulothoracic dissociation, on the other hand, almost always requires some form of immediate surgical procedure; this usually being the repair of a torn or thrombosed axillary or brachial artery.

Flail chest and pulmonary contusion

The term 'flail chest' refers to a clinical condition resulting from the segmental fracture of two or more adjacent ribs in

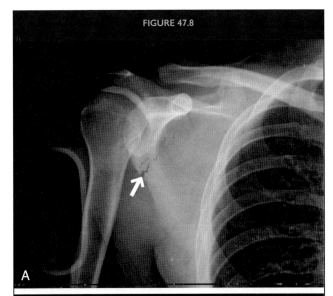

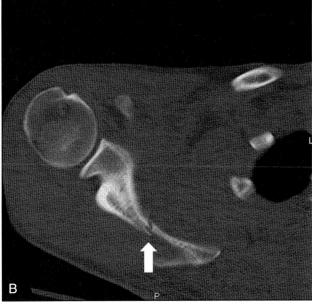

A, Scapular fracture, plain X-ray. **B**, Right scapular fracture, CT scan (glenoid joint is not involved).
Courtesy Dr Caesar Ursic.

two or more places, with associated chest-wall deformation (Fig 47.9). Costochondral joint disruptions associated with rib fractures can also lead to a flail segment. Flail chest results from severe blunt chest trauma, and flail segment of chest wall (Fig 47.10) is no longer mechanically attached to the relatively rigid surrounding bony rib cage. This segment is therefore uncoupled from the mechanical forces that move the chest wall during the breathing cycle. This is not itself dangerous, but is an indicator of severe underlying pulmonary contusion that is present as a result of the original trauma to the chest wall.[45–47]

As discussed above, the pain associated with the rib fractures contributes to poor inspiratory effort, and if an aggressive regimen of analgesia and physiotherapy is not instigated, significant deterioration in respiratory function may result, requiring intubation and mechanical ventilation (see Ch 17, p. 318, for intubation techniques).

FIGURE 47.9 X-ray showing a right-sided flail chest with significant displacement in a 68-year-old female pedestrian hit by a car.

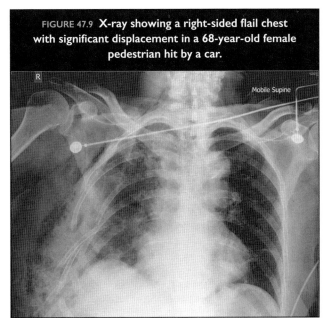

Courtesy Radiology Department, St George Hospital, Sydney.

Assessment

Paradoxical motion of the flail segment may be seen, with the rib segments rising in expiration and falling during inspiration, distinct from the remaining chest wall. This movement of the chest wall is pathognomonic of flail chest (Fig 47.10B). Alternatively, the diagnosis may be a radiographical one if fractures can be seen occurring in two or more places on two or more adjacent ribs.

Pulmonary contusion after blunt chest wall injury can be deduced from progressively increasing respiratory distress and oxygen requirements in a patient with radiographical signs of lung opacification or consolidation. Although it may initially appear normal, the plain CXR soon shows areas of consolidation or opacification corresponding to the underlying contusion. So-called air bronchograms may be evident, where the bronchi are seen as distinctly black 'tubes' or cross-sections surrounded by the dense whiteness of collapsed/consolidated lung tissue. The CT scan is much more sensitive and will demonstrate these changes earlier than will the CXR, usually within the first 6 hours.

PRACTICE TIP

In the patient with multiple rib and scapula fractures, high energy has been transmitted to the thorax. Have a high index of suspicion for lung contusions in these patients, which may not be evident on initial chest X-ray/ computed tomography.

Management

Treatment of the patient with a flail chest will be similar to that of a patient with multiple rib fractures, and will depend on the presence and severity of the underlying pulmonary contusion.[48] Therapy consists of the administration of supplemental oxygen when required, provision of analgesia and aggressive physiotherapy to maintain adequate inspiratory effort and thus

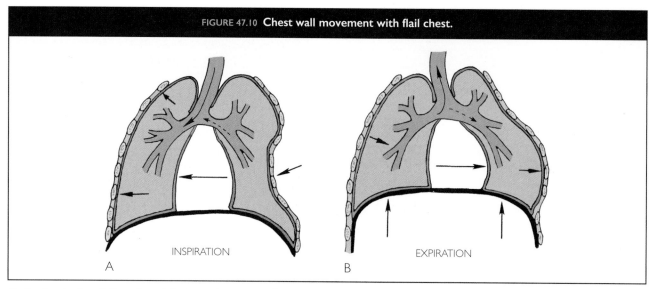

FIGURE 47.10 **Chest wall movement with flail chest.**

A   B

INSPIRATION   EXPIRATION

A, On inspiration flail section sinks in as chest expands, impairing ability to produce negative intrapleural pressure to draw in air. Mediastinum shifts to uninjured side. **B,** On expiration flail segment bulges outwards, impairing ability to exhale. Mediastinum shifts to injured side. Air may shift uselessly from side to side in severe flail chest (broken lines).[44]

minimise retention of airway secretions. This will reduce the probability of respiratory failure or pneumonia.

Patients with multiple rib fractures with flail chest and pulmonary contusions may require endotracheal intubation during the initial days of admission to permit 'splinting' both of the alveoli and of the flail chest wall segment. In addition, if the nurse is concerned by signs of respiratory deterioration in a patient with multiple rib fractures, such as progressive tachypnoea and fatigue, then it is essential that medical review is arranged in a timely manner since these patients often require a period of mechanical ventilation as a prophylactic measure against the development of respiratory failure.

Antibiotics, steroids, diuretics and other anti-inflammatory agents have not been shown to alter the course of pulmonary contusions, which are generally self-limiting and usually resolve gradually over a period of days to weeks. In severe cases, surgical fixation of the segmented ribs has been performed with success, with reports that patients have improved long-term lung function.[49]

Pneumothoraces

When a mechanical breach to the pleural surface occurs after a penetrating or blunt injury, the pleural space may fill with air, blood, or both; forming, respectively, a pneumothorax, haemothorax or haemopneumothorax.

Simple closed pneumothorax

Following blunt trauma, a pneumothorax may result from lacerations to the visceral pleura from the sharp edges of fractured ribs. Penetrating injuries may produce a pneumothorax due to direct pleural laceration, with air entering the thoracic cavity via the chest wall or the lacerated lung (Fig 47.11). If air entry is self-limited, or if air can exit the thoracic space at the same rate at which it enters, this results in a simple pneumothorax.

Assessment

Simple pneumothorax may not produce significant respiratory or haemodynamic instability. In fact, the diagnosis may not be

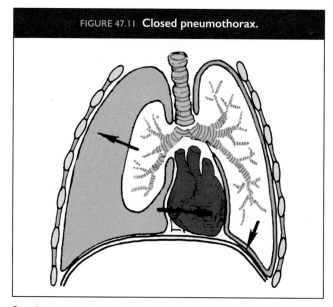

FIGURE 47.11 **Closed pneumothorax.**

Simple pneumothorax is present in right lung with air in pleural cavity and collapse of right lung.[44]

made until the initial CXR is reviewed. In haemodynamically stable patients, the chest wall should be inspected for evidence of blunt or penetrating trauma, which may be subtle. The history of the trauma will provide evidence on which to base the diagnosis; this may subsequently be confirmed on CXR (Fig 47.12). Palpation may reveal not only the tenderness associated with rib fractures, but subcutaneous emphysema from air that has escaped via breaches in the pleura. The presence or absence of breath sounds should be noted on auscultation.

Supine CXR will demonstrate the darker radiolucency of air between the chest wall and lung surface which will be evident in the majority of clinically significant simple pneumothoraces. The edge of the lung, not usually visible when the lung is fully expanded, may be clearly delineated. MDCT is

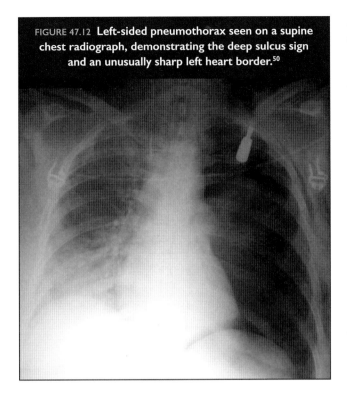

FIGURE 47.12 **Left-sided pneumothorax seen on a supine chest radiograph, demonstrating the deep sulcus sign and an unusually sharp left heart border.**[50]

much more sensitive than CXR and can detect the smallest of pneumothoraces.

Management

In the presence of a simple pneumothorax and signs of respiratory distress, or in patients likely to require positive pressure ventilation, an intercostal catheter should be inserted. Previously assembled kits should be available in the trauma bay along with several sizes of tube. The trauma nurse should know the location of these kits and how to assist with the procedure. There are various techniques for the proper placement of an

intercostal catheter (ICC),[51] but they all have in common several features, as described in Table 47.3.

The thoracostomy tube is usually inserted via the 4th or 5th intercostal space at the mid-axillary line. The largest appropriate tube for the patient's body habitus should be used, typically 32-French or larger in women, 36-French or larger in men.[52] After connecting the tube to an underwater-seal collection bottle, a confirmatory CXR should be performed to document adequate tube placement within the chest. Some clinicians prefer that low continuous suction (3–4 kPa) is applied to the underwater-seal drain (UWSD), so nursing staff should discuss this with the admitting team. See Chapter 17, p. 332, for information on applying a UWSD.

In the vast majority of patients with a simple pneumothorax, tube thoracostomy will be sufficient treatment, and can usually be removed in 1–2 days when the lung is fully inflated on follow-up CXR. A minority will continue to exhibit collapse of the lung on subsequent CXR or persistent air leak as demonstrated by continued bubbling in the drain. These patients will need placement of a second tube to fully re-expand the lung. An even smaller group of patients will require cardiothoracic surgical review for either a formal thoracostomy or a video-assisted thoracoscopic surgery (VATS) procedure to treat a persistent air leak or lung collapse.

Tension pneumothorax

A tension pneumothorax (Fig 47.13) is a less common but much more dangerous variant of the simple pneumothorax, and occurs when air from a laceration in the lung tissue or via an open chest wall injury enters the interpleural space with each breath but cannot escape.[53] The progressive increase in volume of trapped air will compress the adjacent lung, limiting its expansion and leading initially to respiratory distress and hypoxaemia. As the intrathoracic pressure continues to increase, the mediastinal structures, including the venae cavae, the trachea and the heart, are also compressed, and displaced away from the affected

TABLE 47.3 Process for insertion of intercostal catheter	
PATIENT PREPARATION	Mechanical restraint of upper extremities (ipsilateral arm placed behind head whenever possible)
	Wide skin prepping and draping of chest wall with topical antibacterial solution (e.g. povidone–iodine) and sterile towels/drapes
	Minimum of one large-bore intravenous cannula
	Continuous SpO$_2$, blood pressure and cardiac rhythm monitoring
DRUGS	Supplemental oxygen
	1% lignocaine for local anaesthesia
	Parenteral narcotic analgesia and short-acting sedative
	Single dose of prophylactic parenteral antibiotics prior to skin incision should be considered (first-generation cephalosporin, or clindamycin if penicillin-allergic)
EQUIPMENT	Low wall suction
	Closed thoracic drain reservoir device (pre-assembled)
RADIOLOGY	Confirmatory chest X-ray soon after procedure completed

SpO$_2$: partial oxygen saturation pressure

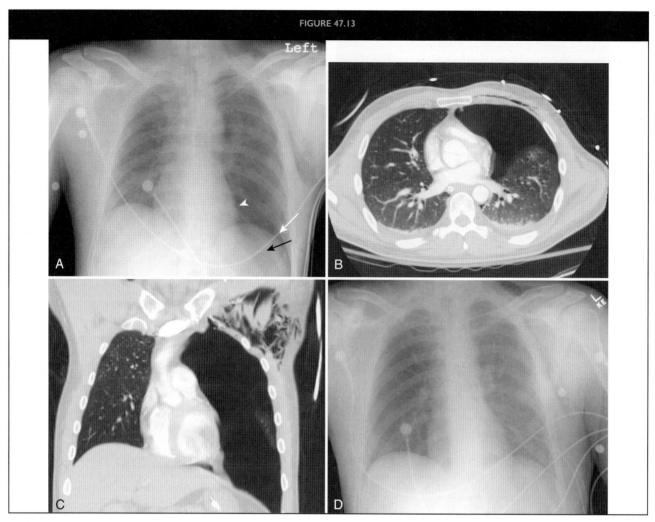

FIGURE 47.13

A, Anteroposterior chest radiograph findings of tension pneumothorax, including the 'deep sulcus' sign (black arrow), sharply outlined cardiac and diaphragmatic border (arrowhead) and depression of the hemidiaphragm (white arrow). Note rightward deviation of the mediastinum consistent with tension. **B**, Axial image from multidetector computed tomography (MDCT) demonstrates air collecting non-dependently in the anterior costophrenic sulcus. Note rightward deviation of the heart, indicating developing tension. **C**, Coronal image demonstrates depression of the hemidiaphragm and rightward deviation of the mediastinum. **D**, Chest-tube placement results in normal positioning of the hemidiaphragm and mediastinum.[28]

side. This results in markedly decreased venous return to the heart with a drop in cardiac preload. The end result is severely compromised cardiac output, which may rapidly progress to cardiogenic shock and eventual cardiac arrest.

Assessment

As previously described, the diagnosis of a tension pneumothorax is a clinical one, not a radiographic one. It is an oft-quoted aphorism that CXR of a tension pneumothorax should never exist. The hallmarks of the condition are the presence of shock and unilaterally absent breath sounds in a patient with clinical or historical evidence of thoracic trauma. The condition may be seen after both blunt and penetrating injury mechanisms, and the patient may present gasping for breath, and may be anxious or even combative due to hypoxia and early shock. A rapid primary survey usually discloses absent or diminished breath sounds on the affected side of the chest and may also reveal signs of chest-wall injury, such as a penetrating wound, bruising and severe tenderness, subcutaneous emphysema or rib fractures. The trachea may be deviated away from the midline

towards the uninjured side. However, this can be an unreliable clinical finding which may only be noted on medical imaging. Distension of jugular veins in the neck may be observed as a result of increased intrathoracic pressures diminishing venous return, but this sign is also unreliable and may be absent in a patient with associated haemorrhagic shock from other injuries. In a patient with early tension pneumothorax without profound shock, where the radiographer responds rapidly to a trauma call, a CXR may in fact be taken which will show complete or almost complete collapse of the affected lung, and shift of the mediastinum away from the lung collapse, dragging the trachea towards the unaffected side.

Management

Urgent decompression of the raised intrathoracic pressure is needed. In the ED in experienced hands, an emergency chest tube is the most appropriate measure unless the patient is in established cardiogenic shock. Then the management is the same as that in the pre-hospital setting. A large-bore (> 16 gauge) cannula should be inserted into the chest via the second intercostal space in the midclavicular line on the affected side.[54,55] This will usually allow sufficient release of the trapped air to permit some increase in cardiac venous return and thereby improve cardiac output. Needle thoracostomy is only a temporary intervention to convert the tension pneumothorax into a simple pneumothorax. The narrow diameter of the cannula imparts resistance to the outflow of the trapped air. In addition, the cannula length must be sufficient to penetrate all layers of the chest wall and enter the interpleural space. A cannula length of at least 4.5 cm is recommended.[56] As soon as practicable, or at the sign of any increase in respiratory distress or circulatory shock, a tube thoracostomy should be placed on the affected side. There is frequently an associated haemothorax, thus a tube of sufficient size should be placed (Fig 47.14).

In the pre-hospital setting, a patient with a tension pneumothorax may not respond to needle thoracostomy, or may deteriorate en route to the trauma centre. Under these circumstances insert another large-bore cannula on the affected side, as the first may be blocked or dislodged. Should this manoeuvre fail then, for appropriately trained personnel, finger thoracostomy may be performed.

An incision is made in the 5th intercostal space, anterior axillary line on the affected side and is deepened through subcutaneous tissue down to muscle. Then using a blunt artery clip or a finger, the pleural cavity is entered. A hiss of air may confirm the position of the finger. The wound is left open and the trapped air leaking from the injured lung tissue escapes through the opening. This is a rapid procedure more suited to the confinement of a moving ambulance or retrieval aircraft than formal chest tube insertion. Once the patient arrives at the trauma centre an intercostal catheter is placed under sterile conditions, but not through the same wound. Bilateral finger thoracostomies may be lifesaving in the field for some patients with massive blunt chest injury.

Occasionally, a patient presenting in extremis with a tension pneumothorax will fail to improve after insertion of

one or more chest drains, remaining tachypnoeic, hypoxaemic and shocked. The chest radiograph will show a persistent lung collapse and there will be a large, continuous air leak. In these cases, serious consideration should be given to the presence of a major tracheobronchial injury (Figs 47.15A and B).[57] This condition will require fibre-optic bronchoscopy for diagnosis and a prompt thoracotomy for direct surgical repair.

Haemothorax

A collection of blood within the interpleural space is termed a haemothorax, and may arise from bleeding from the ends of fractured ribs, lacerated intercostal arteries or pulmonary parenchyma by sharp rib fragments or penetrating objects (knives, bullets, etc.), ruptured or lacerated intrathoracic blood vessels or (rarely) from haemorrhage from a cardiac chamber injury that is decompressing into the chest through a pericardial laceration. Figure 47.16 demonstrates bleeding sources for a haemothorax.

Assessment

A haemothorax should be presumed present in any patient who has diminished or absent breath sounds on auscultation. If the patient is stable and time allows, a confirmatory CXR showing partial or complete opacification of the affected side is diagnostic showing a typical meniscus of layered blood within the chest. This will not be evident on a supine CXR, but the involved thorax will appear hazy. If the volume of blood within the chest is very large (massive haemothorax) complete opacification of the thorax will be noted in comparison to the unaffected side (Fig 47.17). When the patient is in shock and the primary trauma survey does not clearly identify causes for the haemodynamic instability, treatment for haemothorax must proceed based on clinical signs alone without prior radiographical confirmation. The use of portable ultrasound (e-FAST) for rapid bedside confirmation of haemothorax is now routine in many centres.[17]

Management

After blunt injury, small haemothoraces seen on CXR in asymptomatic patients may be managed without drainage, and the patient admitted for observation. Deterioration in respiratory status or repeat CXR after 24–48 hours showing an increase in size of the haemothorax will indicate the need for intercostal catheter placement. However, many of these small blood collections will not increase in size, but will be slowly reabsorbed by the pleura spontaneously without the need for drainage. Larger haemothoraces and those in patients who are hypoxaemic or complaining of shortness of breath require chest tube insertion. If large collections of blood are not drained, the result may be the formation of a 'fibrothorax', which results when fibrin deposition develops in an organised haemothorax and coats both the parietal and the visceral pleural surfaces, trapping the lung. The lung is fixed in position by this adhesive process and is unable to fully expand. Persistent atelectasis of portions of the lung and reduced pulmonary function result from this process. This then compromises respiratory function, especially in individuals with pre-existing pulmonary disease, or in the elderly.[60]

After penetrating injury, most haemothoraces large enough to be seen on CXR should also be drained, since the undrained thoracic blood in these cases has, by definition,

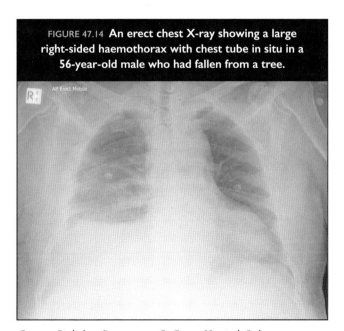

FIGURE 47.14 **An erect chest X-ray showing a large right-sided haemothorax with chest tube in situ in a 56-year-old male who had fallen from a tree.**

Courtesy Radiology Department, St George Hospital, Sydney.

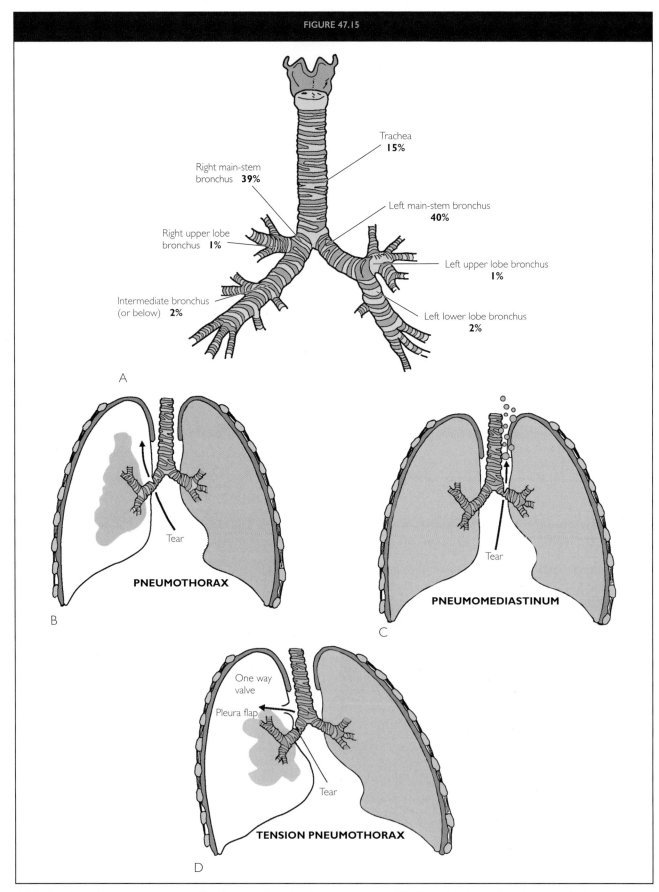

FIGURE 47.15

Trachea **15%**

Right main-stem bronchus **39%**

Left main-stem bronchus **40%**

Right upper lobe bronchus **1%**

Left upper lobe bronchus **1%**

Intermediate bronchus (or below) **2%**

Left lower lobe bronchus **2%**

A

Tear

PNEUMOTHORAX

B

Tear

PNEUMOMEDIASTINUM

C

One way valve

Pleura flap

Tear

TENSION PNEUMOTHORAX

D

A, Tracheobronchial ruptures: general localisations based on literature review[58,59] Complications of tracheobronchial tears: **B**, Pneumothorax[59] **C**, Pneumomediastinum[59] **D**, Progression of pneumothorax.[59]

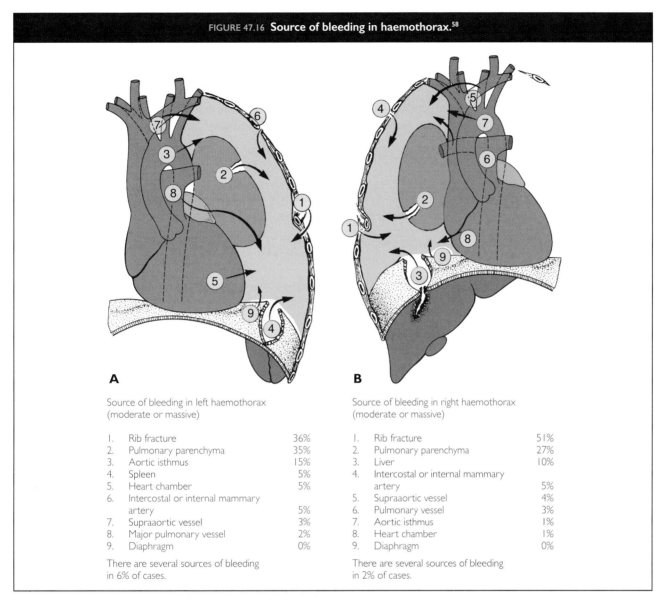

FIGURE 47.16 Source of bleeding in haemothorax.[58]

A

Source of bleeding in left haemothorax
(moderate or massive)

1.	Rib fracture	36%
2.	Pulmonary parenchyma	35%
3.	Aortic isthmus	15%
4.	Spleen	5%
5.	Heart chamber	5%
6.	Intercostal or internal mammary artery	5%
7.	Supraaortic vessel	3%
8.	Major pulmonary vessel	2%
9.	Diaphragm	0%

There are several sources of bleeding
in 6% of cases.

B

Source of bleeding in right haemothorax
(moderate or massive)

1.	Rib fracture	51%
2.	Pulmonary parenchyma	27%
3.	Liver	10%
4.	Intercostal or internal mammary artery	5%
5.	Supraaortic vessel	4%
6.	Pulmonary vessel	3%
7.	Aortic isthmus	1%
8.	Heart chamber	1%
9.	Diaphragm	0%

There are several sources of bleeding
in 2% of cases.

been contaminated by external bacteria and the patient will be at increased risk for the development of an empyema. Most studies recommend only a single pre-procedure dose of an intravenous antibiotic with Gram-positive antimicrobial coverage (e.g. cephazolin), since continued antibiotic administration has not been shown to significantly reduce the incidence of wound infections or empyema in these patients.

In approximately 85% of patients presenting with a haemothorax, no further intervention beyond the tube thoracostomy will be required. However, in a minority, especially following penetrating injury, there will be persistent and ongoing bleeding that will require surgical intervention. The American College of Surgeons Committee on Trauma (ACS COT) via its Advanced Trauma Life Support course (ATLS [EMST in Australia and New Zealand]) advises that initial drainage of 1500 mL of blood or more on insertion of a chest tube will usually dictate the need for surgery in that patient. The nurse assisting with chest tube placement should make note of this initial volume and communicate it to the medical team. Furthermore, even in the absence of an initial large volume of blood drainage,

should the ongoing losses total more than 200 mL/hr over 4 or more hours, this is indicative of persistent haemorrhage which is likely to require surgical intervention to stop. It is crucial to monitor and record all output from the chest tube on a frequent and regular basis (see Ch 44).

Open pneumothorax

Sometimes referred to as a 'sucking chest wound', this is an infrequent but dramatic injury which involves full-thickness loss of chest wall-tissue leading to open and continuous external communication between outside atmospheric pressure and the thoracic cavity (Fig 47.18). In civilian centres it may be seen after close-range shotgun blast injuries, or following wounding by large, rapidly-moving sharp objects, such as watercraft propellers or industrial machinery. In the military setting, open chest wounds may result from blast injury or as a consequence of high-energy gunshot wounds. As a consequence of loss of the negative pressure within the thoracic cavity, the underlying lung completely collapses. If the lung itself has been lacerated there will be air leakage and associated haemorrhage. This leads

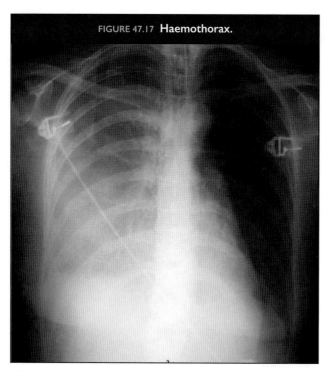

FIGURE 47.17 **Haemothorax.**

Chest radiograph of a 22-year-old female pedestrian hit by a bus. The hazy opacification within the right hemithorax is due to the presence of a large haemothorax caused by a ruptured intercostal artery.[50]

to profound respiratory distress, hypoxaemia and shock, and may progress rapidly to death if not treated.

Management

The communication between the thoracic cavity and atmospheric pressure must be closed to restore negative pressure. In the pre-hospital setting this can be accomplished in a variety of ways: by placing a gloved hand over the hole in order to prevent any further passage of air into/out of the chest; taping an occlusive plastic dressing over the hole or using a dressing designed to allow egress but not ingress of air to prevent tension

pneumothorax while also permitting drainage of any blood that accumulates in the chest cavity (Fig 47.19). If an occlusive taped dressing is used it should only be taped on three sides to allow air to escape during expiration minimising the risk of raised intrathoracic pressure and tension pneumothorax. Eventually a chest tube will be required to restore negative intrathoracic pressure which will re-expand the lung and drain any associated haemothorax. This must be placed through uninjured chest wall and never through the injury itself. For large chest-wall defects, surgical repair with musculocutaneous flaps may be required once the patient has stabilised.

Other thoracic injuries

Diaphragmatic injury

The diaphragm is a thin yet complex sheet of muscle and tendon that separates the abdominal and thoracic cavities, and it is critical to the mechanics of breathing. Its position varies with respect to respiration, rising as high as the 4th intercostal space on forced expiration, and moving as low as the inferior costal margins (T9) on deep inspiration. Diaphragmatic injury is very rare, especially in blunt trauma.[61]

Diaphragmatic rupture after blunt force trauma is more common on the left side because there is little or no liver in the left upper abdomen to absorb energy and thus protect the diaphragm from tearing. Penetrating diaphragmatic injuries occur at any point along the trajectory of the projectile or wounding weapon, and may result from penetration of the abdomen or thorax. Concomitant abdominal visceral injury is not uncommon, especially with gunshot wounds. The diaphragm is more vulnerable on the left again due to the protective bulk of the liver on the right. Injuries to the diaphragm, especially if the defect is small, may cause little clinical effect and may only be diagnosed if the patient needs laparotomy for intra-abdominal trauma.

Diagnosis

Blunt diaphragmatic injury may be suspected when the initial or subsequent CXR shows the presence of a high gastric bubble in the lower left chest (Fig 47.20), suggesting that the

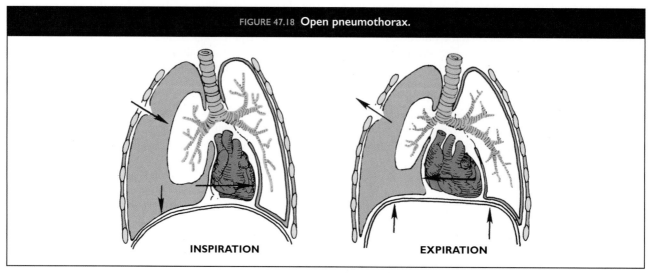

FIGURE 47.18 **Open pneumothorax.**

| INSPIRATION | EXPIRATION |

Collapse of right lung and air in pleural cavity occurs with communication to outside through defect in chest wall. In sucking chest wound, lung volume is greater with expiration.[44]

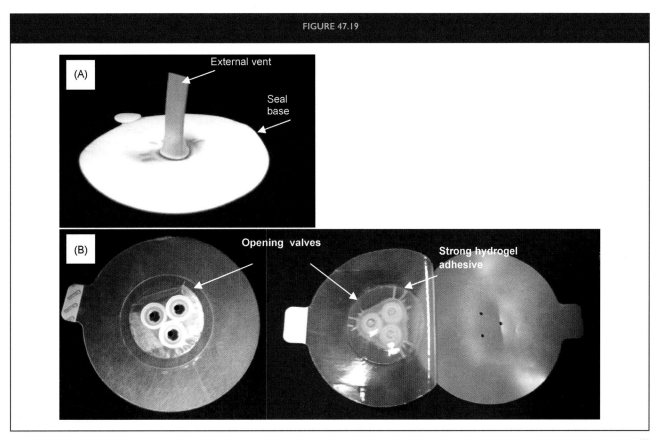

A, Asherman tube chest seal, B, Bolin 3-valve chest seal, both with a 15 cm diameter adhesive base—unopened and opened view.[123]

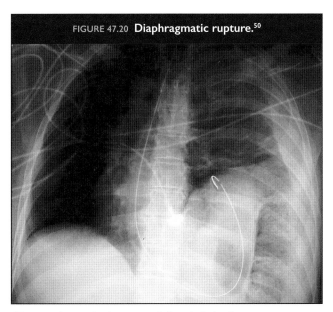

FIGURE 47.20 **Diaphragmatic rupture.**[50]

Chest radiograph showing a left-sided diaphragmatic rupture. Bowel can be seen herniating into the left hemithorax, the mediastinum is displaced to the right and there is a nasogastric tube seen coiled within an intrathoracic stomach.

stomach has herniated through the diaphragmatic defect. The pathognomonic radiographical sign is that of the nasogastric tube coiled in the left lower chest.[62] Occasionally, coils of small bowel or colon may be seen situated in the left thoracic cavity. If the injury is to the right diaphragm, assess the chest

radiograph for an abnormal 'hump' in the lateral diaphragm, which is suggestive of a large laceration of the diaphragm with protrusion of the liver.

Modern CT scanners are sensitive enough to detect often subtle diaphragmatic ruptures after blunt trauma,[62] but even in the absence of CT findings, if the patient has suffered significant blunt force trauma to the thoraco-abdominal area a high index of suspicion must exist that a diaphragmatic injury may have occurred. Additionally, in a retrospective review of registry patients Hammer and colleagues reported that there were specific MDCT signs for diaphragmatic injury that were different between blunt and penetrating injury.[63] The so-called dependent viscera sign, dangling diaphragm sign, the collar sign, elevated abdominal organs and visceral herniation were present only in blunt trauma. The presence of a wound tract traversing the diaphragm was seen virtually exclusively in penetrating trauma. Contiguous injury on both sides of the diaphragm was much more common in the penetrating group.[63] Patients may be asymptomatic, may complain of chest-wall pain due to the presence of associated rib fractures or may even be tachypnoeic and hypoxaemic if the amount of herniated viscera (stomach, colon, small bowel) in the thorax is large enough to compress the adjacent lung.[64] These patients may present in haemodynamic shock as a result of associated intra-abdominal injuries, but the effect of the herniated viscera in compressing the inferior vena cava and thus reducing cardiac preload must also be considered.

Injuries to the diaphragm may also be found at the time of exploratory laparotomy for penetrating trauma. Penetrating injury to the thoraco-abdominal region in an otherwise asymptomatic patient may best be assessed by diagnostic thoracoscopy or laparoscopy, at which time injury to the diaphragm can be detected and in some cases repaired.

Management

Diaphragmatic defects do not spontaneously close, regardless of the size, because of the negative pressure gradient between the thorax and the abdominal cavity caused by respirations. This tends to draw abdominal contents, such as omentum and/or viscera including bowel and stomach, through even small defects in the diaphragm, which subsequently enlarge. If undetected in the early period, non-specific abdominal complaints due to this intermittent herniation may be the subsequent presenting symptom, even well after discharge. Visceral obstruction and incarceration may occur, and visceral ischaemia due to compression of vascular supply by the narrow hernial orifice can result with subsequent bowel necrosis. When patients who have suffered severe blunt thoraco-abdominal injury are intubated and sedated for other injuries, the possibility of such a missed injury or delay in diagnosis may result in serious life-threatening consequences.

As mentioned above, small defects detected at laparoscopy may be repaired at the time. Larger defects are approached via a laparotomy, where care is needed to return the abdominal contents to the peritoneal cavity without causing further injury to the vascular supply. The defect is repaired using heavy non-absorbable sutures. Where there is significant loss of tissue then repair using synthetic or biological mesh may be required. It has previously been suggested that small, right-sided diaphragmatic injuries detected incidentally may be left since the liver protects against herniation of intra-abdominal contents. However, the same negative intrathoracic pressure which draws abdominal contents into the left thorax still acts on the right side. Indeed, there are reports in the literature of delayed herniation of the liver into the right hemi-thorax following right-sided diaphragmatic injury, which may present as a surgical emergency.[65,66] It is advisable that all diaphragmatic injuries are repaired at the time of their detection.

Cardiac injury

Cardiac injury may occur following blunt or penetrating trauma. In clinical series of closed blunt chest trauma, the incidence of cardiac damage, although difficult to determine, is reported to range between 8% and 76%.[67,68] This wide range is mainly due to the variation in diagnostic criteria used, and the fact that there is no gold standard test for this diagnosis. On the other hand, autopsy studies of patients who died after major blunt trauma revealed the incidence of cardiac contusion to range between 14% and 16%.[68] In Australasia, blunt trauma is more commonly seen because of a lower incidence of gun-related injury. High-speed MVCs in which the patient impacts the steering wheel or pre-tensioned seat belt account for the vast majority of cases, with pedestrians struck by vehicles, crush injuries and falls from great heights comprising the other groups of patients with blunt cardiac injury. A slow but steady increase in interpersonal violence in Australasia has seen a parallel rise in the incidence of penetrating cardiac injuries presenting to EDs.

Cardiac injuries can be obvious and catastrophic to patient outcome, but in other cases the injury may be more subtle, making diagnosis challenging. The majority of patients with severe cardiac injuries die at the scene.[69] Those who do survive to reach the hospital present in shock from acute pericardial tamponade, with severe heart failure from myocardial muscle or valve dysfunction, or suffering a wide variety of potentially fatal cardiac dysrhythmias.

Where cardiac damage is less obvious, the mechanism of injury, estimated energy transfer and clinical signs, such as bruising to the chest wall, must alert the treating team to the potential for cardiac injury.

Blunt cardiac injury

There is a wide spectrum of potential injuries to the heart after blunt chest trauma, including cardiac contusion, myocardial rupture, valvular disruptions and injury to the great vessels or the coronary arteries.

Myocardial contusion

Myocardial contusion is the most common injury to the heart after blunt trauma to the chest.[70] It is a well-defined entity with distinct pathological and biochemical abnormalities. However, its manifestation varies widely, making diagnosis and quantification of incidence challenging. In an autopsy study blunt cardiac injury was found to be the cause of death or a significant contributor in 5% of all blunt trauma victims. Although it has been compared to myocardial infarction, there are distinct differences between the two.[71] The position of the right ventricle behind the sternum makes it particularly vulnerable to contusion. Myocardial contusions span a spectrum ranging from asymptomatic and transient elevations of various cardiac enzymes to patchy necrosis and haemorrhage, acute pericardial effusions, isolated tears to the pericardium with the potential for cardiac herniation, malignant dysrhythmias and immediately fatal cardiac chamber ruptures (Table 47.4).

Myocardial rupture

Most patients with uncontained myocardial rupture do not reach the ED alive. Of those who do, hypotension may reduce pressure on the injured myocardium, which may then worsen as fluid resuscitation restores blood pressure. Pericardial tamponade, usually rare following blunt cardiac injury, then develops. In a minority of patients, rapid diagnosis by echo-cardiography or CT scan and operative intervention can be lifesaving. Less severe injuries to the ventricular wall may lead to delayed necrosis and manifest as delayed rupture within several days of admission.

Valvular damage

Disruption of cardiac valves is rare and may present with a spectrum of disorders from new cardiac murmurs to fulminant cardiac failure.

Dysrhythmia

Tachycardia in a trauma patient must always be presumed secondary to haemorrhage until proven otherwise. Only then in the setting of blunt chest trauma should persistent tachycardia, new bundle branch block or mild dysrhythmia raise suspicion of blunt cardiac injury.

TABLE 47.4 Blunt cardiac injury classification and manifestation

ANATOMY/PATHOPHYSIOLOGY OF BLUNT INJURY	CLINICAL MANIFESTATION
Free rupture of cardiac chamber into chest	Immediate death
Contained rupture (by intact pericardium) of cardiac chamber	Acute pericardial tamponade and cardiogenic shock
Rupture of cardiac valve leaflets or chordae tendineae	Acute or delayed valvular insufficiency
Tear of pericardium and cardiac herniation	Cardiogenic shock
Severe contusion of myocardium	Pump failure due to localised myocardial dyskinesis
Mild contusion of myocardium	Electrical conduction disturbances and possibly malignant dysrhythmias
Occlusion of coronary artery	Acute myocardial infarction

Blunt cardiac injury typically occurs in severely injured patients who have associated significant thoracic trauma, such as multiple rib fractures, pulmonary contusions and haemo-pneumothorax.[72] Often none of the clinical features described above manifest until a complication occurs, which can be quite sudden. The injured area of myocardium may then become a focus for dysrhythmias, occasionally resulting in cardiac arrest from ventricular tachycardia or fibrillation. Injury to the conducting system can cause heart block.[73,74] Injury to the myocardium can cause impaired heart contractility with reduced cardiac output, leading to cardiogenic shock and pulmonary oedema. As the pressure within the ventricles increases, a baroreceptor response is initiated to increase the heart rate and stroke volume in an attempt to increase cardiac output. Peripheral vasoconstriction shunts blood from the skin, gut and kidneys towards the brain, heart and lungs. The reduction in kidney blood flow precipitates water retention by way of antidiuretic hormone (ADH) and the renin–angiotensin–aldosterone system, further increasing the load on the heart.

Assessment

Any patient whose history includes a known or potential major transfer of energy to the anterior chest should be considered at high risk for blunt cardiac injury. Examples include sudden decelerations onto a vehicle steering wheel or dashboard, and falls from heights >3 m.[75] The most important test is the ECG. In haemodynamically stable patients, a normal ECG in the ED reliably identifies patients at low risk for cardiac complications who do not need any further cardiac investigations or ongoing cardiac monitoring (see Ch 17, p. 336).[68,72,74,76,77] Virtually any ECG abnormality may indicate cardiac contusion, such as sinus tachycardia, ectopic beats, ST segment deflections or T-wave changes.[74] All of these patients should be monitored

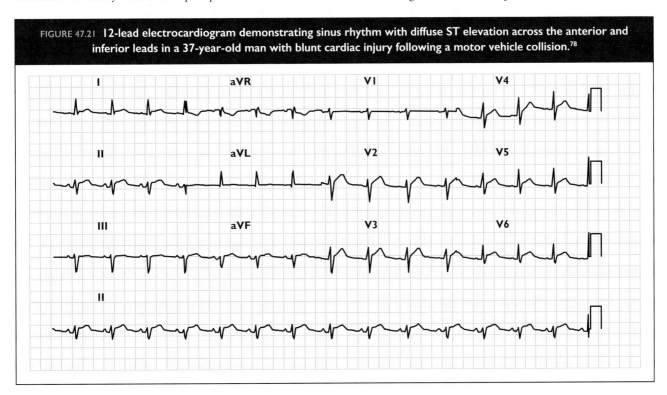

FIGURE 47.21   12-lead electrocardiogram demonstrating sinus rhythm with diffuse ST elevation across the anterior and inferior leads in a 37-year-old man with blunt cardiac injury following a motor vehicle collision.[78]

(Fig 47.21). FAST scan, now performed as an adjunct to primary survey, can assess the presence of pericardial effusion.

Adverse events generally occur within the first 24 hours,[79,80] although, very rarely, serious dysrhythmia may be delayed several days.[81] While elevation of serum troponin and wall motion abnormalities on echocardiography are also associated with adverse events, both of these tests lack adequate reliability for identifying patients who either need to be monitored for complications or can be safely left unmonitored.[74,82–85] If malignant dysrhythmias arise, such as ventricular tachycardia, fibrillation or heart block, they will require prompt pharmacological intervention or electric cardioversion.

Abnormal movement of the heart in response to dysrhythmias can depress cardiac ejection fraction and significantly reduce cardiac output (see Table 47.4). In addition to the ECG, the echocardiogram is very useful in determining both the presence of cardiac dysfunction and the possible aetiology, and should be obtained as soon as the diagnosis is entertained. The most frequent echocardiographic anomaly seen in unstable patients presenting with blunt cardiac injury is a localised or global dyskinesis of the heart chambers. Also seen are acute valvular insufficiencies due to tearing of the valve leaflets or adjacent supporting structures, ruptured interventricular septae and pericardial fluid collections indicating pericardial tamponade due to atrial or ventricular lacerations.

Management

Prehospital providers should manage any patient with potential blunt cardiac injury according to ATLS guidelines with particular focus on airway, breathing and circulation. Rapid transport to the nearest major trauma centre should occur.

In the ED the trauma nurse should ensure that oxygen is applied and that cardiac monitoring leads are in place (see Ch 17, p. 336). Patients with cardiac dysrhythmias who are haemodynamically stable and have no evidence of depressed cardiac function will require no treatment beyond a 24-hour period of continuous ECG monitoring to ensure that there is no progression of their dysrhythmias to more-malignant forms. Malignant dysrhythmias are treated according to their type and severity with pharmacological agents, electric cardioversion, or both. Nursing staff should be aware of clinical signs of deterioration which indicate hypoxaemia, including dysrhythmias, decreased oxygen saturations, tachycardia, hypotension, decreased level of consciousness and increased temperature. The ED nurse should ensure that the patient is admitted to an appropriate acuity ward, that effective hand-over is given so that the receiving nurse is fully aware of the patient's injuries and any potential for deterioration and that a plan is in place for multidisciplinary care, including effective analgesia. If the condition of the patient has deteriorated, nursing staff must ensure timely communication with the treating team, and assist with instigation of treatment and investigation.

Patients with structural heart injuries will generally require admission to an intensive care unit and may require inotropic support for depressed cardiac output.

Penetrating cardiac injury

Any penetrating mechanism to the left and central anterior chest, whether from a low-velocity piercing instrument such as a knife or a higher-velocity handgun missile, should be suspected of producing a cardiac injury until proven otherwise.[86] Entrance wounds located within the praecordial zone of injury, sometimes referred to as 'the box', should be assumed to have produced a cardiac injury and, in the stable patient, the full range of diagnostic measures described must be instigated to look for it. This zone is defined anatomically by an area encompassed superiorly by the clavicles, laterally by the right midclavicular line and the left midaxillary line, and inferiorly by the costal margins.

Assessment

The most widely available and sensitive means to non-invasively diagnose a cardiac injury remains the transthoracic echocardiogram.[87–88] This may be rapidly performed at the bedside by the trauma team as part of the initial FAST examination, or by a dedicated sonographer experienced in the technique of echocardiography if the patient is stable, but in whom there remains a high index of suspicion based on the location of the wound.[89] Transoesophageal echocardiography is also a sensitive tool for this purpose, but is not readily available in most EDs.

Acute pericardial tamponade occurs following penetrating injury to the 'box'. It results when blood from injury to the cardiac chambers or coronary vessels accumulates between the heart and the rigid overlying fibrous pericardium, compressing the cardiac chambers and thus reducing cardiac output as a result of diminished ventricular filling during diastole[90] (Fig 47.22). Clinically, the patient will present with evidence of a diminishing cardiac output which manifests initially by tachycardia, anxiety and agitation as cerebral perfusion decreases, but initially hypotension is rare. As the volume of blood within the pericardial space continues to increase and further compress the heart, the systolic blood pressure eventually drops, resulting in cardiac arrest and death due to compressive heart failure unless immediate action is taken to relieve the tamponade.

Cardiac tamponade is often characterised by a group of findings termed Beck's triad, which consists of hypotension, distant or diminished heart sounds on auscultation and elevated central venous pressure as evidenced by distension of the neck veins. In reality, the complete triad is rarely seen in patients with acute cardiac tamponade after trauma, so the diagnosis of tamponade should never depend on the patient exhibiting all three criteria. A patient exhibiting early to moderately advanced signs of tamponade (tachycardia and only small drops in systemic blood pressure) may be temporarily stabilised by administration of intravenous fluid boluses. This manoeuvre will delay the eventual and inevitable cardiac arrest by temporarily increasing ventricular filling pressures so as to overcome the extrinsic cardiac compression that is preventing normal cardiac output.

Treatment of acute pericardial tamponade requires decompression of the pericardial space around the heart, as well as control and definitive repair of the cardiac injury from which the bleeding originated. This will require direct exposure of the injury via either a median sternotomy or an anterolateral thoracotomy incision. If a patient with a penetrating chest wound presents in pre-arrest or arrests on arrival in the ED, resuscitative thoracotomy (EDT) and decompression of a cardiac tamponade may be life-saving. Otherwise, unstable

FIGURE 47.22

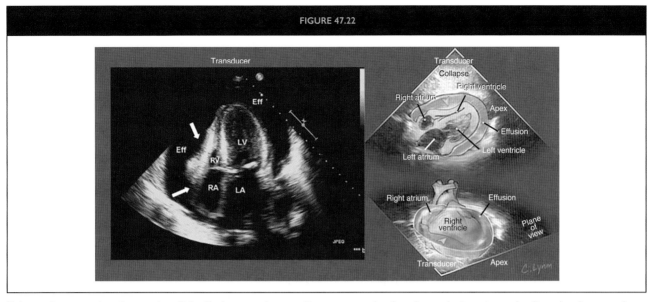

Echocardiogram showing pericardial effusion causing cardiac tamponade. A subcostal view in early diastole shows a large circumferential pericardial effusion compressing the heart, with the right ventricle completely collapsed.[91]

patients with penetrating chest wounds should be rapidly transported to the operating theatre for definitive management.

Historically, needle pericardiocentesis (aspiration of blood from around the heart) has been performed in the emergency setting. However, this technique has been associated with iatrogenic cardiac and liver injury and is rarely effective since the blood is often clotted. Subxiphoid pericardial window is now the recommended, minimally invasive emergency intervention if the expertise to perform definitive EDT is not available.[92]

Management

Any evidence of intrapericardial fluid in a patient with a praecordial penetrating injury usually mandates immediate surgical exploration via either median sternotomy or thoracotomy to detect and repair the injured heart. In the stable patient, this is best done in the controlled environment of the operating theatre where improved lighting, specialised anaesthesia and nursing support and greater instrument availability allow for a safer and definitive operation. However, patients with praecordial penetrating injuries who deteriorate rapidly in the ED or who suffer a cardiac arrest in the field but have undergone less than 10 minutes of closed chest compression resuscitation should undergo a prompt resuscitative ED thoracotomy if the surgical expertise is immediately available.[93] This potentially life-saving technique consists in rapidly opening the chest through a left anterolateral thoracotomy, cross-clamping the descending thoracic aorta, opening the left pericardial sac to evacuate the clot and relieve the compressive tamponade and digitally controlling the site of haemorrhage from the lacerated cardiac chamber while transporting the patient to the operating theatre for definitive repair under more-optimal surgical conditions. Nursing personnel should anticipate transport and monitoring needs for these patients for, if the resuscitation is successful, the patient must be taken directly to the operating theatre if the chances for survival are to be optimised.

The ED resuscitative thoracotomy exposes all involved healthcare personnel to an often frenetic and potentially hazardous environment of splashed blood and sharp objects (instruments, needles, fractured rib ends, etc.) and should only be done when it is most likely to benefit the patient. The highest survival rates for ED thoracotomy are in those patients who sustain cardiac arrest after arrival to the ED from a stab wound to the heart.[94] Patients who have sustained praecordial gunshot injuries have a much lower chance of survival, while those who arrest after a blunt mechanism of injury rarely survive and should not undergo an ED resuscitative thoracotomy (EDT). Detail on the procedure is given in Chapter 44.

Thoracic vascular injury

Blunt thoracic aortic injury is a major cause of death from blunt trauma. In spite of representing less than 1% of injuries in patients involved in MVCs, blunt aortic injury is responsible for 16% of the deaths. It is estimated that 80–85% of patients die before arriving at the hospital.

The thoracic aorta and its major branches, as well as the superior and inferior venae cavae and the azygous veins, carry very large blood flows and significant injury may lead to exsanguinating haemorrhage and death.[95] Because of their relatively fixed position within the chest cavity, these large vessels (aorta, proximal innominate artery, proximal left subclavian and carotid arteries) are vulnerable to sudden decelerative forces after blunt trauma, which may result in the formation of traumatic pseudoaneurysms (i.e. contained partial ruptures of the vessel wall), partial or complete obstructions, lacerations or even total transections that cause massive haemothorax. High-speed MVCs are the most common blunt mechanism producing major intrathoracic vascular injury. Any occupant in the vehicle may sustain this type of injury, and it may occur even from laterally applied forces, such as the so-called left subclavian and carotid arteries, which are vulnerable to sudden decelerative forces. Falls from heights as low as 3 m can sustain this type of injury. Penetrating injuries, such as stab wounds and gunshot wounds, may disrupt the vascular tree at any point within the chest, producing uncontrolled haemorrhage and rapid death if not detected and treated expeditiously (Figs 47.23 and 47.24).

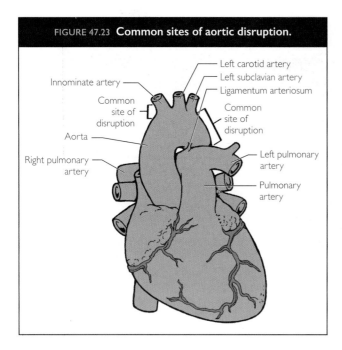

FIGURE 47.23 **Common sites of aortic disruption.**

Assessment

The mechanism of injury and the patient's haemodynamic status will often provide evidence of thoracic vascular injury. Haemodynamically unstable patients with penetrating thoracic trauma who do not respond to resuscitative measures will usually require immediate surgery with a plain film CXR as the only preoperative radiological test. Stable patients with suspected intrathoracic vascular injuries should undergo further radiological evaluation in order to confirm and anatomically stage the injury. If the CXR demonstrates signs suggesting aortic injury then either CT angiography or digital subtraction angiography or both should be performed, a combined approach that allows for more-accurate preoperative localisation of the injury and planning of the operation. As mentioned above, improvements in CT technology and its ready availability have made CT angiography alone the investigation of choice in many centres. CXR signs suggestive of aortic injury are listed in Box 47.1.

Of these findings, the most important one, due to its high positive predictive value, is the 'funny looking mediastinum'. This admittedly imprecise term refers either to a superior mediastinum that appears on the CXR to be widened (more than the oft-quoted 8 cm maximum normal width at the aortic knob) or indistinct or poorly defined, especially along the superolateral border of the aortic knob and descending aorta (Fig 47.24).

Contained aortic ruptures are prone to sudden rupture, which results in exsanguination into the thorax. Therefore, it is imperative that these injuries, when suspected, be diagnosed promptly. It should be remembered, however, that in a haemodynamically unstable patient with a widened mediastinum only, suggesting a contained bleed, other sites of haemorrhage such as the abdomen or the pelvis must be considered. A contained aortic transection will not cause hypovolaemic shock until it ruptures into the thoracic cavity.

Management

Treatment of major thoracic vascular injuries has traditionally been surgical repair via either a sternotomy or a thoracotomy. Pre-hospital personnel should initiate damage control resuscitation protocols. Intravenous fluids should only be administered to maintain a systolic blood pressure around 80–90 mmHg, to avoid disrupting fresh clots and promoting further bleeding, coagulopathy and hypothermia.[95] In the ED the nurse should alert the team leader to any change in haemodynamic parameters or in the conscious state of the patient. Heart rate and systolic blood pressure should be controlled with beta-blockers unless contraindicated. This has been demonstrated to reduce mortality in the ED for those patients awaiting repair.[96] Certain patients with thoracic aortic disruption following blunt trauma may now be suitable to undergo endovascular repair of the injury by percutaneous placement of a stent graft. Where suitable, these injuries are often managed by the vascular surgeons rather than the cardiothoracic surgical team.[97–99]

Oesophageal injury

The oesophagus is a long, muscular organ that begins at the pharyngo-oesophageal junction at the level of the 6th cervical vertebra. It ends at the oesophagogastric junction at the level of the 10th thoracic vertebra near the diaphragm. The surrounding organs and tissues provide protection from external force, therefore oesophageal injury is uncommon. In addition, the clinical symptoms and signs are non-specific, making the diagnosis difficult and often delayed. The risks of delayed diagnosis are high and include retropharyngeal abscess, mediastinitis, empyema, septic shock and death. Penetrating injuries of the oesophagus far outnumber blunt oesophageal injuries. The predominant mechanism of oesophageal trauma or injury is gunshot wounds (70%) or penetration by either a stab injury or another penetrating mechanism (3–5%).[100]

Oesophageal injuries resulting from blunt trauma account for less than 1% of all oesophageal injuries. These injuries are most often located in the cervical oesophagus as the result of an anterior blow with the neck in a hyperextended position. Rarely an acute blow to a distended stomach may produce tears of the distal oesophagus due to a rapid increase in intraluminal pressure. In the same way blast injury can result in oesophageal perforation.

Diagnosis

The rarity of oesophageal injuries means that even busy trauma centres that manage a high percentage of penetrating trauma may see very few. Indeed, a 10-year retrospective multicentre study conducted by the American Association for the Surgery of Trauma (AAST) enrolled only 405 patients with penetrating oesophageal injury from the 34 participating institutions.[101] These injuries do not occur in isolation and many penetrating wounds injure the aorta or heart, resulting in rapid death. Furthermore, since most penetrating injuries occur in the cervical oesophagus, injuries to adjacent structures are common, including the carotid arteries, jugular veins and trachea producing haemorrhage or airway issues that distract from investigation of oesophageal injury. Therefore the keys to prevention of life-threatening complications related to delayed diagnosis is a high index of suspicion based on mechanism and a recognition of injury patterns associated with oesophageal

FIGURE 47.24

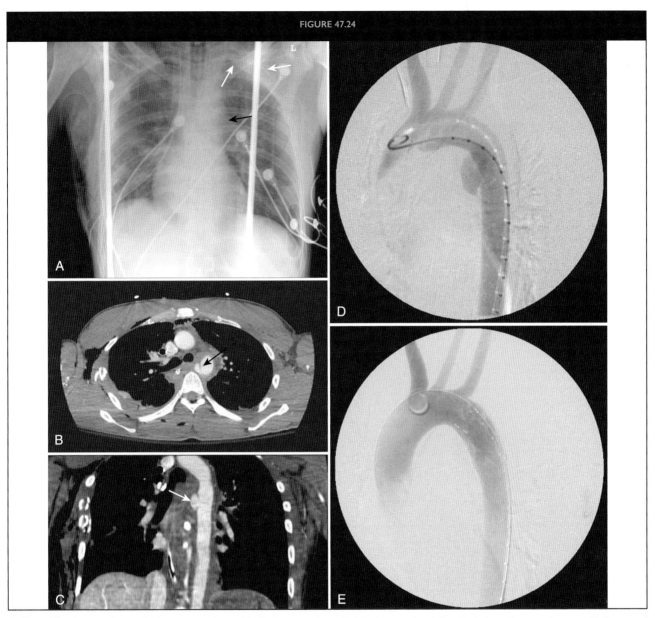

A, Portable chest radiograph shows an enlarged indistinct aortic arch (black arrow), a left apical pleural cap and upper rib fractures (white arrows). **B**, Axial computed tomography demonstrates mediastinal haematoma, intimal flap and pseudoaneurysm (arrow). **C**, Oblique coronal reformation shows the extent of pseudoaneurysm (arrow). **D, E**, Thoracic aortography before and after treatment with an aortic stent.[28]

BOX 47.1 Signs demonstrating potential aortic injury

'Funny-looking mediastinum':
- superior mediastinal width > 8 cm
- indistinct or 'fuzzy' descending aortic margin
- indistinct or 'fuzzy' aortic knob contour

Fracture(s) of first or second rib(s)
Fracture of scapula
Depression of left mainstem bronchus
Deviation of nasogastric tube to right
Deviation of trachea to right
Fractures(s) of upper thoracic vertebra(e)

---

injury. These injuries must be suspected in penetrating neck injuries that violate the platysma, in transmediastinal gunshot wounds, and significant chest trauma with associated tracheobronchial injuries.

Assessment

The clinical symptomatology is non-specific early after perforation. In the AAST study reported above, the majority of patients had no symptoms or signs of oesophageal injury. Dysphagia was present in 29 (7%) and subcutaneous emphysema was found in 78 (19%). Yet other studies have reported pain, located in the chest with cervical perforations and perhaps referred to the abdomen with thoracic perforations, as a frequent complaint by patients with oesophageal perforation, occurring in 70–90% of patients.[102] This pain may intensify with the swallowing of food (odynophagia), and be accompanied by dysphagia, vomiting, low-grade pyrexia and moderate leucocytosis. Tenderness to palpation and with passive motion, dyspnoea and/or hoarseness may be present. Expanding cervical haematoma is concerning, and the subsequent development of fever, cough and stridor may be the first signs of the massive inflammatory response which can result from even minor perforations. Palpable subcutaneous emphysema or air within the soft tissues or a wide pre-vertebral shadow on neck X-ray may also suggest the presence of oesophageal injury, but radiological clues are subtle and may easily be missed. CT scan may detect even small amounts of subcutaneous emphysema in the neck or may demonstrate a pneumomediastinum.

The clinical findings associated with thoracic oesophageal injuries may initially be non-specific or even absent. In thoracic perforations dyspnoea is a common symptom. As mentioned above, pain may be referred to the abdomen and may be associated with abdominal tenderness and/or rigidity. Subcutaneous emphysema may track cranially from the mediastinum leading to cervical crepitus, and Hamman's sign (mediastinal crunch on auscultation). Following penetrating thoracic trauma, the presence of pneumomediastinum and pleural effusion raise suspicion of oesophageal injury (Fig 47.25).

While haemodynamically unstable patients with penetrating neck or thoracic trauma will require surgical exploration for associated wounds, the stable patient may present a diagnostic challenge.

As will be discussed further below, in the past all penetrating neck wounds that breached the platysma underwent routine exploration. Since a more selective approach to the management of penetrating neck wounds is now accepted practice in most trauma centres, a diagnostic algorithm is required to exclude oesophageal perforation.

A water-soluble contrast oesophagram is the preferred first-line approach and can evaluate the entire oesophagus. It can be performed in intubated patients by withdrawing the nasogastric tube into the oesophagus and instilling contrast. If no leakage of

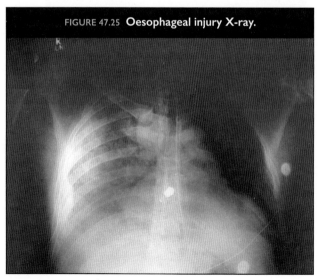

FIGURE 47.25 **Oesophageal injury X-ray.**

Stomach contents have spilled into the thoracic cavity. Post-oesophageal injury caused by a bullet.
Courtesy Kate Curtis.

contrast is seen then dilute barium may be instilled as this adds a measure of safety in excluding injury. However, since contrast studies have a false negative rate reported to be up to 25%, patients regarded as high risk for injury should undergo flexible oesophagoscopy. The specificity of a negative oesophagoscopy combined with negative contrast studies approaches 100%.[103] The value of MDCT in assessing for possible oesophageal perforation is that it allows the tracts of missiles within the chest and mediastinum to be determined, thus potentially excluding oesophageal (as well as vascular) injuries with a high degree of certainty.[21,22] In addition, when combined with oral contrast, MDCT may demonstrate pooling of contrast outside of the oesophageal lumen. Delayed images may be useful in detecting contrast extravasation.

Once an oesophageal injury has been diagnosed, the patient is kept fasted, a nasogastric tube is inserted, broad-spectrum antibiotics are initiated and resuscitation continues according to the patient's haemodynamic status.

Management

Since blunt trauma to the oesophagus is exceedingly rare, management is usually based on the approach to penetrating injuries.

There are divergent views regarding the appropriate management of oesophageal injury, with some authors advocating mandatory exploration while others prefer a conservative approach. The problem with these series and their descriptions of management is that they frequently encompass iatrogenic perforation, spontaneous rupture and chemically-induced perforation as well as external trauma,[104–107] which is least frequently described. The debate over selective versus mandatory neck exploration for penetrating trauma to the cervical oesophagus continues because of lack of data showing conclusively that one approach is superior to, or more cost effective than, the other.[108]

In a retrospective study over 5 years, Mudiba and Muckart reported on a selective approach to the management of penetrating cervical oesophageal injury.[109] All patients with contained extravasation were managed non-operatively, irrespective of the delay from injury to admission. Repair was undertaken in patients with major disruption and those requiring exploration for another reason. Of the 28 patients with confirmed cervical oesophageal injury 17 were managed non-operatively. Sixteen recovered with no complications, while one developed local sepsis. Following an extensive review of the literature Mudiba and Muckart concluded that non-operative management of cervical oesophageal injuries is safe and effective and should always be considered, and stated that the following criteria are essential in deciding between conservative and operative management:

1. It is essential to establish whether the extravasation is contained or not.

2. Operative management is essential in high-velocity injuries, uncontained extravasation and where there are other indications for neck exploration.

3. The decision between debridement and primary repair depends on delay between the time of injury and surgery.

4. Tube feeding and close monitoring are essential during the period of observation.[109]

Where operative exploration is undertaken, the approach is via a neck incision along the anterior border of the left sterno-cleidomastoid muscle for cervical perforations, and via left or right thoracotomy, depending on the proximal or distal location of thoracic oesophageal injury.

In the cervical oesophagus, primary suture repair and drainage is performed. If delayed diagnosis has led to late exploration, then the tissues may be markedly inflamed and friable. Under these circumstances drainage with a penrose or soft silastic drain should be performed with the patient kept fasted and on broad spectrum antibiotics. Oral intake can be commenced once healing is demonstrated on contrast swallow.

For injuries to the thoracic oesophagus primary suture repair may be appropriate if the injury is diagnosed early before a massive inflammatory response and mediastinitis have made the tissues friable. The repair may be buttressed by a pleural or pericardial flap in the mid-oesophagus, or by fundoplication for the lower third. With penetrating trauma multiple injuries may be present and must be looked for.

Where severe mediastinitis and destructive inflammation are found at surgery the safest approach is debridement of the damaged tissue and tube drainage of the affected thorax, with a plan for delayed repair. Only rarely is oesophagectomy indicated.

Neck injuries

Few emergencies pose as great a challenge as neck trauma. Vital anatomical structures (e.g. airway, vascular, neurological, gastrointestinal) are in such close proximity that even a single penetrating wound is capable of causing multisystem injury. Furthermore, seemingly innocuous wounds may not manifest clear signs or symptoms, and potentially lethal injuries could be easily overlooked or discounted. Major neurovascular structures, including the carotid and vertebral arteries and the spinal cord, span the short gap between the head and the torso, and the trachea and oesophagus originate in the neck (Fig 47.26). (Spinal injuries are discussed in Ch 49, and oesophageal injuries are discussed above.)

Neck injuries are classified according to blunt or penetrating mechanism in addition to the structures involved. These injuries may result in exsanguinating haemorrhage or lead to airway occlusion, but often the signs of significant trauma may be far more subtle. Patients presenting with neck trauma should be assessed according to ATLS principles to expeditiously identify life-threatening injuries and appropriately prioritise treatment.

Pre-hospital personnel should be aware of the risk of airway compromise and unless the patient has sustained multiple injuries due to blunt force trauma, thus requiring spinal precautions, the patient should be allowed to sit forward to minimise the risk of aspiration of blood or secretions. In isolated penetrating trauma to the neck, the use of cervical spine protection is not indicated since the risk of cervical cord injury is very low.[111] Semi-rigid collars may also obscure expanding haematomas. Obvious haemorrhage should be controlled by direct manual compression. Impaled objects should not be removed in the field. Intravenous access should be achieved in the extremity contralateral to the injured side in penetrating

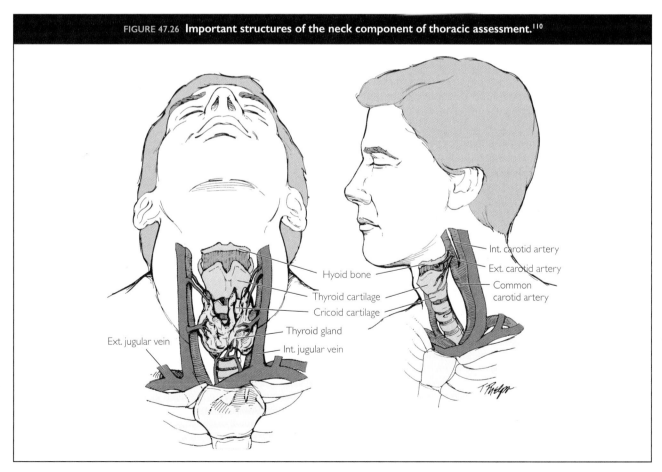

FIGURE 47.26 **Important structures of the neck component of thoracic assessment.**[110]

injury in case the ipsilateral venous system has been damaged, but fluid should only be given in accordance with damage control resuscitation principles (Ch 44).

On arrival in the ED the neck should be inspected after removal of any semi-rigid collars, articles of clothing and jewellery to allow for a complete, circumferential visual and manual examination. The posterior aspect of the neck is best examined during the log-roll. Spinal alignment should be maintained by an assistant performing in-line stabilisation during the examination in any patient at risk of spinal column instability. As mentioned above, the use of cervical spine protection is not required in the ED in patients with isolated stab wounds who do not have neurological deficit at presentation. In the awake patient refrain from oropharyngeal or nasal suction which may cause the patient to gag or cough, potentially dislodging blood clots and precipitating further haemorrhage. The patient may be given a sucker to use.

Penetrating injuries

Assessment

Examination of the neck should look for evidence of underlying injury. A large or expanding haematoma usually indicates an injury to a major underlying vascular structure, typically the carotid arteries or one of their major branches. Tracheal deviation may be seen as a late sign of an expanding haematoma. Its absence does not exclude an underlying haematoma that may rapidly enlarge and occlude the airway. Gurgling or bubbling of air from the neck wound is diagnostic for a pharyngeal or tracheal injury. Signs of cranial nerve deficits may be present, such as tongue deviation caused by injury to the hypoglossal nerve. Haemoptysis is suggestive of injury to the pharynx or trachea, and odynophagia or dysphagia strongly suggests underlying oesophageal injury as described previously. Hoarseness indicates compression or direct injury to the larynx or recurrent laryngeal nerves. A loud 'machinery' bruit over the anterolateral neck is associated with traumatic arteriovenous fistulae between the carotid artery and jugular vein. Although most awake patients will exhibit tenderness over penetrating wounds, diffuse cervical tenderness should raise suspicions for underlying tracheo-oesophageal injury. Haemodynamically unstable patients with penetrating neck trauma or those with evidence of severe injury to the airway, vessels or digestive tract should have the airway secured immediately with an endotracheal tube or, if necessary, a surgical airway (described in Ch 44). Further evaluation and management should take place in the operating theatre where emergency surgical exploration must be undertaken. Patients in this group include those with refractory shock, or who have expansile/pulsatile haematomas, or evidence of severe respiratory injury, the so-called 'hard signs' in neck injuries.

Management

The surface anatomy of the neck has traditionally been divided into three discrete zones for the purpose of evaluating and treating penetrating neck wounds (Fig 47.27).

1. Zone I extends from the inferior border of the cricoid cartilage to the clavicles and contains the trachea, oesophagus, great vessels, upper mediastinum, apices of the lungs and the thoracic duct.

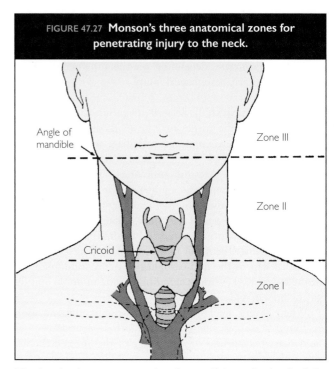

FIGURE 47.27 **Monson's three anatomical zones for penetrating injury to the neck.**

Angle of mandible

Zone III

Zone II

Cricoid

Zone I

The border between zone I and zone II is at the level of the cricoid cartilage. The border between zone II and zone III is at the mandible.[112]

2. Zone II includes the space between cricoid cartilage and the angle of the mandible, and contains the carotid and vertebral vessels, the jugular veins, pharynx, larynx, oesophagus and trachea.

3. Zone III involves the area from the angle of the mandible to the base of the skull and includes extracranial portions of the carotid and vertebral vessels, as well as portions of the jugular veins.

Injuries to Zone II are easily evaluated and operative exposure is more straightforward compared to Zones I and III. Zone II is the most commonly injured, yet injuries to Zone 1 have the highest mortality. The most common cause of death is exsanguination. It should be remembered that trauma to the neck is not necessarily limited to one zone.

As stated above, patients with any of the hard signs of vascular or aerodigestive tract injury should undergo surgical exploration. Prophylactic antibiotics should be administered, usually a cephalosporin, and tetanus immunoglobulin should be given where there is any doubt about the tetanus status of the patient. Blood should be grouped and matched and the trauma nurse should notify the blood bank should the team leader wish to activate the massive transfusion protocol.

Management of haemodynamically stable patients with neck trauma who have no clinical signs warranting immediate intervention has evolved over the last four decades. Classically, Zone II injuries that penetrated deep to the platysma were managed with immediate operative exploration. However, this approach led to a high number of negative neck explorations and in the 1980s and 1990s reports were published detailing non-operative management of these injuries with good outcomes and no missed injuries of clinical significance. This became the accepted approach.[113]

By contrast, Zone I and III injuries, as a result of their anatomic inaccessibility, have traditionally been evaluated more selectively. In some centres these injuries were managed with simple observation, but over time recommended management became routine use of a combination of four-vessel digital subtraction angiography (DSA) and endoscopy to separately examine the vascular and aerodigestive structures of the neck and upper thorax. This approach is both labour intensive and invasive. More recently, based on the high specificity and sensitivity of MDCT and CT angiography to define critical neck structures and identify or exclude injury based on trajectory, Shiroff and colleagues have suggested that the requirement to divide the neck into discrete zones has become outdated.[114] They have proposed a 'No-Zone' algorithm.

Stable patients with no signs of injury should undergo CT angiography and can then be managed with observation only if no injury to vital structures is found.

Blunt injuries

Assessment

Assessment and maintenance of airway patency are the priority in blunt neck injury. The cervical airway, especially the larynx and associated structures, is vulnerable, and developing oedema or expansile haematoma from associated vascular injury can lead rapidly to airway occlusion. The trauma nurse should prepare equipment for intubation and have the difficult airway kit available (see Ch 17, p. 318, for intubation techniques). Vascular structures, including the carotid and vertebral arteries, may be injured by direct trauma, by crushing against bony structures or by hyperextension and rotation of the neck causing intimal tearing. Additionally, the cervical spine and spinal cord are frequently injured following blunt neck trauma and pre-hospital personnel should ensure that the neck is appropriately immobilised during both extrication and transport. Such immobilisation must be continued during all phases of evaluation and treatment of the status of the cervical spine stability can be definitively established (see Ch 49).

The initial physical examination includes assessment of airway patency. Stridor or other changes in phonation are commonly associated with fracture of the larynx, which can promptly progress to localised oedema and complete upper airway obstruction. As stated above, a pulsatile or expansile haematoma places the airway at immediate risk. Patients with any of these findings require prompt intubation since delay may result in an obstructed airway and the need for surgical intervention.

Inspection of the neck may reveal skin bruising or soft-tissue haematomas, indicating possible underlying injuries. Subcutaneous emphysema of the cervical soft tissues may indicate an underlying tear to the distal pharynx or proximal trachea.

Investigations include lateral cervical spine X-ray, which may reveal air outside of the aerodigestive tract, but more commonly MDCT is the investigation of choice. Where a suggestion of vascular injury is visible, CTA (computed tomography angiography) is both sensitive and specific for diagnosis.

Blunt carotid and vertebral artery injuries, collectively termed blunt cerebrovascular injury (BCVI), are uncommon but potentially devastating events. The incidence of blunt cerebrovascular injury in patients sustaining blunt trauma is about 1%. Untreated blunt carotid injury is associated with mortality rates that range from 23–28%, with 48–58% of survivors suffering permanent severe neurological deficits.[115] Partial or complete occlusion of the vessel lumen pseudo-aneurysm formation or complete transection of the carotid or vertebral arteries may result from sudden stretching or buckling of the artery, which leads to localised intimal tears and vascular dissections (Fig 47.28).

Many of these injuries may be occult and initially the patient may be neurologically normal, only to suffer a sudden debilitating or even fatal ischaemic or embolic stroke hours to days later. Where the mechanism of injury or clinical examination raise suspicion of BCVI, it is imperative that appropriate investigations are undertaken. In most modern trauma centres CTA is now the investigation of choice as it is more widely available and has comparable sensitivity and specificity to angiography (Box 47.2).[116–119]

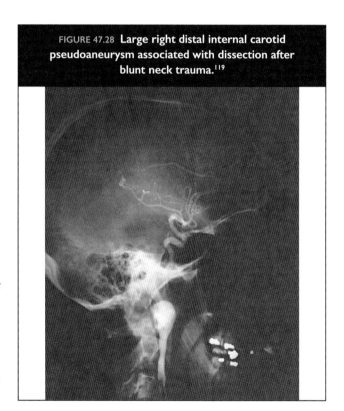

FIGURE 47.28 **Large right distal internal carotid pseudoaneurysm associated with dissection after blunt neck trauma.**[119]

BOX 47.2 **Signs and symptoms associated with blunt cerebrovascular injury**

- Unexplained neurological findings in the face of normal brain computed tomography scan
- Bruising of the lateral neck soft tissues—the 'seat belt' sign of the neck
- Cervical spine fractures, dislocations or ligamentous injuries, especially those involving the first three vertebrae
- Severe maxillofacial fractures

Management

Fractures of the larynx or trachea or ruptures of the oesophagus require surgical repair. Where there is no contraindication such as an intracerebral haemorrhage, small intimal tears of the carotid or vertebral arteries may be successfully treated with systemic anticoagulation, while larger pseudoaneurysms or occlusions are approached surgically and usually undergo re-section and interposition of autologous venous grafts or artificial vascular prostheses. More recently, some of these injuries have been treated successfully by percutaneously-placed endoluminal stents, obviating the need for an open neck exploration. Postoperatively, many of these patients will return to the intensive care unit or ward with surgical drains in situ. Care should be taken to accurately record their outputs, keep their skin exit sites clean and avoid accidental dislodgement during patient turning and transport. Nurses should also be aware of any drain-output parameters that would mandate prompt notification of the surgical team.

SUMMARY

Trauma to the thorax or neck produces some of the most challenging and potentially life-threatening injuries. Injury to major vascular structures or airway compromise may produce death within minutes from shock or hypoxia if not promptly recognised and treated. The mechanism of injury should be determined as accurately as possible since it often guides the diagnostic and therapeutic approach. As with any seriously injured patient, preservation of a patent airway and ensuring adequate oxygenation and ventilation are paramount in the evaluation and resuscitative phases of management.

The clinical examination of the chest as part of the primary survey includes inspection, palpation and auscultation and should provide sufficient information to allow for accurate diagnosis and treatment of immediately life-threatening problems such as tension pneumothorax, pericardial tamponade or massive haemothorax. Chest decompression will often be the mainstay of management in thoracic injury since fewer than 10% of all patients with thoracic trauma will require operative intervention. The plain chest X-ray is performed as part of the trauma series. In many centres e-FAST has become an adjunct to primary survey, but CT scanning is essential in blunt thoracic trauma as it allows assessment of the extent of pulmonary contusions as well as for the assessment of major vessels. CT angiography has a sensitivity similar to that of conventional angiography in the assessment of vascular injury. Adequate analgesia is paramount in thoracic trauma to prevent decreased respiratory effort secondary to pain, which can result in fatigue, atelectasis, hypoxia and subsequent respiratory failure. A multidisciplinary approach to the management of thoracic injuries improves outcomes.

Assessment of injuries to the neck should include examination of both the anterior and the posterior aspects with protection of the cervical spine by in-line stabilisation. CT angiography is an essential part of the assessment of neck trauma, replacing the need to consider the neck in discrete zones. Stable patients with no evidence of occult injury after serial examination or radiological evaluation will often require no operative intervention.

CASE STUDY

A 74-year-old man calls an ambulance following a fall from a ladder while putting up Christmas lights. He is able to walk inside to the telephone and states that the left side of his chest hurt when he breathes.

Questions

1. What initial assessment will you perform on scene?

   His vital signs are:

   heart rate: 64 beats/minute

   respiratory rate: 26 breaths/minute, talking in full sentences

   blood pressure: 140/82 mmHg

   oxygen saturation (SaO$_2$): 94%

   Glasgow Coma Scale (GCS) score: 15 (did not lose consciousness).

   He has left chest-wall tenderness, a small amount of subcutaneous emphysema and a scalp laceration.

2. A. What treatment would you initiate? Why?

   B. If in an urban area, what type of hospital would you transport the patient to? Why?

   C. Given the patient's age, consider what co-morbidities the patient may have that could affect his compensatory response or exacerbate his injury.

En route to the ED in the ambulance, you ascertain the patient's medical history—he has hypertension, takes warfarin for a mitral valve replacement and digoxin for atrial fibrillation. He stopped smoking 15 years ago.

3. A. What triage category would you give this patient? Why?

   B. Where would you place this patient in your department?

The patient arrives on your bed. As the emergency nurse, you perform your initial assessment and find the following:

heart rate: 64 beats/minute

respiratory rate: 32 breaths/minute

blood pressure: 150/84 mmHg

SaO_2: 92%

GCS score: 15.

The patient is in obvious discomfort despite 5 mg intravenous morphine. Air entry is decreased on the left.

4. A. What treatment do you initiate?

   B. What investigations should be performed? Why?

   C. What potential injuries does this patient have?

   D. What potential intervention will you prepare for?

The patient has an intercostal catheter inserted, which has drained 100 mL of blood and the underwater-seal drain is bubbling. His respiratory rate has reduced to 20 breaths/minute, and his SaO_2 increased to 98%. Nil other injuries have been detected at this stage. He has been admitted under the trauma team.

5. A. What type of ward should this patient go to?

   B. What referrals and communication (including medical charts and documentation) should you ensure have been completed prior to transfer?

   C. What potentially could go wrong with this patient, and why?

 Answers to Case Study Questions can be found on evolve
http://evolve.emergencytrauma.curtis

USEFUL WEBSITES

Chest Drain Management Clinical Guideline, Royal Childrens Hospital Melbourne,

www.rch.org.au/rchcpg/hospital_clinical_guideline_index/Chest_Drain_Management/

Pleural Drains in Adults, A Consensus Guideline, NSW Agency for Clinical Innovation,

www.aci.health.nsw.gov.au/__data/assets/pdf_file/0018/201906/ACI-pleural-drain-web-v1-2.pdf

Trauma.org, emergency department thoracotomy procedure, www.trauma.org

Updated evidence-based clinical practice guidelines relating to trauma, www.east.org

REFERENCES

1. Ryan M, Stella J, Chiu H et al. Injury patterns and preventability in prehospital motor vehicle crash fatalities in Victoria. Emerg Med Australas 2004;16(4):274–9.

2. NSW Institute of Trauma and Injury Management. Major trauma in NSW, 2013. NSW Ministry of Health, Sydney; 2014.

3. Kent AL, Jeans P, Edwards JR et al. Ten-year review of thoracic and abdominal penetrating trauma management. Aust N Z J Surg 1993; 63(10):772–9.

4. Bokhari F, Brakenridge S, Nagy K et al. Prospective evaluation of the sensitivity of physical examination in chest trauma. J Trauma 2002; 53(6):1135–8.

5. Rodriguez RM, Hendey GW, Marek G et al. A pilot study to derive clinical variables for selective chest radiography in blunt trauma patients. Ann Emerg Med 2006;47(5):415–18.

6. Chen SC, Chang KJ, Hsu CY. Accuracy of auscultation in the detection of haemopneumothorax. Eur J Surg 1998;164(9):643–5.

7. Roca O, Riera J, Torres F et al. High-flow oxygen therapy in acute respiratory failure. Respir Care 2010;55:408–13.

8. Davis J, Davis I, Benninck L et al. Are automated blood pressure measurements accurate in trauma patients? J Trauma 2003;55(5):860–3.

9. Udeani J. Hemorrhagic shock workup. Medscape 2012. Online. http://emedicine.medscape.com/article/432650-workup; accessed 24th August 2014.

10. MIMMS Online. Penthrox inhalation. www.mimsonline.com.au.acs.hcn.com.au/Search/FullPI.aspx?ModuleName=ProductInfo&search Keyword=methoxyflurane&PreviousPage=~/Search/QuickSearch.aspx&SearchType=&ID=38540001_2

11. Kehlet H, Jensen TS, Woolf CJ. Persistent postsurgical pain: risk factors and prevention. Lancet 2006;367(9522):1618–25.

12. Desborough JP. The stress response to trauma and surgery. Br J Anaesth 2000;85(1):109–17.

13. Mayberry JC. Imaging in thoracic trauma: the trauma surgeon's perspective. J Thorac Imaging 2000;15(2):76–86.

14. Hirshberg A, Thomson SR, Huizinga WK. Reliability of physical examination in penetrating chest injuries. Injury 1988;19(6):407–9.

15. Wilkerson RG, Stone MB. Sensitivity of bedside ultrasound and supine anteroposterior chest radiographs for the identification of pneumothorax after blunt trauma. Acad Emerg Med 2010;17(1):11–17.

16. Dulchavsky SA, Schwarz KL, Kirkpatrick AW et al. Prospective evaluation of thoracic ultrasound in the evaluation of pneumothorax. J Trauma 2001;50(2):201–5.

17. Brooks A, Davies B, Smethhurst M et al. Emergency ultrasound in the acute assessment of haemothorax. Emerg Med J 2004;21(1):44–6.

18. Kirkpatrick AW, Sirois M, Laupland KB et al. Hand-held thoracic sonography for detecting post-traumatic pneumothoraces: the extended focused assessment with sonography for trauma (EFAST). J Trauma 2004;57(2):288–95.

19. Omert L, Yeaney WW, Protetch J. Efficacy of thoracic computerized tomography in blunt chest trauma. Am Surg 2001;67(7):660–4.

20. McGonigal M. Trauma patient stability. The trauma professionals blog. Online. http://regionstraumapro.com/post/4609996532; accessed 24 May 2014.

21. Cook CC, Gleason TG. Great vessel and cardiac trauma. Surg Clin North Am 2009;89(4):797–820, viii.

22. Stassen NA, Lukan JK, Spain DA et al. Re-evaluation of diagnostic procedures for transmediastinal gunshot wounds. J Trauma 2002; 53(4):635–8.

23. Todd SR, McNally MM, Holcomb JB et al. A multidisciplinary clinical pathway decreases rib fracture-associated infectious morbidity and mortality in high-risk trauma patients. Am J Surg 2006;192(6):806–11.

24. Livingston DH, Shogan B, John P et al. CT diagnosis of rib fractures and the prediction of acute respiratory failure. J Trauma 2008; 64(4):905–11.

25. Ziegler DW, Agarwal NN. The morbidity and mortality of rib fractures. J Trauma 1994;37(6):975–9.

26. Sirmali M, Turut H, Topcu S et al. A comprehensive analysis of traumatic rib fractures: morbidity, mortality and management. Eur J Cardiothorac Surg 2003;24(1):133–8.

27. Kent RW, Woods WA, Bostrom O et al. Fatality risk and the presence of rib fractures. Annals of Advances in Automotive Medicine 2008;52:73–84.

28. Soto JA, Lucey BC. Emergency radiology: the requisites. Philadelphia: Mosby; 2009.

29. Holcomb JB, McMullin NR, Kozar RA et al. Morbidity from rib fractures increases after age 45. J Am Coll Surg 2003;196(4):549–55.

30. Flagel BT, Luchette FA, Reed RL et al. Half-a-dozen ribs: the breakpoint for mortality. Surgery 2005;138(4):717–23.

31. Testerman GM. Adverse outcomes in younger rib fracture patients. South Med J 2006;99(4):335–9.

32. Vydareny K, Gober D, Khan A et al. ACR appropriateness criteria: rib fractures. American College of Radiology 2011. www.acr.org; accessed 24 August 2014.

33. Wisner DH. A stepwise logistic regression analysis of factors affecting morbidity and mortality after thoracic trauma: effect of epidural analgesia. J Trauma 1990;30(7):799–805.

34. Bulger EM, Edwards T, Klotz P et al. Epidural analgesia improves outcome after multiple rib fractures. Surgery 2004;136(2):426–30.

35. Kieninger AN, Bair HA, Bendick PJ et al. Epidural versus intravenous pain control in elderly patients with rib fractures. Am J Surg 2005;189(3):327–30.

36. Kernick J, Magarey J. What is the evidence for the use of high flow nasal cannula oxygen in adult patients admitted to critical care units?: a systematic review. Aust Crit Care 2010;23(2):53–70.

37. Knobloch K, Wagner S, Haasper C et al. Sternal fractures occur most often in old cars to seat-belted drivers without any airbag often with concomitant spinal injuries: clinical findings and technical collision variables among 42,055 crash victims. Ann Thorac Surg 2006;82(2):444–50.

38. Recinos G, Inaba K, Dubose J et al. Epidemiology of sternal fractures. Am Surg 2009;75(5):401–4.

39. von Garrel T, Ince A, Junge A et al. The sternal fracture: radiographic analysis of 200 fractures with special reference to concomitant injuries. J Trauma 2004;57(4):837–44.

40. Harston A, Roberts C. Fixation of sternal fractures: a systematic review. J Trauma 2011;71(6):1875–9. doi: 10.1097/TA.0b013e31823c46e8.

41. Denard PJ, Koval KJ, Cantu RV et al. Management of midshaft clavicle fractures in adults. Am J Orthop (Belle Mead NJ) 2005;34(11):527–36.

42. Weening B, Walton C, Cole PA et al. Lower mortality in patients with scapular fractures. J Trauma 2005;59(6):1477–81.

43. Brucker PU, Gruen GS, Kaufmann RA. Scapulothoracic dissociation: evaluation and management. Injury 2005;36(10):1147–55.

44. Rosen P, Barkin RM, Hockberger RS et al. Emergency medicine: concepts and clinical practice. 4th edn. St Louis: Mosby; 1998.

45. Qasim Z, Gwinnutt C. Flail chest: pathophysiology and management. Trauma 2009;11(1):63–70.

46. Velmahos GC, Vassiliu P, Chan LS et al. Influence of flail chest on outcome among patients with severe thoracic cage trauma. Int Surg 2002;87(4):240–4.

47. Athanassiadi K, Gerazounis M, Theakos N. Management of 150 flail chest injuries: analysis of risk factors affecting outcome. Eur J Cardiothorac Surg 2004;26(2):373–6.

48. Davignon K, Kwo J, Bigatello LM. Pathophysiology and management of the flail chest. Minerva Anestesiol 2004;70(4):193–9.

49. Granetzny A, Abd El-Aal M, Emam E et al. Surgical versus conservative treatment of flail chest. Evaluation of the pulmonary status. Interact Cardiovasc Thorac Surg 2005;4(6):583–7.

50. Adam A, Dixon AK. Grainger and Allison's Diagnostic radiology. 5th edn. New York: Churchill Livingstone; 2008.

51. Laws D, Neville E, Duffy J. BTS guidelines for the insertion of a chest drain. Thorax 2003;58(suppl II):ii53–9.

52. Baumann MH. What size chest tube? What drainage system is ideal? And other chest tube management questions. Curr Opin Pulm Med 2003;9(4):276–81.

53. McPherson JJ, Feigin DS, Bellamy RF. Prevalence of tension pneumothorax in fatally wounded combat casualties. J Trauma 2006;60(3):573–8.

54. Cullinane DC, Morris JA Jr, Bass JG et al. Needle thoracostomy may not be indicated in the trauma patient. Injury 2001;32(10):749–52.

55. Davis DP, Pettit K, Rom CD et al. The safety and efficacy of prehospital needle and tube thoracostomy by aeromedical personnel. Prehosp Emerg Care 2005;9(2):191–7.

56. Ball CG, Wyrzykowski AD, Kirkpatrick AW et al. Thoracic needle decompression for tension pneumothorax: clinical correlation with catheter length. Can J Surg 2010;53(3):184–8.

57. Kiser AC, O'Brien SM, Detterbeck FC. Blunt tracheobronchial injuries: treatment and outcomes. Ann Thorac Surg 2001;71(6):2059–65.

58. Besson A, Saegesser F. Chest trauma and associated injuries. Oradell: Medical Economics; 1983.

59. Brenner BE. Comprehensive management of respiratory emergencies. Rockville: Aspen Systems; 1985.

60. Mancini MC. Hemothorax. Emedicine; 2008. Online. http://emedicine.medscape.com/article/425518-overview; accessed 26 May 2010.

61. Chughtai T, Ali S, Sharkey P et al. Update on managing diaphragmatic rupture in blunt trauma: a review of 208 consecutive cases. Can J Surg 2009;52(3):177–81.

62. Sliker CW. Imaging of diaphragm injuries. Radiol Clin North Am 2006;44(2):199–211, vii.

63. Hammer M, Flagg E, Mellnick V, Cummings K et al. Computed tomography of blunt and penetrating diaphragmatic injury: sensitivity and inter-observer agreement of CT Signs. Emerg Radiol 2014;21(2):143–9.

64. Williams M, Carlin AM, Tyburski JG et al. Predictors of mortality in patients with traumatic diaphragmatic rupture and associated thoracic and/or abdominal injuries. Am Surg 2004;70(2):157–62.

65. Kozak O, Mentes O, Harlak A, Yigit T et al. Late presentation of blunt right diaphragmatic rupture (hepatic hernia). Am J Emerg Med 2008;26:e633–5.

66. Peker Y, Tatar F, Kahya MC et al. Dislocation of three segments of the liver due to hernia of the right diaphragm: report of a case and review of the literature. Hernia 2007;11:63–5.

67. Feghali NT, Prisant LM. Blunt myocardial injury. Chest 1995;108:1673–7.

68. Wisner DH, Reed WH, Riddick RS. Suspected myocardial contusion. Triage and indications for monitoring. Ann Surg 1990;212:82–6.

69. Fitzgerald M, Spencer J, Johnson F et al. Definitive management of acute cardiac tamponade secondary to blunt trauma. Emerg Med Australas 2005;17(5–6):494–9.

70. Sybrandy KC, Cramer MJ, Burgersdijk C. Diagnosing cardiac contusion: old wisdom and new insights. Heart 2003;89:485–9.

71. El-Chami M, Nicholson W, Helmy T. Blunt Chest Trauma. The Journal of Emergency Medicine 2008;35(2):127–33.

72. Velmahos GC, Karaiskakis M, Salim A et al. Normal electrocardiography and serum troponin I levels preclude the presence of clinically significant blunt cardiac injury. J Trauma 2003;54(1):45–50; discussion 50–51.

73. Fulda GJ, Giberson F, Hailstone D et al. An evaluation of serum troponin T and signal-averaged electrocardiography in predicting electrocardiographic abnormalities after blunt chest trauma. J Trauma 1997;43(2):304–10; discussion 310–12.

74. Maenza RL, Seaberg D, D'Amico F. A meta-analysis of blunt cardiac trauma: ending myocardial confusion. Am J Emerg Med 1996;14(3):237–41.

75. Turk EE, Tsokos M. Blunt cardiac trauma caused by fatal falls from height: an autopsy-based assessment of the injury pattern. J Trauma 2004;57(2):301–4.

76. Fildes JJ, Betlej TM, Manglano R et al. Limiting cardiac evaluation in patients with suspected myocardial contusion. Am Surg 1995;61(9):832–5.

77. Dowd MD, Krug S. Pediatric blunt cardiac injury: epidemiology, clinical features, and diagnosis. Pediatric Emergency Medicine Collaborative Research Committee: Working Group on Blunt Cardiac Injury. J Trauma 1996;40(1):61–7.

78. Curtis K, Asha S. Blunt cardiac injury as a result of a motor vehicle collision: a case study. Australas Emerg Nurs J 2010;13(4):124–9.

79. Salim A, Velmahos GC, Jindal A et al. Clinically significant blunt cardiac trauma: role of serum troponin levels combined with electrocardiographic findings. J Trauma 2001;50(2):237–43.

80. Rajan GP, Zellweger R. Cardiac troponin I as a predictor of arrhythmia and ventricular dysfunction in trauma patients with myocardial contusion. J Trauma 2004;57(4):801–8; discussion 808.

81. Sakka SG, Huettemann E, Glebe W et al. Late cardiac arrhythmias after blunt chest trauma. Intensive Care Med 2000;26(6):792–5.

82. Ferjani M, Droc G, Dreux S et al. Circulating cardiac troponin T in myocardial contusion. Chest 1997;111(2):427–33.

83. Bertinchant JP, Polge A, Mohty D et al. Evaluation of incidence, clinical significance, and prognostic value of circulating cardiac troponin I and T elevation in hemodynamically stable patients with suspected myocardial contusion after blunt chest trauma. J Trauma 2000;48(5):924–31.

84. Mori F, Zuppiroli A, Ognibene A et al. Cardiac contusion in blunt chest trauma: a combined study of transesophageal echocardiography and cardiac troponin I determination. Ital Heart J 2001;2(3):222–7.

85. Edouard AR, Felten ML, Hebert JL et al. Incidence and significance of cardiac troponin I release in severe trauma patients. Anesthesiology 2004;101(6):1262–8.

86. Thourani VH, Feliciano DV, Cooper WA et al. Penetrating cardiac trauma at an urban trauma center: a 22-year perspective. Am Surg 1999;65(9):811–16; discussion 817–18.

87. Mandavia DP, Joseph A. Bedside echocardiography in chest trauma. Emerg Med Clin North Am 2004;22(3):601–19.

88. Shanmuganathan K, Matsumoto J. Imaging of penetrating chest trauma. Radiol Clin North Am 2006;44(2):225–38, viii.

89. Harris DG, Bleeker CP, Pretorius J et al. Penetrating cardiac injuries: current evaluation and management of the stable patient. S Afr J Surg 2001;39(3):90–4.

90. Humphreys M. Pericardial conditions: signs, symptoms and electrocardiogram changes. Emerg Nurse 2006;14(1):30–6.

91. American College of Cardiology Foundation. Cardiovascular interventions. JACC 2009; 2(8):705–17.

92. Wang RF, Chao CC, Wang TL et al. The effect of different relieving methods on the outcome of out-of-hospital cardiac arrest patients with nontraumatic hemopericardium in the ED. Am J Emerg Med 2008;26(4):425–32.

93. Hunt PA, Greaves I, Owens WA. Emergency thoracotomy in thoracic trauma: a review. Injury 2006;37(1):1–19.

94. Hall BL, Buchman TG. A visual, timeline-based display of evidence for emergency thoracotomy. J Trauma 2005;59(3):773–7.

95. Bickell WH, Wall MJ Jr, Pepe PE et al. Immediate versus delayed fluid resuscitation for hypotensive patients with penetrating torso injuries. N Engl J Med 1994;331(17):1105–9.

96. Fabian TC, Davis KA, Gavant ML et al. Prospective study of blunt aortic injury: helical CT is diagnostic and antihypertensive therapy reduces rupture. Ann Surg 1998; 227:666.

97. Hershberger RC, Aulivola B, Murphy M et al. Endovascular grafts for treatment of traumatic injury to the aortic arch and great vessels. J Trauma 2009;67(3):660–71.

98. Broux C, Thony F, Chavanon O et al. Emergency endovascular stent graft repair for acute blunt thoracic aortic injury: a retrospective case control study. Intensive Care Med 2006;32(5):770–4. Epub 21 Mar 2006.

99. Hirose H, Gill IS, Malangoni MA. Nonoperative management of traumatic aortic injury. J Trauma 2006;60(3):597–601.

100. Christmas AB, Richardson JD. Treatment of Esophageal Injury. In Asensio JA, Trunkey DD eds. Current therapy of trauma and surgical critical care, Mosby, Elsevier; 2008.

101. Asensio JA, Demetriades D, Murray J et al. Penetrating esophageal injuries: Multicenter Study of the American Association for the Surgery of Trauma. J Trauma 2001;50:289–96.

102. Ivatury R, Moore F, Biffl W et al. Oesophageal injuries: Position paper, WSES, 2013 World Journal of Emergency Surgery 2014, 9:9.

103. Weigelt JA, Thal ER, Snyder WH et al. Diagnosis of penetrating cervical esophageal injuries. Am J Surg 1987;154(6):619–22.

104. Wu J, Mattox K, Wall Jr M. Esophageal perforations: new perspectives and treatment paradigms. J Trauma 2007;63:1173–84.

105. Richardson JD, Martin LF, Borzotta AP, Polk HC. Unifying concepts in treatment of esophageal leaks. Am J Surg 1985;149:157–62.

106. Asensio JA, Berne J, Demetriades D et al. Penetrating esophageal injuries: time interval of safety for preoperative evaluation—How long is safe? J Trauma 1997;43:319–24.

107. Symbas PN, Hatcher CR, Vlasis SE. Esophageal gunshot injuries. Ann Surg 1980;191:703–5.

108. McConnell DB, Trunkey DD. Management of penetrating trauma to the neck. Adv Surg 1994;27:97–127.

109. TE Madiba, DJJ Muckart, Ann R. Penetrating injuries to the cervical oesophagus: is routine exploration mandatory? Coll Surg Engl 2003;85:162–6.

110. McQuillan KA, Von Rueden KT, Hartsock RL et al. Trauma nursing from resuscitation through rehabilitation. 3rd edn. Philadelphia: WB Saunders; 2001.

111. Connell RA, Graham CA, Munro PT. Is spinal immobilisation necessary for all patients sustaining isolated penetrating trauma?. Injury 2003;34(12):912–14.

112. Browner BD, Levine AM, Jupiter JB et al. Skeletal trauma. 4th edn. St Louis: WB Saunders; 2008.

113. Atteberry LR, Dennis JW, Menawat SS et al. Physical examination alone is safe and accurate for evaluation of vascular injuries in penetrating Zone II neck trauma. J Am Coll Surg 1994;179(6):657–62.

114. Shiroff AM, Gale SC, Martin ND et al. Penetrating neck trauma: a review of management strategies and discussion of the 'No Zone' approach. Am Surg 2013;79:23.

115. Biffl WL, Moore EE, Ryu RK et al. The unrecognized epidemic of blunt carotid arterial injuries: early diagnosis improves neurologic outcome. Ann Surg 1998;228(4):462.

116. Berne JD, Norwood SH, McAuley CE et al. Helical computed tomographic angiography: an excellent screening test for blunt cerebrovascular injury. J Trauma 2004;57(1):11–19.

117. Biffl WL, Egglin T, Benedetto B et al. Sixteen-slice computed tomographic angiography is a reliable noninvasive screening test for clinically significant blunt cerebrovascular injuries. J Trauma 2006;60(4):745–52.

118. Eastman AL, Chason DP, Perez CL et al. Computed tomographic angiography for the diagnosis of blunt cervical vascular injury: is it ready for primetime? J Trauma 2006;60(5):925–9.

119. Rutherford RB. Vascular surgery. 6th edn. St Louis: Saunders; 2005.

120. Truitt MS et al. Continuous intercostal nerve blockade for rib fractures: Ready for primetime? Journal of Trauma—Injury, Infection and Critical Care 2011;71(6):1548–52.

121. Tighe S, Greene MD, Rajadurai N. Paravertebral block. Continuing Education in Anaesthesia, Critical Care and Pain 2010;10(5):133–7.

122. Standring, S. Thorax: overview and surface anatomy. In: Gray's Anatomy. 40th edn. Elsevier 2008.

123. Arnaud F, Tomori T, Teranishi K et al. Evaluation of chest seal performance in a swine model. Injury 2008;39(9):1082–8.

CHAPTER 48

ABDOMINAL AND GENITOURINARY TRAUMA

KATE KING, JULIE EVANS AND KATE CURTIS

Essentials

- The abdomen should be considered as a possible source of occult bleeding during the primary survey.
- A thorough examination should be repeated at regular intervals in the dynamic trauma patient.
- Late recognition of intra-abdominal injuries can lead to early death from haemorrhage or late death from visceral injuries.
- The management priority should be to stabilise the patient and optimise oxygenation and tissue perfusion.
- Contact a surgeon early if intra-abdominal is suspected.
- Follow local algorithms for blunt and penetrating abdominal injuries where possible to guide management.
- Consider early transfer to a tertiary hospital.

INTRODUCTION

Abdominal injury is a common result of trauma and, if undetected or inappropriately evaluated, can lead to significant morbidity and mortality. Blunt abdominal injury frequently arises as part of multisystem injury following road trauma, high falls, assaults and, much less frequently in Australia and New Zealand, penetrating injury. Accurate assessment, timely resuscitation and appropriate investigations are required to manage patients with abdominal trauma. The last decade has seen many changes in the way abdominal trauma is investigated and managed, and strong team leadership is required to appropriately triage injuries and prioritise investigations and management in the patient with multisystem injuries. In patients where the abdomen is the compelling source of haemorrhage, the priority of the trauma team is to get the patient to the operating room or the interventional radiology suite for definitive treatment as soon as possible.

Epidemiology

Abdominal trauma can be divided in two main mechanisms: blunt and penetrating. The United States, South Africa and some South American countries such as Colombia have a high incidence of penetrating injuries from both stab and gunshot wounds. The majority of hospital admissions in Australia and New Zealand are as a result of blunt trauma, although in certain Australian urban areas penetrating injury has increased significantly in recent years.[1]

Approximately one-third of polytrauma patients have an abdominal injury,[2] and up to 10% of these patients will have some form of genitourinary (GU) trauma, with renal trauma occurring in 1–5% of all traumas.[3] Bladder, urethral, ureter, penile and scrotal trauma make up the remainder of GU trauma. GU trauma is also common in children, but rarely requires surgical management.[4] The kidneys of children have less peritoneal fat, are large in comparison with the abdomen as a whole and have a thinner capsule for protection.[5] Children also have a weaker abdominal musculature and a less ossified rib cage, which offers less kidney protection.[6] Blunt urological injury, the most common form of trauma, accounts for 70–80% of all urological injuries.[7]

Of patients who survive major trauma and are transported to hospital, there are two significant mortality peaks in abdominal trauma patients.

- The first peak occurs early in the emergency department (ED) or operating room (OR), and is a result of significant damage to either abdominal vascular structures or gross injury to vital organ systems. The majority of haemodynamically unstable patients diagnosed with abdominal haemorrhage require emergency abdominal surgery to control bleeding; a small proportion of this population may benefit from interventional radiology treatments such as angioembolisation.[8] It may be necessary to consider damage-control surgery or definitive surgery in these patients, which is discussed later in the chapter.

- The second mortality peak is for patients who survive the initial phase of resuscitation and management but remain susceptible to the sequelae of major trauma. These patients are at risk of developing systemic inflammatory response syndrome (SIRS). If SIRS is associated with infection then sepsis may develop and can progress to multi-organ dysfunction syndrome (MODS). Although MODS is by definition multifactorial, abdominal complications, including anastomotic leaks, peritoneal contamination, abdominal compartment syndrome and haemorrhage are all significant contributing factors.

Anatomy

The abdomen extends from the thoracic diaphragm to the pelvic brim. Organs in the abdominal cavity include the liver, spleen, gallbladder, stomach, pancreas, kidneys, bladder, lower oesophagus and large and small intestines. The spleen, liver and kidneys are solid organs. The stomach and intestines are hollow organs. Solid organs fracture when injured; hollow organs collapse or rupture. The vascular structures in the abdominal cavity include the aorta, vena cava, hepatic vein, iliac artery and the iliac vein. Most of these structures are found in the peritoneal space, and for the purposes of physical assessment are divided into four quadrants (Fig 48.1). Functions of gastrointestinal (GI) and GU system organs are presented in Chapters 24 and 25, and are discussed below in relation to trauma.

Peritoneum

Contained within the peritoneal cavity are the majority of the abdominal organs, including the liver, spleen, stomach, small bowel, parts of the duodenum and parts of the large bowel. The peritoneum is the largest serous membrane in the body, having a surface area about equal to that of the skin, and it is composed of a thin layer of squamous cells resting on a layer of connective tissue. It is made up of the parietal peritoneum, visceral peritoneum, the peritoneal cavity, the retroperitoneal space and the mesentery. The parietal peritoneum lines the abdominal wall. The visceral peritoneum covers the abdominal organs. In females, the peritoneal cavity is continuous with the external environment via the fallopian tubes, the uterus and the vagina. The peritoneal cavity is closed in males.

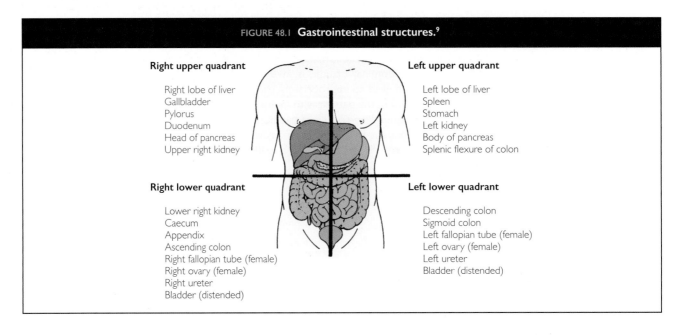

FIGURE 48.1 **Gastrointestinal structures.**[9]

Right upper quadrant

Right lobe of liver
Gallbladder
Pylorus
Duodenum
Head of pancreas
Upper right kidney

Left upper quadrant

Left lobe of liver
Spleen
Stomach
Left kidney
Body of pancreas
Splenic flexure of colon

Right lower quadrant

Lower right kidney
Caecum
Appendix
Ascending colon
Right fallopian tube (female)
Right ovary (female)
Right ureter
Bladder (distended)

Left lower quadrant

Descending colon
Sigmoid colon
Left fallopian tube (female)
Left ovary (female)
Left ureter
Bladder (distended)

The retroperitoneal space is the area posterior to the peritoneum. It contains the kidneys, major blood vessels and the reproductive organs in females. The mesentery consists of a double layer of peritoneum. This layer encloses organs and connects them to the abdominal wall. Folds of the mesentery are known as the greater and lesser omentum.

Vascular structures

The arterial blood supply for the abdominal cavity is the aorta. The abdominal aorta sits to the left of the midline in the abdominal cavity. It bifurcates into the iliac arteries at the pelvic brim. The iliac arteries supply blood to the lower extremities. The abdominal organs are supplied by three arteries originating from the abdominal aorta—the coeliac trunk (which branches into the hepatic, left gastric and splenic arteries), the superior mesentery artery and the inferior mesentery artery (Fig 48.2). The inferior vena cava, formed by the union of the two common iliac veins, is the major vein in the abdomen. Venous drainage is more complex than the arterial supply. Blood is drained from the small intestines, stomach, spleen and pancreas through the superior mesenteric and splenic veins and their tributaries, which join to form the portal vein, ultimately emptying into the hepatic veins and vena cava (Fig 48.3).

Genitourinary system

The GU system consists of the kidneys, ureters, bladder and urethra (Ch 25). Kidneys are retroperitoneal organs that lie high on the posterior abdominal wall. The right kidney, 1–2 cm lower than the left, lies inferior and posterior to the liver and posterior to the ascending colon and duodenum. The left kidney lies posterior to the descending colon and is associated with the tail of the pancreas medially and the spleen superiorly. Ureters are small muscular tubes that are flexible and mobile and drain urine from the kidneys to the bladder. The ureters are rarely injured in blunt abdominal trauma because of their deep location in the retroperitoneal space and added protection from abdominal contents, spine and surrounding muscles. The bladder is an extraperitoneal hollow organ located in the pelvis that is well protected by pelvic bones laterally, urogenital diaphragm inferiorly and the rectum posteriorly. Blood supply is abundant and mainly derived from branches of the internal iliac artery. In the male the prostate gland lies adjacent to the inferior margin and is fixed to the pubis anteriorly by ligaments and inferiorly by the urogenital diaphragm. The female urethra is short and well protected by the symphysis pubis. In the male the urethra is approximately 20 cm long and lies predominantly outside the body. The urogenital diaphragm divides the urethra into posterior and anterior segments.

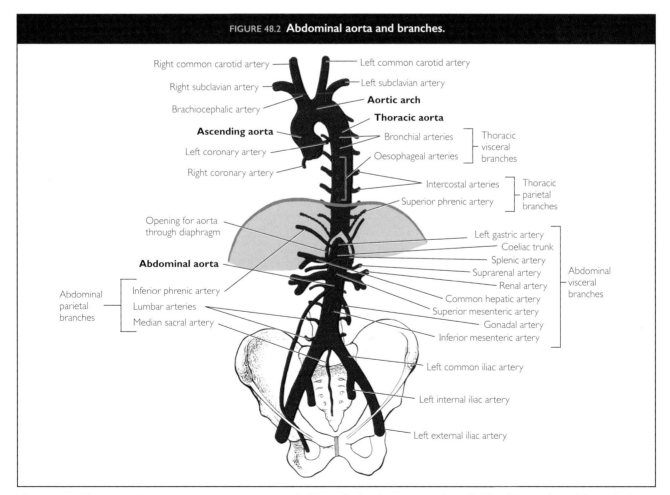

FIGURE 48.2 Abdominal aorta and branches.

The aorta is the main systemic artery, serving as a trunk from which other arteries branch. Blood is conducted from the heart first through the ascending aorta, then the arch of the aorta, then through the thoracic and abdominal segments of the descending aorta.[10]

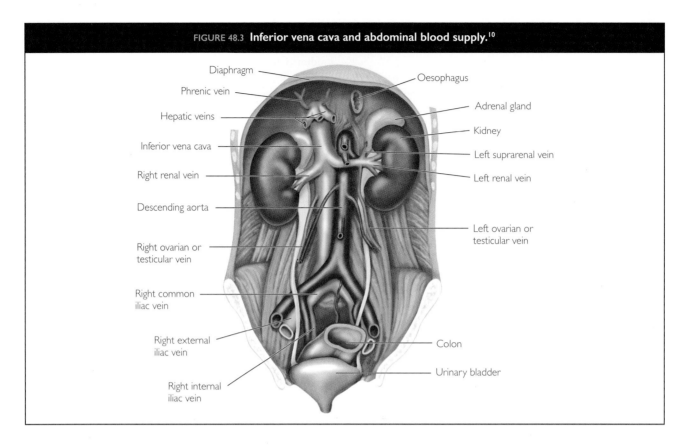

FIGURE 48.3 **Inferior vena cava and abdominal blood supply.**[10]

Mechanism of injury

The most common mechanisms of injury for abdominal injuries are motor vehicle collisions (MVCs), interpersonal violence and falls.[1] Information provided from the pre-hospital scene can assist the emergency department (ED) nurse in predicting injury patterns.

Pre-hospital considerations

The priority of care for the patient with an abdominal injury remains the same: undertake a primary survey and treat any abnormalities according to local protocols before progressing to a secondary survey. The paramedic needs to have a good understanding of the anatomy of the abdomen and the effects of injury.

- If the patient has a solid organ injury they are likely to bleed and therefore demonstrate signs of hypovolaemic shock.
- If the patient has a hollow organ injury they are likely to display signs of peritonism, although this is a later sign, so may not be present in the pre-hospital setting.
- If the patient has injured any of the major vessels of the abdomen, the patient will bleed heavily and is at risk of exsanguination.

Paramedics should have a high index of suspicion for abdominal injury based on mechanism, obvious external trauma to the abdomen, shock with no other identifiable cause, diffuse tenderness over the abdomen or signs of referred pain, such as phrenic nerve pain felt in the shoulder tip. The most reliable signs in the field for abdominal injury are pain and/or deranged vital signs. A rigid abdomen is an unreliable sign. It is not necessary to diagnose the exact injury, as there is little that can

be done in the pre-hospital setting. It is important to treat the clinical signs and transport the patient to the most appropriate hospital, preferably to a trauma centre so the patient can receive definitive treatment. Communication with the receiving hospital will improve hospital trauma team response times. With penetrating injuries, if the object is still impaled leave it in place and secure for transport and consider securing for forensic evidence. If the patient has an open abdomen with evisceration, do not attempt to put the contents back in; just cover with a wet dressing and transport the patient. As with all trauma patients, basic pre-hospital care for those with abdominal injuries should involve maintenance of airway, breathing and circulation (ABC), oxygenation, cannulation and timely transport according to local transport protocols.

PRACTICE TIP

Limit pre-hospital fluids to avoid over-resuscitation sequelae such as coagulopathy and abdominal compartment syndrome.

Initial assessment and management

All trauma patients are assessed using the primary survey, and those fulfilling trauma call criteria should receive trauma team activation (Ch 44). Patients with abdominal injury suspected from the mechanism of injury, the physical signs or associated injuries, should be triaged with a high priority and assessed and treated in the resuscitation room. The trauma team must maintain a high index of suspicion for abdominal injury in all trauma patients and have a low threshold for transfer to a trauma centre for investigation and referral to general/trauma surgeons.

Abdominal assessment

Although a full abdominal assessment is not part of the primary survey, evaluation of the abdomen as a source of bleeding is an integral part of the circulation aspect of the primary survey. The purpose of the initial clinical assessment in the unstable patient is to confirm or exclude the abdomen as a source of concealed bleeding that requires immediate surgery, for example by using focused assessment with sonography for trauma (FAST), which in some practice environments is also being used in the pre-hospital setting.[11] During the secondary survey, the abdominal assessment is systematic and should be repeated throughout all phases of care, preferably by the same clinician to provide the consistency necessary to evaluate changes. On the change-over of shift, the assessment should preferably be conducted together with the relieving staff member, and at the very least thoroughly communicated and documented.

Complaint of abdominal pain from an alert patient is indicative of abdominal injury, although many patients have an altered level of consciousness or distracting injury, and may be unable to provide reliable information. The four-step abdominal assessment, including inspection, auscultation, percussion and palpation, is essential. The initial clinical examination of the abdomen can often be misleading for the unwary. Blood may cause little peritoneal irritation initially; and drugs, alcohol, head injury and other distracting injuries can act to mask abdominal signs. If an abdominal injury is suspected, serial abdominal examinations by one practitioner can assist in early detection of deterioration, especially if radiology capabilities are limited.

Immediate resuscitation considerations

Several evidence-based algorithms guiding the clinician on penetrating and blunt abdominal trauma management have been developed over recent years (Figs 48.4 and 48.5). In the unstable patient with identified abdominal haemorrhage, following the stabilisation of airway and breathing the priority of the trauma team is to expedite the patient's movement to the operating room for surgery. An organised and coordinated team approach is vital to achieve this. Other patients with less-catastrophic injuries may respond rapidly to the initial fluid resuscitation and allow time for more-detailed investigation; however, subsequent cardiovascular deterioration in the light of suspected abdominal injuries requires definitive treatment such as surgery. It is important for the ED nurse to be aware of the indications for laparotomy (Box 48.1) to facilitate rapid transfer to definitive care.

Most institutions follow damage control resuscitation principles (Ch 44), which includes limiting fluid administration to the amount sufficient to maintain perfusion of the vital

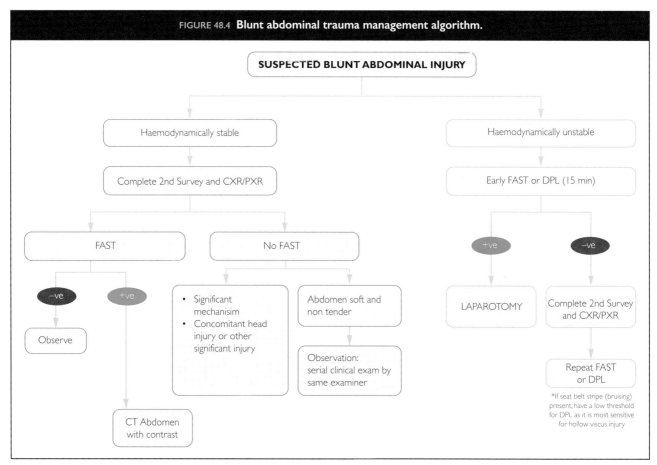

FIGURE 48.4 **Blunt abdominal trauma management algorithm.**

CT: computed tomography; CXR: chest X-ray; DPL: diagnostic peritoneal lavage; FAST: focused assessment sonography for trauma; PXR: pelvic X-ray.

Courtesy Liverpool Hospital Trauma Service, Sydney, NSW.

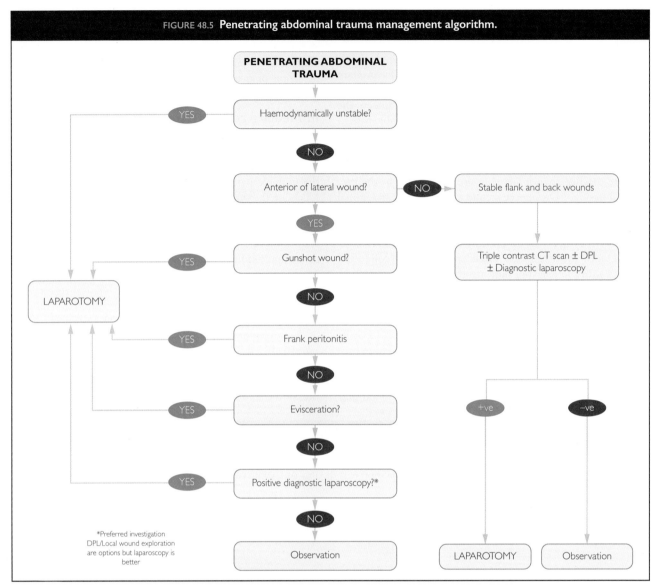

FIGURE 48.5 **Penetrating abdominal trauma management algorithm.**

CT: computed tomography; DPL: diagnostic peritoneal lavage.
Courtesy Liverpool Hospital Trauma Service, Sydney, NSW.

BOX 48.1   Indications for laparotomy[12]

- Gross haemodynamic instability
- Evisceration
- Gunshot wound to abdomen/thorax
- Positive FAST with haemodynamic instability
- Stab wound with peritoneum breached
- Ongoing haemodynamic instability despite correction of estimated blood loss from extra-abdominal sites
- Frank peritonitis (initially or on repeat examination)
- Free gas on plain radiography
- Ruptured diaphragm
- Positive diagnostic peritoneal lavage
- Clinical deterioration during observation of suspected intra-abdominal injury

FAST: Focused assessment with sonography for trauma

---

organs. Robust data on this approach—permissive hypotension in the context of damage control resuscitation (systolic blood pressure 80–90 mmHg)[13,14]—is limited, although some research in penetrating trauma suggests that it confers a survival advantage.[15] There is a theoretical basis for applying this principle to all trauma victims (with the exception of head injuries and blast injuries[16] where it may have a detrimental effect) and resuscitating patients to a blood pressure sufficient to maintain perfusion of vital organs.[17] Hypotensive resuscitation is most likely to benefit those patients who have developed tamponade of their bleeding source. However, the priority in these patients remains rapid transfer of the patient to the operating room for surgical haemorrhage control (Ch 44).

History

The mechanism of injury (Ch 43) is important as it provides information on the likely forces involved and potential injuries. In addition, patient signs and symptoms and response to treatment must be obtained from pre-hospital personnel.

Unconscious patients, or those with obvious injuries above and below the abdomen, have abdominal injury until proven otherwise.

Blunt or penetrating lower chest trauma can result in an abdominal injury, and should therefore be suspected, even in circumstances where the mechanism of injury does not appear to have directly affected the abdomen. The clinician's suspicions should be raised for splenic or liver injury if the patient has lower rib fractures. Seat-belt bruising carries a high association with chance fractures of T12/L1 and bowel injury, although the appearance of bruising can be delayed.[18] Lumbar spine fractures from seat-belt acceleration/deceleration injury also have a high association with bowel perforation. The probability of abdominal injury increases significantly at velocities > 20 kph, age > 75 years or the presence of head, leg or chest injuries, even at low velocities.[19] GU trauma is divided into upper urinary tract, lower urinary tract and genital injuries, and should be considered in patients with severe lower abdominal blunt trauma and pelvic fracture. Urinary tract injury should also be suspected for all patients with penetrating injuries to the abdomen, chest or flank until proven otherwise.

PRACTICE TIP

The two mnemonics that are useful for history-taking are MIST and AMPLE (Ch 14).

Inspection

Inspect the abdomen, flank, back and perineum for contusions, abrasions, lacerations, penetrating injuries, impaled foreign bodies, evisceration and pregnancy. This involves removal of all patient clothing and, as with all trauma patients, conducting a log-roll, keeping in mind the importance of re-covering the patient, preventing heat loss and maintaining patient dignity. Bruising that mirrors location of the seatbelt (seatbelt sign [SBS]) may be evident on admission to the ED, but usually does not occur for several hours after injury. There is some debate about the predictive nature of SBS and abdominal injuries, especially in the paediatric population.[20,21] Distension may be noted; however, it is not a reliable sign (2 L of intraperitoneal fluid increases abdominal girth by only 1.9 cm). Common signs of abdominal injury are listed in Table 48.1.

Consider old scars from previous abdominal surgery; this can provide information about past medical history as well as providing a warning sign for internal scarring and adhesions.

Auscultation

Auscultation of the abdomen can provide helpful information; however, it is usually difficult to hear percussion sounds in the middle of a trauma resuscitation. Auscultation can also provide helpful information about the presence or absence of bowel sounds. Absence of bowel sounds does not confirm intra-abdominal injury; the absence may be due to shock or to the presence of an ileus. Significantly decreased or absent bowel sounds have been reported in more than 50% of documented injuries. On the other hand, absent bowel sounds occur in a significant number (20%) of patients with no injuries at laparotomy.[23] Serial auscultation demonstrating a change in bowel sounds (i.e. diminishing or disappearing) is more diagnostic of abdominal trauma, peritonitis and/or ileus. Bowel sounds in the thorax may indicate a perforated diaphragm with herniation of the stomach or small bowel into the chest.[24]

Percussion

Percussion of the abdomen is also of little practical value in the busy resuscitation room. The aim of percussion of the abdomen is to identify the presence of air, fluid or tissue. Tympanic sounds indicate air-filled spaces such as stomach or gut, and a dull sound is present over organ structures.[25]

Palpation

The abdomen is palpated carefully for pain, rigidity, tenderness and guarding, examining all four quadrants, progressing from light to deep palpation. Tenderness is the most frequent and reliable sign of abdominal injury of the corresponding underlying organs (Fig 48.1). Palpation should commence on the side of no pain. Guarding and rebound tenderness are associated with peritoneal irritation, from either blood or bowel contents. However, even large amounts of blood can cause remarkably little peritoneal irritation and only very subtle signs on examination. The patient may experience referred pain, most commonly Kehr's sign, which is pain in the left shoulder tip secondary to diaphragmatic irritation caused by intra abdominal blood most commonly from splenic rupture (Table 48.1), although alterations in Glasgow Coma Scale (GCS) scores, distracting injury and drugs can mask these subtle signs.

TABLE 48.1 Common signs of abdominal injury[22]		
SIGN	DESCRIPTION	SUSPECTED INJURY
Grey Turner's sign	Bluish discolouration of the lower abdomen and flanks 6–24 hours after onset of bleeding	Retroperitoneal haemorrhage
Kehr's sign	Left shoulder-tip pain caused by diaphragmatic irritation	Splenic injury, although can be associated with any intra-abdominal bleeding
Cullen's sign	Bluish discolouration around the umbilicus	Pancreatic injury, although can be associated with any peritoneal bleeding
Coopernail's sign	Ecchymosis of scrotum or labia	Pelvic fracture or pelvic organ injury

Pelvic springing is controversial. If the pelvis is to be 'sprung', only one clinician should do it. In addition to causing unnecessary pain to the patient, springing can dislodge clots that have tamponaded haemorrhage and cause further damage to muscle, vessels and other structures by bone fragments via a tearing/shearing force. An AP pelvic X-ray will almost always be attended to; therefore, unstable pelvic injuries can be identified without the need for pelvic springing. Haemorrhage from this area needs to be excluded by investigating the retroperitoneum.

Rectal examination includes testing for gross blood and anterior tenderness which can indicate active bleeding or peritoneal irritation. A small group of patients will have an obviously distended or rigid abdomen; however, where the abdominal assessment is equivocal special investigations must be used early and appropriately. A vaginal examination should be conducted if an injury is suspected.

Genitourinary trauma assessment

Rapid diagnosis and treatment of GU trauma can be very difficult because it seldom occurs independently and is often associated with abdominal injuries. The first rule of urological trauma management is to aggressively seek and diagnose urological injury, because many of these injuries are not obvious at the onset. Preexisting renal abnormalities can predispose the kidney to severe injury from even minor trauma, and previous injuries to the GU tract may have caused chronic urological infections and adhesions.

Certain mechanisms of injury carry a higher incidence of GU trauma, such as motor vehicle collisions (MVCs), assaults and high falls.[7] Several patterns of contusion and bruising are specific to GU injuries. Grey Turner's sign is bruising over the flank and lower back that occurs in retroperitoneal haematoma and is frequently present with pelvic fractures (Table 48.1). An oedematous and contused scrotum and perineal bruising may be seen with straddle injuries, pelvic fractures or dissecting retroperitoneal haematomas. Fractures of the 11th and 12th ribs have an increased potential for renal injury. Male genitalia are more easily examined than female genitalia. Laceration and avulsion injuries to the penis[26] and scrotum[27] are immediately apparent.

The abdomen is gently palpated for presence of a distended bladder—an empty bladder is not palpable. It is important to note that a full bladder may indicate the inability to void. If the patient cannot urinate, the urinary meatus should be checked carefully for blood. Blood at the meatus is a cardinal sign for anterior urethral injury. A digital rectal examination provides information on condition of the prostate gland and posterior urethra, as well as spinal cord integrity. A high-riding prostate or boggy mass may indicate a posterior rupture of the urethra, but this is not always a reliable sign in young adult men.[4] Extravasated urine and blood can dislocate the prostate. Haematuria is the best indicator of GU trauma.[28] Radiological tests are discussed later in this chapter relative to specific injuries.

The pregnant patient with abdominal trauma

In Australia and New Zealand, the incidence of abdominal trauma in the pregnant patient is rare and the vast majority suffer no obstetric complication;[29] although worldwide, traumatic injury is the principal non-obstetric cause of maternal death and 7% of pregnant women suffer from trauma.[30,31] Blunt abdominal injury, even with seemingly minor mechanism of injury, can produce placental abruption and may cause uterine rupture.[32,33] Compared with other sites, abdominal trauma is associated more often with uterine contractions, premature labour and a positive Kleihauer-Betke (KB) test (used to detect transplacental haemorrhage enabling Rhesus-negative women to receive appropriate Rh(D) Immunoglobulin (anti-D)). KB testing to predict placental abruption is controversial.[34,35]

Approximately 3–10% of those injured sustain various degrees of damage to the uterus, placenta and fetus secondary to penetrating trauma,[36] with a maternal mortality rate less than 5%.[37–40] This low mortality rate is due to the protective effects of the gravid uterus, which can efficiently absorb projectile energy.[41,42] However, fetal mortality can be as high as 70%, which is a result of direct missile injury or the effects of prematurity.[39,43] Penetrating wounds to the upper abdomen can produce complex injuries because displacement of the small bowel cephalad has been caused by the enlarged uterus. Depending on clinical status and the location of the wound and bullet, the pregnant penetrating trauma patient can be managed non-operatively.[44] However, when surgery is required, laparotomy alone is not an indication for delivery of the fetus, although delivery of the viable fetus by caesarean delivery should occur if the gravid uterus obstructs operative field exposure or evidence of fetal distress is noted.[44] Delivery of a viable fetus within the first 5 minutes of cardiopulmonary resuscitation results in the highest infant survival rate without neurological dysfunction.[37]

Assessment and management

The pregnant trauma patient presents a major challenge to clinicians. The physiological changes that occur during pregnancy may significantly alter the clinical presentation of the patient (see Ch 35). Table 48.2 outlines some of the physiological changes that occur during pregnancy.[45] Pregnancy also distorts maternal anatomy. During the third trimester, the maternal blood volume increases significantly and the pregnant trauma patient may lose up to 35% (1.5–2 L) of their circulating blood volume without showing any overt signs of hypovolaemia.[46,47] Hence, the priority in the management of a pregnant patient who has sustained major trauma must always be maternal stabilisation. Fetal survival is best ensured

TABLE 48.2 Common physiological changes during pregnancy[47]

SYSTOLIC BLOOD PRESSURE	Decreases by 5–15 mmHg
DIASTOLIC BLOOD PRESSURE	Decreases by 5–15 mmHg
HEART RATE	Increases by 10–15 beats/minute
BLOOD VOLUME	Increases by 30–50%
CARDIAC OUTPUT	Increases by 30–50%
OXYGEN CONSUMPTION	Increases by 10%

with maternal resuscitation and adequate perfusion and oxygenation of the placenta; therefore high-flow oxygen should be mandatory until all injuries have been identified.[47]

When the pregnant trauma patient is laid supine, the gravid uterus compresses the inferior vena cava impairing blood flow. To avoid this, the patient should be nursed with a 15-degree angle towards the left. If spinal injury is suspected, a wedge can be placed under the patient's right side without compromising spinal alignment.[45-48] Standard trauma radiological imaging for pregnant trauma patients is the same as for their non-pregnant counterparts. Shielding of the fetus during X-rays and consultation with a radiologist may be beneficial if multiple imaging is required.[47,49]

Fetal distress may occur subtly without overt clinical signs, and obstetric area monitoring should take place for a period of several hours.[50] Patients with viable gestations require at least 6 hours of cardiotocographic monitoring (CTG) after even minor trauma.[31,51] Pregnant trauma patients should be assessed simultaneously where possible by the trauma team and the obstetric team.[52]

Investigations

The abdomen is a major source of missed injury and inadequate recognition of intra-abdominal bleeding.[45] Studies have highlighted the importance of rapid accurate abdominal investigation. The introduction of technology such as focused assessment sonography in trauma (FAST) and further sophisti-cation of computed tomography (CT) in the assessment of the abdomen should allow rapid and accurate diagnosis of injury. The merits of these technologies are summarised in Table 48.3. However, these tools are generally not available in the rural setting and the choice of investigation should be based on technical merit and individual patient circumstances.

Focused assessment sonography in trauma

Focused assessment sonography in trauma (FAST) is a focused ultrasound examination to assess for free intra-abdominal or pericardial fluid, consisting of examination of four areas (Fig 48.6). FAST is a rapid, reproducible, portable and non-invasive bedside test that may be performed simultaneously with ongoing resuscitation.[54-57] These characteristics, along with research demonstrating that trained ED doctors and surgeons can perform FAST accurately,[53,58] have enabled FAST to become accepted as the bedside investigation of choice in abdominal trauma.[59,60] It is also being used in the pre-hospital setting with small portable devices, and some large trauma centres are training their senior nursing staff to perform FAST.[61] It has also been shown to reduce CT and DPL rates in major trauma centres.[62] Modifications in the use of FAST to include assessment of the retroperitoneum and extremities[63] depend on the experience of the operator and have not yet been well evaluated in the literature.[62] In recent years the introduction of the extended focused assessment sonography in trauma (eFAST) has allowed operators to assess the thorax for

---

TABLE 48.3 Comparison of abdominal CT, DPL and ultrasound for investigation of abdominal trauma[12]

ABDOMINAL CT	DPL	ULTRASOUND
Advantages		
Anatomical information	Rapid, cheap, sensitive	Rapid, portable, repeatable
Non-invasive	Minimal training	Non-invasive
Visualises retroperitoneum	Ideal in unstable patients	Ideal in unstable patients
Also views chest, pelvis	Can be done in resuscitation room	Can be done in resuscitation room
		Also views heart, lungs, pelvis
Disadvantages		
Not suitable for unstable patients	Not organ-specific	Requires specific training
Requires transport from resuscitation room	False-negatives	Operator-dependent
Patient safety	Retroperitoneal injuries	False-negatives
Inaccessible while scanning	Hollow viscus injury	Retroperitoneal injuries
Time	Diaphragm injury	Hollow viscus injury
Cost	Iatrogenic injury	Diaphragm injury
False-negatives	Fluid and gas introduced during the procedure interfere with subsequent imaging	False-positives
Hollow viscus injuries		Ascites
IV contrast reactions		
Radiation exposure		

CT: computed tomography; DPL: diagnostic peritoneal lavage; IV: intravenous

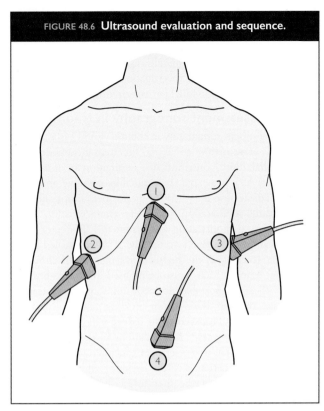

FIGURE 48.6 **Ultrasound evaluation and sequence.**

1, pericardial (subxiphoid); **2**, Morison's pouch (RUQ);
3, splenorenal (LUQ); **4**, pelvis (Douglas' pouch).[58]

pneumothoraces and/or haemothoraces with greater sensitivity than plain radiographs (see Ch 47).[64]

While there is no doubt about the accuracy of FAST in detecting free fluid in the abdominal or pericardial space,[53,54,65–70] limitations to the use of FAST have been recognised.[71–74] The technique does not assess specific organ integrity or function; it is operator-dependent,[75] may miss hollow viscus injury[71,76] and has a low sensitivity between 73% and 88%.[77] An unstable patient with a positive FAST should have an urgent laparotomy; however, a negative FAST either must be repeated or an alternative investigation performed as FAST is unreliable in ruling out injury, especially in penetrating trauma where the sensitivity is only 50%.[64]

> **PRACTICE TIP**
>
> A negative FAST scan does not exclude intra-abdominal injury.

Plain radiograph

While a plain abdominal film is of little use in trauma, an anteroposterior (AP) pelvic X-ray is recommended in the assessment of patients suspected of multisystem blunt trauma.[79] A pelvic X-ray should be conducted as an adjunct to the primary survey. If a pelvic fracture is identified it alerts the clinician to have a higher index of suspicion for occult bleeding, particularly in the retroperitoneum. It is important to obtain a chest film, as thoracic injury is frequently associated with abdominal injury. In patients who

have penetrating injuries and are haemodynamically stable, a plain abdominal film with metal markers at the entry and exit sites can provide information on the trajectory. Trauma patients requiring further abdominal assessment and potential surgery should be transferred to a trauma centre as soon as possible.

Initial radiographic evaluation of penetrating GU wounds consists of plain radiographs of the kidneys, ureters and bladder (KUB) to determine the path and appearance of the projectile. An abdominal X-ray may reveal loss of normal renal outline, loss of psoas muscle shadow on the affected side, scoliosis away from the kidney and a flank mass.[78] The KUB does not rule out renal trauma, but does heighten the examiner's awareness of possible injury.[6] Intravenous pyelogram (IVP) is used in haemodynamically unstable patients with massive haemorrhaging and who require immediate laparotomy. Usually, contrast is injected, then one radiograph is taken. However, an IVP has significant limitations in assessing associated intra-abdominal injuries and staging renal injuries.[79] CT and CT angiogram are the imaging of choice in the haemodynamically stable patient.

Diagnostic peritoneal aspiration and lavage

Diagnostic peritoneal lavage, first developed in 1964, is used to determine the presence of intra-abdominal blood and/or gastric content in the haemodynamically unstable patient requiring emergency abdominal assessment.[80] For example, if the patient requires life-saving neurosurgical intervention and there is suspicion of abdominal injury, a DPL can be conducted in the operating suite; or if the patient is too unstable to be transferred to CT and the abdomen needs to be excluded as a haemorrhage source, a DPL could be conducted in the ED. Insertion of a urinary catheter to empty the bladder and a gastric tube to decompress the stomach are essential to prevent injury to the organs during DPL.

An incision is made through the abdominal wall 2 cm below the umbilicus, and a catheter is introduced. Immediate return/aspiration of fluid or blood when the catheter is inserted is considered positive and the patient is prepared for laparotomy. Otherwise, 1 L of warmed Normal saline or Lactated Ringer's solution is infused into the abdomen. The fluid bag is then placed below the patient to allow gravity drainage of the fluid back into the bag. A positive DPL is indicated by exit of lavage fluid out of other catheters (e.g. intercostal), obvious drainage of intestinal material or bile, or bloodstaining of the lavage fluid.[16] A sample of the fluid is then sent for red and white cell and bacteria counts. Table 48.4 gives parameters for a positive DPL test.

DPL has a 1% complication rate and results in a 10–15% incidence of non-therapeutic laparotomy[82] when surgery is undertaken based on the findings of 100,000 red cells or 500 white cells per mL. A DPL should not be performed in a patient if there is a clear indication for laparotomy. DPL is an invasive procedure with a documented sensitivity of up to 98%.[77] As technology has advanced with the development of high-quality, portable ultrasound machines and the FAST technique, the role of DPL has reduced, although it is still a valuable investigation to confirm a negative FAST in the unstable patient or if ultrasound is not available.

TABLE 48.4 Peritoneal lavage results for blunt trauma[81]

	RESULT	INDICATION
Aspirant	Gross blood >10 mL	Positive
	Pink fluid	Intermediate*
	Clean	Negative
Lavage fluid	Bloody	Positive
	Clear	Negative
Red blood cells	> 100,000 cells/mm³	Positive
	50,000–100,000 cells/mm³	Intermediate*
White blood cells	> 500 cells/mm³	Positive
	100–500 cells/mm³	Intermediate*
Amylase	> 175 U/100 mL	Positive
	75–175 U/100 mL	Intermediate*
	< 75 U/100 mL	Negative
Bacteria	Present	Positive
Faecal material	Present	Positive
Bile	Present	Positive
Food particles	Present	Positive

*Intermediate lavage results require further observation of the patient, possibly repeated lavage, and intervention based on clinical presentation

Diagnostic peritoneal aspiration (DPA) is similar to DPL but without the lavage of 1 L of fluid. A DPA is used when the patient is haemodynamically unstable and the abdomen needs to be excluded as a source of blood loss. It is reported as more sensitive than a FAST scan in predicting blood loss and can be done quickly; often in less than a minute.[83] DPA is a valid option where there is no accredited FAST scan operator available.

Computed tomography

Computed tomography (CT) is the investigation of choice in haemodynamically stable trauma patients. It provides accurate evaluation of the abdomen and retroperitoneum and is increasingly used in both blunt trauma patients and in penetrating ballistic trauma for the evaluation of trajectory and subsequent appropriate surgical approach if required. It is also the best investigative modality to diagnose renal injury, particularly when used with intravenous (IV) contrast. Many institutions have developed CT protocols that encompass scans of the head, cervical spine, chest, abdomen and pelvis in patients with blunt multisystem injury known as a whole body scan or a Pan Scan. Such an approach also allows evaluation of the thoracic and lumbar spine and reformatting of the images for coronal and sagittal views. Whole body CTs have been shown to improve survival in both haemodymically stable and

unstable patients,[84] although clinical assessment should guide the need for the considerable radiation exposure.[85]

CT can demonstrate specific organ injury, allowing non-operative management protocols to be followed for low-grade injuries to the liver, spleen or kidney. In relation to the kidney, it delineates the grade of injury, shows infarcted segments, renal parenchymal injuries such as contusions, lacerations, renal fractures, subcapsular haematomas and renal pedicle injury. It also depicts the size and extent of retroperitoneal haematomas, urine extravasation and evaluates associated intra-abdominal injuries.[79] CT does, however, have varying degrees of sensitivity for hollow viscous injury because it is sometimes difficult to determine the significance of bowel-wall thickening or small pockets of free air.[86] Any patient with a high index of suspicion for abdominal injury with a negative initial CT scan should have serial abdominal clinical exams performed. Diagnostic sensitivity and accuracy may be related to the experience of the technician performing the scan and of the clinician interpreting the scan.[86] Very fast spiral CT provides shorter scanning time, but injury to the renal collecting system may be missed, so delayed scans are needed to rule out urinary extravasation.[4] CT cannot differentiate various causes of traumatic vascular occlusion such as thrombosis, vascular tears, avulsions, intimal tears and spasm.

CT is not appropriate for unstable patients who may rapidly deteriorate while in the scanner. Although modern machines can complete scans in seconds, time is required to transport, load and unload the patient. It is essential that prior to transport, the ED nurse has and is familiar with appropriate, functioning monitoring and transport equipment. Heat loss and excess movement should be minimised. The use of oral contrast has not been demonstrated to increase the diagnostic accuracy of abdominal injury.[88–93] In addition, its administration delays CT scanning and puts the supine, immobilised patient at risk of aspiration.[94,95]

Serial abdominal examination

Serial abdominal examination (SAE), using the four-step approach as previously described, is an alternative approach to assess for the development of abdominal signs and is used in those patients being admitted for observation for potential abdominal injury or conservative injury management, particularly anterior abdominal penetrating wounds.[96,97] SAE is as safe and reliable as diagnostic laparoscopy for predicting the need for therapeutic laparotomy.[98] It is not appropriate to include patients who will be unreliable with a clinical examination due to head or spinal injury or intoxication.[99] There are several requirements for the patient who is admitted for serial clinical examination: the patient needs to be admitted for at least 24 hours, closely monitored from a haemodynamic point of view and have regular abdominal examinations looking for developing signs of peritonitis. It is preferable that the same clinician does the examinations to avoid subjective components; if this is not feasible, then a clear hand-over should be done between the clinicians over the patient so that there is agreement on signs and symptoms.

If the patient does develop any peritonism or haemodynamic instability, the patient requires a laparotomy. If the patient remains stable, they can start eating after the 24-hour mark.

If they have persistent localised symptoms but not peritonitis, they require further investigation; for example, CT, laparoscopy or laparotomy. The clinician should monitor and regularly assess the patient for increasing pain levels, rigidity, nausea, vomiting, increased heart and respiratory rates and temperature, which may indicate an acute abdomen, and ultimately a decreased blood pressure, indicative of septic or hypovolaemic shock, and should communicate any deterioration immediately to the treating medical team.[99,100] There is no role for sequential girth measurements.

Contrast studies

Contrast studies can assist in the diagnosis of specific abdominal injuries if they are suspected. The timing of these studies should be decided by the appropriate specialty. The main studies used include urethrography, cystography, intravenous pyelography and gastrointestinal contrast studies. Urethrography is essential before catheterising a patient who is suspected of having a urethral injury. Both CT cystography and conventional cystography are used to diagnose an intraperitoneal or extra-peritoneal bladder rupture.[101] Intravenous pyelography (IVP) can be used to detect urinary-system injuries if CT is not available. Injuries to retroperitoneal gastrointestinal structures (i.e. duodenum, colon, rectum, etc) may best be imaged using specific GI contrast studies in conjunction with contrast CTs.

Diagnostic laparoscopy

Diagnostic laparoscopy (DL) is emerging as a useful tool in trauma patients to assess the integrity of the peritoneum and avoid non-therapeutic laparotomies.[102] DL does not allow visualisation of the retroperitoneal space or the extent or depth of an organ injury.[103] The majority of the research into this area has involved penetrating injuries, specifically anterior abdominal stab wounds.[97] If penetration is determined, then further assessment at laparotomy is required as it is difficult to exclude all intra-abdominal injuries laparoscopically.[104] Laparoscopy is extremely sensitive in determining peritoneal breach;[105,106] however, more research is required into its role in blunt abdominal trauma.[102,107]

Laboratory tests

Blood samples should be collected as an adjunct to the primary survey when inserting large-bore cannulae. In the acute phase of trauma, the most relevant blood test is either an arterial or a venous blood gas (see Ch 17, p. 332, for information on interpreting test results). They are rapidly available serological markers of shock; lactate and base deficit are highly sensitive in measuring tissue perfusion and demonstrating blood loss (Ch 20).[108] Standard blood tests are sent with each trauma patient, including a full blood count, urea and electrolytes, coagulation studies and cross-matching (Ch 44), and while they may not always be of value in the initial resuscitation, they provide a baseline for ongoing assessment.

Serial haemoglobin and haematocrit are used in conjunction with other clinical signs as an indication of ongoing blood loss. Elevated leucocytes or white blood cell counts are part of the body's normal response to trauma; however, ongoing elevation may indicate an inflammatory process in the peritoneal cavity secondary to hollow viscous injury and, in later phases of patient care, a wound infection or sepsis. Elevated amylase levels may indicate pancreatic or duodenal injury; however, some patients sustain injury to these organs without amylase elevation. The positive predictor of elevated amylase in pancreatic trauma is only 10%.[109] A serum lipase should be obtained if pancreatic injury is suspected, as it is an indicator of pancreatic function, and interpreted in conjunction with other investigative tools. In children, aspartate aminotransferase (AST) levels and physical assessment accurately predict intra-abdominal injury[110] (AST is found in the liver, heart, lungs, muscle tissue, pancreas, spleen and kidneys and is released with damage, becoming elevated after 6–8 hours).

PRACTICE TIPS

- Get a venous blood gas early
- All women of child-bearing age should have a quantitative beta-hCG (human chorionic gonadotrophin) level taken to determine pregnancy status.

Ongoing management

Advances in resuscitation, assessment, new haemostatic agents and fundamental changes in the surgical management of the most severely injured patients have evolved from an improved understanding of the physiological derangements associated with severe injury and may favourably affect the survival of patients with abdominal trauma.[111] Despite initial presentation, haemodynamically stable patients with penetrating abdominal trauma may have significant ongoing haemorrhage and major intra-abdominal injuries. Peritonitis should be a trigger for emergency operation regardless of vital signs, because haemodynamic 'stability' does not reliably exclude significant haemorrhage. Vascular injury, subsequent hypotension, blood transfusion and complicated postoperative course are common in this population.[112] The ED nurse should continue to monitor and assess the patient (Box 48.2).

BOX 48.2 Ongoing abdominal trauma nursing management

- Be aware of patient status, fluid balance, observations.
- Ensure warm fluid administration and prevent heat loss.
- Communicate all findings with trauma team leader.
- Maintain documentation and anticipate requirements, such as preoperative checklist.
- Be familiar with and have appropriate equipment for monitoring for emergency transfer.
- Keep patient and family informed.
- Ensure nurse in charge is aware of progress.
- Facilitate emergency department discharge process to definitive care.
- Monitor for allergic reaction to radiological contrast.
- Regularly reassess the patient for signs of increased pain, blood loss and peritonism.
- When handing over, conduct abdominal assessment with new staff member to ensure consistency of interpretation.
- Ensure police have been notified of firearm injuries as per legislation (Ch 4).

Management techniques

Wounds

All penetrating wounds of the abdomen need to be clearly documented in the patient record. Wounds, especially from ballistic injury and even those apparently distant to the abdomen, need to be thoroughly evaluated for possible communication with the abdomen. Radio-opaque wound markers, such as a paperclip or cardiac monitoring dots, should identify entry and exit sites when plain X-rays are used to evaluate potential injuries.[57] Protruding objects such as a knife should be left in situ and stabilised until operative removal, as they may be adjacent to or penetrating vascular structures. The sudden release of tamponade may result in catastrophic haemorrhage.[16]

Evaluation of penetrating abdominal injuries

Mandatory exploratory laparotomy of all patients sustaining penetrating abdominal injuries will result in an extremely low incidence of delayed diagnoses or missed injuries, but an unacceptably high rate of negative abdominal explorations and potential surgery- and anaesthetic-related complications, especially in patients with low-velocity stab injuries.[113–115] Of course, laparotomy for penetrating abdominal injury is *always* indicated when the patient is unstable or in shock; thus, all such patients should be transported promptly to the operating theatre without any further diagnostic interventions (Table 48.1). Most centres still advocate mandatory exploration for all patients sustaining gunshot wounds to the anterior abdomen irrespective of haemodynamic status, given the high probability of finding visceral (intestinal) injuries in these patients. Researchers from South Africa and the United States[117] have advocated selective non-operative management of these patients with good results, but this practice has yet to spread to other major trauma centres worldwide.[118]

The stable patient with a stab wound to the anterior abdomen who presents without peritonitis, haematemesis, gross rectal bleeding or evisceration of abdominal contents through the wound may be initially managed non-operatively by performing wound exploration under local anaesthesia in the ED. The rationale for this approach is based on the fact that 15–30% of abdominal stab wounds do not actually violate the peritoneal cavity.[119] If the wound is followed through the tissue planes and found to end without violation of the peritoneal layer, then the patient may be discharged from the ED after wound irrigation and closure. The ED nurse should educate the patient on wound healing, maintenance and signs that indicate wound breakdown and the need for intervention. If, however, the wound is found to penetrate the abdominal cavity, or if its depth cannot be determined due to the patient's body habitus, four options exist:

1. Exploratory laparotomy without any further diagnostic interventions, which will reveal no intraabdominal injuries in up to one-third of these stable patients.

2. Diagnostic laparoscopy under general anaesthesia, as previously discussed.

3. Admission for close observation, consisting of frequent (every 2–3 hours) serial abdominal examinations by an experienced clinician and repeated determinations of white blood cell (WBC) count. The nurse should monitor

---

> **BOX 48.3 Delayed clinical manifestations of abdominal injury**
>
> Increasing:
> - pain
> - rigidity
> - bruising
> - heart rate
> - respiratory rate
> - temperature
> - white cell count
> - nausea
> - vomiting.
>
> Decreased:
> - appetite
> - bowel sounds
> - haemoglobin
> - blood pressure
> - urine output.

---

the patient for systemic signs of sepsis such as pyrexia, tachypnoea and tachycardia (Box 48.3),[120] which will lead to laparotomy and repair of injury. If, after 24 hours of observation, the patient does not show any signs of intra-abdominal injury, the likelihood of a missed injury is extremely low. The patient can be fed and, if oral intake is tolerated, discharged.

4. Performance of a diagnostic peritoneal lavage. Patients in whom the DPL is negative should be observed for a period of 24 hours, after which they may be released if no clinical signs of abdominal injury supervene.[121–124] Some have attempted to perform local wound exploration at the bedside using ultrasound rather than the traditional scalpel, with good results.[125–127]

Currently there is no clear evidence either way for the use of prophylactic antibiotics in penetrating abdominal trauma.[128]

Selective non-operative management

Selective non-operative management (SNOM) of solid abdominal organ injury is a technique that was originally described in children, but has rapidly gained acceptance in the management of adult blunt and penetrating trauma.[129,130] A haemodynamically stable patient and accurate imaging by CT are prerequisites for this approach. Isolated injuries to the liver, spleen and kidneys are frequently self-limiting with minimal intra-abdominal blood loss. These patients can be closely observed in a critical care area for any signs of deterioration or bleeding and the vast majority will avoid surgery—and require less blood transfusion and have fewer complications than surgical patients. Unstable patients and those who demonstrate evidence of ongoing bleeding require an urgent laparotomy and haemorrhage control.

SNOM of liver and spleen injury is associated with a small incidence of missed bowel and pancreatic injury; therefore a high index of suspicion, especially with liver injury, should be maintained to detect this. It is thought that the greater amount and/or different vector of energy transfer needed to injure the liver versus the spleen accounts for the greater rate of associated injuries to the pancreas/small bowel.[131] Failure of SNOM is uncommon, typically occurs within the first 12 hours after injury and is associated with injury severity and multiplicity, as well as isolated pancreatic injuries.[132] The nurse should be aware of signs of deterioration and missed injury as previously outlined in Box 48.3.

Interventional radiology

Interventional radiology (IR) has a vital role to play in the management of abdominal trauma by providing therapeutic procedures alternative to surgery,[133] particularly in patients who are bleeding as a result of vascular injury.[22] IR has gained popularity as management option for patients with isolated liver and spleen injuries,[8,134] and it can be used to gain an accurate diagnosis, and to evaluate for and control bleeding from pelvic and other vessels when clinically appropriate.[135] Angiography is also a sensitive modality for staging renal injuries. In penetrating trauma it can be used to identify pseudoaneurysms and arteriovenous fistulas.[22] The technique involves percutaneous access to the vessels, usually in the groin, and a catheter is then introduced under radiological screening. Contrast medium is injected while imaging continues and extravasation of the contrast determines the site and degree of injury.

Various techniques can be attempted to control or stop the bleeding. Embolisation involves the deployment of multiple metallic coils through the catheter into the vessels supplying the injured organ. These act as scaffolding for clot formation, which then leads to occlusion of the damaged vessels. Embolisation can also be achieved by injecting topical haemostatic agents; these agents are absorbed into the body after about 5 days. Alternatively, balloon catheters can be passed either side of a bleeding point in a vessel and inflated to occlude flow to provide temporary control until surgical access is gained. Once again it is essential that the ED nurse have appropriate, functioning monitoring and transport equipment, as well as ensuring that communication with the patient and/or their family has occurred. The intravenous contrast that is administered as part of IR or CT may cause allergic reaction, so the nurse should monitor for signs of rash, hives, flushing of the skin or itching and contact the doctor immediately. Contrast can also impair renal function and so there is a need to monitor urine output and creatinine.

IR techniques may be employed in a number of situations. The presence of a contrast blush in the spleen on abdominal CT suggests ongoing bleeding. Arteriography and coil embolisation can be used to stop the bleeding and avoid surgery. Patients with significant liver injuries that require packing at surgery have a significant risk for ongoing bleeding. Arteriography can be used to define ongoing bleeding and to embolise bleeding vessels before planned return to the operating room. IR is also valuable in the diagnosis and control of pelvic bleeding in open-book pelvic fractures.[136]

PRACTICE TIP

IR suites are often very cold. Remember to continue to actively re-warm your patient with overhead heaters or a Bair-Hugger.

Damage-control surgery

It is well recognised that a combination of hypothermia, coagulopathy and metabolic acidosis is associated with a high

BOX 48.4 Considerations for damage-control surgery

- Multiple penetrating injuries to the torso
- High-energy blunt trauma to the torso
- Multisystem trauma with competing operative/interventional priorities
- Profound haemorrhagic shock at presentation
- Evidence of worsening hypothermia, coagulopathy or metabolic acidosis on presentation or early in evaluation

level of mortality in trauma patients, and the phrase 'the triad of death' has been coined (Ch 44). Damage-control surgery (DCS), as a component of damage control resuscitation (Ch 44), is a concept designed to minimise the time a patient is exposed to this triad and to expedite the patient to a higher care setting where further organ support can be instituted.[137–140] The aim of DCS is to prioritise the restoration of normal physiological parameters versus the normalisation of anatomy.[141] Indications for DCS are summarised in Box 48.4. Preparation is key, and the decision to perform DCS should be made in the ED or at the beginning of the operation. This allows a management strategy to be formulated, and communicated, with the anaesthetist, operating-room staff and critical-care clinicians.

In short, the operating surgeon will initially deal with haemorrhage and contamination only, using a range of abbreviated techniques; the patient is then transferred to the intensive care unit (ICU) for correction of hypothermia, acidosis and coagulopathy due to initial hypovolaemia.[142] The aim is for the patient to return to the operating theatre for definitive surgery within 24–48 hours; this staged surgery allows the patient to be in a physiological state to normalise, giving the patient the best opportunity to recover.[143] The heterogeneous nature of the trauma patient needs to be considered when planning this staged approach. This applies equally to the timing of further investigations or radiological interventions; for example, CT scans. Premature return to theatre will convert what should be a definitive second operation into a second damage-control procedure and result in further physiological insult for the patient. This should be balanced against undue delays, which may increase the risk of abdominal compartment syndrome, intra-abdominal sepsis and the progression of previously unrecognised injuries. The stages of DCS are outlined in Table 48.5.

Specific organ injury

Stomach

The location and relative mobility of the stomach generally protects it from blunt injury. Most trauma of the hollow, pouch-like stomach is penetrating, causing the release of digestive contents and hydrochloric acid into the peritoneal cavity. This may cause severe peritonitis, initially by chemical irritation rather than bacterial.[144] Blunt injuries to the stomach are rare, with the incidence reported between 0.4% and 1.7% of all abdominal trauma; the mechanism is usually high-energy forces to the epigastrium with a full stomach.[145] The stomach has a rich blood supply from the splenic artery, gastroepiploic and short gastric arteries (Fig 48.7).

TABLE 48.5 Stages of damage control			
STAGE 1	Emergency department	Recognition—of the need for damage control surgery (DCS) during the initial evaluation	Assess patient rapidly using ATLS protocol
			Recognise anatomical and physiological patterns
			Plan and prepare for DCS
STAGE 2	Operating room	Operative control—of life-threatening haemorrhage and gastrointestinal contamination	Control haemorrhage by ligation, shunting or repair
			Control contamination, do not perform stomas or anastomoses
			Repair gastrointestinal discontinuity
			Pack solid-organ and pelvic injuries
			Consider IR procedures and mobilise early
			Place temporary abdominal closure
STAGE 3	Intensive care unit	Resuscitation—in the surgical high-dependency or intensive care units, including correction of the triad of death	Assess resuscitation, set endpoints
			Correct acidosis, coagulopathy, hypothermia
			Monitor for abdominal compartment syndrome
			Consider adjunct procedures/studies: X-ray, IR, CT
STAGE 4	Operating room	Return—to operating room for further exploration and definitive management	Identify and repair all injuries
			Assess abdomen for fascial closure
STAGE 5	Operating room	Closure—of surgical and traumatic wounds	Perform definitive wound closure

ATLS: advanced trauma life support; CT: computed tomography; IR: interventional radiology

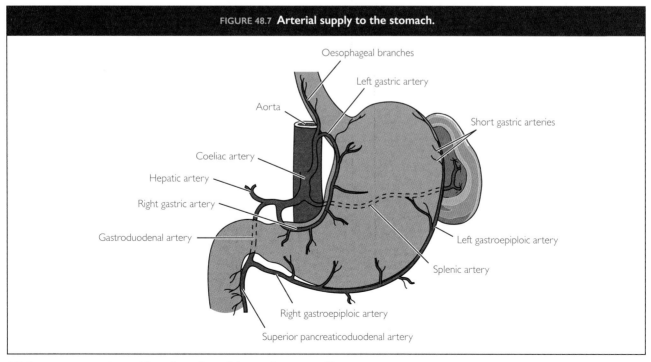

FIGURE 48.7 **Arterial supply to the stomach.**

All the arteries are derived from branches of the coeliac artery.[146]

Symptoms of gastric injury may include severe epigastric or abdominal pain, and signs of peritonitis. Blood loss is indicated by symptoms of hypovolaemia. Blood from a nasogastric tube and the presence of free air on abdominal X-ray may support the diagnosis.[22]

Bowel injuries

Hollow-organ injuries from blunt trauma are rare, but are associated with increased mortality and morbidity. While CT is the imaging modality of choice, its lack of sensitivity and specificity in diagnosing hollow-organ injuries is well reported in the literature. CT findings that are highly suggestive of bowel injury include bowel-wall discontinuity, extraluminal contrast and extraluminal air. However, the absence of these on CT does not completely rule out injury. Regular serial clinical examination in the patient with significant seat-belt injury is vital. Symptoms usually develop slowly and include increased pain, guarding and distention and decreased bowel sounds.

Small bowel

Blunt injury to the small bowel can be caused by direct blows, crushing the intestine between the external force and the spinal column and by shearing forces imposed by rapid deceleration. The presence of abdominal solid organ and lumbar spine injury are predictive of hollow viscus injury and thus the index of suspicion is raised.[147] The ileum and jejunum have a neutral pH and harbour few bacteria, so clinical signs of injury may not be present on initial assessment. It is important for the ED nurse to be aware of the patient's mechanism of injury, the need for reassessment of the abdomen and signs of peritonitis.

Large bowel

The large intestine is about 1.5 m in length and 7 cm in diameter. It is divided into the caecum, colon, rectum and the anal canal. It joins the small intestine at the ileum and exits the rectum. The colon is divided into the ascending, transverse, descending and sigmoid portions. The ascending colon extends from the caecum to the under surface of the liver where it forms the right hepatic flexure. The transverse colon crosses the upper half of the abdominal cavity from right to left, and then curves downwards beneath the lower end of the spleen to form the splenic flexure. The proximity of various parts of the colon to other organs that are injured should raise suspicion of potential colon injury. Trauma causing perforation of the large bowel is lethal if untreated, as a result of faecal contamination of the abdomen.

Management

Early identification and management of bowel injury is essential to control for abdominal contamination and subsequent peritonitis and sepsis. Surgical management of a hollow viscus repair includes either resection or direct repair of the affected segment. Colonic injuries can be resected with primary anastomosis; however, in the face of shock, major blood loss, multiple organ injury, significant faecal contamination and a significant time delay prior to operative management, formation of a stoma may be required. This group of patients is likely to be physiologically challenged postoperatively, leading to poor splanchnic perfusion, increased acidosis and ultimately increased risk of anastomotic breakdown. The patient's physiological status should ultimately determine the extent of any surgical procedure. Complications such as wound infection are related to the extent of contamination and the site of the injury. In addition, other complications such as fistula formation, small bowel obstruction, ischaemic bowel and anastomotic breakdown have been reported.[148]

Liver and gallbladder

The liver's large size and anterior location under the diaphragm and rib cage, occupying most of the right hypochondrium, make it susceptible to injury and that is why it is the most commonly injured solid organ in the peritoneal cavity (Fig 48.8). The most common mechanisms of liver injury are road trauma, falls and assaults.[150] In penetrating or blunt trauma, hepatic injury should be suspected if there is right-sided chest-wall trauma.

Although only 15–20% of the liver is necessary to sustain life, death can occur in less than 12 hours after complete destruction of the liver. The liver has a dual blood supply from the hepatic artery and the portal vein. About 400 mL/min of blood enters the liver through the hepatic artery, and another 1000 mL/min enters through the valveless portal vein making it vulnerable to injury and bleeding.[151]

CT is the imaging modality of choice to diagnose liver trauma in the stable patient. A delayed (venous phase) CT provides more detailed information about the extent of the injury and whether there is any active bleeding.[152] In addition, and particularly in children, elevated blood aspartate aminotransferase (AST; children > 450 IU/L and adults > 360 IU/L) and alanine aminotransferase (ALT) levels are predictive of liver injury.[70,151–155]

Liver injury can be graded on a scale of I to VI (Table 48.6). Non-operative management of all grades of liver injury is now considered the standard of care if the patient is haemodynamically stable, and has been demonstrated to improve outcomes and decrease lengths of stay.[152] However, the higher the grade of liver injury, the higher the incidence

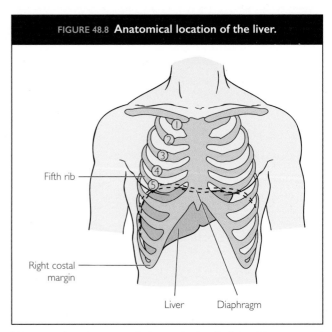

FIGURE 48.8 **Anatomical location of the liver.**

The upper border normally lies at the level of the 4th intercostal space or 5th rib, and the lower border does not normally extend more than 1–2 cm below the right costal margin.[149]

TABLE 48.6 Liver injuries[157]

GRADE	CATEGORY	DESCRIPTION
I	Haematoma	Non-expanding subcapsular haematoma less than 10% of liver surface
	Laceration	Non-bleeding capsular tear less than 1 cm deep
II	Haematoma	Non-expanding subcapsular haematoma covering 10–50% surface area; less than 2 cm deep
	Laceration	Less than 3 cm parenchymal penetration; less than 10 cm long
III	Haematoma	Subcapsular haematoma more than 50% surface area or one that is expanding; ruptured subcapsular haematoma with active bleeding; intraparenchymal haematoma more than 2 cm deep
	Laceration	More than 3 cm deep
IV	Haematoma	Ruptured central haematoma
	Laceration	15–25% hepatic lobe destroyed
V	Laceration	More than 75% hepatic lobe destroyed
	Vascular	Major hepatic veins injured
VI	Vascular	Avulsed liver

of delayed complications causing an increase in morbidity such as multiple organ dysfunction syndrome (MODS) and mortality.[157] If operative management is required, it is usually to control extensive venous haemorrhage. This is often achieved with packing. The operating surgeon will then decide whether a damage-control approach or a definitive repair should be carried out. Both management strategies will include ongoing resuscitation, and postoperatively the patient will require a critical care bed. Some patients may require angiography and embolisation after their initial surgery to assist with haemostasis.[158]

The pear-shaped, hollow muscular gallbladder sac lies directly beneath the right lobe of the liver and stores from 20 to 50 mL of bile. Trauma to the gallbladder is rare, occurring in approximately 2% of all abdominal trauma cases, but when missed or improperly managed it may be associated with significant morbidity.[159,160] It is difficult to diagnose because of its vague symptoms and inconclusive test results and is most often found during laparotomy.[159] In addition, it is often associated with liver, duodenal haematoma or perforation injury.[161] The preferred management is cholecystectomy.[22,160,162]

Pancreas and duodenum

The pancreas, located behind the stomach, is in very close proximity to the duodenum. Blunt pancreatic and duodenal injuries are rare, occurring in approximately 4% of all patients who sustain an abdominal injury.[163,164] Major pancreatic injuries are uncommon, but may result in considerable morbidity and mortality because of the magnitude of associated vascular and duodenal injuries or underestimation of the extent of the pancreatic injury. In addition, pancreatic injury has a high incidence of infectious complications.[165] Neglect of major pancreatic duct injury may lead to life-threatening complications, including pseudocysts, fistulas, pancreatitis, sepsis and secondary haemorrhage.[166,167] Isolated pancreatic

injury would be a relatively unusual finding due to its retroperitoneal location and relative insulation by other organs.

Pancreatic and duodenal injuries are hard to identify on physical examination, but anyone complaining of epigastric pain following blunt or penetrating force to the area should be thoroughly investigated. Pancreatic damage is usually identified on CT scan (85% accurate) or at the time of surgery. Biochemical tests, such as amylase, are non-specific. Any breach of the retroperitoneum should instigate a thorough exploration for pancreatic injury. Debridement of devitalised tissue and drainage can be employed for most cases of pancreatic trauma. Most duodenal injuries can be managed with debridement and primary repair.[168] If there is significant ductal destruction of the body or tail of the pancreas, this damaged area can be resected and a good outcome expected. Destruction of the pancreatic head is often associated with duodenal injury. This may require a Whipple's procedure in the stable patient; the unstable patient may benefit from a damage-control procedure and delayed pancreaticoduodenectomy.

Spleen

This is a relatively large, very vascular organ found in the left upper quadrant behind and in close proximity to ribs 7 to 10, making it vulnerable to injury when those ribs are fractured and at equal risk of damage from both blunt and penetrating injuries to this area. It has a blood flow of 250 mL/min from the splenic artery and a normal volume of approximately 350 mL (Ch 29). Splenic injuries are most commonly associated with blunt trauma. The spleen has a friable capsule leading to rupture from relatively minor trauma, e.g. contact sports. Injury to the spleen may be indicated by Kehr's sign (Table 48.2) and left upper quadrant pain, and is categorised into five grades (Table 48.7). A contrast CT is the radiographic modality of choice for detecting splenic injuries and should include not only a portal venous and delayed phase but also an arterial phase (Fig 48.9).[170]

		TABLE 48.7 Splenic injuries[157]	
GRADE	CATEGORY	DESCRIPTION
I	Haematoma	Subcapsular; involves less than 10% surface area; haematoma does not expand
	Laceration	Non-bleeding capsular tear; less than 1 cm deep
II	Haematoma	Subcapsular haematoma covering 10–50% surface area
		Haematoma does not expand; intraparenchymal haematoma less than 2 cm wide
	Laceration	Capsular tear with active bleeding; intraparenchymal injury 1–3 cm deep
III	Haematoma	Subcapsular haematoma involving more than 50% surface area or one that is expanding; intraparenchymal haematoma less than 2 cm wide or expanding; ruptured subcapsular haematoma with active bleeding
	Laceration	More than 3 cm deep or involving intracellular vessels
IV	Haematoma	Ruptured intraparenchymal haematoma with active bleeding
	Laceration	Segmental laceration or one that involves hilar vessels
		Devascularisation of more than 25% of spleen
V	Laceration	Shattered spleen
	Vascular	Hilar vascular injury; spleen is devascularised

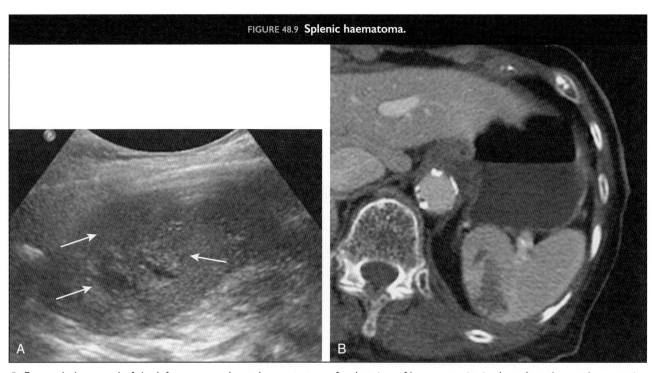

FIGURE 48.9 **Splenic haematoma.**

A, Focused ultrasound of the left upper quadrant demonstrates a focal region of heterogeneity in the spleen (arrows), suggestive of an acute splenic injury. **B,** Computed tomography performed following the initial ultrasound confirms the presence of an acute splenic haematoma.[170]

Historically, an injury to the spleen was treated with a splenectomy. In the last decade there has been a trend change towards SNOM of splenic injuries in selected patients.[171] SNOM patients require close observation in a critical care setting, as re-bleeding 7–14 days post-injury is a recognised complication, usually caused by rupture of a subcapsular haematoma. Furthermore, a period of self-imposed rest at home and avoidance of contact sports for a period of 2 months is also recommended following discharge from hospital. If a splenectomy is performed, the patient will require immunisation against encapsulated organisms including *Pneumococcus* and *Haemophilus*, in an effort to prevent overwhelming post-splenectomy infections (OPSI). Although rare, OPSI can occur from 1 to 5 years after the operation. The illness presents with flu-like symptoms, such as nausea and vomiting, progressing rapidly to confusion, high fever and septic shock, leading to disseminated intravascular coagulation and death.[22] Recent research has demonstrated a benefit in the use of spleen registries in reducing the mortality and morbidity associated with OPSI.[172]

Vascular injury

Major vascular injuries of the abdominal cavity or the retro-peritoneum usually involve the aorta, vena cava, iliac arteries and their major branches, and are often associated with major pelvic fractures or sudden deceleration injuries. They manifest initially by severe or rapidly progressive haemorrhagic shock. The initial evaluation should be brief and directed towards ruling out haemorrhage in these two body compartments, but it is often necessary to embark on an exploratory laparotomy without the benefit of full preoperative localisation of the source of bleeding. If operative facilities are not available, communication to transport the patient to definitive care must be of extremely high priority. The most valuable preoperative intervention in these patients is always definitively controlling the airway via endotracheal intubation (see Ch 17, p. 318). The blood pressure should not be elevated above a systolic value of about 90 mmHg, in keeping with damage control resuscitation principles with permissive hypotension.[12,17]

Most decisions regarding the definitive control of these injuries are made intraoperatively by the surgeons once the actual anatomical injury is visualised. Nursing personnel caring for such patients should ensure that high-flow oxygen is administered, any fluids given are warmed, an accurate record is kept of transfused fluid and vital signs, rapid transfer to the operating suite is facilitated by ensuring transport equipment and documentation are ready, the operating suite is aware of the patient and adequate amounts of blood products are available at all times by liaising with the blood bank. Activation of a massive transfusion protocol is very helpful in these situations (Ch 44).

Abdominal-wall haematoma/retroperitoneal haematoma

Occasionally, a penetrating abdominal injury will result in an abdominal-wall haematoma that requires full exposure under general anaesthesia to evaluate and control. If the haematoma is due to a stab wound or gunshot injury, it is usually explored, as there is a high likelihood of encountering and repairing a major vascular injury in these patients. It is dangerous to simply attempt to treat such injuries by applying local pressure or larger overlying masses of bandages in the hopes of tamponading the bleeding. It is rare that abdominal-wall haematomas due to blunt forces will require surgical intervention, as most resolve spontaneously with time and are self-limiting, although quite painful. The exceptions include internal degloving wounds such as a Morel-Lavallée lesion where the skin separates from the underlying muscular fascia and forms a haemolymphatic mass which may need to be drained.[173]

A general tenet of trauma surgery is that lateral and pelvic retroperitoneal haematomas due to blunt forces are usually left undisturbed (i.e. not surgically explored), unless the patient is unstable or in shock, while central haematomas are explored. If the haematoma is pulsatile or has visibly enlarged during the course of the laparotomy, then exploration is required.

Genitourinary trauma

Renal trauma

The kidneys are retroperitoneal organs that lie high on the posterior abdominal wall. They are enclosed by a strong fibrous capsule and lie within a fatty tissue layer. The perirenal space allows a large amount of blood to accumulate; however, the fascial layer can effectively tamponade renal bleeding in some cases. Normally, the kidneys are mobile within this area and can move vertically up or down three vertebral spaces (Fig 48.10). The kidney is well protected by the vertebral bodies and the back muscles posteriorly and the abdominal viscera anteriorly.

The kidney is the most commonly injured organ in the urinary tract.[175–177] Renal trauma is difficult to assess and early recognition, management and referral is crucial.[175,178] Blunt trauma accounts for up to 90% of renal injuries, and penetrating trauma 5–10%.[179] Blunt injuries are most commonly caused by an MVC, assault or fall from a height. Injury from blunt trauma is due to three mechanisms—direct blow to the flank, laceration of renal parenchyma from a fractured rib or vertebrae or sudden deceleration that causes shearing which leads to renal pedicle injury or parenchymal renal damage (Fig 48.11).[180] Falls from heights are associated with ureteral avulsion at the ureteropelvic junction.

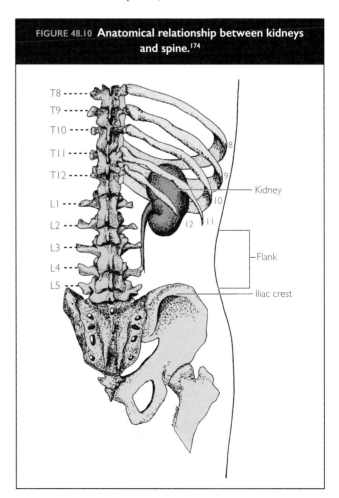

FIGURE 48.10 **Anatomical relationship between kidneys and spine.**[174]

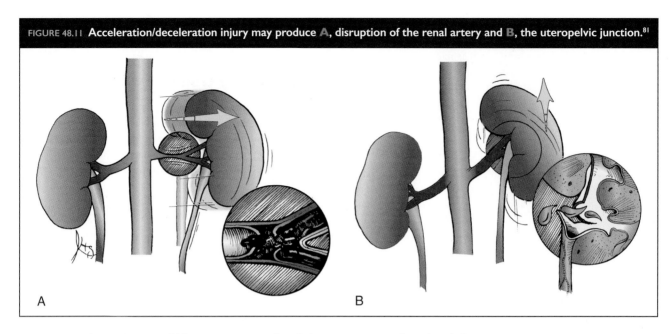

FIGURE 48.11 Acceleration/deceleration injury may produce **A**, disruption of the renal artery and **B**, the uteropelvic junction.[81]

Between 4% and 25% of blunt injuries are classified as major lacerations or vascular injuries, compared with 27–68% of penetrating injuries.[180] Up to 60% of penetrating renal injuries are likely to have adjacent organ damage.[79] Damage to the kidney may be caused by a bullet, bullet fragment or blast effect. The majority of penetrating injuries require surgical intervention. In children, blunt abdominal trauma frequently results in renal injury due to their lack of perirenal fat, relatively larger size of the kidney in relation to other organs and decreased thoracic protection.[5]

Renal injuries have been classified by the American Organ Injury Scaling Committee from grade I (simple contusion) to grade V (complete vascular compromise). They are listed in Table 48.8 and illustrated in Figure 48.12. These classifications have been demonstrated to be a reliable and predictable tool for clinical practice.[183]

Renal pedicle injuries usually occur in a seriously traumatised patient and represent 2% of all renal injuries.[180] The majority of renal pedicle injuries occur in children and young adults, with the left renal vein the most commonly injured vessel. Deceleration injury is the usual mechanism, through which the intimal layer of the renal artery is torn.[179] Renal vascular injuries include a vessel injury, renal artery thrombosis and disruption of the renal artery intimal layer resulting in an aneurysm or thrombosis. No signs or symptoms are specific for renal pedicle injury. Haematuria is absent in one-third of all cases.[79] Early diagnosis and surgical repair of pedicle injury is required to restore blood flow to the ischaemic kidney and salvage renal function.[184] Total avulsion of the renal pedicle with continuing intraoperative haemodynamic instability is often an indication for nephrectomy.[79] Postoperatively, an indwelling catheter is present and bed rest is maintained until gross haematuria clears.

Assessment

In addition to the assessment discussed earlier, clinical indicators of blunt renal injury include history of a direct blow

---

TABLE 48.8 Classification of renal injuries[181,182]

GRADE	TYPE OF INJURY	DESCRIPTION OF INJURY
I	Contusion	Microscopic or gross haematuria, urological studies normal
	Haematoma	Subcapsular, non-expanding without parenchymal laceration
II	Haematoma	Non-expanding perirenal haematoma confined to renal retroperitoneum
	Laceration	< 1.0 cm parenchymal depth of renal cortex without urinary extravasation
III	Laceration	> 1.0 cm parenchymal depth of renal cortex without collecting-system involvement or urinary extravasation
IV	Laceration	Parenchymal laceration extending through renal cortex, medulla and collecting system
	Vascular	Main renal artery or vein injury with contained haemorrhage
V	Laceration	Completely shattered kidney
	Vascular	Avulsion of renal hilum which devascularises kidney

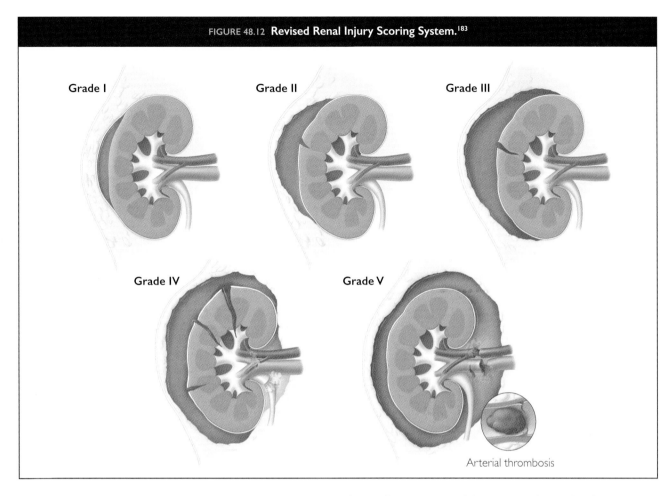

FIGURE 48.12 **Revised Renal Injury Scoring System.**[183]

Grade I

Grade II

Grade III

Grade IV

Grade V

Arterial thrombosis

to the flank, lower thoracic or upper abdomen, and associated intra-abdominal injuries. Renal injury is often associated with costovertebral angle pain on palpation, lower rib fractures, fracture of the lumbar transverse processes, bruising of the body wall, flank mass and flank tenderness. Patients may develop microscopic or gross haematuria, with urine analysis the most important diagnostic investigation used to assess the patient with suspected renal injury.[180] Haematuria is the best indicator of renal injury; however, the degree of haematuria does not always correlate with degree of injury.[174] The gold standard imaging modality to diagnose renal trauma is multislice CT with intravenous contrast.[101,175,176,185] To identify potential injuries to the collecting system excretory phase CT is recommended.[185] The primary role of imaging is to assess the severity and extent of injury and it also enables the clinician to evaluate for underlying disease and assess the function of the opposite kidney.[101] Up to 36% of patients with major lacerations or vascular injury and 6–10% of patients with minor lacerations after penetrating trauma do not have haematuria.[79] Significant renal injury can occur with microhaematuria in the absence of hypotension. Hypovolaemic shock secondary to a major renal laceration can occur.

Management

Surgical exploration is considered in the presence of concomitant injuries, continued haemodynamic instability and the stage and mechanism of the renal injury.[180] Surgical exploration is mandatory in patients with gunshot wounds, life-threatening

haemodynamic instability, expanding/pulsatile perirenal haematoma and grade V vascular injury.[4] Management of stab wounds is different from management of gunshot wounds. Peripheral stab wounds such as flank wounds posterior to the anterior axillary line are more likely to injure non-vital structures.

Most blunt renal injuries, particularly grades I, II and III, can be treated non-operatively with hydration, frequent examinations, serial urinalyses, antibiotics and analgesics. Bed rest is required until gross haematuria resolves. Controversy still exists about whether surgical or conservative management should be used in haemodynamically stable patients with severe renal injury. Absolute indications for surgical exploration are persistent, life-threatening haemorrhage, renal pedicle avulsion and expanding, pulsatile or uncontained retroperitoneal haematoma.[176,101] Unless immediate exploratory laparotomy is indicated for associated injuries or shock, most haemodynamically stable patients with major renal injuries— penetrating or blunt—can be managed by non-surgical treatment and interventional radiology,[187–189] with delayed intervention as needed. However, salvaging the injured kidney does not seem to offer an obvious clinical benefit regarding postoperative renal function.[190]

The nurse should be aware of signs of early complications of renal injury such as delayed bleeding, urinoma, abscess formation, renal insufficiency, urinary extravasation and fistula formation[4] and renal failure post-nephrectomy.[190] Late complications include arteriovenous fistulas, hydronephrosis, stone formation, chronic pyelonephritis and pain. Hypertension can occur after renal artery injury or renal compression injury. Patients may become hypertensive within 24 hours of injury, or onset of hypertension can be delayed up to 10 years after injury. Patients with severe renal injuries are at risk of delayed or secondary haemorrhage, and this can occur anywhere from 2 to 38 days post-injury.[101] These patients require long-term follow-up to identify hypertension, perinephric cysts, arteriovenous fistulas, stones, renal failure and retarded growth in the injured kidney.[79]

Ureteral injuries

Ureteral injuries are rare and account for only 1% of all GU trauma.[4,191] This is due to the protected location, small size and mobility of the ureters. Iatrogenic trauma, often following gynaecological surgery, is the leading cause of ureteral injuries, with penetrating trauma the next most-common mechanism.[192] Diagnosis of ureteral injury is difficult because early signs may not be evident on initial examination, with delayed diagnosis resulting in more significant complications.[192] Blunt trauma usually causes avulsion of the ureteropelvic junction subsequent to major hyperextension of upper lumbar and lower thoracic areas. Penetrating injury can cause partial or complete ureteral transection. With penetrating lower abdominal injury, careful examination of the wound with the ureter in mind is essential.

Assessment and management

Physical findings of ureteral injury are non-specific and usually relate to an associated intra-abdominal injury. The clinician needs to have a high index of suspicion based on the mechanism of injury.[193] Only when the ureter is obstructed and produces pain with classic radiation to the groin is diagnosis easy. Haematuria is an unreliable indicator of ureteral trauma, and is absent in 30–45% of cases.[191] Signs of urine leak, such as prolonged ileus, fever and persistent flank or abdominal pain, are indicators of missed ureteral injury.

Extravasation of contrast media is the hallmark sign of ureteral injury[192] following either an IVP or retrograde ureteropyelography. Delayed spiral CT scanning of the kidney 5–8 minutes or longer after injection of contrast medium (during the excretory phase) should be added to visualise the ureters. Most patients with a ureteral injury require operative exploration for associated abdominal injuries.[192] The type of reconstructive repair procedure depends on the nature and site of the ureteral injury.[191] Untreated ureteral injury can lead to urinoma, abscess or stricture.

Bladder injuries

Bladder injuries occur in less than 2% of blunt abdominal trauma cases, with up to 86% associated with ruptured bladders secondary to motor vehicle crashes.[4] Rupture of the bladder does not usually occur as an isolated injury and is mostly due to direct laceration from a fractured pelvic bone, in particular a widened symphysis and sacroiliac joint fracture,[194] or shearing mechanism.[195] The severity of the pelvic fracture correlates to the likelihood of both bladder and urethral injury.[196] The mechanism of injury in bladder rupture varies with patient population, amount of urine in the bladder at the time of injury and location of injury within the bladder. When the bladder is full it rises into the lower abdomen, making it

more susceptible to injury.[195] The incidence of bladder trauma in children is much lower than in adults, and is more common in boys following a pelvic crush injury and poorly fitting adult seat belts.[197]

Bladder injuries are classified as contusions, extraperitoneal ruptures, intraperitoneal ruptures and combined injuries.[196] Twenty-five per cent are intraperitoneal and usually not associated with pelvic fracture; extraperitoneal bladder ruptures account for 54–56% of bladder trauma (Fig 48.13), and are seen almost exclusively with pelvic fractures.[196] Injuries are usually caused by a suprapubic blow in the presence of a full bladder. The bladder tends to rupture at the weakest point (i.e. dome or posterior wall of the bladder). Intraperitoneal ruptures involve extravasation of blood and urine into the peritoneal cavity. Extraperitoneal bladder rupture involves perforation of the anterolateral bladder with extravasation of blood and urine into the retroperitoneal space. Combined intraperitoneal and extraperitoneal ruptures occur in up to 8% of cases, are associated with severe pelvic injury and are mainly diagnosed during surgery.[197]

Assessment and management

The classic combination of pelvic fracture and haematuria indicates immediate further investigation.[4] Up to 95% of patients will have gross haematuria.[197] Often patients with bladder perforation are unable to void and have suprapubic pain. Haemodynamic instability is common because of extensive blood loss in the pelvis and associated injuries. Late signs and symptoms are abdominal distension, acute abdomen and increased blood urea nitrogen and serum creatinine levels.

Radiographic evaluation consists of retrograde urethrogram and cystogram in all male patients with pelvic fractures associated with gross haematuria, inability to urinate, blood at the meatus, perineal swelling or non-palpable prostate. Addressing haemodynamic instability should remain the priority and non-urgent investigations should be undertaken at an appropriate time. Insertion of an indwelling catheter prior to radiographic imaging remains controversial due to the potential for damage to the associated urethra.[193]

Female patients with a pelvic fracture should undergo careful visual inspection of the urethra. Extraperitoneal bladder rupture is managed conservatively with drainage (via either a Foley or a suprapubic catheter),[193,199,200] antibiotics and close clinical observation for sepsis.[4] A repeat cystogram around day 10 often reveals a healed bladder, although approximately 15% of bladder ruptures may take up to 3 weeks to heal.[197] Intraperitoneal ruptures do not close spontaneously and require surgical repair which has been shown to significantly decrease associated morbidity.[199,200] Bladder injuries can lead to urinary ascites, abscess formation and urinary fistula formation and peritonitis.

Urethral injuries

A urethral injury should be suspected in any patient with a history of perineal or pelvic trauma (Ch 50). Certain fracture locations are associated with increased risk for urethral injury; these are the sacroiliac joint, a widened symphysis and fracture of the inferior pubic ramus.[194,201] Due to the differing lengths of the male and female urethra (4 cm in females versus 20 cm in males), the male urethra is more frequently injured.[177] Urethral

FIGURE 48.13

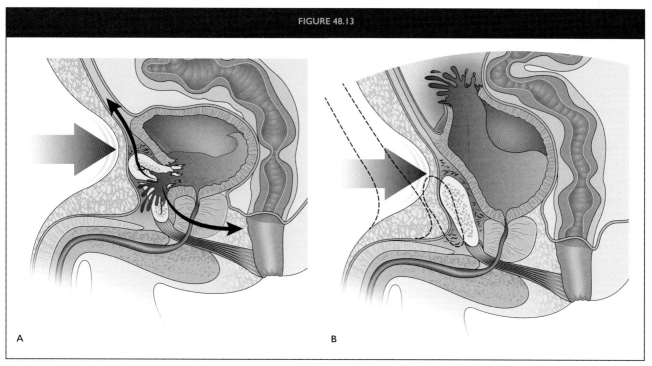

A, Mechanism of extraperitoneal urinary bladder rupture. The public rami are fractured, and the bladder is perforated by a bony fragment. **B**, Mechanism of intraperitoneal vesical rupture. A sharp blow is delivered to the lower abdomen of a patient with a distended urinary bladder. The distensive force is exerted on all surfaces of the bladder, and it ruptures at its weakest point, usually the dome.[198]

injuries in females are rare and are usually associated with a significant pelvic fracture,[177] obstetric injury or anterior vaginal lacerations[4] with labial oedema and haematuria present.[202] Proximal urethral injuries almost invariably occur in men secondary to a MVC (68–84%) or fall from height (6–25%). Iatrogenic injury to the urethra is not uncommon and can occur from traumatic catheter placement or transurethral procedures.

Traumatic urethral injuries are usually caused by shearing rather than direct laceration. If the injury is superior, the prostate can be forced upwards by a developing haematoma. In addition, 5–10% of patients with bladder rupture caused by pelvic trauma have a concomitant urethral injury.[202] Injuries to the anterior urethra can occur as a result of straddle injury, blunt trauma or sharp trauma to the penis caused by passage of a foreign body. Blunt trauma to the posterior urethra causes three general types of injuries, which may be incomplete or complete. With type I injuries, the urethra is stretched but does not rupture. Type II injuries are disruption of the urethra above the urogenital diaphragm; type III injuries are bulbomembranous injuries inferior to the urogenital diaphragm. Injuries to the anterior urethra are classified as contusions or partial or complete lacerations and frequently result from straddle injuries (Fig 48.14).

Assessment and management

Clinical symptoms may be variable. Some patients have a classic triad of blood at the urethral meatus, inability to urinate,

FIGURE 48.14 Mechanism of blunt anterior urethral trauma.

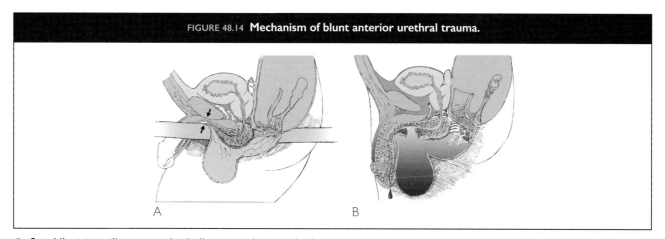

A, Straddle injury illustrating the bulbous urethra crushed against the pubic symphysis. **B**, Resulting urethral disruption with haemorrhage extending along the confines of Colles' fascia. Buck's fascia has been disrupted.[203]

a distended, palpable bladder and perineal bruising.[193,202] However, many patients with partial urethral tears can void. Other signs and symptoms include pain on micturition; perineal, scrotal or penile haematoma or swelling; haematuria; and a 'high-riding' prostate. A digital rectal examination should be performed in all trauma patients to exclude associated rectal injury. Inability to palpate the prostate was previously described as a classic sign of posterior urethral injury; however, it is unreliable due to the significant haematoma that surrounds the prostate following a pelvic fracture[202] and only 34% of male patients will have a displaced prostate.[202] A retrograde urethrogram is the study of choice for evaluation of urethral injuries.[177,204]

A urethral catheter should not be inserted if urethral injury is suspected. Such a procedure can convert a partial urethral disruption into a complete one, raise the risk of contamination and increase the risk of further haemorrhage. Absence of blood at the meatus and a palpable prostate on rectal examination are sufficient evidence to allow passage of a urethral catheter. Diagnostic investigation with a retrograde urethrogram is preferable prior to catheterisation. Postoperatively the patient is allowed to ambulate, but sitting is not advisable, requires intravenous antibiotics and erections are suppressed with diazepam.[204] Impotence, urethral stricture and incontinence are the most severe complications of posterior urethral disruption.[4] With anterior urethral injury, stricture formation is the most common complication. In females, urethral and bladder neck injury can cause significant sexual and lower urinary tract dysfunction.[205]

Genital injuries

Testicular and penile injuries are not common.[206] Injuries to the penis, testes and scrotum are rarely life-threatening, but they do demand prompt attention to avoid long-term sexual and psychological damage.[24] Female genital injuries are associated with severe pelvic fractures and sexual assault.

Penile trauma

Blunt trauma to the erect penis via a direct hit can rupture the tunica albuginea surrounding the corpora cavernosa, causing a penile fracture (Fig 48.15), and accounts for 60% of penile fractures.[4] The patient typically reports a 'cracking or popping sound' during intercourse, sexual play or masturbation, which results in severe pain and immediate detumescence.[23] A haematoma with marked oedema develops in the penile shaft. Diagnosis is frequently made on clinical presentation.[24] Most patients are able to void, but blood at the meatus and inability to void often indicates a lacerated urethra, so urethrography should be considered. Penetrating and degloving injuries of the penis can occur in the workplace. Penetrating injuries mandate exploration and reconstruction with liberal antibiotic coverage.[177] Sexually-related injuries involving strangulation or amputation of the penis have also been reported, and usually occur as a result of assault or self-inflicted wounds.[24] Traumatic amputation requires preservation of the severed penis, as microsurgical reanastomosis is possible.[206]

Early surgical repair gives better outcomes of function and appearance,[207] and is associated with a lower risk of adverse complications that have previously been associated with

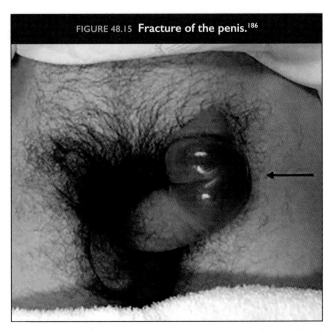

FIGURE 48.15 **Fracture of the penis.**[186]

Traumatic rupture of the corpus cavernosum, usually associated with sexual activity, results in a profound penile haematoma most often requiring operative repair.

non-operative management, i.e persistent penile angulation, longer hospital stay, missed urethral injury and more rapid functional return.[24,177] Adequate analgesia is required until surgery commences.[23] Conservative treatment is only warranted in cases with minimal haematoma and no extravasation during a cavernosography.[4] Treatment includes non-steroidal analgesia, ice packs and elevation of the penis. Other penile injuries may be due to direct trauma from zippers, bites, machines or knives. Treatment is determined by the severity of the injury.

Testicular trauma

Traumatic injury to the testicles is an infrequent occurrence despite their exposed position in the male perineum. Injuries typically occur in young men, usually aged 15–40 years. Blunt trauma to the scrotum, such as from kicking and kneeing during rugby matches,[207] accounts for approximately 85% of cases and can cause testicular rupture.[24] The patient with a scrotal injury may have acute pain, nausea, vomiting, syncope and urinary retention. Patients can have large scrotal haematomas that make examination difficult; therefore, scrotal ultrasound imaging with Doppler studies is the most sensitive and specific imaging modality to assess the vascularity and integrity of the testes.[24]

Minor cases are treated conservatively with scrotal support, non-steroidal analgesia, ice packs, and bed rest for 24–48 hours.[4] Testicular rupture is best diagnosed on ultrasound and, if highly suspected or confirmed, should be repaired immediately as testicular salvage rates of 90% within the first 72 hours have been reported.[177] All penetrating testicular injuries should be explored and repaired. Orchidectomy is necessary in some cases, but rarely indicated unless the entire testis is completely infarcted or shattered.

Avulsion injuries can cause loss of all or part of penile and scrotal skin (Fig 48.16). Industrial or farming accidents are often responsible for such injuries.[206] The penile shaft can be covered with skin grafts; return of function is expected. Partial

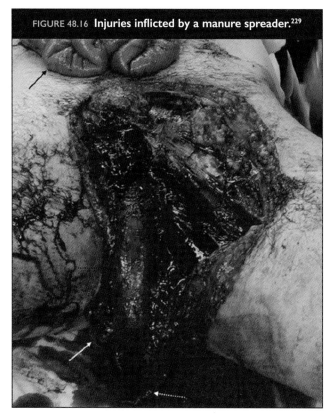

FIGURE 48.16 **Injuries inflicted by a manure spreader.**[229]

The groin laceration resulted in penis degloving (dashed black arrow), left lacerated spermatic cord (dashed white arrow), and right avulsed testicle (white arrow). The eviscerated bowel (black arrow) extrudes through an abdominal laceration (not shown).

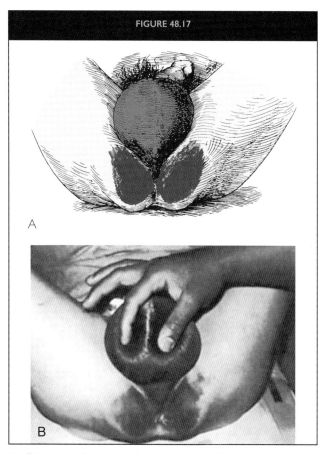

FIGURE 48.17

A, Diagram of a butterfly haematoma. **B**, Appearance of a patient with perineal butterfly haematoma.[198]

scrotal skin loss is managed by primary closure. The scrotum regenerates to accommodate the testicles and spermatic cords. Total skin loss leaves the testicles unprotected, so the testicles are placed temporarily in thigh pouches when immediate grafting is not possible.

Straddle injuries

Straddle injuries occur when a patient falls and takes the brunt of the fall on the perineum.[204] The blow to the perineum compresses the perineal tissues and underlying urethra against the external object and the symphysis pubis.[209] These injuries commonly occur in young patients as they fall onto bicycle bars, motorcycles and fences, and can have a characteristic butterfly-shaped bruised area beneath the scrotum (Fig 48.17). On examination of a female patient, a vulvovaginal laceration with extensive ecchymosis of the perineum may be evident. Straddle injuries in both sexes may result in blood at the meatus; and in men, many are unable to void.[204] Associated urethral injuries and rectal tears should be ruled out. Insertion of urethral catheters should be avoided until after a retrograde urethrogram.[204]

Treatment of straddle injuries involves repair of the laceration with evacuation and drainage of haematomas. A suprapubic and a urethral catheter are required postoperatively for 3–4 days. The urethral catheter is left in situ for 2–3 weeks.[204] The most common complication in the immediate post-

operative period is infection. Erectile dysfunction may also occur long term.

Female genital injuries

Female genital injuries are less common than male genital injuries; however, regardless of the mechanism of injury, all external genital injuries in females increase the suspicion of internal injuries and warrant further investigation. Vaginal bleeding is associated with pelvic fractures and urethral injuries, and requires a urethrogram. Female genital injuries occur in 20–53% of sexual assault victims,[206,210] and nursing support during physical assessment and collection of specimens is required. Vulvar injuries, such as lacerations, can also be due to sports-related straddle-type injuries or from high-pressure water spray during water-based sports, and commonly present as haematomas. These injuries require non-steroidal analgesia and cold packs and, if the laceration or contusion is extensive, vulvar injuries require surgical intervention, drainage and repair and postoperative antibiotics.[4,177] Internal lacerations may require speculum examinations under sedation to repair the laceration.[4] Vaginal packing is used to establish haemostasis. Unrecognised genital injuries in females may result in abscess formation, vesicovaginal fistulae, sepsis and death.[206]

All clinicians should consider sexual abuse as a cause of both female and male genital trauma unless the mechanism is irrefutable.[177] Rarely seen in the Western world is injury from ritual genital surgery, which affects gynaecological, obstetric and sexual health. Given the large numbers of refugees and asylum seekers worldwide, such cases may increase slightly in the future.[211]

Rectal injuries

Rectal injuries can lead to significant complications, and in blunt trauma are most commonly associated with pelvic fractures, in particular the symphysis pubis, even more so when widened, and the sacroiliac (SI) joint.[194] Fractures involving these locations should prompt further work-up for assessment. Diagnosis of these injuries may be difficult, especially in the unconscious or obtunded patient; thus maintaining a high degree of suspicion is vital. Rectal examination should be performed on all pelvic injuries, looking for blood and bone fragments lacerating the rectal wall. If there is any doubt about the diagnosis, rigid sigmoidoscopy should be performed. When identified early and managed appropriately, open pelvic fractures have a mortality approaching that of closed injuries. However, in the presence of a missed rectal injury, the mortality may be as high as 50%.

Penetrating rectal injuries may be caused by injuries to the abdomen, thigh or buttock. Again, any penetrating wound that may have injured the rectum should be fully evaluated with digital examination and proctoscopy/sigmoidoscopy. Even with these examinations it is possible to miss a significant rectal injury.[212] Combined rectal and genitourinary injuries have a significantly higher complication rate than isolated rectal injuries. Complications are increased by distal rectal washout, no pre-sacral drainage, repair of a rectal injury, prolonged suprapubic drainage and failure to adequately separate the GI and GU injuries.[212] As with all trauma patients, the nurse should monitor the patient for signs of sepsis and blood loss.

Foreign bodies and piercing

There are numerous case reports of various types of foreign bodies found in the urethra, bladder and genitalia. In adults, most foreign bodies are inserted for erotic stimulation. However, psychological disorders and drug ingestion are other frequent reasons for such activity. It is unusual for children to present with foreign bodies in the urethra. The most common reason for presentation is dysuria. Other complaints are suprapubic or perineal pain, urethral discharge, haematuria, difficulty urinating, swelling or abscess formation.

The trend of body piercing at sites other than the earlobe has grown in popularity in the past decade and complications of genital body piercing include local and systemic infections, poor cosmesis and foreign-body rejection.[213,214] Piercing sites in men include the penile glans and urethra, foreskin and scrotum; sites in women include the clitoral prepuce or body, labia minora, labia majora and perineum.[215] Jewellery inserted through the glans penis often interrupts urinary flow. Paraphimosis (the inability to replace a retracted foreskin) has been associated with urethral and glans piercings in uncircumcised men.[216,217] The foreskin may be reduced manually after a penile nerve block. Penile rings also can cause engorgement and priapism (i.e. persistent erection), requiring emergency treatment to preserve erectile function. Women with genital piercings can develop bleeding, infections, allergic reactions, keloids and scarring.[214,218]

Clinical diagnosis is based on history and should always be considered in patients with chronic urinary tract infections.

Radiographic studies, including plain X-rays, are usually helpful for radio-opaque objects. Xeroradiography is effective for detecting non-metallic foreign bodies traumatically or deliberately introduced into the genital tissues, including objects made of plastic, glass, rubber, cloth or wood. Foreign bodies below the urogenital diaphragm can usually be palpated and readily removed endoscopically, whereas foreign bodies above the urogenital diaphragm require surgical intervention.[151] The majority of rectal foreign bodies can be removed at the bedside; however, those in the sigmoid colon are more likely to require operative intervention and can cause bowel perforation.[219] In what is usually a very sensitive situation for the patient, the ED nurse should ensure the patient's dignity and privacy.

Postoperative management

The post-laparotomy trauma patient requires close observation and skilled nursing care. Patients with blunt or penetrating injury involving the abdomen are at high risk of developing postoperative complications (atelectasis, pneumonia, intra-abdominal infection). Even when the physiological condition has allowed definitive repair to be performed, at the end of the procedure the patient may be acidotic, cold and have coagulation abnormalities. This automatically necessitates the patient be managed in an ICU/high-dependency unit setting. The postoperative management strategy centres around the avoidance and early detection of complications, reintroduction of oral diet, skin and pressure area care, adequate analgesia, removal of drains, physiotherapy, deep breathing and coughing and rehabilitation. Patients who have undergone damage-control surgery predominantly return to the ICU with an open abdomen. The wound is usually covered by one of two methods, either a 'Bogota bag' (an empty 2 L sterile intravenous bag) or a vacuum-assisted dressing. Both dressings should be attached to suction and monitored.[220]

Postoperative ileus (POI) is frequently experienced by many trauma patients undergoing abdominal operations and other surgical procedures causing physical discomfort. No standardised mode of prevention or treatment exists, and a variety of management approaches have been developed. Combinations of strategies with demonstrated effectiveness such as early feeding, epidural analgesia, laparoscopic surgery and peripherally acting mu-opioid-receptor antagonists aid prevention of POI.[221]

Intra-abdominal pressure and abdominal compartment syndrome

Intra-abdominal pressure (IAP) is the steady-state pressure within the abdominal cavity; the range for a well individual is between sub-atmospheric to 0 mmHg, 5–7 mmHg in critically ill adults and 1–8 mmHg in critically ill children.[222] Intra-abdominal hypertension (IAH) is a sustained or repeated increase in IAP $\geq$ 12 mmHg. Abdominal compartment syndrome (ACS) is caused by untreated IAH where the IAP has an acute increase to 20–25 mmHg and end-organ dysfunction or failure is present.[223]

IAP monitoring can be undertaken directly or indirectly. In Australia and New Zealand, the non-invasive bladder technique is most commonly used. The trauma patients most at risk of developing ACS are those who have multiple injuries, burns or intraperitoneal or retroperitoneal bleeding. Patients who are acidotic, hypothermic and coagulapathic, who have received large volumes of fluid resuscitation, are also at risk. The systemic effects of ACS are listed in Table 48.9, and if left undetected and untreated progress to anuria, hypoxia, hypercapnia and death. The mortality rate associated with ACS is documented to be between 80% and 100% in those who are untreated and remains high in those who have early abdominal decompression.[222]

The nurse should maintain a high index of suspicion, examining for a distended and firm abdomen, monitoring respiratory function (see Ch 17, p. 334) and vital signs, and carry out routine IAP measurements 8-hourly.[225] Absolute criteria for opening the abdomen with raised IAP remain controversial; however, pressures in excess of 20 mmHg with evidence of end-organ dysfunction are candidates for re-opening and conversion to an 'open abdomen'. The nurse should manage the open wound being aware of potential heat and fluid loss and protecting the skin to avoid breakdown.[22]

Other considerations

The volume and contents of drains should be recorded consistently throughout a 24-hour period. Abdominal dressings should be assessed daily for signs of infection (erythema, swelling, discharge, pain) and the dressing changed. Superficial wound infection can be managed by removing the skin sutures or clips. Deep wound infections or dehiscence of the wound requires a return to the operating room. Stomas should be monitored for viability and content of the stoma bag. Ischaemic or obviously necrotic stoma may necessitate a return to the operating room. Patients whose emergency laparotomy is delayed are at significantly higher risk of mortality and complication development.[112,226] Fascial dehiscence after trauma laparotomy is associated with technical failure, wound sepsis or intra-abdominal infection.[227] Malnourishment and malignant obstructive jaundice predispose a patient to wound dehiscence by slowing the healing, and increasing the rate of wound infection.[228]

TABLE 48.9 Systemic effects of abdominal compartment syndrome[224]	
SYSTEM	EFFECTS
Gastrointestinal	Reduced blood flow to abdominal organs
Renal	Reduced renal blood flow and glomerular filtration rate
Cardiovascular	Decreased venous return through pressure on the inferior vena cava and raised intrathoracic pressure, leading to reduced cardiac output
Respiratory	Pressure on the abdominal side of the diaphragm increases abdominal resistance to inspiration. In ventilated patients this is usually demonstrated by elevated peak inspiratory pressures, resulting in reduced tidal and minute volumes as the ventilator cycles off when the preset pressure is reached or pressure alarms are triggered
Central nervous	Reduced cerebral blood flow due to raised intracranial pressure from impaired venous drainage. When this is coupled with a lower cerebral perfusion pressure that results from the reduced cardiac output, it is detrimental to the injured brain
Cytokine	Activation of the stress response, which is seen through raised interleukin (IL) (IL-6 and IL-10), as well as tumour necrosis factor

SUMMARY

Abdominal trauma is a significant cause of morbidity and mortality, and the patient can have life-threatening injuries with minimal evidence of injury or initially obvious clinical signs. This increases the importance of techniques such as FAST and CT in the thorough investigation of potential abdominal injury. The emergency nurse must assume that an injury is present until the possibility is ruled out. Consideration of how the patient was injured can highlight potential injuries and enhance patient assessment. GU trauma can be readily identified clinically and the extent of injury ascertained with radiographic imaging. An injured patient with potential urological injury has a host of general surgical concerns, particularly in conjunction with pelvic fractures; however, life-threatening concerns related to airway control, ventilation and haemodynamic status are still the first priority. Decisions regarding urinary catheterisation are particularly important for these patients.

Ongoing assessment is critical for the patient with abdominal trauma; the patient's condition can change as the patient experiences continued blood loss or responds to bacterial contamination from a perforated intestine. Unstable patients who present with the lethal triad of hypothermia, coagulopathy and metabolic acidosis or show signs of deterioration may benefit from damage-control surgery. Operative management of these patients is often only the beginning of a long recovery phase, much of which is improved by attention to detail and continual reassessment of the patient. Success in returning abdominal trauma patients back to the community requires early recognition of injury and transfer to definitive care, coordination of a multidisciplinary trauma team and early involvement of healthcare professionals experienced in abdominal trauma.

CASE STUDY

It is 1730 hours when the bat phone rings. The following information is provided:

Mechanism: A 30-year-old female motorbike rider has had an unwitnessed motorcycle collision into a tree at high speed, destroying the bike. The patient was wearing full protective gear, including a helmet.

Injuries: LOC, contusion to R side of face, rigid abdomen with tenderness on palpation, ? pelvis

Signs: HR 102, BP 90/50, RR 16, SpO$_2$ 94%, GCS 3,5,6, PEARTL, pale and diaphoretic

1. What would be your priorities in the field?

Treatment: hard collar, pelvic splinting with sheet, Morphine 20 mg IV (in 5 mg increments), Ondansetron 4 mg, Hartmanns 1900 mL

ETA: 30 minutes

2. In the emergency department (ED), you have received pre-hospital notification with a 30-minute estimated time of arrival of the patient. What will you do to prepare for the patient with the information provided by the paramedics?

3. What part of the MIST are you concerned about?

   The patient arrives 30 minutes later. She is triaged as a category 1 and is offloaded into the Resuscitation room where a full trauma team has assembled.

Primary Survey

A: Patent, talking, hard collar in situ

B: Spontaneous, good and equal air entry, trachea midline, SpO$_2$ 100% via PNRB

C: HR 102, BP 100/67, no external sites of bleeding

D: GCS 15, PEARTL, equal limb strength

E: T 33.7°C

4. What is your priority here?

5. What are the adjuncts to the primary survey you would like to see?

   CXR and PXR – NAD

   The patient received an IDC and her βhCG is negative

   FAST scan at 1830 hrs is positive.

6. What does a positive FAST scan indicate?

7. Where are the possible sites of bleeding in the abdomen?

8. Where should this patient go and why?

TIME	TEMP. °C	PULSE BPM	BP mmHg	RR PER MIN	SpO$_2$	FiO$_2$
1800	33.7	102	100/67	20	100%	60%
1815		99	99/70	17	100%	
1830		90	115/73	25	100%	
1845		80	105/62	13	100%	
1900		88	113/57	15	100%	40%
1935	35.5	96	109/62	14	100%	

Observations in the ED

pH	7.236
CO$_2$	62.6
O$_2$	24.8
Hb	91
HCO$_3$	25.6
BD	−0.9
Lac	4.1

VBG on 15L PNRB

9. What does her VBG indicate?

   The patient receives 4 units of packed red blood cells and the first unit of FFP is commenced.

   A – Avocados

   M – Nil

   P – Nil relevant

   L – > 8 hours

   E – Refer to MIST hand-over

   The patient goes from the ED to radiology for a CT head, C-spine, chest and abdomen. The CT demonstrates a small frontal lobe contusion in her head and an extensive laceration to the R lobe of her liver associated with active arterial haemorrhage. Extensive free fluid in upper abdomen and pelvis consistent with blood. Pancreas, spleen and kidneys all NAD.

10. Where should the patient go now and why?

Answers to Case Study Questions can be found on evolve
http://evolve.emergencytrauma.curtis

USEFUL WEBSITES

Eastern Association for the Surgery of Trauma, www.east.org

NSW Institute of Trauma and Injury Management, www.aci.health.nsw.gov.au/networks/itim

Trauma.org, www.trauma.org

Obstetric and gynaecological guidelines:

www.kemh.health.wa.gov.au/development/manuals/O&G_guidelines/sectionb/2/b2.17.pdf

www.osuem.com/downloads/m_m/mirza_fadi_g.pdf

REFERENCES

1. Smith J, Caldwell E, D'Amours S et al. Abdominal trauma: a disease in evolution. Aust N Z J Surg 2005;75(9):790–4.

2. Leenen LP. Abdominal trauma: from operative to nonoperative management. Injury 2009;40(Suppl 4):S62–8.

3. Smith JK, Kenney PJ. Imaging of renal trauma. Radiol Clin North Am 2003;41(5):1019–35.

4. Lynch TH, Martinez-Pineiro L, Plas E et al. EAU guidelines on urological trauma. Eur Urol 2005;47:1–15.

5. Buckley JC, McAninch JW. The diagnosis, management and outcomes of pediatric renal injuries. Urol Clin N Am 2006;33:33–40.

6. Nayduch DA. Genitourinary injuries and renal management. In: McQuillan KA, Von Rueden KT, Hartsock RL et al, eds. Trauma nursing: from resuscitation through rehabilitation. 4th edn. Philadelphia: WB Saunders; 2008.

7. Bariol SV, Stewart GD, Smith RD et al. An analysis of urinary tract trauma in Scotland: impact on management and resource needs. Surgeon 2005;3(1):27–30.

8. Durai R, Ng PC. Role of angio-embolisation in trauma—review. Acta Chirurguca Belgica 2010;110(2):169–77.

9. Stillwell S. Mosby's critical care nursing reference. 4th edn. St Louis: Mosby; 2006.

10. Thibodeau GA, Patton KT. Anatomy and physiology. 7th edn. St Louis: Mosby; 2010.

11. Walcher F, Kirschning T, Muller MP et al. Accuracy of prehospital focused abdominal sonography for trauma after a 1-day hands-on training course. Emerg Med J 2010;27(5):345–9.

12. Cameron P, Jelinek G, Kelly A et al, eds. Textbook of adult emergency medicine. 2nd edn. Edinburgh: Churchill Livingstone; 2004.

13. Revell M, Greaves I, Porter K. Endpoints for fluid resuscitation in hemorrhagic shock. J Trauma 2003;54(5 Suppl):S63–7.

14. Theusinger OM, Madjdpour C, Spahn DR. Resuscitation and transfusion management in trauma patients: emerging concepts. Curr Opin Crit Care 2012;18(6):661–70.

15. Bickell WH, Wall MJ Jr, Pepe PE et al. Immediate versus delayed fluid resuscitation for hypotensive patients with penetrating torso injuries. N Engl J Med 1994;331(17):1105–9.

16. Garner J, Watts S, Parry C et al. Prolonged permissive hypotensive resuscitation is associated with poor outcome in primary blast injury with controlled haemorrhage. Ann Surg 2010;251(6):1131–9.

17. Gruen RL, Brohi K, Schreiber M et al. Haemorrhage control in severely injured patients. The Lancet 2012;380(9847):1099–108.

18. Wilkes GJ. Abdominal trauma. In: Cameron P, Jelinek G, Kelly AM et al, eds. Textbook of adult emergency medicine. 4th edn. Edinburgh: Churchill Livingstone; 2014.

19. Brasel KJ, Nirula R. What mechanism justifies abdominal evaluation in motor vehicle crashes? J Trauma 2005;59(5):1057–61.

20. Sokolove PE, Kuppermann N, Holmes JF. Association between the seat belt sign and intra-abdominal injury in children with blunt torso trauma. Acad Emerg Med 2005;12(9):808–13.

21. Chidester S, Rana A, Lowell W et al. Is the 'seat belt sign' associated with serious abdominal injuries in pediatric trauma? J Trauma 2009;67(1 Suppl):S34–6.

22. Elliot D, Aitken L, Chaboyer W. ACCCN's critical care nursing. Sydney: Elsevier; 2006.

23. Rosen P, Barkin RM, Hockberger RS et al. Emergency medicine: concepts and clinical practice. 4th edn. St Louis: Mosby; 1998.

24. Blank-Reid C. A historical review of penetrating abdominal trauma. Crit Care Nurs Clin North Am 2006;18(3):387–401.

25. Montonye JM. Abdominal injuries. In: McQuillan KA, Von Rueden KT, Hartsock RL et al, eds. Trauma nursing: from resuscitation to rehabilitation. 3rd edn. Philadelphia: Saunders; 2002; 591–619.

26. Cole FL, Vogler RW. Fractured penis. J Am Acad Nurse Pract 2006;18(2):45–8.

27. Morey AF, Metro MJ, Carney KJ et al. Consensus on genitourinary trauma: external genitalia. Br J Urol Int 2004;94(4):507–15.

28. Walsh PC, Retik AB, Vaughan ED et al. Campbell's urology. 8th edn. Philadelphia: Saunders; 2002.

29. Warner MW, Salfinger SG, Rao S et al. Management of trauma during pregnancy. Aust N Z J Surg 2004;74(3):125–8.

30. Mendez-Figueroa H et al. Trauma in Pregnancy: an updated systematic review. AJOG 2013;209(1):1–10.

31. Shah AJ, Kilcline BA. Trauma in pregnancy. Emerg Med Clin North Am 2003;21(3):615–29.

32. Pearlman MD, Tintinalli JE. Evaluation and treatment of the gravida and fetus following trauma during pregnancy. Obstet Gynecol Clin North Am 1991;18(2):371–81.

33. Poole GV, Martin JN Jr, Perry KG Jr et al. Trauma in pregnancy: the role of interpersonal violence. Am J Obstet Gynecol 1996;174(6):1873–8.

34. Muench MV, Baschat AA, Reddy UM et al. Kleihauer-Betke testing is important in all cases of maternal trauma. J Trauma 2004;57(5):1094–8.

35. Marx JA. Abdominal trauma. In: Marx JA, Hockberger RS, Walls RN et al, eds. Rosen's Emergency medicine: concepts and clinical practice. 7th edn. St Louis: Mosby; 2010; 415–36.

36. Oyelese Y, Ananth C. Placental abruption. Obstetrics & Gynecology 2006,108(4):1005–16.

37. Morris JA, Rosenbower TJ, Jurkovich GJ et al. Infant survival after cesarean section for trauma. Ann Surg 1996;223(5):481–91.

38. Esposito TJ, Gens DR, Smith LG et al. Trauma during pregnancy: a review of 79 cases. Arch Surg 1991;126(9):1073–8.

39. Shah KH, Simons RK, Holbrook T et al. Trauma in pregnancy: maternal and fetal outcomes. J Trauma 1998;45(1):83–6.

40. Kissinger DP, Rozycki GS, Morris JA Jr et al. Trauma in pregnancy: predicting pregnancy outcome. Arch Surg 1991;126(9):1079–86.

41. Patterson RM. Trauma in pregnancy. Clin Obstet Gynecol 1984;27(1):32–8.

42. Iliya FA, Hajj SN, Buchsbaum HJ. Gunshot wounds of the pregnant uterus: report of two cases. J Trauma 1980;20(1):90–2.

43. Franger AL, Buchsbaum HJ, Peaceman AM. Abdominal gunshot wounds in pregnancy. Am J Obstet Gynecol 1989;160(5 Pt 1):1124–8.

44. Aboutanos SZ, Aboutanos MB, Malhotra AK et al. Management of a pregnant patient with an open abdomen. J Trauma 2005;59(5):1052–6.

45. Oxford CM, Ludmir J. Trauma in pregnancy. Clin Obstet Gynecol 2009;52(4):611–29.

46. Chames MC, Pearlman MD. Trauma during pregnancy: outcomes and clinical management. Clin Obstet Gynecol 2009;51(2):398–408.

47. Muench MV, Canterino JC. Trauma in pregnancy. Obstet Gynecol Clin North Am 2007;34(3):555–83.

48. Tweddale CJ. Trauma during pregnancy. Crit Care Nurs Q 2006;29(1):53–67.

49. Khandelwal A, Fasih N and Kielar A. Imaging of acute abdomen in pregnancy. Radiologic Clinics of North America 2013; 5(16):1005–22.

50. Kolb JC, Carlton FB, Cox RD et al. Blunt trauma in the obstetric patient: monitoring practices in the ED. Am J Emerg Med 2002;20(6):524–7.

51. Barraco R et al. Practice Management guidelines for the diagnosis and management of injury in pregnant patient: The EAST Practice Management Guidelines Work Group. The Journal of trauma, injury, infection & Crit Care 2010;69(1):211–14.

52. Anderson ID, Woodford M, de Dombal FT et al. Retrospective study of 1000 deaths from injury in England and Wales. Br Med J 1988;296:1305–8.

53. Rozycki GS, Ballard RB, Feliciano DV et al. Surgeon-performed ultrasound for the assessment of truncal injuries: lessons learned from 1540 patients. Am Surg 1998;228(4):557–67.

54. Rozycki GS, Ochsner MG, Jaffin JH et al. Prospective evaluation of surgeons' use of ultrasound in the evaluation of trauma patients. J Trauma 1993;34(4):516–26.

55. Shackford SR. Focused ultrasound examination by surgeons: the time is now. J Trauma 1993;35:181–2.

56. Sirlin CB, Casola G, Brown MA et al. Patterns of fluid accumulation on screening ultrasonography for blunt abdominal trauma: comparison with site of injury. J Ultrasound Med 2001;20(4):351–7.

57. Brooks A, Davies B, Connolly J. Prospective evaluation of handheld ultrasound in the diagnosis of blunt abdominal trauma. J R Army Med Corps 2002;148(1):19–21.

58. Rozycki GS, Feliciano DV, Schmidt JA et al. The role of surgeon-performed ultrasound in patients with possible cardiac wounds. Ann Surg 1996;223(6):737–46.

59. McKenney MG, Martin L, Lentz K et al. 1000 consecutive ultrasounds for blunt abdominal trauma. J Trauma 1996;40(4):607–12.

60. Dolich MO, McKenney MG, Varela JE et al. 2576 ultrasounds for blunt abdominal trauma. J Trauma 2001;50(1):108–12.

61. Henderson SO, Alhern T, Williams D et al. Emergency department ultrasound by nurse practitioners. Journal of the American Academy of Nurse Practitioners 2010;22(7):352–5.

62. Ollerton JE, Sugrue M, Balogh Z et al. Prospective study to evaluate the influence of FAST on trauma patient management. J Trauma 2006;60(4):785–91.

63. Dulchavsky SA, Henry SE, Moed BR et al. Advanced ultrasonic diagnosis of extremity trauma: the FASTER examination. J Trauma 2002;53(1):28–32.

64. Matsushima K, Frankel H. Beyond focused assessment with sonography for trauma: ultrasound creep in trauma resuscitation area and beyond. Curr Opin Crit Care 2011;17:606–12.

65. Rozycki GS, Ochsner MG, Schmidt JA et al. A prospective study of surgeon-performed ultrasound as the primary adjuvant modality for injured patient assessment. J Trauma 1995;39(3):492–500.

66. Boulanger BR, McLellan BA, Brenneman FD et al. Prospective evidence of the superiority of a sonography-based algorithm in the assessment of blunt abdominal injury. J Trauma 1999;47(4):632–7.

67. Rothlin MA, Naf R, Amgwerd M et al. Ultrasound in blunt abdominal and thoracic trauma. J Trauma 1993;34(4):488–95.

68. Boulanger BR, McLellan BA, Brenneman FD et al. Emergent abdominal sonography as a screening test in a new diagnostic algorithm for blunt trauma. J Trauma 1996;40(6):867–74.

69. Kimura A, Otsuka T. Emergency center ultrasonography in the evaluation of haemoperitoneum: a prospective study. J Trauma 1991;31:20–3.

70. Lingawi SS, Buckley AR. Focused abdominal US in patients with trauma. Radiology 2000;217(2):426–9.

71. Stassen NA, Lukan JK, Carrillo EH et al. Examination of the role of abdominal computed tomography in the evaluation of victims of trauma with increased aspartate aminotransferase in the era of focused abdominal sonography for trauma. Surgery 2002;132(4):642–6; discussion 646–7.

72. McGahan JP, Richards J, Gillen M. The focused abdominal sonography for trauma scan: pearls and pitfalls. J Ultrasound Med 2002;21(7):789–800.

73. Miller MT, Pasquale MD, Bromberg WJ et al. Not so fast. J Trauma 2003;54:52–60.

74. Udobi KF, Rodriguez A, Chiu WC et al. Role of ultrasonography in penetrating abdominal trauma: a prospective clinical study. J Trauma 2001;50(3):475–9.

75. Boulanger BR, Brenneman FD, Kirkpatrick AW et al. The indeterminate abdominal sonogram in multisystem blunt trauma. J Trauma 1998;45(1):52–6.

76. Yoshii H, Sato M, Yamamoto S et al. Usefulness and limitations of ultrasonography in the initial evaluation of blunt abdominal trauma. J Trauma 1998;45(1):45–51.

77. Griffin XL, Pullinger R. Are diagnostic peritoneal lavage or focused abdominal sonography for trauma safe screen investigations for hemodynamically stable patients after blunt abdominal trauma? A review of the literature. J Trauma 2007;62(3):779–84.

78. Kaneriya PP, Schweitzer ME, Spettell C et al. The cost-effectiveness of routine pelvic radiography in the evaluation of blunt trauma patients. Skeletal Radiol 1999;28(5):271–3.

79. Alsikafi NF, Rosenstein DI. Staging, evaluation, and nonoperative management of renal injuries. Urol Clin North Am 2006;33(1):13–19, v.

80. Root HD, Hauser CW, McKinley CR et al. Diagnostic peritoneal lavage. Surgery 1965;57:633–7.

81. McQuillan KA, Von Rueden KT, Hartsock RL et al. Trauma nursing: from resuscitation through rehabilitation 4th edn. Philadelphia: WB Saunders; 2008.

82. Nagy KK, Roberts RR, Joseph KT et al. Experience with over 2500 diagnostic peritoneal lavages. Injury 2000;31(7):479–82.

83. Kuncir EJ, Velumahes GC. Diagnostic peritoneal aspiration—the foster child of DPL: a prospective observational study. Int J Surgery 2007;5(3):167–71.

84. Huber-Wagner S, Biberthaler P, Häberle S, Wierer M, Dobritz M et al. Whole-body CT in haemodynamically unstable severely injured patients—a retrospective, multicentre study. PLoS ONE 2013; 8(7):e68880.

85. Asha S, Curtis KA, Grant N et al. Comparison of radiation exposure of trauma patients from diagnostic radiology procedures before and after the introduction of a panscan protocol. Emergency Medicine Australasia 2012;24(1):43–51.

86. Haan J, Kole K, Brunetti A et al. Nontherapeutic laparotomies revisited. Am Surg 2003;69(7):562–5.

87. Wilson RF, Walt AJ. General considerations in abdominal trauma. In: Wilson RF, Walt AJ, eds. Management of trauma: pitfalls and practice. 2nd edn. Baltimore: Williams and Wilkins 1996.

88. Allen TL, Mueller MT, Bonk RT et al. Computed tomographic scanning without oral contrast solution for blunt bowel and mesenteric injuries in abdominal trauma. J Trauma 2004;56(2):314–22.

89. Holmes JH 4th, Wiebe DJ, Tataria M et al. The failure of nonoperative management in pediatric solid organ injury: a multi-institutional experience. J Trauma 2005;59(6):1309–13.

90. Shankar KR, Lloyd DA, Kitteringham L et al. Oral contrast with computed tomography in the evaluation of blunt abdominal trauma in children. Br J Surg 1999;86(8):1073–7.

91. Stafford RE, McGonigal MD, Weigelt JA et al. Oral contrast solution and computed tomography for blunt abdominal trauma: a randomized study. Arch Surg 1999;134(6):622–6; discussion 626–7.

92. Tsang BD, Panacek EA, Brant WE et al. Effect of oral contrast administration for abdominal computed tomography in the evaluation of acute blunt trauma. Ann Emerg Med 1997;30(1):7–13.

93. Clancy TV, Ragozzino MW, Ramshaw D et al. Oral contrast is not necessary in the evaluation of blunt abdominal trauma by computed tomography. Am J Surg 1993;166(6):680–4; discussion 684–5.

94. Federle MP, Peitzman A, Krugh J. Use of oral contrast material in abdominal trauma CT scans: is it dangerous? J Trauma 1995; 38(1):51–3.

95. Shreve WS, Knotts FB, Siders RW et al. Retrospective analysis of the adequacy of oral contrast material for computed tomography scans in trauma patients. Am J Surg 1999;178(1):14–17.

96. Narsaria PH, Edu S, Nicol AJ. Nonoperative management of pelvic gunshot wounds. American Journal of Surgery 2011;201(6):7004–8.

97. Kopleman TR et al. The utility of diagnostic laproscopy in the evaluation of anterior abdominal stab wounds. American Journal of Surgery 2008;196(6):871–7.

98. Sumislawski JJ et al. Diagnostic laparoscopy after anterior abdominal stab wounds. Worth another look? J Trauma and Acute Care Surgery 2013;75(6):1013–17.

99. Velmahos GC, Demetriades D, Toutouzas KG et al. Selective nonoperative management in 1,856 patients with abdominal gunshot wounds: should routine laparotomy still be the standard of care? Ann Surg 2001;234(3):395–402; discussion 402–3.

100. Ertekin C, Yanar H, Taviloglu K et al. Unnecessary laparotomy by using physical examination and different diagnostic modalities for penetrating abdominal stab wounds. Emerg Med J 2005;22(11):790–4.

101. Ramchandani P, Buckler PM. Imaging of genitourinary trauma. Am J Roentgenol 2009;192(6):1514–23.

102. Sauerland S, Agresta F, Bergamaschi R et al. Laparoscopy for abdominal emergencies: evidence-based guidelines of the European Association for Endoscopic Surgery. Surg Endosc 2006;20(1):14–29.

103. Fabian TC, Croce MA. Abdominal trauma, including indications for celiotomy. In: Mattox KL, Feliciano DV, Moore EE, eds. Trauma. 7th edn. New York: McGraw-Hill; 2012.

104. Leppaniemi A, Haapiainen R. Diagnostic laparoscopy in abdominal stab wounds: a prospective, randomized study. J Trauma 2003;55(4):636–45.

105. Villavicencio RT, Aucar JA. Analysis of laparoscopy in trauma. J Am Coll Surg 1999;189(1):11–20.

106. Zantut LF, Ivatury RR, Smith RS et al. Diagnostic and therapeutic laparoscopy for penetrating abdominal trauma: a multicentre experience. J Trauma 1997;42(5):825–31.

107. Johnson JJ et al. The use of laparoscopy in the diagnosis and treatment of blunt and penetrating injuries: 10 year experience at a level 1 trauma centre. The American Journal of Surgery 2013;205(3):317–21.

108. Paladino L, Sinert R, Wallace D et al. The utility of base deficit and arterial lactate in differentiating major from minor injury in trauma patients with normal vital signs. Resuscitation 2008;77(3):363–8.

109. Purtill MA, Stabile BE. Duodenal and pancreatic trauma. In: Naude GP, Bongard FS, Demetriades D, eds. Trauma secrets. Philadelphia: Hanley and Belfus; 1999.

110. Cotton BA, Beckert BW, Smith MK et al. The utility of clinical and laboratory data for predicting intraabdominal injury among children. J Trauma 2004;56(5):1068–74; discussion 1074–5. Comment in: J Trauma 2005;58(6):1306–7.

111. Johnson JW, Gracias VH, Schwab CW et al. Evolution in damage control for exsanguinating penetrating abdominal injury. J Trauma 2001;51:261–71.

112. Brown CV, Velmahos GC, Neville AL et al. Hemodynamically stable patients with peritonitis after penetrating abdominal trauma: identifying those who are bleeding. Arch Surg 2005;140(8):767–72.

113. Conrad MF, Patton JH, Parikshak M et al. Selective management of penetrating truncal injuries: is emergency department discharge a reasonable goal? Am Surg 2003;69(3):266–72.

114. Moore EE, Marx JA. Penetrating abdominal wounds: rationale for exploratory laparotomy. JAMA 1985;253(18):2705–8.

115. Markovchick VJ, Moore EE, Moore J et al. Local wound exploration of anterior abdominal stab wounds. J Emerg Med 1985;2(4):287–91.

116. Demetriades D, Velmahos G, Cornwell E 3rd et al. Selective nonoperative management of gunshot wounds of the anterior abdomen. Arch Surg 1997;132(2):178–83.

117. Velmahos GC, Constantinou C, Tillou A et al. Abdominal computed tomographic scan for patients with gunshot wounds to the abdomen selected for nonoperative management. J Trauma 2005;59(5):1155–61.

118. Pryor JP, Reilly PM, Dabrowski GP et al. Nonoperative management of abdominal gunshot wounds. Ann Emerg Med 2004; 43(3):344–53. Comment in: Ann Emerg Med 2004;44(5):551–2.

119. Rosemurgy AS 2nd, Albrink MH, Olson SM et al. Abdominal stab wound protocol: prospective study documents applicability for widespread use. Am Surg 1995;61(2):112–16.

120. Zubowski R, Nallathambi M, Ivatury R et al. Selective conservatism in abdominal stab wounds: the efficacy of serial physical examination. J Trauma 1988;28(12):1665–8.

121. Sriussadaporn S, Pak-art R, Pattaratiwanon M et al. Clinical uses of diagnostic peritoneal lavage in stab wounds of the anterior abdomen: a prospective study. Eur J Surg 2002;168(8–9):490–3.

122. Gonzalez RP, Turk B, Falimirski ME et al. Abdominal stab wounds: diagnostic peritoneal lavage criteria for emergency room discharge. J Trauma 2001;51(5):939–43.

123. Oreskovich MR, Carrico CJ. Stab wounds of the anterior abdomen. Analysis of a management plan using local wound exploration and quantitative peritoneal lavage. Ann Surg 1983;198(4):411–19.

124. Feliciano DV, Bitondo CG, Steed G et al. Five hundred open taps or lavages in patients with abdominal stab wounds. Am J Surg 1984;148(6):772–7.

125. Bokhari F, Nagy K, Roberts R et al. The ultrasound screen for penetrating truncal trauma. Am Surg 2004;70(4):316–21.

126. Murphy JT, Hall J, Provost DJ et al. Fascial ultrasound for evaluation of anterior abdominal stab wound injury. J Trauma 2005;59(4):843–6.

127. Como JJ, Bokhari F, Chiu WC et al. Practice management guidelines for selective nonoperative management of penetrating abdominal trauma. J Trauma 2010;68(3):721–33.

128. Brand M, Grieve A. Prophylactic antibiotics for penetrating abdominal trauma. Cochrane Database of Systematic Reviews 2013;11: CD007370. DOI: 10.1002/14651858.CD007370.pub3.

129. Landau A, van As AB, Numanoglu A et al. Liver injuries in children: the role of selective nonoperative management. Injury 2006;37(1):66–71.

130. Wise BV, Mudd SS, Wilson ME. Management of blunt abdominal trauma in children. J Trauma Nurs 2002;9(1):6–14.

131. Miller PR, Croce MA, Bee TK et al. Associated injuries in blunt solid organ trauma: implications for missed injury in nonoperative management. J Trauma 2002;53(2):238–42; discussion 242–4.

132. Holmes JF, Offerman SR, Chang CH et al. Performance of helical computed tomography without oral contrast for the detection of gastrointestinal injuries. Ann Emerg Med 2004;43(1):120–8.

133. Pinto F, Bode PJ, Tonerini M et al. The role of the radiologist in the management of polytrauma patients. Eur J Radiol 2006;59(3):315–16.

134. Skattum J et al. Preserved splenic function after the angioembolisation of high grade injury. Injury 2012;43(1):62–6.

135. Madoff DC, Denys A, Wallace MJ et al. Splenic arterial interventions: anatomy, indications, technical considerations, and potential complications. Radiographics 2005;25(Suppl 1):S191–211.

136. Brown CV, Kasotakis G, Wilcox A et al. Does pelvic hematoma on admission computed tomography predict active bleeding at angiography for pelvic fracture? Am Surg 2005;71(9):759–62.

137. Rotondo MF, Schwab CW, McGonigal MD et al. 'Damage control': an approach for improved survival in exsanguinating penetrating abdominal injury. J Trauma 1993;35(3):375–82; discussion 382–3.

138. Johnson JW, Gracias VH, Schwab CW et al. Evolution in damage control for exsanguinating penetrating abdominal injury. J Trauma 2001;51(2):261–9; discussion 269–71.

139. Bose D, Tejwani NC. Evolving trends in the care of polytrauma patients. Injury 2006;37(1):20–8.

140. Schreiber MA. Damage control surgery. Crit Care Clin 2004;20(1):101–18.

141. Jaunoo SS, Harji DP. Damage control surgery. Int J Surg 2009;7(2):110–13.

142. Parr MJ, Alabdi T. Damage control surgery and intensive care. Injury 2004;35(7):713–22.

143. Weber DG, Bendinelli C, Balogh ZJ. Damage control surgery for abdominal emergencies. BJS 2014;10(1):e109–18.

144. Wilson RF, Walt AJ. Injury to the stomach and small bowel. In: Wilson RF, Walt AJ, eds. Management of trauma: pitfalls and practice. 2nd edn. Baltimore: Williams and Wilkins; 1996.

145. Lassandro F, Romano S, Rossi G et al. Gastric traumatic injuries: CT findings. Eur J Radiol 2006;59(3):349–54.

146. Snell RS, Smith MS. Clinical anatomy for emergency medicine. St Louis: Mosby; 1993.

147. Nance ML, Peden GW, Shapiro MB et al. Solid viscus injury predicts major hollow viscus injury in blunt abdominal trauma. J Trauma 1997;43:618–22.

148. Wisner DH. Stomach and small bowel. In: Mattox KL, Feliciano DV, Moore EE, eds. Trauma. 4th edn. New York: McGraw-Hill; 2000.

149. Clochesy JM, Breu C, Cardin S et al. Critical care nursing. 2nd edn. Philadelphia: WB Saunders; 1996.

150. Malhotra AK, Fabian TC, Croce MA et al. Blunt hepatic injury: a paradigm shift from operative to nonoperative management in the 1990s. Ann Surg 2000;231(6):804–13.

151. Herman ML. Gastrointestinal trauma. In: Newberry L, editor. Sheehy's Emergency nursing: principles and practice. 6th edn. St Louis: Mosby; 2009.

152. Lee SK, Carrillo EH. Advances and changes in the management of liver injuries. Am Surg 2007;73(3):201–6.

153. Polanco PM et al. The swinging pendulum: A national perspective of nonoperative management in severe blunt liver injury. J Trauma Acute Care Surg 2013;75(4):590–5.

154. Puranik SR, Hayes JS, Long J et al. Liver enzymes as predictors of liver damage due to blunt abdominal trauma in children. South Med J 2002;95(2):203–6.

155. Karaduman D, Sarioglu-Buke A, Kilic I et al. The role of elevated liver transaminase levels in children with blunt abdominal trauma. Injury 2003;34(4):249–52.

156. Sahdev P, Garramone RR Jr, Schwartz RJ et al. Evaluation of liver function tests in screening for intra-abdominal injuries. Ann Emerg Med 1991;20(8):838–41.

157. Pearl WS, Todd KH. Ultrasonography for the initial evaluation of blunt abdominal trauma, a review in prospective trials. Ann Emerg Med 1996; 27.

158. Polanco P, Leon S, Pineda J et al. Hepatic resection in the management of complex injury to the liver. J Trauma 2008;65(6):1264–9.

159. Jaggard MKJ et al. Blunt Abdominal Trauma Resulting in Gallbladder Injury: A Review with Emphasis on Pediatrics. J Trauma Inj Inf Crit Care 2011;70(4):1005–10.

160. Zellweger R, Navsaria PH, Hess F et al. Gall bladder injuries as part of the spectrum of civilian abdominal trauma in South Africa. Aust N Z J Surg 2005;75(7):559–61.

161. Erb RE, Mirvis SE, Shanmuganathan K. Gallbladder injury secondary to blunt trauma: CT findings. J Comput Assist Tomogr 1994;18(5):778–84.

162. Brennan PM, Welsh FK, Lyness C et al. Avulsion of the gallbladder following trivial injury. Int J Clin Pract 2004;58(3):318–21.

163. Linsenmaier U, Wirth S, Reiser M et al. Diagnosis and classification of pancreatic and duodenal injuries in emergency radiology. Radiographics 2008;28(6):1591–602.

164. Lahiri R, Bhattacharya S. Pancreatic trauma. Annals of the Royal College of Surgeons of England 2013;95(4):241–5.

165. Tyburski JG, Dente CJ, Wilson RF et al. Infectious complications following duodenal and/or pancreatic trauma. Am Surg 2001; 67(3):227–30; discussion 230–1.

166. Krige JE, Beningfield SJ, Nicol AJ et al. The management of complex pancreatic injuries. S Afr J Surg 2005;43(3):92–102.

167. Lopez PP, Benjamin R, Cockburn M et al. Recent trends in the management of combined pancreatoduodenal injuries. Am Surg 2005;71(10):847–52.

168. Rickard MJ, Brohi K, Bautz PC. Pancreatic and duodenal injuries: keep it simple. Aust N Z J Surg 2005;75(7):581–6.

169. Uyeda JW et al. Active hemorrhage and vascular injuries in splenic trauma: utility of the arterial phase in multidetector. Radiology 2014;270(1):99–106.

170. Soto JA, Lucey BC. Emergency radiology: the requisites. Philadelphia: Mosby; 2009.

171. Cadeddu M, Garnett A, Al-Anezi K et al. Management of spleen injuries in the adult trauma population: a ten-year experience. Can J Surg 2006;49(6):386–90.

172. Denholm JT, Jones PA, Spelman DW et al. Spleen registry may help reduce the incidence of overwhelming postsplenectomy infection in Victoria. Med J Aust 2010;192(1):49–50.

173. Shen C, Peng JP, Chen XD. Efficacy of treatment in the peri pelvic Morel-Lavallee leision: a systematic review of the literature. Archives of orthopaedic and trauma surgery 2013;133(5):635–40.

174. Neff JA, Kidd PS, eds. Trauma nursing: the art and science. St Louis: Mosby; 1993.

175. Lee Y, Oh S, Rha S et al. Renal trauma. Radiol Clin N Am 2007;45(3):581–92.

176. Martinez-Pineiro L, Djakovic N, Plas E et al. EAU guidelines on urethral trauma. European Urology 2010;57(5):791–803.

177. Shewakramani S, Reed KC. Urological trauma emergency medicine clinics of North America 2011;29,(3):501–18.

178. Lee S, Thavaseelan J, Low V. Renal trauma in Australian Rules football: an institutional experience. Aust N Z J Surg 2004;74(9):766–8.

179. Cassabaum VD, Bourg PW. The ins and outs of renal trauma. Am J Nurs 2002; S4–7, quiz 25–7.

180. Santucci RA, Wessells H, Bartsch G et al. Evaluation and management of renal injuries: consensus statement of the renal trauma subcommittee. Br J Urol Int 2004;93(7):937–54.

181. Dixon MD, McAninch JW. American Urological Association update series, traumatic renal injuries, part 1: assessment and management. Houston: The Association; 1991.

182. Kidney Injury Scale. The American Association for the Surgery of Trauma. Table 19. Online. www.aast.org/Library/TraumaTools/InjuryScoringScales.aspx; accessed 7 May 2015.

183. Buckley JC, McAninch JW. Revision of Current American Association for the Surgery of Trauma Renal Injury Grading System. J Trauma 2011;70: 35–37.

184. Master VA, McAninch JW. Operative management of renal injuries: parenchymal and vascular. Urol Clin North Am 2006;33(1):21–31, v–vi.

185. Hardee MJ, Lowrance W, Stevens MH, Nirula R, Brant WO, Morris SE, Myers JB. Process improvement in trauma: compliance with recommended imaging evaluation in the diagnosis of high-grade renal injuries. The Journal of Trauma and Acute Care Surgery 2013;74(2):558–62.

186. Minns AB, Sherry Y. Penile fracture in a patient presenting with groin pain. Journal of Emergency Medicine 2011;40(4):441–2.

187. Hagiwara A, Sakaki S, Goto H et al. The role of interventional radiology in the management of blunt renal injury: a practical protocol. J Trauma 2001;51(3):526–31.

188. Shoobridge JJ, Bultitude MF, Koukounaras J et al. Predicting surgical exploration in renal trauma: assessment and modification of an established nomogram. J Trauma and Acute Care Surgery 2013;75(5):819–23.

189. McClung CD, Hotaling JM et al. Contemporary trends in the immediate surgical management of renal trauma using a national database. J Trauma and Acute Care Surgery 2013;75(4):602–6.

190. Velmahos GC, Constantinou C, Gkiokas G. Does nephrectomy for trauma increase the risk of renal failure? World J Surg 2005;29(11):1472–5.

191. Brandes S, Coburn M, Armenakas N et al. Diagnosis and management of ureteric injury: an evidence-based analysis. B J Urol Int 2004;94(3):277–89.

192. Elliott SP, McAninch JW. Ureteral injuries: external and iatrogenic. Urol Clin North Am 2006;33(1):55–66, vi.

193. Bent C, Iyngkaran T, Power N et al. Urological injuries following trauma. Clin Radiol 2008;63(12):1361–71.

194. Aihara R, Blansfield JS, Millham FH et al. Fracture locations influence the likelihood of rectal and lower urinary tract injuries in patients sustaining pelvic fractures. J Trauma 2002;52(2):205–8; discussion 208–9.

195. Harrahill M. Bladder trauma: a review. J Emerg Nurs 2004;30(3):287–8.

196. Corriere JN Jr, Sandler CM. Diagnosis and management of bladder injuries. Urol Clin North Am 2006;33(1):67–71, vi.

197. Gomez RG, Ceballos L, Coburn M et al. Consensus statement on bladder injuries. Br J Urol Int 2004;94(1):27–32.

198. Peters P, Sagalowsky A. Genitourinary trauma. In: Walsh P, Gittes R, Perlmutter A et al, eds. Campbell's Urology. 8th edn. Vol 1. Philadelphia: WB Saunders; 2002.

199. Deibert CA, Spencer BA. The association between operative repair of bladder injury and improved survival: results from the National Trauma Data Bank. The Journal of Urology 2011;186(1):151–5.

200. Pereira BMT, Citatini de Campos CC, Calderan TR et al. Bladder injuries after external trauma: 20 years experience report in a population-based cross-sectional view. World J Urol 2013;31:913–17.

201. Lowe MA, Mason JT, Luna GK et al. Risk factors for urethral injuries in men with traumatic pelvic fractures. J Urol 1988;140(3):506–7.

202. Rosenstein DI, Alsikafi NF. Diagnosis and classification of urethral injuries. Urol Clin North Am 2006;33(1):73–85, vi–vii.

203. Armenakas NA, McAninch JW. Acute anterior urethral injuries: diagnosis and initial management. In: McAninch JW, editor. Traumatic and reconstructive urology. Philadelphia: WB Saunders; 1996.

204. Jordan GH, Virasoro R, Eltahawy EA. Reconstruction and management of posterior urethral and straddle injuries of the urethra. Urol Clin North Am 2006;33(1):97–109.

205. Black PC, Miller EA, Porter JR et al. Urethral and bladder neck injury associated with pelvic fracture in 25 female patients. J Urol 2006;175(6):2140–4; discussion 2144.

206. Wessells H, Long L. Penile and genital injuries. Urol Clin North Am 2006;33(1):117–26.

207. Lawson JS, Rotem T, Wilson SF. Catastrophic injuries to the eyes and testicles in footballers. Med J Aust 1995;163(5):242–4.

208. McAninch JW, Kahn RI, Jeffrey RB et al. Major traumatic and septic genital injuries, J Trauma 1984;24:291–8.

209. Ramchandani P, Buckler PM. Imaging of genitourinary trauma. Am J Roentgenol 2009;192(6):1514–23.

210. Palmer CM, McNulty AM, D'Este C et al. Genital injuries in women reporting sexual assault. Sex Health 2004;1(1):55–9.

211. Momoh C. Female genital mutilation. Curr Opin Obstet Gynecol 2004;16(6):477–80.

212. Brohi K. Injury to the colon and rectum trauma. Trauma.org; 2006. Online. www.trauma.org/archive/abdo/COLONdiagnosis.html; accessed 21 June 2015.

213. Meltzer DI. Complications of body piercing. Am Fam Physician 2005;72(10):2029–34.

214. Nelius T, Armstrong ML, Rinard K et al. Genital piercings: diagnostic and therapeutic implications for urologists. Urology 2011;78(5):998–1007.

215. Koenig LM, Carnes M. Body piercing medical concerns with cutting-edge fashion. J Gen Intern Med 1999;14(6):379–85.

216. Jones SA, Flynn RJ. An unusual (and somewhat piercing) cause of paraphimosis. Br J Urol 1996;78(5):803–4.

217. Hansen RB, Olsen LH, Langkilde NC. Piercing of the glans penis. Scand J Urol Nephrol 1998;32(3):219–20.

218. Muldoon KA. Body piercing in adolescents. J Pediatr Health Care 1997;11(6):298–301.

219. Lake JP, Essani R, Petrone P et al. Management of retained colorectal foreign bodies: predictors of operative intervention. Dis Colon Rectum 2004;47(10):1694–8.

220. McArthur BJ. Damage control surgery for the patient who has experienced multiple traumatic injuries. AORN J 2006;84(6):992–1000.

221. Saclarides TJ. Current choices—good or bad—for the proactive management of postoperative ileus: a surgeon's view. J Perianesth Nurs 2006;21(2A suppl.):S7–15.

222. Carlotti A, Carvalho W. Abdominal compartment syndrome: a review. Pediatric Crit Care Med 2009;10(1):115–20.

223. Malbrain ML, Cheatham ML, Kirkpatrick A et al. Results from the International conference of experts on intra-abdominal hypertension and abdominal compartment syndrome. I. Definitions. Intensive Care Med 2006;32(11):1722–32.

224. Aitken L, Niggemeyer L. Trauma management. In: Elliot D, Aitken L, Chaboyer W, eds. ACCCN's critical care nursing. 2nd ed Sydney: Elsevier; 2011.

225. Sugrue M. Intra-abdominal pressure: time for clinical practice guidelines? Intensive Care Med 2002;28(4):389–91.

226. Choi KC, Peek-Asa C, Lovell M et al. Complications after therapeutic trauma laparotomy. J Am Coll Surg 2005;201(4):546–53.

227. Tillou A, Weng J, Alkousakis T et al. Fascial dehiscence after trauma laparotomy: a sign of intra-abdominal sepsis. Am Surg 2003;69(11):927–9.

228. Waqar SH, Malik ZI, Razzaq A et al. Frequency and risk factors for wound dehiscence/burst abdomen in midline laparotomies. J Ayub Med Coll Abbottabad 2005;17(4):70–3.

229. Ward MA, Burgess PL, Williams DH et al. Threatened fertility and gonadal function after a polytraumatic, life-threatening injury. J Emerg Trauma Shock 2010 Apr–Jun; 3(2):199–203.

CHAPTER 49
SPINAL TRAUMA
JONATHON MAGILL AND KIRSTEN KENNEDY

Essentials

The essential care consideration in the effective management of any level of spinal cord injury (SCI) is to focus on the following:

- Treat your patients with a high level of suspicion of SCI until proven otherwise.
- Adequately maintain spinal alignment from the outset and throughout the course of treatment.
- Through adequate alignment, avoid any progression of neurological deficits in the patient and enhance recovery if deficits exist.
- Through specialist intervention, provide the best opportunity for recovery for the SCI patient.
- If in doubt—always consult.
- Differentiate between neurogenic and hypovolaemic shock.
- Monitor respiratory function closely in high-level injuries.
- Provide regular pressure relief once the patient has been stabilised.

INTRODUCTION

Trauma to the spinal column and the spinal cord can result in devastating injury. Spinal cord injury (SCI) is damage to the spinal cord that results in a loss of function such as mobility or feeling. The effects of SCI depend on the type and level of the injury. Before World War II, most people who sustained SCI died within weeks of their injury due to urinary dysfunction, respiratory infection or bedsores. However, improved resuscitation and long-term management techniques and materials mean that many people with SCI now approach the life span of the general population.[1]

Epidemiology

Flinders University in Adelaide, South Australia, collects statistics for SCI on an annual basis. The most recent report, compiled in 2007–08 and published in January 2010,[2] forms the basis for the Australian statistics in this chapter. The reports in Australia originate from six designated spinal units in five states which specialise in acute management and rehabilitation of SCI patients. In 2007–08, the six units reported 362 new case registrations, of which 285 (79%) had an SCI as a result of a traumatic cause. Traumatic causation is the main focus of the report in general, as shown in Table 49.1. The trend in persisting SCI from traumatic causes was 15.0 new cases per million population for the 2007–08 period. This figure demonstrates a marginal increase on the previous financial year, when there were 14.9 new cases per million of the population.[2]

TABLE 49.1 Case registrations reported to Australian Spinal Cord Injury Register by spinal units; Australia 2007–08[2]

NEWLY INCIDENT SCI CASE CHARACTERISTICS	COUNTS	PERCENTAGE
Traumatic causes		
Australian residents		
Survived 90 days or to discharge, neurological deficit*	266	73
Survived 90 days or to discharge, no neurological deficit	6	2
Died on ward†	6	2
Non-residents		
Survived to discharge, neurological deficit	7	2
Total traumatic causes	285	79
Non-traumatic causes		
Australian residents		
Survived 90 days or to discharge, neurological deficit	75	21
Survived 90 days or to discharge, no neurological deficit	0	0
Died on ward†	—	—
Non-residents		
Survived to discharge, neurological deficit	0	0
Total non-traumatic causes	77	21
Total newly incident SCI cases	362	100

*Includes 23 patients who met the definition of persisting SCI and were inpatients at the time of the report.

†Average age of those who died was 52 years

The New Zealand statistics for the years 2007–09 from the Burwood and Auckland Spinal Units show that 77% of patients had an SCI as a result of a traumatic cause. This represents 30 per million of the population for Traumatic and non-traumatic injury. New Zealand at this point in time does not hold a national SCI register due to the limited sources of data, namely all acute admissions to both spinal units located in the South and North Islands.[3]

Table 49.2 demonstrates the incidence of persisting SCI from traumatic causes in Australia. It shows that the main causative factors in traumatic SCI are land transport involving motor vehicle occupants (*n* = 62, 22%) and land transport involving unprotected road users—motor cyclists, pedal cyclists and pedestrians (*n* = 39, 14%). The incidence of SCI resulting from low falls was 10%, and from high falls 18%. This was inversely the case in New Zealand, where falls accounted for the highest percentage of cases (*n* = 58, 33%) along with, surprisingly, medical causes such as spinal abscess, Guillain-Barré syndrome and metastatic lesions (*n* = 58, 33%). Motorcycle collisions (MBCs) were at 17% (*n* = 30) followed by motor vehicle collisions (MVCs) at 16% (*n* = 29).[3]

There are differences between men and women in the causes of injury. Women tend to have a higher incidence of injuries caused by MVCs whereas men have a higher rate of sports injuries. In Australia, men still score higher than women across all injury groups, with a M:F ratio ranging from a low of 2.9:1 in those aged 75 years and above and a high of 12.0:1 in the 55- to 64-years age range.[2] These trends are not apparent in the New Zealand statistics, with a low of 3.9% (*n* = 7) in the 75-plus age group; the highest, surprisingly, being in the 45- to 54-year age range, sitting at 21% across both sexes (*n* = 38).[3] The steady decline of MVC-related SCI can be partially explained by speed-limit controls on freeways and open roads, stringent drink-driving legislation and increased seatbelt usage. Mandatory seatbelt and child-restraint laws have reduced the incidence, morbidity and mortality associated with SCI. Studies have shown that survivors of an MVC who are wearing a seatbelt are less likely to sustain severe and irreversible disability.[4]

Anatomy and physiology

The vertebral column consists of a series of stacked bones which support the head and trunk, providing the bony case for the spinal cord. It consists of 33 vertebrae: 7 cervical, 12 thoracic, 5 lumbar, 5 fused sacral and usually 4 rudimentary coccyx vertebrae. The anterior column is held in alignment by anterior and posterior longitudinal ligaments, and the posterior column by the nuchal ligament complex (supraspinous, interspinous and infraspinous ligaments), the capsular ligaments and the ligamentum flavum. Apart from the atlas/C1 and the axis/C2, all the vertebrae are anatomically similar, but differ in size and function (Figs 49.1 and 49.2).[5]

The spinal cord is a cylinder, flattened from front to back with the lower end tapering into a cone. Ventrally it possesses a deep midline groove, the anterior median sulcus, and dorsally it shows a shallow sulcus, from which a posterior median glial septum extends into the spinal cord. The posterior median septum within the spinal cord is attached to the incomplete posterior median septum of arachnoid in the subarachnoid space.[5]

TABLE 49.2 Incidence of persisting SCI from traumatic cases by mechanism of injury and neurological level of injury 90 days post admission or discharge; Australia 2007–08 (counts and row percentages)[2]

	NEUROLOGICAL LEVEL 90 DAYS POST ADMISSION OR AT DISCHARGE																	
	TETRAPLEGIA				PARAPLEGIA						NO NEURO-LOGICAL INJURY		NEUROLOGICAL LEVEL NOT AVAILABLE		NEUROLOGICAL LEVEL NOT REPORTED		GROUP TOTAL	
	CERVICAL		THORACIC		LUMBAR		SACRAL		ALL PARAPLEGIA									
MECHANISM	COUNT	%	COUNT	%	COUNT	%	COUNT	%	COUNT	%	COUNT	%	COUNT	%	COUNT	%	COUNT	%
Traffic—motor vehicle occupants	30	48	14	23	7	11	0	0	21	34	0	0	#	#	10	16	62	100
Traffic—unprotected road users*	11	28	20	51	#	#	0	0	23	59					5	13	39	100
Non-traffic—motor vehicle occupants	#	#	#	#	#	#	0	0	#	#	0	0	0	0	0	0	4	100
Non-traffic—unprotected road users*	8	32	12	48	#	#	#	#	16	64	0	0	0	0	#	#	25	100
Low falls	21	72	#	#	5	17	0	0	8	28	0	0	0	0	0	0	29	100
High falls	26	50	13	25	9	17	0	0	22	42	0	0	0	0	4	8	52	100
Struck or collision by person or object	9	36	7	28	#	#	#	#	9	36	0	0	#	#	6	24	25	100
Water-related	26	96	0	0	0	0	0	0	0	0	0	0	0	0	#	#	27	100
Other	#	#	9	41	6	27	0	0	15	68	0	0	0	0	4	18	22	100
All mechanisms	136	48	79	28	35	13	#	1	116	41	0	0	#	1	31	11	285	100

#Cell counts of 3 or fewer, and related percentages, are not shown

*Motorcyclists, cyclists, pedestrians

FIGURE 49.1 **The vertebral column.**[5]

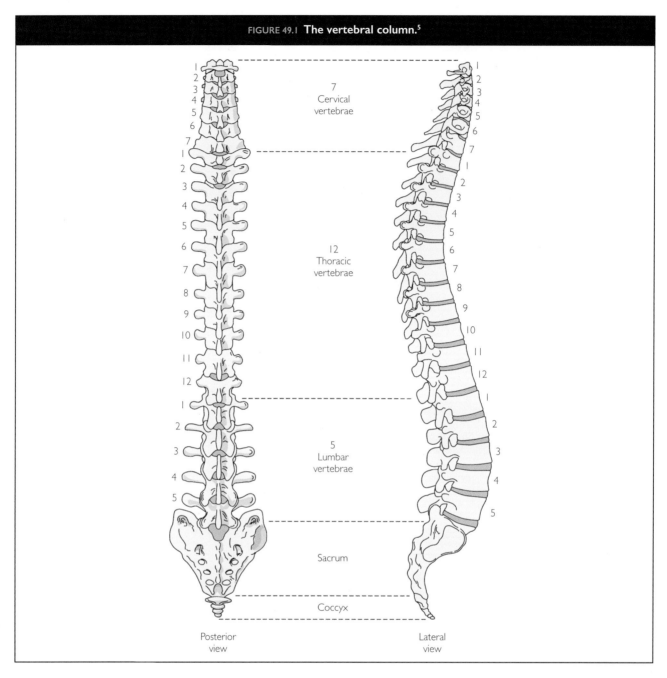

7
Cervical
vertebrae

12
Thoracic
vertebrae

5
Lumbar
vertebrae

Sacrum

Coccyx

Posterior
view

Lateral
view

In the fetus, the spinal cord extends to the lower limit of the spinal dura mater at the level of S2. The spinal dura remains attached at this level throughout life, but the spinal cord becomes relatively shorter: the bony spinal column and the dura mater grow more rapidly than the spinal cord. At birth, the conus medullaris or tip of the spinal cord lies opposite L3 and does not reach its pertinent level adjacent to L1 or L2 until the age of 20 years. The spinal nerve roots, especially those of the lumbar and sacral segments, come to slope more and more steeply downwards as the body matures.[5]

The spinal cord is made up of two symmetrical enlargements (portions), supplying the upper and lower limbs (Fig 49.3). The cervical enlargement supplies the upper limbs and the lumbar enlargement supplies the lower limbs. The spinal levels they occupy are C5 to T1 for the cervical and L2 to S3 for the lumbar enlargement. Both cervical and lumbar enlargements are due to the greatly increased mass of motor cells in the anterior columns of grey matter in these areas.

Spinal nerve roots

Thirty-one pairs of spinal nerves originate from the spinal cord; these are discussed in Chapter 23. The distribution is 8 cervical, 12 thoracic, 5 lumbar, 5 sacral and 1 coccygeal pair of spinal nerves.[6]

Examination of sensory responses to pin-prick and light touch is completed by testing a key point in each of the 28 dermatomes on both sides of the body. A key element of assessment of the extent of injury is demonstrated by a display of a segmental pattern in the alteration of motor, sensory and reflex activity in the extremities.[6] Nerve roots and the muscles they innervate are shown in Figure 49.4.

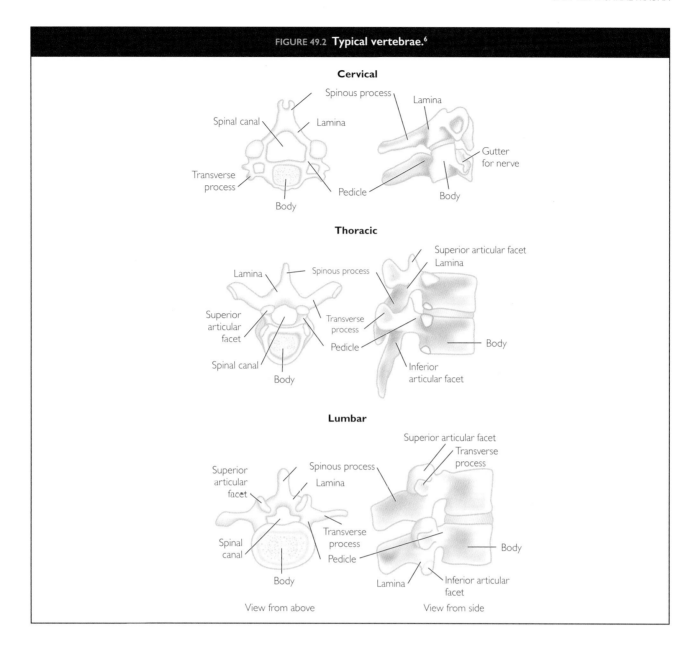

FIGURE 49.2 **Typical vertebrae.**[6]

Cervical

Spinous process

Spinal canal

Lamina

Lamina

Gutter for nerve

Transverse process

Pedicle

Body

Body

Thoracic

Lamina

Spinous process

Superior articular facet

Lamina

Superior articular facet

Transverse process

Body

Spinal canal

Pedicle

Body

Inferior articular facet

Lumbar

Superior articular facet

Transverse process

Superior articular facet

Spinous process

Lamina

Spinal canal

Transverse process

Pedicle

Body

Body

Lamina

Inferior articular facet

View from above

View from side

Vascular supply

The vascular supply to the spinal cord originates from two main sources, namely the anterior and posterior spinal arteries, with a multitude of spinal rami that intercept the intervertebral foramina at successive levels. The anterior artery sits in the median fissure along the length of the spinal cord. The two posterior spinal arteries descend towards the emerging spinal roots. In effect, the anterior artery feeds the ventral two-thirds of the spinal cord, while the posterior arteries feed the remaining dorsal third.[5,7]

If the vascular supply to the cord is damaged, the resulting effect is the deprivation of oxygen and essential nutrients, and ultimately necrosis of surrounding neural tissue. If the arterial supply is compromised, this may lead to ischaemia above the site where the injury has occurred—caused by proximal blood-flow loss. The spinal cord arteries are unable to compensate with collateral circulation in order to preserve neurological function if an injury occurs.[6]

Mechanisms and associated injuries

The majority of injuries to the spinal cord are closed. Four vectors of applied force generally cause SCI: *flexion, extension, compression* and *rotation*.[8] The amount of force exerted to cause an injury depends on the specific area of the spinal cord affected. In most cases, the areas of the spinal column used specifically for mobility, the cervical and lumbar regions, are the areas where most injuries occur. The musculature in the cervical area is less supportive than that in the lumbar area; significant force is required to produce a thoracic spinal injury due to the rigidity of the column in this area and its immobility, largely due to the support from the rib cage.

A flexion-motion injury is most apparent in the patient involved in an MVC, in which the patient has struck their head against the steering wheel or windscreen, forcing the spine into acute hyperflexion and throwing the chin forwards onto the chest. This results in rupture of the posterior ligaments and dislocation of the spine, also known as a burst fracture (Fig 49.5).

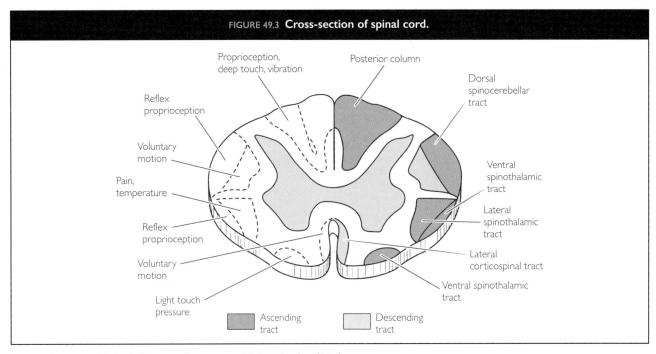

FIGURE 49.3 **Cross-section of spinal cord.**

Marcus Cremonese, Medical Illustration Department, UNSW Faculty of Medicine.

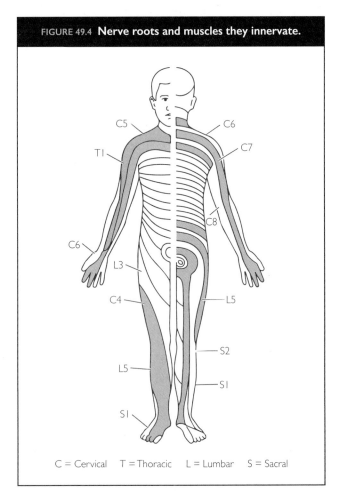

FIGURE 49.4 **Nerve roots and muscles they innervate.**

C = Cervical   T = Thoracic   L = Lumbar   S = Sacral

Marcus Cremonese, Medical Illustration Department, UNSW Faculty of Medicine.

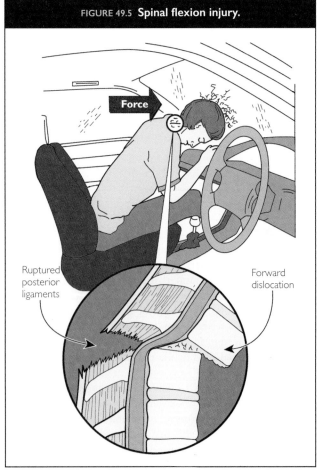

FIGURE 49.5 **Spinal flexion injury.**

Marcus Cremonese, Medical Illustration Department, UNSW Faculty of Medicine.

Extension injuries occur when the chin hits an object and the head is thrown backwards, and is traditionally known as a hangman's fracture. In this instance the anterior ligament is ruptured and the posterior elements of the vertebral body are fractured (Fig 49.6).

Axial load injuries, more commonly referred to as compression-type injuries, are seen in patients who have experienced a fall. The vertebral bodies are wedged and compressed. These burst vertebral shards enter the spinal canal, piercing the cord (Figs 49.7 and 49.8).

FIGURE 49.7 **Spinal compression injury.**

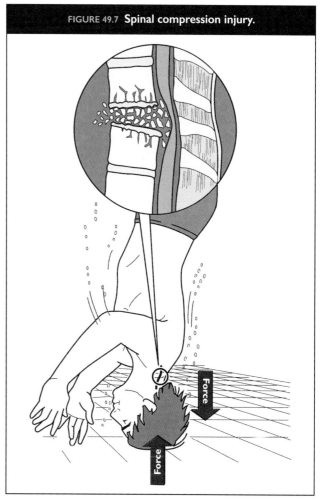

Marcus Cremonese, Medical Illustration Department, UNSW Faculty of Medicine.

FIGURE 49.6 **Spinal extension injury.**

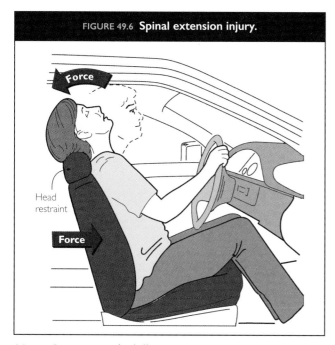

Marcus Cremonese, Medical Illustration Department, UNSW Faculty of Medicine.

FIGURE 49.8 **This 24-year-old man was a victim of a fall from a height, which resulted in a fracture–dislocation at L1–L2 and a complete spinal cord injury.**

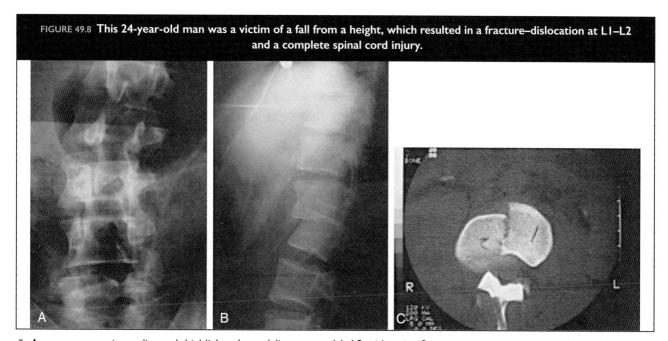

A, An anteroposterior radiograph highlights the malalignment at L1–L2 with a significant rotatory component and lateral slip at this level. **B**, A lateral radiograph confirms the displacement with forward subluxation and overlap at L1–L2. **C**, A computed tomography scan through L1–L2 highlights the displacement and malalignment, resulting in significant canal compromise and spinal cord injury.[9]

Rotational injuries are caused by a number of differing factors. Disruptions of the entire ligamentous structure, fracture and fracture dislocation of the facets occur. Flexion rotation injuries are highly unstable.[9]

The main mechanisms of injury to cause thoracolumbar fractures include:

- falls from a significant height onto the heels, which lead to increased anterior stress concentration
- a significant blow to the back; for example, in mining and construction industries, which causes the spine to bow at the thoracolumbar junction
- flexion and rotation injuries as a result of motor vehicle crashes
- heavy lifting where there are pathological underlying causes.

Penetrating cord injuries are most commonly obtained by stabbing or gunshot injury. If the neural tissue is lacerated, a disruption of blood supply to the cord occurs. Gunshot wounds which have traversed the spinal column may produce incomplete, unstable injuries. Pre-hospital curriculum advocates that it is not necessary to immobilise stab injuries where there is no neurological deficit and the traumatic penetrating injury is affecting the head and neck.[10] Spinal immobilisation devices may interfere with the recognition and management of life-threatening conditions, and research has shown that pre-hospital spinal immobilisation in these cases results in higher mortality.[11]

Pre-hospital assessment and initial management

Pre-hospital management is of the utmost importance. This includes a full patient assessment including identification of any obvious neurological deficit with loss of limb movement, numbness or significant pain to palpation of the cervical region, spinal stabilisation/immobilisation, airway maintenance and cardiovascular support.[12,13]

> **PRACTICE TIP**
>
> Assume that unconscious patients with a high index of suspicion of SCI should be treated as having an SCI until confirmed.

Another good practice point to remember is that airway intervention should always avoid manipulation of the spine, with the cervical spine kept in neutral alignment at all times (see the section below on spinal stabilisation, and Ch 10 on extrication).[12,14] However, airway management always takes precedence over spinal stabilisation and head tilt, and the use of airway adjuncts may be required if the airway is not patent after chin lift with the head in neutral alignment (see Ch 17, p. 314, for airway management techniques).[15,16] As in all trauma patients, indications for intubation in the pre-hospital environment are a threatened airway, hypoxia and hypoventilation.[17] Reviews of causes of adverse airway events due to pre-hospital spinal immobilisation remain unclear. There is a possibility that airway compromise may be attributed to rigid collar size and application; for example, applying a collar too tightly.[18]

All trauma patients should be assessed using the primary and secondary survey methods discussed in Chapter 44. Infor-mation in this chapter is specific to spinal management, SCI or suspected-SCI patients. Spinal immobilisation is a priority in trauma; however, spinal clearance is not. The spine should be assessed and cleared when appropriate, depending on the patient's injury characteristics and physiological state. Primary assessment and survey and treatment with life-saving measures should be carefully controlled, bearing in mind the possibility of SCI, and considering that damage to the spinal cord can mask the painful sensation of associated injuries.

Any indication of hypovolaemia in the SCI patient should be treated as outlined in Chapter 44.

Comfort of the patient should also be considered, as painful distracting injuries can often mask an underlying SCI. Adequate analgesia should be titrated against the patient's pain score and response. When treating moderate to severe pain, morphine is the first choice, followed by fentanyl if the patient was difficult to cannulate (administer intra-nasally) or expressed previous contraindications.[19] The management of mild to moderate pain in SCI could incorporate methoxyflurane as a safe option with minimal side effects.[20]

The risk of aspiration in the SCI patient is a consideration when making transport decisions. The use of a prophylactic antiemetic and insertion of an intragastric tube should be considered, especially for extended road transports or air transfers, although there is no conclusive evidence for the use of this routinely with opiate analgesia.[21]

The prevention of hypothermia is another pre-hospital consideration. Simple measures, such as limiting exposure and scene time, avoiding cold intravenous fluid administration and removing wet items of clothing, can be extremely effective.[22]

Spinal stabilisation

All multi-trauma patients should be treated as having suspected SCI, but the application of definitive immobilisation devices should not take precedence over life-saving procedures.[23] More often than not, the patient arrives at the emergency department (ED) having been suitably immobilised by pre-hospital staff using the methods demonstrated in Figures 49.9 and 49.10.

If the patient is still wearing a helmet, it should be removed as demonstrated in Figure 17.19, p. 326.

Spinal stabilisation for extrication can also be maintained with a Kendrick Extrication Device (KED) (Fig 49.11). A KED is used in conjunction with a cervical collar to help immobilise a patient's head, neck and spine in the normal anatomical position (neutral position). This position helps prevent additional injuries to these regions during vehicle extrication. Sandbags placed beside the patient's head or the use of commercially available head restraints further encourage immobilisation. The KED can also be used for stable patients to remove them from vehicles and confined spaces. A KED wraps the patient's head, back, shoulders and torso in a semi-rigid brace, immobilising the head, neck and spine. It is also used in conjunction with a rigid collar. A typical set-up would consist of two head straps, three torso straps and two leg straps, which are used to adequately secure the KED to the patient. Unlike a backboard, the KED uses a series of wooden or polymer bars in a nylon jacket, allowing responders to immobilise the patient's spine and neck, and remove them from the vehicle or confined space. KEDs can also be used to fully immobilise paediatric patients (Ch 10).[24]

FIGURE 49.9 **Log-rolling the prone patient.**

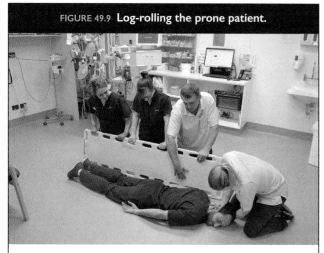

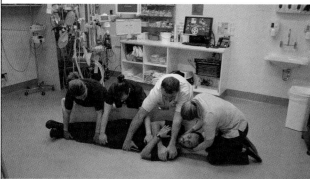

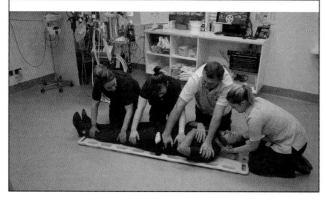

The spine should be protected at all times during the management of the patient with multiple injuries. The ideal position is with the whole spine maintained in a neutral position on a firm surface. This may be achieved manually or with a combination of semi-rigid cervical collar, side head supports and, in the pre-hospital environment, strapping during extrication. Strapping should be applied to the shoulders and pelvis, as well as the head to prevent the neck from becoming the centre of rotation of the body (Fig 49.12). Measuring and application of collars is discussed in Chapter 17, p. 323.

The combative patient and airway management

Patients who are agitated or restless due to shock, hypoxia, head injury or intoxication may be impossible to immobilise adequately. Forced restraints or manual fixation of the head may risk further injury to the spine. It may be necessary to remove immobilisation devices and allow the patient to move unhindered, or anaesthesia and sedation may be necessary to

FIGURE 49.10

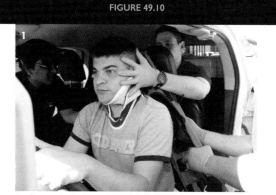

Apply a cervical collar and maintain in-line stabilisation throughout the procedure. Gently slide the KED behind the patient; it may be necessary to rock the patient forwards a few degrees to facilitate placement of the device.

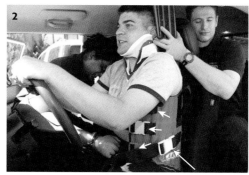

Bring the lateral panels around the chest beneath the patient's shoulders. First secure the thoracic straps (*short arrows*), and then fasten the pelvic support straps (*long arrow*).

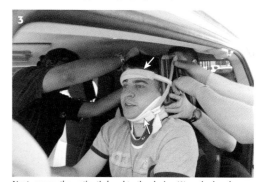

Next, secure the patient's head to the device. Wrap the head panels snugly around the head and neck while another rescuer applies the diagonal head straps (*arrows*).

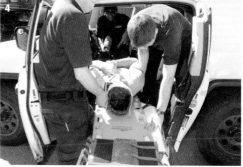

Bring the ambulance stretcher (with a backboard on it) as close to the patient as possible. Rotate the patient out of the vehicle and onto the backboard. Loosen the pelvic straps, and secure the patient to the board.

A, Rapid extrication from a motor vehicle.[24]

Continued

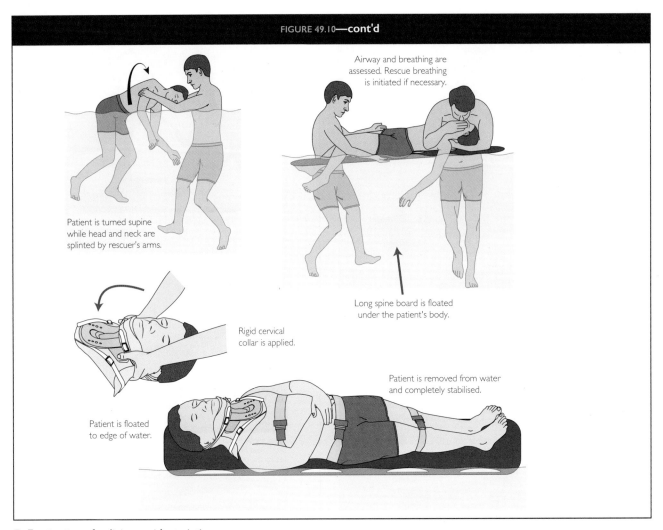

FIGURE 49.10—cont'd

Patient is turned supine while head and neck are splinted by rescuer's arms.

Airway and breathing are assessed. Rescue breathing is initiated if necessary.

Long spine board is floated under the patient's body.

Rigid cervical collar is applied.

Patient is removed from water and completely stabilised.

Patient is floated to edge of water.

B, Extrication of a diving accident victim.

B: Adapted from Sanders M. Mosby's paramedic textbook. 3rd edn. St Louis, Mosby; 2007.

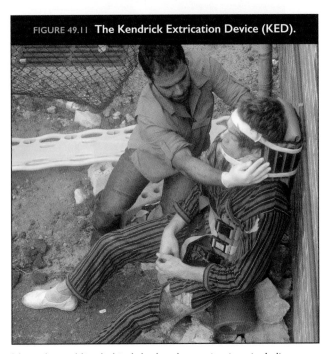

FIGURE 49.11 **The Kendrick Extrication Device (KED).**

Note the padding behind the head to maintain spinal alignment.

allow adequate diagnosis and therapy, based on locally agreed protocols.[25] If the trauma team leader has decided to use anaesthesia, the collar should be removed and manual, in-line protection reinstituted for the manoeuvre (see images in Ch 17, p. 324). The routine use of a gum elastic bougie is recommended, minimising cervical movement by allowing intubation with minimal visualisation of the larynx.[26] However, the introduction and use of laryngoscopes with video capability is becoming more widespread, having been demonstrated to shorten intubation time and be less likely to result in oesophageal intubation in patients with cervical spine immobilisation.[27]

Positioning

In the paediatric trauma patient, a few anatomical considerations are paramount. When supine on a firm surface, the size of the child's head can cause the posterior pharynx to buckle through passive flexion of the cervical spine. This can give rise to difficulties in X-ray interpretation. The maintenance of the sniffing position with a normal alignment of the airway lying in a superior and anterior portion of the mid-face is important, and can be obtained by placing a folded towel or sheet under the patient's shoulders to bring the cervical spine into the neutral position (Fig 49.13). In addition, because of distress, fear and inability

FIGURE 49.12 Long-spine-board immobilisation.[24]

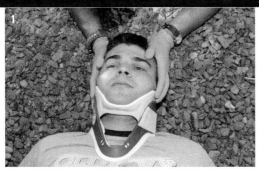

Position one: rescuer at the patient's head to apply manual in-line stabilisation. This rescuer oversees and directs all body movement throughout the procedure.

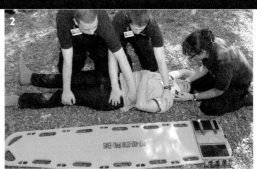

Position the backboard next to the patient's body. Note that a lateral neck stabiliser has been pre-applied to the board.

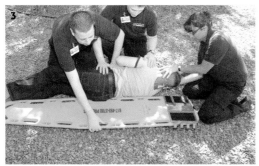

When the rescuer at the patient's head gives the command, roll the patient onto his side, examine the patient's back, and slide the backboard under the patient.

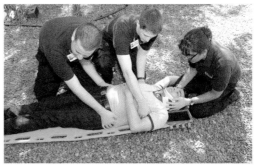

Roll the patient back onto the board when the head rescuer gives the command. Center the patient on the board before applying the straps.

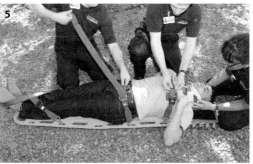

Strap the patient to the board. Proper strap placement (chest, pelvis and legs) and firm contact between the straps and the patient are important in limiting lateral motion.

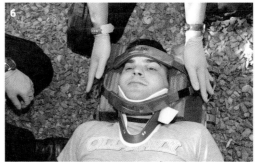

Apply a lateral neck stabiliser, like the Ferno Universal Head Immobiliser shown above, or sandbags.

to comprehend the situation, it may be difficult to immobilise a child adequately. Manual in-line stabilisation can be used instead of a semi-rigid collar. Collar sizing may be difficult and there are no collars that adequately fit infants aged 6 years and below.[28] In the adult population, occipital padding has been demonstrated to improve neutral alignment when compared to no padding, yet the range to achieve optimal alignment varies between 1.3 cm and 5.1 cm in adults making it difficult to ensure the correct alignment with this method alone.[29]

PRACTICE TIP

A simple folded towel placed under the adult patient's head while using in-line immobilisation will generally improve patient comfort and be an effective measure to maintain neutral cervical spine alignment.

Ongoing patient assessment

Once the airway has been secured and spinal precautions are in place, further examination of the patient can proceed. This requires careful removal of the patient's clothing, in such a way that flexion, extension and rotation of the neck or trunk is avoided. The safest method of clothing removal is to cut the clothes off. The clothing that remains under the patient can be removed when the patient is log-rolled. It is important to assess and clear the entire spinal column, as 5% of spinal injuries have a second, possibly non-adjacent, fracture elsewhere in the spine.[27]

Secondary survey and log-roll

One of the aspects of the secondary survey is to fully examine the patient's back. This involves maintaining in-line spinal immobilisation, which requires four members of the emergency team to safely execute (Fig 49.14).[30] This is

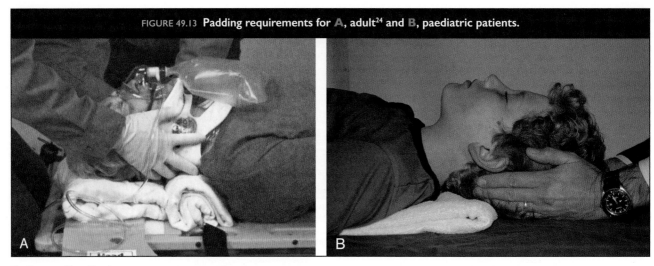

FIGURE 49.13 **Padding requirements for A, adult[24] and B, paediatric patients.**

A

B

B. Courtesy Kate Curtis.

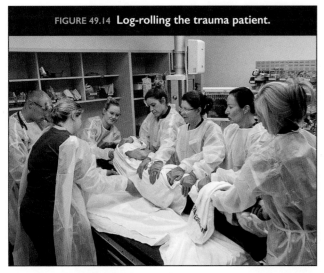

FIGURE 49.14 **Log-rolling the trauma patient.**

Courtesy University of Sydney.

obviously the minimum number and will depend on local resources available at the time. The most senior member of the team not conducting the assessment takes manual control of the cervical spine. It is the person with cervical spine control who is in command of the log-roll at all times. The remaining three members take responsibility for the thorax, pelvis and legs. The person responsible for the legs prevents adduction through maintaining the lateral malleolus in line with the hip. The movement is smooth, well-coordinated and should avoid any rotational movements of individual spinal segments.

Palpation

Palpation of the spine may show point tenderness or deformity, indicating a source of bony injury. A thorough neurological examination of the patient's motor, sensory and reflex functions is of prime importance. Any findings that indicate a presence of sensory or motor function classify the injury as incomplete. The level of sensory deficit is compared with the motor deficits using the standard international neurological classification form.[30] Figure 49.15 shows the American Spinal Injury Association (ASIA) documentation, which facilitates

the communication and referral of the extent of neurological deficit and referral to specialists.

One of the indicators of motor function and the sacral nerves is the rectal examination to ascertain rectal tone.[31] The clinical assessment of rectal tone and sensation indicates the presence of incomplete injury at the sacral level. Rectal tone alone is not an indicative finding of incomplete injury, with positive rectal tone being the common discriminator of the restoration of spinal reflexes and resolution of spinal shock.

Once a full examination of the back has taken place, the person at the head gives the team the command to return the patient to their supine position.

Cervical spine clearance

Spinal clearance is said to have occurred when the relevant clinicians have examined the patient physically and radiographically and have determined that no significant injury exists; at which point, immobilisation procedures are ceased. Spinal clearance involves the use of an assessment framework for the evaluation of the spinal status of patients considered to be at risk of spinal trauma. The assessment process concludes with either the validation of the lack of injury via the appropriate history, examination and investigation, or the diagnosis and subsequent management of an injury.[33] Delay in spinal clearance, or in diagnosis and subsequent injury management, predisposes the unconscious patient to the complications of immobilisation and resultant increase in morbidity, particularly in those cases where the cervical collar is on for longer than 72 hours.[34]

Clinical clearance

Numerous, large, prospective studies have described the high cost and low yield of the indiscriminate use of cervical spine radiology in trauma patients, most notably the NEXUS group study in 2000.[35] Although there are case reports of bony or ligamentous injuries in asymptomatic patients, no asymptomatic patient in the literature has had an unstable cervical spine fracture or suffered neurological deterioration because of the injury.[23] Mechanism of injury alone does not determine the need for radiological investigation. If the NEXUS preconditions are met, as explained in Figure 49.16,

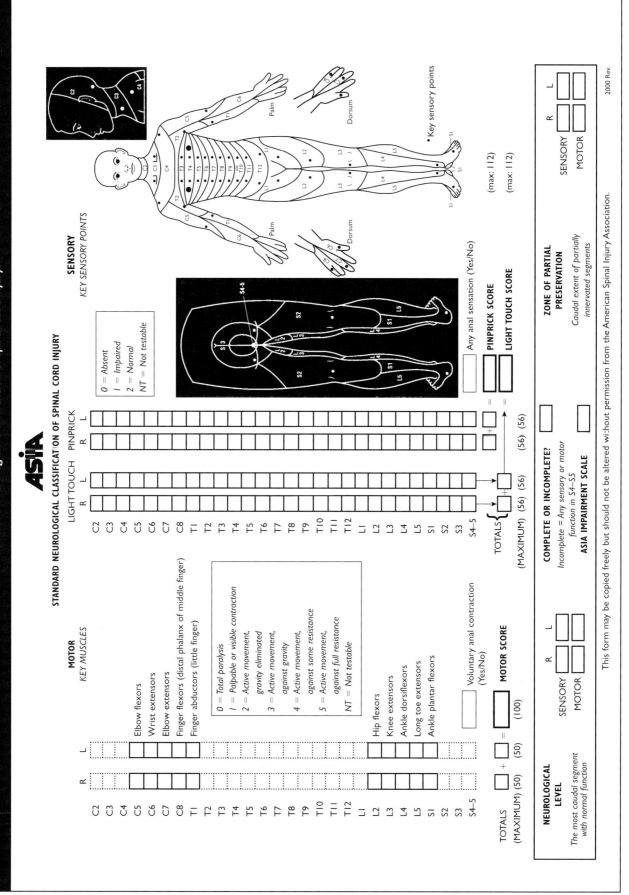

FIGURE 49.15 Standard neurological classification of spinal cord injury.[32]

FIGURE 49.16 NEXUS low-risk criteria.[36]

According to the NEXUS Low-Risk Criteria, cervical
spine radiography is indicated for trauma patients unless
they exhibit ALL of the following criteria:

1. No posterior midline cervical spine tenderness
       and
2. No evidence of intoxication
       and
3. Normal level of alertness
       and
4. No focal neurological deficit
       and
5. No painful distracting injuries

Explanations:
    These are for purposes of clarity only. There are not precise
    definitions for the individual NEXUS Criteria, which are subject
    to interpretation by individual doctors.

1. Midline posterior bony cervical spine tenderness is present if the patient complains of
    pain on palpation of the posterior midline neck from the nuchal ridge to the prominence
    of the first thoracic vertebra, or if the patient evinces pain with direct palpation of any
    cervical spinous process.

2. Patients should be considered intoxicated if they have either of the following: (a) a recent
    history by the patient or an observer of intoxication or intoxicating ingestion; or (b)
    evidence of intoxication on physical examination such as odour of alcohol, slurred
    speech, ataxia, dysmetria or other cerebellar findings, or any behaviour consistent with
    intoxication. Patients may also be considered to be intoxicated if tests of bodily
    secretions are positive for drugs (including but not limited to alcohol) that affect level of
    alertness.

3. An altered level of alertness can include any of the following: (a) Glasgow Coma Scale
    score of 14 or less; (b) disorientation to person, place, time or events; (c) inability to
    remember 3 objects at 5 minutes; (d) delayed or inappropriate response to external
    stimuli; or (e) other.

4. Any focal neurological complaint (by history) or finding (on motor or sensory
    examination).

5. No precise definition for distracting painful injury is possible. This includes any condition
    thought by the clinician to be producing pain sufficient to distract the patient from a
    second (neck) injury. Examples may include, but are not limited to: (a) any long bone
    fractures; (b) a visceral injury requiring surgical consultation; (c) a large laceration,
    degloving injury or crush injury; (d) large burns: or (e) any other injury producing acute
    functional impairment. Doctors may also classify any injury as distracting if it is
    thought to have the potential to impair the patient's ability to appreciate other injuries.

the neck may then be examined. If there is no bruising or deformity, no tenderness and a pain-free range of active movements, the cervical spine can be cleared.

Many alert and stable trauma patients are at extremely low risk for spinal injury and can be clinically cleared without the need for imaging using the Nexus criteria or the Canadian C-Spine Rule. The Canadian C-Spine Rule is an alternative to the NEXUS criteria. It is only to be used in alert and stable adult patients with suspected cervical spine injury. What the rule does is to suggest an X-ray for all high-risk patients. If the patient assessment demonstrates that no high-risk criteria are found, then a single low-risk factor allows safe assessment of the range of motion. On examination, if the patient is able to actively rotate their neck 45° left to right then no X-ray is indicated.[23,35,37] Use of the Canadian C-Spine Rule to clear the cervical spine has been demonstrated to be safe and effective for use by paramedics in the pre-hospital environment[38] and nurses in the ED.[39] The Queensland Ambulance Service (QAS) has been using the Canadian C-Spine Rule since 2011 and has

recently introduced the use of soft cervical collars to replace stiff collars.

If these criteria are not met, radiological evaluation is required and a clinical guideline should be followed (see Fig 49.17 for an example). There is no conclusive evidence in the literature that supports clinical clearance of the spine in the pre-hospital environment, although this appears to be changing.[25] There is enough variation between pre-hospital and in-hospital assessments and circumstance to recommend that pre-hospital removal of spinal immobilisation be avoided. However, there is emerging evidence that considers the efficacy of hard collars in the field and complications associated with their widespread use. The consensus appears to be moving towards optimising appropriate use, that is, more rationed application of the collars in the first place.[25,40] However, the decision to immobilise or not is a component of paramedic practice guidelines based on the NEXUS criteria or Canadian C-Spine Rule, and has been demonstrated to be sensitive in pre-hospital immobilisation selection.[41,42]

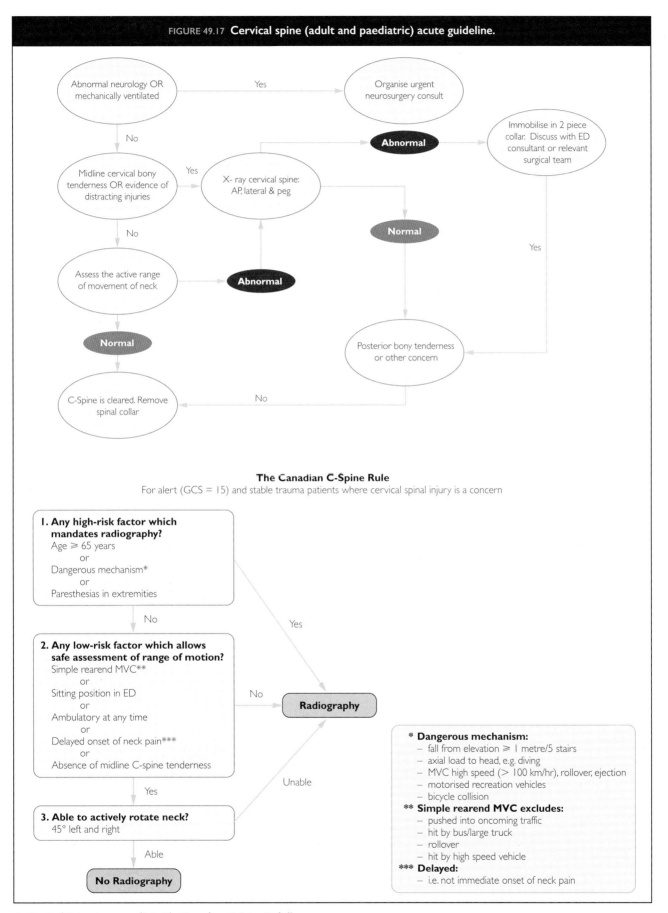

FIGURE 49.17 **Cervical spine (adult and paediatric) acute guideline.**

A. Cervical Spine Assessment.[40] *B. The Canadian C-Spine Rule.*[43]

PRACTICE TIP

If the cervical spine cannot be cleared within 4 hours, then the hard collar should be replaced with a Philadelphia collar (see Ch 17, p. 324).

Radiological investigation

If the patient exhibits any signs of cervical spine tenderness, focal neurological deficit, evidence of intoxication, painful distracting injury or altered mental status, clinical examination is unreliable and radiographical assessment of the cervical spine is advised. Radiological evaluation determines the presence of spinal fractures. For high-risk patients or those with suspicious clinical examinations, the 2009 Eastern Association for the Surgery of Trauma guidelines now recommend computed tomography of the cervical spine (CTC) instead of multiple plain films to identify cervical fractures.[45] This recommendation is based on a number of studies that have demonstrated the inaccuracy of plain films.[46,47]

Traditionally, the cervical spine series consists of anteroposterior (AP), open-mouth (odontoid) and lateral radiographical views. The lateral cervical spine film must include the base of the occiput and the top of the first thoracic vertebra. The lateral view alone is inadequate and will miss up to 15% of cervical spine injuries. The lower cervical spine may be difficult to examine, and gentle traction on the arms should be used to improve visualisation. This can be performed by the ED nurse donning a lead gown, holding the patient's arms, asking them to relax their shoulders and pulling gently. This is redundant if the patient has injuries to their arms and associated structures such as the clavicle. A swimmer's view (one arm raised) is required if the C7/T1 junction is not visualised; however, repeated attempts at plain radiography are usually unsuccessful and waste time. The patient with a normal cervical spine series who has persistent symptoms requires an evaluation of ligamentous injury. Flexion/extension images of the neck are no longer recommended as they are often unable to be completed due to restriction of movement secondary to pain, and can be ambiguous. Magnetic resonance imaging (MRI) should be used when there is high clinical suspicion of injury.[48]

With regard to the management of the unconscious, intubated trauma patient, the extent to which tests are performed in the ED depends mainly on locally defined protocols for spinal management, availability of resources and personnel and the patient's ability to tolerate such procedures. A lateral cervical spine film should be performed if the patient is not proceeding to CT; for example, going to theatre for emergency surgery. Otherwise, the patient should undergo multislice CT scanning. The odontoid radiograph is known to be inadequate in the intubated patient because of the position required to obtain the views: it misses up to 17% of injuries to the upper cervical spine. Overall clinical examination is impossible and plain-film X-ray alone cannot exclude ligamentous instability.[46,47]

Table 49.3 outlines the various diagnostic procedures used to determine spinal column or cord injury.

Thoracolumbar spine clearance

The spine requires radiological investigation for clearance as follows. Clinical signs, such as localised percussion tenderness, back pain following trauma and associated angular kyphosis, indicate that the clinician should have a high index of suspicion for fracture. Pain may also be referred to the chest and abdomen as a result of thoracolumbar injury, which divert attention away from the site of injury. The unconscious trauma patient requires radiological investigation, and if they have undergone CT of the chest and abdomen, spinal column reconstructions should be performed.

Pharmacological management

Clinical trials have produced conflicting evidence regarding the effectiveness of high-dose steroids in SCI. Although the National Acute Spinal Cord Injury Study (NASCIS) II and III shows greater recovery with methylprednisolone initiated within 8 hours of injury, subsequent studies have not reproduced these findings. In addition, it was noted that patients treated with methylprednisolone showed a higher rate of complications than those who weren't.[50] Patients with a penetrating injury who received methylprednisolone had worse outcomes than those not treated with steroids.[51] There is currently no evidence available on the use of steroids in the paediatric population.[51] Side effects of high dose steroids include increased incidence of sepsis, pneumonia, gastrointestinal haemorrhage, hyperglycaemia, hypertension and poor wound healing. Recent guidelines from The Congress of Neurological Surgeons on acute spinal cord injury management do not recommend the use of methylprednisolone due to a lack of supporting evidence.[52]

Additional interventions

Every system of the body is innervated by the spinal cord and during the emergency phase following SCI there are a number of interventions required in order to reduce the risk of further complications, particularly to the urinary, respiratory and integumentary system.

Respiratory

Respiratory function is impaired in the majority of patients following SCI; the extent of dysfunction is dependent upon the level and completeness of injury. The diaphragm, intercostals, abdominal and accessory muscles can all be affected. Autonomic control of respiratory function is disturbed in cervical injuries, which results in additional respiratory complications such as hypersensitive airways and abnormal bronchial secretions.[53]

Damage to the cervical cord causes significant changes in ventilatory control, breathing patterns and respiratory mechanics. This impairment can result in abdominal breathing with inefficient gas exchange and an inability to clear secretions efficiently. Use of accessory muscles causes paradoxical breathing, which is characterised by the abdomen expanding during inspiration while the chest moves inwards. Spastic paralysis of intercostal muscles results following the resolution of spinal shock; this creates a rigid chest wall which ceases to collapse on inspiration and somewhat improves respiratory function.[54]

Injuries at C3 and above require immediate artificial ventilation; those from C3 to C5 have significant respiratory dysfunction with varying amounts of diaphragmatic function remaining intact. These patients remain at high risk of pulmonary complications. Respiratory complications in cervical spine injuries commonly occur within the first 5 days

TABLE 49.3 Diagnostic evaluation procedures for spinal cord injury[49]

PROCEDURE	COMMENTS
Radiography	Able to visualise the entire spine to delineate the exact site and specific nature of bony injuries

Anteroposterior (AP) and lateral views	Views should be examined for:
	  contour and alignment of vertebral bodies according to normal curvature of the spine
	  presence of cervical vertebrae
	  displacement of bone fragments into the spinal canal
	  fracture of the laminae, pedicles, spinous process to determine ligamentous stability
	  spinous process distances
	  degree of soft tissue damage, especially important when no fracture is apparent (SCIWORA)

Swimmer's views	Perform when all cervical vertebrae are not visualised with AP film
Odontoid view	Evaluates integrity of odontoid body and C1 and C2 vertebrae
Computed tomography (CT) scanning	Thin-cut (2 mm) axial CT scanning on specific bone windows, with sagittal and coronal reconstruction should be used to evaluate abnormal, suspicious or poorly visualised areas on plain radiology. With technically adequate studies and experienced interpretation, the combination of plain radiology and directed CT scanning provides a false-negative rate of less than 0.1%. The scan should include the entire vertebral body above and below the region of interest, as these must be undamaged for subsequent internal fixation In recent years, the concept of full cervical spine CT for assessment of spinal injury has emerged. There are several studies that have demonstrated the robustness of the full CT scan, with sagittal and coronal reconstructions, for the exclusion of significant spinal injury. Widening, slippage or rotational abnormalities of the cervical vertebrae suggest soft-tissue injury. An absence of such signs appears to exclude significant instability. If there are abnormal findings on the CT scan, additional modalities, such as MRI, can be employed Helical or multislice CT scanning from the occiput to T1 is performed at 2–3 mm collimation and 1.5 m pitch. Sagittal and coronal reconstructions must be closely examined for indications of ligamentous instability. When whole cervical spine CT scanning is performed, the AP plain film becomes redundant. Further, patients who undergo CT scan of the chest and abdomen can have spinal construction images created which can provide concise detail of the thoracolumbar spine
Magnetic resonance imaging (MRI)	Non-invasive technique Uses radiofrequency radiation in presence of strong magnetic field to provide cross-sectional display of various anatomical structures, including soft tissues Role of MRI during acute care management is becoming the preferred diagnostic test, as it offers greater advantages over other diagnostic methods in terms of sensitivity Difficult in intubated patient
Somatosensory evoked potential (SSEP)	Assists with establishing the extent of injury to the nervous system; often performed within 24–48 hours of admission Used to monitor intraoperative neural function during surgical reduction or instrumentation of the spine

of injury; reasons for this include respiratory muscle fatigue, decreased inspiratory capacity, increased secretion production and impaired cough.[55]

Early intubation and respiratory support in an intensive care unit is recommended for patients who have sustained a high cervical injury; during intubation care should be taken to ensure minimal movement of the cervical spine.[56] Injuries below C5 will cause less respiratory impairment, but the patient will continue to be at risk of respiratory complications such as sputum retention, pneumonia and atelectasis. Refer to Table 49.4 for muscle innervation.

During the phase immediately post injury, loss of respiratory muscle function can result in shallow breaths. An initial increase in respiratory rate can compensate for this shallow breathing pattern, but is not efficient or sustainable. Observation for signs of fatigue and decreased oxygenation is important in order to prevent serious deterioration. Some indicators of respiratory muscle fatigue are excessive use of accessory muscles in the neck, difficulty mobilising secretions, exaggerated abdominal movements, decreased breath sounds and pale or dusky skin.[57]

PRACTICE TIP

Recording baseline and ongoing respiratory function including vital capacity (VC), forced expiratory volume (FEV_1), ABGs and oxygen saturation can provide valuable indicators of respiratory compromise.[56]

TABLE 49.4 Spinal nerve muscle innervation and patient response

NERVE LEVEL	MUSCLES INNERVATED	PATIENT RESPONSE
C4	Diaphragm	Ventilation
C5	Deltoid	Shrug shoulders
	Biceps	Flex elbows
	Brachioradialis	
C6	Wrist extensor	Extend wrist
	Extensor carpi radialis longus	
C7	Triceps	Extend elbow
	Extensor digitorum	Extend fingers
	Flexor carpi radialis	
C8	Flexor digitorum profundus	Flex fingers
T1	Hand intrinsic muscles	Spread fingers
T2 to L1	Intercostals	Vital capacity
	Abdominal	Abdominal reflexes
L2	Iliopsoas	Hip flexion
L3	Quadriceps	Knee extension
L4	Tibialis anterior	Ankle dorsiflexion
L5	Extension hallucis longus	Ankle eversion
S1	Gastrocnemius	Ankle plantar flexion
		Big toe extension
S2 to S5	Perineal sphincter	Sphincter control

Close monitoring is essential for tetraplegic patients, as cord oedema may result in an ascending level of paralysis, which can further compromise respiration. Non-invasive ventilation is often used long-term in tetraplegic patients to support respiratory function.

In addition to SCI, pain and chest trauma, including rib fractures, pneumothorax and pulmonary contusions, can contribute to respiratory impairment, along with patient age and pre-existing conditions. Regular chest physiotherapy, incorporating deep breathing and coughing exercises, can help prevent atelectasis and pneumonia. Assisted coughs can be provided manually or with an insufflation–exsufflation machine.

Circulatory

Acute cervical injuries are often associated with haemodynamic instability. This occurs due to interruption to the sympathetic fibres which exit the spinal cord in the thoracic region, resulting in unopposed parasympathetic outflow, leading to hypotension and potentially cardiac dysrhythmias.

Although hypotension and inadequate tissue perfusion are known to contribute to secondary ischaemic cord injury, the ideal mean arterial blood pressure required to improve spinal cord perfusion and restrict secondary damage is not known.[54,56] Close monitoring of fluid status is important, as aggressive fluid resuscitation of a patient in neurogenic shock can result in pulmonary oedema. Cardiac, haemodynamic and respiratory monitoring will assist in early detection of potential complications and allow initiation of prompt treatment, which can lead to improved patient outcomes and reduced risk of complications.

Poor venous return and immobility place patients with an SCI at an increased risk of venous thromboembolism. Mechanical prophylaxis, including compression stockings, sequential calf compression and regular position changes are not sufficient alone, but their use is recommended in conjunction with anticoagulants.[56,58]

> **PRACTICE TIP**
>
> Prophylactic anticoagulant therapy, preferably administration of low-molecular-weight heparin, should begin as soon as possible, providing there are no contraindications.[56,58,59]

Gastrointestinal

Complete SCI at or above T6 is likely to result in a paralytic ileus.

> **PRACTICE TIP**
>
> Insertion of a nasogastric tube is essential in order to relieve nausea and gastric distension, which can increase the risk of aspiration and further compromise respiratory function. Intravenous fluids are generally required for at least the first 48 hours and the patient needs to remain nil by mouth until bowel sounds return. Acute SCI, particularly cervical injuries, increases the risk of gastric ulcers; ideally, administration of intravenous prophylaxis should be started as soon as possible after injury.[56,60]

Individuals with an acute SCI will present with an acontractile neuropathic bladder.

> **PRACTICE TIP**
>
> Insertion of an indwelling urinary catheter is required in order to facilitate drainage of urine and enable accurate monitoring of fluid balance.

A per rectum examination should be performed daily to ensure the lower bowel is empty. Removal of any faecal material in the lower bowel is necessary to prevent impaction and loss of tone, which can occur if the bowel is left overdistended. A regular bowel regime is required when the patient begins oral intake or enteral feeds. This regime may include aperients, digital stimulation, digital removal, suppositories or enemas, depending on the level of injury.

Other systems

Provision of pain relief throughout the patient journey is an important consideration. In addition to pain at the fracture site and any other region of trauma, neuropathic pain at or below the level of SCI may occur immediately following injury.[54] Neuropathic pain is often described as burning, shooting or electric and can manifest as regions of hypersensitivity with or without a stimulus. There are a number of neuropathic pain mechanisms which are currently not well understood.[61]

The pain relief chosen should not affect respiratory function and needs to take into account neuropathic pain requirements. Neuropathic pain does not respond well to most pain relief agents, including opiates. Medications that have been found to provide effective pain relief are anticonvulsants and tricyclic antidepressants.[62] For further information on pain management, see Chapter 19.

It is essential to monitor and maintain normal body temperature of patients with spinal injuries at or above T6, as they lose the ability to autoregulate body temperature (poikilothermia), and will assume the temperature of their environment. This has significant implications for the haemorrhaging trauma patient. See Chapter 44 for the impact of hypothermia on the trauma patient.

Pressure injuries are largely avoidable and prevention strategies should be implemented as part of the management of acute SCI. Patients with spinal cord injuries are at significant risk of pressure injury as a result of decreased sensation and motor function, coupled with impaired circulation and use of hard support surfaces and cervical collars. Areas at highest risk are bony prominences below the level of injury and the occipital area for those wearing cervical collars. Prolonged immobilisation should be avoided whenever possible, and pressure relief commenced once emergency medical conditions and spinal stabilisation permit. If a hard backboard has been used pre-hospital, it should be removed as part of the log-roll in the secondary survey. Ideally assessment and documentation of the patient's skin condition would happen at this time, with reassessment occurring each time pressure relief is attended.[56] Use of pressure-relieving mattresses as appropriate to the patient condition, along with regular turning or repositioning of individuals with acute spinal cord injury, should be attended every 2 hours if the medical condition allows. It is important to prevent shearing and friction and avoid stretching and folding of soft tissues, when moving and transferring patients.[56] Box 49.1 summarises essential nursing care.

BOX 49.1 Summary of nursing interventions for SCI

- Nasogastric tube
- Indwelling urinary catheter
- Intravenous fluids
- Cardiac monitoring
- Blood pressure monitoring
- Temperature
- Pulse
- Pulse oximetry
- Respiratory rate
- Pressure area care
- Analgesia
- Bowel regimen
- Deep vein thrombosis prophylaxis
- Gastric ulcer prophylaxis
- Arterial blood gases

Definitive care

There are a number of cervical collars available that can be used to stabilise the cervical spine. Most are made of rigid plastic or semi-rigid foam reinforced by plastic struts and secured with Velcro straps. The primary function of these collars is to restrict flexion and extension of the middle and lower cervical spine.

Common collars used include the Philadelphia, Miami J, Aspen and Stiffneck collars. They are available in a range of sizes which cater for a variety of neck circumferences and lengths. Collars need to be fitted and applied correctly in order to provide optimum restriction of movement.

As there are a small number of spinal injuries units in Australia and New Zealand, many patients will be admitted to local and regional hospitals for their initial treatment. Once spinal cord injury is confirmed, the nearest spinal injuries unit should be contacted. Immediate transfer of patients with cervical injuries is ideal, as management in a specialised unit is associated with reduced frequency of respiratory complications.[57]

Transfer to a spinal injury unit should not be delayed for unnecessary diagnostic procedures that will not alter management.

The spine should remain immobilised during transfer, preferably using a split-scoop stretcher or vacuum mattress.[23] Rigid spinal boards are more appropriate for use at the accident site than during transfer.

Cervical tongs and fracture stabilisation/fixation

Treatment of spinal injuries can take the form of surgery or conservative management. Early surgery is the preferred treatment option as it allows earlier mobilisation and reduces the risk of complications from bed rest and immobility. Conservative management is rare as it requires the patient to be maintained on bed rest in spinal alignment for up to 8 weeks. Another less common option is the halo vest, which is the most effective orthotic device for maintaining cervical alignment and preventing movement (Fig 49.18).[63] Cervical traction can be used to reduce fractures or dislocations and relieve pressure on the cord; this is generally used short term prior to surgery (Fig 49.19).

Surgery is performed in order to reduce fractures and dislocations, stabilise injured segments and restore optimal vertebral alignment. Decompression of the spinal cord is often performed during surgery by removing bone and disc fragments impinging on the cord. Surgery can be performed from an anterior or posterior approach; severe injuries may require both anterior and posterior surgery. Depending on the type of surgery performed, a number of internal fixation devices can be used to provide stability. Some factors that influence the surgical approach and type of internal stabilisation device used include the level and type of spinal column injury, the extent of spinal instability, the number of vertebrae requiring stabilisation, the extent of neurological impairment and the preference of the surgeon. Cervical collars, thoracolumbar or thoracolumbosacral braces may be used for 6–8 weeks

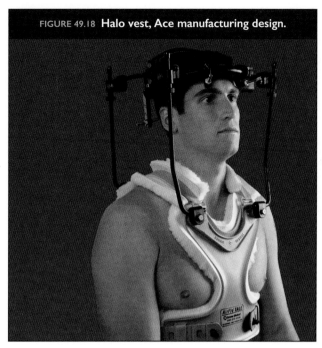

FIGURE 49.18 **Halo vest, Ace manufacturing design.**

Note the rigid shoulder straps and encompassing vest. Various vest sizes are available prefabricated. The halo ring, superstructure and vest are compatible with magnetic resonance imaging.

Courtesy of Acromed Corporation, Cleveland, OH.

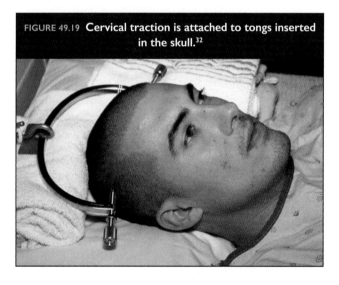

FIGURE 49.19 **Cervical traction is attached to tongs inserted in the skull.**[32]

post surgery to limit movement of the spinal canal and allow optimum healing to occur.

Psychosocial care

SCI is a devastating event with far-reaching psychological, physical and social effects. Immediately following SCI it is common for the patient to struggle to comprehend what this means for them, their family and the rest of their life. Patients often ask questions regarding their long-term prospects, particularly whether they will be able to walk again. These questions are difficult to answer accurately, particularly until the acute phase of injury has passed and spinal shock has resolved. Reassurance, emotional support and honesty are valuable to patients and their family and friends at this time. Common feelings include anxiety, shock, fear and helplessness.

Providing an explanation of all procedures and answering questions can help decrease the distress experienced due to feelings of loss of control in this unfamiliar environment.

Primary and secondary damage

Primary injury is the neurological damage that occurs to the spinal cord at the time of injury and is associated with cord compression, laceration, contusion or disruption due to impact. Secondary and iatrogenic damage occurs over subsequent hours and days. The secondary mechanism encompasses a cascade of biochemical and cellular processes that are initiated by the physical trauma and may cause ongoing cell death or damage (Fig 49.20).

The mechanisms of secondary injury include ischaemia, hypoxia and oedema. Damage is caused by restricted blood flow, excitotoxicity, inflammation, free-radical release and apoptosis, all of which contribute to an increase in the area of damage to the spinal cord. Hypoxia may occur as a result of inadequate airway maintenance and ventilation, while secondary traumatic injury can occur through inadequate spinal stabilisation. Oedema occurs at the site of injury and over time can spread to adjacent areas. It is often first detected by a decrease in function or sensation, and the extent of swelling can be determined on MRI. Prevention or correction of hypotension, shock, decreased arterial oxygen content, catecholamine release, hypercoagulability and hyperthermia is important, as secondary damage is exacerbated by these systemic changes.[56]

Spinal and neurogenic shock

- *Spinal shock* occurs in cervical and upper thoracic injuries at the time of injury and has a duration lasting from days to weeks. It can be defined as a sudden and transient suppression of neural function below the level of SCI. Symptoms include loss of all spinal reflexes below the level of injury and flaccid paralysis, including bladder and bowel. Sustained priapism may also be present. Resolution of spinal shock occurs when the reflex arcs below the level of injury begin to function again; the bulbocavernosus reflex is often the first to return.

- *Neurogenic shock* occurs more commonly in injuries at and above T6 and results from disruption of the sympathetic outflow between T1 and L2. This results in massive vasodilation, a decrease in venous return, cardiac output and tissue perfusion. The loss of sympathetic outflow results in hypotension caused by peripheral vasodilation, bradycardia, loss of cardiac accelerator reflex and the loss of the ability to sweat below the level of injury. Hypothermia may result due to loss of impulses from the temperature regulatory centre in the hypothalamus and the sympathetic nervous system. As the spinal cord loses its ability to autoregulate blood pressure, efforts must be made to regulate the blood pressure, as prolonged hypotension may exacerbate the ischaemia of the injured cord.

PRACTICE TIP

It is important to differentiate between neurogenic and hypovolaemic shock, as they require very different treatment (see Chs 20 and 44).

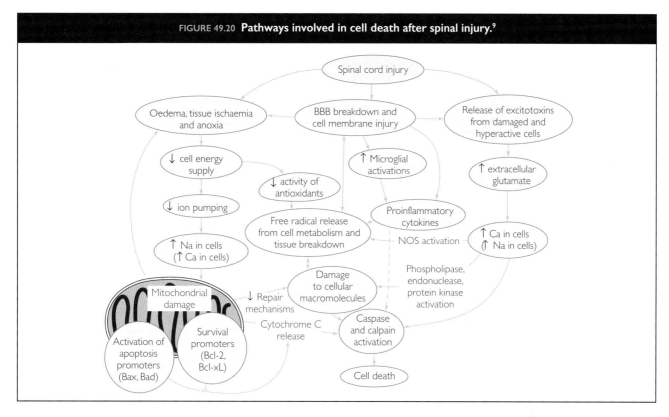

FIGURE 49.20 **Pathways involved in cell death after spinal injury.**[9]

Neurogenic and hypovolaemic shock may co-exist in the multitrauma patient and, in this instance, neurogenic shock exacerbates the effects of hypovolaemic shock by disabling the vasoconstrictive reflexes that ordinarily preserve blood flow to vital organs. Table 49.5 highlights the differences between neurogenic and hypovolaemic shock.

Poikilothermia

Spinal cord injury at T6 and above results in loss of the ability to regulate body temperature. This is referred to as poikilothermia, and is caused by loss of hypothalamic control of the sympathetic nervous system. An inability to maintain body temperature occurs as a result of passive dilation of dermal-level blood vessels.[64] In addition, the ability to shiver and perspire below the level of the injury is lost and the patient will assume the temperature of their environment. As a result, monitoring of body temperature and maintenance of environmental temperature is important.

TABLE 49.5 Differences between neurogenic and hypovolaemic shock	
NEUROGENIC SHOCK	HYPOVOLAEMIC SHOCK
Hypotension	Hypotension
Bradycardia	Tachycardia
Hypothermia	Hypothermia
Dry warm skin	Cool clammy skin
Related to nervous system injury	Related to massive blood or fluid loss

Classification of spinal cord injuries

Classification of spinal cord injuries is determined using the American Spinal Injury Association (ASIA) scale.

- *Tetraplegia* is defined as 'impairment or loss of motor and/or sensory function in the cervical segments of the spinal cord as a result of damage to neural elements within the spinal canal'.[30] Tetraplegia results in decreased function in the arms, trunk, legs and pelvic organs.

- *Paraplegia* is defined as 'impairment or loss of motor and/or sensory function in the thoracic, lumbar or sacral segments of the spinal cord, as a result of damage of neural elements within the spinal canal. Arm function remains intact, but trunk, legs and pelvic organs may be involved',[30] depending on the level of injury. Injuries to the cauda equina and conus medullaris also fall into this category.

- The *neurological level of injury* may differ from the skeletal level of injury. The neurological level is defined as the lowest segment of the spinal cord with normal sensory and motor function on both sides of the body.[30] Using the American Spinal Injury Association (ASIA) impairment scale, injuries are graded from A to E according to motor and sensory function, with A being a complete injury and E normal function (Box 49.2).

The sensory assessment consists of testing pin-prick and light touch using 28 dermatomes. Each side is scored from 0 to 2, with 0 being absent sensation and 2 being normal. The motor assessment involves testing 10 myotomes on each side. Each muscle is graded from 0 to 5, with 0 representing total paralysis and 5 full strength. Dermatomes and myotomes unable to be tested are recorded as NT (not tested).

Complete—no motor or sensory function is preserved in the sacral segments S4–S5
Incomplete—sensory but not motor function is preserved below the neurological level and includes the sacral segments S4–S5
Incomplete—motor function is preserved below the neurological level, and more than half of key muscles below the neurological level have a muscle grade < 3
Incomplete—motor function is preserved below the neurological level, and at least half of key muscles below the neurological level have a muscle grade ≥ 3
Normal—motor and sensory function are normal

Complete spinal cord injury

Complete spinal cord injuries are those with 'an absence of sensory and motor function in the lowest sacral segment; S4–S5'.[30] This is tested by observing for voluntary anal contraction and presence of anal sensation.[30] It is possible to have a zone of partial motor or sensory preservation in complete injuries which is recorded on the ASIA form, but there is very little opportunity for return of function in these injuries. Expected level of function in complete injuries is able to be predicted at an early stage (Table 49.6).

Diagnosis of complete or incomplete injury cannot be made until resolution of spinal shock.

Incomplete spinal cord injury

Incomplete injuries are becoming increasingly common: 72% of tetraplegics and 57% of paraplegics injured in Australia in 2007–08 sustained incomplete injuries.[2] Incomplete injuries result in preservation of varying degrees of motor and/or sensory function below the level of injury, including the lowest sacral segment. This is determined by the presence of anal sensation and voluntary contraction of the anal sphincter. They can often be categorised into one of the following types of injury.

Central cord syndrome

Central cord syndrome occurs as a result of damage to the centrally lying tracts of the spinal cord and occurs predominantly in the cervical region (Fig 49.21).[30] Hyperextension injuries are the primary cause of central cord syndrome and are particularly common in elderly people following falls. Degenerative changes and narrowing of the spinal canal, such as spinal stenosis, can predispose older people to this type of injury. It is possible to sustain central cord damage with no vertebral damage. Neurological loss in central cord syndrome is greater in the upper extremities, with variable bladder, bowel and sexual dysfunction.

Anterior cord syndrome

Anterior cord syndrome occurs due to injury to the anterior section of the spinal cord. This can be a result of decreased blood flow to the anterior spinal artery, which supplies the anterior two-thirds of the cord, resulting in infarction of anterior spinal cord. Other causes include contusion from bone fragments from the vertebral body, disc herniation and fracture dislocation from hyperflexion injuries. Anterior cord syndrome is characterised by variable loss of motor function, pain and temperature perception below the level of injury. Proprioception is maintained.[30]

TABLE 49.6 Guidelines for expected functional outcomes from complete spinal injuries[34]

C1–C3	Loss of motor and sensory function below the neck Require permanent artificial ventilation Mobilise in mouth or head-operated electric wheelchair
C4	Loss of motor and sensory function below the neck Some shoulder movement will remain intact Artificial ventilation may be required during the acute phase Mobilise in chin-operated electric wheelchair
C5	Loss of motor and sensory function below the neck Bicep function present Some shoulder movement will remain intact Mobilise in hand-operated electric wheelchair
C6	Presence of wrist extension Intact sensation extending down the outer arm to the thumb and forefinger Independence in most activities of daily living possible Mobilise in hand-operated electric or manual wheelchair
C7–T1	Intact tricep function Improved finger function Independent in all activities of daily living
T2–T12	Independent in all activities of daily living Sensation, balance and function increase with lower level injuries
L1–L5	Motor and sensory function in hips and upper leg increases with lower level injuries and walking with crutches or leg braces is possible
L2	Hip flexors
L3	Knee extensors
L4	Ankle dorsiflexors
S1–S5	Ankle plantar flexors intact Residual motor weakness in lower limbs but increased control of ankles and feet. May require leg braces to walk

Brown-Séquard's syndrome

Brown-Séquard's syndrome occurs as a result of hemisection of the spinal cord, which is commonly due to knife and bullet wounds or other penetrating injuries (Fig 49.22). Less frequently, flexion and extension injuries cause Brown-Séquard's syndrome. It is characterised by ipsilateral (same side as lesion) motor paralysis with loss of proprioception and vibration sensation below the level of injury due to the severing of corticospinal tracts. Pain and temperature sensation on this side remain intact as the spinothalamic tracts cross over soon after entering the cord. Contralateral (opposite side to lesion) loss of pain and temperature sensation occurs while motor function is retained.[30] That is, poor motor function with good sensation on

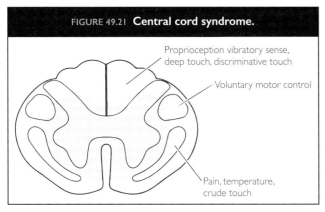

FIGURE 49.21 **Central cord syndrome.**

Proprioception vibratory sense, deep touch, discriminative touch

Voluntary motor control

Pain, temperature, crude touch

Marcus Cremonese, Medical Illustration Department, UNSW Faculty of Medicine.

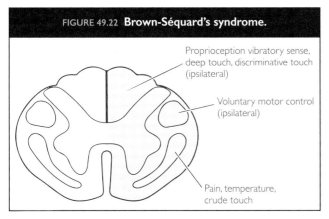

FIGURE 49.22 **Brown-Séquard's syndrome.**

Proprioception vibratory sense, deep touch, discriminative touch (ipsilateral)

Voluntary motor control (ipsilateral)

Pain, temperature, crude touch

Marcus Cremonese, Medical Illustration Department, UNSW Faculty of Medicine.

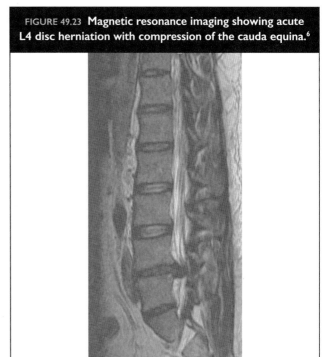

FIGURE 49.23 **Magnetic resonance imaging showing acute L4 disc herniation with compression of the cauda equina.[6]**

the same side as the injury and good motor function with poor sensation on the opposite side.

Nerve root injuries

The collection of nerve roots extending from the conus medullaris are referred to as the cauda equina. Lesions of the lumbar sacral region may involve multiple roots of the cauda equina with a varying pattern of motor and sensory loss. These injuries are classified as lower motor neuron syndromes and result in an areflexic bladder and bowel, sexual dysfunction and flaccid lower limbs. Conus medullaris syndrome is defined by ASIA as an injury of the sacral cord (conus) and lumbar nerve roots within the spinal canal. Cauda equina syndrome is defined as an injury to the lumbosacral nerve roots within the vertebral canal (Fig 49.23).

Penetrating injuries

Penetrating injuries generally arise from gunshot or stab wounds to the spinal column. In most instances there is no structural damage to the vertebrae and therefore no structural instability. These injuries do not require surgery for stabilisation, but may require removal of foreign bodies or repair of vascular damage.

Spinal cord injury without radiographic abnormality (SCIWORA)

It is possible to sustain a spinal cord injury without any bony abnormality being visible on radiological tests. This type of injury is primarily seen in children, as their spinal column is significantly more malleable than the adult spine. As a result, the spine is able to realign itself following a damaging displacement of the vertebrae which has resulted in cord damage.

Autonomic dysreflexia/hyperreflexia

> **PRACTICE TIP**
>
> Autonomic dysreflexia is a potentially life-threatening condition which needs to be recognised and treated immediately.

Autonomic dysreflexia will occur in patients with injuries at or above T6 (above the major splanchnic outflow), after spinal shock has resolved and reflex activity has returned. Autonomic dysreflexia is considered a medical emergency; without prompt treatment the blood pressure can rise to dangerously high levels and result in seizures, cardiac dysrhythmia or intracranial haemorrhage. Stimuli below the level of spinal cord injury causes excessive reflex activity from the sympathetic nervous system. Overactivity of the sympathetic ganglia causes release of noradrenaline and dopamine, which cause severe vasoconstriction leading to a sudden rise in blood pressure, severe headache, skin pallor and piloerection. This activity is uncontrolled due to isolation from the normal regulatory response of the vasomotor centres of the brain. Parasympathetic activity occurs when the rise in blood pressure is detected by the baroreceptors in the carotid bodies and aortic arch. Compensatory bradycardia and vasodilation above the level of injury result but are unable to control the hypertension.

Signs and symptoms of autonomic dysreflexia include hypertension, pounding headache, bradycardia, flushing of skin and sweating above the level of lesion, nasal congestion, blurred vision, shortness of breath, anxiety, skin pallor and piloerection below the level of injury. All or some of these symptoms may be present. The blood pressure of SCI patients needs to be considered in relation to their normal baseline reading. It is common for people with high paraplegia and tetraplegia to have a resting blood pressure of around 90–100/60 mmHg. A blood pressure of 20–40 mmHg above normal resting systolic pressure is considered to be significantly elevated for this group of people, with autonomic dysreflexia likely to occur within the normal blood pressure range for the general population.

PRACTICE TIP

The most common causes of autonomic dysreflexia are an overdistended bladder or bowel. Other causes include tight clothing, burns, kidney stones, urinary tract infection, haemorrhoids, bites, pressure ulcers, fractures and labour. The immediate treatment required is to identify and remove the cause if possible. Nitrates or captopril may be used according to local policy if the cause cannot be identified. Captopril is administered if there is a chance the patient has used erectile dysfunction medication in recent days.

The future

Stem-cell research into treatment of acute and chronic spinal injuries is currently underway but remains in its early stages, with effective treatments likely to be a number of years away.[62,63] Stem cells are under investigation due to the fact that they are able to 'self-renew' to create more stem cells and their ability to develop into specialised cells with a specific function.[65] In order to be effective, large numbers of stem cells need to be available and the donor and recipient need to be a close match to prevent rejection. In addition, a method of instilling the cells into the appropriate part of the body is required, and the cells must be able to integrate and function properly.[64,66] There is concern that experimental studies offered in countries such as China and India 'have not been scientifically proven safe and effective' and may pose significant health risks.[64]

Trials are currently underway to investigate potential neuro-protective and neuroregenerative pharmacological options; however, the outcomes of these trials are not yet known.[67]

Systemic hypothermia appears to be a promising neuro-protective intervention post SCI impacting the rate of tissue damage and extent of neurological deficits.[64] While current evidence is limited, further investigation with a multi-centre trial is planned.[67,68]

SUMMARY

Spinal cord injury is one of the most complex presentations of trauma that a paramedic, ED, intensive care or trauma ward nurse will face, as it impinges on every organ of the body. Highly developed skills of assessment are essential to differentiate between actual and potential problems. Also, a strong pathophysiology knowledge base is needed to cope with the interventions necessary in caring for the patient with an SCI. The goals of care in this setting are the management of life-threatening conditions, stabilisation of the spine to prevent further injury, transfer to a specialist facility, recovery, rehabilitation and reintegration into the patient's community.

CASE STUDY

Ian, an obese male motorbike rider, was out for a Sunday morning ride down the coast, in a National Park. He was involved in a head-on collision at 60 kph with a car travelling at approximately 60 kph. He braked suddenly and was thrown over the car and hit the road behind. He was wearing protective gear.

1. What pre-hospital considerations need to be taken into account when paramedics first arrive on scene?

Ian's observations are Glasgow Coma Scale (GCS) score 15, blood pressure 120 mmHg, heart rate 110 beats/minute. He is given narcotic analgesia and a plan of retrieval is instigated. Research shows that motorcyclists are more likely to sustain head, neck, extremity and thoracic injuries. The majority of the impact of the thoracic spine is from Ian travelling into and over the handlebars and landing onto his back.

2. You receive pre-hospital notification of Ian's arrival. What nursing considerations are needed prior to the patient's arrival in the emergency department?

A trauma call is activated. On arrival at the emergency department (ED), a primary survey and secondary survey takes place. The findings are below.

Primary survey

- Cervical spine immobilisation, no midline tenderness.
- Effectiveness and rate: trachea centred, reduced breath sounds bilaterally.
- Skin temperature, pulse rate: tachycardic, blood pressure down to 90/40 mmHg. Cool peripherally. No active bleeding. FAST negative.
- Neurological deficit: GCS 14, PEARL pin-point from morphine. Unable to move legs bilaterally to T10.
- Temperature 34.8°C, clothes removed, blanket applied.

Secondary survey

- Head: no obvious injury
- Neck: nil tenderness
- Abdomen: left upper quadrant tenderness. No blood at meatus. IDC inserted
- Lower limbs: 2 cm laceration to lower shin on right side
- Right ankle internally rotated/inverted
- Pin-prick sensation lost from umbilicus
- Log-roll of Ian showed haematoma to mid thoracic back on left, very tender; anal tone absent

Plan for Pan scan (head to pelvis): investigations and results showed:

- fracture T6 spinous process
- burst fracture T8/incomplete cord syndrome
- comminuted fracture T12
- cerebral oedema
- fractured scapula
- 2–9 fractures ribs/pulmonary contusion
- right haemopneumothorax.

3. Given the multiple body regions injured, and using a systematic approach, outline your monitoring and ongoing care needs for this patient.

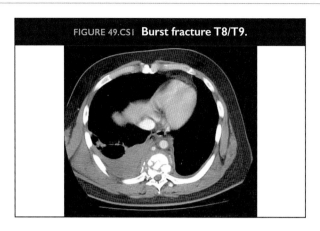

FIGURE 49.CS1 **Burst fracture T8/T9.**

Ian's journey

Ian spent 9 days in the intensive care unit, 5 of which were ventilated. He had an intracranial pressure monitor inserted for cerebral oedema. He then spent 7 days in the high-dependency unit and was transferred to a spinal rehabilitation unit for spinal fusion surgery. His ongoing rehabilitation was performed outside of the tertiary centre as Ian relocated to home in rural NSW. He is still having urinary issues, with recurrent urinary tract infections and a suprapubic catheter as intermittent catheterisation was difficult. Paraplegics with this level of injury are usually self-caring; unfortunately, due to Ian's large size, independent management of his activities of daily living has been impossible, with full-time care instituted. Ian has remained with his partner of 7 years and she is his main carer.

 Answers to Case Study Questions can be found on evolve
http://evolve.emergencytrauma.curtis

REFERENCES

1. Spinal Cord Injuries Australia. 2010. www.scia.org.au; accessed 3 April 2014.
2. Norton L. Spinal Cord Injury, Australia 2007–08. Vol INJCAT 128, Canberra: AIHW; 2010.
3. Derrett S, Beaver M, Sullivan J et al. Traumatic and non-traumatic spinal cord impairment in New Zealand: incidence and characteristics of people admitted to spinal units. Injury Prevention 2012;BMJ(April 29).
4. Gertzbein SD. Scoliosis Research Society. Multicentre spine fracture study. Spine 1992;17(5):528–40.
5. Netter FH. Atlas of human anatomy. 5th edn. Philadelphia: Saunders; 2011.
6. Marx J. Emergency medicine—concepts and clinical practice. 8th edn. St Louis: Mosby; 2014.
7. Rosse C, Gaddum-Rosse P. Hollinshead's textbook of anatomy. 5th edn. Philadelphia: Lippincott-Raven; 1997.
8. McRae R, Esser M. Practical fracture treatment. 5th edn. Edinburgh: Churchill Livingstone; 2008.
9. Browner BD, Jupiter JB, Levine AM et al. Skeletal trauma. 4th edn. Missouri: W.B. Saunders; 2008.
10. Salomone JP, Pons PT, McSwain NE. Prehospital trauma life support. 6th edn. St Louis: Mosby; 2007.
11. Haut E R, Kalish B T, Efron D T et al. Spine immobilisation in penetrating trauma: More harm than good? J Trauma, Injury, Infection Crit Care 2010;68(1):115–21.
12. Sun D, Poon W, Leung C, Lam J. Management of spinal injury. Surgeon 2006;4(5):293–7.
13. Bailes J, Petschauer M, Guskiewicz K, Marano G. Management of cervical spine injuries in athletes. J Athlete Training 2007;42(1):126–34.
14. Davenport M. Fracture, Cervical Spine. eMedicine. 2009. http://emedicine.medscape.com/article/824380-overview; accessed 3 April 2014.
15. Australian Resuscitation Council. Guideline 4—Airway. 2010; www.resus.org.au/; accessed 3 April 2014.
16. Australian Resuscitation Council. Management of Suspected Spinal Injury—Guideline 9.1.6. 2012; www.resus.org.au/; accessed 4 April 2014.
17. Bernhard M, Gries A, Kremer P, Bottiger BW. Spinal cord injury (SCI)—Prehospital management. Resuscitation 2005;66:127–39.
18. Kwan I, Bunn F, Roberts I. Spinal immobilisation for trauma patients. Cochrane Systematic Review. 2001 Updated 2009;2.
19. Ambulance Service New South Wales. Protocols and pharmacology. Sydney: Ambulance Service of New South Wales; 2009.
20. Buntine P, Thom O, Babl F et al. Prehospital analgesia in adults using inhaled methoxyflurane. Emergency Medicine Australasia 2007;19(6):509–14.
21. Bradshaw M, Sen A. Use of a prophylactic antiemetic with morphine in acute pain: randomised controlled trial. Emergency Medicine Journal 2006;23:210–13.
22. Owen R, Castle N. Pre hospital temperature control. Emergency Medicine Journal 2008;25(6):375–6.
23. Trauma.org. Initial assessment of spinal injury. 2002. www.trauma.org/index.php/main/article/380/; accessed 4 April 2014.
24. Roberts JR, Custalow CB, Thomsen TW. Roberts and Hedges' clinical procedures in emergency medicine, 6th edn. Philadelphia, Saunders, Elsevier, Ch 46, 2014:893-922.
25. Connor D, Greaves I, Porter K. Pre-hospital spinal immobilisation: an initial consensus statment. Emerg Med J 2013;30:1067–9.
26. Jabre P, Combes X, Leroux B. Use of gum elastic bougie for prehospital difficult intubation. Am J Emerg Med 2005;23(552):552–5.
27. Gleizes V, Jacquot FP, Signoret F. Combined injuries in the upper cervical spine: clinical and epidemiological data over a 14-year period. Eur Spine J 2000;9(5):386–92.
28. Jones C. Assessment and management of a child with suspected acute neck injury. Nursing Children and Young People 2012;24(3):29–33.

29. American Association of Neurologcal Surgeons. Guidelines for the Management of Acute Cervical Spine and Spinal Cord Injuries. 2002. www.aans.org/Education%20and%20Meetings/~/media/Files/Education%20and%20Meetingf/Clinical%20Guidelines/TraumaGuidelines.ashx; accessed 29 May 2014.

30. Burns S, Biering-Sorenson F, Donovan W et al. ASIA International standards for neurological classification of spinal cord injury, revised 2011. Top Spinal Cord Inj Rehabil 2012;18(1):85–99.

31. Jaworski MA, Wirtz KM. Spinal trauma. In: Kitt S, Selfridge-Thomas J, Proehl JA, eds. Emergency nursing: a physiological and clinical perspective. Philadelphia: WB Saunders; 1995.

32. Lewis SM, Collier IC, Heitkemper MM. Medical–surgical nursing: assessment and management of clinical problems. 7th edn. St Louis: Mosby; 2007.

33. Ackland H. Spinal Clearance Management Protocol. 2009; www.alfred.org.au/Assets/Files/SpinalClearanceManagementProtocol_External.pdf; accessed 3 April 2014.

34. Morris CG, Mullan B. Clearing the cervical spine after polytrauma: implementing unified management for unconscious victims in the intensive care unit. Anaesthesia 2004;59(8):755–61.

35. Hoffman JR, Mower WR, Wolfson AB. Validity of a set of clinical criteria to rule out injury to the cervical spine in patients with blunt trauma. National emergency x-radiography utilisation study group. N Engl J Med 2000;343(2):94–9.

36. Cameron P, Jelinek G, Kelly A et al, eds. Textbook of adult emergency medicine. 3rd edn. Edinburgh: Churchill Livingstone; 2009.

37. Rogers I, Ieraci S. Cervical spine X-rays in trauma; Emergency care evidence in practice series. Melbourne: NICS; 2006. Courtesy of Acromed Corporation, Cleveland, OH.

38. Vaillancourt C, Stiell IG, Beaudoin T et al. The out-of-hospital validation of the Canadian C-Spine Rule by paramedics. Ann Emerg Med 2009;54(5):663–71.

39. Stiell IG, Wells GA, Vandemheen KL et al. The Canadian C-Spine Rule for radiography in alert and stable trauma patients. JAMA. 2001 Oct 17;286(15):1841–8.

40. Royal Children's Hospital Melbourne. Assessment of the cervical spine. www.rch.org.au/clinicalguide/guideline_index/Cervical_Spine_Injury/; accessed 22 June 2015.

41. Domeier RM, Frederiksen SM, Welch K. Prospective performance of an out of hospital protocol for selective spine immobilisation using clinical spine clearance criteria. Annals of Emergency Medicine 2005;46(2):123–31.

42. Vaillancourt C, Steil IG, Beaudoin T et al. The out of hospital validation of the Canadian C-Spine rule by paramedics. Annals of Emergency Medicine 2009;54(5):663–71.

43. Stiell IG, Wells GA, McKnight RD et al. Canadian C-Spine Rule study for alert and stable trauma patients: I. Background and rationale. CJEM 2002;4(2):84–90.

44. Stiell IG, Clement CM, Grimshaw J et al. Implementation of the Canadian C-Spine Rule: A prospective 12 centre cluster randomised trial. BMJ. 2009;339:b4146.

45. Como JJ, Diaz JJ, Dunham CM et al. Practice management guidelines for identification of cervical spine injuries following trauma: update from the eastern association for the surgery of trauma practice management guidelines committee. Journal of Trauma 2009;67(3):651–9.

46. Griffen MM, Frykberg ER, Kerwin AJ et al. Radiographic clearance of blunt cervical spine injury: plain radiograph or computed tomography scan? Journal of Trauma 2003;55(2):222–7.

47. Mathen R, Inaba K, Munera F et al. Prospective evaluation of multislice computed tomography versus plain radiographic cervical spine clearance in trauma patients. Journal of Trauma 2007;62(6):1427–31.

48. Duane TM, Cross J, Scarcella N et al. Flexion-extension cervical spine plain films compared with MRI in the diagnosis of ligamentous injury. American Journal of Surgery 2010;76(6):595–8.

49. Lindsey RW et al. Injury to the vertebrae and spinal cord. In: Feliciano DV, Mattox LV, Moore EE, eds. Trauma. 6th edn. New York: McGraw-Hill; 2008.

50. Hugenholz H. Methylprednisolone for acute spinal cord injury: not a standard of care (commentary). Can Med Assoc J 2003;168(9):1145–6.

51. Schreiber D. Spinal cord injuries: treatment and medication. 2013. http://emedicine.medscape.com/article/793582-treatment; accessed 3 April 2014.

52. Walters BC, Hadley MN, Hurlbert RJ et al. Guidelines for the management of acute cervical spine and spinal cord injuries: 2013 update. Clin Neurosurg 2013;60(S1):82–91.

53. Krassioukov A. Autonomic function following cervical spinal cord injury. Respiratory Physiol Neurobiol 2009;169(2):157–64.

54. Evans LT, Lollis SS, Ball PA. Management of acute spinal cord injury in the neurocritical care unit. Neurosurg Clin N America 2013;24(3):339–47.

55. Berlly M, Shem K. Respiratory management during the first five days after spinal cord injury. J Spinal Cord Med 2007;30(4):309–18.

56. Consortium for Spinal Cord Medicine. Early acute management in adults with spinal cord injury: a clinical practice guideline for health care professionals. USA 2008.

57. Walker J. Spinal cord injuries: acute care management and rehabilitation. Nursing Standard 2009;43:47–50.

58. White JP. Acute spinal cord injury. Orthopedics II: Spine and Pelvis 2012;30(7):326–32.

59. Ploumis A, Ponnappan RK, Maltenfort MG et al. Thromboprophylaxis in patients with acute spinal injuries: an evidence based analysis. Jornal of Bone and Joint Surgery 2009;91(11):2568–76.

60. Weurmser LA, Ho CH, Chiodo AE et al. Spinal cord injury medicine. 2. Acute care management of traumatic and non-traumatic injury. Arch Phys Med Rehabil 2007;88(S1):S55–61.

61. Finnerup NB. Pain in patients with spinal cord injury. Pain 2013;154(S1):S71–6.

62. Middleton J, Siddall P, Nicholson Perry K. Managing pain for adults with Spinal Cord Injury; NSW State Spinal Cord Injury Service; 2008.

63. Looby S, Flanders A. Spine trauma. Radiologic Clinics of North Amercia 2011;49(1):129–63.

64. Didize M, Green BA, Dalton Dietrich W et al. Systemic hypothermia in acute cervical spinal cord injury: a case controlled study. Spinal Cord 2012;51(5):395–400.

65. Australia New Zealand Spinal Cord Injury Network. Stem cell interventions for spinal cord injury. 2009. www.anzscin.org/sites/default/files/file/E_StemCellBroch.pdf; accessed 9 April 2010.

66. National Stem Cell Foundation of Australia & Stem Cells Australia. The Australian stem cell handbook 2013: www.stemcellsaustralia.edu.au/AboutUs/Document-Library/Patient-Information.aspx.

67. Wilson JR, Forgione N, Fehlings MG. Emerging therapies for acute spinal cord injury. CMAJ 2013;185(6):458–91.

68. International Society for Stem Cell Research. Appendix 1 of the guidelines for the clinical translation of stem cells: ISSCR; 2008: www.closerlookatstemcells.org/Patient/ISSCRPatientHandbook.pdf.

CHAPTER 50

MAJOR ORTHOPAEDIC AND NEUROVASCULAR TRAUMA

CELINE HILL

Essentials

- All patients with a suspected fracture should be transported to hospital as quickly as practicable.
- History and understanding of the mechanism of injury is essential in predicting the pattern of fractures and underlying soft-tissue-structure damage; for example, a dislocated knee can tear the popliteal artery or rupture cruciate ligaments.
- Any variation of a neurovascular assessment requires closer observation and potential investigations.
- Splinting of the long bones is essential for reducing pain and attempting to restore anatomical alignment. It will also aid in scene management and transport, making it easier and safer to get the patient on a stretcher.
- All major trauma pelvic fractures should be splinted to decrease haemorrhage and further damage from bone ends, and will assist in transport.
- A combination of pain treatment regimens should be used early to reduce the effects of a stress response and ease the patient of pain, such as opioid analgesia, nerve blocks, ice, elevation, splinting and, in severe circumstances, intubation, which may be required to give adequate analgesia and anaesthesia.
- Any amputated limb should be kept cool and dry.
- All open fractures should be splinted to prevent further breaching of the skin, and a sterile, saline-soaked dressing placed over the breach to prevent bone from drying out.
- Only those who are trained in application should apply skeletal or skin traction. Only the orthopaedic surgeon or registrar should prescribe traction weight.
- The basis for treatment of any patient with suspected fat embolism syndrome is supportive, such as prevention of hypovolaemia, the stress response and hypoxia and stabilisation of fractures.
- All patients with significant soft-tissue trauma or fractures to the lower limbs have a compartment syndrome until proven otherwise. Treatment remains to elevate the limb to heart level, ice, splint and monitor via neurovascular observations and visual examination, including a high index of suspicion and fasciotomy where necessary.

Never elevate an injured limb above the level of the heart, as this will impede venous return and potentially lead to increased risk of compartment syndrome.

INTRODUCTION

This chapter outlines major musculoskeletal trauma incorporating injuries to the bone, muscle and vascular system. Subsequent physiological alterations to these systems are addressed. Extremity trauma is not usually life-threatening, but can result in long-term sequelae that are significantly disabling. Patients with major orthopaedic injuries, especially of the lower limb, have very poor quality of life and functional outcomes.[1] This chapter addresses the major aspects of extremity trauma, associated complications and recommendations for appropriate management and trauma care in the field and in the emergency department (ED) to reduce the chance of long-term disability.

The musculoskeletal system is involved in approximately 66% of all injuries, associated soft-tissue injuries, dislocations and fractures. Consequently, musculoskeletal injuries are widely seen in the healthcare setting, and are becoming a major component of pre-hospital and nursing care.[2]

Mechanism of injury is an important predictive tool and should raise one's index of suspicion of particular injury types when assessing musculoskeletal trauma; however, some research suggests that clinical significance is reduced in the absence of physiological symptoms or injury pattern.[3] The severity of fracture and damage to tissue, nerves, ligaments and muscles will be far greater in a fracture caused by a car travelling at high speeds than a fracture caused by a simple low-energy fall.[4] Mechanism of injury is expanded upon throughout the chapter.

Resuscitation and therapeutic intervention are the basic principles of trauma care for life-threatening injuries. Musculoskeletal trauma seldom falls into this priority category. The exceptions to this rule are injuries which alter haemodynamic status significantly, such as massive pelvic injuries and amputations. Patients with multiple injuries will often have one or more skeletal injuries, and after stabilisation of the neurological and pulmonary systems to maximise patient stability, musculoskeletal injuries require timely recognition and management.[5,6]

Anatomy and physiology

Bone

There are 206 bones in the human skeleton. These bones provide the architectural framework for the body (Fig 50.1).[7]

Other structures, such as tendons, cartilage, ligaments, soft tissue and muscle, allow the bones to perform many functions, such as support, serving as a reservoir for minerals and haematopoietic function (production of red blood cells), shielding internal organs and activities such as protection, work and play, which are coordinated by involuntary and voluntary muscle movement.[7]

Bone is dynamic and can adapt itself when forces are applied to it. Bones can be grouped based on shape, as flat (innominate—pelvis), cuboidal (vertebrae) or long (tibia). Furthermore, bones can be classified as cancellous (spongy or trabecular bone) or cortical (compact). Cortical bone is found where support matters most, in shafts of long bones and outer walls of other bones. Cancellous bone is 'honey-comb' in appearance and makes up the internal network of all bones.[7,9]

Periosteum surrounds bone and contains a substantial network of blood vessels that supply the bone with blood and nutrients. Inside the long bones is the medullary cavity containing yellow marrow (mostly fat) and red marrow (responsible for blood-cell production).[6] Therefore, when the long bone is fractured, blood loss occurs and fat can be released from the medullary cavity, potentially causing fat embolism. See the section on fat embolism for more information.

Injuries to the soft tissue, which includes muscle, skin and subcutaneous fat, can occur in combination with fractures. Sometimes soft-tissue injuries are more significant and have more serious ramifications than the fracture itself. Appreciation of this is essential in preventing complications to healing of a fracture.[5] In understanding soft-tissue damage, it may help to try to envisage the mechanism of injury and the position of the limb at impact when the bone ends are separated. When the patient reaches the ED, soft tissues may have recoiled back to normal position. X-rays give little indication of the extent that soft tissue was stretched.[4]

Healing of an uncomplicated fracture may take from 6 weeks to 6 months. Vascular compromise, infection and other injuries may lengthen the healing process and in some cases non-union may occur.[5]

The five stages of fracture healing do not occur independently, but overlap as progression of the healing process occurs (Table 50.1 and Fig 50.2).[7]

Strength and bone mass change considerably with age. During adolescence, bone mass increases rapidly, reaching a maximum level a decade after skeletal maturity; then it begins to decline. By the eighth or ninth decade, bone mass and strength has decreased to about half its maximum level. Menopause can cause a woman to undergo accelerated bone loss.[10] Age-related osteoporosis is accelerated around menopause. Menopause generally commences between the ages of 45 and 55 years. A sharp decline in oestrogen production leads to accelerated bone loss. Oestrogen, a hormone produced by the ovaries, has been revealed to have protective effects on bone by decreasing bone reabsorption with the reduction and activity of osteoclasts. During menopause, bone loss greatly surpasses that in men. Osteoporosis and osteopenia (low bone mass) occurs when the rate of bone formation is markedly slower than bone reabsorption, resulting in thin, fragile bone and, consequently, fractures.[7,9]

Musculoskeletal tissue

There are two types of tissue in the musculoskeletal system: muscle and connective tissue. Connective tissue is specified as tendon, fascia, ligaments and cartilage. This will be addressed later in the chapter.[7]

Skeletal muscle

Skeletal muscle tissue is a voluntary muscle and has a unique ability to contract, therefore providing the body with the ability to move. Skeletal muscle has high metabolic demands and is provided with a rich blood supply by arteries and veins that penetrate the epimysium (fascia), and are finally embedded in the innermost sheath, the endomysium.[7]

Muscles are enclosed within fascial compartments, which protect the muscle from damaged tissue swelling. Pressure within the compartment can increase so much that muscle ischaemia occurs, resulting in compartment syndrome, which is discussed later.[4]

Skeletal muscle declines with age as a result of decreases in the size and number of muscle cells. Commencing at the age of 25, skeletal muscle mass decreases by as much as 60%. This

FIGURE 50.1 **Skeleton.**[8]

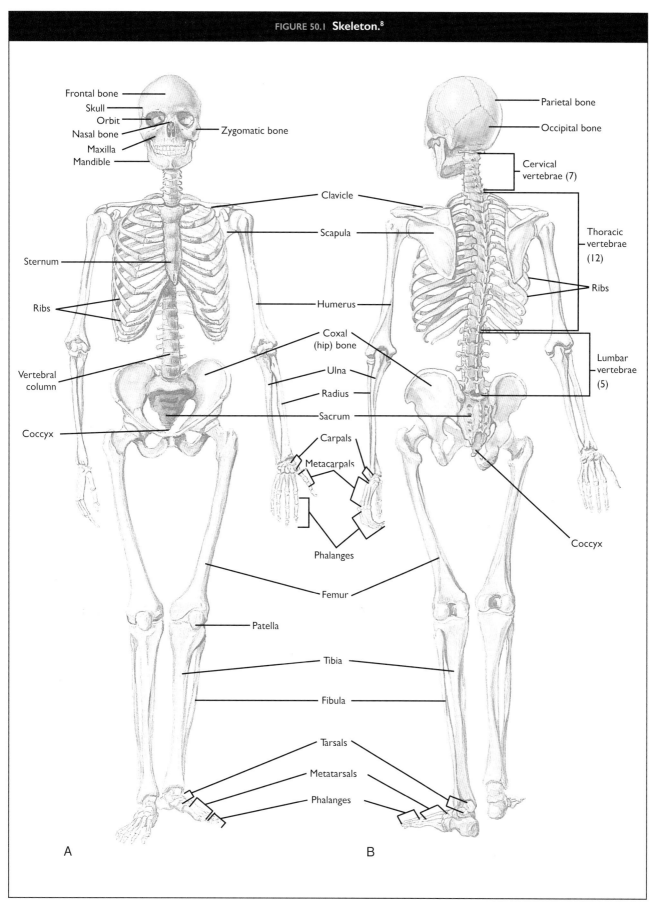

A, Anterior view. **B,** Posterior view.

TABLE 50.1 Stages of fracture healing[4,5,7]

STAGE	DESCRIPTION	LENGTH
I—Haematoma formation	Immediately following fracture, bone ends rub together—called crepitus—causing pain. Amount of haematoma depends on the damage to bone, soft tissue and vessels around the fracture	1–3 days
II—Granulation	Granulation tissue forms after fibroblasts, osteoclasts and chondroblasts invade the haematoma as part of the inflammatory sequelae. Osteoclasts remove dead bone and osteoblasts produce bone	3 days–2 weeks
III—Callus formation	The fracture becomes 'sticky' due to plasma and white blood cells entering the granulation tissue. This material assists in keeping fragments of bone together. PTH increases and calcium is deposited. This is the most important stage; slowing or interruption at this stage means that the last two stages cannot progress, leading to delayed healing or non-union	2–6 weeks
IV—Ossification/ consolidation	Osteoblasts and connective tissue are prolific, bringing the bone ends together. Bridging callus envelops the fracture fragment ends and moves towards the other fragments. Medullary callus bridges the fracture fragments internally thus creating a connection with the marrow cavity and cortices of the fracture fragment. Trabecular bone replaces callus along the stress lines. Unnecessary callus is absorbed. Bony union is thus achieved	3 weeks–6 months
V—Remodelling	Re-establishment of the medullary canal. Fragments of bone are united. Surplus cells are absorbed, bone is remodelled and healing is complete	6 weeks–1 year

PTH, parathyroid hormone

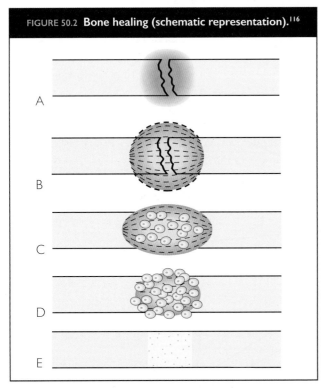

FIGURE 50.2 **Bone healing (schematic representation).**[116]

A, Bleeding at broken ends of the bone with subsequent haematoma formation. **B**, Organisation of haematoma into fibrous network. **C**, Invasion of osteoblasts, lengthening of collagen strands and deposition of calcium. **D**, Callus formation: new bone is built up as osteoclasts destroy dead bone. **E**, Remodelling accomplished as excess callus is reabsorbed and trabecular bone is laid down.

not only limits mobility but increases the risk of falling, thus increasing the probability of injury.[10]

• *Nerve supply*—one or two nerves supply muscle. Each nerve includes efferent (motor) and afferent (sensory) fibres. Nerves provide movement and sensation. Sensory nerves carry impulses to the central nervous system (CNS). Motor nerves carry impulses away from the CNS. Traction, compression, ischaemia, laceration, oedema or burning can damage nerves, resulting in nerve deficit distal to the site of injury.[7,9,11]

• *Vascular supply*—the nutrient artery provides a rich blood supply to bone marrow and some cortex in adult long bones. The large ends of long bones are supplied by the circulus vasculosus (Fig 50.3).[4]

Because of the close proximity of nerves and vessels to bony structures, any musculoskeletal injury can potentially cause vascular and/or neurological compromise (Table 50.2). This is a result of these systems being extremely sensitive to compression or stretch from the fracture, injury or haematoma and impaired circulation. If vascular supply is impaired, tissue perfusion is reduced and ultimately will lead to ischaemia. Irreversible damage to nerves, vascular structures and muscles can occur within 6–8 hours if progression from ischaemia to muscle necrosis occurs.[7] Poor arterial perfusion is evidenced by pallor, and cyanosis is suggestive of venous congestion.[11]

Improper handling of fractures can complicate further care of the patient and increase the degree of injury, as well as causing further bleeding, pain, increased incidence of fat embolism and further damage to soft tissue, nerves and vessels.[5]

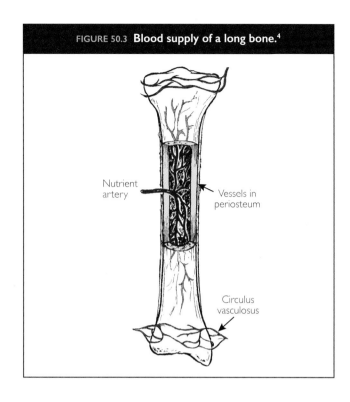

FIGURE 50.3 **Blood supply of a long bone.**[4]

Nutrient artery

Vessels in periosteum

Circulus vasculosus

TABLE 50.2 Joint fractures and dislocations and potential nerve/vessel injury[4,5,7,9,11]

SITE	NERVE/VESSEL INVOLVED
Hip and pelvis	Sciatic nerve
	Iliac arteries and veins and obturator vessels
Knee	Common peroneal or tibial nerve, popliteal artery/vein
Ankle	Posterior tibial nerve, tibial artery
Shoulder	Axillary nerve, brachial plexus, axillary artery
Humeral shaft	Radial nerve
Humeral supracondylar	Radial or median nerve, brachial artery
Elbow	Radial, median or ulnar nerve, brachial artery
Wrist	Median or ulnar nerve

PRACTICE TIP

When handling a fractured limb, always place one hand under the fracture site and the other hand distal to the fracture. This will prevent excessive movement at the fracture site.

Patient assessment

In the pre-hospital environment, initial assessment and management of life-threatening injuries can occur concurrently and in accordance with PHTLS (Pre-Hospital Trauma Life Support)[12] and ITLS (International Trauma Life Support) principles. The priorities of ABC (airway, breathing and circulation) take precedence over orthopaedic injuries, unless the orthopaedic injury is the cause of instability (see Ch 44). While common in trauma, orthopaedic injuries are rarely life-threatening. Extremity injuries are not the primary focus and it is important for paramedics not to become distracted by non-critical extremity injuries, though they may appear painful and horrific.[12] Evaluation of extremities can occur en route to an appropriate trauma centre.[7] If the paramedic suspects a fracture, then neurovascular observations should commence as soon as practicable.[7] The goal of pre-hospital care is to do no further harm and preserve what remains.[7] Adjuncts to assist in further treatment of extremity injuries in the field are the use of splints. Splints can range from a simple cardboard splint and circumferential sheeting to the commercially available traction splints or pelvic binders (see Ch 17, p. 354).[7]

In the ED, immediate attention should be given to assessment and resuscitation as part of the primary survey, in accordance with EMST/ATLS/ITLS (Early Management of Severe Trauma/Advanced Trauma Life Support/International Trauma Life Support) principles.[12] Specific assessment of the extremities is left to the secondary survey in emergency unless active haemorrhage requires controlling.[13,14] Orthopaedic evaluation follows appropriate assessment of airway (A), breathing (B), circulation (C) and neurological status.[14] Severe injuries to the pulmonary, abdominal or neurological systems take precedence over orthopaedic injuries, i.e. life before limb. The caveat to this rule is massive pelvic fractures or traumatic amputations that potentiate haemodynamic instability.[15] Detailed physical examination of the extremities should begin in the ED by taking a comprehensive history, with the patient, paramedic and/or family, regarding mechanism of injury, and presenting symptoms, where appropriate. This may provide important clues to the type and severity of injury. The emergency nurse should then proceed to inspection and palpation. Palpation for pulses, capillary refill examination and colour of the limb is included in the neurovascular assessment, which will be discussed in more detail later in the chapter.

Specific patient groups

- *The obese patient*: Due to the increasing epidemic of obesity, fracture management and treatment in the obese patients poses special challenges. Accurate reduction and fixation will require special considerations and equipment. Obese patients are at higher risk of significant complications, such as nerve injuries, compartment syndrome, medical complications and pressure ulcers. Obese patients may sustain severe fracture patterns from low energy trauma. Due to the large soft tissue covering, open femoral fractures are rare.[16]

- *The paediatric patient*: A child has thicker periosteum, compared to an adult, therefore their fractures heal faster and are generally managed non-operatively. The epiphyseal or growth plate does not fuse until skeletal maturity is reached, after puberty. Fractures through the growth plate can severely affect future growth of the fractured bone or complete physeal arrest. Children's bones are more flexible due to being cartilaginous, therefore greenstick fractures are common.

- *The aged patient:* Generally after the age of 50 years we start to lose skeletal muscle mass. Around this time our bone remodelling is no longer in balance, whereby we resorb more bone than we can produce. This, along with poor calcium intake, will lead to osteoporosis: 'brittle' bones. This will lead to an increased risk of fracture.

Inspection

Initially the patient's clothes should be cut away or removed, taking care not to overexpose the patient and contribute to hypothermia and also taking care to preserve forensic evidence as required. Observing the patient during this procedure for grimacing or guarding when limbs are moved may suggest signs of injury and, if possible, this should be confirmed with the patient. Observe for shortening, deformity/angulation or abnormal rotation.[6,11] Document any evidence in the patient's medical record of impaired skin integrity, potentially due to open fractures, oedema/swelling and ecchymosis due to blood loss into the tissues and muscle spasm due to muscle contracting over the injured part. Observe extremity colour—dusky/cyanosed colour indicates venous congestion and pallor is indicative of insufficient arterial blood supply.[5,6,11]

Palpation and neurovascular assessment

Extremity trauma is multifaceted; it remains a challenge as it can involve both skeletal and arterial injuries. Skeletal trauma accounts for 10–70% of all extremity arterial injuries. There is a substantially higher risk of limb morbidity and limb loss with combined arterial and skeletal trauma, particularly when diagnosis and revascularisation are delayed. Therefore, prompt diagnosis is essential with a high index of suspicion for arterial trauma in all injured extremities. Note whether hard signs of arterial damage are present, such as reduced or absent (late sign) distal pulses, bruit or thrill over wound, active haemorrhage, large, expanding or pulsatile haematoma and signs of distal ischaemia—the five Ps: **p**ain, **p**allor, **p**aralysis, **p**araesthesia, **p**olar (coolness). Angiography is mandatory in the presence of any of these hard signs.[17]

PRACTICE TIP

Distal pulses should be equal and bilateral. Always assess both pulses. For example, dorsalis pedis: assess both feet.

If the injured limb has weak or absent pulses this could be an indication of compromised circulation. Any deviation in pulses should be escalated immediately to the orthopaedic surgeon or the treating team, clearly documented and closely monitored.

Neurovascular assessment examines pain, vascular integrity and neurological integrity. Initial assessment should be thorough to establish a baseline against which further assessment can be compared (Table 50.3).[11]

TABLE 50.3 Parameters for peripheral vascular assessment[7]

	INADEQUATE VENOUS RETURN	INADEQUATE ARTERIAL SUPPLY	NORMAL
Colour	Cyanotic (blue), mottled	White or pale	Pink
Capillary refill	Immediate	> 3 seconds	1–3 seconds
Temperature	Hot	Cool	Warm
Tissue turgor	Distended or tense	Prune-like or hollow	Full

Palpate each bone, observing any disturbance in integrity; this may be difficult as often the only signs of injury are pain, muscle spasm or crepitus. Essential components of palpation are:

- Pain—bones are in essence insensate. Pain is generally caused by injury to periosteum, as periosteum has sensory innervation. Soft-tissue injury, swelling within fascial compartments and muscle spasm will also cause pain.[4,5,7,9,11]
- Muscle spasm—caused by a continuous contraction of the muscle over the injured part.[4,5,7,9,11]
- Crepitus—caused by fractured bone ends moving against each other; usually a grating sound can be heard and felt.[4,5,7,9,11]
- Capillary refill—filling time of more than 2 seconds is abnormal and indicative of arterial injury.[4,5,7,9,11]
- Pulses—presence, quality and absence over the full length of the extremity, rather than just distal to the apparent injury.

The upper extremity has three major pulses that should be palpated: radial, ulnar and brachial (Fig 50.4).

The lower extremity has four major pulses that should be palpated: femoral, popliteal, posterior tibial and dorsalis pedis. Note that 10% of the population will have a congenitally absent dorsalis pedis pulse, called peripheral occlusive arteriosclerosis. If pulse is absent or weak in one limb only, an ankle brachial index may be indicated, as this may be indicative of injury.[4,5,7,9,11]

- Temperature—feel if the skin is warm or cold; this may indicate vascular compromise.
- Sensation—check for variation in sensation to stimuli.[4,5,7,9,11] The conscious patient should be able to recognise numbness and tingling when normal pressure of your finger or slight pressure from your nail is applied (Fig 50.5). Do not use sharp implements that potentially break the skin integrity.
- Movement—do not test range of movement (ROM) on an injured limb, as this may cause further injury to ligaments, muscle and vessel. ROM testing may be passive and active.[4,5,7,9,11] The patient may be able to actively move the injured limb within pain limits.

FIGURE 50.4 Neurovascular structures of the elbow.[22]

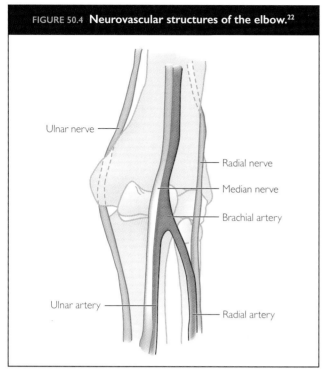

Volar surface of the left elbow is shown.

PRACTICE TIP

Neurovascular status will vary, especially temperature and sensation, particularly if the paitent has peripheral vascular disease or poor peripheral circulation. Always ask the patient about their limb temperature, sensation and movement.

Frequency of neurovascular assessment is dependent on institutional protocols. Generally, in the first few hours after injury, neurovascular/extremity observations should be conducted half-hourly to hourly.[10] When neurovascular status worsens, or after procedures, such as reduction of fractures, dislocations, application of splint, traction, plaster or any other event that may change this status, the orthopaedic surgeon needs to be notified immediately and neurovascular observations should continue hourly for the next few hours until they are deemed stable. These observations should then continue 4-hourly until definitive management occurs, such as internal fixation, then revert to hourly for the postoperative period.

PRACTICE TIP

Use of a dedicated neurovascular observation chart commenced in the ED promotes consistency and the ability to view trends whilst monitoring an injured limb.

Peripheral neurological integrity is checked by assessing sensation and motion. The major nerves in the upper extremity are musculocutaneous radial, ulnar and median, and in the lower extremity sciatic, peroneal and tibial nerves. Initially by touching an area innervated by a specific nerve, ask the patient

what is felt, such as dull, sharp, numb, 'pins and needles'. To assess the motor function, ask the patient to move the affected limb. For lower limb, ask the patient to dorsiflex and/or plantar-flex their foot. For the upper limb, the main motor test is flexion/extension of the wrist, and strength and ability to flex and extend their fingers open and closed (see Fig 50.5).[11]

PRACTICE TIP

If distal pulses are difficult to digitally palpate try using a hand held Doppler.

Clinical interventions

Any obvious or suspected musculoskeletal injury should be properly immobilised and, if applicable, sterile, saline-soaked dressings applied to open wounds. Any immobilised areas should remain splinted (see section on splinting) to prevent further injury. Whenever turning or rolling the patient, one person should assume responsibility for maintaining alignment and immobilisation of the limb.[5,9]

Care should therefore be taken when applying plaster casts, bandages and traction over bony prominences such as the head of the fibula, as compression of the common peroneal nerve can occur, leading to foot drop. With pressure on the radial nerve from humeral fractures or axillary crutches, wrist drop can occur.

PRACTICE TIP

Never elevate an injured limb above the level of the heart; this will impede venous return and potentially lead to increased risk of compartment syndrome.

Radiology

X-ray

In all major trauma patients, an anteroposterior (AP) pelvic X-ray is mandatory, along with AP chest and lateral cervical spine X-rays as part of a standard trauma series. Unstable pelvic fractures require immediate attention and could be the cause of a patient's haemodynamic instability. All unstable or suspected pelvic fractures should be placed in a pelvic binder pre-hospital.

Numerous other X-rays are performed to confirm musculoskeletal injuries. For standard plain films, there should be at least two views of the limb, AP and lateral, to detect displacement and degree of angulation. The exact zone of injury is often not fully appreciated; therefore X-rays of limbs must include areas distal and proximal to any suspected injury. For example, with a mid-shaft tibial fracture, X-rays of joints above and below the fracture are essential to rule out other fractures or dislocations.

Significant force may cause more than one injury on more than one level; for example, with fractures of the calcaneus or femur it is essential to also X-ray the pelvis and the spine.

PRACTICE TIP

Always X-ray joints above and below a fracture.

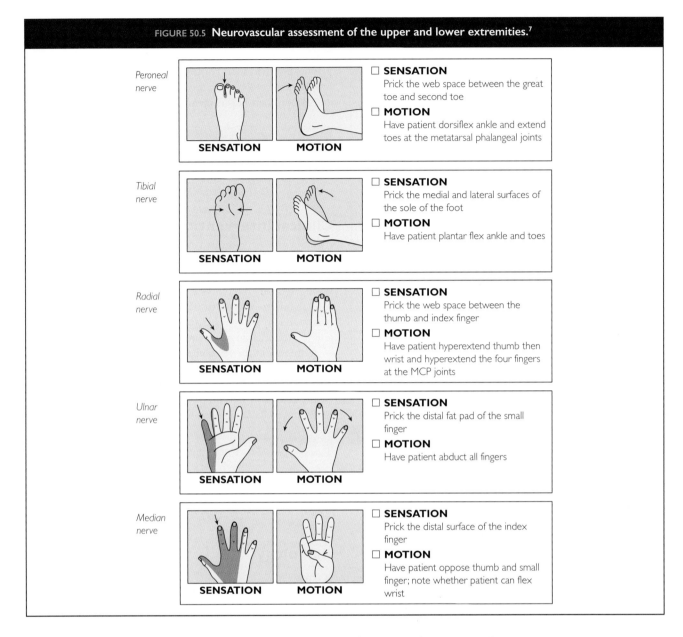

FIGURE 50.5 Neurovascular assessment of the upper and lower extremities.[7]

Peroneal nerve

SENSATION
Prick the web space between the great toe and second toe
MOTION
Have patient dorsiflex ankle and extend toes at the metatarsal phalangeal joints

Tibial nerve

SENSATION
Prick the medial and lateral surfaces of the sole of the foot
MOTION
Have patient plantar flex ankle and toes

Radial nerve

SENSATION
Prick the web space between the thumb and index finger
MOTION
Have patient hyperextend thumb then wrist and hyperextend the four fingers at the MCP joints

Ulnar nerve

SENSATION
Prick the distal fat pad of the small finger
MOTION
Have patient abduct all fingers

Median nerve

SENSATION
Prick the distal surface of the index finger
MOTION
Have patient oppose thumb and small finger; note whether patient can flex wrist

Ultrasound

The use of ultrasound (US) is becoming more widespread in EDs as more practitioners are accredited. The advantages of US over other imaging modalities is that it is portable, repeatable, dynamic, irradiation-free, cheap and allows assessment of soft tissues and musculoskeletal body parts.[18,19] US is a dynamic process that is easily repeatable and provides real time assessment, therefore it can be a good alternative to MRI.[18–20] US has high resolution, enabling detection of nerve compression, foreign bodies, tendon and ligament injury and other soft tissue injury.[19] US has been proven in studies to be accurate to rule in or out extremity fractures.[21] It can also be used for therapeutic guidance, such as post fracture reduction, drainage of collections, nerve blocks, etc.[19] There is still conjecture regarding diagnosing fractures with ultrasound, so it may not replace traditional radiography, but is helpful to rule a fracture in or out.[20]

Computed tomography

Some X-rays may be inadequate in diagnosing fractures in the pelvis, knee and ankle, therefore computed tomography (CT) scans are required to confirm minimally displaced or hidden fractures, and to evaluate the integrity of posterior pelvic structures, haematoma size and visceral injury such as bladder rupture. Three-dimensional CT images are excellent in displaying fracture pattern and extent of injury, particularly in difficult sites such as the acetabulum, calcaneus and vertebral column.[4,5,7,9,11]

Magnetic resonance imaging

Soft-tissue, ligament and tendon injuries are not clearly identified radiologically; magnetic resonance imaging (MRI) should be performed if more-substantial damage is suspected. MRI is regarded as more sensitive than CT on soft-tissue structures. MRI differentiates between muscle, ligaments and tendons, providing anatomical differentiation of structures of the joint. It is particularly useful in visualising anterior and posterior ligaments of the knee.[7,11]

Angiography

Angiography can determine location of arterial occlusion or disruption. Angiographic embolisation is required for persistent haemorrhage from pelvic fractures and severe fracture/dislocations near the knee joint with compromised distal circulation.[5,11] Pelvic fractures can be correlated with significant haemorrhage, largely from pelvic vasculature. Haemorrhage may also originate from abdominal visceral injury. Mortality in patients with haemorrhagic shock and unstable pelvic fracture pattern is higher than 52%, therefore consideration should be given to angiography before laparotomy. Some facilities have the ability to perform 'on-table' interventional angiography in an operating suite. Fundamentally, good coordination between general surgeons, orthopaedic surgeons and the ED in prioritising definitive management is essential to prevent delay in diagnosis and haemostasis, as haemorrhage from unstable pelvic injuries is directly responsible for permanent disability for survivors or death from exsanguination.[22–24]

Retrograde urethrogram/cystography

Evaluation of urethral injuries usually involves retrograde urethrogram. Commonly, fractures of the sacroiliac (SI) joint, symphysis pubis and sacrum are associated with bladder injuries. Fractures of the inferior rami, widened symphysis and SI joint are associated with urethral injuries. There is a 1 in 5 chance of bladder injury in patients with pelvic fractures in both men and women. Bladder distension is directly related to bladder injury; a full bladder is more likely to be injured. Pelvic fractures in combination with blood at the meatus, inability to void, high-riding prostate, scrotal swelling and gross haematuria warrant immediate retrograde urethrogram/cystography to assess the lower urinary tract and bladder.[25–27]

Pain management

There is an enormous stress response produced after major trauma. Inadequate pain relief has been shown to amplify this stress response, with a resultant rise in morbidity.[28] The adverse effects of trauma on ventilation, haemodynamic stability and renal and gastrointestinal function are said to be compounded when pain is untreated. Simple but important measures, such as splinting or immobilising an injured limb, should be instituted initially. These will help avoid further tissue damage and muscle spasm and reduce pain. Elevating the limb promotes venous return, thus reducing venous congestion—elevation above the level of the heart can actually impede venous return and further increase the risk of vascular compromise. As discussed below, cooling via ice packs can decrease swelling and oedema. There are numerous treatments for pain relief available; these include intravenous, oral, inhaled, local and regional anaesthetics.[11,28,29] See Chapter 19 for further information on pain management.

Dislocations and subluxations

A *dislocation* is when the articular (joint) surfaces are no longer in contact, and can be described as anterior/posterior or medial/lateral. A *subluxation* is partial displacement of the articular surfaces. Both injuries occur when the joint is forced beyond its anatomical range of motion. Symptoms of dislocations include loss of normal mobility, pain, change in contour of the joint and discrepancy in length of the extremity.[5,11] Figure 50.6

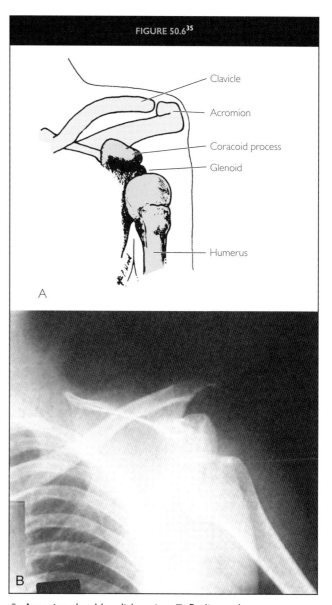

FIGURE 50.6[35]

A, Anterior shoulder dislocation. B, Radiograph.

demonstrates a shoulder dislocation. Ankle, elbow and patella dislocation are discussed in detail in Chapter 18.

If practicable, all dislocations should be X-rayed before reduction to diagnose severity, determine angle of fracture and rule out concomitant fractures, therefore determining whether it is a fracture dislocation pattern. There may be situations where field reduction is warranted, such as in remote locations or in the wilderness. The reduction of anterior dislocations is practised by extended-care paramedics.[30] A dislocation may prove difficult to reduce as fracture fragments could be lodged in the joint. Treatment of fracture dislocations often includes operative fixation.[4]

Motor vehicle trauma is believed to be a key factor in the increased occurrence of traumatic knee dislocations. Knee dislocations frequently damage the nerves and the popliteal artery in 50% of cases, and therefore need to be reduced immediately. A splint, such as a knee immobiliser, should support the knee post reduction to prevent further dislocation. Further investigation of suspected arterial damage is required via a mandatory angiogram, and should be performed immediately. If positive, emergency treatment should be commenced directly. Most dislocations post reduction will benefit from immobilisation with either a sling or a splint.[4,7,9,31]

Prior to reduction, a thorough neurovascular assessment should be completed to provide a baseline, as this will guide monitoring of the neurovascular status post reduction for any changes and adverse effects.

Reduction usually requires intravenous procedural sedation for muscle relaxation and analgesia. Post-reduction X-rays are required to ensure alignment. Patients receiving intravenous sedation require one-on-one nursing for frequent observations, such as respiratory, cardiovascular and neurovascular monitoring.[6]

Common dislocations and management are listed in Table 50.4.

Shoulder dislocations

Background and mechanism

The glenohumeral (shoulder) joint is a ball-and-socket joint that is highly mobile. Loose ligaments provide this mobility, therefore stability is compromised.[33–35] The shoulder is the most commonly dislocated joint, accounting for 50–60% of all joint dislocations.[33,34,36]

There are four types of dislocations represented by the final position of the humeral head: anterior (forward), posterior (backward), inferior (downward) or luxatio erecta and superior (upward).[37]

	TABLE 50.4 Common dislocations[32]		
BODY AREA	TYPICAL MECHANISM OF INJURY	CLINICAL FINDINGS	TREATMENT
Shoulder	Anterior fall on an outstretched arm, or a direct blow to the shoulder	Arm abducted, cannot bring the elbow down to the chest or touch the hand of the affected side to the opposite ear	Splint in a position of comfort; reduce as soon as possible
Posterior	Rare; strong blow to the front of the shoulder; violent convulsions or seizures	Arm held at the side, unable to externally rotate the arm	Same as for shoulder
Elbow: radius and ulna	Fall on an outstretched hand with the elbow in extension	Arm shortened; pain with motion; rapid swelling; nerve injury may occur	Same as for shoulder Surgical repair is required if the dislocation is associated with fracture of the radial head or olecranon
Radial head (children)	Sudden longitudinal pull, jerk or lift on a child's wrist or hand ('nursemaid's elbow')	Pain; patient refuses to use the arm; limited supination; can flex and extend at the elbow; may have no deformity	Reduce; place in a sling; advise parents that this may recur until the age of 5 years
Hip (usually posterior)	Blow to the knee while the hip is flexed and adducted (sitting with crossed knees); common in front-seat passengers in a motor vehicle collision	Hip flexed, adducted, internally rotated and shortened; may have an associated fracture of the femur; sciatic nerve injury (this nerve lies posterior to the femoral head)	Splint in a position of comfort; reduce as soon as possible.
Patella	Spontaneous	The knee is flexed; the patella can be palpated lateral to the femoral condyle	Reduce dislocation (may occur spontaneously) or immobilise with a cast or splint
	Associated with other trauma	Excessive swelling, tenderness and a palpable soft-tissue defect	Surgical repair of soft-tissue injury or fractures is required
Knee (rare)	Severe direct blow to the upper leg or forced hyperextension of the knee	Ligamentous instability; inability to straighten the leg; peroneal nerve and popliteal artery injury are common; assess distal neurovascular function	Immediate neurovascular assessment is necessary; reduce dislocation
Ankle	The ankle is a complex joint, with multiple ligaments providing stability; dislocation is usually associated with other injuries such as fractures and soft-tissue trauma	Swelling, tenderness; loss of alignment and function	Splint ankle; ankle dislocation usually requires open reduction because the joint is complex and must be realigned accurately

- Anterior shoulder dislocations account for the vast majority (90–98%).[33,34,36] Most anterior dislocations are the result of the humeral head slipping off the front of the glenoid.[4,36]

- Posterior shoulder dislocations are uncommon and account for 2–10% of all traumatic shoulder dislocations.[34,36,38] They are generally caused by high-energy trauma, seizures or electrocution.[35,39]

- Inferior and superior dislocations are extremely rare, caused by violent forces due to severe trauma; these will not be discussed.[33,35] Further reading can be found in Browner et al's *Skeletal trauma*, 4th edn,[35] for example. The most common mechanism is extreme external rotation, abduction and extension due to a posterior force against the humerus's internal rotation, usually traumatic.[36] Mechanisms may include sports, assaults, falls, seizures, throwing an object, reaching to catch an object, forceful pulling on the arm, reaching for an object, turning over in bed or combing hair.[40]

Assessment and management

Patients who present with *anterior dislocations* usually have their arm in slight abduction and external rotation. Generally the humeral head can be palpated inferiorly. They have limited adduction and internal rotation; muscle spasms can limit movement and can be very painful.[36] Immediate pre-hospital management should include supporting the patient's arm with a simple broad arm sling, analgesia, and by allowing the patient to assume a position of comfort while maintaining cervical spine immobilisation, if necessary (see Ch 17, p. 323, for cervical spine immobilisation techniques). A pillow between the patient's arm and torso may increase comfort. Neurovascular assessment should be initiated immediately, as complications associated with shoulder dislocations can include axillary nerve or artery injury, rotator cuff and, most commonly, fractures.[40]

Posterior dislocations can be missed. It is estimated that 50% are undiagnosed. The reasons for delayed or missed diagnosis are suboptimal X-ray interpretation, concomitant injuries and multiple injuries.[38,39] Patients generally present with internal rotation and slight adduction. External rotation is significantly reduced. The anterior shoulder is flattened and a posterior prominence is generally palpable.[36] Delayed diagnosis,

complexity and rarity can contribute to significant morbidity.[38] Post reduction, some reduced dislocations can remain unstable. Management in a sling for 3–6 weeks is generally advocated; and preferably a shoulder immobiliser.

Post reduction neurovascular observations should continue for at least 4 hours. The clinician should instruct the patient to not actively use the affected limb.

Radiology

At the very least, the patient should have an AP (antero-posterior) X-ray (Fig 50.7) and an axillary view. Other useful views include the scapular Y view. CT is generally only used if MRI is contraindicated. MRI is useful post reduction in detecting cartilage and rotator cuff tears, biceps injury and capsular abnormalities.[36]

Closed reduction

The ultimate aim is to disengage the humeral head from the glenoid rim. Generally the techniques are classified as leverage or traction techniques.[35] Always examine the X-rays prior to reduction. Reduction is dangerous and not advised if there is an associated fracture.[3] To reduce further trauma to the patient, and increase ease of reduction, adequate analgesia and muscle relaxants to reduce muscle spasm should be administered[35] in a controlled environment where access to cardiac monitoring and intubation equipment are readily available (see Ch 17, for information on cardiac monitoring, p. 336, and intubation techniques, p. 318). Prior to reduction, neurovascular assessment should be conducted and documented.

There are a variety of methods used for shoulder reduction. The technique performed is dependent on the preference and experience of the operator.

Anterior shoulder dislocation reduction methods

- *Kocher method* (Fig 50.8)—the patient is supine and the operator stands at the side. The elbow is held and manual traction applied. The left elbow is held by the left hand and vice versa. 'The humerus is rotated externally and the elbow is moved up towards the chest.'[35] This manoeuvre has been associated with humeral fractures and neurovascular compromise.[35]

- *Traction-countertraction* (Fig 50.9)—the patient lies supine, a sheet is placed around the chest and counter

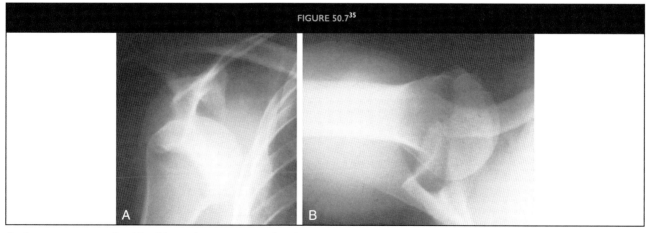

FIGURE 50.7[35]

A, Anteroposterior shoulder X-ray demonstrating glenohumeral dislocation. **B**, The anterior position of the humeral head is confirmed on an axillary lateral X-ray.

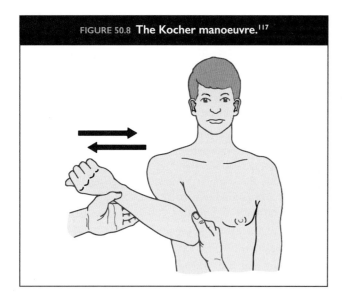

FIGURE 50.8 **The Kocher manoeuvre.**[117]

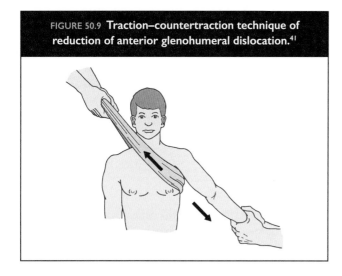

FIGURE 50.9 **Traction–countertraction technique of reduction of anterior glenohumeral dislocation.**[41]

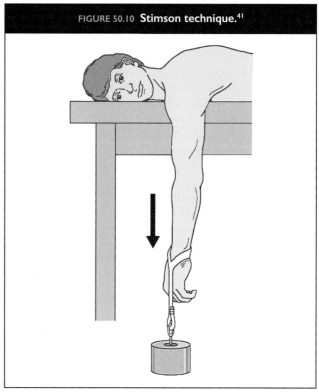

FIGURE 50.10 **Stimson technique.**[41]

traction is applied, the arm is then pulled in the direction of the deformity; sometimes gentle rotation is required to disengage the humeral head.[35]

- *Stimson technique or hanging arm technique* (Fig 50.10)— this involves the patient positioned prone, allowing the arm to hang freely; the weight of the arm produces reduction. Sometimes a weight may need to be applied.[4,35]

Complications

- *Fractures*—Hill–Sachs lesion occurs in 54–76% of patients; this is a compression fracture that produces a groove in the posterolateral part of the humeral head.[33,36] Bankart lesions are fractures of the glenoid rim.[33,36] Greater tuberosity avulsion fractures occur in 10–16% of patients.[33] Coronoid process fractures are uncommon; it is damaged by the humeral head.[33]
- *Neurological damage*—more common than vascular injury, especially axillary neuropraxias which are noted in about 8–10% of patients.[36] Brachial plexus and other isolated nerve damage can occur; the most common nerve damaged is the axillary nerve.[4,33]

- *Vascular injury*—more common in anterior or inferior dislocations. This is rare, but must be considered if the patient has a brachial plexus injury. The axillary artery can rupture causing axillary haematoma, pain, absent pulses and a cool limb.[4,33,36]
- *Irreducibility*—if reduction is not attempted in the first few days, then the shoulder may be impossible to reduce. Open reduction may have to be attempted, but this is difficult and outcomes are uncertain.[4]
- *Rotator cuff injury*—these are rare in young patients but more common in patients > 40 years of age.[36]
- *Joint stiffness*—fibrosis or adhesions of the rotator cuff can severely limit ROM of the shoulder joint.[4]
- *Recurrent dislocation*—younger patients are more likely to suffer from recurrent dislocations due to damage to the glenohumeral ligaments which provide static stabilisation.[4,33]

Conclusions

The initial concern of pre-hospital, ED and orthopaedic services is to use a method that has the lowest risk of morbidity and greatest likelihood of success, bearing in mind that the management route chosen may strongly influence rate of recurrent dislocation and long-term complications. Unfortunately, due to a lack of properly conducted long-term studies, there remains controversy over which is the best method to use.[34]

Traumatic amputations

Traumatic amputations are devastating injuries, whether they are a single digit or a limb. Fingertip amputations are common injuries that generally proceed to surgery for terminalisation. Finger amputations can be a clean transverse cut or contaminated crushing injuries. Management is aimed at producing a useful finger or joint. If the finger is insensate or is exquisitely tender, the patient will not use it. Therefore, it is better to have a useful stump than an ineffective finger. Traumatic amputation of the thumb is serious and disabling, as the thumb is an opposing digit and enables us to complete many tasks; it accounts for 40–50% of the hand's function.[4,6,11] Mechanism of injury is essential in determining the type of amputation.

- Cut- or guillotine-type amputations have wound edges that are well defined, and damage to nerves, tissue and vessels is localised.
- Crush-type amputations involve essentially more soft-tissue trauma, particularly to the vessels.
- Avulsion-type amputation is produced when stretching and tearing forces are produced on the tissues, such as in blast injuries. Stress waves of sufficiently high intensity in blast injuries can produce limb avulsion.[5,42,43] This is discussed in detail in Chapter 51.

Traumatic amputations pose a challenge to the paramedic or emergency nurse in caring for the patient as well as the amputated part. Commonly, amputations are associated with industrial, farming or crush injuries. Although salvage of the limb is important, other life-threatening injuries may need priority care, unless the amputation is the cause for gross haemodynamic instability.[5,11]

Care of the amputated part includes keeping it dry and cool. Gently clean the amputated part, removing gross

contamination, then place the part in a clean, sealed plastic bag and place the bag in iced water, or cold water if there is no ice. Care should be taken to ensure that the part does not become frozen, as freezing will result in irreparable tissue damage. The amputation site should be cleaned with sterile saline and a moist saline dressing applied. Cooling the part slows metabolism, thus making it more resistant to ischaemia. It is extremely helpful for staff and patient in the postoperative phase if a photograph of the wound is placed in the medical record, as often the patient will have a better understanding of the operative management if they can visualise the extent of their injury.[6,11,43]

The emergency nurse and medical officer should clearly document the time and type of amputation, level of amputation, completeness, warm and cold ischaemic time, amount of blood loss, sensation to the stump, previous injuries to the amputated limb and whether (part of) the dominant hand was amputated. Also document injuries to the same extremity at other levels (for example, avulsion amputation of the humeral shaft can cause a shearing/tearing force on the brachial plexus (Fig 50.11), resulting in complete or incomplete loss of function and sensation of the arm) and degree of crush and contamination.

There is a high risk of infection due to contamination, and broad-spectrum antibiotics should be administered early. Administration of tetanus prophylaxis is required, if immunisation history is not up to date or is unknown.[5,6,11,37,42,43] Re-implantation of amputated parts is based on the initial assessment, as stated above. Severely crushed tissue or devascularised tissue is not amenable to re-implantation. Soft tissue is very

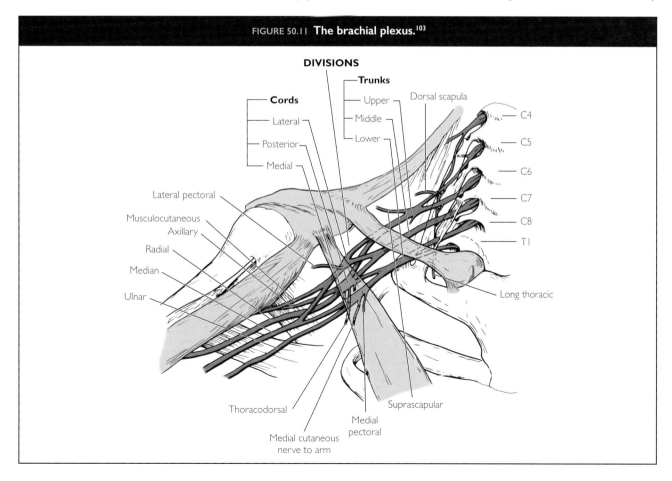

FIGURE 50.11 **The brachial plexus.**[103]

susceptible to ischaemia, so accurate time of warm ischaemia (without cooling) and cold ischaemia (with cooling) should be clearly documented.[6,7,11,44,45]

Fractures

Bone has some degree of elasticity. A fracture results from stress and/or force placed on the bone which it cannot absorb. It may be caused by direct or indirect trauma, stress or weakness of the bone or may be pathological in origin (Fig 50.12).[2,7] The types of force used to cause fractures are direct violence, indirect (generally a twisting injury), pathological (generally a weak bone from tumour or osteoporotic bone) and fatigue (repeated stress on the bone; for example, from military marches).

Classification

Fractures are classified as *stable* or *unstable*. Stable fractures are unlikely to be displaced, whereas unstable fractures are likely to be displaced and require reduction.[11] Fractures are also classified as *open* (see 'Open fractures' for more detail) or *closed*. With closed fractures, there is no penetration of the skin by bone. Conversely, in open fractures the bone breaches the skin or one of the body cavities, or the force that caused the fracture penetrates the soft tissue.[6,9,11]

Type

- *Transverse fractures*—cross the bone at a 90° angle and are generally stable post reduction.[4,7]

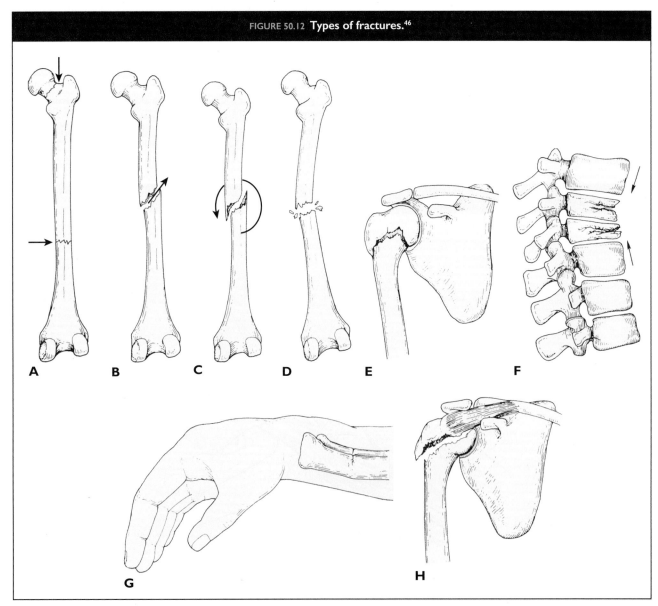

FIGURE 50.12 **Types of fractures.**[46]

A, Transverse fracture. **B**, Oblique fracture. **C**, Spiral fracture. **D**, Comminuted fracture. **E**, Impacted fracture. **F**, Compression fracture. **G**, Greenstick fracture. **H**, Avulsion fracture.

- *Oblique/spiral fractures*—are at a 45° angle to the axis, usually from a twisting force causing upward thrust. Most long-bone fractures are due to violent twisting motions, such as a sharp twist to the leg when the foot is stuck in a hole, producing a spiral fracture. They are difficult to maintain without internal fixation due to malrotation of the fracture.[4,7,11]

- *Comminuted fractures*—high-energy injuries where the bone is splintered in more than two fragments. These are generally associated with significant soft-tissue injury, and reduction and anatomical reconstruction is difficult (Fig 50.13).[4,7,11]

- *Impacted fractures*—occur when one fragment is forced into another. The fracture line may be difficult to visualise.[7,11]

- *Crush fractures*—occur when cancellous bone is compressed or crushed. Reduction is difficult as there are no fragments to manipulate.[4]

- *Avulsion fractures*—occur when soft tissue and bone are torn away from the insertion site.[7,11]

- *Greenstick fractures*—occur when the compressed cortex bends/buckles. If the force persists, the cortex will fracture.[4] These are usually seen in children, as their bones are much more porous and soft.

- *Epiphyseal or growth plate fractures* (Salter-type)—may affect future bone growth because of early closure of the epiphyseal plate and resultant limb shortening. Angulation may occur with partial growth plate fractures because bone growth continues in the non-injured area. Epiphyseal fractures require close orthopaedic follow-up for several months to monitor healing and identify growth abnormalities.

Blood loss from fractures

Blood loss from long bones can be underestimated and is often not appreciated (Table 50.5). A patient with multiple fractures can experience significant blood loss. Third spacing occurs when blood accumulates in surrounding tissue causing fluid shifts into the interstitial space, increasing extremity size. Bleeding may be difficult to assess as it may be slow, as in the shoulder girdle. Blood loss can continue for up to 48 hours and is often greater than expected. Prompt reduction, immobilisation and gentle handling of fractures can limit bleeding. The amount of blood loss is dependent on the type of fracture and location as well as previous medical history of the patient, such as patients on anticoagulants.[48-51]

See Chapter 44 for further reading on shock and fluid resuscitation.

Treatment

Box 50.1 outlines general guidelines for emergency fracture management.

Closed fractures

Closed fractures have no related break in skin integrity. Nursing management includes regular neurovascular observations, pain relief, elevation and ice to reduce swelling, removal of jewellery—particularly in hand injuries (Fig 50.14)—and splinting to reduce movement and prevent soft-tissue damage and pain, and lower the incidence of clinical fat embolism.[6,47]

As part of the advanced practice nursing role in EDs, many centres now have guidelines for ankle injury assessment and X-ray. These are based on the Ottawa ankle rules, which are

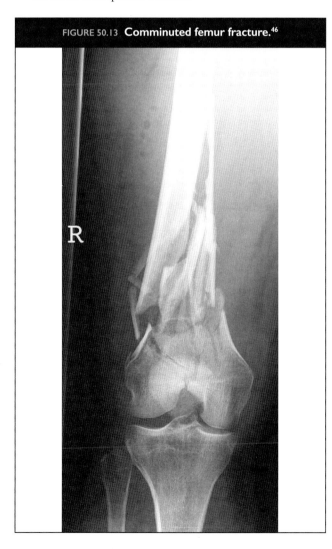

FIGURE 50.13 Comminuted femur fracture.[46]

TABLE 50.5 Estimated blood loss in fractures[4-8,11,47]

FRACTURE	BLOOD LOSS (mL)
Humerus	500–2500
Elbow	250–1500
Radius/ulna	250–1000
Pelvis	750–6000
Hip	1500–3000
Femur	500–3000
Knee	1000–2500
Tibia/fibula	250–2000
Ankle	250–1500
Spine/ribs	1000–3000

BOX 50.1 **General guidelines for fracture management**[83]

- Perform primary survey and initiate appropriate interventions.
- Evaluate neurovascular status of each injured extremity.
- Secure any impaled objects.
- Manage pain.
- Remove rings, other jewellery and tight clothing/shoes from injured extremities.
- Immobilise extremities beyond the joints above and below the site of injury.
- Re-evaluate neurovascular status after repositioning or immobilisation.
- Cover open wounds with a sterile dressing.
- Apply ice packs to areas of swelling.
- Avoid putting cleaning solutions (i.e. hydrogen peroxide, povidone–iodine, chlorhexidine) directly on a wound.
- Elevate injured extremity.
- Obtain radiographs as indicated.
- Assess patient tetanus immunisation status and vaccinate as required.
- Ensure patient maintains nil by mouth status if emergency surgery is probable.
- Repeat radiographs after any manipulation.
- Obtain orthopaedic consultation.

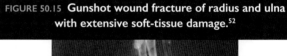

FIGURE 50.14 **Metacarpal fracture.**[52]

evidence-based guidelines used to predict malleolar and foot fractures and are presented in Chapter 18. These rules have been shown to be nearly 100% sensitive, although specificity is low: 77% of patients who meet the Ottawa criteria have no fracture.[53]

Open fractures

An open fracture is where the bone has breached the skin or any of the body cavities, and may result from blunt or penetrating injury (Fig 50.15).

Open fractures generally involve high energy trauma. There can be significant soft tissue stripping and devascularisation of bone and soft tissue and potential for severe contamination.

The risk of compartment syndrome from an open fracture should not be underestimated, with regular patient and neurovascular assessment. Open wounds do not rule out the risk of compartment syndrome.[54]

The most widely cited classification of open fractures is Gustilo's. In 1976 Gustilo and Anderson divided open fractures into three categories: types I, II and III. Gustilo revised this classification in 1984, subdividing type III injuries into IIIA, IIIB and IIIC (see below).[55,56] There is collective agreement that open fractures require urgent surgical debridement and stabilisation. Damage-control orthopaedics are urgent techniques, such as external fixation, which are minimally invasive. Damage control focuses on controlling haemorrhage, managing soft-tissue injuries and provisional skeletal stabilisation, so that the overall condition of the patient is optimised. Damage control avoids additional insults to the patient. Performing major orthopaedic procedures in the initial stages of the patient's surgical management increases

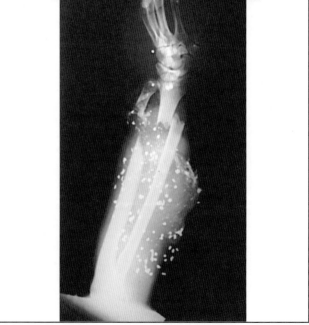

FIGURE 50.15 **Gunshot wound fracture of radius and ulna with extensive soft-tissue damage.**[52]

the incidence of a 'second hit' by inflammatory mediators and potentially increases the risk of developing the trauma triad of death—hypothermia, acidosis and coagulopathy. The damage control concept promotes rapid skeletal stabilisation, generally with external fixation. Studies have shown that early nailing of fractures can lead to worsening systemic inflammatory response and a higher incidence of acute lung injury.[1] Damage control is ideal for the unstable patient or the patient in extremis.[57–59]

Open fracture management basic principles: analgesia/sedation, fracture reduction, wound wash-out with copious amounts of sterile saline, sterile dressing, splinting and antibiotics.

Type I

There is minimal soft-tissue trauma due to a low-energy injury; Type I is characterised by a small wound of less than 1 cm. Typically the bone 'spike' produces an inside-out puncture. There is minimal contamination. Fractures may be transverse or oblique and there is little comminution of the bone.[7]

Type II

This type represents variation of energy between type I (low energy) and type III (high energy). These fractures are associated with lacerations to soft tissue 1–10 cm long. There is moderate contamination, potentially minor periosteal stripping of bone fragments, and slight to moderate comminution/crush of the bone.[7]

Type III

This represents the most severe fracture patterns, divided into IIIA, IIIB and IIIC.

- IIIA—described as having adequate soft-tissue coverage, despite significant soft-tissue trauma. A reflection of the high energy is the presence of extensive flaps or lacerations. The bone may have a segmental fracture or severe comminution. Any open fracture is predisposed to extensive bacterial contamination.[7]
- IIIB—described as having significant soft-tissue damage, necessitating local or distant flap coverage due to areas of exposed bone. These are commonly associated with significant periosteal stripping, exposure of bone, massive contamination and severe comminution (Fig 50.16).[7]

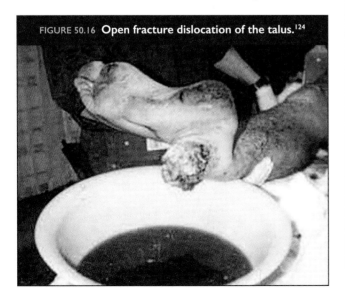
FIGURE 50.16 **Open fracture dislocation of the talus.**[124]

- IIIC—described as an injury with related vascular trauma that requires surgical repair for limb survival, regardless of extent of soft-tissue damage (Fig 50.17).[7]

Assessment and management

Further X-rays of the limb are essential to establish the extent of bony injury. Broad-spectrum antibiotics should commence in the ED. Tetanus prophylaxis needs to be considered if immunisation status is unknown. All open fractures should be examined, irrigated, debrided and stabilised in the operating suite.

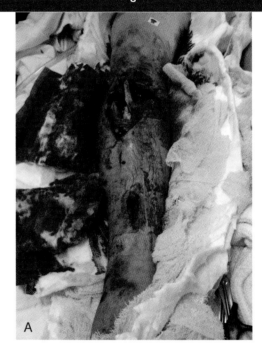
FIGURE 50.17 **Grade IIIC open proximal tibia fracture dislocation following a motorbike crash.**

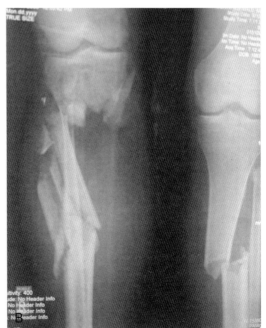

Courtesy Celine Hill.

Open fractures are considered an orthopaedic crisis and represent a limb-threatening and potentially life-threatening emergency.[14] Wounds can be irrigated in ED, generally with copious amounts of sterile saline. This will only get gross contaminants out, such as grass, etc. For optimal wound management a pulse lavage (high pressure) system is used in the operating theatres. Generally, trauma protocols/algorithms state that optimum surgical management of open fractures be carried out urgently, within 6 hours of injury; although the evidence, depending on degree of contamination, supports varied times, up to 24 hours. This is to reduce warm ischaemic time of tissue and infection due to bacteria and devitalised tissue.[1,14,56,58] Initial surgical management includes extensive pulse lavage, thorough debridement and often fracture fixation at another time. Despite these guidelines, in tertiary referral centres surgical delay is common due to patient transfers from other facilities. Skaggs et al[57] state that the single most important factor in treating open fractures is the early administration of antibiotics within 3 hours of injury.

Fracture descriptions by anatomical location are listed in Table 50.6.

PRACTICE TIP

Always apply a sterile, saline-soaked dressing to open fracture wounds. This may assist in preventing the bone from dehydrating. Avoid gauze, as this can leave small fragments behind when removed.

Infection rates of open fractures are listed in Table 50.7.

TABLE 50.6 Fracture names and descriptions by anatomical location[7]			
NAME	DESCRIPTION	COMMON TREATMENT	ILLUSTRATION[61]
Humerus			
Anatomical neck	Two-part fracture of the true neck of the humeral metaphysis at the area of tendon attachment with angulatory or rotational deformity usually less than 45°	Sling and exercise program or collar/cuff and exercise program	
Surgical neck	Fracture occurring below the anatomical neck, usually angulated greater than 45 degrees or malrotated—may have associated non-displaced linear fracture extending into humeral head	Closed reduction with sling and swathe to maintain reduction	
Diaphyseal	Fracture of the humeral shaft; middle third is most common site	Closed—hanging cast or coaptation splint (U-shaped plaster splint with collar/cuff) or sling and swathe

Operative—compression plate and screws, intramedullary rods | |

TABLE 50.6 Fracture names and descriptions by anatomical location[7]—cont'd			
NAME	DESCRIPTION	COMMON TREATMENT	ILLUSTRATION[61]
Elbow			
Condylar	Fracture of medial or lateral articular process of the distal humerus	Lateral: displaced (disrupts joint surface)—open reduction and internal fixation; undisplaced or minimally displaced—immobilisation Medial: displaced—open reduction and internal fixation or pin fixation; undisplaced—aspiration of haemarthrosis and posterior splint application	
Epicondylar	Fracture through the medial or lateral epicondyle	Lateral—immobilisation until pain subsides, displaced over 2–3 cm requires open reduction and internal fixation Medial—open reduction and internal fixation and immobilisation	
Supracondylar	Fracture of distal humeral shaft	Closed reduction under general anaesthesia and posterior splint, or percutaneous pinning Open reduction and internal fixation if reduction is unstable or fails Difficult to treat if displaced—watch for development of compartment syndrome	
Olecranon	Fracture of the olecranon process of the ulna (prominent portion of ulna at the elbow)	Displaced—anatomical reduction and internal fixation or primary excision Undisplaced—long-arm cast with 45–90° elbow flexion	
Forearm and wrist			
Colles'	Fracture through distal radial epiphysis within 13–19 mm (0.5–0.75 inch) of the articular surface with radial displacement and dorsal angulation of the distal fragment	Closed reduction and splint or cast Severely comminuted (uncommon)—external fixator	

Continued

TABLE 50.6 Fracture names and descriptions by anatomical location[7]—cont'd

NAME	DESCRIPTION	COMMON TREATMENT	ILLUSTRATION[61]
Radial head	Fracture of the most proximal part of the radius	Undisplaced—long-arm splint or cast Displaced/single fracture line—open reduction and internal fixation Comminuted—excision with silastic implant	
Hand			
Bennett's	Avulsion fracture of carpometacarpal joint with displacement caused by pull of abduction	Closed—reduction and immobilisation Operative—open reduction and internal fixation under direct visualisation or percutaneous pinning under image intensification	
Boxer's	Fracture of distal metacarpal (usually 4th or 5th) angulated or impacted	Closed reduction and short-arm cast with finger splint; seldom requires closed reduction with percutaneous pin fixation	
Mallet	Avulsion fracture of dorsal articular surface of distal phalanx of any digit involving extensor apparatus insertion, creating dropped flexion of distal segment	Closed reduction and dorsal splint, may require open reduction and internal fixation	

TABLE 50.6 Fracture names and descriptions by anatomical location[7]—cont'd

NAME	DESCRIPTION	COMMON TREATMENT	ILLUSTRATION[61]
Proximal femur			
Femoral neck	Fracture through midportion of femoral neck	Anatomical reduction and stable internal fixation or prosthesis	
Greater trochanter	Avulsion fracture of greater trochanter	Slight displacement—protected weightbearing (as an isolated injury) Displaced—open reduction and internal fixation	
Intertrochanteric	Fracture along a line joining the greater and lesser trochanter	Reduction and internal fixation of proximal femur—fixed or sliding nail/plate device, intramedullary device	
Lesser trochanter	Avulsion fracture of lesser trochanter	Bed rest 2–3 days with hip flexed, then protected ambulation (as an isolated injury)	

Continued

TABLE 50.6 Fracture names and descriptions by anatomical location[7]—cont'd

NAME	DESCRIPTION	COMMON TREATMENT	ILLUSTRATION[61]
Shaft	Fracture between subtrochanteric and supracondylar area	Skeletal traction Cast brace External fixation Intramedullary fixation Closed medullary nailing Interlocking nail, plate and screws	
Subtrochanteric	Transverse fracture between lesser trochanter and a point 5 cm distally (may occur independently or as part of intertrochanteric fracture)	Open reduction and internal fixation Fixed-angle nail and plate AO blade plates Sliding compression hip screw Intramedullary devices	
Distal femur, knee, tibia, fibula			
Bumper (tibial plateau)	Fracture of tibial or fibular condyle resulting from direct blow in the area of the tibial tuberosity	Displaced—open reduction and internal fixation	
Patellar	Fractured kneecap	Undisplaced—cylinder cast Displaced or comminuted—operative fixation or excision	

	TABLE 50.6 Fracture names and descriptions by anatomical location[7]—cont'd		
NAME	DESCRIPTION	COMMON TREATMENT	ILLUSTRATION[61]
Shaft, fibula	Diaphyseal fracture of fibula	As single fracture—cast	
Shaft, tibia	Diaphyseal fracture of tibia	Closed reduction, long-leg cast or pin/plaster or external fixation Open reduction—compression plating or plate and screws	
Supracondylar	Fracture of distal femoral condyle	Open reduction and internal fixation Medullary fixation Blade/plates Skeletal traction	

Continued

TABLE 50.6 Fracture names and descriptions by anatomical location[7]—cont'd

NAME	DESCRIPTION	COMMON TREATMENT	ILLUSTRATION[61]
Tibial plateau	Fracture of proximal tibial articular surface	Soft dressing Cast Traction Closed or open reduction	
Tibial tubercle	Avulsion and proximal dislocation of tibial tubercle	Minimal or nondisplaced—long-leg cast with full knee extension Displaced > 5–7 mm—open reduction and internal fixation	
Ankle, foot			
Boot top	Transverse fracture of distal third of tibia	Stable—closed reduction if possible Unstable—intramedullary fixation	
Paratrooper	Fracture distal tibia and malleolus	Open reduction and internal fixation	

TABLE 50.6 Fracture names and descriptions by anatomical location[7]—cont'd

NAME	DESCRIPTION	COMMON TREATMENT	ILLUSTRATION[61]
Plafond	Fracture of tibial plafond extending in a spiral or longitudinal fashion into tibial shaft	Open reduction and internal fixation	
Pott's	Fracture of distal fibula, usually spiral/oblique, with distal tibial chipping or rupture of surrounding ligaments	Closed reduction or open reduction and internal fixation, followed by cast immobilisation	

TABLE 50.7 Infection rates of open fractures[54]

FRACTURE TYPE	INFECTION RATES %
I	0–2
II	2–5
IIIA	5–10
IIIB	10–50
IIIC	25–50

Mangled limbs

Management of severe lower limb injuries represents an enormous challenge for clinicians. The definitive objective of reconstruction of a mangled lower extremity is salvaging a viable and functional limb. Patients who undergo salvage will endure more-complicated operations, have a longer length of stay and may suffer more complications than primary amputees. Sometimes these complications can be so significant and critical that secondary amputation is required. A number of predictive scoring systems have been developed to assist in the decision of whether to salvage or amputate the mangled extremity. These are: the Mangled Extremity Severity Score (MESS); Predictive Salvage Index (PSI); Hannover Fracture Scale (HFS); Limb Salvage Index (LSI); Nerve injury, Ischaemia, Soft-tissue injury, Skeletal injury, Shock and Age of patient score (NISSSA); and Mangled Extremity Syndrome Index (MESI).

All these scoring systems do not have 100% specificity and sensitivity when tested rigorously. They have limited usefulness and should not be used as a sole criterion for amputation. Other factors that will help in the decision-making are multidisciplinary consultation, age-related factors, co-morbidities, mechanism of injury, fracture pattern, soft-tissue injury, vascular injury, neurological injury, contamination, haemorrhage and hypothermia.[17,62,63]

Pre-hospital and nursing management of the mangled limb is similar to that of open fractures. Immobilise the limb, administer pain relief and ensure wounds are covered with a sterile, saline soaked dressing, and in the ED administer antibiotics, tetanus inoculation and further pain relief.[7,11] Tourniquets can be used to provide rapid haemorrhage control until operative control can be achieved.[64] For wounds that are unsuitable for tourniquet use, consider a commercially available haemostatic dressing to control life-threatening haemorrhage (see Ch 50).[65]

Mangled Extremity Severity Score

The MESS score is a combined vascular and orthopaedic scoring system used to predict lower extremity injuries that may require an amputation. There are four characteristics related to injury: age, shock, injury severity and ischaemia.[66]

Johansen, in 1990, proposed that a MESS score of 7 or more was 100% predictive of amputation.[67] His original retrospective study was of 25 patients only.[66] Bosse et al found that the MESS was only 46–72% sensitive in his retrospective study of 546 high-energy-injury lower extremity injuries.[63] The MESS is still used today, though not as a sole predictor

TABLE 50.8 Mangled Extremity Severity Score (MESS) system[92]	
CHARACTERISTIC	SCORE
A. Skeletal and soft-tissue injury	
Low energy (stabs, simple fracture, pistol, low-energy GSW)	1
Medium energy (open or multiple fractures, dislocations)	2
High energy (close range shotgun, high-energy GSW, crush injury)	3
Very high energy (gross contamination, tissue avulsion)	4
B. Limb ischaemia	
Pulse reduced or absent, perfusion normal	1*
Pulseless, paraesthesias, diminished capillary refill	2*
Cool, paralysed, insensate, numb	3*
C. Shock	
Systolic blood pressure always above 90 mmHg	0
Transient hypotension	1
Persistent hypotension	2
D. Age (years)	
0–30	0
30–50	1
50+	2
Result	
Score < 7 = salvageable extremity	
Score > 7 = non-salvageable extremity	

GSW: gunshot wound

*Double score for ischaemia > 6 hours duration

of management (Table 50.8). See www.hwbf.org/ota/bfc/hersc/mess.htm for an online MESS calculator.

Pelvic fractures

The pelvis is made up of two innominate bones and the sacrum, which combine to form a ring. The ring is held together by the strong iliolumbar and sacroiliac ligaments posteriorly and the weak symphysic joint anteriorly. The pelvis is rigid; therefore a fracture in one point of the ring must be accompanied by a disruption at a second point, unless a direct blow causes an isolated fracture; for example, an acetabular floor fracture.[9]

Significant force is required to fracture a pelvis in young patients. Due to such high energies the patients are often haemodynamically unstable and have concomitant injuries, such as urethral, bladder, vaginal and rectal injuries, torn iliac vessels and neurological deficits.[1] Pelvic fractures can vary

in severity. Isolated pelvic injuries demonstrate a mortality rate of 8–50%. Pelvic fractures can be related to significant haemorrhage from iliac arterial branches, presacral venous plexus and cancellous bone. Other injuries that are potentially prone to haemorrhage due to high-energy trauma are the thorax and abdomen. There are no rapid radiological studies that can swiftly confirm haemorrhage associated with disruption to the pelvic ring.[4,6,22–24,68]

The patient can present with leg length discrepancy, groin, perineal, suprapubic and flank bruising.[11]

Classification

There are many pelvic fracture classifications in the literature. Tile classification is based on the integrity of the sacroiliac ligaments (Fig 50.18A). The most common used is the Young–Burgess classification. This is a system based on mechanism of injury (Fig 50.18B).

- *Lateral compression* (LC)—caused by a blow/compression to the side of the pelvis, causing the ring to buckle and break. In road crashes or falls from a height, it is a side-on impact. On the side of the impact, the pelvis is rotated inwards. Posteriorly, there is significant sacroiliac strain, or a fracture of the ilium or sacrum. Anteriorly, the pubic rami can be fractured on one side, or both. Instability is due to considerable displacement of the sacroiliac joint. Treatment may include bed rest for minor injuries. Major injuries may require open reduction and internal fixation or external fixation at a later date, or bed rest for 6–8 weeks.[5,9]
- *Anteroposterior compression* (APC)—caused by frontal impact to the pelvis. The innominate bones and symphysis pubis are sprung open and the sacroiliac ligaments are torn or the posterior part of the ilium is fractured. Separation of the symphysis pubis is stable when it is less than 2 cm, and unstable when it is greater than 2 cm separation. This disruption is often referred to as an 'open-book' pelvic injury. This injury can cause catastrophic haemorrhage from torn iliac vessels.[4,5,9,14]
- *Vertical shear*—caused typically by falls from a height. One side of the pelvic ring, the hemipelvis, is sheared/displaced vertically, resulting in fractures to the pubic rami and disruption of the sacroiliac joint on the same side. The shearing injury can cause neurological injury and sacral plexus damage. Stabilisation of the pelvis is achieved by reduction of the hemipelvis. This is achieved by traction or external or internal fixation.[4,5,9]
- *Combined*—a combination of mechanisms may produce fracture patterns that do not fit the other categories. These injuries are a combination of ligamentous injuries and forces and are usually unstable.[4,5,9]

Treatment

Not all pelvic fractures are unstable, but for the purpose of this section, treatment of unstable injuries will be addressed.

Initial management should follow the ABCs of trauma management. Attention is then given to stabilisation of the pelvis, initially by using a sheet or commercially available pelvic binder to achieve this rapidly at the scene or in the ED (see Ch 17, p. 354). Other methods include posterior C-clamp and anterior external fixator, which can be used in the resuscitation phase; however, concerns regarding sterility often demand an operating-room environment. Pelvic C-clamps have caused injury to neurovascular structures and intra-abdominal injury; therefore, they should only be applied by clinicians experienced with application of external fixation.[69,70] Pelvic C-clamps are no longer widely used due to the availability of the less invasive pelvic binders.

The theory behind the use of pelvic binders (see section below), sheets and external fixation is to reduce the pelvic volume, which in turn reduces the potential space for bleeding and may aid in the formation of blood clots. Aligning fracture surfaces may reduce bleeding from bones.[68] External fixation should be considered early to allow for rapid restoration of pelvic and haemodynamic stability (Fig 50.19).[24]

Pelvic sheeting is easily accessible, especially in the pre-hospital setting. Application and efficacy is complicated by the ability to apply and maintain a sufficient force in which to reduce the pelvis, and the complication of overcompression.[71] The use of binders or sheets is generally accepted during transport, assessment and imaging.[1]

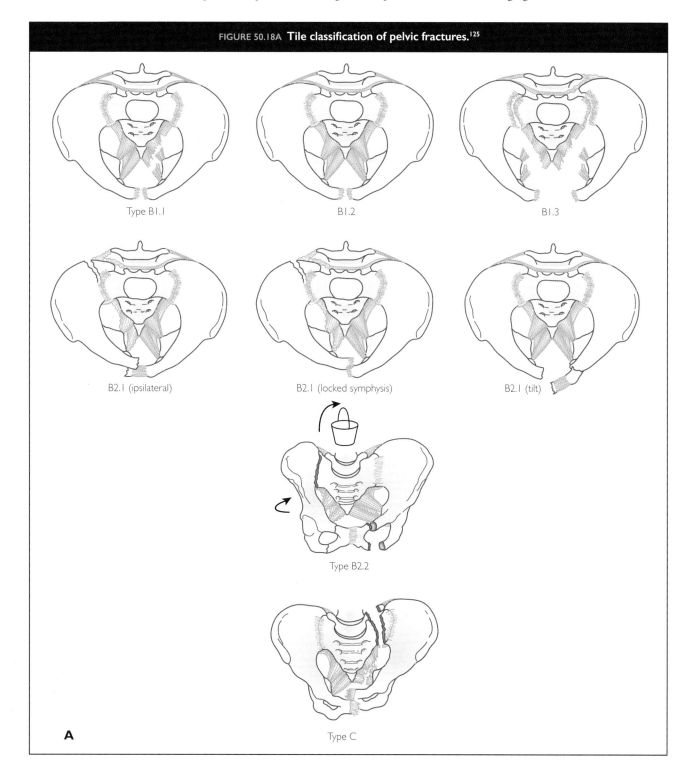

FIGURE 50.18A Tile classification of pelvic fractures.[125]

Type B1.1   B1.2   B1.3

B2.1 (ipsilateral)   B2.1 (locked symphysis)   B2.1 (tilt)

Type B2.2

Type C

A

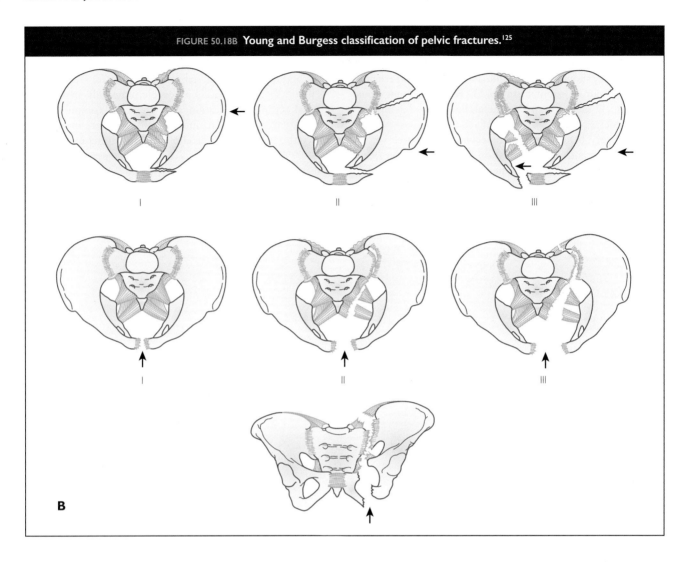

FIGURE 50.18B **Young and Burgess classification of pelvic fractures.**[125]

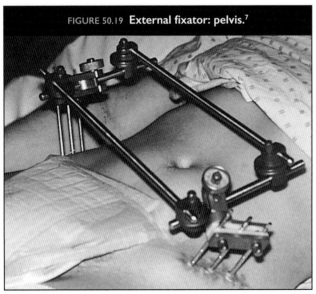

FIGURE 50.19 **External fixator: pelvis.**[7]

Care should be taken when log-rolling unstable pelvic fractures, particularly vertical shear fractures, as these fractures are vertically unstable and can continue to shift upwards when rolled. Log-rolling may cause clot dislodgement and further damage to muscle, vessels and other structures due to bone fragments shifting and causing a shearing/tearing force.

Pelvic springing is controversial. If the pelvis is to be 'sprung', only one person should do it—i.e. only the clinician, such as the orthopaedic surgeon. In addition to causing unnecessary pain to the patient, springing can dislodge clots that have tamponaded haemorrhage and cause further damage to muscle, vessels and other structures by bone fragments via a tearing/shearing force. An AP pelvic X-ray will almost always be attended to; therefore unstable pelvic injuries can be identified without the need for pelvic springing.

As discussed, pelvic fractures have the potential for torrential haemorrhage. These cases will benefit from early angiographic embolisation, bearing in mind that angiography has its own morbidity and mortality risks.[24,68]

Nursing management includes frequent monitoring of haemodynamic status—patients can rapidly exsanguinate—and neurovascular status of both lower limbs. The emergency nurse should anticipate the need for blood transfusion and fluid resuscitation and ensure that a supply of blood and warm fluids is available, and be prepared to urgently transfer the patient to definitive care.[16]

Damage to other structures, such as the rectum, vagina, urethra and bladder, can occur at the time of injury either due to the pelvic fracture, which may indicate an open fracture, or due to direct trauma.[4,11] A rectal and/or vaginal examination must be performed if there is bleeding or suspicion of injury. Rectal and vaginal bleeding is indicative of tears to the walls of these structures. A rectal examination not only evaluates the rectum but also the urogenital tract, assessing for a high-riding prostate which can indicate urethral disruption; although this is an unreliable finding in younger men.[72,74] Blood at the urinary meatus is present in 37–93% of patients with urethral injuries, and this precludes urethral catheterisation until the urethra is adequately imaged.[72,74] Additionally, pain on urination or inability to void with or without haematuria suggests urethral trauma. Initially a suprapubic catheter is required and, depending on extent of urethral damage, various urological surgical options are available to repair the urethra. Injuries to these systems have a high susceptibility to devastating infections, so early diagnosis and treatment is paramount (Box 50.2).[4,9,11]

Lumbosacral plexus or sciatic nerve damage can occur when there is a fracture of the sacrum or displacement of the sacroiliac joint. The sciatic nerve is responsible for dorsiflexion of the foot. Pelvic fractures, whether stable or unstable, require ongoing assessment and observation such as: neurovascular observations, which should continue for days after the injury, daily blood tests (FBC, EUC etc), daily and PRN review by orthopaedics, with any anomaly, however small, escalated and reviewed. Some 7%–14% of stable pelvic fractures with retroperitoneal haemorrhage will require embolisation for haemostasis.[75] Therefore, even if the patient's injury is classified as stable, ambulance and emergency staff need to remain vigilant for signs of haemodynamic instability.

PRACTICE TIP

Pelvic springing is not recommended. If the pelvis is to be 'sprung', then it should only be done by the orthopaedic clinician, and only once.

Pelvic binders

Binders are a commercially available, non-invasive adjunct to unstable pelvic fracture management. The mechanism is simple: 'close the book' and minimise bleeding by reducing pelvic volume, which reduces the amount of space for bleeding, realigning pelvic joints and compression of vasculature.

Binders are often called PCCDs (pelvic circumferential compression devices). In 2002, Bottlang et al[76] determined for the first time the amount of force required to reduce unstable pelvic fractures with a PCCD applied around the trochanters. More importantly, this study demonstrated the efficacy and absence of complications, such as over-compression, from a PCCD. The British Orthopaedic Association recommends the early application of a pelvic binder.[77] Binders are able to be easily applied in the pre-hospital setting, for early and effective stabilisation before and during transport.[78] Binders will not hamper patient assessment and will aid in resuscitation. Binders (Fig 50.20) are preferred over external fixation in the ED because of the ease and rapidity of their application, which is described in Chapter 17, p. 354.[37]

BOX 50.2 Guidelines for retrograde urethrogram[118–120]

Male

A contrast retrograde urethrogram, remains the gold standard for evaluating urethral injuries. It should be performed prior to inserting a Foley catheter in order to exclude injury to the urethra for any blunt injury presenting with *any one or more* of the following:

- Non-palpable or high-riding prostate on digital rectal exam (unreliable finding)
- Perineal or scrotal haematoma/ecchymosis/oedema/pain/tenderness
- Gross haematuria
- Blood at the urethral meatus
- Inability to spontaneously void urine in an alert, cooperative patient
- Any of the following pelvic fractures:
  – diastasis (widening) of the pubic symphysis
  – fracture(s) of one or more pubic rami.

Female

Blunt injuries to the much shorter female urethra are rare. These are most often associated with severe open pelvic fractures after blunt trauma when soft-tissue lacerations extend into the anterosuperior vagina. If upon careful visual inspection such a laceration is felt to be in close proximity to or to involve the urethral orifice, a prompt evaluation by the on-call urologist is mandatory prior to inserting a Foley catheter.

Technique

The retrograde urethrogram can be easily performed in the trauma resuscitation bay as an adjunct to the secondary trauma survey. The patient is positioned supine while a 16 French Foley catheter is inserted (using sterile technique) into the urethral meatus just far enough to admit the uninflated balloon (approx 3–5 cm). The balloon is then slowly inflated with 0.5–1.0 mL of water using the attached syringe. The balloon should *not* be over-inflated, as this will be painful to the patient and may damage the distal urethra by overstretching the mucosa.

An anteroposterior and an oblique X-ray of the lower pelvis are taken while slowly injecting approx 20 mL of full-strength urological contrast material through the catheter using a large urological syringe. If an injury is excluded on the basis of the study, the Foley catheter can then be fully advanced into the bladder after first deflating the balloon. If an injury to the urethra is diagnosed, the Foley catheter should be removed and the urology service contacted, as the patient is likely to require a suprapubic catheter in order to decompress the bladder.

For effective stabilisation, the PCCD should be placed directly over the greater trochanters and not the iliac crests.[78,79] Soft-tissue injuries and pressure sores have occurred due to incorrect fitting of the PCCD or a significantly long length of time left in the binder.[79] There are no clear guidelines on the length of time the patient can remain in the PCCD; suffice it

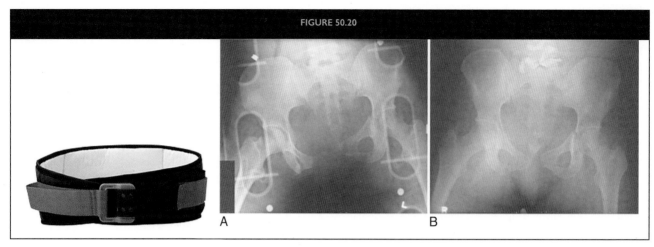

FIGURE 50.20

A

B

A, The SAM Sling. **B,** Open-book pelvis fracture.[112] **C,** After application of the SAM sling.[112]
A Courtesy SAM Medical Products, Portland, Oregon, USA.

to say that definitive management of the unstable pelvis should occur as soon as practicable.

Proximal femur and femoral neck fractures

Proximal femur and femoral neck fractures are commonly referred to as NOF (neck of femur) or hip fractures. For continuity, these will be referred to as hip fractures throughout this section.

Hip fractures are a very common limb injury, particularly in the elderly, encountered by paramedics and EDs.[80] Generally patients will present with a shortening and/or external rotation of the leg, inability to straight-leg-raise and hip pain. There is considerable morbidity and mortality associated with hip fractures; it is estimated that the mortality rate at 1 year is 10–30%.[81]

At the scene and in the ED it is essential to take note of the mechanism of injury, and how long the patient has been on the floor or immobile; it is essential to observe for signs of dehydration, hypothermia, chest infection and pressure sores.[80] The patient will often be in significant pain, so adequate on-scene analgesia, as well as splinting, is essential. Simply tying the legs together with foam padding between the knees along with a blanket around the hips can provide excellent immobilisation.[82]

Classification

There are many classification systems in the literature. For this section we will discuss the most common classifications.

Subcapital fractures are classified by the Garden system, as shown in Figure 50.21. The subcapital fracture is a high transcervical fracture and can interrupt the blood supply to the femoral head, resulting in avascular necrosis (Fig 50.22).

The *intertrochanteric* region of the hip is defined as the region from the extracapsular femoral neck to the area just distal to the lesser trochanter.[83] These type of fractures occur in patients who are more affected by osteoporosis and medical conditions. It has also been reported that these patients are poorer ambulators and more likely to sustain an intertrochanteric fracture. Intertrochanteric fractures are classified into types as shown in Figure 50.23.

Hip fractures in young adults are uncommon, and generally due to high-energy trauma. Hip fractures in the young are associated with higher incidences of non-union and osteonecrosis. This can lead to femoral head collapse and osteoarthritis.[84] Timing of surgery for all hip fractures remains controversial; data are inconclusive as to whether the patient should be operated on as an emergency, urgently or the next day during standard daytime hours.[84,85] It is now considered best practice to operate on hip fractures during standard daytime hours, enabling timely postoperative reviews which have the potential to reduce postoperative complications.[86] The literature states that delayed fixation of hip fractures in young patients can increase the likelihood of osteonecrosis.[84]

Management

The following are recommendations for all hip fractures given by the Scottish Intercollegiate Guidelines Network (SIGN), the British Orthopaedic Association (BOA) standards for trauma and the New Zealand Guidelines Group.[80,81,87,88]

- All patients should be transported to hospital as quickly as possible.
- Early assessment in the ED should include, not in order of priority:
  - vital signs
  - core body temperature
  - pain
  - hydration and nutrition
  - mental state
  - continence
  - pressure sore risk
  - fluid balance
  - co-existing medical conditions
  - previous function
  - previous mobility
  - social circumstances.
- Medical staff should assess patients within 1 hour of arrival.
- All patients at high risk of pressure sores should be placed on a pressure-relieving device.

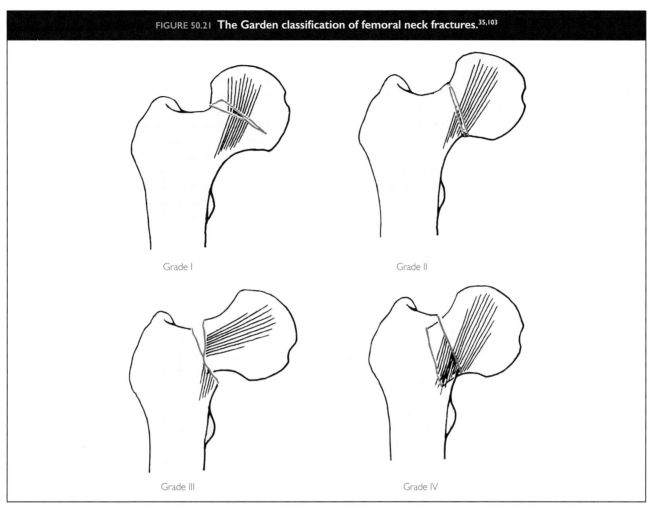

FIGURE 50.21 The Garden classification of femoral neck fractures.[35,103]

Grade I

Grade II

Grade III

Grade IV

Grade I is an incomplete, impacted fracture in valgus malalignment (generally stable). Grade II is a non-displaced fracture. Grade III is an incompletely displaced fracture in varus malalignment. Grade IV is a completely displaced fracture with no engagement of the two fragments. The compression trabeculae in the femoral head line up with the trabeculae on the acetabular side. Displacement is generally more evident on the lateral view in grade IV. For prognostic purposes, these groupings can be lumped into *non-displaced/impacted* (grades I and II) and *displaced* (grades III and IV) because the risk of non-union and aseptic necrosis is similar within these grouped stages.

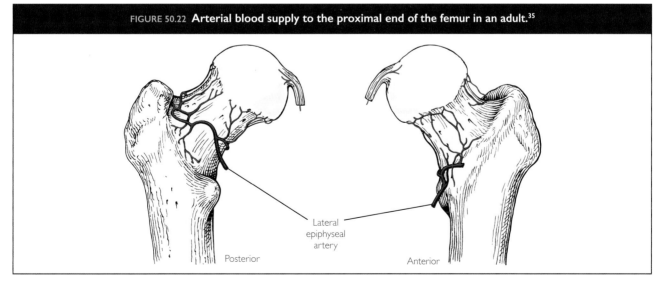

FIGURE 50.22 Arterial blood supply to the proximal end of the femur in an adult.[35]

Lateral epiphyseal artery

Posterior

Anterior

The lateral epiphyseal artery supplies most of the weight-bearing surface of the femoral head in more than 90% of adults. Note the lack of significant arterial supply from the region of insertion of the anterior capsule.

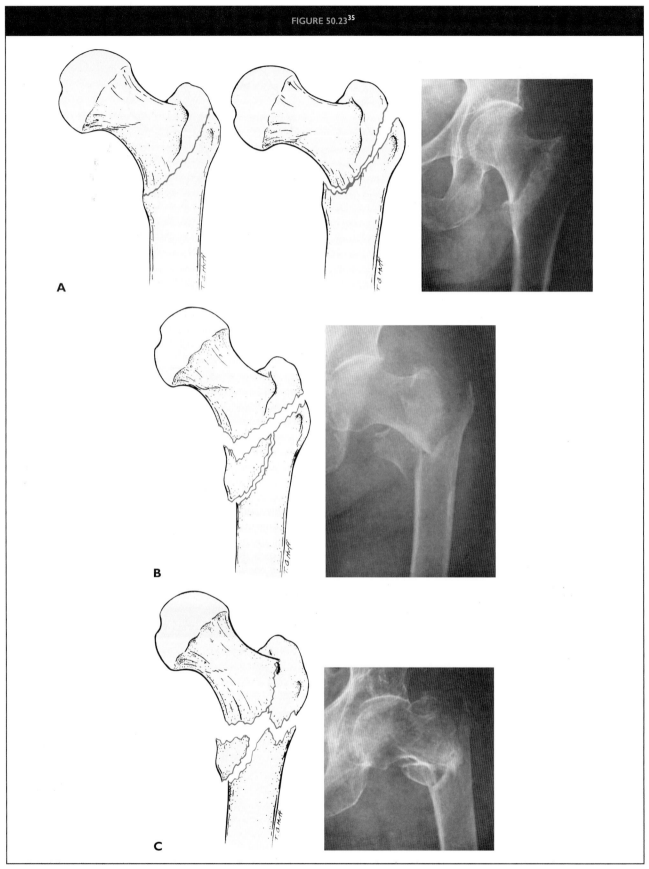

A, Diagrams of a non-displaced and displaced, stable, two-part intertrochanteric fracture, and anteroposterior radiograph of fracture. **B**, Diagram and anteroposterior radiograph of an unstable three-part fracture. **C**, Diagram and anteroposterior radiograph of unstable four-part fracture.

- Patients should be kept warm and have adequate pain relief and pressure-area care.
- Early femoral nerve block can provide effective pain management (Ch 17, p. 358). There is evidence that pain management is poor in Australian EDs and that pre-hospital pain relief has been shown not to influence triage category.[89,90] Essentially, whether the patient has had pain relief or not, the triage category is the same.
- Early radiology should be instigated.
- Measurement and correction of any fluid and electrolyte imbalances should be attended to.
- The consensus of the literature is that indwelling catheters (IDC) should be avoided due to their association with infection; however, their insertion in the ED is standard practice. IDCs are essential for accurate fluid balance and are often used initially to assist with initial pain management until fracture fixation. The IDC should be removed as soon as possible.
- Patients should be transferred to a definitive ward within 2–4 hours of arrival in the ED.
- Oxygen therapy should be administered to maintain tissue oxygenation.[91]
- Reversal of warfarin may commence in the ED.
- Preoperative skin traction has not been shown to be of any benefit, as documented in a 2011 Cochrane review.[3]
- There should be early review by the orthopaedic team, orthogeriatrician and anaesthetist to address medical problems and optimise the patient for surgery.
- Delirium screening should commence in the ED. Untreated pain and dehydration will lead to an increase risk of delirium, which in itself has a significant morbidity and mortality (see Ch 39).
- *ECGs should be obtained early.* These patients will generally all have operative management. ECGs are essential in identifying preexisting cardiac disease that may require reviewing and possible further investigations prior to anaesthesia. They may identify new cardiac changes; if old ECGs are available for comparison, this will direct preoperative care management.

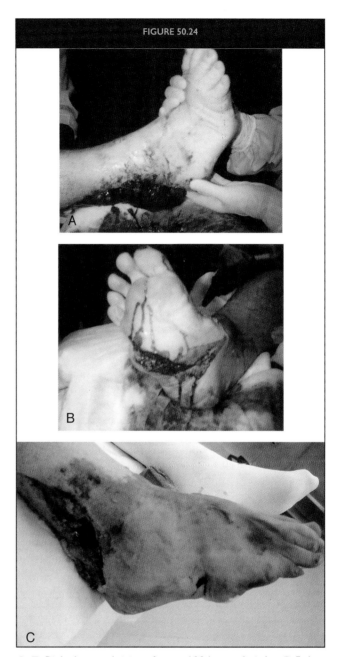

FIGURE 50.24

A, B, Right leg crush injury from a 100 kg steel girder. C, 5 days post crush, patient proceeded to operating suite for below-knee amputation.
Courtesy Celine Hill.

> **PRACTICE TIP**
>
> Get orthopaedics, aged care (or medical registrar) and anaesthetics involved early as this will help to optimise the patient for surgery and address any potentially reversible issues.

Crush injury

Aetiology

Crush injury is prolonged crushing or entrapment, which can occur from a motor vehicle collision where the occupant is trapped by compression, structural collapse of buildings, farming incidents or whenever compression occurs from a traumatic mechanism (Fig 50.24).

Crush syndrome is the result of crush injury. Other trauma patients at risk of crush syndrome are those who have been dragged by a vehicle, struck by a heavy object, suffered massive soft-tissue injury involving muscle mass, have multiple long-bone fractures and compromised local circulation. This syndrome carries a high potential morbidity and mortality for life and limb. Crush syndrome results in rhabdomyolysis, a syndrome of myoglobinuric acute kidney injury (see Ch 25).[5,92]

Crush syndrome is diagnosed initially by mechanism of injury, history and a high index of suspicion. Physical examination should include inspection and palpation of suspected limbs, observing for signs of compression and soft-tissue trauma, and thorough neurovascular assessment. Muscle mass may exhibit signs of erythema, ecchymosis, bullae (large blisters) and abrasions. Neurovascular signs may be a cool, pale, diaphoretic limb, which may be insensate. A weak, thready pulse or the absence of a pulse distal to the injury may indicate compromised circulation or muscle swelling.[92,93]

Pathophysiology

Cellular hypoperfusion and/or hypoxia are a result of prolonged compressive forces. Impaired blood flow and delivery of oxygen to the tissues can occur due to haemorrhage from torn or compressed vessels. Bleeding into an intact compartment may lead to compartment syndrome.[92,93]

When blood flow is re-established to the crushed limb, reperfusion syndrome may ensue, allowing large amounts of myoglobin, phosphorus and potassium to enter the circulation, causing metabolic abnormalities. These abnormalities occur due to disintegrated (lysed) cells releasing inflammatory mediators that cause vascular permeability, vasoconstriction and platelet aggregation, leading to further decreased tissue perfusion and oedema. Lysed cells also release lactic acid, potassium, phosphate, uric acid, thromboplastin, myoglobin and creatine kinase. These metabolic anomalies result in hyperkalaemia, ARF, metabolic acidosis and compartment syndrome.[92,93] Release of potassium from damaged/necrosed cells will increase serum potassium levels leading to cardiac dysrhythmias and/or cardiac arrest.[5] Myoglobin released from damaged cells into plasma is filtered by the glomerulus and may be evident as darkened or reddish-brown ('rust-stained') urine. A low urine pH can be due to hypovolaemia, as well as the release of acid components from injured muscle. Due to low urine pH, myoglobin forms a gel, which blocks the distal nephron resulting in decreased urine output. Calcium deposits in injured muscle and potassium disrupt cardiac rhythm, causing hypocalcaemia and hyperkalaemia—a potentially lethal combination. Death can occur within 3–7 days if anuria, uraemia and hyperkalaemia become evident and are left untreated.[92]

Other systemic symptoms can include profound muscular weakness, pain, swelling, stiffness, cramps, confusion, agitation, delirium, malaise, fever, emesis, nausea and anuria. These symptoms can be a result of electrolyte abnormalities associated with rhabdomyolysis.[93,94]

Rhabdomyolysis is associated with the disintegration of striated muscle, which leads to the release of excessive myoglobin. Trauma is not the only cause of rhabdomyolysis. Other aetiologies may include strenuous exercise (Ch 28), toxicological factors, environmental factors, metabolic abnormalities (Ch 26), infectious risk factors, immunological aetiologies, pharmacological aetiologies and inherited enzyme disorders.[94]

Management

Paramedics should begin treatment as soon as possible. Observe for concomitant injuries such as spinal injuries, solid-organ injuries or fractures. After assessing airway, breathing and circulation, high-flow oxygen should be administered and haemorrhage controlled.[95] Paramedics should consider early aggressive fluid resuscitation at the scene as primary management of an entrapped patient utilising systolic blood pressure as the end point. Fluid administration, generally normal saline, where possible, should be administered before extrication is complete.[94] The paramedic should ensure the patient is on a cardiac monitor, observing for ECG changes, such as peaked T-waves,

QRS widening, no P wave and the presence of life-threatening dysrhythmias, such as sine wave, VT, VF or asystole (see Ch 17, p. 336).[63] Sodium bicarbonate and calcium gluconate may be given pre-hospital.[65] Extrication should be rapid and the patient transported to a definitive facility as quickly as possible.[95]

In the ED crystalloids are continued to achieve a urine output of 100–200 mL/h. The patient should be catheterised and urine measured hourly. Arterial blood gases, electrolytes and myoglobin measurements should be initiated.[95]

Sodium bicarbonate is an agent given to alkalinise the urine. This has been shown to decrease precipitation of myoglobin by minimising myoglobin cast deposits, thus reducing the risk of renal tubular obstruction and therefore improving clearance of myoglobin. Acetazolamide may also be a useful adjunct in forced diuresis. Regular urinary pH testing is essential to monitor the effectiveness of treatment of urinary alkalinisation. Haemodialysis may be required if initial measures fail to control hyperkalaemia, uraemia, fluid overload and metabolic acidosis.[92,93,96]

Electrocardiograms (ECGs) are beneficial in evaluating peaked T-waves, prolonged QRS and P–R intervals and flattening or loss of P waves, all of which may be indicative of hyperkalaemia.[94]

Testing for myoglobin in the urine may be beneficial; however, visible myoglobin pigmentation may be transient, lasting 1–7 days. The primary diagnostic indicator is creatine kinase (CK). When injury to skeletal muscle occurs, CK is secreted into the bloodstream. Normal adult CK levels are 45–260 U/L. A CK level that is elevated at least five times the normal value is an indicator of rhabdomyolysis.

Nursing management should include hourly to 2-hourly monitoring of vital signs, including oxygen saturations, cardiac monitoring, oxygen therapy, hourly measurements of urine output, neurovascular status and urinary pH.[92–94,96] In summary, in the acute phase of rhabdomyolysis, treatment consists of maintaining sufficient circulating volume and adequate diuresis to prevent pulmonary, cardiac and renal complications.[92]

Compartment syndrome

Compartments are classified as closed spaces containing nerves, muscles and vascular structures that are enclosed within bone or fascia (Fig 50.25).

Compartment syndrome is a complication that can occur with any patient who sustains a sprain or fracture, or as a complication from surgery. Compartment syndrome is defined as an increase in pressure within a restricted space. There are 46 anatomical compartments in the body, with 36 of these located in the extremities.[5,97] In the extremities, muscle groups are covered by fascial tissue; fascia is tough and inelastic. In the lower leg, the four compartments most frequently involved in this syndrome are the lateral, posterior, deep posterior and anterior. The forearm contains three compartments: the dorsal, volar and mobile wad. Compartment syndrome can also occur in the upper arm, thigh, gluteal muscles, lumbar paraspinal, shoulder and extraocular compartments and in the foot.[93,97,98]

Aetiology

There are three categories of aetiology:

- *decreased compartment size*—can be due to restrictive splints, casts or dressings, traction or early closure of fascia[100]

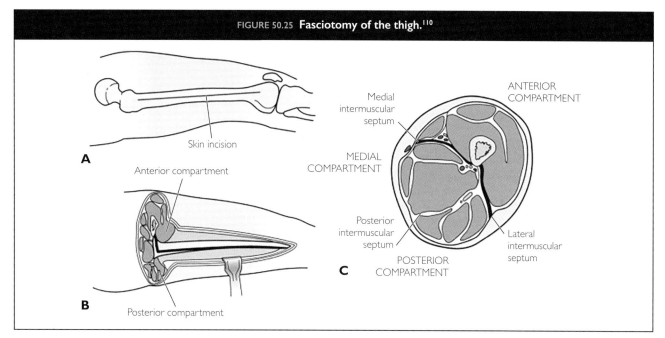

FIGURE 50.25 Fasciotomy of the thigh.[110]

A, The incision extends from the intertrochanteric line to the lateral epicondyle. **B,** The anterior compartment is opened by incising the fascia lata. The vastus lateralis is retracted medially to expose the lateral intermuscular septum, which is incised to decompress the posterior compartment. **C,** Thigh compartments and appropriate incision.

- *increased compartment content*—can be due to bleeding caused by a fracture, or vascular injury. Other aetiologies may include burns, overuse of muscles, envenomation, coagulopathy, venous obstruction or 'tissued' IV site[98]
- *externally applied pressure*—can be due to tight dressings (as previously discussed), or prolonged compression from lying in one position for a significant length of time.[92]

Types

There are three types of compartment syndrome: acute, chronic and crush syndrome. For this section we will only look at acute compartment syndrome.

Pathophysiology

Acute compartment syndrome (ACS) is the rise in interstitial pressure within the closed fascial compartment. This will result in microvascular compromise, neural dysfunction and tissue hypoxia. Local swelling and bleeding results in compressive damage to muscle groups. Due to the inelasticity of fascial compartments, swelling occurs inwards, causing compression and collapse of nerves, muscle cells and blood vessels. If hypoxia continues due to decreased circulation to muscle, the cells will become necrotic.[92] The compartment affected may be distal to the injury, resulting in reduced blood flow, which, in turn, causes the capillaries to lose integrity. Oedema is exacerbated by colloid proteins escaping into soft tissue, pulling fluid with them.

Elevated compartmental pressure is the most significant issue. As the pressure increases within the compartment, vessels begin to collapse as the soft-tissue pressure is greater than the intravascular pressure. Intracompartmental pressures of 30–40 mmHg are high enough to compromise muscle microcirculation. The decrease in blood outflow is directly linked to the collapse of venous structures, which eventually leads to obstructed outflow. If the pressure continues to increase, blood supply can be cut off, and the muscle will become necrotic. In the forearm a pressure of 65 mmHg and in the calf one of 55 mmHg can completely cease tissue circulation in a normovolaemic patient. Normal compartment pressure is 8 mmHg or less. Total cessation of blood flow to the affected extremity is due to the imbalance in pressures between the outflow of venous blood and the inflow of arterial blood. Decreased capillary blood flow, due to tissue-fluid pressure and prolonged periods of microcirculatory ischaemia, will result in irreversible necrosis of intracompartmental tissues, which include nerve tissue and muscle.[93,96]

Signs and symptoms

The symptoms of increased compartment pressure are described in Box 50.3.

Management

The emergency clinican can contribute to prevention of ACS by elevating the limb early and observing closely for early signs of swelling and increasing pain. Elevation above the level of the heart can actually impede venous return and further increase the risk. The emergency nurse must ensure that dressings are applied firmly and are not too tight. Consistent and regular neurovascular assessments are essential. There are a number of pressure monitors on the market that can be used to measure intracompartmental pressures. If the patient is unconscious or unresponsive, continuous monitoring can be used.

If clinical signs and symptoms of compartment syndrome are present, the most important management is to relieve the pressure. This may commence with loosening casts or dressings or proceeding to the operating suite for a fasciotomy to decompress the compartment and halt the ischaemia cycle. Fasciotomies must be done early: within 6 hours and no later

BOX 50.3 Signs of increased compartment pressure and compartment syndrome[5,121–123]

- *Pain*—a critical early sign. The patient may complain of diffuse pain not relieved by analgesia. Pain may be greater during passive motion, and may be out of proportion to the injury. Patients may describe the pain as throbbing, deep or burning: this is due to the ischaemic process of the syndrome.
- *Paraesthesia*—a subtle early sign. Patient may complain of tingling or burning as nerves are very sensitive to pressure. This can lead to numbness.
- *Pallor*—a late sign. Caused by pressure on the artery, it is a late and ominous sign. Skin may look pale, greyish or white. Patients will have a delayed capillary refill of greater than 3 seconds. Skin will feel cool to touch due to decreased capillary perfusion.
- *Paralysis*—a late symptom. Can be caused by either irreversible muscle damage or prolonged nerve compression.
- *Pulselessness*—a very late and ominous sign. The patient may have a very weak pulse or no palpable pulse. This is due to deficient arterial perfusion. This is an indication of tissue death. The pulse will be present until the very late stages.

BOX 50.4 Signs and laboratory diagnosis for fat embolism syndrome (FES)[101,102]

Signs of FES may include:
- petechial rash
- dyspnoea
- cyanosis
- hypoxaemia
- tachypnoea
- loss of consciousness with deepening coma
- fever
- anaemia.

Laboratory tests for diagnosis of FES:
- *Measuring arterial blood gases (ABGs).* This is an essential procedure that should be done early and frequently during the first 48 hours in all patients with significant bony injury.
- *Platelet counts* should be obtained daily for several days after injury. Platelet counts less than 150,000 per mL are indicative of thrombocytopenia and diagnostic of FES.
- *Urine test for lipuria* (the presence of fat in the urine). This test is too sensitive to be of clinical value, because about half of all patients with significant bony injury will have lipuria.
- *Fat in the sputum* is of no significance in the diagnosis of FES.
- *Serum lipase* testing is too sensitive to be of any clinical value, as elevation of serum lipase levels occurs in about half of all patients with fractures.
- *Fat droplets in the circulating blood.* This test is too sensitive to be of clinical value.

than 12 hours from the onset of symptoms. Controversy exists regarding what upper pressure limits mandate a fasciotomy. Several protocols recommend compartment pressures of 30 mmHg or more as the determining level for mandatory fasciotomy.[92–93,97,98] If increased compartment pressure is suspected, the limb should not continue to be elevated as it further decreases venous flow. Post fasciotomy the patient may have a vacuum-assisted wound-closure device, or return to operating suite approximately every 2–3 days for dressing change and potentially further debridement until wound is able to be surgically closed. If the fasciotomy is not able to be surgically closed, a split-skin graft (SSG) may be required.

PRACTICE TIP

If compartment syndrome is suspected, do not elevate the limb, as this will greatly reduce venous return in an already compromised limb.

Fat embolism syndrome

Fat embolism syndrome (FES) results from long-bone fractures, intramedullary manipulation and blunt trauma. Classically, fractures can cause the release of lipid particles (fat emboli) from the bone marrow of fractured long bones, entering the venous circulation and lodging in vital organs.[1,100] It is a potentially serious, life-threatening complication. Fat embolism can produce embolic phenomena from fat within the circulation. FES has identifiable clinical signs and symptoms associated with fat in the circulation; it can also occur with massive soft-tissue injuries, especially adipose tissue, severe burns, severe infections and blunt trauma to fatty organs, particularly fatty livers,[93,101,102] culminating in embolisation of fat in the pulmonary and systemic systems, causing right ventricular failure and cardiovascular collapse.[101]

FES has been the subject of conjecture and controversy, as the syndrome is a series of signs and symptoms that can be common in other critical illnesses. FES is often diagnosed by excluding other injuries/illnesses.[101]

Signs of FES and recommended laboratory investigations for FES diagnosis are listed in Box 50.4. FES can be due to intramedullary reaming during fracture fixation; however, this theory remains controversial. Normal marrow pressure is 30–50 mmHg. During reaming this pressure can increase to up to 600 mmHg. The increase in marrow pressure can cause extravasation of fat emboli from the marrow of bones.[101,103] The incidence of FES has been reported as 1–19%, while a much higher incidence (several times higher) has been noted in postmortem studies. Mortality can reach up to 10–50% in patients with marked respiratory failure and coma.[102,104]

PRACTICE TIP

All other critical illnesses should be ruled out before FES is diagnosed.

Pathophysiology

Mechanical theory

Trauma disrupts fat cells in the marrow. With an increase in marrow pressure, fat droplets escape and are transported to the lung circulation and trapped as emboli. Smaller droplets may reach the kidney, brain, retina and skin. The release of fat is directly related to pressure and the duration of externally applied forces.[93,101,105]

Biochemical theory

Chylomicrons, lipid-containing particles, are released due to haemodynamic changes, such as hypotension and various hormones. This mobilises fat stores, resulting in systemic fat droplet formation and deposition in end-organ vasculature. Free fatty acids are also mobilised due to an elevated concentration of catecholamines as a result of trauma. This chemical process results in aggregation of platelets and formation of fat globules, which leads to acute lung injury, pneumonitis and acute respiratory distress syndrome (ARDS).[93,101,105]

Signs and symptoms

FES is defined as a triad of hypoxia, petechiae and neurological impairment. Signs and symptoms usually occur between 12 and 60 hours, but can occur within a few hours.[93,101,105]

FES signs and symptoms have been divided into major and minor criteria.

Major

- Petechial rash can be transient and occurs in 50–60% of patients. The rash is usually distributed over the chest wall, axilla, conjunctiva and mucous membranes. The rash may be due to stasis, endothelial damage from free fatty acids, loss of clotting factors and platelets, all leading to the rupture of thin-walled capillaries.[93,101,103,105]
- Respiratory and cardiac symptoms with diffuse pulmonary infiltrates on chest X-ray. The lung responds to FES by secreting lipase, turning the fat into free fatty acid. This results in increased capillary bed permeability, destruction of the alveolar architecture and damage to lung surfactant, which leads to immediate and serious impairment of oxygen transfer to haemoglobin (Hb). Hypoxia can be extreme and can result in death. The initial effect of pulmonary microembolism is an increase in perfusion pressure when vessels become engorged, rendering the lung more rigid. The work of breathing increases, which results in the right side of the heart attempting to increase output by dilation, which requires an increase in venous return. An ECG will demonstrate heart strain with prominent S waves, dysrhythmias, right bundle branch block and T wave inversion. The heart is now more susceptible to hypovolaemia with a decrease in central venous return. Death at this point is due to right-sided heart failure.[93,101,105]
- Neurological changes not explained by other medical conditions or trauma and hypoxaemia. Changes can be in the form of restlessness, irritability, headache, anxiety, disorientation, delirium, convulsions and constriction of the pupils.[105]

Minor

- Tachycardia
- Fever < 38°C due to the inflammatory response

- Decreased urine output or fat globules
- Decreasing haematocrit
- Fat globules in the sputum.[105]

Diagnosis

- FES is most likely to occur in patients with multiple long-bone fractures, poor fracture splinting, hypovolaemic shock and rough patient movement.[100]
- There is a variety of diagnostic tools that can be used in the diagnosis of FES. Transoesophageal echocardiography (TOE) can identify circulating embolic particles. It is argued that this has circumspect clinical significance. The best use of TOE is to identify cardiac defects from FES. Other scans such as MRI, CT, chest X-ray and ventilation–perfusion (V/Q) scan tend to be non-specific and have a decreased specificity to FES.[105] Laboratory tests that may diagnose FES are discussed in Box 50.4.

Treatment

Despite technological advances, the treatment of FES remains predominantly supportive—gentle handling and appropriate splinting of fractures, and the prevention and treatment of hypovolaemic shock. Clinicians must support the respiratory system by immediate administration of high-flow oxygen to all patients with significant fractures. In the patient who is intubated and mechanically ventilated, the clinician's main aim is to maintain reasonable ventilatory parameters. Continuous cardiac monitoring, regular arterial blood gas testing and regular analgesia should be performed (see Ch 17 for techniques related to cardiac monitoring, p. 336, and arterial blood gas testing, p. 329). Early fixation of long-bone fractures remains controversial with regard to the type of fixation in the initial stages, i.e. intramedullary nailing versus external fixation. As discussed, early internal fixation may not be advantageous to patients, particularly patients with thoracic trauma.[101,102,104,105]

In summary, the basis of treatment is prevention of hypovolaemic shock, stress response and hypoxia, and then stabilisation of fractures operatively within 24 hours.[101]

Delayed complications

Understanding how a fracture heals is essential in knowing how to treat it (Table 50.1). Factors such as immobilisation and/or internal fixation are important issues in facilitating the healing process. In some cases, the normal healing process is hindered and bone fails to unite, causing delayed union, non-union and malunion. Causes of abnormal fracture healing can be severe damage to soft tissues (which makes union non-viable), abnormal bone, infection, movement at the fracture site and distraction and separation of fragments.[2,4,9]

- *Delayed union* is where the fracture may take a substantial amount of time to heal, between 3 months and 1 year. Delayed union may be due to infection or fracture of the internal fixation device.
- *Non-union* is where the bone fails to complete bony union, usually greater than 6 months. Causes of non-union can be repetitive stress on the fracture site, insufficient blood supply, inadequate or improper immobilisation or infection.
- *Malunion* is where the bone heals in the standard amount of time but in an unacceptable position with residual bony

deformity. Factors that contribute to malunion are gravity on the fracture site, unequal stress forces of muscle pull or improper reduction of the fracture.[2,4,9]

Infection prevention

All patients are at risk of infection when there is a break in the skin. When a fracture is associated with skin trauma, a high risk of infection is possible and may lead to osteomyelitis. This infection is most often attributed to *Staphylococcus aureus*. The emergency nurse's role in infection prevention is to try to prevent the onset. This includes ensuring aseptic technique is used in wound management, administering prophylactic antibiotics and determining requirements for tetanus prophylaxis.[11]

Open fractures are susceptible to wound infections, which can lead to septicaemia, necrotising fasciitis and tetanus. Sepsis in trauma patients carries significantly high mortality. Musculoskeletal infections can be complicated to treat because they are relatively remote to the body's protective macrophages and systemic antibodies.[3,7,106]

Osteomyelitis is a bone infection involving the bone marrow. Bacteria can invade via the blood; via direct introduction, such as in open fractures or penetrating wounds; or during surgery. Treatment includes antibiotic therapy, surgical debridement, irrigation and/or drainage.[4,5,9]

Necrotising fasciitis is an uncommon and rapidly accelerating infectious process. It primarily involves the fascia and subcutaneous tissue. It is a severe infection with toxin-secreting bacteria which leads to life-threatening soft tissue destruction and necrosis. There are a variety of terms used to describe this condition; haemolytic streptococcal gangrene, Fournier gangrene and gas gangrene. Anaerobic bacteria in combination with Gram-negative organisms are most commonly found in necrotising fasciitis. They propagate in an environment of tissue hypoxia. Treatment should include administration of antibiotics, fluid replacement, thorough surgical debridement of necrotic fascia and decompression of compartments. Hyperbaric oxygen has been used to reduce the spread of gangrene, but its use remains controversial due to lack of level one data.[107] The patient may rapidly decline due to toxaemia which, if left untreated, causes coma and death.[4,7,9107] Necrotising fasciitis has a mortality rate of 15–50%.[107]

Traction

Overall, use of traction—a pulling force on a part of the body—has been reduced due to the advances in orthopaedic treatment of fractures. Traction is used for a variety of reasons. It can be applied to maintain alignment of a fracture and to reduce muscle spasms and pain. Most paediatric patients under the age of 6 years are managed in plaster spicas, plaster casts or traction. All patients in traction need regular analgesia, pressure-area care, hydration, bowel regimen, deep venous thrombosis (DVT) prophylaxis and adequate documentation of fluid balance.

Forces used in traction

There are two types of forces that can be used in traction:

- *Balanced traction* is used to suspend a part of the body without pulling on that part, such as Hamilton Russell traction. Balanced traction relies on the patient's bodyweight to provide counter-traction.

- *Inline or running traction* exerts a pull on the axis of the long bone in one plane, such as Buck's skin traction.[7,108]

There are three classifications of traction:

- *Skin traction*, being the most common type of traction, is achieved by the direct application of a pulling force on the skin. It is generally only a temporary measure to maintain immobilisation prior to surgery, and to reduce muscle spasm and therefore pain. Complications from skin traction are blisters, necrosis and compartment syndrome. Generally no more than 2.3–3.6 kg (5–8 lbs) of weight should be applied to skin traction. Hamilton Russell traction has a 'block and tackle' effect; in other words, 2.3 kg (5 lbs) of weight is applied, but the resultant traction pull is 4.5 kg (10 lbs).[7,109]

- *Skeletal traction* is applied directly to the bone and is a strong, steady and continuous pull. A pin or wire is passed through the bone distal to the fracture (Fig 50.26). It is useful in comminuted and complex fractures, as more weight can be applied in skeletal traction, 4.5 kg (10 lbs) or more. Skeletal traction can be the definitive treatment or can precede internal fixation. It is particularly useful in stabilising fractures in patients who are in extremis and too unstable to endure a lengthy orthopaedic procedure.[7,47,108]

- *Manual traction* is applied temporarily by the hands to immobilise an injured limb. Manual traction can be used during application of a plaster of Paris (POP) cast.[7]

Application of skin traction

Skin traction should not be applied to patients who have allergies to tape or have obvious circulatory or vascular disorders, such as varicose veins or ulcers. There is a variety of adhesive or non-adhesive skin traction kits on the market that come prepacked with skin strips, bandage and rope.

Application of the skin strips begins proximal to the malleolus, leaving the foot free for ROM exercises, and should end distal to the head of the fibula. These are areas of risk due to the common peroneal nerve being in close proximity (Fig 50.27). Pressure on this nerve can produce foot drop. Leaving the foot free of bandaging also allows the emergency

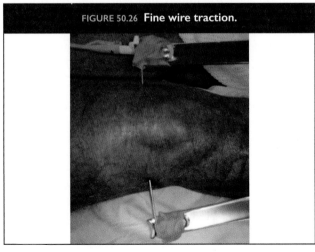

FIGURE 50.26 **Fine wire traction.**

The pin is passed through the tibia to project equally medially and laterally. Points are protected with covers.
Courtesy Celine Hill.

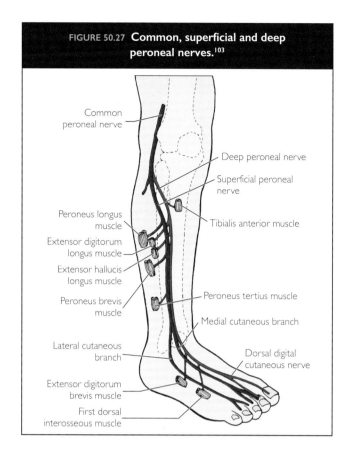

FIGURE 50.27 **Common, superficial and deep peroneal nerves.**[103]

Common peroneal nerve

Deep peroneal nerve

Superficial peroneal nerve

Peroneus longus muscle

Tibialis anterior muscle

Extensor digitorum longus muscle

Extensor hallucis longus muscle

Peroneus brevis muscle

Peroneus tertius muscle

Medial cutaneous branch

Lateral cutaneous branch

Dorsal digital cutaneous nerve

Extensor digitorum brevis muscle

First dorsal interosseous muscle

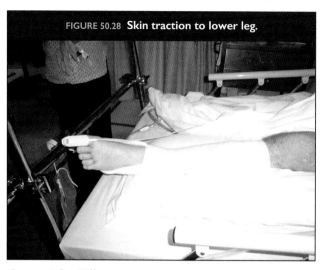

FIGURE 50.28 **Skin traction to lower leg.**

Courtesy Celine Hill.

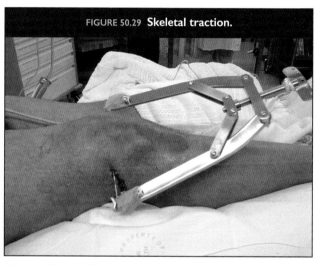

FIGURE 50.29 **Skeletal traction.**

Courtesy Celine Hill.

nurse to assess the neurovascular status regularly. A bandage is provided in the kits and should be applied firmly and in one direction with no twists or creases (Fig 50.28).

The rope is threaded through the pulley and the weight bag is applied. Neurovascular observations must be attended pre-application and at least hourly post application.[8,9,109] Analgesia prior to traction application is essential. The use of opioids or femoral nerve blocks may assist in pain control.

PRACTICE TIP

Do not apply skin traction strips or bandage above the head of the fibula. This will cause compression of the common peroneal nerve, which can potentially lead to foot drop.

Skeletal traction

Skeletal traction can be used for pelvic and femoral fractures. The rationale for traction is to reduce fractures, keep the limb out to length, for pain relief and to decrease haemorrhage. The type of pin used currently is Kirschner's wire (k-wire). The k-wire is easily inserted while the patient is still in the ED. The k-wire should only be inserted by personnel who are trained to do so. Local anaesthetic is used to the periostium. The k-wire is inserted from medial to lateral[35] (to prevent vascular injury). Bend the wire at each end to capture the tensioning device. The k-wire is placed depending on the location of the fracture. Skeletal traction allows substantial weight to be applied directly to the bone.[4,37]

A simple traction set-up will consist of a rope attached to the tensioning device, passing through a pulley at the end of the bed, which is then attached to a hanging weight. The leg should be supported with pillows to reduce deformity and elevate the heel off the bed. A weight of 7–11 kg (15–25 lbs) is generally enough to overcome muscle tension, restoring the femur to length and reducing muscle spasm[37] (Fig 50.29).

Pin-site care is often debated. A 2013 Cochrane review found no evidence for the best technique for pin-site care to minimise complications and infections.[111]

Complications

It is important to understand the complications associated with traction. Traction can cause inadequate alignment of fracture, neurovascular compromise, soft-tissue injury and skin breakdown. Prevention of these problems includes neurovascular observations, regular pressure-area care and maintenance of traction. The application of traction requires a medical order. The order must include type of traction, weight to be applied and whether the traction can be removed for tests, such as CT or MRI.[7]

Because of the infrequent use of traction, emergency nurses' skills have decreased in that area. It is important that nurses are instructed, by an experienced clinician, on application of traction and the essential components of safety of application, assessment and monitoring. The advanced practice emergency nurse should be able to apply skin traction in the ED after education and assessment.

Splints

The purpose of splinting is to reduce pain, risk of fat embolism and risk of further soft-tissue injury due to fracture fragments. The limb must be splinted above and below the fracture site. Some patients may present to the ED with their fracture already splinted by ambulance personnel. Common splints used in the field are the Hare traction splint[112] and the Donway and Sager splints, which are discussed in detail in Chapter 17, p. 352. These splints are bulky and require education and training on use. More commonly used by ambulance and retrieval services are the Kendrick Traction Device or the CT-6 traction splint (see Ch 17, p. 353, and Fig 17.50). They are lightweight and fold down into a pouch. They both provide skin traction.

These devices allow for both immobilisation and traction of the affected limb. Application of the splint requires at least two people experienced in its efficient and effective application, bearing in mind that there is always a risk of applying too much traction. The splinted limb must be continuously monitored for neurovascular compromise and increased pressure from the straps. Straps may need to be loosened and other areas may require further padding to prevent skin breakdown. The traction splint is a temporary measure and should be replaced by more-definitive management, such as traction or internal fixation.[5,7,47]

Other removable splints that can be used include inflatable splints, which are also temporary and should be replaced as soon as practicable. They are useful for fractures of the forearm, wrist and ankle. Caution must be used when inflating them, as pressures above 40 mmHg can reduce or cause cessation of blood flow to the limb. In instances where prefabricated splints are unavailable, anything can be used as a temporary splint; for example, pillows, jumpers, wood or towels. Note that patients with severe fractures should always be splinted to immobilise the limb and prevent further complications.[5,7] Paramedics and emergency nurses should be able to apply these temporary splints, after education and assessment. Chapter 17 covers the application and use of casts (p. 350) and crutches (p. 356).

Psychosocial aspects

The paramedic or emergency nurse is frequently the first person the patient, family or friends see to seek answers to their many questions. In the pre-hospital environment or a busy ED, there are often major pressures on the clinicians' time. It is therefore essential that they are acutely aware of the physiological and psychological impact of trauma, no matter how minor they perceive it to be. Some studies have looked at the psychological consequences of orthopaedic injury, and report that after 2 years at least 20% of patients who sustained a lower extremity injury report severe phobic anxiety and/or depression.[113] With this in mind, the paramedic and emergency nurse's perception of the injury will always be different from that of the patient, family and friends.

SUMMARY

For the paramedic and emergency trauma nurse, musculo-skeletal trauma will continue to be challenging and demanding. Upwards of 70% of trauma patients will have fractures or injured limbs, and with improvements in treatment, medication and surgical management, outcomes for these patients have improved. Research continues to improve options in assessment and management of musculoskeletal injuries. For example, a recent retrospective study found that infection rate from open tibia fractures is not dependent on the time to surgery but is strongly associated with the grade of open fracture, and concluded that delay to theatre may be

justified until optimal and safe operating time is provided.[114] Another recent review of practice in the management of haemodynamically unstable pelvic trauma patients found that haemorrhage-related mortality was extremely high in the laparotomy group and concluded that non-therapeutic laparotomy should be avoided and concentration placed instead on arresting pelvic bleeding.[115] Injury prevention should be the major focus. Further development and funding in the area of injury prevention and research are paramount in reducing and preventing the high morbidity and mortality rates associated with high-energy musculoskeletal trauma.

CASE STUDY

Part 1—Pre-hospital

You are called to a 54-year-old male, who has fallen approximately 10 metres out of a tree, hit a car on the way down and landed on his back on a concrete driveway. The timing is as follows:

- 1013 hours—Ambulance booked
- 1039 hours—Arrival at scene

- 1051 hours—Depart scene
- 1055 hours—Triage
- 1058 hours—Off stretcher.

Using MIST, you note the following:

- Injury—lacerated occipital area. Not responding to verbal commands, conscious but confused. Pupils 5 mm and sluggish to react to light. Chest has

TABLE 50.CS1 Vital signs on initial assessment

TIME	SBP	PR	RR	O₂ SATS	GCS	BREATH SOUNDS	AVPU	O/R	PUPILS
1018	70	145	40	90	9	D	V	R	+ Sluggish
1025	?	101	40	94	12	D	V	O	+ Sluggish
1041	?	93	36	96	12	D	V	O	+ Sluggish

AVPU: Alert, Voice, Pain, Unresponsive; GCS: Glasgow Coma Scale; O₂ SATS: oxygen saturations; PR: pulse rate (beats/minute); RR: respiratory rate (breaths/minute); SBP: systolic blood pressure

decreased air entry on left side, poor tidal volume, decreased oxygen saturations. Tachycardic, hypotensive. Rigid abdomen, not moving limbs. Has externally rotated lower limbs.

- Signs as in Table 50.CS1—note that the patient is dysphasic and is unable to respond verbally due to a pre-existing neurological deficit from a cerebrovascular accident (CVA).

Questions

1. What potential injuries does this patient have?
2. What treatment will you initiate?
3. What type of hospital will you transport the patient to?

Part 2—Emergency department

A trauma call is activated and the patient given a Triage Category 1. A primary and secondary survey are performed (see below). His medical history is further clarified as having had a CVA middle cerebral artery (MCA) in 2003, and being unable to speak; he also has mild left-sided weakness, hypertension and hypercholesterolaemia. There has also been bilateral rotator cuff repair and wrist surgery. He has no known drug allergies.

Primary survey

- Airway: patent, trachea midline, cervical spine collar in situ
- Breathing: oxygen via non-rebreather, 15 L/min
- Circulation: IV Normal saline 3 L and 3 units packed cells. Minimal urine output—100 mL in ED, no in-dwelling catheter (IDC) due to probable pelvic injury.
- Deficit: Normal but does not speak, so usual GCS is 12 (verbal response—incomprehensible sounds).
- Signs—see Table 50.CS2.

Secondary survey

- Head: small occipital head laceration
- Face: NAD
- Neck: possibly tender
- Chest: decreased bibasally. No local tenderness
- Abdomen: distended, upper quadrant guarding. Abrasions right upper quadrant
- Pelvis: tender
- Back: possibly tender, unable to assess thoracic–lumbar spine. No deformity

TABLE 50.CS2 Vital signs after arrival at the ED

TIME	BP	PR	RR	O₂ SATS	GCS	TEMP	PUPILS
1059	99/68	100	20	88%	10	36.8	4+
1100	90/58	90		100%	11		4+
1150	122/70	105	25	100%	12		4+
1215	110/58	105			12		4+
1300	121/60	99	20	100%			
1340					12		4+

GCS: Glasgow Coma Scale; O₂ SATS: oxygen saturations; PR: pulse rate (beats/minute); RR: respiratory rate (breaths/minute); BP: blood pressure; Temp: temperature (°C)

- Upper limbs: no obvious fractures, pulses present
- Lower limbs: pulses present, no obvious fractures.

Adjuncts

- A full range of blood tests was performed, including cross-match.
- Arterial blood gas (ABG) results were: pH 7.15; partial carbon dioxide pressure (pCO$_2$) 54 mmHg, partial oxygen pressure (pO$_2$) 128 mmHg, bicarbonate 18.4 mmol/L, lactate 2.7 mmol/L.
- Chest X-ray: No pneumothorax, no rib fractures
- Cervical spine: no fractures noted
- Pelvis: open-book fracture (Fig 50.CS1)
- FAST scan: negative.

Questions—cont'd

4. Did the patient receive appropriate fluid management?
5. Discuss the concept of damage control resuscitation.
6. What do his ABG results indicate?

Part 3—Management

Initial treatment plan

The patient is admitted under the trauma team with his pelvic binder to remain on (Fig 50.CS2). He undergoes computed tomography (CT) of head, abdomen/pelvis, cervical spine, chest. The patient remains haemodynamically stable during transfer to CT. He is given analgesia of fentanyl 25 μg × 4.

CT scan results

Brain: evidence of old infarct MCA. No intracranial haemorrhage

Chest: Large left pneumothorax; left intercostal catheter (ICC) inserted at 1310

Left posterior rib fracture 4–9, flail segment

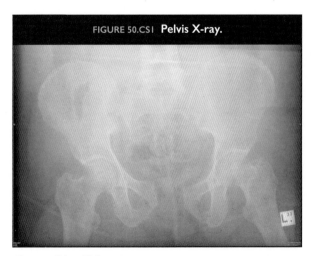

FIGURE 50.CS1 **Pelvis X-ray.**

Courtesy Celine Hill.

Abdomen: NAD

Fracture transverse process T11 and L1–5.

Pelvis: fracture through sacrum into sacroiliac joints bilaterally, left superior pubic ramus fracture, pubic symphysis diastasis. Open-book pelvic fracture

Bilateral retroperitoneal haematoma extending into scrotum on right side.

Orthopaedic surgery review

On review, the patient has palpable dorsalis pedis pulses. His L2 to S5 nerves are intact. A Kirschner's wire (k-wire) is inserted into distal femur for skeletal traction (Fig 50.CS3), and 10 kg (22 lbs) of weight applied for pelvic fracture. He is transferred to the operating theatre at 1530 for open reduction and internal fixation of pelvic fracture.

Operating theatre (1535–2045)

There is a query regarding tension pneumothorax as the patient is cardiorespiratorily unstable. The cardiothoracic registrar reviews the patient and deems a pneumothorax unlikely, clinically, as there is good air entry and a patent left-sided ICC. An anterior ICC is inserted prophylactically. The patient is acidotic: pH 7.28; pCO$_2$ 37 mmHg, pO$_2$ 155 mmHg, Bic 17, Lac 4.4.

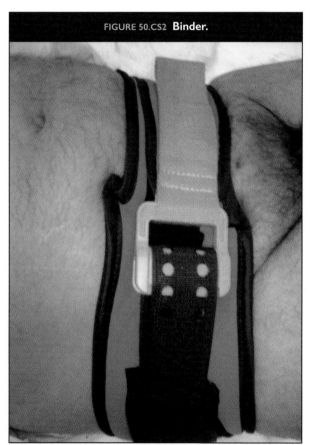

FIGURE 50.CS2 **Binder.**

Courtesy Celine Hill.

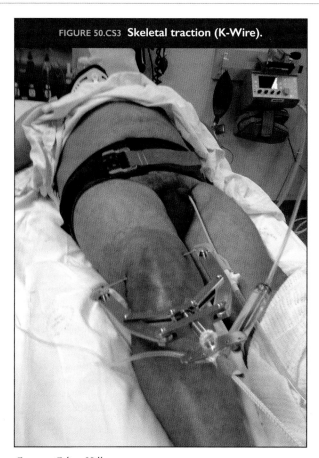

FIGURE 50.CS3 **Skeletal traction (K-Wire).**

Courtesy Celine Hill.

Intensive care

The patient is transferred to the intensive care unit at 2050 hours intubated and ventilated. For the first 48 hours post operation, he requires fluid resuscitation, blood products and pain relief. Ventilation is weaned and the patient is extubated on day 4. ICCs are successfully removed on day 5 and the patient is transferred to the trauma high-dependency unit (HDU) on day 7. There is a delay in transfer to HDU due to bed availability. He remains in the trauma HDU for one day and is stable for transfer to the orthopaedic ward.

Questions—cont'd

7. Explain the complications and risks associated with an open-book pelvic fracture.

8. What processes would you initiate?

Answers to Case Study Questions can be found on evolve
http://evolve.emergencytrauma.curtis

REFERENCES

1. Balogh ZJ, Reumann MK, Gruen RL et al. Advances and future directions for management of trauma patients with musculoskeletal injuries. The Lancet 2012;380(9847):1109–19.

2. Altizer L. Fractures. Orthop Nurs 2002;21(6):51–9.

3. Handoll HHG, Quelly JM, Parker MJ. Pre-operative traction for hip fractures in adults. Cochrane Database Syst Rev 2011;(12); CD000168 Online. http://onlinelibrary.wiley.com/doi/10.1002/14651858.CD000168.pub3/abstract; accessed 17 Jan 2014.

4. Dandy DJ, Edwards DJ. Essential orthopaedics and trauma. 5th edn. Edinburgh: Churchill Livingstone; 2009.

5. McQuillan KA, Makic MBF, Whalen E et al, eds. Trauma nursing: from resuscitation through rehabilitation. 4th edn. Philadelphia: WB Saunders; 2008.

6. Neff JA, Kidd PS. Trauma nursing: the art and science. St Louis: Mosby; 1993.

7. Maher AB, Salmond SW, Pellino TA. Orthopaedic nursing. 3rd edn. Philadelphia: WB Saunders; 2002.

8. Thibodeau GA, Patton KT. Anatomy and physiology. 6th edn. St Louis: Mosby; 2006.

9. Solomon L, Warwick D, Nayagam S. Apley's Concise system of orthopaedics and fractures. 3rd edn. London: Arnold; 2005.

10. Ferri F. Osteoporosis. St Louis: Mosby; 2014.

11. Kitt S, Selfridge-Thomas J, Proehl JA et al. Emergency nursing: a physiologic and clinical perspective. 2nd edn. Philadelphia: WB Saunders; 1995.

12. Mattox KL, Moore EE, Feliciano DV. Trauma. 7th edn. New York: McGraw-Hill; 2012.

13. Giannakopoulos GF, Saltzherr TP, Beenan LF et al. Missed injuries during the initial assessment in a cohort of 1124 level-1 trauma patients. Injury 2012;43(9):1517–21.

14. Olson SA, Rhorer AS. Orthopaedic trauma for the general orthopaedist: avoiding problems and pitfalls in treatment. Clin Orthop Relat Res 2005;(433):30–7.

15. Bongiovanni MS, Bradley SL, Kelley DM. Orthopedic trauma: critical care nursing issues. Crit Care Nurs Q 2005;28(1):60–71.

16. Frykberg ER. Combined vascular and skeletal extremity trauma. Trauma.org 2005;10(5). Online. www.trauma.org/archive/vascular/vascskeletal.html.

17. Streubel PN, Gardner MJ, Ricci WM. Management of femur fractures in obese patients. Orthop Clin N Am 2011;42(1):21–35.

18. Ekinici S, Polat O, Gunalp M, Demirkan A, Koca A. The accuracy of ultrasound in foot and ankle trauma. American Journal of Emergency Medicine 2013;31(11):1551–5.

19. Blankstein A. Ultrasound in the diagnosis of clinical orthopaedics: The orthopaedic stethoscope. World Journal of Orthopedics 2011;2(2):13–24.

20. Bolandparvaz S, Moharamzadeh P, Jamali K et al. Comparing diagnostic accuracy of bedside ultrasound and radiography for bone fracture screening in multiple trauma patients at the ED. American Journal of Emergency Medicine 2013;31(11):1583–5.

21. Joshi N, Lira A, Mehta N et al. Diagnostic accuracy of history, physical examination and bedside ultrasound for diagnosis of extremity fractures in the emergency department: A systemic review. Academic Emergency Medicine 2013;20(1):1–15.

22. Marx J, Hockberger R, Walls R. Rosen's Emergency medicine: concepts and clinical practice. 8th edn. Philadelphia: Saunders; 2014.

23. Grimm MR, Vrahas MS, Thomas KA. Pressure–volume characteristics of the intact and disrupted pelvic retroperitoneum. J Trauma 1998;44(3):454–9.

24. Cullinane DC, Schiller HJ, Zielinski MD et al. Pelvic Fracture Hemorrhage—Update and Systematic Review. EAST Practice Management Guidelines; 2011. Online. www.east.org/resources/treatment-guidelines 16 Jan 2014.

25. Harrahill M. Bladder trauma: a review. J Emerg Nurs 2004;30(3):287–8.

26. Aihara R, Blansfield JS, Millham FH et al. Fracture locations influence likelihood of rectal and lower urinary tract injuries in patients sustaining pelvic fractures. J Trauma 2002;52(2):205–9.

27. Kielb SJ, Voeltz ZL, Wolf JS. Evaluation and management of traumatic posterior urethral disruption with flexible cystourethroscopy. J Trauma 2001;50(1):36–40.

28. Cohen SP, Christo PJ, Moroz L. Pain management in trauma patients. Am J Phys Med Rehabil 2004;83(2):142–61.

29. Ekman EF, Koman LA. Acute pain following musculoskeletal injuries and orthopaedic surgery: mechanisms and management. J Bone Joint Surg Am 2004;86(6):1316–27.

30. Bath T, Lord WA. Risk and benefits of paramedic-initiated shoulder reduction. J Paramedic Practice 2009;1(6):235–40.

31. Miller MD. What's new in sports medicine. J Bone Joint Surg Am 2004;86-A(3):653–61.

32. Kozin S, Berlet A. Pelvis and acetabulum. In: Handbook of common orthopaedic fractures. 4th edn. Chester: Medical Surveillance; 2000.

33. Cunningham NJ. Techniques for reduction of anteroinferior shoulder dislocation. Emerg Med Australasia 2005;17(5–6):463–71.

34. Mattick A, Wyatt JP. From Hippocrates to the Eskimo—A history of techniques used to reduce anterior dislocation of the shoulder. J R Coll Surg Edinb 2000;45(5):312–16.

35. Browner BD, Jupiter JB, Levine AM et al. Skeletal trauma: basic science, management and reconstruction. 4th edn. WB Saunders: Philadelphia; 2008.

36. Welsh S, Veenstra M. Shoulder dislocations. eMedicine; 2012. Online. http://emedicine.medscape.com/article/1261802-overview; accessed 16 Jan 2014.

37. Canale ST, Beatty JH. eds. Campbell's Operative orthopaedics. 12th edn. Philadelphia: Mosby; 2013.

38. Kowalsky MS, Levine WN. Traumatic posterior glenohumeral dislocation: classification, pathoanatomy, diagnosis and treatment. Orthop Clin North Am 2008;39(4):519–33, viii.

39. Robinson CM, Aderinto J. Posterior shoulder dislocations and fracture–dislocations. J Bone Joint Surg Am 2005;87(3):639–50.

40. Wilson S, Price D. Shoulder dislocation in emergency medicine. eMedicine; 2013. Online. http://emedicine.medscape.com/article/823843-overview; accessed 16 Jan 2014.

41. Bucholz RW, Court-Brown CM, Heckman JD. Rockwood and Greens fractures in adults. 6th edn. Philadelphia: Lippincott, Williams & Wilkins; 2005.

42. Covey DC. Blast and fragment injuries of the musculoskeletal system. J Bone Joint Surg Am 2002;84-A(7):1221–34.

43. Langworthy MJ, Smith JM, Gould M. Treatment of the mangled lower extremity after a terrorist blast injury. Clin Orthop Relat Res 2004;(422):88–96.

44. Daniels JM II, Zook EG, Lynch JM. Hand and wrist injuries: part II emergent evaluation. Am Fam Physician 2004;69(8):1949–56.

45. Proehl JA. Accidental amputation. Am J Nurs 2004;104(2):50–3.

46. Cameron P, Jelinek G, Kelly A et al, eds. Textbook of adult emergency medicine. 3rd edn. Edinburgh: Churchill Livingstone; 2009.

47. Simon RR, Sherman SC, Koenigsknecht SJ. Emergency orthopedics: the extremities. 6th edn. New York: McGraw-Hill; 2011.

48. Peerless JR. Fluid management of the trauma patient. Curr Opin Anaesthesiol 2001;14(2):221–5.

49. Pepe PE. Shock in polytrauma: needs better definition and perhaps more selective treatment. Br Med J 2003;327(7424):1119–20.

50. Gillham MJ, Parr MJ. Resuscitation for major trauma. Curr Opin Anaesthesiol 2002;15(2):167–72.

51. Kelley DM. Hypovolemic shock: an overview. Crit Care Nurs Q 2005;28(1):2–19.

52. Frank ED, Long BW, Smith BJ. Merrill's Atlas of radiographic positions and radiologic procedures. 12th edn. St Louis: Mosby; 2011.

53. Wasserman E, Hill S. Ankle injuries in the emergency department: how to provide rapid and cost-effective assessment and treatment. Emerg Med Pract 2002;5(4):1–26.

54. Bennett AR, Smith KD. Open fractures. Orthopaedics and Trauma 2013;27(1):9–14.

55. Gustilo RB, Anderson JT. Prevention of infection in the treatment of one thousand and twenty-five open fractures of long bones: retrospective and prospective analysis. J Bone Joint Surg Am 1976;58(4):453–8.

56. Gustilo RB, Mendoza RM, Williams DN. Problems in the management of type III (severe) open fractures: a new classification of type III open fractures. J Trauma 1984;24(8):742–6.

57. Skaggs DL, Friend L, Alman B et al. The effect of surgical delay on acute infection following 554 open fractures in children. J Bone Joint Surg Am 2005;87(1):8–12.

58. Roberts CS, Pape HC, Jones AL et al. Damage control orthopaedics: evolving concepts in the treatment of patients who have sustained orthopaedic trauma. J Bone Joint Surg Am 2005;87(2):434–49.

59. Neligan PJ, Baranov D. Trauma and aggressive homeostasis management. Anesthesiology Clinics 2013;31(1):21–39.

60. Ozturkmen Y, Karamehmetoglu M et al. Acute treatment of segmental tibial fractures with the Ilizarov method. Injury 2009;40(3):321–6.

61. DePalma A, Connolly J. DePalma's The management of fractures and dislocations. 3rd edn. Philadelphia: WB Saunders; 1981.

62. Hoogendoorn JM, van der Werken C. The mangled leg: decision-making based on scoring systems and outcome. Eur J Trauma 2002;28(1):1–10.

63. Ly TV, Travison TG, Castillo RC, Bosse MJ et al. Ability of lower extremity score to predict functional outcomes after limb salvage. J Bone Joint Surg Am 2008;90(8):1738–43.

64. Cronenwett JL, Johnston KW. Rutherford's vascular surgery. 8th edn. Philadelphia: Saunders; 2014.

65. NSW Ambulance Clinical Governance Unit. Hyperkalaemia—Protocol C9. 2014.

66. Duke Orthopaedics: Wheeless' Textbook of Orthopaedics online. The Mangled Extremity Score (2012). Online. www.wheelessonline. com/ortho/mangled_extremity_severity_score_mess; accessed 25 July 2014.

67. Royal College of Surgeons Edinburgh. The mangled extremity scores. (2004). Online. www.rcsed.ac.uk/fellows/lvanrensburg/classification/trauma%20scores/mangled_extremity_scores.htm; accessed 16 Jan 2014.

68. Wolfgang E, Eid K, Keel M et al. Therapeutic strategies and outcome of polytraumatised patients with pelvic injuries. Eur J Trauma 2000;26(6):278–86.

69. Wong JML, Bucknill A. Fractures of the pelvic ring. Injury 2014 (Article in press).

70. Simpson T, Krieg JC, Heuer F et al. Stabilization of pelvic ring disruptions with a circumferential sheet. J Trauma 2002;52(1):158–61.

71. Krieg JC, Mohr M, Ellis TJ et al. Emergent stabilization of pelvic ring injuries by controlled circumferential compression: a clinical trial. J Trauma 2005;59(3):659–64.

72. Lynch TH, Martinez-Pineiro L, Plas E et al. EAU guidelines on urological trauma. Eur Urol 2005;47(1):1–15.

73. Fitzgerald A, Runciman J, Van Den Driesen M. Royal Melbourne Hospital Trauma Service Guideline: Emergency Trauma Urethrogram. Version 2: 2012. Online. http://clinicalguidelines.mh.org.au/brochures/TRM05.04.pdf; accessed 25 July 2014.

74. Djakovic N, Lynch TH, Martinez-Pinero L et al. Guidelines on urological trauma. Eur Urol 2005;47(1):1–15. Updated on-line 2009, Available: http://www.uroweb.org/gls/pockets/english/19_Urological_Trauma.pdf; accessed 25 July 2014.

75. Fu CF, Wu YT, Liao CH, Kang SC et al. Pelvic circumferential compression devices benefit patients with pelvic fractures who need transfers. American Journal of Emergency Medicine 2013;31(10):1432–6.

76. Bottlang M, Simpson T, Sigg J et al. Non-invasive reduction of open-book pelvic fractures by circumferential compression. J Orthop Trauma 2002;16(6):367–73.

77. British Orthopaedic Association Standards for Trauma (BOAST). BOAST 3: Pelvic and acetabular fracture management. 2008. Online. www.boa.ac.uk/LIB/LIBPUB/Documents/BOAST%203%20-%20Pelvic%20and%20Acetabular%20Fracture%20Management.pdf; accessed 16 Jan 2014.

78. Wayne MA. New concepts in the pre-hospital and ED management of pelvic fractures. Isr J Emerg Med 2006;6(1):39–42.

79. University of Warwick. Trauma emergencies. Major pelvic trauma—new guidance. Online. www2.warwick.ac.uk/fac/med/research/hsri/emergencycare/prehospitalcare/jrcalcstakeholderwebsite/clinicalpracticeupdates/pelvic_trauma_-_final_published_version_issued_21apr2009.pdf; accessed 16 Jan 2014.

80. National Institute for Health and Care Excellence (NICE). 2010 Annual evidence update on hip fracture. Online. www.evidence.nhs.uk/search?q=Annual+evidence+update+on+hip+fracture; accessed 16 Jan 2014.

81. British Orthopaedic Association Standards for trauma (BOAST) 1: Hip fracture in the older person. 2012 Online. www.boa.ac.uk/LIB/LIBPUB/Documents/BOAST%201%20Version%202%20-%20Hip%20Fracture%20in%20the%20Older%20Person%20-%202012.pdf; accessed 16 Jan 2014.

82. University of Warwick. Trauma emergencies—limb trauma. (2006). Online. www2.warwick.ac.uk/fac/med/research/hsri/emergencycare/prehospitalcare/jrcalcstakeholderwebsite/guidelines/limb_trauma_2006.pdf; 16 Jan 2014.

83. Hammond BB, Zimmermann PG, Sheehy SB. Sheehy's manual of emergency care. 7th edn. St Louis: Mosby; 2013.

84. Ly TV, Swiontkowski MF. Treatment of femoral neck fractures in young adults. J Bone Joint Surg Am 2008;90(10):2254–66.

85. Hill CT, Ahmad L et al. The ACI Orthogeriatric model of care: Clinical practice guide 2010. Online. www.aci.health.nsw.gov.au/__data/assets/pdf_file/0013/153400/aci_orthogeriatrics_clinical_practice_guide.pdf; accessed 17 Jan 2014.

86. Leung AH, Lam TP, Cheung WH et al. An orthogeriatric collaborative intervention program for fragility fractures: a retrospective cohort study. J Trauma 2011;71(5):1390–4.

87. Scottish Intercollegiate Guidelines Network. Management of hip fracture in older people guideline no. 111. Online. www.sign.ac.uk/pdf/sign111.pdf; accessed 17 Jan 2014.

88. New Zealand Guidelines Group. Acute management and immediate rehabilitation after hip fracture amongst people aged 65 years and over. (2003). Online. www.health.govt.nz/publication/acute-management-and-immediate-rehabilitation-after-hip-fracture-amongst-people-aged-65-years-and; accessed 17 Jan 2014.

89. Vassiliadis J, Hitos K, Hill CT. Factors influencing prehospital and emergency department analgesia administration to patients with femoral neck fractures. Emerg Med (Fremantle) 2002;14(3):261–6.

90. Holdgate A, Shepherd SA, Huckson S. Patterns of analgesia for fractured neck of femur in Australian emergency departments. Emerg Med Australas 2010;22(1):3–8.

91. Carpenter CR, Stern ME. Emergency orthogeriatrics: Concepts and therapeutic alternatives. Emerg Med Clin North Am 2010;28(4):927–49.

92. Johansen K, Daines M, Howey T et al. Objective criteria accurately predict amputation following lower extremity trauma. J Trauma 1990;30(5):568–73.

93. Stanley JC, Veith FJ, Wakefield TW. Current current therapy in vascular and endovascular surgery. 5th edn. Philadelphia; Saunders; 2014.

94. Adams JG. Emergency Medicine. 2nd edn. Philadelpia; Saunders. 2013.

95. Smith J, Greaves I. Crush injury and crush syndrome: a review. J Trauma 2003;54(5 Suppl):S226–30.

96. Lane R, Phillips M. Rhabdomyolysis. Br Med J 2003;327(7407):115–16.

97. Altizer L. Compartment syndrome. Orthop Nurs 2004;23(6):391–6.

98. Harvey C. Compartment syndrome: when it is least expected. Orthop Nurs 2001;20(3):15–23; quiz 24–6.

99. Pfenninger JL, Fowler GC. Pfenninger and Fowler's procedures for primary care. 3rd edn. St Louis; Mosby. 2011.

100. Kellogg RG, Fontes RB, Lopes DK. Massive cerebral involvement in fat embolism syndrome and intercranial pressure management. J Neurosurg 2013:119(5):1263–70.

101. Mellor A, Soni N. Fat embolism. Anaesthesia 2001;56(2):145–54.

102. Peltier LF. Fat embolism: a perspective. Clin Orthop Relat Res 2004;422:148–53.

103. Jobe MT, Martinez SF. Peripheral nerve injuries. In: Canale ST, Beatty JH (eds). Campbell's operative orthopaedics. 12th edn. Philadelphia: Mosby; 2013.

104. Bone LB, Johnson KD, Weigelt J et al. Early versus delayed stabilization of femoral fractures: a prospective randomized study. Clin Orthop Relat Res 2004;422:11–16.

105. Nastanski F, Gordon WI, Lekawa ME. Posttraumatic paradoxical fat embolism to the brain: a case report. J Trauma 2005;58(2):372–4.

106. Osborn TM, Tracy JK, Dunne JR et al. Epidemiology of sepsis in patients with traumatic injury. Crit Care Med 2004;32(11):2234–40.

107. Kaafarani HMA, King DR. Necrotizing skin and soft tissue infections Surgical clinics of North America 2014;94(1):155–63.

108. Nichol D. Understanding the principles of traction. Nurs Stand 1995;9(46):25–8.

109. Byrne T. The set-up and care of a patient in Buck's traction. Orthop Nurs 1999;18(2):79–83.

110. Chung J, Modrall, J. Compartment syndrome in: Cronenwett JL, Johnston KW. Rutherford's vascular surgery. 8th edn. Philadelphia: Saunders; 2014.

111. Lethaby A, Temple J, Santy J. Pin site care for preventing infections associated with external bone fixators and pins. Cochrane Database of Systemic Reviews 2013; Issue 12. Art. No.: CD004551. DOI: 10.1002/14651858.CD004551.pub3. Online. http://onlinelibrary.wiley.com/doi/10.1002/14651858.CD004551.pub3/full; accessed 16 Jan 2014.

112. Roberts JR, Hedges JR. Clinical procedures in emergency medicine. 6th edn. Philadelphia: Saunders Elsevier; 2013.

113. Cole PA, Bhandari M. What's new in orthopaedic trauma. J Bone Joint Surg Am 2004;86-A(12):2782–95.

114. Sungaran J, Harris I, Mourad M. The effect of time to theatre on infection rate for open tibia fractures. Aust N Z J Surg 2007;77(10):886–8.

115. Verbeek D, Sugrue M, Harris I et al. Acute management of hemodynamically unstable pelvic trauma patients: time for a change? Multicentre review of recent practice. World J Surg 2008;32(8):1874–82.

116. Lewis SM, Collier IC, Heitkemper MM. Medical–surgical nursing. 4th edn. St Louis: Mosby; 1996.

117. Manes, HR. A new method of shoulder reduction in the elderly. Clin Orthop Relat Res 1980;147:200–2.

118. Adapted from Carter CT, Schafer N. Incidence of urethral disruption in females with traumatic pelvic fractures. Am J Emerg Med 1993;11(3):218–20.

119. Koraitim MM, Marzouk ME, Atta MA et al. Risk factors and mechanism of urethral injury in pelvic fractures. Br J Urol 1996;77(6):876–80.

120. Lowe MA, Mason JT, Luna GK et al. Risk factors for urethral injuries in men with traumatic pelvic fractures. J Urol 1988;140:506.

121. Gonzalez D. Crush syndrome. Crit Care Med 2005;33(1 Suppl):S34–41.

122. Walls M. Orthopedic trauma. RN 2002;65(7):52–6, 58.

123. Matsen FA III. Compartment syndromes. New York: Grune & Stratton; 1980.

124. Davis JM et al, eds. Clinical surgery. St Louis: Mosby; 1987.

125. Morrison W, Parvizi W, Weiss J. Pelvic and acetabular fractures in: Presentation, imaging and treatment of common musculoskeletal conditions. Philadelphia: Saunders; 2012.

CHAPTER 51
BLAST INJURY

JANE MATEER

Essentials

- Highly evolved civilian approaches to trauma management do not do justice to the tissue destruction wrought by blast mechanisms.
- The speed, intensity and duration of the pressure wave determine the degree of injury sustained.
- Good blast injury care is a multidisciplinary affair, requiring rapid evacuation, early surgical review and intervention.
- The most severely injured usually arrive after those less injured, because the less injured bypass emergency services and find their own way to hospital.
- Injury patterns in underwater blasts usually reflect severe primary blast injury.
- Body armour protects against fragmentation injury, but not pressure-related injury.
- Auditory pressure injury is inconsistent in predicting pressure injury to lung and gut.
- All fragmentation injuries require thorough exploration.
- All penetrating blast injury should be considered to be contaminated.
- The probability of injury from a blast cannot be adequately assessed in the pre-hospital environment.

INTRODUCTION

Historically military developments in war have advanced technology and practice in a range of disciplines, with absorption into mainstream society. War has informed significant developments in triage, burns management, plastic surgery, gunshot wound (GSW) and chest trauma care. After a period during which war-related injury was rarely seen in many developed countries, recent wars have put blast injury back on the agenda, in both the military and the civilian context, not only in emergency care, but also in the long-term issues faced during rehabilitation. Inherently orientated to the military experience, where blast injury is more prevalent, research over the last decade has advanced military trauma management and sought to consider the application of military lessons to the civilian experience, in terms of both blast trauma and trauma by other means. Thus, while blast injury may have its origins in war, this chapter intersects military and civilian practice as a blast by any means can have a similar effect.

Modern warfare has reminded us that surgery can be integral to the resuscitation process and highly evolved civilian approaches to trauma management do not do justice to the tissue destruction wrought by blast mechanisms. US military surgeons in Iraq initially used civilian trauma criteria in guiding their treatment choices; however, they found them inadequate to manage the appalling damage produced by blast injury and consequently adjusted and essentially simplified their resuscitation techniques.[1] Since then, the evidence gathered during war and from rehabilitation at home has informed research, particularly in surgical advances to both resuscitation and improving long-term outcomes.[2] Consequently, as this chapter will demonstrate, the complexity of blast injury and the way injury can evolve over time should inform our pre-hospital and emergency department (ED) assessment and management with the view to not only what we do as we encounter a victim of a blast, but in consideration of how this treatment and the time we take will impact on their future prognosis. Morbidity and mortality rates in blast injury vary widely and are dependent upon the causative nature and location of the blast, the number of victims, their position relative to the blast, protective equipment, surrounding structures and timelines to appropriate care. Due to the variable, multidimensional and often hidden nature of blast injury, it is difficult to provide clear guidance on its management, and it is essential to understand the pathophysiological differences which can change how we approach blast trauma. However, summaries have been provided to clarify the main points and the chapter provides the detail behind how a presentation may vary. Depending on who first sees the blast-injured patient, on-scene treatment is usually focused on haemorrhage control and minimal intervention to avoid complicating primary blast injury, to hospital environments where more advanced technology allows for a clearer idea of the nature of the trauma sustained, surgical intervention and advanced ventilation support.

Weapons and industry

In recent decades, weapon development and availability has proliferated, with a resurgence of the improvised explosive device (IED), in both known conflict zones and terrorist attacks. In the 21st century, as weapons have developed, so has their level of impact: their design always to maximise killing and maiming capacity. However, the pattern of injury in military and police services has changed, influenced by the more consistent use of body armour. At the same time, the risk of personal harm is greater for non-military personnel affected by terrorist attacks or industrial-style blast events, as they usually have no significant protection. In an industrialised world, explosive incidents occur in factories and vehicles where chemicals and fireworks are stored (B-Double truck carrying ammonium nitrate in Southern Queensland, 2014), mines (Ralph Mine explosion, Waikato, 1914), gas and petroleum facilities, illicit drug laboratories and anywhere compressed gas or fuel can ignite, such as refrigeration trucks or in residential properties. On the international scene, hidden, unexploded mines have been producing limb injury and death for decades.

However, while weaponry has become more effective, so has trauma management and retrieval. Thus, improvements in weapon capacity to injure have been partly countered by advances in health care. Although the rate of those killed in action (KIA) has varied little since World War II (dependent on the war and nature of fighting), now more people survive their injuries. The KIA rate also does not reflect death off the battlefield, from multi-organ failure (MOF) due to prolonged hypoperfusion, infection or other delayed causes. Those who

would have died from uncontrolled haemorrhage at the scene might survive due to improved first aid and evacuation, especially if they are proximal to good medical care. The double edge of advancement is that while we save more lives, the destructive forces of guns and blasts leave many individuals permanently scarred and disabled, from amputation, traumatic brain injury, severe burns, permanent visual impairment or mental health issues. In countries without adequate health and rehabilitation infrastructure, the wounded often live lives of permanent, profound disability.

Blast injury

Blast injury mechanism

An explosion occurs when a liquid or solid is converted into an expanding gas, by chemical, mechanical or nuclear means, resulting in a subsequent rapid release of energy.[3,4] The speed of the conversion reaction governs the velocity of energy release (*detonation velocity*) and therefore overall force and size of the explosion,[4] usually over a period of microseconds. Therefore, a high-performance 'explosion' involves a high-speed conversion reaction, with subsequent rapid energy release and significant blast force. An 'explosive' is a substance such as 2,4,6-trinitrotoluene (TNT) which stores chemical energy for detonation use. Gunpowder is slow to react, whereas TNT is quick.[3,5]

A routine mining blast force (energy release) travels at approximately 3–4 km/s, while common military explosives have a speed of at least 8 km/s.[4] The latter is faster than the speed of sound through air. The blast force displaces air. Where displaced air velocity is greater than the speed of sound it produces a supersonic shock wave, otherwise known as a *blast wave*. This results in overpressure (OP), which is an instantaneous and extremely rapid increase in surrounding atmospheric pressure.[3] In open air, as long as no structural obstruction exists, peak overpressure and duration is directly related to blast energy, a function of the size of the explosive charge. As discussed later, in underwater and enclosed environments, pressure waves act differently, resulting in unpredictable peak overpressure variations. This is followed closely by a *blast wind*, a wave of rapidly moving air and gas. The leading edge of the blast wind is the *blast front*. As soon as the blast wave starts to spread outwards from the epicentre of the explosion, wave intensity declines according to Hopkinson's rule. Hopkinson states that in an unobstructed open air environment, peak OP declines inversely proportionally to the cube of distance from the epicentre.[3,6,7,8] This means a person who is 3 m from an explosion will experience 27 times less OP than a person at the epicentre, while a person at 6 m experiences 216 times less OP compared with the epicentre. The difference in OP between the two distances is a multiplication of 8. Dissipation of OP is often followed by a negative pressure phase (vacuum) at the centre of the blast.[3,9]

The blast wave carries debris and people. Debris is any object between the blast epicentre and outer perimeter of the blast radius, and may include minutely small to large fragments, rocks, glass, dirt, human remains and structural items. Despite the exponential decline in blast wave intensity, in air debris continues to move at rapid rates, particularly small fragments.[10] All explosions produce a degree of heat and fireball, which is usually consumed by the explosion. Adding a volatile fuel to an explosion will increase heat and energy production.[6] Weapons designed to maximise heat load often produce an after-burning phase following detonation, lengthening the OP and fireball duration.[4]

Blast zones and strength

Within the radius of a blast in open air are zones, naturally delineated by the physical characteristics of the blast. Each zone can be superimposed upon others to produce a series of concentric circles lying inside each other. At the centre are all the corollaries: pressure, fragmentation (injury from moving fragments; see the section on secondary blast injury [SBI]), blunt trauma, burns and all range of miscellaneous effects. The radius for burns is usually determined by the outer edge of the fireball. As the fire is usually consumed by the blast, this zone is commonly small. The exception is thermobaric and nuclear weapons, where the effects of heat are enhanced. Death from structural collapse tends to be close to the epicentre at the point of peak OP. The radius for pressure-related injuries overlaps with all except fragmentation and declines over distance. Fragmentation has the greatest potential to injure and kill the greatest number, as fragments can travel several kilometres at 1500 m/s (5400 km/hr), depending on total blast size. In short, each explosion will determine its own specific effects and therefore radii.

It is important to attempt a rough estimate of blast strength, size, type and location. This gives a starting point for expected casualty numbers and risk levels for types of injuries. Structural damage gives an idea of the radius of peak OP. As the blast wave declines with distance, structural damage tends to be focused in the vicinity of highest pressures. Conversely, glass shatters at much lower pressures, thus shattered windows provide an estimate of the outer perimeter to which the blast wave travelled. This can be kilometres. While explosions expand down as well as out, it takes a great force to produce a crater in solid concrete or other hard substances such as compact earth. Therefore, the presence and size of a crater indicates a significant explosion.

Underwater blasts

Water density propagates the movement of the blast wave, allowing it to travel further, unchanged in initial speed (thus faster), in water than in air. The lethal front of an underwater pressure 'wave' is about 3 times further than an equivalent explosion in air.[6,7,11] After the explosion in the underwater environment, the initial blast wave is reflected back from the water–air surface and combines with the initial direct blast load to produce an overall greater blast loading on the victim.[3] The augmentation of blast waves by water tends to occur at less than 1 atmosphere and is greatest near the surface. Water drag reduces the movement of fragmentation. Thus compared to blast zones in open air, water magnifies the pressure wave, and dampens the fireball and fragmentation. Areas of the body in the water are affected the most. Injury patterns reflect severe primary blast injury (PBI), usually without burns, fragmentation or crush injury. Except for the completely submerged diver, people treading water usually suffer abdominal and lower lung field PBI. Injury can also occur where a person is in contact with a hard surface, immediately above the water, such as a boat deck. The blast wave is propagated through the hard structure, producing blunt trauma to the part in contact, commonly heels, leading to calcaneal fractures.

Enclosed spaces and barriers

Solid structures in the environment, including buildings and fortifications, can channel pressure waves and fireballs, allowing fire and pressure to travel around corners, penetrating areas inaccessible to fragmentation.[4] The reflective properties of hard surfaces can exacerbate the total pressure effect. In open air, pressure waves are uniform and decline exponentially in a clear radius. In enclosed spaces, irregular high-pressure waves are produced when the initial wave hits a wall or other hard structure, is deflected and fluctuates. In narrow corridors or tunnels, a pressure wave can be propagated a greater distance unchanged in velocity, compared with open air. Combining the initial energy with the reflected energy produces at least twice the effect and unpredictable injury patterns.[4,9,12] Thus, an individual in an enclosed space may receive a higher total pressure load than if the explosion occurred in the open air the same distance away. Moreover, hiding behind a barrier may protect from fragmentation, but offers no protection from PBI or burns associated with fast-moving pressure waves or fireballs which can travel around a corner or deflect backwards from a wall. Therefore, in addition to concentrated fragmentation and burns (assuming no barrier for protection), confined spaces increase the risk of PBI. For example, in one study, 0.6% of initial survivors of an open air blast had lung PBI, compared with 38% of initial survivors in an enclosed space developing lung PBI.[3,13] There is a demonstrated correlation between the location of the blast to the victim, and survivability, with specific locations such as water or an enclosed space increasing the risk of particular patterns of injury.[14,15]

Explosion characteristics

The characteristics of an explosion are governed by the explosive material, size, container in which the explosive is held, type and speed of the explosive reaction and environment in which the explosion occurs. Thus, the predominating blast effect depends on what explodes (weapon or nonmilitary event) and the location it is deployed in.

In terms of weapons, while lethal in effect, pressure is an unreliable tool for eliciting damage to the human body, because it relies on proximity to the blast. Therefore, increasing the fragmentation load, by adding cut wire, nuts, bolts and other small metal items to the container, will increase the chance of injury and death. Comparison of the first and second Bali bombings demonstrates significant differences in the effects of the blasts, based on different items and tactics. The addition of metal items to explosives in the second bombing significantly increased the incidence of penetrating injury, although the deployment of bombs in a busy enclosed space which collapsed and burned quickly increased the mortality and toll in the first Bali bombing. Thermobaric weapons are designed to maximise the effects of heat and pressure.[4] Some enhanced weapons are designed to trigger a second explosion shortly after the first, propagating a larger and longer pressure wave, increasing the total energy transfer.[9] These devices are more likely to produce a higher incidence of PBI. Explosive-formed projectiles are devices designed to penetrate armoured vehicles, before exploding, producing significant fragmentation, burns and pressure injury in an enclosed space.[13] Table 51.1 outlines the main forms of weaponry and the predominant effects of each type.

Non-military events such as factory explosions are harder to evaluate, because the explosive force varies considerably, highly dependent on the amount and type of fuel available. The effects of an exploding fuel depot, which includes fertiliser (e.g. West Fertilizer Co, Texas, 2013), or a natural gas plant explosion (e.g. Esso Longford, Gippsland, Victoria, 1998), can produce all the effects commonly associated with a military-type explosion. Illicit drug laboratories involve highly volatile and flammable substances, which can lead to an explosion if the fuel combines with an ignition source. The size of the explosion is determined by total fuel load and may involve multiple explosions as each container ignites. In these cases, it is reasonable to assume there is a risk of burns, PBI and some degree of fragmentation injury. In the majority of Australian factory and fuel–chemical tanker fires (e.g. Manly NSW, 2013), the risk of PBI is uncommon, but the risk of burns, structural collapse and toxic inhalation is significant and multiple explosions can occur. However, as the incident in Southern Queensland (2014) demonstrated, PBI can occur if the fuel load (ammonium nitrate) is high enough. Less commonly, explosions occur in residential properties (e.g. Melbourne, 2014) if natural gas is allowed to build up in an enclosed space and is then ignited by a spark (e.g. fire or electrical appliance turns on or off). An explosion will occur, usually with a relatively small force which leaves the structure intact, although large gas build-ups have been known to level buildings. The risk of PBI, blunt trauma and fragmentation is usually low, but there is a high risk of burns due to channelling of the fireball by the surrounding structure.

Classification and physiology of blast injuries

The physics of a blast wave demonstrate a non-linear pattern created by the interaction of multiple characteristics.[3,9] Resulting injury is multidimensional in nature and represents the ultimate challenge, where identifying injury sustained requires understanding of the mechanisms of injury, especially in recognising the occult nature of pressure related injury. This essence of blast injury can tax the judgement of even the most blast injury-experienced trauma and surgical team.[15] This highlights an important aspect of good blast injury care: it is a multidisciplinary affair and there is no room for delayed presentation to hospital (apart from egress delay from the site or unavoidable travel times), nor delay to surgery from the ED where this is critical to survival.[2]

The following classification of blast injuries is a description of the different mechanisms by which blasts injure. While there is consistency in the definition of PBI, differences can be found in both the classifications and the terminology. While a four-part classification system is still in use by many, this chapter includes the more recent inclusion of a fifth classification, which evolved after the destruction of the twin towers in New York. The classification system reflects the non-sequential interactive nature of blast physics[3,7,13,15–17] and the complexities of blast injury.

TABLE 51.1 Types of weapons and their effects[10,13]

WEAPON TYPE	PURPOSE	PATTERNS OF INJURY
Grenades, mortars, rockets	Designed to incapacitate or maim, essentially by cutting effects Blow upwards, dampened by ground	Predominantly penetrating injury with multiple small fragments
Improvised explosive devices (IEDs)	Designed to incapacitate or maim, essentially by cutting effects	Low incidence of PBI, depending on where the device is set off
Vehicle-borne IEDs (VBIEDs)	Blow upwards, dampened by ground Shaped charges can cut through armour Used on suicide missions	Predominantly penetrating injury with multiple small fragments High incidence of traumatic amputation if exploding under or near a vehicle
Antipersonnel mines (landmines)	Designed to incapacitate or maim, essentially by cutting effects Blow upwards, dampened by ground	If stepped on: lower limb, perineal, genital Activated by other/above ground: abdominal, chest, head Handling: facial, upper limb, especially ocular
Enhanced weapons: thermobaric/incendiary fuel–air explosives	Designed to maximise heat and/or pressure Explode in the air	Predominantly burns and PBI
Explosive formed projectiles	Designed to penetrate vehicles and explode in an enclosed space	Burns PBI Fragmentation injury

PBI: primary blast injury

- *Primary blast injury* (PBI) is a direct consequence of the blast wave (pressure) producing a pressure differential at tissue interfaces. It predominantly affects gas-filled organs and contributes to traumatic amputation.
- *Secondary blast injury* (SBI) is the result of projectiles produced by fragmentation and debris. Thus, SBI is a form of ballistic penetrating injury; damage is greatest in soft tissue and it contributes to traumatic amputation. Historically, traumatic amputation was classed as a form of SBI; however this ignores the cutting role of PBI.
- *Tertiary blast injury* (TBI) is the result of wind force, producing victim displacement and structural collapse. This predominantly produces blunt trauma.
- *Quaternary blast injury* covers other effects of blasts, such as burns, crush injury, irritant inhalation, pregnancy complications and aggravation of existing complaints. This category is often referred to as miscellaneous injury.
- *Quinary (Quinternary) blast injury* refers to an immunological response secondary to the toxic effects of a blast.

Primary blast injury (PBI)

In essence, PBI is a form of barotrauma. Rapid OP and under-pressure changes interact directly with internal and external body surfaces, producing extreme pressure differentials at the tissue interface where tissues of different densities meet, with resulting pathophysiological change.[3,8,12–14] At 1 m from an 81 mm mortar detonation, the peak overpressure is approximately 1300 kPa over 2 milliseconds and carries a significantly high risk of producing PBI to lung (blast lung injury, BLI).[11] At 2 m the pressure level falls to 280 kPa, below the usual threshold for BLI.[11] Thus, as a rule, in open air an individual has to be close to the blast centre to be affected by PBI, and this means they are susceptible to all effects of blasts and have a high rate of fatality and severe injury.

Understanding of the effects of pressure waves on body tissues has developed into a clearly defined relationship between tissue stresses, subsequent mechanical failure of organs and related injury.[3,14] The term *blast loading* describes the pressure load received by a body surface from a blast wave travelling at or above the speed of sound. At sea level the speed of sound in air is 343 m/s (1200 km/hr). In the human body the speed of sound in air is 40 m/s (140 km/hr).[3,6,14] Therefore, there is a pressure differential between outside air and internal gas-filled organs of 303 m/s. Furthermore, when a blast load at or above the speed of sound in air reaches a body surface, rapid *acceleration* occurs at the point of contact, coupling the blast wave to the body wall and propagating the wave into the underlying tissue. The high-speed acceleration produces a high-frequency *stress wave*, resulting in application of a significant external force.[3,5] The speed of the acceleration determines the rate of the pressure rise (wave pulse spike) and this directly relates to consequent injury.[11] In a similar way to the behaviour of blast waves in enclosed spaces, stress waves inside the body reflect off body walls, especially corners. This leads to stress concentrations and injuries in acute angles and near structures close to inner surfaces.[11,14] In addition, the point of impact and subsequent energy dispersal to underlying tissue of a pressure wave hitting an individual is affected by their position in relation to the wave. A wave passing over a person lying down is less likely to produce injury than one hitting the upright body. The upright body is at greater risk if in front of a reflecting surface, especially a corner. A reflected wave may be 2–20 times greater than the energy of the initial blast wave.[3,7] In summary, the speed, intensity and duration of the pressure wave determine the degree of injury sustained.

Tissue is stretched, sheared, compressed and disintegrated, depending on individual tissue characteristics and pressure load. Internal organs can be shorn from their vascular supply, contused or lacerated. Stress concentrated in bones results in fractures, with combined soft tissue tearing from blast winds producing traumatic amputation. This largely explains why traumatic amputations from explosions are usually through the shaft rather than the joint.[2,3] However, the greatest density difference occurs between gas-filled organs and their walls, producing unique patterns of injury, with the ear, lung and bowel most at risk.

Otological PBI

PBI trauma to the ear is the most common of all pressure-related injuries, but usually the least serious in terms of immediate risk to health. A pressure of 8–56 kPa above atmospheric pressure is usually required to rupture the tympanic membrane (TM).[3,11,18] Common injuries include temporary deafness without TM rupture, TM rupture and haemotympanum. TM rupture is usually identified by deafness and tinnitus, with occasional vertigo.[18,19] However, it is possible for these signs and symptoms to exist in the presence of an intact TM.[20] Less common are ossicular chain disruptions (an injury which may protect against further inner ear damage), damage to the organ of Corti and traumatic oval window rupture. The latter are both rare and result in permanent deafness. The severity of an isolated auditory injury is affected by orientation of the head in relation to the blast wave and usually decreases with distance from the blast. The exception is enclosed spaces (Kenyan Embassy, 1998) where severe otological injury can occur some distance from the blast epicentre due to wave channelling by the building.[17,20] While the short-term consequences of damage to central auditory function include lost situational awareness and inability to communicate for survival, the longer term effects of hearing loss can be profound.[17,18,21]

Patient assessment and clinical management

During both pre- and hospital-based phases of care, take note of any hearing changes during assessment. Unilateral changes are common, as is the tendency for the victim not to notice mild to moderate hearing changes unless asked. This warrants asking if they hear differently in *either* ear now, compared with before the blast. Unfortunately, hearing problems can make obtaining a history difficult, therefore affecting a person's ability to assess the risk of other PBI. In addition to hearing loss, assess for signs of tinnitus and vertigo, nausea and vomiting. Once in the ED, assessment must include a full visualisation of the canal and TMs. It is important to identify any damage, debris or fluid in the canal and to differentiate bleeding due to direct ear trauma from a fractured base of skull or other penetrating brain injury. Problems with equilibrium may be of either neurological or otological origin. Reactive serous otitis can be difficult to differentiate from a cerebrospinal fluid (CSF) leak.[3]

The presence of TM rupture and/or canal damage warrants frequent wound care and topical antibiotics.[20] Early screening, detection and management are essential to prevent purulence, granulation, cholesteatoma, persistent perforation and permanent deafness.[17,22] Cholesteatoma is a well-documented complication of blast trauma, involving invasion of the middle ear by canal epithelium.[17,20] A steroid taper has been used with some success for sensorineural hearing loss.[21] Referral to an otolaryngologist on admission or prior to discharge for all TM or canal trauma, evidence of 7th cranial nerve dysfunction or vestibular damage and to ensure follow-up for cholesteatoma formation is important.[22,23] Despite normalisation of gross neurological findings, subtle disabilities may persist, affecting performance, which warrants ongoing evaluation by a specialist.[17,21]

Traditionally, TM rupture has been used as a convenient and sensitive predictor of the likelihood of other organ PBI.[5,8,13,17] However, although other organ PBI without associated auditory injury is uncommon, recent research indicates the absence of a ruptured TM does not preclude other PBI and isolated TM rupture is not infrequent.[3,13,17,23] If the victim's ear is not exposed to a direct impact, they may only suffer mild deafness. Therefore, absence of auditory pressure injury has an inconsistent predictive value for PBI of the lung and gut.

Pulmonary PBI (blast lung injury—BLI)

The lung is the second most susceptible area to PBI. A force applied slowly to the chest will expel air naturally via the airway. However, the high-speed impact of a blast wave allows no time for natural air expulsion and equilibrium to be achieved. Energy transfers more quickly through air in the respiratory tract than through pulmonary beds, as lung tissue compresses more slowly. This can result in pressures within the lung parenchyma that are higher than the blast OP producing the initial impact.[3] Pressure differentials disrupt the alveolar–capillary membrane, leading to intra-alveolar haemorrhage and pulmonary contusions.[6,9,24] Intra-alveolar haemorrhage produces a shunt and reduces lung compliance. In open air, damage will be unilateral if the victim was hit on the side by an approaching blast front, bilateral if hit front or rear. Damage is more likely to be bilateral, regardless of orientation, if the blast occurred in a confined space or underwater.[24]

Pleural and subpleural petechiae are the mildest forms of BLI.[7,24] Ecchymoses may appear, often in parallel bands corresponding to intercostal spaces, in larger blast loads.[7,24] Originally known as 'rib markings' when seen on X-ray, they occur in the intercostal spaces, not directly between the ribs and the lung.[3,7] High-energy stress loads are conducted deeper, producing characteristic multifocal haemorrhages portraying the sum of all blast wave movements inside the chest. Haemorrhages are often found under the pleura where a blast front first impacts, and near the diaphragm and mediastinum where the blast wave is reflected.[3,11] Large blast impacts have a tendency to disrupt the pleural wall, producing a range of injuries including pneumothorax, haemopneumothorax, traumatic emphysema and alveolo-venous fistulas. Combined with intra-alveolar damage, these injuries potentially lead to the development of bronchopleural fistulas and arterial air emboli (AAEs). The risk of AAE and pneumothoraces is further aggravated by positive-pressure ventilation (PPV), especially in the presence of high airway pressures or low vascular pressure from haemorrhage.[3,9,13] Systemic AAE from pulmonary interstitial air leaks is a significant concern and is considered to be the most likely form of rapid death as a result of BLI in immediate survivors. Prolonged overpressure may result in hilar structure damage, although this is usually fatal at the scene. If not, the probability of serious abdominal PBI in conjunction with profound BLI offers a poor prognosis.

Patient assessment and clinical management

In the early stages, signs and symptoms of BLI may be subtle, encouraging underestimation of the problem.[13,17] Unless there is massive haemoptysis, airway obstruction is not expected as a direct result of BLI. BLI is significantly greater in patients who demonstrate skull or facial fractures, burns to more than 10% of total body surface area (TBSA) and penetrating head or chest wounds.[23] Rapid shallow respirations are characteristic of BLI, with shortness of breath (SOB), a dry or moist cough, chest pain (often retrosternal) and diminished breath sounds.[5,13] The patient may or may not be wheezing; although if they are, presume BLI until proven otherwise. Consider other causes of wheezing, such as inhalation of irritants or toxins, pulmonary oedema due to myocardial injury or acute respiratory distress syndrome (ARDS).

Depending on the nature and severity of the damage and point of progressive injury reached, cyanosis, haemoptysis, subcutaneous emphysema, dullness to percussion, coarse crepitations and signs and symptoms of a pneumothorax may be present. The combination of dyspnoea, cough and progressive hypoxia are indicative of pulmonary contusion.[3,10] Pulmonary oedema is an ominous sign and is usually accompanied by bilateral lung whiteout on X-ray (ARDS). Fat embolism, an important contributor to the development of ARDS, has been identified postmortem in victims of blast injury and should be considered in the assessment process.[5] Bradycardia and hypotension in the absence of haemorrhage are a combination indicative of post blast wave shock. This is believed to be a unique vagal-nerve-mediated reflex (VMR) form of cardiogenic shock without compensatory vasoconstriction, which occurs immediately and resolves over several hours.[3,25]

An early chest X-ray (CXR) is mandatory in the evaluation of BLI (Fig 51.1A). Any suspicion of thoracic injury, PBI, blunt or penetrating trauma of any degree warrants a CXR. A ruptured TM justifies a CXR. Pulmonary contusions are identified by diffuse pulmonary infiltrates on the affected side, often appearing as a bihilar 'butterfly' pattern on CXR.[26] Infiltrates usually develop within a few hours of injury and maximise between 24 and 48 hours later.[9,26] Therefore, subsequent CXRs are essential.

> ### PRACTICE TIP
>
> The combination of pulmonary infiltrates and hypoxaemia defines BLI.[23]

A CXR will also identify pneumothorax, haemothorax, interstitial and subcutaneous emphysema, pneumomediastinum and air under the diaphragm from ruptured hollow viscera. There is little evidence to suggest the probability of rib fractures as a result of PBI.[3,26] A pressure force great enough to break ribs is usually fatal at the scene. Rib fractures are more likely to result from tertiary injury. A computed tomography (CT) scan will help to identify and quantify interstitial or alveolar fluid, pulmonary laceration and a pneumatocoele (Fig 51.1B). A CT scan is useful for small pneumothoraces and pulmonary lacerations. It is not useful for detecting air in the heart. This requires an echocardiogram. Initial oxygen saturation monitoring is important, although poor perfusion or carbon monoxide poisoning from smoke inhalation may mitigate effectiveness. An arterial blood gas (ABG) analysis is valuable in evaluating gas exchange. Due to the insidious nature of blast-related injury, close assessment for respiratory failure and the development of BLI is essential in the diagnostic process.

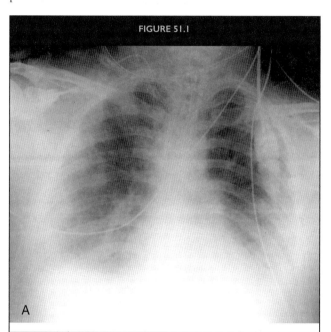

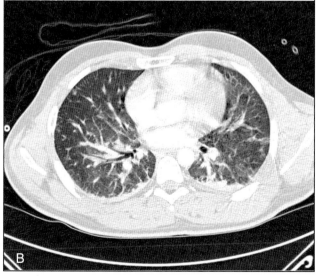

A, Chest X-ray of a patient with blast injury **B**, Chest CT of a patient with blast injury showing the pulmonary consolidations seen in blast lung injury that can potentially be missed on chest X-ray.[74]

The management of BLI is the same as for pulmonary contusions by any other cause, although several important caveats require consideration. BLI has a strong tendency to produce air emboli and persistent pneumothoraces, so keep an eye on repeat CXR, especially after interventions. Mechanical ventilation (MV) needs to be applied judiciously, due to the risk of aggravated barotrauma and inflammation, and AAE. MV in combination with lung contusion, which is the basic pathological response to a blast wave, is believed to potentially aggravate both the pulmonary and the systemic inflammatory responses induced by the contusion.[27] There is also the potential for additional interaction between the contusion and sepsis, leading to a second hit.[27] Consequently, MV strategies need to be protective. Overzealous fluid administration can aggravate evolving contusion, coagulopathy and unidentified cardiac injury.[13]

Ventilation

The focus of management is on gas exchange, using fewer tidal volume (TV) and pressure changes to limit the risk of aggravated barotrauma. Promoting spontaneous respiration reduces the risk of developing AAE. Therefore, where possible, PPV should be avoided until the patient is in a hospital setting capable of treating AAE, delivering the ventilation options described below and effectively maintaining intravascular pressure without aggravating coagulopathy. Like pulmonary contusions, oxygen diffusion is impaired. Therefore, the focus is on delivering oxygen while avoiding a rise in peak inspiratory pressure (PIP), aggravated inflammation and AAE (see Ch 21 for more on contusions and ARDS).[3,7,27] Options for ventilation include[9,10,13,24] positive end-expiratory pressure (PEEP) of 10 cmH$_2$O acceptable initially; PPV with permissive hypercapnia; inverse inspiratory–expiratory (I:E) ratios for refractory hypoxaemia; independent lung ventilation; high-frequency jet ventilation; nitric oxide inhalation and extracorporeal membrane oxygenation (ECMO). ECMO has the ability to enable a fast improvement in oxygenation and correction of acid–base balance, while potentially providing lung-protective ventilation.[28] Research has demonstrated both pump-driven and pumpless ECMO devices, when used in an appropriate tertiary facility, are a suitable treatment option in patients with severe chest injury and acute lung failure.[28] Table 51.2 provides predictors for the use of PPV and PEEP in the management of BLI.[3,29]

As damaged lungs are at high risk of fistula formation, with subsequent AAE, the focus of positioning is to place the damaged lung in the dependent position (injured side down), increasing capillary pressure to reduce emboli entering the vasculature.[10] This often occurs in ICU, where AAE are treated with hyperbaric therapy and positioning. Fowler or Trendelenburg positioning may increase the risk of cerebral or coronary AAE. In the left lateral position, air in the right side of the heart may be decreased, thus reducing the risk of venous emboli.[9] While aspirin is believed to be useful for isolated AAE as a result of diving-related injury, it is contraindicated in acute blast injury (trauma).[8]

If massive haemoptysis occurs, usually a result of significant contusion, recommended management is to block the involved side's main bronchus and unilaterally ventilate the other lung.[3,29]

TABLE 51.2 Severity of pulmonary PBI: predictors for the use of PPV and PEEP[3,29]

	MILD	MODERATE	SEVERE
Infiltrates on X-ray	Unilateral	Patchy and often bilateral	Diffuse bilateral
Bronchopleural fistula	Rare	Possible	Common
Pneumothorax	Possible	Common	Almost universal
SpO$_2$	>75% on room air	>90% on 100% O$_2$	<90% on 100% O$_2$
PPV requirement	Unlikely for lung pathology	Highly probable: using conventional methods	Universal and non-conventional methods common
PEEP requirement	< 5 cmH$_2$O if PPV used	5–10 cmH$_2$O	> 10 cmH$_2$O usual

PBI: primary blast injury; PEEP: positive end-expiratory pressure; PPV: positive-pressure ventilation

Right mainstem intubation is simpler. Rotating the head to the right and rotating the tube 180° before advancing to full depth can achieve left mainstem intubation. If cervical control is required, the tube can be rotated 90° counterclockwise.[3] Pneumothorax and haemothorax are treated as usual. However, short large-bore tubes should be used as large air leaks are associated with bronchopleural fistulas.[3,29]

More often than not, intervention in thoracic trauma involves chest tube placement without the need for operative procedures. Where a massive haemothorax is suspected prior to insertion of the tube, consider an autotransfusion adapter on the chest drainage system.[1] In the absence of penetrating trauma, there is usually time for a CT scan to identify the extent of trauma and need for operative consideration. As with trauma from other causes, penetrating trauma between the nipples and scapulae is associated with a higher probability of injury to great vessels and mediastinal structures (see Ch 44).[1]

An electrocardiogram (ECG) should be performed for all chest pain, although this is not a priority in the first instance of a presenting blast trauma. An ECG should also be performed on all patients experiencing chest trauma, prior to going to surgery, to identify myocardial contusion, which may decompensate under a heavy load of fluid.

Abdominal PBI

The relatively low incidence of explosion injury has resulted in limited and therefore variable data on which to base an accurate probability of abdominal PBI occurring. However, it is generally accepted that abdominal PBI is most likely in victims who are very close to the blast epicentre, are underwater or in enclosed spaces where the blast occurs.[3,11,24] The mechanisms of injury from PBI stress and shear forces is similar to those affecting the lung, with injury occurring at similar overpressures.[3,24] Pathological changes are similar to those affecting the lung, reflecting the blast load and degree of body-wall acceleration secondary to the blast shock wave.[7] The colon (where gas tends to collect) is the most common site for injury.[9,26] Intestinal wall haemorrhage, in the form of small petechiae graduating to larger haemorrhage, occurs at lower pressures. If ischaemia develops, this may lead to necrosis and secondary perforation. Gut-wall rupture and subsequent leakage into the peritoneum requires very high pressures, and therefore implies closer

proximity to the blast and the probability of other significant trauma. Rupture can develop slowly and may occur days after the initial injury, due to stretching or ischaemia, resulting in delayed presentation.[3,9,13] A more likely cause of gut-wall rupture in survivors is fragmentation injury. Importantly, there have been cases of bowel necrosis and perforation secondary to penetrating injury, with no initial obvious peritoneal breach and the majority of large bowel rupture due to PBI involving the right side, with the small bowel the most likely associated organ to be injured.[13]

Solid organs generally do not suffer compression damage, as they have relatively consistent liquid densities.[3] However, they may be susceptible to indirect injuries from abdominal wall displacement where blast loads are high. Acceleration forces may affect organ attachments, separating organs from their vascular supply, while shearing forces can produce subcapsular petechiae, contusions, lacerations or organ rupture.[3,7] In general, injury to abdominal organs, other than the bowel, is more likely to result from conventional blunt or penetrating trauma associated with SBI or TBI. These injuries include testicular rupture, mesenteric and retroperitoneal haematomas and tension pneumoperitoneum.[6,30]

Patient assessment and clinical management

Signs and symptoms of abdominal injury can be extremely vague, despite severe underlying injury and can evolve slowly over time. It is this very vagueness, and the potential for serious underlying evolving injury, that warrants all people complaining of abdominal pain after being hit by a blast wave to be transported to and assessed in hospital. However, in cases of mild abdominal pain without signs or symptoms of other injury, while the victim needs a hospital evaluation, the urgency for transport is not as great. They should, however, have regular, ongoing evaluation of chest and abdomen while awaiting transport. Just as the asthmatic who is wheezing should be considered to be suffering BLI, the person with abdominal pain should be considered to have PBI until proven otherwise.

Assessment of abdominal PBI is the same as for all other abdominal trauma (Ch 48). The purpose of the diagnostic process is to determine a time-frame for treatment, although in blast injury, a normal diagnostic panel does not necessarily equate with no potential for ischaemia, haemorrhage or perforation.[3] A positive FAST is usually followed by a CT, unless surgery is mandated immediately by haemodynamic instability or obvious injury. All acute, distended or tense abdomens with associated hypotension will require exploration.[1,13] Presence of intra-abdominal fluid on FAST is an indication for exploration. In situations where resources are limited or casualty numbers are high, a CT scan of the abdomen can be forgone, as any degree of apparent injury will tend to indicate the need for an exploratory laparotomy, which offers the dual benefit of diagnosis and treatment. While the need for an exploratory laparotomy may be obvious in some, abdominal PBI may be clinically silent until advanced complications exist. Therefore, ongoing evaluation is needed where the probability of abdominal PBI is high or where even vague signs of discomfort exist.[3]

In the management of abdominal injury, damage-control surgery (DCS) is often the first option to provide rapid haemorrhage control and remove contamination. This concept is explained further in the next section on SBI. In the abdominal context, haemorrhage control in the first instance may warrant splenic removal and liver packing. Renal injury management depends on the availability of surgical resources to repair the kidney. Where bleeding is ongoing, nephrectomy is the choice. The high rates of failure for colon repair and the need to rapidly control contamination usually leads to an initial colostomy.[1,13] Following DCS, the abdominal wall is usually closed temporarily, advantageous where there is significant thoraco-abdominal wall loss due to fragmentation injury. In general, notwithstanding the potential need for DCS, when abdominal PBI requires surgical exploration, findings will be managed in the same way as similar injury from other causes of trauma.

When managing hypotension in these patients, maximum fluid resuscitation may be detrimental, necessitating that all fluids are very carefully titrated to response. Aggressive fluid resuscitation for hypotension and low urine output refractory to fluid replacement has been observed to contribute to abdominal compartment syndrome in otherwise healthy individuals. Abdominal compartment syndrome (Ch 48) is possible with pelvic fractures, rectus muscle damage and profound intra-abdominal injury, especially where surgery is required. More is discussed on hypotension in the next section.

Important assessment considerations for PBI

In most military forces around the world, body armour is standard protection to limit fragmentation injury. However, rather than provide a barrier to barotrauma, body armour can increase the risk of PBI. The similarity of the density of materials used for body armour transmits the blast energy directly to the body surface and concentrates it—potentially magnifying the pressure effect inside the armour and into the body. Current research into protective equipment is investigating the use of materials of different densities to reduce stress-wave transmission, disrupting blast wave impact to the chest wall and decoupling wave propagation.[5,12,17] Hearing protection can mitigate blast impact, preventing TM rupture in people who may have received a significant blast loading to other body areas, producing a PBI. Strenuous exercise after a blast loading has previously resulted in increased mortality.[3,7] Thus where practicable, activity levels

| BOX 51.1 | Questions for assessing the mechanism of injury for blast injuries |

- Where did it occur? (e.g. open air, closed space, underwater)
  - Expect more PBI in closed space, underwater explosions
  - Expect more blunt, soft-tissue and crush trauma in structural collapse
  - Expect high numbers of penetrating trauma in open air explosions
  - Expect burns and upper torso and head injury to be complicated by PBI
- What was the cause? (e.g. chemical plant or suicide bombing)
- How big was the explosion?
  - Estimate roughly based on crater size, outer perimeter of window damage
- Number of estimated dead, where this occurred and predominant cause?
  - Where were they? (e.g. centre of blast or distance away)
  - Why: incineration/decimation, building collapse, fragmentation
  - The larger the blast, the greater the number
- Predominant effects? (e.g. burns, structural collapse, fragmentation, toxicity etc.)
  - Fragmentation can injure some distance from the blast
- What is the risk of contamination? (e.g. radiological, chemical, other toxicity)
- Location of victim to blast?
- Where was the victim in relation to surrounding structures?
1. Close equals high risk of PBI till proven otherwise
2. Assess for risk of channelled and magnified blast wave (e.g. down a corridor, behind a table in the corner)
   - How much exercise did they do at the scene? (e.g. assistance with rescue effort, running from scene, etc.)
3. Time of onset of signs and symptoms?
   - Immediate or delayed: which signs or symptoms came first?

should be minimised after a blast and healthcare providers need to include an assessment of activity prior to presentation in history-taking (see Box 51.1).

Less-common PBI

The following injuries are less commonly found as a form of PBI:

- retinal AAE (visual disturbance)[3]
- maxillary sinus implosion—not known whether this is caused by PBI or blunt trauma
- head injury—subarachnoid haemorrhage, subdural (most likely, blunt trauma), although stress waves can penetrate the skull[3]
- cardiac contusions, oesophageal rupture.[7,24]

Secondary blast injury (SBI) (ballistic)

The leading cause of death in a blast, in the absence of building collapse, is SBI.[9] In the absence of body armour, penetrating chest and abdominal injury is a common cause of death. With or without body armour, the most common injury is to the face, neck and limbs. Perineal trauma is uncommon, except where explosions erupt under vehicles, impacting people in a sitting position.

Fragmentation is the disintegration of an object into pieces. In terms of an explosion, fragmentation is loosely used to refer to all debris related to a blast.

- *Primary fragmentation* is produced as a result of the weapon (or other explosive cause).[3] For example, the container in which the explosive was held, or its contents, such as nuts and bolts, will disintegrate with the blast and produce millions of minute to larger sized fragments.
- *Secondary fragmentation* is all other debris energised by the blast from the surrounding environment, including glass, rocks, sticks and vehicle parts.

The word 'shrapnel' has been loosely used to describe all metal fragmentation from weaponry, although it originated as a specific reference to the metal fragmentation from antipersonnel (AP) mines.[3,9]

Traditionally, weapon fragmentation produced larger pieces of inconsistent size. Modern weapons, designed to maximise death and disability, have been developed to produce shrapnel that is small and consistent in size, and can travel great distances, both through the air and into the body. Secondary fragments (not from the weapon) will be more inconsistent in size. Fragments from any blast source (primary or secondary) are usually irregular in shape, sharp and travel at initial speeds of up to 1500 m/s (5400 km/hr).[3,6] Fragments produced and energised close to the blast have the longest penetration range, with lighter objects such as glass able to fly kilometres with big blasts. As flying fragments rely on the blast wave and winds to move them, their speed and ability to penetrate reduce with distance and the exponentially dying force of pressure and air movement. This is especially true for irregular fragments, as they are more greatly affected by aerodynamic drag. Therefore, penetrating damage tends to localise, especially with irregular fragments, which tend to act like low-energy missiles on impact.[26] However, as with most ballistic injuries, there is a degree of cavitation (see Ch 43) and therefore a greater distribution of tissue damage than with a penetrating knife wound. Importantly, it is not the type of projectile and its speed which are the main determinants of injury; rather, it is the characteristics of the projectile and where and how it strikes the victim which are more influential.[31] Large or small, fast or slow, placement is more important when evaluating the severity of an injury and risk it poses to the victim. Further, in blast injury the degree of tissue loss and destruction can be significant, with loss of normal anatomical planes, making repair challenging, even for the most experienced practioner.

Patient assessment

Fragments of all sizes may penetrate the body and the patient will often present with a classic peppered appearance (Fig 51.2). Large fragments are easier to identify and their size usually inhibits movement beyond the body surface. However, ultimately proximity and orientation of the victim to the blast and blast force determines how far and in what direction

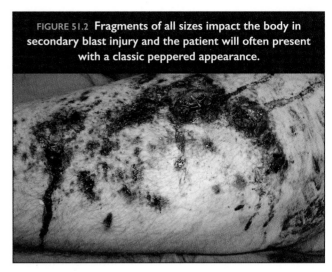

FIGURE 51.2 **Fragments of all sizes impact the body in secondary blast injury and the patient will often present with a classic peppered appearance.**

Jane Mateer, Iraq, 2005.

the fragment penetrates, and therefore the extent of damage. Golfball-size fragments have been known to penetrate the span of the skull or the chest. Smaller fragments are frequently hard to find. Minute ones can travel great distances into and within the body if they track into a blood vessel and embolise, are swallowed or reach the airway and are inhaled. Equally, it is easy to be misled as to the size of a fragment, as large fragments can be well embedded beneath soft tissue, with an apparently small entry hole overlying their position. Prior to X-ray, palpation is initially the best way to estimate the fragment size and whether it is entering or exiting.

Due to the danger posed by the smallest of fragments, all patients must be thoroughly assessed in a hospital. The predominant danger of fragmentation is its cutting effect; for example, a fragment lodged near the carotid may, with future movement, lacerate the artery. Therefore, very careful physical assessment for even the smallest hole is essential. This includes mandatory, thorough radiography of *all* holes, with consideration for internal travel.[32] All X-rays should be repeated prior to surgery if there is a significant delay between the initial X-ray and entering the operating room. Penetrating head wounds are difficult to evaluate without CT scan. On CT scan of the head a 'Milky Way' pattern of a few large and many smaller fragments may be noted. The appearance is similar to that of a disintegrating bullet.

Clinical management

Small fragments can hide in vascular, intestinal and facial structures, producing a high risk of infection and compromise to blood and nerve pathways. Compared to the past, advancements in technology make fragment identification more achievable and surgical practices are more successful at removal if this is required.

Blast penetrating injuries are always contaminated and potential sources for infection. Contamination includes dirt, oil, chemicals, skin flora, car seating or clothes collected prior to penetration; or gastrointestinal flora if the fragment goes through the bowel, mouth or genital tract. Bone from suicide bombers has found its way into victims.[1] The risk of infection is heightened when the time from wounding to treatment is long, cleansing is inadequate, wound size is greater than 1 cm and fractures exist beneath the soft-tissue damage.[10] Cavitation associated with ballistic injuries devitalises tissue, fractures are prone to staphylococcal osteomyelitis[2,10] and multiple fragments penetrating protective muscle sheaths establish deep, dark well-nourished beds for bacterial or fungal growth. Among the multitude of possibilities, the main infective risks include *Clostridium perfringens* (gangrene), beta-haemolytic *Streptococci* and tetanus.

It is essential that blast-injured patients are transported to an ED as urgently as possible, for the provision of excellent wound care, constant re-evaluation and appropriate antibiotics, critical to the prevention of later fatality due to infection.[1] The high risk of infection warrants a three-pronged approach, beginning with tetanus protection and prophylactic antibiotics for all blast-related penetrating trauma. In the first instance, broad-spectrum antibiotics are routine; however, indefinite and excessive use can lead to infections such as pan-resistant acinetobacteria.[1] Examples include ceftriaxone for penetrating head injury, cephalosporins for soft-tissue, bone and organ injury and gentamicin added for open fractures. The third prong in reducing the infection risk is wound management, including early and regular surgery for washout and debridement.

> **PRACTICE TIP**
>
> Never underestimate the risk of infection and need for early wound management.

In general, management of internal trauma is the same as for trauma of other origins, with several caveats on responding to the initial damage, fragment removal and infection. The initial purpose of surgery is damage control, with the intent to stop haemorrhage and control contamination rapidly in order to continue shock resuscitation and restore physiological reserve.[1]

Damage control surgery (DCS) and resuscitation (DCR)

The concept of DCS began life in the abdomen. Against a tradition of completing definitive surgery in one operation, in the US in the 1990s a wave of GSW combined with developing knowledge about physiological tolerance gave rise to a new approach where surgery was simplified and staged, responsibility for resuscitation broadened and the aim was to prevent further physiological degradation and hypoperfusion. The term 'damage control' was coined from a US navy approach to critical ship repair, undertaken during a mission.[33,34]

Severe trauma can lead to a loss of physiological reserve, which refers to the survival parameters of temperature, clotting and acid–base balance. The combination of hypothermia, coagulopathy and acidosis are known as the 'triad of death'. These patients are *in extremis* and will not survive further degradation of physiological limits. Exposure, fluid resuscitation, paralysis and the hypoperfusion associated with severe injury exacerbate hypothermia, acidosis and coagulopathy in a vicious cycle. More than an hour on the operating room table will lead to temperature drops, especially if the abdomen is open. Hypoperfusion has now been demonstrated to have

its own direct driving effect on trauma-induced coagulopathy (TIC), with females at slightly greater risk of developing early TIC.[35–39] Point-of-care testing (POC) for coagulopathy in the pre-hospital environment requires more research to consider factors which may adversely affect POC results, such as ambient temperature, humidity, altitude and electromagnetic interference.[40] See Chapter 44 for more detail on the triad, TIC and management.

DCS can be defined as a series of operations staged around the patient's physiological tolerance and resuscitation.[33,41–48] For the patient *in extremis*, the focus is rapid haemorrhage and contamination control, and return of physiological reserve. In essence, this initially involves a short theatre time focused on the essentials, such as ligating or clamping major vessels, packing cavities and organs, temporarily stapling hollow viscous injuries and performing guillotine amputation of limbs; then transfer to ICU for continued resuscitation and restoration of normal coagulation, acid–base and temperature limits. Few patients, especially those who are victims of blast injury, will be definitively closed at the first operation. In the staged approach, temporary closure allows for regular returns to the OR, washout of contamination and definitive treatment of injury once the wound is clean. Eventually those injuries not considered initially life-threatening will be treated. DCS is also useful where advanced surgical capability is not available but the patient requires intervention to survive to the next level of care, especially if the aeromedical evacuation time to tertiary care is long.

More recently, DCS has been incorporated into a new paradigm for resuscitation, covering the continuum from pre-hospital to ICU, and is part of what is known as damage control resuscitation (DCR).[34,49–52] The tenets of DCS and restoration of physiological reserve stand, but now the ideal DCR process begins at point of wounding, with rapid retrieval, minimal on-scene intervention, early identification of need for hypotensive resuscitation, whole blood reconstitution, limited crystalloid and hypothermia prevention.[15,34,49] CPR at the scene is never indicated.[29] In the UK, civilian retrieval applies a model similar to the one used by British forces in Afghanistan, where medical teams of a doctor, nurse and paramedic retrieve casualties from the front-line to commence early DCR and improve survival.[15,49]

> **PRACTICE TIP**
>
> DCS may be the profoundly shocked patient's only chance of survival. Therefore, urgent transport to an ED and quickly to theatre (as required) is essential.

After DCS, the overall surgical objective is to remove large or compromising fragments. Small, non-compromising fragments are left in place, as the process of removing them may increase damage. Thus systematic removal is not recommended and many people simply live with fragments internally.[3,10] Eventually many fragments will make their way to the surface or seal off. Ketamine has been recommended as a suitable anaesthetic in environments where full surgical capabilities are not available. Ketamine is easier to use, has a wider margin of safety in the management of airway and oxygenation and provides combined analgesia–anaesthesia.[26,53]

In addition to the risk of infection, damage produced by multiple fragmentation wounds and cavitation increases the risks of bleeding and ischaemia, potentially leading to compartment syndrome. Fasciotomy of obvious compartment syndrome needs to occur early and will usually be performed electively in muscles surrounding amputation or other injury (see Ch 50 for compartment syndrome and vascular injury). Amputation rates for late fasciotomies have been shown to be twice the rate of those who have early urgent fasciotomies.[2] Therefore, *all* holes benefit from being surgically washed out to ensure thorough cleansing, with careful incision and drainage of holes containing fragments,[2,10] and formal wound closure delayed for up to 10 days post injury (delayed primary closure). This practice minimises the risk of infection, especially in less-than-sterile environments, allows for determination of muscle viability, permits wound revision where required and, in limbs, helps to avoid unnecessarily high amputations.[2,53] All wounds involving fractures of any kind should be reviewed early by an orthopaedic surgeon and surgically washed out. Subsequent fracture management depends on the break, with all fixations of fractures under open wounds stabilised with an external fixation in the first instance.

Hypotension

As a rule, hypotension is managed as for any other trauma. However, while it is likely to be hypovolaemic in origin, it may also be caused by a tension pneumothorax (potentially missed during evolving BLI), cardiovascular effects of AAE or a VMR (cardiogenic shock). As previously mentioned, consideration also needs to be given to the effects of fluid resuscitation on evolving BLI and abdominal compartment syndrome. The application of permissive hypotension as discussed in Chapter 44 is useful.

Limb injury—traumatic amputation

Fragmentation injury significantly affects the limbs, particularly the legs. Apart from a broad range of soft tissue injuries and fractures, traumatic amputation is the main concern. Traumatic amputations occur most commonly as a combination of direct pressure (blast wave) application and the effects of fragmentation. The latter is particularly common with mine injury. Traumatic amputation (Fig 51.3) is indicative of a high-impact force and should be viewed as a predictor of severe PBI elsewhere in the body. When the blast wave hits the body, energy impacting bone can produce a stress concentration in the shaft. Subsequently the bone fractures and the blast wind following the blast front tears soft tissue, amputating the limb. Consequently the limb is torn apart, stripping tendons, blood vessels and nerves from some distance up the limb and rupturing the bone through the shaft. This establishes a very high risk of infection and makes haemorrhage control and repair exceedingly difficult.

Patient assessment and clinical management

Unless the limb is completely removed by the blast, assessment of a mutilated limb can be extremely difficult. In the pre-hospital setting, the focus of limb assessment should be solely on bleeding and applying a rapid tourniquet, as the nature of the tissue destruction, including multiple fractures, usually makes direct pressure ineffective.

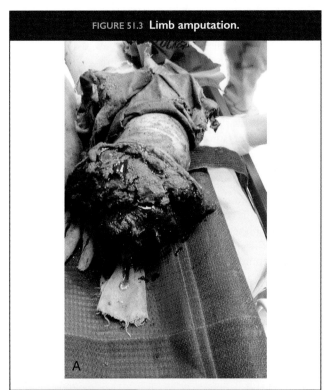
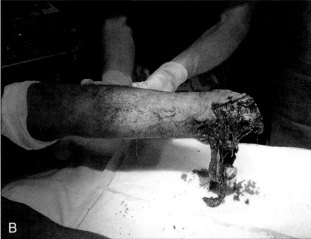

FIGURE 51.3 **Limb amputation.**

A, Upper limb amputation. Traumatic amputation is indicative of a high impacting force and should be viewed as a predictor of severe PBI elsewhere in the body. **B**, Lower limb amputation.
A, Jane Mateer, Iraq, 2005. B, Dr Adam Brooks, Iraq, 2005.

PRACTICE TIP

Traumatic amputation is one situation in which an arterial tourniquet offers the best chance of survival. A well applied tourniquet saves lives if used in the right way at the right time for the right patient.

Tourniquet use

Where direct pressure, elevation and wound-packing fail to stem bleeding, there is an obvious partial or complete limb amputation or the patient is in shock (with an obvious source of bleeding not stemmed by other means), the use of an arterial tourniquet (TQ) is indicated and must be considered. As previously discussed, coagulopathy in trauma is aggravated by a shocked state. It is critical to stop bleeding and avoid haemodilution caused by replacing what is lost.

Traditionally, TQs have been taboo in the civilian environment, due to concerns over limb loss secondary to ischaemia; however, recent military experience has demonstrated that with rapid retrieval, the use of TQ for partial or complete amputation or exsanguinating penetrating injury does not increase the risk of unnecessary limb loss.[54–58]

Application of a TQ involves the following:[54,55]

- Placement above the site of bleeding (3–5 cm), as low down a single bone limb as is possible to stem bleeding and not over clothing, joints or impaled objects.

- It is tightened far enough to stop bleeding.

- Once in place, it is **never** covered up, the patient is marked on the torso to indicate location and time of application (e.g. TQ 1545) and it is **not** removed by anyone other than a surgeon when evaluating the wound. A TQ is placed for a purpose—to stem uncontrolled bleeding, so there is no value in removing or loosening the TQ till vascular integrity can be examined. Life comes before limb and arterial laceration with an amputation will result in limb ischaemia anyway.

- Evacuation is a priority, for vascular review and probable surgery.

- A TQ may also be used as a rapid form of haemorrhage control where there is an urgent need to move the victim to safety, before further assessment can be undertaken, such as in an explosion or building fire.

- There is a 6-hour time window from injury to revascularisation, before a limb cannot be salvaged. If this has passed, leave the TQ in place until a surgeon can remove it.

The exception to a TQ is a limb removed at the shoulder or hip, where direct pressure is the only option. Attempting any other form of bleeding control can be fatal, as it is time-consuming to find the bleeding artery and the patient continues to lose blood. Surgery is usually the only option for saving the patient's life. This mandates rapid transport to hospital.

To evaluate neurovascular status in a damaged, non-amputated limb, a Doppler study may be required to find a distal pulse. X-ray of the limb is mandatory, as the decision to repair is made on the prognosis of both bone and vascular repair. It is critical to determine the exact time injury occurred and when a tourniquet, if applied, went on.

Risks to life include ongoing bleeding, acidosis, toxicity from devitalised tissue (rhabdomyolysis) and infection. Risks to the limb include infection, compartment syndrome and nerve damage. Traumatic amputations from blast injury are highly prone to all of these, with profound blood loss occurring before a dressing or tourniquet is applied. Limbs shredded by fragmentation and pressure-stress concentrations are riddled with soot, explosive residue, dirt, shrapnel and other forms of contamination. In addition to the amputation, intact muscle compartments (except for minor fragmentation wounds) are

highly prone to compartment syndrome, because of contusions resulting from dissipation of the blast energy force.[2,13,53] Careful ongoing assessment is required. A high surgical amputation to prevent ongoing bleeding in a patient *in extremis* post exsanguination, or where contamination and tissue destruction is extensive, is not uncommon.[59] As vascular repair is time intensive and requires heparin administration to maintain blood flow integrity and prevent clotting of an anastomosis, a shocked patient is a poor candidate for an attempt to salvage the limb. Limb salvage will be attempted if orthopaedic repair is possible and vascularisation can be achieved without compromising the patient's life.

The surgical approach is thorough washout, debride dead or dying tissue, perform vascular and orthopaedic repair if possible, or remove the limb. If not, the wound may be left open, packed lightly to allow for drainage and covered with loose dressings to allow for swelling of the limb.[1,10] The wound will be reassessed daily, washed out and debrided at least every 48 hours until it is determined the tissue will remain viable. At this point, usually 7–10 days post injury, the wound will be closed.[2,53,59] As with all significant long-bone trauma there is a risk of fat emboli (Ch 50), demonstrated by sudden hypoxaemia and central nervous system (CNS) changes. Ongoing neurovascular damage will be assessed at a later stage, after the life of the limb (bone and vascular) is confirmed as viable. See Chapter 50 for more information on neurovascular and musculoskeletal trauma.

Tertiary blast injury (TBI)

Tertiary blast injuries are the result of blunt trauma from blast-wind-induced human body displacement or collapsing, flying structures. A peak overpressure of 35 kPa, which is enough to rupture half the TMs exposed to this force, can produce a blast wind of up 70 m/s.[3] This is a wind speed equal to a category 4–5 tropical cyclone (e.g. Cyclone Tracy) and capable of propelling a body. A blast wind capable of producing BLI may exceed 400 m/s (1400 km/hr).[3] Channelled by surrounding structures, the blast wind may be substantially magnified, applying greater force and body displacement. The displacement distance is an important question in the history process. The most common injuries are the same as for falls or ejection from a vehicle, with blunt head, spinal and pelvic injury, abrasions and contusions. Impalement is less common.

As indicated by several high-profile civilian blast incidents, collapsing structures are a high cause of fatality. In Oklahoma City, 1995, the chance of dying in the blast was 16 times greater for people located in the federal building, than if they were outside at the time of detonation.[3]

Children are particularly susceptible to tertiary blast injury, due to their smaller body mass. A high incidence of TM rupture and head injury[8,17] can be partly attributed to the larger head-to-body ratio, which results in young children often landing head first. Consideration needs to be given to the effect on development of being exposed to a blast. Assessment, diagnosis and management of tertiary blast injuries in both adults and children are the same as for blunt trauma from any other cause, bearing in mind that they may be suffering other blast-related effects.

Quaternary blast injury

A broad, miscellaneous category, this includes pregnancy, crush injury, asphyxiation and any pre-existing condition potentially aggravated by a blast, resulting in increased morbidity and mortality.

Crush injury (see Ch 50) is caused by entrapment in collapsed structures for long periods. In conjunction with engineering safety concerns, security problems can prevent rapid retrieval. Crush injury is assessed and managed as for crush injury of any other cause, keeping in mind any specific blast-related problems, such as PBI or fragmentation injury.

Asphyxiation is predominantly due to toxic inhalation of carbon monoxide or cyanide, produced from incomplete combustion during the blast; however, it can also occur as a result of oxygen deficiency at the centre of the blast, particularly with high fire load and after-burning. Management principles include oxygenation, ventilation and treatment of relevant toxicity, bearing in mind associated BLI.

Radiation fallout can occur as a result of a nuclear reactor explosion which would lead to immediate injury and a greater radius of radiation fallout than a meltdown. A 'dirty bomb' is one which is attached to any radioactive substance producing radiation contamination on detonation.

Pregnancy

The relatively low incidence of blast injury and limited research into the effects on pregnancy offer little information. However, amniotic fluid, like water, is relatively incompressible. Therefore, while a few cases of fetal skull fractures in women with pelvic fractures have been reported,[17] direct injury to the fetus is uncommon. Placental injuries are more likely to occur with shearing forces at the change in density between endometrium and placenta, and placental abruption should be considered.[9,17] See Chapters 35 and 48 for management of the pregnant trauma patient.

Burns

The initial fire and heat produced by an explosion are usually consumed by the blast. The result is incineration of victims very close to the blast and relatively small numbers of burn victims who were in close proximity to it, except where structures burn and collapse (Bali, 2002). Burns tend to accompany other severe injury, particularly PBI.[6,60] The intensity of the heat-producing burns can reach several thousand degrees, producing extensive damage. Certain situations will promote a higher fire and heat load, such as: large blasts with a fireball fuelled by a high chemical load, where a building ignites, aircraft fuel is involved or specialised weapons are deployed. Incendiary bombs are designed to maximise heat. Thermobaric weapons are designed to maximise heat and pressure. Napalm—a mixture of powdered aluminium, soap and petrol—was designed to stick on impact and prolong the burning time. In addition to thermal burns, there is always the possibility of radiation and chemical burns.

The assessment and management of burns follows the same processes outlined in Chapter 52. However, blast-related trauma is multidimensional and presents additional unique challenges. For any injury presenting with a dressing, the dressing should be taken down for a full evaluation of not only the extent of the burn, but any accompanying fragmentation injury. Further, experience in Bali and Iraq shows that burnt limbs, initially appearing to be well perfused, may become compromised over time.[1,2,60] It is important to continually re-evaluate neurovascular status and to ensure early hospital management.

Quinary (quinternary) blast injury

Quinary blast injury is a relatively recent term describing toxic absorption, either by inhalation or through wounds, producing an immunological response and unique early hyper inflammatory state.[17,61] Biohazard contamination (see Ch 12) can occur from a variety of sources, including radiation (see quaternary injury), chemical and toxic smoke from burning plastics, chemicals, petroleum products and metal. Irritant inhalation includes asbestos, coal and dust. The World Trade Center 2001 attack produced pulverised clouds of building dust channelled by streets kilometres from the epicentre, leading to asphyxiation, respiratory distress and significant subsequent respiratory disease. Biological contamination is unlikely, as the blast would incinerate microorganisms.

White phosphorus

Contact with white phosphorus (WP) can produce potentially lethal electrolyte disturbances and pulmonary irritation. WP is used in some military weapons, especially hand grenades. On contact with air, WP ignites producing intense heat, phosphorus pentoxide gas and a fine, whitish phosphorus powder, which can be inhaled or absorbed through the skin. It is a significant pulmonary irritant and WP absorption can lead to hypocalcaemia, hypokalaemia and hyperphosphataemia, producing ECG changes and lethal dysrhythmias.[8]

Be aware of the combustive effects of oxygen and flammable gases around WP before it is treated. Management involves initial and timely removal of all obvious particles of WP. Using a Wood's lamp in a darkened room may highlight the particles, making them easier to remove.[8] Follow gross particle removal with a rinse of 1% copper sulfate ($CuSO_4$) solution; after the $CuSO_4$ turns black, rinse off with copious saline or conventional soap and water. Removing the $CuSO_4$ is important to avoid intravascular haemolysis and renal failure, which can occur if $CuSO_4$ is absorbed.[8] Intravenous calcium may be required if calcium levels drop dangerously. Electrolyte disturbances are managed conventionally.

Specific anatomical areas

Head and spine

The head is prone to injury as armour does not protect against blunt trauma, the concussive effects of blast pressure or penetration via the face. Traditionally blast induced traumatic brain injury (bTBI) has reflected the original four-phase blast classification system, with TBI resulting from primary, secondary tertiary and quaternary effects.[62] Most are 'primary' causes of brain injury (see Ch 45). Secondary (SBI) effects reflect TBI as a result of penetrating fragmentation, the signature injury of recent US war deployment. Tertiary (TBI) effects represent the type of blunt trauma seen in civilian settings, for example, from a blow to the head. Quaternary effects (incorporating the new quinary category) include a miscellaneous range of causes, many of them fitting the 'secondary' brain injury category such as hypoxia.

Current evidence on mechanisms of bTBI is limited, with most opinions on the likely mechanisms extrapolated from shock wave research. Research has demonstrated pathological findings as a result of blast wave impact (blunt trauma) consistent with findings in TBI and include haemorrhage, oedema, pseudoaneurysm formation, vasoconstriction and induction of apoptosis.[62] The extent of TBI as a result of a pressure wave is influenced by the pressure differentials between brain tissue, skull shape and response to the shear and tensile stress forces, cavitation formation and the pathways of blast wave entry to the brain—via the openings in the cranial vault and direct coupling impact.[64] Data suggests oxidative stress and neuronal cell damage from blast exposure may be responsible for concussive dysfunction considered to be mild TBI (mTBI).[13] Further, the temporal lobe is susceptible to axonal shearing at relatively minor levels of trauma and biochemical systems in the brain are believed to be altered by a blast impact, especially cholinergic fibres.[15] Diffusion tensor imaging (DTI), an advanced form of MRI, has been used in the US to detect blast-related mTBI in US military personnel with clinical signs of mTBI, demonstrating axonal injury in 60%, with persistent abnormality consistent with evolving injury up to 12 months later.[63]

Little has been done to investigate the role of altered cerebral blood flow (CBF) in bTBI.[64] As discussed in Chapter 45, the secondary effects of hypoxia and hypotension on brain injury are well known; however, their role in bTBI has not been established. Thus the risk to the brain of injury from OP damage to the lung producing hypoxia and hypotension secondary to haemorrhage should not be underestimated. Blast injury may also contribute to impaired cerebral vascular function, through production of superoxide radicals that impair cerebral vascular compensatory responses to hypoxia and hypotension, leaving the brain vulnerable to secondary insults.[64] Consequently, CBF may not respond to attempts to raise it by conventional physiological or treatment means, leading to aggravated secondary injury.

The continuum of bTBI is from mild to severe and includes concussion, epidural and subdural haemorrhages, intracerebral bleeds and foreign objects, axonal injury and a range of neuropsychiatric responses. AAE is an indirect effect of PBI. Spinal injury can occur from penetration, blunt trauma, concussion and abnormal range of movement. As a consequence of blast exposure some people will develop stress-related neurobehavioral disorders, which have overlapping pathology and functional outcomes with bTBI, and evidence suggests bTBI increases the risk of developing post traumatic stress disorder (PTSD).[65–67] Persistent impairment after a blast may be due to a stress disorder; however, a link between repeated mTBI and chronic traumatic encephalopathy has not been confirmed.[66]

mTBI was defined by the American Congress of Rehabilitation Medicine (1993) as injury characterised by altered LOC no greater than 30 minutes and a period of post traumatic amnesia (PTA) lasting up to 24 hours.[67] GCS is typically 13 to 15 and symptoms include the neurological range; for example, acute such as headache, cognitive such as poor concentration and memory, and emotional, such as anxiety or depression. The mTBI definition underwent review by the WHO (2004), although consensus across all disciplines remains elusive. The key points to note are: neuroimaging is adjunctive and often normal, neuropsychological testing evaluates the consequences of bTBI, not necessarily its evolution and the initial diagnosis is primarily on LOC and PTA, with the potential for neurological signs.[68] Memory problems after blast concussion are common. Reduced concentration, personality changes and other neuropsychological sequelae are increasingly recognised as a result of blast OP exposure.[13]

Identifying the difference between stress-related disorders and bTBI on initial presentation is not possible. Ideally detection begins on the 'battlefield', in the pre-hospital environment, where initial assessment provides valuable evidence and a baseline for establishing the presence of potential concussion. All possible concussive events require follow-up in ED for further assessment, as the cognitive sequelae post blast concussion can be significant and rehabilitation is required.

Injury is identified through the usual neurological assessment tools and physical examination. This includes a number of screening methodologies and their value to identifying TBI, listed in Table 51.3. When assessing a patient, consider causes of altered mental state, such as hypoxaemia from lung injury, cardiocompressive shock, haemorrhage, myocardial infarction, conventional blunt or penetrating head injury or AAE. Focal deficits are usually indicative of an intracerebral bleed or AAE. Other signs of AAE, including air in the retinal vessels and demarcated tongue blanching, are insensitive.[3]

For the spine, look for signs of minute penetrating trauma in the patient complaining of sensory or motor deficits. Partial transection has occurred with millimetre-wide fragments. Consider axonal loading resulting in spinal injury, in patients thrown significant distances from a blast or in patients who have received an impact to the base of the spine while sitting in a vehicle. A force great enough to push someone towards the roof of a vehicle is significant, producing injury anywhere along the spine. Assessment and management is otherwise according to the principles outlined in Chapter 49.

Skull X-rays are of little value in penetrating trauma, as they will only give a gross idea of the fragmentation path. CT scans are mandatory for all patients with an altered mental state, penetrating trauma of any size and significant blunt force trauma. Facial CT scan cuts may be required for predominant facial injury. Cervical spine is usually included, but neck studies need to be considered for all penetrating trauma. However, in mTBI a CT scan is frequently normal (see Table 51.3). The same is true of MRI.

The crux of good management is good screening and referral. Neurosurgical consultation should be obtained as soon as possible for all intracranial or spinal injury and the patient transferred as required for the level of care needed. Any patient with an altered LOC at any stage post blast, PTA or

TABLE 51.3 Screening methodologies for the diagnosis of acute, blast-related mild TBI[65]

Military Acute Concussions Evaluation (MACE)	The Standardised Assessment of Concussion is used in MACE, and also in assessment of sports concussion. Use The Sport Concussion Assessment Tool (SCAT3) as an equivalent assessment tool to MACE
Automated Neuropsychological Assessment Metrics	Computer-assisted cognitive testing—more useful if a baseline is available to measure post blast TBI against
Eye tracking	Not fully evolved for use, but promising as an adjunct
Balance testing	Useful, as vestibular and otolith dysfunction produces balance disturbance
CT and MRI	Usually normal, so of little value in diagnosing mTBI. Useful for more severe TBI injury determination
Diffusion tensor imaging (DTI)	Not useful for early diagnosis of mTBI Frequently normal early in injury, more useful sometime after injury
PET and functional MRI	Not useful for early diagnosis of mTBI Currently under investigation for use in later diagnosis of blast related mTBI
Biomarkers	No reliable serum biomarker is available for blast-related TBI—they are dependent on time since injury, so not useful outside of specific hospital settings
Blast dosimeters	Small detectors for blast dose, which may have applicability if placed on helmets or clothing. Currently under investigation. Not useful in the civilian setting.

other neurological or behavioural signs should be referred to neurology for follow-up.

Management of TBI is described in Chapter 45, and it is currently believed the rehabilitation from bTBI is similar to TBI from non-blast means.[67] However, as with all blast injury, there are additional considerations. For a decade in Iraq and Afghanistan, the choice for fragment and contamination removal in severe penetrating TBI was decompressive craniectomy (DECRA). The skull had already been significantly breached and DCS was often mandated by the patient's instability or large patient numbers. However, as a result of subsequent research, neurological debridement in the military setting is now controversial. It is generally not recommended to perform DECRA or debride,[13] although all penetrating wounds will need some degree of cleaning and temporary closure of the skull. Like all wounds, they will be contaminated due to the nature of blast destruction.

Ocular

Ocular injuries are uncommon in personnel who wear protective goggles. When injuries do occur, they are usually of pressure and blunt force trauma origin, including retinal AAE, ruptured globe, hyphaema and serous retinitis. Penetrating injury usually involves corneal and scleral laceration or abrasion, orbital fracture, lid laceration, traumatic cataracts and a lacerated globe.

All victims of blast trauma should have an ocular examination during initial ED care as per Box 51.2. All identified ocular injuries (except for corneal abrasions) should be covered with a patch and shield and referred to an ophthalmologist as soon as possible. Most corneal abrasions (not including full-thickness corneal laceration) can be treated locally. Due to

---

BOX 51.2 Assessment and management of ocular blast trauma[1,68,69]

- Check each eye for vision.
- Check for eye pain or sensation of a foreign body. Instil local anaesthetic eye drops, stain with fluorescein and check for foreign bodies or injury.
- Check reactivity and equality of pupils.
- Check for relative afferent pupil defect.
- Check ability to close eyes. If there are any injuries preventing lid closure (including 7th cranial nerve palsy), instil antibiotic ointment and cover eye (from brow to cheek) with clear plastic foodwrap, using white soft paraffin to adhere plastic to skin.

The unconscious patient
- Check reactivity and equality of pupils.
- Evert lids, stain with fluorescein and check for foreign bodies or injury.
- If the lids are shut, instil antibiotic ointment, or if open, instil antibiotic ointment and cover with plastic wrap as above.

Ocular perforation
- Apply eye pad and shield (a shield of any kind is important).
- Administer IV antibiotics and tetanus.

---

the high risk of *Pseudomonas*, the patient should be examined daily.[1,69] If the abrasion is not improving or an infiltrate develops, then the patient should be referred immediately to ophthalmology. Gentamicin is not recommended as it is often used inappropriately and causes corneal epithelial toxicity, which confounds ocular examination.[1] Steroids should never be used without consultation with an ophthalmologist. Due to the relatively unknown medium- to long-term effects of blast-related injury, ideally all eye injuries or visual disturbances should be referred to an ophthalmologist or ophthalmic surgeon. Evacuation of all eye injuries related to blast trauma should ideally avoid flights above 1000 m to avoid the risk of barotrauma and retinal ischaemia. For further information on eye trauma see Chapter 33.

Maxillofacial

The face is not protected by armour and is thus exposed to injury in all victims of blast injury, potentiated by the upward movement of a blast wave. The damage to soft tissue and bone can be devastating, removing normal anatomical landmarks and challenging repair. Multiple fragments aggravate the extent of damage and large cavitation injuries are not uncommon.[1,70–72] The primary risk to the life of the patient is airway compromise, and intervention can be profoundly challenged in complete mid-third facial injury with segmented mandibles and severe dental injury. A cricothyroidotomy or tracheostomy is often required if neck involvement is extensive. The second risk to life is carotid or jugular injury. While injury is managed according to principles outlined in Chapter 46, in blast injury surgical management is focused on irrigation, ligation, packing and delayed primary closure.

Neck

The neck is highly susceptible to both blunt and penetrating trauma, with penetrating injuries common.[1] For neck assessment see Chapter 47. The airway is the greatest problem of significant blunt injury to the neck, including the risk of a fractured larynx or cricotracheal separation. Thus, regardless of whether the injury is pharyngeal, laryngeal or tracheal, to the carotid sheath, the oesophagus or the vagus nerves, the airway is the primary focus. Following ABC resuscitation, which may require a tracheostomy, a CT scan of the neck with contrast is required, ideally with thin cuts through the larynx,[1] to assess the extent of injury and determine the location of fragments. This includes the patient who has a patent airway but some voice changes or dysphagia. In general, it is agreed that injury to zones I and III warrant imaging of the blood vessels to determine the need for exploration. Controversy exists regarding mandatory exploration of the neck versus selective neck exploration for zone II injury. The risk of missing a laryngopharyngeal defect on a CT scan tends to justify exploration of injury to anterior zone II. In posterior zone II wounds where the fragment is deeply embedded in the muscle and away from the carotid sheath, the patient may be observed without exploration, as long as the CT scan is otherwise normal.[1]

Vascular extremity injury

Vascular extremity injury as a result of penetrating or blunt force trauma is common. The most important concern is the proximity of tissue destruction and large fragments to major vessels.[1] See Chapter 50 for general management of vascular injury. Active, uncontrolled bleeding mandates urgent surgery. Regular neurovascular assessment at least every 15 minutes is critical to identifying deterioration. Pulses may be intact with partial injury to an artery. If not, use Doppler to establish the state of the pulse. Thoroughly assess sensory and motor function, even in the presence of a pulse. The severity of extremity injury often results in profound bleeding. A limb blown or torn off at the hip or shoulder is difficult to stem bleeding in and usually warrants clamping of blood vessels. Rapid transfer to a facility capable of repairing the damage is essential.[1]

> **PRACTICE TIP**
>
> After application of an arterial TQ for amputation, or if direct application of pressure is the only option, transfer should not be delayed by an inability to stem bleeding, as surgery may be the only chance the patient has for survival.

This is true for all severe trauma, where bleeding can only be definitively stopped by surgery and holding the patient in either the pre-hospital or ED environment results in aggravated coagulopathy and shock with mortality outcomes.

In the presence of vascular injury, all surrounding compartments in a limb require fasciotomy. This usually involves four compartment fasciotomies of the lower limb and consideration of forearm fasciotomy for the upper limbs.[1,2,13] The sum effects of time, resuscitation and severe tissue destruction necessitated this practice in all extremity vascular injuries treated in the Iraq and Afghanistan wars. Vascular repair is often challenged by the severity of soft-tissue destruction and the need for multiple fasciotomies preventing good tissue coverage of blood vessels and anastamosis. Combined with concurrent muscle injury and fractures requiring fixation, vascular repair can be impaired. Further, despite successful re-vascularisation, amputation is often necessary.[1,13] Particularly in the lower leg, anatomically intact nerves may not lead to positive neurological outcomes, with subsequent amputation because the limb cannot be used (moved).

General considerations

Within the context of the trauma assessment and management framework described in Chapter 44, blast trauma requires consideration of the difficulties associated with assessing and identifying underlying trauma, the time-critical nature of obvious profound injury, re-evaluation for insidious PBI development, the unique complications associated with blast trauma and, potentially, the challenge of large casualty numbers.[3,15] See Box 51.3 for general management principles, Table 51.4 for specific blast primary considerations and Table 51.5 for secondary survey considerations in the blast-injured patient. This must be carried out bearing in mind potential issues with communication system failures, triage, forensics, safety and security, which arise with blast trauma and apply in all disaster and large casualty settings. See Chapter 12 for more on disaster preparedness and response.

Security and safety

Blast injury has several unfortunate corollaries for healthcare providers. The first of these is the risk of a security breach. In known or potential terrorist situations, be aware of the tactic of dual explosions, where a second explosion is planned in the direction most people will flee or be taken. As the intent

BOX 51.3 General blast trauma management principles[8,9]

- Have a very high index of suspicion.
- Presentation in full cardiac arrest or with greater than 90% burns have a poor prognosis, aggravated by the almost certain presence of severe PBI.
- Always conduct a thorough primary and secondary survey on every patient.
- Assess TMs early to guide evaluation for other PBI and subsequent blast injury management.
- Assess lungs, abdomen and TMs for *all* blast victims, no matter how insignificant the apparent injury. Repeat all assessments prior to discharge.
- Inspect *all* penetrating trauma, no matter how small.
- View all fragmentation wounds as low velocity GSW.
- A period of observation is essential for all blast victims, as pulmonary and abdominal injury can evolve slowly.
- Give clear discharge information on when to return if any subtle or more obvious signs of respiratory or abdominal discomfort develop.
- Admit the patient with persistent abdominal signs.
- Obtain accurate history and mechanism of injury in order to identify probable blast effects (see Box 51.1).
- Always obtain a chest X-ray.

is to maximise civilian casualties and overwhelm existing resources, do not underestimate the risk of an attack on pre-hospital providers or a direct hospital attack, especially once casualties start arriving. Security is mandatory and all patients and visitors (or bystanders) should be checked for weapons. Checks include unknown staff, staff not wearing ID badges, women, children and *all* non-hospital personnel as, in this type of situation, no uniform is safe without a supporting ID. Follow standard bomb protocols for all packages left lying around. Be aware of the risk of chemical, radioactive or biological contamination and follow standard protocols for protecting staff and other patients.

PRACTICE TIP

Do not trust anyone you do not know, who has no identification. Ensure security is strict.

Consider the risk of unexploded ordnance (an explosive device which failed to detonate) embedded in a patient. This will require the patient to be left outside until the right equipment is located and a plan of action for safe removal is determined. This can happen occasionally with fireworks. Security also includes protecting all patients from the media and mobile phones with photographic capability. Strict control

TABLE 51.4 Blast injuries: Primary Survey—problems and considerations for management[3]

PROBLEM	CONSIDERATIONS FOR MANAGEMENT
Airway	
Altered mental status	While intubation is considered for a GCS less than 9, consider the ramifications of subsequent ventilation—spontaneous breathing is the preferred method for avoiding high airway pressures and reducing risk of AAE
	Oxygenation is the priority
Facial injury: oedema, direct injury obstruction	Manage as for non-blast trauma
Massive haemoptysis	Unilateral ventilation of the unaffected lung
Cervical spine	Immobilisation
	When checking the cervical spine, check the TMs
Breathing	
Tension pneumothorax	Needle thoracocentesis and manage as for non-blast trauma
Open pneumothorax	Manage as for non-blast trauma
Haemothorax	Manage as for non-blast trauma and consider auto-transfusion
Refractory hypoxaemia: pulmonary contusion (PBI)	PPV ± PEEP of > 10 cmH$_2$O
	Unconventional ventilation methods may be required: see section on BLI
	Permissive hypotensive fluid management reduces aggravation of contusions by high fluid loads
Persistent pneumothorax	Bronchopleural fistulas are more common with blast injury

TABLE 51.4 Blast injuries: Primary Survey—problems and considerations for management[3]—cont'd

PROBLEM	CONSIDERATIONS FOR MANAGEMENT
Ruptured diaphragm	Additional ICC may be required, or unilateral ventilation in severe cases
	Surgical repair
Apnoea	All apnoea requires ventilation
Wheezing	Wheezing is pulmonary contusion until proven otherwise, even in the known asthmatic
Circulation	
Hypotension	Is most likely due to hypovolaemia
	Also consider: tension pneumothorax, VMR, AAE. Sudden hypotension is a tension pneumothorax until proven otherwise
	Fluids should be given judiciously, titrated to response—focus is rate and quantity required to just correct tissue perfusion. Suggested physiological endpoints are BP 100 systolic, pulse rate of < 120 beats/minute and normal mentation
	Instead of standard 20 mL/kg fluid boluses, an approach of re-evaluation of physiological endpoints after 5 mL/kg boluses is recommended (exception: obvious exsanguinations, although re-evaluate with every litre)
	Rapid fluid administration may adversely aggravate lung injury, inhibit cardiac activity and cerebral perfusion or promote abdominal compartment syndrome
Shock	Evaluation for internal haemorrhage is the same as for non-blast trauma: check all spaces for fine fragments or contusions
	Management of external haemorrhage is the same as for non-blast trauma: check all wounds, no matter how small
	Non-compressible haemorrhage may require a TQ or clamping.
	TQ are lifesaving in traumatic amputation and stay on until evaluated by a vascular or orthopaedic surgeon. They should be checked for effectiveness
	Incidence of AAE is reduced with normalising preload
	Use blood early for obvious haemorrhage. Consider a haematocrit goal of 27%
	Whole blood reconstitution needs to start early—give component therapy according to massive transfusion protocols
	Other fluids are useful when blood loss is not ongoing
	Burns formula remains the same, although focus is on achieving physiological endpoints, rather than delivering the calculated volume
Cardiocompressive shock	Check for the rare potential of a cardiac tamponade
	Most likely AAE or, less commonly, cardiac contusion: evaluate as for non-blast MI
Myocardial ischaemia, infarction, cardiogenic shock	Position lying left lateral for AAE and consider hyperbaric treatment
	Thrombolytics, vasodilators and nitrates are contraindicated
	Usually the result of blunt or penetrating spinal trauma, although occasionally AAE
Neurogenic shock	Position lying semi-left lateral for AAE and consider hyperbaric treatment
	Usually occurs 24–72 hours post trauma in the patient with multiple injuries and massive tissue injury, prolonged oxygen debt and massive transfusion
Systemic inflammatory response syndrome (SIRS)	Occurs with fat emboli from long bone and pelvic trauma, embolised fragments, as a response to MV in patients with pulmonary contusions and with toxic exposure

Continued

TABLE 51.4 Blast injuries: Primary Survey—problems and considerations for management[3]—cont'd

PROBLEM	CONSIDERATIONS FOR MANAGEMENT
Pulmonary embolism (PE)	CT scan and manage as for PE of any other cause
Disability	
Altered mental status, seizures, focal neurological signs	Usually due to blunt or penetrating trauma
	Less commonly due to AAE or a VMR
	Treat AAE with positioning and hyperbaric therapy. VMR will self-resolve
	Consider blast induced concussion (mild TBI)
Visual defects	Blunt or penetrating eye injury is a common cause, although retinal AAE may occur
	Blunt or penetrating head injury may produce papillary changes and visual disturbance
	Treat retinal AAE with positioning and hyperbaric therapy
Hearing loss	Common in blast injuries, may be unilateral or bilateral
Environment	
Prevent hypothermia	This is critical to coagulopathy prevention and management

AAE: arterial air emboli; BP: blood pressure; CT: computed tomography; GCS: Glasgow Coma Scale; ICC: intercostal catheter; MI: myocardial infarction; MV: mechanical ventilation; PBI: primary blast injury; PEEP: positive end-expiratory pressure; PPV: positive-pressure ventilation; TBI: tertiary blast injury; TM: tympanic membrane; TQ: tourniquet; VMR: vagal-nerve-mediated reflex.

of personnel according to the principles of disaster management will maximise outcomes.

Triage

The challenge is PBI and hidden, but dangerous, fragments. If they are hard of hearing, consider PBI. Even small holes can be dangerous. Apply a high index of suspicion. If the explosion was yesterday and they present a day later with abdominal pain, get them seen urgently. Check pulses on all immobile limbs and burns, even if they otherwise look okay.

> **PRACTICE TIP**
>
> If they were close to the blast, but look okay, they probably are not. Give them a minimum ATS 2 category.

Forensics

Forensic evidence should be preserved. Keep all clothes, body armour, eye protection, footwear, body parts or fragments which may fall off or are otherwise removed, and any items carried by the patient. Manage as per standard forensic evidence protocols. Do not wash the body unless you have to for aseptic reasons prior to surgery, or to clean the eyes, as gunpowder or explosive residue may be present. If teeth are removed as penetrating objects, they are forensic evidence of someone else's identity—process them accordingly and note who they came out of.

Dressings and wound management

Wounds bleeding excessively should be packed; all others should be covered with damp saline dressings where bleeding is not a concern. Avoid compressive bandages, which may aggravate contused muscle compartments, unless they are required for haemorrhage control. To avoid excessive wound disturbance and further damage when dressings are regularly removed for wound assessment, use only what is needed for wound coverage and bleeding control. All wounds, including those dressed prior to presentation, should be assessed on arrival and daily for the presence of infection, including the smell of all wounds more than 24 hours old.[1] For further information on wound assessment see Chapter 18. All wounds involving fragmentation injury require X-ray.

Laboratory investigations

Full blood count (FBC) with cross-match should be mandatory and early for all victims of an explosion: blood transfusion and clotting requirements will be determined on the results. Expect significantly altered clotting factors for patients with severe trauma and those who have received fluid management prior to arrival, especially where transfer to hospital has been delayed. Carboxyhaemoglobin measurement is recommended for explosions in an enclosed space or where a fire is known to have occurred. An international normalised ratio is useful for evaluating the effect of previous fluid resuscitation and determining some clotting factor requirements. Urea and electrolytes are important for an initial renal assessment and acid–base balance. Cardiac enzymes may be required where severe burns, crush injury or compartment syndrome exist. Calcium and phosphate levels are needed if white phosphorus has been used in deployed weapons. Specific toxicity levels are decided upon where contamination with specific substances is suspected, urinalysis or specific blood testing or use of hazardous materials personnel is required. Always conduct a routine urinalysis for blood.

TABLE 51.5 Blast injuries: Secondary Survey—problems and considerations for management[1,9,23]

PROBLEM	CONSIDERATIONS
General considerations	The insidious and occult nature of PBI and some fragmentation injury warrants thorough secondary surveys on everyone who suffers any degree of blast wave impact
	There is a high probability of combined primary, secondary, tertiary, quaternary and quinary injury: the greater the multiplicity of effects, the greater the risk of morbidity
	BLI is significantly greater in patients who demonstrate skull or facial fractures, burns to more than 10% TBSA and penetrating head or chest wounds
	The combination of traumatic amputation, open fractures and burns carries a high risk of death.
	Compartment syndrome is a high probability in fragmentation limb injury
	Rectal bleeding is an important and ominous sign of abdominal injury
Radiography	A CXR is mandatory in all patients potentially exposed to a blast wave, who have any penetrating trauma (no matter how small) to the neck, chest or upper abdomen, who have a ruptured TM or who demonstrate any signs of respiratory compromise
	Abdominal supine and upright films may be useful for identifying free air or fluid
	A FAST scan is a rapid and useful tool, although a negative FAST does not preclude significant injury
	A CT is not required prior to laparotomy in the unstable patient
Tympanic membrane Hearing, balance and vision	Despite being an inconsistent predictor of other PBI, *early* TM assessment is recommended, to guide evaluation and management: assess the TMs early, for blast wave impact and fluid
	If the TM is intact and there are no signs of respiratory distress or abdominal injury, it is acceptable to conditionally exclude PBI during initial treatment. Further evaluation involving CXR and ABG (if not done for other reasons) should be conducted later
	If the TM is ruptured, the presence or development of other PBI should be expected and evaluated
	Treat conditions as found, observe and monitor SpO_2 for at least 6 hours, discharging only if SpO_2, CXR and other assessments remain normal
	Hearing, balance and vision play an important role in determining the presence of PBI
Altered mental state—behaviour	Identify possible blast-induced concussion early, with referral. See Table 51.3.
Pain relief/sedation	Apply the same principles of analgesia assessment and management as for other trauma, bearing in mind haemodynamic instability
	Propofol is generally not an appropriate choice for sedation post intubation, as it has a greater tendency to precipitate hypotension: use has been demonstrated to precipitate PEA in the blast-injured patient with significant injury
Dressings/wounds	Take everything down: even the smallest hole is potentially covering a dangerous injury
	Check the smell of all wounds more than 24 hours old
	Take the time to look at every wound and every dressing on every patient, every day
	Where other methods fail, pack excessively bleeding wounds, cover all else with damp saline dressings and where bleeding is not a concern, avoid compressive bandages, which may aggravate contused muscle compartments

ABG: arterial blood gas; CXR: chest X-ray; FAST: focused assessment with sonography for tumour; PEA: pulseless electrical activity; SaO_2: oxygen saturation in arterial blood; TBSA: total body surface area; TM: tympanic membrane

Disposition

All victims of a blast should be examined in a hospital, due to the potential complexity and evolving nature of blast injury. The decision to admit or discharge is based on the likelihood of PBI developing or worsening.[3] Several studies have tried to determine the risk of developing PBI sequelae after discharge, with inconclusive results.[3] Anecdotal evidence suggests that patients surviving within the first hour usually have a positive outcome, and lung PBI is most likely to develop within the first couple of hours.[3,73] However, some patients have been observed to develop BLI and ARDS after being admitted for surgery for severe limb trauma. The conservative recommendation in the civilian setting is to admit and observe for 48 hours[11] anyone who fulfils the criteria in Box 51.4. In the military setting, this may be 24 hours. These criteria are not exclusive and have been adapted and developed according to identified problems with blast trauma.

Following a 4- to 6-hour period of observation for development of pneumothoraces or AAE, discharge may be considered for patients who meet the criteria outlined in Box 51.4. Because of the insidious nature of blast-related injury, patients should seek advice if they develop or have ongoing pain or other new signs or symptoms. In addition, all patients being discharged must be provided with advice on how to seek support and counselling for psychological issues.

BOX 51.4 Admission and discharge criteria[3,8]

Admission criteria
- Unconscious for any period, at any time after the blast
- Physically moved by a blast wave, knocked over, thrown, etc
- In an enclosed space or even partially underwater where a blast occurred
- Signs of blast wave impact, e.g. TM rupture, small fragmentation wounds
- Abnormal vital signs, lung injury, WP contamination, burns, suspected AAE, renal impairment or penetrating injury to the thorax or head

In addition, admit for 48 to 72 hours:
- Anyone with any complaint of abdominal pain, indications of potential abdominal injury, regardless of clear diagnostic studies
- Anyone requiring hyperbaric therapy, ventilation, surgery, etc

- All children and pregnant women; for both groups the consequences of blast trauma are less well known; they may develop late signs and the psychological impact is potentially greater

Discharge criteria following a 4- to 6-hour period of observation
- Open-air explosions with no apparent injury, normal vital signs, no complaints of chest or abdominal pain, discomfort or otherwise, normal CXR and normal ABG. Discharge with advice to return if there is any SOB, pain, vomiting or any abdominal symptoms or signs occur.
- Isolated TM rupture may go home with the following advice: antibiotics are not recommended in the absence of infection and all patients with a ruptured TM must have ENT referral for follow-up on cholesteatoma formation.

AAE: arterial air embolism; ABG: arterial blood gas; CXR: chest X-ray; ENT: ear, nose, throat; SOB: shortness of breath; TM: tympanic membrane; WP: white phosphorus

---

SUMMARY

Blast injury is complex. This chapter offers an initial guide to blast mechanism of injury, assessment, resuscitation and definitive care. Due to the multidimensional nature of blast injury, it is essential that all patients are evaluated in a hospital as quickly as possible and pre-hospital care is judicious, taking into consideration the effects PPV and fluid resuscitation can have on developing injury and the not infrequent need for life-saving surgery. In the DCR timeline, pre-hospital care prioritises rapid bleeding control and evacuation. Once in the ED, to evaluate the risk of PBI and other occult blast injuries, it is critical to take a very detailed history, including the victim's relative position to the blast, the type of blast and the location in which it occurred. The speed, intensity and duration of the pressure wave determine the degree of sustained injury. As with all trauma, assessment needs to be thorough and ongoing and the healthcare provider should always maintain a high index of suspicion, being wary of insidious injury development producing injury at a later stage, which was not apparent on first presentation.

CASE STUDY

It is 1430 hours on a Saturday afternoon in spring in Melbourne, Australia. The usual Saturday afternoon influx of Spring Racing Carnival over-indulgences and sporting injuries has been constantly streaming in.

A dull thud is heard by people in the waiting room and a small vibration is felt by all in the emergency department

(ED). An elderly gentleman sitting in the waiting room starts looking agitated and his daughter comments that he is always like that since 'the war', whenever he feels what reminds him of an explosion. Outside is now unusually quiet and someone walking into the triage area comments that they can see a large plume of smoke rising to the south of the area. They think a factory or something has gone up in flames.

Business continues as usual, until suddenly a man walks into the ED carrying a young girl, covered in blood. He claims a bomb has gone off in the local shopping centre and he simply picked up his daughter and ran. He can barely speak, does not seem to be able to hear what you are saying and is extremely agitated. No other notification has been received. A car pulls up at the same time, carrying several severely injured people missing limbs (makeshift tourniquet applied) and with skin hanging off, and one with a profound head injury. Someone in the waiting room takes a mobile call from a friend, confirming the story about a bomb. The local shopping centre has partially collapsed, shops opposite have been destroyed and are on fire, a 50 m crater is now where the road was, windows have shattered for up to a kilometre away and there are bodies everywhere. Apparently many people are making their way out by the only route and your department is only 3 km away.

At the same time, a call comes in stating that a bomb has gone off, emergency services are on their way to the scene and there is no idea as to how many are wounded. Your hospital activates its internal disaster plan as, regardless of what is happening externally, you are faced with waves of severely injured people, including children, who you do not normally see.

Questions

1. What are the risks for emergency services going to the scene?
2. What circumstances may delay egress from the scene?
3. What do pre-hospital services need to consider when assessing and managing the injured?
4. Should people who do not look injured be sent home by pre-hospital services? Give a reason for your answer.
5. What safety and security procedures should pre-hospital services conduct with all personnel removed from the scene as patients?
6. What information about the blast could pre-hospital services gather to provide to ED staff?
7. What is the pre-hospital role in the DCR continuum?
8. In the ED, what security considerations need to be implemented, and why?
9. How can you gather a reasonable idea of the severity of the blast and what minimum number of questions should you ask pre-hospital services to get this information?
10. What additional considerations need to be made at triage when assessing patients from the blast scene?
11. What injuries do you need to evaluate all the injured for, and how will you do this?
12. What clinical manifestations might make you think of BLI?
13. How would you manage BLI in terms of ventilation and fluid management?
14. In a severely injured patient with multiple amputations, what is the role of damage-control surgery and why might it be necessary?
15. What are the key considerations for good wound care post blast injury?
16. If someone with multiple lower limb fragmentation injuries needs to wait for up to 24 hours for theatre because it is so busy, what do you need to assess regularly and why?
17. When would you consider mild TBI in a patient exposed to a blast?
18. Under what circumstances would someone who has been near the explosion and been mildly injured be allowed to go home?
19. If a patient returns the next day with abdominal pain after being exposed to the blast, what assessment do they require and why?

 Answers to Case Study Questions can be found on evolve
http://evolve.emergencytrauma.curtis

USEFUL WEBSITES

There are not many professional websites on this topic that add research based value, although there are many with lots of general non-validated information. A few which may be useful are:

American College Emergency Physicians, www.acep.org/blastinjury/

American Trauma Society, www.amtrauma.org/?page=BlastInjuries

American Speech, Language, Hearing Association, www.asha.org/aud/articles/CurrentTBI/

Australian Psychological Society, www.psychology.org.au/publications/inpsych/2012/april/ponsford/

Centre for Blast Injury Studies, Imperial College, London, www3.imperial.ac.uk/blastinjurystudies

UK Doctor, www.patient.co.uk/doctor/Blast-Injury.htm

REFERENCES

1. Gawande A. Casualties of war: military care for the wounded from Iraq and Afghanistan. N Engl J Med 2004;351(24):2471–5.

2. Ramasamy A, Cooper G, Sargeant ID et al. An overview of the pathophysiology of blast injury with management guidelines. Ortho Trauma; 2013:27(1):49–55.

3. Wightman JM, Gladish SL. Explosions and blast injuries. Ann Emerg Med 2001;37(6):664–78.

4. Wildegger-Gaissmaier AE. Aspects of thermobaric weaponry. ADF Health 2003;4(1):3–6.

5. Tsokos M, Paulsen F, Petri S et al. Histologic, immunohistochemcial and ultrastructural findings in human blast lung injury. Am J Respir Crit Care Med 2003;168(5):549–55.

6. Hogan DE, Burstein JL. Disaster Medicine. Wolters Kluwer: LWW; 2007.

7. Bellamy RF, Zajtchuk R, eds. Conventional warfare: ballistic, blast and burn injuries. Washington, DC: Office of the Surgeon General of the US Army; 1991.

8. Pennardt A. Blast injuries. eMedicine. Online. http://emedicine.medscape.com/article/822587-overview; 29 Apr 2013.

9. DePalma RG, Burris DG, Champion HR et al. Blast injuries. N Engl J Med 2005;352:1335–42.

10. Bersten AD, Soni N, eds. Oh's Intensive care manual. 6th edn. London: Butterworth–Heinemann; 2009.

11. Cooper GJ, Dudley HA, Gann DS et al, eds. Scientific foundations of trauma. Oxford: Butterworth-Heinemann; 1997.

12. Cooper GJ. Protection of the lung from blast overpressure by thoracic stress wave decouplers. J Trauma 1996;40(3 suppl):S105–10.

13. Plurad DS. Blast injury. Mil Med 2011;176(3):276–82.

14. Mellor SG. The relationship of blast loading to death and injury from explosion. World J Surg 1992;16(5):893–8.

15. Kashuk J, Halperin P, Caspi G et al. Bomb explosions in acts of terrorism: evil creativity challenges our trauma systems. J Am Coll Surg 2009:134–40.

16. Mellor SG, Dodd KT, Harmon JW et al. Ballistic trauma: clinical relevance in peace and war. London: Arnold; 1997.

17. Finlay S, Earby M, Baker D, Murray V. Explosions and human health: the long-term effects of blast injury. Prehospital Disaster Med 2012;27(4):385–91.

18. Dougherty A, MacGregor A, Han P et al. Blast related ear injuries among US military personnel. JRRD 2013:50(6):893–904.

19. Sylvia FR, Drake AI, Wester DC. Transient vestibular balance dysfunction after primary blast injury. Mil Med 2001;166(10):918–20.

20. Goldfarb A, Eliashar R, Gross M et al. Middle cranial fossa cholesteatoma following blast trauma. Ann Otol Rhinol Laryngol 2001;110(11):1084–6.

21. Gallun F, Lewis S, Fomer R et al. Implications of blast exposure for central auditory function: a review. JRRD 2013;49(7):1059–74.

22. Helling ER. Otologic blast injuries due to the Kenya embassy bombing. Mil Med 2004;169(11):872–6.

23. Almogy G, Luria T, Richter E et al. Can external signs of trauma guide management? Lessons learned from suicide bombing attacks in Israel. Arch Surg 2005;140(4):390–3.

24. Mayorga MA. The pathology of primary blast overpressure injury. Toxicology 1997;121(1):17–28.

25. Irwin RJ, Lerner MR, Bealer JF et al. Shock after blast wave injury is caused by a vagally mediated reflex. J Trauma 1999;47(1):105–10.

26. Hare SS, Goddard I, Ward P et al. The radiological management of bomb blast injury. Clin Radiol 2007;62(1):1–9.

27. van Wessem K, Hennus M, van Wagenberg L et al. Mechanical ventilation increase the inflammatory response induced by lung contusion. JSR 2013:183:377–84.

28. Reid M, Bein T, Philipp A et al. Extracorporeal lung support in trauma patients with severe chest injury and acute lung failure: a 10 year institutional experience. Crit Care 2013;17:R110.

29. Stewart C. Blast injuries: true weapons of mass destruction. 2010. Online. www.az1dmat.org/dmat_blast_injuries.pdf Emerg Med Prac; accessed 2 Feb 2014.

30. Cameron GR, Short RH, Wakely CP. Abdominal injuries due to underwater explosion. Br J Surg 1943;31:51–66.

31. Powers D, Delo R. Characteristics of ballistic and blast injuries. Atlas Oral Maxillofac Surg Clin N Am 2013;21:15–24.

32. Khan MS, Kirkland PM, Kumar R. Migrating foreign body in the tracheobronchial tree: an unusual case of firework penetrating neck injury. J Laryngol Otol 2002;116(2):148–9.

33. Germanos S, Gourgiotis S, Villias C et al. Damage control surgery in the abdomen: an approach for the management of severe injured patients. Int J Surg 2008;6:246–52.

34. Chovanes J, Cannon J, Nunez T. The evolution of damage control surgery. Surg Clin N Am 2012;92:859–75.

35. Hess J, Brohi K, Dutton R et al. The coagulopathy of trauma: a review of mechanisms. J Trauma 2008;65(4):748–54.

36. Brohi K, Cohen M, Ganter M et al. Acute coagulopathy of trauma: hypoperfusion induces systemic anticoagulation and hyperfibrinolysis. J Trauma 2008;64(5):1211–17.

37. Engels P, Rezende-Neto J, Mahroos A et al. The natural history of trauma-related coagulopathy: implications for treatment. J Trauma 2011;71(5):S448–55.

38. Simmons J, White C, Ritchie J et al. Mechanism of injury affects acute coagulopathy of trauma in combat casualties. J Trauma 2011;71(1):74–7.

39. Hess JR. Blood and coagulation support in trauma care. Hematology Am Soc Hematol Educ Program 2007:187–91.

40. Hagemo J. Prehospital detection of traumatic coagulopathy. Transfusion 2013:53.

41. Jaunoo S, Harji D. Damage control surgery. Int J Surg. 2009;7:110–13.

42. Mylankal K, Wyatt M. Control of major haemorrhage and damage control surgery. Emerg Surg 2013;31:11.

43. Cirocchi R, Montedori A, Farinella E et al. Damage control surgery for abdominal trauma (review). The Cochrane collaboration. 2013.

44. Blackbourne L. Combat damage control surgery. Crit Care Med 2008;36(7).

45. Sambasivan C, Underwood S, Cho S et al. Comparison of abdominal damage control surgery in combat versus civilian trauma. J Trauma 2010;69(1).

46. Dutton R. Resuscitative strategies to maintain homeostasis during damage control surgery. Brit J Surg 2012;99(1):21–8.

47. Gentilello LM, Pierson DJ. Trauma critical care. Am J Respir Crit Care Med 2001;163(3 Pt 1):604–7.

48. Morrison J, Ross J, Poon H et al. Intra-operative correction of acidosis, coagulopathy and hypothermia in combat casualties with severe haemorrhagic shock. Anaesthesia 2013;68:846–50.

49. Chewter M. From point of wounding: damage control resuscitation. J Periop Prac 2013:23(7):163–6.

50. Jansen J, Thomas R, Loudon M, Brooks A. Damage control resuscitation for patients with major trauma. BMJ 2009:338.

51. Holcomb J, Jenkins D, Rhee P et al. Damage control resuscitation: directly addressing the early coagulopathy of trauma. JIICC 2007:62.

52. Frauenfelder C, Raith E, Griggs W. Damage control resuscitation of the exsanguinating trauma patient: pathophysiology and basic principles. J Mil Vet Hea 2011;19(2).

53. Parr RR, Providence BC, Burkhalter WE et al. Treatment of lower extremity injuries due to antipersonnel mines: blast resuscitation and victim assistance team experiences in Cambodia. Mil Med 2003;168(7):536–40.

54. Rasmussen T, Clouse D, Jenkins D et al. Echelons of care and the management of wartime vascular injury: a report from the 332nd EMDG/Air Force Theater Hospital, Balad Air Base, Iraq. Perspectives Vasc Surg Endovasc Ther 2006;18(19).

55. Richey S. Tourniquets for the control of traumatic haemorrhage: a review of the literature. World J Emerg Surg 2007;2:28.

56. Niven M, Castle N. Use of tourniquets in combat and civilian trauma situations. Emerg Nurse 2010;18(3):32–6.

57. Kragh J, O'Neill M, Walters T et al. Minor morbidity with emergency tourniquet use to stop bleeding in severe limb trauma: research, history, and reconciling advocates and abolitionists. Mil Med 2011;176(7):817–23.

58. Kragh J. Use of tourniquets and their effects on limb function in the modern combat environment. Foot Ankle Clin 2010;15(1):23–40.

59. Dickens J, Kilcoyne K, Kluk M et al. Risk factors for infection and amputation following open, combat-related calcaneal fractures. J Bone Joint Surg Am 2013;95:1–8.

60. Southwick GJ, Pethick AJ, Thalayasingam P et al. Australian doctors in Bali: the initial medical response to the Bali bombing. Med J Aust 2002;177(11–12):624–6.

61. Mayo A, Kluger Y. Blast induced injury to air containing organs. ADF Health 2006;7:40–4.

62. MacDonald C, Johnson A, Cooper D et al. Detection of blast-related traumatic brain injury in US military personnel. NEJM 2011;364(22):2091–100.

63. Nakagawa A, Manley G, Gean A et al. Mechanism of primary blast-induced traumatic brain injury: insights from shock-wave research. J Neurotrauma 2011;28:1101–19.

64. Rosenfeld J, McFarlane A, Bragge P et al. Blast-related traumatic brain injury. Lancet 2013;12:882–93.

65. DeWitt D, Prough D. Blast-induced brain injury and post traumatic hypotension and hypoxemia. J Neurotrauma 2009;26:877–87.

66. Kamnaksh A, Kovesdi E, Kwon SK et al. Factors affecting blast traumatic brain injury. J Neurotrauma 2011;28:2145–53.

67. Bogdanova Y, Verfaellie M. Cognitive sequelae of blast-induced tramatic brain injury: recovery and rehabilitation. Neurpsychol Rev 2012;22:4–20.

68. Ruff R, Iverson G, Barth J et al. Recommendations for diagnosing a mild traumatic brain injury: A national academy of Neuropsychology education paper. Archives of Clin Neuropsych 2009;24:3–10.

69. Crompton J. Ocular and adnexal injuries in the Bali bombing. ADF Health Australia 2003;4:2.

70. Shuker S. The effect of a blast on the mandible and teeth: transverse fractures and their management. Br J Oral Maxillofac Surg 2008;46(7):547–51.

71. Shuker S. Mechanism and emergency management of blast eye/orbital injuries. Ophthalmol 2008;3(2):229–45.

72. Shuker S. Maxillofacial air-containing cavities, blast implosion injuries and management. J Oral Maxillofac Surg 2010;68:93–100.

73. Leibovici D, Gofrit ON, Shapira SC. Eardrum perforation in explosion survivors: is it a marker of pulmonary blast injury? Ann Emerg Med 1999;34(2):168–72.

74. Wolf SJ, Bebarta VS, Bonnett CS et al. Blast injuries. The Lancet 2009;374(9687):405–15.

CHAPTER 52
BURNS TRAUMA

LINDA QUINN AND ANDREW HOLLAND

Essentials

- Burns remain a common, potentially life-threatening injury in both adults and children.
- While visually dramatic, burns may occur in association with other forms of trauma.
- Appropriate first aid, which includes stopping the burning process and the application of at least 20 minutes of cold running water while avoiding hypothermia, may reduce the depth of the burn injury.
- Major burns (greater than 10% total body surface area (TBSA) in children and 20% TBSA in adults), although appearing to involve only the skin, lead to a generalised increase in vascular permeability, in association with an intense and sustained metabolic response.
- All patients with major burns require supplementary oxygen, which should be warmed and humidified, together with intravenous fluids in proportion to the area of the burn. Children will also require maintenance fluids based on their weight.
- Oedema may result in rapid loss of the airway in patient with facial, neck and inhalational burns, or distal ischaemia in those with limb burns. Early, elective intubation must be considered, together with escharotomy, prior to transfer.
- Appropriate temporary burn wound dressings should be discussed with the receiving burns unit.
- Scarring and contracture formation remain important long-term sequelae in those patients with deep burns.

INTRODUCTION

'Burn' derives from the Old English word *baernan* for an injury as a result of heat, or a chemical, radiological or mechanical force simulating the action of heat. Despite improvements in prevention, either through legislation or education or a combination of the two, a burn remains one of the most devastating forms of injury in all ages. In the United States there were 450,000 patients in 2010 who required medical treatment for burn injuries and in 2008 3,400 deaths.[5] This comparatively high mortality rate reflects a combination of the systemic inflammatory consequences of major burn injury, the increased risks of sepsis, together with the impact of any associated inhalational injury. While the majority of burns occur in adults, children and the elderly appear uniquely at risk as a result of a combination of their thin skin and different responses to burn injury. In Europe, a systematic literature review in 2010 identified an incidence of severe burns of between 0.2 and 2.9/10,000, with over 50% in the paediatric age group.[6] Worldwide, in 1997 burns caused the loss of 11.9×10^6 disability-adjusted life years (DALYs), resulting in a greater loss than that of diabetes, HIV and asthma.[1] Furthermore, these injuries are not evenly distributed geographically, with a much higher proportion occurring in low- to middle-income countries, especially

South-East Asia.[1] Between 1990 and 2004, of the 505,276 children with burn injuries reported in the literature, 57% were located in Asia.[6]

From 1 July 2011 to 30 June 2012 there were 2772 cases that required admission to a burns unit in Australia and New Zealand, however only 15 of the 17 burns units entered data.[7] Fortunately, Australia and New Zealand have a lower percentage of major burns in both paediatric and adult cases when compared to the United States. However, over half of these burn admissions (57%), occurred in rural and remote areas with significant implications for transport and pre-hospital care.[7]

For those clinicians dealing with burns patients, however, these numbers represent only part of the whole picture.[5] Increasing survival translates to a higher frequency of morbidity, with a very great burden on the patient, their family, clinicians and the healthcare system.[8] Perhaps this feature, together with the need for excellent teamwork to acheive an optimal outcome, explains in part the esprit de corps that typically exists in burn units.[9] Certainly, burn injury may represent one of the best examples of trauma care in which the provision of ideal pre-hospital treatment may directly affect the patient's final outcome, especially in relation to the depth of burn injury and the need for subsequent operative intervention.[10,11]

Epidemiology and aetiology of burns

Although there appears to be some conflicting data in the literature, several key facts remain. First, burns, like nearly all forms of trauma, generally affect males more commonly than females, with an average ratio of 1.6 : 1.[12] Second, while the overall incidence of burns requiring hospital admission has decreased over at least the last two decades in high-income countries, approximately 1% of the population in Australia and New Zealand will sustain some form of burn injury per annum.[12–14] In certain high-risk groups, such as children in South-East Asia and Australasia, the prevalence of burn injury may in fact be rising.[6,15,16] In part, these apparently conflicting data may reflect a failure to adequately account for differences between high-income and middle- to low-income countries.[6,17] A lack of agreement on age definitions and the increased use of ambulatory versus inpatient care in the management of burn injuries in many units makes accurate comparison and analysis of trends difficult.[6,16,18]

The mechanism of burn injury also would seem both more complex and more dynamic than might at first appear: historically, flame burns have accounted for the majority of burns in adults, followed by scalds and then contact burns.[13] In contrast, in children this order has been transposed, with scalds predominating, trailed by flame and then contact burns.[13] Depths of burn injuries are demonstrated in Figure 52.1.

Some studies have suggested a rise in the proportion of scald burns in adults, perhaps in parallel with a greater proportion of the elderly as part of the adult population, although this may also reflect the inclusion of paediatric data.[19–21] In the paediatric age group, there appears to have been a rise in the number of contact burns, which may now have replaced flame burns as the second most-common cause of burn injury in childhood after scalds.[22]

Knowledge of the likely aetiology of the burn injury remains important to pre-hospital, nursing and allied health personnel involved in the care of that patient, as it enables both understanding and provision of optimal burns first-aid treatment and provides an opportunity for advice on prevention.[10,16,23,24]

Pathophysiology

A burn injury has an effect on all of the five major functions of the skin:

- thermoregulation
- fluid and electrolyte imbalance
- immune response
- protection from bacterial invasion
- neurosensory interface.

Local response

To assist in understanding the pathophysiology of a burn it is useful to look to Jackson's burn wound model (Fig 52.2), first described in 1953.[1]

1. *Zone of coagulative necrosis*—this is the site of injury where the heat source is at its greatest, and rapid cell death occurs. This central zone of tissue death becomes deeper and wider as the heat intensifies and length of exposure increases. The damage in this zone is irreversible.

2. *Zone of stasis*—this area surrounds the zone of coagulation and the tissue damage is less severe; however, there is damage to the microcirculation. Sluggish circulation makes this area susceptible to additional insult and may potentially extend into the zone of coagulation. This area is viable given appropriate fluid resuscitation and wound care, avoiding excessive oedema and infection.

3. *Zone of hyperaemia*—surrounding the zone of stasis is one of limited cellular damage, and complete recovery usually prevails. The inflammatory mediatory response causes widespread vasodilation and this increased blood flow brings necessary nutrients to support the zone of stasis.[14,25,26]

The final depth and area of the burn wound is dependent on the fate of the zone of stasis, and treatment is centred on facilitating the recovery of this area. The true extent of injury may take 3–5 days, as areas that acutely appear to be perfused often go on to show delayed healing. This is seen clinically as burn wound progression.

Recovery of the zone of stasis can be supported by:

- adequate burns first aid
- prevention of hypothermia
- good fluid resuscitation
- elevation of affected limbs
- prevention of infection
- covering of the burn wound
- analgesia.

Systemic response

A burn injury induces changes in every organ system in the body, especially in those injuries greater than 20% TBSA. These are caused by the release of inflammatory mediators and neural stimulation, with the most profound and immediate

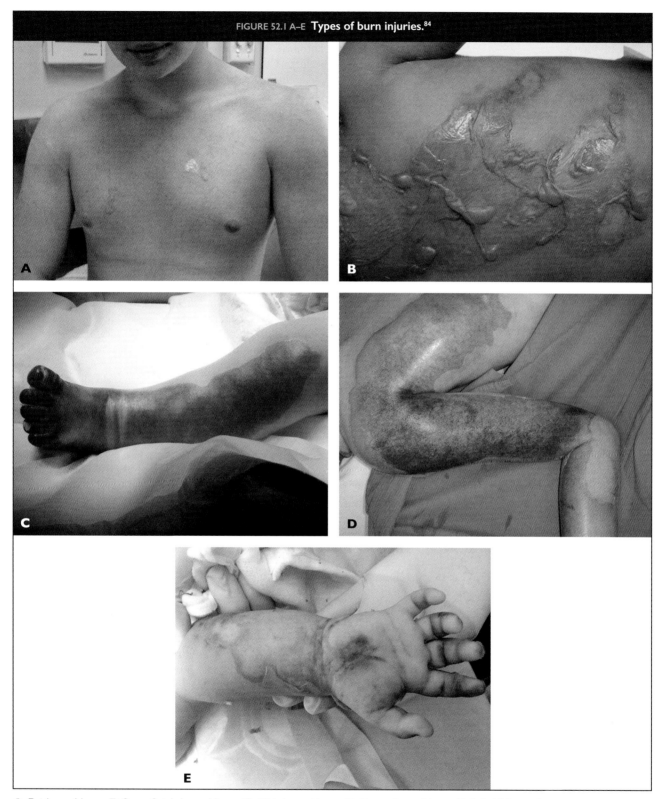

FIGURE 52.1 A–E **Types of burn injuries.**[84]

A, Epidermal burn. **B**, Superficial dermal burn. **C**, Mid dermal burn. **D**, Deep dermal burn. **E**, Full thickness burn.

effect on the circulation.[13] Vasodilation occurs, along with an increase in capillary permeability and a lowering of intercellular pressure. This causes mass movement of albumin out of the circulation and into the interstitial space, producing oedema. Changes in cell permeability result in an abnormal exchange of sodium. Sodium shifts into the cells in exchange for potassium,

which results in further depletion of intravascular sodium. The decreased interstitial hydrostatic pressure is thought to be the predominant mechanism responsible for the initial rapid development of oedema. The generalised oedema seen in non-injured skin and organs of patients with injuries greater than 25% TBSA is due to the circulatory mediators.

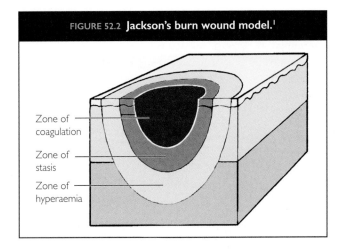

FIGURE 52.2 **Jackson's burn wound model.**[1]

Zone of coagulation

Zone of stasis

Zone of hyperaemia

Simple ways to assist with minimising oedema and increasing perfusion include:

- nurse with head of bed at 30°
- elevation of limbs
- careful observation of adequacy of fluid resuscitation
- active or passive range of motion exercises.

Hypermetabolic state and nutrition

As a result of a severe burn injury, stress hormones, such as cortisol, catecholomines and glucagon, are released, which in turn sets up a hypermetabolic state. The patient's metabolic rate can increase as much as two to three times the normal rate, far in excess of that seen in any other disease state, including other major traumas.[27] The stress response causes the suppression of anabolic hormones (growth hormones, insulin and anabolic steroids), which results in considerable catabolism including muscle protein breakdown.[9] We see these changes clinically as tachycardia, hyperthermia and protein wasting. This protein breakdown leads to the depletion of glycogen stores within 24 hours post injury, along with depletion of visceral and muscle protein stores. All patients with a significant burn injury consequently require aggressive high-protein, high-carbohydrate nutritional support. This is generally ideally provided via enteral feeding, with parenteral feeding held in reserve for those with a prolonged ileus or intolerance to enteral feeding.[13,27] There is now a considerable volume of literature to support pharmacological modification of this hypermetabolic state, especially the use of propranolol, a non-selective β1 and β2 receptor blocker, to reduce the elevated resting heart rate, decrease the basal metabolic rate and reduce lipolysis.[9,28]

Depression of the immune mechanism causes immuno-suppression, and consequently infection is still the leading cause of mortality in burn patients. The diffuse capillary leakage, hypovolaemia and release of vasoconstrictive agents following a severe burn injury cause a decrease in mesenteric blood flow.[29] This leads to mucosal ischaemia, breakdown, impaired gut barrier function, and an increase in bacterial translocation; another rationale for the early commencement of enteral feeds.[13,27]

The lungs commonly suffer from a post burn systemic inflammatory response, resulting in acute respiratory distress syndrome (ARDS), even when not associated with an inhalation injury.

There are also widespread and long-term growth changes in the seriously burn-injured patient, which may never be restored. This may have special long-term consequences in children who sustain a major burn, particularly during their pubertal growth spurt.

Paramedic emergency and first aid treatment

While burn injuries appear visually dramatic to patients, relatives and care providers, the general immediate care and management remains the same for any patient with trauma. It is vital that those tasked with the pre-hospital care of burns patients not allow themselves to be distracted by either the initial appearances of the injury or the apparent general wellbeing of the victim. Appropriate measures in relation to both provision of burns first-aid treatment (BFAT) and application of general trauma care principles in relation to management of airway, ventilation and circulatory support may have a profound impact on the patient's final outcome.

For all patients, it is crucial that the first-responder/paramedic should initially ensure their own safety. It is certainly not uncommon that in providing first aid, the first-responder will themselves sustain a burn injury, especially in the setting of flame, chemical, radiation or electrical burns, doubling the number of victims and therefore resources required for treatment. If the patient is still alight, the correct approach remains to 'stop, drop and roll'.[13] A blanket, towel or similar item may be used to smother the flames. In the case of an electrical burn, the first-responder should exercise caution and ensure that the source of any current has been disconnected before approaching the patient, and use a non-conductor to separate the patient from the source.[30] Extensive chemical or radiological burns require the first-responder to seek additional resources before providing effective care safely.

The second step in stopping the burning process is cooling the burn, while avoiding hypothermia.[31] Australian and New Zealand Burn Association (ANZBA) guidelines define this as the application of cool (but not iced) running tap water to the burn wound for at least 20 minutes within 3 hours of the burn injury.[13] Children and the elderly would appear most at risk of hypothermia, especially with a greater than 20% TBSA burn cooled in a bath or shower. This may be avoided by warming the general environment and/or by the use of warm towels or a space blanket over that part of the patient that has not been burnt.

In addition to the analgesic action of cool running water, there now exists considerable experimental and epidemiological evidence to support the efficacy of this regimen in reducing burn wound depth.[32–34] Based on experimental data from a scald burn wound model, not only does cool running water appear the most effective treatment when used for 20 minutes, but it also remains effective even when its use has been delayed for up to 1 hour post injury.[33–36] Future studies may provide scientific evidence to support the efficacy of cool running water for up to 3 hours post injury.

While apparently straightforward in the case of a contact burn involving the hand, the provision of optimal BFAT often proves challenging in the setting of more-extensive burns or outside the hospital environment. Several studies in both adults and children have identified the very low number of patients provided with optimal BFAT.[16,37,38] While knowledge remains an issue, even among healthcare providers, there also would appear to be practical barriers to the use of cool running water outside the domestic or hospital environments.[23] This has led to the development of a variety of commercial products based on a foam dressing combined with water and melaleuca oil. Their effectiveness in the provision of BFAT, however, remains unproven by independent trials and they are likely to be less effective than cool running water.[34,39,40]

Further, as with the use of cold running water, special care should be taken with these products to avoid the risk of hypothermia.

BFAT should be continued at the scene by paramedics as long as management of the airway, breathing and circulation (ABCs) are not compromised.

PRACTICE TIP

Always check that the patient has had optimal burns first aid: cold running water for 20 minutes within 3 hours of the burn injury, avoiding hypothermia.

Immediate treatment

A standard approach to the management of airway, breathing and circulation was given in Chapter 44 (see also Ch 17, p. 314). Several specific issues in relation to management of the burns patient require emphasis. First, any burn injury might be associated with other forms of trauma, including a cervical fracture or thoracic injury. The paramedic needs to recall this and avoid being distracted by the burn injury in isolation. Second, the airway may initially be readily maintained by the patient but may be rapidly lost as a result of a combination of oedema secondary to the burn injury itself, compounded by the use of intravenous (IV) fluids. Particular caution is advised in the patient with an inhalational burn. Early indications of a potential airway burn include facial burns, stridor, hoarse voice with a brassy cough and tachypnoea. While not necessarily requiring intubation at the scene, the airway requires careful monitoring to avoid a more complex, emergent intubation with the patient in transit. Supplementary oxygenation should always be given; preferably 100% humidified oxygen via a non-rebreathing Hudson mask.

In relation to breathing, a circumferential or near-circumferential burn of the chest and upper abdomen may restrict ventilation, acting as a cuirasse or tight 'binding'. This rarely occurs in the first 2–4 hours post burn injury, but may develop insidiously especially after the patient has been commenced on IV fluids. If combined with an inhalational burn, it may be rapidly fatal as a result of the combination of impaired chest-wall compliance, airway and pulmonary oedema, alveolar collapse and vessel shunting, and systemic toxicity from compounds such as carbon monoxide and cyanide.[13]

Finally, circulatory support in the form of resuscitation with IV fluids will be required for 'large' or major burns, defined as > 10% TBSA in children and > 15% TBSA in adults.[13] These fluids should be commenced as soon as practical by the paramedic, to help support the circulation, in addition to the benefits of helping reduce the potential depth of the burn as a result of prompt resuscitation. Monitoring resuscitation of the burn patient in the pre-hospital setting may prove problematic, as both blood pressure and pulse rate may be difficult to measure and inaccurate as a result of limb oedema. External monitoring of the heart rate, if available, may therefore be the most effective option.[41] Intravenous or intra-nasal opioids should be given as required for analgesia.

It is often useful to document at this point the time and mechanism of injury, and what first aid (including its duration) and any other care has been provided. Often this information will otherwise be lost once the patient has been transferred to their definitive care location.

PRACTICE TIP

Optimal management of the patient's airway, breathing and circulation will assist in ensuring optimal management of the burn injury.

Transportation and transfer

There appears to be clear evidence in the literature that, with the exception of a small minority of patients with life-threatening problems identified in the primary survey or those injured in a rural setting, optimal care for the major burns patient may be best provided by direct transfer to a hospital with a burns unit.[42,43] ANZBA referral criteria have been summarised in Box 52.1.

For patients with minor burns, initial consultation with the local burns unit may avoid an unnecessary transfer or, equally, an inappropriately delayed referral. Each emergency department (ED) should have their region's burns transfer protocols clearly displayed and readily available online. Despite increasing numbers of referrals to centres with a burns unit, there remain instances of stable patients having secondary transfers from hospitals without a burns unit.[44,45] As well as representing poor use of resources, this delays the provision of optimal, definitive care.

For those patients requiring transfer, careful consideration should be given in consultation with the receiving burns unit as to the ideal timing and mode of transfer.[13] During this consultation with the medical and nursing staff of the receiving burns unit, joint decisions over the current management of the patient can be made to assist in the patient receiving the best possible care prior to and during their transfer (Box 52.2).

- Burn > 10% TBSA
- Full-thickness burn > 5% TBSA
- Burns of special areas:
  - face
  - hands
  - feet
  - genitalia and perineum
  - major joints
- Electrical burns
- Chemical burns
- Inhalational burn
- Circumferential burn of limb or torso
- Burns in children or the elderly
- Burns in patients with pre-existing illness
- Any burn with associated injuries

TBSA: total body surface area

BOX 52.2 **Preparation for transfer**

- Airway and breathing
- Secure airway
- 100% humidified oxygen
- Cervical spine protection if appropriate
- Circulation
- Two, secure large-bore intravenous cannulae
- Appropriate resuscitation fluids
- Monitor blood pressure, pulse and urine output
- Burn wound
- Cleaned chlorhexidine 0.1% or Normal saline
- Appropriate dressing
- Review need for tetanus prophylaxis
- Nutrition and support
- Gastric tube
- Consider enteric feeding if > 10% TBSA in child or > 15% TBSA in adult
- Keep the patient warm
- Analgesia and documentation
- Should be a narcotic, given intravenously
- Document management
- Copies of radiographs and other investigation results

TBSA: total body surface area

Many centres now offer the option of submitting photographs of the patient's burn wound so that a better-informed decision of the need and timing of transfer, or advice on immediate management, can be made. In addition to planning the transfer, advice can be given in relation to adequate BFAT, resuscitation, the need for escharotomies and use of dressings. Accurate determination of the TBSA of the burn remains crucial to assist in determining optimal resuscitation and fluid management, with both the more common overestimation and the less frequent underestimation equally deleterious

to overall management of the patient and their burn wound.[44,46,47] For other principles relating to interhospital transfer of patients, such as communication and transport type, see Chapter 16.

PRACTICE TIPS

- If in doubt, always discuss referral with a burns unit.
- A digital photograph from a mobile phone or digital camera facilitates communication.

Burns shock and fluid resuscitation

Adequate fluid resuscitation is critical to the survival of a severely burn-injured patient. Prior to the understanding of the massive fluid shifts and vascular changes that occur during burn shock, the leading cause of death after burn injury is from hypovolaemic shock or shock-induced renal failure. Combined with the fluid loss from the exudating wound, there is insufficient blood flow throughout the body to maintain adequate tissue perfusion. Burn shock is both hypovalaemic shock and cellular shock, and is characterised by specific haemodynamic changes, including decreased cardiac output, extracellular fluid, plasma volume and oliguria. As in the treatment for other forms of shock, the primary goal is to restore and preserve tissue perfusion and ultimately avoid ischaemia. In burn shock, resuscitation is complicated by burn oedema and major fluid shifts. These fluid shifts are caused by the increase in capillary permeability and alteration in cell membranes, which in a severe burn can occur in areas that have not been heat-injured.[48] Correction of this hypovolaemia is a life-saving task in the first hours following a major thermal injury,[25,48,49] and the aim is to give the least amount of fluid necessary to maintain adequate organ perfusion.

Estimating the fluid requirements is based on the extent of injury (TBSA), the patient's weight and by using a fluid resuscitation formula. The volume infused should be continually titrated so to avoid both under- and over-resuscitation.

PRACTICE TIPS

- The best measure of tissue perfusion in the major burns patient remains urine output.
- Over-resuscitation is more common and is as dangerous as under-resuscitation, especially in children and the elderly with major burns.

Extent of injury

Burn assessment tends to be done poorly, even by those who are experts.[50] There are three commonly used methods used to estimate burn size, and it is important that simple erythema is not included. This is a common error, and overestimation can occur and consequently fluid resuscitation is overcalculated.

- *Palmar method*: the surface area of a patient's palm (including fingers) is approximately 1% of TBSA. Relatively small burns can be assessed this way, but it is inaccurate for more-significant burns.

- *Rule of nines*: the body is divided into areas of 9% (Fig 52.3) and is a good, quick method to calculate adult burns. It is inaccurate for children because they have a different ratio of body to surface area. Children have proportionately smaller hips and legs, and larger shoulders and heads than adults. This may seriously under- or overestimate the size of the burn if used.
- The *Lund and Browder chart* (Fig 52.4) takes these considerations into account. If used correctly, it is the most accurate method. To make an accurate assessment, all of the burn must be exposed while keeping the environment warm. Pigmented skin can be difficult to assess, and if loose epidermal layers are not removed prior to estimation, the estimate will be undercalculated.[50]

PRACTICE TIPS

- Study a burns chart before you meet your first burns patient.
- Consider a commercial application (such as uBurn) available for smartphones to assist with calculation of the area of the burn.[51]

Estimating fluid requirements

The commonly used formula as approved by ANZBA is the Parkland formula:

- 3–4 mL crystalloid (e.g. Hartmann's solution or Normal saline)/kg bodyweight/percentage burn

These fluid requirements are required for children with burns > 10% TBSA and adults with burns > 15% TBSA. (See the section on burns in children for additional requirements.)

The calculation of fluid requirements commences from time of burn, not time of presentation. The calculated volume is that estimated for the first 24 hours. This is divided into two phases: half the calculated volume is given in the first 8 hours and the remaining half given over the succeeding 16 hours.[13,49]

Example: 70 kg man with a 40% burn

Parkland formula 4 × 70 × 40 = 11,200 for first 24 hours

Half this amount = 5,600 given from the time of burn,
   i.e. if 1 hour from injury, this is given over 7 hours =
   800 mL/hour

Second half is given over the next 16 hours = 350 mL/hour

The most reliable method of monitoring fluid resuscitation is by closely following urine output. Adequate organ perfusion is maintained if urine output is kept near the following ranges:

- Adults 0.5 mL/kg/h
- Children (< 30 kg) 1.0 mL/kg/h

A urinary catheter is essential for accurately monitoring urine output, and should be inserted for burns that require intravenous fluid resuscitation.

Fluids need to be titrated, as large urine output indicates excessive fluid resuscitation with gratuitous oedema formation; low urine output indicates poor tissue perfusion.[13,49]

Pain relief

A burn injury is extremely painful and in all but the most minor cases should be given narcotic analgesia intravenously. Taking

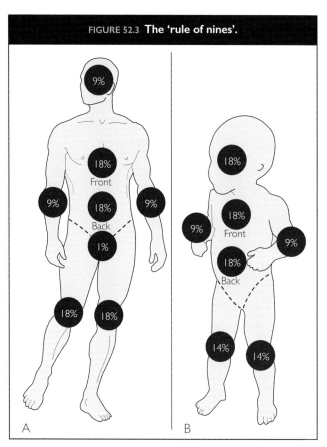

FIGURE 52.3 **The 'rule of nines'.**

A, Adult. **B**, Child.[2]

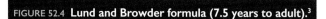

FIGURE 52.4 **Lund and Browder formula (7.5 years to adult).**[3]

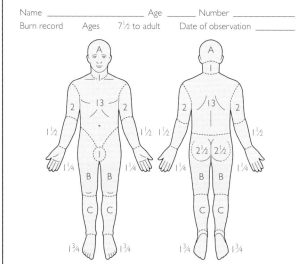

Relative percentages of areas affected by growth

Area	Age 10	15	Adult
A = ½ of head	5½	4½	3½
B = ½ of one thigh	4¼	4½	4¾
C = ½ of one leg	3	3¼	3½

% Burn by areas

Lund and Browder Chart
Estimation of extent of burn (7½ yrs–adult)

into account any pre-existing disease or associated injury, IV morphine 0.05–0.1 mg/kg should be administered as soon as possible. Further doses are often required, but must be titrated against pain and sedation, followed by early commencement of narcotic infusion.

Inhalational injury

Inhalation injuries, whether seen in conjunction with a cutaneous injury or in isolation, are one of the most critical injuries following a thermal injury and are strongly linked to an increase in mortality.[52,53] Inhalation injury requires early diagnosis and treatment and is classified according to the site of injury:

1. Airway injury above the larynx.
2. Airway injury below the larynx.
3. Systemic intoxication injury.

A patient may have one or more of the above types of injury. See Box 52.3 for clinical indicators of an inhalation injury and Figure 52.5 for facial and inhalation injury.

Upper airway injuries

These are caused by the inhalation of hot gases and are most likely to occur in an enclosed space (if trapped in a fire) or with the inhalation of steam. As in thermal injury to skin, inhalation injuries above the larynx produce inflammatory mediators to cause oedema and loss of the protective functions of the mucosa. This leads to respiratory obstruction, which may not occur until 12–36 hours post injury as the body responds to the injury, oedema progresses and fluid resuscitation fluid is given.

The upper respiratory tract has a tremendous ability to reflect heat; it is only after extreme heat exposure that pure heat damage to the lower respiratory tract occurs.[52,54,55]

Lower airway injuries

Burns to the airway below the larynx are produced by inhalation of the products of combustion. Fires produce by-products, which include carbon monoxide and dioxide, cyanide, esters and complex organic compounds, ammonia, phosgene and hydrogen chloride. When these compounds dissolve in the water contained in the respiratory mucous membranes they produce strong acids and alkalis, which cause irritation, bronchospasm,

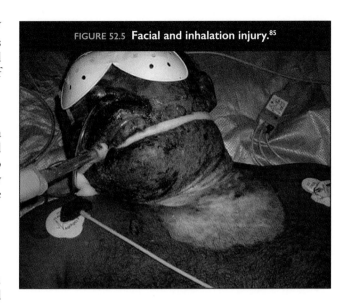
FIGURE 52.5 **Facial and inhalation injury.**[85]

ulceration and oedema. Laryngospasm and breath-holding are protective mechanisms against irritation in a conscious patient. An unconscious patient loses these mechanisms, however, resulting in a more severe injury.[54–56]

Systemic toxins

Carbon monoxide (CO) intoxication is the most common systemic intoxication associated with burns.[54,55] Oxygen is utilised during combustion and in turn CO is released due to incomplete oxidation of carbon. CO is a colourless and odourless gas which binds 200 times more readily with haemoglobin than oxygen, forming carboxyhaemoglobin (COHb). This reduces the oxygen-carrying capacity of the blood, and tissue anoxia occurs. CO can go on to bind with the intracellular cytochrome system, leading to further cell death.

Patients with CO intoxication are often misdiagnosed with alcohol intoxication as they often display similar symptoms. Therefore, CO intoxication must be ruled out prior to a diagnosis of alcohol intoxication.

Patients with an altered state of consciousness after a burn injury have CO intoxication unless proven otherwise. The majority of deaths occurring at the scene of a fire are due to CO intoxication; what we often hear reported as 'being overcome by the fumes'.

A thorough history is required, as burns in an enclosed space, such as a house, motor vehicle or aircraft, or burns with an associated explosion from petrol or gas fire or from a bomb, are likely to be associated with an inhalation injury. Symptoms of CO poisoning include cherry-red skin, tachypnoea, headache, dizziness and nausea, but commonly do not manifest until COHb levels are greater than 20% (Table 52.1).

Assessment and treatment

Maximum tissue oxygenation for all burn injuries during the initial assessment is facilitated by the administration of humidified oxygen at 10 L/min. This is especially imperative in those with a suspected inhalation injury. Intubation may be necessary in injuries above the larynx if increasing airway obstruction is detected, and without delay. In injuries below the larynx, intubation may be necessary to clear secretions,

---

BOX 52.3 Clinical indicators of an inhalation injury

- Burns to the mouth, nose and pharynx
- Sputum containing soot
- Change of voice
- Hoarse, brassy cough
- Inspiratory stridor
- Tracheal tug
- Singed nasal hairs
- Productive cough
- Respiratory distress
- Rib retraction
- Flaring of alae nasae
- Restlessness

TABLE 52.1 Carbon monoxide intoxication	
CARBOXYHAEMOGLOBIN (COHb) %	SYMPTOMS
0–15	None (smokers, long-distance truck drivers)
15–20	Headache, confusion
20–40	Nausea, fatigue, disorientation, irritability
40–60	Hallucinations, ataxia, syncope, convulsions, coma
> 60	Death

along with intermittent positive-pressure ventilation. (See Ch 17, p. 318, for details on intubation.)

The clinical indicators of an inhalation injury evolve over time, as with all traumas; therefore, repeat evaluation is critical. Constant observation of a change in these signs can detect the complications of an inhalation injury, which include airway obstruction, deteriorating consciousness, retained secretions, deteriorating oxygenation and respiratory failure. In assessing for an inhalation injury, one of the most useful tools is the fibre-optic bronchoscope, which allows for direct visualisation of the supraglottic airway and tracheobronchial tree.[55,56]

Treatment of systemic intoxication includes respiratory support as described above, along with protection of the unconscious patient and allowing for the natural washout effect with time.[54,55,57] The use of inhaled beta-agonists, such as salbutamol, can assist in the severe bronchospasm resulting from the inhalation of irritants.[57] There has also been a reported benefit of using aerosolised heparin, which acts as a mucolytic to help prevent the build-up of secretions.[54,58] Fibre-optic bronchoscopy can also be effective in lavaging when physical therapy and pharmacological agents still fail to expectorate secretions.[54]

It must be noted that several studies have shown that the patient's fluid requirement is increased when an inhalation injury is present.[13,54]

PRACTICE TIP

- Always consider the possibility of airway injury.
- Warmed, humidified, supplemental oxygen will benefit most patients, especially those with a major burn injury.

Burn wound assessment and management

Depth

Burn depth is classified in Australia and New Zealand via the following system, depending on the depth of tissue damage:

- epidermal
- superficial dermal
- mid-dermal
- deep dermal
- full thickness.

It is important to remember, however, that all burns are a mixture of different depths. Refer to Table 52.2 and Figure 52.6 for diagnosis of burn depth.

Wound management

The fundamental aim of all burn care management is to achieve wound closure in a timely fashion with minimal complications. This is dependent on wound care, good nutrition, maintenance of function, oedema reduction, prevention of infection and adequate analgesia (see Ch 17, p. 372, for a discussion on types of wound management).

Wound care should promote spontaneous healing, prevent further tissue loss, prevent infection, provide optimal conditions for surgery if required and be as painless as possible.[59,60]

Debridement of the burn wound removes devitalised tissue from the wound and is an important measure in the promotion of wound healing. It reduces the wound's biological burden, clearing the debris that slows cellular movement necessary for healing and minimising infection.[59,60]

TABLE 52.2 Diagnosis of burn depth[87]					
DEPTH	COLOUR	BLISTERS	CAPILLARY REFILL	SENSATION	HEALING
Epidermal	Red	No	Present	Present	Yes
Superficial dermal	Pale pink	Small	Present	Painful	Yes
Mid-dermal	Dark pink	Present	Sluggish	±	Usual
Deep dermal	Blotchy red	±	Absent	Absent	No
Full thickness	White	No	Absent	Absent	No

±: may or may not be present

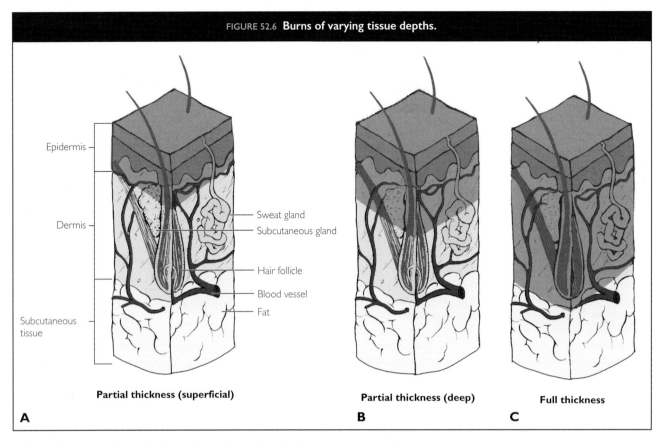

FIGURE 52.6 **Burns of varying tissue depths.**

Epidermis

Dermis

Sweat gland

Subcutaneous gland

Hair follicle

Blood vessel

Fat

Subcutaneous
tissue

Partial thickness (superficial)

Partial thickness (deep)

Full thickness

A

B

C

A, Superficial dermal burn. **B**, Deep dermal burn. **C**, Full-thickness burn injury.[4]

Warm and moist wound-healing principles are well supported; a burn dressing aims to protect the wound, provide patient comfort and function and reduce evaporative losses. There are many varieties of dressings available, including: silver dressings, foams, hydrofibres, calcium alginates, hydrocolloids, hydrogels, polyurethrane-membrane-supported gels, film dressings and biological dressings. Different products seem to work in different centres, with contributing factors including patient demographics, local environment and product availability. The important factors that need to be considered when selecting a suitable dressing are:

- depth of the burn (determines amount of exudate)
- site of the burn
- extent of the burn
- possibility of removing dressing without traumatising tissue
- type of burn first aid (e.g. cooling of burn in dirty river water may increase the risk of infection)
- cause of the burn (burns caused by flammable liquids or hot oil have a high risk of infection)
- whether it protects against mechanical trauma
- how functional and manageable it is by the patient (or caregiver), especially if managed in an ambulatory setting
- cost.

In the case of a patient who requires transfer to a burns unit, the wounds should be gently washed with chlorhexidine solution or Normal saline and covered with cling wrap or a clean, dry sheet. Care must be taken not to wrap cling wrap around circumferential burns; lay it lengthways so as not to further restrict circulation. Advice on burn wound management will be discussed by consultation with the receiving burns unit, especially if transfer is going to be delayed. Advice on burn wound treatment for all burns can be gained through contact with your referral burns unit irrespective of the need for transfer.

Specific burn management

Epidermal/superficial dermal burns

The very superficial burn or epidermal burn that has no epidermal loss requires no dressing management. Sunburns or flash injuries typically fall into this category, and can be treated with a moisturising cream and pain relief as they are extremely painful.

Superficial dermal burns that involve skin loss can be treated with a variety of wound-care products that aim at encouraging re-epithelisation. These include hydocolloids, polyurethane-membrane-supported gels and film dressings. An antimicrobial may need to be considered if infection is present or suspected.

Partial-thickness burns

Burns in this category include mid-dermal and deep dermal, depending on the extent of injury. After initial wound debridement—removing all devitalised skin, including blisters—these burns can be managed with products from the following groups:

- hydrocolloids
- polyurethane films
- foam dressings
- calcium alginates
- silver dressings.

Specialised burn units may also utilise temporary skin substitutes such as Biobrane for mid- to deep dermal burns.

Full-thickness burns

Full-thickness burn injuries involve both the epidermal and the dermal layers, extending to the subcutaneous fat, and consequently require antibacterial dressings. The most common antibacterial dressings used in burn care contain silver, and there are several varieties available. The choice of product is guided by the same principles for any dressing. Full-thickness burn injuries require surgical intervention unless they are of limited size, and require referral to a specialised burn unit for ongoing treatment.

Circumferential burns

A deep dermal or full-thickness burn loses the ability to expand as oedema progresses. When the burn involves the whole of a limb or the chest, it may become necessary to release the burn wound surgically by incising the burned skin down to the subcutaneous fat. This procedure is known as an escharotomy (see Fig 52.7). If transfer to a burns unit is going to be delayed, this may have to be performed by the referral centre following consultation and advice.

Limbs

When a limb is burned circumferentially the rigid burned skin may interfere with circulation. Affected limbs must be elevated to limit swelling and closely observed for:

- deep pain at rest
- pain on passive movement of distal joints
- loss of distal circulation
- pallor
- decrease of capillary return
- coolness
- loss of palpable pulses
- numbness
- decrease in oxygen saturations.

> **PRACTICE TIP**
>
> - Initial appearances can be very deceiving: never reassure patients or relatives that the burn is 'just superficial and will heal in a few days'.
> - Early escharotomy can be limb saving.

Electrical burns

Electrical burns account for between 2% and 10% of all burn injuries.[61,62] As a result of occupational exposure they remain more common in adults.[62,63] Traditionally these burns have been classified by voltage, whether high (greater than 1000 V, including lightning burns) or low (less than 1000 V), although this may not necessarily reflect injury severity.[64] High-voltage injuries may be associated with cardiac or respiratory arrest at the scene.[13,62] In a number of cases, reported electrical burns may in fact represent a flash or flame burn as a result of a short-circuit or blown fuse.[65]

True electrical burns are characteristically full thickness and associated with an entry and exit site. A careful examination of the patient should be performed to determine the location of

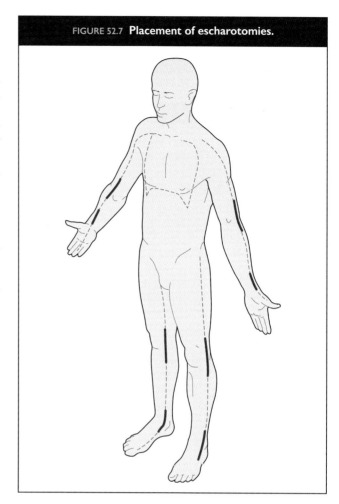

FIGURE 52.7 **Placement of escharotomies.**

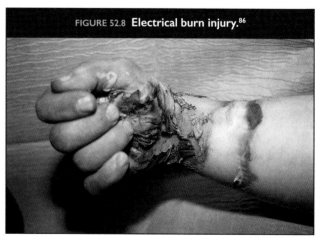

FIGURE 52.8 **Electrical burn injury.**[86]

both sites, as this provides important information on the likely path of the electrical current (Fig 52.8). Those that have passed along a limb or across the torso have a greater risk of injury to deeper structures, compartment syndrome and myocardial dysrhythmias.[64,66]

While ECG monitoring has been generally recommended for 24 hours post injury in patients with electrical burns, the risk of haemodynamically significant dysrhythmias would appear very low after 4 hours.[13,61,62] As a result of the greater heating effect of the electrical current on high-resistance structures such as bone, termed the Joule effect, apparently minor superficial electrical burns may be associated with extensive muscle oedema leading to compartment syndrome and, potentially, renal failure from secondary myoglobinuria.[13,62,64] As the risk of complications and associated injuries remains high, all patients with an electrical burn injury should be transferred to a burns unit.[13]

Chemical burns

Chemical burns make up a small number of burn injuries seen, particularly in children. Chemical burns, like all burn injuries, cause a denaturation of cell protein. The denaturation in burn injury may be due to heat, changes in pH or dissolution of lipids. Chemical burns can cause progressive damage until the chemical is inactivated. The severity of this type of burn depends on the type of chemical, strength of the agent, quantity, length of exposure, amount of tissue involved and the mechanism of action. Skin damage can range from erythema through to necrosis. There are three categories of chemical agents:

1. alkalis—producing liquefaction necrosis and loosening of tissue
2. acids—producing coagulative necrosis and precipitation of protein
3. organic compounds—causing chemical and systemic effects.[67,68]

Alkaline agents generally cause more tissue damage than acids, although paradoxically acid burns are at least initially more painful, with the destructive effects of alkali burns occurring more slowly over time. The first aid for chemical burns involves removing the agent from contact with the patient. It is important to ensure the protection of the first-aid providers. Caution must be exercised so as not to cause damage to uninjured tissue by an inadvertent spread of the chemical agent. Dry powders should be brushed off before irrigation is commenced. Chemical burns require copious lavage and irrigation may need to continue anywhere from 30 minutes to 2 hours, or until pain resulting from the chemical injury ceases. Alkali burns particularly require prolonged irrigation, generally for at least 1 hour.[13]

Hydrofluoric acid, an industrial cleaning agent occasionally used in a domestic setting on alloy wheels, requires special mention because of its unique and rapid toxicity, even when only a very small TBSA has been involved.[69] The fluorine binds calcium ions, causing a profound hypocalcaemia, which leads to dysrhythmias and death. While irrigation with water should still be performed, calcium gluconate is a specific antidote, preferentially binding the free fluoride ions. It may be used topically as a gel, or given IV, with complete relief of pain the best indicator that adequate treatment has been provided.[13,69]

Interestingly, petrol may cause a chemical burn even when ignition has not occurred. While these burns are typically only partial-thickness, they may be readily avoided by prompt irrigation of all areas exposed.

Ingestion or aspiration of corrosive agents is really beyond the scope of this text, but fortunately has become much less frequent in Australasia as a result of improvements in prevention through the use of child-proof containers.[70] While such injuries remain more common in children, typically they now occur when an adult has elected to store a usually alkaline corrosive agent in a recycled drinks container. As with all alkaline burns, the severity of the injury will usually not initially be appreciated. All such patients should be carefully evaluated clinically and should have both chest and abdominal radiography performed to exclude free air from a perforation. Subsequent endoscopy to assess the pharynx, oesophagus and stomach should be performed, as the absence of intraoral burns does not necessarily exclude a clinically important injury of the aerodigestive tract. While IV steroids may be of benefit in reducing the inflammatory element of inhalational chemical burns, they appear to be of no proven benefit following caustic ingestion.[71]

Bitumen and friction burns

Hot bitumen burns typically occur as an occupational injury. Immediate BFAT with cold running water should be applied, but no attempt made to physically remove the bitumen in the field, as this may cause further injury.[13] Subsequently, paraffin oil should be applied and the bitumen removed mechanically as part of a surgical debridement.

Friction burns may be seen in both adults and children, often as a result of falls from bicycles onto the road, pedestrian versus motor vehicle trauma or entrapment in a home treadmill.[72] The depth of these burns is often very difficult to appreciate initially and there may be underlying neurovascular or tendon involvement, especially in children. Wound management for these injuries is dependent on depth assessment and other considerations, as with all burn wounds.

Eyes

Unless the mechanism of injury can rule out eye damage, e.g. an isolated contact burn, all facial burns need to undergo an eye examination.[13] This is especially imperative in chemical injuries, which require copious irrigation with water for up to 3 hours. Contact lenses, if worn, should be removed, as chemicals can track behind the lens and damage the cornea. Irrigation should continue after lens removal. Early eye examination using staining with fluorescein eye drop can detect any corneal damage before the resultant oedema makes it difficult and even impossible to perform.

Burns in children

Burns in children remain distinct from those in adults as a result of physiological differences, psychological aspects in relation to the response to the injury, and important variations in aetiology and their impact on likely outcomes (see Ch 36).[14,15] While the overall approach and management strategies remain the same, an understanding of the differences will facilitate improved outcomes in this important group of patients for whom the consequences of the injury may be lifelong

Aetiology and prevention of burns in children

The predominance of scald injuries in children has been well documented, reflecting the propensity of toddlers exploring the home environment to sustain burn injuries while poorly supervised.[73,74] Approximately two-thirds of burn injuries in children will involve toddlers or preschool-age children with scald burns to the head, neck, upper torso and arms

(Fig 52.9).[22,31,73,74] Typically these burns will be mixed depth, with the child's relatively thin skin predisposing them to a proportionally deeper burn in relation to that suffered by an adult following exposure to the same hot liquid for the same time.[16] These same differences make accurate prediction of burn wound outcome problematic in children, stimulating the development of new technologies to determine the need for operative surgical intervention in deep burns.[75] Great caution should be exercised by first-responders and all clinicians involved in the initial care of these patients regarding falsely reassuring parents or carers over the likely depth of the burn.

In addition to their propensity for scald burns, children remain at risk of several specific forms of burn injury infrequently seen in adults; in addition, sadly, to burns as a result of non-accidental injury. These include friction burns from home treadmills, hot noodle burns and those resulting from contact with inadequately insulated reflective oven doors, all recently identified as major sources of morbidity in the paediatric age group.[72,76–79] As with scald burns, prevention has been shown to be effective but remains only sporadically applied and requiring constant re-enforcement.[73,79–82] Nursing and allied health professionals remain uniquely positioned to influence the approach of parents and older children to this important issue.[24]

Health professionals need to show that it is understood how difficult it is to watch a child constantly and how demanding it is to keep children safe.

It is not the task of health professionals to evaluate the probability of abuse and neglect. It is part of the burns assessment, however, to attempt to fully understand how the injury happened so as to help reduce the risks of similar injuries to other children.

Any suspicion of neglect or an inflicted injury requires reporting to the appropriate mandatory body.

Indicators for a possible non-accidental burn

- Delay in seeking help
- Different accounts of history of injury over time
- Injury inconsistent with history or with the development capacity of the child
- Past abuse or family violence
- Inappropriate behaviour/interaction of child or caregivers.
- Obvious immersion patterns, e.g. glove or sock patterns
- Symmetrical burns of uniform depth

- Restraint injuries on upper arms
- Other signs of abuse or neglect such as numerous healed wounds.

Response to burn injury in children

The normal response in an adult would be to first avoid an obvious source of burn injury. Second, if suffering a burn, the adult would immediately withdraw and instinctively cool the burn. These three responses remain at best infrequent in children: in addition to unguarded exploration of their environment, preschool-age children will often simply cry out when sustaining a burn rather than withdraw from the painful stimulus. This predisposes them to a longer duration and therefore a deeper burn. These behavioural differences highlight the special importance of the first-responder and paramedic in applying optimal BFAT for the paediatric burns patient.[10,16,37]

Management of burn injuries in children

As a result of their greater ratio of surface area to bodyweight, children have a proportionally greater metabolic rate and higher rates of water and heat loss than adults. A greater proportion of their total body water remains extracellular, further increasing fluid losses in burn injury. In addition, their compensatory mechanisms, such as shivering, are either reduced or much less effective, especially in the infant and toddler age groups. As a result, they are more likely to suffer hypothermia following a burn injury, and require resuscitation with IV fluids and nutritional support. Thus children with > 10% TBSA burns will require IV fluids and nutritional supplementation, usually initially via a gastric tube.[13] In addition to resuscitation fluids, children will require maintenance fluids with glucose to avoid hypoglycaemia (see Box 52.4).[13,83] The predominantly diaphragmatic nature of breathing in children increases the likelihood of the need for an escharotomy of a chest or upper abdominal burn to permit adequate ventilation.

Just as there are differences in treatment, there are several differences in relation to monitoring the paediatric burn patient. Due to their usually normal cardiovascular system and enhanced reserves, but potentially rapid decline into shock, assessment of hypovolaemia requires a multimodal approach rather than a reliance on blood pressure and pulse alone.[13,41] In particular, skin colour, temperature and capillary refill should be frequently assessed in addition to urine output as a guide to the patient's status and response to resuscitation.[13,41]

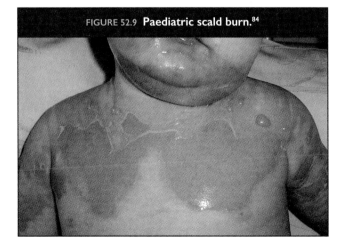

FIGURE 52.9 Paediatric scald burn.[84]

BOX 52.4 IV fluids in paediatric burns

- Give resuscitation and maintenance fluids if the burn is > 10% TBSA
- Resuscitation fluids follow adult formula
- Maintenance fluids of 4% dextrose in 1/4 or 1/5 Normal saline over the first 24 hours:
    - 100 mL/kg up to 10 kg
    - plus 50 mL/kg from 10 to 20 kg
    - plus 20 mL/kg for each kg over 20 kg
- Monitor blood pressure, pulse and capillary refill
- Aim for urine output of 1.0 mL/kg/h

TBSA: total body surface area

SUMMARY

Burns represent a potentially devastating form of trauma with important long-term consequences. Optimal first aid and initial medical management, including securing the airway and ensuring appropriate fluid resuscitation, may make a significant positive impact in reducing the need for operative intervention and subsequent scarring. Just as a major burn may involve every organ system, so too will patients benefit from optimal management through the coordinated efforts of a multi-disciplinary care team.

CASE STUDY 1

You have been called to the scene of a 20-year-old man weighing 80 kg after he sustained a flame burn. The injury occurred when his older brother threw petrol onto a camp fire. He has burns to the front and backs of both legs and his abdomen.

Questions

1. Outline your initial examination of this patient.

2. Using the information below, calculate the total body surface area of this burn injury. You may want to use a body chart to assist you.

   Both legs; whole fronts of thigh and leg = 18%

   Backs of leg to mid-thigh = 18%

   Abdomen; below umbilicus to groin = 9%

3. Use your answer above to calculate the fluid requirements of this patient. How do you monitor the adequacy of the fluids?

4. During your examination you note circumferential burns to both legs. What does this indicate? What observations need to be carried out?

5. Your secondary survey reveals no further injury, and transfer to a burns unit is advised. Outline the reasons for transfer.

6. What wound care is required prior to transfer?

 Answers to Case Study Questions can be found on evolve
http://evolve.emergencytrauma.curtis

CASE STUDY 2

Using the Parkland formula calculate the fluid resuscitation required for a 12 kg 17-month-old who sustained a 25% scald to her face, neck, chest, abdomen and thighs when she pulled a kettle of hot water onto herself this morning at 0930. You are called to the scene immediately. When you arrive the mother is in the shower with the child.

Questions

1. Outline your initial response.

2. Calculate the fluid resuscitation using the Parkland formula.

3. Calculate the maintenance fluids with % dextrose and 0.45% Normal saline.

 Answers to Case Study Questions can be found on evolve
http://evolve.emergencytrauma.curtis

USEFUL WEBSITES

Australian and New Zealand Burn Association, www.anzba.org.au/
International Society for Burn Injuries, www.worldburn.org/

REFERENCES

1. Jackson DM. The diagnosis of the depth of burning. Br J Surg 1953;40:588–96.
2. Elliot D, Aitken L, Chaboyer W, eds. ACCCN's critical care nursing. Sydney: Elsevier; 2006.
3. Hawley R, King J. Australian nurses' dictionary. 3rd edn. Sydney: Ballière Tindall; 2004.

4. Edlich R, Bailey T, Bill T. Thermal burns. In: Marx T, Hockenberger R, Walls R, eds. Rosen's emergency medicine: concept and clinical practice. 5th edn. St. Louis: Mosby; 2002.

5. Meyer AA. Death and disability from injury: a global challenge. J Trauma: Injury, Infec Crit Care 1998;44:1–12.

6. Burd A, Yuen C. A global study of hospitalized burn patients. Burns 2005;31:432–8.

7. Team B-NBRP. Bi-National Burns Registry Annual Report. Melbourne: Monash University;2013.

8. Keswani MH. The cost of burns and the relevance of prevention. J Burn Care Rehabil 1996;17:485–90.

9. D'Cruz R, Martin HCO, Holland AJA. Medical management of paediatric burn injuries: Best practice part 2. J Paediat Child Health 2013.

10. Allison K. The UK pre-hospital management of burn patients: current practice and the need for a standard approach. Burns 2002;28(2):135–42.

11. Allison K, Porter K. Consensus on the pre-hospital approach to burns patient management. Injury 2004;35(8):734–8.

12. Pruitt BA Jr, Goodwin CW, Mason AD Jr. Epidemiological, demographic, and outcome characteristics of burn injury. In: Herndon D, ed. Total burn care. Vol 2. London: Saunders; 2002:16–30.

13. Committee TE. Emergency manual of severe burns course manual. In: Association AaNZB, 15th edn. Albany Creek: ANZBA; 2011.

14. Spinks A, Wasiak J, Cleland H et al. Ten-year epidemiological study of pediatric burns in Canada. J Burn Care Res 2008;29:482–8.

15. Tse T, Poon CHY, Tse K et al. Paediatric burn prevention: An epidemiological approach. Burns 2006;32(2):229–34.

16. Holland AJA. Pediatric burns: the forgotten trauma of childhood. Can J Surg 2006;49(4):272–7.

17. Forjuoh SN. Burns in low- and middle-income countries: a review of available literature on descriptive epidemiology, risk factors, treatment, and prevention. Burns 2006;32:529–37.

18. Foglia RP, Moushey R, Meadows L et al. Evolving treatment in a decade of pediatric burn care. J Pediatr Surg 2004;39(6):957–60.

19. Forjuoh SN. The mechanisms, intensity of treatment, and outcomes of hospitalized burns: issues for prevention. J Burn Care Rehab 1998;19(5):456–60.

20. den Hertog PC, Blankendaal FA, ten Hag SM. Burn injuries in The Netherlands. Accid Anal Prev 2000;32(3):355–64.

21. Hettiaratchy S, Dziewulski P. ABC of burns. Introduction. BMJ 2004;328(7452):1366–8.

22. Abeyasundara SLR, Lam L, Harvey JG et al. The changing pattern of pediatric burns. J Burn Care Res 2011;32(2):178–84.

23. Rea S, Kuthubutheen J, Fowler B, Wood F. Burns first aid in Western Australia—do healthcare workers have the knowledge? Burns 2005;31:1029–34.

24. Grant EJ. Burn prevention. Crit Care Nurs Clin North Am 2004;16(1):127–38.

25. Rutan RL. Physiological response to cutaneous burn injury. In: Carrougher GJ, ed. Burn care and therapy. Missouri: Mosby; 1998:1–34.

26. Williams WG. Pathophysiology of the burn wound. In: Herndon D, ed. Total burn care. Vol 2. London: Saunders; 2002:514–22.

27. Norbury WB, Herndon DN. Modulation of the hypermetabolic respose after burn injury. In: Herndon D, ed. Total Burn Care. Philadephia: Saunders Elsevier; 2007:420–33.

28. Williams FN, Herndon DN, Kulp GA, Jeschke MG. Propranolol decreases cardiac work in a dose-dependent manner in severely burned children. Surgery 2011;149(2):231–9.

29. Beierle EA, Chung DH. Surgical management of complications of burn injury. In: Herndon D, ed. Total burn care. Philadephia: Saunders Elsevier; 2007:502–12.

30. Mlcak RP, Buffalo MC. Pre-hospital management, transportation, and emergency care. In: Herndon DN, ed. Total burn care. Vol 3. Philadelphia: Saunders Elsevier; 2007:81–92.

31. Kim LKP, Martin HCO, Holland AJA. Medical management of paediatric burn injuries: best practice. J Paediat Child Health 2012;48(4):290–5.

32. Nguyen NL, Gun RT, Sparnon AL, Ryan P. The importance of immediate cooling—a case series of childhood burns in Vietnam. Burns 2002;28(2):173–6.

33. Yuan J, Wu C, Holland AJA et al. Assessment of cooling on an acute burn wound in a porcine model. J Burn Care Res 2007;28:514–20.

34. Cuttle L, Pearn J, McMillan JR, Kimble R. A review of first aid treatments for burn injuries. Burns 2009;35(6):768–75.

35. Bartlett N, Yuan J, Holland AJ et al. Optimal duration of cooling for an acute scald contact burn injury in a porcine model. J Burn Care Res 2008;29:828–34.

36. Rajan V, Bartlett N, Harvey JG et al. Delayed cooling of an acute scald contact burn injury in a porcine model: is it worthwhile? J Burn Care Res 2009;30(4):729–34.

37. McCormack RA, La Hei ER, Martin HC. First-aid management of minor burns in children: a prospective study of children presenting to the Children's Hospital at Westmead, Sydney. Med J Aust 2003;178(1):31–3.

38. O'Neill AC, Purcell E, Jones D et al. Inadequacies in the first aid management of burns presenting to plastic surgery services. Ir Med J 2005;98(1):15–16.

39. Cuttle L, Kempf M, Kravchuk O et al. The efficacy of Aloe vera, tea tree oil and saliva as first aid treatment for partial thickness burn injuries. Burns 2008;34:1176–82.

40. Price J. Burnaid. Burns 1998;24(1):80–2.

41. DeBoer S, O'Connor A. Prehospital and emergency department burn care. Crit Care Nurs Clin North Am 2004;16(1):61–73.

42. Sanchez JL, Pereperez SB, Bastida JL, Martinez MM. Cost-utility analysis applied to the treatment of burn patients in a specialized center. Arch Surg 2007;142(1):50–7.

43. Wong K, Heath T, Maitz P, Kennedy P. Early in-hospital management of burn injuries in Australia. ANZ J Surg 2004;74(5):318–23.

44. Greenwood JE, Tee R, Jackson WL. Increasing numbers of admissions to the adult burns service at the Royal Adelaide Hospital 2001–2004. ANZ J Surg 2007;77(5):358–63.

45. Holland AJ, Jackson AM, Joseph AP. Paediatric trauma at an adult trauma centre. ANZ J Surg 2005;75(10):878–81.

46. Freiburg C, Igneri P, Sartorelli K, Rogers F. Effects of differences in percent total body surface area estimation on fluid resuscitation of transferred burn patients. J Burn Care Res 2007;28(1):42–9.

47. Chan QE, Barzi F, Cheney L et al. Burn size estimation in children: still a problem. Emerg Med Australas 2012;24(2):181–6.

48. Kramer GC, Lund T, Beckum OK. Pathophysiology of burn shock and burn oedema. In: Herndon D, ed. Total burn care. Philadelphia: Saunders Elsevier; 2007:93–106.

49. Warden GD. Fluid resuscitation and early management. In: Herndon D, ed. Total burn care. Philadelphia: Saunders Elsevier; 2007.

50. Hettiaratchy S, Papini R. Initial management of a major burn: II—assessment and resuscitation. Br Med J 2004;329:101–3.

51. Morris R, Javed M, Bodger O et al. A comparison of two smartphone applications and the validation of smartphone applications as tools for fluid calculation for burns resuscitation. Burns 2014;40(5):826–34.

52. Woodson LC. Diagnosis and grading of inhalation injury. J Burn Care Res 2009;30(1):143–5.

53. Palmieri TL. Inhalation injury consensus conference: conclusions. J Burn Care Res 2009;30(1):209–10.

54. Toon MH, Maybauer MO, Greenwood JE et al. Management of acute smoke inhalation injury. Crit Care Resusc 2010;12(1):53–61.

55. Fidkowski CW, Fuzaylov G, Sheridan RL, Cote CJ. Inhalation burn injury in children. Paediatr Anaesth 2009;19 Suppl 1:147–54.

56. Palmieri TL, Warner P, Mlcak RP et al. Inhalation injury in children: a 10-year experience at Shriners Hospitals for Children. J Burn Care Res 2009;30(1):206–8.

57. Palmieri TL. Use of beta-agonists in inhalation injury. J Burn Care Res 2009;30(1):156–9.

58. Palmieri TL, Enkhbaatar P, Sheridan R et al. Studies of inhaled agents in inhalation injury. J Burn Care Res 2009;30(1):169–71.

59. Kavanagh S, McRae S. Burns nursing study guides. Adelaide: The University of Adelaide; 2005.

60. Alsbjorn B, Gilbert P, Hartmann B et al. Guidelines for the management of partial-thickness burns in a general hospital or community setting—recommendations of a European working party. Burns 2007;33(2):155–60.

61. Tomkins KL, Holland AJ. Electrical burn injuries in children. J Paediatr Child Health. 2008.

62. Rai J, Jeschke MG, Barrow RE, Herndon DN. Electrical injuries: A 30-year review. J Trauma Inj Infec Crit Care 1999;46:933–6.

63. Arnoldo B, Klein M, Gibran NS. Practice guidelines for the management of electrical injuries. J Burn Care Res 2006;27:439–47.

64. Lee RC. The pathophysiology and clinical management of electrical injury. In: Lee RC, Cravalho EG, Burke JF, eds. Electrical trauma: the pathophysiology, manifestations and clinical management. Cambridge: Cambridge University Press; 1992:33–79.

65. Fordyce TA, Kelsh M, Lu ET et al. Thermal burns and electrical injuries among electric utility workers, 1995–2004. Burns 2006;26:379–81.

66. Maghsoudi H, Adyani Y, Ahmadian N. Electrical and lightning injuries. J Burn Care Res 2007;28(2):255–61.

67. Palao R, Monge I, Ruiz M, Barret JP. Chemical burns: pathophysiology and treatment. Burns 2010;36(3):295–304.

68. Hardwicke J, Hunter T, Staruch R, Moiemen N. Chemical burns—an historical comparison and review of the literature. Burns 2012;38(3):383–7.

69. Wang X, Zhang Y, Ni L et al. A review of treatment strategies for hydrofluoric acid burns: Current status and future prospects. Burns 2014.

70. Riffat F, Cheng A. Pediatric caustic ingestion: 50 consecutive cases and a review of the literature. Dis Esophagus 2009;22(1):89–94.

71. Fulton JA, Hoffman RS. Steroids in second degree caustic burns of the esophagus: a systematic pooled analysis of fifty years of human data: 1956–2006. Clinical toxicology (Philadelphia, Pa) 2007;45(4):402–8.

72. Wong A, Maze D, La Hei E et al. Pediatric treadmill injuries: a public health issue. J Pediatr Surg 2007;42(12):2086–9.

73. Eadie PA, Williams R, Dickson WA. Thirty-five years of paediatric scalds: are lessons being learned? Br J Plast Surg 1995;48(2):103–5.

74. Dewar DJ, Magson CL, Fraser JF et al. Hot beverage scalds in Australian children. J Burn Care Rehabil 2004;25(3):224–7.

75. Holland AJA, Martin HC, Cass DT. Laser Doppler imaging prediction of burn wound outcome in children. Burns 2002;28(1):11–17.

76. Jeremijenko L, Mott J, Wallis B, Kimble R. Paediatric treadmill friction injuries. J Paediatr Child Health 2008;45:310–12.

77. Choo KL, Wallis B, Jain A et al. Too hot to handle: instant noodle burns in children. J Burn Care Res 2008;29(2):421–2.

78. Yen KL, Bank DE, O'Neill AM, Yurt RW. Household oven doors: a burn hazard in children. Arch Pediatr Adolesc Med 2001;155(1):84–6.

79. Atiyeh BS, Costagliola M, Hayek SN. Burn prevention mechanisms and outcomes: pitfalls, failures and successes. Burns 2009;35(2):181–93.

80. Cagle KJ, Davis JW, Dominic W, Gonzales W. Results of a focused scald-prevention program. J Burn Care Rehabil 2006;27(6):859–63.

81. Spallek M, Nixon J, Bain C et al. Scald prevention campaigns: do they work? J Burn Care Res 2007;28(2):328–33.

82. Durand MA, Green J, Edwards P et al. Perceptions of tap water temperatures, scald risk and prevention among parents and older people in social housing: a qualitative study. Burns 2012;38(4):585–90.

83. Mlcak R, Cortiella J, Desai MH, Herndon DN. Emergency management of pediatric burn victims. Pediatr Emerg Care 1998;14(1):51–4.

84. South Australia Health—Women and Children's Hospital Network, 2014.

85. Medhat EH. Initial burn management. Austin J Surg 2014;1(2):1010.

86. Barret JP, Herndon DN, eds. Color atlas of burn care. St Louis: WB Saunders; 2001.

87. Australia and New Zealand Burns Association. Emergency Manual of Severe Burns Course Manual (pamphlet). 10th edn. ANZBA; 2006.

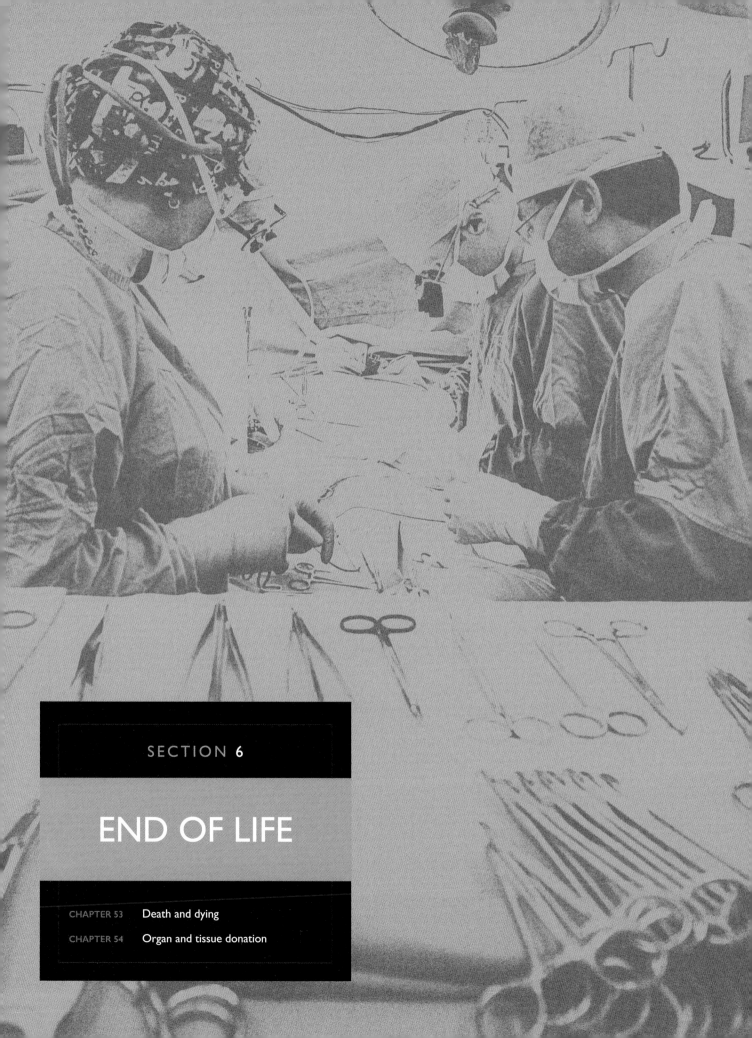

SECTION 6

END OF LIFE

CHAPTER 53
DEATH AND DYING
LINDA ORA AND DWIGHT ROBINSON

Essentials

- Appreciate the impact of culture on the patient and their family's experience through trauma, death and grief; and the impact of emergency organisational culture on the experience of the individual and their family.
- Understand the skills and processes that are required to facilitate appropriate care of patient and family in both expected and sudden or unexpected death situations.
- Ensure that emergency clinicians understand their role in the Advance Care Planning process, to respect and safeguard the patient's wishes for care at the end of life.
- Palliative care involves a full and active approach to comfort, and is the collective responsibility of all clinicians involved in a patient's care.
- Ensure emergency clinicians understand the legislation and guidelines in relation to management of death and dying in the country, state or territory they work in.

INTRODUCTION

The primary focus of emergency departments (EDs) and paramedic services is to minimise morbidity and mortality.[1] Despite this, life and death sit firmly alongside one another in the ED.[2] Providing care for a person who is dying or who has died, and supporting the person's family (both biological and non-biological significant others) during this difficult time are core components of the emergency clinician's role. Managing the practical and emotional aspects of a person's death in the ED and paramedical settings can be confronting for even the most experienced emergency clinician. There are two broad categories of death in the emergency setting that will be referred to in this chapter: the death of a person from a known chronic life-limiting illness, categorised as an *expected* death. The other category is a *sudden* or *unexpected* death, which can be traumatic or violent in nature. Irrespective of the nature or cause of the death, the emergency clinician's ability to communicate compassion and provide individualised care for the patient and their grieving family can have a lasting impact on the lives of all concerned.

PRACTICE TIP

Emergency clinicians are in a privileged position to be at the front-line of care for people who are dying either from an expected illness or from a sudden or traumatic death. Clinicians must never underestimate the impact of their care on people at this time, memories of which will remain with the survivors for life.

Cultural considerations

When members of the pre-hospital or emergency clinical team are faced with a death, irrespective of the cause, self-awareness and cultural awareness are driving factors in how clinicians respond to the situation. Hence, cognisance of one's personal beliefs and culture in relation to death and dying is crucial. Australia is defined as a multicultural society, with 29.1% of Australians born in countries outside Australia.[3] Similarly in New Zealand, just over one-quarter of the population was born overseas.[4] Culture permeates all aspects of the human experience, and while people from culturally and linguistically diverse (CALD) backgrounds may have particular needs, no individual can or should be reduced to a simplistic set of expected cultural norms, values or practices. The emergency clinician must ensure they are culturally competent to meet the needs of CALD patients and families, acknowledging that EDs and paramedic services have their own organisational culture, expectations and practices. Furthermore, culturally safe service delivery[5] relies on the emergency clinician's ability to encourage empowerment, share respect and foster a safe environment for Indigenous communities of Australia and New Zealand, in order to promote meaningful pathways to self-determination. It is crucially important that clinicians have the ability to understand and respond to the unique cultural needs of both their workplace and a diversity of people facing death and grief in the emergency care setting.

There are several models to guide clinicians on how to deliver culturally competent and culturally safe care,[5,6,7] and more information on cultural considerations in emergency care can be found in Chapter 5. The following steps provide some guidance on how to begin to provide cultural support in the context of death and dying:

- Have an awareness of one's own attitudes, beliefs, values about death and dying and how this can impact on the patient and family.
- Ask clear and concise questions about patient and family culture, beliefs and rituals around death and dying.
- Show respect for nationality, culture, age, sex, political and religious beliefs.
- Establish trust and open, non-threatening relationships, often in a short period of time.
- Use effective communication skills to elicit family members' understanding about what is happening to the patient in the situation at hand.
- Provide practical support for CALD families, such as offering to assist with arranging interpreters, spiritual or community leader support.
- Communicate with family to ascertain if there are any specific cultural needs and and/or if particular rituals need to be observed when the patient has died.

PRACTICE TIP

Each individual clinician, patient or family member will cope with death and dying based on his or her own situation, emotion, culture and experience.

Different cultures may require specific management of the deceased. A resource such as an outline of different cultural beliefs at the time of death can be helpful as a general guide for clinicians.[6,7]

Expected death

Of the 144,000 people who die each year in Australia, up to half are clinically expected deaths from known chronic life-limiting conditions.[7,8] Furthermore, older people are the fastest growing demographic in developed countries and with this comes increased prevalence of life-limiting, chronic conditions such as cardiovascular, cerebrovascular and respiratory disease and dementia.[9] While many emergency clinicians feel comfortable managing a dying patient and report they find the experience rewarding, an Australian study highlighted that approximately 70% of clinicians felt that the ED was 'not the right place to die'.[1] This is largely due to the busy nature of the ED environment and poor structural design that does not allow for adequate privacy or time to provide appropriate end-of-life care.[9,10] In addition, emergency clinicians can have significant issues communicating with patients' usual care teams, particularly out-of-hours.[2] Nonetheless, this patient cohort is known to use inpatient and ED services extensively in the last year of life and, while many presentations are warranted, EDs should not be expected to substitute for a lack of appropriate in- and out-of-hours community-based services.[8,11]

Patients living with life-limiting illness will often present to EDs for management of symptoms, such as gastrointestinal problems, breathing difficulties and pain.[11] The skills that palliative care specialist teams use to effectively communicate and engage with patients and families, and palliate such symptoms, are (and ought to be) transferrable to emergency clinicians. However, it has been recognised that more needs to be done to increase the skill capacity of emergency clinicians by fostering partnerships between specialties, and ensuring palliative care is integrated in the emergency education curriculum.[12]

While the main role of paramedics in Australasia is perceived to be answering emergency calls to provide life-saving treatment, these emergency clinicians in particular have frequent contact with palliative care patients who require optimal symptom management and end-of-life care at home, in order to avoid unnecessary ED presentation.[13,14] Likewise, there is a need for more education specifically for paramedics in palliative care.[14] Recently, some progress has been made to empower paramedics to effectively manage people who are dying from expected deaths, and this will be discussed later in this chapter with advance care planning.

Palliative care

At times emergency clinicians confront a major dilemma relating to whether an accurate prediction of appropriate active treatment is possible and whether decisions about a transition to palliation can or should be made.[15] When heroic life-saving measures—also known as taking full or 'active measures'—transition to 'comfort measures', the emergency clinician has an opportunity to provide not 'just' comfort measures. Rather, *not* escalating treatment means a full, active approach can be taken to promote comfort and alleviate suffering. As the goals of care or a *treatment ceiling* are established, through good communication and advance care planning where possible, it becomes the responsibility of all generalist and specialist clinicians to effectively palliate and provide comfort to those who are dying and their families.

> ### PRACTICE TIP
>
> A 'goals of care' discussion with the patient and their family is the appropriate way to begin the advance care planning process.

While the best efforts may be made to keep palliative care patients at home, the paramedical and emergency services stand at the 'front door' of hospital services where patients can receive high-level care when it is needed. Though it is acknowledged that the ED is not the ideal place to provide end-of-life care due to lack of space, privacy and specialist palliative care trained staff, emergency clinicians have the opportunity to provide skilled and attentive care to patients in the last hours of life to enable a 'good death', with a focus on relief of symptoms and suffering, and support for grieving families.[9,10] Forero et al cite the Institute of Medicine Framework, which encapsulates the definition of a 'good death' succinctly: 'A decent or good death is the one that is: free from avoidable distress and suffering for patients, families, and caregivers; in general accord with patients' and families' wishes; and reasonably consistent with clinical, cultural, and ethical standards.'[15] To help achieve this goal, emergency clinicians can benefit from training in basic symptom management[16] to effectively manage common end-of-life symptoms such as pain, terminal delirium, restlessness, anxiety and respiratory distress. It is acknowledged that these are a distinct skill set, different from those needed to stablise non-palliative patients in ED.[15] For particularly complex or challenging symptoms, early palliative care consultation in the ED is recommended.[17]

Advance care planning

Advance care planning (ACP) is a worldwide trend that recognises the importance of integrating patient's wishes into the holistic management of their chronic life-limiting illness treatment.[18] ACP begins with a 'goals of care' discussion, whereby the person is supported to discuss their life goals, values and personal views and choices about their preferred outcomes of care with a trained professional, family and close friends[18] in a conversation that is ongoing and may change over time.[1] It is recommended that ACPs be incorporated in all electronic health records.[19]

Delays in appropriate end-of-life care planning can result in:[18]

- continued aggressive, unwanted and/or unwarranted life-sustaining measures instigated for those approaching end of life, including even those who are imminently dying
- poor experiences for families where distraught family members are called on at a time of grieving to engage in end-of-life decisions, and who often experience distress observing life-sustaining measures in their dying loved one

- potentially avoidable conflicts between families and the healthcare team, or within the health care team, about the best course of treatment and care for the dying patient
- care being delivered in acute settings when better patient outcomes could be delivered in supported community or home environments
- stress for health professionals balancing their obligation to act in the best interests of dying patients, sometimes differing views amongst treating clinicians and families about what that entails, and good stewardship of health resources.

An advance care directive (ACD) is a type of advance planning tool that can only be completed by a person with decision-making capacity to direct care when they lose the capacity to do so. These were formerly known as 'living wills'.[19] ACDs should not be confused with 'Not for Resuscitation' or 'No CPR' orders or 'palliative care pathways' which are clinical care plans written to guide clinical care of the patient and are applicable to the patient's current admission. It is appropriate that clinical care plans be put in place irrespective of whether a person has made an ACD.[19,20] Such clinical care plans, however, should be guided by the patient's documented preferences and/or an ACD if one has been provided.

A substitute decision-maker (SDM) is appointed or identified by law to make substitute decisions on behalf of a person whose decision-making capacity is impaired. An SDM may be appointed by the person, appointed for (on behalf of) the person, or identified as the default decision-maker by guardianship legislation. More than one SDM can be appointed under an ACD.

There are three categories of SDMs:[19]

1. SDMs *chosen by* the person (e.g. one or more enduring guardians appointed under a statutory ACD or a nominated SDM in a common law ACD)
2. SDMs *assigned to* the person by the law in the absence of an appointed SDM (e.g. family member, carer or 'person responsible')
3. SDMs *appointed for* the person (e.g. a guardian appointed by a guardianship tribunal).

In Australia and New Zealand, national framework documents[18–20] and advance care planning websites (see 'Useful websites') can be accessed to guide clinicians, as well as local policy between states and territories.

The Australian national framework recognises:[19]

- that under common law the terms of an ACD must be respected whether or not the person was medically informed of the consequences when the ACD was written
- that a person (or the SDM) can consent to treatment options that are offered, and refuse such treatment, but cannot demand treatment that is not medically indicated
- the need to protect health and aged care professionals from civil and criminal liability if they abide by the terms of an ACD that they believe, in good faith, to be valid
- that voluntary euthanasia and physician-assisted suicide are currently illegal in Australia and New Zealand.[19,20]

In 2014, a new innovation was announced within the NSW Ambulance Service, in conjunction with local health districts, the Ambulance Authorised Adult Palliative Care Plan protocol and information kit.[21] The kit gives general practitioners (GPs) the option to authorise NSW ambulance paramedics to deliver tailored treatment to their palliative care patients should they need assistance after hours. This model empowers paramedics to provide treatment to the patient in line with the patient's preferences and established end-of-life care plan, and potentially avoid unnecessary hospital admission. The Ambulance Authorised Adult Palliative Care Plan[22] outlines the patient's history, diagnosis and current medications and gives GPs tick box procedures for the paramedics to follow, for example, in the event the patient is in cardiac arrest or death has occurred. An Authorised Paediatric Palliative Care Plan[23] is also available in NSW.

The culture of EDs and paramedic services can be at odds with the palliative approach[14,16] and non-escalation of treatment, for many reasons previously discussed in this chapter. Furthermore, some doctors in emergency settings feel it is not their duty to initiate goals-of-care discussions with patients who are not known to them.[14] At the same time, palliative care teams are under pressure to ensure their often-limited resources are used for appropriate patients with high-level, complex physical, psychological and or social needs.[9] Therefore, it is the collective responsibility of all clinicians involved in the patient's health management to ensure that the treatment and care that is given is guided by the person's wishes and preferences.

Sudden and unexpected death

A *sudden* death implies the death occurred usually within 24 hours of the first symptoms. Sudden death may also refer to those resuscitated from cardiac arrest who die during the same hospital admission. Most sudden deaths occur over a few seconds or minutes. *Unexpected* death refers to knowledge of prior circumstances, such as someone who was believed to have been in good health or who had a stable chronic condition (e.g. cardiomyopathy, epilepsy or a respiratory condition such as asthma) in whom sudden death was not expected. A person's death may be considered unexpected if it occurred in the presence of an illness that would not be expected to cause death.[24]

The responsibility of notifying the family of a death may fall to the emergency clinician, particularly in rural areas. How, when and where the family is notified can have a significant impact on their bereavement outcomes.[25] For emergency clinicians, the emotional toll of communicating death notification and providing emotional support to the family cannot be underestimated. Emergency clinicians report feeling uncomfortable communicating death notifications and these experiences can be very stressful, particularly for inexperienced clinicians.[26] Formal training for how to notify someone of a death varies and many learn through experience.[25] The following is a brief outline of the 'steps' in the death notification process:[25]

1. *Preparation*: choose the appropriate individual to attend the notification who is fully aware of the situation.
2. *Initiating contact*: confirm identity of the person to be notified; do not delay notification; allow for privacy in a safe and comfortable environment.
3. *Delivering bad news*: give chronology of events; avoid euphemisms such as 'passed away'; be compassionate and humanistic.

4. *Responding to the survivor's reaction and providing support*: constantly monitor for emotional and physical support needs; allow time for expression of emotions; offer the person the opportunity to spend time with the deceased; allow customs and rituals; provide anticipatory guidance.
5. *Provision of ongoing support*: provide written information and information about resources; attend/arrange follow-up contact.
6. *Dealing with notifier's response*: provide adequate information and education about death notification; provide opportunities for supportive discussion for those staff involved.

The sudden or unexpected death of a person leaves family members unprepared and, most often, emotionally distraught. Emergency clinicians have an important role to play in supporting grieving family members, even if notification of death falls to other health team members such as medical staff or chaplains.[25] Genuineness, warmth, empathy, active listening and openness[27] are central qualities and skills that are required to provide essential bereavement support to families at a very difficult time.

> ### PRACTICE TIP
>
> Genuineness, warmth, empathy, active listening and openness are central qualities and skills that are required by emergency clinicians to provide support to dying people and their families.

Sudden death of a child

As with adult deaths, good bereavement care provided after the death of a child can have positive long-term effects on the bereavement outcomes of parents and siblings. For emergency clinicians, the death of a child in the emergency setting may be one of the most distressing and stressful events that can occur.[28] Adequate training and education to prepare staff for how to manage these events is essential. The following are key practice points from Lawrence's[28] guidelines for best practice in supporting parents after the death of their child:

- An emergency-trained clinician or appropriately trained staff member should immediately be allocated to support the parents, particularly through the resuscitation process. The allocated staff member should learn the names and roles of family members present and the child should always be referred to by their name.
- Allow time for parents to hold the child and offer the opportunity for them to assist with washing or dressing the child if this is permitted by the coroner.
- Understand that siblings should be told of the death by their parent or a person they know and trust, and offer some supportive literature to parents to help siblings make sense of their loss and grief.
- If permitted by the coronial process, parents may be offered mementoes such as photographs, imprints of hands and feet or a lock of hair. Details of what is given to the parents should be clearly documented. If this cannot be accommodated within the particular health facility

due to the coronial process, medical examiners acting on behalf of the coroner can facilitate this at a later time.

- Reassure parents that their child will continue to receive care and attention after they have left the ED.
- Be aware of multiagencies who may need to be notified after a child's death and advise parents of who they may be required to speak to.
- Ensure appropriate after-care, possibly including a condolence card from the ED staff.
- Ensure debriefing for staff, both formal and informal, to allow reflection on this highly emotionally demanding aspect of the emergency clinician's role.

Family presence during resuscitation

The presence of family during resuscitation was first explored in the United States in the 1980s, after a survey revealed that relatives would have preferred to have been present.[29] Since then, a significant amount of anecdotal and research evidence has been and continues to be published providing reasons to support or not support relatives' presence. Reasons given to support family presence include:[29–36]

- better communication between family and staff, which can also reduce the risk of liability
- family can realise the seriousness of the situation and that everything was done to try to save their loved one
- family are better able to cope with the outcome of the resuscitation and have a sense of closure, knowing the death was real.

Reasons not to allow family members to be present include:[29–36]

- witnessing resuscitation could be more traumatic for the family
- increases the stress or distraction for staff
- could increase litigation and breach patient confidentiality
- the family may interfere during the resuscitation.

Both the Australian and New Zealand Resuscitation Councils[37] and the Emergency Nursing Association (ENA) recommend family members be offered the opportunity to be present during resuscitation. The following practical recommendations are given by the ENA[35] for organisations that are considering implementing the practice of relatives' presence during resuscitation:

- Provide an environment that is suitable for the implementation of the program.
- Provide chairs for family to sit on, to ensure that there is less potential for injury of family members while they are witnessing the resuscitation.
- Educate staff on how to work with grieving families.
- Prepare the family with a clear explanation of what to expect when they are in the resuscitation room.
- Provide a support person to accompany the relatives during their presence in the resuscitation room.

Evidence for a designated emergency clinician to support the family looking on in a resuscitation situation is highly recommended in the literature.[36] However, a designated family support person is not always evident in practice due to staff shortage,[28] and was considered in one study to be 'low on the priority list'.[36] The decision to allow family to be present during resuscitation remains controversial and, ultimately, culturally defined.[29–36] Evidence generally suggests that while family presence at resuscitation is recommended, and can reduce the risk of Post Traumatic Stress Disorder (PTSD) in family members[31,32] it is not widely observed in practice, therefore more research is needed.[34]

Viewing/identification of a deceased relative or friend

Where there are no legal implications, preparing the body for viewing can include sponging, slightly elevating the head of the deceased, placing hands above the sheet for ease of access for family and providing a quiet place for family to view and grieve. In the event of a suspicious or 'reportable death' (see following section), sponging the body is generally not permitted. In the pre-hospital setting where resuscitation has been withheld or withdrawn, it may be appropriate to move the deceased to a more appropriate location to enable viewing by family members. For example, a patient who has died on the property outside their home may be brought inside the home and placed on a bed once resuscitation has been determined to be futile. The exception to this is a suspicious or reportable death, where the scene and deceased should not be disturbed to preserve evidence for police. It is implicit that staff caring for deceased patients should follow standard precautions for infection control. In situations where the infection risk is high, additional precautions may be required and should be extended to include family.

Each jurisdiction may have different requirements for the identification of a deceased relative or friend. Usually the coroner will require identification of the body by the family to be attended in the presence of a police officer. Sometimes this can be done with an intermediary, namely an emergency clinician who acts as a witness to the identification by the family, then signs a form and hands over this identification to the police officer after the family have left the hospital. This may assist in reducing the time the family is required at the hospital following the death of their relative. During the identification process, the body should be prepared for viewing as described above. There are a number of legal aspects that emergency clinicians need to take into consideration that legislation will vary across Australia and New Zealand; issues relating to emergency care and the law is explored in Chapter 4.

Reportable deaths

A 'reportable death' is a death that should be brought to the attention of the coroner.[38] The coronial process and criteria for reportable deaths will vary across states and territories, so emergency clinicians should familiarise themselves with the relevant legislation. Categories of death that meet this requirement are generally sudden, violent or accidental deaths.[38] Other criteria include (but are not limited to) the following:

- If the person's identity is unknown.
- If the person died under suspicious or unusual circumstances.
- If the person was held, or temporarily absent from a care facility, mental health facility or was in custody.
- Where the death occurred unexpectedly after a medical procedure.

- If a medical practitioner had not seen the person within 6 months of the death.
- To assist with determining the circumstance and cause of death, the coroner may request a post mortem examination.

Post mortem examination

The topic of post mortem examination (PME) may be equally awkward for the emergency clinician as it is upsetting for the family of the deceased. A request for a PME may seem insensitive, and it comes, of necessity, at an extremely difficult time. Families may also request a PME if they have reasonable grounds for making such a request. A PME involves a procedure (autopsy) where a detailed examination of the body's external surfaces and internal organs is undertaken to establish the cause of death. Other samples or organs may be taken from the body for further examination.[39,40] Family members often have questions about the autopsy procedure and its effects on funeral arrangements. The practice of autopsy may be a source of added distress for families whose religious views place a strong emphasis on the inviolability of human remains and where anything more than ritual cleaning of the body could be viewed as a desecration.[39] Emergency clinicians should be prepared to address the family's queries on the PME process. PME information booklets for families[40] can be sourced through the coroner's office in each state or territory.

Deaths for review by the Coroner and management of evidence

When a person dies and a death certificate cannot be completed, the death will be referred to the relevant coroner for further investigation. As previously outlined, variances exist between different state and territory jurisdictions and internationally between Australia and New Zealand. Links to relevant local resources are provided for further review at the end of this chapter. Local health organisations should also further refine specific local procedures to guide clinicians in managing potential cases for referral to the coroner.

A Coroner will investigate a suspicious or unexpected death with the aim of providing answers to the following questions (of which some or all may never be known):

- The identity of the deceased.
- The cause of death.
- The circumstances in which the death occurred.

On occasion, the coroner may be satisfied that there is enough evidence to answer these questions without requesting a PME. If a PME is undertaken, and the above questions are still not answered, then a coronial process may be initiated, whereby further investigations may be conducted and explored through formal court proceedings. If applicable, at the conclusion of this coronial process, the coroner may go on to make recommendations that include:

- suggesting criminal or professional misconduct proceedings be commenced by the applicable authorities
- mitigation steps to reduce the likelihood of similar occurrences in the future
- returning an 'open finding' where there is not enough evidence to answer the three questions above (but may be re-examined in the future if further information is uncovered).

The investigations by the Coroner can extend from a simple review of the medical record and discussion with the local investigating police, which could be completed in days, to a full judicial investigation through a coronial court, which could take several years. It is beyond the scope of the paramedic or the hospital clinician to determine the likely breadth and depth of the coroner's investigations. As such, all deaths where a death certificate is not going to be written must be treated as a potential 'coroner's case'. For clarification of coronial reporting processes, a call to the local coroner's office can provide helpful assistance, both in and out of business hours. It is prudent for clinicians, whether in the pre-hospital or ED setting, to assume that they may be called as a witness in the coronial investigation process. It is essential that medical records are accurate, and chain of evidence protocols are adhered to and documented correctly.

For all coroner's cases, the principles of 'chain of possession' (or chain of evidence) and evidence preservation must be maintained.[41] The chain of possession ensures that there is a record of all who come into contact with a particular piece of evidence.[41] For a piece of clothing, this could include the paramedic who touched the patient to place them on a stretcher, the nurse who cut off the piece of clothing and placed the item in a paper bag, the police officer who took custody of the evidence and the lab technician who examined the piece of evidence. *Evidence preservation* refers to the handling and treatment of pieces of evidence in a way that preserves physical macro and micro evidence such as DNA, hair, chemical and paint samples.[41] General principles that maintain the chain of possession and evidence preservation when someone will be referred to the coroner include the following:

- All medical records must be up to date. This includes pathology, medical imaging and the like. It also includes noting the names of treating and assisting clinicians (anyone who came into contact with the patient or items that may be used as evidence).
- All medical devices or equipment that were in situ should not be removed. This would include (but is not limited to) endotracheal tubes, catheters, cannulas and gastric tubes.
- The body should not be washed or otherwise tampered with once life has been declared extinct. In this way, any trace evidence is preserved.
- Any bodily fluids should be preserved and stored in a clearly marked and sealed container. This allows possible testing of ingested substances.
- All items removed from the patient during medical interventions/resuscitation, including clothing, jewellery and suchlike, should be placed into separate paper bags to preserve DNA and other trace materials. (Plastic bags should be avoided due to condensation that may degrade the evidence.)
- Sharps related to the above should be stored or secured in a way that maintains safety for all staff involved with the chain of evidence.

Certification of death

New Zealand and each state or territory in Australia have resources available to guide clinicians on the legislative requirements on the process for 'certification as to the cause of death', a medical form completed by a registered medical officer at the time of a person's death for deaths which are not required to be referred to the Coroner for investigation. The form details the medical cause of death and the doctor who certifies a patient's death is also required to separately notify the Registrar of Births, Deaths and Marriages within a designated period after the death.

Establishing that a person is deceased—also referred to as 'verification of death' or 'extinction of life assessment'—can be attended by a medical officer; it can be a registered nurse or a paramedic in some jurisdictions in New Zealand and Australia. This process involves a clinical assessment of the body only to establish that death has occurred. For example, relevant policies exist in New Zealand and some states of Australia outlining that a registered nurse or a paramedic can attend an extinction-of-life assessment on a patient known to palliative care services who has died an expected death at home, in the case where a medical officer cannot immediately attend. The medical officer is contacted at the time of death and is then required to complete the certification as to the cause of death within 48 hours.

Care of the deceased bariatric patient

Increasing numbers of morbidly obese patients are being managed in pre-hospital and ED settings.[42] This has resulted in emergency clinicians, hospital staff and funeral service staff experiencing manual handling challenges during collection, transport, preparation, funeral service and burial of the deceased bariatric patient. The approximate weight and girth of the patient should be known, as this will need to be communicated to hospital and funeral services staff involved in transporting the deceased bariatric patient. EDs should have ready access to bariatric beds and trolleys for care and transportation of the deceased bariatric patient. It is important that the appropriate bariatric equipment be used, if it is available. To ensure that the patient's dignity is maintained, transport through public areas and access should be closed to the public. If this is not possible, or the patient is required to remain on the hospital bed for transfer, the clinician could place an oxygen mask on the patient so as not to draw attention from the public that the person is deceased.[42] At times, the facility's mortuary refrigerator may not be the appropriate size to accommodate the deceased bariatric patient. In this case, clinicians or hospital staff could arrange funeral services to collect the body directly from a private area within the facility such as a viewing room or mortuary room.

Organ donation

Organ donation is the process of transplanting one or more organs or tissues from a 'donor' to a recipient. The organ and tissue donation process is covered in detail in Chapter 54. The primary source of organ donation is from donors who have died. Both Australian and New Zealand health authorities provide guidelines and clinical triggers that outline when to initiate discussions with families about organ and tissue donation. For the emergency clinician, this discussion may be initiated when restorative treatment measures are no longer viable and end-of-life treatment planning has commenced. When organ donation is set to occur, the dying person receives care that is aimed at preserving organ function. These treatments may include artificial ventilation to promote oxygenation, inotropic support to promote perfusion and strict temperature and blood glucose control.

Mass fatalities

Whether in the pre hospital or ED environment, mass fatalities in the context of mass casualty incidents and disasters, by their definition, will overwhelm existing resources. Examples include catastrophic events such as a major earthquake, or an insidious public health issue like the 2014 West African Ebola outbreak.[43,44] While the same principles of emergency care should be maintained where possible, differences will inevitably exist. The ways in which the dying, the dead and family and friends are managed may need to be adjusted to match the specifics of the catastrophic event. For example, those that are imminently dying may be triaged lower than those seriously injured. Local, state, national and international protocols and guidelines exist to guide management in such situations (see Useful websites). Most health entities offer specific training to emergency clinicians in mass casualty incidents where management of the dead and dying are covered in detail.

Staff support

Emergency clinicians, namely nurses and paramedics, are routinely confronted with human suffering, trauma and death, often in the midst of a hectic work environment. In addition, they are expected to assess, manage, treat and transport critically ill patients and manage both their own emotions and the emotions of others who are potentially in distress.[45] It is not surprising then that emergency clinicians are highly vulnerable to post traumatic stress disorder (PTSD) symptoms including anxiety, depression, nightmares, intrusive thoughts and loss of concentration.[46] Clearly, this can have a significant impact on the clinician, but also can impact on the quality of patient care. Williams'[45] research into the paramedic experience of managing workplace trauma recognised that the focus is on technical education and training under the biomedical model, which fails to adequately address the 'emotional labour' expended by paramedics in their day-to-day work. Furthermore, literature in the area of emotion work is deficient. Williams also recommends that emotion work be a core component of the paramedic educational curriculum.

Critical incident stress debriefing (CISD) allows those involved in an incident to reflect and process the event; and sessions should be led by adequately trained staff. Although most emergency clinicians believe that CISD is important, many EDs have no formal structures, such as guidelines or policies, in place to ensure this practice is followed.[47] Ongoing debriefing programs such as clinical supervision, as well as CISD, have been found to reduce occupation stress in emergency settings.[46] Positive workplace environments encourage:[46–48]

- 'talking it through' with colleagues and maximising existing resources of social support
- using reflective practice
- leadership that is supportive, communicative, empathic and anticipatory
- clinical mentorship programs
- using humour to 'offload' emotion, and see the 'lighter side of things'.

It is clear that organisations should take preventive measures to ensure that staff have means to foster and maintain professional resilience.[49] In addition, emergency clinicians are responsible for developing their personal resilience by taking active measures to participate in self-care strategies to 're-fuel' physically, socially, psychologically and spiritually. Such activities could include enjoyable exercise; going out with friends and family; keeping a reflective journal; or participating in meaningful rituals. Collectively, these professional and personal strategies can assist emergency clinicians to ensure their physical and emotional wellbeing, and enable them to provide the best-quality patient care.

SUMMARY

Emergency clinicians have the privilege of being at the front-line of emergency care settings and are involved with people's lives at significant times of trauma, loss and grief. These highly skilled clinicians must provide end-of-life care across a continuum that ranges from patients who have made their wishes clear as they come to the end of a struggle with illness, to those for whom death was entirely unforeseen. Emergency clinicians are tasked with providing the highest quality care to critically ill patients in a highly demanding clinical environment and ensuring the requirements of law in their relevant country, state or territory are met. In addition, emergency clinicians are required to meet the needs of families that often can be in a state of distress and emotional suffering. The ongoing impact of a compassionate and individualised approach to care for families who have suffered a loss cannot and should not be underestimated.

CASE STUDY 1

Brian is a 68-year-old male who has just been transported to the emergency department (ED). He collapsed while having lunch with his family. CPR was being done by family members when paramedics arrived. The attending paramedics continued CPR, as well as initiating protocols for airway management and a shockable cardiac rhythm. On arrival to the ED, Brian was found to be in asystole. Advanced life support resuscitation efforts continued for another 15 minutes. After a cardiac ultrasound revealed no cardiac movement, 'cardiac standstill', resuscitation was ceased and Brian was pronounced dead.

Questions

1. The doctor assumes that the cause of death was probably a sudden cardiac arrest or maybe Brian choked on some food. Which of the following is true?
   A. A death certificate can be written because cause of death is known.
   B. All tubes, lines and the like can be removed because the cause of death is known.
   C. The police must be informed because the death will be referred to the coroner.
   D. The family will not be able to see Brian because the death will be referred to the coroner.

2. In providing psychosocial support to Brian's family members, what might be helpful?
   A. Provide the family with information about death, dying and the coronial process.
   B. Discuss organ donation because Brian had an organ donor card in his wallet.

   C. Organise a minister of religion because you heard one of Brian's family praying.
   D. Provide the family with information about screening for cardiac risk factors now they have a family history of cardiac arrest.

3. Which of the following is true in relation to Brian and the coronial process?
   A. Family members are not to be left alone with Brian's body; they must be supervised by hospital staff or police at all times.
   B. All lines, tubes and the like must be left in place to assist in the coronial investigation.
   C. An autopsy will be carried out only if the coroner requires it to be completed or the family requests it.
   D. All of the above.

4. The senior medical officer has suggested that the resuscitation team, including the paramedics, meet for debriefing. The purpose of this debrief would best be described as an opportunity to:
   a. review the treatment of Brian and comment on the performance of individual team members so they can improve next time.
   b. screen all team members for symptoms of post traumatic stress response and organise referral to a councillor.
   c. allow team members to reflect on and discuss what happened during the resuscitation and ask questions that may arise.
   d. attend something that must be done after every unexpected death.

Answers to Case Study Questions can be found on evolve
http://evolve.emergencytrauma.curtis

CASE STUDY 2

Harriet is a 19-year-old woman who has been battling leukaemia since she was 15. Over the last 6 weeks she has transitioned to palliative care with the goal of maximising her quality of life. Harriet called the ambulance due to increased, uncontrolled pain. When she arrived in the ED she deteriorated quickly, became unconscious and died a short time later.

Questions

1. A large number of Harriet's family and school friends are arriving at the hospital and are understandably very upset. Which of the following strategies do you think would work best for this situation?

   A. Limiting bedside visitors to two at a time in line with the ED visitor policy.

   B. Restricting bedside visitors to immediate family and Harriet's closest friends.

   C. Providing an area where the family and friends can congregate separate to the ED waiting room.

   D. Appointing a family spokesperson who can be a point of contact for both ED staff and other family and friends.

2. The ED medical officer is not willing to write a death certificate because they have not seen Harriet before. Which of the following actions are indicated in this situation?

   A. Try to contact the relevant palliative care doctor to provide further information on Harriet's medical history.

   B. Consult any available previous medical records to provide further information on Harriet's medical history.

   C. Treat this death as a Coroner's case until a death certificate is completed.

   D. Inform Harriet's next of kin that a death certificate will not be written at this stage.

3. Harriet's parents have requested that no males be left alone with her as it is in line with their cultural practices. On reflection, this is:

   A. A reasonable request for the parents to make in line with their cultural belief.

   B. An unreasonable request because this can not be guaranteed by hospital staff.

4. A staff member is upset by Harriet's death. An empathic response would include:

   A. Encouraging the staff member to move on as it was an expected death.

   B. Expressing understanding about how sad Harriet's death is and how 'only the good die young'.

   C. Discouraging the staff member to express their feelings because it is unprofessional for emergency clinicians.

   D. Allowing the staff member to express their thoughts and feelings without judgement.

 Answers to Case Study Questions can be found on evolve
http://evolve.emergencytrauma.curtis

USEFUL WEBSITES

Advance Care Planning

Advance Care Planning Australia, http://advancecareplanning.org.au/

Advance Care Planning New Zealand, www.advancecareplanning.org.nz

Department of Birth Deaths and Marriages

Births Deaths and Marriages Registries, http://australia.gov.au/topics/law-and-justice/births-deaths-and-marriages-registries

Department of Internal Affairs, New Zealand, http://www.dia.govt.nz/Births-deaths-and-marriages

Mass Fatality Incident Management

New Zealand Ministry of Health, www.health.govt.nz/our-work/emergency-management

Australian Emergency Management, www.em.gov.au/Pages/default.aspx

Organ donation

Australian Government Organ and Tissue Authority, www.donatelife.gov.au/

Organ Donation New Zealand, www.donor.co.nz/

Palliative care

Palliative Care Australia, www.palliativecare.org.au

Palliative Care New Zealand, www.hospice.org.nz

REFERENCES

1. Marck CH, Weil J, Lane H et al. Care of the dying cancer patient in the emergency department: finding from a National survey of Australian emergency department clinicians. Intern Med J 2014;44(4):362–8.

2. Ieraci S. Palliative care in the emergency department. Emerg Med Australas 2013;25:112–13.

3. Australian Bureau of Statistics. 2011 Census Quickstats: Australia. Commonwealth of Australia. Online. www.censusdata.abs.gov.au/census_services/getproduct/census/2011/quickstat/0; accessed 1 June 2014.

4. Statistics New Zealand. 2013 Census quickstats about national highlights: Cultural diversity. New Zealand Government. Online. www.stats.govt.nz/Census/2013-census/profile-and-summary-reports/quickstats-about-national-highlights/cultural-diversity.aspx; accessed 7 June 2014.

5. Human Rights Commission. 2011. Cultural safety and security: Tools to address lateral violence: Social Justice Report. Online. www.humanrights.gov.au/publications/chapter-4-cultural-safety-and-security-tools-address-lateral-violence-social-justice#Heading56; accessed 1 October 2014.

6. Stein K. Moving cultural competency from abstract to act. J Am Diet Assoc 2010;110(5):s21–7.

7. Loddon Mallee Regional Palliative Care Consortium. 2011. An outline of different cultural beliefs at the time of death. Online. http://lmrpcc.org.au/admin/wp-content/uploads/2011/07/Customs-Beliefs-Death-Dying.pdf; accessed 7 June 2014.

8. Commonwealth of Australia. 2010. The national palliative care strategy: Supporting Australians to live well until the end of life. Online. www.health.gov.au/internet/main/publishing.nsf/Content/A87BC5583161BEBFCA257BF0001D3AF6/$File/NationalPalliativeCareStrategy.pdf; accessed 7 June 2014.

9. Rosenwax LK, McNamara BA, Murray K et al. Hospital and emergency department use in the last year of life: a baseline for future modifications to end of life care. Med J Aust 2011;194(11):570–3.

10. Peters L, Cant R, Payne S et al. Emergency and palliative care nurses' levels of anxiety about death and coping with death: A questionnaire survey. Australas Emerg Nurs J 2013;16:152–9.

11. Bailey CJ, Murphy R, Porock D. Dying cases in emergency places: Caring for the dying in emergency departments. Soc Sci Med 2011;72:1371–7.

12. Hjermstad MJ, Kolflaath J, Lokken AO et al. Are emergency admissions in palliative cancer care always necessary? Results from a descriptive study. Br Med J 2013;3:e002515.

13. Lukin W, Douglas C, O'Connor. Palliative care in the emergency department: An oxymoron of just good medicine? Emerg Med Australas 2012;24:102–4.

14. Lord B, Recoche K, O'Connor M et al. Paramedics perceptions of their role in palliative care: Analysis of focus group transcripts. J Palliat Care 2012;28(1):36–40.

15. Forero R, McDonnell G, Gallego B et al. A Literature review on care at the end of life in the emergency department. Emerg Med Int 2011;2012:1–11.

16. Grudzen CR, Richardson LD, Hopper SS. Does palliative care have a future in the emergency department? Discussions with attending emergency physicians. J Pain Symptom Manage 2012;43(1):1–9.

17. Smith AK, Schonberg MA, Fisher J et al. Emergency department experiences of acutely symptomatic patients with terminal illness and their family caregivers. J Pain Symptom Manage 2010;39(6):972–81.

18. Ministry of Health NSW. 2013. Advance planning for quality care at end of life: Action plan 2013–2018. Online. www.health.nsw.gov.au/patients/acp/Publications/acp-plan-2013-2018.pdf; accessed 8 June 2014.

19. The Clinical, Technical and Ethical Principal Committee of the Australian Health Ministers' Advisory Council. A National Framework for Advance Care Directives. 2011. Online. http://www.ahmac.gov.au/cms_documents/AdvanceCareDirectives2011.pdf; accessed 6 June 2014.

20. Ministry of Health New Zealand. 2011. Advance Care Planning: A guide for the New Zealand health workforce. Online. www.health.govt.nz/system/files/documents/publications/advance-care-planning-aug11.pdf; accessed 8 June 2014.

21. Ambulance Service of NSW. 2014. Authorised Adult Palliative Care Plan. General Practitioner Information Kit. Online. www.snswml.com.au/images/stories/documents/Primary%20Care%20Support/GP_Info_Palliative_Care_Plan.pdf; accessed 8 June 2014.

22. Medicare Local Southern NSW. Authorised Adult Palliative Care Plan. Online. www.snswml.com.au/primary-care-support/palliative-care.html; accessed 7 June 2014.

23. Ambulance Service of NSW. Authorised Paediatric Palliative Care Plan. Online. www.nsml.com.au/for-health-professionals/resource-centre/palliative-care/paediatricpalliative-care-plan-application-protocol-p1_20140313171039.pdf; accessed 7 June 2014.

24. Trans-Tasman Response Against Sudden Death in the Young. 2008. Post-mortem in sudden unexpected death in the young: Guidelines on autopsy practice. Online. www.cidg.org/webcontent/LinkClick.aspx?fileticket=DO9YIQWqegl%3D&tabid=161; accessed 8 June 2014.

25. Roe E. Practical strategies for death notification in the emergency department. J Emerg Nurs 2012;38(2):130–4.

26. Douglas L, Ratnapalan S, Cheskes S, Feldman M. Paramedics' experiences with death notification: A qualitative study. J Paramed Prac 2012;4(9):533–9.

27. Scott T. Sudden death in emergency care: Responding to bereaved relatives. Emerg Nurs 2013;21(8):36–9.

28. Lawrence N. Care of bereaved parents after sudden infant death. Emerg Nurs 2010;18(3):22–5.

29. Doyle CJ, Post H, Burney RE et al. Family participation during resuscitation: an option. Ann Emerg Med 1987;16(6):673–5.

30. Norton CK, Hobson G, Kulm E. Palliative and end of life care in the emergency department: Guidelines for nurses. J Emerg Nurs 2011;37(3):240–5.

31. Jabre P, Belpomme V, Azouley E et al. Family presence during cardiopulmonary resuscitation. N Engl J Med 2013;368:1008–18.

32. Jacques H. Family presence at resuscitation attempts. Nurs Times 2014;110(10):20–1.

33. Fernandes AP, de Souza Carnerio C, Goecze L et al. Experiences and opinions of health professionals in relation to the presence of the family during in-hospital cardiopulmonary resuscitation: An integrative review. J Nurs Ed Prac 2014;4(5):85–94.

34. Sak-Dankosky N, Adndruszkiewicz P, Sherwood PR, Kvist T. Integrative review: Nurses and physicians experiences and attitudes towards inpatient-witnessed resuscitation of an adult patient. J Adv Nurs 2013;70(5):957–74.

35. ENA Emergency Nursing Resources Development Committee. Clinical practice guideline: Family presence during invasive procedures and resuscitation. 2012. Online. www.ena.org/practice-research/research/CPG/Documents/FamilyPresenceCPG.pdf; accessed 6 June 2014.

36. Porter JE, Cooper SJ, Taylor B. Emergency resuscitation team roles: What constitutes a team and who's looking after the family? J Nurs Ed Prac 2014;4(3):124–32.

37. Australian Resuscitation Council & New Zealand Resuscitation Council. 2012. Guideline 10.5 Legal and Ethical Issues Related To Resuscitation. Online. http://www.resus.org.au/policy/guidelines/section_10/guideline-10-5-%20july-2012.pdf; accessed 10 October 2014.

38. Forrester K, Griffiths D. Essentials of law for health professionals. 3rd edn. Marrickville: Mosby; 2010.

39. Burton EC, Gurevitz, SA. Religions and autopsy. 2010. Online. http://emedicine.medscape.com/article/1705993-overview; accessed 8 June 2014.

40. NSW Government Justice and Attorney General Department. 2009. NSW Coroners Court: A guide to services. Online. www.coroners.lawlink.nsw.gov.au/agdbasev7wr/_assets/coroners/m40160111/coroners%20ct%20brochure_guide%20to%20services.pdf; accessed 7 June 2014.

41. Barnes M. Preserving evidence when a 'reportable death' occurs in a health care setting. 2007. Online. www.courts.qld.gov.au/__data/assets/pdf_file/0004/92875/m-osc-scene-preservation.pdf; accessed 15 October 2014.

42. Australian Safety and Compensation Council. Manual handling risks associated with the care, treatment and transportation of bariatric (severely obese) patients in Australia. 2009. Online. www.safeworkaustralia.gov.au/sites/swa/about/publications/Documents/314/ManualHandlingRisks_CareTreatmentTransportation_fBariatricSeverelyObesePatients_Australia_2009_PDF.pdf; accessed 10 October 2014.

43. Cheng AC, Kelly H. Are we prepared for Ebola and other viral haemorrhagic fevers? Aust N Z J of Public Health 2014;38(5):403–4.

44. Tovaranonte P, Cawood TJ. Impact of the Christchurch Earthquakes on Hospital Staff. Prehospital Disaster Med 2013;28(3):245–50.

45. Williams A. Emotion work in paramedic practice: The implications for nurse educators. Nurs Ed Today 2012;32:368–72.

46. Adriaenssens J, de Gucht V, Maes S. The impact of traumatic events on emergency room nurses: Findings from a questionnaire survey. Int J Nurs Stud 2012;49(11):1411–22.

47. Healy S, Tyrrell M. Importance of debriefing following critical incidents. Emerg Nurs 2013;20(10):32–7.

48. Williams A. The strategies used to deal with emotion work in student paramedic practice. Nurs Ed Prac 2013;13:207–12.s

49. De Boer J, Lok A, Van't VE et al. Work-related critical incidents in hospital based health care providers and the risk of post traumatic symptoms, anxiety and depression: A meta-analysis. Soc Sci Med 2011;73(2):316–26.

CHAPTER 54
ORGAN AND TISSUE DONATION

CARRIE ALVARO, LEIGH MCKAY, MYRA SGORBINI AND
JANE TRELOGGEN

Essentials

- It is important to stay up to date with changing donation practices to maintain high standards of care within the required legal, procedural and ethical frameworks.
- Rapid and early referral of patients meeting the clinical trigger allows staff to explore their suitability to donate and provides an opportunity to plan the family donation conversation.
- Medical suitability of potential donors should be determined by the respective tissue banks and organ and tissue donation service.
- Proactive donor management optimises solid-organ function following consent to donation.
- Consistent and appropriate bereavement support for families of organ and tissue donors moves them to find meaning in their loss.
- Collaborative efforts between emergency department clinicians, intensive care clinicians and hospital administrators develop mutual accountability and responsibility that leads to improved outcomes.
- Maintaining open channels of communication between hospital clinicians, tissue banks and the organ and tissue donation service will build strong partnerships for success.

INTRODUCTION

Human organ and tissue transplantation has become a very effective treatment option for irrevocable failure of vital organs.[1,2] Retrieval and transplantation of organs and tissues from the deceased has been occurring in Australia since 1911 when a portion of pancreas was transplanted unsuccessfully at the Launceston General Hospital in Tasmania. This was followed by the first reported corneal transplant in 1941, kidneys in 1956 and liver and heart in 1968.[3,4]

Transplantation began in New Zealand with the commencement of corneal grafting in the 1940s and the first organ to be transplanted was the kidney in 1965. Bone tissue and hearts were first successfully transplanted in the 1980s and the 1990s saw the commencement of skin, lung, liver and pancreas transplantations.[5,6,7]

Long-term graft survival became possible with the discovery and use of immuno-suppressive agents in the 1960s,[8,9] and the current era of organ and tissue transplantation in Australia (1982) and New Zealand (1964) began with the enactment of legislation that defined death and addressed the retrieval and use of tissue from living and deceased persons. Since then, programs have commenced for solid-organ transplantation, i.e. heart, lung, liver, kidney, pancreas, islet cell and intestinal, and corneal, cardiac and musculoskeletal tissues.[3,4]

Organ and tissue donation is a component of end-of-life care, and the variables of how, when and where the person dies will influence which organs and tissues they can donate. With a focus on paramedics, emergency care clinicians and nurses, this chapter will detail the process and clinical implications of deceased organ and tissue donation in Australia and New Zealand with reference to best-practice evidence from the literature. Useful websites are listed at the end of the chapter.

Donation and transplantation in Australia and New Zealand

Legislation governing organ and tissue donation in Australia is state and territory based. The Australian Organ and Tissue Authority (OTA) was established in 2009 to implement A World's Best Practice Approach to Organ and Tissue Donation for Transplantation.[9] OTA is the peak body that works with all sectors to maximise the potential for organ and tissue donation in Australia. Organ and tissue donation services (OTDS) are based in each Australian state and two territories and are known as the DonateLife network. State-based tissue banks facilitate tissue retrieval in partnership with their local OTDS. National legislation on organ and tissue donation is enforced in New Zealand. Organ Donation New Zealand (ODNZ) is the national organisation with primary responsibility for coordinating the donation of organs and tissues from deceased donors in New Zealand.

Quality and safety processes involved in tissue retrieval, manufacture and transplantation are governed by the Australian Therapeutic Goods Administration (Australian Code of Good Manufacturing Practice—Human Blood and Tissues) and the New Zealand Medicines and Medical Devices Safety Authority (New Zealand Code of Good Manufacturing Practice for Manufacture and Distribution of Therapeutic Goods). The process of potential organ and tissue donor identification and management in the critical care environment is guided by the Australian and New Zealand Intensive Care Society (ANZICS) Statement on Death and Organ Donation Edition 3(2) 2013. Donor selection, eligibility and allocation criteria were developed by the Transplantation Society of Australia and New Zealand (TSANZ) and the National Health and Medical Research Council (NHMRC) to ensure that there are equitable and transparent processes in place.

The Australia and New Zealand Organ Donation Registry (ANZOD) records and reports on a wide range of statistics that relate to organ and tissue donation following death, and the Australia and New Zealand Dialysis and Transplant Registry (ANZDATA) collects a wide range of statistics that relate to the outcomes of treatment of those with end-stage renal failure (see Table 54.1).

A professional education package has been developed for Australian health professionals working within critical care areas and includes ADAPT (Australasian Donor Awareness Program) and the Family Donation Conversation (Core and Practical) workshops. This package is funded by OTA and endorsed by the Australian College of Critical Care Nurses (ACCCN), the College of Intensive Care Medicine (CICM) and ANZICS. ADAPT is also offered in New Zealand. Professional associations in organ and tissue donation and transplantation

TABLE 54.1 Summary of solid-organ donations 2005–2014[11]

	AUSTRALIA	NEW ZEALAND
2005	204 (10)	29 (7)
2006	202 (10)	25 (6)
2007	198 (9)	38 (9)
2008	259 (12)	31 (7)
2009	247 (11)	43 (10)
2010	309 (14)	41 (9)
2011	337 (15)	38 (9)
2012	354 (15.6)	38 (9)
2013	391 (16.9)	36 (8)
2014	378 (16.1)	46 (10.2)

Donors per million population reported in brackets

include the Australasian Transplant Coordinators Association (ATCA), the Transplant Nurses' Association (TNA), the Biotherapeutics Association of Australasia (BAA) and the Eye Bank Association of Australia and New Zealand (EBAANZ).

'Opt in' system of donation

There are two general systems of approach to consent for deceased organ and tissue donation around the world. Some countries have an 'opt-out' or presumed consent system (e.g. Spain, Singapore and Austria), where eligible persons are considered for organ and tissue retrieval at the time of their death if they have not indicated their explicit objection. In Australia, New Zealand, United States, United Kingdom and most other common-law countries, the approach is to 'opt in', with specific consent required from the potential donor or their next of kin.[12,13] In Australia, a person may indicate their consent for organ and tissue donation on the Australian Organ Donor Register and on their driver's licence (South Australia only). New Zealand is the only nation where indicating one's donation decision is compulsory in order to obtain a driver's licence.[14] In Singapore, the *Human Organ Transplant Act* of 1987 combines a presumed consent system with a required consent system for the Muslim population. In other parts of Asia, the informed-consent legislation of Japan and Korea came into force in 1997 and 2000 respectively.[15,16]

Legislation

Legislation governing organ and tissue donation in Australia and New Zealand takes the form of an Act that addresses the retrieval and use of human tissue before and after death. The legislation enables a person to choose to be a donor, and organ and tissue donation can proceed unless revoked or objected to by the family. If the deceased's wishes are not known, consent for donation rests with the next of kin. The *New Zealand Human Tissue Act 2008* governs the practice in New Zealand; however, this does not include a statutory definition of death, but it is defined in the New Zealand Code of Practice for

Transplantation of Cadaveric Organs.[17] Each Australian state and territory enacts its own legislation or Human Tissue Act and these can be found on state government websites. Australian legislation defines death as the:

- irreversible cessation of all function of the brain of the person, or
- irreversible cessation of circulation of blood in the body of the person.[18]

Pathways of donation

Organ and tissue may be donated by a living or deceased person. Organ and tissue donation from a living person is divided into the categories of *regenerative* and *non-regenerative* tissue. Regenerative tissue includes blood and bone marrow, while non-regenerative tissue includes cord blood, kidneys, liver (lobe/s), lungs (lobe/s), tendon and femoral heads. The implications of consent differ for each type of tissue. For example, the collection of bone marrow or the retrieval of a kidney, the lobe of a liver or a lung are invasive procedures that could potentially put the health and wellbeing of the donor at risk.[19] In contrast, the donation of a femoral head could be the end-product of a total hip replacement where the bone is otherwise discarded. Similarly, cord blood from the umbilical cord would be discarded if not retrieved immediately after birth.

After death, organ and tissue donation is clinically dependent on the variables of medical, surgical and social history, and how, when and where the person died. Legally and ethically, organ and tissue donation is dependent on informed decision-making and consent by the donor and their family. The most common form of donation after death in Australia and New Zealand is tissue donation.

Tissue-only donation

Many people can be tissue donors after their death. Eyes (whole or corneal button) are retrieved for corneal and scleral transplantation. Musculoskeletal tissue is used for bone grafting (long bones of upper and lower limbs and hemipelvis), urology procedures and treatment of sports injuries (ligaments, tendons, fascia and meniscus). Heart tissue (bicuspid and tricuspid valves, aortic and pulmonary tissue) is used for heart valve replacement and cardiac reconstruction. Skin is used for the treatment of burns.[20]

The potential tissue-only donor

The most influential component of the tissue-only donation process is the early notification of the potential donor's death to the relevant tissue bank or OTDS, ideally within hours of circulatory standstill. All deceased persons can be considered potential donors, with assessment for clinical suitability completed on a case-by-case basis.

The process of tissue-only donation

In general, local health, palliative and aged-care facilities notify the tissue bank or OTDS of any death. People who die in their home are not routinely notified, due to logistical issues and the length of time elapsed since circulatory standstill. However, the family may raise the issue of donation and this may be facilitated directly through the funeral home with the tissue bank and OTDS. The determining factors are age, cause of death, serology results, presence of infection, risk assessment of social and medical history, and time elapsed since circulatory standstill.[21] The legal requirements of obtaining consent mirror those of the multi-organ donor discussed later in the chapter.

Following medical suitability assessment and relevant donor registry checks, the tissue bank coordinator or other trained personnel will approach the next of kin with the possibility of tissue donation. Eyes can be retrieved from 12 to 24 hours after circulatory standstill depending on the techniques used when processing the tissue after retrieval; heart tissue, skin and musculoskeletal tissue can be retrieved up to 24 hours after circulatory standstill. Of note, eye donors can be up to 99 years of age, heart tissue donors up to 60 years and musculoskeletal donors up to 90 years of age in Australia and New Zealand.

Following tissue retrieval, every effort is made to restore anatomical appearance. Incisions are sutured, closed and covered with surgical dressings as appropriate, limbs given back their form and the eye shape is restored with the lids kept closed with eye caps.[21,22]

Support requirements for the families of tissue-only donors share many of the aspects of programs provided for the families involved in donation after circulatory and brain death, as discussed later in the chapter. A sensitive approach, provision of adequate information to assist informed decision-making, offers of formal bereavement support and follow-up information of recipient outcomes are proven aspects of successful programs.[23,24] A possibility for some potential donor families is solid-organ donation, as confirmation of death using circulatory criteria does not necessarily preclude solid-organ retrieval. See the section on donation after circulatory death.

Clinical trigger

The use of clinical triggers in the emergency department (ED) and the intensive care unit (ICU) facilitates the early identification and referral of potential donors.[25] A clinical trigger is a tool used as part of a systematic approach to organ and tissue donation and is based on established international best practice.[26] A new nationally consistent clinical trigger is under development by Australia's OTA to optimise the identification and referral of all potential organ, eye and tissue donors.

> **PRACTICE TIP**
>
> Early notification about a potential donor should take place, as it allows for medical suitability assessment by donation and transplant experts, and provides staff with the opportunity to plan the family donation conversation.[25,27] ED and ICU staff are asked to contact the hospital-based donation team (where available), OTDS or tissue bank when a patient meets the trigger criteria whereby no further treatment options are available or appropriate, and a family discussion regarding end-of-life care has or is to be conducted.

Donation after circulatory death

Donation after circulatory death (DCD), previously known as non-heart-beating donation and donation after cardiac death, is now an established pathway to multi-organ donation in patients with irreversible neurological conditions who do not fulfill the brain death criteria or in patients with a catastrophic and irreversible cardio-respiratory condition where withdrawal of cardio-respiratory support (WCRS) is considered appropriate. Prior to brain death legislation in the late 1960s and early 1970s, DCD was the source of cadaveric kidneys for transplantation.[28,29]

Initially, long-term success of transplantation from organs procured from DCD donors was limited due to prolonged warm ischaemic time, ineffective immunosuppression, unrefined surgical technique and underdeveloped organ preservation methods.[28] However, DCD programs around the world were re-established following evidence to suggest that organs from DCD provide relatively equivalent outcomes when compared with organs from donation after brain death (DBD) donors.[30]

The renewed focus on DCD in Australia and New Zealand has been driven, in part, by stagnant donation rates and greater indications for transplantation. DCD forms part of a broad approach to expand the donor pool and the availability of organs for transplantation. In 2010, Australia's OTA released the National Protocol for DCD, ensuring clinical consistency, effectiveness and safety for both the donor and the recipient.[31] In New Zealand, the ODNZ developed a national protocol for DCD in consultation with intensive care and transplant professionals that was released in 2007.[32] DCD allows the families of patients who do not meet the brain death criteria the opportunity to donate solid organs and tissue after death.

The potential DCD donor

With consideration of the lessons learnt from the DBD program, a successful DCD program is founded on evidence-based ethical and clinical grounds that aim to maintain the dignity of the donor at all times and provide the donor family with support and information to ensure informed decision-making.[33]

Four categories of potential DCD donors have been identified, and are known as the Holland–Maastricht categories:[34,35]

- Category 1: Dead on arrival—unknown warm ischaemic time (uncontrolled)
- Category 2: Unsuccessful resuscitation—known warm ischaemic time (uncontrolled)
- Category 3: Awaiting cardiac arrest after planned withdrawal of cardio-respiratory support—known and limited warm ischaemic time (controlled)
- Category 4: Cardiac arrest after confirmation of brain death but prior to organ retrieval—known and potentially limited warm ischaemic time (uncontrolled).

Categories 1, 2 and 4 are unpredictable and present logistical difficulties in limiting the length of warm ischaemic time; present legal and ethical restrictions in the management of the potential donor; and do not allow enough time for informed decision-making by the potential donor's family.

Category 3 is the only option that is able to be controlled. The category 3 potential DCD donor is a person ventilated and monitored in ED or ICU who has suffered an irrecoverable condition that is not likely to deteriorate to brain death, and the decision has been made that further treatment is no longer

of benefit to the person and current interventions are to be withdrawn.

Transplant outcomes from this form of donation are influenced by the length of warm ischaemia, which is the time taken from cessation of ventilation and treatment to the certification of death, and then to the commencement of infusion of cold perfusion fluid and/or organ retrieval. The cold perfusion fluid is an electrolyte-specific solution that is used to flush the organs and temporarily halt the demand for oxygen by decreasing the temperature and stabilising the cell walls.[36]

> **PRACTICE TIP**
>
> The decision to withdraw cardio-respiratory support must be made independent of any decision to donate organs for transplantation and must be agreed to by the family and the treating healthcare team.[37]

The process of donation after circulatory death

The clinical suitability assessment for solid-organ retrieval replicates that of a multi-organ DBD donor (as discussed later in the chapter), with medical, surgical and social history, serology and organ function information collected prior to WCRS. The legal requirements for obtaining consent are the same as in DBD. Families will be informed that retrieval may not take place due to a number of variables, including the length of time from WCRS to circulatory standstill.[33,35]

DCD is deemed not appropriate if, in the judgement of the treating medical practitioner, it is anticipated that the patient is likely to survive after WCRS for significantly longer than the allocated time limit. The time limit ensures a respectful approach to managing the patient's death where the possibility of DCD might complicate an unexpectedly prolonged dying process.[38] Furthermore, the longer the warm ischaemic time, the greater the risk of irreparable damage to the organ due to hypotension and hypoxaemia.[39] Transplant units determine the specific time limits for the warm ischaemic period, for example: no more than 30 minutes from WCRS for liver, 60 minutes for kidney and pancreas; and 90 minutes for lungs.[40] Research into the potential for heart transplantation from DCD donors is currently being undertaken.

It should be noted that the ability to accurately predict the timing of death is difficult and the use of predictive algorithms to assess the likelihood of the patient dying within the time limit should be at the discretion of the treating medical practitioner. The University of Wisconsin criteria for predicting asystole following WCRS assigns a numerical value to clinical parameters to generate a score predicting the likelihood of death occurring within 90 minutes.[28] The UNOS tool (United Network for Organ Sharing) also uses a set of criteria for identifying potential DCD patients.[38] While these tools are commonly used within the United States, widespread validation of their effectiveness has not yet occurred in Australia or New Zealand. Clinical indicators (such as ventilator support, use of inotropes and sedation, body mass index, Glasgow Coma Scale, (GCS)) can be used as an 'informal' guide for predicting death; however, the decision to proceed with DCD is generally at the discretion of the patient's treating medical practitioner. If the time-frames are not met following WCRS in a potential DCD donor, the organ retrieval process is abandoned, usual end-of-life care continues and tissue donation pursued following death if indicated.

DCD retrieval process alternatives

WCRS in a potential DCD donor most commonly occurs in the ICU, but may also take place in the ED or operating theatre. The location of WCRS is generally dependent upon family requests and hospital policy. Consideration should also be given to logistical constraints which may have an impact on organ viability. Rapid transfer of the patient to theatre must occur following the certification of death to ensure that warm ischaemic time is kept to a minimum. The operating room is prepared well ahead of the scheduled WCRS and the procurement team and other operating room staff are kept updated until death is certified.[41]

If the patient is donating lungs, an anaesthetist will re-intubate prior to moving the patient on to the operating table to prevent aspiration. For multi-organ procurement (involving both abdominal and thoracic organs), a super-rapid laparotomy is performed in tandem with a sternotomy. The aim is to cannulate the aorta and, if necessary, the pulmonary artery to initiate the rapid infusion of cold preservation solutions. The thoracic aorta is cross-clamped and the right atrium vented. Topical cooling of the thoracic and abdominal viscera with icy saline slush is also performed. Once organ flushing with preservation solution has occurred, the surgical procedure continues as for a standard multi-organ procurement, or as a renal-only procurement depending on the circumstances.

If WCRS occurs in the operating theatre and circulatory standstill does not occur, the patient is transferred back to the ED or ICU or another appropriate area.[33] The priority at all times is the provision of high-quality end-of-life care, and the donation process should not compromise this aim.[43]

Donation after brain death

In Australia and New Zealand, the most common pathway to deceased donation is DBD, which is more likely to occur in the ICU than in the ED. There are four main factors that directly influence the number of donors after brain death:

- the incidence of brain death
- identification of potential donors
- brain death confirmation and informed consent for donation
- clinical management after confirmation of brain death.

Brain death

The diagnosis of brain death is now widely accepted, and most developed countries have legislation governing the definition of death and the retrieval of organs and tissues for transplantation. In Australia and New Zealand, the most common cause of brain death is spontaneous intracranial haemorrhage, which has implications for the organs and tissues retrieved as the donors may be older and often have cardiovascular and other co-morbidities.[42,43] There is no legal requirement to formally confirm brain death if organs and tissues are not going to be retrieved for transplantation.[18]

Brain death is only observed clinically when the patient is supported with mechanical ventilation, as the respiratory reflex

TABLE 54.2 Conditions associated with brain death[44]

Hypotension
Diabetes insipidus
Disseminated intravascular coagulation
Dysrhythmias
Cardiac arrest
Pulmonary oedema
Hypoxia
Acidosis

that is lost due to cerebral ischaemia will result in respiratory and cardiac arrest. Mechanical ventilation maintains the oxygen supply to the natural pacemaker of the heart, which functions independently of the central nervous system. Brain death results in hypotension due to loss of vasomotor control of the autonomic nervous system, loss of temperature regulation, reduction in hormone activity and loss of all cranial nerve reflexes. Table 54.2 lists the common conditions associated with brain death. Irrespective of the degree of external support, circulatory standstill will mostly occur in a matter of hours to days once brain death has occurred.[18,45]

Brain death testing methods

The aim of testing for brain death is to determine irreversible cessation of brain function. Testing does not demonstrate that every brain cell has died, but that a point of irreversible ischaemic damage involving cessation of the vital functions of the brain has been reached. Two senior medical practitioners with relevant and recent experience and no involvement with transplant recipient selection participate in this process. In Australia, one of the medical staff must be a designated specialist appointed by the governing body of their health institution.[18]

There are a number of steps in the process, the first being the observation period. ANZICS recommends that the observation period is a minimum of 4 hours from onset of no response observed until formal testing commences (with the patient being mechanically ventilated, a GCS score of 3, non-reacting pupils, absent cough and gag reflexes and no spontaneous respiratory effort).[18]

The second step is to consider the preconditions (see Box 54.1). Once the observation period has passed, during which time the patient receives ongoing treatment, and the preconditions have been met, formal testing can occur. Formal testing for brain death in Australia and New Zealand is undertaken using either clinical testing of brainstem function or cerebral blood flow studies.[21] The most common form of testing is clinical testing of the brainstem, involving assessment of the cranial nerves and the respiratory centre (see Table 54.3). Brain death is confirmed if there is no response to stimulation of all of these reflexes, with the respiratory centre tested last and only if the other reflexes prove to be absent. If the patient demonstrates no response to the first set of tests, the testing is replicated to demonstrate irreversibility. It is recommended

BOX 54.1 Preconditions of brain death testing[18]

- Definite clinical or neuro-imaging evidence of acute brain pathology consistent with irreversible loss of neurological function
- Normothermia (core temperature > 35°C)
- Normotension (systolic blood pressure > 90 mmHg, mean arterial pressure > 60 mmHg in an adult)
- Exclusion of effects of sedative drugs

- Absence of severe electrolyte, metabolic or endocrine disturbances
- Intact neuromuscular function
- Ability to adequately examine the brainstem reflexes (at least one ear and one eye)
- Ability to perform apnoea testing

TABLE 54.3 Clinical brain death testing[18,46]

		CRANIAL NERVES	TEST TECHNIQUE	OUTCOME
1	Response to noxious stimuli	Trigeminal V (sensory), facial VII (motor)	Stimulus within the cranial nerve distribution, e.g. firm pressure over supraorbital region	If reflex is absent the patient will not grimace or react
2	Pupillary response to light	Optic II, occulomotor III	Use torch to shine bright light into eye	If reflex is absent the pupils are fixed; may or may not be dilated
3	Corneal reflex	Trigeminal V (sensory), facial VII (motor)	Use wisp of cotton wool to touch the cornea	If the reflex is absent the eyes will not react or blink
4	Gag reflex	Glossopharyngeal IX, vagus X	Use a tongue depressor on the oropharynx or move ETT	If reflex is absent there is no gag or pharyngeal response
5	Cough reflex	Glossopharyngeal IX, vagus X	Use suction catheter down ETT to deliberately stimulate the carina	If reflex is absent there is no cough response
6	Occulovestibular reflex	Vestibulocochlear VII, occulomotor III, abducens VI	Check first that both tympanic membranes are intact or not obstructed. Then slowly irrigate both ears with 50 mL of iced water while eyes are held open	When the reflex is absent the eyes remain fixed rather than deviating towards the stimulus
7	Apnoea test	Medulla respiratory centre	The last test to be performed when all other reflexes have proven to be absent. The patient is pre-oxygenated on 100% oxygen, an ABG analysis is performed to ascertain the baseline carbon dioxide, and then the patient is disconnected from mechanical ventilation but supplied with oxygen via catheter or T-piece. The patient is observed for signs of respiratory effort	The period of time disconnected from the ventilator must be long enough for the arterial carbon dioxide level to rise to a threshold high enough to normally stimulate respiration; i.e. an arterial carbon dioxide pressure greater than 60 mmHg and an arterial pH of less than 7.30

ABG: arterial blood gas; ETT: endotracheal tube

that the two sets of tests be performed separately and independently.[18]

PRACTICE TIPS

- When testing for corneal reflex, take care not to cause corneal abrasion which might prevent the cornea being transplanted if the patient is an eye donor.
- Invite the next of kin to observe the second set of clinical tests to assist their comprehension of brain death.[47]

If the preconditions listed in Box 54.1 cannot be met, brain death can be confirmed using cerebral blood flow imaging to demonstrate absent blood flow to the brain, either by four-vessel angiography or radionuclide imaging. A four-vessel angiography is performed by direct injection of contrast medium into both carotid arteries and both vertebral arteries.[18] Brain death is confirmed if there is no blood flow above the level of the carotid siphon or above the foramen magnum (Fig 54.1).[18,48,49]

The radionuclide imaging is performed by administering a bolus of short-acting radionuclide isotope intravenously while

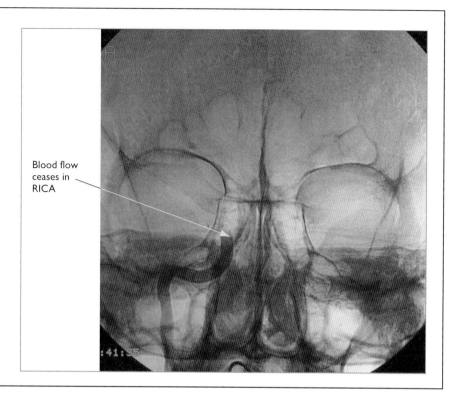

FIGURE 54.1

Brain death study—four-vessel cerebral angiography. Frontal cranial view of contrast flow in right internal carotid artery (RICA).

Blood flow ceases at the carotid siphon (arrow). Conclusion: if blood flow shown to have ceased in all the vessels there is no functioning cerebrum/cerebellum.

Courtesy Radiology Department, St George Hospital, Sydney.

Blood flow ceases in RICA

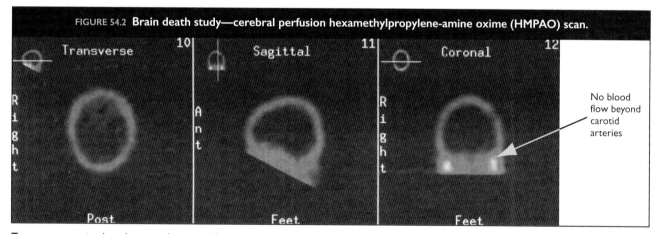

FIGURE 54.2 Brain death study—cerebral perfusion hexamethylpropylene-amine oxime (HMPAO) scan.

No blood flow beyond carotid arteries

Transverse, sagittal and coronal views. No uptake is seen in the cranial vault within the cerebrum or cerebellum. Blood flow is present in the sagittal and coronal views only to the carotid siphon (arrow). Conclusion: there is no functioning cerebrum/cerebellum within the cranial vault.

Courtesy Nuclear Medicine Department, St George Hospital, Sydney.

imaging the head using a gamma camera. No intracranial uptake of the radionuclide isotope confirms absent blood flow to the brain (Fig 54.2).[18,48]

The time of death is recorded as the time the second clinician determines that brain death has occurred, whether this is by clinical examination or imaging to confirm the absence of intracranial blood flow, and this should be documented accordingly.[18]

The potential donor after brain death

A potential DBD donor is someone who is suspected of or has been confirmed as being brain dead. The inclusion and exclusion criteria for organ and tissue donation are constantly reviewed and amended.[50] In Australia, advice regarding medical

suitability for organ and tissue donation is available 24 hours a day, 7 days a week from the OTDS. This advice can be sought at any stage of the process and there is no expectation that the treating clinician and nursing staff at the bedside would have to make this decision.[51]

Obtaining consent

An important factor that influences the number of donors is the consent process. It is common practice in Australia and New Zealand that the treating medical practitioner will either initiate or be involved in approaching the next of kin after death has been confirmed or anticipated.[52] Approaching the next of kin to discuss organ and tissue donation is part of the duty of care to that patient, who may have indicated their wish to be a donor at the time of their death.[18,53,54] The act of offering information about donation could also be considered part of the duty of care to the family. This view is supported by a survey of donor families who have indicated that donation has brought some long-term meaning to their loss, knowing that their loved one helped others through transplantation.[55] Similarly, a study of Australian donor families revealed that 86% of the respondents felt that being approached about organ and tissue donation did not add to their distress; 99% believed that they had made the right decision by granting consent; and 86% felt that it provided some comfort in their loss.[56]

There are three elements involved when discussing organ and tissue donation with the family:

- the knowledge, beliefs and attitudes they bring to the situation
- the in-hospital experience they have received[57]
- the biases and beliefs of the health professional/s conducting the conversation.[58]

The outcome of the conversation should not be predicted or anticipated, as it may affect the 'spirit' in which the approach is made. Evidence to support this statement can be found in the results of a large study undertaken in the United States. Evanisko et al[59] endorsed a non-presumptive approach because they found that clinical staff asked to predict the response of the next of kin were incorrect 50% of the time.

Influence of knowledge, beliefs and attitudes

Attitudes towards organ and tissue donation are influenced by spiritual beliefs, cultural background, prior knowledge about donation, views on altruism and prior healthcare experiences (see cultural considerations in Ch 5).[60] The next of kin need to consider two aspects associated with existing attitudes and knowledge:

- the thoughts and feelings of the decision-maker(s)
- the previous wishes and beliefs of the person on whose behalf they are making the decision.

There is evidence of a link between consent rates and prior knowledge of the positive outcomes of organ and tissue donation.[61–64]

Delivery of relevant information

An important detail to be considered by all health professionals is that families may have a diminished ability to receive and understand information because they are often emotionally and physically overwhelmed at this time of family crisis.[56,65] Randhawa[66] suggests that interviews held with the family are the foundation of the entire organ and tissue donation process. The discussion about brain death or impending death must be clear and emphatic, using language that is free of medical terminology, and includes an explanation of the physical implications.[46,67] The use of diagrams, analogies, scans and written materials have been suggested as useful aids for enhancing understanding by next of kin.[53,61,68] For example, Haddow[68] relates the effective use of the analogy of brain death being described as a jigsaw puzzle with a piece missing to illustrate the relationship of the brain to the rest of the body. The opportunity to provide intensive training to health professionals in sensitive communication with accredited education programs improves the likelihood of meeting the needs of the family.[46,69–71]

As the time of confirmation of brain death is the person's legal time of death, a discussion would then be held with the family to discuss the subsequent plan and implications. As death has been confirmed, ventilation will be ceased to allow circulatory standstill to occur. However, if donation is to occur, ventilation and haemodynamic support will be provided to facilitate organ and tissue donation. The donation process must be fully explained, in a sensitive manner, to ensure an informed decision, while not overburdening the next of kin.[52,72] Box 54.2 lists some of the aspects of the organ and tissue donation process that may be included in such a discussion. The family should be given information on the benefits of donation, the right of the family to decline, the donation process and the inability to guarantee that the organs will be transplanted.[72] Of note, a best-practice approach to this discussion aims to assist the family to make the decision that is 'right' for them and not necessarily to result in gaining consent.[41]

Meetings with the family

Common to all pathways of donation after death, the timing, location, content and process of discussions with the family are all important considerations. An effective protocol for communicating with the family of the potential donor must include:

- frequent and honest updates on the patient's prognosis
- clear explanation of cause of death
- the possibility of organ and tissue donation not to be raised until the family accepts that the patient is likely to die or has already been confirmed as brain dead
- conversations held in a private and quiet setting[60,63,74–76]
- involvement of an organ and tissue donation specialists with clearly defined roles.[60]

There is compelling evidence that the meeting confirming the diagnosis of brain death should be held separately or de-coupled from the conversation about organ and tissue donation.[59,62,63,74–76] In reality, the pace of the discussions should be assessed on a case-by-case basis, as there may be circumstances when the discussion about donation is appropriately held prior to the confirmation of death.[18,42,53]

Other influential components of this process have been identified from insightful surveys completed with donor and non-donor families. The first is the use of inappropriate terms like 'harvest' to describe the organ retrieval surgery and 'life support' to describe the ventilator. The first term is considered extremely harsh and undignified, while the second term could perpetuate the hope of a chance of survival or recovery.[54,56,68,77] Another component is the attire of the personnel involved. Haddow[68] suggests that staff wearing clothing other than the standard uniform, e.g. surgical scrubs or plastic aprons, made the families wonder what was being done to their relative to require the health professional to be wearing such a garment. Another component is the timing or use of the information sourced from organ-donor registers and the driver's licence. Careful consideration must be taken when introducing this information in the family donation conversation.[68]

Staff roles, delineation and involvement

The process of organ and tissue donation within the emergency and critical care environments is significant for all concerned.

BOX 54.2 Information about the deceased donation and retrieval, to assist informed decision-making[73]

Ensure that the next of kin have understanding of:

- brain death or impending death
- time of death
- eventual organ failure if kept ventilated in critical care (DBD)
- organ and tissue donation.

If they choose to donate:

- In DBD, they will not be with the donor at time of circulatory standstill
- The donor will remain in critical care monitored and ventilated until transfer to theatre for retrieval
- Explain the organ retrieval surgery—including presence of anaesthetist
- Discuss which organs and tissue would be potentially medically suitable for retrieval
- Next of kin can give specific consent—not obliged to grant global consent
- Only named organs and tissues with consent are retrieved
- Advise regarding expected length of process
- Explain reason for bloods being taken and stored
- Advise that a donor specialist will be present through the entire process
- Explain how the donor will look after the retrieval
- Organ donation will not delay funeral plans
- Explain consent form
- Privacy implications of Human Tissue Act and similar legislation—for donor family and transplant recipients
- Explain reasons why donation may not proceed
- Explain organs may be transplanted interstate

- In the event of an abnormality/diseases, organs will not be retrieved
- Explain consent for research
- The site designated officer will also sign the consent form.

If a coronial case:

- Coroner's authorisation required
- Police identification
- Possible autopsy, brain retrieval
- Deceased will go to the coroner's mortuary after retrieval
- Explain contact with Coroner's Court.
- If organs are retrieved and not able to be transplanted:
  - Offer options—uses for research if consent provided, will be returned and placed with donor, or respectfully disposed of as medical waste.

Support services:

- Offer of viewing the patient and a telephone call after the retrieval
- Offer lock of hair and/or hand print
- Provide contact details of donation specialist and family support coordinator (if applicable)
- Provide printed information
- Offer social work or pastoral support
- Explain other support services available.

Follow-up information:

- Outcome of retrieval
- Recipient outcomes
- Written material and letters

When death is confirmed, it marks the end of an episode that has been catastrophic for the patient and their family and a potentially stressful and draining experience for the staff.[78–82]

Supporting a potential donor family is very much a multi-disciplinary team effort. As noted earlier, the ANZICS guidelines[18] encourage the treating medical staff to continue their involvement with the patient and their family after death is confirmed for continuity of care. Nursing staff involvement in the process of organ and tissue donation is intrinsic. This includes the practicalities of the process and care of the potential donor and their family during the decision-making process.[83] Donor families have identified nurses as being the most helpful health professionals in providing information and emotional support.[55,77,84]

A holistic approach for supporting families includes the involvement of social workers and pastoral-care workers. Often these health professionals have been working with the family for a number of days, and act as confidants and a resource for information on matters like the implications of a coronial enquiry and the stance a religious denomination has on organ and tissue donation. It is timely to note that the majority of primary religions are supportive of organ and tissue donation for transplantation, and most would instruct the family to make the decision that they felt was right for them.[56,85]

The organ and tissue donation specialist acts as a resource and is invited into the emergency or critical care area when appropriate.[73] A health professional who is an expert in donation, has had training in sensitive communication and has the time to spend with the family could be the best person to conduct a family donation conversation.[76] Findings of a large US study found that the combination of separating the conversations about death and donation, holding the conversations in a private setting and the involvement of an organ and tissue donation specialist improved consent rates.[75]

PRACTICE TIP

All staff and management must be aware of the possibility of experiencing grief reactions when involved in the organ and tissue donation process and the personal drain it can cause when trying to maintain professional boundaries. Compassion fatigue is a well-recognised phenomenon and staff must be sensitive to their own limitations.[81,82]

Role of designated officers

Under Australian law, a designated officer is appointed by the governing body of the institution to authorise non-coronial postmortems and the removal of tissue from a deceased person for transplantation or other therapeutic, medical or scientific purposes.[18] The designated officer must be satisfied that all the necessary inquiries have been made and that the necessary consent has been obtained before granting authority. Medical, nursing and administrative staff can be appointed to the role; however, they must not act in a case in which they have a clinical or personal involvement.

The term designated officer is not used in New Zealand legislation. The person with equivalent authority under the *Human Tissue Act 1964* is the person lawfully in possession of the body.[86] In the case of a hospital, this person is specified as the medical officer in charge and in practice, the treating clinician undertakes this consultation with the family.

Consent-indicator databases

The most influential contribution that an individual can make to the decision-making process of their family is the existence of an advance care directive or prior indication of consent. Some authors have reported that the existence of such information has made the decision-making 'easier';[87,88] it preserves patient autonomy[63,89] and could mean that the wishes of the patient are followed even when family decision-makers would have made the opposite decision.[90] Table 54.4 lists prospective donation databases available in Australia and New Zealand.

Documentation of consent

Consent is sought for the individual organs and tissues rather than a 'global' approach. If granted, the individual organs and tissues are indicated on the consent form, or named if the consent is being recorded over the telephone, and only those organs and tissues will be retrieved. The donation specialist staff might also seek permission to retrieve organs and tissues for approved research projects.

Definition of next of kin

In Australia, the definition of next of kin for adults and children is listed in strict order (see Table 54.5). In New Zealand, there is no stated hierarchy of next of kin, with a surviving spouse or relative able to act in this role.[18,86] In both countries, the next of kin can object on ethical grounds to grant consent, but experience shows that the family rarely disagrees if the wishes of the deceased are known.[18]

Role of Coroner and forensic pathologists

Because of the nature of their death, many donors are subject to coronial inquiry. If this is the case, permission to undertake organ and tissue retrieval is sought from the respective forensic pathologist and coroner according to local policy and procedure as part of the authorisation process. The coronial system is very supportive of donation for transplantation; in Australia 48% of donors in 2013 were subject to Coronial inquiry compared to 43% in 2012. In New Zealand it was 28% for 2013 compared to 50% in 2012.[43]

TABLE 54.4 Consent-indicator databases in Australia and New Zealand[91,92]

DATABASE NAME	HOST	ACCESS TO DATABASE INFORMATION	AVAILABILITY TO JOIN
Australia			
Australian Organ Donor Register	Medicare Australia	Limited to coordinators nominated by state donation agencies and tissue banks	Via Medicare offices, internet or phone 1800 777 203
Driver's licence	SA Department of Planning, Transport and Infrastructure	Limited to coordinators nominated by state donation agencies and tissue banks	Driver's licence application and renewal form
New Zealand			
Driver's licence	Land Transport Safety Authority	Limited to coordinators nominated by the National Transplant Donor Coordination Office	Driver's licence application and renewal form

TABLE 54.5 Definition of next of kin for children and adults in Australian legislation[73]

DONOR	ORDER OF SENIORITY	RELATIONSHIP
Child	1	Parent
	2	Adult sibling (over 18 years of age)
	3	Guardian (immediately before death)
Adult	1	Spouse or de facto (at time of death)
	2	Adult offspring (over 18 years of age)
	3	Parent
	4	Adult sibling (over 18 years of age)

Referral of potential donor after brain death

If consent is obtained, the referral process usually commences immediately. To ensure organ viability for transplantation, the time from brain death confirmation to retrieval of the organs is kept to a minimum. The longer the time delay, the more likely organ-failure-related complications will occur.[44]

The referral process starts with the donation specialist collating the past and present medical, surgical and social history of the potential donor, and relaying this information to the relevant local transplant units (see Table 54.6). Using this information, local transplant teams allocate the organs to the most suitable and appropriate recipient/s. If the local transplant team does not have a suitable recipient, the offer is extended to another team within Australia or New Zealand on rotation using TSANZ guidelines.[51]

Tissue typing and cross-matching

A vital component of the assessment and referral process is the tissue typing, cross-matching and serology testing of the potential donor's blood. Blood is drawn from the potential donor and sent to the relevant accredited laboratory for testing (see Table 54.7). Tissue typing identifies the human leucocyte antigen (HLA) phenotype from the genes on chromosome 6. The HLA molecules control the action of the immune system to differentiate between 'self' and 'foreign' tissue, and initiate an immune response to foreign matter. A transplanted organ will always be identified as foreign tissue by the recipient's body, hence the use of immunosuppressive drugs to suppress the immune response. A test routinely used to predict the level of this response is the cross-match. Lymphocytes from the potential donor are added to the potential recipient's serum to test if the recipient has an antibody that is specific to the HLA antigens of the donor. A reaction where the recipient's serum destroys the donor's cells is a positive cross-match, and is a contraindication for transplantation.[73]

Pre-hospital care

Before organ and tissue donation can be considered, paramedics have a duty of care to act in the immediate best interest of their patient. Therefore, paramedics should aim to provide optimal physiological support for the patient to enable the establishment of a diagnosis and assessment of prognosis upon arrival in the ED. Immediate and effective physiological support also preserves the opportunity for organ donation. It allows for the determination of brain death, ensures best possible organ function for potential recipients and, most importantly, it allows time for the family to make a decision about organ and tissue donation.[18]

Donor management

Another important factor that influences the number of actual donors is the clinical management the donor receives after confirmation of death according to brain death criteria. The ANZICS[18] guidelines recommend that 'it is reasonable to continue providing extracranial physiological support, while awaiting the determination of brain death or very severe irreversible brain damage'. If consent for organ and tissue retrieval is given, the aim of donor management is to support and optimise organ function until the procurement commences, while maintaining the dignity and respect for the donor and support for the family.

Ideal parameters for biochemistry, vital signs, urine output and clinical management are detailed in Table 54.8.

PRACTICE TIP

When managing a potential multi-organ donor after confirmation of brain death, continuation of eye care, chest physiotherapy, suctioning and positioning is vitally important, and can influence which organs and tissues are able to be retrieved.

TABLE 54.6 Donor referral information[73]

SECTION	DETAILS
Personal details	Address, phone number, gender, age, date of birth, height, weight, race, religion, build
Cause of death	Date and time of hospital admission, intubation, critical care admission, other trauma
Brain death confirmation	Date, time, method
Consent details	Specific organs and tissues, Designated Officer details, forensic pathologist and coroner details, police details, next of kin and databases accessed
Donor history	Family history, medical, surgical, travel, social and sexual history
Blood results	Blood group, biochemistry and haematology on admission and within last 12 hours, microbiology, gas exchange
Test results	Chest X-ray including lung field measurements, electrocardiogram, echocardiogram, bronchoscopy and sputum
Haemodynamics	Blood pressure, mean arterial pressure, heart rate, central venous pressure, urine output and temperature
Admission history	Cardiac arrest, temperature, renal and hepatic function, nutrition, drug and fluid administration
Physical examination	Scars, trauma, lesions, needle marks, tattoos, etc

TABLE 54.7 Blood tests required for organ donation[94,95]

	TEST	RESPONSE TIME FOR RESULTS
Serology	HBsAg, HBsAB, Anti-HBcAb, HBcAB IgM Anti-HIV-1/2 Anti-HCV Anti HTLV-I/II CMV IgG, CMV IgM EBV IgG, EBV IgM EBNA Toxo Ab IgG, Toxo AB IgM Chagas WNV Syphilis (next day)	3–3.5 hours
	Nucleic acid testing (NAT) NAT HIV NAT HCV NAT HBV	High-risk donor—done prior to referral Low-risk donor—next day
Tissue typing	Cross-matching with the blood of potential recipients for relevant ABO blood groups	5 hours

HBsAg: hepatitis B surface antigen; HBc: hepatitis B core; HIV: human immunodeficiency virus; HCV: hepatitis C virus; HTLV: human T-cell lymphotrophic virus; CMV: cytomegalovirus; EBV: Epstein-Barr virus

TABLE 54.8 Donor management care plan[44,45,96]

MANAGEMENT AIMS	VARIATION IN BRAIN DEATH	CAUSES AND CONSIDERATION	TREATMENT
pH 7.35–7.45 PaO_2 > 300 mmHg on FiO_2 100% and PEEP 5 (if lungs for Tx) $PaCO_2$ 35–45 mmHg	No cough or respiratory drive Hypoxaemia Orthostatic pneumonia Neurogenic pulmonary oedema	Optimise tissue oxygenation Prevent lung injury including over-expansion Aim to reduce atelectasis	Ventilate to normocarbia Lowest FiO_2 PEEP 5 cmH$_2$O ± bronchodilators Regular suctioning and repositioning 2–3 times in 24 hours Regular ABGs + when treatment or ventilation changed Regular physiotherapy Strict asepsis Broad-spectrum antibiotics (if necessary) CXR within last 12 hours
MAP > 60 mmHg HR < 120 bpm CVP 6–12 mmHg	Decrease in MAP Decrease in CVP Dysrhythmias Hypertension	Blood loss Deliberate dehydration to decrease cerebral oedema Polyuria—diabetes insipidus (DI), diuretics Electrolyte and acid–base disturbance, hypotension, hypothermia Common during herniation Dysrhythmias are usually self-limiting	Optimise intravascular volume as guided by CVP Physical assessment and FBC Choice of replacement fluid depends on fluid loss Consider ceasing contributing medications (diuretics, mannitol and barbiturates) Use of inotropes if not hypertensive, consider using agent with a short half-life Hormone resuscitation for persistent instability

TABLE 54.8 Donor management care plan[44,45,96]—cont'd

MANAGEMENT AIMS	VARIATION IN BRAIN DEATH	CAUSES AND CONSIDERATION	TREATMENT
Temperature > 35°C	Decrease in temperature Increase in temperature	Non-functioning hypothalamus Depressed metabolism Inability to shiver or vasoconstrict Cold IV fluid/blood administration Sepsis/infection	Avoid long exposure Active warming Warmed IV fluids Cooling blanket
Electrolytes within normal range	Increase in Na Decrease in K Decrease in Mg Decrease in Ca	Commonly encountered secondary to urinary losses in uncontrolled DI Increase in Na: DI Decrease in K: dysrhythmias Decrease in Mg: dysrhythmias	Frequent serum electrolytes Electrolyte replacement Correct hypernatraemia ECG within last 12 hours Control urine output, i.e. DI
Urine output 1 mL/kg/hr	Decrease in U/O Increase in U/O (> 300–400 mL/h)	Hypovolaemia DI (lack of ADH leads to an inappropriate and large U/O)	Restore circulating volume Consider correcting 'free water' deficit and replace electrolytes Consider the use of DDAVP in small amounts to decrease urine output
Blood glucose level	Increase in BGL	Insulin resistance–stress response + circulation of catecholamines IV fluids containing dextrose	Insulin infusion Avoid dextrose
Good general nursing care and infection control Maintain patient's dignity and respect	Some may consider unnecessary as patient has been confirmed dead	Demonstrate continuum of care Act as a patient advocate Optimise success of donation and transplantation	2-hourly eye care (for eye retrieval) 2-hourly repositioning 2-hourly mouth care General hygiene

ABG: arterial blood gas; ADH: antidiuretic hormone; BGL: blood glucose level; BP: blood pressure; Ca: calcium; CVP: central venous pressure; CXR: chest X-ray; DDAVP: desmopressin; DI: diabetes insipidus; ECG: electrocardiogram; FBC: full blood count; FiO_2: fraction of inspired oxygen; Hb: haemoglobin; HR: heart rate; IV: intravenous; K: potassium; MAP: mean arterial pressure; Mg: magnesium; Na: sodium; $PaCO_2$: arterial pressure of carbon dioxide; PaO_2: arterial pressure of oxygen; PEEP: positive end-expiratory pressure; Tx: transplant; U/O: urine output

The procurement process

The procurement surgery occurs in the hospital where the donor is located and the local operating theatre staff are involved in this process. The donor is transferred to theatre after routine pre-operative checks and documentation is completed, including death confirmation and consent for organ and tissue retrieval. Depending on which organs are to be retrieved, the procurement teams will be tasked to abdominal organs and thoracic organs, and will bring most of their specialised equipment with them. An anaesthetist will be present in DBD to monitor haemodynamics, ventilation and administer medications, but will not deliver anaesthetic agents. The local operating theatre staff will work with the visiting surgical teams and a donation specialist will be present to document the procedure and its outcomes, and act as a resource for everyone present.

The surgery takes 5–7 hours, depending on the extent of the retrieval. In DBD, once the surgeons have identified all the various anatomical points, the aorta is cross-clamped with vascular clamps below the diaphragm and at the aortic arch, the heart is stopped and ventilation is ceased. Before the organs are removed, the procurement teams administer a cold perfusion fluid with an electrolyte-specific mix to the organs. Upon removal, the organs are bagged with sterile slush and perfusion fluid, and transported in ice by the procurement teams to the transplanting hospitals. Some procurement teams use ex-vivo perfusion technology that allows normothermic preservation of organs such as lungs and hearts. This portable technology pumps warm, oxygenated, nutrient-rich blood through the organ, thus allowing more time between donation and transplant; hence the ability to assess the organ before transplant for better overall outcomes.[96,97]

The incision that extends from the sternal notch to the pubic symphysis is closed by the surgeons in a routine manner and covered with a surgical dressing. If the donor is not a coroner's case, the remaining lines, catheter and drains are removed according to local policy, the donor is washed and arrangements made to transfer them to a specified location for a viewing with the family or to the mortuary. The musculoskeletal tissue, skin and eye retrieval can occur at the end of the solid-organ retrieval in theatre or later in the mortuary.[40,98,99]

Donor family care

Family support begins from the time their loved one is admitted to hospital and continues well beyond organ and tissue retrieval. In addition to individual considerations, such as religion, culture, family dynamics, coping skills and prior experiences with loss, that may influence the grieving process, the family of an organ and tissue donor will be dealing with a number of unique factors. The death of their family member was likely to have been sudden and unexpected; brain death can be difficult to understand when their loved one looks like they are asleep rather than dead; the opportunity of donation might mean having to make a decision on behalf of their loved one if their wishes are not known; in DCD, the decision to withdraw cardio-respiratory support might set off feelings of

guilt and thoughts of prematurely withdrawing treatment; and in DBD, the process might mean they may not be able to be with their loved one when their heart stops.[100]

Donor families benefit from emotional and physical support throughout and following the donation process. In the critical care area, support can take the form of open visiting times, privacy for meetings, clear and precise information, and regular contact with the treating clinical team and the donation specialist. After retrieval, the ongoing care of a donor family can include contact with a bereavement specialist, written resource material, telephone support, private or group counselling and correspondence from recipients.[23,101] Organ Donation New Zealand and the Australian DonateLife network have cost-free, structured aftercare and follow-up programs that offer these features.[51] Holtkamp[77] states that trained personnel involved with a donor family through this process have the unique opportunity to positively influence the family's grief journey (Ch 53).

SUMMARY

In summary, organ and tissue donation is a routine component of end-of-life care. Along with age, medical, surgical and social history, the location, cause and mechanism of the death are determining factors of which donation pathway is possible. Every potential donor is assessed on a case-by-case basis to determine medical suitability for organ and tissue retrieval for transplantation. In Australia and New Zealand, consent for organ and tissue donation is required in writing, which can be indicated by the person themselves before their death or by their next of kin after their death. In some instances, verbal consent can be recorded over the phone. Only the organs and tissues with specific consent will be retrieved.

Notification of the person's impending or confirmed death and participation in the assessment and referral process is seen as a component of end-of-life care by the treating clinical staff. Support and guidance to the process of organ and tissue donation is available 24 hours a day from the tissue banks and donation services in both countries. There is no expectation that the treating clinicians and nursing staff would have to make decisions about medical suitability and are therefore encouraged to contact the relevant tissue bank or donation service at any stage of the process. The organ and tissue donation referral and retrieval process has legal, practical and ethical components that must be observed, but the overriding aim is to treat the donor and their family with the care and dignity they deserve.

CASE STUDY

It is 10.15 am and Tony, a 19-year-old electrician, has collapsed on a building site. On arrival, the paramedics find him lying unconscious and surrounded by his work-mates, who have placed him in the recovery position. On examination, Tony has a Glasgow Coma Scale (GCS) score of 5 and is spontaneously breathing. He reportedly complained of a severe headache and vomited just prior to collapsing. Tony is intubated and transferred to hospital.

Questions

1. During the transfer, the aim of treatment is to:
   A. Resuscitate and optimise oxygenation and organ function for potential organ and/or tissue donation.
   B. Resuscitate and optimise oxygenation and organ function for assessment of cause of injury and prognosis.

   C. Limit resuscitation as Tony is likely to have suffered a life-ending event.

2. On arrival at the emergency department, Tony's GCS is 3, his pupils are fixed and dilated, and he has stopped spontaneously breathing. The next intervention should be:
   A. Brain death testing
   B. Wait for family to arrive before withdrawing treatment.
   C. Cerebral computed tomography.

3. Transferred to the intensive care unit (ICU), Tony is kept intubated and ventilated, sedated and inotropes are titrated to maintain his blood pressure. After 3 days, the sedation is weaned and ceased. Tony is triggering spontaneous breaths, but only scoring a GCS of 5. After a further 3 days, Tony's condition

has not changed. The neurosurgical and ICU team meet with his parents to explain that he is unlikely to survive this incident or deteriorate to brain death, and that withdrawal of treatment is appropriate. After consideration, Tony's parents agree to withdrawal of treatment and ask if organ and tissue donation would be possible.

Is this possible?

A. No, Tony is not brain-dead.

B. Only tissue donation is possible after circulatory death is confirmed.

C. Donation of both solid organs and tissues is possible via the donation-after-circulatory-death pathway (DCD).

4. If organ and tissue donation is possible, does Tony have to be transferred to a tertiary referral centre?

A. Yes, smaller hospitals will not have the specialised equipment necessary for the donation coordination and retrieval.

B. No, the donation coordination staff and procurement team can travel to regional and metropolitan sites.

 Answers to Case Study Questions can be found on evolve
http://evolve.emergencytrauma.curtis

USEFUL WEBSITES

Australasian Transplant Coordinators Association, www.atca.org.au

Australian and New Zealand Intensive Care Society, Statement on Death and Organ Donation Ed 3.2 [1]2013, www.nepeanicu.org/pdf/Organs%20Donation/ANZICSstatementondeathandorgandonation.pdf

Australian Code of Good Manufacturing Practice—Human Blood and Tissues, www.tga.gov.au/publication/australian-code-good-manufacturing-practice-human-blood-and-blood-components-human-tissues-and-human-cellular-therapy-products

Australian Donor Awareness Program, www.donatelife.gov.au/

Australian Organ Donor Register, www.medicareaustralia.gov.au/public/services/aodr/index.jsp

Australian Tissue Banking Forum, www.bioaa.org.au/

Eye Bank Association of Australia and New Zealand, www.ebaanz.org

New Zealand Code of Good Manufacturing Practice for Manufacture and Distribution of Organ Donation New Zealand, www.donor.co.nz

Therapeutic Goods, www.medsafe.govt.nz/regulatory/Guideline/code.asp

Transplantation Society of Australia and New Zealand, www.tsanz.com.au

Transplant Nurses' Association, www.tna.asn.au

REFERENCES

1. Chapman J, New B. Transplantation. In: Chapman JR, Deierhoi M, Wight C, eds. Organ and tissue donation for transplantation. London: Arnold; 1997:1–22.

2. Mathew TH, Chapman JR. Organ donation: a chance for Australia to do better. Med J Aust 2006;185(5):245–6.

3. Chapman JR. Transplantation in Australia—50 years in progress. MJA Monograph no. 3 1993:3–6.

4. McBride M, Chapman JR. An overview of transplantation in Australia. Anaesth Intensive Care 1995;23(1):60–4.

5. George C. Caring for kidneys in the Antipodes: how Australia and New Zealand have addressed the challenge of end-stage renal failure. American Journal of Kidney Diseases 2009;53(3):536–45.

6. Roake J. Editorial: Liver transplantation in Australia and New Zealand. ANZ Journal of Surgery 2008;78:628–9.

7. Australian Organ and Tissue Authority, Donatelife. History of organ and tissue transplantation; Australian Government, Canberra, October 2009, http://www.donatelife.gov.au/sites/default/files/History_of_Organ_and_Tissue_Donation.pdf; accessed 18 May 2015.

8. Borel JF, Feurer C, Gubler HU et al. Biological effects of cyclosporin-A: a new antilymphocytic agent. Agents Actions 1976;6:468–75.

9. Russ GR. Immunosuppression in transplantation. MJA Monograph no. 3; 1993:4–19.

10. Australian Government Organ and Tissue Authority, A world's best practice approach to organ and tissue donation for transplantation. 2008. Online. www.donatelife.gov.au.

11. Australia and New Zealand Organ Donor (ANZOD) Registry. Annual reports. Online. www.anzdata.org.au/anzod/updates/anzod1989toCurrent.pdf; accessed 23 June 2015.

12. Kelly M. 'Opting-out' vs 'Hot Pursuit': organ donation and the family. Bioethics Outlook. John Plunkett Centre for Ethics in Health Care 1996;7(2):1–6.

13. Dickens BC, Fluss SS, King AR. Legislation on organ and tissue donation. In: Chapman JR, Deierhoi M, Wight C, editors. Organ and tissue donation for transplantation. London: Arnold; 1997:95–119.

14. Rosenblum A, Li A, Roels L et al. Worldwide variability in deceased organ donation registries. Transplant International 2012;25:801–11.

15. Kita Y, Aranami Y, Aranami Y et al. Japanese organ transplant law: a historical perspective. Prog Transplant 2000;10(2):106–8.

16. Kim JR, Elliott D, Hyde C. The influence of sociocultural factors on organ donation and transplantation in Korea: findings from key informant interviews. J Transcult Nurs 2004;15(2):147–54.

17. New Zealand Ministry of Health. A code of practice for transplantation of cadaveric organs. Wellington: MOH; 1987.

18. Australian and New Zealand Intensive Care Society. The ANZICS statement on death and organ donation. 3.2 edn. Melbourne: ANZICS; 2013.

19. Gleeson G. Organ transplantation from living donors. Plunkett Centre for Ethics in Health Care. Bioethics Outlook 2000;11(1):5–8.

20. Pearson J. Tissue donation. Nurs Stand 1999;13(45):14–15.

21. Cordner S, Ireland L. Tissue banking. In: Chapman JR, Deierhoi M, Wight DC, eds. Organ and tissue donation for transplantation. London: Arnold; 1997:268–303.

22. Haire MC, Hinchliff JP. Donation of heart valve tissue: seeking consent and meeting the needs of donor families. Med J Aust 1996;164(1):28–31.

23. Beard J, Ireland L, Davis N et al. Tissue donation: what does it mean to families? Prog Transplant 2002;12(1):42–8.

24. Rodrigue JR, Cornell DL, Howard RJ. Organ donation decision: comparison of donor and non-donor families. Am J Transplant 2006;6(1):190–8.

25. Zavotsky KE, Tamburri LM. A case in successful organ donation: emergency department nurses do make a difference. J Emerg Nurs 2007;33(3):235–41.

26. Graham JM, Sabeta ME, Cooke JT et al. A system's approach to improve organ donation. Prog Transplant 2009;19(3):216–20.

27. Murphy PG, Logan L. Clinical leads for organ donation: making it happen in hospitals. J Intensive Care Soc 2009;10(3):174–8.

28. Lewis J, Peltier J, Nelson H et al. Development of the University of Wisconsin donation after cardiac death evaluation tool. Prog Transplant 2003;13(4):265–73.

29. Levvey B, Griffiths A, Snell G. Non-heart beating organ donors: a realistic opportunity to expand the donor pool. Transplant Nurses J 2004;13(3):8–12.

30. Bell MDD, Bodenham AR. Non-heart beating organ donation: can we balance duty of care, the law and recipient need? Care Critically Ill 2004;20:1–2.

31. Australian Government Organ and Tissue Authority. National protocol for donation after cardiac death. 2010. Online. www.donatelife.gov.au.

32. Organ Donation New Zealand. Protocol for donation after cardiac death. 2007. Online. www.donor.co.nz.

33. American College of Critical Care Medicine, Society of Critical Care Medicine, Ethics Committee. Recommendations for non-heartbeating organ donation. Crit Care Med 2001;29:1826–31.

34. Kootstra G, Daemen JH, Oomen AP. Categories of non-heart-beating donors. Transplant Proc 1995;27(5):2893–4.

35. Brook NR, Waller JR, Nicholson ML. Nonheart-beating kidney donation: current practice and future developments, Kidney Int 2003;63:1516–29.

36. Deierhoi M. Organ recovery from cadaveric donors. In: Chapman JR, Deierhoi M, Wight C, editors. Organ and tissue donation for transplantation. London: Arnold; 1997:152–61.

37. Steinbrook R. Organ donation after cardiac death. N Engl J Med 2007;357:209–13.

38. Coleman N, Brieva J, Crowfoot E. Identification of a realistic donation after cardiac death (DCD) donor: predicting time of death within 60 minutes following withdrawal of futile life sustaining treatment. Transplant Nurses J 2008;17(2):22–5.

39. DeVita MA, Snyder JV, Arnold RM et al. Observations of withdrawal of life-sustaining treatment from patients who become non-heart-beating organ donors. Crit Care Med 2000;28(6):1709–12.

40. Bernat JL, D'Alessandro AM, Port FK et al. Report of a national conference on donation after cardiac death. Am J Transplant 2006;6(2):281–91.

41. Shemie SD, Baker AJ, Knoll G et al. National recommendations for donation after cardiocirculatory death in Canada. CMAJ 2006; 175(8 Suppl):S1–24.

42. Streat S, Silvester W. Organ donation in Australia and New Zealand—ICU perspectives. Crit Care Resusc 2001;3(1):48–51.

43. Australia and New Zealand Organ Donation Registry. ANZOD Registry Report. Adelaide: ANZOD; 2009. Online. Available: www.anzdata.org.au/anzod/v1/AR-2009.html.

44. Kutsogiannis D, Pagliarello G, Doig C et al. Medical management to optimize donor organ potential: review of the literature. Can J Anesth 2006;53(8):820–30.

45. Power BM, Van Heerden PV. The physiological changes associated with brain death—current concepts and implications for treatment of the brain dead organ donor. Anaesth Intensive Care 1995;23(1):26–36.

46. Dobb GJ, Weekes JW. Clinical confirmation of brain death. Anaesth Intensive Care 1995;23(1):37–43.

47. Siminoff LA, Mercer MB, Arnold R. Families' understanding of brain death. Prog Transplant 2003;13(3):218–24.

48. Monsein LH. The imaging of brain death. Anaesth Intens Care 1995;23:44–50.

49. Tortora GJ, Grabowski SR. The principles of anatomy and physiology. 9th edn. New York: Wiley; 2000.

50. Transplantation Society of Australia and New Zealand. Updates. Online. www.tsanz.com.au; accessed 11 Jan 2010.

51. NSW/ACT Organ Donation Network. Area donor coordinator; clinical pathway. Sydney: NSW/ACT ODN; 2008.

52. Thompson JF, Hibberd AD, Mohacsi PJ et al. Can cadaveric organ donation rates be improved? Anaesth Intensive Care 1995; 23(1):99–103.

53. Raper RF, Fisher MM. Brain death and organ donation—a point of view. Anaesth Intens Care 1995;23:16–19.

54. Streat S. Clinical review: moral assumptions and the process of organ donation in the intensive care unit. Critical care 2004;8:382–8. Online. http://ccforum.com/inpress/cc2876; 24 Jan 2005.

55. Pelletier ML. The needs of family members of organ and tissue donors. Heart Lung 1993;22(2):151–7.

56. Australasian Transplant Coordinators Association. National donor family study. Melbourne; 2008.

57. Beasley C. Maximizing donation. Transplant Reviews 1999;13:31–9.

58. Verble M, Worth J. Biases among hospital personnel concerning donation of specific organs and tissues: implication for the donation discussion and education. J Transpl Coord 1997;7(2):72–7.

59. Evanisko MJ, Beasley CL, Brigham LE et al. Readiness of critical care physicians and nurses to handle requests for organ donation. Am J Crit Care 1998;7(1):4–12.

60. Verble M, Worth J. Fears and concerns expressed by families in the donation discussion. Prog Transplant 2000;10(1):48–55.

61. Pearson IY, Zurynski Y. A survey of personal and professional attitudes of intensivists to organ donation and transplantation. Anaesth Intensive Care 1995;23(1):68–74.

62. DeJong W, Franz HG, Wolfe SM et al. Requesting organ donation: an interview study of donor and nondonor families. Am J Crit Care 1998;7(1):13–23.

63. Siminoff LA, Gordon N, Hewlett J et al. Factors influencing families' consent for donation of solid organs for transplantation. JAMA 2001;286(1):71–7.

64. Rodrigue JR, Scott MP, Oppenheim AR. The tissue donation experience: a comparison of donor and nondonor families. Prog Transplant 2003;13(4):258–64.

65. Douglass GE, Daly M. Donor families' experience of organ donation. Anaesth Intensive Care 1995;23(1):96–8.

66. Randhawa G. Specialist nurse training programme: dealing with asking for organ donation. J Adv Nurs 1998;28(2):405–8.

67. Coyle MA. Meeting the needs of the family: the role of the specialist nurse in the management of brain death. Intensive Crit Care Nurs 2000;16(1):45–50.

68. Haddow G. Donor and nondonor families' accounts of communication and relations with health professionals. Prog Transplant 2004;14(1):41–8.

69. Redfern S. Organ donation: how do we ask the question? J R Coll Nurs Aus Collegian 1997;4(2):23–5.

70. Sutton RB. Supporting the bereaved relative: reflections on the actor's experience. Med Educ 1998;32(6):622–9.

71. Morton J, Blok GA, Reid C et al. The European donor hospital education programme (EDHEP): enhancing communication skills with bereaved relatives. Anaesth Intensive Care 2000;28(2):184–90.

72. Verble M, Worth J. Adequate consent: its content in the donation discussion. J Transpl Coord 1998;8(2):99–104.

73. Australasian Transplant Coordinators Association. National guidelines for organ and tissue donation. 4th edn. Sydney: ATCA; 2008.

74. Edwards J, Hasz R, Menendez J. Organ donors: your care is critical. RN 1997;60(6):46–51.

75. Gortmaker SL, Beasley CL, Sheehy E et al. Improving the request process to increase family consent for organ donation. J Transpl Coord 1998;8(4):210–17.

76. Ehrle RN, Shafer TJ, Nelson KR. Referral, request and consent for organ donation: best practice—a blueprint for success. Crit Care Nurse 1999;19(2):21–36.

77. Holtkamp S. Wrapped in mourning: the gift of life and organ donor family trauma. New York: Brunner-Routledge; 2002.

78. Johnson C. The nurse's role in organ donation from a brainstem dead patient: management of the family. Intensive Critical Care Nurs 1992;8(3):140–8.

79. Duke J, Murphy B, Bell A. Nurses' attitudes toward organ donation: an Australian perspective. Dimens Crit Care Nurs 1998; 17(5):264–70.

80. Pelletier-Hibbert M. Coping strategies used by nurses to deal with the care of organ donors and their families. Heart Lung 1998;27(4):230–7.

81. Pearson A, Robertson-Malt S, Walsh K et al. Intensive care nurses' experiences of caring for brain dead organ donor patients. J Clin Nurs 2001;10(1):132–9.

82. Ainsworth K, Sgorbini M. Compassion fatigue: who cares for the carers? Transplant J Australas 2010;19(2):21–2, 24–5.

83. Kiberd MC, Kiberd BA. Nursing attitudes towards organ donation, procurement, and transplantation. Heart Lung 1992;21(2):106–11.

84. McCoy J, Argue PC. The role of critical care nurses in organ donation: a case study. Crit Care Nurse 1999;19(2):48–52.

85. Australian Organ and Tissue Authority. Organ donation and your religion, fact sheet. Online. www.donatelife.gov.au/Media/docs/religion_web_040210-243f32ec-aedf-4f91-8590-d35a6cfae2d8-2.pdf; accessed 6 Aug 2010.

86. New Zealand Government. Human Tissue Act 1964. Section 2.

87. Wheeler MS, O'Friel M, Cheung AHS. Cultural beliefs of Asian-Americans as barriers to organ donation. J Transpl Coord 1994; 4:146–50.

88. Thompson TL, Robinson JD, Kenny RW. Family conversations about organ donation. Prog Transplant 2004;14(1):49–55.

89. Richter J, Eisemann MR. Attitudinal patterns determining decision-making in severely ill elderly patients: a cross-cultural comparison between nurses from Sweden and Germany. Int J Nurs Stud 2001;38(4):381–8.

90. Pearson IY, Bazeley P, Spencer-Plane T et al. A survey of families of brain dead patients: their experiences, attitudes to organ donation and transplantation. Anaesth Intensive Care 1995;23(1):88–95.

91. New Zealand Ministry of Health. Organ donation fact sheet. 2004. Online. www.moh.govt.nz/moh.nsf; accessed 25 Jan 2005.

92. Australian Government. Health Insurance Commission. Australian organ donor register. Online. www.humanservices.gov.au/customer/services/medicare/australian-organ-donor-register?utm_id=9; accessed 23 June 2015.

93. Electronic Donor Record: Standard operating procedure and user guide. Australian Government Organ and Tissue Authority, Version 4.01, December 2013.

94. Moyes K. Improving organ donation rates with standard nucleic acid testing on all potential donors. Transplant Nurses J 2002;11:15–16.

95. Australian Red Cross Blood Service. Blood testing: safety and testing. 2008. Online. www.donateblood.com.au/all-about-blood/safety-and-testing.

96. Rosendale JD, Kauffman HM, McBride MA et al. Aggressive pharmacologic donor management results in more transplanted organs. Transplantation 2003;75:482–7.

97. Warnecke G, Moradiellos J, Tudorache I et al. Normothermic perfusion of donor lungs for preservation and assessment with the Organ Care System Lung before bilateral transplantation: a pilot study of 12 patients. The Lancet 2012;380:1851–8.

98. Prastein D, Poston R, Gu J, Gage F. Viability markers to assess nonheartbeating donor hearts during ex vivo perfusion. Transplantation 2004;78(2):642.

99. Lilly KT, Langley VL. The perioperative nurse and the organ donation experience. AORN J 1999;69(4):779–91.

100. Regehr C, Kjerulf M, Popova SR et al. Trauma and tribulation: the experiences and attitudes of operating room nurses working with organ donors. J Clin Nurs 2004;13:430–7.

101. Holtkamp SC. The donor family experience: sudden loss, brain death, organ donation, grief and recovery. In: Chapman JR, Deierhoi M, Wight C, eds. Organ and tissue donation for transplantation. London: Arnold; 1997:304–22.

102. Verble M, Worth J. Cultural sensitivity in the donation discussion. Prog Transplant 2003;13(1):33–7.

BOX, FIGURE AND TABLE CREDITS

Section 1 background image Shutterstock/Monkey Business Images.

Section 2 background image Courtesy the University of Sydney.

Section 3 background image Courtesy NSW Ambulance.

Section 4 background image Courtesy University of Sydney.

Section 5 background image Roberts JR MD. Roberts and Hedges' Clinical Procedures in Emergency Medicine, Elsevier; 2013.

Section 6 background image Courtesy Marco Sacchi.

Table 1.1 Adapted from: Australian Health Workforce Advisory Committee: Health workforce planning and models of care in emergency departments. Canberra: National Health Workforce Secretariat; 2006.

Box 1.1 ACEM: Role delineation for emergency departments. Emergency Medicine 1998;10:65–69.

Box 1.2 Hewitt A, Roos R, Baldwin K. Emergency Department use 2011/12. Wellington: New Zealand Ministry of Health, 2012.

Figs 2.1, 2.2, 2.3 Courtesy NSW Ambulance.

Table 2.1 Data from the statutory ambulance services in Australia/New Zealand, Queensland Ambulance Service, Field Reference Guide 2011, Paramedicine Role Descriptions, Paramedic Australasia. Online. www.paramedics.org/content/2009/07/PRD_211212_WEBONLY.pdf.

Table 2.2 Adapted from Caffey, M. Paramedic and Emergency Pharmacology Guidelines, 2013.

Box 3.1 Nursing and Midwifery Board of Australia. Code of ethics for nurses in Australia. Online. http://www.nursingmidwiferyboard.gov.au/Codes-Guidelines-Statements/Codes-Guidelines.aspx#codesofethics.

Box 3.2 Paramedics Australasia Code of Conduct from https://www.paramedics.org/our-organisation/who-we-are/code-of-conduct/.

Box 3.3 Beauchamp T, Childress J. Principles of biomedical ethics. 5th edn. New York: Oxford University Press; 2001.

Box 3.4 Kerridge I, Lowe M, Stewart C. Ethics and law for the health professions. 3rd edn. Sydney: Federation Press; 2013; Milligan E, Winch S. Practical ethics in clinical care. In: Psychosocial dimensions in medicine. J Fitzgerald, G Byrne eds. Melbourne: IP Communications, 2015.

Table 6.1 Wren DA, Bedeian AG, Breeze JD. The foundations of Henry Fayol's administrative theory. Management Decision 2002;40(9):906–18.

Table 6.2 Mintzberg H. Mintzberg on management: inside our strange world of organizations. New York: Free press; 1989.

Table 6.3 Robbins SP, Bergman R, Stagg I et al. Management. Sydney: Prentice Hall; 2000.

Fig 8.1 Graham ID, Logan J, Harrison MB et al. Lost in knowledge translation. J Contin Educ Health Prof 2006;26:13–24.

Box 8.1 Burns N, Grove S. The practice of nursing research, conduct, critique and utilization. 4th edn. London: Saunders; 2001; Kerlinger FN. Foundations of behavioral research. New York: Holt, Reinhart and Winston; 1986; Yin RK. Case study research: design and methods. 3rd edn. Thousand Oaks, CA: Sage Publications; 2002.

Box 8.2 National Health and Medical Research Council, Australian Research Council, Committee AVCs. National statement on ethical conduct in human research 2007. Canberra: Commonwealth of Australia; 2014.

Box 8.3 National Health and Medical Research Council. A guide to the development, implementation and evaluation of clinical practice guidelines. In: NHMRC, ed. Canberra: NHMRC: Commonwealth of Australia; 1999.

Box 8.4 Schneider Z, Elliott D, LoBiondo-Wood G, Haber J. Nursing research: methods, critical appraisal and utilisation. 2nd edn. Sydney: Mosby; 2004; Glaser B, Strauss A. The discovery of grounded theory: strategies for qualitative research. New York: Aldine; 1967; Hart E, Bond M. Action research for health and social care: a guide to practice. Philadelphia: Open University Press; 1995; Munhall PL. Philosophical ponderings on qualitative research methods in nursing. Nursing Science Quarterly 1989;2(1):20.

Box 9.1 Silverman J, Kurtz S, Draper J. Skills for communicating with patients. 3rd edn. London: Radcliffe Publishing; 2013; Clark NM, Gong M, Schork A et al. Impact of education for physicians on patient outcomes. Paediatrics 1998;101:831–6.

Box 9.3 Weiss BD, Health literacy and patient safety: Help patients understand: Manual for clinicians, American Medical Association Foundation, ed. 2007: Chicago; Rudd RE, Guidelines for creating materials. In: Health Literacy Studies. Harvard School of Public Health; 2010; The United Kingdom Department of Health, Toolkit for producing patient information. NHS, United Kingdom; 2002.

Fig 10.1 Courtesy NSW Ambulance and Kate Curtis.

Figs 10.2, 10.3 Courtesy NSW Ambulance.

Figs 10.4, 10.5 Courtesy PM Middleton.

Figs 10.6, 10.7 Courtesy Signs of Safety, www.signsofsafety.net.au.

Figs 10.8, 10.9, 10.10, 10.11, 10.12, 10.13, 10.14, 10.15 Courtesy NSW Ambulance.

Fig 10.16 Courtesy K Harbig, NSW Ambulance.

Figs 10.17, 10.18, 10.19 Courtesy NSW Ambulance.

Fig 10.20 Courtesy Dr Jason Bendall.

Figs 10.21, 10.22, 10.23, 10.24, 10.25, 10.26 Edgar C SCAT (Special Casualty Access Training) reference text. NSW Ambulance; 2006.

Fig 10.27 Courtesy NSW Ambulance.

Box 10.2 Naval Sea Systems Command. Protective Clothing—Hazmat Gear Online. Available: www.dcfp.navy.mil/library/dcnews/PPETip001.htm; 4 Dec 2010.

Box 10.3 Greaves I, Hodgetts T, Porter K. Emergency care. A textbook for paramedics. London: WB Saunders; 1997.

Box 10.4 EMS Safety: Techniques and Applications. Federal emergency management agency. United States Fire Administration. Online. www.usfa.dhs.gov/downloads/pdf/publications/fa-144.pdf.

Box 10.6 Hodgetts TJ, Abraham K, Homer T, eds. Major incident medical management and support. The practical approach (Australian supplement). Sydney: SWSAHS Staff Development Unit; 1995.

Box 10.7 Moore R. Vehicle rescue life cycle. In: Moore R, ed. Vehicle rescue and extrication. 2nd edn. Mosby: JEMS; 2003.

Boxes 10.8, 10.10 Edgar C SCAT (Special Casualty Access Training) reference text. NSW Ambulance; 2006.

Box 10.11 Adapted from Caroline N Nancy. Caroline's Emergency care in the streets. 6th edn. Sudbury, MA: Jones and Bartlett; 2008.

Fig 11.4 Shaban RZ. Paramedic clinical judgment of mental illness: a case study of accounts of practice [PhD]. Brisbane: Arts, Education and Law Group, Griffith University; 2011.

Table 11.1 Council of Ambulance Authorities. CAA Annual Report Data Dictionary 2011–2012.

Table 11.3 Wong MC, Yee KC, Turner P. Clinical Handover Literature Review. eHealth Services Research Group, University of Tasmania, Australia; 2008.

Box 11.1 Shaban RZ. Theories of judgment and decision-making: a review of the theoretical literature. Journal of Emergency Primary Health Care. 2005;3:1–2.

Fig 12.1 Gabriel-Flickr: 20110224-DSC_0467.jpg. CC BY 2.0.

Fig 12.2 Lithgowlights, http://commons.wikimedia.org/wiki/File:Fire_in_Lithgow.jpg, CC BY 3.0.

Fig 12.3 International Labour Organisation, Flickr CC BY 2.0.

Fig 12.4 Shutterstock/Michael Muraz.

Fig 12.5 AAP/AFP.

Fig 12.6 Corbis/epa/Peter Macdiarmid.

Fig 12.8 © TSG Associates LLP, www.smartmci.com.

Figs 12.9, 12.10 Adapted from Cato D, Health Aspects of Dealing With Disasters in Australia, DCBiomed; 2002.

Figs 12.13, 12.14, 12.15, 12.16, 12.17, 12.18, 12.19 Courtesy Emergency Department, Royal North Shore Hospital, St Leonard's NSW 2065 Australia, 2014.

Fig 12.20 Adapted from Health Aspects of Chemical Biological and Radiological Hazards, Australian Emergency Series part 111, Emergency Management Practice Volume 2—specific issues manual 3; 2000.

Fig 12.21 Courtesy NSW Ambulance, Martin Ward and David Koop.

Fig 12.22 Flickr/US Navy, CC BY 2.0.

Fig 12.23 Courtesy Safety Equipment Australia.

Table 12.1 Brennan RJ, Bradt DA, Abrahams J. Medical issued in disasters. In: Cameron P, Jelinek G, Kelly A et al, eds. Textbook of adult emergency medicine. 2nd edn. Edinburgh: Churchill Livingstone; 2004:694.

Table 12.3 Adapted from Advanced Hazmat life Support (AHLS) Instructor manual. 2nd edn, 2000, University of Arizona Emergency Medicine Research Center, American Academy of Clinical Toxicology.

Table 12.5 Adapted from Center for Biological Defense WMD agent quick reference guide. Online. www.bt.usf.edu/files/WMD.pdf; 8 January 2010 (Bio chart); Centers for Disease Control and Prevention. Emergency preparedness and response: bioterrorism agents/diseases Department of Health and Human Services. Online. www.bt.cdc. gov/agent/agentlist-category.asp; January 2010; Klein R, Walter GW et al. Advanced HAZMAT Life support instructor manual. 2nd edn. University of Arizona Emergency Medicine Research Center, American Academy for Clinical Toxicology 2000; Ch 23:290–2; Potential biological agent operational data charts; FM8–9: NATO handbook the medical aspects of NBC defensive operations. AMedP–6(B). Online. www.cbwinfo.com/biological/FM9Table.html.

Table 13.1 Adapted from the ACEM Australasian Triage Scale.

Table 13.2 Australasian College for Emergency Medicine (ACEM). The Australasian Triage Scale. Emergency Medicine 2002;14:335–6; District Health Board: DHB Hospital Benchmark Information. Wellington: New Zealand Ministry of Health; 2010.

Fig 14.1 Adapted from Curtis K, Murphy M, Lewis MJ. The emergency nursing assessment process—a structured framework for a systematic approach. Australas Emerg Nurs J 2009;12:130–6.

Fig 14.2 Adapted from Berman A, Snyder S, Kozier B et al. Kozier and Erb's techniques in clinical nursing. 5th edn. Prentice Hall; 2003.

Fig 14.3 Adapted from Timby B. Fundamental skills and concepts in patient care. 7th edn. Philadelphia: Lippincott Williams & Wilkins; 2002.

Figs 14.4, 14.6 Cox C. Examination of the cardiovascular system. Physical assessment for nurses. Oxford: Blackwell Publishing; 2008:46–72. Reproduced with permission.

Fig 14.5 Adapted from Timby B. Fundamental skills and concepts in patient care. 7th edn. Philadelphia: Lippincott Williams & Wilkins; 2002.

Table 14.2 Adapted from Horswill, MS et al. Detecting abnormal vital signs on six observation charts: An experimental comparison. 2010. www.safetyandquality.gov.au/wp-content/uploads/2012/01/35983-DetectingAVS.pdf; NSW Health, Child Health Networks. Paediatric resuscitation reference chart 2012.

Table 14.4 Teasdale G, Maas A, Lecky F et al. The Glasgow Coma Scale at 40 years: standing the test of time. The Lancet 2014;13(8):844–54.

Table 14.5 James HE, Ana NG, Perkins RM. Brain insults in infants and children: pathophysiology and management. Elsevier; 1985.

Table 14.9 Rudolf M, Malcolm I. Milestones that it is essential to memorise. In: Paediatrics and child health. London: Blackwell Science; 1999:42.

Table 14.11 Grealy B, Chaboyer W. Essential nursing care of the critically ill patient. In: Elliot D, Aitken L, Chaboyer W. ACCCN's Critical Care Nursing 2nd edn. Sydney: Elsevier. 2012.

Table 14.12 Fulbrook P, Grealy B. Essential nursing care of the critically ill patient. In: Elliot D, Aitken L, Chaboyer W, eds. ACCCN Critical Care Nursing. Sydney: Elsevier; 2006.

Box 14.6 Ellis RB, Gates RJ, Kenworthy N, eds. Interpersonal communication. In Nursing: theory and practice. 2nd edn. New York: Churchill Livingstone; 2003.

Box 14.8 Courtesy Studer Group.

Box 14.9 Frank AW. Just listening: narrative and deep illness. Families, Systems & Health 1998;16(3):197–212; Lee LY, Lau YL. Immediate needs of adult family members of adult intensive care patients in Hong Kong. J Clin Nurs 2003;12(4):490–500; Mitchell M, Wilson D, Wade V. Psychosocial and cultural care of the critically ill. In: Elliot D, Aitken L, Chaboyer W, eds. ACCCN Critical care Nursing. Sydney: Elsevier; 2006; Saunders K. A creative new approach to patient satisfaction. Top Emerg Med 2005, Oct–Dec;27(4):256–7.

Box 14.10 Lewis SM, Collier IC, Heitkemper MM et al, eds. Medical–surgical nursing: assessment and management of clinical problems. 7th edn. St Louis: Mosby; 2007.

Fig 15.1 Australian Resuscitation Council. Guideline 4: Airway. Melbourne: Australian Resuscitation Council. Online. www.resus.org.au.

Fig 15.2 Australian Resuscitation Council. Guideline 8: Cardiopulmonary Resuscitation. Melbourne: Australian Resuscitation Council. Online. www.resus.org.au; 2011.

Figs 15.3, 15.4 Reproduced with permission of the Australian Resuscitation Council.

Fig 15.5 Photo courtesy Armstrong Medical Industries, Inc.

Tables 15.2, 15.3 Australian Resuscitation Council. Guideline 11.4: Electrical Therapy for Adult Advanced Life Support. Melbourne: Australian Resuscitation Council. Online. www.resus.org.au; 2011; Australian Resuscitation Council. Guideline 11.2: Protocols for Adult Advanced Life Support. Melbourne: Australian Resuscitation Council; www.resus.org.au; 2011. Aehert B. ECGs made easy. 4th edn. Elsevier Science; 2009.

Table 15.4 Krieser D, Nguyen K, Kerr D et al. Parental weight estimation of their child's weight is more accurate than other weight estimation methods for determining children's weight in an emergency department? Emergency Medicine Journal 2007;24:756–9.

Table 15.6 Australian Resuscitation Council. Guideline 11.6: Equipment and Techniques in Adult Advanced Life Support. Melbourne: Australian Resuscitation Council. www.resus.org.au; 2011; Australian Resuscitation Council. Guideline 12.4: Medications and Fluids in Paediatric Advanced Life Support. Melbourne: Australian Resuscitation Council. www.resus.org.au; 2011.

Table 15.7 British Paramedic Association. Nancy Caroline's Emergency Care in the streets. Sudbury/US: Jones and Bartlett Publishers; 2009.

Box 15.1 Australian Resuscitation Council. Guideline 11.2: Protocols for adult advanced life support. Melbourne: ARC. Online. www.resus.org.au.

Box 15.2 Australian Resuscitation Council. Guideline 11.4: Electrical therapy for adult advanced life support. Melbourne: Australian Resuscitation Council. www.resus.org.au; 2011; Maguire J. Advanced life support. In: Cameron P, Jelinek G, Kelly A, Murray L, Heyworth J, eds. Adult textbook of emergency medicine. 3rd edn. Sydney: Churchill Livingstone; 2009.

Box 15.4 Bessman ES. Emergency cardiac pacing. In: Roberts JR, Hedges JR, eds. Clinical procedures in emergency medicine. 4th edn. Philadephia: Sanders; 2004; Colquhoun M, Handley A, Evans T, eds. ABC of resuscitation. 5th edn. Bristol: BMJ Publishing Group; 2004.

Figs 16.3, 16.4 Based on MedSTAR emergency medical retrievals. Agency overview. SA Health: SA Ambulance Service. South Australia: Government of South Australia; 2007.

Table 16.1 Taylor CB, Stevenson M, Jan S et al. A systematic review of the costs and benefits of helicopter emergency medical services. Injury 2010;41(1):10–20.

Table 16.2 Harding J, Goode D. Physical stresses related to the transport of the critically ill: optimal nursing management. Aust Crit Care 2003;16(3):93–100.

Tables 16.3,16.5 Based on MedSTAR Emergency Medical Retrievals. Agency overview. SA Health: SA Ambulance Service. South Australia: Government of South Australia; 2007.

Table 16.4 Data from http://www.boc-healthcare.com.au/internet.lh.lh. aus/en/images/HCD070B_Oxygen_data_sheet350_72384.pdf.

Box 16.1 Ellis D, Hooper M. Cases in pre-hospital and retrieval medicine. Sydney: Churchill Livingstone; 2010.

Figs 17.1, 17.2, 17.8, 17.9 Reardon RF, Mason PE, Clinton JE. Basic airway management and decision-making. In: Roberts JR, Hedges JR, eds. Clinical procedures in emergency medicine. 5th edn. Philadelphia: WB Saunders; 2010.

Figs 17.3, 17.4, 17.5, 17.6, 17.7 Skillings KN, Curtis BL. Oropharyngeal airway insertion. In: Wiegand DJ, Carlson KK, eds. AACN procedure manual for critical care. 5th edn. St Louis: WB Saunders; 2005.

Fig 17.10 Auerbach PS. Wilderness medicine. 5th edn. St Louis: Mosby; 2007.

Fig 17.11 Dargin J, Medzon R. Emergency Department Management of the Airway of Obese Adults. Annals of Emergency Medicine 2010; 56(2); 95–104.

Fig 17.12 López AM, Valero R, Bovaira, P et al. A critical evaluation of four disposable laryngeal face masks in adult patients. Journal of Clinical Anesthesia 2008;20(7):514–20.

Figs 17.13, 17.14 Day MW. Laryngeal mask airway. In: Wiegand DJ, Carlson KK, eds. AACN procedure manual for critical care. 5th edn. St Louis: Saunders; 2005.

Fig 17.15 A, Zuidema GD, Rutherford RB, Ballinger WF. Management of trauma. 4th edn. Philadelphia: WB Saunders; 1996; B, Courtesy Liverpool Hospital Trauma Service, Sydney, NSW.

Fig 17.16 Courtesy Emergency Department, Prince of Wales Hospital, Sydney.

Figs 17.17, 17.18 Roberts JR, Hedges JR, eds. Clinical procedures in emergency medicine. 5th edn. Philadelphia: WB Saunders; 2010.

Fig 17.19 Reproduced with permission from Norman E. McSwain Jr, MD, FACS, and Richard L. Garnnelli, MD, FACS—American College of Surgeons Committee on Trauma, April 1997.

Fig 17.20 Frakes M. Measuring end-tidal carbon dioxide: clinical applications and usefulness. Crit Care Nurse 2001;21(5):23.

Fig 17.21 Barbara J Aehlert RN. Paramedic practice today: above and beyond; Elsevier; 2009.

Fig 17.22 Davey AJ. Ward's Anaesthetic equipment. Elsevier Ltd. 2012. All rights reserved.

Fig 17.23 Chulay M. Suctioning: endotracheal or tracheostomy tube. In: Wiegand DJ, Carlson KK, eds. AACN procedure manual for critical care. 5th edn. St Louis: WB Saunders; 2005.

Fig 17.24 OSCE, CC BY 2.0.

Fig 17.25 May JL. Emergency medical procedures. New York: John Wiley and Sons; 1984.

Figs 17.26, 17.28 Urden LD, Stacy KM, Lough ME. Thelan's critical care nursing: diagnosis and management. 5th edn. St Louis: Mosby; 2006.

Fig 17.27 Kirsch TD. Tube thoracostomy. In: Roberts JR, Hedges JR, eds. Clinical procedures in emergency medicine. 5th edn. Philadelphia: WB Saunders; 2010.

Fig 17.29 Friedman HH: Diagnostic electrocardiography and vectorcardiography. New York, McGraw-Hill, 1985; In: Reich et al. Essentials of cardiac anesthesia, Elsevier; 2008.

Figs 17.30, 17.31 Courtesy Life in the Fast Lane, http://lifeinthefastlane.com/education/lead-positioning.

Fig 17.32 Courtesy ZOLL Medical Corporation.

Figs 17.33, 17.34, 17.37, 17.38 Potter PA, Perry AG. Fundamentals of nursing. 5th edn. St Louis: Mosby; 2001.

Figs 17.39, 17.40, 17.41, 17.42, 17.43 Deitch K. Intraosseous infusion. In: Roberts JR, Hedges JR, eds. Clinical procedures in emergency medicine. 5th edn. Philadelphia: WB Saunders; 2010.

Fig 17.47 Roberts JR. Chapter 34, Roberts and Hedges' clinical procedures in emergency medicine. 6th edn, Philadelphia: WB Saunders; 2014.

Fig 17.48 Chudnofsky CR, Byers SE. Splinting techniques. In: Roberts JR, Hedges JR, eds. Clinical procedures in emergency medicine. 5th edn. Philadelphia: WB Saunders; 2010.

Figs 17.49, 17.50 Marx JA, ed. Rosen's emergency medicine: concepts and clinical practice. 7th edn. Philadelphia: Mosby; 2009.

Figs 17.51, 17.52, 17.53, 17.54 Roberts JR, Hedges JR, eds. Clinical procedures in emergency medicine. 6th edn. Philadelphia: WB Saunders; 2014.

Fig 17.57 Fleisher LA, Gaiser R, eds. 2008 Anesthesia procedures consult. Elsevier, Philadelphia, PA. Online. www.proceduresconsult.com/medicalprocedures/anesthesia-specialty.aspx.

Fig 17.58 Drake R, Vogl AW, Mitchell AWM et al. Gray's atlas of anatomy. Philadelphia, Churchill Livingstone/Elsevier; 2008.

Fig 17.59 Waldman SS. Atlas of interventional pain management. 4th edn; 2015 by Saunders, an imprint of Elsevier Inc.

Fig 17.60 Roberts and Hedges' clinical procedures in emergency medicine, 6th edn, Philadelphia: WB Saunders; 2014.

Figs 17.61, 17.62 Kelly JJ, Spektor M. Nerve blocks of the thorax and extremities. In: Roberts JR, Hedges JR, eds. Clinical procedures in emergency medicine. 5th edn. Philadelphia: WB Saunders; 2010.

Fig 17.63 Roberts JR. Intravenous regional anesthesia. In: Roberts JR, Hedges JR, eds. Clinical procedures in emergency medicine, 6th edn. Philadelphia: WB Saunders; 2014.

Fig 17.64 Browner B, Fuller R. Musculoskeletal emergencies, Elsevier 2012.

Fig 17.65 Adapted from Green DP, Hotchkiss RN, Pederson WC, Wolfe SW (eds). Green's operative hand surgery, 5th edn. Philadelphia: Churchill Livingstone; 2005. Copyright Elizabeth Martin. Miller M, Hart J, MacKnight J. Essential orthopaedics. © 2010 by Saunders, an imprint of Elsevier Inc.

Fig 17.66 Fleisher LA, Gaiser R, eds. Bier Block, 2008 Anesthesia procedures consult. Elsevier, Philadelphia, PA. Online. www.proceduresconsult.com/medicalprocedures/anesthesia-specialty.aspx.

Figs 17.67, 17.68, 17.69, 17.70 Roberts JR, Hedges JR, eds. Clinical procedures in emergency medicine. 6th edn. Philadelphia: WB Saunders; 2014.

Fig 17.71 Meeker MH, Rothrock JC. Alexander's care of the patient in surgery. 11th edn. St Louis: Mosby; 1999.

Figs 17.74, 17.75, 17.76, 17.77, 17.78, 17.79 Roberts JR, Hedges JR, eds. Clinical procedures in emergency medicine. 6th edn. Philadelphia: WB Saunders; 2014.

Table 17.1 Laryngeal Mask Airway (LMA) Classic™, Flexible™ and Unique™ Sizing Guide 15. The Laryngeal Mask Company. LMA instruction manual. Online. http://www.lmaco.com/products/LMA%20Airway%20Management™.

Table 17.3 Vincent, JL, Abraham, E, Moore FA, et al. Textbook of critical care, 6th edn. 2011 by Saunders, an imprint of Elsevier Inc.

Table 17.4 Adams BD, Lyon ML, DeFlorio PT. Central venous catheterization and central venous pressure monitoring. In: Roberts JR, Hedges JR, eds. Clinical procedures in emergency medicine. 5th edn. Philadelphia: WB Saunders, 2010; Arrow International. Central venous catheter: nursing care. Guideline 1996.

Table 17.5 Australian Medicines Handbook 2015. Table 2-3 Comparison of local anaesthetics. Australian Medicines Handbook Pty Ltd; Adelaide. p 33.

Table 17.6 Swanson NA, Tromovitch TA. Suture materials 1980s: properties, uses and abuses. Int J Dermatol 1982;21:373–8.

Box 17.1 Walls RM, Murphy MF, eds. Manual of emergency airway management. 3rd edn. Philadelphia: Lippincott Williams & Wilkins; 2008.

Box 17.2 Adapted from www.airwayregistry.org.au RSI checklist.

Box 17.3 Moore T. Suctioning techniques for the removal of respiratory secretions. Nurs Stand 2003;18(9):47–53.

Box 17.4 Pedersen CM, Rosendahl-Nielsen M, Hjermind J et al. Endotracheal suctioning of the adult intubated patient—what is the evidence? Intensive Crit Care Nurs 2009;25(1):21–30.

Box 17.6 Urden LD, Stacy KM, Lough ME. Thelan's Critical care nursing: diagnosis and management. 5th edn. St Louis: Mosby; 2006.

Box 17.7 Johns DP, Pierce R. Spirometry: the measure and interpretation of ventilatory function in clinical practice. Online. www.nationalasthma.org.au; 2008. Booker R. Simple spirometry measurement. Nurs Stand 2008;22(32):35–9.

Box 17.9 Garretson S. Haemodynamic monitoring: arterial catheters. Nurs Stand 2005;19(31):55–64. Becker DE. Arterial catheter insertion (perform) AP. In: Wiegand DJ, Carlson KK, eds. ACCCN procedure manual for critical care. 5th edn. St Louis: WB Saunders; 2005.

Box 17.10 Munro N. Central venous catheter insertion (assist). In: Wiegand DJ, Carlson KK, eds. AACN procedure manual for critical care. 5th edn. St Louis: WB Saunders; 2005.

Box 17.11 Woodrow P. Central venous catheters and central venous pressure. Nurs Stand 2002;16(26):45–51; Munro N. Central venous/right atrial pressure monitoring. In: Wiegand DJ, Carlson KK, eds. AACN procedure manual for critical care. 5th edn. St Louis: WB Saunders; 2005.

Box 17.12 Scales K. Central venous pressure monitoring in clinical practice. Nurs Stand 2010;24(29):49–55; Munro N. Central venous/right atrial pressure monitoring. In: Wiegand DJ, Carlson KK, eds. AACN procedure manual for critical care. 5th edn. St Louis: WB Saunders; 2005.

Box 17.17 Roberts JR, Hedges JR, eds. Clinical procedures in emergency medicine. 6th edn. Philadelphia: WB Saunders; 2010.

Figs 18.1, 18.2 Moses K, Banks JC, Nara PB et al. Atlas of clinical gross anatomy. St Louis: Mosby; 2005.

Fig 18.3 McRae R, Esser M. Practical fracture treatment. 5th edn. Edinburgh: Elsevier; 2008.

Fig 18.5 Cameron P, Jelinek G, Kelly A et al. Textbook of adult emergency medicine. 2nd edn. Edinburgh: Churchill Livingstone; 2002.

Fig 18.8 Canale ST, Beaty JH. Campbell's operative orthopaedics. 11th edn. St Louis: Mosby; 2007.

Figs 18.9, 18.10 Lammers RL. Methods of wound closure. In: Roberts JR, Hedges JR, eds. Clinical procedures in emergency medicine. 5th edn. Philadelphia: Saunders; 2010.

Fig 18.11 Moses K, Banks JC, Nara PB et al. Atlas of clinical gross anatomy. St Louis: Mosby; 2005.

Fig 18.13 Bachmann LM, Kolb E, Koller MT, et al. Accuracy of Ottawa ankle rules to exclude fractures of the ankle and mid-foot: systematic review. Br Med J 2003;326(7386):417.

Fig 18.15 Mandell GL, Bennett JE, Mandell, DR. Douglas and Bennett's Principles and practice of infectious diseases, 7th edn. Philadelphia: Churchill Livingstone; 2010. (From Postlethwaite RW. Principles of operative surgery: Antisepsis, technique, sutures, and drains. In: Sabiston DC, ed. Davis-Christopher Textbook of surgery. 12th edn. Philadelphia: WB Saunders; 1981.)

Fig 18.16 Lammers RL. Methods of wound closure. In: Roberts JR, Hedges JR, eds. Clinical procedures in emergency medicine. 5th edn. Philadelphia: Saunders; 2010.

Fig 18.17 Canale ST, Beaty JH. Campbell's Operative orthopaedics. 11th edn. St Louis: Mosby; 2007.

Fig 18.18 Simon B, Hern HG Jr. Wound management principles. In: Marx JA, ed. Rosen's emergency medicine. 7th edn. Philadelphia: Mosby; 2009.

Fig 18.19 Lammers RL. Methods of wound closure. In: Roberts JR, Hedges JR, eds. Clinical procedures in emergency medicine. 5th edn. Philadelphia: Saunders; 2010.

Fig 18.20 Kliegman RM, Behrman RE, Jenson HS, et al. Nelson textbook of pediatrics. 18th edn. Philadelphia: Saunders; 2007.

Table 18.1 Doughty DB, Sparks-Defriese B. Wound healing physiology. In: Bryant RA, Nix DP, eds. Acute and chronic wounds. 3rd edn. St Louis: Mosby; 2007.

Table 18.2 Anon. Local anaesthetics. Therapeutic guidelines: analgesic version 13. West Melbourne: Therapeutic Guidelines; 2007. Murtagh JE. Managing painful pediatric procedures. Aust Prescr 2006;29:94–6.

Table 18.3 Cameron P, Jelinek G, Kelly A et al. Textbook of adult emergency medicine. 2nd edn. Edinburgh: Churchill Livingstone; 2002; Wilson R. Wound management. In: Curtis K, Ramsden C, Friendship J, eds. Emergency and trauma nursing. Marrickville: Mosby; 2007.

Table 18.4 Wilson R. Wound management. In: Curtis K, Ramsden C, Friendship J, eds. Emergency and trauma nursing. Marrickville: Mosby; 2007; Lewis SM, Heitkemper MM, Dirksen SR. Medical–surgical nursing: assessment and management of clinical problems. 5th edn. St Louis: Mosby; 2000.

Table 18.5 Table 3.21.1 from Australian Immunisation Handbook. 10th edn. Australian Government; 2014.

Fig 19.1 Brown D, Edwards H, eds. Lewis's medical-surgical nursing. 3rd edn. Sydney: Elsevier; 2011.

Fig 19.2 Brown D, Edwards H, eds. Lewis's medical-surgical nursing. 4th edn. Sydney: Elsevier; 2014.

Table 19.1 McCaffery M, Pasero C. Pain: clinical manual. 2nd edn. St Louis: Mosby; 1999.

Table 19.2 Hockenberry MJ, Wilson D, eds. Wong's essentials of pediatric nursing. 8th edn. St Louis: Mosby; 2009; Merkel SI, Voepel-Lewis T, Shayevitz JR, Malviya S. The FLACC: a behavioral scale for scoring postoperative pain in young children. Pediatr Nurs 1997;23(3):293–7.

Tables 19.3, 19.4 Brown D, Edwards H, eds. Lewis's Medical-surgical nursing. 4th edn. Sydney: Elsevier; 2014.

Table 19.5 Macintyre PE, Schug SA. Acute pain management: a practical guide. 4th edn. CRC press; 2015.

Table 19.6 Australian Medicines Handbook 2015. Online. Adelaide: Australian Medicines Handbook Pty Ltd; 2015 January. www.amh.net.au.

Table 19.7 Bryant B, Knights K, Salerno E. Pharmacology for health professionals. 4th edn. Sydney: Mosby; 2014.

Boxes 19.1, 19.2 Macintyre PE, Schug SA. Acute pain management: a practical guide. 4th edn. CRC press; 2015.

Fig 20.1 Porth CM, Curtis RL. Cell and tissue characteristics. In: Porth CM, ed. Pathophysiology concepts and altered states. 4th edn. Philadelphia: JB Lippincott; 1994.

Fig 20.4 Guyton AC, Hall JE. Textbook of medical physiology. 11th edn. Philadelphia: Elsevier; 2005.

Fig 20.5 Gas Exchange across the Alveoli. Boundless Biology. Boundless, 03 Jul. 2014. https://www.boundless.com/biology/textbooks/boundless-biology-textbook/the-respiratory-system-39/gas-exchange-across-respiratory-surfaces-220/gas-exchange-across-the-alveoli-836-12081/.

Figs 20.6, 20.9 Guyton AC, Hall JE. Textbook of medical physiology. 11th edn. Philadelphia: Elsevier; 2005.

Fig 20.7 Frakes M. Measuring end-tidal carbon dioxide: clinical applications and usefulness. Crit Care Nurse 2001;21(5):23.

Figs 20.10, 20.11, 20.13, 20.14 Lewis SM, Collier IC, Heitkemper MM. Medical–surgical nursing: assessment and management of clinical problems. 7th edn. St Louis: Mosby; 2007.

Fig 20.12 Gruen RL, Brohi K, Schreiber M et al. Haemorrhage control in severely injured patients. The Lancet 2012;380(9847):1099–108.

Table 20.2 Cameron P, Jelinek G, Kelly A-M et al. Textbook of adult emergency medicine. 4th edn. Sydney: Elsevier; 2014.

Table 20.3 Lewis SM, Collier IC, Heitkemper MM. Medical–surgical nursing: assessment and management of clinical problems. 7th edn. St Louis: Mosby; 2007.

Table 20.5 Newberry L, ed. Sheehy's emergency nursing. 5th edn. St Louis: Mosby; 2003.

Fig 21.1 McCance KL, Huether SE. Understanding pathophysiology. 4th edn. St Louis: Mosby; 2010.

Fig 21.3 Sztrymf B, Messika J, Mayot T et al. Impact of high-flow nasal cannula oxygen therapy on intensive care unit patients with acute respiratory failure: A prospective observational study. Journal of Critical Care 2012;27(3):324.e9–13, © 2012 Elsevier Inc.

Tables 21.1, 21.2 Brashers V. Alterations of pulmonary function. In: McCance KL, Huether SE, eds. Pathophysiology: the biological basis for disease in adults and children. 4th edn. St. Louis: Mosby; 2010.

Table 21.3 Simpson H. Respiratory assessment. Br J Nurs 2006;15(9):484–8. Rempher K, Morton P. Patient assessment: respiratory system. In: Morton P, Fontaine D, Hudak C et al, eds. Critical care nursing: a holistic approach. 8th edn. Philadelphia: Lippincott Williams & Wilkins; 2005; Kelly A-M. Asthma. In: Cameron P, Jelinek G, Kelly A-M et al. eds. Textbook of adult emergency medicine. 2nd edn. Sydney: Churchill Livingstone; 2004. Bradley R. Improving respiratory assessment skills. JNP 2007:3(4):276–7.

Table 21.4 Saposnick A, Hess D. Oxygen therapy: Administration and management. In: Hess DR, MacIntyre NR, Mishoe SC et al, eds. Respiratory care: principles and practice. Philadelphia: WB Saunders; 2002.

Table 21.5 Hill NS. Non-invasive ventilation. In: MacIntyre NR, Branson RD, eds. Mechanical ventilation. 2nd edn. St Louis: Saunders; 2009. Saatci E, Miller DM, Stell IM, et al. Dynamic dead space in face masks used with noninvasive ventilators: a lung model study. Eur Respir J 2004;23(1):129–35.

Table 21.6 Hill NS. Noninvasive mechanical ventilation. In: MacIntyre NR, Branson RD, eds. Mechanical ventilation. 2nd edn. St Louis: Saunders; 2009.

Table 21.9 Holets S, Hubmayr RD. Setting the ventilator. In: Tobin M, ed. Principles and practice of mechanical ventilation. 2nd edn. New York: McGraw-Hill; 2006. Huang Y-CT, Singh J. Basic modes of mechanical ventilation. In: Papadakos PJ, Lachmann B, eds. Mechanical ventilation: clinical applications and pathophysiology. Philadelphia: Saunders; 2008.

Tables 21.12, 21.13 Adapted from the Australian asthma handbook, quick reference guide, version 1.1. National Asthma Council Australia, Melbourne, 2015. http://www.asthmahandbook.org.au.

Table 21.14 Urden LD, Stacy KM, Lough ME. Thelan's critical care nursing: diagnosis and management. 5th edn. St Louis: Mosby; 2006.

Table 21.15 Wolf S, McCubbin T, Feldhaus K et al. Prospective validation of Wells criteria in the evaluation of patients with suspected pulmonary embolism. Annals of Emergency Medicine 2004;44(5):503–10.

Tables 21.16, 21.17 Cruise DC. Carbon monoxide. In: Cameron P, Jelinek G, Kelly A et al, eds. Textbook of adult emergency medicine. 2nd edn. Edinburgh: Churchill Livingstone; 2004.

Box 21.1 Johns D, Pierce R. Spirometry: The measurement and interpretation of ventilatory function in clinical practice. The Thoracic Society of Australia and New Zealand; 2008. Online. www.nationalasthma.org.au/images/stories/manage/pdf/spirometer_handbook_naca.pdf.

Boxes 21.2, 21.3 Marini JJ, Hotchkiss JR, Bach JR. Non-invasive ventilation in the acute care setting. In: Bach JR, ed. Non-invasive mechanical ventilation. Philadelphia: Hanley & Belfus; 2002; Gramlich T. Basic concept of non-invasive positive pressure ventilation. In: Pilbeam SP, Cairo JM, eds. Mechanical ventilation: physiological and clinical applications. 4th edn. St Louis: Mosby; 2006; Hill NS. Non-invasive ventilation. In: MacIntyre NR, Branson RD, eds. Mechanical ventilation. 2nd edn. St Louis: Saunders; 2009.

Fig 22.1 Atkinson LJ, Fortunato NM. Berry & Kohn's Operating room technique. 8th edn. St Louis: Mosby; 1996.

Fig 22.2 Thompson JM et al. Mosby's clinical nursing. 5th edn. St Louis: Mosby; 2002.

Figs 22.3, 22.4, 22.14 Urden LD, Stacy KM, Lough ME. Thelan's critical care nursing: diagnosis and management. 5th edn. St Louis: Mosby; 2006.

Fig 22.CS1 Jowett N, Thompson D. Comprehensive coronary care. 4th edn. Edinburgh: Elsevier/Baillière Tindall; 2007.

Table 22.1 Newberry L, Barret G, Ballard N. A new mnemonic for chest pain assessment. J Emerg Nurs 2005;31:84–85.

Table 22.8 Newberry L, ed. Sheehy's emergency nursing: principles and practice. 6th edn. St Louis: Mosby; 2005.

Box 22.1 Newberry L, ed. Sheehy's emergency nursing principles and practice. 6th edn. St Louis: Mosby; 2005.

Box 22.4 Jowett N, Thompson D. Comprehensive coronary care. 4th edn. Edinburgh: Elsevier/Baillière Tindall; 2007.

Boxes 22.5, 22.6 Urden LD, Stacy KM, Lough ME. Thelan's critical care nursing: diagnosis and management. 5th edn. St Louis: Mosby; 2006.

Fig 23.1 Adapted from MedicineNet, Inc., http://www.emedicinehealth.com/hematoma/page3_em.html.

Fig 23.2 Koeppen BM, Stanton, BA. Berne and Levy physiology. 6th edn. St. Louis: Mosby; 2010.

Fig 23.3 Lewis SM, Collier IC, Heitkemper MM. Medical–surgical nursing: assessment and management of clinical problems. 8th edn. St Louis: Mosby; 2011.

Figs 23.4, 23.5 Rund DA, Barkin RM, Rosen P. Essentials of emergency medicine. 2nd edn. St Louis: Mosby; 1996.

Fig 23.6 Davis JH, Drucker WR. Clinical surgery. vol 1. St Louis: Mosby; 1987.

Figs 23.7, 23.8, 23.9, 23.10 Lewis SM, Collier IC, Heitkemper MM. Medical–surgical nursing: assessment and management of clinical problems. 7th edn. St Louis: Mosby; 2007.

Table 23.1 Lewis SM, Collier IC, Heitkemper MM. Medical–surgical nursing: assessment and management of clinical problems. 7th edn. St Louis: Mosby; 2007.

Table 23.3 Brown D, Edwards H. Lewis' Medical–Surgical Nursing. Sydney: Mosby; 2005; Thibodeau GA, Patton KT. Anatomy and physiology. 5th edn. St. Louis: Mosby; 2003.

Table 23.4 Cameron P, Jelinek G, Kelly A et al. Adult textbook of emergency medicine. 3rd edn. Sydney: Churchill Livingstone; 2009; Sawin P, Loftus C. Diagnosis of spontaneous subarachnoid hemorrhage. American family physician 1997;55:145–56.

Table 23.5 Lewis SM, Collier IC, Heitkemper MM. Medical–surgical nursing: assessment and management of clinical problems. 7th edn. St Louis: Mosby; 2007.

Table 23.6 Cameron P, Jelinek G, Kelly A et al. Adult textbook of emergency medicine. 3rd edn. Sydney: Churchill Livingstone; 2009.

Table 23.7 Lewis SM, Collier IC, Heitkemper MM. Medical–surgical nursing: assessment and management of clinical problems. 7th edn. St Louis: Mosby; 2007.

Box 23.1 Cameron P, Jelinek G, Kelly A et al. Adult textbook of emergency medicine. 3rd edn. Sydney: Churchill Livingstone; 2009.

Box 23.2 Morton P, Tucker T. Patient assessment: Cardiovascular system. In: Morton PG, Fontaine DK, Hudak CM, Gallo BM, eds. Critical care nursing: a holistic approach. 8th edn. Philadelphia: Lippincott Williams & Wilkins; 2005.

Box 23.4 McGillivray B, Considine J. Implementation of evidence into practice: development of a tool to improve emergency nursing care of acute stroke. Australasian Emergency Nursing Journal 2009;12:110–19.

Fig 24.1 © 2015 medicalartstudio.com

Figs 24.2, 24.3, 24.4, 24.5, 24.7 Seeley R, Stephens T, Tate P, eds. Anatomy and physiology. 2003. McGraw Hill.

Fig 24.6 Marx J, Hockberger R, Walls R et al, eds. Rosen's emergency medicine: concepts and clinical practice, Vol. 1. 7th edn. St. Louis: Mosby; 2010.

Fig 24.8 Society of Gastroenterology Nurses and Associates. Gastroenterology nursing: a core curriculum. St. Louis: Mosby; 1993.

Figs 24.9, 24.10, 24.11, 24.12, 24.13 Lewis S, Heitkemper M, Dirksen S, eds. Medical–surgical nursing: assessment and management of clinical problems. 5th edn. St. Louis: Mosby; 2000.

Fig 24.14 Liechty R, Soper R. Fundamentals of surgery. 6th edn. St. Louis: Mosby; 1989.

Fig 24.15 Marx J, Hockberger R, Walls R et al, eds. Rosen's emergency medicine: concepts and clinical practice, vol. 1. 7th edn. St. Louis: Mosby; 2010.

Fig 24.16 Mettler F, Guibertereau M, Voss C, Urbina C. Primary care radiology. Philadelphia: WB Saunders; 2000.

Fig 24.17 Dettenmeier P. Radiographic assessment for nurses. St. Louis: Mosby; 1995.

Table 24.1 Lewis S, Heitkemper M, Dirksen S, eds. Medical–surgical nursing: assessment and management of clinical problems. 5th edn. St. Louis: Mosby; 2000.

Table 24.2 Adapted from Colucciello S, Lukens T, Morgan D. Assessing abdominal pain in adults: a rational, cost-effective, and evidence-based strategy. Emergency Medicine Practice 1999;1(1):1–20.

Table 24.6 Bennett D, Tambeur L, Campbell W. Use of cough test to diagnose peritonitis. British Medical Journal 1994;308(6940):1336; Golledge J, Toms A, Franklin I et al. Assessment of peritonism in appendicitis. Annals of the Royal College of Surgeons of England 1996;78(1):11–14; Jahn H, Mathiesen F, Neckelmann K et al. Comparison of clinical judgment and diagnostic ultrasonography in the diagnosis of acute appendicitis: experience with a score-aided diagnosis. European Journal of Surgery 1997;163(6):433–43; Fenyö G, Lindberg G, Blind P et al. Diagnostic decision support in suspected acute appendicitis: validation of a simplified scoring system. European Journal of Surgery 1997;163(11):831–8; Mahadevan M, Graff L. Prospective randomized study of analgesic use for ED patients with right lower quadrant abdominal pain. American Journal of Emergency Medicine 2000;18(7):753–6; Hallan S, Asberg A, Edna T. Estimating the probability of acute appendicitis using clinical criteria of a structured record sheet: the physician against the computer. European Journal of Surgery 1997;163(6):427–32; Mookadam F, Cikes M. Cullen's and Turner's signs. New England Journal of Medicine 2005;353(13):1386; Markle G. Heel-drop jarring test for appendicitis. Archives of Surgery 1985;120(2):243; Markle G. A simple test for intraperitoneal inflammation. American Journal of Surgery 1975;125:721–2; Lane R, Grabham J. A useful sign for the diagnosis of peritoneal irritation in the right iliac fossa. Annals of the Royal College of Surgeons of England 1997;79:128–9. Andersson R, Sward A, Tingstedt B, Akerberg D. Treatment of acute pancreatitis: focus on medical care. Drugs 2009;69(5):505–14. Fernandes J, Lopez P, Montes J, Cara M. Validity of tests performed to diagnose acute abdominal pain in patients admitted at an emergency department. Revista Española de Enfermedades Digestivas 2009;101(9):610–18. Singer A, McCracken G, Henry M et al. Correlation among clinical, laboratory, and hepatobiliary scanning findings in patients with suspected acute cholecystitis. Annuals of Emergency Medicine 1996;28(3):267–72. Adedeji O, McAdam W. Murphy's sign, acute cholecystitis and elderly people. Journal of the Royal College of Surgeons of Edinburgh 1996;41(2):88–9. Mills LM, Mills T, Foster B. Association of clinical and laboratory variables with ultrasound findings in right upper quadrant abdominal pain. Southern Medical Journal 2005;98(2):155–61. Berry J, Malt R. Appendicitis near its centenary. Annals of Surgery 1984;200(5):5575–676; Wagner J, McKinney M, Carpenter J. Does this patient have appendicitis? Journal of American Medical Association 1996;276(19):1589–94; Izbicki J, Knoefel W, Wilker D et al. Accurate diagnosis of acute appendicitis: a retrospective and prospective analysis of 686 patients. The European Journal of Surgery 1992;158(4):227–231; John H, Neff U, Keleman M. Appendicitis diagnosis today: clinical and ultrasound deductions. World Journal of Surgery 1993;17(2):243–49. Alshehri M, Ibrahim A, Abuaisha N, et al. Value of rebound tenderness in acute appendicitis. East African Medical Journal 1995;72(8):504–6. Andersson R, Hugander A, Ghazi S et al. Diagnostic value of disease history, clinical presentation, and inflammatory parameters of appendicitis. World Journal of Surgery 1999;23(2):133–40.

Table 24.7 Brown D, Edwards H, eds. Lewis's medical–surgical nursing: assessment and management of clinical problems. Sydney: Elsevier; 2005.

Table 24.8 Marx J, Hockberger R, Walls R et al eds. Rosen's emergency medicine: concepts and clinical practice, Vol 1. 7th edn. St. Louis: Mosby; 2010.

Table 24.9 Victorian Government Department of Health Services. The blue book: guidelines for the control of infectious diseases. 2005, reproduced with kind permission of the Victorian Government.

Tables 24.10, 24.11, 24.12 Lewis S, Collier I, Heitkemper M, eds. Medical–surgical nursing: assessment and management of clinical problems. 7th edn. St. Louis: Mosby; 2007.

Tables 24.13, 24.14 Sargent S. Pathophysiology, diagnosis and management of acute pancreatitis. British Journal of Nursing 2006;15(18):999–1005; Lewis S, Collier I, Heitkemper M, eds. Medical–surgical nursing: assessment and management of clinical problems. 7th edn. St. Louis: Mosby; 2007.

Table 24.15 Marx J, Hockberger R, Walls R et al, eds. Rosen's emergency medicine: concepts and clinical practice, vol 1. 7th edn. St. Louis: Mosby; 2010.

Table 24.16 Lewis S, Collier I, Heitkemper M, eds. Medical–surgical nursing: assessment and management of clinical problems. 7th edn. St. Louis: Mosby; 2007; Marx J, Hockberger R, Walls R et al, eds. Rosen's emergency medicine: concepts and clinical practice, vol 1. 7th edn. St. Louis: Mosby; 2010.

Tables 24.17, 24.18, 24.19, 24.20 Lewis S, Collier I, Heitkemper M, eds. Medical–surgical nursing: assessment and management of clinical problems. 7th edn. St. Louis: Mosby; 2007.

Box 24.1 Lewis S, Collier I, Heitkemper M, eds. Medical–surgical nursing: assessment and management of clinical problems. 7th edn. St. Louis: Mosby; 2007.

Box 24.3 Marx J, Hockberger R, Walls R et al, eds. Rosen's emergency medicine: concepts and clinical practice, volume 1. 7th edn. St. Louis: Mosby; 2010.

Box 24.4 Lewis S, Collier I, Heitkemper M, eds. Medical-surgical nursing: assessment and management of clinical problems. 7th edn. St. Louis: Mosby; 2007.

Box 24.5 Victorian Government Department of Health Services. The blue book: guidelines for the control of infectious diseases. 2005; http://docs.health.vic.gov.au/docs/doc/FE2665DB66894C46CA2578B0001BE87E/$FILE/bluebook.pdf; Therapeutic Guidelines. Antibiotics: gastrointestinal tract infections. 2011.

Figs 25.1, 25.2, 25.3 McCance KL, Huether SE. Pathophysiology: the biologic basis for disease in adults and children. 6th edn. St Louis: Mosby; 2010.

Fig 25.4 Adapted from Herlihy B, Maebius N. The human body in health and illness. 2nd edn. Philadelphia: Saunders; 2003.

Figs 25.5, 25.6, 25.7 Thibodeau GA, Patton KT. Anatomy and physiology. 4th edn. St Louis: Mosby, 1999.

Fig 25.8 Brundage DJ. Renal disorders. St Louis: Mosby, 1992.

Figs 25.9, 25.10, 25.11 Brown D, Edwards H, eds. Lewis's medical–surgical nursing, 4th edn, Sydney: Elsevier; 2014.

Fig 25.12 Brown D, Edwards H, eds. Lewis's medical–surgical nursing: Sydney: Elsevier; 2008.

Fig 25.13 Thompson JM, McFarland GK, Hirsch JE et al. Mosby's clinical nursing. 5th edn. St Louis: Mosby; 2001.

Fig 25.14 Brown D, Edwards H, eds. Lewis's medical–surgical nursing. 4th edn. Sydney: Elsevier; 2014.

Fig 25.15 Soto JA, Lucey BC. Emergency radiology: the requisites. Philadelphia: Elsevier; 2009.

Fig 25.16 Roberts and Hedges' clinical procedures in emergency medicine, 6th edn. Saunders; 2014.

Fig 25.17 Price SA, Wilson LM. Pathophysiology: clinical concepts of disease processes. 5th edn. St Louis: Mosby; 1997.

Tables 25.1, 25.2, 25.3, 25.4, 25.5, 25.6, 25.7 Brown D, Edwards H, eds. Lewis's Medical–surgical nursing. 4th edn. Sydney: Elsevier; 2014.

Box 25.1 Fogazzi GB, Verdesca S, Garigali G. Urinalysis core curriculum 2008. Am J Kidney Dis 2008;51(6):1052–67; Patel JV, Chambers CV, Gomella LG. Hematuria: etiology and evaluation for the primary care physician. Can J Urol 2008;15(suppl 1):54–62.

Boxes 25.2, 25.3, 25.4, 25.5 Brown D, Edwards H, eds. Lewis's medical–surgical nursing. 4th edn. Sydney: Elsevier; 2014.

Figs 26.2, 26.3 Thompson JM, McFarlance GK, Hirsch JE et al. Mosby's clinical nursing. 5th edn. St Louis: Mosby; 2001.

Fig 26.4 Davis JH, et al. Surgery: a problem-solving approach. Vol 2. 2nd edn. St Louis: Mosby; 1995.

Fig 26.7 Kozak G, ed. Clinical diabetes mellitus. Philadelphia: WB Saunders; 1982.

Table 26.1 Brown D, Edwards H, eds. Lewis's medical–surgical nursing. 4th edn. Sydney: Elsevier; 2014.

Table 26.4 Ellenberg M, Rifkin H, eds. Diabetes mellitus: theory and practice. New York: Medical Examination Publishing; 1983.

Table 26.7 Kozak G, ed. Clinical diabetes mellitus. Philadelphia: WB Saunders; 1982.

Fig 27.2 National Health and Medical Research Council. Australian guidelines for the prevention and control of infection in healthcare.

In: Australian Commission on Safety and Quality in Healthcare, ed. Canberra: Australian Government; 2010.

Fig 27.4 World Health Organization. WHO guidelines on hand hygiene in health care. Geneva, Switzerland: WHO; 2009.

Table 27.1 Curson P. Epidemics and pandemics in Australia. Sydney: University of Sydney; 2010.

Tables 27.2, 27.3 National Health and Medical Research Council. Australian guidelines for the prevention and control of infection in healthcare. Australian Commission on Safety and Quality in Healthcare, ed. Canberra: Australian Government; 2010.

Table 27.4 Porter R, ed. Merck Manual Professional Version. Copyright 2006 by Merck Sharp & Dohme Corp., a subsidiary of Merck & Co, Inc, Kenilworth, NJ. Online. www.merckmanuals.com/professional/.

Box 27.1 Australian Commission on Safety and Quality in Health Care. Standard 3—Preventing and Controlling Healthcare Associated Infections—Safety and Quality Improvement Guide Sydney: Australian Commission on Safety and Quality in Health Care, 2012.

Box 27.2 National Health and Medical Research Council. Australian guidelines for the prevention and control of infection in healthcare. Australian Commission on Safety and Quality in Healthcare, ed. Canberra: Australian Governement; 2010.

Fig 28.1 Marx J, Hockberger R, Walls R. Rosen emergency medicine, 8th edn. Saunders; 2014.

Fig 28.2 Lewis SM, Collier IC, Heitkemper MM. Medical–surgical nursing: assessment and management of clinical problems. 7th edn. St Louis: Mosby; 2007.

Fig 28.3 Rosen P, Barkin RM, Hockberger RS et al. Emergency medicine: concepts and clinical practice, vol. 1. 3rd edn. St Louis: Mosby; 1992.

Tables 28.4, 28.6 Cameron P, Jelinek G, Kelly A, et al. eds. Textbook of adult emergency medicine. 3rd edn. Edinburgh: Churchill Livingstone; 2009.

Table 28.7 Lewis SM, Collier IC, Heitkemper MM. Medical–surgical nursing: assessment and management of clinical problems. 7th edn. St Louis: Mosby; 2007.

Box 28.1 Rogers I, Williams A. Heat related illness. In: Cameron P, Jelinek G, Kelly AM et al, eds. Textbook of adult emergency medicine. 3rd edn. Edinburgh: Churchill Livingstone; 2009; Bucher L, Parkinson S. Emergency care situations. In: Brown D, Edwards H, eds. Lewis's medical–surgical nursing: assessment and management of clinical problems, 2nd edn. Sydney: Elsevier; 2008.

Fig 29.1 Modified from Patton KT, Thibodeau GA. Anatomy and physiology, 8th edn, St Louis: Mosby; 2013; Brown D, Edwards H, eds. Lewis's Medical–surgical nursing. 4th edn, Sydney: Elsevier; 2014.

Figs 29.2, 29.3 Lewis SM, Collier IC, Heitkemper MM. Medical–surgical nursing: assessment and management of clinical problems. 7th edn. St Louis: Mosby; 2007.

Fig 29.4 Clinical Excellence Commission, © New South Wales Ministry of Health for and on behalf of the Crown in right of the State of New South Wales, http://www.cec.health.nsw.gov.au/programs/sepsis/sepsis-tools.

Table 29.2 Lewis SM, Collier IC, Heitkemper MM. Medical–surgical nursing: assessment and management of clinical problems. 7th edn. St Louis: Mosby; 2007; Newberry L, ed. Sheehy's emergency nursing. 5th edn. St Louis: Mosby; 2003.

Table 29.4 Shelton BK, Rome SI, Lewis SL. Nursing assessment: haematological system. In Brown D, Edwards H, eds. Lewis's medical–surgical nursing. 4th edn. Sydney: Elsevier; 2008.

Box 29.1 Kitchen G. Immunology and haematology. Edinburgh: Mosby; 2012.

Box 29.2 Brack S. Nursing management of haematological problems. In: Lewis SM, Collier IC, Heitkemper MM, eds. Medical–surgical nursing: assessment and management of clinical problems. 7th edn. St Louis: Mosby; 2007; Maclaren H. Anaemia. In: Cameron P, Jelinek G, Kelly A et al, eds. Textbook of adult emergency medicine. 3rd edn. Edinburgh: Churchill Livingstone; 2009.

Box 29.4 Ariyan CE, Sosa JA. Assessment and management of patients with abnormal calcium. Crit Care Med 2004;32(4 Suppl):S146–54.

Box 29.8 ACCP/SCCM. American College of Chest Physicians/Society of Critical Care Medicine Consensus Conference: definitions for sepsis and organ failure and guidelines for the use of innovative therapies in sepsis. Crit Care Med 1992;20(6):864–74.

Box 29.9 Australian and New Zealand Society of Blood Transfusion. Guidelines for the administration of blood components. Australia: ANZSBT; 2004. Online. www.anzsbt.org.au/publications/documents/AdminGiudelinesOct2004.pdf; van der Meer PF, Gulliksson H, AuBuchon JP et al. Interruption of agitation of platelet concentrates: effects on in vitro parameters. Vox Sang 2005;88:227.

Box 29.10 Australian and New Zealand Society of Blood Transfusion. Administration of Blood Products. December 2011.

Box 29.11 Gillies D, O'Riordan L, Carr D et al. Gauze and tape and transparent polyurethane dressings for central venous catheters. Cochrane Database Syst Rev 1. Most recent update 29 Aug 2003; Kuter DJ. Thrombotic complications of central venous catheters in

cancer patients. Oncologist 2004;9:207–16; Stevens LC, Haire WD, Tarantolo S et al. Normal saline versus heparin flush for maintaining central venous catheter patency during apheresis collection of peripheral blood stem cells (PBSC). Transfus Sci 1997;18:187–93.

Table 30.4 Adapted from McCoubrie D, Murray L, Daly FF, et al. Toxicology case of the month: ingestion of two unidentified tablets by a toddler. Emerg Med J 2006;23(9):718–20.

Boxes 30.1, 30.6 Murray L, Daly F, Little M, et al. Toxicology handbook. Sydney: Elsevier; 2006.

Fig 31.1 Shutterstock/Kristian Bell.

Fig 31.2 Shutterstock/mroz.

Fig 31.3 Flickr/F Delventhal/CC BY 2.0.

Fig 31.4 Flickr/Stephan Ridgway/CC BY 2.0.

Fig 31.5 Wikipedia/Sputniktilt/CC BY-SA 3.0.

Fig 31.6 Shutterstock/Peter Waters.

Fig 31.7 Shutterstock/ ChameleonsEye.

Fig 31.8 Copyright Dr David Wachenfeld/AUSCAPE. All rights reserved.

Tables 31.1, 31.2 Murray L, Daly F, Little M, et al. Toxicology handbook. 2nd edn. Sydney: Elsevier; 2011.

Box 31.3 White J. CSL Antivenom Handbook. CSL: Parkville, Melbourne, Victoria; 2001.

Fig 32.1 Epstein O, Perkin GD, Cookson J, et al. Ear, nose and throat. In: Clinical examination. 4th edn. Sydney: Elsevier; 2008:82–104.

Fig 32.2 Marx J, Hockberger RS, Wallia R et al: Rosen's emergency medicine, 8th edn, Elsevier; 2014.

Fig 32.3 Wilson SF, Thompson JM: Respiratory disorders, St Louis, 1990, Mosby.

Figs 32.4, 32.5, 32.6, Epstein O, Perkin GD, Cookson J et al. Ear, nose and throat. In: Clinical examination. 4th edn. Sydney: Elsevier; 2008.

Fig 32.7 Marx J, Hockberger RS, Wallia R et al: Rosen's emergency medicine, 8th edn, Elsevier; 2014.

Fig 32.8 Barkauskas V, Pender NJ, Hayman L et al. Health and physical assessment. 2nd edn. St Louis: Mosby; 1998.

Fig 32.13 Skapetis T, Naim A. Dental infections management flowchart. General Practice Training Tasmania; 2009. Online. http://aci.moodlesite.pukunui.net/pluginfile.php/1581/mod_resource/content/2/Skapetis%20et%20al%202012.pdf.

Fig 32.19 Courtesy Dr Tony Skapetis.

Fig 32.29 Courtesy Dr Tony Skapetis.

Fig 32.30 Courtesy Mr Simon A Hickey.

Fig 32.31 Epstein O, Perkin GD, Cookson J et al. Ear, nose and throat. In: Clinical examination. 4th edn. Sydney: Elsevier; 2008.

Figs 33.1, 33.2 Batterbury M, Bowling B. Ophthalmology: an illustrated colour text. 2nd edn. Sydney: Elsevier; 2005.

Figs 33.3, 33.5 Lewis SM, Collier IC, Heitkemper MM. Medical–surgical nursing: assessment and management of clinical problems. 7th edn. St Louis: Mosby; 2007.

Fig 33.4 Rudy EB. Advanced neurological and neurosurgical nursing. St Louis: Mosby; 1984.

Fig 33.6 Guyton AC, Hall JE. Textbook of medical physiology. 11th edn. Philadelphia: WB Saunders; 2006.

Figs 33.7, 33.8 Batterbury M, Bowling B. Ophthalmology: an illustrated colour text. 2nd edn. Sydney: Elsevier; 2005.

Figs 33.9, 33.10 Lewis SM, Collier IC, Heitkemper MM. Medical–surgical nursing: assessment and management of clinical problems. 7th edn. St Louis: Mosby; 2007.

Figs 33.12, 33.13 Batterbury M, Bowling B. Ophthalmology: an illustrated colour text. 2nd edn. Sydney: Elsevier; 2005.

Fig 33.14 Webb LA. Manual of eye emergencies—diagnosis and management. 2nd edn. Edinburgh: Butterworth–Heinemann; 2004.

Fig 33.15 Stein HA, Slatt BJ, Stein RM. The ophthalmic assistant. 7th edn. St Louis: Mosby; 2000.

Fig 33.16 McQuillan KA, Von Rueden K, Hartsock R et al, eds. Trauma nursing: from resuscitation through rehabilitation. 3rd edn. Philadephia: WB Saunders; 2002.

Figs 33.17, 33.18 Webb LA. Manual of eye emergencies—diagnosis and management. 2nd edn. Edinburgh: Butterworth–Heinemann; 2004.

Fig 33.19 Abrams D. Ophthalmology in medicine: an illustrated clinical guide. St Louis: Mosby; 1990.

Fig 33.20 McQuillan KA, Von Rueden K, Hartsock R et al, eds. Trauma nursing: from resuscitation through rehabilitation. 3rd edn. Philadephia: WB Saunders; 2002.

Fig 33.21 Bhavsar AR. Surgical techniques in ophthalmology: Retina and vitreous surgery. © 2009, Elsevier Inc.

Figs 33.23, 33.25 Batterbury M, Bowling B. Ophthalmology: an illustrated colour text. 2nd edn. Sydney: Elsevier; 2005.

Table 33.1 Batterbury M, Bowling B. Ophthalmology: an illustrated colour text. 2nd edn. Sydney: Elsevier; 2005.

Table 33.2 Adapted from New South Wales Health. Eye emergency modules. Online. www.health.nsw.gov.au/resources/gmct/ophthalmology/pdf/eye_manual.pdf.

Table 33.4 Lewis SM, Collier IC, Heitkemper MM. Medical–surgical nursing: assessment and management of clinical problems. 7th edn. St Louis: Mosby; 2007.

Box 33.1 Lewis SM, Collier IC, Heitkemper MM. Medical–surgical nursing: assessment and management of clinical problems. 7th edn. St Louis: Mosby; 2007.

Box 33.2 Ambulance Service of New South Wales. Protocols and pharmacologies. 2001. Online. www.ciap.health.nsw.gov.au/specialties/CDA/.

Figs 34.1, 34.2, 34.3, 34.4, 34.5 Fraser D, Cooper M, eds. Myles' textbook for midwives. 15th edn. Edinburgh: Churchill Livingstone; 2009.

Fig 34.6 LifeART image, © 2006; Lippincott Williams & Wilkins. Callahan T, Caughey A. Blueprint's obstetrics and gynaecology. 6th edn. Philadelphia: Lippincott Williams & Wilkins; 2013.

Table 34.1 Donovan B, Bradford DL, Cameron S, et al. The Australasian contact tracing manual. 3rd edn. Australasian Society of HIV Medicine (ASHM). Canberra: Commonwealth of Australia; 2006. Online. www.ashm.org.au/images/publications/aust-contact-tracing.pdf; Bradford D, Hoy J, Matthews G. HIV, viral hepatitis and STIs: a guide for primary care. Australasian Society for HIV Medicine (ASHM); 2008. Online. Available: www.ashm.org.au/images/publications/monographs/HIV_viral_hepatitis_and_STIs_a_guide_for_primary_care/hiv_viral_hepatitis_and_stis_whole.pdf.

Box 34.2 Donovan B, Bradford DL, Cameron S, et al. The Australasian contact tracing manual. 3rd edn. Australasian Society of HIV Medicine (ASHM). Canberra: Commonwealth of Australia; 2006. Online. www.ashm.org.au/images/publications/aust-contact-tracing.pdf; Bradford D, Hoy J, Matthews G. HIV, viral hepatitis and STIs: a guide for primary care. Australasian Society for HIV Medicine (ASHM); 2008. Online. www.ashm.org.au/images/publications/monographs/HIV_viral_hepatitis_and_STIs_aguide_for_primary_care/hiv_viral_hepatitis_and_stis_whole.pdf.

Box 34.3 Callahan T, Caughey A. Blueprint's obstetrics and gynaecology. 6th edn. Philadelphia: Lippincott Williams & Wilkins; 2013; Brown A, Cadogan M. Emergency medicine: diagnosis and management. 6th edn. London: Hodder Arnold; 2011.

Box 34.4 Weston G, Vollenhoven B. Menstrual and other disorders. In: McDonald S, Thompson C, eds. Women's health: a handbook. Sydney: Elsevier; 2005.

Box 34.5 Cook K. Pelvic pain in females. In: Bourke S, ed. National management guidelines for sexually transmissible infections. SHSOV; 2008.

Box 34.6 Huffam S, Haber P, Wallace J et al. Talking with the patient: risk assessment and history taking. In: Bradford D, Hoy J, Matthews G, eds. HIV, viral hepatitis and STIs: a guide for primary care. Australasian Society for HIV Medicine (ASHM); 2008.

Fig 35.1 Personal drawings Allison Cummins.

Fig 35.2 Photograph taken by Allison Cummins.

Table 35.1 Adapted from American Heart Association Guidelines for Cardiopulmonary Resuscitation and Emergency Cardiovascular Care (American Heart Association 2010).

Box 35.1 Adapted from the Guidelines for the management of hypertensive disorders of pregnancy from the Society of Obstetric Medicine of Australia and New Zealand (SOMANZ); Lowe S, Bowyer L, Lust K et al. The management of hypertensive disorders of pregnancy. Society of Obstetric Medicine of Australia and New Zealand (SOMANZ). 2014. Online. www.somanz.org/documents/HTguideline2014ConsultationDraft120214.pdf.

Box 35.2 Lewis, G, ed. The Confidential Enquiry into Maternal and Child Health (CEMACH). Saving mothers' lives: reviewing maternal deaths to make motherhood safer – 2006–2008. The Eighth Report on Confidential Enquiries into Maternal Deaths in the United Kingdom. London: CEMACH; 2011.

Box 35.3 Adapted from Oates et al. Back to basics. In: Lewis G. Saving mothers' lives: Reviewing maternal deaths to make motherhood safer 2006–08. The Eighth Report of the Confidential Enquiries into Maternal Deaths in the United Kingdom. BJOG 2011;118(Suppl. 1):1–203.

Fig 36.2 Cambridge University Hospitals. Infant with nasal cannula [image]. www.cuh.org.uk/resources/images/rosie/neonatal/nicu/how_we_care/vital_needs/nasal_cannula_131008.jpg.

Fig 36.3 Brierley J et al. Clinical practice parameters for hemodynamic support of pediatric and neonatal septic shock: 2007 update from the American College of Critical Care Medicine. Critical Care Medicine 2009;37(2):666–88.

Fig 36.4 Adapted from Royal Children's Hospital, Melbourne. Clinical practice guidelines—afebrile seizures. www.rch.org.au/clinicalguide/cpg.cfm?doc_id=12322.

Fig 36.6 From the Merck Manual Professional Version, edited by Robert Porter. © 2014 by Merck Sharp & Dohme Corp., a subsidiary of Merck & Co, Inc, Kenilworth, NJ. www.merckmanuals.com/professional/injuries_poisoning/fractures_dislocations_and_sprains/pediatric_physeal_growth_plate_fractures.html.

Fig 36.7 Hicks CL et al. The Faces Pain Scale-Revised: toward a common metric in pediatric pain measurement. Pain 2001; 93(2):173–83; with permission from IASP®.

Fig 36.8 Courtesy Teleflex Medical.

Table 36.4 Starte D, Meldrum D. Developmental surveillance and assessment. In: Roberton MD, South M, eds. Practical paediatrics. Churchill Livingstone: Edinburgh; 2006.

Table 36.5 © Ministry of Health New Zealand, http://www.health.govt.nz/our-work/preventative-health-wellness/immunisation/new-zealand-immunisation-schedule; © Commonwealth of Australia, http://www.immunise.health.gov.au/internet/immunise/publishing.nsf/Content/national-immunisation-program-schedule.

Table 36.6 Adapted from Hockenberry M, Wilson D. Wong's nursing care of infants and children. 8th edn. St Louis, Mosby; 2007.

Table 36.7 Advanced Life Support Group, Advanced Paediatric Life Support: The practical approach. 5th edn. London: Wiley-Blackwell; 2007.

Table 36.8 Davis RJ, et al. Head and spinal cord injury. In: Rogers MC, ed. Textbook of pediatric intensive care. Baltimore: Williams & Wilkins, 1987; James H, Anas N, Perkin RM. Brain insults in infants and children. New York: Grune & Stratton; 1985; Morray JP, et al. Coma scale for use in brain-injured children. Crit Care Med 1984;12:1018–20.

Table 36.9 Considine J, LeVasseur S, Charles A. Consistency of triage in Victoria's emergency departments: Literature Review, 2001, Monash Institute of Health Services Research. Report to the Victorian Department of Human Services: Melbourne.

Table 36.12 Henning R. Assisted ventilation. In: Care of the Critically Ill Child. Macnab A, Macrae D, Henning R, eds. Churchill Livingstone: Edinburgh; 1999.

Table 36.13 Royal Children's Hospital. Clinical Practice Guideline: Bronchiolitis guideline. 2011. Online www.rch.org.au/clinicalguide/guideline_index/Bronchiolitis_Guideline/; Fitzgerald DA, Kilham HK. Bronchiolitis: assessment and evidence-based management, Med J Aust 2004;180(8):399–404.

Table 36.15 Friedman JN et al. Development of a clinical dehydration scale for use in children between 1 and 36 months of age. Journal of Pediatrics 2004;145(2):201–7. Goldman RD, Friedman JN, Parkin PC. Validation of the clinical dehydration scale for children with acute gastroenteritis. Pediatrics 2008;122(3):545–9

Table 36.16 Gastanaduy AS, Begue RE. Acute gastroenteritis. Clinical pediatrics 1999;38(1):1–12; Hahn S, Kim S, Garner P. Reduced osmolarity oral rehydration solution for treating dehydration caused by acute diarrhoea in children. Cochrane Database of Systematic Reviews 2002(1):Art No:CD002847.

Table 36.18 Beasley S. Abdominal pain and vomiting in children. In: Roberton DM, South M, eds. Practical paediatrics. Churchill Livingstone: Edinburgh; 2007.

Table 36.20 Phillips R, Orchard D, Starr M. Dermatology. In: Cameron P et al, eds. Textbook of paediatric emergency medicine. Churchill Livingstone: Edinburgh; 2006.

Table 36.22 Merkel SI et al. The FLACC: a behavioral scale for scoring postoperative pain in young children. Pediatric Nursing 1997;23(3): 293–7.

Boxes 36.1, 36.2 Advanced Life Support Group, Advanced Paediatric Life Support: The practical approach. 5th edn, London: Wiley-Blackwell; 2007.

Box 36.3 Gorelick M, Shaw K, Murphy K. Validity and reliability of clinical signs in the diagnosis of dehydration in children. Pediatrics 1997;99:E6.

Table 37.1 Adapted from Victorian Government Department of Health. Ambulance transport of people with a mental illness protocol 2010. Melbourne; 2010. Online. www.health.vic.gov.au/mentalhealth/publications/amb-transport0910.pdf.

Table 37.2 Adapted from Mental Health and Drug and Alcohol Office. Mental Health for Emergency Departments – a reference guide. Sydney, Australia: NSW Department of Health, 2009. Online. www0.health.nsw.gov.au/resources/mhdao/pdf/mhemergency.pdf.

Box 37.1 Adapted from Davies T. ABC of mental health: mental health assessment. Br Med J 1997;314(7093):1536–9.

Boxes 37.2, 37.5 Adapted from Paquette M, Rodemich C. Psychiatric nursing diagnosis care plans for DSM-IV. Sudbury: Jones and Bartlett; 1997.

Box 37.10 Adapted from Rogers I, Williams A. Heat related illness. In: Cameron P, Jelinek G, Kelly AM et al, eds. Textbook of adult emergency medicine. 3rd edn. Edinburgh: Churchill Livingstone; 2009.

Box 37.11 Adapted from SANE Australia Factsheet 14a. Suicidal behaviour and self harm. Online. Available: www.sane.org/information/factsheets-podcasts/211-suicidal-behaviour-and-self-harm; 08 Jan 2011.

Box 37.12 Adapted from Brooks JG. The violent patient. In: Cameron P, Jelinek G, Kelly AM et al, eds. Textbook of adult emergency medicine. 2nd edn. Edinburgh: Churchill Livingstone; 2004.

Fig 38.1 Regnard C, Reynolds J, Watson B et al. Understanding distress in people with severe communication difficulties: developing and assessing the Disability Distress Assessment Tool (DisDAT). J Intellect Disabil Res 2007;51(Pt 4):277–92.

Table 38.1 Jansen DE, Krol B, Groothoff JW et al. People with intellectual disability and their health problems: a review of comparative studies. J Intellect Disabil Res 2004;48(2):93–102.

Table 38.2 Grossman SA, Richards CF, Anglin D et al. Caring for the patient with mental retardation in the emergency department. Ann Emerg Med 2000; 35(1):69–76.

Table 38.3 Cheetham T, Lovering JS, Telch J et al. Physical health. In: Brown I, Percy M, eds. A comprehensive guide to intellectual and developmental disabilities. 2nd edn. Baltimore: Paul H Brookes; 2007.

Table 38.4 Brown I, Percy M, eds. A comprehensive guide to intellectual and developmental disabilities. 2nd edn. Baltimore: Paul H Brookes; 2007.

Box 38.1 Radford JP, Park DC. Historical overview of developmental disabilities in Ontario. In: Brown I, Percy M, eds. Developmental disabilities in Ontario. 2nd edn. Toronto: Ontario Association on Developmental Disabilities; 2003.

Box 38.2 Centre for Developmental Disability Studies. Health care in people with intellectual disability—guidelines for general practitioners. North Sydney: CDDS for NSW Health; 2006. Reproduced by permission, NSW Ministry of Health © 2015.

Fig 39.1 Lach MS. Functional decline. In: Sanders AB, ed. Emergency care of the elder person. St Louis: Beverly Cracom Publications; 1996.

Fig 39.2 Department of Human Services Victoria. Clinical practice guidelines for the management of delirium in older people. Victorian Government; 2006. Online. www.health.vic.gov.au/acute-agedcare.

Fig 39.3 Australian Institute of Health and Welfare. Australian hospital statistics 2007–08. Health services series no. 33. Cat. no. HSE 71. Canberra: AIHW; 2009.

Fig 39.4 Morgan TK, Williamson M, et al. A national census of medicines use: a 24-hour snapshot of Australians aged 50 years and older. Med J Aust 2012;196(1):50–3. © 2012 The Medical Journal of Australia—reproduced with permission. The Medical Journal of Australia does not accept responsibility for any errors in translation.

Fig 39.5 Brown D, Edwards H, eds. Lewis's medical–surgical nursing: assessment and management of clinical problems. Sydney: Elsevier; 2005.

Table 39.1 Wooding Baker M, Heitkemper MM, Chenoweth L. Older adults: Age-related physiologic changes. In: Brown D, Edwards H et al, eds. Medical–surgical nursing: assessment and management of clinical problems. 3rd edn. Chatswood: Elsevier Australia; 2012.

Box 39.2 Katz S, Ford AB, Moskowitz RW et al. Studies of illness in the aged: the index of ADL: a standardized measure of biological and psychosocial function. JAMA 1963;185:914–19; Lawton MP, Brody EM. Assessment of older people: self-maintaining and instrumental activities of daily living. Gerontologist 1969;9(3):179–86.

Box 39.3 Garratt S. Assessment of patterns of body defence and healing. In: Koch S, Garratt S, eds. Assessing older people: a practical guide for health professionals. Sydney: MacLennan and Petty; 2001.

Box 39.6 Sanders AB, ed. Emergency care of the elder person. St. Louis: Beverly Cracom Publications; 1996.

Box 39.7 Brown D, Edwards H, eds. Lewis's Medical–surgical nursing: assessment and management of clinical problems. Sydney: Elsevier; 2005.

Box 39.8 Sanders AB. The elder patient. In: Tintinalli JE, Kelen GD, Stapczynski JS, eds. Emergency medicine: a comprehensive study guide. 6th edn. McGraw-Hill; 2004.

Fig 41.1 Thorley A. The effects of alcohol. In: Plant M, ed. Drinking and problem drinking. London: Junction Books; 1982; de Crespigny C, Talmet J, eds. Alcohol, tobacco and other drugs: Clinical guidelines for nurses and midwives. Version 3. 2012. The University of Adelaide School of Nursing and Drug and Alcohol Services SA. www.sahealth.sa.gov.au/wps/wcm/connect/9087368041793eefa6e1ef67a94f09f9/ATOD+Clinical+Guidelines+for+Nurses+and+Midwives+V3+2012-DASSA-April2014.pdf?MOD=AJPERES&CACHEID=9087368041793eefa6e1ef67a94f09f9.

Fig 41.2 de Crespigny C, Talmet J, eds. Alcohol, tobacco and other drugs: Clinical guidelines for nurses and midwives. Version 3. 2012. The University of Adelaide School of Nursing and Drug and Alcohol Services SA. www.sahealth.sa.gov.au/wps/wcm/connect/9087368041793eefa6e1ef67a94f09f9/ATOD+Clinical+Guidelines+for+Nurses+and+Midwives+V3+2012-DASSA-April2014.pdf?MOD=AJPERES&CACHEID=9087368041793eefa6e1ef67a94f09f9.

Fig 41.3 Courtesy Department of Radiology, St George Public Hospital, Sydney.

Fig 41.4 Alcohol treatment guidelines for Indigenous Australians from Department of Health and Ageing; 2007.

Fig 41.5 de Crespigny C, Talmet J, eds. Alcohol, tobacco and other drugs: clinical guidelines for nurses and midwives. Version 3. 2012. The University of Adelaide School of Nursing and Drug

and Alcohol Services SA. www.sahealth.sa.gov.au/wps/wcm/connect/9087368041793eefa6e1ef67a94f09f9/ATOD+Clinical+Guidelines+for+Nurses+and+Midwives+V3+2012-DASSA-April2014.pdf?MOD=AJPERES&CACHEID=9087368041793eefa6e1ef67a94f09f9.

Table 41.1, 41.5 Lewis SM, Collier IC, Heitkemper MM. Medical–surgical nursing: assessment and management of clinical problems. 7th edn. St Louis: Mosby; 2007.

Table 41.2, 41.4, 41.6 de Crespigny C, Talmet J, eds. Alcohol, tobacco and other drugs: clinical guidelines for nurses and midwives. Version 3. 2012. The University of Adelaide School of Nursing and Drug and Alcohol Services SA. www.sahealth.sa.gov.au/wps/wcm/connect/9087368041793eefa6e1ef67a94f09f9/ATOD+Clinical+Guidelines+for+Nurses+and+Midwives+V3+2012-DASSA-April2014.pdf?MOD=AJPERES&CACHEID=9087368041793eefa6e1ef67a94f09f9.

Table 41.3 South Australian Drug and Alcohol Services Council material. Parkside: DASC; 1996.

Boxes 41.2, 41.3, 41.4, 41.5, 41.7, 41.8, 41.9, 41.10, 41.11, 41.12, 41.13, 41.14, 41.16 de Crespigny C, Talmet J, eds. Alcohol, tobacco and other drugs: clinical guidelines for nurses and midwives. Version 3. 2012. The University of Adelaide School of Nursing and Drug and Alcohol Services SA. www.sahealth.sa.gov.au/wps/wcm/connect/9087368041793eefa6e1ef67a94f09f9/ATOD+Clinical+Guidelines+for+Nurses+and+Midwives+V3+2012-DASSA-April2014.pdf?MOD=AJPERES&CACHEID=9087368041793eefa6e1ef67a94f09f9.

Box 41.6 Baker A, Lee NK, Jenner L, eds. Models of intervention and care for psychostimulant users. 2nd edn. National Drug Strategy Monograph Series No 51. Commonwealth of Australia. Canberra: Australian Government Department of Health and Ageing; 2004; Australian Department of Health and Ageing. Alcohol treatment guidelines for indigenous Australians. Canberra: Department of Health and Ageing; 2007. Allison MG, McCurdy MT. Alcoholic Metabolic Emergencies. Emergency Medicine Clinics of North America 2014;5;32(2):293–301.

Box 41.15 de Crespigny C, Talmet J, eds. Alcohol, tobacco and other drugs: clinical guidelines for nurses and midwives. Version 3. 2012. The University of Adelaide School of Nursing and Drug and Alcohol Services SA. www.sahealth.sa.gov.au/wps/wcm/connect/9087368041793eefa6e1ef67a94f09f9/ATOD+Clinical+Guidelines+for+Nurses+and+Midwives+V3+2012-DASSA-April2014.pdf?MOD=AJPERES&CACHEID=9087368041793eefa6e1ef67a94f09f9; Latt N, White J, McLean S et al, Central nervous system stimulants, In: Hulse G, White J, Cape G, eds. Management of alcohol and drug problems. Melbourne: Oxford University Press; 2002.

Box 41.17 de Crespigny C, Talmet J, eds. Alcohol, tobacco and other drugs: clinical guidelines for nurses and midwives. Version 3. 2012. The University of Adelaide School of Nursing and Drug and Alcohol Services SA. www.sahealth.sa.gov.au/wps/wcm/connect/9087368041793eefa6e1ef67a94f09f9/ATOD+Clinical+Guidelines+for+Nurses+and+Midwives+V3+2012-DASSA-April2014.pdf?MOD=AJPERES&CACHEID=9087368041793eefa6e1ef67a94f09f9; Hulse G, White J, Cape G, eds. Management of alcohol and drug problems. Melbourne: Oxford University Press; 2002.

Fig 42.1 Lozano R, Naghavi M, Foreman K et al. Global and regional mortality from 235 causes of death for 20 age groups in 1990 and 2010: A systematic analysis for the Global Burden of Disease Study 2010. The Lancet 2012;380(9859):2095–128.

Fig 42.2 Global Road Safety Facility, The World Bank, Institute for Health Metrics and Evaluation. Transport for Health: The Global Burden of Disease from Motorized Road Transport. In: The Institute for Health Metrics and Evaluation (ed.). Seattle: University of Seattle; 2014. http://documents.worldbank.org/curated/en/2014/01/19308007/transport-health-global-burden-disease-motorized-road-transport. The contents of this publication may be reproduced and redistributed in whole or in part, provided the intended use is for noncommercial purposes, the contents are not altered, and full acknowledgment is given to the World Bank and IHME. This work is licensed under the Creative Commons Attribution-NonCommercial-NoDerivatives 4.0 Unported License. To view a copy of this license, please visit: http://creativecommons.org/licenses/by-nc-nd/4.0/.

Fig 42.3 Lyons RA, Finch CF, et al. The injury list of all deficits (LOAD) framework—conceptualising the full range of deficits and adverse outcomes following injury and violence. Int J Injury Control Safety Promotion 2010;17(3):145–59.

Fig 42.4 Australian Bureau of Statistics. Causes of Death, Australia, 2012. Commonwealth of Australia; 2014 [25/04/2014]; www.abs.gov.au/ausstats/abs@.nsf/Lookup/by%20Subject/3303.0~2012~Main%20Features~Key%20Characteristics~10009.

Fig 42.5 Ministry of Health and Accident Compensation Corporation. 2013. Injury-related health loss: A report from the New Zealand Burden of Diseases, Injuries and Risk Factors Study 2006–2016. Wellington: Ministry of Health. www.health.govt.nz/system/files/documents/publications/injury-related-health-loss-aug13_0.pdf.

Fig 42.6 Australian Institute of Health and Welfare. www.aihw.gov.au/WorkArea/DownloadAsset.aspx?id=1073742216.

Table 42.1 Australian Transport Council. National Road Safety Strategy 2011–2020, 2011.

Table 42.2 National Public Health Partnership. The National Injury Prevention and Safety Promotion Plan: 2004–2014. Canberra: NPHP; 2004; Cooper DJ, McDermott FT, Cordner SM, et al. Quality assessment of the management of road traffic fatalities at a level 1 trauma centre compared to other hospitals in Victoria, Australia. J Trauma 1997A;45(4):1–8; Sampalis JS, Denis R, Frechette P et al. Direct transport to tertiary trauma centers versus transfer to lower level facilities: impact on mortality and morbidity among patients with major trauma. J Trauma 1997;43(2):288–96.

Table 42.3 Walter E, Curtis K. The role and impact of the specialist trauma nurse: an integrative review. Journal of trauma nursing 2015;22:153–69.

Box 42.1 Danne PD. Trauma management in Australia and the tyranny of distance. World J Surg 2003;27(4):385–9; Australian Transport Safety Bureau (ATSB). Road crash casualties and rates, Australia, 1925 to 2005. Canberra: ATSB; 2007. Online. www.infrastructure.gov.au/roads/safety/publications/2008/pdf/1925_05_casualties.pdf.

Box 42.2 Adapted from Gordon C. Driver distraction: an initial examination of the 'attention diverted by' contributory factor codes from crash reports and focus group research on perceived risks. Paper presented to the Institute of Professional Engineers Technical Conference. Auckland: New Zealand; 2005. Online. www.ipenz.org.nz/ipenztg/papers/2005_pdf/04_Gordon.pdf.

Box 42.3 Adapted from National Public Health Partnership. The National Injury Prevention and Safety Promotion Plan: 2004–2014. Canberra: NPHP; 2004.

Box 42.4 Baker SP, O'Neill B, Ginsburg MJ et al. The injury fact book. 2nd edn. New York: Oxford University Press; 1992. Haddon W Jr. The basic strategies for preventing damage from hazards of all kinds. Hazard Prevent 1980;16:8–12.

Box 42.6 Royal Australasian College of Surgeons. The Australasian trauma verification program manual. Melbourne: RACS; 2009.

Figs 43.5, 43.6 Neff JA, Kidd PS. Trauma nursing: the art and science. 2nd edn. St Louis: Mosby; 1993.

Fig 43.7 McSwain NE, Paturas JL. The basic EMT: comprehensive prehospital patient care. 2nd edn. St Louis: Mosby; 2001.

Fig 43.8 Courtesy KidSafe WA.

Fig 43.10 Neff JA, Kidd PS. Trauma nursing: the art and science. 2nd edn. St Louis: Mosby; 1993.

Fig 43.11 Adapted from Committee of the National Association of Emergency Medical Technicians in cooperation with the Committee on Trauma of the American College of Surgeons. Prehospital trauma life support: basic and advanced prehospital trauma life support. 4th edn. St Louis: Mosby; 1999.

Fig 43.12 Riggle A, Bollins J, Konda S et al. Penetrating pediatric trauma owing to improper child safety seat use. J Ped Surg 2010;45(1):245–8.

Fig 43.13 Neff JA, Kidd PS. Trauma nursing: the art and science. 2nd edn. St Louis: Mosby; 1993.

Table 43.1 Australian Road Rules. Part 16: Rules for persons travelling in or on vehicles. National Transport Commission, February 2009. Online. www.ntc.gov.au/filemedia/Reports/ARR_February_2009_final.pdf.

Table 43.2 Revere CJ. Mechanism of injury. In: Newberry L, ed. Sheehy's emergency nursing principles and practice. St Louis: Mosby; 2003; Choo KL, Hansen JB, Bailey DM. Beware the boogie board: blunt abdominal trauma from body boarding. Med J Aust 2002;176(1):326–7. Fong CP, Hood N. A paediatric trauma study of scooter injuries. Emerg Med Australas 2004;16(2):139–44; Orchard J, James T, Alcott E et al. Injuries in Australian cricket at first class level 1995/1996 to 2000/2001; Br J Sports Med 2002;36(4):270–5; Pringle RG, McNair P, Stanley S. Incidence of sporting injury in New Zealand youths aged 6–15 years. Br J Sports Med 1998;32(1):49–52; Falvey EC, Eustace J, Whelan B et al. Sport and recreation-related injuries and fracture occurrence among emergency department attendees: implications for exercise prescription and injury prevention. Emerg Med J 2009;26(8):590–5.

Box 43.3 Cole E. Trauma care: Initial assessment and management in the emergency department. Oxford: Blackwell; 2009.

Box 43.4 Revere CJ. Mechanism of injury. In: Newberry L, ed. Sheehy's emergency nursing principles and practice. St Louis: Mosby; 2003.

Fig 44.1A based on diagram from The Royal Melbourne Hospital, Victoria.

Figs 44.1B, 44.3 Courtesy The Royal Melbourne Hospital, Melbourne, Victoria.

Fig 44.2 Victoria State Trauma Committee. Adult pre hospital major trauma criteria. About the VSTS. Online. www.health.vic.gov.au/trauma/about.htm.

Fig 44.4 Gruen RL, Brohi K, Schreiber M et al. Haemorrhage control in severely injured patients. The Lancet 2012;380(9847):1099–108.

Fig 44.5 Curtis K, Fraser M, Grant N et al. Adding insult to injury, hypothermia in the trauma patient: a trauma centre's experience in monitoring temperature. Achiev Nurs 2004;6:30–5; Kirkpatrick AW, Chun R, Brown R et al. Hypothermia and the trauma patient. Can J Surg 1999;42(5):333–43. Lewis AM. Trauma triad of death: emergency! Nursing 2000;30(3):62–4.

Fig 44.6 Zuidema GD, Rutherford RB, Ballinger WF, eds. The management of trauma. 4th edn. Philadelphia: WB Saunders; 1985; B, Courtesy Liverpool Hospital Trauma Service, Sydney, NSW.

Fig 44.7 Roberts J, Hedges J eds. Clinical procedures in emergency medicine. 3rd edn. Philadelphia: WB Saunders; 1998.

Fig 44.8 Cameron P, Jelinek G, Kelly AM et al, eds. Textbook of adult emergency medicine. 3rd edn. Edinburgh: Churchill Livingstone; 2009.

Fig 44.10A Republished, with permission, from resources at The Royal Children's Hospital, Melbourne, Australia. www.rch.org.au/clinicalguide/guideline_index/Intraosseous_Access/

Fig 44.10B Courtesy Teleflex Incorporated.

Fig 44.11 Adapted from Victorian Department of Human Services.

Table 44.1 Newberry L, ed. Sheehy's emergency nursing: principles and practice. 5th edn. St Louis: Mosby; 2003; Hotz H, Henn R, Lush S et al. Advanced trauma care for nurses. Instructor manual. Sante Fe: Society of Trauma Nurses; 2003.

Table 44.2 Newberry L, ed. Sheehy's emergency nursing: principles and practice. 5th edn. St Louis: Mosby; 2003. American College of Surgeons Committee on Trauma. Advanced trauma life support for doctors. ATLS student course manual. 9th edn. Chicago: American College of Surgeons; 2012.

Table 44.3 Newberry L, ed. Sheehy's emergency nursing: principles and practice. 5th edn. St Louis: Mosby; 2003.

Table 44.4 American College of Surgeons Committee on Trauma. Advanced trauma life support for doctors. ATLS student course manual. 9th edn. Chicago: American College of Surgeons; 2012; McQuillan KA, Makic MB, Whalen E, eds. Trauma nursing: from resuscitation through rehabilitation. 4th edn. Philadelphia: WB Saunders; 2008; Hotz H, Henn R, Lush S et al. Advanced trauma care for nurses. Instructor manual. Sante Fe: Society of Trauma Nurses; 2003; Curry N, Davis P. What's new in resuscitation strategies for patients with multiple trauma? Injury 2012;43(7):1021–8.

Table 44.5 American College of Surgeons Committee on Trauma. Advanced trauma life support for doctors. ATLS student course manual. 9th edn. Chicago: American College of Surgeons; 2012.

Table 44.6 Boffard K. Manual of definitive surgical trauma care. London: Hodder Arnold; 2011; Wise D, Davies G, Coats T et al. Emergency thoracotomy: 'how to do it'. Emerg Med J 2005;22(1):22–4; Doll D, Bonanno F, Smith MD et al. Emergency department thoracotomy (EDT). Trauma 2005;7:105–8; Hopson LR, Hirsh E, Delgado J et al. Guidelines for withholding or termination of resuscitation in pre-hospital traumatic cardiopulmonary arrest: a joint position paper from the National Association of EMS Physicians Standards and Clinical Practice Committee and the American College of Surgeons Committee on Trauma. Prehosp Emerg Care 2003;7(1):141–6.

Table 44.7 Newgard CD, Schmicker RH, Hedges JR et al. Emergency medical services intervals and survival in trauma: assessment of the 'golden hour' in a North American prospective cohort. Ann Emerg Med 2010;55(3):235–46; Kidd PS, Sturt PA, Fultz J. Mosby's emergency nursing reference. 2nd edn. St Louis: Mosby; 2000.

Table 44.8 Newberry L, ed. Sheehy's emergency nursing: principles and practice. 5th edn. St Louis: Mosby; 2003.

Table 44.9 Moore EE, Feliciano DV, Mattox KL. Trauma. 7th edn. New York: McGraw-Hill; 2012. Newberry L, ed. Sheehy's emergency nursing: principles and practice. 5th edn. St Louis: Mosby; 2003. American College of Surgeons Committee on Trauma. Advanced trauma life support for doctors. ATLS student course manual. 9th edn. Chicago: American College of Surgeons; 2012; McQuillan KA, Makic MB, Whalen E, eds. Trauma nursing: from resuscitation through rehabilitation. 4th edn. Philadelphia: WB Saunders; 2008; Hotz H, Henn R, Lush S et al. Advanced trauma care for nurses. Instructor manual. Sante Fe: Society of Trauma Nurses; 2003; Einsiedel P, Gumm K, Judson R. Trauma TACo. TRM 08.07 X-ray Imaging During Pregnancy V3. Melbourne: The Royal Melbourne Hospital Trauma Service; March 2014; Gumm K, Kennedy M, Oats J et al. TRM05.01 The Pregnant Trauma Patient Guideline V3.0. 3.14: The Royal Melbourne Hospital Trauma Service; March 2014. Mendez-Figueroa H, Dahlke J, Vrees R, Rouse D. Trauma in pregnancy: an updated systematic review. American Journal of Obstetrics & Gynecology 2013;209(1):1–10.

Table 44.10 Newberry L, ed. Sheehy's emergency nursing: principles and practice. 5th edn. St Louis: Mosby; 2003; Hotz H, Henn R, Lush S et al. Advanced trauma care for nurses. Instructor manual. Sante Fe: Society of Trauma Nurses; 2003.

Table 44.11 ROTES. Review of trauma and emergency services: Victoria 1999. Final report of the Ministerial Taskforce on Trauma and Emergency Services and the Department Working Party on Emergency and Trauma Service. Melbourne: Department of Human Services; 1999. Bevan C. Pre-hospital criteria for paediatric major trauma patients. Melbourne: The Royal Children's Hospital; 2005.

Box 44.1 Newberry L, ed. Sheehy's emergency nursing: principles and practice. 5th edn. St Louis: Mosby; 2003. American College of Surgeons Committee on Trauma. Advanced trauma life support for doctors. ATLS student course manual. 9th edn. Chicago: American College of Surgeons; 2012.

Box 44.2 American College of Surgeons Committee on Trauma. Advanced trauma life support for doctors. ATLS student course manual. 9th edn. Chicago: American College of Surgeons; 2012.

Box 44.3 DiDomenico PB, Pietzsch JB, Paté-Cornell ME. Bayesian assessment of overtriage and undertriage at a level I trauma centre. Philos Transact A Math Phys Eng Sci 2008;336(1874):2265–77; Cox S, Currell A, Harris L et al. Evaluation of the Victorian State adult pre-hospital triage criteria. Injury 2012;42(5):573–81; Advisory Committee on Trauma. TRM08.03 Trauma Team Activation: Trauma Call, Version 6.0. The Royal Melbourne Hospital; 2013. http:// clinicalguidelines.mh.org.au/brochures/TRM08.03.pdf; Advisory Committee on Trauma. TRM08.02 Trauma Team Activation: Trauma Alert, Version 6.0 The Royal Melbourne Hospital; 2013. http:// clinicalguidelines.mh.org.au/brochures/TRM08.02.pdf; Victoria State Trauma Committee. Adult pre hospital major trauma criteria. About the VSTS. Online. www.health.vic.gov.au/trauma/about. htm; Teixeira PG, Inaba K, Hadjizacharia P, et al. Preventable or potentially preventable mortality at a mature trauma center. J Trauma 2007;63(6):1338–46.

Box 44.5 Newberry L, ed. Sheehy's emergency nursing: principles and practice. 5th edn. St Louis: Mosby; 2003.

Box 44.6 Cameron P, Jelinek G, Kelly AM et al, eds. Textbook of adult emergency medicine. 3rd edn. Edinburgh: Churchill Livingstone; 2009.

Box 44.7 Cohen SS. Trauma nursing secrets: questions and answers reveal the secrets to safe and effective trauma nursing. Philadelphia: Hanley and Belfus; 2003; Kirkpatrick AW, Chun R, Brown R et al. Hypothermia and the trauma patient. Can J Surg 1999;42(5):333–43; Lewis AM. Trauma triad of death: emergency! Nursing 2000;30(3):62–4.

Box 44.8 ATLS manual. American College of Surgeons, Committee on Trauma. Initial Assessment and Management. In: Advanced Trauma Life Support® for Doctors. 9th edn. Chicago, IL: 2012.

Figs 45.1, 45.2 Lindsay DT. Functional human anatomy. St Louis: Mosby; 1996.

Fig 45.3 Rangel-Castilla L, Gasco J, Nauta HJ et al. Cerebral pressure autoregulation in traumatic brain injury. Neurosurg Focus 2008;25(4):E7.

Fig 45.4 O'Shea RA. Principles and practice of trauma nursing. Edinburgh: Churchill Livingstone; 2005.

Fig 45.5 Adam A, Dixon AK. Grainger and Allison's diagnostic radiology. 5th edn. New York: Churchill Livingstone; 2008.

Fig 45.6 Soto JA, Lucey BC. Emergency radiology: the requisites. Philadelphia: Mosby; 2009.

Fig 45.7 Courtesy Dr Ken Harrison, CareFlight, Sydney.

Fig 45.9 Ravi Sunder, Kevin Tyler. Basal skull fracture and the halo sign. 2013. CMAJ. JAMC.

Figs 45.10, 45.11, 45.12, 45.14 O'Shea RA. Principles and practice of trauma nursing. Edinburgh: Churchill Livingstone; 2005.

Fig 45.13 Jallo J, Loftus CM, eds. Neurotrauma and critical care of the brain. New York: Thieme Medical Publishers; 2009.

Figs 45.15, 45.16 Haaga J, Dogra VS, Forsting M et al, eds. CT and MRI of the whole body. 5th edn. Philadelphia: Mosby; 2009.

Fig 45.18 Huether SE, McCance KL. Understanding pathophysiology. 2nd edn. St Louis: Mosby; 2000.

Fig 45.20 Thelan LA et al. Critical care nursing: diagnosis and management. 3rd edn. St Louis: Mosby; 1998.

Table 45.1 Heron R, Davie A, Gillies R et al. Interrater reliability of the Glasgow Coma Scale scoring among nurses in sub-specialties of critical care. Aust Crit Care 2001;14(3):100–5; Mayer SA, Chong JY. Critical care management of increased intracranial pressure. J Intensive Care Med 2002;17(2):55–67.

Box 45.1 Le TH, Gean AD. Neuroimaging of the traumatic brain injury. Mt Sinai J Med 2009;76(2):145–62.

Box 45.2 Minardi J, Crocco TJ. Management of traumatic brain injury: first link in chain of survival. Mt Sinai J Med 2009;76:138–44.

Box 45.3 Le TH, Gean AD. Neuroimaging of the traumatic brain injury. Mt Sinai J Med 2009;76(2):145–62; Reed D. Adult trauma clinical practice guidelines: initial management of closed head injury in adults. NSW Institute of Trauma and Injury Management; 2007.

Box 45.4 Cameron P, Jelinek G, Kelly A et al. Textbook of adult emergency medicine. 2nd edn. Edinburgh: Churchill Livingstone; 2004.

Fig 46.1 Drake RL, Vogl AW, Mitchell AWM. Gray's basic anatomy. Churchill Livingstone, Elsevier, 2012.

Fig 46.2 Hansen, John T. Netter's clinical anatomy, Elsevier; 2014.

Fig 46.3 Moses, KP. Atlas of clinical gross anatomy. © 2013, 2005, by Saunders, an imprint of Elsevier Inc.

Fig 46.4 Bogart BI. Elsevier's integrated anatomy and embryology © 2007 Mosby, an affiliate of Elsevier Inc.

Fig 46.5 Mayersak, Ryanne J. Rosen's emergency medicine. © 2014 Saunders, an imprint of Elsevier Inc.

Fig 46.6 Burton JH, Kuehl KN. Emergency medicine. © 2013, 2008 by Saunders, an imprint of Elsevier Inc.

Figs 46.7, 46.9 Perry M, Dancey A, Mireskandari K et al. Emergency care in facial trauma—a maxillofacial and ophthalmic perspective. Injury 2005;36:875–96.

Fig 46.8 Edibam C, Robinson H. Oh's Intensive Care Manual © 2014 Elsevier Ltd.

Fig 46.11 Burton, John H., Emergency Medicine © 2013, 2008 by Saunders, an imprint of Elsevier Inc.

Fig 46.13 Cunningham LL, Khader R. Oral and maxillofacial trauma, © 2013, 2005, 1997, 1991 by Saunders, an imprint of Elsevier Inc, Courtesy Dr. Daniel Plank.

Fig 46.14 Reddy LV. Oral and maxillofacial surgery © 2009, 2000 by Saunders, an imprint of Elsevier Inc.

Fig 46.15 Burton JH, Kuehl KN. Emergency medicine © 2013, 2008 by Saunders, an imprint of Elsevier Inc.

Fig 46.16 Engelstad, M. Current therapy in oral and maxillofacial surgery, © 2012 Saunders, an imprint of Elsevier Inc. Fig 46.17 Rosen P et al. Emergency medicine. 6th edn. St Louis: Mosby; 2006.

Fig 46.18 Steed MB, Bagheri SC. Clinical review of oral and maxillofacial surgery: a case-based approach © 2014 by Mosby, Inc., an affiliate of Elsevier Inc.

Fig 46.19 Marx J, Hockberger R, Walls R. Rosen's emergency medicine. 8th edn. St Louis: Mosby; 2014.

Fig 46.20 Sheehy SB, Jimmerson CL. Manual of clinical trauma care. 2nd edn. St Louis: Mosby; 1994.

Fig 46.21 Winegar B, Murillo H, Tantiwongkosi B. Spectrum of critical imaging findings in complex facial skeletal trauma. Radiographics 2013;33:3–19. http://pubs.rsna.org/doi/figure/10.1148/rg.331125080.

Fig 46.22 Papageorge MB, Oreadi D. Oral and maxillofacial trauma. © 2013, 2005, 1997, 1991 by Saunders, an imprint of Elsevier Inc.

Fig 46.23 Burton JH, Kuehl KN. Emergency medicine © 2013, 2008 by Saunders, an imprint of Elsevier Inc.

Fig 46.24 Adam A, Dixon AK. Grainger and Allison's diagnostic radiology. 5th edn. New York: Churchill Livingstone; 2008.

Fig 46.25 Bell RB, Al-Bustani SS. Current therapy in oral and maxillofacial surgery, © 2012 Saunders, an imprint of Elsevier Inc.

Table 46.2 Rosen P et al. Emergency medicine. 6th edn. St Louis: Mosby; 2010.

Table 46.5 Trunkey DD, Lewis FR. Current therapy of trauma. 2nd edn. Toronto: BC Decker; 1986.

Fig 47.1 Image IDs: 67620 and 4595. © 2015 Elsevier Inc. All rights reserved. www.netterimages.com.

Fig 47.2 Susan Standring, ed. Thorax: overview and surface anatomy. In: Gray's Anatomy, 40th edn. © Elsevier; 2008.

Figs 47.3, 47.7, 47.8 Dr Caesar Ursic.

Fig 47.4 Soto JA, Lucey BC. Emergency radiology: the requisites. Philadelphia: Mosby; 2009.

Figs 47.5, 47.9, 47.14 Courtesy Radiology Department, St George Hospital, Sydney.

Fig 47.6 Soto JA, Lucey BC. Emergency radiology: the requisites. Philadelphia: Mosby; 2009.

Figs 47.10, 47.11, 47.18 Rosen P, Barkin RM, Hockberger RS et al. Emergency medicine: concepts and clinical practice. 4th edn. St Louis: Mosby; 1998.

Figs 47.12, 47.17, 47.20 Adam A, Dixon AK. Grainger and Allison's diagnostic radiology. 5th edn. New York: Churchill Livingstone; 2008.

Fig 47.13 Soto JA, Lucey BC. Emergency radiology: the requisites. Philadelphia: Mosby; 2009.

Figs 47.15A, 47.16 Besson A, Saegesser F. A Colour Atlas of Chest trauma and associated injuries. Oradell: Medical Economics; 1983.

Fig 47.15B Brenner BE. Comprehensive management of respiratory emergencies. Rockville: Aspen Systems; 1985.

Fig 47.19 Arnaud F, Tomori T, Teranishi K et al. Evaluation of chest seal performance in a swine model. Injury 2008;39(9):1082–8.

Fig 47.21 Curtis K, Asha S. Blunt cardiac injury as a result of a motor vehicle collision: a case study. Australas Emerg Nurs J 2010;13(4):124–9.

Fig 47.22 © American College of Cardiology Foundation. Cardiovascular interventions. JACC 2009; 2(8):705–17.

Fig 47.24 Soto JA, Lucey BC. Emergency radiology: the requisites. Philadelphia: Mosby; 2009.

Fig 47.25 Kate Curtis.

Fig 47.26 McQuillan KA, Von Rueden KT, Hartsock RL et al. Trauma nursing from resuscitation through rehabilitation. 3rd edn. Philadelphia: WB Saunders; 2001.

Fig 47.27 Browner BD, Levine AM, Jupiter JB, et al. Skeletal trauma. 4th edn. St Louis: WB Saunders; 2008.

Fig 47.28 Rutherford RB. Vascular surgery. 6th edn. St Louis: Saunders; 2005.

Fig 48.1 Stillwell S. Mosby's critical care nursing reference. 2nd edn. St Louis: Mosby; 1996.

Figs 48.2, 48.3 Thibodeau GA, Patton KT. Anatomy and physiology. 4th edn. St Louis: Mosby; 1999.

Fig 48.4, 48.5 Courtesy Liverpool Hospital Trauma Service, Sydney, NSW.

Fig 48.6 Rozycki GS, Ballard RB, Feliciano DV et al. Surgeon-performed ultrasound for the assessment of truncal injuries: lessons learned from 1540 patients. Am Surg 1998;228(4):557–67.

Fig 48.7 Snell RS, Smith MS. Clinical anatomy for emergency medicine. St Louis: Mosby; 1993.

Fig 48.8 Clochesy JM, Breu C, Cardin S et al. Critical care nursing. 2nd edn. Philadelphia: WB Saunders; 1996.

Fig 48.9 Soto JA, Lucey BC. Emergency radiology: the requisites. Philadelphia: Mosby; 2009.

Fig 48.10 Neff JA, Kidd PS, eds. Trauma nursing: the art and science. St Louis: Mosby; 1993.

Fig 48.11 McQuillan KA, Von Rueden KT, Hartsock RL et al. Trauma nursing: from resuscitation through rehabilitation. 3rd edn. Philadelphia: WB Saunders; 2002.

Fig 48.12 Buckley JC, McAninch JW. Revised Renal Injury Scoring System. Revision of Current American Association for the Surgery of Trauma Renal Injury Grading System. J Trauma 2011;70:35–7.

Fig 48.13 Peters P, Sagalowsky A. Genitourinary trauma. In: Walsh P, Gittes R, Perlmutter A et al, eds. Campbell's urology. 5th edn. vol 1. Philadelphia: WB Saunders; 1986.

Fig 48.14 Armenakas NA, McAninch JW. Acute anterior urethral injuries: diagnosis and initial management. In: McAninch JW, ed. Traumatic and reconstructive urology. Philadelphia: WB Saunders; 1996.

Fig 48.15 Minns AB, Sherry Y. Penile fracture in a patient presenting with groin pain. Journal of Emergency Medicine 2011;40(4):441–2. © 2011.

Fig 48.16 Ward MA, Burgess PL, Williams DH et al. Threatened fertility and gonadal function after a polytraumatic, life-threatening injury J Emerg Trauma Shock 2010;3(2):199–203.

Fig 48.17 Peters P, Sagalowsky A. Genitourinary trauma. In: Walsh P, Gittes R, Perlmutter A, et al, eds. Campbell's Urology. 5th edn. vol 1. Philadelphia: WB Saunders; 1986.

Table 48.1 Elliot D, Aitken L, Chaboyer W. ACCCN's critical care nursing. Sydney: Elsevier; 2006.

Table 48.2 Muench MV, Canterino JC. Trauma in pregnancy. Obstet Gynecol Clin North Am 2007;34(3):555–83.

Table 48.3 Cameron P, Jelinek G, Kelly A et al, eds. Textbook of adult emergency medicine. 2nd edn. Edinburgh: Churchill Livingstone; 2004.

Table 48.4 McQuillan KA, Von Rueden KT, Hartsock RL et al. Trauma nursing: from resuscitation through rehabilitation. 3rd edn. Philadelphia: WB Saunders; 2002.

Tables 48.6, 48.7 Pearl WS, Todd KH. Ultrasonography for the initial evaluation of blunt abdominal trauma, a review in prospective trials. Ann Emerg Med 1996;27(3):353–61.

Table 48.8 Dixon MD, McAninch JW. American Urological Association update series, traumatic renal injuries, part 1: assessment and management. Houston: The Association; 1991. Kidney Injury Scale. The American Association for the Surgery of Trauma. Online. www.aast.org/Library/TraumaTools/InjuryScoringScales.aspx.

Table 48.9 Aitken L, Niggemeyer L. Trauma management. In: Elliot D, Aitken L, Chaboyer W eds. ACCCN's critical care nursing. Sydney: Elsevier; 2006.

Box 48.1 Cameron P, Jelinek G, Kelly A et al, eds. Textbook of adult emergency medicine. 2nd edn. Edinburgh: Churchill Livingstone; 2004.

Fig 49.1 Netter FH. Atlas of human anatomy. 5th edn. Philadelphia: Saunders; 2011.

Fig 49.2 Marx J. Rosen's emergency medicine: Concepts and Clinical Practice. 8th edn. St Louis: Mosby; 2014.

Figs 49.3, 49.4, 49.5, 49.6, 49.7 Marcus Cremonese & UNSW Faculty of Medicine.

Fig 49.8 Browner BD, Levine AM, Jupiter JB et al. Skeletal trauma. 4th edn. Philadelphia: WB Saunders; 2008.

Fig 49.10A Roberts JR, Hedges JR. Roberts and Hedges' clinical procedures in emergency medicine. Elsevier; 2013.

Fig 49.10B Adapted from Sanders M. Mosby's paramedic textbook. rev 3rd edn. St Louis, Mosby 2007.

Fig 49.12, 49.13A Roberts JR. Roberts and Hedges' clinical procedures in emergency medicine. Elsevier; 2013.

Fig 49.13B Kate Curtis.

Fig 49.14 Courtesy University of Sydney.

Fig 49.15 Lewis SM, Collier IC, Heitkemper MM. Medical–surgical nursing: assessment and management of clinical problems. 7th edn. St Louis: Mosby; 2007.

Fig 49.16 Cameron P, Jelinek G, Kelly A et al, eds. Textbook of adult emergency medicine. 3rd edn. Edinburgh: Churchill Livingstone; 2009.

Fig 49.17A Adapted from the Royal Children's Hospital Cervical Spine Assessment Guideline, www.rch.org.au/clinicalguide/guideline_index/Cervical_Spine_Injury/; B: Stiell IG, Wells GA, Vandemheen KL et al. The Canadian C-spine rule for radiography in alert and stable trauma patients. JAMA 2001;286(15):1841–8; Stiell IG, Clement CM, Mcknight RD et al. The Canadian C-spine rule versus the NEXUS low-risk criteria in patients with trauma. N Engl J Med 2003;349(26):2510–18; Stiell IG, Clement CM, Grimshaw J, et al. Implementation of the Canadian C-Spine Rule: A prospective 12 centre cluster randomised trial. BMJ 2009;339:b4146.

Fig 49.18 Courtesy Acromed, DePuy Inc.

Fig 49.19 Lewis SM, Collier IC, Heitkemper MM. Medical–surgical nursing: assessment and management of clinical problems. 7th edn. St Louis: Mosby; 2007.

Fig 49.20 Browner BD, Levine AM, Jupiter JB et al. Skeletal trauma. 4th edn. Philadelphia: WB Saunders; 2008.

Figs 49.21, 49.22 Marcus Cremonese & UNSW Faculty of Medicine.

Fig 49.23 Marx J. Rosen's emergency medicine—concepts and clinical practice. 8th edn. St Louis: Mosby; 2014.

Tables 49.1, 49.2 Norton L. Spinal cord injury, Australia 2007–08. Injury research and statistics series no. 52. Cat. no. INJCAT 128. Canberra: Australian Institute of Health and Welfare; 2010.

Table 49.3 Lindsey RW, et al. Injury to the vertebrae and spinal cord. In: Feliciano DV, Mattox LV, Moore EE, eds. Trauma. 6th edn. New York: McGraw-Hill; 2008.

Fig 50.1 Thibodeau GA, Patton KT. Anatomy and physiology. 6th edn. St Louis: Mosby; 2006.

Fig 50.2 Lewis SM, Collier IC, Heitkemper MM. Medical–surgical nursing. 4th edn. St Louis: Mosby; 1996.

Fig 50.3 Dandy DJ, Edwards DJ. Essential orthopaedics and trauma. 5th edn. Edinburgh: Churchill Livingstone; 2009.

Fig 50.4 Marx J, Hockberger R, Walls R. Rosen's emergency medicine: concepts and clinical practice. 7th edn. St Louis: Mosby; 2010.

Fig 50.5 Maher AB, Salmond SW, Pellino TA. Orthopaedic nursing. 3rd edn. Philadelphia: WB Saunders; 2002.

Figs 50.6, 50.7 Browner BD, Jupiter JB, Levine AM et al. Skeletal trauma: basic science, management and reconstruction. 4th edn. WB Saunders: Philadelphia; 2008.

Fig 50.8 Manes HR. A new method of shoulder reduction in the elderly. Clin Orthop Relat Res 1980;147:200–2.

Figs 50.9, 50.10 Bucholz RW, Court-Brown CM, Heckman JD. Rockwood and Greens fractures in adults. 6th edn. Philadelphia: Lippincott, Williams & Wilkins; 2005.

Fig 50.11 Jobe MT, Martinez SF. Peripheral nerve injuries. In: Canale ST, Beatty JH eds. Campbell's Operative orthopaedics. 12th edn. Philadelphia: Mosby; 2013.

Figs 50.12, 50.13 Cameron P, Jelinek G, Kelly A et al, eds. Textbook of adult emergency medicine. 3rd edn. Edinburgh: Churchill Livingstone; 2009.

Figs 50.14, 50.15 Frank ED, Long BW, Smith BJ. Merrill's atlas of radiographic positions and radiologic procedures. 12th edn. St Louis: Mosby; 2011.

Fig 50.16 Davis JM, et al, eds. Clinical surgery. St Louis: Mosby; 1987.

Fig 50.17 Permission granted by author C Hill.

Fig 50.18AB Morrison W, Parvizi W, Weiss J. Pelvic and acetabular fractures. In: Presentation, imaging and treatment of common musculoskeletal conditions. Philadelphia: Saunders; 2012.

Fig 50.19 Maher AB, Salmond SW, Pellino TA. Orthopaedic nursing. 3rd edn. Philadelphia: WB Saunders; 2002.

Fig 50.20 Roberts JR, Hedges JR. Clinical procedures in emergency medicine. 6th edn. Philadelphia: Saunders Elsevier; 2013. Courtesy SAM Medical Products, Portland, Oregon, USA.

Fig 50.21 Adapted from Browner BD, Jupiter JB, Levine AM, et al. Skeletal trauma: basic science, management and reconstruction. 4th edn. WB Saunders: Philadelphia; 2008; Jobe MT, Martinez SF. Peripheral nerve injuries. In: Canale ST, Beatty JH eds. Campbell's operative orthopaedics. 12th edn. Philadelphia: Mosby; 2013.

Figs 50.22, 50.23 Browner BD, Jupiter JB, Levine AM et al. Skeletal trauma: basic science, management and reconstruction. 4th edn. WB Saunders: Philadelphia; 2008.

Fig 50.24 Permission granted by author C Hill.

Fig 50.25 Chung J, Modrall, J. Compartment Syndrome. In: Cronenwett JL, Johnston KW. Rutherford's vascular surgery. 8th edn. Philadelphia: Saunders; 2014.

Fig 50.27 Jobe MT, Martinez SF. Peripheral nerve injuries. In: Canale ST, Beatty JH eds. Campbell's Operative orthopaedics. 12th edn. Philadelphia: Mosby; 2013.

Figs 50.26, 50.28, 50.29, 50.CS1, 50.CS2, 50.CS3 Permission granted by author C Hill.

Table 50.1 Descriptions from Maher AB, Salmond SW, Pellino TA. Orthopaedic nursing. 3rd edn. Philadelphia: WB Saunders; 2002 and Illustrations from DePalma A, Connolly J. DePalma's The management of fractures and dislocations. 3rd edn. Philadelphia: WB Saunders; 1981.

Table 50.2 Adapted from Dandy DJ, Edwards DJ. Essential orthopaedics and trauma. 5th edn. Edinburgh: Churchill Livingstone; 2009; McQuillan KA, Makic MBF, Whalen E et al, eds. Trauma nursing: from resuscitation through rehabilitation. 4th edn. Philadelphia: WB Saunders; 2008; Maher AB, Salmond SW, Pellino TA. Orthopaedic nursing. 3rd edn. Philadelphia: WB Saunders; 2002; Solomon L, Warwick D, Nayagam S. Apley's concise system of orthopaedics and fractures. 3rd edn. London: Arnold; 2005; Kitt S, Selfridge-Thomas J, Proehl JA et al. Emergency nursing: a physiologic and clinical perspective. 2nd edn. Philadelphia: WB Saunders; 1995.

Table 50.3 Maher AB, Salmond SW, Pellino TA. Orthopaedic nursing. 3rd edn. Philadelphia: WB Saunders; 2002.

Table 50.4 Kozin S, Berlet A. Pelvis and acetabulum. In: Handbook of common orthopaedic fractures. 4th edn. Chester: Medical Surveillance; 2000.

Table 50.5 Adapted from Dandy DJ, Edwards DJ. Essential orthopaedics and trauma. 5th edn. Edinburgh: Churchill Livingstone; 2009; McQuillan KA, Makic MBF, Whalen E, et al, eds. Trauma nursing: from resuscitation through rehabilitation. 4th edn. Philadelphia: WB Saunders; 2008; Neff JA, Kidd PS. Trauma nursing: the art and science. St Louis: Mosby; 1993; Maher AB, Salmond SW, Pellino TA. Orthopaedic nursing. 3rd edn. Philadelphia: WB Saunders; 2002; Solomon L, Warwick D, Nayagam S. Apley's Concise system of orthopaedics and fractures. 3rd edn. London: Arnold; 2005; Kitt S, Selfridge-Thomas J, Proehl JA et al. Emergency nursing: a physiologic and clinical perspective. 2nd edn. Philadelphia: WB Saunders; 1995; Simon RR, Sherman SC, Koenigsknecht SJ. Emergency orthopedics: the extremities. 6th edn. New York: McGraw-Hill; 2011.

Table 50.6 Descriptions from Maher AB, Salmond SW, Pellino TA. Orthopaedic nursing. 3rd edn. Philadelphia: WB Saunders; 2002. Illustrations from DePalma A, Connolly J. DePalma's The management of fractures and dislocations. 3rd edn. Philadelphia: WB Saunders; 1981.

Table 50.7 Bennett AR, Smith KD. Open fractures. Orthopaedics and trauma 2013;27(1):9–14.

Table 50.8 Johansen K, Daines M, Howey T et al. Objective criteria accurately predict amputation following lower extremity trauma. J Trauma 1990;30(5):568–73.

Box 50.1 Hammond BB, Zimmermann PG, Sheehy SB. Sheehy's manual of emergency care. 7th edn. St Louis: Mosby; 2013.

Box 50.2 Adapted from Carter CT, Schafer N. Incidence of urethral disruption in females with traumatic pelvic fractures. Am J Emerg Med 1993;11(3):218–20; Koraitim MM, Marzouk ME, Atta MA et al. Risk factors and mechanism of urethral injury in pelvic fractures. Br J Urol 1996;77(6):876–80; Lowe MA, Mason JT, Luna GK, et al. Risk factors for urethral injuries in men with traumatic pelvic fractures. J Urol 1988;140:506.

Box 50.3 Adapted from McQuillan KA, Makic MBF, Whalen E et al, eds. Trauma nursing: from resuscitation through rehabilitation. 4th edn. Philadelphia: WB Saunders; 2008. Gonzalez D. Crush syndrome. Crit Care Med 2005;33(1 Suppl):S34–41. Walls M. Orthopedic trauma. RN 2002;65(7):52–6, 58. Matsen FA III. Compartment syndromes. New York: Grune & Stratton; 1980.

Box 50.4 Adapted from Mellor A, Soni N. Fat embolism. Anaesthesia 2001;56(2):145–54; Peltier LF. Fat embolism: a perspective. Clin Orthop Relat Res 2004;422:148–53.

Fig 51.1 Chest radiograph of a patient with blast injury and Chest CT of a patient with blast injury. In: Wolf SJ, Bebarta VS, Bonnett CJ. Blast injuries. The Lancet 2009;374(9687):405–15.

Fig 51.2 Jane Mateer, Iraq, 2005.

Fig 51.3A, Jane Mateer, Iraq, 2005. B, Dr Adam Brooks, Iraq, 2005.

Table 51.1 Bersten AD, Soni N, eds. Oh's intensive care manual. 6th edn. London: Butterworth–Heinemann; 2009. Plurad DS. Blast Injury. Mil Med 2011;176(3):276–82.

Table 51.2 Wightman JM, Gladish SL. Explosions and blast injuries.

Ann Emerg Med 2001;37(6):664–78; Stewart C. Blast injuries: true weapons of mass destruction. 2010. www.az1dmat.org/dmat_blast_injuries.pdf Emerg Med Prac.

Table 51.3 DeWitt D, Prough D. Blast-induced brain injury and post traumatic hypotension and hypoxemia. J Neurotrauma 2009;26:877–87.

Table 51.4 Wightman JM, Gladish SL. Explosions and blast injuries. Ann Emerg Med 2001;37(6):664–78.

Table 51.5 Gawande A. Casualties of war: military care for the wounded from Iraq and Afghanistan. N Engl J Med 2004;351(24):2471–5; DePalma RG, Burris DG, Champion HR et al. Blast injuries. N Engl J Med 2005;352:1335–42; Almogy G, Luria T, Richter E et al. Can external signs of trauma guide management? Lessons learned from suicide bombing attacks in Israel. Arch Surg 2005;140(4):390–3.

Box 51.2 Gawande A. Casualties of war: military care for the wounded from Iraq and Afghanistan. N Engl J Med 2004;351(24):2471–5; Ruff R, Iverson G, Barth J, et al. Recommendations for diagnosing a mild traumatic brain injury: A national academy of Neuropsychology education paper. Archives of Clin Neuropsych 2009;24:3–10. Crompton J. Ocular and adnexal injuries in the Bali bombing. ADF Health 2003;4:2, Australia.

Box 51.3 Pennardt A. Blast injuries. eMedicine. Online. http://emedicine.medscape.com/article/822587-overview; DePalma RG, Burris DG, Champion HR, et al. Blast injuries. N Engl J Med 2005;352:1335–42.

Box 51.4 Wightman JM, Gladish SL. Explosions and blast injuries. Ann Emerg Med 2001;37(6):664–78. Pennardt A. Blast injuries. eMedicine. Online. http://emedicine.medscape.com/article/822587-overview.

Fig 52.1A–E South Australia Health—Women and Children's Hospital Network 2014.

Fig 52.2 Jackson DM. The diagnosis of the depth of burning. Br J Surg 1953;40(164):588–96.

Fig 52.3 Elliot D, Aitken L, Chaboyer W eds. ACCCN's critical care nursing. Sydney: Elsevier; 2006.

Fig 52.4 Hawley R, King J. Australian nurses' dictionary. 3rd edn. Sydney: Ballière Tindall; 2004.

Fig 52.5 Medhat Emil Habib. Initial burn management. Austin J Surg. 2014;1(2):1010.

Fig 52.6 Edlich R, Bailey T, Bill T. Thermal burns. In: Marx J, Hockenberger R, Walls R, eds. Rosen's emergency medicine: concepts and clinical practice. 5th edn. St Louis: Mosby; 2002.

Fig 52.8 Barret JP, Herndon DN, eds. Color atlas of burn care. St Louis: WB Saunders; 2001.

Fig 52.9 South Australia Health—Women and Children's Hospital Network 2014.

Table 52.2 Australia and New Zealand Burns Association. Emergency Manual of Severe Burns Course Manual (pamphlet). 10th edn. ANZBA; 2006.

Fig 54.1 Courtesy Radiology Department, St George Hospital, Sydney.

Fig 54.2 Courtesy Nuclear Medicine Department, St George Hospital, Sydney.

Table 54.1 Data from ANZOD Registry, website, accessed 23 June 2015 http://www.anzdata.org.au/anzod/updates/anzod1989toCurrent.pdf.

Table 54.2 Kutsogiannis D, Pagliarello G, Doig C et al. Medical management to optimize donor organ potential: review of the literature. Can J Anesth 2006;53(8):820–30.

Table 54.3 Australian and New Zealand Intensive Care Society. The ANZICS statement on death and organ donation. 3rd edn. Melbourne: ANZICS; 2008; Dobb GJ, Weekes JW. Clinical confirmation of brain death. Anaesth Intensive Care 1995;23(1):37–43.

Table 54.4 New Zealand Ministry of Health. Organ donation fact sheet. 2004. Online. Available: via www.moh.govt.nz/moh.nsf; 25 Jan 2005. Australian Government. Health Insurance Commission. Australian organ donor register. Online. www.humanservices.gov.au/customer/services/medicare/australian-organ-donor-register?utm_id=9.

Table 54.7 Moyes K. Improving organ donation rates with standard nucleic acid testing on all potential donors. Transplant Nurses J 2002;11:15–16; Australian Red Cross Blood Service. Blood testing: safety and testing. 2008. Online. www.donateblood.com.au/all-about-blood/safety-and-testing.

Table 54.8 Kutsogiannis D, Pagliarello G, Doig C et al. Medical management to optimize donor organ potential: review of the literature. Can J Anesth 2006;53(8):820–30; Power BM, Van Heerden PV. The physiological changes associated with brain death—current concepts and implications for treatment of the brain dead organ donor. Anaesth Intensive Care 1995;23(1):26–36; Rosendale JD, Kauffman HM, McBride MA et al. Aggressive pharmacologic donor management results in more transplanted organs. Transplantation 2003;75:482–7.

Box 54.1 Australian and New Zealand Intensive Care Society. The ANZICS statement on death and organ donation. 3rd edn. Melbourne: ANZICS; 2008.

Box 54.2 Australasian Transplant Coordinators Association. National guidelines for organ and tissue donation. 4th edn. Sydney: ATCA; 2008.

INDEX